AF322856

LATEST APPROVED METHODS OF TREATMENT
FOR THE PRACTICING PHYSICIAN

Edited by

ROBERT E. RAKEL, M.D.

Professor and Chairman, Department of Family Medicine
Associate Dean for Academic and Clinical Affairs
Baylor College of Medicine, Houston, Texas

W.B. SAUNDERS COMPANY
A Division of Harcourt Brace & Company
Philadelphia   London   Toronto   Montreal   Sydney   Tokyo

1997

Conn's Current Therapy

W.B. SAUNDERS COMPANY
A Division of Harcourt Brace & Company

The Curtis Center
Independence Square West
Philadelphia, Pennsylvania 19106

Library of Congress Cataloging-in-Publication Data

Current therapy; latest approved methods of treatment for the practicing physician.

Editors: H. F. Conn and others.

v. 28 cm. annual.

ISBN 0–7216–8674–5

1. Therapeutics.   2. Therapeutics, Surgical.   3. Medicine—Practice.
  I. Conn, Howard Franklin, 1908–1982 ed.

RM101.C87   616.058   49–8328 rev*

CONN'S CURRENT THERAPY 1997   ISBN 0–7216–8674–5

Copyright © 1997 by W.B. Saunders Company

All rights reserved. No part of this publication may be reproduced or transmitted in any form or by any means, electronic or mechanical, including photocopy, recording, or any information storage and retrieval system, without permission in writing from the publisher.

Printed in the United States of America.

Last digit is the print number: 9   8   7   6   5   4   3   2   1

Contributors

G. DAVID ADAMSON, M.D.
Clinical Professor, Stanford University School of Medicine, Stanford, California; Clinical Associate Professor, University of California, San Francisco; Active Staff, Columbia Good Samaritan Hospital, San Francisco, California; Active Staff, Stanford University Hospital, Stanford, California; Director Fertility Physicians of Northern California, Palo Alto, California
Endometriosis

CARLOS A. AGUDELO, M.D.
Professor of Medicine, Acting Chief, Rheumatology, Emory University; Chief of Rheumatology, VA Medical Center; Staff, Emory University, Atlanta, Georgia
Hyperuricemia and Gout

HAGOP S. AKISKAL, M.D.
Professor of Psychiatry and Director of the International Mood Clinic, University of California, San Diego; Medical Director, Outpatient Psychiatric Services, VA Medical Center, San Diego, California
Mood (Affective) Disorders

A.N. ALAM, M.B., PH.D.
Consultant Physician, International Centre for Diarrhoeal Disease Research, Dhaka, Bangladesh
Cholera

JORGE E. ALBINA, M.D.
Professor of Surgery, Brown University School of Medicine; Director, Nutritional Support Service; Director, Surgical Research, Rhode Island Hospital, Providence, Rhode Island
Parenteral Nutrition in Adults

A. LOREN AMACHER, M.D.
Director, Department of Neurosurgery, Geisinger Medical Center, Danville, Pennsylvania
Pediatric Head Injury

MAMMO AMARE, M.D.
Former Professor of Medicine, Department of Medicine, Division of Hematology, University of Kansas Medical Center, Kansas City, Kansas; Texas Oncology P.A. and Methodist Medical Center, Dallas, Texas
Vitamin K Deficiency

JAYASEELAN AMBROSE, M.B.
Fellow, Cardiovascular Medicine, University of California, San Diego, San Diego, California
Infective Endocarditis

EZRA A. AMSTERDAM, M.D.
Director, Coronary Care Unit, University of California, Davis, Medical Center, Sacramento, California
Premature Beats

KARL E. ANDERSON, M.D.
Professor, Departments of Preventive Medicine and Community Health, Internal Medicine, and Pharmacology and Toxicology, University of Texas Medical Branch at Galveston; Member of Medical Staff, University of Texas Medical Branch, Galveston, Texas
The Porphyrias

ROBERT J. ANDERSON, M.D.
Professor of Medicine, Creighton University School of Medicine; Chief, Section of Endocrinology, Diabetes and Metabolism, VA Medical Center, Omaha, Nebraska
Adrenocortical Insufficiency

MARY–MARGARET ANDREWS, M.D.
Instructor of Clinical Medicine, Dartmouth Medical School, Hanover, New Hampshire; Clinical Fellow in Infectious Diseases, Dartmouth-Hitchcock Medical Center, Lebanon, New Hampshire
Toxic Shock Syndrome

BAHA M. ARAFAH, M.D.
Associate Professor of Medicine, Case Western Reserve University, School of Medicine; Physician, University Hospitals of Cleveland, Cleveland, Ohio
Hypopituitarism

GERARD V. ARANHA, M.D.
Professor of Surgery, Loyola Stritch School of Medicine; Chief, General Surgery Section and Section of Surgical Oncology, Hines VA Hospital; Chief, Section of Surgical Oncology, Loyola University Medical Center, Maywood, Illinois
Gastric Tumors

DONALD ARMSTRONG, M.D.
Professor of Medicine, Cornell University Medical College; Chief, Infectious Disease Service; Director, Microbiology Laboratory, Memorial Sloan-Kettering Cancer Center, New York, New York
Brain Abscess

STEVEN E. ARNOLD, M.D.
Assistant Professor, Departments of Psychiatry and Neurology, School of Medicine, University of Pennsylvania; Attending Physician, Hospital of the University of Pennsylvania, Philadelphia, Pennsylvania
Alzheimer's Disease

BASIM I. ASMAR, M.D.
Associate Professor of Pediatrics, Wayne State University School of Medicine; Associate Director, Division of Infectious Diseases, Children's Hospital of Michigan; Attending Physician, Children's Hospital of Michigan, Detroit, Michigan
Mumps

MARK WAYNE AUSTIN, M.D.
Instructor, Eastern Virginia Medical School, Norfolk, Virginia
Uterine Leiomyoma

J. MICHAEL BACHARACH, M.D.
Section Head, Vascular Medicine and Vascular Intervention, North Central Heart and Vascular Institute, Sioux Falls, South Dakota
Deep Venous Thrombosis of the Extremities

WILLIAM C. BAILEY, M.D.
Professor, University of Alabama at Birmingham School of Medicine; Staff Physician, University Hospital, TB Control Officer of VA, Birmingham, Alabama
Tuberculosis and Nontuberculous Mycobacterial Diseases

HUGH BARBER, M.D.
Director, Department of Obstetrics/Gynecology, Lenox Hill Hospital, New York, New York
Urinary Incontinence

ARIEL BARKAN, M.D.
Professor, University of Michigan Medical School; DVA Medical Center, University of Michigan Medical Center, Ann Arbor, Michigan
Hyperprolactinemia

WILLIAM M. BARRON, M.D.
Professor of Medicine and Obstetrics and Gynecology, Loyola University, Stritch School of Medicine; Director, Division of General Internal Medicine, Loyola University Medical Center, Maywood, Illinois
Hypertensive Disorders of Pregnancy

SHANNON M. BATES, M.D.
Clinical Scholar, Department of Medicine, Faculty of Health Sciences, McMaster University, Hamilton, Ontario, Canada
Platelet-Mediated Bleeding Disorders

DAVID E. BECK, M.D.
Chairman, Department of Colon and Rectal Surgery, Ochsner Clinic, New Orleans, Louisiana
Hemorrhoids, Anal Fissure, and Anorectal Abscess and Fistula

JAMES R. BERENSON, M.D.
Associate Professor of Medicine, University of California, Los Angeles; Chief, Medical Oncology, West Los Angeles VA Medical Center; Staff Physician, University of California, Los Angeles, Center for the Health Sciences, Los Angeles, California
Multiple Myeloma

PAULOS BERHANU, M.D.
Associate Professor of Medicine, University of Colorado Health Sciences Center, Division of Endocrinology and Diabetes; University Hospital of the University of Colorado Health Sciences Center, Denver, Colorado
Diabetes Mellitus in Adults

RUSTIN BERLOW, M.D.
Fellow in Psychobiology and Psychopharmacology, Clinical Research Center for Affective Disorders, University of California, San Diego, San Diego, California
Mood (Affective) Disorders

KARL R. BEUTNER, M.D., PH.D.
Associate Clinical Professor of Dermatology, University of California, San Francisco, San Francisco, California; Department of Medicine, Sutter Solano Medical Center; Solano Dermatology, Vallejo, California
Genital Warts

FRANK J. BIA, M.D., M.P.H.
Professor of Medicine and Laboratory Medicine, Yale School of Medicine; Yale–New Haven Hospital, New Haven, Connecticut; West Haven VA Hospital, West Haven, Connecticut
Amebiasis

DAVID R. BICKERS, M.D.
Carl Truman Nelson Professor and Chairman, Department of Dermatology, Columbia University, College of Physicians and Surgeons; Director of Service and Attending Dermatologist, Department of Dermatology, The Presbyterian Hospital, New York, New York
Sunburn

JOSÉ BILLER, M.D.
Professor and Chairman, Department of Neurology, Indiana University School of Medicine; Chief, Neurology Services, Department of Neurology, University Hospital, Indiana University Medical Center, Indianapolis, Indiana
Intracerebral Hemorrhage

DAVID G. BORENSTEIN, M.D.
Professor of Medicine, The George Washington University Medical Center, Washington, DC
Connective Tissue Disease (Systemic Lupus Erythematosus, Dermatomyositis, Other Myopathies, and Scleroderma)

WILLIAM Z. BORER, M.D.
Associate Professor, Department of Pathology and Cell Biology, Thomas Jefferson University; Director, Clinical Chemistry Section, Thomas Jefferson University Hospital, Philadelphia, Pennsylvania
Reference Intervals for the Interpretation of Laboratory Tests

SANSERN BORIRAKCHANYAVAT, M.D.
Resident in Urology, University of California, San Francisco, San Francisco, California
Erectile Dysfunction

DENNIS N. BOURDETTE, M.D.
Associate Professor of Neurology, Oregon Health Sciences University; Acting Chief of Neurology, Veterans Affairs Medical Center, Portland, Oregon
Multiple Sclerosis

GENE D. BRANUM, M.D.
Assistant Professor, Department of Surgery, Division of Gastrointestinal Surgery, Emory University School of Medicine; Director of General Surgery, Atlanta Veterans Affairs Medical Center; Associate Chief, Gastrointestinal Surgery, Emory Clinic, Atlanta, Georgia
Acute Pancreatitis and Its Complications

MAYER BREZIS, M.D.
Professor of Medicine, Hadassah University Hospital; Chief Physician, Hadassah University Hospital, Jerusalem, Israel
Acute Renal Failure

JOHN W. BRICE, M.D.
Associate Professor of Medicine, University of South Carolina School of Medicine; Chief, Pulmonary and Critical Care Section, W.J.B. Dern VA Medical Center, Columbia, South Carolina
Acute Respiratory Failure

DAVID R. BROOKER, M.D.
Assistant Professor of Medicine, University of Medicine and Dentistry of New Jersey/Robert Wood Johnson Medical School at Camden; Attending Physician, Cooper Hospital/University Medical Center, Camden, New Jersey
Diabetes Insipidus

DALE BROWN, JR., M.D.
Clinical Professor, Department of Obstetrics and Gynecology, Baylor College of Medicine; Chief of Staff, Chief of Obstetrics, and Associate Chief of Obstetrics/Gynecology, St. Luke's Episcopal Hospital, Houston, Texas
Neoplasms of the Vulva

RUTH DOWLING BRUUN, M.D.
Clinical Associate Professor of Psychiatry, Cornell University Medical College, New York, New York; Senior Consultant, Movement Disorders Center, North Shore University Hospital; Assistant Attending Psychiatrist, North Shore University Hospital, Manhasset, New York
Gilles De La Tourette Syndrome

CATHY L. BUDMAN, M.D.
Assistant Professor of Psychiatry and Neurology, Cornell University Medical College, New York, New York; Coordinator, Movement

Disorders Center, North Shore University Hospital; Assistant Attending Psychiatrist, North Shore University Hospital, Manhasset, New York
Gilles De La Tourette Syndrome

THOMAS W. BURKE, M.D.

Associate Professor of Gynecologic Oncology, University of Texas M.D. Anderson Cancer Center, Houston, Texas
Cancer of the Endometrium

JOSEPH J. BURRASCANO, JR., M.D.

Attending, Southampton Hospital, Southampton, New York
Lyme Disease

JOHN B. BUSE, M.D., PH.D.

Associate Professor of Medicine, University of North Carolina School of Medicine; Director, Diabetes Care Center, University of North Carolina Hospitals, Chapel Hill, North Carolina
Diabetic Ketoacidosis

THOMAS BUTLER, M.D.

Professor, Texas Tech University Health Sciences Center; Attending Physician, University Medical Center, Lubbock, Texas
Typhoid Fever

FERNANDO CABANILLAS, M.D.

Professor of Medicine; Chief, Section of Lymphoma, M.D. Anderson Cancer Center, Houston, Texas
Non-Hodgkin's Lymphoma

JOHN W. CALDWELL, PHARM.D.

Director of Clinical Research, Kern Medical Center; Associate Professor of Medicine, University of California at Los Angeles, Los Angeles, California
Coccidioidomycosis

WALTER L. CALMBACH, M.D.

Associate Professor, Department of Family Practice, University of Texas Health Science Center at San Antonio; University Hospital, San Antonio, Texas
Common Sports Injuries

G. DOUGLAS CAMPBELL, JR., M.D.

Professor of Medicine; Chief of Division of Pulmonary and Critical Care, Louisiana State University School of Medicine; Louisiana State University Medical Center; Overton Brooks Veterans Affairs Medical Center, Shreveport, Louisiana
Bacterial Pneumonia

LAURA C. CAMPBELL, M.D.

Instructor of Medicine, Louisiana State University School of Medicine–Shreveport (Division of Hematology/Oncology); Overton Brooks Veterans Affairs Medical Center; Louisiana State University Medical Center, Shreveport, Louisiana
Bacterial Pneumonia

ROBERT C. CANBY, M.D.

Instructor, Internal Medicine, Division of Cardiology, Clinical Electrophysiology and Pacing, University of Texas, Southwestern Medical Center; UT Southwestern Affiliated Hospitals (Parkland Memorial Hospital, Dallas VA Medical Center, St. Paul Hospital, Zale-Lipshy University Hospital), Dallas, Texas
Tachycardias

DAVID E. CARNOVALE, M.D.

Assistant Professor, Reproductive Endocrinology and Infertility, Department of Obstetrics and Gynecology, James H. Quillen College of Medicine, East Tennessee State University, Johnson City, Tennessee
Amenorrhea

THOMAS R. CARACCIO, PHARM.D.

Assistant Professor of Emergency Medicine, State University of New York at Stony Brook, Stony Brook, New York; Assistant Professor of Pharmacology/Toxicology, New York College of Osteopathic Medicine, Old Westbury, New York; Assistant Professor of Clinical Pharmacy, St. John's University College of Pharmacy, Jamaica, New York; Assistant Director of Long Island Regional Poison Control Center, Winthrop-University Hospital, Mineola, New York
Acute Poisonings

R. DUANE CESPEDES, M.D.

Clinical Instructor, Division of Urology, University of Texas–Houston Medical School; Clinical Fellow—Incontinence and Voiding Dysfunction, Hermann Hospital, Houston, Texas
Childhood Enuresis

PARAMJIT S. CHANDHOKE, M.D., PH.D.

Associate Professor of Surgery and Medicine, University of Colorado Health Sciences Center, Denver, Colorado
Renal Calculi

KAY W. CHANG, M.D.

Otolaryngology Resident, University of Washington, Seattle, Washington
Sinusitis

JOHANNA CHAPEL, M.D.

Department of Medicine, Section of Dermatology, Oakwood Hospital, Dearborn, Michigan
Granuloma Inguinale (Donovanosis); Lymphogranuloma Venereum

THOMAS A. CHAPEL, M.D.

Clinical Professor of Dermatology and Syphilology, Wayne State University, Detroit, Michigan; Chief, Section of Dermatology, Oakwood Hospital, Dearborn, Michigan
Granuloma Inguinale (Donovanosis); Lymphogranuloma Venereum

GLENN M. CHERTOW, M.D., M.P.H.

Instructor in Medicine, Harvard Medical School; Assistant Director of Dialysis, Brigham and Women's Hospital, Boston, Massachusetts
Chronic Renal Failure

CHING SHIANG CHI, M.D.

Associate Professor, China Medical College; Clinical Associate Professor, National Yang-Ming University School of Medicine; Clinical Associate Professor, National Defense Medical Center; Director of Pediatrics, Department of Pediatrics, Taichung Veterans General Hospital, Taichung, Taiwan, Republic of China
Reye's Syndrome

NEEOO W. CHIN, M.D.

Clinical Assistant Professor, University of Cincinnati College of Medicine; Co-Director, Greater Cincinnati Institute for Reproductive Health at The Christ Hospital, Cincinnati, Ohio
Dysfunctional Uterine Bleeding

MICHELLE CHOUCAIR, M.D.

Dermatology Fellow, Boston University Medical Center, Boston, Massachusetts
Venous Stasis Ulcers

KEVIN C. CHUNG, M.D.

Attending Hand and Plastic Surgeon, Robert Wood Johnson Scholar, Section of Plastic and Reconstructive Surgery, Department of Surgery, University of Michigan Medical Center; Lecturer, Department of Surgery; Lecturer, Department of Internal Medicine, University of Michigan Hospital, Ann Arbor, Michigan
Keloids

CHRISTOPHER M. CLARK, M.D.

Director, Memory Disorders Clinic, Department of Neurology, School of Medicine, University of Pennsylvania; Director, Memory Disorders Clinic, Hospital of the University of Pennsylvania, Philadelphia, Pennsylvania
Alzheimer's Disease

RICHARD F. CLARK, M.D.

Assistant Professor of Clinical Medicine, University of California, San Diego; Medical Director, San Diego Regional Poison Center; Director, Division of Medical Toxicology, UCSD Medical Center, San Diego, California
Spider Bites and Scorpion Stings

BART L. CLARKE, M.D.

Assistant Professor of Medicine, University of Chicago Pritzker School of Medicine; Director, Outpatient Endocrinology Clinic, University of Chicago Medical Center, Chicago, Illinois
Paget's Disease of Bone

MARY H. CLENCH, Ph.D.

Research Scientist, Division of Gastroenterology, Department of Internal Medicine, The University of Texas Medical Branch, Galveston, Texas
Irritable Bowel Syndrome

MICHAEL COBURN, M.D.

Assistant Professor of Urology, Baylor College of Medicine; Chief of Urology, Ben Taub General Hospital, Houston, Texas
Trauma to the Genitourinary Tract

D.W. COCKCROFT, M.D.

Professor, University of Saskatchewan; Active Staff, Royal University Hospital; Consultant Staff, St. Paul's Hospital; Consultant Staff, Saskatoon City Hospital, Saskatoon, Saskatchewan, Canada
Asthma in Adolescents and Adults

CHARLES C. CODDINGTON, M.D.

Professor, Obstetrics and Gynecology, Eastern Virginia Medical School, Norfolk, Virginia
Uterine Leiomyoma

RICHARD F. CODY, Jr., M.D.

Research Fellow, Department of Neurological Surgery, University of Washington School of Medicine, Seattle, Washington
Acute Head Injuries in Adults

LAWRENCE S. COHEN, M.D.

The Ebenezer K. Hunt Professor of Medicine, Yale University School of Medicine; Attending Physician, Yale–New Haven Medical Center, New Haven, Connecticut
Hypertrophic Cardiomyopathy

DANIEL G. COIT, M.D.

Associate Professor of Surgery, Cornell University Medical School; Associate Attending Surgeon, Memorial Sloan-Kettering Cancer Center, New York, New York
Malignant Melanoma

JOHN W. COWDEN, M.D.

Professor and Chairman, Department of Ophthalmology, Mason Institute of Ophthalmology, University of Missouri–Columbia; Active Staff, University Hospital and Clinics; Active Staff, Harry S Truman Memorial VA Hospital, Columbia, Missouri
Conjunctivitis

TRACY COWLES, M.D.

Clinical Associate Professor, Department of Obstetrics and Gynecology, University of Missouri; Overland Park Regional Medical Center, Research Medical Center, Kansas City, Missouri
Postpartum Care

JOHN V. COX, D.O.

Hematology/Medical Oncology, Texas Oncology, P.A.; Clinical Faculty, Internal Medicine, Methodist Hospitals of Dallas; Clinical Instructor, University of Texas Southwestern, Dallas, Texas
Vitamin K Deficiency

GARY L. CRAIG, M.D.

Assistant Clinical Professor, Faculty, Internal Medicine, University of Washington, Spokane; Staff, Sacred Heart Medical Center and Deaconess Hospital, Spokane, Washington
Osteoarthritis

LARRY D. CROOK, M.D.

Chief, Department of Internal Medicine, Gallup Indian Medical Center, Gallup, New Mexico
Plague

VANESSA E. CULLINS, M.D., M.P.H.

Assistant Professor, Johns Hopkins University, School of Medicine, Department of Gynecology and Obstetrics; Johns Hopkins Bayview Medical Center, Baltimore, Maryland
Dysmenorrhea

GREGORY A. DASCH, Ph.D.

Microbiologist, Viral and Rickettsial Diseases Program, Infectious Diseases Department, Naval Medical Research Institute, Bethesda, Maryland
The Typhus Fevers

RICHARD A. DAVIDSON, M.D., M.P.H.

Associate Professor of Internal Medicine, University of Florida, College of Medicine; Clinical Internal Medicine Physician, Shands Hospital, Gainesville, Florida
Giardiasis

IRA DAVIS, M.D.

Assistant Professor of Dermatology, New York Medical College; Assistant Attending Physician, Westchester County Medical Center, Valhalla, New York; Active Attending Physician, Bayley Seton Hospital, New Rochelle, New York
Premalignant Skin Lesions

CATHERINE L. DEAN, M.D., M.P.H.

Clinical Instructor, Washington University School of Medicine; Barnes-Jewish Hospital, Missouri Baptist Hospital, and Christian Hospital Northwest, St. Louis, Missouri
Contraception

ANTONIO DE LA CRUZ, M.D.

Clinical Professor of Otolaryngology/Head and Neck Surgery, University of Southern California School of Medicine, and House Ear Clinic, Inc.; St. Vincent's Medical Center and USC County General Hospital, Los Angeles, California; University of California; Irvine, Hospital, Irvine, California
Meniere's Disease

TOM R. DeMEESTER, M.D.

Professor and Chairman, Department of Surgery, University of Southern California School of Medicine, Los Angeles, California
Gastroesophageal Reflux Disease

CHRISTINE J. DEMPSEY, M.D.

Clinical Assistant, University of Massachusetts Medical School; Department of Medicine, University of Massachusetts Medical Center, Worcester, Massachusetts
Acute Bronchitis

RICHARD D. deSHAZO, M.D.

Professor of Medicine and Pediatrics, Chairman, Department of Internal Medicine, College of Medicine, University of South Alabama; University of South Alabama Hospitals and Clinics, Mobile, Alabama
Allergic Reactions to Drugs and Biologic Agents

NICHOLAS D. D'ESOPO, M.D.

Clinical Professor of Medicine, Yale School of Medicine, New Haven, Connecticut; Formerly, Chief of Pulmonary Diseases Service, VA Hospital, West Haven, Connecticut
Primary Lung Abscess

J.L. DÍAZ-PÉREZ, M.D., Ph.D.

Professor of Dermatology, University of the Basque Country; Chairman, Department of Dermatology, Cruces Hospital, Bilbao, Spain
Polyarteritis Nodosa

MARIANNE DIETERICH, M.D.

Professor of Neurology, Department of Neurology, University of Munich; Department of Neurology, Klinikum Grosshadern, University of Munich, Munich, Germany
Episodic Vertigo

MONICA E. DOERR, M.D.

Fellow, Division of Endocrinology, Department of Medicine, University of North Carolina, Chapel Hill, North Carolina
Diabetic Ketoacidosis

ELEN CASSO DONAHUE, M.D.

Resident, Department of Dermatology, Medical College of Pennsylvania and Hahnemann University, Philadelphia, Pennsylvania
Viral Diseases of the Skin

JANE M. DOYLE, M.D.

Assistant Professor of Medicine, University of Massachusetts Medical School; Division of Pulmonary Medicine, St. Vincent Hospital, Worcester, Massachusetts
Acute Bronchitis

MICHAEL V. DRAKE, M.D.

Professor of Ophthalmology, Associate Dean, University of California, San Francisco; Attending Physician, Moffitt/Long Hospitals, University of California; San Francisco General Hospital, San Francisco, California
Glaucoma

IVO DRURY, M.B., B.Ch.

Associate Professor, Department of Neurology, University of Michigan Medical School; Director, Clinical Neurophysiology Laboratories and Epilepsy Program, University of Michigan Medical Center, Ann Arbor, Michigan
Epilepsy in Adolescents and Adults

MICHAEL C. DUFFY, M.D.

Clinical Assistant Professor of Medicine, Wayne State University School of Medicine, Detroit, Michigan; GI Fellowship Program Director, William Beaumont Hospital, Royal Oak, Michigan
Gastritis

NANCY E. DUNLAP, M.D., Ph.D.

Associate Professor of Medicine, Division of Pulmonary and Critical Care Medicine, University of Alabama at Birmingham School of Medicine, University of Alabama Hospital, Birmingham, Alabama
Tuberculosis and Nontuberculous Mycobacterial Diseases

DENNIS E. DURIEX, M.D.

Methodist Hospital and St. Mary of the Plains Hospital, Lubbock, Texas
Psittacosis

SAMUEL F. DWORKIN, D.D.S., Ph.D.

Professor, University of Washington Schools of Dentistry and Medicine; Attending Clinical Psychologist, University Hospital, Seattle, Washington
Temporomandibular Disorders

WALTER DZIK, M.D.

Assistant Professor of Medicine, Harvard Medical School; Director, Transfusion Medicine, Deaconess Hospital, Boston, Massachusetts
Therapeutic Use of Blood Components

LIBBY EDWARDS, M.D.

Clinical Associate Professor (Dermatology), Bowman Gray School of Medicine, Winston-Salem, North Carolina; Chief of Dermatology, Carolinas Medical Center, Charlotte, North Carolina
Pruritus Ani and Vulvae

GARY S. EGLINTON, M.D.

Associate Professor and Chief, Division of Maternal Fetal Medicine, Georgetown University School of Medicine, Washington, D.C.
Vaginal Bleeding in Late Pregnancy

ANDERS G. EKLUND, M.D., Ph.D.

Associate Professor of Pulmonary Medicine, Karolinska Institute; Deputy Chairman, Department of Medicine, Karolinska Hospital, Stockholm, Sweden
Sarcoidosis

URI ELKAYAM, M.D.

Professor of Medicine, Director of Heart Failure Program, University of Southern California School of Medicine, Los Angeles California
Congestive Heart Failure

C. GREGORY ELLIOTT, M.D.

Professor of Medicine, University of Utah School of Medicine; Chief, Pulmonary Division, LDS Hospital, Salt Lake City, Utah
Acute Pulmonary Embolism

DEAN A. EMANUEL, M.D.

Director Emeritus, National Farm Medicine Center, Marshfield Clinic, Marshfield, Wisconsin
Hypersensitivity Pneumonitis (Extrinsic Allergic Alveolitis)

CHARLES H. EMERSON, M.D.

Professor of Medicine, University of Massachusetts Medical Center; Staff Physician, University of Massachusetts Medical Center, Worcester, Massachusetts
Goiter

ANTHONY L. ESPOSITO, M.D.

Associate Professor of Medicine, University of Massachusetts School of Medicine; Director, Division of Infectious Diseases; Associate Chief, Department of Medicine, Saint Vincent Hospital, Worcester, Massachusetts
Acute Bronchitis

E. DALE EVERETT, M.D.

Professor of Medicine, Director, Infectious Diseases Division, University of Missouri Health Sciences Center, Columbia, Missouri
Mycoplasmal and Viral Pneumonias

R. WESLEY FARR, M.D.

Assistant Professor of Medicine, Section of Infectious Diseases, Robert C. Byrd Health Sciences Center of West Virginia University, Morgantown, West Virginia
Relapsing Fever

S. HOSSEIN FATEMI, M.D., Ph.D.

Associate Professor of Psychiatry, University of Minnesota School of Medicine, Minneapolis, Minnesota
Schizophrenia

JEROME M. FELDMAN, M.D.

Associate Professor of Medicine, Duke University Medical School; Duke University Hospital and Durham VA Medical Center, Durham, North Carolina
Pheochromocytoma

JO-DAVID FINE, M.D., M.P.H.

Professor of Dermatology and Clinical Professor of Epidemiology, University of North Carolina at Chapel Hill; Attending Physician, University of North Carolina Hospitals; Principal Investigator and Head, National Epidermolysis Bullosa Registry, Chapel Hill, North Carolina
Bullous Diseases

LORRAINE A. FITZPATRICK, M.D.

Professor of Medicine, Mayo Medical School; Consultant, Endocrinology and Metabolism, Mayo Clinic and Mayo Foundation, Rochester, Minnesota
Hyperparathyroidism and Hypoparathyroidism

D. PRESTON FLANIGAN, M.D.

Clinical Professor of Surgery, University of California, Irvine, California
Acquired Diseases of the Aorta

SCOTT E. FLETCHER, M.D.

Assistant Professor of Pediatrics, Joint Division of Pediatric Cardiology, Creighton University and University of Nebraska, Childrens Hospital, Omaha, Nebraska
Congenital Heart Disease

SHIRLEY A. FLOYD-REISING, PH.D.

Assistant Professor of Pediatrics, Division of Infectious Diseases, Children's Hospital Medical Center, University of Cincinnati College of Medicine; Director, Clinical Microbiology and Virology/Infectious Disease Serology, Cincinnati, Ohio
Rubella and Congenital Rubella

HARALD FODSTAD, M.D., PH.D.

Associate Professor of Neurosurgery, New York Hospital–Cornell Medical Center, New York, New York; Chief of Neurosurgery, New York Methodist Hospital, Brooklyn, New York
Hiccup

FRANCINE M. FOSS, M.D.

Associate Professor of Medicine and Dermatology, Director, Cutaneous Lymphoma Program; Section of Hematology-Oncology, Department of Medicine, Boston University Medical Center, Boston, Massachusetts
Cutaneous T Cell Lymphoma

LAWRENCE S. FRIEDMAN, M.D.

Associate Professor of Medicine, Harvard Medical School; Associate Physician, Gastrointestinal Unit, Massachusetts General Hospital, Boston, Massachusetts
Acute and Chronic Viral Hepatitis

CHRISTOPHER J. GALLANT, M.D., M.Sc.

Assistant Professor, Department of Medicine (Dermatology), Dalhousie University Faculty of Medicine; Queen Elizabeth Health Science Center, Halifax, Nova Scotia, Canada
Contact Dermatitis

NELSON M. GANTZ, M.D.

Clinical Professor of Medicine, Pennsylvania State University School of Medicine, Hershey, Pennsylvania; Chairman, Department of Medicine, Chief, Division of Infectious Diseases, Pinnacle Health System, Harrisburg, Pennsylvania
Chronic Fatigue Syndrome

J. GARDEAZABAL, M.D.

Assistant Professor of Dermatology, University of the Basque Country; Consultant in Dermatology, Cruces Hospital, Bilbao, Spain
Polyarteritis Nodosa

JAMES A. GARRITY, M.D.

Associate Professor, Mayo Medical School; Consultant, Department of Ophthalmology, Mayo Foundation, Rochester, Minnesota
Optic Neuritis

BRUCE GENOVESE, M.D.

Clinical Instructor, Medicine (Cardiology), University of Michigan School of Medicine; Medical Director, Coronary Care Unit, St. Joseph Mercy Hospital, Ann Arbor, Michigan
Heart Block

ANDREW J. GHIO, M.D.

Adjunct Assistant Professor of Medicine, Duke University Medical Center; Durham VA Medical Center, Durham, North Carolina
Silicosis

ROMA GIANCHANDANI, M.D.

Lecturer, University of Michigan Medical School, Ann Arbor, Michigan
Hyperprolactinemia

JONATHAN GLASS, M.D.

Professor of Medicine, Chief, Section of Hematology/Oncology, Director, Cancer Center, Louisiana State University Medical School–Shreveport; Attending Physician, Louisiana State University Medical Center, Shreveport, Louisiana
Iron Deficiency Anemia

MICHAEL A. GLASS, M.D.

Resident, Division of Urology, University of Colorado Health Sciences Center, Denver, Colorado
Renal Calculi

ANDREW W. GODDARD, M.D.

Assistant Professor of Psychiatry, Yale University School of Medicine; Director, Yale Anxiety Clinic at Connecticut Mental Health Center, New Haven, Connecticut
Panic Disorder

JOSEPH GOLBUS, M.D.

Associate Professor of Medicine, Section of Arthritis and Connective Tissue Diseases, Northwestern University Medical School, Chicago, Illinois; Senior Attending Physician and Head, Division of Rheumatology, Evanston Hospital, Evanston, Illinois
Rheumatoid Arthritis

STANLEY M. GOLDBERG, M.D.

Clinical Professor of Surgery, University of Minnesota Medical School; Attending Physician, Fairview Southdale Hospital, Hennepin County Medical Center, University of Minnesota Hospitals, Minneapolis, Minnesota
Tumors of the Colon and Rectum

MITCHELL GOLDMAN, M.D.

Assistant Professor of Medicine, Division of Infectious Diseases, Indiana University School of Medicine; Director, Immunocompromised Infectious Diseases Clinical Service, Indiana University Hospital, Indianapolis, Indiana
Infectious Mononucleosis

JORGE L. GOMEZ, M.D.

Clinical Instructor, Department of Obstetrics and Gynecology, New York University Medical Center; Fellow in Maternal-Fetal Medicine, New York University Medical Center, New York, New York
Antepartum Care

STEVEN D. GORE, M.D.

Assistant Professor of Oncology, Johns Hopkins Oncology Center, Johns Hopkins University School of Medicine; Active Staff, Johns Hopkins Hospital, Baltimore, Maryland
Acute Leukemia in Adults

M. SEAN GRADY, M.D.

Associate Professor of Neurological Surgery, University of Washington School of Medicine; Harborview Medical Center, Seattle, Washington
Acute Head Injuries in Adults

JANE M. GRANT–KELS, M.D.

Professor and Chief, Division of Dermatology; Director of Dermatopathology, University of Connecticut Health Center, Farmington, Connecticut
Acne Vulgaris and Rosacea

ROBERT P. GREEN, M.D.

Associate Clinical Professor of Otolaryngology, Mount Sinai School of Medicine; Attending, Mount Sinai Hospital, New York, New York
Tinnitus

BARRY H. GREENBERG, M.D.

Professor of Medicine, University of California, San Diego; Director, Heart Failure/Transplant Cardiology Program, University of California, San Diego, San Diego, California
Infective Endocarditis

DAVID G. GREENHALGH, M.D.

Associate Professor of Surgery, University of Cincinnati College of Medicine; Assistant Chief of Staff, Shriners Burns Institute; Attending Staff, University Hospital; Attending Staff, Children's Hospital Medical Center, Cincinnati, Ohio
Burns

JOSEPH GREENSHER, M.D.

Professor of Pediatrics, State University of New York at Stony Brook, Stony Brook, New York; Medical Director and Associate Chairman, Department of Pediatrics, Winthrop-University Hospital; Associate Director, Long Island Regional Poison Control Center, Winthrop-University Hospital, Mineola, New York
Acute Poisonings

FRANK L. GREENWAY, M.D.

Professor and Medical Director, Pennington Biomedical Research Center, Louisiana State University, Baton Rouge, Louisiana; Clinical Professor of Medicine, Louisiana State University School of Medicine, New Orleans, Louisiana
Obesity

DIRK K. GREINEDER, M.D., Ph.D.

Assistant Clinical Professor, Department of Ambulatory Care and Prevention, Harvard Medical School; Chief of Allergy, Harvard Community Health Plan, Boston, Massachusetts
Asthma in Children

H. BARTON GROSSMAN, M.D.

Professor, Departments of Urology and Cell Biology, W. A. "Tex" and Deborah Moncrief, Jr., Chair in Urology, The University of Texas M. D. Anderson Cancer Center, Houston, Texas
Malignant Tumors of the Urogenital Tract

JAMES C. GROTTA, M.D.

Professor of Neurology and Director of the Stroke Program, University of Texas, Houston; Attending Neurologist, Hermann Hospital, Houston, Texas
Ischemic Cerebrovascular Disease

RICHARD L. GUERRANT, M.D.

Professor of Medicine, Thomas Hunter Professor of International Medicine; Chief, Division of Geographic and International Medicine, University of Virginia School of Medicine, Charlottesville, Virginia
Food-Borne Illness

DAVID A. HAAKE, M.D.

Assistant Professor of Medicine, University of California, Los Angeles, School of Medicine; Staff Physician, West Los Angeles Veterans Affairs Medical Center, Los Angeles, California
Tularemia

ANN E. HALLSTONE, M.D.

Assistant Clinical Professor of Medicine and Surgery, University of California, Davis, California; Staff Gastroenterologist, VA Northern California System of Clinics, Martinez, California
Nausea and Vomiting

LAWRENCE H. HANAU, M.D., Ph.D.

Assistant Professor of Medicine, Albert Einstein College of Medicine; Director, Infectious Diseases Clinic, Montefiore Medical Center, Bronx, New York
Rat-Bite Fever

ECKART HANEKE, M.D., Ph.D.

Chairman and Professor of Dermatology, Department of Dermatology, Ferdinand-Sauerbruch Hospital, Academic Teaching Hospital of the University of Düsseldorf, University of Witten/Herdecke Health Center, Wuppertal, Germany
Diseases of the Nails

CATHLEEN A. HANLON, V.M.D., Ph.D.

Deputy Public Health Veterinarian, New York State Department of Health, Division of Epidemiology, Albany, New York
Rabies

GEORGE P. HANNA, M.D.

Senior Cardiology Fellow, Hermann Hospital, Houston, Texas
Angina Pectoris

PHILIP M. HANNO, M.D.

Professor and Chairman, Department of Urology, Temple University School of Medicine; Chief of Urology, Temple University Hospital, Philadelphia, Pennsylvania
Prostatitis

JAMES M. HARIG, M.D., M.S.

Clinical Associate of Medicine, University of Illinois Medical Center, Chicago, Illinois
Constipation

RICHARD L. HARVEY, M.D.

Assistant Professor of Physical Medicine and Rehabilitation, Northwestern University Medical School; Director, Center for Stroke Rehabilitation, The Rehabilitation Institute of Chicago, Chicago, Illinois
Rehabilitation of the Stroke Patient

RODRIGO HASBUN, M.D.

Postdoctoral Fellow in Infectious Diseases, Yale University School of Medicine; Fellow in Infectious Diseases, Yale—New Haven Hospital, New Haven, Connecticut; Admitting Officer of the Day, West Haven VA Medical Center, West Haven, Connecticut; House Physician, Hospital of Saint Raphael, New Haven, Connecticut
Amebiasis

WILLIAM S. HAUBRICH, M.D.

Clinical Professor of Medicine, University of California, San Diego, San Diego, California; Senior Consultant Emeritus, Scripps Clinic and Research Foundation, La Jolla, California
Diverticula of the Alimentary Tract

GRANVIL L. HAYS, D.D.S., M.S.

Associate Professor, Department of General Dentistry, Dental Branch; Associate Professor, Department of Family Practice and Community Medicine, Medical School; University of Texas–Houston, Health Science Center, Houston, Texas
Diseases of the Mouth

JEFFERY E. HECK, M.D.
Associate Professor, Department of Family Medicine, University of Cincinnati; Residency Director, University of Cincinnati–Providence Hospital Family Medicine Program, Cincinnati, Ohio
Acute Infectious Diarrhea

JONATHAN D. HEILICZER, M.D.
Associate Professor of Pediatrics, University of Illinois College of Medicine; Co-Director, Children's Kidney Center of Illinois, University of Illinois Medical Center, Chicago, Illinois
Parenteral Fluid Therapy for Infants and Children

P. S. HELLIWELL, D.M., P.H.D.
Senior Lecturer, University of Leeds, Leeds, England, United Kingdom; Honorary Consultant Rheumatologist, Bradford NHS Trust, Bradford, England, United Kingdom
Ankylosing Spondylitis

WAYNE J. G. HELLSTROM, M.D.
Associate Professor of Urology, Tulane University School of Medicine; Chief of Urology, Medical Center of Louisiana, New Orleans, Louisiana
Nongonococcal Urethritis

REX T. HOFFMEISTER, M.D.
Retired Assistant Clinical Professor of Medicine, University of Washington School of Medicine, Spokane, Washington
Osteoarthritis

N. WILSON HOLLAND, M.D.
Assistant Professor of Medicine, Rheumatology, Emory University; Emory University Hospital and Emory Clinic, Atlanta, Georgia
Hyperuricemia and Gout

W. KEITH HOOTS, M.D.
Associate Pediatrician and Associate Professor of Pediatrics, University of Texas M.D. Anderson Cancer Center; Associate Professor of Pediatric and Internal Medicine, University of Texas Medical School at Houston; Pediatrician, Hermann Children's Hospital and St. Joseph's Hospital, Houston, Texas
Hemophilia and Related Conditions

LINTON C. HOPKINS, M.D.
Professor of Neurology, Emory University School of Medicine, Atlanta, Georgia
Myasthenia Gravis

IFFATH ABBASI HOSKINS, M.D.
Associate Professor, Department of Obstetrics and Gynecology, New York University Medical Center; Attending (Maternal Fetal Medicine), New York University Medical Center (Tisch Hospital and Bellevue Hospital), New York, New York
Antepartum Care

RICHARD J. HOWARD, M.D., PH.D.
The Robert H. Axline Professor of Surgery, University of Florida School of Medicine; Attending Surgeon, Chief, Division of Transplantation, Shands Hospital, Gainesville, Florida
Necrotizing Soft Tissue Infections

PATRICIA A. HUGHES, D.O.
Assistant Professor of Pediatrics, Section of Infectious Disease, Albany Medical College; Assistant Professor of Pediatrics, Albany Medical Center, Albany, New York
Measles (Rubeola)

DONALD B. HUNNINGHAKE, M.D.
Professor of Medicine and Pharmacology, Director, The Heart Disease Prevention Clinic, University of Minnesota, Minneapolis, Minnesota
Hyperlipoproteinemias

DAVID L. HURT, M.D.
Resident, Department of Dermatology, University of Iowa Hospitals and Clinics, Iowa City, Iowa
Papulosquamous Diseases

EDSEL ING, M.D.
Clinical Fellow, Medical College of Pennsylvania, Philadelphia, Pennsylvania; Lecturer, University of Pittsburgh; Clinical Fellow, Allegheny General Hospital, Pittsburgh, Pennsylvania
Optic Neuritis

ANDREW F. INGLIS, JR., M.D.
Associate Professor of Otolaryngology–Head and Neck Surgery, University of Washington; Active Staff, Children's Hospital and Medical Center, University of Washington Medical Center, and Harborview Medical Center, Seattle, Washington
Sinusitis

ADRIAN P. IRELAND, M.D.
Research Fellow, Department of Surgery, University of Southern California, Los Angeles, California
Gastroesophageal Reflux Disease

ROBERT R. ISACKSEN, M.D.
Chief Resident in Urology, Loyola University Medical Center, Maywood, Illinois
Benign Prostatic Hyperplasia

IVOR M.D. JACKSON, M.D.
Professor of Medicine, Director, Division of Endocrinology, Brown University School of Medicine; Physician-in-Charge, Division of Endocrinology, Rhode Island Hospital, Providence, Rhode Island
Acromegaly

ALAN C. JACOBSON, M.D.
Rheumatology Fellow, The George Washington University Medical Center, Washington, D.C.
Connective Tissue Disease (Systemic Lupus Erythematosus, Dermatomyositis, Other Myopathies, and Scleroderma)

ROBERT J. JACOBSON, M.D.
Medical Director, Cancer Institute, Good Samaritan Medical Center, West Palm Beach, Florida; Consulting Associate, Duke University Medical Center, Durham, North Carolina
Pernicious Anemia and Other Megaloblastic Anemias

EDWARD JAROSZEWSKI, M.D.
Assistant Professor of Psychiatry, University of Connecticut School of Medicine, Farmington, Connecticut; Director, Emergency Psychiatry; Associate Director of Psychiatric Consultation; Medical Director of the Institute of Living Assessment Center, Hartford Hospital, Hartford, Connecticut
Drug Abuse

KAJ JOHANSEN, M.D., PH.D.
Professor of Surgery, University of Washington School of Medicine; Director, Surgical Education, Providence Medical Center, Seattle, Washington
Bleeding Esophageal Varices

JAMES R. JOHNSON, M.D.
Associate Professor, Department of Medicine, University of Minnesota; University of Minnesota Hospital and Clinic, Minneapolis, Minnesota
Bacterial Infections of the Urinary Tract in Women

LARRY E. JOHNSON, M.D., PH.D.
Assistant Professor of Family Medicine, University of Cincinnati Medical Center; Medical Director, Pro-Health Patient Services, Franciscan Health System of the Ohio Valley, Cincinnati, Ohio
Vitamin Nutrition

LIVETTE JOHNSON, M.D.

Assistant Professor of Clinical Medicine, New York Medical College, Valhalla, New York; Attending Physician, Metropolitan Hospital Center, New York, New York
Acquired Immune Deficiency Syndrome (AIDS)

STEVEN C. JOHNSON, M.D.

Assistant Professor of Medicine, Division of Infectious Diseases, University of Colorado Health Sciences Center; University Hospital and Veterans Administration Medical Center, Denver, Colorado
Syphilis

KEITH A. JOINER, M.D.

Professor of Medicine, Epidemiology and Public Health and Cell Biology; Chief, Infectious Diseases Section; Yale–New Haven Hospital; Yale University School of Medicine, New Haven, Connecticut
Toxoplasmosis

MARK A. KALLGREN, M.D.

Pain Management Consultant, Advanced Pain Management Group (St. Vincent's Hospital), Portland, Oregon
Pain

ATTALLAH KAPPAS, M.D.

Sherman Fairchild Professor, The Rockefeller University; Physician-in-Chief Emeritus, The Rockefeller University Hospital, New York, New York
The Porphyrias

JAMES H. KAPPLER, M.D.

Clinical Instructor, University of Michigan School of Medicine; Consultant in Cardiology and Clinical Electrophysiology, St. Joseph Mercy Hospital, Ann Arbor, Michigan
Heart Block

CAROL A. KAUFFMAN, M.D.

Professor of Internal Medicine, University of Michigan Medical School; Chief, Infectious Diseases Section, Ann Arbor Veterans Affairs Medical Center, Ann Arbor, Michigan
Histoplasmosis

MAUREEN KAYS, M.D.

Clinical Instructor, Department of Pediatrics, University of Florida; Shands Hospital and North Florida Regional Hospital, Gainesville, Florida
Pertussis

DAVID J. KEARNEY, M.D.

Gastroenterology Fellow, University of California, San Francisco, San Francisco, California
Gaseousness and Indigestion

JOHN G. KELTON, M.D.

Professor of Medicine and Pathology, McMaster University, Faculty of Health Sciences; Chief of Medicine, Chedoke-McMaster Medical Centre, Hamilton, Ontario, Canada
Platelet-Mediated Bleeding Disorders

EKKEHARD KEMMANN, M.D.

Professor, Department of Obstetrics, Gynecology and Reproductive Sciences, UMD–Robert Wood Johnson Medical School, New Brunswick, New Jersey
Ectopic Pregnancy

CHARLES D. KENNARD, M.D.

Chief, Dermatologic Surgery, Wilford Hall Medical Center, Lackland Air Force Base; Assistant Clinical Professor of Medicine (Dermatology), University of Texas Health Science Center, San Antonio, Texas
Urticaria

DAVID J. KESSLER, M.D.

Electrophysiology Fellow, Division of Cardiology, Clinical Electrophysiology and Pacing, University of Texas Southwestern Medical Center; University of Texas Southwestern Affiliated Hospitals—Parkland Memorial Hospital and Dallas VA Medical Center, Dallas, Texas
Tachycardias

JAY S. KEYSTONE, M.D.

Professor of Medicine and Microbiology, University of Toronto; Director, Tropical Disease Unit, The Toronto Hospital, University of Toronto, Toronto, Ontario, Canada
Intestinal Parasites

ZAFAR KHAN, M.D.

Attending, Department of Urology, Beth Israel Medical Center, New York, New York
Urinary Incontinence

DONALD G. KIM, M.D.

Resident, Colon and Rectal Surgery, Department of Surgery, Division of Colon and Rectal Surgery, University of Minnesota Medical School, Minneapolis, Minnesota
Tumors of the Colon and Rectum

KAREN E. KIM, M.D., M.S.

Associate in Medicine, University of Illinois Medical Center; Associate in Medicine, University of Illinois, Chicago, Illinois
Constipation

CHARLES E. KING, M.D.

Formerly Associate Professor and Director of Endoscopy, University of Florida College of Medicine, Gainesville, Florida, Digestive Disorders Associates, Annapolis and Glen Burnie, Maryland; Anne Arundel Medical Center, Annapolis, Maryland; North Arundel Hospital, Glen Burnie, Maryland
Malabsorption

CRAIG S. KITCHENS, M.D.

Professor and Vice-Chairman, Department of Medicine, University of Florida; Chief, Medical Service, Department of Veterans Affairs Medical Center, Gainesville, Florida
Snakebite

RONALD E. KLEINMAN, M.D.

Associate Professor of Pediatrics, Harvard Medical School; Chief, Division of Pediatric Gastroenterology and Nutrition, Combined Program in Pediatric Gastroenterology and Nutrition, Associate Chief, Children's Service, Massachusetts General Hospital, Boston, Massachusetts
Normal Infant Nutrition

TIMOTHY K. KNILANS, M.D.

Assistant Professor of Pediatrics and Medicine, University of Cincinnati College of Medicine; Director, Clinical Cardiac Electrophysiology and Pacing, Children's Hospital Medical Center, Cincinnati, Ohio
Cardiac Arrest: Sudden Cardiac Death

RONALD T. KODAMA, M.D.

Assistant Professor, Department of Surgery, Division of Urology, University of Toronto; Sunnybrook Health Science Centre, Toronto, Ontario, Canada
Urethral Strictures

RONALD J. KOENIG, M.D., PH.D.

Professor, Division of Endocrinology and Metabolism, Department of Internal Medicine, University of Michigan Medical Center, Ann Arbor, Michigan
Hypothyroidism

HILARY KOPROWSKI, M.D.

Professor, Department of Microbiology and Immunology, Thomas Jefferson University, Philadelphia, Pennsylvania
Rabies

STEPHEN M. KORBET, M.D.

Professor of Medicine, Section of Nephrology, Department of Medicine, Rush Medical College; Rush–Presbyterian–St. Luke's Medical Center, Chicago, Illinois
Primary Glomerular Diseases

JOYCE A. KORVICK, M.D.

Department of Infectious Disease, Veterans Administration Medical Center, Washington, D.C.
Legionellosis (Pontiac Fever and Legionnaires' Disease)

HENRY R. KRANZLER, M.D.

Associate Professor of Psychiatry, University of Connecticut School of Medicine; Associate Scientific Director, Alcohol Research Center, University of Connecticut Health Center, Farmington, Connecticut
Alcoholism

STEPHEN J. KRAUS, M.D.

Director, Georgia Clinical Research; Staff Physician, West Paces Medical Center; Staff Physician, St. Joseph's Hospital; Staff Physician, Northside Hospital, Atlanta, Georgia; Staff Physician, Newton General Hospital, Covington, Georgia
Chancroid

JOHN N. KRIEGER, M.D.

Professor, Department of Urology, University of Washington School of Medicine; University of Washington Medical Center, Harborview Medical Center, Seattle VA Medical Center, and Childrens Orthopedic Hospital, Seattle, Washington
Epididymitis

RICHARD W. KROUSKOP, M.D.

Associate Professor of Pediatrics, Louisiana State University Medical Center; Neonatologist, Louisiana State University Medical Center, Shreveport, Louisiana
Care of the High-Risk Neonate

FAITH H. KUNG, M.D.

Associate Professor of Pediatrics, UCSD School of Medicine; Associate Professor of Pediatrics, UCSD Medical Center, San Diego, California
Acute Leukemia in Children

LINDA LACROIX, M.D.

Assistant Professor of Medicine, McGill University; Associate Physician–Hematologist, Division of Hematology, The Montreal General Hospital, Montreal, Quebec, Canada
Thrombotic Thrombocytopenic Purpura

MARK D. LACY, M.D.

Fellow in Infectious Diseases, Robert C. Byrd Health Sciences Center of West Virginia University, Morgantown, West Virginia
Relapsing Fever

THOMAS J. LANE, M.D.

Associate Professor of Clinical Medicine, University of Connecticut School of Medicine, Farmington, Connecticut; Director, Section of General Medicine and Geriatrics, New Britain General Hospital, New Britain, Connecticut
Cough

PEARON G. LANG, Jr., M.D.

Professor, Medical University of South Carolina; Attending, Medical University of South Carolina; Consultant, VA Hospital, Charleston, South Carolina
Cutaneous Vasculitis

W. ROBERT LANGE, M.D., M.P.H.

Assistant Professor of Medicine, Johns Hopkins School of Medicine; Assistant Professor, Department of International Health, Johns Hopkins School of Public Health; Associate Physician, Johns Hopkins Hospital, Greater Baltimore Medical Center, Baltimore, Maryland
Underwater Medicine

J. MICHAEL LAZARUS, M.D.

Associate Professor of Medicine, Harvard Medical School; Senior Vice President/Medical Director, National Medical Care, Inc., Boston, Massachusetts
Chronic Renal Failure

JACQUES R. LECLERC, M.D.

Associate Professor of Medicine, McGill University; Director, Division of Hematology, The Montreal General Hospital, Montreal, Quebec, Canada
Disseminated Intravascular Coagulation; Thrombotic Thrombocytopenic Purpura

I.M. LEIGH, M.D.

The London Hospital Medical College and Medical School of St. Bartholomew's Hospital; Royal London Hospital, London, England
Erythema Multiforme

MARTHA L. LEPOW, M.D.

Professor of Pediatrics, Chair, Department of Pediatrics, Albany Medical College; Professor of Pediatrics, Albany Medical Center, Albany, New York
Measles (Rubeola)

ROSEMARIE A. LEUZZI, M.D.

Clinical Assistant Professor of Medicine, Division of Internal Medicine, Thomas Jefferson University Hospital, Philadelphia, Pennsylvania
Thromboembolic Disease in Pregnancy

ROBERT A. LEVINE, M.D.

Associate Professor of Medicine, Harvard Medical School; Director, Cardiac Ultrasound Laboratories, Massachusetts General Hospital, Boston, Massachusetts
Mitral Valve Prolapse

NATALIE LEWIS, M.B., B.S.

Assistant Professor of Clinical Medicine, University of Connecticut School of Medicine, Farmington, Connecticut; Associate Director, Section of General Medicine and Geriatrics, New Britain General Hospital, New Britain, Connecticut
Cough

PHILIP L. LIEBERMAN, M.D.

Clinical Professor of Medicine, University of Tennessee College of Medicine, Memphis, Tennessee
Anaphylaxis and Serum Sickness

KEITH D. LILLEMOE, M.D.

Professor, Department of Surgery, The Johns Hopkins University School of Medicine; Active Staff, The Johns Hopkins Hospital, Baltimore, Maryland
Cholelithiasis and Cholecystitis

FRANK W. LING, M.D.

Faculty Professor and Chairman, Department of Obstetrics and Gynecology, University of Tennessee, Memphis, Memphis, Tennessee
Pelvic Inflammatory Disease

BENJAMIN A. LIPSKY, M.D.

Associate Professor; Department of Medicine, University of Washington School of Medicine; Director, General Internal Medicine

Clinic; Hospital Epidemiologist, VA Puget Sound Health Care System, Seattle, Washington
Bacterial Infections of the Urinary Tract in Men

BENJAMIN LIPTZIN, M.D.

Professor and Deputy Chair of Psychiatry, Tufts University School of Medicine, Boston, Massachusetts; Chairman, Department of Psychiatry, Baystate Medical Center, Springfield, Massachusetts
Delirium

JEFFREY R. LISSE, M.D.

Associate Professor of Medicine and Pathology, Director, Division of Rheumatology, University of Texas Medical Branch, Galveston, Texas; Active Staff, St. Johns Hospital, Nassau Bay, Texas
Polymyalgia Rheumatica and Giant Cell Arteritis

N. SCOTT LITOFSKY, M.D.

Assistant Professor of Surgery (Neurosurgery), University of Massachusetts Medical Center, Worcester, Massachusetts
Brain Tumors

IRAKLIS LIVAS, M.D.

Post-Doctor Clinical Fellow, Johns Hopkins Asthma and Allergy Center, Baltimore, Maryland
Allergic Rhinitis Caused by Inhalant Factors

GERALD L. LOGUE, M.D.

Professor of Medicine, Head, Division of Hematology, State University of New York at Buffalo; Chief of Staff, VA Medical Center, Buffalo, New York
Autoimmune Hemolytic Anemia

SORNCHAI LOOAREESUWAN, M.D.

Professor of Medicine and Head of Division of Critical Care for Tropical Diseases, Department of Clinical Tropical Medicine, Faculty of Tropical Medicine, Mahidol University; Deputy Director of the Hospital for Tropical Diseases, and Head of Division of Critical Care for Tropical Diseases, Hospital for Tropical Diseases, Faculty of Tropical Medicine, Mahidol University, Bangkok, Thailand
Malaria

DIRK LUCAS, PHARM.D.

Clinical Manager, CMS/Spectrum Owen Healthcare, Houston, Texas
Drugs Approved in 1995; Top 200 Drugs Prescribed in the United States

TOM F. LUE, M.D.

Professor of Urology, University of California, San Francisco; Attending Urologist, UCSF/Mt. Zion Hospital, San Francisco Veterans Affairs Medical Center, San Francisco, California
Erectile Dysfunction

CHRISTINA LUEDKE, M.D., PH.D.

Fellow in Pediatrics, Harvard Medical School; Fellow in Medicine (Endocrinology), Children's Hospital; Clinical Associate in Pediatrics, Massachusetts General Hospital, Boston, Massachusetts
Diabetes Mellitus in Children and Adolescents

VELIMIR A. LUKETIC, M.D.

Assistant Professor of Medicine, Medical College of Virginia, Virginia Commonwealth University, Richmond, Virginia
Cirrhosis

PAULA LUTZ, M.D.

Instructor in Pathology, Harvard Medical School; Assistant Director, Transfusion Medicine, Deaconess Hospital, Boston, Massachusetts
Therapeutic Use of Blood Components

J. DICK MacLEAN, M.D.

Associate Professor, McGill University; Senior Physician, Montreal General Hospital; Director, McGill University Centre for Tropical Disease, Montreal, Quebec, Canada
Trichinellosis

ROBERT D. MADOFF, M.D.

Clinical Associate Professor of Surgery, Director of Research, Division of Colon and Rectal Surgery, University of Minnesota Medical School, Minneapolis, Minnesota
Tumors of the Colon and Rectum

MICHAEL L. MARKEL, M.D.

Associate Professor of Medicine, Assistant Professor of Pediatrics, Director of Electrophysiology, University of Cincinnati, and University of Cincinnati Medical Center; Staff Physician, University of Cincinnati Medical Center, Cincinnati VA Hospital, and Consulting Physician, Cincinnati Children's Hospital, Cincinnati, Ohio
Cardiac Arrest: Sudden Cardiac Death

PAULA MARLTON, M.B., B.S.

Senior Lecturer in Pathology, University of Queensland; Assistant Director of Haematology, Princess Alexandra Hospital, Brisbane, Australia
Non-Hodgkin's Lymphoma

ANDREW T. MARSHALL, M.D.

Fellow in Gastroenterology, Division of Gastroenterology, Department of Medicine, Beth Israel Hospital, Boston, Massachusetts
Ulcerative Colitis

G. ROBERT MASON, M.D.

Professor and Chairman, Department of Thoracic and Cardiovascular Surgery, Loyola University School of Medicine; Chief of Thoracic and Cardiovascular Surgery, Loyola University Medical Center and Hines VA Hospital, Maywood, Illinois
Gastric Tumors

JOHN R. MATHIAS, M.D.

Professor of Medicine, The University of Texas Medical Branch, Galveston, Texas
Irritable Bowel Syndrome

KEVIN D. MAUPIN, M.D.

Instructor, Department of Pediatrics, University of Alabama at Birmingham; Fellow in Pediatric Pulmonary Medicine, The Children's Hospital of Alabama, Birmingham, Alabama
Tuberculosis and Nontuberculous Mycobacterial Diseases

JAMES S. McCARTHY, M.B.B.S.

Visiting Associate, Laboratory of Parasitic Diseases, National Institute of Allergy and Infectious Diseases, National Institutes of Health, Bethesda, Maryland
Parasitic Diseases of the Skin

BETSY LOVE McCLUNG, R.N., M.N.

Associate Director, Oregon Osteoporosis Center, Providence Portland Medical Center, Portland, Oregon
Osteoporosis

MICHAEL R. McCLUNG, M.D.

Associate Professor of Medicine, Oregon Health Sciences University; Director, Oregon Osteoporosis Center, Providence Portland Medical Center, Portland, Oregon
Osteoporosis

GEOFFREY M. McCULLEN, M.D.

Instructor of Orthopedic Surgery, University of California, San Diego; Naval Medical Center, San Diego; University of California, San Diego, Medical Center; Veterans Administration Medical Center, San Diego, California
Low Back Pain

JAMES A. McGREGOR, M.D., C.M.

Professor and Vice Chair, Department of Obstetrics and Gynecology, University of Colorado School of Medicine, Denver, Colorado
Vulvovaginitis

KENNETH E. McINTYRE, JR, M.D.

Professor of Surgery, Chief, Vascular Surgery Section, University of Texas Medical Branch; Attending Staff Surgeon, John Sealy Hospital, Galveston, Texas
Peripheral Arterial Disease

JOSEPH S. McLAUGHLIN, M.D.

Professor of Surgery and Head, Division of Thoracic and Cardiovascular Surgery, University of Maryland School of Medicine; Director, Thoracic and Cardiovascular Surgery, University of Maryland Medical Center, Baltimore, Maryland
Atelectasis

KENNETH R. McQUAID, M.D.

Associate Professor of Clinical Medicine, University of California, San Francisco; Director of GI Endoscopy, San Francisco VA Medical Center, San Francisco, California
Gaseousness and Indigestion

HERBERT Y. MELTZER, M.D.

Professor of Psychiatry and Pharmacology, Vanderbilt University School of Medicine, Nashville, Tennessee
Schizophrenia

NANCY PRICE MENDENHALL, M.D.

Professor and Chairman, Department of Radiation Oncology, University of Florida College of Medicine; Shands Teaching Hospital, Gainesville, Florida
Hodgkin's Disease: Radiation Therapy

MARY GAIL MERCURIO, M.D.

Assistant Professor of Clinical Dermatology, Attending Physician, Columbia University College of Physicians and Surgeons, New York, New York
Sunburn

GENO J. MERLI, M.D.

Clinical Professor of Medicine, Jefferson Medical College; Deputy Chairman, Department of Medicine; Director, Division of Internal Medicine, Thomas Jefferson University Hospital, Philadelphia, Pennsylvania
Thromboembolic Disease in Pregnancy

HENRY S. MILLER, JR., M.D.

Professor of Medicine/Cardiology, Bowman Gray School of Medicine, Wake Forest University; Medical Director, Cardiac Rehabilitation, North Carolina Baptist Hospital and Wake Forest University, Winston-Salem, North Carolina
Cardiac Rehabilitation

MARIE E. MINNICH, M.D.

Director, Obstetric Anesthesia; Associate, Department of Anesthesiology, Geisinger Medical Center, Danville, Pennsylvania
Obstetric Anesthesia

KATHERINE MINNICK, M.D.

Fellow in Infectious Diseases, University of Virginia School of Medicine, Roanoke–Salem Program in Infectious Diseases; Section of Infectious Diseases, Veterans Affairs Medical Center, Salem, Virginia
Rocky Mountain Spotted Fever

AYESHA MIRZA, M.D.

Fellow in Pediatric Infectious Diseases, Louisiana State University School of Medicine and Tulane University School of Medicine; Active Staff, Children's Hospital, University Hospital, and Tulane Medical Center, New Orleans, Louisiana
Diphtheria

CLIFFORD O. MISHAW, M.D.

Assistant Professor, Baylor College of Medicine; Texas Children's Hospital, Houston, Texas
Immunization Practices

HOWARD C. MOFENSON, M.D.

Professor of Pediatrics and Emergency Medicine, State University of New York at Stony Brook, Stony Brook, New York; Professor of Pharmacology and Toxicology, New York School of Osteopathy, Old Westbury, New York; St. John's University College of Pharmacy, Jamaica, New York; Director, Long Island Regional Poison Control Center; Winthrop-University Hospital and Nassau County Medical Center, Mineola, New York
Acute Poisonings

MANOJ MONGA, M.D.

Senior Resident in Urology, Chief, Section of Andrology and Male Infertility, Tulane University Medical Center; Medical Center of Louisiana, New Orleans, Louisiana
Nongonococcal Urethritis

MIGUEL MONTEJO, M.D., PH.D.

Faculty Associate Professor of Medicine, University of Basque Country, School of Medicine; Infectious Diseases, Internal Medicine, Hospital de Cruces, Bilbao, Spain
Brucellosis

TERRY L. MOORE, M.D.

Professor of Pediatrics and Internal Medicine, Director, Division of Rheumatology, St. Louis University Health Sciences Center; St. Louis University Hospital and Cardinal Glennon Children's Hospital, St. Louis, Missouri
Juvenile Rheumatoid Arthritis

LEWIS B. MORGENSTERN, M.D.

Assistant Professor of Neurology, University of Texas, Houston; Attending Neurologist, Hermann Hospital, Houston, Texas
Ischemic Cerebrovascular Disease

MAUREEN MORIARITY–SHEEHAN, R.N.

Adjunct Faculty, University of Maryland School of Nursing; Greater Baltimore Medical Center, Baltimore, Maryland
Underwater Medicine

VICKI A. MORRISON, M.D.

Assistant Professor of Medicine, Sections of Hematology/Oncology and Infectious Disease, University of Minnesota; Staff Physician, Medicine Service, Sections of Hematology/Oncology and Infectious Disease, Veterans Affairs Medical Center, Minneapolis, Minnesota
Chronic Leukemias

MONICA MORROW, M.D.

Associate Professor of Surgery, Northwestern University Medical School; Director, Lynn Sage Comprehensive Breast Program, Northwestern Memorial Hospital, Chicago, Illinois
Diseases of the Breast

ABRAHAM MORSE, M.D.

Resident, The Johns Hopkins Hospital, Baltimore, Maryland
Dysmenorrhea

JOSEPH F. MORTOLA, M.D.

Associate Professor, Harvard Medical School; Director, Division of Reproductive Endocrinology, Beth Israel Hospital, Boston, Massachusetts
Premenstrual Syndrome

STEPHEN MUELLER, M.D.

Assistant Professor of Psychiatry, Tufts University School of Medicine, Boston, Massachusetts; Medical Director, Department of Psychiatry, Baystate Medical Center, Springfield, Massachusetts
Delirium

AUGUSTINE D. MUNOZ, M.D.

Associate Professor of Medicine, University of California, Los Angeles, Los Angeles, California; Chief, Pulmonary and Critical Care Medicine, Kern Medical Center, Bakersfield, California
Coccidioidomycosis

MAURICE MURPHY, M.B.

Fellow, Infectious Disease Service, Department of Medicine, Memorial Sloan-Kettering Cancer Center, New York, New York
Brain Abscess

ATTILA NAKEEB, M.D.

Senior Resident, Department of Surgery, The Johns Hopkins Hospital, Baltimore, Maryland
Cholelithiasis and Cholecystitis

FELIPE NAVARRO, M.D.

Clinical Associate, Cleveland Clinic Foundation, Cleveland, Ohio
Deep Venous Thrombosis of the Extremities

TABINDA NAZIR, M.D.

Senior Resident, Department of Primary Care Internal Medicine, Elmhurst Hospital Center, Elmhurst, New York
Urinary Incontinence

BRETT R. NEUSTATER, M.D.

Gastroenterology Fellow, University of Miami School of Medicine, Miami, Florida
Crohn's Disease

PETER E. NEWBURGER, M.D.

Professor of Pediatrics and Molecular Genetics/Microbiology, University of Massachusetts Medical School; Director, Pediatric Hematology/Oncology and Associate Director, Cancer Center, University of Massachusetts Medical Center, Worcester, Massachusetts
Neutropenia

KRISTIN L. NICHOL, M.D., M.P.H.

Associate Professor of Medicine, University of Minnesota Medical School; Acting Chief, Medicine Service, Minneapolis VA Medical Center, Minneapolis, Minnesota
Influenza

CLAUS NIEDERAU, M.D.

Professor of Medicine, Heinrich-Heine University School of Medicine; Department of Medicine, Gastroenterology Unit, Heinrich-Heine University, Düsseldorf, Germany
Hemochromatosis

LYNNETTE K. NIEMAN, M.D.

Clinical Director and Senior Investigator, National Institute of Child Health and Human Development, National Institutes of Health; Attending Physician, Warren Grant Magnusen Clinical Center, National Institutes of Health, Bethesda, Maryland
Cushing's Syndrome

THOMAS B. NUTMAN, M.D.

Head, Helminth Immunology Section, Laboratory of Parasitic Diseases, National Institute of Allergy and Infectious Diseases, National Institutes of Health, Bethesda, Maryland
Parasitic Diseases of the Skin

ANGELA OGDEN, M.D.

Assistant Professor, Department of Pediatrics, Division of Hematology/Oncology, Baylor College of Medicine; Medical Director, Bone Marrow Transplant Unit, Texas Children's Hospital, Houston, Texas
Polycythemia Vera

KATHERINE A. O'HANLAN, M.D.

Assistant Professor, Department of Gynecology and Obstetrics, Stanford University School of Medicine; Associate Director, Division of Gynecologic Oncology; Director, Dysplasia Clinic, Stanford University, Stanford, California; Chief of Gynecology Service, Palo Alto Veterans Hospital, Palo Alto, California
Carcinoma of the Cervix Uteri

ELISE A. OLSEN, M.D.

Associate Professor of Medicine, Division of Dermatology, Director, Duke Dermatopharmacology Study Center, Duke University Medical Center, Durham, North Carolina
Hair Disorders

E. MARY O'NEILL, M.D.

Medical Director, American Red Cross Blood Services, Dedham, Massachusetts
Adverse Reactions to Blood Transfusion

ROBERT H. OSSOFF, D.M.D., M.D.

Guy M. Maness Professor and Chairman, Vanderbilt University Medical Center; Attending Physician, Vanderbilt University Hospital, VUMC; Attending Physician, St. Thomas Hospital; Attending Physician, Veterans Administration Hospital, Nashville, Tennessee
Hoarseness and Laryngitis

JUDITH A. OWENS–STIVELY, M.D., M.P.H.

Assistant Professor of Pediatrics, Brown University School of Medicine; Member, Division of Ambulatory Pediatrics and Community Medicine, Hasbro Children's Hospital; Director, Behavioral Pediatrics Clinic, Hasbro Children's Hospital, Providence, Rhode Island
Attention Deficit Hyperactivity Disorder (ADHD)

RICHARD L. PAGE, M.D.

Associate Professor of Medicine; Director, Clinical Cardiac Electrophysiology, University of Texas Southwestern Medical Center; Director of Clinical Cardiac Electrophysiology, Parkland Memorial Hospital and Zale-Lipsky University Hospital, Dallas, Texas
Tachycardias

PETER G. PAPPAS, M.D.

Associate Professor, Division of Infectious Diseases, University of Alabama at Birmingham School of Medicine, Birmingham, Alabama
Blastomycosis

JEFFREY PARSONNET, M.D.

Associate Professor of Medicine and of Microbiology, Dartmouth Medical School, Hanover, New Hampshire; Staff Physician, Infectious Disease Section, Dartmouth-Hitchcock Medical Center, Lebanon, New Hampshire
Toxic Shock Syndrome

DAVID S. PARSONS, M.D.

Professor of Surgery and Pediatrics, University of Missouri School of Medicine; The Children's Hospital, University Hospital and Clinics, Columbia, Missouri
Otitis Externa

JEFFREY F. PEIPERT, M.D., M.P.H.

Assistant Professor of Obstetrics and Gynecology, Brown University School of Medicine; Physician-in-Charge, OB/Gyn Emergency Services, Women and Infants' Hospital of Rhode Island, Providence, Rhode Island
Chlamydia trachomatis Infection

MYLES L. PENSAK, M.D.

Professor of Otolaryngology, Head and Neck Surgery; Director, Division of Otology, Neurotology, and Skull Base Surgery, University of Cincinnati College of Medicine, Cincinnati, Ohio
Otitis Media

MARK A. PEPPERCORN, M.D.
Associate Professor of Medicine, Harvard Medical School; Director, Center for Inflammatory Bowel Disease, Division of Gastroenterology, Department of Medicine, Beth Israel Hospital, Boston, Massachusetts
Ulcerative Colitis

EDITH A. PEREZ, M.D.
Associate Professor of Medicine, Mayo Medical School; Consultant, Division of Hematology and Oncology, Mayo Clinic Jacksonville, Jacksonville, Florida
Nausea and Vomiting

CLAUDE H. PERRET, M.D.
Professor of Pathophysiology, University of Lausanne Faculty of Medicine; Head of Intensive Care Service and Head of Clinical Pathophysiology Institute, University Hospital of Lausanne, Lausanne, Switzerland
Disturbances Due to Cold

RONALD F. PFEIFFER, M.D.
Professor of Neurology; Director, Division of Neurodegenerative Diseases, Department of Neurology, University of Tennessee; Baptist Memorial Hospital, Regional Medical Center at Memphis, UT Bowld Hospital, and Veterans Administration Medical Center, Memphis, Tennessee
Parkinson's Disease

HANS WALTER PFISTER, M.D.
Professor of Neurology, Ludwig-Maximilians University, Munich, Germany
Bacterial Meningitis

ELIZABETH J. PHILLIPS, M.D.
Medical Microbiology Resident, The Toronto Hospital, University of Toronto, Toronto, Ontario, Canada
Intestinal Parasites

TANIA J. PHILLIPS, M.B.B.S.
Associate Professor, Dermatology Department, Boston University Medical Center; Attending Physician, Boston University Medical Center Hospital and Boston UM Hospital, Boston, Massachusetts
Venous Stasis Ulcers

MICHAEL E. PICHICHERO, M.D.
Professor of Microbiology and Immunology, Professor of Pediatrics and Professor of Medicine, University of Rochester, Strong Memorial Hospital, Rochester, New York
Pertussis

WARREN W. PIETTE, M.D.
Professor, University of Iowa College of Medicine, Iowa City, Iowa
Papulosquamous Diseases

PHILLIP M. PINELL, M.D.
Assistant Professor, Department of Pediatrics, Baylor College of Medicine; Columbia Woman's Hospital of Texas, The Methodist Hospital, St. Luke's Episcopal Hospital, and Ben Taub General Hospital, Houston, Texas
Pyelonephritis

ALFONS POMP, M.D.
Associate Professor of Surgery, University of Montreal; Attending Surgeon, Hôtel-Dieu de Montréal Hospital, Montreal, Quebec, Canada
Parenteral Nutrition in Adults

MARK A. POPOVSKY, M.D.
Clinical Professor, Department of Pathology and Laboratory Medicine, Boston University School of Medicine; Department of Laboratory Medicine, Beth Israel Hospital, Boston, Massachusetts
Adverse Reactions to Blood Transfusion

GREGORY N. POSTMA, M.D.
Fellow in Laryngology and Care of the Professional Voice and Instructor, Department of Otolaryngology, Vanderbilt University Medical Center, Nashville, Tennessee
Hoarseness and Laryngitis

ARUN K. PRAMANIK, M.D.
Professor of Pediatrics, Louisiana State University Medical Center; Chief, Section of Neonatology, Louisiana State University Medical Center, Shreveport, Louisiana
Care of the High-Risk Neonate

JULIE S. PRENDIVILLE, M.B.
Clinical Assistant, Professor in Pediatrics, University of British Columbia; Head, Division of Pediatric Dermatology, British Columbia's Children's Hospital, Vancouver, British Columbia; Canada
Atopic Dermatitis

RICHARD L. PYLE, M.D.
Associate Professor of Psychiatry, University of Minnesota Medical School; Attending Physician, University of Minnesota Hospital and Clinic, Minneapolis, Minnesota
Bulimia Nervosa

RONALD P. RAPINI, M.D.
Professor and Chairman, Department of Dermatology, Professor of Pathology, Texas Tech University, Lubbock, Texas
Nevi

ROBERT W. REBAR, M.D.
Professor and Director, Department of Obstetrics and Gynecology, University of Cincinnati College of Medicine; Chief of Obstetrics and Gynecology, University Hospital and Children's Hospital, Cincinnati, Ohio
Menopause

LAWRENCE D. RECHT, M.D.
Professor of Neurology and Surgery (Neurosurgery), University of Massachusetts Medical Center, Worcester, Massachusetts
Brain Tumors

BARBARA R. REED, M.D.
Assistant Clinical Professor, University of Colorado; University of Colorado Health Science Center and Rose Medical Center, Denver, Colorado
Specific Dermatoses of Pregnancy

MARY KATHRYN REEVES–HOCHÉ, PH.D.
Director of Research, Respironics, Inc., Murrysville, Pennsylvania; Consultant, VA Medical Center, Lebanon, Pennsylvania
Sleep Apnea Syndrome

JEFFREY D. REICH, M.D.
Instructor in Urology, Temple University School of Medicine; Resident in Urology, Temple University Hospital Program, Philadelphia, Pennsylvania
Prostatitis

JIM REICHMAN, M.D.
Chief Resident in Medicine, Hadassah University Hospital, Jerusalem, Israel
Acute Renal Failure

DOUGLAS K. REX, M.D.
Professor of Medicine, Indiana University School of Medicine; Director of Endoscopy, Indiana University Hospital, Indianapolis, Indiana
Peptic Ulcer

JAMES P. RICHARDSON, M.D., M.P.H.
Associate Professor, Departments of Family Medicine, and Epidemiology and Preventive Medicine, University of Maryland School of Medicine; Attending Physician, University of Maryland Hospital, Baltimore, Maryland
Tetanus

M. JOYCE RICO, M.D.
Associate Professor of Dermatology, New York University; Chief, Dermatology Service, New York, VA Medical Center, New York, New York
Specific Dermatoses of Pregnancy

FRANK G. RIEGER III, M.D.
Assistant Professor, Mason Institute of Ophthalmology, University of Missouri–Columbia; Active Staff, University Hospital and Clinics; Active Staff, Harry S Truman Memorial VA Hospital, Columbia, Missouri
Conjunctivitis

MICHAEL L. RITCHEY, M.D.
Associate Professor, Department of Surgery and Pediatrics, University of Texas–Houston Medical School; Chief of Pediatric Urology, Hermann Hospital, Houston, Texas
Childhood Enuresis

DONALD D. ROBERTSON, M.D.
Assistant Professor of Otolaryngology, Department of Surgery, McMaster University; Staff Otolaryngologist, St. Joseph's Hospital, Hamilton, Ontario, Canada
Meniere's Disease

ENRIQUE ROCHE, PH.D.
Research Assistant, Department of Nutrition, University of Montreal, Montreal, Quebec, Canada
Disturbances Due to High Altitude Sickness

GRIFFIN P. RODGERS, M.D., M.M.SC.
Chief, Molecular Hematology Section, National Institute of Diabetes, Digestive and Kidney Diseases, National Institutes of Health, Bethesda, Maryland
Thalassemia

ARVEY I. ROGERS, M.D.
Professor of Medicine, University of Miami School of Medicine; Chief, Gastroenterology Division, University of Miami School of Medicine; Chief, Gastroenterology Section, VA Medical Center; Attending Physician, Jackson Memorial Hospital and University of Miami Hospital and Clinics, Miami, Florida
Crohn's Disease

DAVID ROMERO–ALVIRA, PH.D., M.D.
Staff, Service Cardiology, Hospital Miguel Servet, Zaragoza, Spain
Disturbances Due to High Altitude Sickness

DOUGLAS S. ROSS, M.D.
Assistant Professor of Medicine, Harvard Medical School; Associate Physician and Co-Director, Thyroid Associate, Massachusetts General Hospital, Boston, Massachusetts
Hyperthyroidism

JONATHAN H. ROSS, M.D.
Section of Pediatric Urology, Cleveland Clinic Foundation, Cleveland, Ohio
Bacterial Infections of the Urinary Tract in Girls

RICARDO L. ROSSI, M.D.
Professor of Surgery, Pontificia Catholic University of Chile; Attending Physician, Catholic University Hospital, Clinica Alemana, Santiago, Chile
Chronic Pancreatitis

MARTI JILL ROTHE, M.D.
Associate Professor, Department of Medicine, Division of Dermatology, University of Connecticut Health Center, Farmington, Connecticut
Acne Vulgaris and Rosacea

I. JON RUSSELL, M.D., PH.D.
Associate Professor of Medicine; Director, University Clinical Research Center; Editor, Journal *Musculoskeletal Pain,* The University of Texas Health Science Center; Staff Physician, Attending Physician, Medical Center Hospital, San Antonio, Texas
Soft Tissue Pain Syndromes

ROBERT S. RUST, M.D.
Director of Child Neurology, Assistant Professor of Neurology and Pediatrics, University of Wisconsin School of Medicine; University of Wisconsin Hospital and Clinics, Madison, Wisconsin
Viral Meningitis and Encephalitis

NEIL S. SADICK, M.D.
Clinical Assistant Professor, Cornell University Medical College, New York, New York; Attending Physician, New York Hospital, New York, New York; North Shore University Hospital, Manhasset, New York
Bacterial Diseases of the Skin

J. SAGRISTÀ–SAULEDA, M.D.
Associate Professor of Cardiology, Universitat Autonoma, Barcelona, Spain
Pericarditis

WILLIAM SALZER, M.D.
Associate Professor of Clinical Medicine, Division of Infectious Diseases, University of Missouri Health Sciences Center, Columbia, Missouri
Mycoplasmal and Viral Pneumonias

BENJAMIN U. SAMUEL, M.D.
Fellow, Infectious Diseases Section, Yale–New Haven Hospital; Yale University School of Medicine, New Haven, Connecticut
Toxoplasmosis

MARIE–DENISE SCHALLER, M.D.
Associate Professor in Intensive Care Medicine, Faculty of Medicine, University of Lausanne; Head Associate, Intensive Care Medicine, Department of Medicine, University Hospital of Lausanne, Lausanne, Switzerland
Disturbances Due to Cold

GARY SCHILLER, M.D.
Assistant Professor of Medicine, University of California, Los Angeles; Staff Physician, University of California, Los Angeles, Center for the Health Sciences, Los Angeles, California
Multiple Myeloma

CHARLES J. SCHLEUPNER, M.S., M.D.
Professor of Internal Medicine, University of Virginia School of Medicine, Charlottesville, Virginia; Chief, Medical Service, Veterans Affairs Medical Center, Salem, Virginia
Rocky Mountain Spotted Fever

SANDRA SCHNALL, M.D.
Associate Professor of Medicine, Division of Hematology-Oncology, Temple University School of Medicine, Philadelphia, Pennsylvania
Hodgkin's Disease: Chemotherapy

LORI A. SCHUH, M.D.
Clinical Assistant Professor, Department of Neurology, University of Michigan Medical School; Director, Adult Epilepsy Laboratory, University of Michigan Medical Center, Ann Arbor, Michigan
Epilepsy in Adolescents and Adults

KONRAD S. SCHULZE-DELRIEU, M.D.

Professor, Department of Internal Medicine, Division of Gastroenterology and Hepatology, University of Iowa College of Medicine; Staff, University of Iowa Hospitals and Clinics and Veterans Affairs Medical Center, Iowa City, Iowa
Dysphagia and Esophageal Obstruction

HOWARD J. SCHWARTZ, M.D.

Clinical Professor of Medicine, Case Western Reserve University; Associate Physician, University Hospitals; Chief, Allergy and Clinical Immunology, Meridia Hillcrest Hospital, Cleveland, Ohio
Allergic Reactions to Insect Stings

LAWRENCE E. SCHWARTZ, M.D.

Clinical Instructor, Tacoma Family Medicine Residency Program; Consultant in Infectious Diseases, Infections Limited, Tacoma, Washington
Streptococcal Pharyngitis

JOHN D. SEIGNE, M.B.

Junior Faculty Associate, Department of Urology, The University of Texas M.D. Anderson Cancer Center, Houston, Texas
Malignant Tumors of the Urogenital Tract

LYLE L. SENSENBRENNER, M.D.

Professor of Internal Medicine and Pediatrics, University of Maryland School of Medicine; Director, Bone Marrow/Stem Cell Transplantation Program, University of Maryland Medical System, Baltimore, Maryland
Aplastic Anemia

MITESH V. SHAH, M.D.

Assistant Professor, Department of Neurological Surgery, Indiana University School of Medicine; Assistant Professor, Department of Neurological Surgery, University Hospital, Indiana University Medical Center, Indianapolis, Indiana
Intracerebral Hemorrhage

KAUSHIK A. SHASTRI, M.D.

Assistant Professor of Medicine, State University of New York at Buffalo; Staff Hematologist, VA Medical Center, Buffalo, New York
Autoimmune Hemolytic Anemia

MITCHELL L. SHIFFMAN, M.D.

Associate Professor of Medicine, Chief, Hepatology Section; Medical Director, Liver Transplant Program, Medical College of Virginia, Richmond, Virginia
Cirrhosis

STANFORD T. SHULMAN, M.D.

Professor of Pediatrics and Associate Dean for Academic Affairs, Northwestern University Medical School; Chief, Division of Infectious Diseases, Children's Memorial Hospital, Chicago, Illinois
Rheumatic Fever

LEONARD SHVARTZMAN, M.D.

Resident, Department of Dermatology, University of Texas Southwestern Medical Center, Dallas, Texas
Cancer of the Skin

MICHAEL E. SHY, M.D.

Associate Professor of Neurology and Molecular Medicine, Wayne State University School of Medicine; Co-Director, Division of Neuromuscular Diseases, Harper Hospital/Detroit Receiving Hospital, Detroit, Michigan
Peripheral Neuropathies

M. A. SIDDIQUI, M.D.

Resident, Department of Internal Medicine, Wayne State University, Detroit, Michigan
Hypertension

ERIC A. F. SIMOES, M.D., D.C.H.

Assistant Professor, Department of Pediatrics, Division of Infectious Diseases, University of Colorado Health Sciences Center; The Children's Hospital, Denver, Colorado
Viral Respiratory Infections

NEAL P. SIMON, M.D.

Assistant Professor, Department of Pediatrics; Director, Developmental Continuity Program, Emory University School of Medicine, Atlanta, Georgia
Resuscitation of the Newborn Infant

GARY R. SIMONDS, M.D.

Assistant Professor of Surgery, Uniform Services University of the Health Sciences, Bethesda, Maryland; Associate, Department of Neurosurgery, Geisinger Medical Center, Janet Weis Memorial Children's Hospital, Danville, Pennsylvania
Pediatric Head Injury

MICHAEL J. SISACK, M.D.

Chief Resident, Dermatology Department, University of Virginia Health Science Center, Charlottesville, Virginia
Pruritus (Itching)

CHRISTIAN SITTEL, M.D.

Resident, ENT Department, Cologne University, Cologne, Germany
Acute Peripheral Facial Paralysis (Bell's Palsy)

MORTON SKORODIN, M.D.

Professor of Medicine, University of Oklahoma–Tulsa Medical College, Tulsa, Oklahoma; Staff Physician, Veterans Affairs Medical Center, Muskogee, Oklahoma
Chronic Obstructive Pulmonary Disease

RICHARD W. SMALLING, M.D., Ph.D.

Professor of Medicine and Co-Director, Division of Cardiology, University of Texas Medical School at Houston; President of the Medical Staff and Director of the Hermann Heart Center, Hermann Hospital, Houston, Texas
Angina Pectoris

DAVID J. SMITH, Jr., M.D.

Section Head, Plastic and Reconstructive Surgery, University of Michigan Medical Center; Professor, Department of Surgery; Associate Chairman, Department of Surgery, University of Michigan Medical Center, Ann Arbor, Michigan
Keloids

STEPHEN T. SMITH, M.D.

Associate Director, Cardiac Intensive Care Unit, Henry Ford Hospital; Director, Cardiology, Edsel Ford Pavilion, Henry Ford Hospital Clinic, Detroit, Michigan
Acute Myocardial Infarction

STEVEN A. SMITH, M.D.

Division of Internal Medicine and Endocrinology, Mayo Clinic; Assistant Professor of Medicine, Mayo Medical School; Saint Mary's Hospital and Rochester Methodist Hospital, Rochester, Minnesota
Thyroiditis

PETER SO, M.D.

Senior Resident, Department of Medicine, Metropolitan Medical Center, New York, New York
Acquired Immune Deficiency Syndrome (AIDS)

J. SOLER–SOLER, M.D.

Professor of Cardiology, Universitat Autonoma of Barcelona, Barcelona, Spain
Pericarditis

GLEN D. SOLOMON, M.D.

Associate Professor of Medicine, Ohio State University; Head, Section of Headache, Department of General Internal Medicine, Cleveland Clinic Foundation, Cleveland, Ohio
Headache

KEYOUMARS SOLTANI, M.D.

Professor and Chair, Section of Dermatology, University of Chicago, Chicago, Illinois
Pigmentary Alterations

SUSAN SOLYMOSS, M.D.

Assistant Professor of Medicine, McGill University; Hematologist, Montreal General Hospital and St. Mary's Hospital Center, Montreal, Quebec, Canada
Disseminated Intravascular Coagulation

JAMES R. SOWERS, M.D.

Professor of Medicine and Physiology, Wayne State University, School of Medicine; Director, Division of Endocrinology, Metabolism and Hypertension, Wayne State University, Harper Hospital, Detroit, Michigan
Hypertension

RICHARD L. SPIELVOGEL, M.D.

Professor and Chair, Dermatology, and Professor of Pathology of Laboratory Medicine, Medical College of Pennsylvania and Hahnemann University, Philadelphia, Pennsylvania; Dermatologist in Chief, Allegheny Health, Education, and Research Foundation, Pittsburgh, Pennsylvania
Viral Diseases of the Skin

CATHERINE Y. SPONG, M.D.

Clinical Instructor, Georgetown University Medical Center; Perinatal Research Branch, National Institutes of Health, Bethesda, Maryland; Georgetown University Medical Center, Washington, D.C.
Vaginal Bleeding in Late Pregnancy

LAWRENCE R. STANBERRY, M.D., PH.D.

Professor of Pediatrics, Director, Division of Infectious Diseases, University of Cincinnati College of Medicine, Children's Hospital Medical Center, Cincinnati, Ohio
Rubella and Congenital Rubella

MARSHALL S. STANTON, M.D.

Associate Professor of Medicine, Mayo Graduate School of Medicine, Mayo Clinic, Rochester, Minnesota
Atrial Fibrillation

RUSSELL W. STEELE, M.D.

Professor and Vice-Chairman of Pediatrics and Director, Division of Infectious Diseases, Louisiana State University School of Medicine; Active Staff, Children's Hospital, University Hospital, and Tulane Medical Center, New Orleans, Louisiana
Diphtheria

EBERHARD STENNERT, M.D.

Chair of the Department of Otolaryngology/Head and Neck Surgery, University of Cologne, Cologne, Germany
Acute Peripheral Facial Paralysis (Bell's Palsy)

JAMES B. STEWART, JR., M.D.

Assistant Professor, Department of Dermatology, University of Oklahoma Health Sciences Center; HCA Presbyterian, University Hospitals, OUHSC, Oklahoma City, Oklahoma
Superficial Fungal Infections of the Skin

JANET A. STOCKHEIM, M.D.

Instructor, Northwestern University Medical School; Fellow, Division of Infectious Diseases, The Children's Memorial Hospital, Chicago, Illinois
Rheumatic Fever

GEORG STROHMEYER, M.D.

Professor Emeritus, School of Medicine, Heinrich-Heine University; Department of Medicine, Gastroenterology Unit, Heinrich-Heine University, Düsseldorf, Germany
Hemochromatosis

DAVID W. STRYKER, M.D.

Clinical Associate, University of New Mexico; Active Staff, Presbyterian Hospital and St. Joseph's Hospital, Albuquerque, New Mexico
Q Fever

BRIAN J. SWANSIGER, M.D.

Gastroenterology Fellow, William Beaumont Hospital, Royal Oak, Michigan
Gastritis

PAUL S. SWERDLOW, M.D.

Associate Professor of Medicine, Wayne State University School of Medicine; Director, Red Cell Disorders, Harper Hospital, Detroit Medical Center, Detroit, Michigan
Sickle Cell Disease

RONALD W. SWINFARD, M.D.

Associate Professor and Associate Chairman for Clinical Affairs, Department of Internal Medicine (Dermatology), University of Missouri–Columbia, School of Medicine; University of Missouri Health Sciences Center and Harry S Truman VA Hospital, Columbia, Missouri
Warts (Verruca Vulgaris)

DAMIEN TAGAN, M.D.

Chief Resident, Intensive Care Service, Department of Medicine, University Hospital, Lausanne, Switzerland
Disturbances Due to Cold

MANUEL E. TANCER, M.D.

Associate Professor of Psychiatry and Behavioral Neurosciences, Wayne State University School of Medicine; Director, Psychiatry Research, Detroit VA Medical Center, Detroit, Michigan
Anxiety Disorders

KENZABURO TANI, M.D., PH.D.

Associate Professor, Department of Hematology/Oncology, The Institute of Medical Science, The University of Tokyo; Associate Professor, Research Hospital, The Institute of Medical Science, The University of Tokyo, Tokyo, Japan
Nonimmune Hemolytic Anemia

F. M. TATNALL, M.D.

Consultant Dermatologist, Mount Vernon and Watford Hospitals Trust, Hertfordshire, England
Erythema Multiforme

MARTIN G. TÄUBER, M.D.

Assistant Professor of Medicine and Neurology, School of Medicine, University of California, San Francisco; Attending Physician, San Francisco General Hospital, San Francisco, California
Bacterial Meningitis

R. STAN TAYLOR, M.D.

Assistant Professor, University of Texas Southwestern Medical Center; Attending Staff, St. Paul Medical Center, Children's Medical Center, Zale Lipshy Medical Center, Veterans Memorial Medical Center, and Parkland Memorial Hospital, Dallas, Texas
Cancer of the Skin

NATHAN M. THIELMAN, M.D., M.P.H.

Assistant Professor of Research in Internal Medicine, Divisions of Geographic and International Medicine and Infectious Diseases, University of Virginia School of Medicine, Charlottesville, Virginia
Food-Borne Illness

CHESNEY THOMPSON, M.D.

Assistant Professor, Department of Obstetrics and Gynecology, University of Colorado School of Medicine, Denver, Colorado
Vulvovaginitis

EDWIN M. THORPE, JR., M.D.

Clinical Associate Professor, Department of Obstetrics and Gynecology, University of Tennessee, Memphis, Tennessee
Pelvic Inflammatory Disease

ALAN D. TICE, M.D.

Clinical Assistant Professor, Department of Medicine, University of Washington, Seattle, Washington
Streptococcal Pharyngitis

ALKIS TOGIAS, M.D.

Associate Professor of Medicine, Johns Hopkins Asthma and Allergy Center; Attending Physician, Johns Hopkins Hospital and Johns Hopkins Bayview Medical Center, Baltimore, Maryland
Allergic Rhinitis Caused by Inhalant Factors

EDMOND L. TRUELOVE, D.D.S., M.S.D.

Professor, Department of Oral Medicine, University of Washington; University of Washington Medical Center and University Hospital, Seattle, Washington
Temporomandibular Disorders

JOSEPH A. TRUSZKOWSKI, M.D.

Assistant Professor, Division of Gastroenterology and Hepatology, Department of Internal Medicine, University of Iowa Hospitals and Clinics, Staff, University of Iowa Hospitals and Clinics and Veterans Affairs Medical Center, Iowa City, Iowa
Dysphagia and Esophageal Obstruction

DEAN T. TSUKAYAMA, M.D.

Assistant Professor, Department of Medicine, University of Minnesota Medical School; Medical Director, Musculoskeletal Sepsis Unit, Hennepin County Medical Center, Minneapolis, Minnesota
Osteomyelitis

THOMAS W. UHDE, M.D.

Professor, Departments of Psychiatry and Behavioral Neurosciences and Pharmacology; Chairperson, Department of Psychiatry and Behavioral Neurosciences, Wayne State University, Detroit, Michigan
Anxiety Disorders

ARVID E. UNDERMAN, M.D.

Clinical Professor of Medicine, Microbiology and Immunology, University of Southern California School of Medicine, Los Angeles, California; Assistant Director, Internal Medicine Training Program, Huntington Memorial Hospital, Pasadena, California
Salmonellosis

RODRIGO L. VALDERRAMA, M.D.

Professor of Medicine, The University of Chile; Attending Physician, San Juan De Dios Hospital, Clinica Alemana, Santiago, Chile
Chronic Pancreatitis

WILLIAM M. VALENTI, M.D.

Clinical Associate Professor of Medicine, University of Rochester School of Medicine and Dentistry; Founding Medical Director, Community Health Network, Rochester, New York
Bacteremia and Sepsis

R. NEIL VAN LEEUWEN, M.D.

Resident Physician, University Hospital and Clinics, Columbia, Missouri
Otitis Externa

ROBERT A. VESCIO, M.D.

Assistant Professor of Medicine, University of California, Los Angeles; Staff Physician, University of California, Los Angeles, Center for the Health Sciences, Los Angeles, California
Multiple Myeloma

EILEEN P. G. VINING, M.D.

Associate Professor of Neurology and Pediatrics, The Johns Hopkins Medical Institutions; Johns Hopkins Hospital, Baltimore, Maryland
Epilepsy in Infants and Children

HENRY WAGNER, JR., M.D.

Associate Professor of Radiology, University of South Florida; Director of Thoracic Oncology, H. Lee Moffitt Cancer Center, Tampa, Florida
Carcinoma of the Lung

MICHAEL P. WAINSCOTT, M.D.

Associate Professor, Division of Emergency Medicine, Department of Surgery; Director of Undergraduate Education, University of Texas Southwestern Medical School; Attending Faculty, Parkland Hospital Emergency Department, Dallas, Texas
Disturbances Due to Heat

PHILIP D. WALSON, M.D.

Professor of Pediatrics, Pharmacology, Pharmacy and Allied Health; Chief, Division of Clinical Pharmacology/Toxicology, Ohio State University College of Medicine; Children's Hospital and The Ohio State University Hospitals, Columbus, Ohio
Fever

MARK A. WARD, M.D.

Assistant Professor of Pediatrics, Baylor College of Medicine; Texas Children's Hospital, Houston, Texas
Varicella

M.F.R. WATERS, M.B.

Honorary Senior Clinical Lecturer, London School of Hygiene and Tropical Medicine, and University College London Joint Medical School; Consulting Leprologist, Hospital for Tropical Diseases, London, England
Leprosy (Hansen's Disease)

GUILLERMO S. WATKINS, M.D.

Fellow of Gastrointestinal Surgery, Pontificia Catholic University of Chile; Catholic University Hospital, Santiago, Chile
Chronic Pancreatitis

CHARLES G. WATSON, M.D.

Professor and Vice Chairman, Department of Surgery; Chief, Division of Endocrine Surgery, University of Pittsburgh School of Medicine; Active Staff, University of Pittsburgh Medical Center, Pittsburgh, Pennsylvania
Thyroid Cancer

MYRON H. WEINBERGER, M.D.

Professor of Medicine; Director, Hypertension Research Center; Indiana University School of Medicine; Indiana University and Affiliated Hospitals, Indianapolis, Indiana
Primary Aldosteronism

CARL WEINER, M.D.

Professor and Chairman, Department of Obstetrics, Gynecology and Reproductive Sciences, University of Maryland School of Medicine; Director, Center for Advanced Fetal Care, University of Maryland Medical System, Baltimore, Maryland
Hemolytic Disease of the Fetus and Newborn

LAWRENCE S. WEISBERG, M.D.

Associate Professor of Medicine, University of Medicine and Dentistry of New Jersey/Robert Wood Johnson Medical School at Cam-

den; Attending Physician, Cooper Hospital/University Medical Center, Camden, New Jersey
Diabetes Insipidus

ROBERT G. WESTPHAL, M.D.

Clinical Professor of Medicine, University of Vermont College of Medicine, Burlington, Vermont; American Red Cross Blood Services, Dedham, Massachusetts
Adverse Reactions to Blood Transfusion

JOHN S. WHEELER, Jr., M.D.

Professor of Urology, Loyola University, Chicago, Illinois; Staff Urologist, Loyola University Medical Center and Hines Veterans Administration Hospital, Maywood, Illinois
Benign Prostatic Hyperplasia

RICHARD I. WHYTE, M.D.

Assistant Professor, Section of Thoracic Surgery, Department of Surgery, University of Michigan School of Medicine; Attending Physician, Hospitals of the University of Michigan; Consulting Physician, Ann Arbor, VA Medical Center, Ann Arbor, Michigan
Pleural Effusion and Empyema Thoracis

POLRAT WILAIRATANA, M.D.

Assistant Professor, Department of Clinical Tropical Medicine, Faculty of Tropical Medicine, Mahidol University; Attending Physician, Division of Critical Care for Tropical Diseases, Hospital for Tropical Diseases, Faculty of Tropical Medicine, Mahidol University, Bangkok, Thailand
Malaria

ROBERT H. WILKINS, M.D.

Chief, Division of Neurosurgery, Duke University Medical Center, Durham, North Carolina
Trigeminal Neuralgia

BARBARA BRAUNSTEIN WILSON, M.D.

Associate Professor, University of Virginia Medical School; Attending Physician, University of Virginia Health Sciences Center, Charlottesville, Virginia
Pruritus (Itching)

STEPHEN L. WINBERY, Ph.D., M.D.

Education Director, University of Tennessee Medical Group, Department of Emergency Medicine; Attending Physician, Regional Medical Center, Memphis, Tennessee
Anaphylaxis and Serum Sickness

ANDREW WINOKUR, M.D., Ph.D

Professor, Departments of Psychiatry and Pharmacology, University of Pennsylvania School of Medicine; Associate Director, Center for Sleep and Respiratory Neurobiology, University of Pennsylvania Medical Center, Philadelphia, Pennsylvania
Insomnia

JOSEPH I. WOLFSDORF, M.B., B.Ch.

Associate Professor of Pediatrics, Harvard Medical School; Clinical Director of Endocrinology, Children's Hospital; Chief of Pediatrics, Joslin Diabetes Center, Boston, Massachusetts
Diabetes Mellitus in Children and Adolescents

MICHELLE H. WOODARD, M.D.

Clinical Assistant Professor, University of Florida College of Medicine; Shands Hospital, Park Avenue Internal Medicine Clinic, Gainesville, Florida
Giardiasis

SCOTT W. WOODS, M.D.

Associate Professor of Psychiatry, Yale University School of Medicine; Director, Treatment Research Program, Connecticut Mental Health Center, New Haven, Connecticut
Panic Disorder

DEREK B. WOOLNER, M.D.

Dermatopathology Fellow, University of Chicago, Chicago, Illinois
Pigmentary Alterations

V. WRIGHT, M.D.

Emeritus Professor of Rheumatology, University of Leeds, Leeds, England
Ankylosing Spondylitis

GARY M. YARKONY, M.D.

Clinical Professor, Section of Orthopaedic Surgery and Rehabilitation Medicine, Department of Surgery, Clinical Professor of Neurology; Chief of Rehabilitation Services, University of Chicago Hospitals, Rehabilitation Center; Vice President, Clinical Program Development, Schwab Rehabilitation Hospital, Chicago, Illinois
Pressure Ulcers

HANSEN A. YUAN, M.D.

Professor of Orthopedic and Neurologic Surgery, State University of New York Health Science Center, Syracuse; SUNY Health Science Center; Crouse-Irving Memorial Hospital, Syracuse, New York
Low Back Pain

ALAN ZACHARIAS, M.D.

Instructor in Neurology, Emory University School of Medicine; Instructor in Neurology, Emory University Hospital, Atlanta, Georgia
Myasthenia Gravis

HOWARD A. ZACUR, M.D., Ph.D.

Theodore and Ingrid Baramki Professor, Johns Hopkins Medical Institutions; Director, Reproductive Endocrinology, Johns Hopkins Medical Institutions, Baltimore, Maryland
Amenorrhea

JEROME B. ZELDIS, M.D., Ph.D.

Director, Janssen Research Foundation; Clinical Assistant Professor of Medicine, Cornell Medical School; Assistant Physician, New York Hospital, New York, New York
Acute and Chronic Viral Hepatitis

JONATHAN M. ZENILMAN, M.D.

Associate Professor, Johns Hopkins University School of Medicine; Attending Physician, Johns Hopkins Hospital, Baltimore, Maryland
Gonorrhea

ED E. ZIJLSTRA, M.D., Ph.D.

Assistant Professor, Institute of Endemic Diseases, University of Khartoum, Khartoum, Sudan
Leishmaniasis

Preface

This is the 49th edition of *Current Therapy,* continuing the same format established by Howard Conn in 1949. The intent is to provide the busy practitioner with up-to-date information on recent advances in medicine in a concise and easy to read manner.

Experts who frequently see these problems are invited to present their method of treatment. Often these treatments are recently developed and are not yet approved by the FDA; for many, approval is never requested. It is estimated that half of the prescriptions written by doctors are "off-label," meaning they are prescribed to treat conditions for which there is no official approval.

Each year, this is an entirely new book with new authors presenting their favorite treatment methods. Often, a problem is approached differently than the previous year's author, giving the reader a variety of options to choose from. Although we try to obtain 100% new authors each year, this may never be possible because of the tight deadlines required for an annual publication. This year, we came close, with 95% new authors; the remaining 5% updated their material from the previous edition. This extensive annual updating is necessary to remain current with the rapidly changing technical and therapeutic advances in medicine.

Our goal is to focus on problems frequently encountered in practice and those less common conditions that could have serious consequences if not managed properly. New topics are added annually to keep pace with new diseases and developments. This year there are six new topics: *chronic fatigue syndrome,* focusing on the diagnosis and management of this increasingly prominent and perplexing disorder; *high altitude sickness,* a problem most skiers and rock climbers encounter at some time, best managed by prevention and early diagnosis; *giardiasis,* the most common pathogenic parasitic infection in the United States and a common cause of diarrhea; *erectile dysfunction,* focusing on new treatments available to the 15 million men in the United States with impotence; *attention deficit hyperactivity disorder,* one of the most common behavioral disorders in childhood; and *hypertrophic cardiomyopathy,* discussing diagnosis and treatment that ranges from beta blockers to surgery.

Contributors are authorities who see these problems frequently and often are those who have conducted research leading to changes in therapy. Many of these are from countries other than the United States. For example, changes in the treatment of cholera are presented by an expert in Bangladesh, and new therapies in managing sarcoidosis are given by a physician in Sweden. In addition to these, 30 topics are presented by authors in Germany, Spain, The Netherlands, Thailand, the United Kingdom, Canada, Japan, Israel, Chile, Switzerland, and the Republic of China.

Special credit for the ongoing quality of this annual publication goes to Ray Kersey and the excellent editorial staff at W.B. Saunders, and to Caroline Kosnik, my editorial assistant who manages the flow of manuscripts and ensures that deadlines are met. My special thanks as well to the physicians who use the book in their practice and provide suggestions for changes.

ROBERT E. RAKEL, M.D.

NOTICE

Medicine is an ever-changing field. Standard safety precautions must be followed, but as new research and clinical experience broaden our knowledge, changes in treatment and drug therapy become necessary or appropriate. The editors of this work have carefully checked the generic and trade drug names and verified drug dosages to ensure that the dosage information in this work is accurate and in accord with the standards accepted at the time of publication. Readers are advised, however, to check the product information currently provided by the manufacturer of each drug to be administered to be certain that changes have not been made in the recommended dose or in the contra-indications for administration. This is of particular importance in regard to new or infrequently used drugs. It is the responsibility of the treating physician, relying on experience and knowledge of the patient, to determine dosages and the best treatment for the patient. The editors cannot be responsible for misuse or misapplication of the material in this work.

THE PUBLISHER

Contents

SECTION 1. SYMPTOMATIC CARE PENDING DIAGNOSIS

SECTION 2. THE INFECTIOUS DISEASES

SECTION 3. THE RESPIRATORY SYSTEM

SECTION 4. THE CARDIOVASCULAR SYSTEM

CONTENTS

SECTION 5. THE BLOOD AND SPLEEN

SECTION 6. THE DIGESTIVE SYSTEM

SECTION 7. METABOLIC DISORDERS

SECTION 8. THE ENDOCRINE SYSTEM

SECTION 9. THE UROGENITAL TRACT

SECTION 10. THE SEXUALLY TRANSMITTED DISEASES

SECTION 11. DISEASES OF ALLERGY

SECTION 12. DISEASES OF THE SKIN

SECTION 13. THE NERVOUS SYSTEM

SECTION 14. THE LOCOMOTOR SYSTEM

SECTION 15. OBSTETRICS AND GYNECOLOGY

SECTION 16. PSYCHIATRIC DISORDERS

SECTION 17. PHYSICAL AND CHEMICAL INJURIES

SECTION 18. APPENDICES AND INDEX

Symptomatic Care Pending Diagnosis

PAIN

method of
MARK A. KALLGREN, M.D.
Portland, Oregon

Pain is ubiquitous in medical practice, and the principles of its treatment are critical for all clinicians. An accepted definition of pain is "an unpleasant sensory and emotional experience associated with actual or potential tissue damage, or described in terms of such damage." The physiologic sequelae of acute pain may lead to hyperactivity of the sympathetic nervous system, potentially resulting in tachycardia, hypertension, increased peripheral vascular resistance, and decreased intestinal motility. Historically, pain has been greatly undertreated because of fear of analgesic side effects, ignorance of the existence of deleterious aspects of pain, or unavailability of needed medications or technologies. Recent studies, for example, have shown that 75% of patients receiving parenteral opioids for moderate to severe pain fail to achieve complete relief.

Medical etiologies producing pain can be conveniently divided into three entities: acute (e.g., trauma, renal colic), chronic (e.g., postherpetic neuralgia), and cancer (e.g., metastatic adenocarcinoma). Although the specific strategies used for each category are different, many of the treatment principles are consistent and can be utilized regardless of the underlying diagnosis. This article mainly addresses the frontline therapies, particularly pharmacologic, in pain management, realizing that more disease-specific techniques are found elsewhere in this text.

PATHOPHYSIOLOGY

Four primary physiologic events act in concert in the conduction of pain impulses: transduction, transmission, modulation, and perception. Therefore, the processing and ultimate perception of a noxious stimulus involve a complex process with many modulating factors, interconnections, and various chemical mediators. The importance of this system's complexity is that the goal of achieving analgesia must be considered multidimensionally to best achieve success. Clinically, one frequently benefits from the synergism that is obtained by combining different medi-cation classes, doses, and routes of delivery to overcome obstacles to analgesia.

The conscious realization of pain is a phenomenon that integrates not only the aforementioned pathways but also the psychologic milieu of the patient. Social, cultural, and personality factors all interact to affect the perception of pain. Recognizing and understanding these "nonphysiologic" aspects are crucial and will go a long way toward helping to achieve relief of suffering.

PAIN ASSESSMENT

Recognition and measurement of pain are imperative in order to detect its presence and avoid undertreatment. The initial pain assessment typically coincides with a detailed history and physical examination. Descriptive characteristics such as onset, intensity, location, and mitigating factors should be noted and compared with subsequent evaluations. A 0 to 10 numeric pain intensity score is an easily obtainable way to objectively record and follow a patient's course and response to therapy. Alternatively, a visual analog score (VAS), which consists of a 10-cm line with verbal anchors at either end, can serve as a good self-report assessment tool. Frequent updates of pain assessment need to take place and be documented, with responsible practitioners changing therapies as needed.

TREATMENT

Opioid Analgesics

The opioids represent the mainstay of drugs available to relieve pain and include naturally occurring alkaloids of opium and synthetic/semisynthetic derivatives. The opioids can be classified as agonist, antagonist, or mixed agonist-antagonists. These classifications are based on the existence of different opioid receptors in the central nervous system and periphery: mu, kappa, and delta. Research supports that mu receptors, which are predominantly supraspinal in location, are linked to analgesia, respiratory depression, euphoria, and physical dependence. Kappa receptors, found within the spinal cord, mediate spinal analgesia, miosis, and sedation. Delta receptors are thought to be mostly involved in affective behavior. Table 1 lists commonly used opioid compounds and pertinent pharmacologic data.

In general, the delivery route for a given opioid depends on the routes available, the rapidity needed, and the anticipated time a drug will be used. For example, a patient with severe pain from a new fracture may initially require a strong opioid parenterally, changing to a scheduled dose of an oral medication later. For long-term use of analgesics (e.g., cancer pain), the following principles hold true: oral is the preferred route when available and effective, drugs should be given on a scheduled basis rather than "as needed," and analgesic strength and dosing should be titrated in relationship to each patient. Additionally, physical dependence and opioid tolerance are expected with long-term use and should not be confused with addiction. Meperidine (Demerol), because of the toxicity of its normeperidine metabolite, should not be used for prolonged treatment and used with caution if moderate to high doses of opioids are needed. The agonist-antagonist drugs should not be given to patients receiving opioid agonists, as they may precipitate a withdrawal syndrome. In general, the agonist-antagonist drugs are very limited in their usefulness and are not appropriate for long-term use.

Recently, tramadol hydrochloride (Ultram) has been released in the United States. This medication is truly an opioid, yet because of unique receptor-binding sites has not been shown to be a significant drug of abuse in Europe. Part of its benefit may result from an ill-defined non-opioid analgesic effect that appears novel to this particular drug. Clinical studies conducted thus far demonstrate it to be an effective medication for many mild pain problems.

Patient-Controlled Analgesia (PCA)

PCA, first described in the early 1970s, has the advantage of being able to bypass individual variations in pharmacokinetics and pharmacodynamics. The PCA pump is an infusion device integrated with a microprocessor, connected to a push button that the patient activates, delivering a predetermined dose of narcotic. PCA devices can be used to safely deliver drug via the intravenous, epidural, intrathecal, or subcutaneous routes. Intravenous PCA is the most widely used setup, and numerous studies have documented the safety, efficacy, and high patient satisfaction found with this analgesic technique. Morphine, meperidine (Demerol), and hydromorphone (Dilaudid) are all easily used for intravenous PCA. Typical orders specify a given dose (e.g., morphine, 1 mg) and a lockout period (e.g., 10 minutes) during which the patient must wait in order to receive another dose on demand. Generally, continuous basal infusions should not be routinely ordered unless the patient has been on a narcotic analgesic previously. Standard preprinted PCA orders, with instructions for the management of side effects, should be policy at institutions using PCA.

TABLE 1. **Opioid Medications**

Drug	Approximate Equianalgesic Dose		Usual Starting Dose for Moderate to Severe Pain	
	Oral	*Parenteral*	*Oral*	*Parenteral*
OPIOID AGONIST				
Morphine	30 mg q 3–4 h	10 mg q 3–4 h	30 mg q 3–4 h	10 mg q 3–4 h
Morphine, sustained-release (MS Contin, Oramorph)	90–120 mg q 12 h	N/A	90–120 mg q 12 h	N/A
Hydromorphone (Dilaudid)	7.5 mg q 3–4 h	1.5 mg q 3–4 h	6 mg q 3–4 h	1.5 mg q 3–4 h
Levorphanol (Levo-Dromoran)	4 mg q 6–8 h	2 mg q 6–8 h	4 mg q 6–8 h	2 mg q 6–8 h
Meperidine (Demerol)	300 mg q 2–3 h	100 mg q 3 h	Not recommended	100 mg q 3 h
Methadone (Dolophine, other)	20 mg q 6–8 h	10 mg q 6–8 h	20 mg q 6–8 h	10 mg q 6–8 h
Oxymorphone (Numorphan)	N/A	1 mg q 3–4 h	N/A	1 mg q 3–4 h
COMBINATION OPIOID/NSAID PREPARATIONS				
Codeine (with aspirin or acetaminophen)	180–200 mg q 3–4 h	130 mg q 3–4 h	60 mg q 3–4 h	60 mg q 3–4 h (IM/SC)
Hydrocodone (in Lorcet, Lortab, Vicodin, others)	30 mg q 3–4 h	N/A	10 mg q 3–4 h	N/A
Oxycodone (Roxicodone, also in Percocet, Percodan, Tylox, others)	30 mg q 3–4 h	N/A	10 mg q 3–4 h	N/A
MIXED OPIOID AGONIST/ANTAGONIST				
Buprenorphine (Buprenex)	N/A	N/A	N/A	0.3–0.4 mg q 6–8 h
Butorphanol (Stadol)	N/A	N/A	N/A	2 mg q 3–4 h
Nalbuphine (Nubain)	N/A	N/A	N/A	10 mg q 3–4 h
Pentazocine (Talwin)	N/A	N/A	50–100 mg q 6–8 h	60 mg q 3–4 h
NOVEL OPIOIDS				
Tramadol HCl (Ultram)	N/A	N/A	50–100 mg q 6–8 h	N/A
OPIOID ANTAGONISTS				
Naloxone (Narcan)	N/A	N/A	N/A	0.4 mg (for life-threatening events only)
Naltrexone (ReVia)	N/A	N/A	4–100 mg q 24 h	N/A

Neuraxial Opioids

Narcotic agents may be injected directly into the epidural or subarachnoid spaces via single percutaneous injections or continuous catheter techniques. Either route provides a path for diffusion of drug into the cerebrospinal fluid (CSF), where the drug has immediate access to spinal cord opiate receptors. Neuraxial narcotics have the advantage of providing intense analgesia without motor autonomic blockade. Addition of even low concentrations of local anesthetics allows enhanced analgesia, with less narcotic needed and concomitant sympathetic blockade of some degree. This combination of opioid drugs with local anesthetics, used in epidural infusions, has been shown to significantly improve patient outcome after intra-abdominal surgery, as well as to decrease length of hospital stay.

Transdermal Opioids

Use of the highly potent narcotic fentanyl citrate in a transdermal delivery system (Duragesic) offers some advantages for selected patients. This route provides for slow absorption and sustained release, and can give fairly constant serum drug levels over time. This system is very useful for patients who cannot tolerate oral medications but who need potent analgesia by a noninvasve means. The patch's slow onset (typically 2 hours or more) and prolonged effect after discontinuation (elimination half-life being greater than 20 hours) definitely warrant caution when considering the drug's use.

Opioid Side Effects

Although the opioid analgesics act principally to decrease pain, they have obvious pharmacologic effects throughout the body. As is the case with drug onset and potency, the more direct routes, such as neuraxial and intravenous, have the potential for more rapid development of side effects. However, all drugs in this class can cause serious problems in any given patient and with any given dose. Extremes of age, pre-existing medical conditions, and concomitant medications all influence the effects of a given dose of narcotic.

The most common side effect of opioids that must be anticipated is constipation. Activity, dietary fiber, stool softeners, and laxatives should all be utilized as appropriate. Prevention and anticipation of constipation are mandated and lead to less frustration by patients.

Other side effects include sedation, nausea, and pruritus. Tolerance to most opioid side effects typically develops with persistent use and is often idiosyncratic, so one may decrease the incidence of side effects by switching to alternate drugs. The most serious complication of opioid analgesics is their direct depressant effect on the brain stem respiratory centers. Clinically, respiratory depression is rare, particularly when reasonable doses of opioids are

started and observation is done by family members, nursing staff, or clinicians. Patients who do develop mild respiratory depression usually only require closer observation and mild stimulation. If a patient should develop severe respiratory depression, support of ventilation and naloxone (Narcan), 0.1 to 0.4 mg intravenously, given slowly, are usually rapidly effective. When naloxone has been used, one must remember that it has a short half-life (approximately 1 hour), and be wary of "re-narcotization" due to the longer half-lives of the opioid agonist drugs.

For patients taking opioid analgesics for ongoing pain problems, the risk of iatrogenic addiction is exceedingly small. Drug tolerance and need for increased dosing should not be confused with psychologic addiction and are to be expected. The pure opioid agonist drugs, such as morphine, actually do not have a therapeutic ceiling dose, unlike many other medications. In end-stage cancer pain, one often may need to increase narcotic dosing by 20 to 50% per hour until effective analgesia is achieved. Fear of addiction and misunderstanding of tolerance are two common, but misguided, causes of inadequate patient analgesia.

Nonopioid Analgesic Medications

Acetaminophen (Tylenol), particularly when used in conjunction with other analgesics, is an important medication and should not be forgotten as a useful tool. A nonsalicylate, acetaminophen is similar to aspirin in its analgesic and antipyretic properties but has no antiplatelet effects and minimal demonstrated anti-inflammatory effects. Avoidance of excessive dosing must be done to prevent hepatotoxicity, particularly if one is prescribing larger amounts of combination drugs (e.g., Tylenol No. 3, Lorcet, Percocet, and others) that contain acetaminophen.

Aspirin and the nonsteroidal anti-inflammatory drugs (NSAIDs) represent a large class of very effective nonopioid analgesic medications. NSAIDs work by preventing the synthesis and release of prostaglandins via inhibition of cyclooxygenase. Prostaglandins, released in response to cell trauma, sensitize C fiber nociceptors and lower the pain threshold in the periphery ("hyperalgesia"). Indeed, several studies have shown that NSAIDs given preoperatively will decrease the amount of postoperative pain and the subsequent opioid medications used. There are literally dozens of NSAIDs available, and it is recommended that clinicians become thoroughly familiar with a few agents from each different class and prescribe based on the individual patient. Important factors to consider when prescribing an NSAID include cost of the medication, side-effect profile, drug interactions, long-term safety record, and documented efficacy for given conditions. In general, many older medications that are now generic or less expensive are equal to if not better than some of the newer NSAIDs released. Responses to NSAIDs tend to be idiosyncratic, and a therapeutic failure or side effects with one NSAID does not predict the success with a different NSAID.

Ketorolac tromethamine (Toradol) was the first parenteral NSAID released and certainly can be useful for many acute pain settings. Studies indicate that its potency is comparable with low-dose morphine; however, ketorolac's dosing range is limited. This drug does not have opioid side effects but raises the usual concerns when using any NSAID medication. Toradol should not be used continuously for more than a few days, and it should be used cautiously in the elderly, renal patients, and those with active peptic ulcer disease or bleeding problems. Because of the considerable cost, one should not use Toradol in a setting where another, oral NSAID might serve the purpose desired.

Useful specifically for migraine headaches, sumatriptan succinate (Imitrex) is rapid acting and offers a unique therapeutic option. Sumatriptan has been demonstrated to be a selective agonist for a vascular 5-hydroxytryptamine (serotonin) subtype, causing constriction of intracranial vasculature. Sixty to 80% of patients with migraine pain are said to get relief with a single injection of this medication. Sumatriptan is available as a 6-mg subcutaneous injectable or in 25- and 50-mg oral tablets. Failure to achieve any relief from this medication should alert practitioners to possible nonvascular sources of headache pain. In a chronic pain clinic setting, a large percentage of "migraine" headache patients are found to have headaches that meet criteria for diagnoses other than migraine (e.g., analgesic rebound headache). Many times, once other sources of headaches have been addressed and treated, "standard" migraine treatments, including Imitrex, may be effective.

There are many other nonopioid adjunctive medications that are very effective in given clinical situations. Some of the options available with specific examples would include the following:

Anticonvulsants for neuropathic pain; carbamazepine (Tegretol), 200 to 1600 mg orally, for trigeminal neuralgia.

Antidepressants for neuropathic pain and as prophylaxis for migraine headaches; amitriptyline (Elavil),* 25 to 150 mg orally.

Antihistamines for opioid synergy and relief of symptoms including anxiety, pruritus, and nausea; hydroxyzine (Vistaril), 50 to 100 mg orally or parenterally.

Corticosteroids for bony metastases in cancer or used as epidural injection for acute nerve root pain; dexamethasone (Decadron), 16 to 24 mg/day orally or intravenously, for pain due to brachial or lumbar plexopathy caused by tumor compression.

Radiopharmaceuticals for pain due to bony metastases; strontium 89 can provide relief in 60 to 80% of appropriately selected cancer patients.

The Multidisciplinary Pain Approach

Rapid advances in many diverse areas of basic science and clinical research have greatly enhanced the armamentarium in the battle against pain. Likewise, increased appreciation of the widespread undertreatment of pain has led to the concept of multidisciplinary pain teams. The organization of such teams is variable, but their goal is to diagnose and treat pain problems by using the skills of anesthesiologists, neurosurgeons, psychologists, physical therapists, and others in a cost-effective and complementary fashion. Expert consultation from pain management specialists can be highly gratifying for both the affected patient and the referring clinician.

NAUSEA AND VOMITING

method of
EDITH A. PEREZ, M.D.
Mayo Clinic Jacksonville
Jacksonville, Florida

and

ANN E. HALLSTONE, M.D.
Veterans Administration Northern California
System of Clinics
Martinez, California

Nausea and vomiting are among the most common symptoms in medicine. They are associated with a wide variety of disorders, some of which are relatively trivial, others of which may be serious and debilitating. Nausea and vomiting may be evoked by disorders of the gastrointestinal tract, but they also may reflect neurologic, psychogenic, endocrine, metabolic, iatrogenic, or toxic conditions and are common manifestations of pediatric illness (Table 1). Serious consequences of nausea and vomiting include electrolyte depletion, acid-base disorders, malnutrition, Mallory-Weiss syndrome, aspiration pneumonia, or esophageal rupture (Boerhaave's syndrome). Three recognized components of vomiting are nausea, retching, and emesis. Nausea refers to the urge to vomit. Retching is the rhythmic movement of vomiting without effect. Emesis is the forceful expulsion of gastric contents from the mouth. Nausea and its physical signs of pallor, flushing, tachycardia, diaphoresis, decreased gastric and pyloric tone, and increased duodenogastric reflux are under autonomic nervous system control, whereas retching and vomiting require coordinated effort of the somatic nervous system.

Control of vomiting involves two anatomically and functionally distinct components: a vomiting center (VC) and a chemoreceptor trigger zone (CTZ). The exact location of the vomiting center in humans has not been identified, but current evidence suggests that it lies within the lateral reticular formation adjacent to medulla oblongata areas involved in respiration, salivation, cardiovascular response, and cranial nerves VIII and X. This area is directly excited by visceral afferent nerve impulses in the gastrointestinal tract and elsewhere. The CTZ, located in the area postrema of the fourth ventricle, is responsive to blood- and cerebrospinal fluid–borne chemical agents. Although direct stimulation of the CTZ does not result in vomiting, it is responsive to chemical stimuli via the circulatory system and an emetic response requires an intact VC.

Once the VC is stimulated directly or via the CTZ, efferent pathways bring about vomiting via somatic phrenic,

---

*Not FDA-approved for this indication.

TABLE 1. Differential Diagnosis of Nausea and Vomiting

Central Nervous System

Abscess
Epilepsy
Head injury
Labyrinthitis
Malignancy
Meniere's disease
Meningitis
Migraine
Motion sickness
Pseudotumors
Vestibular disorder

Endocrine

Adrenal insufficiency
Diabetic acidosis
Hypercalcemia
Hyperparathyroidism
Pregnancy
Thyrotoxicosis

Gastrointestinal

Adhesions
Appendicitis
Biliary tract disease
Carcinoid tumor
Cholecystitis
Constipation, fecal impaction, obstipation
Food poisoning (toxins)
Gallstone ileus
Gastroparesis
Hepatitis
Hernias
Infectious gastroenteritis (Norwalk agent, Hawaii agent,
    salmonella)
Inflammatory bowel disease
Intussusception
Malignancy
Meckel's diverticulum
Motility disorders
Pancreatitis
Parasitosis
Peritonitis
Pseudo-obstruction
Peptic ulcer disease
Superior mesenteric artery syndrome
Visceral pain
Zollinger-Ellison syndrome

Iatrogenic

Chemotherapy
Radiation therapy
Surgery
Medications (narcotics, aminophylline, analgesics, antibiotics,
    cardiac glycosides, copper, mercury, ammonium chloride)

Miscellaneous

Alcoholism
Asthma
Graft-versus-host disease
Myocardial infarction

Pediatric

Atresia
Feeding disorder
Foreign body
Gastroenteritis
Gastroesophageal reflux
Hirschsprung's disease
Intussusception
Meconium-ileus
Meningitis
Necrotizing enterocolitis
Pancreatitis
Peritonitis
Pyloric stenosis
Reye's syndrome
Subdural hematoma
Tracheoesophageal fistula
Volvulus/malrotation of gut

Psychogenic

Anorexia nervosa
Anticipatory
Anxiety
Bulimia
Cyclic vomiting
Depression
Eating disorders (self-induced)

vagus, and spinal nerves to the respiratory and abdominal musculature and organs. Changes in stomach tone and motility during vomiting are mediated by visceral vagal efferent nerves. Somatic efferent nerves coordinate muscles of respiration responsible for retching and expulsion of gastric contents. The areas of the brain controlling nausea and vomiting, as well as the gastrointestinal tract, contain neurotransmitters such as serotonin, dopamine, histamine, acetylcholine, and endorphins. The evaluation of the patient with nausea and vomiting and the pharmacologic approach to treatment must take into consideration the etiology of symptoms. A thorough physical examination and medical history are essential. The history should include the character of the emesis; relation to meals; association with pain, fever, diarrhea, constipation, or vertigo; acute or chronic nature; if there has been exposure to anyone else with a similar illness; emotional state; weight loss; history of biliary, pancreatic, or renal disease; possibility of pregnancy; surgical history; and medications. Laboratory studies should include serum electrolytes, glucose,

calcium, amylase, lipase, creatinine, liver panel, and beta–human chorionic gonadotropin if the patient is female and of childbearing age. Depending on the findings, radiologic imaging with chest x-ray or abdominal flat plate or brain CT/MRI may be helpful.

GENERAL MANAGEMENT

Supportive measures, such as correction of electrolyte or acid-base imbalance, hydration, and appropriate medications, should be offered, preferably tailored to the etiology of vomiting.

The clinical management of emesis includes pharmacologic mediation, patient support, and behavioral or psychological mediation. Improved understanding of the neurochemistry of the emetic reflex has been instrumental in the development and applicability of newer antiemetic agents. Table 2 describes some commonly used antiemetic agents, their proposed

TABLE 2. **Antiemetic Agents**

Agent	Mechanism of Action	Standard Doses and Schedule of Administration	Type of Emesis Used For
5-HT 3 Antagonists			
Ondansetron (Zofran)	5-HT$_3$ receptor blockade	32 mg IV × 1 OR	Chemotherapy
Granisetron (Kytril)		0.15 mg/kg × 3	Radiation
		8 mg PO tid	Postoperative
		10 μg/kg IV OR	
		1 mg PO bid	
Substituted benzamides			
Metoclopramide (Reglan)	Dopamine receptor blockade, 5-HT$_3$ receptor blockade	1–2 mg/kg IV q 2 h × 2–4 doses OR 10 mg PO 30 min ac and hs	Chemotherapy Gastroparesis Gastroesophageal reflux
Phenothiazines			
Prochlorperazine (Compazine)	Dopamine receptor blockade	2.5–10 mg PO IM OR IV q 3–4 h OR 25 mg bid rectally	Carcinomatosis Uremia
Perphenazine (Trilafon)		8–24 mg PO daily	Radiation
Promethazine (Phenergan)		12.5–25 mg PO OR IM q 4–6 h	Drug-induced
Thiethylperazine (Torecan)		10 mg PO, IM, OR rectally bid OR tid	Postoperative
Chlorpromazine (Thorazine)		50–100 mg q 6–8 h	
Corticosteroids			
Dexamethasone*	Unclear	10–20 mg IV × 1 dose	Chemotherapy
Benzodiazepines			
Lorazepam (Ativan)*	Anxiolytic amnesic	0.5–1 mg IV q 4 h OR 30 min before chemotherapy	Chemotherapy
Butyrophenones			
Haloperidol (Haldol)*	Dopamine receptor blockade	1–3 mg IV OR 5 mg PO q 2–6 h	Chemotherapy
Droperidol (Inapsine)		0.5–2 mg IV q 4 h OR 1–2 mg PO OR IM q 8 h	
Cannabinoids			
Dronabinol (Marinol)	Central psychotropic action	5–10 mg PO q 3–4 h	Chemotherapy
Nabilone†		2 mg PO q 6–12 h	
Anticholinergics			
Scopolamine (Transderm-Scōp)	Cholinergic blockade	1 patch behind ear 4 h before travel	Motion sickness Postoperative
Antihistamines			
Diphenhydramine (Benadryl)	H$_1$ receptor antagonism	50 mg PO q 4–6 h	Motion sickness
Hydroxyzine (Atarax)*		25–100 mg PO OR IM q 6–8 h	
Meclizine (Antivert)		20–50 mg PO 1 hr before travel	
Prokinetic Agents			
Cisapride (Propulsid)*	Increase postganglionic acetylcholine release	10 mg PO 30 min ac and hs	Gastroparesis

*Not FDA-approved for this indication.
†Not yet approved for use in the United States.

mechanism of action, appropriate doses, and types of emesis they are used for. Anticholinergic medications, such as scopolamine, are centrally acting and do not work on the CTZ. They are the most effective medications for motion sickness. Antihistamines, such as hydroxyzine (Atarax),* meclizine (Antivert), and diphenhydramine (Benadryl) also do not work on the CTZ but are effective in treating motion sickness and vestibular disturbances. Delta-9-tetracannabinate (dronabinol [Marinol]) inhibits intestinal motility and may be effective in some cases of chemotherapy-induced emesis. Prokinetic agents, such as cisapride (Propulsid)* and metoclopramide (Reglan),

increase intestinal contractile force and accelerate transit, increase acetylcholine, and, in the case of metoclopramide, inhibit dopamine receptors; these agents may be useful in chemotherapy-induced emesis, as well as in intestinal pseudo-obstruction and functional or diabetic gastroparesis. Neuroleptic agents, such as chlorpromazine (Thorazine), prochlorperazine (Compazine), perphenazine (Trilafon), promethazine (Phenergan), and thiethylperazine (Torecan), inhibit the central dopamine receptors and affect the CTZ and are therefore effective in uremia, drug-induced emesis, carcinomatosis, or radiation sickness. The nausea and vomiting of pregnancy usually abate after the first trimester, although hyperemesis gravidarum may require supportive care.

*Not FDA-approved for this indication.

There are no currently approved drugs for treatment of nausea and vomiting during pregnancy.

Patients with malignancies require special consideration because their treatment as well as complications of their diseases may contribute to development of nausea and vomiting. Specifically, brain metastases, surgery, pain medications, bowel stasis, and abdominal distention may all contribute to nausea and vomiting in addition to chemotherapy treatment.

CHEMOTHERAPY-INDUCED EMESIS

Control of chemotherapy-induced nausea and vomiting is an important component in the overall treatment of patients with neoplastic disease.

Chemotherapy-induced emesis is a complicated, multifactorial event. There are numerous neurotransmitters (histamine, acetylcholine, dopamine, serotonin) involved in the emetic reflex. Receptors for these neurotransmitters have been identified in the area postrema, the CTZ, in other areas of the brain, and in gastrointestinal mucosa. A proposed mechanism of chemotherapy-induced emesis involves the rapid release of serotonin from enterochromaffin cells in the small intestinal mucosa. Serotonin may stimulate 5-hydroxytryptamine (5-HT$_3$) receptors on vagal afferent neurons in the gut and in the nucleus tractus solitarius of the VC in the brain. The VC is activated by afferent impulses from the chemoreceptor trigger zone, vestibular apparatus, midbrain, limbic system, or periphery (pharynx or gastrointestinal tract). Following integration of the afferent impulses that can potentially result in vomiting, output to the nearby medullary control centers occurs with subsequent activation of somatic and visceral efferent impulses to the effector organs.

Phases

Chemotherapy-induced emesis is categorized as anticipatory, acute (early-and late-onset), or delayed emesis (Table 3). These categories of emesis are unique pathophysiologic events and give rise to different therapeutic problems. Failure to control acute emesis can lead to the activation of anticipatory and delayed emesis and to worsening of subsequent acute emesis.

Whereas acute phase emesis is mediated through the release of serotonin, the pathophysiology and pharmacology of delayed emesis are still unclear. Although delayed emesis is usually less severe in the frequency of emetic episodes, delayed emesis continues to result in significant morbidity.

No drug treatment has proved clearly and consistently effective in delayed emesis. Therefore, drug therapy tends to be empirical and remains based on customary practice. The most important aspect of treatment in patients who are at risk of delayed emesis is clearly to achieve optimal control during the first 24 hours; poor control during the acute phase is the primary risk factor for delayed emesis.

Factors Affecting Emesis Control

Antiemetic therapy may fail in some patients due to the psychological effects of antineoplastic therapy, previous emetic experiences, disease factors, or additional, unknown mechanisms.

Three risk factors have been identified that influence the ability of the clinician to control chemotherapy-induced emesis: patient characteristics, chemotherapy regimen, and antiemetic regimen. Of the various patient types, women and children usually achieve poorer control of emesis than men and older patients on a regular basis; patients with poor control of emesis during previous chemotherapy are also at increased risk of anticipatory and acute emesis during subsequent chemotherapy cycles. Chemotherapeutic agents are classified according to their potential to induce emesis (Table 4).

Management of Chemotherapy-Induced Emesis

In view of the undesirable consequences of poor antiemetic management, choosing an effective antiemetic agent and determining the optimal dosing regimen are critical. Antiemetic regimens should be tailored to the specific patient population and emetogenicity of the chemotherapy to be administered (Table 5). In general, the potential for acute nausea and vomiting increases as doses of chemotherapy are increased. In addition, combination chemotherapy treatments are more likely to cause nausea and vomiting than are single drugs.

The discovery and clinical application of the 5-HT$_3$ receptor antagonists has transformed the treatment of emesis induced by anticancer therapies and as a result has dramatically improved the quality of life of a significant portion of those patients. The currently

TABLE 3. **Phases of Chemotherapy-Induced Emesis**

Type of Emesis	Time of Occurrence	Mechanism	Best Therapy
Anticipatory	Pre-chemotherapy	Learned response	Benzodiazepines
Acute—early onset	1–6 hours after chemotherapy	Rapid release of serotonin	5-HT$_3$ receptor antagonism plus dexamethasone
Acute—late onset	7–24 hours after chemotherapy	Gradual release of serotonin	Unknown, probably 5-HT$_3$ receptor antagonism plus dexamethasone
Delayed	16 hours–6 days after chemotherapy	Undefined	Prevention of acute and late-onset acute emesis

TABLE 4. **Emetogenicity of Commonly Used Chemotherapeutic Agents**

Low (<30%)	Moderate (30–60%)	Moderately High (60–90%)	High (>90%)
Bleomycin	Asparaginase	Actinomycin D	Cisplatin
Busulfan	Azacytidine	Carmustine $\geq$100 mg/m²	Cytarabine >500 mg/m²
Chlorambucil	Carboplatin	Cyclophosphamide $\geq$600 mg/m²	Dacarbazine
Cladribine	Carmustine <100 mg/m²	Dactinomycin >50 mg/m²	Ifosfamide >1.5 gm/m²
Corticosteroids	Cyclophosphamide <600 mg/m²	Doxorubicin >50 mg/m²	Mechlorethamine
Cytarabine $\leq$500 mg/m²	Daunorubin <50 mg/m²	Lomustine	Streptozocin
Docetaxel	Doxorubicin $\leq$50 mg/m²	Methotrexate >200 mg/m²	
Etoposide	5-Fluorouracil	Procarbazine	
Fludarabine	Hexamethylmelamine	Semustine	
Gemcitabine	Idarubicin		
Hydroxyurea	Ifosfamide $\leq$1.5 gm/m²		
Melphalan	Methotrexate >500 mg/m²		
Mercaptopurine	Mitomycin C		
Methotrexate	Mitoxantrone		
Paclitaxel			
Pentostatin			
Plicamycin			
Thioguanine			
Thiotepa			
Topotecan			
Vinblastine			
Vincristine			
Vinorelbine			

available 5-HT₃, receptor antagonists, granisetron (Kytril) and ondansetron (Zofran), have been shown to be as or more effective and have an improved therapeutic ratio compared with other antiemetic regimens in preventing chemotherapy-induced nausea and vomiting. Comparative clinical trials of granisetron and ondansetron given intravenously demonstrate similar efficacy and safety in patients receiving cisplatin- or cyclophosphamide-containing regimens. Due to the relative high cost of 5-HT₃ receptor antagonists, appropriate dosing and schedules have been investigated. While the Food and Drug Administration–approved doses for intravenous ondansetron are 32 mg × 1 or .15 mg/kg every 4 hours × 3 for cisplatin (Platinol) and 32 mg IV × 1 for moderately emetogenic regimens, doses lower than 32 mg in the later subgroup have been utilized (in combination with dexamethasone) with good efficacy. However, these patients received intravenous doses of granisetron, 10 μg/kg × 1, on the day of either cisplatin or moderately emetogenic chemotherapy; doses less than 10 μg/kg IV were not given.

Antiemetic prophylaxis with intravenous 5-HT₃ receptor antagonists during chemotherapy has now become well established.

While chemotherapy-induced emesis can be very effectively controlled with intravenous antiemetic agents, oral therapy may be more convenient and acceptable to patients. An effective oral 5-HT₃ receptor antagonist would allow administration in ambulatory and outpatient settings, which is particularly important for patients in whom the onset of emesis may be delayed, such as women with breast cancer receiving treatment with cyclophosphamide. Outpatient administration would also reduce the requirement for medical resources, and the convenience of the dose form would benefit both patients and staff, translating into a reduction in the overall cost of chemotherapy and associated treatments. The oral antiemetics approved by regulatory agencies for chemotherapy-induced emesis include 3-day ondansetron (at a dose of 8 mg three times daily) treatment for patients receiving moderately emetogenic chemotherapy and granisetron (at a day of 1 mg twice a day) on the day of either moderately or highly emetogenic chemotherapy. Studies have also demonstrated that a single daily dose of 2 mg of oral granisetron is as effective as the divided dose given on the day of chemotherapy. Of note is that oral granisetron is the only oral 5-HT₃ receptor antagonist approved for emetic prophylaxis in patients receiving cisplatin-based chemotherapy. The oral form of ondansetron is used for prophylaxis only in patients receiving moderately emetogenic chemotherapy.

Corticosteroids have not been approved by regulatory agencies for use as antiemetic agents; however, their efficacy (primarily that of dexamethasone)* has been extensively documented. Although effective as a single agent, dexamethasone, 10 to 20 mg intravenously, when used in combination, has been shown to increase the efficacy of conventional antiemetics, such as metoclopramide, and recently the 5-HT₃ receptor antagonists, ondansetron and granisetron.

The mechanisms by which dexamethasone inhibits cytotoxic-induced emesis are not clearly understood, although several have been proposed. These include reduction of prostanoid turnover by inhibition of arachidonic acid release, modulation of substances derived from arachidonic acid metabolism (e.g., lipoxygenase products), reduction of the amount of

---

*Not FDA-approved for this indication.

TABLE 5. Guidelines for Selecting Antiemetic Treatment

1. Determine the relative emetogenic potential of the antineoplastic drugs (high, moderate, low). For moderate to highly emetogenic chemotherapy, a combination regimen of a 5-HT$_3$ receptor antagonist and a corticosteroid is generally effective in controlling emesis; for low emetogenic chemotherapy, either corticosteroid or phenothiazines such as prochloprazine therapy is recommended.
2. Determine ease of administration (duration of intravenous infection, oral versus intravenous availability and efficacy). The ease and convenience of using the particular antiemetic are important selection considerations, hopefully allowing patients to continue their normal daily activities and thus maintain their quality of life.
3. Efficacy, duration of action, as well as absolute and relative cost should also be considered.
4. Understanding of potential adverse reactions. It is sometimes difficult to evaluate the safety profile of an antiemetic in cancer patients, since cancer patients are generally polysymptomatic. The adverse events may be a result of the cancer rather than the treatment. Of importance to cancer patients, the 5-HT$_3$ receptor antagonists are not associated with the dystonia and akathisia observed with use of dopaminergic antagonists such as metoclopramide. The most common side effects observed with the 5-HT$_3$ antagonists are mild constipation, headache, asthenias, diarrhea, and abdominal pain.
5. The 5-HT$_3$ receptor antagonists have clearly altered the choices available to oncologists, due to their excellent safety profile, flexibility, and efficacy. In an effort to reduce the cost of a particular antiemetic regimen, antiemetic agents should only be used in proven indications. Physicians need to identify and target those patient groups for whom clinical benefits of receiving 5-HT$_3$ antagonists are legitimate and explain the additional expenses arising from 5-HT$_3$ antagonist therapy. The significant health gain and low incremental cost incurred by 5-HT$_3$ receptor antagonist therapy clearly indicates its use for acute-phase emesis in patients receiving moderately high to highly emetogenic chemotherapy. The physiologic basis for the use of serotonin antagonists in the prevention of acute-phase emesis appears confirmed, but their role in delayed emesis is not clear.

available serotonin by activation of tryptophan pyrrolase (shunting metabolism away from serotonergic synthetic pathways), and modulation of vagal depolarization. Further studies to elucidate the pathophysiologic mechanisms of dexamethasone are warranted.

Compared with the excellent control of acute nausea and vomiting achieved in most patients receiving chemotherapy ($\geq$60%), the treatment of delayed emesis remains a significant problem. Delayed emesis may occur in 30 to 70% of patients receiving cisplatin-based chemotherapy. Recommended treatments include prochlorperazine plus dexamethasone or metoclopramide plus dexamethasone; the role of 5-HT$_3$ receptor antagonists in the management of delayed emesis has not been established.

Radiotherapy and High-Dose Chemotherapy–Induced Emesis

Serotonin is released from the gastrointestinal tract in response to various insults, including radiation therapy to the abdomen. The onset, incidence, and severity of radiation-induced emesis vary with the dose per fraction, field size, and the site irradiated. Many studies have shown that 5-HT$_3$ receptor antagonists are active in preventing radiotherapy-induced emesis. However, their superiority over conventional antiemetics has not been proven, as the comparators have never reached an accepted standard, such as has been reached in chemotherapy-induced nausea and vomiting. In view of this problem and the cost of these agents, combined with the lack of adequate data on their superiority over conventional agents, it is not yet possible to recommend first-line use of 5-HT$_3$ receptor antagonists for all types of abdominal radiation therapy.

Treatment with high-dose alkylating agents requiring stem cell rescue by peripheral blood stem transplant (PBST) or bone marrow transplantation (BMT) administered over 3 to 5 consecutive days and the use of total body irradiation (TBI) lead to marked nausea and vomiting. Vomiting in this setting has been particularly difficult to manage, due to both the simultaneous use of potent emetogenic chemotherapeutic agents and the high radiation dose (8 to 11 Gy). The antiemetic failure rate in this group is greater than 50% over the first week of treatment, in spite of continuous infusion of the 5-HT$_3$ receptor antagonists.

GASEOUSNESS AND INDIGESTION

method of
DAVID J. KEARNEY, M.D., and
KENNETH R. McQUAID, M.D.
University of California–San Francisco
San Francisco, California

GASEOUSNESS

Excessive gaseousness is an extremely common complaint among patients presenting to primary care physicians. Patients may use the complaint of gaseousness as a descriptor for many different gastrointestinal complaints, including excessive bloating, borborygmi, abdominal pain, belching, cramping, and flatulence.

BELCHING

The major source of upper intestinal gas is swallowed air. Each time swallowing occurs (particularly during drinking), a few milliliters of air is deposited in the stomach. Excessive air swallowing is often promoted by chewing gum, smoking, and rapid eating or drinking habits. This may result in prominent complaints of belching and occasionally excessive flatus. More forceful air swallowing (termed aerophagia) may be achieved voluntarily or involuntarily and is sometimes seen in patients with anxiety or major psychiatric diagnoses.

Belching results when the air swallowed by one of the preceding mechanisms is passed retrograde across the lower and upper esophageal sphincters and out of the oral cavity. This is a normal phenomenon that occurs following eating and should not prompt a diagnostic evaluation. If associated symptoms such as dysphagia, odynophagia, significant abdominal pain, vomiting, or weight loss are present, an investigation should be undertaken. Behavioral modification is the mainstay of therapy for patients with excessive belching. This may include measures such as a change to a slower pace of eating, avoidance of drinking with a straw, and avoidance of chewing gum.

FLATULENCE

Intraluminal gas is present due to the combined effects of air swallowing and intraluminal gas production. Nitrogen usually accounts for approximately 80 to 90% of gas within the intestinal lumen, whereas oxygen is readily absorbed into the bloodstream and surrounding tissues. The remainder of intestinal gas is accounted for by the intraluminal production of carbon dioxide, hydrogen, and methane as the products of bacterial metabolism. The average amount of gas passed per rectum ranges from 500 to 1500 mL per day, with an average of 14 episodes of gas passage per day.

Bacterial fermentation of carbohydrates normally occurs in the colon and results in the production of hydrogen, methane, and carbon dioxide. The presence of excessive quantities of carbohydrate within the colon may result in excessive gas production by bacterial metabolism and an increased volume of flatus. This may occur during small bowel disease with malabsorption (e.g., celiac sprue) or, more commonly, due to a genetic deficiency of lactase. Bacterial fermentation of carbohydrates may also occur in the small bowel if bacterial overgrowth is present. In addition, the ingestion of poorly absorbable carbohydrates such as stachyose and raffinose (contained in beans) or sugars such as fructose and sorbitol (in fruits) may also lead to increased gas production within the colon.

The clinical evaluation of patients with excessive flatulence should include a thorough dietary history. The patient should be questioned regarding the ingestion of specific foods, including beans, apples, cauliflower, Brussels sprouts, cabbage, broccoli, onions, red wine, beer, prunes, and raisins. Gum, candy, and diet foods may also contain significant amounts of sorbitol, and a history of ingestion of these items should be ascertained. The usual initial therapy for patients with excessive flatulence involves a trial of elimination of potentially offending foods. If lactase deficiency is suspected, the diagnosis may be confirmed by a hydrogen breath test, although a simple elimination trial of lactose-containing foods may be adequate to make this diagnosis presumptively. Ingestion of small quantities of milk (8 ounces of 2% milk fat daily) does not appear to increase the severity of abdominal symptoms as compared with a similar quantity of milk not containing lactose. "Beano"

(alpha-galactosidase) has been shown to be useful in decreasing gas production after ingestion of baked beans.

INDIGESTION

The term indigestion is synonymous with *dyspepsia* and may be defined as epigastric pain or discomfort (including bloating, fullness, belching, nausea, and early satiety) located in the upper abdomen (between the xiphoid process and umbilicus). Dyspepsia is extremely common in the general population, with prevalence studies indicating that up to one fourth of the population is affected, depending upon the criteria used. It is one of the most common reasons that patients seek the advice of a physician, and studies have indicated that direct and indirect costs of the evaluation and treatment of dyspepsia are enormous.

Differential Diagnosis

A wide variety of disorders may account for the symptoms of dyspepsia. These may include medication-induced dyspepsia, endocrine/metabolic disturbances, luminal GI tract disease, and pancreatic/biliary disease (Table 1). *Helicobacter pylori*–associated gastritis has *not* been shown to be a cause of chronic dyspepsia. Gallbladder disease is also typically con-

TABLE 1. **Causes of Dyspepsia**

Luminal GI Tract

Peptic ulcer disease
Gastroesophageal reflux disease
Gastric malignancy
Gastroparesis
Malabsorption
Chronic intestinal ischemia
Irritable bowel syndrome
Parasites *(Giardia, Strongyloides)*

Pancreatic/Biliary Disease

Chronic pancreatitis
Pancreatic cancer
Cholelithiasis, choledocholithiasis
Sphincter of Oddi dysfunction
Hepatobiliary neoplasms

Medications

Digitalis
NSAIDs
Iron supplements
Oral antibiotics
Potassium supplements
Theophylline

Endocrine/Metabolic

Diabetes mellitus
Hyperparathyroidism
Pregnancy
Collagen vascular disease
Hyper- or hypothyroidism

Other

Coronary ischemia
Intra-abdominal malignancy
Alcohol use

sidered in the differential diagnosis of dyspepsia, although evidence from clinical studies implicating cholelithiasis as a cause of constant epigastric discomfort is lacking. Large endoscopic series have shown that when patients lacking an obvious cause of dyspepsia (e.g., medication-related or associated with systemic conditions) undergo endoscopy, the percentage of patients having each diagnosis is as follows: peptic ulcer disease (20 to 25%), gastroesophageal reflux disease (25%), gastritis/duodenitis or normal (50 to 60%), and malignancy (2%). Patients with normal or near-normal endoscopies (which constitute 50 to 60% of cases) are commonly classified as having *nonulcer dyspepsia*.

Clinical Evaluation

The history should clarify the chronicity, location, and quality of the discomfort, as well as rule out the presence of certain "alarm" symptoms. These alarm symptoms may include weight loss, persistent vomiting, dysphagia, anemia, and bleeding. The presence of any of these signs or symptoms should prompt investigation by barium studies or preferably endoscopy. Potentially offending medications should be identified (see Table 1) and discontinued if possible. Intermittent, severe symptoms localized to the upper abdomen warrant abdominal ultrasonography to rule out cholelithiasis. The physical examination is rarely helpful but may identify abdominal mass lesions, guaiac positivity, ascites, or organomegaly. Laboratory studies should include a complete blood count, electrolytes, calcium, and liver function tests.

The symptom profile is unable to reliably differentiate between nonulcer dyspepsia, peptic ulcer disease, gastroesophageal reflux disease, and malignancy. For example, a patient with predominant complaints of belching or bloating may have peptic ulcer disease, gastroesophageal reflux disease, or nonulcer dyspepsia, and a patient with epigastric pain may not necessarily have peptic ulcer disease. Malignancy almost invariably occurs in patients 45 years of age or older. A complaint of *heartburn* (epigastric burning with substernal radiation) in association with epigastric pain or bloating has a low sensitivity and specificity for the diagnosis of gastroesophageal reflux. However, when the complaint of heartburn is the single dominant complaint, it is approximately 90% specific for acid reflux disease.

Management

The appropriate initial approach to the evaluation of patients with dyspepsia is controversial. A strategy of empiric treatment of younger patients and investigation by endoscopy of older patients (>45 years old) has been advocated by the American College of Physicians. With this treatment strategy, younger patients would undergo a limited treatment course of 6 to 8 weeks of H_2 antagonist therapy, with endoscopic evaluation if symptoms worsen or fail to improve. This strategy is aimed at empirical treat-

ment (with H_2 antagonists) of underlying peptic ulcer disease or gastroesophageal reflux disease (which together comprise approximately 50% of cases of dyspepsia). Unfortunately, the vast majority of patients with peptic ulcer disease, gastroesophageal reflux disease, and nonulcer dyspepsia treated with only a limited course of H_2 antagonists will experience symptomatic recurrences within a year, resulting in repeat visits with high costs and low levels of patient satisfaction. Available evidence indicates that patient satisfaction is greater when managed with initial endoscopy as compared with empirical H_2 blocker therapy, while costs are approximately equivalent. Since there appears to be little difference in cost on long-term follow-up, patient preference should play an important role in the choice of initial investigation versus an empirical trial of medical therapy.

An additional consideration in the initial management of patients with dyspepsia is the role of testing for the presence of *Helicobacter pylori* infection. *H. pylori infection* may be diagnosed by noninvasive means (IgG serology, urea breath test) with sensitivities and specificities of greater than 90% for each of these tests. Studies have shown that a negative *H. pylori* serology in conjunction with the absence of a history of nonsteroidal anti-inflammatory (NSAID) use virtually excludes the possibility of peptic ulcer disease. A strategy of not performing endoscopy on younger patients (<45 years old) with negative *H. pylori* serologies and absence of NSAID use has been advocated as a means of significantly reducing endoscopy workload. The vast majority of these *H. pylori*–negative patients will have nonulcer dyspepsia and may benefit from empirical treatment with a promotility agent (see later). Empiric treatment of *H. pylori* infection for those patients testing positive by serology should result in effective treatment of dyspeptic symptoms in the approximately 20 to 25% of dyspeptic patients with underlying peptic ulcer disease. A dyspepsia management strategy based upon testing for *H. pylori* remains to be validated by clinical trials, although computer modeling indicates that it may be the most cost-effective approach. In contrast to therapy with a limited course of H_2 antagonists, treatment of peptic ulcer disease with anti–*H. pylori* regimens prevents recurrence of peptic ulcer disease and may decrease repeat visits in the subset of dyspeptic patients with underlying peptic ulcer disease. A possible management algorithm incorporating the preceding concepts is shown in Figure 1.

Nonulcer dyspepsia (also termed functional dyspepsia) may be defined as chronic dyspepsia for which no structural abnormality or biochemical abnormality can be found to account for the symptom profile. Approximately 50% of patients presenting with dyspepsia will be classified as having nonulcer dyspepsia following endoscopic evaluation. *H. pylori–associated* gastritis has not been shown to be a cause of nonulcer dyspepsia, and routine testing and treatment for *H. pylori* is not indicated at this time. H_2 antagonists have been shown to be effective only in a small subset of patients with nonulcer dyspepsia.

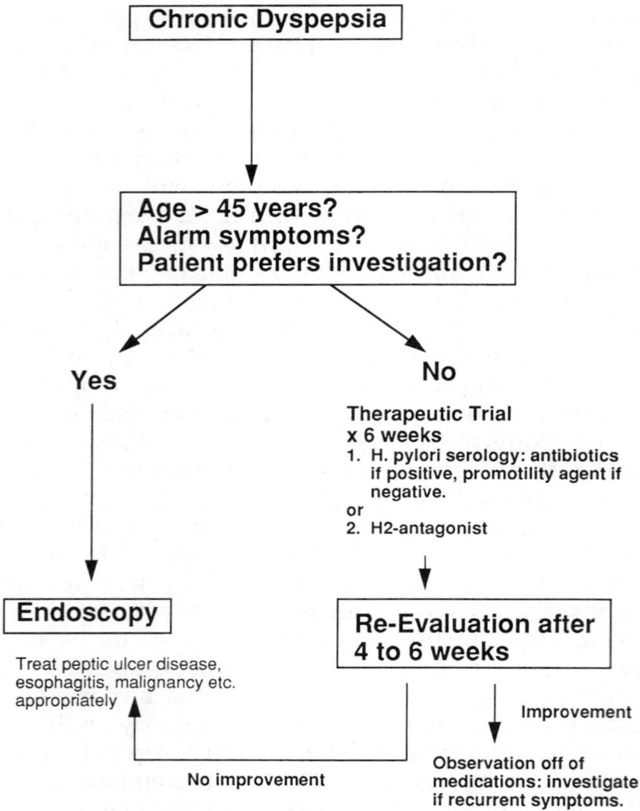

Figure 1. Management of dyspepsia.

Prokinetic agents (cisapride, metoclopramide) have been evaluated in multiple placebo-controlled trials and appear to be significantly better than placebo as treatment for nonulcer dyspepsia. These agents may be considered the agents of choice for nonulcer dyspepsia. Symptom improvement with prokinetic agents correlates poorly with abnormalities on gastric emptying studies, and measurement of gastric emptying is not indicated routinely prior to initiating one of these agents.

HICCUP

method of
HARALD FODSTAD, M.D., PH.D.
New York Methodist Hospital
Brooklyn, New York

Hiccup (hiccough, hoquet diabolique, singultus) is a repeated involuntary, spasmodic, and short-lasting contraction of the diaphragm, accompanied by sudden closure of the glottis. The hiccup spasm may occur from 40 to 100 times per minute. The diaphragm is innervated by the phrenic nerves, which arise in the neck on each side, chiefly from the fourth cervical segment, but they also receive filaments from the third, fifth, and sixth segments. In its route to its distribution on the undersurface of the diaphragm, each nerve is in close relationship to the deep musculature of the neck, the first portion of the subclavian artery, subclavian vein, internal mammary artery, the root of the lung, and the pericardium and peritoneum. There is also communication with the sympathetic system in the chest, the superior and inferior sympathetic ganglia, and the spinal accessory and hypoglossal nerves. An accessory phrenic nerve may be present in 20 to 75% of cases.

The great majority of hiccup spasms have been reported to be unilateral and confined to the left hemidiaphragm, and men are more often affected than women. The sensation leading to hiccup is mediated by sensory branches of the phrenic and vagus nerves as well as dorsal sympathetic afferents. The principal efferent limb and spasms of the diaphragm are mediated by motor fibers of the phrenic nerve. The hiccup reflex mechanism is demonstrated in Figure 1.

HISTORICAL BACKGROUND

The recognition of hiccup or singultus dates back to the time of Hippocrates, who in his *Aphorisms* concluded that "a convulsion of singultus supervening on excessive purging is a bad sign." In the dialogues of Plato, Eryximachus says to Aristophanes, who during dinner is suffering from singultus, "Let me advise you to hold your breath and if this fails, then gargle with a little water and if the hiccup still continues, tickle your nose with something and sneeze, and if you sneeze once or twice, even the most violent hiccup is sure to go."

Paulus Aegineta discussed the possible role of fullness of the stomach, presence of "acrid or pungent humors in the stomach," and "rigors." As therapy against singultus, he suggested emetics or retaining of the breath. Celsus (25 B.C.–50 A.D.) in Rome believed frequent hiccups to be a symptom of liver inflammation, whereas the Greek physician Galen (A.D. 129–199) stated that hiccup was caused by excitement that aroused the stomach to violent emotions and might be cured by sneezing. In Aetius' work *Tetrabiblion* (A.D. 500), hiccups were attributed to be a sign of inflammation of the stomach and adjacent structures. In severe cases, heated cupping instruments were applied to the breast, stomach, and back.

In 1627, Thomas Lupton in London published *A Thousand Notable Things of Sundrie Sortes*, in which he proposed: "Stop both your ears with your fingers and the hickops will go away within a while after. Proved." He also

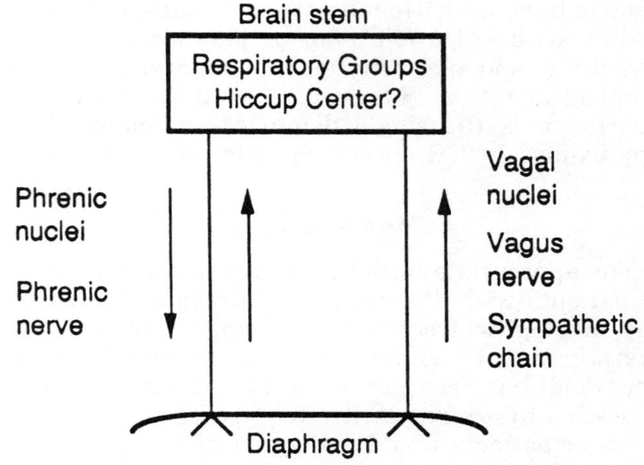

Figure 1. The hiccup reflex mechanism. (From Fodstad H, Nilsson S: Intractable singultus: A diagnostic and therapeutic challenge. Br J Neurosurg 7:255–260, 1993.)

stated, "It is proved and a secret: that if you give to them that have a hickop every morning three hours before meate, one roote of green ginger and immediately after drinking two draughts of Malmesey, you shall see that he will become cured."

According to the *Guiness Book of Records*, Jack O'Leary of Los Angeles, California, hiccupped more than 160 million times in an attack that lasted from 1948 to 1956. He received 60,000 suggestions for cures, of which only one worked: a prayer to Saint Jude, the patron saint of lost causes. The world record of persistent hiccup is probably held by Charles Osborne (1894–1991) from Iowa, who between 1922 and 1990 hiccupped every 1½ seconds. He contracted the hiccup when slaughtering a hog and was unable to find a cure. Nevertheless, he was said to have led a reasonably normal life and fathered eight children.

ETIOLOGY

Hiccups may be classified as either *transient* (self-limited) or *persistent* (intractable). Conditions associated with transient hiccup are gastric distention, alcohol ingestion, smoking, sudden temperature changes, and emotional stress or excitement.

The etiology of persistent hiccup is obscure. The causes have been localized to the central nervous system (CNS), neck, thorax, and abdomen, e.g., along the pathways of the phrenic and vagus nerves. Generally speaking, hiccups may be triggered by CNS lesions or irritation of the phrenic and vagus nerves. Numerous reports have described trauma, infections, inflammations, chemicals, vascular disease, demyelinating disease, arteriovenous malformations, tumors, and hysteria as causative factors. Drugs, blood disease, and cardiac pacemakers may also trigger hiccups. Persistent hiccups have been considered a form of mild myoclonic encephalitis or brain stem encephalitis. They have also presented as a symptom of brain stem tumors. Causes of transient and intractable hiccup are presented in Table 1.

PATHOPHYSIOLOGY

The neuroanatomic locus for hiccup is not known, but the central connection probably consists of an interaction among the brain stem respiratory centers, phrenic nerve nuclei, medullary reticular formation, and the hypothalamus. The existence of a "hiccup center" in the brain stem or in the cervical cord between C3 and C5 has been postulated by several authors. Visceral reflexes such as hiccup, coughing, sneezing, swallowing, and vomiting are invariably connected with the vagus nerve and are considered to follow similar reflex arcs. Hiccup has been classified as a respiratory reflex similar to coughing and as a gastrointestinal phenomenon more similar to the vomiting reflex. Fetal hiccups, which are relatively common, are similar to the gasping reflex. It is well known that hiccups in young infants may affect breathing in clinically significant ways.

Hiccup has been provoked by altering the metabolism of the respiratory center in guinea pigs during histamine shock. Subcortical electrostimulation in dogs, cats, and monkeys has resulted in spasmodic forceful expirations resembling sneezing and coughing and inspiratory movements resembling sniffing when stimulating the olfactory tract, rostral piriform cortex, and amygdaloid nuclei. Stimulation in the amygdaloid complex produced arrest of respiration. Stereotactic electrostimulation of the amygdaloid nuclei in humans has produced the same phenomenon as well as mastication, swallowing, or chewing.

TABLE 1. **Causes of Transient and Intractable Hiccup**

Central Nervous System	**Peripheral Nerve Involvement**
Neoplasms	
Surgery	Postoperative states
Trauma	Gastric distention
Infection (e.g., meningitis, encephalitis)	Myocardial infarction
	Pericarditis
Cerebrovascular accident	Hiatal hernia
Multiple sclerosis	Esophagitis
Parkinson's disease	Hepatitis
Hydrocephalus	Gallbladder disease
Syringomyelia	(e.g., cholecystitis)
Arteriovenous malformation	Subdiaphragmatic
Metabolic	abscess
	Pancreatitis
Toxic (alcohol, medications)	Tympanic membrane
Uremia	irritation
Diabetes mellitus	Infections (e.g.,
Electrolyte imbalance	pneumonia, pleurisy)
Hypocapnia (hyperventilation)	Neoplasms
Gout	Pulmonary
Psychological	Cervical
	Ear, nose, and throat
Excitement	Abdominal
Hysteria	Mediastinal
Stress	Gastritis
Malingering	Ulcer disease
Idiopathic	Peritonitis
Anorexia nervosa	
Enuresis nocturna	
Pharmacologic	
Steroids	
Barbiturates	
Diazepam (Valium)	
Alpha-methyldopa (Aldomet)	
Chlordiazepoxide (Librium)	

These clinical observations and animal experiments demonstrate the complexity of the visceral reflexes rather than pointing at a specific "hiccup center" in the brain or medulla. It has been postulated that the hiccup is served by a supraspinal mechanism largely distinct from that generating rhythmic breathing, and that the principal site of interaction of the hiccup discharge with other descending drives to the respiratory motoneuron is at the spinal level.

REMEDIES

The first person to associate the diaphragm and phrenic nerve irritation with hiccup was probably Dr. Shortt of Edinburgh, who in 1833 advised blistering the skin along the course and origin of the phrenic nerve in the neck until the attack stopped. In 1897, galvanic stimulation of the phrenic nerves to treat hiccup was described by Reges and Debedat, and in 1904 the famous German surgeon Ferdinand Sauerbruch performed phrenectomies to cure hiccups. His countryman Fritz Kroh in 1922 observed that diaphragmatic paralysis following bilateral section of the phrenic nerves was only temporary and of little discomfort to the patient. A celebrated case of persistent hiccup is one of Pope Pius XII (1876–1958). He was successfully treated by Dr. Paul Niehans from Switzerland with injections of animal tissue suspensions as well as local anesthetics to the phrenic nerves in the neck. Dr. Janet G. Travell, White House physician for President John F. Kennedy, reportedly cured hiccups by pulling hard on the tongue, thereby inducing a gag. She also used noxious agents such as ammonia, which causes either a gasp or a gag reflex.

The different therapeutic approaches to hiccup are equally impressive in their magnitude and variation. Transient hiccups that last only a few minutes rarely require any treatment, but some simple measures may be of help: holding the breath, breathing into a paper bag, drinking water, sucking on sugar or candy, compressing the nose while swallowing, pulling on the tongue, putting a finger in the throat, coughing, and sneezing (Table 2).

Most hiccups will stop when the presumed underlying cause is successfully treated. When the hiccups become persistent or intractable, a variety of pharmacologic agents are available for trial (Table 3). Among these, baclofen seems to be the most promising at the present time.

Baclofen (Lioresal)* is an antispastic drug that exerts its therapeutic effect by acting as a GABA (gamma-aminobutyric acid) agonist at GABA-B receptors. The effect probably occurs through inhibition or release of the excitatory amino acid neurotransmitter glutamate and aspartate and/or is mediated through an increase in K^+ fluxes in neurons. The

---

*Not FDA-approved for this indication.

TABLE 2. **Mechanical Methods for Treating Hiccups**

Stimulation of Uvula or Nasopharynx

Forcible traction of the tongue
Lifting the uvula with a spoon
Catheter stimulation
Gargling with water
Sipping ice water
Drink water while turning the cup
Sucking on hard candy
Swallowing dry granulated sugar
Swallowing hard bread
Noxious taste (vinegar, angostura bitters)
Instillation of irritants (ammonia, ether)

Interruption of Respiratory Rhythm

Valsalva maneuver
Coughing
Gasping
Sneezing
Continuous positive airway pressure
Compression of the thyroid cartilage

Respiratory Center Stimulants

Breathing 5% carbon dioxide
Hyperventilation
Breath holding
Rebreathing into a paper bag

Counterirritation of the Diaphragm

Pulling the knees up to the chest
Leaning forward to compress the chest
Applying pressure at points of diaphragmatic insertion

Relief of Gastric Distention

Gastric lavage
Nasogastric aspiration
Emetic-induced vomiting

TABLE 3. **Pharmacotherapy of Hiccup**

Major tranquilizers
  Chlorpromazine hydrochloride (Thorazine),* 25–50 mg IV q 6 h; if successful, switch to PO at the same dose
  Haloperidol (Haldol), 2–12 mg/day PO
Anticonvulsants
  Phenytoin (Dilantin),* 200 mg IV bolus, then 100 mg PO qid
  Valproic acid (Depakene),* 15 mg/kg/day PO or rectally
  Carbamazepine (Tegretol),* 200 mg PO qid
  Magnesium sulfate (magnesium sulfate inj. USP), 2 mL of a 50% solution IM
Central nervous system stimulants
  Methylphenidate hydrochloride (Ritalin),* 6–20 mg IV bolus
  Amphetamine sulfate (Adderall),* 10–20 mg PO bid
  Ephedrine sulfate (Marax),* 25 mg PO tid
Anesthetic
  Lidocaine hydrochloride (Xylocaine),* 2–4 mg per min continuous IV infusion, (Anestacon) jelly used topically in the mouth
Antispastic
  Baclofen (Lioresal),* 5–20 mg PO q 6–12 h
Calcium channel blocker
  Nifedipine (Adalat),* 10 mg PO bid (escalated to 20 mg tid)
Antidepressant
  Amitriptyline hydrochloride (Elavil),* 10 mg PO tid
Serotonin antagonist
  Ondansetron hydrochloride (Zofran),* 4–32 mg IV bolus or 8 mg PO tid
Dopamine antagonist
  Metoclopramide hydrochloride (Reglan),* 10 mg PO q 6 h or 5–10 mg IM or IV q 8 h
Dopamine agonist
  Amantadine hydrochloride,* 100 mg PO daily
Parasympathomimetic
  Edrophonium chloride (Tensilon),* 5 mg IV
Parasympatholytics
  Atropine sulfate (atropine sulfate inj. USP),* 1 mg IV
  Quinidine sulfate (quinidine sulfate),* 200 mg PO q 8 h

---

*Not FDA-approved for this indication.

end result is a suppression of both mono- and polysynaptic reflexes. The effect of baclofen on persistent hiccup may indicate that its neuroanatomic locus is in the brain stem and that the underlying cause could be brain stem seizures. Since baclofen has strong synergistic effect with carbamazepine, the combined treatment may be tried in those cases where baclofen alone is not effective.

Besides a multitude of exotic remedies and pharmaceuticals, the following therapeutic modalities have been tried and recommended with varying results: acupuncture, hypnosis, continuous positive air-

TABLE 4. **Neuromodulation for Hiccup**

Phrenic Nerve

Blocks with local anesthetics or alcohol
Electrostimulation
Phrenic crush or transection

Vagus Nerve

Supraorbital pressure
Carotid sinus massage
Microvascular decompression

way pressure (CPAP), paravertebral block of C3–5 or epidural blockade below C5, pharyngeal stimulation, faradic and galvanic currents, continuous electrophrenic stimulation, blockade, crush and transection of the phrenic nerves, as well as posterior fossa microvascular decompression of the vagus nerve (Table 4).

For centuries, trial and error has brought us but a little closer to an effective remedy for persistent hiccups. There is probably no disease that has had more forms of treatment and fewer results from treatment than has intractable hiccups. Sixty-five years ago, Charles W. Mayo made a statement on persistent hiccups that still seems valid:

The amount of knowledge on any subject such as this can be considered as being in inverse proportion to the number of different treatments suggested and tried for it.

ACUTE INFECTIOUS DIARRHEA

method of
JEFFERY E. HECK, M.D.
*University of Cincinnati College of Medicine and
Providence Hospital Family Medicine*
Cincinnati, Ohio

Worldwide, there are an estimated 3 to 5 billion episodes of diarrhea annually, causing considerable morbidity, lost productivity, high medical costs, and mortality. Diarrheal diseases are responsible for 3 million deaths per year among children under the age of 5 in developing countries. Many of these deaths could be prevented by the use of oral rehydration therapy (ORT), which is the mainstay of treatment for diarrhea and costs on average just .07 U.S.$ per liter. Although mortality from diarrhea has decreased significantly, the incidence has not declined to nearly the same degree. For example, there were almost 500,000 cases during the recent cholera epidemic in South America. However, as a result of the widespread distribution and promotion of ORT, the mortality rate was less than 0.5%, a remarkable reduction from as much as 50% in previous epidemics. New advances in understanding the pathophysiology of diarrhea, the promotion of cereal-based feedings, and the development of vaccines continue to provide hope that the incidence and overall mortality from diarrhea will fall.

ETIOLOGY AND PATHOPHYSIOLOGY

For practical and therapeutic purposes, the pathophysiology of acute infectious diarrhea can be divided into two general categories: inflammatory and noninflammatory diarrhea. Inflammatory diarrhea is caused by the invasion of the colonic mucosa by enteropathogens and is characterized clinically by bloody stools and the presence of fecal leukocytes. Noninflammatory diarrhea occurs as the result of toxin-producing pathogens that stimulate the secretion of excess fluid in the small bowel by inhibiting sodium reabsorption from the lumen into the enteric cells, resulting in large-volume, non-bloody diarrhea.

The clinical and laboratory differences are illustrated in Table 1.

The etiology of acute infectious diarrhea can also be suspected on the basis of the epidemiologic setting. For example, bacterial causes are much more likely to be present in patients living in or returning from developing countries than in patients living in developed countries. Table 2 lists the most common organisms seen in the general population and in the most common epidemiologic settings.

DIAGNOSIS

For practical purposes, diarrhea can be defined as three or more loose stools in 24 hours. Infectious diarrhea is often accompanied by other symptoms such as nausea, vomiting, abdominal cramps, tenesmus, blood in the stool, and fever. However, in many cases diarrhea is the only symptom. Infectious causes should be suspected in all patients with diarrhea, especially in children. Noninfectious causes of diarrhea can be difficult to distinguish from infectious causes and are usually suspected after a thorough history. There are many causes of noninfectious diarrhea, but these are not discussed in this article.

Dehydration is the most common and the potentially most serious effect of diarrhea. All patients should be assessed for symptoms and signs of significant dehydration. If severe dehydration is present, it will increase the urgency of making an accurate diagnosis and possibly deciding the form of treatment. (See algorithim in Figure 1.)

Since most otherwise healthy patients with community-acquired diarrhea who present to the physician's office have mild disease that will resolve spontaneously, a laboratory evaluation is usually not

TABLE 1. **Assessment by Pathophysiology of Diarrhea**

	Diarrhea Type	
	Inflammatory	**Noninflammatory**
Pathophysiology	Invasion of intestinal mucosa	Abnormal secretion of fluid into the small bowel
Clinical presentation	Bloody, small-volume diarrhea Left lower quadrant cramping pain May be febrile or even toxic	Large-volume, watery diarrhea May have nausea and vomiting Cramps
Fecal leukocytes	Present	Absent
Causes	*Shigella* *Salmonella* Amebic dysentery *Campylobacter* *Yersinia* Enteroinvasive *E. coli* *Clostridium difficile*	Viruses *Vibrio cholerae* *Giardia* Enterotoxigenic *E. coli* Enterotoxin-producing bacteria Food-borne gastroenteritis
Evaluation	Directed laboratory evaluation	Usually no laboratory evaluation needed

TABLE 2. **Most Common Causes of Diarrhea by Epidemiologic Setting**

Acquired in the U.S. by Healthy Host	Traveler's Diarrhea	AIDS Patient	Institutional Diarrhea (Day Care, Hospitals, Extended Care Facilities)
Viruses (especially *Rotavirus*)	Enterotoxigenic *E. coli*	Cytomegalovirus	Rotavirus (younger infants)
Shigella	*Shigella*	*Cryptosporidium*	*Giardia lamblia* (toddlers)
Campylobacter sp	*Campylobacter jejuni*	Microsporidia	*Clostridium difficile* (hospitalized patients)
Giardia lamblia	*Salmonella* sp	*Mycobacterium* sp	*Campylobacter jejuni*
Clostridium difficile		*Entamoeba histolytica*	*Shigella*
		Giardia lamblia	
		Salmonella sp	

necessary (see Figure 1). Patients without severe dehydration, fever, or blood in the stool can be treated with oral rehydration therapy (ORT) until the symptoms are resolved. Most will do so within 5 days. However, patients presenting with severe dehydration, fever, or blood in the stool, or whose diarrhea is not resolved after 5 to 7 days, should have a directed laboratory evaluation. Such patients should initially have a stool examination for WBCs.

To examine the stool for the presence of fecal leukocytes, a small sample of stool is obtained from a collected specimen or by performing a rectal examination followed by smearing a small amount of fecal material on a glass slide. The slide is prepared using a few drops of methylene blue or a Gram stain. If three or more leukocytes are seen in more than four high-power fields, an inflammatory diarrhea is suspected. Rare scattered leukocytes can be normal. The presence of fecal leukocytes can also occur from conditions other than infectious diarrhea, such as Crohn's disease, ulcerative colitis, radiation colitis, and ischemic colitis.

A patient with acute infectious diarrhea and a fresh stool examination that is positive for the presence of fecal leukocytes should be suspected of having an infection caused by *Salmonella*, *Shigella*, or *Campylobacter*. Once these organisms are suspected as the etiology of the diarrhea, a directed stool culture for these three organisms should be obtained. At this point, it is also reasonable to treat the diarrhea empirically with antibiotics. Since it is not cost effective to include other organisms in this "standard" stool culture, most laboratories will look for these three organisms only unless requested otherwise. *Clostridium difficile*, enteroinvasive *Escherichia coli*, and *Entamoeba histolytica* should also be considered in certain epidemiologic settings. In addition, the absence of fecal leukocytes does not exclude any of these organisms.

Patients with bloody diarrhea may also be infected with a new and particularly virulent enteropathogen, *Escherichia coli* O157:H7, which should especially be considered in young children and the elderly. *E. coli* O157:H7 produces cytotoxins similar to those of the most virulent *Shigella* strains and has recently been associated with outbreaks of fatal hemorrhagic colitis after hamburger patties were consumed at a national restaurant chain. Young children, especially those in day care centers, and the elderly, particularly those in nursing homes, with bloody diarrhea should have their stools specifically examined for *E. coli* O157:H7.

Diarrhea caused by viruses and bacteria, treated or not, generally resolves spontaneously within 5 to 7 days or rarely up to 2 weeks. Because of this, diarrhea that persists beyond 2 weeks is considered chronic and the etiology is rarely detected by a stool culture for *Salmonella*, *Shigella*, and *Campylobacter*. At this point, examination of the stool for parasites is a more effective test. In the normal host, infections with parasites cause diarrhea that is mild, and patients often present after they have had symptoms for a week or more. One of the more common parasitic causes of diarrhea in the United States, *Giardia lamblia*, presents as mild diarrhea with foul-smelling, light-colored stools, abdominal bloating, and gas. Since the organism will be detected by a single stool examination only half the time, this clinical scenario should prompt empirical therapy before more extensive, and expensive, diagnostic testing is performed. Results are often dramatic and therefore highly supportive of the diagnosis.

SPECIAL EPIDEMIOLOGIC SETTINGS

Figure 1 highlights a clinical algorithmic approach that takes into account five special epidemiologic settings, aiding the evaluation and treatment of the patient with acute infectious diarrhea. These five settings are described in more detail in the following sections.

Child Less than 5 Years: Winter Season (*Rotavirus*)

Rotavirus is the most frequently identified pathogen in children admitted to the hospital for diarrhea and dehydration in both developed and developing countries. In temperate zones in the Northern Hemisphere, the peak incidence occurs from November to March. The reason for this seasonal variation is not

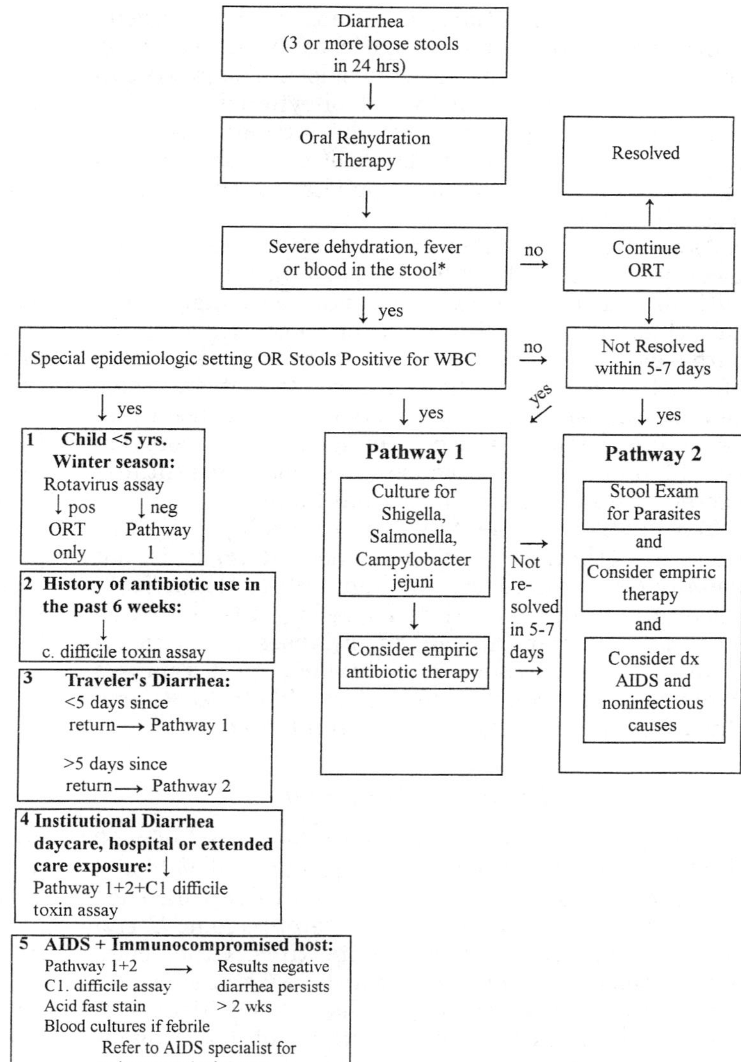

Figure 1. Management algorithm for acute diarrhea of less than two weeks. ORT = oral rehydration therapy.

known. Children between the ages of 3 and 15 months are most vulnerable to infection, but infection commonly occurs in children up to age 5. The initial infection is usually most severe; subsequent infections are milder, implying partial immunologic protection. Children less than 3 months of age are not generally affected, likely due to protection from transplacental antibodies.

Rotavirus infections are frequently asymptomatic. Symptomatic individuals often have vomiting, early in the infection. They may also have low-grade fever. The incubation period is 1 to 3 days, and the illness typically is resolved within 5 days. Between 16 and 32% of parents of children with rotaviral infection have symptoms of mild diarrhea. A wide variety of assays are available to detect the pathogen in the stool. Because large numbers of viruses are shed in the stool, assay detection is both specific and sensitive. Treatment is directed toward fluid replacement, preferably with oral rehydration. Antidiarrheal agents are generally unnecessary.

History of Antibiotic Use in the Past 6 Weeks: *Clostridium difficile*

C. difficile is responsible for virtually all cases of pseudomembranous colitis and 20% of cases of antibiotic-associated diarrhea. Infections occur following disruption of the normal bacterial flora of the colon, colonization by *C. difficile,* and release of toxins that cause mucosal damage and inflammation. It can be caused by any antibiotic but is most common with broad-spectrum penicillins and clindamycin. Symptomatic infection usually begins during or shortly after antibiotic therapy but may be delayed for up to 6 weeks. Suspicion of *C. difficile* colitis should be especially high in patients recently hospitalized or exposed to an extended care facility.

Clinical manifestations in patients with *C. difficile* colitis vary from asymptomatic to life-threatening colonic perforation and/or septic shock. Diagnosis can be made most accurately by a stool-cytotoxin test, but the specimen requires overnight incubation. Rapid immunoassay for the detection of *C. difficile* toxins is less sensitive but yields immediate results and is less expensive.

Asymptomatic patients require no treatment, and most patients with mild diarrhea improve simply with discontinuation of antibiotics. Oral metronidazole (Flagyl) is the first drug of choice for patients with severe or persistent diarrhea or those whose antibiotics cannot be discontinued. If metronidazole cannot be used or is ineffective, oral vancomycin (Vancocin) should be used. Intravenous vancomycin should not be used because it is not substantially excreted into the gastrointestinal lumen.

Ten to 20% of patients will have a relapse of diarrhea once therapy is discontinued. Relapse is not usually from resistance, but from failure to eradicate the organism or reinfection. Therefore, it is not necessary to use vancomycin in relapses of patients treated with metronidazole. In fact, most relapses resolve spontaneously and are less likely to recur a third time if no treatment is administered.

Traveler's Diarrhea

Bacteria are the etiologic agents responsible for 50 to 80% of traveler's diarrhea acquired in developing countries, as compared with 5% of traveler's diarrhea acquired in the United States. Enterotoxigenic *E. coli* is the specific cause over half the time. Other common pathogens include *Shigella* and *Campylobacter jejuni*. Many other pathogens have been identified. Cholera is an extremely uncommon etiologic agent in travelers. Even without specific treatment, most individuals with traveler's diarrhea will improve within 3 to 5 days. If diarrhea lasts beyond 2 weeks, other causes must be considered, especially noninfectious and parasitic causes.

Traveler's diarrhea can be defined as the passage of three or more unformed stools in 24 hours accompanied by abdominal cramps, fever, nausea, or the presence of blood in the stools. Fifteen percent of patients will present with vomiting. Traveler's diarrhea is not a life-threatening illness and rarely requires intravenous fluid replacement. If fluid loss is treated promptly, it is seldom a problem and can almost always be corrected by oral replacement.

Because toxin-producing *E. coli* cannot be easily or quickly detected, treatment for bacterial causes must be empirical and directed toward a wide range of organisms. Since resistance to ampicillin and doxycycline is widespread, these antibiotics should not be considered first-line therapy. The most effective empirical therapy is with trimethoprim/sulfamethoxazole (Bactrim DS or Septra DS) or the quinolones (Cipro or Noroxin). The quinolones may be preferable because there is less resistance and they are more effective against *Campylobacter*. Antimotility agents are also effective (Imodium or Lomotil), as is bismuth

subsalicylate (Pepto-Bismol); but antibiotics should be the mainstay, if not sole form, of therapy. Antibiotics should be given for 3 days, but several studies have shown a single dose of antibiotics with or without an antimotility agent to be as effective. Travelers should be given a prescription for therapy to fill and take with them while traveling, since treatment is most effective when instituted promptly.

Prevention of diarrhea is most effectively accomplished by careful avoidance of potentially contaminated food or water. Avoiding tap water, ice cubes, raw fruits and vegetables, salads, and undercooked foods is very effective. Prophylactic antibiotics for traveler's diarrhea is controversial. Nonetheless, both trimethoprim/sulfamethoxazole and the quinolones have been shown to be highly effective with minimal side effects in travelers whose trip is less than 2 weeks' duration. It should be reserved for travelers whose trips are critical in nature or in persons with underlying health problems that may increase their susceptibility to diarrhea or increase the severity of the illness.

Institutional Diarrhea (Day Care, Hospital, or Extended Care Exposure)

Children in day care centers are, in general, at higher risk for infectious diarrhea. The spread of organisms through fecal-oral contamination is substantially greater when there are many children who are still in diapers. Special needs children in extended care facilities are similarly at risk. Commonly encountered organisms include *Shigella* spp, *Campylobacter jejuni*, *Cryptosporidium*, *Giardia lamblia*, rotavirus, and *Clostridium difficile*. Treatment should be directed toward the specific causative agent.

The most commonly encountered cause of hospital-acquired diarrhea is infection with *Clostridium difficile*. In addition to an increased prevalence of the organism in the environment, patients are at greater risk because of antibiotic or chemotherapy use while in the hospital. Therefore, patients who develop diarrhea while hospitalized should be evaluated with a single test: a stool examination for *C. difficile*. However, other, noninfectious causes such as drug side effects, narcotic withdrawal, and fecal impaction should also be considered.

AIDS and Immunocompromised Hosts

Diarrhea occurs in 30 to 60% of patients with acquired immune deficiency syndrome (AIDS). Opportunistic organisms such as cytomegalovirus (CMV), *Cryptosporidium*, Microsporidia, and *Mycobacterium* spp are the most common causes. However, there is a substantial number of patients in whom no causative microbial pathogen is found. Almost 60% of patients with AIDS and diarrhea will respond to diphenoxylate hydrochloride (Lomotil); therefore, all such patients should receive a trial of therapy.

The evaluation of diarrhea in patients with AIDS should initially proceed as with any other patient.

However, when diarrhea is chronic (greater than 2 weeks) and associated with weight loss of at least 10% of premorbid weight, it is defined as the AIDS diarrhea/wasting syndrome. This condition may or may not be associated with an enteric pathogen. Nonetheless, it is important to search for opportunistic enteric pathogens because in many cases treatment can be effective.

If diarrhea lasts for longer than 2 weeks in a patient with AIDS, and initial stool studies (routine bacterial cultures, *C. difficile,* and examination for parasites) are negative, an acid-fast stain of the stool should be performed to detect the presence of mycobacteria, cyptosporidia, and *Isospora belli.* In febrile patients, blood cultures should be obtained for bacteria, mycobacteria, and CMV. When no pathogen is detected, a colonoscopy should be performed to detect CMV. One should especially consider CMV colitis in AIDS patients with lower abdominal pain, fever, frequent stools of smaller volume, hematochezia, fecal leukocytes, and/or thickened colonic mucosa on CT scanning. Upper endoscopy should be performed to detect cryptosporidia or Microsporidia, especially in patients with higher volume diarrhea occurring in the early morning, not associated with fecal blood, fecal leukocytes, or fever.

TREATMENT

Fluid and Electrolyte Replacement

The morbidity and mortality associated with acute infectious diarrhea are related to the fluid and electrolyte losses that commonly accompany severe diarrhea. Fluid losses range from 10 to 200 mL per kg per day, resulting in dehydration, tissue hypoperfusion, and circulatory collapse if the losses are not corrected promptly. High-volume secretory diarrhea can result in an isotonic dehydration and metabolic acidosis secondary to bicarbonate losses in the stool. Oral rehydration solutions (ORS) are appropriate for correcting the fluid and electrolyte losses in most patients. However, when fluid losses exceed 10% of the body weight, patients may have alterations in their sensorium affecting their ability to consume fluids. These patients are more appropriately rehydrated with nasogastric or intravenous fluids and electrolytes.

TABLE 3. **Antibiotic Therapy of Diarrhea**

Organism	Adult Recommendations	Notes
Therapy for Diarrhea Caused by Bacteria		
Campylobacter jejuni	Erythromycin, 250 mg q 6 h × 5 days or Ciprofloxacin (Cipro), 500 mg bid × 5 days	In most cases, rehydration alone is sufficient.
Clostridium difficile	Metronidazole (Flagyl), 250 mg tid × 10 days or Vancomycin 250 mg q 6 h × 10 days	Stop the implicated antibiotic. Isolate infected patient and reinforce infection control practices.

Escherichia coli
  Entertoxigenic
  Enterohemorrhagic
    (O157:H7)
	Ciprofloxacin (Cipro), 500 mg bid × 5 days
	or
	Norfloxacin (Noroxin), 400 mg bid × 5 days
	or
	TMP-SMX (Bactrim DS, Septra DS), 160 mg/800 mg bid × 5 days
		Uncertain if antibiotics help in enterohemorrhagic *E. coli.*
		Immune globulin may contain antibodies to the Shiga-like toxin elaborated by enterohemorrhagic *E. coli* and ameliorate the course of hemolytic-uremic syndrome.

Salmonella	Ciprofloxacin (Cipro), 500 mg bid × 5 days or Norfloxacin (Noroxin), 400 mg bid × 5 days or TMP-SMX (Bactrim DS, Septra DS), 160 mg/800 mg bid × 5 days	Antibiotic therapy may prolong the duration of bacterial shedding in stools. If associated with enteric fever: chloramphenicol, 50 mg/kg/day in 4 doses × 2 weeks.
Shigella	Ciprofloxacin (Cipro), 500 mg bid × 5 days or Norfloxacin (Noroxin), 400 mg bid × 5 days or TMP-SMX (Bactrim DS, Septra DS), 160 mg/800 mg bid × 5 days	Antimotility agents may worsen symptoms and predispose to toxic megacolon. Resistance to TMP-SMX in travelers to developing countries is common.
Vibrio cholerae	Tetracycline 500 mg qid × 2 days or Doxycycline, 300 mg in a single dose or TMP-SMX (Bactrim DS, Septra DS), 160 mg/800 mg bid × 3 days	Aggressive fluid replacement with oral rehydration therapy is the most important therapy.

Table continued on following page

TABLE 3. **Antibiotic Therapy of Diarrhea** *Continued*

Organism	Adult Recommendations	Notes
Therapy for Diarrhea Caused by Parasites		
Cryptosporidium	Metronidazole (Flagyl), 250 mg tid × 5 days or Paromomycin (Humatin), 500 mg qid × 14 days	Metronidazole is not an FDA-approved drug for treatment of *Cryptosporidium*.
Entamoeba histolytica		In areas where *E. hystolytica* is endemic, asymptomatic patients are not treated.
Asymptomatic cysts	Paromomycin (Humatin), 500 mg tid × 7 days or Iodoquinol (Yodoxin), 650 mg tid × 20 days or Diloxanide furoate (Furamide),† 500 mg tid × 10 days	Alternative treatment for symptomatic patients include tinidazole and ornidazole; however, they are not available in the United States. They are as effective as metronidazole and better tolerated.
Symptomatic	Metronidazole (Flagyl), 750 mg tid × 10 days and Paromomycin (Humatin), 500 mg tid × 7 days or Iodoquinol (Yodoxin), 650 mg tid × 20 days	Treatment for an hepatic abscess is the same as for symptomatic diarrhea.
Giardia lamblia	Metronidazole (Flagyl), 250 mg tid × 5 days or Furazolidone (Furoxone), 100 mg qid × 7 days	Tinidazole is an alternative treatment but is not available in the U.S. Quinacrine hydrochloride (Atabrine) is no longer available in the U. S.
Microsporidia	Metronidazole (Flagyl), 250 mg tid × 5 days or Paromomycin (Humatin), 500 mg qid × 14 days	Metronidazole is not an FDA-approved drug for treatment of Microsporidia.
Stronglyloides stercoralis	Thiabendazole (Mintezol), 22 mg/kg bid × 2 days or Ivermectin,* 200 µg/kg qd × 2 days	
Other Causes		
Cytomegalovirus (CMV)	Fluid replacement, nutritional support	Some studies indicate that octreotide (Sandostatin), a somatostatin analogue, may be effective in controlling diarrhea.
Mycobacterium avium	Clarithromycin (Biaxin) or azithromycin (Zithromax) with other antimycobacterial drugs	*M. avium* is resistant to many drugs, and effectiveness of treatment is controversial.
Rotavirus	Fluid replacement only	

*Not available in the United States.
†Available only from the CDC.

ORS were developed to provide simple, inexpensive replacement of fluid and electrolytes in patients with diarrhea. Because common home remedies contain inadequate quantities of electrolytes, they are not suitable preparations for fluid replacement therapy. Oral rehydration should be accomplished with WHO (World Health Organization) ORS (only in developing countries) or one of the many commercially available products (e.g., Pedialyte, Rehydralyte, Resol, and Ricelyte). Controversy exists concerning the best concentration of sodium in ORS. Currently, WHO ORS contain a higher concentration of sodium (90 mmol/L) than most commercially available U.S. products (45 to 50 mmol/L). Higher concentrations of sodium are most appropriate for initial rehydration in severe diarrhea when stool sodium losses are highest, and lower concentrations are better for maintenance therapy.

Cereal-based ORS, e.g., Ricelyte, may be the most efficacious rehydration solutions and are becoming more widely used. Grains yield complex polymers that are hydrolyzed to provide glucose and amino acids to aid in the co-transport of sodium out of the gut lumen, increasing the absorption of sodium and water into the enterocyte.

Nutrition During Diarrhea

Recent studies fail to support the practice of withholding solid foods during diarrheal illness. In fact, children especially are likely to benefit from continued feeding. As much as 95% of dietary carbohydrates and 70% of dietary fats and proteins will continue to be absorbed during a diarrheal episode, not only sustaining nutrition but also shortening the duration of the diarrhea. Infants should continue breast-feeding or, if taking lactose-based formula, should continue taking it diluted by half during the first 2 days of the diarrhea. Older children and adults should continue eating foods, but perhaps avoid eating fruits and vegetables (because they are hard to digest), diluted soups (because of the high sodium concentration), and foods with high sugar content (because of the high osmolarity, which may worsen the diarrhea). Finally, there is no evidence that avoiding milk will benefit the course of acute diarrhea.

Antibiotics

Antibiotics are the mainstay of treatment of acute bacterial diarrhea. Stool cultures are positive in only 50% of adult patients with acute diarrhea of presumed infectious etiology. Therefore, patients with moderate or severe diarrhea often require empirical therapy based on the epidemiologic setting as discussed previously. When possible, antibiotics should be directed toward specific organisms either identified by culture or clinically suspected (Table 3). Because the most common bacterial enteropathogens in the United States are *Campylobacter*, *Salmonella*, and *Shigella* species, empirical therapy should be directed against all three. As with traveler's diarrhea, the quinolone antibiotics (Cipro and Noroxin) are the most effective drugs.

Non-antibiotic Antidiarrheal Agents

There are many commercial preparations sold for the symptomatic relief of diarrhea. Controlled clinical trials have not proved the safety or efficacy of most of them. Table 4 summarizes the commonly

TABLE 4. **Nonantibiotic Antidiarrheal Agents**

Category	Examples	Summary of Efficacy
Adsorbents	Kaolin and pectin (Kaopectolin, Kaopectate), Attapulgite (Parepectolin)	Kaolin and pectin have not been shown to be effective in reducing diarrheal symptoms. Although attapulgite has more adsorbent capacity, it has only been shown to increase stool consistency but does not decrease stool water content.
Anticholinergics	Dicyclomine hydrochloride (Bentyl) Hyoscyamine sulfate (Levsin, Anaspaz) Belladonna Many others	Can relieve cramps by reducing contractile activity but has no effect on diarrhea.
Bismuth subsalicylate	Pepto-Bismol	Binds toxins and prevents bacteria from attaching to intestinal epithelium. Has been shown to effectively reduce symptoms of traveler's diarrhea but not to the same degree as antibiotics.
Bulk agents	Metamucil Citrucel	Have been shown to increase consistency and, occasionally, the frequency of stools, but only in mild diarrhea.
Cholestyramine	Questran	Has been shown to effectively bind *Clostridium difficile* toxins and perhaps other bacterial toxins. Probably most helpful for a recurrence of *C. difficile* diarrhea after a course of an effective antibiotic.
Lactobacillus acidophilus	Bacid Lactinex	Theoretically promotes the growth of normal intestinal flora, but there are no well-designed studies to show that it is an efficacious agent for treating diarrhea.
Octreotide acetate	Sandostatin	Stimulates sodium and water reabsorption but must be given subcutaneously. Has been shown to effectively reduce stool volume and frequency in pathogen-negative AIDS-related diarrhea.
Opiates	Loperamide (Imodium) Diphenoxylate hydrochloride with atropine (Lomotil) Camphorated opium tincture (Paregoric)	These agents have a profound effect on mobility. Loperamide also may have significant antisecretory effects and increases anal sphincter tone. These agents are generally contraindicated in dysentery, but loperamide has been shown to be effective in relieving symptoms of traveler's diarrhea, including dysentery.

used available agents. In addition to those listed, there are many other combination agents. In general, these nonspecific antidiarrheal agents are not efficacious and should not be used as a substitute for oral rehydration and directed antibiotics.

CONSTIPATION

method of
KAREN E. KIM, M.D., M.S, and
JAMES M. HARIG, M.D., M.S.
University of Illinois at Chicago
Chicago, Illinois

Constipation is an extremely common gastrointestinal condition encountered by practicing physicians. Although there are a number of criteria for identifying constipation, no uniform definition exists to diagnose this entity, since constipation is a symptom, not a disease. Generally, symptoms of constipation are accompanied by a decrease in average daily stool weight. The difficulty in understanding the pathogenesis and treatment of constipation lies in the absence of objective criteria and the need to rely on patient subjectivity to define normal and abnormal bowel habits. Despite the absence of a single definition for constipation, certain categories are commonly used as general guidelines for clinical practice. Bowel frequency of less than two times a week, unusual straining with defecation, stool consistency and caliber, and incomplete evacuation are often used as objective criteria, combined with the patient's subjective complaints. This discussion provides guidelines for the evaluation of constipation and acute and chronic management strategies for the practicing clinician.

EVALUATION

The initial evaluation of a patient with constipation involves a careful review of the patient's general medical condition, including pre-existing illnesses and signs and symptoms of underlying organic diseases (Table 1). The history should include details of the patient's bowel habits, the duration and onset of constipation, and a chronologic assessment of symptoms. A history of constipation from birth suggests a congenital origin, while onset in later life is suggestive of an acquired process. A recent change in bowel habits may indicate an acute process such as a mechanical obstruction (e.g., malignancy) and should be evaluated promptly, while chronic constipation often suggests a functional disorder. A review of all prescribed and over-the-counter medications, including laxatives, is essential, as these can interfere with normal bowel motility (e.g., anticholinergic agents, narcotics, nonsteroidal anti-inflammatory agents, and others) or increase stool water absorption (steroids). Dietary habits should be reviewed with attention to daily fiber intake, dairy products (lactose consumption), and organic diets.

Physical examination is often not as helpful as the history in defining the etiology of constipation. Nongastrointestinal processes can often be defined through a careful examination, such as thyroid disorders, and especially neurologic deficits. Since the gastrointestinal system is highly innervated, autonomic neuropathies as seen with patients suffering from diabetes mellitus, for example, often result in constipation. The abdomen should be examined for the presence of previous surgical scars, palpable masses (re-

tained stool), and abnormal bowel sounds. Rectal examination should particularly focus on pain during examination, rectal tone, stool consistency in the vault, and, of course, occult blood testing.

Laboratory evaluation should complement the history and physical examination. Routine laboratory data such as a complete blood count, electrolytes, calcium, and liver function should accompany more specific studies as indicated. The presence of endocrinopathies should be excluded, as these can cause, exacerbate, or aggravate constipation. In particular, the presence of thyroid disease and diabetes mellitus should be determined.

TABLE 1. **Etiology of Constipation**

Systemic

Drugs

Antacids (aluminum or calcium)
Analgesics
Anticholinergics
Antidepressants
Antihypertensives
Anticonvulsants
Barium
Diuretics
Sympathomimetics
Iron
Nonsteroidal anti-inflammatory drugs (NSAIDs)

Metabolic/Endocrine

Diabetes mellitus
Hypo/hyperthyroidism
Addison's disease
Cushing's syndrome
Hypercalcemia
Hypokalemia
Uremia
Pregnancy
Hyperparathyroidism

Gastrointestinal

Colonic Disorders

Malignancy
Intussusception
Strictures
Scleroderma
Hernia
Volvulus
Amyloidosis
Diverticular disease

Anorectal Disorders

Anal stenosis
Pelvic floor dysfunction
Rectocele
Anal fissure
Ulcerative proctitis
Hirschsprung's disease

Neurologic

Multiple sclerosis
Spinal cord tumors
Cerebrovascular accident
Autonomic neuropathy
Parkinson's disease
Intestinal pseudo-obstruction
Cerebral tumors

Other

Idiopathic
Irritable bowel disease
Inactivity
Visceral myopathies

Other diagnostic studies should be initiated based upon the previously cited history and physical examination. Flexible sigmoidoscopy or colonoscopy with deep rectal biopsy may be necessary to exclude an obstructive, inflammatory, and/or neurogenic lesion in the colon. X-ray examination may further assist the localization or presence of anatomic abnormalities or irregularities. With severe refractory constipation, a variety of studies can be used to assess colonic and anorectal function. Rectal manometry is utilized to investigate rectal tone, coordination, and anal sphincter function. Colonic transit studies using ingestible radiopaque markers are useful in the evaluation of patients complaining of infrequent bowel movements. Defecography may be used to study patients with complaints of excess straining during defecation. A combination of studies is often used to evaluate and categorize patients with constipation and require exclusion of reversible and acute processes. Obviously, diagnostic work-up should be cost effective as directed by the information gleaned from the office visit. Often, nothing need be done diagnostically if the cause is obvious (drugs) or symptoms are mild.

MANAGEMENT

The management of constipation requires a stepwise approach involving behavior modification, dietary intervention, drug therapy, and, rarely, surgical correction of anatomic defects. Primary medical conditions and drugs that cause constipation need to be corrected prior to initiation of more aggressive therapy. Patients must be instructed to address behavioral patterns that might influence regular bowel habits, such as suppressing the urge to defecate. Habit training has proved to be effective in children with idiopathic constipation, where regular evacuation is encouraged to prevent stool build-up. A similar approach can be used in elderly patients, those with neurogenic constipation, and debilitated patients. Biofeedback has been used with success in patients with pelvic floor dyssynergia. Regular exercise to increase mobility, especially in the geriatric population, can facilitate normal bowel patterns. Dietary intervention consists mainly of an increase in fiber intake and adequate hydration. Thirty grams per day of natural fiber is the recommended intake for the general American diet. Foods such as bran cereal, legumes, and fresh fruit can be used to provide dietary fiber. In addition to dietary fiber, adequate water consumption (at least 64 ounces per day) is recommended.

Despite compliance with diet, patients often require pharmacologic therapy. Laxatives are widely used and are categorized by their mode of action. The five main groups are bulk-forming agents, emollient laxatives, saline laxatives, hyperosmolar agents, and stimulant laxatives.

Bulk-Forming Laxatives. This group of laxatives is often used as a first line of therapy in those patients unable to consume adequate fiber in their normal diet. They increase stool water content as well as stool bulk. Patients need to increase daily water intake while using bulk-forming agents to avoid obstruction and fecal impaction, especially in the elderly population.

Emollient Agents. Docusate sodium and mineral oil are the main medications used in this category. They reduce surface tension, thereby softening the stool and allowing intestinal fluid penetration. These agents are most helpful in situations in which excess straining must be prevented, such as postoperatively and during recovery from myocardial infarction. Elderly patients and those with esophageal dysmotility should avoid the use of mineral oils, as aspiration can cause lipoid pneumonia. Additionally, long-term use can lead to malabsorption of fat-soluble vitamins.

Saline-Based Laxatives. These agents are nonabsorbable cations and anions that create an osmotic gradient to increase intraluminal water absorption. Systemic absorption of these substances can lead to electrolyte imbalance and therefore needs to be avoided in patients with renal insufficiency. These agents are used mainly for bowel preparation prior to radiologic and endoscopic procedures.

Hyperosmolar Agents. Nonabsorbable sugars (sorbitol and lactulose) and polyethylene glycol are the substances used in this category of medications. Colonic bacteria metabolize these nonabsorbable sugars, producing short chain fatty acids that increase the acidity and osmolarity of stool and increase colonic peristalsis. These laxatives need to be titrated to the desired effect and to reduce associated cramping and bloating. They are useful in those patients who fail to respond to bulk-forming agents.

Stimulant Laxatives. Anthraquinones and diphenylmethanes are the most commonly used over-the-counter stimulant agents. Short-term use is preferred, as side effects with long-term usage are often seen. Melanosis coli is a benign, reversible pigmentation of the colonic mucosa seen with anthraquinones. Chronic use can cause smooth muscle atrophy and myenteric plexus damage leading to worsening of constipation. Diphenylmethanes can produce erythema multiforme, hyperaldosteronism, and vitamin malabsorption.

Other Agents. Other pharmacologic therapy includes the use of prokinetic agents such as cisapride (Propulsid).* Although this medication is approved for use in gastroesophageal reflux, it is effective in those patients with delayed colonic transit.

Surgical Treatment. Surgical treatment for constipation is rare and usually unwarranted with the exception of Hirschsprung's disease, where the aganglionic segment is removed.

---

*Not FDA-approved for this indication.

FEVER

method of
PHILIP D. WALSON, M.D.
The Ohio State University
Columbus, Ohio

Fever is the single most common symptom for which patients are seen by primary care physicians, and in the majority of instances these patients receive medications. Numerous studies have increased our knowledge about the pathophysiology as well as the risks and benefits of treating fever. However, many members of both the general public as well as many health care professionals harbor misconceptions about the dangers of, and the need to treat, fever. This can result in much unnecessary diagnostic and therapeutic intervention.

Fever is a common manifestation of many medical conditions, both trivial and serious. Only in very rare situations, and only when extremely high (i.e., above 106° C), can elevated body temperature cause harm, and it may even be protective. Treatment of fever can prolong recovery from disease or cause delay in seeking needed, disease-specific treatment. However, fever treatment can also have benefits, providing patients comfort, improving oral intake, allowing for sleep, as well as discouraging unnecessary diagnostic evaluation or dangerous therapeutic interventions.

PATHOPHYSIOLOGY OF FEVER

Both the decision whether to treat fever or not and the choice of methods used to lower body temperature require an appreciation of the pathophysiology of fever. There are multiple causes of elevated body temperature. Infectious causes of fever are the most common and are the only causes associated with an altered "set point" of the central "thermostat," located in the preoptic anterior hypothalamic region. It is important clinically to distinguish these infectious causes of fever from hyperthermia. Hyperthermia results from excessive heat production, altered heat dissipation, or pharmacologic or physiologic alterations in homeostatic temperature regulatory mechanisms. A risk/benefit analysis of lowering temperature depends on the underlying cause(s) of temperature elevation. True hyperthermia should be treated only by external cooling, whether caused by chemicals (e.g., salicylates, nitrophenol, anticholinergics, stimulants, anesthetics), dehydration, elevated environmental temperature or wrapping, excessive exercise, head trauma, neurosurgery, etc. Other noninfectious causes of fever such as malignancy, hyperthyroidism, autoimmune diseases, and so forth should receive disease-specific treatment.

This discussion deals with the symptomatic treatment of infection-associated fever, caused by increases in inflammatory mediators (i.e., cytokines such as interleukin-1, interleukin-8, and tumor necrosis factor) that are released from cells, especially white blood cells, in response to infection. These mediators act on the central "thermostat" to reset the body temperature by causing production of prostaglandin E_2. There are many patient-specific factors that alter the response to these mediators. For example, patients who are very young or very old, malnourished, treated with certain drugs (i.e., steroids or nonsteroidal anti-inflammatory drugs [NSAIDs]), or have renal diseases can all have altered fever responses.

DEFINITION OF FEVER

The definition of fever is arbitrary, in part because temperature variability, both between and within individuals, is rather large. "Normal," baseline temperatures differ during the day by almost 2° C (from 36 to 37.8° C) in the same individual, with highest temperatures at night. Some temperature variability is the result of differences in measurement techniques, patient age, environmental temperature, dress, body composition, exercise, and metabolic state. In older children and adults, an oral temperature above 37.5° C, a rectal temperature above 38° C, or an axillary temperature above 37.2° C is generally accepted to constitute a fever.

Tympanic membrane temperature measurements are said to be capable of predicting core, or rectal temperatures, but not all studies have validated the accuracy of tympanic measurements, especially in inexperienced hands. Accurate measurement of body temperature is not trivial, especially in ill or uncooperative patients. The site of measurement, the equipment used, the ambient temperature, the skill of the observer, and the cooperation of the subject all can have major effects on the accuracy of temperature measurements. For example, consumption of liquids, location and duration of the thermometer in the mouth, and mouth breathing have all been found to alter oral temperature measurements, especially if electronic temperature devices are used without disabling their automatic timing devices. Electronic temperature probes that are ingested orally and transmit core temperatures to a radio receiver device have even been used experimentally to obtain accurate measurements. Fortunately, there is seldom any need to obtain very accurate temperatures in the vast majority of clinical situations.

RISKS AND BENEFITS OF FEVER

Fever has been associated with some harmful clinical effects such as fetal damage from fever in pregnancy, increased metabolic needs in malnutrition, and increased cardiac demand with borderline cardiac function. However, most of the misconceptions concerning fever are the result of other, weak, noncausal associations. There is sound evolutionary theory that fever is beneficial, and despite some contrary opinions, there are also some data to support this theory. Fever has been shown in animal studies to enhance the immune response to many infectious agents and some malignancies. Use of antipyretic drugs to lower fever has been shown to increase both morbidity and mortality in infected laboratory animals, as well as to prolong varicella infection in humans. Much of the fear of fever is the result of concern that high fever can cause "brain damage." There are simply no data to support these fears, which appear to be perpetuated by the common association between fever and conditions such as brain trauma, CNS infections, neurosurgery, hyperthermia, and febrile convulsions. Febrile convulsions are a special cause of fear. Yet, almost all simple febrile convulsions, in previously normal children, are associated with neither recurrence of seizures (febrile or otherwise) nor with any "brain damage." Most, if not *all*, children who are found to have "brain damage" after a high fever, with or without convulsions, were either suffering from a disease known to cause damage (i.e., meningitis) or had abnormal brain development prior to the onset of fever and convulsions. It is the presence of abnormal development preceding the seizure, not the recurrence of high fever or the clinical characteristics of the febrile seizures themselves, that is most predictive of seizure recurrence or "brain damage." There is also no evidence that parents can prevent recurrent febrile convulsions with the use of antipyretic drugs. Prescribing or using such therapy leads to failure, frustration, and parental guilt.

CLINICAL ASPECTS OF TREATMENT DECISIONS

In addition to the risks of symptomatic therapies (see later), the major risk of fever treatment involves delay in diagnosis and initiation of specific treatment. The physician must always first attempt to diagnose the cause of the fever and determine what benefit, if any, would come from specific or nonspecific therapy.

Treatment of hyperthermia requires cooling and specific therapy as mentioned previously. Fevers from drugs or toxins require specific toxicologic management. Malignancies and autoimmune diseases need specific drug therapy. Symptomatic therapy may also be used but can be dangerous. For example, shock can occur in Hodgkin's lymphoma patients given antipyretics. In infectious causes of fever, treatment decisions involve the type and seriousness of the infection and which, if any, specific and nonspecific therapy is needed. The assessment of the febrile patient is a critically important, complicated, clinical decision that is often transparent to the patient or parent. The need for therapy depends on a clinical assessment of how ill the patient is, rather than how high the temperature is. This is especially true in patients known to have decreased ability to generate a febrile response or to tolerate delay in specific treatment (i.e., elderly, malnourished, immunocompromised, newborn, or renal patients). In all patients, the decision to treat and what to use are based on the patient's history, physical findings, and occasionally on laboratory test results.

There is a general misconception that trivial causes of fever respond more readily to antipyretic medication than do serious infections. In fact, there is no difference in the response of fever to symptomatic therapy between children with serious as opposed to trivial illnesses. Whether symptomatic therapy is given or not, the physician must continually assess the patient's overall clinical condition and not just whether the temperature decreases.

NONPHARMACOLOGIC THERAPY

A number of nondrug therapies are available. If used, they should make the patient more comfortable rather than just lower the reading on a thermometer. Over-wrapped patients should have extra clothing removed. Activities that raise the body temperature such as shivering, crying, and excessive motor activity should be minimized. Excessive environmental temperature (i.e., above 20° C, or 68° F) should be avoided, but the child should not become chilled enough to shiver. Extra fluids should be encouraged to prevent dehydration. Sponge bathing is controversial. If attempted, only comfortable temperature water should be used, only small portions of the body exposed to the water, the sponging stopped if the child becomes too upset or inconsolable, and the child should be held and comforted by a competent adult at all times. Ice water and alcohol bathing must *not* be used. Alcohol is absorbed through the skin and lungs and can cause a chemical pneumonitis or ketosis; both ice water and alcohol can cause shivering, discomfort, and increased motor activity.

Antipyretics/analgesics are commonly used for the symptomatic treatment of fever. Their major advantage is their ability to control pain. They may make patients more comfortable even when the fever is not controlled. Studies in adults have demonstrated that there is only a modest correlation between improvement in subjective feelings of wellness and temperature decrease. Parents and patients should be encouraged to think of these drugs as pain killers rather than as fever reducers. The goal of therapy with antipyretic/analgesics is to make patients more comfortable. If this were understood, caretakers would be less likely to treat thermometer readings and less likely to awaken quietly sleeping patients in order to dose them again or to continue to dose comfortable, awake patients with minimally elevated temperatures.

There are two general classes of antipyretics/analgesics: acetaminophen (paracetamol) and nonsteroidal anti-inflammatory drugs (NSAIDs) (i.e., salicylates, ibuprofen, and others).

The choice of drug is based on a number of things, including the clinical situation, cost, availability, dosage forms, patient age, drug allergies, and other patient characteristics that influence the relative safety of the individual agents.

There are a number of prescription and over-the-counter NSAIDs that are effective antipyretics/analgesics; some have specific benefits such as parenteral dosage forms (i.e., ketorolac) or prolonged durations of action (i.e., naproxen). While the drugs are useful in selected clinical situations, the relative safety and efficacy of these alternatives have not yet been sufficiently studied to recommend them for routine symptomatic fever therapy.

PHARMACOTHERAPEUTIC AGENTS

Acetaminophen

Acetaminophen (paracetamol—Tylenol, Panadol, Bayer, multiple others) can be very inexpensive and is available in a wide variety of brands and dosage forms. While it does have the ability to inhibit certain peripheral prostaglandin synthetic enzymes, it is not generally classified as an NSAID. It has been available chemically for over a century and used clinically for almost 50 years. It is rapidly and well absorbed orally and rectally. Parenteral dosage forms are available in some European but not North American countries. It is a very effective antipyretic and analgesic, but its anti-inflammatory activity is weak. There is a 1- to 3-hour delay between the attainment of maximal plasma concentrations and therapeutic effects. Clearance is largely by hepatic metabolism to inactive and nontoxic metabolites. However, in overdose its usual metabolic pathways can be saturated and a toxic quinone produced. This metabolite can be detoxified by endogenous glutathione. However, when production of the toxic metabolite exceeds glutathione stores, such as in malnourished patients or in patients whose hepatic metabolizing enzymes are induced (by cigarettes, anticonvulsants, etc.), these detoxification mechanisms can be overwhelmed, leading to hepatic or even renal toxicity. Except for rare reports of hepatotoxicity in alcoholic patients who took therapeutic doses chronically, the drug appears to be very safe in patients taking usual therapeutic doses. Even in overdose, if diagnosed and treated within 12 to 24 hours, the use of acetylcysteine (Mucomyst) (as a glutathione substitute) is remarkably effective in preventing serious morbidity or mortality. However, if the diagnosis of overdose is delayed, especially in patients taking enzyme-inducing drugs, pregnant women, and malnourished patients, serious or fatal hepatic or renal toxicity can occur. Yet, despite its potential to produce toxicity in overdose, acetaminophen is by far the safest analgesic/antipyretic drug to use therapeutically, especially in patients with GI ulcers, bleeding problems, allergies, asthma, or renal diseases and in pregnant or elderly patients. Therapeutic acetaminophen use can be problematic only in patients at risk for chronic, accidental, or intentional overdose, such as patients who have liver dysfunction, alcoholism, malnutrition, or who smoke, take inducing drugs, or are pregnant. Dosing is generally 10 to 15 mg per kg every 4 to 6 hours, with ample evidence that at least 15 mg per kg and probably 20 mg per kg can be given safely and be effective for up to 8 hours (therefore not changing the total daily mg per kg exposure). Doses in adults are from 325 to 650 mg every 3 to 4 hours. There are multiple dosage forms available, including drops, elixirs, syrups, tablets, capsules, caplets, chewable tablets, and suppositories. Recently, prolonged-release preparations that would allow for less frequent dosing have been made available. It is not known whether double-dosing of a rapid-release preparation would be more effective or less safe than use of these less frequent, higher dose, prolonged-release products.

Ibuprofen

Ibuprofen (Advil, Motrin, Nuprin, multiple others) is a classic NSAID that works as a reversible inhibitor of prostaglandin synthesis. Of note, it is available as a racemic mixture of two optical (R and S) isomers, which differ in pharmacokinetics as well as therapeutic and toxic effects. The R isomer is converted enzymatically in the body to the more active and less toxic S isomer. It is unclear whether the use of pure S isomer would improve the therapeutic ratio, and this could increase costs significantly. While used for decades as an anti-inflammatory and analgesic, ibuprofen has only recently been widely used as an antipyretic. It is rapidly absorbed, but the percentage absorbed can differ between preparations and be decreased by food. Ibuprofen at the doses used for antipyresis produces a more rapid temperature fall and longer duration of action (usually 5 to 6 and up to 8 hours) than acetaminophen after the first dose, especially in children with higher (i.e., above 102.5° F) temperatures. This advantage may not be maintained with repeated dosing.

The toxicity of ibuprofen is similar to that of all NSAIDs. GI upset is much more common than with acetaminophen but is usually minor. Serious GI, renal, pulmonary, allergic, and bone marrow toxicity can also occur. Patients with hypovolemia or renal disease can develop renal failure after taking ibuprofen. Asthmatic patients can develop bronchospasm. If taken by a mother in the third trimester, fetal toxicity can occur (i.e., closure of the ductus arteriosus, delayed labor, decreased fetal urine output, oligohydramnios, bleeding, etc.). Sudden, previously silent, life-threatening GI hemorrhage (especially in the elderly), GI ulcers, hepatic damage, platelet dysfunction, hypertension, rashes, worsening of psoriasis, bone marrow suppression, headaches, confusion, and even aseptic meningitis all can occur. Toxicity is much more common than with acetaminophen but apparently less common than with other NSAIDs, including salicylates or naproxen. The risk of Reye's syndrome is unknown. The major advantage of ibuprofen, in addition to its longer duration of action and excellent efficacy, is its safety in overdose. While ibuprofen can produce life-threatening toxicity in certain susceptible populations (i.e., ulcer or renal patients, pregnant women, or asthmatics), it appears to be incredibly safe when taken in overdose by most of the general population. Except for mild acidosis and some CNS changes, there have been few reports of serious, nonidiosyncratic, acute, or long-term toxicity after even massive overdoses.

Ibuprofen is available both by prescription and over the counter in a number of liquid and solid dosage forms from a number of manufacturers at a variety of prices. Over-the-counter dosing recommendations result in about 5 to 10 mg per kg per dose, which is given every 6 to 8 hours. Higher temperatures may respond better to the higher dosages, but after the first dose repeat doses as little as 2.5 mg per kg may be equally effective. The adult over-the-counter dose is 200 to 400 mg given every 4 to 6 hours.

Salicylates

Aspirin, acetylated salicylic acid, is the classic NSAID. While still important analgesic and antiplatelet drugs, the salicylates are seldom used as only antipyretics because of safety concerns. Use is especially rare in children. Fear of drug-induced Reye's syndrome has stopped their use in all but very rare childhood diseases (e.g., for Kawasaki disease, arthritis, or inflammatory bowel diseases) or as components of various preparations (e.g., topical methylsalicylate and bismuth subsalicylate preparations).

All salicylates are rapidly and well absorbed and both metabolized and excreted renally as both metabolites and unchanged drug. The metabolism and distribution of salicylates are saturable as well as time, dose, duration, and pH-dependent processes. This is part of the reason that toxicity is so problematic. The onset of different effects are variable. Noncompetitive antiplatelet effects occur very rapidly; platelet prostaglandin synthetase is irreversibly acetylated when aspirin is rapidly deacetylated (half-life about 15 minutes). This results in inhibition of platelet function that persists for the life of the affected platelet, since platelets cannot resynthesize the prostaglandin synthetase. The antipyretic and additional antiplatelet effects of salicylates are reversible, last only about 3 to 4 hours, and are slower in onset.

Aspirin and other salicylates are very inexpensive and effective antipyretics, analgesics, and anti-inflammatory drugs. They are probably the standard in terms of efficacy against which other drugs (at least in adults) should be compared. Toxicity rather than cost or efficacy limits their more widespread use. Adverse effects from salicylates are common and can be serious after both therapeutic use and with accidental and intentional overdose. They produce the same GI, hepatic, renal, allergic, platelet, fetal, and pulmonary toxicity as ibuprofen. Aspirin additionally produces irreversible platelet dysfunction. Salicylate toxicity from therapeutic, accidental, or suicidal overdose is both common and often life-threatening. Because there are safer, inexpensive, equally effective drugs available, use of salicylates for symptomatic antipyresis cannot be recommended.

Combinations

Use of combinations of two antipyretics for fever, while a common clinical practice, is mentioned only to question this approach. The combination of aspirin and acetaminophen was historically shown to be more effective at lowering temperature than either drug alone. However, there is no reason to believe that it is necessary to lower temperature more than can be done with a single drug, nor is it expected that further lowering of temperature correlates with comfort provided. It is also not known whether the current practice of alternating usual therapeutic doses of acetaminophen with ibuprofen is either more effective or as safe as use of a single drug alone at usual, or at increased doses. Combining drugs is expensive, adds toxicity, could delay proper diagnosis or therapy, and contributes to the impression that lowering temperature, rather than controlling symptoms, is the primary goal of therapy. This practice perpetuates what has been called "fever phobia."

ACKNOWLEDGMENT

Supported in part by NICHD Pediatric Pharmacology Research Unit HD31316.

COUGH

method of
NATALIE LEWIS, M.B., B.S., and
THOMAS J. LANE, M.D.
New Britain General Hospital
New Britain, Connecticut

Cough is the most frequent chief complaint presented to physicians in the United States, accounting for 3.6% of all office visits. Cough is a "top five" chief complaint in all age groups and is the most common symptom presented to family physicians, pediatricians, and internists. In half of all presentations, the cough is chronic. About $600 million is spent annually on prescription and over-the-counter medications for the treatment of cough in the United States. Patients typically seek medical attention for chronic cough because they fear that they have a serious disease, such as cancer, AIDS, or tuberculosis, or because the cough results in a change in their lifestyle. They are also usually looking for symptom relief.

Cough is defined as a sudden explosive release of air following forceful expiration against a closed glottis. The cough reflex is an important mechanism that removes excess secretions and foreign material from the lungs and airways. The afferent receptors for the cough reflex are found mainly in the larynx, trachea, and bronchi; other sites include the tympanic membrane, pleura, nose, sinuses, pharynx, stomach, and diaphragm. The receptors respond to mechanical, inflammatory, or irritant stimuli. The efferent pathways include the somatic nervous system, the respiratory muscles, the lungs, and the airways.

Cough can be either acute or chronic, and the differential diagnosis and hence the treatment vary for these two entities. Five of the 10 most frequent morbidity-related diagnoses made during physician office visits in the United States are common causes of acute or chronic cough. These are acute upper respiratory infections, chronic sinusitis, asthma, bronchitis, acute pharyngitis, and allergic rhinitis. A chronic cough is defined as one that has persisted for longer than 3 weeks. A cutoff point of 3 weeks effectively eliminates patients with self-limited viral upper respiratory infections. One study on cough and the common cold has shown that cough had disappeared in 77% of patients, and was regressing in severity and frequency in the remaining patients, by 2 weeks. However, it has also been suggested that 8 weeks may be a more appropriate upper limit for acute cough, as bronchial hyper-reactivity in normal subjects with viral upper respiratory infections may persist and cause cough for up to 7 weeks. The treatment of cough can be definitive, i.e., specific therapy for the underlying etiology, or purely symptomatic. This article presents a diagnostic algorithm for cough and discusses both definitive and symptomatic treatment.

ACUTE COUGH

The most common cause of acute cough is a viral upper respiratory infection. The cough is triggered by acute inflammation and/or mild bronchospasm of the airways and is usually self-limited. Occasionally, acute cough is caused by a bacterial infection, such as sinusitis, pharyngitis, bronchitis, or pneumonia, or by aspiration of a foreign body. Acute cough may also be caused by allergic rhinitis or exacerbation of asthma. The cause of acute cough is usually obvious after a brief history and physical. Treatment of acute cough secondary to a viral upper respiratory infection is symptomatic.

CHRONIC COUGH

In the community, chronic cough is most commonly related to cigarette smoking. Smoking triggers the cough reflex by direct bronchial irritation, and by inducing inflammatory changes and mucus production, stimulating a self-propagating productive cough. Chronic bronchitis may eventually develop. Cough rates increase with the number of cigarettes smoked. The prevalence of chronic cough is

25% in ½ pack per day smokers, 50% in 1 pack per day smokers, and greater than 50% in heavy smokers. Fortunately, smoking cessation results in complete resolution of the cough in 77%, while a further 17% experience considerable improvement. However, the majority of patients complaining of chronic cough are nonsmokers. In nonsmokers, the prevalence of chronic cough is 8 to 14% but has been reported to be as high as 22% in males.

The clinical approach to chronic cough has been advanced by the use of anatomic diagnostic protocols. Protocols are based on the anatomy and distribution of cough receptors and afferent nerves and are designed to encourage physicians to consider extrapulmonary as well as pulmonary conditions as potential causes of chronic cough. Anatomic protocols have been used in five studies of chronic cough in adults and children, based in tertiary hospital and community pulmonary practices. A specific diagnosis has been made in 88 to 100% of cases, and cough has responded to specific therapy, when adhered to, in 89 to 98% of cases.

In protocol-based studies, postnasal drip is the most common cause of a chronic cough (27 to 41%), followed by asthma (24 to 29%), gastroesophageal reflux (6 to 21%), bronchitis (5 to 12%), and miscellaneous causes (5 to 6%). Miscellaneous causes in various studies have included bronchogenic carcinoma, congestive heart failure, sarcoidosis, interstitial lung disease, and drugs. Drugs implicated as possible causes of cough include beta blockers, L-dopa, and angiotensin-converting enzyme (ACE) inhibitors. ACE inhibitors were judged to be the cause of cough in 2% of patients in one study; this may increase as their use becomes more widespread. ACE inhibitors cause cough by increasing the activity of the bradykinin system. The newer angiotensin II antagonist agents (e.g., losartan) do not cause cough. Multiple diagnoses underlying cough are common; in one study, there were two cough-associated diagnoses in 23% of patients, and three diagnoses in 3% of patients. In many cases, cough was the sole presentation for both asthma (28%) and gastroesophageal reflux disease (GERD) (43%).

Figure 1 presents a diagrammatic representation of the authors' recommended method of evaluating chronic cough. History, physical examination, methacholine challenge testing, and prolonged esophageal pH monitoring are the

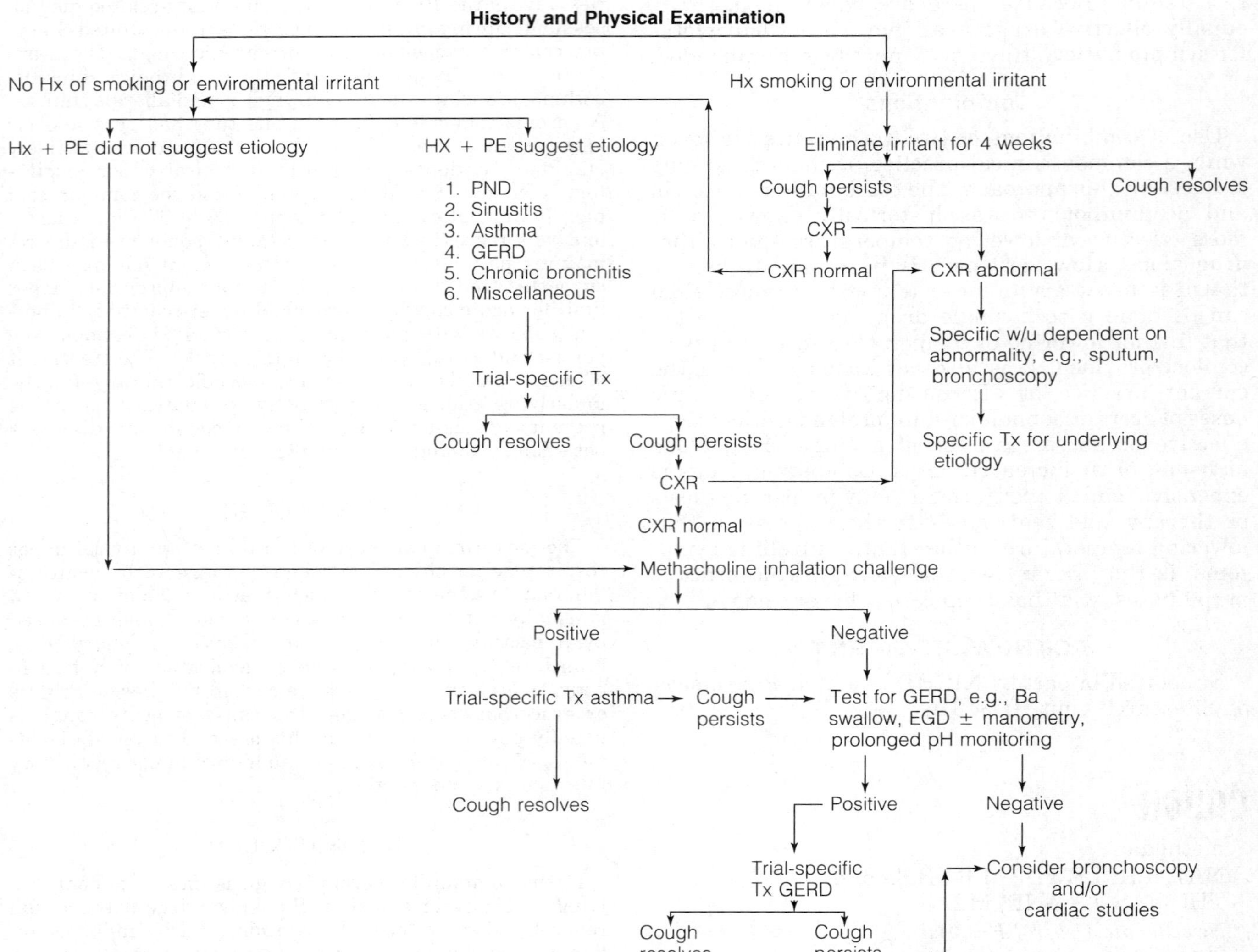

Figure 1. Evaluation of chronic cough. *Abbreviations:* PND = postnasal drip; GERD = gastroesophageal reflux disease; EGD = esophagogastroduodenoscopy.

TABLE 1. **Specific Therapy for Cough**

Etiology	Generic Name	Trade Name	Dosage and Route
Postnasal drip	Beclomethasone dipropionate *or*	Vancenase AQ Nasal	Intranasal, 1 puff each nostril bid
	Dexbrompheniramine maleate + pseudoephedrine sulfate	Drixoral Cold & Allergy	Sustained release 1 PO bid
Sinusitis	Antibiotic plus oxymetazoline hydrochloride *and*	Afrin	Intranasal 2–3 sprays each nostril bid (max 3 days)
	Dexbrompheniramine maleate + pseudoephedrine sulfate	Drixoral Cold & Allergy	Sustained release 1 PO bid
Asthma	Beclomethasone inhaler	Beclovent inhaler	2 puffs tid–qid
	Albuterol inhaler	Proventil inhaler	2 puffs q 4–6 h prn
	Albuterol tablets	Proventil Repetabs oral	4–8 mg PO q 12 h
Gastroesophageal reflux disease (GERD)	Metoclopramide	Reglan	PO 5–15 mg qid 30 min ac and hs
	Cisapride	Propulsid	PO 10 mg qid 15 min ac and hs
	Cimetidine	Tagamet	PO 800 mg bid
	Omeprazole	Prilosec	PO 20 mg qd
Chronic bronchitis	Antibiotic of choice		

most productive components of the diagnostic evaluation. Specific therapy is almost always successful, regardless of the underlying etiology for chronic cough. Some patients, however, have recurrent cough within 3 months, suggesting a chronic or recurrent problem, which is often GERD. Another approach emphasizes initial empirical treatment of all nonsmoking patients with a course of an antihistamine-decongestant combination. This is often effective and reduces the need for diagnostic evaluations.

TREATMENT

Specific Treatment of Cough

Recommendations for therapy of cough due to specific etiologies are listed in Table 1. Coughs due to postnasal drip, which is caused by allergic, perennial nonallergic, postinfectious, vasomotor, or irritative rhinitis, are best treated with intranasal steroids or decongestant-antihistamine combinations. Environmental precipitants should be avoided. Vasomotor rhinitis that fails to respond to these interventions can be treated with intranasal ipratropium bromide. Coughs due to sinusitis should be treated with a combination of an appropriate antibiotic, decongestant nasal spray, and oral decongestant-antihistamine preparation. Coughs due to asthma or chronic bronchitis are treated with smoking cessation, elimination of irritants, inhaled bronchodilators, inhaled corticosteroids, or oral corticosteroids, in stepwise fashion depending on response. Coughs due to GERD

TABLE 2. **Effective Nonspecific Therapies for Cough**

Generic	Brand	Dosage and Rate
Antitussive		
Ipratropium bromide*	Atrovent	Aerosol 2 puffs qid × 7 wk
Dexbrompheniramine maleate + pseudoephedrine sulfate	Drixoral	PO 1 bid × 7 d
Codeine		PO 20 mg bid × 3 d or 30–60 mg × 1 dose syrup 10 mL q 4–6 h × 3 d
Dextromethorphan		PO 60 mg × 1 dose, 10–20 mg qid × 10 d, 20 mg bid × 3 d Syrup (30 mg in 5 mL)
Diphenhydramine	Benadryl	PO 25–50 mg q 4 for 16 h available in syrup
Antitussive combination preparations		
Codeine + pseudophedrine	Nucofed	PO 1 cp q 6 h PO 5 mL q 6 h
Dextromethorphan + pseudoephedrine + dexbrompheniramine	Bromfed-DM	PO 10 mL q 4 h
Protussive		
Hypertonic saline		Aerosol bid × 3 d

*Not FDA approved for this indication.

are managed with lifestyle changes, including a high-protein, low-fat, antireflux diet; not eating for 2 to 3 hours prior to lying down; avoidance of large meals; elevation of the head of the bed; and with metoclopramide or cisapride, along with anti-acid therapy, such as H_2 blockers or proton pump inhibitors.

Nonspecific Treatment of Cough

In circumstances where it is not possible to ascertain or effectively treat the underlying cause of the cough, it may be necessary to provide nonspecific therapy. This most commonly occurs in the treatment of an acute cough caused by a viral upper respiratory tract infection. As these are self-limited, there are other therapeutic options aside from pharmacologic intervention. One can suggest that the patient try tea with honey, licorice, or lozenges to help relieve that annoying tickle. One can also advise that the patient rest, use simple analgesics or antipyretics, drink adequate fluids, humidify the air, use nasal saline drops, and take hot showers to relieve symptoms. It is also an opportunity to encourage smokers to consider stopping. Medications for the nonspecific treatment of cough are classified as either antitussive or protussive. Recommendations for effective nonspecific pharmacotherapy of cough are given in Table 2. Patients often expect medications for cough in the form of a syrup and may gain some psychological benefit from receiving it as such.

Antitussive Therapy

Antitussive therapy is appropriate when the cough is annoying, may lead to complications, and is not performing any useful function. Nonspecific antitussives are proven to be effective if they have been shown to significantly decrease cough frequency, intensity, or both, by objective cough counting or standardized questionnaires used in randomized, double-blind, placebo-controlled studies performed in patients with pathologic cough. Antitussive drugs that meet these criteria for effectiveness are arranged by mechanism in the following outline.
A. Drugs that alter mucociliary factors.
   1. Ipratropium bromide (Atrovent) in chronic bronchitis.
   2. Guaimesal* in acute and chronic bronchitis.
   3. Dexbrompheniramine maleate plus pseudo-ephedrine sulfate (Drixoral) in the common cold.
B. Drugs that increase threshold or latency of cough center.
   1. All narcotics of the phenanthrene alkaloid group—e.g., morphine and codeine.
   2. Non-narcotics: dextromethorphan, diphenhydramine, caramiphen,* viminal p-hydroxybenzoate,* and levodropropizine.*
C. Drugs that may increase the threshold or latency of the efferent limb of the cough reflex.

---

*Not available in the United States.

   1. Ipratropium bromide aerosolized in chronic bronchitis.

Protussive Therapy

When cough performs a useful function (e.g., clearing secretions) but is not effective, protussive therapy may be indicated.

Protussives are proven effective if they have been shown to significantly increase the clearance of particles from the lower airways during coughing in randomized, double-blind, placebo-controlled studies performed in patients with pathologic cough. Effective protussive drugs include aerosolized amiloride* (in cystic fibrosis) and aerosolized hypertonic saline (in bronchitis).†

---

*Not available in the United States.
†Clinical significance of improvement must await further studies to assess short term and long term effects on the patient's condition.

HOARSENESS AND LARYNGITIS

method of
ROBERT H. OSSOFF, D.M.D., M.D., and
GREGORY N. POSTMA, M.D.
Vanderbilt University Medical Center
Nashville, Tennessee

"Hoarseness" is a generic term used to describe any unnatural change in an individual's voice. It results from a wide range of disease processes and is the most common symptom of any laryngeal disorder. Otolaryngologists use the word "dysphonia" to denote any abnormal voice regardless of the cause. Hoarseness may be described in many ways. It may be harsh, raspy, rough, breathy, or refer to a change in pitch or volume. It may be used to describe vocal fatigue or the need for increased effort during phonation. The underlying cause may range from something as mild as viral laryngitis to a life-threatening neoplastic process.

Voice production results from a complex interplay of a number of factors. A source of air, forcefully propelled past the true vocal folds, begins the process. The vocal folds vibrate passively in response to air passing between their opposed surfaces. The degree of laryngeal closure, control of vocal fold length and tension, normal vocal fold mucosal movement, and mucus serving as a lubricant are all necessary for normal phonation. The resonators are the pharynx, oral cavity, and nose, which modify the sound resulting in a normal voice. Alteration of any part of the larynx changes the vibratory character of the vocal folds. This alters the smooth, periodic vibration of the mucosal cover layer of the folds, which in turn results in turbulent air flow that we perceive as hoarseness.

A key concept to understand when evaluating someone with hoarseness is that regardless of the etiology of the vocal disturbance, an individual will attempt to compensate for the dysphonia. In this fashion, harmful or maladaptive speech patterns may develop in an attempt to speak in a normal voice. These vocal habits can lead to further laryngeal mucosal damage, which then results in greater hoarseness. In this way, the original insult, and attempts at compensation, perpetuate and exacerbate each other. It is critical that such habits be identified and steps taken to retrain the patient in proper vocal techniques.

HOARSENESS IN CHILDREN

The initial consideration of hoarseness or any airway changes in a child is whether or not significant airway compromise is present. Suspicion of airway compromise should lead to immediate evaluation in an emergency room by experienced providers. It is imperative that the individual evaluating the child ensure that the patient's hoarseness is not actually stridor. Stridor is a moderate to high-pitched sound produced by airflow through a significantly obstructed airway, usually at the glottic or subglottic level. It may occur during any phase of the respiratory cycle.

Nodules

The most common cause of hoarseness in a child is vocal nodules. These "screamer's nodules" are common in school-age children and are a sign of vocal abuse. Vocal abuse is the exuberant overuse of one's voice or the development of habits that cause forceful glottic closure resulting in vocal fold damage. Such habits include excessive shouting or singing, chronic coughing or throat clearing, excessive whispering, attempting to speak over loud noise, or conversing with hard-of-hearing individuals. These bilateral lesions are usually located at the junction of the anterior and middle one third of the vocal folds. This is the central portion of the membranous vocal fold and is the point of maximal amplitude during phonation. Speech therapy and behavioral modification are the keys to treatment. Identification of the abusive vocal behavior and then its control or elimination are critical. Surgery is indicated only if the nodules are extremely large or if they do not resolve with long-term therapy. The nodules will almost certainly recur if the patient's vocal habits are not altered.

Recurrent Respiratory Papillomatosis

Recurrent respiratory papillomatosis (RRP) is the most common laryngeal tumor in children. Although benign, it is potentially life-threatening due to its propensity for relentless growth and recurrence. These are wartlike lesions believed to be due to the human papillomavirus. Hoarseness is almost always the initial symptom and is usually progressive. Approximately 15% of patients will have disease persisting into adulthood. Treatment involves repeated endoscopic excision using the microscope and CO_2 laser. This is performed at periodic intervals depending upon the severity of the symptoms, as well as the location and rapidity of recurrence. Great care is taken to avoid damaging the vocal folds. Tracheotomy is avoided, owing to the risk of spreading papilloma into the trachea and distal bronchi. Biopsies are taken due to the small incidence of malignant transformation over many years. Various types of systemic therapy have been used. Interferon, methotrexate, and photodynamic therapy have shown some promise, but further work is needed.

Laryngomalacia

Laryngomalacia is the most common laryngeal abnormality seen in a neonate or young child. It often presents as a hoarse cry or weak voice a few months after birth. Laryngomalacia is believed to be due to neurologic immaturity of the larynx. This causes a floppy supraglottis that can be literally "sucked" into the larynx with forceful inspiration. This causes turbulence and possible airway obstruction. The symptoms are usually worse when the patient is supine, feeding, or having a concurrent upper respiratory infection (URI). Treatment is conservative, with positional changes of the patient during feeding and sleeping. The child will usually outgrow this within 6 to 18 months. Patients with severe disease manifested by failure to thrive, obstructive sleep apnea, right-sided heart failure, or severe stridor may benefit from CO_2 laser excision of a portion of the supraglottic tissue. Only the most severely affected patients require tracheotomy.

Laryngeal Paralysis

Vocal fold paralysis is the second most common laryngeal abnormality in young children. In contrast to adults, unilateral vocal fold paralysis can result in airway obstruction and therefore requires prompt evaluation (Table 1). A chest x-ray and barium swallow should be obtained. Both flexible fiberoptic laryngoscopy and direct laryngoscopy are performed as part of the examination.

Bilateral vocal cord paralysis will probably require tracheotomy. It is important to rule out a central lesion as the etiology of the bilateral paralysis. Both the Arnold-Chiari malformation and hydrocephalus can cause this disorder. After the airway is stabilized, further surgery is usually deferred until the patient reaches the age of 4 to 5.

TABLE 1. **Indications for Otolaryngology Consultation**

Stridor/airway obstruction
Suspected vocal fold paralysis
Hoarseness with significant dysphagia
New-onset hoarseness lasting greater than 2 weeks
Any voice change after head and neck trauma
Hoarseness in a smoker
Chronic hoarseness
Hoarseness with neck mass
Hoarseness lasting greater than 2 days after extubation
Sudden voice change or hoarseness after extreme vocal use or abuse
Professional vocal performer with vocal complaint
Foreign body sensation in throat for greater than 3 weeks
Throat pain lasting greater than 2 weeks

Hemangioma

Subglottic hemangiomas may present with a hoarse cry or stridor. This will often worsen with crying or an URI. These usually present a few months after birth. The diagnosis is made upon direct laryngoscopy. Fifty percent of these children will have cutaneous hemangiomas. These subglottic hemangiomas regress in 10 to 18 months, and therefore no treatment is required if the symptoms are not severe. Steroids provide temporary improvement; however, laser surgery or tracheotomy is required in severe cases.

Inflammation

Inflammatory causes of hoarseness can usually be easily differentiated from other etiologies due to their associated symptoms. Supraglottitis is seen in children between 2 and 6 years of age. It is characterized by a rapid clinical course with a severe sore throat, fever, drooling, stridor, and a muffled voice. The patients often sit with their head held forward and neck extended. The diagnosis must be made promptly and the airway controlled. The child is kept calm with a parent in attendance and taken to the operating room for intubation and direct laryngoscopy. This will confirm the diagnosis and allow cultures of the blood and epiglottis to be taken. The offending organism is usually *Haemophilus influenzae,* and appropriate antibiotic treatment is initiated pending culture results. Extubation can normally be attempted within 48 to 72 hours.

Laryngotracheobronchitis (LTB) is far more common and less severe. The child is usually less than 3 years old and presents with a URI progressing to stridor over a 2- to 3-day period. A seal-like barking cough is classic. This is often viral and is treated supportively with nebulized racemic epinephrine, humidified oxygen, and steroids. Close monitoring of the airway is needed for moderate to severe cases. Progression of symptoms and fever suggest a bacterial LTB. This requires intravenous antibiotics and frequently intubation for airway control and suctioning of secretions.

HOARSENESS IN ADULTS

Acute Laryngitis

Acute laryngitis is defined as an inflammation of the laryngeal mucosa and is the primary cause of hoarseness in adults. This is usually associated with a routine URI. Eighty-five percent of these are presumed to be viral, with the rhinovirus as the predominant virus. Primary or secondary bacterial infections after a viral laryngitis are often due to *Moraxella catarrhalis, Haemophilus influenzae,* or the pneumococcus.

The patient will usually complain of hoarseness with a sore throat or pain when speaking. Occasionally the patient may be aphonic. Examination will show erythema and edema of the vocal folds. This swelling results in hoarseness due to the increased mass of the folds. Due to the self-limited nature of this illness, treatment is supportive. An increase in fluids, humidification of the room, and the use of an antitussive, if the patient has a significant cough, are important. Of greatest benefit is voice rest. This is not complete cessation of speaking, but rather a relative voice rest in which the patient speaks only when it is absolutely necessary. The patient should speak in a normal, unforced voice without whispering or shouting. Antibiotics may be given in cases associated with fever, adenopathy, or purulent sputum or rhinorrhea.

Vocal fold hemorrhage should be suspected when an individual complains of a sudden change or loss of voice after extreme vocal effort or a Valsalva maneuver. This patient should be seen immediately by an otolaryngologist. This injury may lead to scarring and polyp formation. It is usually seen in premenstrual women or patients on anticoagulant therapy or aspirin. Treatment is complete voice rest.

Hoarseness from laryngeal candidiasis is not uncommon in patients suffering from AIDS. However, it can also be seen in immunocompetent patients using steroid inhalers. The treatment is nystatin (Mycostatin) troches to be used orally three or four times per day.

Chronic Laryngitis

Chronic laryngitis is very common. Causative and exacerbating factors include gastroesophageal reflux (GER), voice abuse, allergies, rhinitis, sinusitis, chemical exposures, chronic throat clearing and cough, tobacco and alcohol abuse, and airline travel. Nasal obstruction acts via the drying effect mouth breathing has on the larynx, resulting in decreased lubrication with consequent increased vocal fold irritation. Allergies are normally an indirect offender, via sneezing, coughing, and throat clearing. Airline travel creates hoarseness due to the dry recirculated air on airplanes. In addition, individuals are tempted to speak louder to be heard over engine noise.

There is normally little or no pain associated with chronic laryngitis, just long-standing dysphonia or vocal fatigue. Patients often try to overcome vocal changes by increased effort during phonation, which compounds the problem.

A spectrum of findings are noted on examination. The folds may be erythematous and edematous. This may progress to gross thickening or polyp formation. At the other end of the spectrum are hyperkeratosis and leukoplakia. Leukoplakia is a descriptive term for white patches on mucosal surfaces and is considered premalignant. This requires biopsy to rule out carcinoma.

Treatment requires the removal of the offending agent, habit, or condition. In addition, improved vocal hygiene by increasing fluids, avoiding tobacco or alcohol, use of mucolytic agents, and voice therapy is valuable (Table 2). The treatment of GER is usually necessary. Antibiotics and steroids are occasionally

TABLE 2. **General Treatment of Hoarseness**

Most cases of acute hoarseness will resolve spontaneously, but a number of measures can be employed to hasten the process and decrease the chance of either recurrent problems or chronic sequelae.

1. Voice rest: Voice rest avoids a self-perpetuating cycle of laryngitis. Mucosal injury followed by even normal talking may lead to further irritation that will delay healing. This is not aphonia, but rather using the fewest words in a comfortable pitch and volume. At no time should the patient whisper, yell, or talk in areas with high ambient noise levels.
2. Hydration: Adequate hydration is very important in order to produce thin, watery mucus to properly lubricate the vocal folds. Some consider it the key defense mechanism of the larynx. Individuals should drink at least 2 quarts of water or caffeine-free liquid per day. A number of situations exist when an individual should increase water intake. These include an increase in exercise, febrile illness, use of antihistamines, drinking alcohol, and airline travel.
3. Thinning secretions with a mucolytic such as guaifenesin (Humibid L.A.), 1200 mg twice daily, has proven beneficial in many patients.
4. Treatment of gastroesophageal reflux: Reflux can be treated in four ways: dietary/lifestyle modification, acid suppression, enhancement of gastric emptying, and surgery. The first two modalities are usually used together.
   a. This includes head of bed elevation and dietary modifications (see Table 3).
   b. Acid suppression: Ranitidine (Zantac), 150 mg two to four times daily, or omeprazole (Prilosec), 20 mg once or twice daily.
   c. Promoting gastric emptying: Metoclopramide (Reglan), 10 to 15 mg before meals and at bedtime, or cisapride (Propulsid), 10 to 20 mg 15 minutes before meals and at bedtime, may be effective in selected patients.
   d. Fundoplication in those cases in which maximal medical therapy fails.
5. No throat clearing: Vocal fold irritation is often perceived as something in the throat or postnasal drip. Throat clearing leads to forceful closure of the glottis, further irritating the damaged mucosa.
6. Cough suppression: Coughing is very traumatic to the larynx, and if the cough is irritative in nature, and not infectious, it should be suppressed. Over-the-counter preparations may be used.
7. Increased humidification in bedroom: This helps to avoid drying of the laryngeal mucosa.
8. Gargling: Gargling has long been a "home remedy" for hoarseness. In general, it is of very little benefit and can be harmful. If one gargles with anything other than physiologic saline, the solution may act as a chemical irritant on the delicate mucosa of the vocal folds and epiglottis.
9. Decongestants: Nasal obstruction can lead to mouth breathing, which bypasses the humidification and filtration process the nose provides. Topical nasal sprays, such as oxymetazoline (Afrin), 2 to 3 sprays per nostril twice a day for 2 or 3 days, is a good acute-acting nasal decongestant. Beclomethasone (Beconase AQ), 2 sprays each nostril twice a day, is outstanding for long-term usage, as is fluticasone nasal spray (Flonase).
10. Coffee and alcohol: Eliminate or decrease caffeine and alcohol usage due to their diuretic effect and promotion of gastroesophageal reflux.
11. Avoid medication side effects: A number of drugs have deleterious effects on the larynx. Antihistamines result in a drying and thickening of the mucous blanket as well as decreasing the mucociliary action of the upper respiratory tract, which will affect the passive vibration of the vocal folds. In addition, tranquilizers and antidepressants often have anticholinergic side effects, also resulting in drying of the vocal folds. Aspirin and nonsteroidal anti-inflammatory drugs may increase the change of hemorrhage from dilated vessels on an erythematous vocal fold.
12. Avoid irritants: Nearly any irritant can alter mucociliary flow and thicken the mucous blanket, rendering the vocal folds more susceptible to injury. These include dust, smoke, chemical fumes, gas, paints, household cleansers, solvents, and insecticides.
13. NO SMOKING.

---

used. Biopsy of any lesions should be performed in an atraumatic fashion under microscopic visualization. Microflap surgical techniques, which preserve mucosa and avoid vocal fold damage, should be employed.

Gastroesophageal Reflux

Gastroesophageal reflux (GER) is one of the most common problems seen in otolaryngology practice. Although some patients will have the classic findings of heartburn, belching, or even peptic ulcer disease, a number of patients do not present with classic symptoms. These patients with silent reflux may complain of chronic or nocturnal cough, hoarseness in the morning, or a persistent sore throat. A foreign body sensation or the need to constantly clear one's throat is often seen. On examination, erythema or edema of the posterior glottis and the arytenoid mucosa is seen. In severe cases, ulcers or granulomas are seen. In long-standing disease, a thickened polypoid posterior glottis may be present.

GER must be considered a major cofactor for chronic laryngitis along with voice abuse. A normal mucosal surface may be able to resist a small amount of acid reflux, but even with minor damage to the mucosa, the vulnerability to acid is increased and further pathologic changes of the vocal folds may then occur. In addition to its effect on phonation, some evidence suggests that reflux may play a role in laryngeal carcinogenesis.

Smoking is both a direct mechanical and chemical irritant to the mucosa of the vocal folds. In addition, nicotine relaxes the gastroesophageal sphincter and increases gastric acid production, both of which worsen GER. Reflux treatment is summarized in Tables 2 and 3. Similar handouts may be given to patients.

Polypoid Corditis

Polypoid corditis may develop secondary to chronic laryngitis or smoking. This so-called Reinke's edema is a deposition of mucoid material in the superficial lamina propria of the vocal folds. Redundant, fluid-filled, baglike vocal folds are seen. The treatment is

TABLE 3. **Dietary and Lifestyle Modification for Reflux Treatment**

Lifestyle

Lose weight if you are overweight
Do not lie down after eating
Avoid exercise and straining after eating
Stop smoking
NPO 2 hours before bedtime
Head of bed elevated 6–12 inches
Avoid tight pants or belts

General Diet

Avoid caffeine (coffee; tea; chocolate; many carbonated beverages, particularly colas and other soft drinks with caffeine)
Eat small, frequent meals
Avoid or limit fatty and fried foods
Avoid or limit alcohol consumption, particularly in the evening
Avoid overeating

surgical with intensive voice therapy. During surgery, the mucoid material is removed by raising the vocal fold mucosa, dissecting and aspirating the material, then trimming and redraping the redundant mucosa. Voice therapy and GER treatment are critical to eliminate those factors that initially caused the problem. Failure to perform adequate speech therapy will probably result in return of the lesions.

Granuloma

Contact ulcers and vocal process granulomas are a difficult problem to manage. These are often due to trauma from endotracheal tube intubation or prolonged voice abuse. GER is also a major factor. The initial injury results in damage to the delicate mucosa over the vocal process of the arytenoid cartilage in the posterior larynx. This leads to inflammation and ischemic changes over the cartilage. Ulcers may develop, with possible perichondritis. In severe cases, chondritis itself may occur. This can induce the formation of granulation tissue, further increasing the patient's dysphonia. The patient will often complain of a sore throat or discomfort when speaking in addition to the hoarseness. Pain referred to the ipsilateral ear is not uncommon. The patient's voice changes are due to the thickened tissue, the mass effect on the vocal fold, and the interposition of the granuloma between the vocal folds preventing closure.

Treatment involves speech therapy and aggressive treatment of GER. Surgery is avoided unless the granuloma is large, refractory to medical management, or there is a suspicion of malignancy. If surgery is performed, a minimal amount of mucosa is removed. Speech therapy must follow the surgery.

Nodules

Vocal nodules also occur in adults. As is common with phonatory disorders, these are a sign of voice abuse, and not the problem itself. These nodules cause painless hoarseness. The nodules hinder vocal fold closure and vibration, resulting in breathiness, decreased pitch, and an occasional foreign body sensation. This sensation leads to coughing and repetitive throat clearing, worsening the problem. Nodules are seen at the point of maximal vibration of the vocal folds, as in children. Speech therapy, with the elimination of voice abuse, is the appropriate treatment. It is hoped that the progression of damage in the vocal fold, leading to fibrosis and scarring, can be interrupted and surgery avoided.

Polyps

Polyps, like nodules, are limited to the superficial lamina propria of the vocal fold. However, these are usually unilateral and soft and fleshy in appearance. These are believed to be the result of a single significant abusive episode, such as yelling at a sporting event. Further injury occurs as one attempts to compensate for the incomplete vocal fold closure, resulting in inflammation and enlargement of the polyp. Treatment is microsurgical excision with mucosal preservation in those cases in which speech therapy and medical management fail.

Carcinoma

Laryngeal cancer, primarily squamous cell carcinoma, is a major problem worldwide. It is usually seen in older individuals with a history of tobacco and alcohol use. Hoarseness is often the initial complaint and is constant and slowly progressive. Dysphagia or a sore throat may be the predominant complaint in patients with a cancer of the larynx located above the vocal folds. The key to treatment of laryngeal cancer is early diagnosis. One should consider cancer in any adult with hoarseness, particularly if the patient has a history of tobacco use. All smokers with hoarseness should be referred for a complete head and neck examination. Even small lesions may cause hoarseness, as they disrupt the mucosal wave of the vocal fold. Evaluation of patients with laryngeal carcinoma includes a chest x-ray and liver function tests to screen for metastatic disease. Endoscopic examination of the larynx, trachea, bronchi, and esophagus is performed to stage the cancer and search for possible synchronous lesions. With early diagnosis and treatment, squamous cell carcinoma has a high cure rate with surgery and/or radiation therapy. Small to moderate-size lesions on the vocal folds can be treated with endoscopic laser excision or conservation laryngeal surgery. Larger lesions usually require a near-total or total laryngectomy with possible postoperative radiation therapy. In some instances, laryngeal preservation can be attempted using combined radiation and chemotherapy. Major strides have been made in the last 10 years with postlaryngectomy vocal rehabilitation, in which the majority of patients have a strong functional voice following surgery.

Trauma

Laryngeal trauma may have a number of different causes. Improper or difficult intubation may cause injuries to the larynx, such as abrasions, lacerations, or a hematoma. Damage to the vocal process may lead to granuloma formation. Such problems can result in compensatory attempts at phonation that cause the individual to be hoarse long after the initial injury has healed.

Arytenoid dislocation after intubation is an uncommon problem but disastrous if not diagnosed early. Patients will usually have hoarseness with pain after extubation and should be referred for early evaluation. Patients with hoarseness lasting longer than 2 days after extubation should also be seen promptly. Dislocation results in an immobile vocal fold. Endoscopic reduction of the dislocation may result in a normal voice.

Laryngeal surgery itself may cause chronic hoarseness. The loss of large amounts of vocal fold mucosa or damage to the underlying vocal ligament may cause scarring with resultant dysphonia. Working anteriorly on both vocal folds during the same operation can result in web formation at the area of the anterior commissure. Such injuries are very difficult to remedy, even for the experienced laryngologist.

External laryngeal trauma is usually not a diagnostic problem for the physician. The patient may have tenderness over the larynx, hoarseness, airway compromise, subcutaneous emphysema, or dysphagia. Hoarseness after laryngeal trauma may be delayed. External trauma may result in minor damage, such as edema, or major problems with subcutaneous air and palpable deformities of the thyroid cartilage. These patients require otolaryngologic evaluation. Minor injuries are treated with voice rest, humidification, antireflux measures, steroids, and observation. Serious injuries may require open reduction and internal fixation of fractures with closure of mucosal lacerations and possible stenting of the larynx. It is critical to remember that endotracheal intubation could be disastrous due to the possibility of causing further damage to the laryngeal mucosa as well as possibly precipitating airway obstruction. Whenever possible, a tracheotomy under local anesthesia should be performed.

Laryngeal Paralysis

Vocal fold paralysis in adults in usually due to a nonlaryngeal malignancy in the lungs, mediastinum, thyroid, or skull base. Other causes of paralysis include thyroid surgery (iatrogenic) and central nervous system abnormalities. Approximately 20 to 30% of cases are idiopathic and are presumed to be of viral origin.

Unilateral paralysis presents with a breathy voice, poor cough, and possible aspiration. The evaluation must include a complete head and neck examination and a chest x-ray. A computed tomographic scan is obtained from the skull base to the midchest to follow the entire course of the vagus and recurrent laryngeal nerves. These patients may compensate for the immobile fold or regain function over 6 to 12 months. They may eventually achieve vocal fold closure but will often have some breathiness to their voice and decreased pitch. When it is critical to maintain the patient's voice or because of aspiration, medialization injections may be performed with fat, Gelfoam, or collagen. Medialization thyroplasty and arytenoid adduction may be performed and are the standard of care at this time.

Bilateral vocal fold paralysis is primarily due to neck surgery, usually total thyroidectomy. These patients have airway obstruction and a strained voice. The diagnosis is readily apparent upon laryngeal examination. The initial concern is to establish an airway by oral intubation followed by tracheotomy. After approximately a year, if cord mobility has not returned, an endoscopic laser arytenoidectomy or cordotomy may be performed. There is a trade-off between an adequate voice and an adequate airway. Reinnervation surgery using neuromuscular pedicles anastomosed into the lone abductor of the larynx, the posterior cricoarytenoid (PCA) muscle, have been performed. The results are not encouraging enough to justify routine usage.

Neurologic

A host of neurologic problems cause hoarseness. Cerebrovascular accidents involving the brain stem may result in unilateral vocal fold paralysis. This can be disastrous in a patient after a stroke due to decreased communication and swallowing. It may also cause aspiration. The treatment is often vocal fold injection or thyroplasty under local anesthesia. Amyotrophic lateral sclerosis often leads to progressive cranial nerve weakness. This causes a weak voice with dysarthria due to tongue fasciculations. This is progressive, resulting in eventual aphonia and aspiration. Essential laryngeal tremor is manifested by a rhythmic quivering voice. Treatment to date has been suboptimal; the use of botulinum toxin A or methazolamide (Neptazane)* has been efficacious on occasion. Myasthenia gravis is a readily treatable cause of hoarseness. Edrophonium (Tensilon), given 1 mg intravenously, is both diagnostic and therapeutic. Patients with Parkinson's disease often have a weak, monotonal, low-pitched voice. They talk slowly and have trouble initiating speech. They usually develop progressive articulation difficulties. Multiple sclerosis patients may develop a vocal tremor and scanning speech.

Spasmodic Dysphonia

Spasmodic dysphonia is a fascinating laryngeal dystonia that may be associated with other generalized and regional dystonias. Two types affect the

---

*Not FDA-approved for this indication.

larynx. In the more common, adductor dysphonia, patients have a characteristic strained, choking, or strangled voice with numerous speech breaks. This is treated by the percutaneous injection of botulinum toxin A into the patient's thyroarytenoid muscles. The less common, abductor dysphonia, results in a weak, breathy voice. This is treated with unilateral botulinum toxin injections into the PCA muscle. Botulinum toxin treatment requires repeated interval injections due to its temporary effectiveness of only 3 to 4 months.

Systemic Disease

A number of systemic diseases may affect the larynx. The most well-known is hypothyroidism that results in edematous changes to the laryngeal mucosa. This edema and thickening of the folds results in a decreased pitch of the voice. Treatment is thyroid replacement therapy.

Rheumatoid arthritis may affect the cricoarytenoid joint. This is a synovial joint that can become inflamed and limit vocal fold motion. This condition is treated with systemic steroids or, occasionally, local steroid injection. Other causes of hoarseness include pemphigus vulgaris, systemic lupus erythematosus, sarcoidosis, Wegener's granulomatosis, amyloidosis, tuberculosis, and fungal infections.

Intracordal Pathology

Disorders that usually can only be diagnosed with specialized instruments include intracordal cysts and sulcus vocalis. These may present with hoarseness and a completely normal routine laryngeal examination. The diagnosis is made by laryngovideostroboscopy. These conditions are treated using microlaryngeal surgical techniques.

Functional Dysphonia

Individuals with an altered voice due to abuse or misuse without any evidence of laryngeal disease are defined as having functional dysphonia or muscular tension dysphonia (MTD). These individuals have no organic pathology or psychiatric problems, and their hoarseness is usually due to poor vocal habits. The best example of such hoarseness is "postviral dysphonia." This is seen when an individual recovers from a routine episode of viral laryngitis but continues to have hoarseness. This is due to habitual misuse of the voice in an effort to compensate for the hoarseness originally caused by the viral infection. Speech therapy is of great benefit in re-educating the laryngeal and cervical muscles in these patients.

Psychogenic

Because the voice is a major avenue of emotional expression, it is not surprising that psychiatric disorders can lead to voice changes. The best known of these conversion disorders is hysterical aphonia. The treatment of such individuals involves a cooperative effort between the psychiatrist or psychologist and speech language professionals.

Repeated vomiting associated with bulimia may produce chronic laryngitis. This should be considered in thin adolescent women with hoarseness.

Aging Voice

Vocal changes due simply to aging—presbylarynges—are occasionally seen in patients over 60 years of age due to atrophy of the thyroarytenoid muscle. A number of elderly individuals may have voice changes as a result of diseases or conditions associated with aging, such as degenerative nervous system diseases, poor pulmonary function, or cancer, but few due to aging per se.

Presbylarynges in men is manifested by a loss of elasticity of the vocal fold, as well as thyroarytenoid muscle atrophy. This increase in stiffness and lack of bulk result in the increased pitch seen in some elderly men. Women undergo the same changes, but, in addition, at menopause women often develop submucosal edema or polypoid changes of the vocal folds. This results in the overall decrease in pitch often seen in older women. Attempts at compensation may worsen the voice. The atrophy of the thyroarytenoid muscle results in incomplete closure and sometimes bowing of the vocal folds. This causes a weak or breathy voice during attempted adduction of the folds. Treatment begins with speech therapy, particularly in patients who may lack abdominal breath support, in order to increase their volume. Injection of Gelfoam, fat, or collagen may be beneficial. Some patients have had dramatic improvement with bilateral medialization thyroplasty.

Professional Voice Users

Professional voice users are not simply opera singers and country music stars. Any individual who uses the voice as a major component of his or her job is dependent on it and is therefore considered a professional voice user. This includes teachers, football coaches, physicians, lawyers, salespersons, and people who frequently speak on the telephone. Such people may require evaluation and care by laryngologists familiar with the sophisticated management of voice problems. In the case of vocalists, performing even with "simple" laryngitis may be career-threatening.

If a performance or a speech must be given while hoarse, this individual must be seen by an otolaryngologist. The patient's vocal folds must be examined to rule out hemorrhage, varices, or a hemorrhagic polyp. Further voice use in this setting could result in tremendous damage to the folds. If no such lesions are seen and a performance must be given, the standard regimen of hydration, reflux treatment, and relative voice rest should be followed. Steroids may be given for a brief period of time. Ten milligrams of intramuscular dexamethasone acetate (Decadron-

LA) is given if the performance is 12 to 24 hours away. If the performance is within the next 2 to 4 hours, 5 mg of dexamethasone acetate and 5 mg of dexamethasone sodium phosphate are given intramuscularly. Systemic steroids will decrease the swelling but will not enhance wound healing and may allow more damage to occur.

INSOMNIA

method of
ANDREW WINOKUR, M.D., PH.D.
Center for Sleep and Respiratory Neurobiology,
University of Pennsylvania School of Medicine
Philadelphia, Pennsylvania

Insomnia is a commonly encountered clinical problem that is responsible for considerable anguish and anxiety in patients seen in a variety of medical practice settings. Insomnia is associated with and complicates a number of medical and psychiatric disorders and is responsible for a significant cost to society in terms of financial impact in lost work time and productivity and in serious injuries and fatalities related to automobile crashes and industrial accidents caused by impaired functioning secondary to sleepiness. While complaints of insomnia are common in family practice settings, the majority of patients with significant sleep problems do not report these symptoms to their physician, and recognition of clinically significant insomnia is frequently not achieved during routine office visits. This article begins with a definition of insomnia and a discussion of the public health significance of this problem. The next section reviews the clinical evaluation of insomnia, including consideration of differential diagnostic possibilities and evaluation strategies. Finally, a discussion of treatment options, both pharmacologic and nonpharmacologic, is presented.

OVERVIEW

It should be clearly noted at the outset that the term *insomnia* does not represent a specific diagnosis, but rather a description of a symptom or set of symptoms of unsatisfactory quality of sleep. Typically, complaints of insomnia relate to problems falling asleep (impaired sleep onset), problems waking up frequently during the night (impaired sleep maintenance), waking up too early in the morning (early morning awakening), or a subjective perception of unsatisfactory sleep. The subjective nature of dissatisfaction with sleep represents a significant component of the total insomnia problem. In studies comparing subjective reports by the patient of total sleep time to objective scoring of a laboratory sleep record, many instances have been observed of substantial mismatch between these parameters. Thus a patient may report having slept only an hour during the previous night, yet be recorded by polysomnographic techniques as having been asleep for 6 hours. This fairly common situation in patients with insomnia is referred to as the *sleep state misperception syndrome*. Other clinical complaints associated with poor quality sleep include reports of excessive daytime sleepiness and impaired daytime functioning. When a patient reports any of these complaints in the context of an office visit, it is important to undertake a more detailed investigation to delineate the nature of the sleep problem and to develop an appropriate differential diagnosis, implement a suitable strategy for further diagnostic evaluation, and, finally, tailor a specific treatment plan.

EPIDEMIOLOGIC ASPECTS OF INSOMNIA

A number of epidemiologic studies of insomnia have been carried out in recent years, with findings consistently indicating that approximately one-third of adults experience some difficulty with sleep during the course of the year. Strikingly, about half of these individuals (i.e., approximately 17%) describe their sleep difficulties as being prominent and persistent. Several studies carried out both in the United States and in Europe have specifically examined complaints of insomnia in patients attending general medical clinics and observed comparable or even higher incidences of insomnia than has been reported in general population surveys. Yet, as reported in a recent Gallup Poll survey involving 700 patients with insomnia, most patients with sleep difficulties do not discuss these problems with their physician, and very few patients schedule office visits specifically because of concerns about insomnia. This limited detection of the widespread problem of insomnia is particularly distressing when considered in the context of recent estimates of the cost to society of untreated insomnia. From strictly economic perspectives, the cost of insomnia has been estimated to be approximately $100 billion per year, with sleepiness-related motor vehicle accidents accounting for a cost of some $50 billion annually. Moreover, such financial estimates do not take into account the cost in terms of human suffering and lost potential in productivity of this treatable yet commonly undiagnosed medical problem.

RECOGNITION AND ASSESSMENT OF INSOMNIA

Based on the prevalence and importance of insomnia as a public health problem, it seems appropriate to propose that physicians in primary care settings routinely include specific questions about sleep in all clinical interviews. It is advisable to follow up a general inquiry about a patient's satisfaction with sleep by asking about problems falling asleep, about awakenings during the night, about feeling rested and refreshed upon arising in the morning, and about level of alertness during the day. If the patient reports problems with any or several of these symptoms, more detailed investigation regarding possible significant sleep-related problems is warranted, as discussed later. For example, it is important to define the *chronicity* of the sleep symptoms. Recent convention in the sleep field has involved classifying the duration of insomnia into categories of *transient, short-term,* and *chronic* (Table 1).

ESTABLISHING THE ETIOLOGY OF INSOMNIA

Once a significant manifestation of insomnia has been established, it is important to attempt to identify the underlying etiology rather than simply prescribing a sedative-hypnotic medication to treat the symptoms. In cases

TABLE 1. **Classification of Insomnia on the Basis of Duration of Symptoms**

Transient insomnia: up to several days
Short-term insomnia: up to 3 weeks
Chronic insomnia: greater than 3 weeks

TABLE 2. **Causes of Insomnia**

Stress
Sleep schedule
Indiscretions of sleep hygiene guidelines
Medical disorders
Medications and ingested substances
Lifestyle and circadian rhythm factors
Psychiatric disorders
Primary sleep disorders

of transient or short-term insomnia, acute situational stresses may often be identified that provide adequate explanation for the development of the sleep problem. Moreover, identification of such situational stresses often leads to the formulation of relatively straightforward strategies for effectively coping with the sleep disorder. For patients with chronic insomnia, on the other hand, precipitating stresses may not be readily identifiable, and even in cases in which an initiating stress can be identified, many subsequent physiologic and psychological factors may have intervened to maintain and even amplify the sleep difficulties.

Many factors may be associated with the initiation or perpetuation of chronic insomnia (Table 2). For example, careful assessment of the patient's daily schedule and customary patterns may shed light on the origin of the sleep problems. Violation of good sleep hygiene guidelines (as reviewed in Table 3) can lead to chronically disrupted sleep patterns. Specific examples of common sleep hygiene deficiencies include irregular sleep schedule, daytime napping, eating a heavy or spicy meal close to bedtime, and exercising vigorously late in the day. Additionally, many medical problems may be associated with sleep disruption, including thyroid disorders, gastritis or peptic ulcer disease, and any medical condition associated with chronic pain. Various drugs used to treat other medical problems may produce disrupted sleep patterns, significant examples including sympathomimetic agents, beta blockers, and selective serotonin reuptake inhibitors. It is also important to ask about consumed agents that may alter sleep patterns, including caffeine-containing substances, alcohol, and various recreational drugs. Disturbances in circadian rhythms can also underlie complaints of insomnia or nonrestorative sleep. Contemporary lifestyles include numerous situations in which circadian rhythms may be severely strained, such as shift work and jet travel across time zones. Environmental stimuli may also jeopardize well-consolidated sleep patterns. Thus, it is important to inquire about conditions in the bedroom, such as noise, excessive light, or uncomfortable ambient temperature.

An important category to consider in the differential diagnosis of insomnia is psychiatric disorders. Recalling that insomnia is a symptom, not a diagnosis, it must be emphasized that insomnia is a common symptom associated with many psychiatric disorders. In one study involv-

TABLE 3. **Sleep Hygiene Guidelines**

Maintain a regular sleep-wake schedule
Avoid naps during the day
Exercise earlier in the day, not in the evening
Avoid alcohol or caffeine consumption in the evening
Avoid heavy or spicy meals too close to bedtime
Have some time for winding down and relaxing before bedtime
Evaluate the conditions of the bedroom to optimize the
  environment for sleep

ing over 800 patients with insomnia, 40% were found to have a psychiatric disorder as well, most commonly an anxiety disorder (26%) or depression (14%). From a different perspective, patients with depression usually demonstrate insomnia as a prominent clinical feature. While *early morning awakening* has been cited as the most distinctive sleep complaint of depression, initial insomnia (prolonged sleep latency) and middle insomnia (increased number of awakenings during the night) are often observed in depression as well. Moreover, depressed patients often describe sleep as being nonrestorative. In a general practice setting, a vitally important diagnostic challenge is to identify the presence of coexisting depression in the context of insomnia, since some patients focus on their sleep complaints and deny or minimize symptoms of mood disorder per se. In such circumstances, the physician may prescribe a sedative-hypnotic drug but may not recommend appropriate treatment for the mood disorder itself. This scenario can lead to a situation in which the insomnia portion of the patient's symptoms is reduced, but effective treatment for the depressive disorder is not initiated. Since clinical depression can be associated with a substantial risk for suicide, potentially tragic consequences can ensue from a treatment approach that is not appropriately broad and well integrated.

A final category that must be considered in the evaluation of insomnia involves a range of primary sleep disorders that are commonly associated with complaints of insomnia, nonrestorative sleep, or excessive daytime sleepiness. Foremost among these primary sleep disorders are *obstructive sleep apnea syndrome* and *periodic leg movement disorder* (formerly referred to as *nocturnal myoclonus*). In the case of both of these disorders, it may be appropriate to have the patient undergo polysomnographic studies in order to confirm a diagnosis that can be suspected only on the basis of clinical history alone.

TREATMENT OF INSOMNIA

General Comments

As discussed earlier, the foundation of appropriate treatment for insomnia involves making a concerted effort to establish a specific etiologic basis for the sleep problem. In many cases, establishing a causative foundation for the insomnia can then lead to the implementation of a specific and effective treatment strategy. For example, if the sleep problem is found to represent a complication of a medical disorder such as hyperthyroidism, correction of the primary endocrinologic disorder may lead to restoration of normal sleep patterns. When insomnia represents a symptom of underlying major depressive disorder, appropriate antidepressant therapy may lead to improved sleep consolidation in conjunction with elevated mood state. To provide another example, insomnia occurring as a result of sleep hygiene violations or circadian rhythm disruptions (e.g., shift work, jet lag, etc.) may respond readily to behavioral modification interventions to remedy these specific circumstances.

It must also be acknowledged that no specific causative factor may be identified in a substantial number of patients with insomnia (perhaps in 50% of cases). In such cases, it is necessary to undertake a treatment plan for a problem that may be viewed as

TABLE 4. **Nonpharmacological Treatments for Insomnia**

Sleep hygiene guidelines	Cognitive therapy
Stimulus control	Sleep restriction therapy
Relaxation techniques	Psychotherapy

idiopathic insomnia, both to provide some symptomatic relief to the individual suffering with this condition and to break a potentially escalating cycle of sleep disturbance. In general, treatment approaches for idiopathic insomnia are grouped under categories of nonpharmacologic therapy techniques and medication approaches, as discussed in the following sections.

Nonpharmacologic Therapy Techniques for Insomnia

A variety of therapy approaches have been proposed for relief of insomnia (Table 4). While some of these approaches are probably most appropriately implemented by a specialist in the field of sleep disorders medicine, aspects of several of these techniques can readily be utilized in a family practice setting.

Sleep Hygiene Guidelines. Reviewing with a patient some of the basic elements of proper sleep hygiene can often help to elicit some behavioral changes that may favorably effect sleep patterns. Discussion of sleep hygiene practices can often be carried out in the context of asking a patient with complaints of insomnia to keep a detailed sleep diary for a limited period of time (e.g., 2 weeks) and then reviewing the information in the diary with the patient. A patient may not be aware of or may have a blind spot about certain behavioral patterns (e.g., irregular bedtime schedule, excess caffeine consumption) that may lead to significant sleep disruption. It often makes sense to attack a complicated sleep disorder by focusing initially on discrete and readily correctable components of the problem.

Stimulus Control. This approach involves some straightforward behavior modification strategies designed both to help reduce the likelihood of experiencing insomnia and to provide the patient with some easily implemented coping methods to help reduce the severity and frustration of episodes of insomnia. Basic elements of the stimulus control method are listed in Table 5. These techniques can

TABLE 5. **Stimulus Control**

Go to bed only when sleepy
Get out of bed and go to a different room and engage in a quiet relaxing activity if unable to fall asleep within a reasonable time interval (e.g., 20 minutes)
Do not watch television in the bedroom
Get up at a consistent time each morning
Do not nap during the day
Use the bed only for sleep and sexual relations

From Bootzin RR, Perlis MD: J Clin Psychiatry 53(6, Suppl):37–41, 1992. Copyright 1992, Physicians Postgraduate Press. Reprinted by permission.

effectively be integrated with practical advice about sleep hygiene practices and may be quite useful for some patients. However, for patients with more severe degrees of insomnia, the contributions of sleep hygiene, behavior modification, and stimulus control techniques may be useful components but, by themselves, not sufficiently effective therapeutic modalities.

Relaxation Techniques. A variety of methods, including biofeedback techniques, meditation, and deep muscle relaxation techniques, contain elements in common of attempting to foster the individual's ability to maintain and enhance a sense of relaxation in the face of potentially increased arousal levels. While some patients may benefit from working formally with a therapist trained in relaxation techniques, many patients may be able to benefit from a largely self-directed course of relaxation therapy carried out under the general supervision of the primary physician. A variety of self-help materials (i.e., books and tapes) are available to guide an individual in the use of relaxation techniques. While relaxation techniques are generally not effective in directly inducing sleep in patients with insomnia, these techniques can be quite helpful in allowing the patient to obtain a sense of mastery in inducing a state of heightened relaxation.

Cognitive Therapy. Cognitive therapy was originally developed for application in the treatment of depression, and this modality has been widely accepted as an effective intervention for this indication. In recent years, cognitive therapy techniques have been utilized with good results in the treatment of other disorders as well, most notably for various anxiety disorders. The elements of cognitive therapy involve first helping the patient to identify the negatively skewed thought patterns (i.e., cognitions) that typically accompany depression, such as thoughts of helplessness, hopelessness, and low self-esteem. It is believed that the ongoing flood of such negative cognition actually becomes an important component in sustaining and exacerbating the depressive phase. Once the patient has become adept at recognizing the negative cognitions, the next stage in the application of cognitive therapy involves teaching the patient strategies to counter these cognitions, thus neutralizing their pervasive impact.

The use of at least a modified form of cognitive therapy is helpful for virtually all patients suffering with significant insomnia. Most patients with insomnia have some exaggerated and negative cognitions about the meaning of their sleep problem in terms of dire health consequences, the potential for developing even more severe problems (e.g., "I might go crazy"), or other catastrophizing thoughts. Teaching a patient with insomnia to recognize and balance out these distressing negative cognitions often represents a critical step in undoing the potentially vicious cycle of insomnia. Frequently, elements of cognitive therapy will be integrated with one or more of the other intervention strategies reviewed in this article. In some cases, referral for a specific, concentrated course of cognitive therapy (often lasting 10 to 12 sessions) is appropriate.

Sleep Restriction Therapy. This is a recently developed technique for insomnia that is quite demanding but that may be highly effective for some patients. In the application of sleep restriction therapy, the patient and therapist agree upon an initial period of time, set to be deliberately short, that the patient will spend in bed. For example, the starting schedule may require the patient to go to bed at 1:00 A.M. and to get up at 6:00 A.M., allowing a maximum of 5 hours of sleep. Through the rest of the day, the patient is expected to be up and active, with no napping allowed. This expectation is maintained regardless of how much sleep the patient actually obtains in the 1:00 A.M. to 6:00 A.M. period. The efficacy of sleep restriction therapy rests upon the well-established physiologic need for sleep and the recognition that exposure to sleep deprivation strikingly increases the need for sleep (increases *sleep pressure*). In the context of a sleep restriction therapy paradigm, many of the psychological barriers that typically prevent sleep from occurring in a tired individual with insomnia are removed. Once the individual has developed solid sleep patterns (e.g., sleeping at least 90% of the time) on the initial sleep schedule, the allowed sleep interval is gradually increased. While this treatment approach requires a high degree of patient compliance and persistence and can be rather stressful, it has been found to be quite effective in many individuals with otherwise treatment-refractory insomnia.

Psychotherapy. For some individuals, insomnia occurs in the context of significant psychosocial stressors or personality problems. In such cases, referral for psychotherapy may represent a critical component of the overall treatment strategy. It is quite evident that failing to identify and deal with underlying stresses and psychological problems is likely to make the patient susceptible to repeated patterns of sleep difficulties.

Pharmacologic Treatment Option for Insomnia. A number of classes of pharmacologic agents have been utilized in the treatment of insomnia, including barbiturates, antipsychotic agents, antihistaminic compounds, chloral hydrate, and the sedating antidepressants (e.g., amitriptyline [Elavil], doxepin [Sinequan], trazodone [Desyrel]). However, many of these drugs have not been demonstrated to have efficacy in the treatment of insomnia, are associated with unacceptable side effects, or both. In recent years, much publicity has been directed at the use of melatonin to treat insomnia and some circadian rhythm disorders. Few studies to date have characterized the efficacy of melatonin in the treatment of insomnia, and this compound has not yet been approved for this indication by the FDA. Moreover, the use of at least higher doses of melatonin could be associated with some significant side effect problems, such as suppression of the gonadotropic axis. There

does appear to be interesting potential for melatonin or melatonin analogues in the treatment of insomnia or circadian rhythm disorders.

To date, the most widely employed pharmacologic treatments for insomnia have included several of the benzodiazepine compounds and the imidazopyridines. Five benzodiazepines have been evaluated specifically for the treatment of insomnia (triazolam [Halcion], temazepam [Restoril], quazepam [Doral], estazolam [ProSom] and flurazepam [Dalmane]). These drugs differ primarily on the basis of half-life (e.g., triazolam is very short acting, while flurazepam has a markedly long duration of action) and presence or absence of active metabolites. Familiarity with information about such pharmacokinetic properties of the various benzodiazepine sedative-hypnotics may help the physician select one of these options that best suits the needs of a particular patient. To date, only one compound is available in the imidazopyridine category: the short half-life drug zolpidem (Ambien). All of these sedative-hypnotic compounds have been demonstrated to be effective in the treatment of insomnia, both by reducing sleep latency (time to fall asleep) and improving sleep continuity (reduction in nocturnal awakenings).

In general, the sedative-hypnotic compounds cited previously all have a relatively benign side effect profile, with the most commonly reported side effects being daytime sedation and ataxia. Caution should be given to the combined use of alcohol and a benzodiazepine sedative-hypnotic drug. Additionally, since the benzodiazepines have the potential to suppress respiration, these compounds should be avoided in patients with obstructive sleep apnea. In recent years, long-term use of benzodiazepine compounds has been reported to be associated with problems with dependence and withdrawal. Thus, it is preferable to limit the duration of treatment with the benzodiazepines. Some suggestions have appeared that zolpidem has lower abuse liability, but further studies are needed to evaluate this possibility.

Conventional guidelines suggest that sedative-hypnotic therapy should be limited to a duration of 4 weeks. It should be noted, however, that some patients with chronic, severe insomnia expect and may require treatment over a considerably longer period of time. In such cases, the physician must make a considered judgment about the advisability of recommending long-term sedative-hypnotic therapy. In a patient who is being treated with a benzodiazepine sedative-hypnotic drug for a prolonged period, care must be taken to avoid abrupt discontinuation of the drug regimen.

In summary, the hallmark of effective treatment for insomnia is the identification of symptoms of a sleep problem, careful evaluation of factors underlying the insomnia, development of a specific diagnosis, and then implementation of a treatment program that may involve integration of pharmacologic and other treatment modalities.

PRURITUS
(Itching)

method of
MICHAEL J. SISACK, M.D., and
BARBARA BRAUNSTEIN WILSON, M.D.
University of Virginia Health Sciences Center
Charlottesville, Virginia

Pruritus, or itching, can be defined as the sensation that provokes the desire to scratch. It can be an extremely frustrating, almost maddening problem for the patient and physician alike. What makes pruritus and scratching as a behavior so difficult to treat is that scratching itchy skin is often inherently pleasurable. Chronic scratching often leads to skin changes that initiate a vicious itch/scratch cycle that is very hard to break. The neurophysiology of pruritus is incompletely understood. Although the sensations of itch and pain are both transmitted via unmyelinated C fibers, itch is best considered a primary sensory modality rather than subthreshold pain. The complex neurochemistry that peripherally mediates itch includes histamine as well as opioid peptides, leukotrienes, prostaglandins, serotonin, and vasoactive and neuroactive peptides. Ineffective treatment of pruritus can lead to substantial morbidity. Excoriated skin is prone to secondary infection and bleeding, and the chronic trauma leads to lichenification and prurigo nodule formation. Irritability, fatigue, and loss of sleep are also frequently experienced.

DIAGNOSIS

When treating the symptom of pruritus, it is important to make as accurate a diagnosis as possible. As with most conditions, the key to solving the problem lies in the directed history and physical. Although personal stress can accentuate a person's perception of itching, stress should not be diagnosed as the primary cause of pruritus. In broad terms, pruritus can be caused by primary dermatologic conditions (Table 1) and underlying systemic disease (Table 2). Many medications can cause pruritus with a drug-induced rash. Opiates, CNS stimulants, and gold compounds are some examples of medications that can cause pruritus with no obvious cutaneous manifestations. Duration and characteristics of the itch, along with initiating, exacerbating, and relieving factors, are often important clues to glean from an interview. Nocturnal worsening of pruritus is described with scabies infestation but is also seen in many other conditions and probably relates more to the relative lack of other competing stimuli at that time. Two common primary dermatologic conditions that may be

TABLE 1. Selected Dermatologic Conditions Associated with Pruritus

Allergic/irritant contact dermatitis
Eczematous dermatitis
Psoriasis
Xerosis
Insect bites
Mycosis fungoides
Bullous pemphigoid
Scabies
Urticaria
Dermatographism
Dermatitis herpetiformis

TABLE 2. Selected Systemic Conditions Associated with Pruritus

Lymphoma and other internal malignancy
Polycythemia vera
Chronic renal failure
Hepatobiliary disease
Hyper- or hypothyroidism
HIV infection
Pregnancy

subtle and easily overlooked as a cause for pruritus are xerosis (dry skin), especially in the elderly, and dermatographism. If no dermatologic condition is present to explain persistent pruritus, a work-up for underlying systemic disease should be performed. In addition to a thorough history and physical examination, studies that may be helpful include CBC with differential, sedimentation rate, routine chemistries including renal and liver function, thyroid function tests, serum protein electrophoresis, and a chest x-ray. A skin biopsy is rarely helpful when performed on normal-appearing skin.

TREATMENT

Topical Therapy

Primary dermatologic conditions, when present, should be appropriately treated, and steroid-responsive dermatoses should be treated with appropriate strength topical steroids. Topical therapy of pruritus is often effective and avoids the potential side effects of systemic therapy. It is hard to overestimate the role of skin moisturization because dry skin frequently initiates pruritus or exacerbates other itchy conditions such as eczema or psoriasis. The authors recommend limiting the use of harsh soaps and substituting mild cleansing bars or lotions like fragrance-free Dove, Purpose, Basis, or Cetaphil. Double-rinsing clothes in the washing machine can be helpful as well. The authors advocate soaking in a tub of lukewarm water containing approximately 30 mL of fragrance-free bath oil once or twice daily. Patients should be cautioned about getting into and out of slippery tubs. Alternatively, bath oil can be manually applied to the skin following a shower or sponge bath. Soaking must be followed immediately by the generous application of a moisture-sealing ointment or cream like Eucerin, Aquaphor, or petroleum jelly. An over-the-counter product containing menthol like Sarna is often soothing and can be used ad lib. Asking a pharmacist to add ¼% menthol to a standard ointment or cream vehicle is similarly helpful. Compounds containing pramoxine, a topical anesthetic (Prax, PrameGel, Pramosone), are sometimes effective as well. The use of the topical antihistamine diphenhydramine (Benadryl) and topical anesthetic benzocaine is generally discouraged because of a significant incidence of allergic contact sensitization. A useful newer antipruritic agent, topical doxepin (Zonalon), has potent antihistamine qualities. It is applied up to four times per day to affected skin. It is indicated for short-term use and is limited somewhat by its cost and its potential to cause significant sedation when used over extensive areas. Another frustrating problem, pruritus ani, can often be improved with gentle meticulous cleansing after bowel movements, followed by the application of zinc oxide ointment. If pruritus persists, application of 3% clioquinol (Vioform)/1% hydrocortisone cream mixture may be helpful.

Systemic Therapy

Once again, accurate diagnosis is paramount. The use of systemic steroids without a clear indication rarely justifies the long-term risk. Oral antihistamines are the mainstay of symptomatic therapy for pruritus. The H_1 histamine antagonist hydroxyzine (Atarax) is frequently beneficial. The usual dose is 10 to 25 mg up to four times daily but can be titrated higher based on response and degree of sedation. Other H_1 blockers, including diphenhydramine (Benadryl), 25 to 50 mg every 6 hours, and cyproheptadine (Periactin), 4 mg every 8 hours, can also be tried. The tricyclic antidepressant doxepin (Sinequan) has potent H_1 and H_2 histamine antagonist qualities and can be very effective for itching. Doses of 10 to 25 mg every 8 hours or in one nighttime dose can be effective but again can be carefully titrated upward as side effects allow. Doses above 100 mg a day may require periodic ECGs to look for QT interval prolongation. Use of antihistamines in the elderly should be done cautiously to avoid potentially dangerous side effects such as mental status changes and urinary retention. Nonsedating antihistamines including terfenadine (Seldane, 60 mg every 12 hours), astemizole (Hismanal, 10 mg once daily), and loratadine (Claritin, 10 mg once daily) may be effective for chronic urticaria and other pruritic conditions, especially when sedation is not desired. H_2 blockers have been used for urticaria, but in the authors' experience, they add little to the previously described therapies. Itching caused by underlying malignancy is recalcitrant to therapy but usually resolves following successful treatment of the cancer. Recurrent itching may herald recurrent disease. Oral cholestyramine (Questran),* 4 grams twice daily, can be tried for pruritus related to hepatobiliary disease. Decompression of the biliary system via percutaneous drainage or stent placement can have great palliative value when malignancy is involved. Ultraviolet B phototherapy has demonstrated effectiveness in treatment of pruritus associated with many dermatologic conditions, chronic renal insufficiency, hyperbilirubinemia, and HIV disease. As with all complex or recalcitrant cases of pruritus, consultation with a dermatologist regarding use of ultraviolet therapy should be considered.

---

*Not FDA-approved for this indication.

TINNITUS

method of
ROBERT P. GREEN, M.D.
Mount Sinai School of Medicine
New York, New York

Tinnitus is an abnormal perception of sound that is localized within the head or ears. Tinnitus can range from a minor annoyance to a disabling symptom complex. Often patients are fearful of the presence of a brain tumor, and this, in fact, may not be unfounded. It is estimated that over 12 million Americans suffer from severe tinnitus that is disabling in quality. Some degree of tinnitus is common in many millions more.

Two general types of tinnitus may be defined.

1. *Objective tinnitus* may be heard by an observer, often with a stethoscope, as well as by the patient. The cause is often vascular or neuromuscular. Vascular lesions such as glomus tumors, arteriovenous malformations, and turbulent venous or arterial flow must be considered and appropriate radiographic and vascular studies performed. Besides computed tomography (CT) scanning with contrast, magnetic resonance angiography (MRA) can be very helpful in defining vascular lesions that may be a source of objective tinnitus. Traditional angiography may be appropriate when a vascular lesion appears to be present. Myoclonic contractions of the palate, stapedius, or tensor tympani muscles may also present as objective tinnitus but are easily distinguished by the lack of correlation to the arterial pulse. Therapy is often successful and is generally surgical and directed at eliminating the offending lesion.

2. *Subjective tinnitus* (that heard only by the patient) is unfortunately far more common and less amenable to treatment. Establishing the cause, however, is paramount in providing reassurance and, at times, therapeutic intervention. Conductive hearing deficits will often be associated with tinnitus. The correction of these problems, thus improving hearing, will often mask out an underlying tinnitus, making it imperceptible. Therefore, correction of a cerumen impaction, drainage of a middle ear effusion, or performance of a stapedectomy in an otosclerotic patient will often provide dramatic relief.

The most difficult cases, however, are those associated with inner ear hearing loss or no identifiable hearing loss at all. Benign, age-related hearing loss, ototoxicity, noise-induced hearing loss, and Meniere's disease must be distinguished from cerebellopontine angle tumors.

In addition to obtaining routine audiometry, it cannot be emphasized too strongly that a detailed neuro-otologic work-up is essential, including a CT scan or magnetic resonance imaging (MRI) to rule out a cerebellopontine angle tumor. At present, auditory brain stem response represents an accurate and useful screening examination, particularly if routine audiometry reveals asymmetrical hearing loss or retrocochlear signs. There should, however, be no hesitation to obtain an MRI scan with the infusion of intravenous gadolinium, as this is highly accurate in detecting even small acoustic neuromas or related lesions. A detailed blood work-up should include at least a Venereal Disease Research Laboratory-fluorescent treponemal antibody (VDRL-FTA) and serologic tests to help identify those patients with neurosyphilis or autoimmune sensorineural hearing loss, both of which can be helped with conventional medical therapy. Lyme titers, thyroid function tests, and serum glucose complete an appropriate evaluation.

TREATMENT

Most often, the tinnitus patient has an identifiable sensorineural hearing loss caused by age, noise, or ototoxicity. Tinnitus can often be relieved by amplifying environmental sounds to mask out the perception of tinnitus. A hearing aid during the day may be effective in this regard, and the use of an FM radio tuned between stations may help patients fall asleep. Mixed success has been obtained using the tinnitus masker. This device, worn like a hearing aid, provides a band of noise that masks out the tinnitus without interfering with the speech frequencies. Biofeedback has proved to be a useful technique by shifting body awareness away from the tinnitus.

It is becoming increasingly clear that certain forms of tinnitus represent spontaneous neural activity probably originating at the brain stem level. With this in mind, limited success has been obtained using a variety of centrally acting medications, including anticonvulsants, antidepressants, and anxiety-reducing agents. There is unquestionably a strong association of depression with severity of tinnitus. At times, therefore, the help of a psychiatrist may be in order.

Pharmacotherapy at present consists of conventional trial doses of phenobarbital,* carbamazepine (Tegretol),* amitriptyline (Elavil),* or benzodiazepines such as alprazolam (Xanax).* Carbamazepine may be given as a starting dose of 100 mg at night to a maximum of 200 mg three times a day, increasing by 100 mg each week. Complete blood counts as well as renal and hepatic function must be monitored. Alprazolam may be given as 0.5 mg at night, increasing to 0.5 mg three times a day in gradual increments.

The converse of administering centrally acting medications is the elimination of medications that may be likely causes of tinnitus. Included for consideration would be salicylates, quinine, psychoactive drugs, and any other medication whose initiation coincides with the onset of tinnitus.

When all is said and done, many patients respond to simple reassurance following a thorough investigation to rule out a serious problem. A referral to the American Tinnitus Association (503-248-9985) can provide additional support via newsletters and up-to-date literature.

---

*Not FDA-approved for this indication.

LOW BACK PAIN

method of
GEOFFREY M. McCULLEN, M.D.
University of California, San Diego
Naval Medical Center, San Diego, California

and

HANSEN A. YUAN, M.D.
State University of New York
Syracuse, New York

Acute low back pain is an expected and even "normal" part of life. It is the fifth most common reason for visits to physicians. Only rarely will the pain last longer than 2 weeks. One to 2 percent of patients will have a "radicular" component with pain traveling down the lower extremity following a specific nerve root distribution (e.g., "sciatica").

Currently, there are approximately 2.6 million Americans considered "disabled" from chronic low back pain. The combined direct and indirect costs of this condition are staggering: $50 billion each year. Seventy-five percent of these costs are consumed by only 5% of those with back pain. Psychosocial factors are believed to play a significant role in chronic disability. Those with poor health habits, job dissatisfaction, and a compensatory injury have the worst prognosis. By classifying and treating chronic low back pain within the medical paradigm, physicians may have unwittingly assisted in creating a dependent environment with "epidemic" proportions of disability.

STRUCTURE AND FUNCTION

The spine serves two distinct roles. It provides the body's mobile, central axis and protects the neural tissues. The proper blending of flexibility and stability is required to simultaneously fulfill these functions. This is accomplished by a linked structure containing 24 mobile vertebral bones connected by 75 stable articulations that control motion. Adjacent vertebrae meet at three articulations known as the "triple joint complex," a tripod-shaped array with the discovertebral joint anteriorly and paired facet joints posteriorly. The intervertebral disk is a composite structure with the nucleus pulposus core surrounded by the multilayered fibers of the anulus fibrosus.

Most of the structures of the spine are innervated (A delta and C fibers), with the exception of the nucleus and the inner layers of the anulus. The outer layers of the anulus are richly supplied by branches of the sinuvertebral nerve, which arborize to supply several contiguous levels. Stimulation of a specific nerve results in generalized low back pain that is not well localized.

THE DEGENERATIVE CASCADE

The intervertebral disc nucleus is 80% water in youth and desiccates with age. The lower lumbar segments face loads of up to four times body weight, especially with sitting, forward bending, and lifting. Under these stresses, by 30 to 40 years of age, fissures may develop within the retaining anulus, allowing the nucleus to migrate from the center of the disk to the periphery, thereby stimulating the sinuvertebral nerve and causing diffuse low back pain.

A "herniated disk" occurs when the nucleus transgresses all of the retaining layers of the anulus. The nuclear material may mechanically compress or chemically irritate the adjacent nerve root, creating radicular symptoms: leg pain, tingling, numbness, or weakness.

After 3 years of age, there is no blood supply directly to the center of the disk. Nutrients must pass by diffusion after release from capillaries in the vertebral end-plates. Thus, healing capacity of the disk is poor.

A disk without a competent nucleus is unable to function properly. The loss of disk height means less space for the exiting nerve root within the neuroforamen. The facets, which normally experience only 16% of the compressive load, must take on an increased proportion, resulting in facet joint arthropathy. Increased motion between vertebrae is allowed. The end-plates become sclerotic and less porous, thereby restricting the transfer of water and nutrients. Products of metabolism accumulate, creating an acidic environment. The local formation of immunoglobulins and prostaglandins is among the chemical factors that can produce back pain.

To maintain mechanical stability with aging, the components of the spine, including ligament, bone, and facet joint, thicken and hypertrophy. The result is "spinal stenosis," a narrowing of the room available for the neural elements. "Neurogenic claudication" may occur in elderly patients with stenosis and mimic the symptoms of vascular claudication. The lower extremities "ache," "burn," or "fatigue" with walking. Symptoms are relieved by assuming a forward, flexed posture at the waist, which increases spinal canal dimensions.

DIFFERENTIAL DIAGNOSIS

The diffuse, nonspecific nature of low back pain creates a diagnostic challenge for the clinician. Up to 85% of patients with back pain will never be given a definitive diagnosis. It is, however, critical to consider a broad differential: developmental, infectious, inflammatory, metabolic, neoplastic, degenerative, and referred mechanisms of pain (Table 1).

Most episodes of acute low back pain will arise from "overuse" and are usually the consequence of the degenerative process. In a primary care setting, evaluation of those with low back pain will reveal approximately 4% compression fractures, 0.7% spinal neoplasms, 0.3% ankylosing spondylitis, and 0.01% spinal infections. A systematic search for each of the "red flags" in the history and physical examination is essential to avoid missing these rare etiologies, which are best served by early diagnosis and treatment (Table 2).

TABLE 1. **Differential Diagnosis of Low Back Pain**

Developmental

Stenosis

Infectious

Diskitis
Vertebral osteomyelitis

Inflammatory

Seronegative spondyloarthropathies
Polymyalgia rheumatica

Traumatic

Osteoporotic compression fracture

Metabolic

Osteomalacia
Hyperparathyroidism
Iatrogenic (steroid use)

Neoplastic

Primary
Metastatic

Degenerative

Herniated disk
Degenerative disk disease
Facet arthropathy
Spinal stenosis
Spondylolisthesis

Referred

Vasculogenic
    Aortic aneurysm, ischemia
Viscerogenic
    GI, GU, pancreas
Hip osteoarthritis

Unknown

Musculoligamentous overuse
Psychosocial factors

TABLE 2. **The "Red Flags" of Low Back Pain**

Age <15 or >50 years
Known malignancy
Known propensity for infection
Severe, unrelenting pain
Worsening despite rest
Increased pain at night and with recumbency
Fevers, chills
Constitutional symptoms
Weight loss
Sustained early morning stiffness
Neurologic abnormalities

PHYSICAL EXAMINATION

Examination begins with a review of the vital signs. Hypertension may draw attention to a vascular etiology. An elevated temperature suggests infection. However, not all patients with vertebral osteomyelitis will have fever or other constitutional signs.

The spine is assessed in a standing position for malalignment and paraspinal mass, swelling, erythema, warmth, or spasm. The sacroiliac joint and sciatic notch are evaluated for localized tenderness. Limitations of lumbar motion are noted.

A head-to-toe examination is warranted on any patient presenting with a "red flag" finding. A thorough abdominal examination may detect the source of referred pain. Forty percent of those with vertebral osteomyelitis will have an identifiable extraspinal source of infection. The most common locations for primary infection include the genitourinary tract, skin, and respiratory tract, and with intravenous drug abuse. The seven most common primary sites for spinal metastasis are breast (31%), lung (21%), prostate (20%), kidney (7%), colon (5%), bladder (3%), and head and neck (2%). Primary tumors of the spine are rare.

Compromise of neurologic structures seen in those with radicular symptoms can be detected by a detailed evaluation of motor, reflex, and sensory functions in the lower extremities. A tethered root lacks the normal excursion that occurs with extremity motion. Tension signs (straight leg raising and femoral stretch test) elicit radicular pain. Bowel and bladder findings with decreased rectal tone and diminished perianal sensation and an elevated postvoid residual (>50 mL) indicate a surgical emergency ("cauda equina syndrome").

Nonorganic (Waddell) signs may assist in identifying psychologic distress. These include superficial tenderness, pain with simulated loading and axial rotation, inconsistent straight leg raising (sitting vs. supine), nonanatomic distribution of sensory and motor findings, and over-reaction.

LABORATORY STUDIES

A complete blood count and erythrocyte sedimentation rate assist in distinguishing those cases due to infection or inflammation. A normal white cell count does not exclude osteomyelitis. A screening chemistry profile (electrolytes, blood urea nitrogen, creatinine, calcium, phosphorus, and alkaline phosphatase) will detect metabolic anomalies. Serum protein electrophoresis (SPEP) identifies multiple myeloma. HLA typing is occasionally helpful, as 90% of those with ankylosing spondylitis will be HLA-B27 positive.

RADIOLOGIC STUDIES

Plain radiographs are performed after traumatic events in the presence of any "red flags" and with pain lasting more than 6 to 8 weeks. At minimum, orthogonal views of the lumbar spine (anteroposterior [AP] and lateral) should be obtained. An AP view of the pelvis is added to evaluate the sacroiliac joint in the spondyloarthropathies. The hip joint is evaluated in cases of anterior thigh and groin pain, possibly referable to hip pathology.

A systematic inspection of the radiograph includes evaluation of soft tissue shadows, bone quality, and alignment. The findings of osteophytes, lumbarization or sacralization, disk space narrowing, and spina bifida occulta are nonspecific and occur with the same frequency whether symptoms are present or absent.

Spondylolysis, a lucency across the pars interarticularis (usually L5), is best visualized on 45-degree oblique radiographs. This finding occurs in approximately 5 to 7% of the population and is very rarely symptomatic. Those undergoing hyperextension activities (gymnastics, football linemen) appear to be predisposed.

A spondylolisthesis, the forward slide of one vertebra on its adjacent vertebra, occurs in 2 to 3%. In adolescence, this is most typically due to a spondylolysis and affects the L5–S1 level ("isthmic spondylolisthesis"). Elderly females preferentially develop degenerative spondylolisthesis at the L4–L5 level as a result of degenerative change. Low-grade "slips" (<25% translation) are most frequently asymptomatic and nonprogressive. Greater than 50% translation is associated with an increased frequency of pain and neurologic findings.

In osteoporosis, plain radiographs demonstrate relative accentuation of the vertical trabeculae with loss of horizontal trabeculae. Disk expansion into weakened endplates leads to the appearance of "codfish" vertebrae.

To be detected on plain radiographs, tumors or loci of infection require destruction of approximately 50% of the vertebra. Thus, relying solely on plain radiographs to confirm such diagnoses will lead to a critical delay in recognition. A compression fracture without a history of trauma suggests an underlying pathologic process (osteoporosis, metabolic bone disease, infection, or tumor).

If plain radiographs are normal and there is a clinical suspicion of tumor or infection, a bone scan is obtained to detect any areas of increased osteoblastic activity. Sites of multiple myeloma are frequently "cold" and are missed on bone scan. A vertebra with increased radionucleotide uptake should be further evaluated with either computed tomography (CT) (CT-directed biopsy and culture) or magnetic resonance imaging (MRI). Bone detail is best assessed with the CT scan. MRI emphasizes the soft tissues including disk and neural elements.

MRI has emerged as the most sensitive and specific diagnostic modality for spinal disorders. It is attractive because it is noninvasive, avoids radiation exposure, and has no known side effects. Despite this, physicians should engage in selective use and interpretation of this device. Altered morphology on the MRI does not always correlate with the clinical signs and symptoms. One third of asymptomatic subjects have been found to have an MRI abnormality (herniated disk, stenosis).

MRI is capable of demonstrating changes within the nucleus pulposus with loss of signal on T2 images indicating a disk desiccation. Focal, angular extension of the disk beyond the vertebral margin indicates a disk protrusion. Osteophytes are poorly visualized.

Gadolinium-DTPA may be injected intravenously to serve as a contrast agent, localizing within well-vascularized granulation tissue. This enables the distinction between scar and a recurrent disk herniation and is effective in differentiating benign from malignant compression fractures.

THERAPEUTICS

Prevention of injury is the best means of limiting the degenerative cascade and avoiding disability. "Back schools" have evolved to provide the necessary instruction to modify the work environment and encourage ongoing fitness, smoking cessation, and weight loss.

Most acute back pain is treated successfully with a short course of activity modification. Bed rest should be limited to less than 2 days, as rapid cardiovascular deconditioning occurs. Bracing with a lumbar corset to assist in "unloading" the spine should also be temporary, to prevent disuse muscle atrophy. Activities requiring repetitive bending, twisting, lifting greater than 10 pounds, and prolonged sitting should be avoided for approximately 6 weeks.

With the physician's encouragement, the patient should be made an active participant in a treatment program. Passive modalities such as traction, acupuncture, trigger point injections, heat, ultrasound, and transcutaneous electrical nerve stimulation (TENS) units, when used in isolation, are of limited and unproven benefit. Active programs, including either McKenzie's extension or Williams' flexion exercises, should be individually tailored and monitored by a well-trained physical therapist. Muscle relaxants and narcotics are best avoided or, if used, limited to 7 to 10 days' duration. Epidural steroids occasionally provide long-standing relief of radicular pain arising from a herniated disk or mild stenosis.

Surgical methods for lumbar conditions include decompression (relieving pressure on the neural elements), fusion for spinal instability and deformity, and both decompression and fusion. Elective surgical intervention is considered after nonoperative methods have failed.

Section 2

The Infectious Diseases

ACQUIRED IMMUNE DEFICIENCY SYNDROME (AIDS)

method of
PETER SO, M.D., and
LIVETTE JOHNSON, M.D.
Metropolitan Hospital Center
New York, New York

Acquired immune deficiency syndrome (AIDS) was first recognized in the summer of 1981, when unusual clusters of *Pneumocystis carinii* pneumonia and Kaposi's sarcoma were reported in young, previously healthy homosexual men in Los Angeles and New York. In 1983, the human immunodeficiency virus (HIV) was isolated from persons with AIDS with chronic lymphadenopathy, and in 1984, this retrovirus of the lentivirus family was clearly demonstrated to be the causative agent of AIDS. A serologic test was developed in 1985 to detect HIV infection. Since that time, clinicians and researchers have become very familiar with the pathogens, syndromes, and neoplasias that accompany infections with the virus that causes AIDS.

DEFINITION

The Centers for Disease Control and Prevention (CDC) surveillance case definition for AIDS was established originally for surveillance purposes, where the presence of opportunistic infections and neoplasms in the absence of known causes of underlying immune defects was indicative of severe HIV-related immune suppression and disease. Upon the availability of a sensitive and specific diagnostic test for HIV, the case definition of AIDS has undergone several revisions. The 1993 surveillance case definition is shown in Table 1.

ETIOLOGY AND PATHOPHYSIOLOGY

The etiologic agent of AIDS is HIV, an RNA virus that belongs to the family of human retroviruses and the subfamily of lentiviruses. It is closely related to two other human retroviruses, the human T cell lymphotropic viruses, HTLV I and HTLV II. HIV is primarily a cytopathic virus, whereas the HTLV I and HTLV II viruses are notable for their ability to transform infected cells. The most common cause of HIV disease in the United States and throughout the world is HIV-1. HIV-2 was first identified in 1986 in West Africa. A number of cases of HIV-2 have been reported in Europe, South America, Canada, and the United States; however, the virus continues to be found mostly among heterosexual persons in West Africa. HIV-2 can result in severe immune suppression and development of serious opportunistic diseases that are indistinguishable from those caused by HIV-1. Modes of transmission of HIV-1 and HIV-2 are similar, although HIV-2 is not as readily transmitted from mother to infant. Preliminary observations indicate that the incubation period from the time of initial infection to the development of AIDS may be longer for HIV-2.

The critical step in infection with HIV is the binding of the viral envelope protein gp 120 to the cellular CD4 receptor molecule, found predominantly on a subset of T lymphocytes responsible for helper or inducer function in the immune response. This binding is both specific and highly efficient. The receptor molecule is also expressed on the surface of the monocyte/macrophage (M/M) lineage. Following binding and fusion with the host cell membrane, the HIV genomic RNA is uncoated and internalized. The reverse transcriptase enzyme catalyzes the reverse transcription of the genomic RNA into double-stranded DNA. The DNA is then integrated into the host cells' chromosomes as a "provirus" that either remains inactive (latent) or manifests high levels of gene expression with active production of virus. Cellular activation results in transcription and translation of the viral proteins from proviral DNA and the subsequent packaging of these proteins into virions that are then released by budding from the cell and the subsequent spread of infection.

As the virus enters the the bloodstream, it is cleared from the circulation to the lymphoid organs, where it replicates to a critical level and then leads to a burst of viremia. The high level of viremia leads to acute mononucleosis–like symptoms or the "acute viremia syndrome." The development of the HIV-specific immune response (both humoral and cell mediated) and the trappings of virions in the lymph node germinal centers lead to curtailment of viremia, disappearance of symptoms, and the beginning of clinical latency, which lasts for variable periods, (median duration 10 years). Most patients are asymptomatic during the clinical latency period with gradual decline in the $CD4^+$ T cell count. As the $CD4^+$ T cell count falls below critical levels (<200 cells per mm^3), the patient becomes highly susceptible to opportunistic diseases.

TRANSMISSION

There are three primary modes of transmission: sexual contact; exposure to blood, largely through injection drug use and transfusion; and perinatal transmission from infected mothers to their infants. There is no evidence that HIV is transmitted by casual contact or that the virus can be spread by insects such as by a mosquito bite.

Sexual Transmission

Sexual contact is the major mode of transmission worldwide. Heterosexual transmission is the major mode of transmission particularly in developing countries, whereas in the United States and Europe, homosexual contact is the most common modality of transmission, with heterosexual transmission increasing in frequency. HIV has been demonstrated in the semen, in cervical smears, and in vaginal

TABLE 1. **CDC Surveillance Case Definition for AIDS (1993)**

A. Definitive evidence of indicator diseases without laboratory evidence of HIV infection:
1. Candidiasis of esophagus, trachea, bronchi, or lungs
2. Cryptococcosis, extrapulmonary
3. Cryptosporidiosis with diarrhea persisting > 1 month
4. Cytomegalovirus disease of any organ, excluding liver, spleen, and lymph node in a patient > 1 month of age
5. Herpes simplex virus esophagitis, bronchitis, pneumonitis; or mucocutaneous disease persisting > 1 month
6. Kaposi's sarcoma in a patient < 60 years of age
7. Lymphoma of the brain (primary) in a patient < 60 years of age
8. Lymphoid interstitial pneumonia in a child < 13 years of age
9. *Mycobacterium avium* complex or *M. kansasii* disease (disseminated)
10. *Pneumocystis carinii* pneumonia
11. Toxoplasmosis of the brain in a patient > 1 month of age

B. With laboratory evidence of HIV infection and:
1. Any disease listed in Section A
2. Bacterial infections (multiple or recurrent) in children < 13 years of age caused by *Haemophilus, Streptococcus,* or other pyogenic bacteria
3. Coccidioidomycosis, disseminated at a site other than, or in addition to, the lungs or cervical or hilar lymph nodes
4. HIV encephalopathy
5. Histoplasmosis, disseminated at a site other than, or in addition to, the lungs or cervical or hilar lymph nodes
6. Isosporiasis with diarrhea persisting > 1 month
7. Kaposi's sarcoma
8. Non-Hodgkin's lymphoma of B cell or unknown phenotype and having the histologic type of small noncleaved lymphoma or immunoblastic sarcoma
9. Any mycobacterial disease, disseminated, excluding *M. tuberculosis* at a site other than or in addition to lungs, skin, or cervical or hilar lymph nodes
10. *M. tuberculosis,* extrapulmonary
11. *Salmonella* (nontyphoid) septicemia, recurrent
12. HIV wasting syndrome
13. Invasive cervical cancer
14. Isosporiasis with diarrhea persisting > 1 month
15. Recurrent salpingitis
16. Recurrent pneumonia within a 12-month period

C. Presumptive diagnosis of indicator diseases in the presence of laboratory evidence of HIV infection:
1. Candidiasis of the esophagus
2. Cytomegalovirus retinitis with loss of vision
3. Kaposi's sarcoma
4. Lymphoid interstitial pneumonia in a child < 13 years of age
5. Mycobacterial disease, disseminated (no culture)
6. *Pneumocystis carinii* pneumonia
7. Toxoplasmosis of the brain in a patient > 1 month of age

D. The 1993 expanded definition includes:
1. All HIV-infected persons who have < 200 CD4$^+$ T lymphocyte counts per mm^3, or a CD4$^+$ T lymphocyte % of total lymphocytes < 14
2. Pulmonary tuberculosis
3. Pneumonia, recurrent—bacterial
4. Invasive cervical cancer

---

fluid. Factors that are associated with increased infectiousness of the source partner include advanced disease stage as measured by diseases indicative of AIDS or decreased numbers of peripheral CD4$^+$ T lymphocytes; the presence of genital ulcer disease in the source partner; the presence of nonulcerative sexually transmitted diseases such as gonorrhea, chlamydial infections, and trichomoniasis; and traumatic sexual practices that result in rectal mucosal disruption, as in receptive anal intercourse.

Blood and Blood Products

Transmission through blood and blood products is either through sharing of contaminated needles for injection drug use or through transfusions of blood and blood products. Factors that have been associated with HIV infection among injection drug users include the duration of injecting drug use, the frequency of needle sharing, the number of needle-sharing partners, the number of injections, the median numbers of injections in "shooting galleries," and the prevalence of HIV infection in the area of residence.

HIV has been transmitted through receipt of whole blood, blood cellular components, plasma, and clotting factors. The likelihood of a person becoming infected with HIV after a single donor blood product documented to be HIV positive approaches 100%. Other blood products such as hepatitis B immune globulin, immune serum globulin, Rh(D) immune globulin, and hepatitis B vaccine have not been associated with transmission of HIV infection. The procedures involved in the processing of these products either inactivates or removes the virus. Currently, in the United States and in most other developed countries, the combination of screening of all blood for HIV antibody by enzyme-linked immunosorbent assay (ELISA) and confirmatory Western blot assay, the self-deferral of donors on the basis of risk behavior, and the screening out of HIV-negative individuals with positive surrogate laboratory parameters for HIV infection such as hepatitis B and C and syphilis has made the risk of transmission of HIV infection by transfused blood or blood products extremely small. Since the screening of blood was instituted, the risk of HIV transmission through transfusion of blood screened as HIV-negative has been estimated to be 1 in 36,000 to 1 in 225,000 per unit transfused. Such rare transmissions are due to donations from recently infected donors who have not developed detectable antibody. This "window period" is estimated to last an average of 1.5 to 2.1 months, with 95% of persons developing detectable antibody within 6 months.

HIV transmission by organ transplantations such as liver, heart, kidney, pancreas, bone, and skin has been documented. Avascular tissues such as corneas have not been associated with transmission. Therefore, donors of such tissues or organs are now screened for HIV infection prior to transplantation.

Perinatal Transmission

HIV can be transmitted from an infected mother to her fetus during pregnancy or during delivery or during the postpartum period through the colostrum and breast milk. Maternal transmissions to the fetus/infant occur most commonly in the perinatal period. Higher rates of transmission have been associated with mothers at both extremes of the clinical spectrum of HIV infection with either the acute, primary infection or the advanced, symptomatic disease due to higher levels of viremia. Prospective studies of infants born to women with HIV infection have found rates of transmission ranging from 13 to 40%.

Occupational Transmission Among Health Care and Laboratory Workers

Percutaneous, mucous membrane, and cutaneous exposures to blood and contaminated body fluids can occur in the health care setting. Studies have indicated that the risk of HIV transmission following skin puncture from a needle or other sharp objects that are contaminated with blood from a person with documented HIV infection is approximately 0.3%. There have been reports of transmission of HIV after mucous membrane and cutaneous exposures to blood; however, the risk is much smaller than that of needle puncture. Transmission of HIV from a health care worker to patients has been documented in only one instance, in a dental practice in Florida. Transmission of HIV from patient to patient through improper sterilization or reuse of contaminated needles and syringes has been reported in Romania and the former Soviet Union.

EPIDEMIOLOGY

As of October 31, 1995, a total of 501,310 persons with AIDS had been reported to the Centers for Disease Control and Prevention (CDC) in the United States, with 311,387 (62%) reported to have died. During the same time period, the World Health Organization (WHO) estimates that 18 million adults and 1.5 million children have been infected with HIV, resulting in approximately 4.5 million AIDS cases worldwide, with over 80% from the Third World. In sub-Saharan Africa, the major mode of transmission is through heterosexual contact; this is in contrast to the United States and Europe, where approximately 90% of cases are transmitted through homosexual contact and among injection drug users (IDUs). In the United States, the majority of cases are among men who have had sex

with men (56%). Over the past few years, the incidence of AIDS among IDUs has been increasing. In addition, the relative number of cases among heterosexuals, women, and children is also increasing. HIV infection and AIDS have disproportionately affected the minority populations in the United States, where the majority of IDUs in the inner cities are African Americans and Hispanics. The National Center for Health Statistics reports that in 1990, AIDS was the leading cause of death for men and women aged 25 to 44 in several cities in the United States. In fact, in 1993, HIV infection was the eighth leading cause of death for all ages in the United States.

DIAGNOSIS AND LABORATORY MONITORING

The diagnosis of HIV infection is dependent on the detection of antibodies against the viral antigens. Direct detection of viral antigens and culture of the virus in cell culture are also possible; however, the former is relatively insensitive and the latter is expensive. Other methods like the use of polymerase chain reaction (PCR) assays to detect genomic DNA or RNA is possible. The use of the enzyme-linked immunosorbent assay (ELISA) for HIV antibodies is an extremely good screening test, highly sensitive (99%) and specific (95 to 99%). A number of conditions, including collagen vascular diseases, chronic hepatitis, and malaria, have been associated with false-positive results on ELISA. Serum samples that are reactive by ELISA should be retested; if repeatedly positive, samples should be confirmed with a highly specific test such as the Western blot method or by an immunofluorescence assay (IFA). If the sample is positive with IFA or Western blot, the specimen is considered a true positive. Patients with a positive or indeterminate ELISA after being tested repeatedly and having a negative result on Western blot are considered negative and the ELISA reaction as false positive. If the Western blot test is indeterminate, one should proceed to a PCR assay and repeat the Western blot assay in 1 month. If the PCR is negative and the Western blot does not show progression, HIV infection is ruled out. If the PCR is positive and/or the Western blot shows progression, a diagnosis of HIV infection is made. Antibodies to HIV generally appear in the circulation 4 to 8 weeks following infection. Shortly after exposure to the virus and prior to the development of an immune response, there is a period of viremia and p24 antigenemia. HIV antigen (p24) testing is indicated in patients suspected of having acute HIV syndrome prior to the development of HIV antibodies.

The $CD4^+$ T cell count is the only laboratory test generally accepted as a reliable indicator of the progression of HIV infection. This cell count correlates well with clinical progression. Patients with $CD4^+$ T cell counts of less than 200 per mm^3 are at risk of infection with *Pneumocystis carinii*, and patients with a $CD4^+$ T cell count of less than 100 per mm^3 are at high risk of infection with cytomegalovirus (CMV) and *Mycobacterium avium* complex (MAC). The $CD4^+$ T cell count should be measured approximately every 6 months and more frequently if a declining trend is noted. Once the $CD4^+$ T cell count is less than 200 per mm^3, patients should be placed on a regimen for PCP prophylaxis. Other markers of HIV disease progression include serum beta$_2$ microglobulin, neopterin, soluble $CD8^+$ T lymphocytes, low concentrations of anti-p24 antibodies, elevated anti-cytomegalovirus antibodies, the conversion of a patient's viral phenotype from non–syncytium inducing (NSI) to syncytium inducing (SI), and the ability to culture the virus. Beta$_2$ microglobulin is a low-molecular-weight immune globulin that forms the light chain of the class I major histocompatibility center (MHC) receptor. It is elevated in HIV infection, particularly in patients with advanced disease, and levels of beta$_2$ microglobulin have a predictive value for progression to AIDS. Serum and urine neopterin concentrations are elevated with advanced disease and in asymptomatic patients are associated with an increased risk of progressing to AIDS. Thus, the combination of a CD4$^+$ T cell count and either a beta$_2$ microglobulin or a neopterin level may provide the best prediction about the risk of progression to AIDS.

CLINICAL MANIFESTATIONS

The clinical spectrum of HIV infection ranges from an acute mononucleosis–like syndrome associated with primary infection to a prolonged asymptomatic state to the advanced immunodeficient state with opportunistic infection. HIV disease can be empirically divided on the basis of the degree of immune suppression into an early stage (CD4$^+$ T cell count 500 per mm^3), an intermediate stage (CD4$^+$ T cell count between 200 and 500 per mm^3), and an advanced stage (CD4$^+$ T cell count <200 per mm^3). Most AIDS-defining opportunistic infections and malignancies occur during the advanced stage. Several systems were proposed to classify HIV infection. The 1986 CDC classification separates HIV-infected persons into four categories: Group I, acute infection; Group II, asymptomatic seropositive; Group III, persistent generalized lymphadenopathy; Group IV, symptomatic HIV disease. This system has limited prognostic utility and has been supplanted with the 1993 CDC classification (Table 2), which categorizes HIV-infected persons according to clinical symptoms and CD4 cell level groupings.

The Acute Retroviral Syndrome

The initial manifestation of 50 to 70% of recently infected individuals is a mononucleosis-like syndrome, referred to as the acute retroviral syndrome, which occurs approximately 3 to 6 weeks following primary infection. The clinical features of the acute retroviral syndrome are nonspecific and variable. Symptoms usually last for 1 to 2 weeks and gradually subside as an immune response to HIV develops. This stage is accompanied by a burst of viremia and p24 antigenemia. Signs and symptoms of the acute retroviral syndrome are fever, malaise, myalgias, anorexia, nausea, vomiting, diarrhea, weight loss, nonexudative pharyngitis, lymphadenopathy, and headache. Neurologic symptoms occur in some patients, including encephalitis, aseptic meningitis, peripheral neuropathy, and ascending polyneuropathy (Guillain-Barré syndrome). Two-thirds of the patients may have a truncal exanthema appearing as a maculopapular roseola-like rash.

Laboratory evaluation of patients reveals a reduced total lymphocyte count, elevated sedimentation rate, negative heterophil antibody test, and elevated transaminase and alkaline phosphatase levels. Total lymphocyte count, both CD4$^+$ and CD8$^+$ T lymphocytes, is initially reduced, with a normal ratio of CD4 to CD8 cells. An inversion of the CD4 to CD8 ratio occurs within several weeks due to a relative rise in CD8 cells. The ratio of CD4 to CD8 cells remains inverted as the acute illness resolves. Following the onset of symptoms, humoral and cellular immune responses are detected and coincide with the disappearance of symptoms and the decrease and/or disappearance of plasma viremia and p24 antigenemia. Most patients recover spontaneously from this syndrome, followed by a prolonged period of clinical latency.

The Asymptomatic Stage: Clinical Latency

After immune clearance and sequestration of the virus in the lymph nodes during the acute retroviral syndrome stage, patients enter a prolonged clinical latency period prior to the development of clinical disease. The clinical latency period varies among individuals; the median time is approximately 10 years. During this period, active viral replication continues. Some patients develop persistent generalized lymphadenopathy; other patients experience intermittent symptoms of malaise, lethargy, weakness, and/or anorexia.

Persistent Generalized Lymphadenopathy

After seroconversion, approximately 50 to 70% of infected individuals develop persistent generalized lymphadenopathy (PGL). PGL is defined as the presence of two or more extrainguinal sites of lymphadenopathy (1 cm) for a minimum of 3 to 6 months for which no other explanation can be found. The pathogenesis of PGL is related to the rapid infection of CD4 cells in lymph nodes by HIV after the initial infection leading to marked follicular hyperplasia. The most frequently involved node groups are the posterior and anterior cervical, submandibular, occipital, and axillary chain of nodes. Differential diagnosis includes mycobacterial infection, Kaposi's sarcoma, and lymphoma. Lymph node biopsy is not indicated unless patients have clinical findings suggestive of opportunistic diseases.

Neurologic Disease

Neurologic complications of HIV infection may be primary due to the direct, immunologic sequelae of the HIV infection, or secondary to the opportunistic infections or neoplasms. Neurologic complications may involve both the central (CNS) and peripheral nervous systems. Table 3 shows the neurologic complications of HIV infection.

TABLE 2. **1993 CDC AIDS Surveillance Case Definition and Staging System**

CD4 Categories		Clinical Categories		
CD4 (Number)	CD4 (Percent)	Asymptomatic or Acute HIV, PGL	Symptomatic, Not A or C	AIDS Indicator Conditions
>499	>29	A1	B1	C1
200–499	14–28	A2	B2	C2
<200	<14	A3	B3	C3

Abbreviation: PGL = persistent generalized lymphadenopathy. AIDS indicator conditions for 1993 are listed in Table 1.

TABLE 3. **Neurologic Complications of HIV Infection**

Aseptic meningitis
Guillain-Barré syndrome
Chronic inflammatory demyelinating polyneuropathy
Multiple mononeuropathy
Peripheral predominantly sensory neuropathy
HIV encephalopathy
Vascular myelopathy
Opportunistic infection of CNS
  Toxoplasmosis
  Cryptococcosis
  Progressive multifocal leukoencephalopathy
  Cytomegalovirus
  Syphilis
  Mycobacterium tuberculosis
  Human T cell lymphotropic virus Type I (HTLV I)
Neoplasms of CNS
  Primary CNS lymphoma
  Kaposi's sarcoma

Peripheral Neuropathy

Peripheral neuropathies are common (20 to 40%) in patients with HIV infection. Symptoms may occur at any time during the course of HIV infection. The most common peripheral neuropathy is a distal, predominantly sensory polyneuropathy. It presents as chronic, symmetrical, painful dysesthesias in the feet and lower extremities, particularly the soles. Patients complain of numbness and painful burning sensations, and pain even when lightly touched. This polyneuropathy is due to HIV-mediated axonal degeneration, and electrophysiologic studies show combined sensory and motor neuropathy. This is almost always a late complication of HIV disease. Therapy is predominantly symptomatic using analgesics and tricyclic antidepressants.

Acute inflammatory, demyelinating polyneuropathy (Guillain-Barré syndrome) usually occurs early in the course of HIV infection. Patients report progressive motor weakness with minimal sensory symptoms. On examination, areflexia and weakness are noted. CSF reveals pleocytosis with an elevated protein level; a nerve biopsy may reveal mononuclear cell infiltration and demyelination. The clinical course waxes and wanes.

Differential diagnosis of peripheral neuropathy in HIV infection includes polyneuropathies secondary to cytomegalovirus infection and drug-associated peripheral neuropathy including that caused by didanosine, zalcitabine, stavudine, and isoniazid.

Aseptic Meningitis

During the acute retroviral syndrome, one-quarter to one-third of patients may experience a syndrome of headache, photophobia, and sometimes frank encephalitis. Meningeal signs may be minimal. CSF examination reveals slight lymphocytic pleocytosis, elevated protein, and normal glucose. Cranial neuropathies may be present. This syndrome is rarely seen in the late stage of HIV infection. Clinically, signs and symptoms may wax and wane for months but usually resolve spontaneously.

HIV Encephalopathy

HIV encephalopathy or AIDS dementia complex is a late complication of HIV infection. The etiology remains unclear; it may represent the direct effects of HIV infection on the CNS. Patients have neurocognitive deterioration manifested as decline in cognitive ability, impaired concentration, memory loss, mental slowness, and progressive deterioration in performing complex tasks. Patients also have motor and behavioral changes. Motor complaints include ataxia, tremors, unsteady gait, hyper-reflexia, and profound weakness in later stages. Behavioral changes include apathy and lack of initiative with progression to a vegetative state in some instances. In most instances, there is no significant change in the level of alertness. Seizures have been reported occasionally as a late complication.

There are no specific criteria for diagnosis of AIDS dementia complex. Laboratory and clinical evaluation is necessary to rule out opportunistic diseases, depression, and other causes of mental status changes. Diagnosis requires the demonstration of a decline in cognitive function using a neuropsychiatric test or the Folstein mini-mental status examination on serial assessments. Cranial imaging studies, such as computed tomography (CT) and magnetic resonance imaging (MRI), demonstrate generalized cerebral atrophy inconsistent with the patient's age. Lumbar puncture reveals nonspecific findings in the CSF, a slight pleocytosis with normal glucose, and elevated CSF protein. Lumbar puncture is of value to rule out opportunistic diseases. Markers of immune activation such as beta$_2$ microglobulin, CSF quinolinic acid, and neopterin are elevated in the CSF of patients with AIDS dementia complex. However, these findings are nonspecific. Brain biopsy demonstrates nonspecific findings of gliosis, focal necrosis, demyelination, myelin pallor, and multinucleated giant cells scattered throughout the cerebral cortex and white matter. There is no specific treatment for HIV encephalopathy; antiretroviral agents may be of benefit. There were reports of zidovudine or didanosine resulting in improvement of cognitive function.

ANTIRETROVIRAL THERAPY

Antiretroviral therapy has been shown to decrease viral load and delay immunologic decline; however, it does not kill the virus. Nucleoside derivatives, such as zidovudine (ZDV) (Retrovir), didanosine (ddI) (Videx), zalcitabine (ddC) (Hivid), and lamivudine (3TC) (Epivir), cause premature termination of the viral DNA chain. The exact mechanism by which these nucleoside compounds inhibit HIV reverse transcriptase is unclear. Antiretroviral therapy in symptomatic patients has been shown to delay the development of opportunistic infections and prolong survival.

The question of when to initiate antiretroviral therapy and how many drugs to use remains controversial. Initial studies conducted with zidovudine had mixed results. Some U.S. studies showed a survival benefit in patients with CD4$^+$ T lymphocyte counts between 200 and 500 cells per mm^3. However, a European study did not. Because of the definite delay in progression of disease with early therapy regardless of CD4$^+$ T lymphocyte cell count, early initiation of antiretroviral therapy seems appropriate.

Early therapy usually means initiating treatment when the CD4 counts approach 500 cells per mm^3; many experts view this approach as an actual delay in therapy. To begin treatment when the disease is diagnosed will prevent ongoing viral replication and cell death and possibly some immunologic damage. A collaborative European–Australian study showed benefit with ZDV in patients with CD4 counts greater than 400 cells per mm^3. With our current armamentarium of drugs with activity against the virus that causes AIDS, many combinations are available to treat patients in all stages of infection. Treatment strategies should be individualized based on patient lifestyle, initiative, opportunistic infections, and toxicities of available agents. A review of currently available agents follows:

Zidovudine (3'-azido-2',3'-dideoxythymidine; AZT or ZDV [Retrovir]) was the first retroviral agent approved for the treatment of HIV infection. It is well absorbed orally. Plasma elimination half-life is approximately 1 hour, but the intracellular half-life of the active triphosphate is about 3 to 4 hours. Hence, the dosing regimen may be given three to five times daily. Clinical trials have shown that ZDV increases total lymphocyte count, including CD4+ T cell counts, and causes a decline in the circulating levels of p24 antigen resulting in weight gain and improvement in neurologic function.

When given to pregnant HIV-infected women, ZDV reduces transmission of the virus to their offspring by two-thirds (from 28% to 8%). Toxicities include neutropenia, anemia, and myopathy. Most of these toxicities are dose dependent and also related to the severity of the HIV infection. Other side effects such as nausea, vomiting, diarrhea, fatigue, malaise, and headache may subside. ZDV-related anemia, usually of the macrocytic type, can be treated with either the administration of recombinant erythropoietin or blood transfusion. ZDV-associated neutropenia can be reversed by reducing the dose or by administration of granulocyte colony-stimulating factor (G-CSF). ZDV myopathy is characterized by weakness, muscle wasting, and elevated creatine kinase. Bluish discoloration of the nails is particularly noticeable among black patients. The development of in vitro ZDV resistance occurs during the course of therapy, usually in patients receiving ZDV for 12 months or longer and in patients with advanced HIV infection. This development of resistance has been shown to be related to the development of mutations in the reverse trancriptase enzymes. Isolates resistant to ZDV are usually sensitive to ddI. Hence, there are proposals of the early use of combination regimens.

Didanosine (ddI) (Videx) therapy is usually given to patients who have received prolonged ZDV therapy, and who show clinical or laboratory decline while receiving ZDV. The plasma half-life of ddI is about 1.6 hours, but the intracellular half-life is about 8 to 24 hours. Didanosine is given as a twice-daily regimen. The drug should be administered on an empty stomach because bioavailability of the drug is reduced when taken with food. Toxicities associated with ddI include painful sensory peripheral neuropathy, mouth ulceration, and pancreatitis. Neuropathy is reversed with discontinuation of the drug. Pancreatitis occurs in about 4 to 5% of patients receiving ddI. Patients with pancreatitis present with abdominal pain, with or without associated elevation of amylase level. Concomitant use of drugs that are associated with drug-induced pancreatitis and alcohol abuse increase the frequency of ddI-induced pancreatitis. Didanosine is contraindicated in patients with prior history of pancreatitis, regardless of etiology. Didanosine has a minimal effect on the bone marrow. This absence of hematologic toxicity allows ddI to be used in combination with ZDV. Cross-resistance exists between ddI and ddC.

Zalcitabine (ddC) (Hivid) is the third drug approved for treatment of HIV infection. However, in contrast to ZDV and ddI, zalcitabine is not approved for monotherapy; it is licensed only for use as part of a combination regimen with ZDV. Zalcitabine is well absorbed orally and given as a three-times-a-day regimen. Toxicities associated with ddC include peripheral neuropathy, pancreatitis, and penile ulcers. As with ddI, neuropathy is reversible, but pancreatitis is less frequent compared with ddI.

Stavudine (d4T) (Zerit), a nucleoside derivative, has an antiretroviral activity comparable with that of ZDV. It is well absorbed orally. Toxicities associated with d4T include peripheral neuropathy, pancreatitis, and elevations of alanine aminotransferase (ALT). Hematologic complications are minimal. Stavudine, when used as monotherapy, is associated with decreased levels of resistance when compared with other available agents. Stavudine is available only directly from the manufacturer.

Lamivudine (3TC) (Epivir) is another analogue of HIV reverse transcriptase. Concurrent use of ZDV and 3TC suppresses HIV resistance to ZDV, decreases viral load, and increases and maintains CD4+ cell counts. Studies of 3TC alone have shown only transient increases in CD4+ cell counts and decreases in viral load, with rapid development of resistance. Toxicities are similar to those of ZDV.

Protease inhibitors are a new class of drugs that inhibit HIV protease activity and prevent HIV replication in vitro; they are active against viral strains resistant to reverse transcriptase inhibitors. Two of these agents are currently available: saquinavir (Invirase) and ritonavir (Norvir). The third, indinavir (Crixivan),* is currently available in limited quantities in expanded access programs. Saquinavir plus ZDV increased and sustained CD4 cell counts more than either drug alone. Indinavir alone or with ZDV was more effective and had a more sustained effect than ZDV alone in lowering serum HIV RNA levels and increasing CD4 counts. Triple therapy with a protease inhibitor and two nucleoside analogues may be more effective than treatment with two drugs. Resistance to the new agents can develop. Early studies have not found severe toxicity, but nephrolithiasis has occurred with indinavir. Some protease inhibitors may have extensive drug interactions, and this should be taken into consideration when pre-

---

*Investigational drug in the United States.

scribing these drugs. Doses of available antiretroviral agents are found in Table 4.

OPPORTUNISTIC INFECTIONS

Patients with HIV infections are susceptible to opportunistic infection, which occurs in later stages of the disease usually in patients with less than 200 CD4[+] T lymphocyte cell count. Opportunistic infections are the leading cause of morbidity and mortality in patients with HIV infection. The development of opportunistic infection is related to the degree of immunosuppression (CD4[+] T lymphocyte count) and to the exposure of the patient to the pathogens. For example, patients with CD4[+] T lymphocyte count greater than 200 cells per mm³ rarely have *Pneumocystis carinii* pneumonia, and patients with CD4[+] cell counts more than 75 to 100 cells per mm³ rarely have disseminated *Mycobacterium avium* complex (MAC). Opportunistic infections may represent reactivation of latent infection, primary infection, or exogenous reinfection. Hence, HIV-associated opportunistic infections vary geographically and depend on the specific behavior pattern of the individual.

Fungal Infections

Pneumocystis carinii

Pneumocystis carinii has recently been reclassified as a fungus based upon molecular genetic data.

Infection with *Pneumocystis carinii* is one of the most common infections in HIV-infected individuals in North America; approximately 70 to 80% of patients will have at least one bout of *Pneumocystis carinii* pneumonia (PCP) at some point during the course of their disease. With prophylaxis, the prevalence of PCP has markedly declined. However, PCP continues to be a substantial cause of morbidity and mortality. PCP is listed as the immediate cause of death in 15 to 20% of patients with AIDS. Patients with elevated alveolar arterial gradient (30 mmHg), severely abnormal chest radiographs, high numbers of organisms detected on lavage or biopsy, severe immunologic dysfunction and the presence of concomitant pathogens have poor prognosis. Thus, drug therapy is more likely to be successful if therapy is started when pulmonary dysfunction is mild, and other opportunistic infections are absent. The risk of PCP infection increases as the CD4[+] T cell count

declines (200 cells per mm³) and in patients with previous bouts of PCP. Therefore, HIV-infected individuals with a history of previous bouts of PCP and a CD4[+] T cell count less than 200 per mm³ should receive some form of prophylaxis.

Patients with PCP present with fever and a cough that is usually nonproductive (80%). Fever may be absent in patients who are severely immunodeficient. Patients may have chest tightness, dyspnea on exertion or exercise intolerance, fatigue, and weight loss. Physical findings are minimal. Breath sounds are usually clear, and chest radiographs reveal a variety of patterns; the most common finding is either a normal chest radiograph or bilateral interstitial infiltrate. Patients receiving aerosolized pentamidine for prophylaxis present with upper lobe cavitary lesions resembling tuberculosis. Other, less common findings on chest x-ray include lobar infiltrates and, in few instances, pleural effusions. Pneumothorax complicates PCP in patients with prior episodes of PCP and in patients receiving aerosolized pentamidine for prophylaxis.

Pathologically, PCP causes air-space consolidation due to the protein-rich exudates consisting of numerous *P. carinii* trophozoites that fill the alveoli and cause intrapulmonary right-to-left shunt and arterial hypoxemia. Parenchymal inflammation and edema and interstitial fibrosis occur. Laboratory findings are nonspecific; patients may have leukocytosis or present with leukopenia, especially in the severely immune deficient. The serum lactate dehydrogenase is often elevated, and arterial blood gases reveal hypoxemia with a decline in PaO_2 and an increase in the alveolar-arterial (A-a) gradient. Definitive diagnosis of PCP requires demonstration of the trophozoite or cyst forms of the organism (using modified Giemsa stain, silver methenamine, and toluidine blue O) from induced sputum, bronchoalveolar lavage, transbronchial biopsy, or open lung biopsy. Induced sputum examination by well-trained laboratory personnel provides a sensitive and low-cost method for diagnosis of PCP. Recently, polymerase chain reaction (PCR) assay has been used to identify specific DNA sequences for *Pneumocystis carinii* in clinical specimens. Patients whose induced sputum does not have a demonstrable PCP should undergo a bronchoscopic evaluation. Bronchoalveolar lavage (BAL) alone has a sensitivity of 85 to 95%. The combination of BAL and transbronchial biopsy has a diagnostic yield of more than 95%. Because of the cost of diagnostic evaluation, sometimes it may be appropriate to treat mild cases of presumptive PCP empirically.

Extrapulmonary *Pneumocystis carinii* infection occurs occasionally, particularly in patients receiving aerosolized pentamidine for prophylaxis. Common sites of extrapulmonary pneumocystosis include the middle ear, mastoid, retina, liver, lymph nodes, spleen, and bone marrow.

Trimethoprim/sulfamethoxazole (TMP/SMX) (Bactrim, Septra) is the treatment of choice for PCP, which is effective for 90% of the cases. No other agent

TABLE 4. **Dose of Antiretrovirals**

Zidovudine (Retrovir)	200 mg PO tid or 100 mg PO 5 times daily
Didanosine (Videx)	200 mg PO bid for patients > 60 kg 100 mg PO bid for patients < 60 kg
Zalcitabine (Hivid)	0.75 mg PO tid
Lamivudine (Epivir)	40 mg PO bid
Stavudine (Zerit)	30 mg PO bid for patients <60 kg 40 mg PO bid for patients >60 kg
Saquinavir (Invirase)	600 mg PO tid + AZT or ddC
Ritonavir (Norvir)	600 mg PO bid
Indinavir (Crixivan)	800 mg PO q 8 h

has shown higher efficacy than TMP/SMX. Clinical improvements are noted within 4 to 8 days of initiation of therapy in terms of fever, respiratory rate, alveolar-arterial gradient, and dyspnea. There may be worsening of the patient's condition during the first 48 to 72 hours of treatment because of inflammatory response resulting from the death of large numbers of the organisms in the lung. This inflammatory response can be markedly reduced by the adjunctive use of glucocorticoids. Steroids are indicated in patients with severe PCP in whom the PaO_2 is less than 70 mmHg or an A-a gradient of over 35 mmHg. The disadvantage of using TMP/SMX is the relative high incidence of side effects, which include skin rash, nausea, vomiting, granulocytopenia, transaminase elevations, nephritis, and hyperkalemia. Serious hypersensitivity reactions such as Stevens-Johnson syndrome are rare but fatal. The development of skin rash and other side effects does not indicate the discontinuation of this drug regimen. Adverse reactions can be reduced without sacrificing efficacy by lowering the recommended dose of TMP/SMX by 25%. If patients are unable to tolerate TMP/SMX, several options are available (Table 5).

Parenteral pentamidine isethionate (Pentam 300) is effective therapy for PCP. It is administered by intravenous route only. Intramuscular administration is associated with sterile abscess. Aerosolized pentamidine is used only for prophylaxis. Adverse reactions include renal toxicity, hypoglycemia, hyperglycemia, granulocytopenia, cardiac arrhythmias, hypotension, and pancreatitis. Hypotension is related to the rate of infusion; the drug should be administered over a 60-minute period. Renal dysfunction can be minimized by discontinuation of other nephrotoxic drugs such as foscarnet and by dose reduction of 20 to 50%.

Less effective alternative agents for the treatment of PCP such as dapsone plus trimethoprim tend to be associated with fewer toxicities. One side effect of dapsone is the development of methemoglobinemia, and its use is contraindicated in patients with glucose-6-phosphate dehydrogenase deficiency.

Atovaquone (Mepron) is a hydroxynaphthoquinone that interferes with the mitochondrial electron transport in the microorganisms, and thus has a mechanism of action distinct from TMP/SMX or pentamidine. Skin rash and neutropenia are common side effects. Compared with TMP/SMX, it has a lower incidence of side effects but has lower overall response rate and higher relapse rate; hence, it is used as a second-line therapy for mild to moderate PCP.

Clindamycin (Cleocin)* and primaquine have been used successfully in patients with mild, moderate, and severe PCP. Toxicity associated with this regimen includes rash, elevation of transaminases, diarrhea, and hemolysis.

Trimetrexate (NeuTrexin), a potent inhibitor of dihydrofolate reductase, is effective against PCP when used alone or in combination with a sulfonamide. It is given in conjunction with high-dose leucovorin to minimize the suppressive bone marrow side effects of trimetrexate. Adverse effects include leukopenia and skin rash. Trimetrexate is associated with high rate of poor response and a high relapse rate.

In an AIDS patient with PCP who has failed to improve while receiving conventional therapy (after 7 to 10 days of therapy), or if the patient is deteriorating rapidly, a repeat bronchoscopy and possible transbronchial biopsy is considered to determine whether there is another pathogen present like cytomegalovirus, fungal, or mycobacterial infection. If *Pneumocystis carinii* is the only identifiable pathogen, and the patient has failed to improve after 7 to 10 days of therapy, one should consider switching to another drug regimen like parenteral pentamidine, adding corticosteroids to conventional therapy if steroids have not been already added, or using two specific therapies concurrently (TMP/SMX and pentamidine).

Prevention of PCP plays a major role in the management of the HIV-infected patient. Prophylactic (primary prophylaxis) measures are indicated in patients with a CD4+ T lymphocyte count less than 200 cells per μL or in those patients, regardless of the CD4+ T lymphocyte count, with otherwise unexplained persistent fever or oropharyngeal candidiasis. Secondary prophylaxis (the prevention of second or subsequent episodes of PCP) is indicated for any patient with a documented previous bout of PCP. TMP/SMX is a preferred prophylactic agent, given as one double-strength tablet per day. Trials have shown that TMP/SMX is more effective than aerosolized pentamidine (NebuPent) for either primary or

TABLE 5. **Recommended Therapy for *Pneumocystis carinii* Pneumonia (PCP)**

Drug	Dose	Route	Duration
Trimethoprim (TMP) with sulfamethoxazole (SMX) (Bactrim, Septra)	TMP 15–20 mg/kg/d SMX 95–100 mg/kg/d in 3–4 divided doses	PO, IV	21 days
or			
Trimethoprim plus dapsone	5 mg/kg/d q 8 h 100 mg qd	PO PO	21 days
or			
Pentamidine	4 mg/kg qd	IV	21 days
or			
Atovaquone (Mepron)	750 mg suspension bid	PO	21 days
or			
Clindamycin (Cleocin) plus primaquine	300–450 mg q 6 h 600 mg q 6–8h 15 mg qd	PO IV PO	21 days
or			
Trimetrexate (NeuTrexin) plus leucovorin	45 mg/m² q 24 h 20 mg/m² q 6 h	IV PO, IV	21 days
Prednisone (adjunct for severe episodes)	40 mg bid for 5 d, then 40 mg/d for 5 d, then 20 mg qd to the end of therapy	PO	

---

*Not FDA-approved for this indication.

secondary prophylaxis, has the benefit of also reducing the frequency of toxoplasmosis, and reduces the frequency of pneumococcal and *Haemophilus* infections. A disadvantage of TMP/SMX as prophylaxis is the frequency of side effects. Reducing the dose of TMP/SMX to a single-strength tablet daily or to a double-strength tablet two to three times per week lowers the toxicity and appears to be equally efficacious.

Aerosolized pentamidine, 300 mg monthly, delivered by the Respirgard nebulizer, is an alternative to patients who are unable to tolerate TMP/SMX. Aerosolized pentamidine is not as effective (higher relapse rate) as TMP/SMX and has a higher incidence of pneumothorax and disseminated pneumocystosis. The patient should be screened for pulmonary tuberculosis before using aerosolized pentamidine because of environmental contamination with respiratory secretions, which has considerable potential of spreading tuberculosis. Other alternative prophylactic regimens include dapsone-pyrimethamine, dapsone alone (100 mg orally every day), atovaquone, and clindamycin-primaquine.

Other Fungal Infections

Infection by *Candida* species is the most common fungal infection in HIV-infected individuals, usually seen in relatively early stages of the disease. Almost all HIV-infected patients experience *Candida* infections over the course of their illness. *Candida* may cause mucocutaneous infections that are generally easy to control or may cause systemic invasion secondary to indwelling catheters. The incidence of candidiasis increases as HIV infection progresses. As $CD4^+$ T cell counts decline to less than 100 cells per μL, infection may involve the esophagus, trachea, bronchi, or lungs.

Oral candidiasis (thrush) is very common and may involve the hard and soft palates, buccal mucosa, tongue, pharynx, and hypopharynx. It appears as white, cottage cheese plaques on the mucosal surface that are easily scraped off. Sometimes, it appears as flat, erythematous plaques without the white exudate (atrophic candidiasis). Diagnosis is made on the basis of physical examination alone. Demonstration of branching pseudohyphae on wet-mount KOH preparations is diagnostic. Cultures are not usually necessary . A therapeutic trial of antifungal agents also helps establish the diagnosis.

Candidal esophagitis is common; presenting symptoms are odynophagia or dysphagia, often associated with persistent or intermittent burning or retrosternal pain. The presence of concomitant oral candidiasis strongly suggests esophageal candidiasis, but it may be absent, especially in those patients receiving topical oral antifungal agents. Upper GI contrast radiography shows a classic pattern of diffuse ulcerations and plaques. Patients who do not have oral thrush and do not respond to empirical antifungal therapy need upper endoscopy for definitive diagnosis and to detect other causes of esophagitis.

Oral and vaginal candidiasis often responds to topical antifungal agents (nystatin, clotrimazole). Systemic therapy with oral ketoconazole (Nizoral), itraconazole (Sporanox), or fluconazole (Diflucan), is more convenient, albeit expensive, and probably more effective than topical therapy. Ketoconazole is less expensive than fluconazole and itraconazole, but both ketoconazole and itraconazole can cause adrenal suppression and are poorly absorbed in the presence of high gastric pH, which is common in patients with advanced HIV infection. Stomatitis, esophagitis, and proctitis often recur when therapy is discontinued. Fluconazole may have to be continued for life if recurrences are frequent and severe. In recurrent cases, severely immnosuppressed patients may require low-dose intravenous amphotericin B.

Cryptococcus neoformans is a leading cause of meningitis in patients with AIDS, generally occurring in advanced stages of the disease. Cryptococcal infections are acquired by inhaling the organism into the lungs. The primary pulmonary infection is often asymptomatic and rapidly disseminates to the brain and meninges. Approximately 80% of patients with cryptococcal disease have CNS infection. Cryptococcal meningitis presents with fever, malaise, dull headache, nausea and vomiting, and altered mental status; only about 25% of patients have meningeal signs. Focal neurologic deficits and seizures are rare. Symptoms are usually mild, and a high index of suspicion is essential in order to make an early diagnosis. Extraneural sites include pulmonary disease, skin involvement resembling molluscum contagiosum, fungemia, and prostatitis. Pulmonary involvement is seen in 40% of patients, 90% of whom will have CNS infection. Cyptococcal pneumonia presents with fever, night sweats, malaise, cough, and dyspnea, and, in some cases, hemoptysis. Chest radiograph shows focal lobar infiltrates and, rarely, cavitary disease. Fungemia occurs in more than 80% of patients with cryptococcal meningitis. The prostate gland may serve as a reservoir for smoldering infection and cause relapse in patients who do not take suppressive therapy.

The diagnosis of meningeal involvement is made by demonstration of the organisms in spinal fluid on India ink examination, by the presence of cyptococcal antigen in blood and CSF, and/or by isolation of *Cryptococcus* from the CSF. CSF findings in cryptococcal meningitis are usually benign, with slight pleocytosis (5 to 50 mononuclear cells per mm^3), slightly elevated protein, and low or normal glucose. India ink examination reveals the organism 50 to 90% of the time, and cryptococcal antigen is positive 90 to 95% of the time. CSF cultures are invariably positive in primary disease but may be negative in patients who have relapse from previously treated cryptococcal infection. In this setting, a rising titer of cryptococcal antigen suggests relapse.

The most potent therapy for cryptococococcal meningitis consist of combined amphotericin B (Fungizone) 0.3 to 1.25 mg/kg intravenously every day and flucytosine (Ancobon) 100 to 150 mg/kg orally every day in divided doses. Flucytosine can cause granulocytopenia, thrombocytopenia, and hepatitis. Chronic suppressive therapy is necessary after acute therapy. Fluconazole (200 mg to 400 mg orally every day) is recommended and is as effective as once-weekly intravenous amphotericin B. Relapse occurs in 50 to 60% of the patients without suppressive therapy.

Histoplasma capsulatum is a dimorphic fungus endemic in the Mississippi and Ohio River valleys, the south-central United States, Puerto Rico, Dominican Republic, and South America and parts of Mexico. The organism exists in mycelial form in soil and yeast form in homeothermic animals. Organisms are found in soil enriched with bird guano and bat droppings. The pathogenesis of histoplasmosis is similar to tuberculosis; up to 80% of the population in endemic areas are positive for the skin test for histoplasma antigen, but the majority are asymptomatic. Conidia are inhaled and deposited in pulmonary alveoli as yeast forms, either viable or dead, and often persist within the granulomatous lesions for many years without consequence. However, in patients with HIV infection who have gradual impairment of cell-mediated immunity, it leads to reactivation and dissemination of the organisms. The CD4+ T cell count of patients with histoplasmosis is usually less than 200 cells per μL, indicating a late manifestation of the HIV infection. Patients usually present with fever, headache, malaise, weight loss, anorexia, and nonproductive cough. Radiographic findings in patients with pulmonary histoplasmosis include diffuse interstitial infiltrates, with nodular infiltrates and less frequently, focal disease. Extrapulmonary histoplasmosis involves the liver, spleen, bone marrow, gut, adrenals, and central nervous system. Mucocutaneous manifestations appear as erythematous, maculopapular eruptions that are widely distributed on the face, trunk, and extremities that may be mistaken for molluscum contagiosum or other viral eruptions.

Diagnosis requires growth of the fungus from samples of body fluids or tissues. *Histoplasma* polysaccharide antigen testing of blood or urine is highly sensitive and specific; however, this test is not available in commercial laboratories. Histoplasmin skin test is of great value for epidemiologic studies, but useless for diagnosis because most of the population living in endemic areas are positive.

Treatment consists of amphotericin B 0.5 to 1.0 mg/kg daily intravenously to a total dose of 35 to 40 mg/kg followed with chronic maintenance therapy of amphotericin B 0.5 to 0.8 mg per kg intravenously every week or itraconazole 200 mg orally twice a day. Serum and urine *Histoplasma capsulatum* polysaccharide antigen titers are useful for monitoring chronic suppressive therapy and predicting relapse.

Coccidioides immitis infection (coccidioidomycosis), also known as San Joaquin Valley fever, is a common complication of HIV infection in endemic areas of the southwestern part of the United States. Coccidioidomycosis in HIV infection probably represents reactivation usually in late stages of HIV infection. Pulmonary disease is the most common manifestation of the infection (70%). Patients present with nonspecific symptoms of fever, chills, anorexia, cough, sputum production, malaise, and weight loss. Chest radiographic findings show diffuse pulmonary reticulonodular disease in 40%. Extrapulmonary disease includes meningitis, hepatic involvement, and cutaneous involvement. Diagnosis is made by culture from involved tissues. Serologic testing is helpful; rising titers indicate a poor prognostic sign. Treatment consists of amphotericin B, 0.5 to 1.0 mg per kg intravenously every day to a total dose of 1 gram, followed with lifelong suppression with itraconazole (100 to 200 mg orally twice daily) or ketoconazole (400 mg orally every day).

Protozoal Infections

Toxoplasma gondii

Toxoplasmosis is the most common opportunistic CNS infection in patients with AIDS. It is usually a late complication of HIV infection, usually in patients with CD4+ T cell counts less than 100 cells per μL. Toxoplasmosis represents reactivation rather than primary infection in most cases. Patients usually have IgG antibodies against *Toxoplasma*, indicating prior infection. About 5 to 10% of cases are seronegative for *Toxoplasma gondii*; hence a negative antibody titer does not eliminate a diagnosis of toxoplasmosis.

Toxoplasmosis in HIV-infected patients usually presents as a space-occupying cerebral lesion manifested as fever, headache, and focal neurologic deficits. Patients may present with seizure, aphasia, lethargy, dementia, confusion, and progression to coma. Definitive diagnosis requires brain biopsy, which is frequently associated with morbidity and a diagnostic yield of only 50%. Radiologic findings are sensitive (MRI is more sensitive than double-contrast CT) for diagnosis of cerebral toxoplasmosis. Findings include single or multiple ring-enhancing lesions usually involving the basal ganglia. Pathologically, these lesions represent central necrosis resulting in a ring-enhancing appearance on contrast CT and MRI. The abscess center contains scant organisms; most of the *T. gondii* organisms are seen on the periphery of the abscess. Differential diagnosis includes tuberculosis, cryptococcosis, nocardiosis, pyogenic brain abscess, lymphomas, and progressive multifocal leukoencephalopathy (PML). Primary CNS lymphoma usually presents as a single, hyperdense lesion, while PML causes diffuse, nonenhancing, hemispheric white matter lesions without edema or mass effect. If cranial imaging studies reveal no mass effect, a lumbar puncture can be performed for bacterial, fungal, and mycobacterial culture and for cryptococcal antigen assay.

Because of the high frequency of cerebral toxoplasmosis and rapid response to antimicrobial therapy and the morbidity associated with brain biopsy, patients with intracranial mass lesions and radiologic findings consistent with cerebral toxoplasmosis will benefit from empirical therapy with pyrimethamine (Daraprim), 200 mg orally the first day followed by 50 mg pyrimethamine orally every day, plus sulfadiazine, 1 to 2 grams orally every 6 hours. If there is no clinical and radiographic improvement within 10 to 14 days of treatment, a definitive diagnostic procedure (brain biopsy) is indicated to establish whether the etiology is an infectious or a neoplastic process other than toxoplasmosis. Side effects of this regimen include leukopenia, which may be ameliorated with concomitant use of folinic acid, 10 to 20 mg orally or intravenously every 6 hours; fever; rash; thrombocytopenia; and renal failure due to sulfadiazine crystalluria. Alternative therapy for patients unable to tolerate sulfadiazine includes clindamycin (Cleocin), 600 mg every 6 hours orally or intravenously, plus pyrimethamine, 75 mg orally every day; atovaquone, 750 mg orally every 6 hours, plus pyrimethamine; and macrolide antibiotics such as clarithromycin (Biaxin), 1 gram orally every 12 hours, and azithromycin (Zithromax), 1 gram orally loading, then 500 mg orally every day.

For patients who respond to anti-*Toxoplasma* therapy, a lifelong suppressive regimen is indicated, because relapses occur in the same sites of the initial disease if therapy is discontinued. For primary prophylaxis TMP/SMX (one double-strength tablet orally every day) is efficacious.

Cryptosporidium in HIV-infected individuals presents as a self-limited or intermittent diarrhea in the relatively early stages of the HIV infection to a severe, voluminous, life-threatening diarrhea in late-stage AIDS. This is accompanied by crampy abdominal pain, sometimes nausea and vomiting. *Cryptosporidium* may also cause biliary tract disease presenting as cholecystitis with or without accompanying cholangitis. Diagnosis is made by stool examination for the presence of oocysts that stain with acid-fast dyes. The use of sucrose flotation technique helps to separate the cyst from other particles. Therapy for cryptosporidiosis has been disappointing. Agents that have shown some success include octreotide (Sandostatin), 50 µg subcutaneously every 8 hours for 48 hours; if no response is seen, increase the dose stepwise to 500 µg every 8 hours and add paromomycin and azithromycin.

Microsporidium is an obligate intracellular parasite found within the cytoplasm of enteric cells. It causes watery diarrhea and abdominal pain. It is difficult to detect because of the small size of the organisms. Definitive diagnosis depends on the electron microscopic examination of the stool sample, intestinal aspirate, or biopsy specimen. There is no proven therapy at present, although high-dose albendazole has been reported to be effective in preliminary reports. Treatment is purely supportive.

Isospora belli is a coccidian parasite; it also appears as acid-fast structures in the stool as with *Cryptosporidium*. It usually infects an HIV patient of Haitian or African origin. It also causes watery diarrhea; however, this infection can be treated with TMP/SMX, one double-strength tablet orally every 6

hours for 7 to 10 days, but the relapse rate is high and chronic suppression with TMP/SMX is necessary. Pyrimethamine may be an alternative for patients with severe intolerance to TMP/SMX.

Entamoeba histolytica and *Giardia lamblia* are seen with increasing frequency in HIV-infected individuals, usually associated with conventional risk factors for diarrhea such as sexual practices and travel. These protozoal infections often respond to standard therapeutic regimens.

Mycobacterial Infections

Mycobacterium tuberculosis has been included in the 1993 CDC expanded list for AIDS-defining opportunistic infections. There has been an increase in cases of *M. tuberculosis* infection since the HIV epidemic. The majority of tuberculosis cases in patients who are HIV infected represent reactivation of latent infection, but acute infection and reinfection has been seen as well as an increase in the number of multidrug-resistant (MDR) tuberculosis. The risk of developing active tuberculosis in a positive tuberculin skin test in HIV-infected patients is approximately 8% annually, compared with a risk of 0 to 0.02% annually for immunologically intact individuals. Tuberculosis is common in patients of ages 25 to 44, among African Americans and Hispanics, in patients in New York City and Miami, and in patients in developing countries. Active tuberculosis may occur early in the course of HIV infection and may be among the earliest clinical signs of HIV infection.

Clinical features of tuberculosis in HIV-infected individuals are quite varied, depending on the degree of immunosuppression. In patients with relatively high CD4+ T cell counts, the usual presenting symptoms of fever, night sweats, weight loss, dyspnea on exertion, and chest radiographic findings of apical cavitary lesions of the upper lobes are seen. In patients with low CD4+ T cell counts, the chest radiographic findings are usually atypical, with diffuse infiltrates consistent with miliary spread, intrathoracic adenopathy, more frequent extrapulmonary dissemination, and *M. tuberculosis* bacteremia. Pathologic findings in severely immunosuppressed individuals become atypical with poorly formed granulomas without caseation.

Definitive diagnosis is made by culture of the organism from an involved site; a presumptive diagnosis is made with positive acid-fast bacilli on smears and consistent presentation while awaiting the culture results.

Tuberculosis in HIV-infected individuals responds well to chemotherapy unless the organism is drug resistant. Initial therapy consists of four drugs unless the likelihood of resistance is extremely small. Isoniazid (INH), rifampin, pyrazinamide (25 mg per kg orally every day) and ethambutol (25 mg per kg orally every day) are recommended initially. If the organism is susceptible to the drugs being used, INH and rifampin and pyrazinamide should be continued to complete an initial 2 months of therapy; INH and rifampin may then be continued for a total course of at least 9 months or 6 months after sputum culture becomes negative. Drug-resistant strains are increasing; the MDR strains of tuberculosis are associated with higher mortality. Thus, in areas where MDR tuberculosis is common, a four- or five-drug regimen is initiated while awaiting sensitivity results.

Chemoprophylaxis is given to HIV-infected individuals with a positive tuberculin test (at least 5 mm diameter in induration). HIV-infected patients should receive chemoprophylaxis regardless of the tuberculin skin test status if they meet the following criteria: (1) those with a history of a positive tuberculin test who were not adequately treated, (2) those who have close contacts with a patient with active tuberculosis, and (3) a chest radiograph that is consistent with previous untreated tuberculosis. Recommended prophylaxis is INH for 12 months. If patients are unable to tolerate INH, or if there is a possibility of drug-resistant strains, a prophylactic combination regimen of at least two of these three drugs— rifampin, pyrazinamide, or a quinolone—is an alternative.

Atypical mycobacteria, particularly *Mycobacterium avium* complex (MAC), are present in approximately 40% of HIV-infected patients. MAC infections account for more than 95% of the atypical mycobacterial infections in HIV-infected patients. Other atypical or nontuberculous mycobacteria include *M. kansasii, M. xenopi, M. gordonae,* and *M. haemophilum,* which account for 3 to 5% of infections. MAC is a common environmental saprophyte, found in water, soil, vegetables, and unpasteurized milk and milk products and can be acquired orally or inhaled from aerosols. MAC infection is a late complication of HIV infection, usually in patients with CD4$^+$ T cells of less than 100 per μL. Common manifestations of MAC infections include fever, night sweats, and weight loss. MAC can infect the liver, spleen, gut, lymph nodes, lungs, skin, brain, adrenals, kidneys, and bone marrow. About 85% of patients have mycobacteremia, and large numbers of the organisms are demonstrated on bone marrow biopsy. The recovery of MAC from pulmonary specimens is often an incidental finding and does not necessarily imply systemic infections because MAC seldom causes invasive pulmonary disease. Gastrointestinal symptoms such as abdominal pain and persistent diarrhea and, in patients with liver involvement, hepatosplenomegaly and elevated alkaline phosphatase, are common. Laboratory findings are nonspecific, but anemia and leukopenia are usually pronounced. Diagnosis depends on the demonstration of acid-fast bacilli in direct smears and confirmed by cultures from the involved tissues.

Drugs used to treat MAC include ethambutol (Myambutol), rifabutin (Mycobutin), rifampin (Rifadin), clofazimine (Lamprene), quinolones, aminoglycosides, and macrolides like clarithromycin (Biaxin) and azithromycin (Zithromax). Combination regimens of four or five drugs are beneficial and reduce or eliminate bacillemia and reduce the likelihood of development of drug-resistant organisms. These multidrug regimens are associated with a higher incidence of toxicities. Because MAC infection is a source of substantial morbidity, prophylactic measures are given to HIV-infected patients with CD4$^+$ T cell counts less than 100 per mm^3. Rifabutin, 300 mg orally every day, clarithromycin, 500 mg orally twice daily, or azithromycin 1250 mg orally every week is recommended and has been shown to delay the onset of bacillemia.

Bacterial Infections

Patients with HIV infections are prone to bacterial infections frequently manifested as respiratory tract infections, sepsis, skin and soft tissue infections, and gastroenteritis. Patients with HIV infections are prone to infections with encapsulated organisms such as *Streptococcus pneumoniae* and *Haemophilus influenzae* as a consequence of altered B cell activation and/or defects in neutrophil function secondary to the disease itself or secondary to drugs. Bacterial pneumonia in AIDS patients is often bacteremic (80% in patients with *Streptococcus pneumoniae* pneumonia). Hence, all HIV-infected patients should receive pneumococcal polysaccharide vaccine.

Other bacteria associated with HIV infection include *Pseudomonas aeruginosa* and *Moraxella catarrhalis,* which may cause sinusitis. *Rhodococcus equi* and *Nocardia* and *Legionella* species may cause pulmonary disease.

Enteric pathogens such as *Salmonella, Shigella,* and *Campylobacter* species are more common in homosexual men and are often severe and more prone to relapse. *Clostridium difficile*–associated colitis is also a common cause of enterocolitis in HIV-infected patients, particularly in those who were receiving antimicrobial therapy. Salmonellosis is bacteremic in about 50% of cases, and enteric symptoms may be minimal. Bacteremia with *Shigella* and *Campylobacter* species has also been reported. Therapy for these enteric pathogens follows standard treatment; however, *Salmonella* and sometimes *Shigella* tend to relapse. Long-term suppressive therapy is usually recommended.

Treponema pallidum (syphilis) in HIV-infected patients usually has a typical presentation, but the formerly rare clinical syndromes are encountered more frequently (i.e., neurosyphilis). Serologic testing (Venereal Disease Research Laboratory [VDRL]) may reveal false-positive results secondary to polyclonal B cell activation or may have false-negative results because of severe immune suppression. Treatment of HIV-infected patients with syphilis follows the standard guidelines. However, standard treatment may not be adequate to cure CNS infection or to prevent systemic relapses. High-dose intravenous penicillin is preferred over benzathine penicillin.

Bacillary angiomatosis is attributed to *Rickettsia*-like organisms *Bartonella (Rochalimaea) henselae* and *B. quintana.* It usually presents with cutaneous lesions that appear as single or multiple or disseminated erythematous nodules or plaques that resemble cutaneous Kaposi's sarcoma or basal cell carcinomas.

Visceral involvement is common, such as hepatitis (bacillary peliosis), osseous lesions, pneumonitis, and lymph node and CNS infection. Bacillary peliosis is a characteristic illness that presents with fever, right upper quadrant pain, and hepatomegaly and elevated liver enzymes. It appears as multiple, cystic lesions on imaging studies. Diagnosis is made by demonstration of perivascular accumulation of bacilli with Warthin-Starry stain and confirmed by electron microscopy. Treatment with prolonged courses of macrolides or tetracycline has been successful.

Viral Infections

Cytomegalovirus (CMV) infection is common among HIV-infected individuals; as much as 95% of patients are seropositive for CMV. With progressive immunosuppression as a result of HIV infection, CMV activity increases. CMV infection probably represents activation of latent infections as well as superinfection by additional strains from repeated exposure. CMV retinitis is the most common manifestation of CMV infection; it also involves the macula and optic disk rapidly and causes retinal detachment. The disease is usually bilateral, affecting one eye more than the other. Patients complain of painless, progressive loss of vision, scotoma, and ultimately blindness. Diagnosis is generally made clinically by an experienced ophthalmologist; it appears as white granular exudates superimposed with patches of perivascular hemorrhages. Therapy is urgent and may be started based on the ophthalmologic appearance of CMV retinitis even without histologic or virologic diagnosis. CMV retinitis responds to either ganciclovir (Cytovene) at a dose of 5 mg per kg intravenously every 12 hours or foscarnet (Foscavir) at 60 mg per kg intravenously every 8 hours or 90 mg per kg intravenously every 12 hours as induction therapy for a period of 14 to 21 days, followed with chronic suppressive therapy of single daily infusion for both drugs at a dose of 5 to 6 mg per kg intravenously every day or 1000 mg orally three times daily with food for ganciclovir and 90 to 120 mg per kg intravenously every day for foscarnet. Maintenance therapy does not prevent relapse from occurring, but it will serve to prolong the interval until relapse by several weeks or months. If relapse occurs, patients usually respond to reinduction with ganciclovir or foscarnet. Toxicities associated with ganciclovir include bone marrow suppression with neutropenia and thrombocytopenia, confusion, nausea, vomiting, and transaminase elevation. Patients unable to tolerate ganciclovir may either use intravitreal injections and intravitreal implants of ganciclovir, which appear to be effective and relatively safe, or may use parenteral foscarnet. Patients with neutropenia associated with ganciclovir will benefit from the use of G-CSF (filgrastim [Neupogen]). Foscarnet is nephrotoxic and can cause nausea, vomiting, seizures, hypocalcemia, hypomagnesemia, and penile ulcers. To prevent nephrotoxicity, foscarnet should be infused over 60 minutes following a 60-minute infusion of saline solution. Foscarnet therapy is associated with a longer patient survival period than patients treated with ganciclovir in a large prospective study. The reason for this finding is unclear, but it may be due to the antiretroviral activity of foscarnet.

Aside from retinitis, CMV can also cause esophagitis, enteritis, colitis, adrenalitis, pneumonitis, and myelitis. CMV esophagitis is symptomatically indistinguishable from *Candida* or herpes simplex esophagitis. Endoscopy usually reveals a single, large shallow ulcer in the distal esophagus; multiple ulcers may rarely be seen. CMV colitis is associated with small volume diarrhea, cramping and bloating, pain, fever, and tenesmus. Severe CMV colitis may result in perforation of the colon. CMV may also cause papillary stenosis and acalculous cholecystitis. Pulmonary pneumonitis is associated with fever, nonproductive cough, and dyspnea with hypoxia. It usually appears as interstitial infiltrate on chest x-ray. For these syndromes, a specific diagnosis requires a histologic demonstration of the characteristic intranuclear and intracytoplasmic inclusion bodies from suspected tissues. Culture of CMV from secretions and excretions is not sufficient to indicate that the CMV is causing the disease, given the fact that most patients with advanced HIV infection have CMV viremia. Histologic and clinical data should be correlated before concluding that CMV infection warrants specific antiviral therapy. Disease outside the retina may not require lifelong suppressive therapy; however, an aggressive search for retinal involvement should occur.

The current guidelines for prophylactic measures against CMV infection are changing with the availability of oral ganciclovir; clinical studies are ongoing.

Herpes simplex virus (HSV) is a frequent cause of morbidity in patients with HIV infection. As CD4[+] T cell counts decline, HSV infection recurs more frequently and for prolonged periods and with more severity. Transmission is by direct contact of infected secretions (oral or genital). Lesions of herpes appear first as painful erythematous papules; later they vesiculate and ulcerate, and pustular formation occurs when the lesions are superinfected. Oral/labial lesions may be caused by either HSV-1 or HSV-2. Lesions may involve the lips, buccal mucosa, gingiva, soft palate, and tongue. HSV-2 often causes outbreaks in the genitals and anal lesions. In advanced AIDS, extragenital involvement is common, including esophagitis, colitis, pneumonitis, retinitis, and encephalitis. Diagnosis is by the typical appearance and distribution of the lesions and by culture. Tzanck preparations show multinucleated giant cells. Some physicians base their diagnosis on how the patient responds to empirical therapy with acyclovir. Oral acyclovir (Zovirax), 400 mg orally three times per day, is effective for perirectal lesions, proctitis, esophagitis, oral lesions, and digital lesions. Intravenous therapy (10 to 12.4 mg per kg every 8 hours for 14 to 21 days) may be indicated in patients with more serious conditions such as disseminated or central nervous system HSV infections. The response to therapy is usually prompt and occurs within 3 to 10 days. Refractory herpetic lesions to acyclovir therapy may be related to acyclovir-resistant strains; these strains are usually also resistant to ganciclovir. Foscarnet has been used successfully against these strains. Toxicities associated with acyclovir include disorientation, hallucinations, tremors, seizures, and reversible renal dysfunction. Topical acyclovir has not shown beneficial results in patients with HIV infection. Relapse occurs with high frequency; chronic suppression may be indicated if relapses occur quite often. Acyclovir at a dose of 200 mg orally three times daily or 400 mg orally twice daily may be used for maintenance therapy.

Varicella-zoster virus (VZV) infection, or shingles, in HIV-infected individuals occurs as a result of reactivation of latent infection. Dermatomal outbreaks are common, and in advanced stages of HIV infection, they may involve several dermatomes; extracutaneous involvement (VZ retinitis, encephalitis) has been reported. VZV infection is characterized by radicular pain and pruritus several days prior to the appearance of erythematous papules, and later vesicle formation. Secondary bacterial infections are common. Involvement of the ophthalmic branch of the trigeminal nerve results in corneal lesions, leading to scarring and opacification of the cornea, resulting in visual impairment. Postherpetic neuralgia is common. Chronic herpes zoster is reported in HIV-infected patients, probably associated with acyclovir resistance. Chronic herpes zoster presents as sustained new lesion formation and nonhealing existing lesions. Visceral involvement is rare, even in HIV-infected patients with extensive disseminated cutaneous lesions. Treatment of dermatomal herpes zoster is not required, but it helps in the reduction of time to resolution of the lesions. Patients with persistent or recurrent lesions or zoster ophthalmicus are treated with high-dose oral acyclovir (800 mg orally five times daily or 10 to 12.4 mg per kg intravenously every eight hours). Patients with acyclovir-resistant VZV may benefit from foscarnet.

Epstein-Barr virus (EBV) is associated with oral hairy leukoplakia, which presents as a raised, white lesion on the surface of the tongue and buccal mucosa. Oral hairy leukoplakia consists of epithelium of keratinized cells. These lesions may be confused with *Candida*, but in contrast to *Candida*, oral hairy leukoplakia cannot be scraped off with a tongue blade. Oral hairy leukoplakia is usually asymptomatic, but it may impair taste and hinder eating if the lesion is large. Treatment is not indicated for oral hairy leukoplakia; it has a relatively high spontaneous remission rate (25 to 50%).

JC virus, a papovavirus, is the etiologic agent of progressive multifocal leukoencephalopathy (PML), which is an AIDS-defining illness and occurs in the late stage of HIV infection. In the United States, PML is reported in fewer than 1% of the patients with AIDS. PML is a demyelinating disease characterized by multiple, discrete foci of disease involving the cerebral white matter and sometimes the cerebellum and brain stem. Histologic findings result from direct infection of the oligodendrocytes with the JC virus leading to decreased myelin production and demyelination. Symptoms include headache, ataxia, confusion, visual field deficits, aphasia, and focal deficits without changes in mental status. CT scans reveal nonenhancing, low-density lesions of the periventricular white matter. MRI reveals high-signal-intensity lesions without enhancement. Definitive diagnosis requires brain biopsy. JC virus can be identified by electron microscopy, by immunofluorescence staining, or by PCR. Clinically, patients deteriorate progressively and death usually occurs within 3 to 6 months from the onset of symptoms. No effective therapy is currently available, but there have been reports that cytosine arabinoside and zidovudine may be beneficial.

Neoplastic Diseases

Kaposi's sarcoma (KS) is the most common neoplasm in HIV-infected patients. For unknown reasons, it occurs predominantly in HIV-infected homosexual men. The etiology of KS is still unknown. Current epidemiologic data and molecular evidence indicate the possibility of a infectious agent that is sexually transmitted may play a role in the development of KS. This evidence includes the association of KS with certain sexual practices such as anal sex among homosexual men, the decline in incidence of KS with changes in sexual behavior like practicing safe sex, and the identification of unique herpes-like virus DNA sequences in tissue samples from patients with KS. The tumor may be seen at any stage of HIV infection, even in patients with normal CD4$^+$ T lymphocyte cell counts. It is considered to be an endothelial neoplasm of either capillary or lymphatic origin. Histologically, the tumor consists of proliferation of vascular structures with malignant-appearing endothelial cells. Grossly, the KS lesions appear as nodular, reddish purple pigmentation and may appear simultaneously in widely scattered areas of the body and, in HIV-infected patients, involvement of visceral structures are common. The lesions may vary in size from a few millimeters to several centimeters.

Cutaneous KS is easily diagnosed by the appearance of the typical cutaneous lesions, but should be confirmed by biopsy. A punch biopsy is usually sufficient and safe and can be performed in the ambulatory setting with local anesthesia. Oral KS is common and usually involves the hard palate, posterior pharyngeal wall, gingiva, and tongue. Oral KS is usually asymptomatic. Large lesions cause obstruction and difficulty in swallowing, and with superficial necrosis lead to pain and bleeding.

Gastrointestinal involvement is the most common visceral KS. Any segment of the GI tract may be involved, but the stomach, duodenum, and rectum are the most common sites affected. Gastrointestinal Kaposi's is usually asymptomatic but may cause intestinal obstruction, enteropathy, and bleeding. Biliary tract involvement may lead to a clinical picture of obstructive jaundice. Diagnosis is made by endoscopy, visualizing the typical lesions. The tumor may be located subcutaneously and easily missed by biopsy.

Pulmonary KS is less common than GI involvement; however, it is usually symptomatic. Patients with pulmonary KS present with cough, chest tightness, and shortness of breath. Chest x-ray shows bilateral lower lobe infiltrates or interstitial infiltrates that obscure the margins of the mediastinum and diaphragm. Pleural effusions are seen in 70% of pulmonary KS. These effusions are frequently bloody, and cytologic examination is usually nondiagnostic. Gallium scanning shows no uptake, in contrast to those with infectious pneumonias. Diagnosis is made by bronchoscopy or open lung biopsy. When endobronchial lesions are visualized, transbronchial biopsy is contraindicated because lesions are vascular and hemorrhage is common.

Poor prognosis is associated in patients with multiple lesions; those with visceral and extensive oral lesions; patients with constitutional symptoms such as unexplained fever, night sweats, and weight loss; patients with low CD4$^+$ T cell counts and high p24 antigenemia; and patients with concurrent opportunistic infections.

Treatment should be individualized. Lesions that remain indolent do not require treatment. Patients with bulky and disfiguring lesions, facial lesions, or lesions subject to repeated trauma (i.e., overlying joints) can be managed by local treatment such as surgical excision or local radiation therapy, or topical and intralesional treatment. Radiation therapy shrinks the KS lesions and also reduces KS-associated lymphedema; however, it is associated with local toxicity such as radiation-induced mucositis and cutaneous erythema. Lesions tend to recur despite intensive radiation therapy. Topical or intralesional treatment such as cryotherapy with liquid nitrogen or intralesional injections of small amounts of dilute vinblastine have been associated with remarkable results.

Systemic chemotherapy is indicated for patients with multiple and extensive lesions and those with visceral lesions. Disadvantages of systemic chemotherapy include toxicities and side effects associated with the chemotherapeutic agents, further suppression of the immune system, and susceptibility to opportunistic infections. Vincristine, vinblastine, bleomycin, doxorubicin, etoposide, and interferon-α (IFN-α) are the chemotherapeutic agents available for use in the treatment of KS. Chemotherapeutic agents may be used singly or in combination. Response rate depends on the CD4$^+$ T cell count, especially when using IFN-α, where the response rate for patients with CD4$^+$ T cell counts of greater than 600 cells per μL is approximately 80% compared with a response rate of less than 10% for patients with CD4$^+$ T cell counts less than 150 cells per μL. Objective tumor response with IFN-α can be seen in 4 to 8

weeks. Because of its delayed response, IFN-α is not desirable for use during urgent and life-threatening situations such as laryngeal and extensive pulmonary KS. IFN-α has an added advantage because of its antiretroviral activity.

Non-Hodgkin's lymphoma (NHL) is the second most common neoplasm associated with HIV infection. It is seen in all risk groups and is usually a late manifestation of HIV infection. Approximately 90% are of B cell phenotype and of poor histologic types, either large cell, undifferentiated, or immunoblastic type. Etiology of HIV-associated NHL is still unknown. Genetic variants, derangement of immune systems, and infectious agents (particularly EBV) have been proposed.

Primary CNS lymphoma is one of the AIDS-defining diseases, usually a late manifestation of the HIV infection at CD4$^+$ T cell count less than 50 cells per μL. Patients with CNS lymphomas are EBV positive in most cases. Patients present with motor deficits and cranial nerve deficits, headache, and seizures. Imaging studies with either contrast-enhanced CT or MRI usually reveal a single, hyperdense lesion. The presence of multiple lesions does not rule out CNS lymphoma. MRI is more sensitive and is indicated if head CT is negative and there are clinical findings suggestive of intracranial mass lesions. If empirical therapy for toxoplasmosis (after 1 to 2 weeks of treatment) fails to show clinical improvement and fails to regress the size of the CNS lesions, a brain biopsy is indicated to establish the diagnosis of CNS lymphoma. NHL may involve any organ system, the GI tract, bone marrow, liver, or lungs. The GI tract is the second most common site of extranodal lymphomas; the disease may affect any segment. Patients present with obstructive symptoms or abdominal pain. Constitutional symptoms of fever, weight loss, diarrhea, and night sweats are common in patients with extranodal disease. Bone marrow involvement occurs in about 20% of patients and usually manifests as pancytopenia.

Diagnosis of NHL is made by biopsy. Clinical staging is indicated after diagnosis is made. Investigations include imaging of the head, chest, and abdomen; bone marrow aspiration with biopsy; and lumbar puncture. After staging is completed, therapy should be coordinated with the oncologist and initiated promptly. Prognosis is usually poor because most of the lymphomas in HIV-infected patients are of an aggressive histologic type. Patients with CNS NHL have median survival of 2 to 3 months after diagnosis, while patients with systemic lymphomas have a median survival of about 10 months.

There are no definitive or established guidelines for the treatment of HIV-associated NHL. Combinations of drug regimens are used; however, response rates are low and relapse rates are high. Mortality may be a direct result of lymphoma itself, a result of AIDS-related infections, or a result of chemotherapy-associated infections.

Other Neoplasms

Hodgkin's lymphoma is relatively common in HIV-infected patients. Hodgkin's disease is usually diagnosed at an advanced stage and is usually of mixed cellular or lymphocyte-depleted histology. It responds well to conventional therapy, but relapses are common.

Cervical and anal cancer are also common in HIV-infected patients. They are associated with human papillomavirus infection. Periodic rectal and routine annual pelvic examinations with Papanicolaou smears are indicated for patients with HIV infection for early detection of cellular dysplasia.

AMEBIASIS

method of
RODRIGO HASBUN, M.D., and
FRANK J. BIA, M.D., M.P.H.
Yale University School of Medicine
New Haven, Connecticut

Amebiasis is a disease process resulting from infections caused by the enteric protozoan *Entamoeba histolytica*. It is one of the major parasitic diseases of humans, affecting approximately 10% of the world's population, with the potential for approximately 50 million cases of invasive amebiasis and up to 100,000 deaths yearly. Amebiasis has a worldwide distribution, but it is more prevalent in countries with low levels of sanitation. High rates of amebiasis occur in India, Africa, the Far East, and in both Central and South America. In more developed countries, amebiasis is concentrated within certain high-risk groups, including travelers and immigrants from endemic regions, migrant workers, institutionalized and mentally retarded individuals, and promiscuous male homosexuals. *E. histolytica* is found in either its trophozoite or its cyst form. Infection is acquired most commonly by ingestion of food or water contaminated with cysts that are resistant to the acidic pH of the stomach. Trophozoites do not transmit this infection because they rapidly degenerate outside the body, and they are susceptible to the acid pH of the stomach. Person-to-person transmission through fecal-oral contact also occurs.

There are two distinct species of *Entamoeba* that are morphologically identical. *Entamoeba dispar,* the more prevalent species, is apparently associated only with an asymptomatic carrier state. The pathogenic species, now referred to as *E. histolytica,* clearly has the capacity to cause invasive disease. The two species are distinguished in the following ways: (1) the presence of ingested erythrocytes within *E. histolytica*; (2) an analysis of zymodemes, which are patterns of electrophoretic mobility of certain parasitic isoenzymes; (3) RNA and DNA probes; (4) presence of serum antiameba antibodies, indicating *E. histolytica* infection; and (5) the use of polymerase chain reaction (PCR) amplification in the detection of parasitic DNA from serum and feces is also under investigation. *E. dispar* infections are approximately 10-fold more common than those caused by *E. histolytica.* Symptomatic invasive amebiasis develops in approximately 10% of individuals with *E. histolytica* infection. Therefore, disease will develop in approximately 1% of individuals who are determined to be in any way infected with *Entamoeba* species by stool microscopy.

The major clinical manifestations of amebiasis are primarily evident in the colon and the liver, but other organs can be involved (Table 1). Intestinal amebiasis develops when *E. histolytica* invades the colonic epithelium and lyses mucosal cells. In approximately 10% of cases, pathogenic amebae enter the mesenteric circulation and reach the liver, causing an hepatic abscess to form, the most common extraintestinal manifestation of amebiasis.

INTESTINAL AMEBIASIS

As noted earlier, approximately 10% of individuals infected with amebae harbor the pathogenic strain, *E. histolytica,* and about 10% will develop invasive disease. The spectrum of intestinal disease ranges from mild diarrhea to fulminant colitis and death (see Table 1). Patients with acute amebic dysentery present with a 1- or 2-week history of crampy abdominal pain, tenesmus, and frequent, watery stools containing blood and mucus. About 30% of such patients have a low-grade fever. Fulminant colitis is an unusual complication of amebic dysentery, and it is associated with a high mortality rate, at times exceeding 50%. Such patients present with severe bloody diarrhea, high fever, rapid onset of abdominal pain, intestinal perforation, and peritoneal signs. This is a rare condition and is more likely to affect children, especially neonates, pregnant women, or patients who are malnourished, on chronic corticosteroid therapy, or have an underlying malignancy. *Chronic nondysenteric amebiasis can resemble inflammatory bowel disease, and a clear distinction between these conditions must be made before instituting corticosteroid therapy for presumed inflammatory bowel disease.*

Diagnosis

A diagnosis of intestinal amebiasis is made by detecting *E. histolytica* trophozoites, cysts, or both, in stool samples using light microscopy. Prior administration of bismuth-containing compounds, laxatives, antacids, hypertonic enemas, or antibiotics, such as tetracycline and erythromycin, will interfere with the detection of amebae in stools and should be avoided. Light microscopy cannot differentiate between *E. histolytica* (pathogenic) and *E. dispar* (non-pathogenic), unless the visualization of ingested erythrocytes clearly indicates infection with *E. histolytica.* Occult

TABLE 1. **Clinical Syndromes Associated with** *Entamoeba histolytica* **Infection**

Intestinal Disease

Asymptomatic infection
Symptomatic noninvasive infection
Acute rectocolitis (amebic dysentery)
Fulminant colitis with perforation
Toxic megacolon
Chronic nondysenteric colitis
Ameboma (inflammatory colonic mass mimics carcinoma)
Perianal ulceration

Extraintestinal Disease

Liver abscess
Liver abscess complicated by peritonitis
Liver abscess complicated by empyema
Liver abscess complicated by pericarditis
Lung abscess
Brain abscess
Genitourinary disease
Enterocutaneous fistula
Hepatopulmonary fistula

Modified from Ravdin JI: Clin Infect Dis 20:1457, 1995.

blood in stool can be detected in almost 100% of patients with amebic colitis, thus making it an effective screening test for invasive disease. Despite the presence of deep mucosal ulcerations and occult blood in stools, fecal leukocytes may not be found because they are lysed by parasites. Amebic serology is a useful diagnostic adjunct because serum antibodies develop only in the presence of *E. histolytica* infection; *E. dispar* does not elicit the production of detectable serum antiamebic antibodies. Detectable serum antibody levels usually appear about 1 week after the initiation of intestinal infections. Moreover, in endemic areas, the presence of antiamebic antibodies may not reflect active disease, because serum antibodies may persist for several years following both infection and its treatment.

TREATMENT OF INTESTINAL AMEBIASIS

Treatment of amebic infection is a complex issue, and the clinician may find it necessary to prescribe multiple agents to eradicate the parasite from both the bowel lumen and tissues. Therapy can be divided into two types: (1) eradication of cysts or lumen-dwelling trophozoites with a lumen-active agent, and (2) treatment of invasive disease with a tissue-active agent.

Treatment of Asymptomatic Cyst and Trophozoite Passers

Asymptomatic cyst passers who do not produce detectable antibodies to amebae are likely to have an infection with *E. dispar*. However, if serology is not available, in nonendemic areas, treatment of these individuals is advised. All individuals with *E. histolytica* infection should be treated, although in the developing world, where infection is endemic, the general accepted practice is to neither evaluate nor treat asymptomatic patients harboring amebae, given the cost and the high infection rate within the population. There is also a high risk of reinfection. Diloxanide furoate (Furamide) is the preferred agent for eradicating intraluminal infection. It is relatively nontoxic, and a 10-day course has an 85% success rate. In the United States, this agent is available from the Centers for Disease Control and Prevention (CDC: telephone 404-639-3670 or 404-639-2888); in Canada, it is available only with authorization of the Bureau of Drugs, Health Protection Branch, Ottawa (Table 2). Paromomycin (Humatin) is an oral nonabsorbable aminoglycoside agent that is also highly effective. It is safe to use in pregnancy, and the major side effect is mild diarrhea. Iodoquinol (diiodohydroxyquin [Yodoxin]) is equally effective as diloxanide furoate but must be administered for 20 days. In addition to gastrointestinal side effects, it may interfere with thyroid function tests because of its high iodine content. It has rarely been associated with neurotoxicity if given in high doses or for a prolonged time. Metronidazole (Flagyl) should not be used to treat asymptomatic cyst or trophozoite passers in general, because it often fails to completely eradicate all cysts from the bowel lumen.

TABLE 2. **Treatment of the Asymptomatic Cyst Passer**

Drug	Adult Dosage (PO)	Pediatric Dosage (PO)
Diloxanide furoate* (Furamide)	500 mg tid × 10 days	20 mg/kg/day† × 10 days (maximum 1500 mg/day)
Paromomycin (Humatin)	30 mg/kg/day† × 7 days	25 mg/kg/day† × 7 days (maximum 2 g/day)
Iodoquinol (Yodoxin)	650 mg tid × 20 days	30–40 mg/kg/day† × 20 days (maximum 2 g/day)

*In the United States, available only through the Centers for Disease Control and Prevention: telephone 404-639-3670; nights and emergencies, 404-639-2888. In Canada, authorized through the Bureau of Drugs, Health Protection Branch, Ottawa.
†Administered in three divided doses.
From Gamble K, Keystone JS: Amebiasis. *In* Rakel RE (ed): Conn's Current Therapy 1995. Philadelphia, WB Saunders Co, 1995, pp 53–55.

Treatment of Invasive Disease

Amebic Colitis

Metronidazole is the drug of choice for patients with invasive intestinal disease and/or an amebic liver abscess (Tables 3 and 4). It has a cure rate of 90%, and despite widespread use, metronidazole-resistant *E. histolytica* trophozoites have not been reported. The recommended duration of therapy for amebic colitis is 7 to 10 days, but recent studies indicate that 2.5 gm of metronidazole given orally once daily for 3 days is equally effective. Metronidazole is not recommended during pregnancy. Although

TABLE 3. **Treatment of Invasive Disease***

Drug	Adult Dosage	Pediatric Dosage
Metronidazole (Flagyl)†	750 mg tid × 5–10 days **Alternative** 2.5 gm once daily × 3 days	30–50 mg/kg/day‡ × 10 days (maximum 2250 mg/day)
Tinidazole (Fasigyn)‖	2 gm once daily × 3 days	50 mg/kg/day (max. 2 grams) × 3 days
Alternative Dehydroemetine§ (Mebadin)	1–1.5 mg/kg/day IM × 5 days (maximum 90 mg/day)	1–1.5 mg/kg/day IM × 5 days (maximum 90 mg/day)

*Treatment of intestinal disease is followed by a complete course of a luminal agent (e.g., diloxanide furoate) to eliminate intestinal colonization using the regimen in Table 2.
†May be administered intravenously if patient unable to take by mouth.
‡Administered in three divided doses.
§In the United States, available only through the Centers for Disease Control and Prevention: telephone 404-639-3670; nights and emergencies, 404-639-2888. In Canada, authorized through the Bureau of Drugs, Health Protection Branch, Ottawa.
‖Marketed outside of the United States and Canada.
From Gamble K, Keystone JS: Amebiasis. *In* Rakel RE (ed): Conn's Current Therapy 1995. Philadelphia, WB Saunders Co, 1995, pp 53–55.

TABLE 4. Treatment of Amebic Liver Abscess*

Drug of Choice	Adult Dosage	Pediatric Dosage
Metronidazole†	750 mg tid × 10 days or 2.5 gm orally stat	30–50 mg/kg/day‡ × 10 days
Alternative Dehydroemetine§ (Mebadin)	1–1.5 mg/kg/day IM × 5 days (maximum 90 mg/day)	1–1.5 mg/kg/day IM × 5 days (maximum 90 mg/day)

*Treatment of amebic liver abscess is followed by a complete course of a luminal agent (e.g., diloxanide furoate) to eliminate intestinal colonization using the regimen in Table 1.

†May be administered intravenously if patient unable to take by mouth.

‡Administered in three divided doses.

§In the United States, available only through the Centers for Disease Control and Prevention: telephone 404-639-3670; nights and emergencies, 404-639-2888. In Canada, authorized through the Bureau of Drugs, Health Protection Branch, Ottawa.

From Gamble K, Keystone JS: Amebiasis. *In* Rakel RE (ed): Conn's Current Therapy 1995. Philadelphia, WB Saunders Co, 1995, pp 53–55.

a long-term follow-up study of several thousand women inadvertently treated with metronidazole during pregnancy for trichomoniasis did not reveal any drug-related problems, adequate and well-controlled studies in humans have not been conducted (FDA pregnancy category B). Therapy of invasive amebic disease during pregnancy is warranted because of the risk of severe complications if therapy is withheld.

Up to one-third of the patients receiving metronidazole develop gastrointestinal symptoms such as nausea, metallic taste, and abdominal discomfort. Other side effects include headache, dark-colored urine, ataxia, confusion, and paresthesias. Patients taking metronidazole must avoid ingesting alcoholic beverages because of its disulfiram-like properties. Metronidazole can be administered orally or intravenously. For the treatment of invasive disease such as colitis or amebic abscess, a lumen-active agent should always be given, in conjunction with, or following therapy with metronidazole.

Outside the United States and Canada, tinidazole (Fasigyn)* is the preferred drug for the therapy of invasive disease because it has fewer gastrointestinal side effects. The recommended dose is 2 gm, or 50 mg per kg (max. 2 grams) orally, once daily, for 3 days, but a one-dose regimen has been shown to also be effective in the therapy of amebic liver abscess Tinidazole also must be followed by treatment with a lumen-active agent. Tetracycline or erythromycin, when combined with another lumen-active agent, has been an effective alternative for treating mild cases of amebic colitis in patients who are intolerant of metronidazole. This combination, however, will not eradicate trophozoites in the liver. Dehydroemetine (Mebadin) is rapidly amebicidal, but it is highly toxic, and up to 50% of patients develop gastrointestinal side effects; neuromuscular complaints and cardio-

toxicity are not uncommon. In the United States, it is available only through the CDC. Dehydroemetine must be given in a controlled and monitored hospital setting. Follow-up stool examinations should be performed after completing therapy to screen for treatment failures.

Amebic Liver Abscess

Patients with amebic liver abscess can either present acutely or subacutely. The acute presentation is characterized by a syndrome of less than 10 days' duration consisting of fever, right upper quadrant abdominal pain that can radiate to the shoulders, and painful hepatomegaly. Some patients present subacutely with a duration of more than 2 weeks. This syndrome consists of weight loss, hepatomegaly, and anemia; fever is less likely to occur. The diagnosis is suspected upon finding a space-occupying lesion in the liver either by ultrasound or CT scan. Amebic serology is positive in 94% of such patients but may be negative during the first week of symptoms. An antecedent history of diarrhea is present in less than 30% of the patients.

Amebic liver abscess is usually managed by medical therapy alone (see Table 4). Metronidazole is the drug of choice, but it should be followed by diloxanide furoate or another lumen-active agent. The mortality rate due to an uncomplicated amebic liver abscess is less than 1%. In uncomplicated mild to moderate cases, single-dose therapy with 2.5 gm of metronidazole has been effective. The recommended duration of therapy is 5 to 10 days, and the majority of patients have symptomatic improvement within 3 to 5 days. Patients who do not improve in 3 days, as evidenced by persistence of fever, right upper quadrant pain, and constitutional symptoms, should undergo aspiration of the abscess for diagnostic and therapeutic indications. Drainage is also indicated for a ruptured abscess, as is drainage of any left hepatic lobe abscess that has the potential for involving the pericardium, or if any abscess is so large as to risk rupture due to a thin capsule of liver. Aspiration can be accomplished either at surgery or percutaneously. Chloroquine phosphate (Aralen) has amebicidal properties and achieves high levels in hepatic tissue. It has been used in conjunction with metronidazole for therapy of critically ill patients with an amebic abscess. There are, however, no controlled studies indicating improved outcome when compared with other agents. Patients should be followed for at least 6 months. A residual cavity can persist in up to 20% of patients, yet this is not an indication for repeated therapy or aspiration if the patient is asymptomatic. Antiamebic antibodies may persist for 2 or more years following effective therapy.

---

*Not available in the United States.

GIARDIASIS

method of
MICHELLE H. WOODARD, M.D., and
RICHARD A. DAVIDSON, M.D., M.P.H.
University of Florida
Gainesville, Florida

The intestinal protozoan *Giardia lamblia* poses both diagnostic and therapeutic challenges for medical practitioners. Giardiasis is typically a small intestine disease caused by the flagellate protozoan *Giardia lamblia,* alternatively known as *G. duodenalis* and *G. intestinalis.* While giardiasis is the most common pathogenic parasitic infection in the United States, there is wide variation in its geographic distribution, making it difficult to estimate a worldwide prevalence. Some developing countries have reported overall population infection rates as high as 40%, and in the United States, attack rates in day care centers have ranged from 15% to 50%. High-density populations and overcrowding appear to contribute to an increased prevalence of giardiasis.

EPIDEMIOLOGY AND PATHOGENESIS

Transmission of giardiasis has been associated with ingestion of ineffectively filtered or pretreated surface water; person-to-person contact (fecal-oral transmission in day care centers, and transmission between male homosexual contacts), exposure to beavers, muskrats, and domestic animals; and ingestion of contaminated foods such as unwashed raw vegetables.

The pathogenesis of giardiasis remains poorly understood. Host factors such as nutritional status, and both mucosal and systemic immunity, contribute to the degree of tissue damage, which ranges from minimal mucosal changes to enterocyte damage, villous atrophy, and crypt hyperplasia. Other mechanisms of pathogenesis may include toxin secretion, superinfection, and inflammation. All the tissue changes identified in association with giardiasis reverse with therapy.

Trophozoites (the intestinal dwelling stage) attach securely to host intestinal epithelium and undergo mitosis within the intestinal lumen; they detach from the epithelium every 72 hours by villous sloughing. A few become encysted and are passed in the host feces, where they can be transmitted to a new host by ingestion. New organisms emerge from these cysts in the new host's duodenum and mature by an arrested mitotic division.

Trophozoites can be detected in the duodenum and proximal jejunum of infected patients; in patients who develop vitamin B_{12} malabsorption, it has been hypothesized that the terminal ileum may also be infected. The onset of symptoms follows an incubation period of 12 to 19 days.

DIAGNOSIS

Clinical manifestations vary widely. For reasons that are unclear, many people living in endemic areas are asymptomatic carriers who pass cysts in their stools. Acute, symptomatic infection can be transient or persistent and is characterized by diarrhea, flatulence, eructation, abdominal cramps, distention, fatigue, anorexia, nausea, steatorrhea, and weight loss.

Subacute or chronic infection of the intestine can result in recurrent episodes of frothy stools alternating with normal stools or even constipation, abdominal distention, fla-

tus, mid to upper epigastric or substernal burning, and sulfuric eructation. This infection can involve the stomach, gallbladder, urinary tract, and, rarely, the pancreas and can mimic peptic ulcer disease, biliary colic, bacterial cystitis, and pancreatitis.

Acute diarrhea due to *Giardia* must be differentiated from that caused by other bacterial, viral, and protozoal agents. The absence of blood or mucus in the stool, presence of upper abdominal cramping, distention, and foul odor of feces and gas suggest giardiasis. Chronic diarrhea due to giardiasis must be differentiated from that caused by other intestinal parasites, inflammatory bowel disease, celiac disease, other malabsorptive illnesses, and the irritable bowel syndrome.

Diagnosis has traditionally been based on examinations of several stool samples, but if stool studies are negative and clinical suspicion is high, examination of duodenal aspirate (collected by endoscopy or the "string test") or biopsy material may be necessary. Some practitioners treat giardiasis empirically if stool studies are unrevealing and clinical suspicion is high.

Recent advances that appear to be more sensitive than stool examination include direct detection of the entire organism or one of its antigens by indirect immunofluorescence or enzyme-linked immunosorbent assays, and the use of markers such as DNA probes in the diagnosis of some cases of *Giardia lamblia.* These methods fail to identify other parasites that may be simultaneously infecting an individual and may be best utilized in tandem with stool studies for ova and parasites.

TREATMENT

The World Health Organization advocates the use of the nitroimidazoles metronidazole (Flagyl), tinidazole, ornidazole, and nimorazole for giardiasis based on their efficacy and tolerability. Metronidazole is the only nitroimidazole currently available in the United States. Drugs available in the United States for monotherapy of *Giardia lamblia* infection include metronidazole, furazolidone (Furoxone), albendazole, and paromomycin (Humatin) (Table 1). Both metronidazole and furazolidone have been associated with hemolysis in glucose-6-phosphate dehydrogenase–deficient individuals.

TABLE 1. **Dosages of Antigiardial Agents Available in the United States**

Drug	Adult Dose	Pediatric Dose
Metronidazole* (Flagyl)	250 mg tid for 5 d	15 mg/kg/d in 3 doses for 5 d
Furazolidone (Furoxone)	100 mg qid for 7 d	5 mg/kg/d in 4 divided doses for 10 d
Albendazole†	400 mg/d for 5 d	400 mg/d for 5 d
Paromomycin‡ (Humatin)	30 mg/kg/d in 3 divided doses for 7 d	—

*Considered investigational by the FDA for this usage.
†Available for compassionate use only from manufacturer.
‡Safe in first trimester of pregnancy.

Metronidazole, while still not FDA approved for treatment of giardiasis in the United States, is relatively well tolerated. Side effects include a metallic taste, lassitude, nausea, drowsiness, rare peripheral neuropathy, and a disulfiram-like interaction with alcohol. The usual adult dosage is 250 mg three times daily for 5 days. Single-dose courses of metronidazole have been associated with high failure rates and are not recommended.

Furazolidone, a derivative of nitrofurantoin, is minimally absorbed, available in suspension form, and therefore useful in pediatric populations. A mild monoamine oxidase inhibitor, its side effects include nausea, vomiting, diarrhea, and lassitude. Adult dosage is 100 mg four times daily for 7 days. Pediatric dosage is 5 mg per kg per day in four divided doses for 10 days.

At a pediatric dosage of 400 mg per day for 5 days, albendazole, a broad-spectrum anthelmintic, was shown to be as effective as metronidazole, but it is available in the United States only for compassionate use. Its most common side effects are loose stools and the passage of worms in patients concomitantly infected with intestinal nematodes.

Paromomycin, a nonabsorbable aminoglycoside, has some antigiardial activity but is not as efficacious as the aforementioned agents. Its utility has been primarily as an agent safe in the first trimester of pregnancy, if treatment is absolutely required. Dosage is 30 mg per kg per day in 3 divided doses for 7 days. It has been suggested that pregnant women delay antigiardial therapy until after delivery, if possible. For cases requiring therapy when paromomycin has failed in the pregnant population, metronidazole is recommended.

Quinacrine sulfate, the first clearly effective antigiardial medication, is no longer available in the United States; in other parts of the world it is not as widely used as it once was, largely due to its common side effects of nausea, vomiting, and abdominal cramping; its occasional side effects of yellow discoloration of the skin, sclera, and urine; and its rare side effects of exfoliative dermatitis and toxic psychosis.

Alternative medications widely used worldwide but not available in the United States include tinidazole and ornidazole, which are effective in single-dose regimens. Combination therapy, while not commonly used, may be an option for recalcitrant giardiasis. Azithromycin-furazolidone and doxycycline-mefloquine have shown promise in vitro by virtue of their ability to inhibit adherence of trophozoites to Dacron fiber microcolumns. Recently it has been shown that tricyclic antidepressant drugs bind to a *Giardia* protein and inhibit growth in vitro ten times more effectively than metronidazole, suggesting a possible role for these drugs as novel therapeutic agents against giardiasis.

Asymptomatic Carriers

Controversy exists as to the treatment of asymptomatic cyst passers. Treatment has been recommended where good sanitation exists and reinfection is unlikely, largely to avoid development of symptomatic infection in the individual and outbreaks of giardiasis in those exposed to the carrier, especially if the carrier is a food handler. In the day care center population, if strict handwashing and treatment of symptomatic children fail to eradicate infection, treatment of all infected children is a consideration.

TREATMENT FAILURE

For giardial infections that do not appear to respond to appropriate therapy, confirmation of ongoing infection may be necessary. Postinfection lactose intolerance due to disacchacharidase deficiency can mimic continuing infection. The recurrence of symptoms after re-exposure, 10 to 12 days after therapy has been completed, suggests reinfection, whereas symptom recurrence closer to therapy cessation suggests treatment failure. Although reinfection can be treated with the same drug, failure of therapy due to apparent drug resistance warrants switching to another class of therapeutic agents. Hypogammaglobulinemia should be considered in patients failing repeated courses of therapy. These patients may require combination therapy or chronic suppressive therapy. A few strains of *Giardia* found to be resistant to metronidazole and furazolidone have been treated successfully with azithromycin, but its wide variation in efficacy among different strains precludes its use in general.

PREVENTION

Proper treatment of community water supplies, good personal hygiene, and appropriate disposal of human and animal wastes are important in preventing the spread of giardiasis. Wilderness hikers and overseas travelers can disinfect small volumes of water for personal consumption by boiling for at least 10 minutes (longer at higher altitudes). If boiling is not possible, kits are available for halogenating water with either iodine or chlorine, and filters can eliminate *Giardia* and enteric bacteria if the pore size is less than 2 μm.

To eliminate fecal-oral transmission, strict attention to handwashing should be observed, especially for those who change diapers. Exclusion of infected children from day care centers has not been shown to decrease rates of infection. Venereal transmission can be decreased by avoiding oral-anal or oral-genital contact.

BACTEREMIA AND SEPSIS

method of
WILLIAM M. VALENTI, M.D.
Rochester, New York

BACTEREMIA

Bacteremia occurs in a variety of clinical settings and may be transient, intermittent, or sustained.

The portal of entry can be the skin, oral cavity, genitourinary tract, respiratory tract, mucous membranes of the gastrointestinal tract, or medical devices (intravascular catheters, shunts, etc). Transient bacteremia is of short duration, is self-limited, and can be of little clinical significance. It can occur after brushing teeth, dental procedures, bowel movements, sexual intercourse in women, or after procedures such as upper or lower endoscopy or cystoscopy. The precise duration of transient bacteremia is hard to define, but it is generally agreed that this time is measured in minutes (≤ 15 minutes) rather than hours or days.

Intermittent bacteremias are those with multiple, intermittently positive blood cultures in the absence of therapy. They are usually due to a definable cause such as obstruction of infected urinary or biliary tracts, presence of abscess, or repeated manipulation or procedures in a contaminated area.

Sustained bacteremia is a continuous bacteremia with multiple positive blood cultures taken over several hours or days. The classic sustained bacteremias are intravascular infections, involving arteries, veins, arteriovenous shunts, or heart valves. Sustained bacteremias will often involve one of the numerous types of intravascular catheters. Bacteremia can be either primary or secondary. Primary bacteremia refers to bacteremia without any infected focus outside the bloodstream. Secondary bacteremias are those that are the result of some identifiable focus, such as an abscess or intravascular catheter.

When bacteria enter the bloodstream, a rapid systemic response occurs with phagocytosis, usually involving polymorphonuclear cells, to contain the infection. The host response of ingestion and killing of bacteria can be augmented by immunoglobulins or complement, or both.

In some patients, depending on a variety of patient factors, including the immune response, severity of underlying illness, and nutritional state, among others, bacteremia may also evolve to sepsis and shock. Sepsis refers to the physiologic manifestations of bacteremia. Fever, shaking chills, apprehension, hyperventilation with associated respiratory alkalosis, changes in mental status, and leukocytosis are a part of the clinical picture of sepsis. On occasion, patients will be hypothermic.

In septic shock, there will also be evidence of hypoperfusion, including a drop in blood pressure (<90 mmHg systolic or a one-third decrease over previous systolic measurements) and decreased urine output. Decreased platelet count and evidence of bleeding are also seen.

When bacteremia is suspected, it requires sound clinical judgment and a quick response for evaluation and treatment.

Evaluation of the Patient

A careful physical examination is an important part of the evaluation of the patient with proven or suspected bacteremia and may provide some clues that will help direct treatment and further evaluation. The skin is a good place to start, paying careful attention to skin or soft tissue infections, needle injection marks, lacerations, abrasions, or other disruptions of the integument.

In addition, some types of bacteremia will occasionally manifest with secondary manifestations on the skin. The classic ecthyma gangrenosum of *Pseudomonas aeruginosa* presents as an ulcerated central lesion with an area of erythema around it.

Meningococcemia and *Staphylococcus aureus* occasionally have similar petechial lesions that may appear ecchymotic or purpural. Scrapings of these lesions may show bacteria on Gram's stain. In infective endocarditis, peripheral manifestations such as splinter hemorrhages in nail beds; Roth's spots, hemorrhagic retinal lesions; Janeway's lesions, painless plaques of the palms or soles; and conjunctival petechiae may be seen.

Any medical devices should also be considered as the portal of entry for bacteria. In particular, intravascular catheters should be inspected for evidence of infection at the exit site and tunnel. Peripheral vessels should be examined for evidence of erythema, tenderness, and pus. However, bacteremia may be due to intravascular devices in the absence of these signs.

Blood cultures should be obtained to assist in diagnosis. The traditional method involves taking one set of cultures, usually consisting of two bottles (an aerobic bottle and anaerobic bottle), on at least two occasions, 30 minutes or so apart. In addition, when the possibility of intravascular catheter infection exists, one set of cultures should also be drawn through the catheter itself. Blood culture sets should be labeled with the date and time drawn, as well as the source of the culture (peripheral blood, catheter, etc.). This will allow for easier interpretation of results later on.

A single blood culture set has a sensitivity of 80 to 90%. Three sets of blood cultures approach 100% sensitivity. Sensitivity will be determined by the amount of blood taken. The recommended volume is 10 mL per culture set. In general, not more than three sets of blood cultures drawn in a 24-hour period are needed to diagnose bacteremia, except in cases in which antibiotics have been used prior to obtaining cultures. Cultures will become positive within 24 hours about 66% of the time, and will be positive within 72 hours about 90% of the time.

In the febrile patient with AIDS and a low CD4 count (i.e., ≤ 50), one should suspect infection with nontuberculous mycobacteria (e.g., *Mycobacterium avium* complex [MAC]). Blood cultures that are plated on solid media such as the Dupont or Bactec systems are necessary if MAC is suspected. In the case of MAC, bacteremia is most often sustained and it is customary to draw only one tube for MAC isolation, in addition to the routine aerobic and anaerobic cultures.

The so-called isolator blood culture systems also support the growth of fungi and certain gram-negative rods, most notably *Salmonella* species. While fungi and gram-negative bacteria can be isolated within the time frame noted previously for routine aerobic and anaerobic blood cultures, mycobacteria may take as long as several weeks.

Interpretation of Blood Culture Results

A careful analysis of blood culture data can help with accurate clinical assessment and appropriate treatment decisions. When interpreting blood culture results, it is necessary to have complete information on Gram's stain characteristics and/or organism identification, which bottles were positive (aerobic, anaerobic, or both), the source of culture (peripheral blood or catheter), and the date and time of collection. Complete data will help with treatment decisions, support the diagnosis of true bacteremia, and help rule out contamination. It is also helpful to know which bottles remain negative, in order to better distinguish between patterns of bacteremia (transient, intermittent, continuous) and contamination. Contamination of blood cultures, which usually occurs at the time of collection, is most often attributed to gram-positive organisms such as coagulase-negative *Staphylococcus* or a variety of *Staphylococcus* species, including *Staphylococcus epidermidis*. With contamination, the most common pattern of blood culture positivity is one or two bottles positive for one or more species of coagulase-negative *Staphylococcus*.

However, the patient with an infected intravascular catheter is likely to have bacteremia with these organisms, presenting a diagnostic dilemma in terms of the distinction between true infection and contamination. In general, the likelihood of true bacteremia is increased as the number of bottles that are positive (aerobic and anaerobic) increases, as the same organisms are found in blood cultures drawn from different sites and/or at different times, and with increasing amounts of bacteria found in quantitative or semiquantitative blood cultures. In addition to intravascular devices, common scenarios in which bacteremia is seen include bacteremia secondary to meningitis, upper respiratory infection (e.g., otitis media, sinusitis), pneumonia, intra-abdominal infection, skin or soft tissue infection, or urinary tract infection.

Treatment

Therapy for bacteremia is often empirical, since the diagnosis, when suspected, requires prompt, empirical intervention. Such empirical therapy can be life-saving. Once the diagnosis of bacteremia is confirmed and the organism(s) and sensitivities are identified, antibiotic management will be more precise and less empirical.

Initiation of therapy for possible bacteremia requires a high index of suspicion in the patient with a change in clinical status, as noted previously. Empirical therapy for bacteremia will be guided by the patient's clinical history and physical examination. Specific information regarding the patient's age, un-

derlying illness, recent surgical or other invasive procedures, travel history, life habits (use of injection drugs, nutritional habits), possible risks for HIV infection, and recent antibiotic use should be obtained. Suggestions for empirical management are shown in Table 1. Recent medication changes should also be noted as part of the evaluation for drug fever. In some cases, the patient may not be able to provide this history because of confusion or obtundation, and these data may need to be obtained from other sources, such as the medical record or family members. History of underlying illnesses can also provide clues to the nature of bacteremia and provide direction for antibiotic management (Table 2).

During the empirical phase of treatment for bacteremia, it is important to provide coverage that is as broad as possible to ensure that the most likely bacterial etiologies are covered (see Table 1). It is also important to select antibiotics that take into account the possibility of antibiotic resistance. Later, when bacterial etiologies are determined, therapy can be adjusted more precisely, often by discontinuing antibiotics that are believed to be unnecessary. Finally, completed blood culture reports will allow for focused therapy based on identification of the offending bacteria and sensitivity patterns.

In addition to blood cultures, other appropriate laboratory studies should be performed prior to initiating therapy. These studies include complete blood count; urinalysis; chest roentgenogram; and cultures of urine, sputum, and cerebrospinal fluid, if clinically indicated. Imaging scans by computed tomography (CT), magnetic resonance imaging (MRI), or gallium scans may also be helpful in identifying abscesses. Collection or drainage of abscesses for Gram's stain examination and culture should also be performed prior to initiating therapy, if possible. However, in severely ill patients, it is important not to withhold treatment while awaiting the results of these diagnostic procedures.

As shown in Table 1, in patients without an obvious site of infection, empirical coverage should cover both gram-positive and gram-negative bacteria, since it is not possible to distinguish between the two groups of organisms clinically. Broad coverage, in these cases, includes more than one antibiotic. This approach will maximize coverage for both gram-positive and gram-negative organisms, and antibiotic-resistant bacteria. This is especially important when treating suspected hospital-acquired infections, suspected intra-abdominal sepsis, and when treating the immunocompromised host. Combination therapy is also essential when treating patients with suspected bacteremia who have more than one possible source of infection (e.g., the patient with possible abdominal sepsis and an intravascular line in place). Other helpful information in antibiotic selection includes organisms and sensitivities isolated previously from cultures in the same patient or, in hospitalized or recently hospitalized patients, bacteria endemic to the facility (e.g., oxacillin-resistant *Staphylococcus aureus* [ORSA]). In the less severely ill patient, it

TABLE 1. **Empirical Antibiotic Therapy for Bacteremia Based on Suspected Site of Primary Infection***

Meningitis†		
Adult	*Streptococcus pneumoniae, Neisseria meningitidis*	Ceftriaxone (Rocephin), cefotaxime (Claforan)
Postneurosurgical	*Enterobacteriaceae, Pseudomonas aeruginosa, Staphylococcus aureus, Staphylococcus epidermidis*	Ceftazidime (Fortaz) or antipseudomonal penicillin‡ plus aminoglycosides§ plus vancomycin (Vancocin)
Pneumonia†		
Community acquired	*Streptococcus pneumoniae, Haemophilus influenzae,* mouth anaerobes, *Legionella* and other atypical bacteria	Cefuroxime or cefotaxime plus erythromycin if atypical pneumonia is suspected
Hospital acquired	*Enterobacteriaceae, Pseudomonas aeruginosa, Staphylococcus aureus*‖	Ceftazidime or antipseudomonal penicillin plus aminoglycoside
Endocarditis		
Native valve (acute)	*Enterococcus, Staphylococcus aureus, Streptococcus pneumoniae*	Vancomycin or penicillin plus nafcillin‖ plus gentamicin
Native valve (subacute)	*Enterococcus, Streptococcus bovis, Streptococcus viridans*	Penicillin G or ampicillin‖ plus gentamicin
Prosthetic valve (early)	*Enterobacteriaceae, Staphylococcus aureus, Staphylococcus epidermidis*	Vancomycin plus gentamicin plus third-generation cephalosporin¶
Intravenous drug user	*Enterobacteriaciae, Staphylococcus aureus*	Nafcillin‖ plus gentamicin plus antipseudomonal third-generation cephalosporin**
Urinary Tract†		
Community acquired	*Enterobacteriacae, Enterococcus*	Ampicillin plus gentamicin (trimethoprim/sulfamethoxazole or third-generation cephalosporin or quinolone†† if no gram-positive cocci on Gram's strain)
Hospital acquired or recurrent	*Enterobacteriaceae, Pseudomonas aeruginosa, Enterococcus*	Third-generation cephalosporin or antipseudomonal penicillin plus aminoglycoside
Gastrointestinal Tract		
Bowel or hepatobiliary	*Enterobacteriaceae,* anaerobes, *Enterococcus*	Clindamycin (Cleocin) or metronidazole (Flagyl) plus aminoglycoside
Primary peritonitis	*Enterobacteriaceae, Streptococcus pneumoniae,* group A streptococci	Aminoglycoside plus ampicillin; or cefoxitin (Mefoxin), or ampicillin/sulbactam (Unasyn), alone
Skin and Soft Tissue		
Wound infection	*Staphylococcus aureus, Enterobacteriaceae, Staphylococcus epidermidis*	Vancomycin plus aminoglycoside or third-generation cephalosporin
Primary cellulitis	*Staphylococcus aureus, Streptococci*	Nafcillin or first-generation cephalosporin (Mefoxin),
Gynecologic Infection		
Endometritis	Enterobacteriaceae, Groups A and B streptococci, *Bacteroides* sp., esp. *Bacteroides bivivus*	Clindamycin or metronidazole plus aminoglycoside or third-generation cephalosporin
Pelvic inflammatory disease	*Neisseria gonorrhoeae, Chlamydia trachomatis, Bacteroides* sp., Enterobacteriaceae, streptococci	Cefoxitin or ampicillin/sulbactam plus doxycycline
Neutropenic Host	*Enterobacteriaceae, Pseudomonas aeruginosa*	Antipseudomonal third-generation cephalosporin or antipseudomonal penicillin plus aminoglycoside
Catheter-Related Sepsis	*Staphylococcus epidermidis, Staphylococcus aureus,* Enterobacteriaceae, *Pseudomonas aeruginosa*	Vancomycin plus antipseudomonal third-generation cephalosporin
Unidentified Site	Enterobacteriaceae, *Staphylococcus aureus,* streptococci	Aminoglycoside plus third-generation cephalosporin, ± clindamycin or metronidazole

*Initial therapy should be modified and simplified if possible when culture results are known.
†Base therapy on Gram's stain when possible.
‡Antipseudomonal penicillins and related compounds include ticarcillin (Ticar), pipericillin (Pipracil), mezlocillin (Mezlin), imipenem/cilastatin (Primaxin), ticarcillin/clavulanate (Timentin), and piperacillin/tazobactam (Zosyn).
§Aminoglycosides include gentamicin, tobramycin (Nebcin), amikacin (Amikin).
‖Use vancomycin if high risk for methicillin-resistant *S. aureus* or penicillin allergic.
¶Third-generation cephalosporins and related compounds include ceftazidime, cefoperazone (Cefobid), ceftriaxone (Rocephin), ceftizoxime (Cefizox), and cefotaxime (Claforan).
**Antipseudomonal third-generation cephalosporins and equivalents include ceftazidime, cefoperazone (Cefobid), aztreonam (Azactam), quinolones.
††Parenteral quinolones include ciprofloxacin (Cipro) and ofloxacin (Floxin).
Modified from Horowitz HW, Marisiddiah H: Bacteremia. *In* Rakel RE (ed): Conn's Current Therapy 1995. Philadelphia, WB Saunders Co, 1995, p 57.

TABLE 2. **Epidemiologic and Immunologic Risks for Specific Organisms Causing Bacteremia**

Bites	
Human	*Eikenella corrodens*
Cat	*Pasteurella multocida*
Dog	*Capnocytophagia canimorus*
After splenectomy	*Streptococcus pneumoniae, Neisseria meningitidis, Haemophilus influenzae*
Sickle cell anemia	*Haemophilus influenzae, Salmonella* sp., *Streptococcus pneumoniae*
Neutropenia	*Corynebacterium jekeium, Clostridium tertium, Clostridium septicum*
Late component complement deficiency	*Neisseria meningitidis*
Chronic granulomatous disease	*Staphylococcus aureus*
Multiple myeloma and other humoral immune deficiencies	*Streptococcus pneumoniae, Haemophilus influenzae, Neisseria meningitidis, Escherichia coli*
Cellular immune deficiencies	*Listeria monocytogenes, Salmonella* sp.
AIDS	*Salmonella* sp., *Staphylococcus aureus, Haemophilus influenzae, Streptococcus pneumoniae, Pseudomonas aeruginosa, Mycobacterium avium* complex (MAC)
Rheumatoid arthritis	*Staphylococcus aureus*
Burn	*Pseudomonas aeruginosa, Staphylococcus aureus,* Enterobacteriaceae
Toxic shock	*Staphylococcus aureus,* Group A streptococcus
Pregnancy	Group B streptococci, *Listeria monocytogenes*
Achlorhydria/postgastrectomy	*Salmonella* sp.
Exposure to raw shellfish or brackish water	*Vibrio* sp.
Flea bite or contaminated meat ingestion	*Yersinia pestis*
Contact with body fluid or tissue of infected mammal or bite by infected arthropod (tick)	*Francisella tularensis*
Ingestion of unpasteurized milk or cheese, direct contact with contaminated tissues of cattle or swine	*Brucella*
Ingestion of unpasteurized milk or cheese	*Listeria monocytogenes, Salmonella*

Abbreviation: AIDS, acquired immune deficiency syndrome.
Modified from Horowitz HW, Marisiddiah H: Bacteremia. *In* Rakel RE (ed): Conn's Current Therapy 1995. Philadelphia, WB Saunders Co, 1995, p 58.

may be appropriate to use a very broad spectrum agent, such as carbapenem imipenem-cilastatin (Primaxin).

Because of the urgent nature of treatment, intravenous therapy is required for initial management of bacteremia. Other considerations in choosing therapy include the following:

1. The need for synergistic combination therapy. In these cases, the additive effects of combination therapy are greater than that achieved by either drug alone. Infections due to enterococcus or *Pseudomonas aeruginosa* require synergistic combinations of appropriate penicillins (e.g., ampicillin and anti-*Pseudomonas* penicillins, respectively) to weaken the cell wall, and an aminoglycoside, which acts at the ribosomal level.

2. Induction of resistance with single-agent therapy. This is commonly seen with infections due to *P. aeruginosa, Serratia*, and *Enterobacter* spp. In these cases, combination therapy is preferred to minimize the induction of resistance.

3. Epidemiology of antibiotic sensitivity and resistance that are unique to a particular health facility. Most microbiology laboratories will have this information available as a part of their ongoing monitoring of bacterial susceptibilities.

4. Differences in offending organisms and antibiotic susceptibility between hospital-acquired (nosocomial) and community-acquired infections. Nosocomial infections are more likely to involve organisms that are resistant to multiple antibiotics, as well as a higher frequency of infections due to gram-negative bacilli and methicillin/oxacillin-resistant *Staphylococcus aureus.*

5. Limitations in penetration of antibiotics. For example, first- and third-generation cephalosporin and aminoglycoside antibiotics penetrate the cerebrospinal fluid poorly. Second-generation cephalosporins such as cefuroxime (Ceftin) and cefoperazone (Cefobid) are exceptions.

6. Combination therapy to shorten the duration of treatment. Infective endocarditis with highly sensitive *Streptococcus viridans* (minimal inhibitory concentrations ≤ 0.1 μg per mL) can be treated with penicillin and an aminoglycoside for 2 weeks instead of 4 weeks.

Once antibiotic therapy has been started, the patient should be monitored for signs of clinical response. Treatment failure includes lack of clinical improvement and persistence of positive blood cultures despite therapy. Persistence of bacteremia suggests that there is a source of infection that has not been identified, requires drainage or removal, or that antibiotic coverage is inadequate.

Peak and trough antibiotic levels should be monitored, usually after the third dose, and adjusted as necessary. Aminoglycoside drugs and vancomycin are usually monitored this way because of their renal clearance and tendency to accumulate to toxic doses if left unmonitored. In recent years, continuous infusion of aminoglycoside drugs has become another method of aminoglycoside use and may avoid the peak and valley phenomenon of intermittent dosing. Monitoring for other possible drug toxicities should also be performed; these include rashes, cytopenias, nephrotoxicity, and diarrhea (e.g., *Clostridium difficile* and others).

Part of the therapy for bacteremia may also include débridement of devitalized tissue, drainage of abscesses or other areas of localized infection, and removal of any offending devices, most commonly an infected intravascular catheter. The longer intravascular devices are left in place, the more likely they are to be a cause of infection. The risk of infection with standard peripheral catheters (e.g., heparin locks or similar devices) increases significantly after 3 days in place. Other lines that are designed to be in place for longer periods—peripheral intravenous central catheters (PICC lines) or central lines, Hickman catheters, and central port access devices—can stay in place considerably longer than 3 days without risk of infection (i.e., weeks to months). In some cases, especially in patients with limited intravascular access, it may be possible to treat bacteremia with the intravascular device left in place. However, most clinicians experienced at treating device-related bacteremias will attempt to remove the offending device and move it to another site.

Duration of therapy will be determined by the organism isolated, severity of underlying illness, severity of bacteremia, and its complications. Treatment of primary bacteremia usually differs from that of secondary bacteremias. In uncomplicated primary bacteremia, intravenous therapy is continued for 1 to 2 weeks. *S. aureus* bacteremia, with or without an indwelling device, is usually treated for 4 weeks because of the possibility of development of infective endocarditis with shorter courses of treatment, even on normal heart valves. In some cases of uncomplicated *S. aureus* catheter-associated bacteremia, if the catheter is removed and the patient has an appropriate clinical response and defervescence within 3 days, 10 to 14 days of antibiotic therapy is appropriate.

In some uncomplicated cases of primary bacteremia, it may also be possible to complete therapy in an ambulatory setting (i.e., at home). This requires careful evaluation of the patient in terms of adequate response to inpatient therapy. In addition, ambulatory follow-up therapy requires that the patient be clinically stable and afebrile for 72 or more hours in hospital. Home antibiotics also require a convenient regimen (e.g., drugs given no more than twice daily), good intravenous access, a compliant patient with demonstrated ability to administer antibiotics, a home care agency experienced with home infusion therapy, and regular medical follow-up.

Secondary bacteremias, because of the need to treat the underlying source of infection, may require more prolonged therapy. In the neutropenic host, treatment is usually continued for the duration of neutropenia or until a specific infection has been treated, whichever is longer. In some neutropenic patients, therapy may be discontinued earlier if the patient remains clinically stable, afebrile, and has negative blood cultures. However, such patients still require close medical surveillance in the event that bacteremia recurs later on.

Occasionally, oral therapy may be used after the patient becomes clinically stable and afebrile for 72 hours. This is often done after treatment of urosepsis using the quinolone group of antibiotics (ciprofloxacin [Cipro] or ofloxacin [Floxin]), which are well absorbed and have a suitably broad spectrum of antibacterial activity.

SEPSIS

Sepsis is a clinical term that describes the physiologic consequences of severe bloodstream infection. Bacteremia is usually, but not always, documented. Positive blood cultures are documented in at least 80% of clinically septic patients. Approximately 300,000 to 500,000 cases of sepsis occur in the United States each year, with a mortality rate ranging from 30 to 50%, even with antibiotic treatment.

The manifestations of sepsis are varied and may involve many or all organ systems. Although gram-negative organisms generally cause septic shock, it is not possible to distinguish clinically between sepsis caused by gram-negative and gram-positive bacteria. Viable bacteria and their cell components, such as endotoxin, induce a complex series of physiologic events leading to sepsis and/or septic shock, the so-called systemic inflammatory response syndromes (Figure 1). Release of bacterial products such as endotoxin, exotoxin, and teichoic acid antigen leads to synthesis of macrophage polypeptides or cytokines, including cachectin or tumor necrosis factor. These substances act as mediators of multiple organ system responses in sepsis, along with endogenous pyrogens, which are responsible for fever.

Some patients may develop more severe illness with hypotension (systolic blood pressure < 90 mmHg or decrease in systolic pressure of one-third over previous readings), hypoperfusion, and organ dysfunction with lactic acidosis. Septic shock develops in about 50% of patients with sepsis and is a major cause of adult respiratory distress syndrome. As the patient's status deteriorates, multiple organ dysfunction develops, despite supportive therapy.

Presumably, early antibiotic intervention will prevent the progression to septic shock in 50% of patients with bacteremia. Other supportive measures are important in the management of sepsis and may help prolong survival. Optimal management requires treatment of the myriad of physiologic abnormalities in individual patients. In general, this care is best provided in an intensive care unit because of complex medical care needs and the need for ongoing patient monitoring of parameters such as pulmonary artery wedge pressures to better manage fluid replacement in hypotensive patients.

During the early phases of the systemic inflammatory response syndrome of sepsis, systemic vascular resistance falls and cardiac output is elevated. Rapid fluid replacement with large volumes of fluid is required. If hypotension persists despite this massive

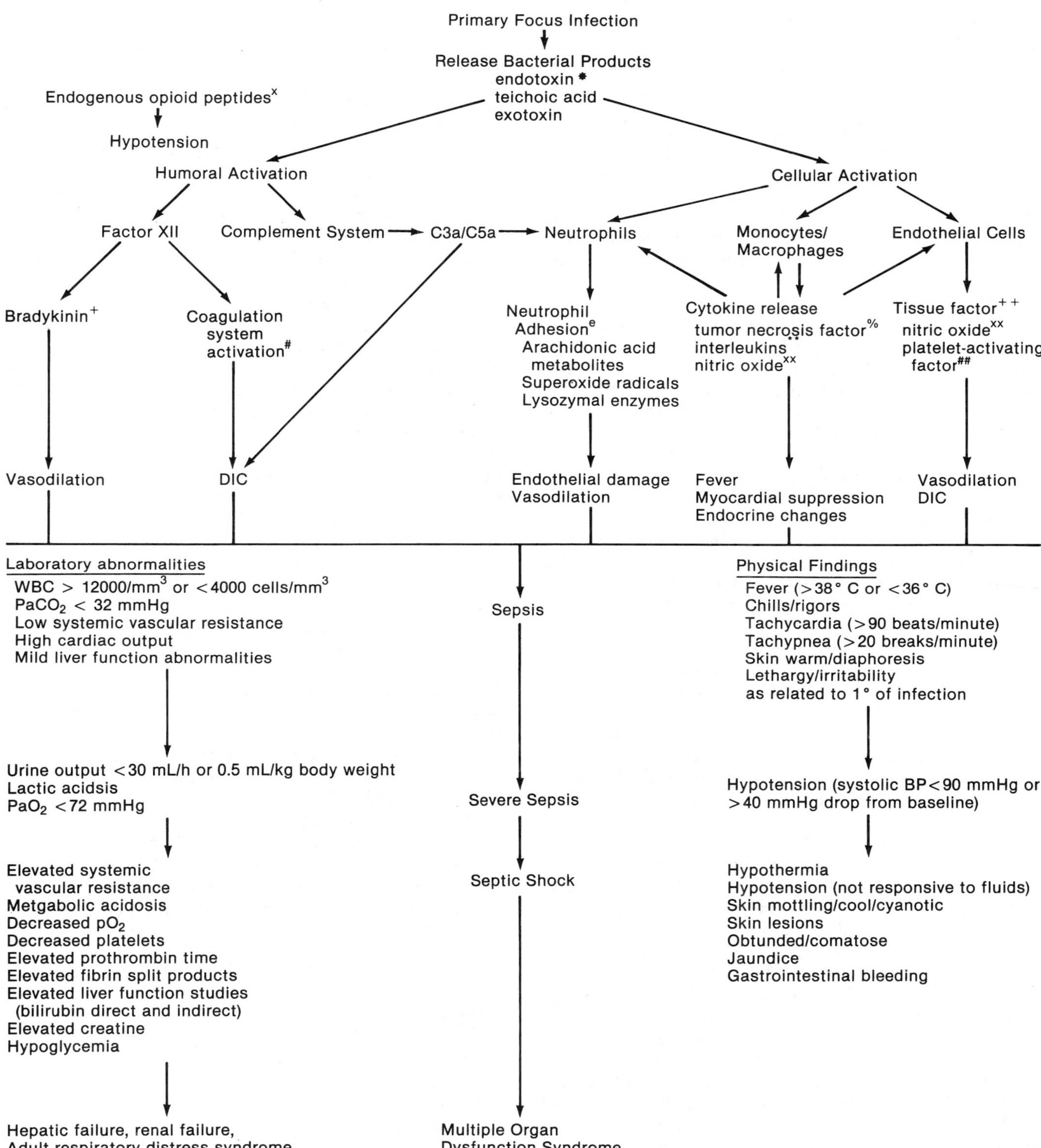

Figure 1. Pathogenesis of sepsis: Symbols represent specific therapeutic interventions in trial: *, antiendotoxin antibodies; ×, naloxone; +, bradykinin antagonists; #, antithrombin 3; e, cyclooxygenase inhibitors, antiphospholipase antibodies; %, tumor necrosis factor antibodies or receptor infusion; **, interleukin-1 receptor antagonist, anti-interleukin-6 antibodies, interleukin 10 infusion; ××, nitric oxide inhibitors; ++, tissue factor inhibitor; ##, platelet-activating factor antagonist, platelet-activating factor receptors, thromboxane synthetase inhibitors, thromboxane receptor blockers. (From Horowitz HW, Marisiddiah H: Bacteremia. *In* Rakel RE [ed]: Conn's Current Therapy 1995. Philadelphia, WB Saunders Co, 1995, p 61.)

fluid replacement, and pulmonary artery wedge pressures remain 15 to 18 mmHg, a vasopressor agent such as dopamine is indicated, in a dosage of 2 to 20 µg per kg per minute. In patients who are unresponsive to this single-drug regimen or require higher titrations to maintain systolic blood pressures greater than 90 mmHg, a second pressor agent should be added. Drugs such as dobutamine or isoproterenol should be added to dopamine. Metabolic acidosis may develop due to tissue hypoperfusion in the systemic inflammatory response syndrome. If metabolic acidosis is severe enough, it may impair the patient's response to sympathomimetic agents and also contribute to myocardial depression. While bicarbonate is not usually required, it should be considered, especially when the arterial pH is less than 7.1. If supplemental oxygen cannot maintain a Po_2 higher than 50 to 60 mmHg, ventilatory assistance with positive end-expiratory pressure (PEEP) may also be required. The need for ventilatory support is an ominous sign and is often associated with the development of the adult respiratory distress syndrome.

Several additional supportive measures have also been used to improve outcome, most notably corticosteroids. While controlled studies have not shown a survival advantage for steroids in the systemic inflammatory response syndrome, they are often used as adjunctive therapy with methylprednisolone (Solu-Medrol) in a dosage of 40 to 60 mg every 6 hours. Despite failure to show this survival advantage, the use of steroids to improve oxygenation and to avoid ventilatory support is still open to question. Monoclonal antiendotoxin antibodies* have been tested but with debatable efficacy and high cost. The drug's manufacture has been discontinued and it is not available at the time of this writing, although a phase III trial for use in meningococcemia has been completed and data are under review.

A variety of other therapies designed to interrupt the cascade of events related to the endotoxin-mediated inflammatory response have been studied to alter the outcome of sepsis. Currently, a number of novel strategies to neutralize the biologic effects of two of the principal mediators of the sepsis syndrome, TNF-alpha and IL-1, are under investigation. These compounds include (1) monocolonal antibodies (MoAbs) directed against cytokines, (2) soluble receptors to bind extracellular cytokines, and (3) proteins or antibodies directed against the cell surface cytokine receptors. Some of these agents are soluble TNF receptor, IL-1 receptor antagonist, and soluble IL-1 receptor. Although neutralizing the effects of TNF-alpha or IL-1 has been associated with reduced mortality in some animal and human trials of sepsis, there are several limitations to this form of therapy. Because IL-1 and especially TNF-alpha are synthesized and secreted very rapidly in response to endotoxin, anticytokine therapy must be administered early in the course of illness. Delays in treatment may render anticytokine therapy ineffective. In addition, many of the immune events in sepsis, such as complement activation and mediator release, can occur as a direct result of endotoxin exposure, bypassing the need for TNF-alpha or IL-1 mediation. Also, some studies have suggested that anticytokine treatment can increase patient mortality among those without evidence of clinical shock, or who have shock due to causes other than gram-negative bacteria. Finally, these therapies are very costly.

Further drug development activity is needed to isolate compounds that may benefit patients with sepsis syndrome, and clinical trials are required to determine which patient groups or subgroups might really benefit from these compounds.

The best management for sepsis at the present time involves prevention whenever possible. In some situations, sepsis may not be preventable, such as that secondary to intra-abdominal sepsis or meningitis. However, there are multiple opportunities for prevention of nosocomial or hospital-acquired colonization, which include such "low-technology" maneuvers as handwashing to minimize colonization with potentially invasive and/or antibiotic-resistant organisms, and proper maintenance of invasive devices and equipment. These strategies become even more important as hospitals begin to deal with emerging pathogens, such as vancomycin-resistant enterococci and *S. aureus*, which have no known effective treatment. Equally important is the judicious use of antibiotics, such as vancomycin (Vancocin), to also help prevent the development of antibiotic-resistant pathogens. Since the management of suspected bacteremia and/or sepsis requires broad coverage, many antibiotics will be overused out of necessity. It is important to balance the clinical need for broad-spectrum coverage based on clinical impression with the discontinuation of unnecessary drugs once bacteriologic information is available.

It is inevitable that preventive strategies cannot be applied to all bacteremias. Therefore, it is important to maintain a high index of suspicion for bacteremia, with prompt clinical assessment and empirical treatment in an effort to minimize morbidity and improve outcome.

BRUCELLOSIS

method of
MIGUEL MONTEJO, M.D., PH.D.
Hospital de Cruces
Vizcaya, Spain

Brucellosis is a disease of domestic animals that is transmissible to humans. There are six species of *Brucella* genus: *B. melitensis, B. suis, B. abortus, B. canis, B. neotomae,* and *B. ovis.* Only the first four produce illness in humans. The microorganism is a gram-negative coccobacillus with slow growth; nutritional requirements are media enriched with blood or serum. Each *Brucella* species has a

---

*Investigational drug in the United States.

preference for different hosts (*B. melitensis* for goat and sheep; *B. abortus* for cattle; *B. suis* for hogs; and *B. canis* for dogs).

The disease exists worldwide: it is a health problem in developing countries and in Mediterranean areas, especially *B. melitensis*. The incidence of *Brucella* in the United States is 200 cases per year (that includes *B. abortus* and *B. suis*). It mainly affects men between the ages of 30 and 40 years. The incidence in children is low. Most cases are due to ingestion of unpasteurized milk or milk products. Inhalation and skin or conjunctival inoculation are less frequent ways of acquisition. Transmission person to person is very rare. Occupational forms occur in developing countries.

The clinical signs associated with *Brucella* are high fever, chills, sweats, malaise, headache, arthralgia, and myalgia; less common are cough, diarrhea, and skin rash. Sepsis and coagulopathy are very uncommon complications. Hepatomegaly is reported in 20 to 60% of patients, splenomegaly in 20 to 30%, and mild lymphadenopathy in 10 to 20%.

Laboratory findings include leukopenia, lymphocytosis (50%), and thrombocytopenia (33%). Anemia is rare. Hepatic dysfunction with increased ASAT and ALAT occurs in 50% of patients.

Epidemiologic data, such as exposure to animals and the patient's occupation, may support clinical suspicion. In infections due to *B. melitensis*, blood culture is positive in up to 90% of patients, and half this number in those with *B. abortus*. The microorganism can be isolated from other organic fluids or tissues. The rose Bengal method is a rapid agglutination test with value in nonendemic areas; false-negative results may be seen in long-term infections or in the first few days of disease. Most cases of active infections will have titers of 1/80 or greater in the serum agglutination test (SAT), but titers below this do not rule out the disease. The Coombs' test may be complementary to the serum agglutination test. The enzyme-linked immunosorbent assay (ELISA) is useful in detecting relapses because it has better sensitivity and specificity than indirect immunofluorescence and immunoglobulin quantification by radioimmunoassay. Bone marrow and liver biopsies are not recommended except in special situations.

TREATMENT

Streptomycin, 1 gram intramuscularly daily for 2 weeks, plus doxycycline (Vibramycin), 200 mg per day orally for 6 weeks, is effective and results in very few relapses. Rifampin (Rifadin), 600 to 900 mg daily plus doxycycline, 200 mg, both for 6 weeks, is as effective as the just-mentioned regimen except in patients with spondylitis, in whom the association of streptomycin and doxycycline is more effective. Each case must be individualized with respect to the presence of spondylitis, adverse effects of streptomycin, and the advantage of oral administration.

Relapses are usually associated with immunologic factors and could be treated with the same antimicrobial regimen initially used. The antimicrobial of choice in children younger than 8 years and pregnant women is rifampin in combination with trimethoprim-sulfamethoxazole (Bactrim, Septra) for 4 to 6 weeks. In children, the dose of rifampin is 10 mg per kg per day once daily orally; the dose of trimethoprim is 10 mg per kg per day; and that of sulfamethoxazole is 50 mg per kg per day orally as two equal portions given every 12 hours.

Fluoroquinolone compounds (ciprofloxacin [Cipro] and ofloxacin [Floxin]) have been used as monotherapy although with a high relapse rate. Nevertheless, the combination of ofloxacin plus rifampin for 6 weeks has proved to have high efficacy. Ceftriaxone (Rocephin) results in many relapses.

Most patients with infective endocarditis need valve replacement and antimicrobial treatment. Combinations of doxycycline, streptomycin, rifampin, and trimethoprim-sulfamethoxazole have been used. The treatment duration after valve replacement has not been established yet. Doxycycline plus rifampin or doxycycline plus trimethoprim-sulfamethoxazole for more than 6 to 8 weeks has been recommended.

The treatment of neurologic complications of brucellosis is not defined. The majority of cases do not need intrathecal administration of antimicrobials. The efficacy of corticosteroids remains unproved. The length of therapy will be more than 6 weeks or until the CSF glucose level returns to normal, with mononuclear pleocytosis below 100 and lowered antibody titer.

In general, patients with sacroiliitis or spondylitis do not need longer periods of treatment.

Other uncommon complications: liver, spleen, scrotal, and epidural abscesses may require needle aspiration or surgical drainage. Spleen rupture also requires surgery.

With appropriate treatment, most patients recover within weeks to months. Relapse (3 to 5%) generally occurs within weeks to months after therapy ends.

Prevention of brucellosis in humans depends on the control or eradication of the disease in domestic animals.

CONJUNCTIVITIS

method of
FRANK G. RIEGER III, M.D., and
JOHN W. COWDEN, M.D.
Mason Institute of Ophthalmology
University of Missouri–Columbia
Columbia, Missouri

The conjunctiva is a mucous membrane that covers the inner surface of the eyelids and the anterior sclera. It is divided into three anatomic divisions: palpebral, forniceal (cul-de-sac), and bulbar. The conjunctiva is very elastic and allows free movement of the eye without the need of redundant tissue. Like most mucous membranes, the conjunctiva has an epithelial layer and a deeper substantia propria.

Conjunctivitis is an inflammation of the conjunctiva that may have infectious or noninfectious etiologies. Noninfectious entities include allergic/immunologic, toxic, and infectious agents, including bacteria, viruses, and chlamydia.

OPHTHALMIA NEONATORUM (Table 1)

This particular entity requires special attention since it can have devastating effects on the eye and vision along with systemic manifestations. It is defined as conjunctival inflammation occurring during the first 30 days of life.

The clinical signs and the age at presentation can be variable, making it imperative to use laboratory methods to assist in the differential diagnosis. An ophthalmologist should be consulted to participate in the management of these patients.

Chemical conjunctivitis has been reported in 10% to 100% of neonates treated with topical prophylactic agents at birth. Although it is 2.5 to 12 times more common when silver nitrate 1% is used, it has been reported with the use of topical erythromycin and tetracycline derivatives. Mild conjunctival erythema and lid edema present within the first 24 hours of life, and the Gram stain shows neutrophils with no organisms. This is a self-limited condition that resolves spontaneously in 48 hours in most cases.

Conjunctival cultures of vaginally delivered neonates reflect the flora of the vaginal canal, whereas the conjunctiva of neonates delivered by C-section within 3 hours of membrane rupture are culture negative. Therefore, the conjunctival flora of the neonate is correlated with the method of delivery. The most common organism isolated in bacterial ophthalmic neonatorum is *Staphylococcus aureus*, followed in frequency by *Haemophilus* sp., *Streptococcus pneumoniae*, enterococcus, *Pseudomonas aeruginosa*, and *Neisseria gonorrhoeae*. Gram stain and cultures are needed to make the diagnosis. With the exception of *Neisseria gonorrhoeae* and *Pseudomonas aeruginosa*, sight-threatening complications such as corneal ulcers, infiltrates, and endophthalmitis are rare, and topical therapy is adequate. Topical gentamicin drops are recommended for gram-negative organisms and erythromycin ointment for gram-positive organisms.

Pseudomonas aeruginosa is a very virulent organism that is rarely seen in healthy neonates but may be seen as a nosocomial pathogen in sick neonates. Corneal perforation and endophthalmitis can result from this organism, and an ophthalmologist should be consulted to participate in the management of these patients. These neonates should be hospitalized, isolated, and treated with fortified topical antibiotics, applying 1 drop every hour to the involved eye for the first 3 days. Systemic antibiotics are indicated only if other foci of infection are identified.

Gonococcal conjunctivitis in the neonate presents suddenly with marked eyelid edema and hyperpurulence. If left untreated the gonococcal organism can perforate the intact cornea within 24 hours and can disseminate causing arthritis and meningitis, making this condition a medical emergency. Therapy must be started immediately based on a presumptive diagnosis made from the Gram stain that shows gram-negative intracellular diplococci. The neonate should be hospitalized in an isolation unit for systemic therapy (a single intramuscular dose of kanamycin [Kantrex], 100 mg, cefotaxime [Claforan], 100 mg per kg, or ceftriaxone [Rocephin], 125 mg, plus topical erythromycin ointment 0.5% applied four times a day) initiated with frequent saline irrigation of the conjunctiva for several days until the purulence improves. An ophthalmologist should be con-

TABLE 1. **Differential Diagnosis and Treatment of Ophthalmia Neonatorum**

Etiology	Microscopic Features of Conjunctival Smears	Culture Media	Other Diagnostic Tests	Treatment
Chemical	Neutrophils, occasional lymphocytes (Gram)	None necessary		None necessary
Bacterial	Bacteria, neutrophils (Gram)	Reduced blood agar, thioglycolate broth, chocolate agar in CO_2, Thayer-Martin media	Drug sensitivity testing	Gram-positive organisms: erythromycin ointment Gram-negative organisms: gentamicin drops *Pseudomonas*-fortified topical antibiotics *N. gonorrhoeae:* IV penicillin G PCN-resistant gonorrhea: IM (Kantrex), cefotaxime (Claforan), or ceftriaxone (Rocephin) + topical erythromycin or tetracycline
Chlamydial	Neutrophils, lymphocytes, plasma cells (Gram)	McCoy cell culture	ELISA, rapid fluorescent antibody test, in situ DNA hybridization	PO erythromycin estolate (Ilosone) or ethylsuccinate (EES) + topical tetracycline, erythromycin, or sulfacetamide drops
Herpetic	Lymphocytes, plasma cells, multinucleate giant cells (Gram) Eosinophilic intranuclear inclusions in epithelial cells (Papanicolaou)	Viral cultures	Virus particle identification on EM, antigen detection tests	Intravenous acyclovir (Zovirax) + topical trifluridine (Viroptic)

From O'Hara MA: Ophthalmia neonatorum. Pediatr Clin North Am *40*:715–725, 1993.

sulted to monitor the status of the eyes. The child's mother and her sexual contacts should be evaluated and treated.

Chlamydia trachomatis is a modified bacterium that is an obligate intracellular parasite that can infect the genital tract. Neonatal conjunctivitis will result in 50% of the babies born to an infected mother, making the incidence in the United States 8.2/1000 live births or about 73,800 cases per year. It presents as mild to moderate erythema of the conjunctiva that is more apparent on the palpebral rather than the bulbar conjunctiva. No preauricular lymph nodes or follicles are present owing to the immaturity of the neonate's immune system. Treatment is with systemic erythromycin and topical erythromycin or tetracycline (oral erythromycin estolate [Ilosone], 10 mg per kg three times daily, or erythromycin ethylsuccinate [E.E.S.], 50 mg per kg in divided doses daily for 14 days; topical tetracycline or sulfacetamide drops or erythromycin ointment q.i.d. for 2 to 3 weeks). The mother should be treated systemically, avoiding the use of tetracycline in the mothers who are breast feeding.

Viral conjunctivitis in the neonate is almost always herpetic and is seen in 40% to 60% of infants born to mothers with active genital infections. These infections are usually herpes type II; however, type I has been isolated. There is erythema of the conjunctiva and edema of the lids on presentation, with a nonpurulent discharge. This entity can be associated with central nervous system herpes or disseminated disease. The diagnosis is confirmed by the characteristic vesicular skin lesions or a corneal dendrite if present, otherwise a maternal history of herpes is helpful in making the diagnosis. Conjunctival scrapings can be cultured and evaluated with the Papanicolaou technique, which shows eosinophilic intranuclear inclusion bodies. Antigen detection methods are also available. Treatment is with intravenous acyclovir (Zovirax), 10 mg per kg every 8 to 10 hours, and topical trifluridine (Viroptic), 1 drop five times per day. Ophthalmic consultation is recommended.

CONJUNCTIVITIS IN OLDER CHILDREN AND ADULTS (Table 2)

Hyperacute Bacterial Conjunctivitis

This entity presents with copious amounts of purulent discharge associated with marked lid swelling and conjunctival edema. The globe can be very tender, and a preauricular node is usually present. The causative organism is commonly *Neisseria gonorrhoeae*; however, other organisms such as *Neisseria meningitidis* have been reported. Gram stain and cultures on Thayer-Martin and chocolate agar should be performed, followed by systemic and topical therapy.

Acute Bacterial Conjunctivitis

This presents with modest mucopurulent discharge and diffuse conjunctival hyperemia and a small or absent preauricular node. The most common organisms are *Staphylococcus aureus, Haemophilus influenzae, and Streptococcus pneumoniae.* Even though some cases may resolve spontaneously, topical treatment is recommended with a broad-spectrum topical antibiotic such as Neosporin or Polytrim, 1 drop four times a day for 10 days. Fluoroquinolones are very potent broad-spectrum antibiotics but are best reserved for specific indications or resistant

TABLE 2. **Conjunctivitis in Other Age Groups**

Etiology	Signs/Symptoms	Treatment
Bacterial	Discharge with lids sealed shut in A.M., conjunctival injection	Erythromycin 0.5% or polymyxin B/trimethoprim compound (Polytrim), 4 times daily
Gonococcal	Hyperpurulent conjunctivitis Beefy-red conjunctival injection	Topical bacitracin, 500 U/gm 8 times daily PLUS Ceftriaxone, 1 gm IM every 24 hours for 5 days
Chlamydial	Chronic unilateral or bilateral mucopurulent conjunctivitis	Tetracycline 500 mg, or erythromycin stearate, 500 mg, orally 4 times daily for 3 weeks
Viral	Serous discharge starting unilaterally, then spreading bilaterally, mild itching, conjunctival injection	Artificial tears, cold compresses, fomite precautions
Allergy	Bilateral itching, increased lacrimation, conjunctival injection, associated systemic allergy	Topical antihistamine 4 times daily Consider prophylactic treatment with lodoxamide 0.1% 4 times daily in patients with documented seasonal allergic conjunctivitis Artificial tears 4 to 6 times daily Levocabastine (Livostin) Ladoxamide tromethamine (Alomide) Cold compresses prn
Toxic	Unilateral/bilateral irritation with associated conjunctival injection	Artificial tears Removal of inciting agent

From Frangie JP, Leibowitz HM: Conjunctivitis. *In* Rakel RE (ed): Conn's Current Therapy 1995. Philadelphia, WB Saunders Co, 1995, p 66.

cases. It is felt that topical therapy shortens the course and prevents complications such as corneal ulceration and permanent conjunctival changes.

Chronic Bacterial Conjunctivitis

Staphylococcus aureus is the most common organism identified due to its ability to colonize the eyelids. Topical antibiotic therapy is directed toward *Staphylococcus aureus*, with lid hygiene being indicated in many cases.

Viral Conjunctivitis

Many cases of conjunctivitis, or pink eye, are caused by adenoviruses. Epidemic keratoconjunctivitis is a common form of conjunctivitis that is extremely infectious and caused by adenovirus serotypes 8 and 19. Preauricular nodes are present in most cases, and the patient complains of the eyelids sticking together in the morning. This follicular conjunctivitis runs a 2-week course, often followed by subepithelial corneal opacities. The diagnosis is made by clinical signs and rarely by the use of cultures, Gram stain, or immunofluorescent techniques. Other adenoviral infections are pharyngoconjunctival fever and hemorrhagic conjunctivitis. The treatment is supportive with the use of artificial tears and topical decongestants and the prophylactic use of topical antibiotics. Topical steroids are controversial and should not be used without consultation with an ophthalmologist.

Primary herpetic conjunctivitis is follicular in nature and usually indistinguishable from an adenoviral infection unless the typical vesicular skin lesions are present in the periorbital region or a corneal dendrite is seen.

Adult Inclusion Conjunctivitis

This entity is caused by *Chlamydia trachomatis* and is characterized by a chronic follicular conjunctivitis associated with an enlarged preauricular lymph node. The diagnosis is made by a direct fluorescent antibody assay or an enzyme immunoassay, since a Giemsa stain of the conjunctival scrapings has a very low sensitivity. Treatment is with systemic tetracycline or erythromycin, and topical therapy is optional. Also, the patient's sexual contacts should be treated with systemic therapy.

Allergic Conjunctivitis

Seasonal allergic conjunctivitis (SAC) is an acute process characterized by conjunctival edema, erythema, and itching. It has been proved to be IgE-mediated and triggered by airborne allergens such as pollen, dander, mold, and house dust, resulting in the degranulation of conjunctival mast cells. Other more severe forms of allergic conjunctivitis are associated with giant papillary reaction. They are vernal keratoconjunctivitis (VKC) and atopic keratoconjunctivitis (AKC).

SAC is controlled by avoidance of the offending allergens if possible. A topical antihistamine/decongestant can be used for treatment of the acute symptoms. Levocabastine (Livostin) is a newer antihistamine that is very effective at eliminating symptoms. Cromolyn sodium 4% (Crolom) and lodoxamide (Alomide) are mast cell stabilizers and can be used prior to exposure to the offending allergen. Topical steroids can be very effective in controlling the symptoms of SAC; however, because of the side effects of cataract formation and secondary glaucoma they should be used with the involvement of an ophthalmologist. Patients with VKC and AKC should be referred to an ophthalmologist for management.

Irritative Conjunctivitis

Many agents in the environment can cause irritation of the conjunctivitis by direct contact. They include drugs, chemicals, foreign bodies, pollutants, and organic matters. The treatment usually involves removal of the toxic agent if possible. Topical therapy can include artificial tears, topical antibiotics to prevent secondary infection, and topical steroids in a weak concentration in consultation with an ophthalmologist. If the agent cannot be removed from the environment, measures must be taken to reduce the exposure, such as use of occlusive goggles.

VARICELLA

method of
MARK A. WARD, M.D.
Baylor College of Medicine
Houston, Texas

Varicella-zoster virus is a member of the herpesvirus family. Like other members of this family, varicella-zoster virus establishes latency after the primary infection. Periodic reactivation of latent virus may occur. The clinical expression of this biological behavior is two distinct syndromes: chickenpox and herpes zoster (shingles). Chickenpox is the clinical manifestation of primary varicella zoster infection, whereas herpes zoster represents the reactivation of latent virus.

CLINICAL

Chickenpox

Chickenpox occurs year round, but the incidence peaks during late winter and early spring. In temperate climates, such as in the continental United States, most people experience chickenpox during childhood. In contrast, the incidence of infection in children residing in tropical climates is much lower, resulting in a large proportion of susceptible adults in these regions. Transmission of infection is person-to-person via the airborne route.

Virtually all primary varicella-zoster virus infections are symptomatic, resulting in the clinical syndrome known as chickenpox. The incubation period is 10 to 21 days, after which patients may experience a prodrome of fever and mild, nonspecific symptoms. The rash characteristically begins on the trunk and scalp and spreads centrifugally. Occasionally, the mucous membranes are involved. Individual lesions begin as erythematous macules that rapidly evolve into papules and then vesicles. The vesicles subsequently become pustular, rupture, and crust. New lesions continue to erupt for several days; therefore, lesions in various stages of evolution will be present at any given time. Associated symptoms include fever, pruritus, general malaise, and anorexia.

Although most cases of chickenpox resolve uneventfully, complications may occur. The most common is secondary bacterial infection of the skin lesions. Less frequent complications include pneumonitis, encephalitis, keratitis, hepatitis, and Reye's syndrome. The frequency of complications is increased in adults, immunocompromised patients, pregnant women, and newborn infants of women experiencing peripartum varicella.

The diagnosis of chickenpox is usually based on the presence of the characteristic rash. If confirmation is required, lesions can be cultured. However, results may require 5 to 10 days to return from the laboratory. Rapid confirmation is most easily made using a direct immunofluorescent-antibody stain of lesion scrapings. Less sensitive, but more readily available, is the Tzanck preparation, a method of staining scrapings of the base of a skin lesion with Giemsa or Wright stain. The presence of multinucleated giant cells indicates the presence of a herpesvirus infection but does not distinguish varicella from herpes simplex virus infection. Serology is also available but is generally useful only to confirm a diagnosis retrospectively.

Herpes Zoster

Herpes zoster (shingles) is the clinical syndrome resulting from the reactivation of latent varicella-zoster virus. Because latency is maintained in the dorsal root ganglia, reactivation produces cutaneous lesions in a dermatomal distribution. Thoracic and lumbar dermatomes are involved most frequently. Occasionally, more than one dermatome may be involved, but generally the affected dermatomes are contiguous. The eruption consists of grouped vesicles on an erythematous base. Systemic symptoms are uncommon.

Complications of herpes zoster include dissemination (rare in immunocompetent patients), secondary bacterial infection, acute neuritis, and postherpetic neuralgia. Postherpetic neuralgia is more common and more severe in older patients (older than 50 years of age). Groups at increased risk of developing complications are similar to those for chickenpox, except that complications of herpes zoster do not appear to be more frequent in pregnant women or their offspring.

Diagnosis is generally made by physical examination. Confirmatory tests include direct immunofluorescent-antibody stain, Tzanck preparation, and viral culture, as described for chickenpox.

TREATMENT
Chickenpox

Normal Host

Treatment of chickenpox in healthy children is primarily symptomatic. Antihistamines (e.g., diphenhy-dramine [Benadryl] and hydroxyzine [Atarax]) are useful in managing pruritus. In addition, topical therapy with colloidal oatmeal (Aveeno) baths and calamine lotion or similar products may alleviate itching. The child's fingernails should be trimmed short to minimize excoriation of lesions and the potential for secondary infection. Frequent bathing may also be useful in reducing the risk of secondary bacterial infection. Fever may be treated with acetaminophen or ibuprofen. Aspirin should not be used because of the association with Reye's syndrome in patients with varicella.

Specific antiviral treatment of chickenpox is possible. Acyclovir (Zovirax) started within 24 hours of rash onset has been shown to decrease the number and hasten the resolution of cutaneous lesions. However, the clinical significance of this difference remains controversial. Because of this and the practical difficulty in getting treatment started within 24 hours of rash onset (the only period when any benefit has been demonstrated), routine use of acyclovir for otherwise healthy children younger than 13 years of age is not recommended. On the other hand, oral acyclovir is routinely indicated for treatment of chickenpox in adolescents (13 years of age and older) and adults because of their increased risk for severe and complicated disease. The recommended dose is 20 mg per kg per dose (maximum of 800 mg), four times daily for 5 days.

Treatment of complications of chickenpox is often problematic. Secondary bacterial skin infections are treated with antibiotics active against *Staphylococcus aureus* and group A *Streptococcus*. Ocular involvement confined to the conjunctiva is relatively common, is not associated with complications, and does not require specific therapy. If more serious ocular involvement (e.g., keratitis) is suspected, consultation with an ophthalmologist is advised. Treatment of most other complications is primarily supportive. Evidence is strong that some complications (e.g., cerebellar ataxia) are immune mediated rather than due to active viral replication. Antiviral therapy in this setting is not likely to be of benefit. When the pathogenesis is unclear and may involve direct viral infection, the use of antiviral agents is certainly reasonable.

High-Risk Host

All immunocompromised hosts with chickenpox should be treated with antiviral agents. Both cytosine arabinoside* (Cytosar-U) and acyclovir have been found effective in reducing the severity of disease in these patients. Acyclovir is preferred because of its ease of administration, requirement for less fluid, fewer side effects, and evidence in some studies of greater efficacy. It should be administered intravenously at 500 mg per M^2 per dose every 8 hours. Maintenance of adequate hydration and slow (1-hour) infusion of acyclovir are important to prevent crystallization of the drug in the renal tubules. Al-

---

*Not FDA-approved for this indication.

though oral acyclovir has been used in small numbers of immunocompromised patients with chickenpox, it has not been studied adequately enough to allow recommending its use in this setting.

Patients on steroids for conditions that are not immunocompromising (e.g., asthma) pose a special problem. Those receiving physiologic doses (e.g., children with congenital adrenal hyperplasia) may be treated as normal hosts. Those receiving inhaled steroids or short courses of oral steroids do not appear to be at high risk for complications, but reports of severe disease do exist. Therefore, I would treat these patients with oral acyclovir, as described for the normal host. When feasible, the steroids should be discontinued. Those patients receiving prolonged high doses of steroids should be considered at high risk for severe disease and treated as just described for high-risk hosts.

Herpes Zoster

Normal Host

Herpes zoster in normal children is most often a benign, self-limited disease. Rarely is it complicated by dissemination or postherpetic neuralgia. Therefore, treatment is symptomatic, as described for chickenpox. There is no demonstrated benefit to the use of acyclovir in this group. I would make an exception for those children with involvement of the ophthalmic branch of the trigeminal nerve. I routinely treat these patients with oral acyclovir in the same dose as for chickenpox for 7 days because of the risk of serious ocular complications, even though such treatment is of unproved benefit. If ocular involvement beyond simple conjunctivitis is suspected, an ophthalmologist should also be involved in the evaluation and management.

Adults who suffer from herpes zoster are at risk for postherpetic neuralgia. The effect of antiviral treatment on the incidence of this complication is controversial. Acyclovir has been studied most extensively; many, but not all, investigators have concluded that it is beneficial in reducing the incidence and/or duration of postherpetic neuralgia. Two newer antiviral agents, famciclovir (Famvir) and valacyclovir (Valtrex), have been approved for use in the treatment of herpes zoster in adults. Both have been shown to reduce the duration of postherpetic neuralgia in patients older than 50 years of age. The recommended dose of famciclovir is 500 mg orally three times daily for 7 days and of valacyclovir is 1 gram orally three times daily for 7 days. Note that neither famciclovir nor valacyclovir has been approved or studied in immunocompromised patients and children. Management of herpes zoster involving the ophthalmic branch of the trigeminal nerve in adults is the same as for children.

High-Risk Host

All immunocompromised hosts with herpes zoster should be treated with acyclovir. Because the degree of immunocompromise varies from patient to patient, depending on the underlying condition and treatment, this approach is very conservative. Many less severely compromised patients do well with no therapy. Because it is difficult to predict which patient will develop severe disease, I begin therapy in all. For the same reason, I generally initiate therapy with intravenous, rather than oral, acyclovir in the same doses as described earlier for chickenpox. For less severely compromised patients who demonstrate a prompt response to intravenous therapy, treatment may be completed with oral acyclovir.

Unlike the case in chickenpox, pregnancy does not appear to be a risk factor for complicated zoster or to place the fetus at any risk. Therefore, acyclovir is not routinely indicated for pregnant women.

PREVENTION

Primary Prevention

Primary prevention of varicella is now possible with the use of varicella vaccine. It is a live attenuated virus vaccine and is indicated as part of routine childhood immunization at 12 to 18 months of age. Adolescents (13 years of age and older) and adults should be given two doses of vaccine 4 to 8 weeks apart. The second dose is necessitated by the decreased immunogenicity of the vaccine in these age groups. Immunocompromised patients, including those with human immunodeficiency virus infection, should not be immunized. Although some shedding of virus has been shown to occur in immunized patients, secondary spread does not occur. Therefore, household contacts of immunocompromised patients may safely be given the vaccine.

Secondary Prevention

Secondary prevention (i.e., prophylaxis after exposure to disease) is possible by two methods. First, the patient may be given varicella-zoster immune globulin (VZIG). The dose is 1 vial (125 units) per 10 kg body weight (minimum 1 vial/maximum 5 vials). This treatment is indicated for most susceptible persons with increased risk of severe or complicated disease, including pregnant women. Despite their increased risk, otherwise normal adolescents and adults need not receive VZIG because acyclovir is available for treatment should disease develop. An additional group of patients for whom VZIG prophylaxis is indicated is newborn infants of women who experience the onset of varicella between 5 days before and 2 days after delivery. These infants are at high risk for severe or fatal chickenpox. They should be given VZIG (1 vial). Term neonates exposed to varicella after 2 days of life need not receive VZIG, even if born to a nonimmune mother.

A second potential method of prophylaxis is the use of acyclovir. In immunocompetent patients, this has been shown to be highly effective in preventing chickenpox after household exposure to varicella. However, the efficacy of this type of prophylaxis in immunocompromised patients has not been established. Therefore, the use of acyclovir in this fashion is to be discouraged. With the advent of routine immunization, the need for postexposure prophylaxis should decline.

CHOLERA

method of
A.N. ALAM, M.B., PH.D.
*International Centre for Diarrhoeal Disease
    Research
Dhaka, Bangladesh*

Cholera is an acute dehydrating diarrheal illness caused by infection due to *Vibrio cholerae* serogroup 1. *Vibrio cholerae* passes through the gastric barrier, attaches to and colonizes the mucosal lining of the proximal small intestine, and liberates a potent enterotoxin (cholera toxin). The toxin is composed of an active A subunit and five B subunits arranged in a circular form. The A subunit penetrates the cell membrane, activates adenylate cyclase, and causes massive outpouring of fluid and electrolytes into the bowel, resulting in secretory diarrhea.

Cholera is one of the most feared epidemic illnesses to threaten mankind. Disregarding the geographic boundaries of nations and continents, it can rapidly spread through contaminated water and foodstuffs, causing epidemics and pandemics. The highest attack rates occur in populations living in crowded environments where safe water supplies and sanitation facilities are limited or virtually nonexistent. Mostly it causes a minor illness with no symptoms or only mild diarrhea that is indistinguishable from other forms of acute watery diarrhea. In a minority of cases, however, it may rapidly lead to severe dehydration, loss of electrolytes, circulatory collapse, and death in hours, even in a healthy adult. Acute cholera is equally dramatic in its response to treatment. A severely ill patient in profound shock with distantly audible heart sounds could be back on his feet within hours of timely and appropriate rehydration therapy.

A typical cholera patient experiences an abrupt onset of profuse, watery diarrhea leading to dehydration and loss of electrolytes. Severe, effortless vomiting follows soon after because of metabolic acidosis. The volume of fluid lost through stools and vomitus can be large: 100 to 200 mL per kg or more in the first 24 hours. This leads to dehydration characterized by decreased skin turgor, sunken eyes, depressed fontanelle in infants, dry mucous membranes, cold and clammy extremities with wrinkled hands and feet ("washerwoman's hands"), and weak or absent peripheral pulses. Blood pressure may be unobtainable, and the patient remains well-oriented but apathetic. Patients are extremely thirsty and will drink fluids eagerly. Painful cramps in the arms and legs may occur. Oliguria and even anuria may ensue if the dehydration is not corrected. In a typical case, the stool rapidly becomes clear without fecal matter, with a mild fishy odor, and contains only flecks of mucus (rice water stool). In children, the presence of hypoglycemia may be associated with convulsions and coma.

A new epidemic strain of cholera, *Vibrio cholerae* 0139 Bengal, was first detected in October 1992 in Madras in Southern India. The epidemic spread very rapidly through India and reached Southern Bangladesh in December the same year. So far, 10 countries in Asia have reported a severe, cholera-like diarrheal disease caused by the new strain. The strain did not react with any antisera to other 138 serotypes, but closely resembled El Tor vibrios and produced cholera toxin in quantities similar to that produced by *V. cholerae* 01. The clinical presentation and the response to treatment were identical to those of cholera. Adults over 15 years of age were mostly affected, indicating that the population was virgin to the organism.

Hemoconcentration due to fluid loss results in raised plasma specific gravity, hematocrit, plasma protein concentration, serum creatinine, and urea nitrogen. Severe metabolic acidosis manifested by depression of arterial blood pH and plasma bicarbonate values with an increased serum anion gap can occur due to stool bicarbonate losses and lactic acidosis associated with dehydration. Marked potassium deficits are not reflected in serum potassium values due to the presence of uncorrected acidosis. The diagnosis of cholera can be established by isolating *V. cholerae* 01 from the stool or rectal swab on selective media.

TREATMENT

It is the complication of dehydration that kills the majority of patients with cholera, and the provision of adequate intravenous or oral rehydration—until diarrhea ceases—remains the cornerstone of therapy in cholera. Rehydration is achieved in two phases: initial rehydration by rapid replacement of water and salts already lost and maintenance of normal hydration by replacing ongoing losses, preferably on a volume-to-volume basis as long as diarrhea persists.

Oral rehydration therapy as a safe, powerful, and inexpensive tool has revolutionized the treatment of cholera; the World Health Organization (WHO)-recommended glucose-based oral rehydration salt (ORS) solution (Table 1) alone can successfully be used for both the initial rehydration and the maintenance phase in 80% to 90% of cholera patients not in shock. For patients with some dehydration, WHO recommends 50 to 100 mL of ORS solution to be given within the first 4 hours (the approximate amount can be calculated by multiplying the patient's weight in kg by 75).

Rice-based oral rehydration salt solution significantly reduces the rate of stool output in patients with cholera by 32% to 36% in comparison with glucose-ORS. To prepare a rice-based ORS solution, 50 gm of rice powder replacing 20 gm of glucose (Table

TABLE 1. **World Health Organization–Recommended Oral Rehydration Salt Solution**

	Grams/L		Mmol/L
Sodium chloride	3.5	Sodium	90
Trisodium citrate, dihydrate	2.9	Chloride	80
OR			
Sodium bicarbonate	2.5	Potassium	20
Potassium chloride	1.5	Citrate	10
		OR	
Glucose (anhydrous)	20.0	Bicarbonate	30
		Glucose	111

1) should be boiled in 1100 mL of water for about 7 to 8 minutes, should be cooled, and then salts as recommended for the WHO-ORS solution should be added and mixed well before being served. Rice-based ORS solution should be used within 6 to 8 hours. Vomiting subsides within 2 to 3 hours as acidosis is corrected, and this should never contraindicate successful use of ORS solution in achieving rehydration as most patients retain enough fluid to become rehydrated.

It is extremely important to understand the rapidity and the severity of volume depletion in cholera. So it is essential to start oral rehydration therapy vigorously at the first sign of diarrhea, as a cholera patient might lose as much as 8% to 10% of body fluid within 3 to 4 hours of the onset of illness. The amount of fluid required in the first 24 hours could be large, as much as 350 mL per kg, although the average requirement is about 200 mL per kg of body weight. During the maintenance phase, stool losses are replaced with an equivalent amount of ORS solution.

In about 10% of cholera patients who may present with severe dehydration and/or hypovolemic shock, prompt intravenous rehydration is mandatory to avert death. Prompt intervention with effective rehydration can drastically reduce mortality from 50% to less than 1%. However, ORS solution should be used immediately after the initial fluid and salt deficits have been corrected in 1 to 4 hours. Ideally, appropriate intravenous fluids should replace the electrolyte losses in cholera stool (Table 2), which is almost isotonic with that of plasma. Commercially available Ringer's lactate (Hartmann's) solution or specially prepared polyelectrolyte solution, such as cholera saline (Dhaka solution), is the preferred fluid for intravenous rehydration. Ringer's lactate does not have sufficient potassium, and so potassium chloride (10 to 15 mL per L) can be added to the solution. Normal saline solution, although less effective, can be used for initial rehydration if suitable solutions are not available, but ORS solution should be started as soon as the patient can drink and tolerate oral fluids to replace the potassium and base deficits. Plain dextrose in water is ineffective and should not be used. For severely dehydrated patients who are in profound shock or cannot drink, intravenous fluids should be given as rapidly as possible to restore the circulating volume quickly.

With an estimated deficit of about 10% of body weight, an adult weighing 60 kg will require 6 liters (i.e., 100 mL per kg) of rehydration fluids to correct the existing fluid and electrolyte deficit. For patients aged 1 year and older, WHO recommends that 30 mL per kg of body weight be given as swiftly as possible in the first half hour, and then 70 mL per kg in the next 2.5 hours. Similarly, in patients less than 1 year old, an initial 30 mL per kg can be given within the first hour and then 70 mL per kg in the next 4 to 5 hours. The patient should be monitored frequently, and oral rehydration therapy should be started soon after initial rehydration. However, ORS solution can be offered as soon as the patient can drink, even when the initial fluid and salt deficits are being corrected. Plain water should be offered ad libitum in addition to ORS solution. Once the patient is fully hydrated, the radial pulse should be strong and the blood pressure normal, and skin turgor should return to normal. A severely dehydrated patient should also gain about 8% to 10% of body weight. Urine output resumes 6 to 8 hours after starting rehydration. Cholera patients are conveniently treated on a "cholera cot" on which a plastic sheet with a central hole is placed. A sleeve fits into the hole to channel the diarrhea stool into a calibrated bucket placed underneath. A simple intake and output chart should be maintained at the bedside showing the amounts of intravenous and oral solutions given and the volume of stool output and vomitus.

As an adjunct to effective oral rehydration therapy, antimicrobials are started as soon as the initial rehydration is completed in 4 to 6 hours. Appropriate antibiotic therapy, although not essential, significantly reduces the stool volume, duration of diarrhea, and duration of vibrio excretion in feces and thus reduces the cost of treatment and hospitalization. Although the emergence of multiple antibiotic-resistant isolates of *V. cholerae* 01 has been reported, tetracycline still remains the drug of choice for the treatment of cholera. The dose is 500 mg every 6 hours in adults and 12.5 mg per kg of body weight every 6 hours in children for 3 days. Doxycycline should be used when available in a single dose of 300 mg for adults and 4 mg per kg of body weight for children, given with food to avoid nausea and vomiting. The drug is preferred particularly in situations like rural treatment centers and refugee camps where patient compliance is difficult to obtain. Erythromycin, 500 mg every 6 hours or 30 mg per kg per day in three divided doses in children for 3 days, is a safe alternative for patients with tetracycline-resistant strains of *V. cholerae*. Trimethoprim-sulfamethoxazole (5 mg of trimethoprim and 25 mg of sulfamethoxazole per kg per day in two divided doses for 3 days) is the antibiotic of choice in children, and

TABLE 2. **Electrolyte Composition of Cholera Stool and Intravenous Solutions in Use**

	Mean Concentration (mmol/L)			
	Na$^+$	K$^+$	Cl$^-$	HCO$_3$
Cholera stool				
Adults	135	15	100	45
Children	105	25	90	30
Ringer's lactate*	131	4	109	28
(Hartman's solution)				
Dhaka solution†	133	13	98	48
Normal saline‡	154	0	154	0

*Best commercially available solution to be used in all age groups; its lactate is converted to bicarbonate.

†In use to treat cholera at the International Centre for Diarrhoeal Disease Research, Bangladesh.

‡Can be used for initial rehydration only if suitable solutions are not available.

furazolidone (Furoxone), 100 mg every 6 hours for 3 days is the preferred antibiotic for pregnant women. Antibiotic susceptibility patterns of local strains of vibrio should ideally be known before the antibiotic is chosen. Chloramphenicol is usually not recommended for use in cholera. Mass chemoprophylaxis is not recommended as it does not prevent spread of epidemic cholera and may, on the other hand, contribute to the emergence of antibiotic resistance.

Diet

Food should be offered to cholera patients as soon as acidosis is corrected and vomiting has stopped after initial rehydration. Early liberal feeding should be encouraged to assist rapid nutritional recovery.

Complications

Prompt and effective case management based on rehydration therapy can prevent most complications due to cholera. Acidosis is normally corrected within hours of appropriate use of rehydration fluids. Dyselectrolytemias, such as hyponatremia, hypernatremia, and hypokalemia should be corrected by optimal use of oral rehydration therapy. Early resumption of a normal diet and sustained feeding usually prevent the development of hypoglycemia, although any child presenting with convulsions or coma should promptly be given intravenous glucose solution.

PREVENTION

Water and food contaminated with *V. cholerae* are the main vehicles of transmission of cholera. Use of plenty of clean water for drinking, washing utensils, and other purposes; washing hands with soap and water; and sanitary disposal of feces are the most effective preventive measures. The two-dose WC/BS (killed whole-cell/B subunit [Cholera Vaccine]) vaccine providing short-term protection, even in persons with blood group O and in those who lack natural immunity to cholera, can currently be considered for prevention and control of cholera when dealing with actual or threatened outbreaks during acute emergencies. A single-dose vaccine, such as CVD 103-HgR,* is more desirable but not yet recommended as its efficacy in the field and safety in HIV-infected people are being evaluated. Ideally, a universal cholera vaccine should include antigens of both 01 (serotypes Inaba and Ogawa and biotypes El Tor and classical) and newly appeared 0139 vibrios. At present, no cholera vaccine is recommended for public health use to control endemic cholera.

---

*Not available in the United States.

DIPHTHERIA

method of
AYESHA MIRZA, M.D., and
RUSSELL W. STEELE, M.D.
Louisiana State University School of Medicine
and Children's Hospital
New Orleans, Louisiana

Diphtheria is a potentially severe illness caused by the bacterium *Corynebacterium diphtheriae,* with a case fatality rate that ranges from 1.5% to 10% among unimmunized populations. The last outbreak in the United States affected 201 persons in San Antonio, Texas, from December 1969 to December 1970; there were three deaths. Since 1980, five or fewer cases have been reported each year, and since 1988 all reported culture-confirmed cases have been imported. Diphtheria continues to be a major health issue in other parts of the world. During 1994, a provisional total of 47,802 cases and 1746 deaths from diphtheria were reported throughout the new independent states of the former Soviet Union.

The incubation period for diphtheria is 1 to 6 days, and it may present in a number of clinical forms. Diagnosis is confirmed by culture of material from beneath the pharyngeal membrane. Treatment, however, must be based on clinical suspicion rather than awaiting culture results. The treatment prescribed varies with severity of disease as well as duration of symptoms prior to starting treatment. Prognosis depends on the patient's age, the location and extent of the diphtheritic membrane, and the promptness with which antitoxin is given.

Systemic complications due to the diphtheria toxin are primarily cardiac and neurologic. Subtle evidence of myocarditis may be detected in as many as two thirds of the patients. Changes in the electrocardiogram (ECG), particularly ST-T wave changes and first-degree heart block, can progress to severe degrees of block, atrioventricular dissociation, and other arrhythmias. Neurologic complications include development of neuropathies involving both cranial and peripheral nerves. Oculomotor and ciliary paralysis or lower extremity peripheral neuritis may manifest 2 to 8 weeks after the onset of illness. Mechanical airway obstruction and myocarditis account for most diphtheria-related deaths.

TREATMENT

Patients with suspected respiratory diphtheria should be treated on clinical grounds until bacteriologic confirmation is available since they may deteriorate rapidly. Treatment of suspected cases includes administration of diphtheria hyperimmune equine antitoxin, antibiotics, and diphtheria toxoid (Table 1). Because antitoxin neutralizes only circulating toxin that is not as yet bound to tissue, prompt administration is critical. The preferred route of administration is intravenous. The site and size of the diphtheritic membrane, the degree of toxicity, and the duration of illness are guides for estimating the dose of antitoxin. The presence of soft, diffuse cervical lymphadenitis ("bull neck") suggests moderate-to-severe toxin absorption.

Before intravenous administration, tests for sensitivity should be performed with 1:10 antitoxin dilu-

TABLE 1. **Treatment of Diphtheria**

Drug/Support	Dosage/Duration
Antitoxin	Dilute 1:20 in isotonic sodium chloride and infuse IV not exceeding 1 mL/min
Symptom duration <48 h with mild pharyngeal, laryngeal, or nasopharyngeal symptoms	40,000 U antitoxin
Symptom duration >48 h, severe symptoms, or diffuse swelling of the neck	80,000 U antitoxin
Extremely severe or malignant diphtheria	100,000–120,000 U antitoxin
Diphtheria toxoid	First dose at end of 1st week of illness Second dose 1 mon later Third dose 1 mon after second dose

Antibiotics
  Penicillin
  OR
  Erythromycin
	100,000 U/kg/d IV divided q 6 h for 10 d
	
	20–50 mg/kg/d IV divided q 6 h for 10 d

Supportive intensive care	Airway protection with endotracheal intubation as needed to assure patent airway and prevent aspiration Mechanical ventilation for respiratory failure associated with paralysis of muscles of respiration Support for failing circulation Bedrest (minimum 2–3 wk) until risk of myocarditis passes Prednisone 1–1.5 mg/kg/d for 2 wk for myocarditis Provision for nutrition and hydration (enteral or parenteral) Isolation after completion of antibiotic therapy until two cultures of nose and throat taken 24 h apart are negative for toxigenic diphtheria bacilli

tion for conjunctival testing or 1:100 dilution for intradermal testing. Desensitization is necessary for 10% of patients who are sensitive to equine toxin (Table 2). Antibiotics must be given to eradicate the organism, terminate toxin production, and decrease the likelihood of transmission. Antimicrobial therapy is not a substitute for antitoxin administration.

For cutaneous diphtheria, thorough cleansing of the lesion with soap and water and 10 days of antimicrobials are recommended. Antitoxin is probably of little value, although some authorities recommend up to 20,000 to 40,000 U of antitoxin since toxic sequelae have been reported. The patient should receive active immunization with diphtheria toxoid during convalescence since clinical infection does not always induce protective levels of antitoxin.

TABLE 2. **Desensitization Schedule for Diphtheria Equine Antitoxin**

Dose	Amount (mL)	Dilution	IV Route	ID/SC/IM Route
1	0.10	1:1000	All IV	ID
2	0.30	1:1000		ID
3	0.60	1:1000		SC
4	0.10	1:100		SC
5	0.30	1:100		SC
6	0.60	1:100		SC
7	0.10	1:10		SC
8	0.30	1:10		SC
9	0.60	1:10		SC
10	0.10	undiluted		SC
11	0.20	undiluted		SC
12	0.60	undiluted		IM
13	1.0	undiluted		IM

Abbreviations: IV = intravenous; ID = intradermal; SC = subcutaneous; IM = intramuscular.

Antibiotics are recommended for contacts of index cases regardless of vaccination status, as soon as samples are obtained for culture (Table 3).

Supportive Care

Supportive care is also important. Bedrest during the acute phase of the infection and intubation of the patient to avoid aspiration or obstruction by the pharyngeal membrane are generally recommended. Close ECG monitoring of the patient is also essential. Steroids have shown to be of no benefit during the acute phase of the illness except for mycocarditis. Careful attention should be paid to providing adequate hydration and nutrition throughout the entire course.

Isolation

For pharyngeal diphtheria, patients and carriers of toxigenic strains should be placed in strict isola-

TABLE 3. **Management of Contacts in Diphtheria**

Contact	Management
Immunized household contacts	Schick test, observation
Greater than 3 doses of DT, DTP, or dT and last dose > 5 yr ago	Booster dose of DT, DPT, or dT
3 or more doses of vaccine and last dose < 5 yr ago	No booster except children who have not received their 4th (12–15 mon) or 5th (4–6 yr) booster doses
Nonimmunized household	Benzathine penicillin, 1.2 × 10⁶ U IM OR Erythromycin, 40 mg/kg/d for 7 d Culture before and after treatment Observation daily for 7 days Diphtheria toxoid Less than 3 doses of DT, DPT, or dT or unknown: administer immediate dose of diphtheria toxoid and complete primary series according to schedule

tion until two cultures from both the nose and throat are negative. Patients with cutaneous diphtheria should be placed in contact isolation until two cultures of the skin are negative. Material for the cultures should be obtained at least 24 hours apart after cessation of the antibiotics.

Identification of Secondary Cases and Carriers

In view of the short incubation period of diphtheria and the delays in diagnosis, the primary means of detecting cases is to identify and monitor close contacts for at least 7 days. Asymptomatic carriers should also be identified because they may transmit the organism. Erythromycin, 40 mg per kg per day given orally for 7 days, is preferred over penicillin, as several reports have demonstrated its increased efficacy for carriers.

Prevention

Universal immunization remains the most effective control measure. However, although vaccination protects against the effects of the toxin, it does not protect against carriage or local disease. Therefore, effective treatment of patients with pharyngitis and of carriers is essential to eradicate both toxigenic organisms and those strains that may revert if left untreated.

FOOD–BORNE ILLNESS

method of
NATHAN M. THIELMAN, M.D., M.P.H., and
RICHARD L. GUERRANT, M.D.
University of Virginia School of Medicine
Charlottesville, Virginia

Diverse pathogenic microorganisms, toxins, and chemicals ingested with food may lead to varied gastrointestinal, neurologic, and systemic syndromes. Evaluation of the patient with a suspected food-borne illness should include careful attention not only to presenting symptoms and signs but also to a detailed food history and timing of symptoms in relation to food ingestion, recent travel, season, and the presence of similar symptoms among those who have shared similar meals (Figure 1). Although a food-specific attack rate is important for those who ate the suspected food, the most important additional figure is the attack rate among those who did not eat the suspected food to help implicate that food. Laboratory testing for suspected microorganisms or their toxins may help to establish the definitive etiology and enable directed therapy.

For many food-borne illnesses, appropriate treatment is primarily supportive because the toxic insult is generally short-lived and reversible. Patients with food-borne gastroenteritis caused by certain bacterial pathogens may, however, benefit from additional antimicrobial therapy (Table 1 and see text later). The cornerstone of therapy for patients with diarrheal illnesses is replacement of lost fluid and electrolytes. In most cases, this is best accomplished with the simple and inexpensive oral rehydration therapy (ORT) recommended by the World Health Organization (WHO). This lifesaving, simple, and cost-effective formulation can be reconstituted from packets (Jianas Brothers Packaging Co., Kansas City, Missouri), or approximations of this formulation can be made at home (Table 2). In addition, food or cereal-based ORT can be prepared as noted in Table 2; rice powder–based ORT packets can also be purchased inexpensively (Cera Products, Inc., Columbia, Maryland). A number of more expensive commercially available products (such as Pedialyte and Lytren) vary from the WHO formulation but remain safe and effective alternatives. Regardless of which solution is used, therapy should be prompt and aimed at replacing both the existing fluid deficit and the continuing fluid losses resulting from diarrhea and basal metabolism. Uncontrolled vomiting, ileus, severe fluid deficit with obtundation or toxicity, or severe monosaccharide malabsorption are contraindications to ORT and mandate intravenous fluid resuscitation.

Most food-borne diarrheal illnesses are self-limited and brief. With more prolonged illnesses not associated with inflammatory colitis, symptomatic therapy with loperamide (Imodium) for adults, 4 mg initially, followed by 2 mg after each loose stool, not to exceed 16 mg per day, usually provides significant relief. Bismuth subsalicylate (Pepto-Bismol), although in general not as effective as loperamide, has shown modest efficacy in treating traveler's diarrhea.

Protracted nausea and vomiting associated with food-borne illnesses may be controlled with an antiemetic agent. Prochlorperazine (Compazine), 5 to 10 mg orally, 25 mg per rectal suppository, or 10 mg intramuscularly; promethazine (Phenergan), 12.5 to 25 mg orally, intramuscularly, or per rectum; or trimethobenzamide (Tigan), 250 mg orally, or 200 mg intramuscularly or per rectum, may help to control nausea and vomiting in adults. Trimethobenzamide can be used in children over 2 years of age.

MICROBIAL FOOD POISONING SYNDROMES

Early-Onset Nausea and Vomiting

Food poisoning characterized primarily by nausea and vomiting within 1 to 6 hours of ingestion is typically caused by preformed enterotoxins of *Staphylococcus aureus* or *Bacillus cereus*. If symptoms occur within 5 to 60 minutes of ingestion, and are associated with a metallic taste, heavy metal poisoning should also be considered (see later).

Staphylococcal food poisoning typically follows ingestion of foods such as ham, cream-filled cakes, poultry, and egg salads—all of which favor the growth of staphylococci following contamination by an infected or colonized food handler and improper

84

Figure 1 presents the characteristics of infectious food poisoning syndromes as a branching chart linking clinical syndromes, incubation periods, fecal leukocytes, and etiologic agents, with attributes listed below. The content is transcribed as a table.

Etiologic Agent	Clinical Syndrome	Incubation Period	Fecal Leukocytes	Frequently Associated Foods/Situations	Other Clinical Features	Duration of Illness	Season	Laboratory Diagnosis
Staph. aureus	Nausea & Vomiting	1–6 h	−	Ham, Poultry, Pastries, Egg salads	Diarrhea 68%	<24 h	Summer	Egg-yolk–tellurite–glycine–pyruvate agar or mannitol salt; phage-type isolates; enterotoxin testing
Bacillus cereus "emetic syndrome"	Nausea & Vomiting	1–6 h	−	Fried rice, Meats, Vegetables, Cream	Diarrhea 33%	<12 h	Year-round	>10⁵ colonies on peptone-beef extract egg-yolk agar; need controls for stool analysis (may be normal flora)
Clostridium perfringens	Abdominal Cramps & Diarrhea	6–24 h	−	Beef, Poultry, Gravy, Mexican food	Vomiting & fever <10%	<24 h	Fall, winter, spring	Egg-yolk–free tryptose–sulfite–cyclo-serine agar; Hobbs or bacteriocin typing
B. cereus "diarrhea syndrome"	Abdominal Cramps & Diarrhea	6–24 h	−	Meats, Vegetables, Soups, Puddings, Sauces	Vomiting 33%	<24 h	Year-round (?)	Same as "emetic syndrome"
Norwalk Virus	Watery Diarrhea	16–72 h	−	Shellfish, Salads	Vomiting >50%	24–48 h	Year-round	Immune EM; ELISA, RIA, and PCR in research laboratories
ETEC	Watery Diarrhea	16–72 h	−	Travel	Rare fever & vomiting	72–96 h	Summer	ELISA for LT/ST; tissue culture assay, DNA probes
Vibrio cholerae	Watery Diarrhea	16–72 h	−	Shellfish	Rare fever & vomiting	5 days	Variable	TCBS agar
*Vibrio parahaemolyticus**	Watery Diarrhea	16–72 h	+	Seafood	Vomiting 35–80%	3–5 days	Spring, summer, fall	TCBS agar
Salmonellae*	Fever, Tenesmus, & Dysenteric Diarrhea	16–72 h	±	Eggs, Poultry, Beef, Dairy	Vomiting 35–80%	3–5 days	Summer	Salmonella-Shigella (SS) medium; deoxycholate citrate, Hektoen enteric or xylose-lysine-deoxycholate media
Shigellae & EIEC	Fever, Tenesmus, & Dysenteric Diarrhea	16–72 h	+	Eggs, Vegetables, Dairy	Vomiting 35–80%	3–5 days	Summer, fall	Salmonella-Shigella (SS) medium; deoxycholate citrate, Hektoen enteric or xylose-lysine-deoxycholate media; EIEC by Sereny test or DNA probe only
Campylobacter jejuni[1]	Fever, Tenesmus, & Dysenteric Diarrhea	16–72 h	+	Poultry, Milk, Pets, Beef	Vomiting 15–25%	5–7 days	Spring, summer, fall	Skirrow, Butzler, Campy-BAP and others grown in reduced oxygen
Yersinia enterocolitica	Fever, Abdominal Pain	16–72 h	±	Milk, Tofu, Pork	Vomiting 25–40%	24 h to 4 weeks	Winter	Cold enrichment, alkali treatment, or selective CIN agar increases yield
Clostridium botulinum	Paralysis ± Vomiting, Diarrhea	12–36 h	−	Vegetables, Fruits, Fish	Constipation later in illness	Weeks to months	Summer, fall	Toxin detection by mouse bioassay and special media by CDC
EHEC	Bloody Diarrhea	1–8 days	−[2]	Beef, Dairy, Cider	Fever usually absent; leukocytosis[3]	1–12 days (uncomplicated)	Variable	Sorbitol-MacConkey medium and serotyping

·Incubation periods for *V. parahaemolyticus* and Salmonellae may rarely be as short as 5 h.

[1]Incubation periods for *C. jejuni* may be as long as 7 days.

[2]Fecal leukocytes are present in approximately 30% of patients with EHEC.

[3]Systemic leukocytosis may herald the onset of hemolytic uremic syndrome.

Figure 1. Characteristics of infectious food poisoning syndromes. *Abbreviations*: ETEC = enterotoxic *Escherichia coli*; EIEC = enteroinvasive *E. coli*; EHEC = enterohemorrhagic *E. coli*; EM = electron microscopy; ELISA = enzyme-linked immunosorbent assay; RIA = radioimmunoassay; PCR = polymerase chain reaction; LT/ST = labile toxin/stable toxin; TCBS = thiosulfate citrate bile salts sucrose; BAP = blood agar plate; CIN = cefsulodine-irgasan-novobiocin; CDC = Centers for Disease Control and Prevention.

TABLE 1. **Antibiotics for Acute Bacterial Food-Borne Illnesses***

Pathogen	Drug	Usual Adult Dosage	Notes
Shigella	**Ciprofloxacin** (Cipro)†	500 mg PO bid × 3–5 days	A single 1-gram dose of ciprofloxacin may be as effective as a 5-day/10-dose course in patients with *Shigella* other than *S. dysenteriae* type 1
	Norfloxacin (Noroxin)†	400 mg PO bid × 3–5 days	
	TMP-SMX (Bactrim, Septra)	1 DS PO bid × 3–5 days	Increasingly resistant strains are reported in many developing regions
	Ampicillin	500 mg PO or 1 gm IV q 6 h × 3–5 days	Increasingly resistant strains are noted in many developing regions
	Nalidixic acid (NegGram)	1 gm q 6 h × 3–5 days	Like 4-fluoroquinolones, causes arthropathy when given in high doses to immature animals
Nontyphoid *Salmonella*‡	**Ciprofloxacin**†	500 mg PO bid or 400 mg IV q 12 h until patient is free of fever for at least 24 h	Antimicrobial therapy may prolong intestinal shedding of *Salmonella* spp
	TMP-SMX	1 DS PO bid	
	Amoxicillin	500 mg PO tid	
	Ampicillin	1–2 gm IV q 4–6 h	
	Cefoperazone (Cefobid)	2 gm IV q 12 h	
	Ceftriaxone (Rocephin)	1 gm IV q 12 h	
Campylobacter jejuni§	**Erythromycin**	250–500 mg PO qid × 5–7 days	Increased rates of resistance reported in Thailand
	Ciprofloxacin†	500 mg PO bid × 7 days	Increased resistance in Thailand; rarely resistance and associated clinical relapse has developed during therapy
	Tetracycline‖	500 mg PO qid × 7 days	Higher resistance rates (~30%)
Travelers' diarrhea¶	**Ciprofloxacin**†	1 gm once or 500 mg PO bid × 3–5 days	
	Norfloxacin†	800 mg once or 400 mg PO bid × 3–5 days	
	Ofloxacin (Floxin)	600 mg once or 300 mg PO bid × 3–5 days	
	TMP-SMX	2 DS once or 1 DS PO bid × 3–5 days	Loading dose regimen followed by standard doses for 3 days may be more effective
	Furazolidone (Furoxone)	100 mg PO qid × 7 days	
*Vibrio cholerae***	**Tetracycline**‖	500 mg qid or 2 gm q day × 2 days	Tetracycline-resistant outbreaks have been reported in Africa and Asia
	Doxycycline‖	300 mg PO × 1 day	
	TMP-SMX	1 DS PO bid × 3 days	
	Furazolidone	100 mg PO qid × 3 days	Alternative for treatment of children and pregnant women

*Preferred antibiotics are listed in **bold;** directed antibiotic therapy should also take into account local sensitivity patterns if available.

†Quinolones in immature animals can cause arthropathy, and their safety and efficacy has not been established in persons <18 years of age, pregnant women, and nursing mothers.

‡Treatment is particularly recommended for bacteremia prophylaxis in patients at extremes of age, with prosthetic material(s) present, or immunocompromised hosts (see text).

§Studies in which antibiotic treatment is initiated early in the course of illness (≤4 days) demonstrate clinical benefit.

‖Should not be used in children <7 years of age.

¶Most common bacterial enteropathogens include enterotoxigenic, enteroadherent, and enteroinvasive *Escherichia coli* as well as *Shigella, C. jejuni,* and *Salmonella.*

**Although the mainstay of therapy should be volume replacement, antibiotics diminish volume and duration of diarrhea and volume replacement requirements.

Abbreviations: TMP-SMX = trimethoprim-sulfamethoxazole; DS = double strength.

storage at room temperature. About 75% of patients present with nausea and vomiting, and a slightly lower percentage of patients will subsequently develop diarrhea. Fever and other systemic symptoms are rare. Definitive diagnosis can be established by culturing the stool or vomitus of a patient or the implicated food itself.

Ingestion of a preformed emetic toxin produced by *B. cereus* causes an acute emetic syndrome similar to that seen with staphylococcal food poisoning. The strong association of *B. cereus* emetic syndrome with consumption of fried rice has been attributed to germination of heat-resistant spores on cooling boiled rice to room temperature; flash-frying does not pro-

TABLE 2. **Oral Rehydration Formula**

WHO Formula		Home Recipe	
Ingredient	*Amount**	*Ingredient*	*Amount**
NaCl	3.5 gm	Table salt	¾ tbsp
NaHCO$_3$	2.5 gm	Baking soda	1 tsp
KCl	1.5 gm	Orange juice	1 cup
Glucose	20 gm	Table sugar†	4 level tbsp

*Per 1 liter (1.05 quarts) of clean water.
†Food-based oral rehydration formulations, prepared by replacing table sugar with 50–60 gm of cereal flour or 200 gm of mashed boiled potato, may help to reduce fluid output.
Abbreviation: WHO = World Health Organization.

duce sufficient heat to inactivate the heat-stable emetic toxin.

Because the duration of both staphylococcal and *B. cereus* emetic illnesses is usually less than 12 to 24 hours, therapy aimed at correcting fluid and electrolyte abnormalities is generally sufficient. Antibiotic therapy is not indicated.

Noninflammatory Diarrhea

Early Onset (6–24 Hours)

Profuse watery diarrhea and abdominal cramping occurring 6 to 24 hours after ingestion of contaminated food is frequently caused by the in vivo production of either a heat-labile toxin from *Clostridium perfringens* or by the diarrheogenic toxin of *B. cereus*. Although nausea may occur, vomiting is usually not seen, and fever is rare. In most patients, symptoms resolve within 24 hours. Typically *C. perfringens* food poisoning occurs when meat products are allowed to sit at temperatures between 15° and 60° C for 2 to 3 hours or more, thereby allowing clostridial spores (commonly present in raw meats and vegetables) to germinate and multiply. In outbreaks of *C. perfringens* food poisoning, around 50% of individuals consuming the contaminated food will develop symptoms. The diarrheal syndrome of *B. cereus* has been associated with ingestion of proteinaceous foods, sauces, puddings, and vegetables.

Later Onset (16–72 Hours)

Norwalk virus and other small, round, structured viruses (SRSVs) cause diarrhea after a longer incubation period of 24 to 48 hours. Poorly cooked or raw shellfish, salads, and contaminated drinking water have all been implicated in point-source outbreaks caused by this organism. Secondary cases among close contacts not initially exposed to the contaminated food suggests Norwalk virus as a possible cause. Clinically, infection is usually manifest first by abdominal cramping and nausea, followed by myalgias with diarrhea and/or vomiting. Malaise and headaches are not uncommon; low-grade fevers occur in close to 50% of patients. Various tests are available to diagnose Norwalk infection definitively (see Figure 1), but these are not practical in most clinical situations. Treatment with bismuth subsalicylate has been shown to decrease gastrointestinal symptoms in Norwalk-induced disease in human volunteers.

Enterotoxigenic *Escherichia coli* (ETEC) is the leading identifiable cause of diarrhea among travelers from industrialized regions to the developing world and has been rarely associated with food-borne outbreaks in the United States. Like cholera, ETEC causes a profuse watery diarrhea unaccompanied by fevers or vomiting. The incubation period for each of these illnesses is between 16 and 72 hours. Although symptoms rarely last longer than 5 days, the severe dehydration caused by ETEC may be life-threatening. ORT is the mainstay of therapy in mild-to-moderate disease; in severely dehydrated patients, intravenous therapy may be necessary. Early antimicrobial therapy further reduces fluid losses and the duration of diarrhea. ETEC infections typically respond to ciprofloxacin (Cipro), norfloxacin (Noroxin), or trimethoprim-sulfamethoxazole (TMP-SMX) (Bactrim, Septra), although resistance to all of these agents is increasing globally. Occasionally food-borne diarrhea associated with *Vibrio cholerae* has been reported in the United States. Tetracycline is the drug of choice for most patients with cholera; doxycycline, TMP–SMX, and furazolidone (Furoxone) are also effective.

Inflammatory Diarrhea

Food-borne diarrheal illnesses associated with fever, tenesmus, mucoid stools, severe dehydration, or prolonged duration should prompt examination for fecal leukocytes or fecal lactoferrin (a sensitive and specific surrogate marker for leukocytes in adults). Such syndromes usually occur within 16 to 72 hours of ingesting contaminated food (or water) and are characteristically caused by invasive pathogens including *Salmonella*, *Shigella*, and *Campylobacter*.

Salmonellosis is the single leading identified cause of food-borne disease in the United States, with approximately 1% of the population becoming infected each year. In 1994, a single outbreak linked to contaminated ice cream was responsible for more than 200,000 estimated cases of *Salmonella enteritidis* gastroenteritis. Improperly prepared poultry, eggs, beef, pork, and dairy products are the most common sources for food-borne salmonella infections. Taking antimicrobials in the month prior to illness has been identified as a risk factor for salmonellosis. In most patients, the illness is usually self-limited with resolution of fever within 2 days and resolution of diarrhea after 3 to 5 days. Among human immunodeficiency virus (HIV)–infected patients the disease is frequently more severe, and bacteremia is more common. The diagnosis is readily made by culturing the organism from freshly passed stools onto a variety of standard enteric laboratory media. Although some antibiotics (particularly ciprofloxacin) may reduce the duration of symptoms in *Salmonella* gastroenteritis, they may prolong the intestinal carriage state and have been associated with clinical relapse. Thus, the routine use of antibiotics in the uncomplicated patient is controversial. However, patients with *Salmonella* gastroenteritis who are younger than 12 weeks of age or older than 50 years; those with lymphoproliferative disorders, malignancies, hemoglobinopathies (including sickle cell disease), or acquired immune deficiency disease (AIDS); transplant recipients; those with vascular grafts, artificial joints, marked degenerative joint disease, valvular heart disease; and those on steroids should receive antibiotics until afebrile for at least 24 hours. All bacteremic patients should be treated for 7 to 14 days (longer if a metastatic focus is present). Fluoroquinolones or a third-generation cephalosporin are reasonable initial antibiotic choices until culture sensitivity results become available.

Recent estimates suggest that the annual incidence of food-borne *Campylobacter* gastroenteritis in the United States may rival that of *Salmonella*-induced disorders. Common food sources include poultry, milk, and beef, and infection usually occurs in nonwinter months. The gastrointestinal symptoms associated with inflammatory diarrhea are often preceded by a 12- to 24-hour prodrome of headache, fever, and malaise; diarrhea generally lasts for 5 to 7 days. Routine stool cultures often do not detect campylobacter organisms; thus, selective media (such as Skirrow, Butzler, Campy-Bap) should be used when this organism is suspected. Because the illness is short-lived and self-limited, antibiotics generally do not alter the course of disease unless administered early. Erythromycin has been shown to eradicate *Campylobacter* from stool but does not alter the natural course of the disease when initiated 4 days or longer after the onset of symptoms. Increasing erythromycin resistance is being reported in developing regions. Ciprofloxacin is also usually effective, although resistant organisms are increasing (two-thirds of isolates in U.S. troops in Thailand were recently reported to be resistant), and clinical relapses occasionally occur. In general, if the patient presents soon after the onset of symptoms, appears toxic, or is immunocompromised, antimicrobial therapy is indicated.

Shigellosis, also a relatively common cause of food-borne disease, occurs most frequently in the summer and fall. As ingestion of fewer than 200 *Shigella* organisms readily causes disease, transmission of shigellosis is very efficient, rendering direct person-to-person contact a common means of infection. Food-borne transmission, when it occurs, tends to be associated with large outbreaks coupled with cases of secondary transmission. Fever is documented in 33% of cases and grossly bloody stools are seen in 40%; tenesmus and abdominal pain are frequent. As with *Salmonella, Shigella* can be cultured on routine enteric media. Microbiologic recovery of the organism is best accomplished early in the illness when higher concentrations of viable organisms are present. For shigellosis acquired in the United States, either TMP-SMX or a fluoroquinolone is a reasonable initial antimicrobial choice; shigellosis acquired in developing regions (where trimethoprim resistance is common) should be treated with a fluoroquinolone (the newer agents are not approved for use in children; see Table 1), pending susceptibility testing.

Rarely in the United States, but more frequently in Japan, *Vibrio parahaemolyticus* has been implicated in food-borne infections. Illness is characterized by the sudden onset of watery diarrhea associated with ingestion of seafood. In some patients the disease appears to be more inflammatory and is characterized by fever, chills, and bloody dysentery. Because of the short duration of illness, treatment beyond supportive measures generally is not necessary.

Yersinia enterocolitica is also a relatively rare cause of food-borne disease in the United States; it is more prevalent in Europe. Children under 5 years of age are particularly susceptible to *Yersinia* food poisoning, which occurs primarily during the winter months and is associated with improperly prepared meat or dairy products. In addition to causing diarrhea, *Y. enterocolitica* infection may be complicated by mesenteric adenitis or a reactive polyarthritis, the latter particularly in adults. There are no data to support the use of antibiotics in uncomplicated *Y. enterocolitica* gastroenteritis; in complicated illnesses, treatment should be guided by in vitro susceptibility data.

Hemorrhagic Diarrhea

Enterohemorrhagic *E. coli* (EHEC) (particularly *E. coli* serotype O157:H7) and *Shigella* are the most common food-borne causes of bloody diarrhea and colitis. EHEC infections have been linked to the consumption of rare hamburgers, unpasteurized dairy products, fresh-pressed apple cider, and contaminated water—usually 72 to 120 hours prior to the onset of symptoms. Most patients with hemorrhagic colitis remain afebrile, and fecal leukocytes are seen in only 30 to 40% of cases. The potentially devastating complication, hemolytic uremic syndrome (HUS), a constellation of microangiopathic hemolytic anemia, thrombocytopenia, and acute renal failure, occurs most frequently in children between 1 and 4 years of age and in elderly people; it may be heralded by the onset of fever and leukocytosis during the acute illness. When EHEC is suspected, stool should be plated on sorbitol-MacConkey medium, and any sorbitol-negative *E. coli* isolates should be serotyped. In addition, serologic testing for *E. coli* O157 infections is a potentially useful clinical diagnostic tool.

The role of antibiotics in treating EHEC infections has not been clearly established. Some potentially biased epidemiologic data have associated TMP–SMX administration with the development of HUS in some patients, and in vitro clinical EHEC isolates have been found to secrete more toxin in response to TMP-SMX and other antibiotics. Other studies, however, have found that prolonged antibiotic therapy either had no effect on or decreased the incidence of progression to HUS. Currently, supportive care with particular attention toward maintaining euvolemia and monitoring for signs of HUS (by following platelet counts, blood smears, and renal function) remains the mainstay of management of EHEC infections.

NEUROLOGIC SYMPTOMS (FOOD–BORNE BOTULISM)

A rare but serious food-borne disease manifested primarily as a symmetrical descending paralysis is caused by toxins produced by *Clostridium botulinum*. Among adults, the disease usually occurs after ingestion of improperly canned foods or fish contaminated with botulinum toxin, whereas among infants under 1 year of age disease has been associated with in vivo toxin production after ingesting honey contaminated with *C. botulinum* spores. Early symptoms include blurred vision and photophobia, dry mouth, dysphagia, dysphonia, nausea and vomiting, and generalized weakness. This may be followed by constipation, postural hypotension, and paralysis with respiratory compromise. Major considerations in the differential diagnosis of botulism includes Guillain-Barré syndrome, myasthenia gravis, poliomyelitis, stroke, and drug reaction. The diagnosis may be supported by specific electromyographic findings; definitive diagnosis may be established by a mouse bioassay for the toxin in the patient's stool or serum or in the suspected food. Intensive monitoring and aggressive respiratory support are mandatory in any patient with suspected botulism. Patients with suspected botulism should be reported immediately to state health department officials and to the Centers for Disease Control and Prevention (404-639-2206) from whom trivalent equine antitoxin may be obtained. Antitoxin therapy does not reverse pre-existing paralysis, but it does prevent its progression. It is associated with hypersensitivity reactions in nearly 10% of patients.

Syndromes Associated with Seafood Ingestion

Ciguatera Fish Poisoning

Ciguatera fish poisoning results from ingestion of fish contaminated with ciguatoxin, a neurotoxin originating from dinoflagellates and propagated through the aquatic food chain. More than 400 species of fish (restricted to oceans within a 30-degree latitude on either side of the equator) have been noted to harbor ciguatoxin; grouper, red snapper, and barracuda have been most frequently implicated. Nausea, vomiting, and diarrhea may be followed by pruritus, paresthesias, dry mouth, photophobia, and blurred vision. In severe cases, cranial nerve palsies, bradycardia, hypotension, and respiratory paralysis may occur.

If the patient presents within 4 hours of ingestion, emesis induction or gastric lavage may prevent further toxin absorption, and in severe cases, atropine may be useful to control symptomatic bradycardia. Mechanical ventilation may be necessary if the patient develops respiratory failure secondary to paralysis.

Scombroid Fish Poisoning

Ingestion of spoiled fish, most commonly from the families Scombridae and Scomberesocidae (which include tuna, mackerel, skipjack, mahi-mahi, and bonito) may lead to scombrotoxicosis, a syndrome resembling a histamine reaction. Typically within 10 minutes to 3 hours after ingesting the contaminated fish, patients will develop symptoms including sudden onset flushing, headache, nausea, vomiting, diarrhea, and in severe cases, respiratory distress. The diagnosis is confirmed by demonstrating greater than 100 mg of histamine per gram in the suspected fish. Antihistamines and bronchodilators may provide symptomatic relief, although most symptoms usually resolve within 6 hours.

Puffer Fish Poisoning

Ingestion of improperly prepared puffer fish may lead to tetrodotoxin intoxication. Such poisoning is characterized by the rapid onset of weakness, paresthesias, and abdominal pain, which may be followed by a general flaccid ascending paralysis with respiratory failure and death. In Japan, where most cases are described, mortality rates as high as 60% have been reported.

Paralytic Shellfish Poisoning

Paralytic shellfish poisoning is caused by eating mussels, clams, or oysters containing concentrated saxitoxin, a potent neurotoxin that causes nausea, vomiting, diarrhea, and facial paresthesias. In severe cases, dysphonia, dysphagia, paralysis, and respiratory compromise may occur. Most illnesses occur in the summer and early fall and may be associated with a red tide event that reflects high concentrations of potentially toxin-producing dinoflagellates. The incubation period is probably inversely related to the amount of toxin ingested, ranging from 30 minutes to 10 hours; symptoms last from a few hours to a few days. If not contraindicated by the presence of an ileus, enemas or cathartics may be used in an attempt to remove unabsorbed toxin from the intestinal tract.

Neurotoxic Shellfish Poisoning

Neurotoxic shellfish poisoning usually occurs within 4 hours of eating shellfish harvested during the spring or fall from the Gulf Coast or Florida's Atlantic coast. Much like paralytic shellfish poisoning, illness is characterized by nausea, vomiting, and paresthesias; however, paralysis does not occur, and symptoms are usually milder in neurotoxic shellfish poisoning.

Amnesic Shellfish Poisoning

Described in a 1987 outbreak in Canada, amnesic shellfish poisoning (also called "toxic encephalopathic shellfish poisoning") was associated with ingesting mussels contaminated with domoic acid. Clinical features of amnesic shellfish poisoning include initial nausea, vomiting, and diarrhea, often followed by confusion, anterograde amnesia, coma, and cardio-vascular instability in severe cases.

Mushroom Poisoning

Toxic mushroom ingestion may lead to a variety of clinical syndromes, depending on the type of mushroom ingested (Table 3). Although many mushroom intoxication syndromes are self-limited and require only supportive therapy, others may be fatal. If mushroom poisoning is suspected, a local poison control center should be contacted promptly. Thirty minutes to 2 hours after ingestion of the muscarine-containing mushrooms *Clitocybe* spp and *Inocybe*

spp, patients develop an anticholinergic syndrome of sweating, salivation, lacrimation, and bradycardia, among other indications of parasympathetic hyperactivity. Although symptoms usually resolve within 24 hours, severe cases may be fatal and thus should be treated with parenteral atropine sulfate, up to 1 to 2 mg every 2 to 6 hours as warranted for bradycardia.

Most fatal mushroom poisonings occur with ingestion of *Amanita phalloides* and several other species that produce amatoxins and phallotoxins. The resultant illness is characteristically biphasic with abdominal pain, vomiting, and diarrhea occurring 6 to 12 hours after ingestion and usually resolving within 24 hours. After appearing well for 1 to 2 days, the pa-

TABLE 3. **Seafood, Mushroom, and Plant Poisoning Syndromes**

Food	Toxic Compound	Incubation Period	Syndrome
Seafood			
Ciguatera fish poisoning (grouper, red snapper, barracuda)	Ciguatoxin	1–6 h	Nausea, vomiting, diarrhea, pruritus, paresthesias
Scombroid poisoning (tuna, mackerel, bonito, skipjack, mahi-mahi)	Scombrotoxin	Within 30 min	"Histamine-like" reactions: headache, flushing, pruritus, urticaria, nausea, vomiting
Puffer fish poisoning	Tetrodotoxin	5–30 min	Paralysis, respiratory failure
Paralytic shellfish poisoning	Saxitoxin and others	1–10 h	Paresthesias (face, extremities), nausea, vomiting, diarrhea, paralysis in severe cases
Neurotoxic shellfish poisoning	Several neurotoxins	Within 3 h	Paresthesias, nausea, vomiting, diarrhea
Amnesic shellfish poisoning	Domoic acid	15 min–6 h	Vomiting, cramps, diarrhea—sometimes followed by confusion, amnesia, coma, cardiovascular instability
Mushrooms			
Clitocybe and *Inocybe* groups	Muscarinic compounds	30 min–2 h	Anticholinergic syndrome: sweating, salivation, lacrimation, bradycardia, vomiting
Amanita spp	Ibotenic acid and isoxazole derivatives	20–90 min	Confusion, restlessness, visual disturbances
Psilocybe or *Panaeolus* spp	Psilocybin, psilocin, and related indoles	30–60 min	Mood elevation, hallucination, hyperkinetic activity, and muscle weakness
Coprinus spp	Coprine	Up to 5 days	Disulfiram-like reaction within 30 min after alcohol ingestion
Amanita phalloides	Amatoxins and phallotoxins	6–24 h	Initially: abdominal pain, vomiting, diarrhea 2–3 days later: renal failure, hepatic failure
Gyromitra spp	Gyromitrin	2–12 h	Nausea, vomiting, hemolysis, methemoglobinemia, hepatic failure
Corinarius spp	Orellanine	3–5 days	Thirst, nausea, headache, abdominal pain, visual disturbance
Plants			
Favism (fava bean)	Vincine and convincine	5–24 h	Acute hemolytic crisis in patients with G6PD deficiency
Lathyrism (chickling vetch, sweet peas)	Possibly neurolathyrogen	Prolonged; insidious	Muscle spasm, cramps, leg weakness, signs of degeneration in posterolateral tract of spinal cord
Solanine poisoning (potato tubers, vines, leaves, new sprouts; tomato plant stems, leaves)	Solanine	8–12 h	Headache, abdominal pain, diarrhea, confusion
Acute cyanide poisoning (lima beans, manioc, unripe sorghum, bitter almonds, apricot kernels, apple seeds)	Cyanogenetic glycosides	Within 1 h	Hyperventilation, headache, paralysis, seizures, respiratory arrest
Chronic cyanide poisoning (cassava)	Cyanogenetic glycosides	Prolonged; insidious	Ataxic neuropathy, goiter, possibly amblyopia

Abbreviation: G6PD = glucose-6-phosphate dehydrogenase.

tient develops both renal and hepatic failure. Despite intensive supportive care, the mortality rate may be as high as 30 to 50%. Hemoperfusion may be useful to help remove circulating toxin. A similar syndrome without renal failure may occur after ingestion of mushrooms of the genus *Gyromitra* containing gyromitrin, an inhibitor of pyridoxal phosphate. In addition to hepatic failure, hemolysis and methemoglobinuria are seen in the later phases of the illness. Intravenous pyridoxine hydrochloride may be useful for treatment of neurologic symptoms.

Other Food-Related Illnesses

Acute food-related syndromes rarely result from ingestion of various plant-derived foods that contain high levels of endogenous toxicants. Consumption of fava beans (*Vicia faba*), particularly by individuals who are glucose-6-phosphate dehydrogenase–deficient, may lead to an acute hemolytic crisis within 5 to 24 hours after ingestion. The acute illness typically lasts for 24 to 48 hours, although support with blood transfusions may be necessary. Solanine poisoning, primarily associated with potato tubers, causes abdominal pain, diarrhea, and confusion typically 8 to 12 hours after ingestion. Rarely, acute cyanide poisoning may result from ingestion of a number of different plant-derived foodstuffs. Chronic cyanide poisoning from high consumption of cassava, particularly in some African cultures, may lead to tropical ataxic neuropathy, tropical amblyopia, and possibly goiters. Lathyrism, an insidious neurologic illness progressing from muscle spasm and cramps to weakness and paralysis, and associated with degeneration of the posterolateral tracts of the spinal cord, results from chronic ingestion of large quantities of legumes of the genus *Lathyrus*. Lathyrism is generally confined to Africa and Asia and is particularly associated with increased consumption of *L. sativus* (sweet peas).

Monosodium glutamate (MSG) ingestion, particularly on an empty stomach, may cause nausea, headache, flushing, and a burning sensation in the skin. Symptoms typically occur soon after beginning the meal and resolve within 4 hours. Because MSG is commonly used in Chinese foods (particularly won ton soup) the syndrome associated with its ingestion has been called the "Chinese restaurant syndrome."

Heavy metal poisoning with copper, zinc, iron, tin, or cadmium is known to cause nausea, vomiting, diarrhea, and a metallic taste within 5 to 60 minutes after ingestion. In addition, cadmium may be associated with increased salivation and cadmium and zinc may cause myalgias. Heavy metal contamination often occurs when acidic (especially citric or carbonated) beverages are allowed to come in contact with metal containers or tubing for prolonged periods of time.

NECROTIZING SOFT TISSUE INFECTIONS

method of
RICHARD J. HOWARD, M.D.
University of Florida
Gainesville, Florida

Necrotizing soft tissue infections are a group of diverse diseases characterized by infection-induced, extensive, rapidly progressive necrosis of the soft tissues: skin, subcutaneous tissue, fascia, and muscles. These necrotizing infections most commonly affect tissues of the lower parts of the body including the lower extremities, perineum, perianal area, and abdomen, although any soft tissue can be affected.

Classification systems for necrotizing soft tissue infections range from a simple one of including all necrosis due to infectious causes under the name necrotizing soft tissue infection to complicated schemes based on the site of infection and the etiology. Some of these latter classifications include bacterial synergistic gangrene, necrotizing fasciitis, streptococcal gangrene, gas gangrene, clostridial cellulitis, nonclostridial cellulitis, monomicrobic necrotizing fasciitis, polymicrobic necrotizing fasciitis, clostridial myonecrosis, nonclostridial myonecrosis, necrotizing cutaneous mucormycosis, and gangrenous cellulitis. Attempts have been made to differentiate among these necrotizing infections based on predisposing conditions, the amount of pain, toxicity, presence or absence of fever, presence or absence of crepitus, appearance of the wound, and etiology. These complicated classification schemes are of little clinical usefulness. In practice it is difficult to differentiate among bacterial etiologies based on location or appearance of the wound. Furthermore, these complicated classification schemes do not help the clinician treat the patient. Because necrotizing infections frequently involve more than one layer of tissue, necrotizing fasciitis, necrotizing cellulitis, or necrotizing myonecrosis is seldom seen in pure form. Thus, including all necrotizing infections under one simple disease entity—necrotizing soft tissue infections—seems to be the most clinically useful and is by far the simplest classification.

PREDISPOSING CAUSES

Necrotizing soft tissue infections usually occur as a result of previous operation, after injury, or as a complication of inadequately treated or unrecognized minor infections such as perianal abscess, infected sebaceous cyst, infected Bartholin's duct cyst, or fistula-in-ano. Occasionally these infections can be primary, resulting from the spread of bacteria by the bloodstream to skin or other soft tissues where the bacteria proliferate and cause necrotizing infections. Necrotizing soft tissue infections can also be due to burns, bites, pre-existing cutaneous ulcers, or injections. They can even occur without any apparent predisposing cause.

Conditions that favor growth of anaerobic organisms such as *Clostridium* or mixed anaerobic and aerobic bacteria are commonly found in necrotizing soft tissue infections of the perineum and abdomen. These pathophysiologic factors include devitalization of tissue, foreign bodies, extensive contamination, improperly or poorly cared for wounds, blunt or penetrating trauma, burns, animal bites, and intravenous or subcutaneous injections. Even apparently clean operative incisions can be the initiating site of these infections. They also can develop because of previous ulcerative lesions such as ischemic leg ulcers, decubitus ulcers, perirectal or Bartholin's cyst abscesses, or inappropriate closure of contaminated wounds. Certain host factors also predispose patients to necrotizing soft tissue infections such as immunosuppression and chronic systemic diseases like diabetes mellitus.

Streptococcal and staphylococcal necrotizing infections tend to occur in individuals with chronic diseases such as diabetes or in immunosuppressed patients. But they can occur in apparently healthy individuals. Similarly, necrotizing infections due to *Vibrio* species occur primarily in individuals with severe liver disease but can also occur in those who are diabetic or in immunosuppressed cancer patients. They can also occur in apparently normal individuals. These infections are either a result of bloodborne bacteria after eating raw oysters or are due to contamination of apparently insignificant extremity wounds with marine waters.

It is good to remember that while many individuals have some predisposing cause, many cases of necrotizing soft tissue infections are found in otherwise apparently healthy individuals.

MICROBIOLOGY

Most necrotizing soft tissue infections are polymicrobial and are caused by common aerobes and anaerobic intestinal bacteria. These infections most commonly originate in the perineum or abdomen following abdominal operations or penetrating abdominal trauma. Commonly cultured bacteria include *Escherichia coli, Klebsiella, Pseudomonas, Bacteroides, Clostridium, Peptostreptococcus*, and *Peptococcus*. Gram-positive aerobic bacteria such as enterococci, staphylococci, and streptococci can also be identified in these mixed infections. In most series both anaerobic and aerobic intestinal bacteria can be cultured from approximately 75% of patients with necrotizing soft tissue infections.

Monomicrobic necrotizing infections are usually due to *Streptococcus pyogenes, Staphylococcus aureus*, or *Clostridium* species. *Vibrio* species can also cause necrotizing infections in individuals who eat raw oysters or those exposed to marine waters.

In certain susceptible individuals such as diabetics, Phycomycetes (*Rhizopus, Mucor*, and *Absidia*) can produce slowly progressive necrotizing infections. These infections are commonly found in the oropharyngeal cavity and frequently involve the hard and soft palate or nasal sinuses.

DIAGNOSIS

The diagnosis of necrotizing soft tissue infections is obvious when it involves the skin. Necrotic areas of skin may reflect only a small amount of the underlying necrotic tissue. The diagnosis is less obvious when necrosis involves subcutaneous tissue, fascia, or muscle without skin involvement. In these latter patients, signs and symptoms of necrotizing soft tissue infections include severe pain out of proportion to the local physical findings, marked edema, tenderness beyond the extent of cutaneous erythema, and crepitus. Skin vesicles and bullae may provide the outward signs of underlying necrotic tissue.

Patients can develop systemic signs of infection at any time during the course of the infection, such as fever, tachycardia, hypotension, and mental status changes that can range from mild confusion to delirium. With *Clostridium* especially, confusion can be the first sign of infection. If the infection is untreated, patients progress to severe sepsis with multiple-system organ failure, rhabdomyolysis in patients with myonecrosis, disseminated intravascular coagulation, and ultimately, death.

The diagnosis of necrotizing soft tissue infections is usually made clinically. Soft tissue roentgenograms can be helpful if they demonstrate gas in the subcutaneous tissues. Soft tissue gas and its clinical counterpart, crepitus, are usually late findings and may reflect a more advanced infection. Gas is released by many organisms in the course of respiration and metabolism and does not mean the patient has a clostridial infection. In fact, if gas is present, it is more likely that the patient has a mixed anaerobic/aerobic infection, since bacteria such as *E. coli* and other aerobes also release gas into the soft tissue and are much more common than clostridia.

Other visualization methods such as computed tomography and magnetic resonance imaging can also demonstrate soft tissue gas. They can also identify asymmetric edema within tissue planes, but edema is not diagnostic of infection, nor is edema diagnostic of necrosis in patients with infection. Soft tissue gas, however, is unusual in the absence of necrotizing infections in most series, especially when examined with standard roentgenograms.

Patients with myonecrosis can have elevated creatine phosphokinase levels. A normal CPK level virtually excludes muscle necrosis. Myoglobinuria can also be identified in patients with necrotic muscle. Laboratory tests, however, are rarely used to establish or exclude the diagnosis of necrotizing soft tissue infection.

It has been suggested that any of the following findings are indications for an open biopsy: local changes such as epidermal gangrene, cyanosis, blistering or bronzing of skin, severe pain or spreading area of anesthesia, wounds with thin reddish drainage and undermined edges, cellulitis with extensive surrounding edema, cellulitis that progresses despite antibiotics, cellulitis adjacent to any surgical wound or hematoma, abscess with multiple tracts, crepitus or radiographic evidence of gas, and systemic findings such as confusion, tachycardia, tachypnea, ketoacidosis, and hypoglycemia. Some have recommended early biopsy and frozen-section examination in suspicious cases to speed diagnosis and treatment. The dilemma for the surgeons is to identify as early as possible tissue necrosis in the presence of cellulitis. One is naturally reluctant to make incisions in every patient with cellulitis only because necrosis may be found. Nevertheless, because these necrotizing soft tissue infections are so lethal, it is frequently better to make what turns out to be unnecessary incisions than to let a necrotizing soft tissue infection go undiagnosed.

TREATMENT

Necrotizing soft tissue infections should be operated on as soon as possible once the disease is recognized and the patient has been adequately resuscitated and prepared for surgery. Patients who are operated on soon after necrotizing soft tissue infections are recognized to have a lower mortality rate than those in whom surgery is delayed. The mortality rate is also high when initial treatment is inadequate. The highest rate of survival occurs among patients in whom the necrotizing infection can be resolved with the first operation. But patients with necrotizing soft tissue infections usually require multiple débridements, on average 2.4 to 3.4 operations per patient.

The initial goal of operative therapy is débridement of all necrotic tissue, drainage of abscesses, control of the source of the infection if possible, antibiotic therapy, and possibly hyperbaric oxygen.

In patients in whom there is a high index of suspicion of tissue necrosis due to infection, it may be necessary to incise through normal tissue to examine the underlying tissue for viability. It is helpful to make skin incisions parallel to nerves or blood vessels to attempt to minimize injury to these structures. It is tempting for the surgeon not to remove all necrotic tissue at the initial therapy, because reconstructive surgery may be extremely difficult with large tissue defects. It is well to remember that unless total removal of all necrotic tissue is carried out there will be no reconstruction, because the patient will die.

Tissue specimens, abscess contents, and any other drainage or exudate should be sent to the laboratory for Gram stain, culture, and antimicrobial sensitivity testing. Cultures must be done aerobically and anaerobically. The specimen should also be cultured for fungi.

In patients with necrotizing soft tissue involving the extremities, fasciotomies are frequently necessary to prevent compartment syndrome. For patients with full-thickness necrotizing infections of the abdominal wall, prosthetic mesh may be required to prevent evisceration.

Colostomy may be required in patients with necrotizing soft tissue infection involving the perineum to prevent continuing contamination of the wound. In certain cases primary amputation may be life saving in patients with necrotizing soft tissue infection of the extremities.

It is not surprising that the surgeon may be reluctant to remove large amounts of soft tissue because of the disability that may ensue. Furthermore, extensive débridement always leads to large, unsightly scars and defects. Despite these drawbacks of extensive soft tissue removal, the surgeon should not be at all concerned about the eventual reconstruction of the wound. Only when the patient has completely stabilized and the infection controlled should reconstruction be reconsidered.

It can be difficult to differentiate viable from nonviable tissues. There is little difficulty with differentiating viable skin and subcutaneous fatty tissue from nonviable tissue. But muscle can present problems. Naturally, the surgeon is reluctant to remove tissue that may be viable. Difficulty in differentiating viable and nonviable muscle and fascia is one reason that reoperation for necrotizing soft tissue infection is usually required.

Virtually all patients should be reoperated on within 24 hours to make sure that all necrotic tissue has been removed. These wounds are so large and dressing changes are so painful initially that frequently general anesthesia is required anyway just to change the dressings. With few exceptions, re-

exploration should not be done in the intensive care unit because of the lack of adequate lighting and surgical equipment. Occasionally, however, with small necrotizing wounds, re-exploration can be done there if adequate anesthesia can be provided. Since these patients are frequently on respirators, a short-acting intravenous anesthetic can be given. Reoperation should be carried out frequently until the surgeon is assured that no more necrotic tissue remains.

Dressings should be applied to wounds to promote drainage. The term "packing" is unfortunate since frequently it becomes a contest to see how much dressing one can get into the wound. One should try to place as *little* dressing as possible so that drainage is maximally encouraged. Dressings can initially be soaked with saline or applied dry. They will become wet with wound exudate. Many surgeons like to apply dressing soaked in various solutions such as povidone-iodine, acetic acid, sodium hypochlorite solution, or hydrogen peroxide. These antiseptics do little to inhibit bacterial growth and kill human fibroblasts at lower concentrations than they kill bacteria. Their use should generally be discouraged.

Antibiotic Therapy

Because of the wide range of microorganisms that can cause necrotizing soft tissue infections and because of the rapidly fatal clinical course, initial antibiotic therapy should be broad-spectrum so that it covers virtually all the bacteria that can potentially cause these infections. Once culture results and Gram stain results have been obtained, more specific antibiotic therapy can be used. Initially, antibiotic therapy should include penicillin G because *Clostridium* and most *Streptococcus* species are sensitive to this antibiotic. Because many necrotizing soft tissue infections are due to mixed aerobic and anaerobic intestinal flora, broad-spectrum antibiotic regimens similar to those used to treat patients with peritonitis should be used. An aminoglycoside that covers gram-negative aerobic enteric bacteria and either metronidazole or clindamycin that is active against anaerobic bacteria should be initially administered. There are several other choices, such as imipenem/cilastatin (Primaxin) and extended-spectrum penicillin with a beta-lactamase inhibitor such as piperacillin/tazobactam (Zosyn), ticarcillin/clavulanic acid (Timentin), or ampicillin/sulbactam (Unasyn). Other combinations can also be used to treat these infections, such as metronidazole and a third-generation cephalosporin.

If the patient has a necrotizing soft tissue infection and a history of eating raw oysters or exposure to seawater, so that marine *Vibrio* bacteria are likely to be the causative organisms, antibiotics to which these bacteria are sensitive should be used. These antibiotics include cephalosporins, erythromycin, and tetracycline.

There is no clear indication of how long antibiotic therapy should be continued. We generally stop antibiotics when a patient is afebrile, the white count is returning toward normal, and the invasive infection is eradicated. Indications that invasive infection is eradicated include absence of systemic toxicity, cellulitis, and fever, decreasing or normal white blood cell count, and no further tissue necrosis. Prolonged antibiotic therapy may be required.

Hyperbaric Oxygen

Hyperbaric oxygen (HBO) has long been advocated as an adjunctive measure in treating necrotizing soft tissue infection, especially those due to *Clostridium* species. Despite strong feelings by advocates for the use of HBO in treating these infections, there are no data that clearly indicate it leads to a lower mortality rate or earlier resolution of the infection. Although HBO can clearly reduce the mortality rate in experimental clostridial infections, and despite the fact that several clinical studies suggest a decreased mortality rate when HBO therapy is used, there still remains no strong evidence that HBO therapy leads to a lower mortality rate or an earlier recovery rate in patients with either clostridial or other necrotizing soft tissue infections. No doubt HBO will be controversial in the future as well. It is unlikely that efficacy will ever be proved. No randomized studies are likely to be performed. The surgeon must ensure that its use does not delay surgical intervention or cause a surgeon to compromise on the adequacy of surgical débridement thinking that HBO will make questionable tissues come back to life. If HBO is to be administered, the patient should be treated after the initial débridement.

INFLUENZA

method of
KRISTIN L. NICHOL, M.D., M.P.H.
Minneapolis VA Medical Center and University of Minnesota Medical School
Minneapolis, Minnesota

THE VIRUS

Influenza viruses are single-stranded RNA viruses of the orthomyxovirus family. The three types of influenza viruses, A, B, and C, are determined by their nuclear material. Influenza A viruses are further classified into subtypes on the basis of the hemagglutinin (H1, H2, and H3) and neuraminidase (N1 and N2) surface antigens. All three types of influenza viruses may cause infections in humans, but only types A and B are significant causes of human illness. Over time, the influenza viruses can display remarkable antigenic variation. Because immunity to one viral subtype may confer little or no protection against viruses of other subtypes, major epidemics of respiratory disease continue to occur. In temperate climates, these influenza epidemics typically peak during the months of December through March.

EPIDEMIOLOGY

Influenza is truly a major though often unrecognized cause of illness, suffering, and death in the United States and worldwide. Each year, 10% to 20% of the American population develops influenza, which is characterized by the abrupt onset of fever, sore throat, nonproductive cough, myalgias, headaches, and malaise. Up to half of people with influenza may not present with these classic symptoms, especially in elderly populations. Although the typical episode resolves within 3 to 5 days, influenza may also be associated with profound malaise that persists for several weeks. Because of the substantial morbidity associated with illness, influenza is a cause of millions of school and work loss days among the 25 to 50 million persons in this country who develop influenza in any given year. The complications of influenza include not only pneumonia (typically secondary bacterial pneumonia) but also exacerbations of underlying respiratory and cardiac conditions, such as chronic obstructive lung disease and congestive heart failure, and even death. These complications occur most frequently and are most devastating among elderly people and account for hundreds of thousands of hospitalizations, tens of thousands of excess deaths, and billions of dollars in health care costs each year. In children, another rare complication of influenza B (and varicella-zoster) is Reye's syndrome, which may be associated with the use of aspirin to treat these illnesses.

DIAGNOSIS

Influenza is usually diagnosed on the basis of clinical findings, particularly when there are known community outbreaks. It may also be confirmed through laboratory means including viral culture (throat or nasopharyngeal swabs obtained within 3 days of onset of illness), serologic confirmation from acute and convalescent antibody titers, and rapid direct antigen testing for influenza A. Laboratory confirmation may be particularly useful for surveillance and for outbreak identification and control in closed populations like nursing homes.

VACCINE

The major means of preventing influenza is through the use of inactivated influenza virus vaccine. Current formulations of the vaccine (either whole virus or split virus) contain antigens from three virus strains (two type A and one type B) likely to circulate during the coming influenza season. Because these component strains may change from year to year, annual immunization is recommended. The Advisory Committee on Immunization Practices (ACIP) of the U.S. Public Health Service strongly recommends that persons at increased risk for complications from influenza and also persons who may transmit influenza to high-risk persons receive the vaccine each year (Table 1). Other groups may also benefit from vaccination, including pregnant women during their third trimester who may be at increased risk of serious complications from influenza, persons infected with human immunodeficiency virus, foreign travelers, and all other people wishing to avoid illness. Because the vaccine contains only inactivated, noninfectious viruses, it cannot cause influenza and is safe for use in immunocompromised persons. People who have a history of severe egg allergy or allergies (i.e., immediate hypersensitivity reactions) to other vaccine components, including thimerosal, may

TABLE 1. **Groups Specially Targeted for Annual Influenza Vaccination**

Groups at increased risk for complications from influenza
    Persons ≥ 65 years of age
    Residents of nursing homes and other chronic-care
        facilities
    People with chronic cardiopulmonary conditions,
        including children with asthma
    People with other serious chronic medical conditions,
        including diabetes mellitus, renal dysfunction,
        immune compromise
    People ages 6 months to 18 years who are receiving
        chronic aspirin therapy and therefore might be at
        risk for developing Reye's syndrome after influenza

Groups that can transmit influenza to high-risk persons
    Physicians, nurses, and other health care workers
    Employees of nursing homes and other chronic-care
        facilities
    Providers of home care to high-risk persons
    Household members of persons in high-risk groups

Adapted from the Centers for Disease Control and Prevention: Prevention and control of influenza: Recommendations of the Advisory Committee on Immunization Practices (ACIP). MMWR Morb Mortal Wkly Rep *44* (RR-3): 1–22, 1995.

experience an immediate hypersensitivity reaction to the vaccine. They should not receive the vaccine, or they should be given it only after appropriate desensitization. The recommended doses according to age group are listed in Table 2.

Recent studies have clearly demonstrated the effectiveness of influenza vaccination in a variety of populations. In young, healthy persons, influenza vaccination may prevent influenza illness in 70% or more and may significantly reduce work absenteeism. For community-living seniors, vaccination has been shown to reduce influenza illness by approximately 50%; hospitalizations for pneumonia by 30% to 50% or more; hospitalizations for all acute and chronic respiratory conditions by 20% to 40%; and deaths from all causes by 30% to 50%. Vaccination is also cost saving (including direct medical costs for complications from influenza after taking into account program costs for vaccination) in this population. Among nursing home residents, vaccination reduces influenza illness by 30% to 40%; pneumonia

TABLE 2. **Influenza Vaccine Doses (1995–1996 U.S. Vaccine)**

Age Group	Vaccine Type*	Dosage (ml)	No. Doses†
6–35 mo	split virus	0.25	1 or 2
3–8 yr	split virus	0.50	1 or 2
9–12 yr	split virus	0.50	1
>12 yr	whole or split virus	0.50	1

*Because of lower rates of febrile reactions and other side effects, only the split virus form of the vaccine is recommended for children.

†Two doses of vaccine at least 1 month apart are recommended for children <9 years of age who have not been previously vaccinated. For people of all ages, the intramuscular route of injection is recommended.

Adapted from the Centers for Disease Control and Prevention: Prevention and control of influenza: Recommendations of the Advisory Committee on Immunization Practices (ACIP). MMWR Morb Mortal Wkly Rep *44* (RR-3): 1–22, 1995.

by 50% to 60%; and deaths by 70% to 80%. When considering the results of many of these studies, it should be noted that the underlying efficacy of the vaccine is undoubtedly considerably higher than the observed clinical effectiveness. For example, with an observed clinical effectiveness of 30% in reducing all pneumonias, if only 40% of these pneumonias were actually related to influenza, then the underlying true efficacy of the vaccine would be 75%.

Immunization with influenza vaccine is well tolerated. Current formulations of the vaccine have been shown in randomized, placebo-controlled trials in elderly people and in healthy working adults to be associated with systemic symptom rates that are no different from those observed in placebo recipients. Thus, systemic symptoms experienced during the week following immunization are most likely due not to the vaccine but rather to a coincidental illness or heightened somatic awareness after the injection. However, recipients of the vaccine may experience mild, local reactions such as tenderness or swelling at the injection site. This occurs in about 20% to 25% of elderly persons and in up to 50% or more of healthy adults under age 65 years.

Another potential adverse event related to immunization that is of concern to health care providers and vaccine recipients is Guillain-Barré syndrome. The 1976 swine influenza vaccine was associated with rare occurrences of Guillain-Barré syndrome, at a rate above background of slightly less than 1 per 100,000 vaccinations. Subsequent influenza vaccines have not clearly been associated with this syndrome. Even if the syndrome were related to influenza vaccination, the increased risk would be less than that of contracting a severe case of influenza. Persons who have previously had Guillain-Barré syndrome, however, may have a substantially higher risk for subsequently developing the syndrome following vaccination. A decision whether or not to vaccinate in this situation should be made after weighing the risks of severe influenza and its complications, given the patient's overall risk status, against the risk of contracting Guillain-Barré syndrome.

Vaccine Delivery

Despite the availability of a safe and effective vaccine, 50% or more of targeted persons fail to receive influenza vaccine each year. For patients, important considerations include concerns about vaccine safety and efficacy, uncertainty about their personal risk for influenza and its complications, convenience, and cost. One of the strongest predictors of vaccination behavior is a physician's recommendation. For health care providers, knowledge of "the facts" regarding influenza and the vaccine is important. But even more important for successful vaccine delivery are effective administrative and organizational strategies in the clinical practice setting that promote vaccination. Components of successful strategies are listed in Table 3. These strategies should be implemented in outpatient and inpatient settings, nursing

TABLE 3. Administrative and Organizational Strategies to Promote and Enhance the Delivery of Influenza Vaccine

Ensure the systematic and automatic offering of vaccine
  Patient identification, recall, and tracking system
  Reminders to patients and providers
Facilitate vaccine administration
  Standardized documentation and information forms
  Standing orders for nurses
  Walk-in clinics
Develop a durable program
  Maximize program efficiency and minimize additional
    workload burden on involved personnel
Educate patients, addressing their concerns about
  vaccine safety and efficacy, and emphasize provider
  recommendation
Educate health care providers
Monitor and evaluate the program's success
  Pharmacy logs for number of doses utilized
  Chart audits/patient surveys to assess vaccination
    rates, especially in high-risk groups

Adapted from Nichol KL: Preventing influenza: The physician's role. Semin Respir Infect 7: 71–77, 1992.

homes, and other places where high-risk persons may have contact with health care providers.

ANTIVIRALS

Whereas immunization is the mainstay of prevention for influenza, the antiviral agents amantadine (Symmetral) and rimantadine (Flumadine) also play a significant role in preventing influenza. These agents interfere with the replication of influenza A viruses and therefore have activity only against influenza A and not influenza B. Chemoprophylaxis should always be considered an adjunct to immunization and is used primarily for persons at greatest risk for complications from influenza. Antivirals are most often prescribed for high-risk patients at the time of vaccination to provide protection against influenza until they have developed a protective antibody response to vaccination (usually 2 weeks for adults, or until 2 weeks following the second dose of vaccine in young children receiving influenza vaccine for the first time). Amantadine and rimantadine are also commonly used in the context of outbreak control activities in nursing homes and other closed-population settings.

Antivirals may also be used to treat influenza A. Certainly the mainstay of treatment for acute influenza is conservative management with fluids, adequate rest, antipyretics/analgesics (aspirin should be avoided especially in children because of the risk of Reye's syndrome), and decongestants. Amantadine and rimantadine can also reduce the severity and duration of influenza A among healthy adults when administered within 48 hours of the onset of illness. Antiviral therapy for influenza illness should be discontinued as soon as clinically indicated to reduce the risk of possible induction of drug-resistant viruses. Generally, treatment can be stopped after 3 to 5 days or within 24 to 48 hours of the disappearance of the clinical signs and symptoms of infection. It is unknown whether treating high-risk patients will reduce the risk of complications from influenza A.

Decisions regarding the use of antiviral agents should be made only after careful consideration of the benefits, costs, and risks associated with their use. Despite their chemical and therapeutic similarities, these two drugs have different pharmacokinetic properties and side effect profiles. Amantadine is primarily excreted unchanged by the kidneys while 75% of rimantadine is metabolized by the liver, and amantadine is more often associated with certain side effects, including those of the central nervous system. Elderly people and persons with impaired renal function are especially susceptible to side effects following amantadine, and great care should be taken to ensure appropriate dosing. The package insert should always be reviewed before prescribing these agents, and dosages selected should take into account the patient's age, weight, renal function, underlying medical conditions, other medications, and reason for use (i.e., treatment or prophylaxis).

LEISHMANIASIS

method of
ED E. ZIJLSTRA, M.D., PH.D.
University of Khartoum
Khartoum, Sudan

The leishmaniases are a group of diseases that result from the inoculation of *Leishmania* parasites by the bite of a female sandfly (*Phlebotomus* species in the Old World, *Lutzomyia* species in the New World). In most areas, it is a zoonosis with humans as an accidental host; however, in other areas it is anthroponotic with a cycle between sandflies and man. After inoculation in the skin, the injected spindle-shaped flagellated promastigotes transform into oval amastigotes that multiply within cells of the mononuclear-macrophage lineage.

Leishmania causes three important clinical syndromes, depending on the species of *Leishmania* involved and the host's immune response: (1) visceral leishmaniasis (VL), also known as kala-azar, with systemic involvement that runs a fatal course if untreated; (2) cutaneous leishmaniasis (CL), with chronic skin ulcers that have a slow tendency to heal and leave a typical scar; and (3) mucocutaneous leishmaniasis (MCL) with involvement of the nasal, oral, pharyngeal, or laryngeal mucosa, with severe disfigurement and sometimes a fatal course in severe cases. There is no specific prophylaxis for leishmaniasis. Insect repellents may be advised; bednets should have a particularly fine mesh as sandflies can penetrate standard mosquito nets. A vaccine is not yet available, but several are currently being tested.

The leishmaniases affect thousands of people in endemic areas; large epidemics of both visceral and cutaneous leishmaniasis occur. Travelers or expatriates in endemic areas are at the same risk of contracting the infection as the indigenous population and may present with leishmaniasis upon return, in particular with CL.

CLINICAL SYNDROMES

Visceral Leishmaniasis. VL occurs in Asia (India, Bangladesh, Pakistan, southern Russia, China), Africa (Sudan, Ethiopia, Somalia, Kenya), the Middle East, along the Mediterranean basin, and Central and South America. The classic syndrome consists of fever, hepatosplenomegaly, and wasting; other clinical features may include epistaxis, diarrhea, cough, weakness, and lymphadenopathy. Laboratory investigation reveals pancytopenia and hypergammaglobulinemia; immunologically, *Leishmania*-specific immunosuppression can be demonstrated: in vivo by skin anergy for the leishmanin skin test (LST) and in vitro by absence of response in lymphocyte proliferation tests (LPT) after stimulation with *Leishmania* antigen. Differential diagnosis depends on the geographic area and may include malaria, brucellosis, tuberculosis, typhoid, histoplasmosis, and African trypanosomiasis (sleeping sickness). The incubation period is usually 4 to 6 months, but may vary from 2 weeks to several years.

There is a spectrum of disease; after inoculation by a sandfly bite, a subclinical infection may occur as evidenced by seroconversion or conversion in the LST without clinical signs. Some patients may develop a skin ulcer from which *L. donovani* may be isolated (leishmanioma), before proceeding to self-cure or visceral disease. Among American soldiers who were found infected with *Leishmania* upon returning from the Persian Gulf after Operation Desert Storm in 1990–1991, some developed a mild, mononucleosis-like illness, and some self-healed. Most patients, however, are ill and present with visceral disease that is considered to run a fatal course if untreated. The reasons for this variation of presentation are unknown, but such factors as nutritional state, intercurrent illness, genetic factors, and parasite virulence may play a role.

VL can occur as an opportunistic infection in immunosuppressed individuals (e.g., following organ transplantation and/or during use of steroids) and is increasingly found among HIV-infected patients, in particular in Mediterranean countries. Diagnosis may be difficult as patients may be asymptomatic and the classic clinical signs may be absent. Patients may present with unusual sites of infection (gastrointestinal tract, skin, lungs). Conversely, pancytopenia and hypergammaglobulinemia may be the result of other diseases or drug therapy and may not immediately lead to considering the diagnosis of VL in these patients.

In the Old World, *L. donovani* and *L. infantum* are the most important species involved; *L. tropica* is also reported to cause VL in the Middle East, Kenya, and India. In the New World, the parasite involved is *L. chagasi*, which is closely related to *L. infantum*.

Post–Kala-Azar Dermal Leishmaniasis (PKDL). This condition is mainly found in India and follows in 20% of kala-azar cases after 2 to 5 years; it was thought to be uncommon in Africa, but it was reported to be frequent in the Sudan (in around 50% of kala-azar cases), occurring 0 to 6 months after treatment. Some patients do not have a history of kala-azar. PKDL is characterized by the occurrence of macules, papules, or nodules in the skin, in particular of the face, although spread over the whole body may occur. In contrast to VL, the patient is usually well, and parasites are demonstrated only in the skin lesions but no longer in the bone marrow or spleen. Mild cases may self-cure; more severe cases need treatment. Cases with longstanding PKDL may play an important role in transmission in certain areas.

PKDL is mainly found in areas where *L. donovani* is the causative parasite of kala-azar (India, Sudan) and is rare in areas where *L. infantum* or *L. chagasi* occur. Other parasites associated with PKDL are *L. amazonensis* and *L. tropica*. PKDL may be confused with a number of diseases of which leprosy is the most important.

Cutaneous Leishmaniasis. CL occurs in the Old World along the Mediterranean coast, in Middle and Central Asia, India, Pakistan, and Africa (in particular East Africa); in the New World it is found in South and Central America; there is an endemic area in southern Texas. The typical CL lesion is a volcano-shaped ulcer that develops out of a papule occurring at the site of inoculation. The nonpainful ulcer typically follows the skin creases, and satellite papules at the edge may be found. Regional lymph node involvement may be found, and lymphatic spread may occur with metastatic lesions (sporotrichoid-like). Depending on the species of *Leishmania* involved, most lesions will heal after several months to years. In the Old World, *L. major* and *L. tropica* are by far the most common parasites involved. *L. major* usually causes multiple wet ulcers; dry ulcers with *L. major* are less common. The ulcers heal in 6 months. *L. tropica* usually forms a single dry ulcer and heals within 1 year. In both, secondary infection may occur, in particular in lesions involving the feet and legs. Leishmaniasis recidivans (LR) is an uncommon condition caused by *L. tropica*, in which the mainly facial lesions run a chronic relapsing course. It is mainly reported from Iran. *L. infantum* forms small papules, nodules, or plaques with late or little ulceration; the lesions may last for years if left to self-heal. *L. aethiopica* is less common and is limited to Ethiopia and Kenya; the lesions are mainly single and show late or absent ulceration; they are slow to heal (years). *L. aethiopica* may also cause diffuse cutaneous leishmaniasis (DCL); there are multiple papules, nodules, or plaques, usually symmetric, in particular on the face, producing a leonine facies, and on the extensor surfaces of the limbs; it resembles lepromatous leprosy. Ulceration does not occur; there is no tendency to spontaneous cure.

In the New World, CL is caused by several subspecies of *Leishmania*. *L. braziliensis* is the most important, and the ulcers are single or multiple with involvement of the regional lymph nodes and lymphatic spread. Metastatic (hematogenous) spread to the nasopharyngeal mucosa is the most feared complication and may lead to mucocutaneous leishmaniasis. *L. mexicana* usually gives a single ulcer on the face or ears (Chiclero's ulcer) and has a tendency to self-heal. *L. guyanensis* may cause multiple lesions (Pian-bois or bush yaws) with spread along the lymphatics and little tendency to spontaneously heal. In Panama, *L. panamensis* causes single or few ulcers (ulcera de Bejuco) with frequent lymphatic spread and little tendency to self-heal. In Peru, *L. peruviana* causes single or few lesions (Uta) that may self-heal; mucosal damage may occur but only by contiguity. In the New World, DCL is associated with *L. amazonensis*; there is also a focus in the Dominican Republic, where the parasite involved has not been characterized satisfactorily.

Mucocutaneous Leishmaniasis. This is a condition typically seen in endemic areas; occasionally cases may be seen outside these areas in immigrants. There are several reports of mucosal involvement in HIV-infected patients. A nasal ulcer develops that may cause nasal obstruction, perforation of the nasal septum, and collapse of the nose; further spread may involve the upper lip, palate, and the pharyngeal and laryngeal mucosa, leading to severe mutilation. Death may occur from laryngeal closure or secondary bacterial infections such as pneumonia.

MCL mainly occurs in the New World where it is known

as espundia; it follows in fewer than 10% of patients who had CL caused by *L. braziliensis*. Also, *L. panamensis* and *L. guyanensis* may cause MCL. In 50% of patients, MCL occurs after 2 years of the primary CL; others may have longer intervals. In the Old World, MCL mainly occurs in the Sudan and is caused by *L. major* or *L. donovani*; in the latter case, it can be seen as a post–kala-azar manifestation. There is no preceding cutaneous lesion as in New World MCL. *L. infantum* and *L. aethiopica* have also been described in association with mucosal disease.

DIAGNOSIS

Visceral Leishmaniasis. Diagnosis should be sought by demonstration of the parasite, usually in a bone marrow aspirate. A splenic aspiration is more sensitive and is safe if the platelet count is not below 40×10^9 per L and the prothrombin time is normal. If lymphadenopathy is present as in African VL, an inguinal lymph node, even if moderately enlarged, may be aspirated with a 20- to 22-gauge needle and 2-mL syringe. A smear is made and, simultaneously, some of the material should be used for culture; several media are suitable of which NNN (Nicolle's modification of Novy and McNeal's medium) and Schneider's drosophila medium are most commonly used. Apart from confirming the diagnosis, a positive culture may be used for species parasite characterization by isoenzyme analysis. In patients co-infected with HIV, parasites may be found in a peripheral blood smear; less frequently parasites may be found in immunocompetent individuals, but examination of the peripheral blood is not a reliable method for diagnosis.

A number of serologic tests have been developed, of which the direct agglutination test (DAT), enzyme-linked immunosorbent assay (ELISA), and indirect fluorescent antibody test (IFAT) have been most evaluated. Their usefulness in an endemic area is limited as they do not discriminate between past (sub) clinical infection and active disease. A positive result in a traveler suspected of VL who is returning from an endemic area would strongly suggest the disease.

Newer molecular biologic techniques such as monoclonal antibodies, the polymerase chain reaction, and DNA hybridization can identify parasites as *Leishmania* to the species level; these techniques are still being developed and are not yet available for routine use.

Tests for cell-mediated immunity include the leishmanin skin test (LST); 0.1 mL of a solution containing 5×10^6 per mL of *Leishmania* promastigotes is injected intradermally in the skin of the forearm and the induration is read after 48 to 72 hours. The test is typically negative during active disease; it will become positive in 80% of cases 6 months after treatment. A positive test strongly argues against VL but does not exclude it, as the test may be positive in some (relapse) cases. Lymphocyte proliferation tests (LPT) are only done in well-equipped laboratories and are of no use in routine diagnosis.

PKDL. The diagnosis of PKDL is suggested clinically by the appearance of skin lesions in a patient with a history of (recent) VL; occasionally patients may not give a history of manifest kala-azar. Parasites may be demonstrated in smears or biopsies. Parasites may be scanty, in particular in early papular or macular lesions. Culture is successful in Indian PKDL, but not in the Sudan. Serology is of little use; the LST may be positive or negative.

Cutaneous Leishmaniasis. Diagnosis is made by demonstration of parasites in a skin slit smear or fine-needle aspirate; some material is used for culture. Alternatively, a biopsy can be taken for impression smears, culture, and histology. Serologic reactions are of little use as titers are usually low. The LST will be positive in most cases and is useful in travelers who come from an endemic region. In people from an endemic area, a positive test could simply point to a previous infection, as the test most likely will remain positive for life. As in VL, the new molecular biologic techniques are promising but not yet widely available or evaluated for routine diagnosis. In diffuse cutaneous leishmaniasis (DCL), parasites can be easily demonstrated in smears or biopsies; serologic tests such as ELISA will show high titers of antibodies. Cell-mediated immunity is absent, as shown in a negative LST and absent responses in LPT. In leishmaniasis recidivans (LR), parasites are scanty and the LST is strongly positive.

Mucocutaneous Leishmaniasis. Diagnosis is attempted by demonstration of parasites in smears and culture, but parasites may be scanty and *L. braziliensis* does not grow well in culture. Hamster inoculation may be tried. Alternatively, a biopsy can be taken; serologic tests, including IFAT and ELISA, may be useful. The LST is (strongly) positive. New molecular biologic techniques would be particularly useful in MCL in view of the paucity of parasites.

TREATMENT

For most forms of leishmaniasis, pentavalent antimony is still the drug of choice. Two preparations are available: sodium stibogluconate* (Pentostam, Wellcome Laboratories, UK) is used in most English-speaking countries, including the United States, and is available as bottles of 100 mL, with 100 mg of antimony per mL. Meglumine antimoniate† (Glucantime, Rhone-Poulenc, France) is used in French-, Spanish-, and Portuguese-speaking countries and is available in ampules of 5 mL, containing 85 mg of antimony per mL. The drug is given intramuscularly or intravenously. As the volume that must be administered is rather large, the intravenous route is preferred. The drug is added to 50 mL of 5% dextrose in water and given over 10 to 15 minutes. The drug does not have acute toxicity as it is rapidly excreted by the kidney (60 to 80% of an injected dose is excreted within 6 hours). Depending on dose and duration, cumulative toxicity may occur.

Side Effects of Antimony

Locally, intravenous injection may cause thrombophlebitis that can be avoided by giving the drug diluted in dextrose and over 10 to 15 minutes as described. Systemic side effects include leukopenia, thrombocytopenia, hepatotoxicity, pancreatitis, cardiac toxicity, and arthralgias. Hematologic abnormalities are rare. Antimony may cause hepatocellular damage and hepatic functional impairment with elevation of liver enzymes up to tenfold of the upper limit of normal; these abnormalities will decrease despite continuation of treatment and are completely reversible. However, in patients with pre-existing liver disease, an alternative drug should be considered.

---

*Investigational drug in the United States.
†Not available in the United States.

Antimony causes elevations of pancreatic enzymes, in particular lipase, in most patients; half of these are symptomatic. Treatment can be continued in cases with mild symptoms, but stopping treatment is advised in those with severe symptoms (nausea, vomiting, abdominal pain) or a severe rise of lipase (greater than 15 times the upper limit of normal) or a rise in amylase (more than 4 times the upper limit of normal). After clinical improvement or after a substantial decrease of enzymes, treatment may be continued. Cardiac toxicity is demonstrated in electrocardiographic changes such as T-wave flattening or inversion, and nonspecific ST segment changes occur in most patients and are of no clinical importance. Prolongation of the QT interval is serious but is unlikely to occur during the recommended doses and duration of treatment. However, there are few data on elderly individuals receiving antimony treatment, and sudden unexplained deaths have occurred. Arthralgias may occur and are usually mild and easily controlled by analgesics; in rare instances, however, these may be severe and debilitating and arthropathy with effusions has been described, necessitating discontinuation of treatment. Lastly, idiosyncratic reactions may occur unrelated to the dose regimen used.

Visceral Leishmaniasis. All patients with confirmed VL should be treated; although limited data are available on the effects of antimony in pregnancy, both the mother and the fetus may die if adequate treatment is withheld.

There is no clear standard for treatment of VL, but a regimen of 20 mg per kg per day for 30 days without a maximum daily dose is safe and probably the best choice for most cases. In every endemic area, however, adjustments should be made according to local experience. In India, resistance to antimony is increasingly encountered, and treatment should be extended to 40 days. In Mediterranean countries and Brazil, treatment for 20 days should be sufficient.

The most important new development in chemotherapy of leishmaniasis is the introduction of liposomal amphotericin B* (AmBisome, Vestar, San Dimas, CA, USA), which proved very effective with few side effects; it is, however, expensive. The optimal regimen is not yet established for all areas, but a total dose of 20 to 30 mg per kg should be given in 10 to 21 days, in six or more doses of 3 to 4 mg per kg intravenously. Another liposomal formulation is Amphotericin B Cholesterol Dispersion* (Amphocil, Liposome Technology Inc., Menlo Park, CA, USA) that was shown effective in a dose of 2 mg per kg per day for 7 days in two studies; however, it is not advised for young children under 6 years of age because of side effects (chills, fever, respiratory distress); in older patients, premedication should be considered. Other alternative therapy includes conventional amphotericin B, which is much more effective in vitro than antimony but also more toxic. The dose is 0.5 to 1.0 mg per kg per day or on alternate days intravenously for a total of 1 to 2 grams. The lowest and shortest effective regimen was reported from India: 0.5 mg per kg of amphotericin B on alternate days for a total of 14 doses showed excellent results with a cure rate of 100% without serious side effects.

There are few studies on aminosidine* (Gabbromycin) as monotherapy; in one study from Kenya, aminosidine was more effective than antimony (79% and 55% cure, respectively) and had less toxicity, although nephrotoxicity and ototoxicity may occur. The dose is intravenous or intramuscular administration over 90 minutes of 15 mg per kg for at least 3 to 4 weeks. In combination with antimony, cure rates of more than 90% may be reached. Pentamidine isethionate† (Pentam 300) may be used in a dose of 4 mg per kg intramuscularly three times weekly for 5 to 25 weeks depending on the response; side effects include nephrotoxicity and hypo- and hyperglycemia. Ketoconazole (Nizoral) and itraconazole (Sporanox) cannot be recommended because of insufficient and conflicting data. In case of relapse, the patient may be retreated with antimony for 4 to 8 weeks. In case of further relapse or unresponsiveness to antimony, (liposomal) amphotericin, aminosidine, or pentamidine may be considered. Cases that relapse or are drug-refractory may benefit from combined treatment with antimony and gamma-interferon† (Actimmune).

There is no consensus on the treatment of HIV co-infected patients; antimony (with or without gamma-interferon), amphotericin B or liposomal amphotericin B, pentamidine, or aminosidine may be used as a first-line treatment, but toxicity is greater than in immunocompetent patients. In a study from France, amphotericin B (20 or more mg per kg total dose) was superior to antimony (20 mg per kg per day for 20 days), with initial response rates of 100% and 50% respectively, but with frequent relapses in both groups and no significant difference in survival time. Relapses are frequent as cell-mediated immunity is required to clear or control the parasites. Maintenance therapy is advisable; however, all maintenance regimens that were tried so far, including pentamidine, liposomal amphotericin B, ketoconazole, itraconazole, and allopurinol, have shown failures, and no definite recommendation can be made. Intravenous pentamidine isethionate, 4 mg per kg two to four times weekly may be tried; an alternative would be intravenous AmBisome, 2 mg per kg every 2 weeks.

MONITORING TREATMENT. Initial and weekly electrocardiograms, a full blood count, and liver and pancreatic enzyme levels should be obtained. Measurement of amylase and lipase should be more frequent if clinically indicated.

AFTER TREATMENT. A test of cure is recommended, and a bone marrow or spleen aspiration should be done 2 weeks after the end of treatment as parasites may be cleared at a slow rate from the viscera. If parasites are still found, treatment is considered to

---

*Investigational drug in the United States.

*Investigational drug in the United States.
†Not FDA-approved for this indication.

have failed. If the test of cure is negative, patients should be followed up at 3-month intervals for 1 year and repeatedly investigated if clinically suspect for a relapse.

ADDITIONAL TREATMENT. Patients should be investigated for iron and folic acid deficiency and treated accordingly. Concurrent infections (pneumonia, tuberculosis, gastrointestinal infections) should be actively sought and treated. Adequate nutrition is essential, in particular in patients who are malnourished. Subcutaneous administration of granulocyte-macrophage colony-stimulating factor* (GM-CSF [Leukine, Prokine]) simultaneously with antimony was reported to reverse the neutropenia and reduce secondary bacterial and viral infections and deserves further study before it may be recommended for routine use.

PKDL. In India, PKDL is treated with at least 4 months of antimony, 20 mg per kg per day; in the Sudan, early and mild lesions may be left untreated to self-heal. More severe cases should be treated with antimony, 20 mg per kg per day for 1 to 2 months. Liposomal amphotericin B (AmBisome) may be a promising alternative. Ketoconazole in standard doses is ineffective as is a combination of itraconazole and terbinafine.

Cutaneous Leishmaniasis. The treatment of CL is complicated by a number of issues. First, a number of CL patients may cure spontaneously, in particular those infected with *L. major*. Second, many reports on various treatment modalities lack a control group and adequate follow-up and are therefore difficult to interpret. Third, there is a plethora of treatment modalities to choose from, including systemic treatment, topical application of drugs by ointment or intralesional injection, curettage, heat, freezing, and irradiation. Fourth, there are undoubtedly differences in capacity of self-healing and response to treatment between species from different areas in the Old World and New World; a beneficial result in one area in lesions caused by a specific parasite may not be effective in another area where a different parasite is involved.

In Old World CL, simple lesions caused by *L. major* and *L. tropica* may be left untreated and observed. Systemic treatment with antimony, 20 mg per kg for 20 days, is advised for lesions that are multiple, chronic, in the face, or over large joints. After the end of treatment, lesions may still further regress, and evaluation after 6 weeks is advised. In case of failure, a repeated course of antimony may be given. Alternative regimens may be tried but experience is often local and may not necessarily be the same in other areas or parasites. They include oral ketoconazole, 600 mg for 30 days in *L. major* infection or itraconazole, 100 to 200 mg per day for 6 to 8 weeks. In India, these two azole drugs were ineffective, but dapsone cured 82% of patients, in a dose of 200 mg per day for 4 weeks. In a study from Israel, topical application of paromomycin 15 and 12% methylben-

zethonium chloride (MBCL) was effective in 77% of patients with *L. major* infection, whereas 27% of a placebo group were cured. MBCL, however, may cause severe local inflammation. Another preparation of paromomycin 15 and 10% urea was not better than placebo in a study in Tunisia (also *L. major* as the causative parasite). DCL should be treated with pentamidine,* 4 mg per kg once weekly; aminosidine,† 15 mg per kg per day, is an alternative. Duration of treatment is guided by the clinical response. Combination therapy of antimony, 10 mg per kg per day, and aminosidine, 14 mg per kg per day, proved effective in a limited number of patients. Combination therapy with antimony and gamma-interferon seems promising. Treatment of LR consists of 4 to 8 weeks of antimonial treatment, but relapses are frequent.

New World CL tends to be more severe and difficult to treat than Old World CL. First-line treatment should be systemic antimony, 20 mg per kg for 20 days, and a cure rate of over 90% should be reached; recently, in one study in Guatemala, it was shown possible to reduce the duration of treatment to 10 days of antimony with equal results. In case of failure, the same regimen may be repeated. The most attractive alternative treatment is intramuscular injection of pentamidine,* 2 mg per kg for 7 days every other day or 3 mg per kg for 4 days every other day; these studies from Colombia await confirmation from other areas. Injectable aminosidine† as monotherapy is less effective than antimony. Speciation of the causative parasite is important; alternative treatment with oral ketoconazole, 600 mg for 30 days, may be considered for *L. mexicana* and *L. panamensis* infections but is less effective in CL caused by *L. braziliensis*. Itraconazole was not more effective than placebo in Colombia.

Topical treatment as monotherapy cannot be recommended at present, in particular when *L. braziliensis* infection is a possibility. However, a combination regimen consisting of a topical formulation of 15% paromomycin/5% methylbenzethonium chloride twice a day for 10 days and parenteral meglumine antimoniate,‡ 20 mg per kg per day for 7 days, cured 90% of patients with CL caused by *L. panamensis* in Colombia. Allopurinol cannot be recommended as a single agent in the treatment of CL as evidence on its efficacy is inconsistent. Immunotherapy with antimony and gamma-interferon or with a vaccine consisting of live BCG and killed *L. mexicana* promastigotes has shown good results; its place in treatment is not yet well described.

Mucocutaneous Leishmaniasis. Treatment of New World MCL is unsatisfactory. The standard treatment regimen as advised by WHO is with antimony, 20 mg per kg for 30 days. Patients should be evaluated 3 months after treatment, and follow-up should be for at least 3 years. With this regimen,

---

*Not FDA-approved for this indication.

†Investigational drug in the United States.

‡Not available in the United States.

75% of patients with nasal lesions will be cured. The response in patients with nasal and oral lesions is less satisfactory, with cure rates of 10 and 63% reported in two studies, respectively. Extension of treatment to 40 days does not increase the cure rate. Alternative therapy with (liposomal) amphotericin B may be considered, but conclusive studies on dose and duration are not yet available. Combined treatment with antimony and gamma-interferon may also be successful. During treatment, severe inflammation and swelling of the lesion may occur because of antigen release from killed parasites. Corticosteroids should be given for this reaction.

In contrast, in the Old World, response to treatment with antimony is excellent. Ketoconazole was shown to be effective in a limited number of cases.

As all types of leishmaniasis are rare as imported diseases and the response to therapy varies with the geographic location, it is advisable to seek consultation with a center in which experience with these diseases has been accumulated. In the United States, the Centers for Disease Control and Prevention, Atlanta, may be consulted (Tel: 404-639-3670), through which stibogluconate may be obtained.

LEPROSY
(Hansen's Disease)

method of
M. F. R. WATERS, M.B.
Hospital for Tropical Diseases
London, United Kingdom

Leprosy is a chronic infectious disease, occurring widely in the tropics and subtropics, caused by the intracellular acid-fast bacillus (AFB) *Mycobacterium leprae*. Although this bacillus was discovered in 1873, it still cannot be grown in vitro, despite the development of a complete gene library and the recent mapping of about two thirds of its genome. Grown in the foot pads of mice or in armadillos, the leprosy bacillus has a generation time of 11 to 12 days. Therefore, the incubation period is usually of the order of years; leprosy is very rare in infancy, and like *Mycobacterium tuberculosis*, the organism can remain apparently dormant for decades in the host's body before causing clinical disease. It is thought that the main method of spread is airborne, as large numbers of bacilli are excreted from the upper respiratory tract of untreated lepromatous patients, although the attack rate is in general less than that of tuberculosis.

The World Health Organization (WHO) estimates that there are now only about 1.8 million leprosy patients worldwide requiring or receiving chemotherapy, the leading six countries being India, Brazil, Bangladesh, Myanmar, Indonesia, and Nigeria. Approximately 550,000 new cases are diagnosed each year, and there are perhaps 3 million patients suffering from significant residual deformities. The majority of cases in First World countries occur among immigrants, whether recent or long-term. In the United States, about 200 new cases are reported per annum, of which the great majority are immigrants, only around 15% being native-born Americans.

CLINICAL MANIFESTATIONS

Leprosy displays a wide clinical "spectrum" related to the host's ability to develop and maintain specific cell-mediated immunity (CMI). In high-resistant polar tuberculoid (TT) leprosy, asymmetrical localized signs are restricted to skin and peripheral nerve, whereas low-resistant polar lepromatous leprosy (LL) is a generalized bacteremic disease involving many systems, with widespread lesions of the skin, upper respiratory tract, peripheral nerves, reticuloendothelial system, testes, and anterior part of the eyes. The unstable middle part of the spectrum is known as borderline leprosy, and in the Ridley-Jopling classification it is subdivided into borderline tuberculoid (BT), mid-borderline (BB), and borderline lepromatous (BL) leprosy; in the absence of treatment, such patients may "downgrade" across the spectrum towards lepromatous leprosy (LL).

Common complications of "spectrum" leprosy include immunologically mediated inflammatory episodes—"reactions"—of which there are two major varieties. Deformities—which may occur on the hands, feet, and face, either from primary involvement of tissues, especially motor nerves, or from secondary inflammation in the anesthetic areas that result from peripheral or dermal nerve damage—include claw hand and foot, foot drop, lagophthalmos, exposure keratitis, trophic ulcers of the feet, and loss of digits.

Child contacts of lepromatous cases may develop an early form, indeterminate (Ind) leprosy, usually consisting of a single hypopigmented macule; although only a quarter of these patients evolve to spectrum leprosy, the majority curing themselves, the condition is always treated if diagnosed.

Diagnosis is based on the clinical findings of typical skin lesions (which in TT and BT leprosy are routinely anesthetic to light touch, pain, and temperature) and/or of nerve lesions, the involved nerve(s) (which may include the ulnar, median, common peroneal, posterior tibial, radial cutaneous, and great auricular) being thicker than normal, and the finding of acid-fast bacilli either in the histology of biopsied lesions or in skin smears. These last are taken from the dermis of both ear lobes and up to four active skin sites. In untreated diseases, AFB are so scanty that on examination of 100 oil immersion fields they are not detected in skin smears from TT, almost all indeterminate, and many BT patients; such "smear-negative" patients are classified by the WHO as suffering from paucibacillary leprosy (PBL). All LL, BL, BB, and those borderline tuberculoid patients who are skin-smear positive for AFB are classified as suffering from multibacillary leprosy (MBL). It is assumed that in PBL a patient's total bacterial load will not exceed 10^7 *M. leprae*, and of these many bacilli may be killed naturally, as such patients are allergic (lepromin-positive) to *M. leprae*. Therefore, spontaneously occurring rifampin-resistant mutant bacilli are unlikely to be present. In MBL the bacterial load is assumed to be $>10^7$, most patients are anergic (lepromin-negative), and subpopulations of drug-resistant bacilli are likely to be present. Indeed, in advanced LL leprosy a patient's total bacterial load of *M. leprae* may be as high as 10^{11} to 10^{12}, with the skin smear sometimes containing more than 1000 bacilli in a single oil-immersion field.

GENERAL TREATMENT

Although leprosy is now an eminently treatable disease with excellent results, especially if diagnosed early and treated well, its old stigma dies hard. Therefore it is essential to maintain patient confidentiality. The drug clofazimine (discussed later), used routinely in the chemotherapy of MBL patients, is a lipid-soluble orange dye, which both gives a reddish color to the skin and causes increased melanin production, especially in light-exposed areas. Many light-skinned patients dislike the resulting color change and are very fearful that it will lead to their diagnosis being detected by neighbors and acquaintances; therefore, the choice of treatment regimen may have to be discussed openly with the patient, who should also be informed of the duration of chemotherapy. Patients need warning, in simple terms, of the possibility of developing reactions, so that if reactions occur, they return quickly for appropriate treatment. Those who at diagnosis give a recent history (less than 6 months) of nerve damage require additional initial anti-inflammatory treatment. Patients with permanent nerve damage to hand, foot, or face should be taught self-protection to avoid increasing disability, and appropriate reconstructive surgery may be planned.

Antileprosy Drugs

At present, three drugs are used routinely to treat leprosy: rifampin,* dapsone, and clofazimine. Rifampin is rapidly and highly bactericidal against *M. leprae*, so that a single dose of 600 mg results in a 99.9% kill. Clofazimine and dapsone individually take 3 to 4 months to produce the same kill, although perhaps slightly faster in combination. Ofloxacin,* minocycline,* and clarithromycin* each take about 4 weeks for an equivalent kill, and a single combined dose has a significant bactericidal action; therefore these three drugs are already included in alternative regimens recommended by the WHO. They have replaced the hepatotoxic ethionamide and prothionamide that are no longer recommended.

Rifampin

Rifampin (Rifadin, Rimactane) acts by inhibiting mycobacterial DNA-dependent RNA polymerase. It is rapidly absorbed from the gastrointestinal tract and has a half-life of 3 to 4 hours after a single dose of 600 mg. It is available as 150- and 300-mg capsules. Initially, it was given in the dosage of 600 mg daily, which occasionally proved hepatotoxic or caused thrombocytopenia, the "flu syndrome," drowsiness, pruritus, rashes, eosinophilia, or kidney damage. It induced microsomal enzyme production, resulting in increased metabolism of a number of important drugs, including oral contraceptives. In addition, it caused a reddish discoloration of the urine and sometimes of saliva, sweat, and tears. Sub-

sequently it was found that a dosage of 600 mg on two successive days every 4 weeks was equally effective in LL over 2 years, and a single 600-mg dose every month was virtually as good, presumably because of the very long generation time of *M. leprae*. This intermittent dosage is rarely toxic, very occasionally causes transient erythema and mild fever about 2 hours after ingestion, has little effect on drug metabolism, is much cheaper (important in Third World countries), and makes supervision of drug intake possible. However, as even daily rifampin, when given as monotherapy to new or relapsed cases of LL leprosy, can result in the development of drug resistance within 4 years, the drug should always be given in combination drug regimens.

Clofazimine

Clofazimine (Lamprene) is a rimino-phenazine derivative, available in 50-mg and 100-mg capsules. Being water-insoluble, it is only slowly absorbed from the gut and is best taken after a main meal; the standard preparation of microcrystalline drug in an oil-wax base gives about 70% absorption, and with a half-life of 10.6 days, it takes about 30 days for the full blood level to be reached. Clofazimine's mode of action is uncertain, but it binds to mycobacterial DNA. It is surprising that no independently confirmed case of clofazimine resistance has yet been reported.

The routine dosage of clofazimine is 50 mg daily, with a loading dose of 300 mg monthly. Some change in skin color is detectable by 8 weeks, and on skin biopsy the subcutaneous fat is orange. Increased melanin production is visible within 3 months. Failure to develop pigmentation may indicate poor compliance. With time in LL, the skin color fades slightly, associated with resolution of the dermal lepromatous infiltrate, but full return to normal implies failure to continue taking the drug. After stopping clofazimine, the pigmentation takes 6 to 18 months to fade completely.

In standard dosage, clofazimine causes few important side effects, save rarely some gastrointestinal discomfort or diarrhea, although xerosis and ichthyosis, especially of the legs, is common, particularly in anesthetic areas in LL. In higher dosage, clofazimine also has an anti-inflammatory action that is particularly valuable in suppressing the immunologic reaction of LL known as erythema nodosum leprosum (ENL). However, this increases the risk of gastrointestinal symptoms, and if high dosage is continued for many months or years the drug will crystallize out in the gut submucosa and mesenteric lymph nodes, eventually leading to severe chronic diarrhea. Therefore the WHO recommends that the dose should not be raised above 300 mg daily, nor continued for more than about 3 months before reduction. Even in the dosage of 50 mg daily, clofazimine appears to lower the incidence of ENL reactions.

Dapsone

Dapsone, used since 1946 for treating leprosy, inhibits dihydrofolic acid synthesis. The dose is 1 to 2

---

*Not FDA-approved for this indication.

mg per kg, the usual adult dosage being 100 mg daily, or 50 mg in small adults. It is available in 50-mg and 100-mg tablets. Dapsone is well absorbed and has an average half-life of 27 hours; the peak blood level attained after ingestion of a single dose of 100 mg is 500 times the minimal inhibitory concentration for fully sensitive *M. leprae*. This partly explains why dapsone resistance, which develops in a stepwise fashion, was not detected until a full decade after the drug's introduction as monotherapy. However, since 1960, dapsone resistance has become increasingly common worldwide, necessitating the introduction of multidrug therapy (MDT) comparable to that used for tuberculosis.

Dapsone is generally well tolerated and is not teratogenic. It is mildly hemolytic, which usually is unimportant, but in those rare patients with gross glucose-6-phosphate dehydrogenase (G6PD) deficiency, severe anemia may develop within a few days. It occasionally causes methemoglobinemia, fixed drug eruptions, peripheral neuropathy, nephritis, and rarely agranulocytosis. However, about 1 patient in 500 develops drug allergy; between 15 and 50 days after commencing dapsone, the patient develops pruritus, dermatitis, and fever, and if the dapsone is not stopped immediately, the patient may proceed to exfoliative dermatitis, lymphadenopathy, hepatitis, and psychosis. Severe dapsone allergy is potentially fatal, requiring treatment with steroids; in the First World, plasmapheresis should be considered because of the slow rate of elimination of the drug.

Fortunately, most primary dapsone resistance is only low grade, and dapsone is retained in standard MDT because of its low cost, general safety, acceptability, and effectiveness.

Ofloxacin

Ofloxacin (Floxin) is a fluorinated quinolone that inhibits the bacterial enzyme DNA gyrase. Other effective quinolones include pefloxacin and sparfloxacin, but not ciprofloxacin. Although shown to be highly bactericidal against *M. leprae* in animals and, since 1990, in short-term clinical trials, it is still too early for long-term relapse rates to be known for regimens combining ofloxacin and rifampin. Ofloxacin is already included in some WHO standard alternative regimens.

Ofloxacin is available in 200- and 400-mg tablets, the standard dose being 400 mg daily. Its main side effects are gastrointestinal; those affecting the central nervous system, including headaches, dizziness, insomnia, and mild psychosis; and (rarely) agranulocytosis. Because it causes cartilage damage in immature animals, its use is not recommended in children.

Minocycline

Minocycline (Minocin) a semisynthetic tetracycline that inhibits protein synthesis by binding to the 30S ribosome. Although introduced in 1972 so that its adverse side effects are well identified, it was only in 1990 shown to be effective against human leprosy in a short-term clinical trial. It is the most lipophilic tetracycline and the only one bactericidal for *M. leprae*.

Minocycline is available in 50-mg and 100-mg tablets. The standard dosage is 100 mg daily. Its main side effects include gastrointestinal and vestibular disturbances, especially vertigo (which may occur in 5% of patients), and skin rashes. Like other tetracyclines, it discolors teeth, and its use is not recommended in children or during lactation.

Clarithromycin

Clarithromycin (Biaxin) is a macrolide antibiotic, less toxic than erythromycin, that binds to the microsomal 70S ribosome. It is available in 250- and 500-mg tablets. The standard dosage is 500 mg daily. Its side effects include nausea, dermal hypersensitivity, and rashes. It is not contraindicated in children.

TREATMENT REGIMENS

Following the discovery of secondary dapsone resistance in LL and BL patients in 1964, many different combination regimens were investigated. The only MDT regimens generally accepted are the two recommended by the WHO Study Group on the chemotherapy of leprosy for control programs in 1981. To date more than 6.5 million patients have been treated, and the prima facie relapse rates (likely to be overestimates, especially in PBL) are approximately only 0.1% per annum. Strains of *M. leprae* tested from relapse cases have been shown to have developed no new drug resistances.

The WHO MBL regimen consists of:

Rifampin: 600 mg monthly (or every 4 weeks), supervised;

Clofazimine: 50 mg daily, unsupervised, plus 300 mg (supervised) every month or 4 weeks;

Dapsone: 100 mg daily, unsupervised.

When regular monthly supervision is not possible, blister packs are available (including in appropriate dosage for children). In First World countries, regular supervision of drug intake may be socially unacceptable, and cost is much less of a consideration. It has been my practice in London to double the dose of rifampin, prescribing 600 mg on two consecutive days, preferably the first two days of each month (which is easy to remember), and to check compliance by testing the patient's urine for rifampin on one such day once or twice a year, with the "supervised" 300-mg dose of clofazimine being omitted. In the Third World, treatment is now stopped after a minimum period of two years, but in the First World the original advice to continue longer until the patient becomes skin-smear negative for AFB is still maintained, as it decreases the risk of relapse in highly bacilliferous LL and BL patients. Smear-positive BT and most BB patients are negative at 2 years, but BL patients may take 4 to 5 years and LL patients 7 to 10 years to reach smear negativity. To date, there is no convincing evidence that daily rifampin has significant advantage over monthly dosage.

Patients who refuse clofazimine may receive instead either ofloxacin or minocycline or, in children, clarithromycin. Those rare patients who suffer from rifampin-resistant leprosy are given clofazimine, 50 mg, plus two of the three "new" drugs daily for 6 months, and thereafter clofazimine plus either minocycline or ofloxacin daily for the full duration of treatment.

PBL patients are treated with the standard WHO-MDT regimen of rifampin, 600 mg once a month (supervised) for 6 months, plus dapsone, 100 mg daily (unsupervised) for 6 months. Should a PBL patient develop dapsone toxicity, then clofazimine is substituted in the same dosage as in the MBL regimen; MBL patients who develop dapsone toxicity continue treatment with rifampin and clofazimine.

TREATMENT OF COMPLICATIONS

Neuritis

Patients who present with signs of nerve damage that, from the history, occurred within 6 months of diagnosis, warrant additional treatment with corticosteroids to attempt to regain some nerve function. There are no standard courses, and dosage is influenced by the acuteness of the history and the degree of nerve tenderness present. I usually commence with prednisolone, 40 mg daily, and start slowly to reduce the dosage once any nerve tenderness has subsided, to a maintenance level of around 20 mg daily. This is continued for about 3 months and then slowly tailed off, giving a total duration of around 6 months. Some workers prefer higher initial dosages of 60 to 80 mg of prednisolone daily, although I have seldom found this necessary.

Neuritis can occur after commencing treatment, either in association with a reaction (which determines the overall treatment) or by itself. It may sometimes occur in the absence of nerve pain or tenderness, and therefore patients should undergo regular sensory and motor testing throughout chemotherapy. Early detection and rapid treatment with prednisolone will prevent further nerve damage and enable considerable recovery of function to occur.

REACTIONS

About one third of patients with leprosy develop immunologically mediated reactive episodes of varying degrees of severity during the course of the disease, although they appear to be less common in those treated with clofazimine. The two major varieties, namely erythema nodosum leprosum (ENL) (Type 2 reaction) and reversal reaction (Type 1 reaction), are related to the destruction of the bacilli and the release of bacterial antigens, usually as a result of chemotherapy although they may sometimes occur in untreated patients. Most occur during the first year of treatment, though occasionally much later.

It is important to continue chemotherapy, the reaction being suppressed by additional therapy. A third type of reaction, Lucio's phenomenon, occurs only in patients suffering from diffuse lepromatous leprosy, usually untreated, from Central and northern South America and occasionally in the United States. It consists of vasculitis with dermal infarcts especially on the legs and requires immediate chemotherapy plus corticosteroids.

Erythema Nodosum Leprosum

ENL, which develops in LL and occasional BL patients, usually consists of febrile crops of painful erythema nodosum–like nodules on the face and extensor surfaces of trunks and limbs, but peripheral neuritis, iridocyclitis, lymphadenitis, orchitis, arthritis, and nephritis may also occur. Some patients have only a few crops of nodules with little fever, others may have high fever, with repeated crops over months or years, and if the ENL is inadequately suppressed, they develop secondary amyloidosis. Mild espisodes may be controlled with aspirin. Severe episodes and all those involving body systems other than skin need treatment in one of three ways.

1. Corticosteroids suppress ENL rapidly. Usually an initial dose of prednisolone, 40 to 60 mg daily, is sufficient, and it can then be tailed off over a few weeks, but severe ENL usually becomes chronic. It may last for some years until the bacterial load has fallen to a low level before it gradually dies out; break-through episodes occur as the dose is cut, the maintenance dosage may rise gradually with time, and steroid-associated side effects become a major problem.

2. In men and postmenopausal women, thalidomide,* which suppresses production of tumor necrosis factor alpha, is as effective as prednisolone, with few side effects. The initial dosage is 200 mg twice daily, and once the reaction is controlled, I usually start reducing the morning dose first because of the associated drowsiness. Thalidomide peripheral neuropathy has not been reported in ENL, although regular checks every 3 to 6 months are necessary, and ENL neuritis is well suppressed. It may be necessary to continue treatment for 1 to 7 years, but the maintenance dose tends gradually to fall, usually being initially 200 mg nightly, falling eventually to 50 mg every second night. If the supply of thalidomide runs out, prednisolone can immediately take over ENL suppression, but it may take 6 weeks to wean a patient off steroids onto thalidomide; therefore I prefer not to give both drugs simultaneously apart from during the change-over period. Patients must be warned precisely what the drug is and that it must never be given to anyone else.

3. Clofazimine, though less powerful and slower acting, is also useful in controlling ENL. The dose is raised to 100 mg three times daily for 3 months but must then be reduced to 200 mg daily for 3 months and thereafter to 100 mg daily indefinitely. Moder-

---

*Investigational drug in the United States.

ately severe ENL will be controlled in 6 to 10 weeks; in severe ENL, clofazimine is steroid-sparing. If a rapid action is required, high-dose clofazimine plus prednisolone may be commenced together. The patient must be warned of the marked pigmentation effect.

Reversal Reactions

These reactions can occur in any part of the spectrum save in extreme polar TT and LL leprosy. They are evidenced by erythema and edema of lesions; peripheral edema may occur, new lesions may erupt, and/or neuritis can be very acute, although fever is mild. If there is any nerve pain or tenderness, any danger of motor or sensory deficit, or any skin ulceration, corticosteroids should be started immediately. I usually give 40 to 60 mg of prednisolone daily for the first five to 10 days; some workers give even higher dosages. Once the reaction is well suppressed, the dosage is gradually cut. Corticosteroids may be required for 3 to 6 months in dermal reactions, but for up to 12 months in neuritis; in general, reactions in BL need longer treatment than in BT patients.

Iridocyclitis

Iridocyclitis is usually associated with ENL in LL patients. In addition to systemic treatment with thalidomide or prednisolone, atropine and corticosteroid eye drops are essential, under the care of an ophthalmologist.

CONTROL MEASURES

Isolation of LL patients is scarcely necessary, as rifampin renders them noninfectious within a few days. Short-term admission to hospital may be helpful for patient education, initial treatment of neuritis and reactions, or for secondary injury or infection.

In endemic countries, the WHO does not recommend chemoprophylaxis, although the Centers for Disease Control and Prevention advises 3 years of dapsone prophylaxis for household contacts of MBL patients who are aged less than 25 years. My own practice is to offer chemoprophylaxis with rifampin (dose according to age and body weight) once monthly for six doses to child household contacts of infectious LL and BL patients, together with bacille Calmette-Guérin (BCG) vaccination. Close contacts should be examined and any suspicious lesions should be smeared. The contacts are either invited to attend annually for 5 years, or given simple education concerning the disease, so that they return as soon as they detect any suspicious signs or symptoms.

FUTURE PROSPECTS

The introduction of the three new groups of bactericidal antileprosy drugs has raised the hope of shorter and/or simpler regimens, but because of the long time scale of the disease and of relapses, these new regimens will take years to evaluate.

If protective antigens of *M. leprae* can be identified, second-generation vaccines could be developed relatively quickly through genetic engineering, although they too would take years to evaluate.

MALARIA

method of
SORNCHAI LOOAREESUWAN, M.D.,
   D.T.M.&H., and
POLRAT WILAIRATANA, M.D.
Mahidol University
Bangkok, Thailand

Malaria is one of the oldest infections, mentioned in ancient writings from Egypt, India, and China. Clinical symptoms were described by Hippocrates 400 years before the Christian era. It has been a major cause of morbidity and mortality since prehistory. It is estimated that between 300 and 500 million people suffer from malaria, and there are approximately 1 to 2 million deaths each year, mostly African children aged less than 2 years. Although the *Plasmodium* life cycle was discovered more than 100 years ago, control of malaria in endemic areas is still far from being achieved. Problems of politics, economics, movement of nonimmune people, short-term traveling, and changes in vector behavior all interfere with the success of control. In addition, parasite resistance to antimalarial drugs is increasing, and a malaria vaccine is unlikely to be used successfully in humans in the near future. Imported malaria in tourists, travelers, and immigrants is common.

ETIOLOGY

Four *Plasmodium* species cause human malaria: *Plasmodium vivax*, *P. malariae*, *P. ovale*, and *P. falciparum*, but only *P. falciparum* is a major cause of death. The infective agent is the sporozoite, which is injected into humans by the bite of an infected female anopheline mosquito as the mosquito feeds. Sporozoites disappear from the blood within 1 hour and enter liver cells where they proliferate into pre-erythrocytic schizonts (exoerythrocytic phase). Development in liver cells requires 1 to 2 weeks, depending upon the species. In *P. vivax* and *P. ovale*, some sporozoites remain dormant (hypnozoites) for months or years before proliferation (relapse). Merozoites emerge from a liver cell containing a mature schizont and invade red blood cells in the circulation, beginning the erythrocytic development.

Intra-erythrocytic parasite development can follow two pathways. First, asexual parasites develop from young ring forms through trophozoites and schizonts, which subsequently rupture, and merozoites reinvade new red cells. The erythrocytic cycle of schizogony is repeated over and over again, thus continuing the cycle of symptomatic or oligosymptomatic malaria infections. However, some intraerythrocytic parasites differentiate into male and female gametocytes, thus entering the sexual pathway. When male and female gametocytes are ingested by female mosquitoes during a blood meal, fertilization occurs, resulting in a zygote. After transformation into a motile ookinete, the parasite penetrates the mosquito midgut wall to form an oocyst containing sporozoites. When oocysts mature (8 to 30 days), they rupture, and sporozoites invade the salivary glands and are ready to be injected into humans, completing the malaria life cycle.

Other modes of transmission do occur rarely; they include blood transfusion, transplantation, re-use of blood-contaminated syringes, laboratory accidents, and congenital transmission from mother to fetus.

EPIDEMIOLOGY

Malaria is a tropical disease occurring in more than 100 countries. *P. falciparum* and *P. vivax* are the two most common species and are found side by side in most malarious areas outside tropical Africa (*P. falciparum* is the predominant species in the highly endemic areas of Africa, New Guinea, Haiti, the Amazon region of South America, and parts of Asia and Oceania, whereas *P. vivax* is more common in the Indian Subcontinent and Central America and nearly absent in tropical Africa). *P. malariae* is widely distributed but outside tropical Africa less common than the other two species. *P. ovale* occurs almost exclusively in tropical Africa. The epidemiology of malaria has changed in recent years with the spread of parasite resistance to antimalarial drugs, increasing international travel, immigration, and movement of nonimmune populations into malarial endemic areas.

P. falciparum malaria has developed resistance to nearly all available antimalarial drugs except possibly artemisinin derivatives. The earliest description of drug resistance dates back to 1910 when resistance of *P. falciparum* to quinine was reported from Brazil. Resistance to dihydrofolate reductase inhibitors such as pyrimethamine was noted soon after their introduction at the end of the second World War. However, resistance to these drugs was of little consequence as other synthetic antimalarials were readily available and effective. Drug resistance became a major problem with the appearance of resistance in *P. falciparum* (the most dangerous species of malaria parasite) to the most potent and widely used synthetic antimalarial drug chloroquine. The first evidence came almost simultaneously from Colombia, South America, Thailand, and Southeast Asia in the late 1950s.

Grading of drug response (*P. falciparum*) to schizontocidal drugs (chloroquine [Aralen]) is defined as: S: clearance of asexual parasitemia within 7 days of initiation of treatment without subsequent recrudescence. RI: clearance of asexual parasitemia as in sensitivity, followed by recrudescence. RII: marked reduction of asexual parasitemia, but no clearance. RIII: no marked reduction of asexual parasitemia.

Many mechanisms have been put forward to explain these phenomena. These include selection of resistant parasites from heterogeneous but predominantly sensitive populations, physiologic adaptation, spontaneous mutation, and selection of resistance in gene expression via resistance transfer factors or plasmids, which would manifest themselves under drug pressure (treatment with subtherapeutic dose) both in humans and in the mosquito vector. Of these mechanisms, selection of resistant individuals and spontaneous gene mutation are considered to be the most likely explanation for drug-resistant malaria. Some of the processes underlying chloroquine resistance are related to the drug concentration in the food vacuole; resistant parasites do not concentrate chloroquine sufficiently in the food vacuole because they are able to pump the drug out of the cell. The process that pumps quinoline antimalarial drugs out of the resistant parasites is similar to the multiple drug resistance mechanism in tumor cells. Resistance to dihydrofolate reductase inhibitors is mainly ascribed to gene amplification and changes in the affinity between drug and enzyme. Simultaneous resistance to pyrimethamine (Daraprim) or cycloguanil* in one area might not be true for other areas. In some countries, proguanil or cycloguanil can still be used in the treatment of falciparum malaria despite resistance to pyrimethamine. However, studies in Thailand revealed that all antifolates (pyrimethamine, proguanil, cycloguanil) are associated with therapeutic failure.

Drug failure in falciparum malaria may be divided into three main categories: due to parasite, host, and drug factors. True resistance results from genetic determination in the parasite but also from abnormal handling of antimalarial drugs by the host (even though they were given a therapeutic dose). Variations in antimalarial drugs may be responsible for therapeutic failure. Parasite factors include intrinsic resistance, which occurs from the presence of resistant subpopulations, or mutation of the parasites. The host factors include immunity, parasite burden, vomiting of oral drugs, abnormalities in drug absorption, drug elimination, and drug metabolism. Finally, the antimalarial drug factors include use of suboptimal doses, reduced drug bioavailability, decreased drug absorption due to different kinds of food intake (for example, halofantrine [Halfan]* and hydroxynapthoquinone (atovaquone [Mepron]) have more absorption with fatty meals), differences in drug plasma protein–binding, and differences in drug disposition.

Antimalarial drug concentrations in blood plasma are undoubtedly important, but as malaria is an intraerythrocytic parasite, it has been suggested that concentrations within infected red cells may be more relevant. However, this hypothesis overlooks important features in drug partition. Moreover, there is variation in drug susceptibility during various stages of parasite development. Most of the antimalarial drugs act on the growing trophozoites, whereas very young and mature forms are least sensitive to drugs. Primaquine acts on hypnozoites of *P. vivax* and *P. ovale*, on pre-erythrocytic schizonts, and on mature gametocytes of *P. falciparum*.

The relationship between antimalarial drug concentrations and treatment failure has been studied in few clinical trials. In Thai children patients who were infected with falciparum malaria and were treated with quinine, recrudescent infections occurred if serum quinine concentrations fell below 10 mg per liter in the latter half of the treatment course. In Thailand, where mefloquine (Lariam) resistance is increasing rapidly, the cure rates of mefloquine at a 15-mg per kg dose increased from 40% to 88% when a 25-mg per kg dose was used. Resistance has developed to some drugs such as halofantrine even though the medication has not been widely used in Thailand, obviously due to cross-resistance with mefloquine. Hydroxynaphthoquinone (atovaquone), the use of which was so far restricted to clinical trials, showed insufficient activity on its own since it was first used. This drug requires combination with other antimalarials such as tetracyclines or proguanil to obtain adequate activity and to inhibit/slow down the occurrence of resistance. These phenomena could not be explained easily by cross-resistance or genetic development of drug-resistant parasites and need to be investigated further.

P. vivax malaria resistance to chloroquine has been reported recently from Indonesia, Papua New Guinea, Myanmar, and India. However, many questions need to be prop-

---

*Not available in the United States.

erly answered in this condition. These include early release of hypnozoites from liver cells (early relapse), missed diagnosis of ring forms of *P. falciparum* from *P. vivax* in mixed infections treated initially with chloroquine (early recrudescence), reinfection with *P. vivax*, and failure of primaquine treatment or use of subtherapeutic doses of chloroquine or primaquine. With these unclear conditions, no changes in therapy for *P. vivax* are recommended at present.

PATHOGENESIS

Fever and malaise in malaria are believed to result from the release of endogenous cytokines (e.g., interleukin 1, 6, and 8 and tumor necrosis factor [TNF]) in response to parasite antigens. Signs and symptoms of malaria are associated with the rupture of parasitized red cells. In severe malaria, tissue hypoxia is believed to play an important role leading to organ dysfunction. However, the pathophysiologic mechanisms are still not clearly understood, especially in cerebral malaria. It is thought that microvascular obstruction from sequestration of parasitized erythrocytes, the phenomenon of cytoadherence, rosette formation, and reduced red cell deformability described next, all contribute to tissue hypoxia.

Sequestration

The discrepancy between the microscopic examination of the peripheral blood and the cerebral vessels of patients dying from cerebral malaria has been observed for a century. The cerebral capillaries and venules are packed with red cells containing mature forms of *P. falciparum* and pigment. This phenomenon is described as sequestration. It is believed to be an essential pathophysiologic feature of severe malaria. The degree of sequestration varies among organs, being greatest in the brain, particularly the white matter; prominent in the heart, liver, kidneys, and intestine; and least in the skin. In patients who die without having cerebral malaria, sequestration is less significant in the brain. These findings suggest a relationship between the organ distribution of sequestration and pathology. Pathologic events in severe malaria are believed to result from tissue ischemia and hypoxia.

Cytoadherence

The main cause of sequestration appears to be cytoadherence of parasitized erythrocytes (PRBC) to vascular endothelium, which requires an intact spleen. Parasitized erythrocytes do not cytoadhere in splenectomized monkeys. Electron microscopic examination of parasitized erythrocytes reveals electron-dense, knoblike protrusions of erythrocytic membrane at the point of contact between the parasitized erythrocytes and endothelial cells. These knobs were considered essential for cytoadherence. However, recently it has been demonstrated that knobless (K−) parasites can also cytoadhere in vitro through the same molecular mechanism as the parasites with knobs (K+).

Cytoadherence between the parasitized erythrocytes and endothelial cells involves specific parasite ligands and host receptors. Thrombospondin (TSP), leukocyte differentiation antigen (CD36), and intercellular adhesion molecule 1 (ICAM-1) are candidate receptor molecules for cytoadherence.

Thrombospondin (TSP) is an adhesive glycoprotein produced by activated platelets. Cytoadherence was specifically inhibited by anti-TSP monoclonal antibodies. However, further work has revealed that these phenomena are not consistent.

Leukocyte differentiation antigen (CD36) is a membrane glycoprotein that is also expressed on the surface of monocytes and platelets, and PRBC have also been shown to cytoadhere to these cells. A monoclonal antibody to CD36, OKM5, was shown to inhibit and reverse the cytoadherence of PRBC to epithelial cells and C32 melanoma cells in vitro.

Intercellular adhesion molecule 1 (ICAM-1), or CD54, is a glycoprotein and has a role in mediating cellular immune responses by acting as a ligand for lymphocyte function antigen 1 (LFA-1). Cytoadherence can be inhibited by specific monoclonal antibodies.

More recently VCAM, E-selection and chondroitin sulfate have all been shown to mediate cytoadherence in laboratory-adapted parasites.

The clinical correlation of cytoadherence with the three receptor molecules is still under investigation. The degree of binding to C32 melanoma cells and purified CD36 was positively correlated with biochemical indicators of disease severity, but there was no correlation between cytoadherence and the presence of cerebral symptoms in adult Thai patients.

Putative parasite cytoadherence ligands are parasite-derived proteins that have been detected on infected erythrocytes. One potential candidate for the parasite ligand is *P. falciparum* erythrocyte membrane protein (PfEMP 1). This molecule undergoes antigenic variation and is the major population-defining antigen in vivo. Inhibition or reversal of cytoadherence by immune sera occurs in a strain-specific manner.

Rosetting

Erythrocytes containing mature parasites adhere to uninfected erythrocytes. This phenomenon is called rosetting and appears both in vitro and in vivo. Rosetting shares many of the characteristics of cytoadherence. It occurs only with parasite species that sequester. Both phenomena occur with mature stages of *P. falciparum*. Rosetting can be reversed by immune sera that also reverse cytoadherence. However, unlike cytoadherence, rosetting is inhibited by heparin and calcium chelators and cannot be prevented by antimalarial drug exposure of the young ring form parasites. Rosetting is associated with cerebral malaria. Parasites obtained from Gambian children with cerebral malaria showed a significantly greater degree of rosetting than those from children with uncomplicated malaria. Cytoadherence and rosette formation properties are probably intrinsic to the parasites.

Reduced Red Cell Deformability

In normal microcirculatory flow, red cells (diameter: 8 microns) must change their shape in order to pass through capillaries (diameter: 4 microns). It has been shown that reduced deformability of red cells infected with *P. falciparum* is directly proportional to the maturity of the parasite; the older the parasite, the more rigid is the infected cell. Several possible factors contribute to reduced red cell deformability. These include reduced sphingomyelin and phosphatidylcholine in the infected red cell membrane, increased membrane stiffness, increased cytoplasmic viscosity, and relative parasite mass.

CLINICAL MANIFESTATIONS

Rupture of intraerythrocytic schizonts coincides with paroxysms of fever, and this has led to the traditional categorization of the different types of human malaria.

1. Tertian malaria (fever every third day) for *P. vivax* and *P. ovale*.

2. Quartan malaria (fever every fourth day) for *P. malariae*.

3. Subtertian malaria, or sometimes called malignant tertian (fever more often than every third day, and the disease is lethal) for *P. falciparum*.

Nowadays, these terms are not recommended, because patterns of fever are variable, especially during primary attack, and some patients die from *P. falciparum* although they never develop periodic fever, particularly in nonimmune patients and during the early stage of illness. Symptoms and signs of malaria are vague, including fever, headache, malaise, lassitude, fatigue, muscle pain, and loss of appetite. These are not specific for malaria and are similar to symptoms of flu or viral infections. It is advised to make a blood examination for malaria.

In severe malaria (Table 1), alteration of consciousness is the most prominent manifestation. The patient usually presents with a history of fever for several days and loss of consciousness that may be sudden following one or more grand mal seizures. In approximately 50% of patients over 6 years of age, coma follows a convulsion. In young children with cerebral malaria, the history may be very short. Vomiting may also occur, which is important to know because aspiration pneumonia could develop before admission to hospital. In many countries in the tropics, empirical antimalarial or antibacterial treatment and antipyretics have often been given before admission to the hospital. This may explain some reports of patients with cerebral malaria in whom no parasites were demonstrated on a peripheral blood smear. On examination, most patients are usually febrile and in unarousable coma. A few patients who have very severe infections have a subnormal temperature. Admission temperature usually exceeds 38.0° C in most cases and rises above 39.0° C during the first 2 days of hospitalization. There is no classic pattern of fever in cerebral malaria. Rigors are rare in comatose patients, but a sustained high fever resistant to antipyretic treatment is commonly found. The skin temperature is cool relative to the rectal temperature in hypoglycemic or shocked patients.

TABLE 1. **Definition of Severe Malaria and Complicated Falciparum Malaria**

1. Cerebral malaria
2. Severe anemia (hematocrit <15%)
3. Renal failure (no urine or urine output <400 mL in 24 h, or 12 mL/kg/24 h after rehydration, or serum creatinine >3 mg%)
4. Pulmonary edema or adult respiratory distress syndrome
5. Hypoglycemia (blood sugar <40 mg%)
6. Shock (systolic BP <70 mmHg in adults or <50 mmHg in children age 1–5 y)
7. Spontaneous bleeding and disseminated intravascular coagulation
8. Repeated convulsions
9. Acidosis (arterial pH <7.25 or plasma HCO_3 <15)
10. Macroscopic hemoglobinuria
11. Hyperparasitemia (>5% parasitemia in nonimmunes)
12. Hepatic dysfunction
13. Hyperpyrexia (T >40° C)

Jaundice is common in adult patients, and anemia develops rapidly in severe malaria. The chest is usually normal on clinical examination, although aspiration pneumonia or pulmonary edema may develop. Changes in respiration can be a warning sign of hypoglycemia, metabolic acidosis, pneumonia, and pulmonary edema, but then may occur as a result of high fever alone. Therefore, careful examination and proper investigation should be performed in all patients.

Hepatosplenomegaly is common. Massive splenomegaly is most unusual in severe malaria. Abdominal pain and tenderness are prominent in some patients. In children, the physical signs are similar to those in adults except that convulsions are more common, hepatomegaly may be prominent, and anemia is common; however, jaundice and renal failure are relatively less frequent.

Retinal hemorrhages may occur in 15% of cerebral malaria patients in Thailand, but in Papua New Guinea they were detected in 28% of consecutive admissions to hospital. Hemorrhages may occur anywhere in the retina. Some appear similar to Roth's spots, which are associated with endocarditis. Exudates are unusual, and papilledema is rare (less than 1%). The hemorrhages resolve rapidly in survivors and do not interfere with vision after recovery of consciousness. Systemic bleeding due to disseminated intravascular coagulation (DIC) is present in a few patients (less than 5%). Abnormal eye movements, such as divergence of the eyes or nystagmus, are seen occasionally. Pupillary responses to light, and the oculocephalic and oculovestibular reflexes, are always normal. Corneal reflexes are usually present. There may be passive resistance to head flexion, but other signs of meningeal irritation are absent. Ankle clonus is present in one third of patients. The abdominal reflexes are almost absent. There is no other clinical evidence of autonomic dysfunction in cerebral malaria. The duration of coma is 48 to 72 hours in most adult patients in Thailand. After treatment, most of the survivors have complete recovery (90%).

DIAGNOSIS

The diagnosis of malaria is made by demonstration of asexual forms of *Plasmodium* species in Giemsa-stained blood smears. On some occasions, the parasites can be demonstrated in necropsy or biopsy tissues from brain, liver, heart, muscle, and tissue fluid taken from bone marrow, umbilical cord, and skin puncture fluid. In clinically suspected malaria with negative slides, blood films should be taken frequently (at 6- to 8-hour intervals) irrespective of fever, until 3 to 6 smears of thick films have been obtained. The diagnosis may be difficult in (1) patients who have been previously or partially treated with antimalarial drugs or who have taken prophylactic drugs; and (2) patients whose blood films have been poorly prepared or stained.

Other methods for malaria diagnosis include special staining (QBC), enzyme-linked immunosorbent assay (ELISA), and radioimmunoassay (RIA) to detect malaria antigen; hybridization (DNA) probes or polymerase chain reaction (PCR) techniques to detect parasite DNA. However, these techniques have certainly no greater value in clinical management than the microscopic examination of blood smears.

DIFFERENTIAL DIAGNOSIS

The most common differential diagnoses include influenza, enteric fever, typhus, leptospirosis, pneumonia, cholangitis, and pyelonephritis. Other differential diagnoses in severe malaria include hepatitis, bacterial or viral meningoencephalitis, psychosis, cerebrovascular accidents, hepatic, diabetic, or uremic comas, epilepsy, eclampsia, heat stroke, and drug intoxications (Table 2). Therefore, blood smears have to be taken in all febrile patients who have been exposed to malaria risk or received a blood transfusion. Cerebrospinal fluid should be taken for examination in comatose patients.

TREATMENT

Symptomatic Treatment

Supportive treatment and symptomatic treatment of malaria are equally important to antimalarial drugs since most patients have headache, nausea, vomiting, diarrhea, and high fever and cannot take any food while they are ill. Therefore, rehydration and the use of antipyretic and antiemetic drugs might be necessary in those patients. Antipyretic and antiemetic drugs should be administered a few hours before antimalarials are given to reduce the occurrence of vomiting and to comfort the patients. After antimalarial drug administration, it is advisable to keep patients under observation for an hour or let the patients lie down to make sure that they have retained the drugs and did not vomit. If they vomit within an hour of antimalarial drug administration, repeat medication should be given. Some important points on the management of falciparum malaria are shown in Table 3.

Specific Treatment with Antimalarial Drugs

Antimalarial drugs used for treatment depend upon the species of malaria and its severity. General recommendations are shown in Table 4. In some areas, especially in Thailand, falciparum parasites resist all commonly used drugs, as shown by a yearly decline of the cure rate (Figure 1).

TABLE 2. **Differential Diagnosis of Severe Falciparum Malaria**

Fever	Enteric fever, brucellosis, influenza
Hyperpyrexia	Heat stroke, sepsis
Jaundice	Viral hepatitis, leptospirosis, relapsing fevers, yellow fever, drug-induced or toxic hepatitis
Hypoglycemia	Severe septicemia, liver failure, Reye's syndrome
Acute hemolytic anemia	Drug-induced, due to toxic substances, autoimmune diseases, blood diseases—e.g., inheritable red cell abnormalities, or G6PD deficiency
Gastrointestinal symptoms	Peptic ulcer, gastroenteritis, salmonellosis, traveler's diarrhea
Abnormal bleeding	Hepatic failure, poisons, viral hemorrhagic fevers, leptospirosis
Convulsions	Febrile confusions, epilepsy, cerebrovascular accidents
Encephalopathy	Viral, fungal, bacterial, protozoal encephalitis; eclampsia; toxic substances

TABLE 3. **Important Points in Management of Falciparum Malaria**

1. Parenteral antimalarial drugs should be administered to patients with severe infections and those whose condition deteriorates after being treated with oral preparations. The IV route is preferred to IM injection, particularly in severely ill patients or those in shock, to secure absorption. In remote areas where facilities are not available, IM or rectal adminstration can be used. Severe malaria may be complicated by coma, pulmonary edema, acute renal failure, hypoglycemia, lactic acidosis, liver dysfunction, anemia, intravascular hemolysis, and concurrent systemic bacterial infections. Supportive treatment of these complications is essential to reduce mortality.
2. Recurrent fever during the first 2 months after treatment for malaria should be reinvestigated. Treatment failures can occur in any treatment regimens as falciparum malaria is becoming progressively more resistant to all existing drugs. In addition, mixed infection with *P. vivax* occurs in about one third of patients, which usually becomes manifest within 2 months after being treated for falciparum malaria.
3. Malaria patients may have other diseases that they contract in the malarious areas (e.g., scrub typhus, filariasis, amebiasis, leptospirosis, typhoid). If fever persists after treatment of malaria, other causes of infection should be sought.

The development of antimalarial drugs is summarized in Table 5. Pharmacokinetic data of oral antimalarial drugs are shown in Table 6. Dose (salt/base) of the drugs is shown in Table 7. The most important antimalarial compounds are divided into those in current use and those currently undergoing development.

The following compounds are in current use:

1. 4-aminoquinolines (chloroquine, amodiaquine)
2. Cinchona alkaloids (quinine, quinidine)
3. 8-aminoquinolines (primaquine)
4. Diaminopyrimidines (pyrimethamine)
5. Sulfonamides and sulfones (sulfadoxine, sulfalene, dapsone)
6. Tetracyclines (tetracycline, doxycycline, minocycline)
7. Biguanides (proguanil, chlorproguanil)
8. 4-quinoline methanols (mefloquine)
9. Phenanthrene methanols (halofantrine)

The following compounds are undergoing development:

1. Sesquiterpene lactones (artemisinin derivatives include crude plant extract, artemisinin, artemether, artesunate, dihydroartemisinin, artelinic acid, arteether).
2. Hydroxypiperaquine
3. Hydroxynaphthoquinones
4. Pyronaridine
5. Benflumetol

Chloroquine (Aralen)

Chloroquine was the first synthetic antimalarial, introduced 50 years ago, and for many years was the mainstay of antimalarial treatment for all four types of human malaria. Because of increasing chloroquine

TABLE 4. **Recommended Antimalarial Drugs**

Type	Clinical	Recommended	Alternative
P. falciparum			
A. Chloroquine-sensitive	Not severe	chloroquine (Aralen) PO[1]	sulfadoxine/pyrimethamine (Fansidar) PO[2]
	Severe	chloroquine IV[3]	chloroquine IM[4]
B. Chloroquine-resistant but sensitive to sulfadoxine/ pyrimethamine	Not severe	sulfadoxine/pyrimethamine PO[2]	quinine PO[5]
	Severe	quinine (Quinamm) IV[6]	quinine IM[7]
C. Chloroquine-resistant and resistant to sulfadoxine/ pyrimethamine	Not severe	quinine PO[5]	mefloquine (Lariam) PO[8]
	Severe	quinine IV[6]	quinidine (Quinalan) IV[9] quinine IM[7]
D. Multidrug-resistant	Not severe	quinine PO[5] plus tetracycline	See 5.1 below
	Severe	quinine IV[6] artesunate IV[10] artemether IM[11]	quinine IV[9] quinine IM[7]
P. vivax		chloroquine PO,[1] followed by PO primaquine[12]	mefloquine PO[8] followed by primaquine PO[12]
P. ovale			
P. malariae		chloroquine PO[1]	mefloquine PO[8]
Mixed Infections or Species Unknown	Not severe Severe	Treat as if *P. falciparum,* then treat other species as indicated[13]	

Note: Doses are given as base except those marked salt.
1. Adults: 300 mg × 3, 1st day; 300 mg, 2nd and 3rd day
   Children: 5 mg/kg × 3, 1st day; 5 mg/kg on 2nd and 3rd days
2. Adults: 3 tablets, single dose
   Children: <5 years: 0.5 tablet; <9 years, 1 tablet; <15 years, 2 tablets (1 tablet = sulfadoxine, 500 mg, or sulfalene, 500 mg, plus pyrimethamine, 25 mg)
3. Chloroquine: 10 mg/kg rate-controlled IV over 8 h, followed by 15 mg/kg over 24 h (total dose: 25 mg base/kg)
4. Chloroquine: 3.5 mg/kg IM or sq injection every 6 h to a total dose of 25 mg/kg
5. Adults: 600 mg salt (2 tablets) every 8 h for 7 d
   Children: 10 mg salt/kg every 8 h for 7 d
5.1   *In areas of quinine resistance (e.g., Thailand), add tetracycline, 250 mg qid for 7 days except children under 7 years and pregnant women. Quinidine tablet or quinidine slow-release preparation at the same dose of quinine can be used in place of quinine.*
6. Quinine: 20 mg salt/kg (loading dose) IV infusion over 2 h, followed by 10 mg salt/kg IV infusion over 2 h, given 8 hourly until the patient can swallow, then quinine tablets to complete 7 d of treatment
   Loading dose must not be used if patient had already started quinine or mefloquine treatment.
7. Quinine: The same dose as (6) given deep IM to the anterior thigh (not the buttock). The loading dose is split and given to both legs.
8. Mefloquine: 15 mg/kg single dose or 25 mg/kg divided into 2 doses 6 h apart in areas where mefloquine resistance is emerging (e.g., Thailand).
9. Quinidine 10 mg base/kg infusion over 1 h followed by 0.02 mg/kg/min under ECG monitoring until the patient can swallow, then quinine or quinidine tablets to complete 7 d of treatment.
10. Artesunate:* 2 mg/kg IV injection in 3 min followed by 1 mg/kg IV injection every 12 h until the patient can swallow, then artesunate tablets to complete 5–6 d of treatment (total dose: 600–750 mg), with the consideration of adding mefloquine, 15–25 mg/kg at the end of artesunate treatment to avoid recrudescence.
11. Artemether:* 3.2 mg/kg IM followed in 12 h by 1.6 mg/kg, then 1.6 mg/kg IM qd until the patient can swallow, then artemether tablets to complete 5–6 d of treatment (total dose: 600–750 mg) with the consideration of adding mefloquine, 15–25 mg/kg, at the end of artemether treatment to avoid recrudescence.
12. Primaquine: Adult: 15 mg once daily for 14 d (0.25 mg/kg once daily)
13. If *P. vivax* or *P. ovale* is positive or clinical evidence is indicated, primaquine should be added.

*Not available in the United States.

resistance in *P. falciparum* in most malaria-endemic areas in recent years, chloroquine can be recommended at present only for treating nonimmunes with falciparum malaria acquired in some parts of West Africa and Central America. However, chloroquine is still the drug of choice in the treatment of *P. vivax, P. malariae*, and *P. ovale* infections.

Amodiaquine*

Amodiaquine is similar to chloroquine and was once used as a substitute for chloroquine. However, the potential toxicity of amodiaquine leading to agranulocytosis may limit the use of this drug for the treatment of malaria.

*Not available in the United States.

Quinine (Quinamm)

Quinine is the most commonly used and available drug in treating falciparum malaria. Recently, its effectiveness has declined when used alone. Quinine resistance is appearing in several parts of the world, including Tanzania, Vietnam, and Thailand; however, most of the resistance is at the RI level. Minimal inhibitory concentrations (MIC) of quinine for *P. falciparum* parasites have risen above 10 mg/liter in some areas. In this situation, and in severe malaria, a loading dose of 20 mg of quinine dihydrochloride per kg body weight, and maintenance doses of 10 mg per kg given every 8 hours, are required. Persistent parasitemia after a loading dose of quinine is not uncommon. It is believed that the MIC of quinine must be maintained for 7 days to effect complete cure

Percentage cure (Thailand)

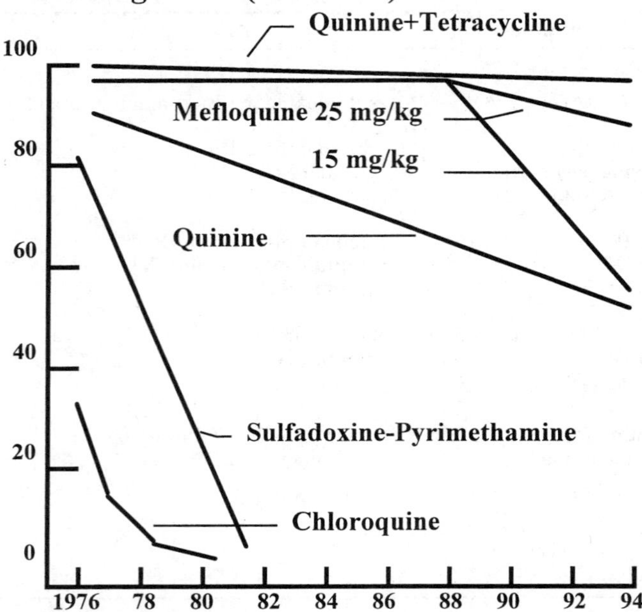

Figure 1. Yearly cure rates of antimalarial drugs for falciparum malaria in Thailand. It shows declining of antimalarial drug efficacy since 1976. Quinine alone (10 mg per kg) given every 8 hours for 7 days reveals a cure rate of 50% in 1994, but maintains a cure rate over 90% when tetracycline (20 mg per kg for 7 days) is added. Mefloquine (15 mg per kg single dose) cures 50% in 1994, but its cure rate increases to 80% when high-dose mefloquine (25 mg/kg divided into 2 doses, 15 and 10 mg per kg, 6 hours apart) is used.

of *P. falciparum* infections. Therefore, quinine must be given for at least 7 days or longer. In quinine-resistant areas, a second drug such as tetracycline or doxycycline has been added to increase cure rates, which approached 100% in 1986 but have declined to 90% in 1991. For children, in whom tetracycline is contraindicated, increasing the individual dose of quinine to 15 mg per kg in the second half of the treatment period improves the cure rate.

In severe malaria, if the patient has not received quinine or mefloquine in the previous 24 hours, an initial loading dose of 20 mg per kg of quinine dihydrochloride salt should be infused over 4 hours, followed by maintenance doses of 10 mg per kg at 8-hour intervals until the patient can take oral medication, for a total treatment course of 7 days. The initial doses should never be reduced; the maintenance doses should be reduced by one third if by the third day of treatment there has been no clinical improvement, or if there is established acute renal failure. Hypoglycemia is the most serious and frequent adverse effect of cinchona alkaloids.

Quinidine (Quinalan)

Quinidine, the diastereomer of quinine, has a lower MIC for *P. falciparum*. It is as effective as or perhaps more effective than quinine for the treatment of falciparum malaria, as shown in open trials of oral quinidine sulfate and parenteral quinidine gluconate in both acute uncomplicated and severe falciparum malaria in Thailand. Quinidine bisulfate and quinidine slow-release formula were tested in uncomplicated falciparum malaria in Thailand in 1983–1984. They proved effective (with a cure rate of 100%), were well tolerated, and had few side effects. They should be considered as alternative antimalarial drugs in the treatment of uncomplicated falciparum malaria.

Where quinine is not available, as in Japan; or not in stock, as occasionally occurs in America, or in Europe, quinidine may be used in place of quinine. It is more effective but also more cardiotoxic than quinine. The electrocardiogram shows consistent dose-related prolongation of the Q-Tc interval. In severe malaria, an initial loading dose of 15 mg base per kg is given over 4 hours, followed by 7.5 mg base per kg given over 2 hours at 8-hour intervals. Quinine should be substituted when it becomes available to complete a 7-day treatment course. Hypotension is a serious side effect, particularly when the infusion is given over a period less than 2 hours.

Combination of Quinine, Quinidine, and Cinchonidine.* In vitro testing against fresh isolates of

---

*All are investigational drugs in the United States.

TABLE 5. Antimalarial Drug Development and Trials

1630	Cinchona (quinine)	Countess of Chinchon in Peru was treated by an extract of the cinchona bark. The "Jesuit's" or "Peruvian" bark was named after Jesuit priests who introduced it to Europe for treating malaria.
1928	8-Aminoquinoline	Pamaquine (one of the 8-aminoquinoline series) was first synthesized, and it was discovered in India that it reduced the relapse rates in vivax malaria. Later, primaquine was synthesized in the USA in 1950.
1934	Mepacrine	Synthesized in the 1930s and was the most commonly used antimalarial during World War II.
1941	Chloroquine	Synthesized in 1934 and introduced for use in 1941 during World War II. It was the drug of choice for treatment of malaria in replacement of quinine.
1945	Proguanil	Synthesized during World War II.
1952	Pyrimethamine	Developed during World War II.
1972	Qinghaosu	Used in treating fever, presumably malaria, 2000 years ago. However, its structure was discovered in 1972.
1984	Mefloquine	Developed by the United States Army and registered for use in the treatment of malaria.
1988	Halofantrine	Developed by the United States Army and registered for use in the treatment of malaria in the US and most countries in Africa.
1992	Hydroxynaphthoquinone	Developed by the Wellcome Research Laboratories. The drug has been tested worldwide in combination with proguanil (atovaquone) with good results.

TABLE 6. **Pharmacokinetic Data of Oral Antimalarial Drugs**

	t $^{1/2}$	Vd (L/kg)	CL (mL/kg/min)	Tmax (h)	PPB (%)
Chloroquine (Aralen)	30 d	100–1000	2	3–6	55
Halofantrine (Halfan)*	110 h	?	1.5	16	>90
Mefloquine (Lariam)	20 d	20	0.5	6–20	>90
Primaquine	<6 h	3	6	2	?
Proguanil*	16 h	24	20	2–4	?
Pyrimethamine (Daraprim)	80 h	3	0.5	4	?
Quinine (Quinamm)	10–15 h	1	1.5	2–4	>90
Quinidine (Quinalan)	10 h	1.3	2	1–2	>80

*Not available in the United States.
Abbreviations: t $^{1/2}$ = half-life (d = day, h = hour); Vd = total apparent volume of distribution; CL = total clearance; Tmax = time to peak concentration; PPB = plasma protein binding.

P. falciparum suggested that the combination containing equal parts of the three drugs was more potent than the individual drugs. In clinical trials, the combination preparations in both oral and intravenous preparations were studied in uncomplicated falciparum malaria in Thailand. The combination drug was given every 8 hours in the dose of 11.4 mg base per kg per dose for 7 days. The results reveal that the oral or intravenous preparation of the three drugs is not toxic and is effective in the treatment of chloroquine-resistant falciparum malaria. However, this combination is not generally available.

8-Aminoquinolines (Primaquine). Primaquine is an 8-aminoquinoline derivative. It has gametocytocidal activity for all species of human malaria. It is a poor blood schizonticide but is highly effective against the exoerythrocytic stages of all species and prevents relapses due to *P. vivax* and *P. ovale*. In Thailand, the use of primaquine, 15 mg daily for 14 days, in adults infected with *P. vivax* produces a radical care of 80%, and the cure rate increased to 90% if 22.5 mg of primaquine was given daily for 14 days.

Other 8-aminoquinoline derivatives are being developed by the Walter Reed Army Institute for Research as an alternative to primaquine for radical cure of relapse malaria. Several new 5-phenoxy-compounds (WR 225448, WR 233195, WR 238605, WR 242471)* were synthesized and tested in animal malarias. WR 238605 will soon be tested in human malaria. The 8-aminoquinoline derivatives were found to be five times more active than primaquine in animal malarias.

Pyrimethamine (Daraprim)

Pyrimethamine (dihydrofolate reductase DHFR inhibitor) alone is now used rarely in treatment or prophylaxis because resistance is widespread. Potentiating combinations of pyrimethamine with long-acting sulfonamides (sulfadoxine/sulfalene†) are still used for the treatment of malaria where the parasites are sensitive to the combinations. At present, prophylactic use of the combinations is not recommended because of the potential toxicity of long-acting sulfonamides.

Sulfonamides and Sulfones

Sulfonamides and sulfones (PABA [para-aminobenzoic acid] inhibitor) are moderately effective blood schizonticides for *P. falciparum* malaria but are less active against the asexual blood forms of other malarial parasite species. Their action is too slow to kill the parasites if used alone. The combination of pyrimethamine with sulfonamides has been shown to potentiate antimalarial activity and to produce complete cure of malaria infections. This combination (sulfadoxine and pyrimethamine [Fansidar]) was effective when it was first introduced as a single-dose treatment for acute uncomplicated falciparum malaria. Over the years, resistance has developed in many parts of the world, including South America. Increasing treatment failures are reported from tropical Africa, Indonesia, Malaysia, Papua New Guinea, Kenya, Myanmar, and Thailand. In some parts of Thailand, it is totally ineffective. The use of intramuscular sulfadoxine and pyrimethamine in severe malaria is now questioned since absorption is slow and peak blood concentrations are lower than following oral administration.

TABLE 7. **Salt and Base Equivalents of Antimalarial Drugs**

	Base (mg)	Salt (mg)
Amodiaquine dihydrochloride*	400	522
Chloroquine sulfate	300	204
Chloroquine diphosphate	300	484
Chloroquine hydrochloride	300	368
Primaquine phosphate	30	52
Quinine sulfate	300	363
Quinine bisulfate	300	508
Quinine dihydrochloride	300	367
Quinidine bisulfate	300	351
Quinidine gluconate	300	433

*Not available in the United States.

*All are investigational drugs in the United States.
†Not available in the United States.

Tetracycline

Tetracycline has a very slow blood schizonticidal activity. Action against tissue schizonts of chloroquine-resistant *P. falciparum* has been reported. Doxycycline (Vibramycin) and minocycline (Minocin) are as effective as tetracycline, but minocycline is more expensive. These drugs are reported to have synergistic activity with quinine, mefloquine, and artemisinin derivatives.

Biguanides

Proguanil* and chlorproguanil* are prodrugs for the active triazine metabolites cycloguanil and chlorcycloguanil, respectively. They are considered the safest of all antimalarials. Their action is based on DHFR inhibition. Proguanil is used for prophylaxis and often in combination with chloroquine. Chlorproguanil is used in combination with dapsone as a treatment of *P. falciparum* infections in Africa. However, the combinations of proguanil or chlorproguanil with dapsone are not sufficiently effective in the treatment of uncomplicated falciparum malaria in Thailand. The antimalarial activities of these compounds are due to their active metabolites, which require enzyme cytochrome P-450 for their formation. This enzyme shows marked genetic polymorphism. It is estimated that 3% of Africans and Whites and 15% of Asians fail to convert the parent compounds to their active metabolites. However, the combination of proguanil and hydroxynaphthoquinone (atovaquone) is synergistic, is proved safe, and produced a 100% cure rate in multidrug-resistant falciparum malaria in Thailand and other areas of the world.

Mefloquine (Lariam)

Mefloquine, a synthetic 4-quinolinemethanol, was developed by the United States Army antimalarial drug development program. It was initially thought to be the ideal antimalarial. Its action is rapid, and it is effective against all species of human malaria parasites, including chloroquine-resistant *P. falciparum*. In an effort to delay development of resistance to mefloquine, a combination of mefloquine and sulfadoxine-pyrimethamine (Fansimef)* was advocated. This drug has been registered for use in Thailand since 1984. The evidence that the combination may delay development of drug resistance came mainly from a mouse model and has not been generally accepted. In patients with acute falciparum malaria, the combination (Fansimef)* has not prevented the development of resistance to mefloquine. Furthermore, severe adverse effects have resulted (presumably from the sulfadoxine component) when the combination was used for malaria prophylaxis. It now seems unequivocal that mefloquine should be used as a single agent.

Treatment failures have been reported in many parts of the world, caused either by true parasite resistance (intrinsic) or inadequate dosing. In Thailand, Fansimef* with the dose of mefloquine at 15 mg per kg gave a cure rate of over 98% of uncomplicated falciparum malaria in 1983 to 1986, which subsequently fell to 71% by 1990. However, a higher dose of mefloquine, 25 mg per kg given in two divided doses 6 hours apart, achieved a cure rate of 81% in 1991. In children, mefloquine alone, in doses ranging from 18 to 25 mg per kg, has also shown a decrease in cure rates from 98% in 1986 to 73% in 1990. At present, mefloquine has been used successfully in combinations with artemisinin derivatives or in sequential treatment of multidrug-resistant falciparum malaria. These combinations or sequential treatments proved safe and produced higher efficacy.

Halofantrine (Hafan)*

Halofantrine, a phenanthrene methanol, is another product of the United States Army antimalarial drug development program. Initial studies showed it to be effective against multidrug-resistant *P. falciparum* both in Thailand and Africa. However, subsequent studies in Thailand in 1988 and 1991 have shown that halofantrine (total dose of 1500 mg given in three doses) cured only 58% and 70% of patients respectively, even though this drug had not been widely used. Higher doses of halofantrine were tested at different regimens in Thailand and showed increased cure rates. However, some electrocardiogram changes have been observed in a study in Karen patients living in the western part of Thailand. Halofantrine was licensed by the Food and Drug Administration (FDA) in 1992 for use at a dose of 8 mg per kg given every 8 hours on day 1 and day 7. However, it should not be used in patients with underlying cardiac abnormalities.

Qinghaosu (Artemisinin) Derivatives

Qinghaosu is a sesquiterpene lactone peroxide extracted from the qinghao plant (*Artemisia annua*). It has been used in Chinese traditional medicine for over 2000 years, to treat the chills and fever associated with malaria. The active constituent, artemisinin, was isolated in 1972. Qinghaosu derivatives are highly effective in killing parasites; however, recrudescence rates are high. Attempts have been made to reduce the high recrudescence rates by increasing the dosage, lengthening the period of drug administration, or using drug combinations. Two derivatives (artemether and artesunate) are now widely used and have been licensed in Thailand.

Artesunate*

Artesunate is formulated either as tablets (50-mg tablet) or as a dry powder of artesunic acid for injection (supplied in a 60-mg vial with an ampule of 1 mL 5% sodium bicarbonate). The powder is dissolved in the sodium bicarbonate and then further diluted in 1 mL of normal saline and used immediately as an intravenous or intramuscular injection.

---

*Not available in the United States.

*Not available in the United States.

Artesunate is manufactured by Guilin No. 2 Pharmaceutical Factory, Guangxi, China. It has rapid antimalarial activity, with clearance of over 90% of parasitemias within 24 hours. However, recrudescence rates are high, ranging from 10% to 100% depending upon the dose and duration of treatment and severity of disease; the more severe, the higher the probability of recrudescence. To reduce the high recrudescence rate, the optimum dose of artesunate in combination with other drugs such as mefloquine or tetracycline or doxycycline is currently being investigated in Thailand (see Table 4).

Recently, artesunate, in both oral (200-mg tablet) and rectal suppository (200 mg) forms, has been developed by Mepha Ltd., Aesch-Basel, Switzerland. These formulations proved safe and well-tolerated in acute uncomplicated and severe falciparum malaria.

Artemether*

Artemether (80-mg ampule), manufactured by Kunming Pharmaceutical Factory, Kunming, China, is formulated in peanut oil for intramuscular injection. Oral artemether (tablet and capsule of 50 mg) is undergoing clinical trials. As with artesunate, the parasiticidal effect is rapid, with clearance of over 90% of parasitemias within 24 hours. Unfortunately, recrudescence rates are also high. The optimum dose of artemether, combined with other drugs such as mefloquine, tetracycline, or doxycycline, is under study in Myanmar, Vietnam, and Thailand.

Arteether*

Arteether, a more recent semisynthetic derivative of artemisinin, has been developed by the World Health Organization Special Programme for Research and Training in Tropical Diseases in collaboration with the Walter Reed Army Institute of Research, Washington, D.C. In addition, with funds provided by the Netherlands Ministry of Development Cooperation, the registration and manufacturing of arteether injection is being pursued by a Dutch company, ACF Beheer B.V. Because of the investment in development of arteether by public sector agencies, the cost of arteether is expected to be substantially lower than that of artemether, and this may benefit malaria-endemic developing countries. The dose used is the same as that of artemether, 9.6 mg per kg total dose given in 5 to 7 days, and the main indication for use of arteether injection will be for the the treatment of severe malaria. Comparative clinical trials of arteether versus other antimalarial drugs in severe malaria are ongoing.

Dihydroartemisinin*

All artemisinin derivatives are metabolized to a biologically highly active metabolite, dihydroartemisinin, once they are absorbed into the body. This compound is simpler and cheaper to manufacture than artesunate or artemether, both of which use dihydroartemisinin as an intermediate in synthesis.

In vitro, it is two to three times more active than the derivatives. Dihydroartemisinin (Cotecxin), manufactured by Beijing Sixth Pharmaceutical Factory, China, has proved safe and effective in the treatment of acute uncomplicated falciparum malaria in China and Thailand.

Hydroxypiperaquine*

Hydroxypiperaquine, an analogue of piperaquine, was synthesized in China. It has been shown to have blood schizontocidal activity similar to that of chloroquine in both *P. falciparum* and *P. vivax*. Field studies in China indicate that the drug is active against chloroquine-resistant falciparum malaria, but laboratory studies suggest that there is some degree of cross-resistance.

Hydroxynaphthoquinones (Atovaquone [Mepron])†

At the Wellcome Research Laboratories, research has been conducted for many years on the development of hydroxynaphthoquinones as potential antimalarial drugs. These drugs have blood schizontocidal activity but very variable oral bioavailability. Atovaquone has proved safe and effective against multidrug-resistant malaria in Thailand. It is one of the most promising compounds; when given together with proguanil, it gave a 100% cure rate. The combinations of hydroxynaphthoquinone with tetracycline, doxycycline, or proguanil have shown synergistic effects both in vitro and in vivo. Atovaquone has been registered for use in the treatment of *Pneumocystis carinii* infection. It is also effective in the treatment of toxoplasmosis in patients with acquired immunodeficiency syndrome (AIDS).

Pyronaridine*

Compounds of the pyronaridine series have been shown to be highly active blood schizontocides, effective against chloroquine-resistant strains of animal and human malaria. They were developed in China. The drug has been used successfully in the treatment of *P. falciparum* malaria in China in combination with sulfadoxine-pyrimethamine. However, a clinical trial in Thailand with oral pyronaridine alone showed a cure rate of 63% and 88%, with the total dose of 1200 mg and 1800 mg (300 mg given twice in the first day, then 300 mg once daily) given over 3 days and 5 days, respectively.

Benflumetol*

Benflumetol was synthesized in the 1970s by the Academy of Military Medical Sciences, Beijing, and registered for use in China as an antimalarial drug in 1987. It is formulated for oral administration and used together with artemether for the treatment of *P. falciparum* malaria. Phase III clinical trials are being performed in Thailand and elsewhere.

---

*Not available in the United States.

*Not available in the United States.
†Not FDA-approved for this indication.

COMPLICATIONS

In severe malaria, especially in cerebral malaria, intensive care of the unconscious patient and treatment of life-threatening complications such as pulmonary edema, metabolic acidosis, renal failure, hypoglycemia, bacterial septicemia, and aspiration pneumonia are essential for the management of severe malaria. Cerebral malaria is an emergency condition that requires much effort during the first 48 hours of admission. It was calculated that nearly 80% of all fatalities occurred during this period.

Hyperthermia

The condition of patients with severe malaria usually deteriorates while they have high fever. Temperatures above 38.5° C are associated with an increased incidence of convulsions, especially in children. Temperatures between 39.5° C and 40° C are associated with delirium, and above 42° C, with coma. High body temperatures may cause permanent severe neurologic damage. In pregnant women with malaria, high fever is associated with fetal distress. In the severely ill patient, cooling blankets, fanning, and tepid sponging are necessary. In the tropics, clinicians often accept the risk of agranulocytosis and use parenteral antipyretics such as dipyrone.

Acute Pulmonary Edema

Although pulmonary edema may develop at any stage of the acute illness, it tends to occur later than the other acute manifestations of malaria. Central venous pressure is a useful measure of hydration. A permeability edema associated with normal pulmonary wedge pressure measurements may develop at any time in the first few days of treatment and is difficult to treat. There is no specific therapy, and management should be the same as that for adult respiratory distress syndrome occurring in other conditions. Malaria in pregnancy usually has a high risk of pulmonary edema, particularly after delivery.

Acute Renal Failure

This results from acute tubular necrosis. Some impairment of renal function is common in adults with cerebral malaria and is also associated with hemoglobinuria; some patients go on to develop established renal failure. Hypercatabolic acute renal failure should be managed with hemodialysis or, if unavailable, peritoneal dialysis. Fluid balance should be strictly monitored.

Hepatic Dysfunction

This is manifested by jaundice, raised serum enzyme levels, prolonged prothrombin time, decreased serum albumin concentration, and lactic acidosis. Bilirubinemia is predominantly of the unconjugated type, but some patients show an increase in conjugated bilirubin indicating hepatocellular damage.

Hypoglycemia

Hypoglycemia should be reversed by intravenous dextrose and the plasma glucose maintained between 80 and 120 mg%. Frequent monitoring is essential. This condition should be suspected in any patient whose consciousness is deteriorating, who develops convulsions, or who has a changed respiratory pattern.

Shock (Algid Malaria)

This is most commonly the result of hypovolemic status or complicating septicemia. Other causes are endotoxemia, hypoglycemia, lactic acidosis, hemorrhage (disseminated intravascular coagulation [DIC], gastrointestinal bleeding, drugs, ruptured spleen), myocardial failure, or cardiac arrhythmias.

Severe Anemia

Anemia develops very rapidly in cerebral malaria, and blood transfusion is often required. Anemia results from a combination of bone marrow suppression and accelerated red cell destruction of both parasitized and unparasitized red cells. Blood should be cross-matched on admission and transfused to maintain the hematocrit over 21%. Fresh blood is preferable as thrombocytopenia and clotting factor depletion may coexist with anemia. Transfusion rates should be slow to avoid volume overload, and it may be necessary to give a potent diuretic such as furosemide intravenously at the same time.

Metabolic Acidosis

This condition is serious and rapidly fatal. Lactic acidosis and renal impairment both contribute to hydrogen ion retention. Lactic acidosis results from the parasite, increased anaerobic glycolysis, and a failure of hepatic gluconeogenesis. Sodium bicarbonate provides temporary restoration of acidosis, but its use is controversial. Dichloroacetate has proved safe and effective in decreasing the degree of acidosis. However, it did not reduce the mortality rate in a double-blind controlled study in adult patients suffering from other diseases. Its use in malaria remains to be investigated.

Hyperparasitemia

In nonimmune patients with severe falciparum malaria, mortality increases with the degree of parasitemia. Exchange transfusion might reduce the burden of parasitemia more rapidly than chemotherapy alone and might also remove harmful toxic products, e.g., toxins and cytokines. This technique offers an opportunity to replace blood, plasma, platelets, and clotting factors and to correct other abnormalities, e.g., fluid, electrolytes, and acid base imbalance. Exchange transfusion should be considered in nonimmune patients who have parasitemias exceeding 10%, whose condition has deteriorated under conventional chemotherapy, and who have at least two complications of severe falciparum malaria (cerebral malaria, renal failure, jaundice, acute pulmonary edema). When total exchange transfusion is not possible, partial exchange transfusion with 4 to 6 units of fresh blood, performed manually either alternately venesecting and transfusing the patient, is still use-

TABLE 8. **Drugs Used in the Prophylaxis of Malaria**

Drug	Adult Dose	Pediatric Dose	Main Protection
Chloroquine (Aralen)	300 mg base PO, once a wk	5 mg/kg base PO, once a wk	All species (if *P. falciparum* is still sensitive to chloroquine)
Mefloquine (Lariam)	250 mg base PO once a wk	5–6 mg/kg PO, once a wk	All species (if *P. falciparum* is still sensitive to mefloquine)
Doxycycline (Vibramycin)	100 mg PO, once a d	Contraindicated	Mainly for multi-drug–resistant *P. falciparum*
Proguanil*	200 mg PO, once a d; better is 100 mg twice a d	Adjusted according to body surface area	All species (if parasites are still sensitive to proguanil)

*Not available in the United States.

ful. Monitoring of central venous pressure, vital signs, and blood pressure must be done frequently during exchange transfusion.

Bacterial Infections

Gram-negative septicemia, aspiration pneumonia, and urinary tract infections may complicate cerebral malaria and should be treated with appropriate antibiotics. Any patient who develops shock at any stage should be investigated, because nearly 40% of such patients have positive blood cultures.

Coagulopathy

Using sensitive measures, activation of the coagulation cascade can be detected in all patients with acute symptomatic malaria, but significant disseminated intravascular coagulation occurs in less than 5% of patients with severe disease. Replacement therapy (not heparin) is essential, and in the tropics fresh blood is preferable.

PROGNOSIS

Factors indicating a poor prognosis in severe falciparum malaria include deep coma, repeated convulsions with signs of decerebration, high parasitemia (>5% in nonimmunes), peripheral schizontemia, clinical jaundice or serum enzyme concentrations elevated more than threefold, uremia (creatinine more than 3.0 mg% and blood urea nitrogen more than 60 mg% after rehydration), metabolic acidosis (elevated plasma and/or cerebrospinal fluid lactate, or arterial blood gas pH <7.2), leukocytosis (>15,000/μl), retinal hemorrhages, and hypoglycemia (clinical hypoglycemia or blood glucose <40 mg%).

PREVENTION AND CONTROL

Although a global control program for malaria was started in 1957 with the support of the World Health Organization, the eradication of malaria has not been achieved because of many obstacles, such as resistance of parasites to drugs, resistance of mosquitoes to insecticides, and extremely intensive malaria transmission in some parts of the world. Therefore a revised strategy of malaria control was introduced in 1969.

There is no good chemoprophylaxis for malaria at present. Guidelines for the prevention of malaria must take into account the risk of exposure to malaria, including chloroquine-resistant *P. falciparum*, the efficacy and safety of drugs, the effectiveness of personal protective measures, and the availability of adequate medical care for treatment of malaria infections. Preventive measures are warranted in nonimmune visitors (short-term or long-term), children, pregnant women, soldiers, and residents in malaria-endemic areas. The choice of chemoprophylaxis might not be the same in all cases, and it may not be easy to make decisions. Drugs generally used in the prophylaxis of malaria are shown in Table 8, and they should be taken 1 or 2 weeks before a person travels to endemic areas, while staying there, and continued for 6 weeks after the person leaves an endemic area. The use of personal protective measures is also very important. These include general precautions to reduce mosquito bites, covering exposed skin in the evenings, the use of insect repellents, and the use of an efficient, impregnated mosquito net.

BACTERIAL MENINGITIS

method of
H. WALTER PFISTER, M.D.
Ludwig-Maximilians-Universität
Munich, Germany

and

MARTIN G. TÄUBER, M.D.
University of California, San Francisco
San Francisco, California

CLINICAL ASPECTS

Bacterial meningitis is clinically characterized by stiff neck, headache, fever, photophobia, malaise, vomiting, alteration of consciousness, seizures, confusion, irritability, and, rarely, acute psychosis. Cerebrospinal fluid (CSF) usually reveals an elevated white blood cell count of more than 1000 white blood cells per μL, consisting of more than 60% polymorphonuclear leukocytes, an elevated total protein content, and a decreased CSF/serum glucose ratio. A CSF white blood cell count of less than 1000 cells/μL may be found early in the disease, in partially treated bacterial meningitis, in overwhelming bacterial meningeal

TABLE 1. **Common Pathogens of Bacterial Meningitis, According to Age of Patient, and Empirical Antimicrobial Therapy**

Age	Typical Microorganisms	Recommended Antibiotic Regimen
<1 month	Gram-negative Enterobacteriaceae (*Escherichia coli, Klebsiella, Enterobacter, Proteus, Pseudomonas aeruginosa*) Streptococci, in particular group B streptococci *Listeria monocytogenes*	Cefotaxime (Claforan) plus ampicillin
1 month–6 years	*Haemophilus influenzae** *N. meningitidis* *S. pneumoniae*, streptococci	Third-generation cephalosporin
>6 years	*N. meningitidis* *S. pneumoniae* Streptococci, *H. influenzae, Listeria*, staphylococci, gram-negative Enterobacteriaceae (incl. *Pseudomonas aeruginosa*)	Third-generation cephalosporin plus ampicillin

*Incidence has declined since the introduction of *H. influenzae* type b vaccine.

infection ("apurulent bacterial meningitis"), and in immunosuppressed and leukopenic patients. The spectrum of meningeal microorganisms causing bacterial meningitis is strongly influenced by the age of the patient, predisposing factors, and underlying diseases (Tables 1 and 2).

The incidence of bacterial meningitis is estimated at 5 to 10 cases per 100,000 persons per year. There are approximately 25,000 cases of bacterial meningitis annually in the United States. Due to the introduction of *Haemophilus influenzae* type b conjugate vaccines, the incidence of *H. influenzae* disease among children age younger than 5 years has declined in the United States from 41 cases per 100,000 in 1987 to 2 cases per 100,000 in 1993. Bacterial meningitis is much more common in developing countries and in specific geographic areas, such as the meningitis belt of Africa, where there is an estimated incidence of 70 cases per 100,000 persons per year.

With the introduction of antimicrobial agents into clinical practice, mortality rates of bacterial meningitis were markedly reduced. Mortality rates of meningitis due to *H.*

TABLE 2. **Bacterial Microorganisms and Predisposing Factors of Bacterial Meningitis**

Sinusitis, mastoiditis, otitis media	*Str. pneumoniae, N. meningitidis, H. influenzae*
Traumatic head injury, dural fistula	*Str. pneumoniae, S. aureus, H. influenzae*, gram-negative Enterobacteriaceae
Nosocomial meningitis (e.g., after neurosurgical procedure)	Gram-negative Enterobacteriaceae, *Pseudomonas aeruginosa*, staphylococci
Ventriculitis due to external ventricular drainage, shunt infection	*S. epidermidis, S. aureus*, gram-negative Enterobacteriaceae
Pneumonia	*Str. pneumoniae*, streptococci, *H. influenzae*
Endocarditis	*S. aureus, Str. pneumoniae*
Recurrent meningitis	*Str. pneumoniae, H. influenzae*
Petechial rash	*N. meningitidis, Str. pneumoniae*
Immunosuppression	*Listeria monocytogenes*, gram-negative Enterobacteriaceae
Splenectomy, alcoholism	*Str. pneumoniae, Listeria*
Intravenous drug abuse	Staphylococci, *Pseudomonas aeruginosa, Candida*

influenzae type b are less than 7%, and those of meningitis due to *Neisseria meningitidis* are 6 to 14%. With the advent of third-generation cephalosporins, the mortality of gram-negative bacillary meningitis has decreased from 40 to 80% to 10 to 20%. However, despite further progress in antimicrobial therapy and improvements in intensive care medicine, the mortality rate of meningitis due to *Streptococcus pneumoniae*, the organism most often responsible for bacterial meningitis in adults, has remained relatively unchanged during the last few decades and is still unacceptably high (approximately 20%). Neurologic and neuropsychologic sequelae resulting from bacterial meningitis are found overall in 10 to 30% of patients. Cerebral and systemic complications arising during the acute phase of the disease are responsible for both the mortality and the long-term sequelae caused by bacterial meningitis. The major acute complications involving the central nervous system include cerebrovascular insults, brain edema, and hydrocephalus. Cerebrovascular involvement, both of arteries (arteriitis, vasospasm) and veins (septic sinus venous thrombosis), may lead to infarction with severe irreversible cerebral damage and an increase of intracranial pressure due to cytotoxic edema. In addition to edema, increased intracranial blood volume due to disturbed cerebrovascular autoregulation or to septic venous sinus thrombosis may lead to life-threatening elevation of intracranial pressure with the risk of herniation. There is a risk of cortical necrosis when cerebral perfusion pressure (defined as the difference between systemic mean arterial blood pressure and intracranial pressure) decreases as a result of increased intracranial pressure and systemic hypotension. Interstitial edema may occur due to transependymal movement of CSF from the ventricular system into the surrounding brain parenchyma as a consequence of obstructive hydrocephalus. Systemic complications of bacterial meningitis include sepsis, including septic shock, disseminated intravascular coagulation, adult respiratory distress syndrome, and inappropriate secretion of antidiuretic hormone.

PATHOPHYSIOLOGY

Experiments in animal models and cell culture systems have substantially improved our understanding of the complex pathophysiologic mechanisms of bacterial meningitis. Once bacteria have entered the subarachnoid space, subcapsular bacterial surface components (e.g., cell wall components of gram-positive pathogens and lipopolysaccharide of gram-negative pathogens) induce the local production of several inflammatory mediators within the CSF, including platelet-activating factor and certain cytokines, e.g., interleukin-1 and tumor necrosis factor. The action of these cytokines may lead to an increased expression of adhesion molecules on both the endothelium and neutrophils. These processes result in an enhanced adhesion of leukocytes to the cerebral endothelium and finally in transmigration of leukocytes into the subarachnoid space. Leukocytes in the subarachnoid space are thought to be more harmful than beneficial; they are ineffective in the eradication of the infection within the subarachnoid space. Phagocytosis of encapsulated microorganisms, the major defense function of leukocytes, is inefficient in the cerebrospinal fluid due to low concentrations of anticapsular antibodies and complement. Some potentially toxic mediators such as oxygen free radicals, nitric oxide, peroxynitrite, and excitatory amino acids seem to be involved in alterations of the permeability of the blood-brain barrier and neuronal injury. As the disease progresses, loss of cerebrovascular autoregulation and a reduction of cerebral blood flow occur with the risk of secondary cerebral brain damage.

TREATMENT

General Management of a Patient with Bacterial Meningitis

In patients with severe, life-threatening meningitis, the most important aspect of management is the immediate institution of empiric antibiotic therapy (see later for selection of antibiotics). The authors recommend that patients suspected of having bacterial meningitis, who present with a rapidly progressive course (1 to 2 days of symptoms) and severe alteration of mental status/coma, receive an initial antibiotic dose immediately after a single blood culture, prior to any other diagnostic procedures. In this patient population, the authors also advocate the use of dexamethasone as adjunctive therapy, to be initiated at the same time as antibiotics (see later discussion for details). In less acutely ill patients with clinical signs and symptoms suggesting acute bacterial meningitis, and in the acutely ill patient after initiation of therapy, a lumbar puncture should be performed immediately after the initial clinical examination. In patients who are unconscious and have focal neurologic deficits, a CT scan should be performed prior to lumbar puncture. Contraindications to lumbar puncture are clinical signs of cerebral herniation (e.g., unconsciousness, a unilaterally dilated and unreactive pupil, decerebrate movements) or a focal mass lesion (e.g., large, space-occupying brain abscess) on CT. If there are CT findings indicating brain edema and raised intracranial pressure, hyperosmolar agents (e.g., 250 mL 20% mannitol) may be infused intravenously just before the lumbar puncture. However, there is no scientific proof of the efficacy of this type of management in this situation. If a CT scan cannot be performed immediately and a lumbar puncture is deemed dangerous, empirical antibiotic therapy should be initiated after blood cultures have been sent. CT scanning and CSF exami-

nation should be performed afterwards as soon as possible. The presence of a parameningeal infectious focus such as sinusitis or mastoiditis should also be investigated by CT, including the bone window technique. In addition, clinical examination by an otolaryngologist should be performed. If a parameningeal focus (e.g., otitis, mastoiditis, sinusitis) is identified as a possible origin of bacterial meningitis, drainage is required as soon as possible. In contrast, surgical correction of CSF dural leaks (e.g., in patients with previous head trauma) is usually performed when the meningeal infection is treated, typically after 10 to 14 days, rather than during the very acute stage of meningitis. If the patient's clinical condition does not improve despite antibiotic therapy, the possibility of complications of bacterial meningitis should be investigated (e.g., repeated CT or MRI scanning) and additional sources of infection sought (e.g., endocarditis). Importantly, the sensitivity of the causative pathogen against the antibiotic regimen administered must be confirmed by in vitro testing, and antibiotic coverage must be adjusted to the sensitivity results. If the causative organism has not been isolated, broadening of the antibiotic coverage should be considered in patients who fail to respond to the initial therapy.

Initial Empirical Antibiotic Therapy

If antibiotic therapy has to be started without microbiologic confirmation, empirical therapy is initiated under consideration of the patient's age, predisposing factors, underlying diseases, and the most probable meningeal pathogens (Tables 1 and 2). Repeat lumbar punctures should be performed within 24 hours, if the patient fails to respond promptly to antibiotic therapy.

The most common bacterial microorganisms in **neonates** with bacterial meningitis are enteric gram-negative bacilli, group B streptococci, and *Listeria monocytogenes* (Table 1). Therefore, a third-generation cephalosporin (e.g., cefotaxime [Claforan]) plus ampicillin is recommended as empirical therapy in this age group. Alternatively, some authors recommend ampicillin combined with an aminoglycoside. As third-generation cephalosporins are inactive against *L. monocytogenes,* antibiotic therapy with a third-generation cephalosporin alone should not be used in this age group.

In **infants and children** (over 2 months of age), initial empirical antibiotic therapy usually includes the administration of one of the third-generation cephalosporins, which have been shown in clinical controlled studies to be equally effective as ampicillin plus chloramphenicol. In addition, resistance of *H. influenzae* to ampicillin is an emerging problem, resistant isolates reaching a rate of 25% in most countries. Moreover, resistance of pneumococci to ampicillin is also increasing.

The initial antibiotic treatment of healthy, immunocompetent **adults** for community-acquired bacterial meningitis, most often caused by *S. pneumoniae* or *N. meningitidis*, consists of the administration of a third-generation cephalosporin (most commonly cefotaxime [Claforan] or ceftriaxone [Rocephin]). In patients with risk factors for *Listeria* meningitis (immunosuppression, alcoholism, corticosteroids, pregnancy), a combination of a third-generation cephalosporin and ampicillin is recommended, the latter being added to cover *L. monocytogenes*. CSF isolates of *S. pneumoniae* or *N. meningitidis* should be tested for penicillin G and cephalosporin susceptibility. Penicillin G should not be given as monotherapy until it is confirmed that the CSF isolates of *S. pneumoniae* or *N. meningitidis* are sensitive to penicillin G. In recent years, an increasing number of penicillin-resistant strains of *S. pneumoniae* have been reported from several countries around the world, particularly in Spain, Hungary, Australia, New Guinea, South Africa, and some areas of the United States. Furthermore, penicillin-resistant strains of *N. meningitidis* are also emerging in some regions of the world (e.g., Spain, South Africa). For penicillin-resistant meningococci or relatively penicillin-resistant pneumococci, a third-generation cephalosporin is recommended. Highly resistant pneumococci typically also have reduced sensitivity or resistance to third-generation cephalosporins, and in areas where these highly resistant organisms are commonly isolated, the addition of vancomycin (Vancocin) or rifampin (Rifadin) needs to be considered, until the organism and its antibiotic susceptibilities are known (Table 3).

Empirical antibiotic therapy of a patient with bacterial meningitis after a recent head trauma or a neurosurgical procedure should include a third-generation cephalosporin combined with an antistaphylococcal antibiotic (e.g., nafcillin, flucloxacillin,* vancomycin, or fosfomycin*) plus an aminoglycoside. Ventriculitis associated with an external intraventricular drainage device or a ventriculoperitoneal shunt should be treated with antibiotics that cover *Staphylococcus epidermidis*, *S. aureus*, and enteric gram-negative bacilli. In this clinical setting, a combination of a third-generation cephalosporin plus vancomycin (plus an aminoglycoside) is often recommended. In ventriculoperitoneal shunt infections caused by enteric gram-negative bacilli susceptible to aminoglycosides, gentamicin may be given intraventricularly in addition to intravenous administration. Intraventricular vancomycin is used in some centers for catheter-associated ventriculitis caused by staphylococci. A combination of a third-generation cephalosporin plus ampicillin is usually recommended for immunocompromised adults to cover *Listeria monocytogenes*, *Streptococcus pneumoniae*, and gram-negative Enterobacteriaceae.

Specific Antibiotic Therapy

Once the infecting pathogen has been identified and sensitivity tests performed, antibiotic coverage should be adjusted to provide highly active but narrow coverage against the microorganism causing meningitis (Table 4). High systemic doses of all anti-

---

*Not available in the United States.

TABLE 3. **Recommended Antibiotics for the Treatment of Bacterial Meningitis**

Causative Organism	Drug of Choice	Alternatives
N. meningitidis	Penicillin G	Third-generation cephalosporin,[1] ampicillin, chloramphenicol
S. pneumoniae		
Penicillin-susceptible	Penicillin G	Third-generation cephalosporin,[1] chloramphenicol, vancomycin
Intermediate sensitivity (MIC 0.1–1 µg/ mL)	Third-generation cephalosporin[1]	Vancomycin
Penicillin-resistant (MIC > 1 µg/mL)	Ceftriaxone (Rocephin) + vancomycin (Vancocin) or rifampin (Rifadin)	Vancomycin + third-generation cephalosporin,[1] high-dose cefotaxime[6]
H. influenzae	Third-generation cephalosporin[1]	Ampicillin plus chloramphenicol
Streptococci (group B)	Ampicillin plus gentamicin	Third-generation cephalosporin,[1] vancomycin
Gram-negative Enterobacteriaceae (e.g., *Klebsiella*, *E. coli*, *Proteus*)	Third-generation cephalosporin[1] plus aminoglycoside[2, 3]	Extended-spectrum penicillin[4] plus aminoglycoside[2, 3]
Pseudomonas aeruginosa	Ceftazidime plus aminoglycoside[2, 3]	Piperacillin (Pipracil) plus aminoglycoside[2, 3]
Staphylococci (methicillin-susceptible)	Nafcillin (Unipen) or flucloxacillin[5]	Fosfomycin[5] or vancomycin
Staphylococci (methicillin-resistant)	Vancomycin	Trimethoprim-sulfamethoxazole (Bactrim, Septra) (if susceptible)
Listeria monocytogenes	Ampicillin (plus aminoglycoside[2])	Trimethoprim-sulfamethoxazole
Bacteroides fragilis	Metronidazole (Flagyl)	Chloramphenicol

[1]Cefotaxime, ceftriaxone, or ceftizoxime.
[2]Gentamicin or tobramycin (Nebcin).
[3]Confirmation of activity by in vitro tests necessary.
[4]Piperacillin or mezlocillin (Mezlin).
[5]Not available in the U.S.
[6]20–24 gm per day.

TABLE 4. **Recommended Dosing Regimens of Selected Antimicrobial Agents for the Treatment of Bacterial Meningitis**

Antimicrobial Agent (Trade Name)	Individual Doses and Schedule by Age Group[a]					
	≤7 days[b]		8–30 days[b]		Children >1 month[b]	Adults
	≤2 kg[c]	>2 kg[c]	≤2 kg[c]	>2 kg[c]		
Aminoglycoside						
Gentamicin[d] (Garamycin)	2.5 mg[c] q 12 h	2.5 mg[c] q 12 h	2.5 mg q 8 h	2.5 mg q 8 h	2.5 mg q 8 h	1.5–2 mg[e] q 8 h
Tobramycin[d] (Nebcin)	2 mg q 12 h	2 mg q 12 h	2 mg q 8 h	2 mg q 8 h	2–2.5 mg q 8 h	1.5–2 mg[e] q 8 h
Penicillins						
Penicillin G	50,000 U q 12 h	50,000 U q 8 h	50,000 U q 8 h	50,000 U q 6 h	50,000 U q 4 h	4,000,000 U q 4 h
Ampicillin	50 mg q 12 h	50 mg q 8 h	50 mg q 8 h	50 mg q 6 h	50 mg q 4 h	2 mg q 4 h
AS penicillins						
Nafcillin (Unipen)	50 mg q 12 h	50 mg q 8 h	50 mg q 8 h	50 mg q 6 h	50 mg q 6 h	1.5–2 gm q 4 h
Flucloxacillin[g]	50 mg q 12 h	50 mg q 8 h	50 mg q 8 h	50 mg q 6 h	50 mg q 6 h	1.5–2 gm q 4 h
E-S penicillins						
Piperacillin (Pipracil)	—	—	—	—	50–75 mg q 4 h	3–4 gm q 4 h
Cephalosporin 3						
Cefotaxime (Claforan)	50 mg q 12 h	50 mg q 12 h	50 mg q 8 h	50 mg q 6–8 h	50 mg q 6 h	2 gm q 4–6 h
Ceftriaxone (Rocephin)	—	—	—	—	40–50 mg q 12 h	2–4 gm q 24 h
Ceftizoxime (Cefizox)	50 mg q 12 h	50 mg q 12 h	50 mg q 8 h	50 mg q 8 h	50 mg q 6 h	3 gm q 6–8 h
Rifampin (Rifadin)	—	—	—	—	10–20 mg q 24 h	600 mg q 24 h
TMP/SMX (Bactrim)	—	—	—	—	5 mg[f] q 6 h	5 mg[f] q 6 h
Vancomycin[d] (Vancocin)	10 mg q 12 h	10 mg q 12 h	10 mg q 8 h	10 mg q 8 h	10–15 mg q 6 h	500 mg q 6 h

Abbreviations: AS = antistaphylococcal; E-S = extended-spectrum; cephalosporin 3 = third-generation cephalosporins; TMP/SMX = trimethoprim-sulfamethoxazole.

[a] All doses given intravenously, based on normal renal and hepatic function.
[b] All pediatric doses are per kg body weight. Total daily dose should not exceed maximum daily dose for adults.
[c] Birthweight.
[d] Monitoring of serum concentrations is recommended and may require change in dosing.
[e] Doses are per kg body weight.
[f] Doses are per kg body weight based on trimethoprim component.
[g] Not available in the United States.

Modified from Townsend GC, Scheld WM: Bacterial meningitis. *In* Rakel RE (ed): Conn's Current Therapy 1995. Philadelphia, WB Saunders Co, 1995, pp 98–103.

biotics used for the treatment of meningitis are needed in order to provide adequate CSF concentrations, since the blood-brain barrier limits access of antibiotic to the site of infection, and other factors, such as the acidic environment in the inflamed CSF and the slow rate of bacterial growth, may also reduce antibiotic efficacy. Experimental and clinical studies have suggested that the best therapeutic response is achieved with CSF-antibiotic concentrations that exceed by 10- to 20-fold the in vitro minimal bactericidal concentration for a particular organism.

Duration of Antibiotic Treatment

Treatment of bacterial meningitis due to *Streptococcus pneumoniae, N. meningitidis, H. influenzae,* and group B streptococci usually consists of intravenous administration of antibiotics for 10 to 14 days. However, some clinical observations have suggested that shorter courses of 7, 5, or even 4 days may be adequate for meningococcal meningitis. For antibiotic treatment of meningitis due to *L. monocytogenes* and gram-negative Enterobacteriaceae, a treatment duration of 3 to 4 weeks may be required.

Adjunctive Therapy

Dexamethasone has shown beneficial effects in animal models of bacterial meningitis. It inhibits the synthesis or release of inflammatory mediators involved in the pathophysiologic processes of bacterial meningitis. In prospective, placebo-controlled clinical studies in children with bacterial meningitis (most suffering from *H. influenzae* type b meningitis), intravenous dexamethasone given for 4 days reduced the incidence of bilateral hearing loss and neurologic sequelae. Furthermore, another study in children with bacterial meningitis showed that 2 days of dexamethasone treatment was as effective as a 4-day dexamethasone regimen. The beneficial effect of dexamethasone in pneumococcal meningitis was suggested when (1) in a retrospective data analysis of children with pneumococcal meningitis, neurologic sequelae were less frequently detected in children treated with dexamethasone plus antibiotics than in those treated with antibiotics alone; and (2) in an open, randomized Egyptian study, dexamethasone reduced mortality of pneumococcal meningitis in adults. Based on the available clinical and experimental data, the use of dexamethasone in *H. influenzae* meningitis in children (0.15 mg per kg body weight intravenously every 6 hours for 2 to 4 days) and in pneumococcal meningitis in children and adults (8 to 10 mg intravenously every 8 hours for 2 to 4 days) seems to be justified. The American Academy of Pediatrics recommends consideration of dexamethasone therapy in infants and children 2 months of age and older with proven or suspected bacterial meningitis. It may be most beneficial to administer the first dexamethasone dose several minutes before the first antibiotic dose in order to achieve maximal inhibition of the inflammatory cascade, which is initiated by antibiotic-induced bacteriolysis and the release of cell wall components. In the authors' practice, they administer dexamethasone immediately before intravenous antibiotic therapy to all adult patients with suspected, severe bacterial meningitis, but do not use it routinely, if patients are only mildly ill without altered mental status or neurologic deficits.

In animal models of penicillin- and cephalosporin-resistant pneumococcal meningitis, the penetration of both ceftriaxone and vancomycin into the CSF was reduced with dexamethasone therapy, resulting in a delay in CSF sterilization. When rifampin was used with ceftriaxone, bacteriologic cure occurred promptly, irrespective of therapy with dexamethasone or not. Thus, it was recommended that in areas with high rates of resistant pneumococcal strains, initial empirical therapy should include two antibiotics, ceftriaxone and either rifampin or vancomycin. When dexamethasone is used in this situation, ceftriaxone combined with rifampin is preferred.

Experimental or clinical data have not proven the efficacy of dexamethasone in meningococcal meningitis. Corticosteroids are not recommended for the therapy of meningitis following infective endocarditis, or in newborns with bacterial meningitis.

Increased intracranial pressure may be managed by *elevation of the head* of the bed to 30 degrees, *hyperventilation* to maintain a Pco_2 concentration between 25 and 30 torr, and the intravenous *administration of hyperosmolar agents* (e.g., 20% mannitol). Stuporous or comatose patients may benefit from intracranial pressure monitoring to control this therapy. If meningitis-associated hydrocephalus is diagnosed by computed tomography, CT scan follow-up investigations or ventricular drainage should be performed, depending on the patient's level of consciousness and the degree of ventricular dilatation on CT. Angiographic studies in patients with bacterial meningitis and focal neurologic deficits may reveal vasospasm of the large arteries at the base of the brain resembling vasospasm following subarachnoid hemorrhage. In these patients, *hypervolemic therapy* or *nimodipine* (Nimotop) (e.g., 1 to 2 mg per hour intravenously in adults) therapy should be considered; however, these therapeutic approaches have not been investigated systematically in clinical trials. *Anticoagulation* of septic venous sinus thrombosis in bacterial meningitis is controversial. There are no prospective controlled clinical studies, but anticoagulation with dose-adjusted intravenous heparin should be considered in patients with meningitis-associated septic venous sinus thrombosis proven by MRI or cerebral angiography. *Anticonvulsants* are given to treat seizures, e.g., rapid intravenous phenytoin administration (e.g., 20 mg per kg, no faster than 50 mg per minute in adults). Sterile subdural effusion usually resolves spontaneously and does not require surgical therapy. CT-guided stereotactic aspiration is recommended initially for cases of subdural empyema, but open surgical procedures may be necessary.

Experimental Approaches. Several therapeutic agents, which may limit meningeal inflammation, have shown beneficial effects in animal models of bacterial meningitis (in particular, the rat and the rabbit). Aside from dexamethasone, these anti-inflammatory agents include nonsteroidal anti-inflammatory drugs (e.g., indomethacin),* pentoxifylline (Trental),* antagonists of leukocyte-endothelial cell adhesion molecules, monoclonal antibodies against cytokines, platelet-activating factor receptor antagonists, free radical scavengers, and nitric oxide synthase inhibitors. Aside from dexamethasone, these agents have not yet been investigated in humans with bacterial meningitis, but some show promising beneficial effects in experimental models. Further experimental studies are needed to clarify whether some of these approaches may be applied to clinical practice.

---

*Not FDA-approved for this indication.

INFECTIOUS MONONUCLEOSIS

method of
MITCHELL GOLDMAN, M.D.
Indiana University School of Medicine
Indianapolis, Indiana

Infectious mononucleosis is a common clinical syndrome resulting from symptomatic infection with Epstein-Barr virus (EBV). The illness is most often diagnosed in late adolescence and early adulthood. The clinical manifestations of infectious mononucleosis include the triad of sore throat, fever, and lymphadenopathy, although other frequently described symptoms include malaise, headache, anorexia, myalgias, chills, and nausea. In addition to lymphadenopathy, pharyngitis, and fever, physical examination may reveal splenomegaly, hepatomegaly, palatal petechiae, jaundice, and/or rash. The diagnosis can usually be made on clinical grounds and confirmed by the laboratory findings of atypical lymphocytosis and a positive heterophil test. Infection is transmitted through intimate contact between those shedding the virus in the oropharynx and susceptible individuals. The incubation period is approximately 4 to 6 weeks.

DIAGNOSIS

The most frequent presenting complaint is a sore throat, which may be severe. Cervical lymphadenopathy is present in 80 to 90%, and splenomegaly may be detected in about half of patients during the illness. Fever is experienced by over 90% of patients and in most cases resolves over 10 to 14 days. Rash develops in about 5% of patients not treated with antimicrobials and in 90 to 100% of those treated with ampicillin.

Laboratory tests reveal a positive heterophil test in 90% of cases, although young children less often have a positive test. Atypical lymphocytosis is seen in about 70% of individuals at presentation, and thrombocytopenia may be seen in half of patients. Elevations in hepatocellular enzymes and lactic dehydrogenase are common. For patients with syndromes compatible with EBV-induced infectious mononucleosis and a negative heterophil antibody test, a determination of EBV antibodies may help to establish the diagnosis. It is important to note that heterophil-negative mononucleosis may also be caused by several other agents, including cytomegalovirus; hepatitis A, B, and C; acute HIV infection; *Toxoplasma gondii*; mumps; rubella; and human herpesvirus 6 (HHV-6).

Most patients with infectious mononucleosis have a self-limited illness and recover uneventfully in 2 to 3 weeks. Complications include autoimmune hemolytic anemia, thromboctyopenia, and neutropenia, which are usually mild although may rarely be severe and life-threatening. Splenic rupture, although rare, should be suspected if abdominal pain occurs or if shock and falling hematocrit are seen. Neurologic complications occur in less than 1% of cases and include encephalitis, aseptic meningitis, Guillain-Barré syndrome, seizures, transverse myelitis, as well as other conditions. Pericarditis and myocarditis have also been described.

Death is rare and may occur from either overwhelming EBV infections or due to complications of the disease. In otherwise healthy individuals, neurologic complications, splenic rupture and upper airway obstruction are the most frequent fatal complications of infectious mononucleosis. Overwhelming and fatal infections are best described for those with the Duncan X-linked recessive immunodeficiency syndrome, although such infections may also be seen in those without known immunodeficiency.

TREATMENT

Spontaneous recovery without specific therapy over 2 to 3 weeks is the rule for the majority of patients with infectious mononucleosis. There are no data showing that the use of high-dose acyclovir (Zovirax), vidarabine* (adenine arabinoside), or interferon-alpha† is of sufficient clinical benefit to recommend their use for treatment of uncomplicated EBV-related infectious mononucleosis. Likewise, there are insufficient data supporting the use of antivirals for the treatment for complications of the illness. As there is no effective antiviral therapy at present, treatment is largely supportive. Acetaminophen, 650 to 1000 mg every 4 to 6 hours (maximum, 4 grams per 24 hours), can be used for relief of fever, sore throat, myalgias, and arthralgias. For most, the level of activity should be tailored to what an individual can comfortably tolerate. Because of concern for splenic rupture, contact sports or other excessive physical activity such as heavy lifting should be avoided during the first 2 to 3 weeks of the illness, particularly in those with splenomegaly. For similar reasons, constipation, if present, should be treated with a gentle laxative.

The use of corticosteroids in uncomplicated cases is generally not encouraged. Corticosteroids are recommended for the treatment of impending airway obstruction from tonsillar enlargement. For life-threatening airway obstruction, intravenous methylprednisolone (Solu-Medrol), 60 mg every 6 hours, should be used initially with rapid taper over 1 to 2 weeks. In severe cases, tracheotomy may be required. For those with severe thrombocytopenia and hemolytic anemia, treatment with an equivalent dose of corticosteroids to prednisone at an initial dose of 60 to 80 mg per day in divided doses followed by a taper over 1 to 2 weeks is considered appropriate. Corticosteroids have been used for the treatment of severe CNS involvement, myocarditis, and pericarditis, although such treatment cannot be routinely recommended because data are lacking. For those with the rare complication of splenic rupture, splenectomy is recommended. Early plasmapheresis is indicated for patients who suffer from the Guillain-Barré syndrome.

PREVENTION

EBV infection is ubiquitous, with 90 to 95% of populations studied having demonstrable antibodies by adulthood. As is the case with other herpesviruses, infection with EBV persists for life. EBV has been cultured from the oropharyngeal washing of patients for up to 18 months after clinical recovery. The virus can be isolated from 10 to 20% of normal healthy adults and an even greater number of patients who are immunocompromised. As only 6% of those with infectious mononucleosis have a history of contact with a known case of the illness, most are infected through contact with asymptomatic individuals. The majority of cases are believed to occur as a result of intimate contact with spread of virus through saliva. Sexual transmission may be possible, as there is evidence that the cervix can be a source of viral shedding. The oral secretions of an individual with acute illness should be considered infectious. However, because the spread of EBV requires intimate contact, isolation of patients with infectious mononucleosis is not necessary. As EBV may be

---

*Not available in the United States.

†Not FDA-approved for this indication.

spread by transfusion, blood donations should be postponed for at least 6 months after onset of illness. At present, there remains no effective vaccine, although work in this area is ongoing.

CHRONIC FATIGUE SYNDROME

method of
NELSON M. GANTZ, M.D.
Pennsylvania State University College of
*   Medicine*
Hershey, Pennsylvania

Fatigue is a common complaint in patients seeking primary care and accounts for about 20% of office visits. In most cases, the fatigue is of limited duration and resolves. In some patients, fatigue can be chronic and debilitating. Fatigue is the hallmark of the chronic fatigue syndrome (CFS). Interest in CFS occurred in the mid 1980s when reports erroneously linked Epstein-Barr virus to chronic fatigue. The disorder was formally defined in 1988 by a group of investigators convened by the Centers for Disease Control and Prevention. A revised case definition was published in 1994 and is listed in Table 1.

The diagnosis of CFS is based on the patient's history and on excluding other illnesses. In evaluating a patient with suspected CFS, a mental status examination is essential in addition to a detailed history and physical examination. Any abnormalities noted on the mental status examination require a psychiatric, psychologic, or neurologic consultation. Screening laboratory tests to exclude other disorders should include a complete blood count, erythrocyte sedimentation rate, alanine aminotransferase, total protein, albumin, globulin, alkaline phosphatase, glucose, electrolytes, creatinine, thyroid-stimulating hormone, and urinalysis. Other tests should be obtained based on epidemiologic clues from the history and physical examination to exclude other diagnoses.

Patients are classified as having idiopathic chronic fatigue if fewer than four of the symptoms listed in Table 1 are present. Certain chronic disorders that could cause chronic fatigue exclude a diagnosis of CFS. Examples of exclusionary illnesses include untreated hypothyroidism, sleep apnea, chronic active hepatitis, major depression with psychotic features, schizophrenia, dementia, bipolar affective disorder, anorexia nervosa, bulimia, recent substance abuse, and severe obesity. Certain disorders do not exclude a diagnosis of CFS, such as anxiety, nonpsychotic depression, or adequately treated thyroid or Lyme disease. Fibromyalgia, a disorder that is similar to CFS, should be included under the framework of fatiguing illnesses. Patients may be labeled as having CFS by one doctor and fibromyalgia by a rheumatologist since the features of both of these conditions overlap.

In evaluating a patient with suspected CFS, it is important to note that there is no laboratory test to establish the diagnosis. Serologic tests for viruses and fungi, as well as measurements of immunologic function, are not indicated. Similarly, imaging studies of the head using magnetic resonance imaging or positron emission tomography are of no value in diagnosis. In one report, patients with CFS were noted to have neurally mediated hypotension as shown by having an abnormal tilt test. In an uncontrolled study, symptoms of some of the patients improved with therapy of the hypotension using fludrocortisone with or without a beta blocker such as atenolol. Patients with neurally mediated hypotension should not restrict their sodium intake. Further studies are needed to define the importance of hypotension as a cause of fatigue in patients with CFS.

MANAGEMENT OF THE PATIENT WITH CFS

Table 2 lists an approach to be used in managing a patient with CFS. CFS is a chronic illness in which the course waxes and wanes. The objectives of therapy are to help the patient develop realistic goals and expectations through education, to provide symptomatic relief, and to preserve and improve the patient's ability to function. At the outset, it is very important to acknowledge the sense of illness and debility expressed by these patients. Although expressions such as "Nothing is wrong" may be intended to provide reassurance, they can lead the patient to believe that the physician does not believe the patient feels ill. Patient support groups can play

---

TABLE 1. **Definition of Chronic Fatigue Syndrome**

Classify as chronic fatigue syndrome (CFS) if both of the following criteria are met:

Unexplained persistent or relapsing fatigue of new or definite onset that is not due to ongoing exertion, is not relieved by rest, and results in a substantial reduction in previous levels of activity

Four or more of the following symptoms are concurrently present for 6 months or longer:

(1) Impaired memory or concentration that impairs everyday activities
(2) Sore throat
(3) Tender cervical or axillary lymph nodes
(4) Muscle pain
(5) Multijoint pain
(6) New headaches lasting more than 24 hours
(7) Unrefreshing sleep
(8) Postexertion malaise

From Fukuda K, et al: Ann Intern Med *121*:953–959, 1994.

TABLE 2. **Steps in Managing the Patient with Chronic Fatigue Syndrome**

Establish the diagnosis
Symptomatic treatment
   Medications for depression, anxiety, pain, sleep, allergies
   Avoid exotic untested remedies
   Cognitive behavior therapy
Provide reassurance and emotional support
   Acceptance of symptoms
   Avoid confrontational approach
   Referral to support groups and counseling
Lifestyle management
   Apply stress reduction techniques
   Restructure activities
   Make realistic goals
Prevent further disability
   Graded exercise program
   Physical therapy
Regular follow-up
Continue to R/O other medical problems

a key role in helping both the patient and family cope with a frustrating chronic illness. Since the etiology of CFS is unknown, no specific therapy is available. The key to managing a patient with CFS is using symptomatic therapy for depression, anxiety, pain, sleep disorder, and allergic symptoms.

Nonpharmacologic Therapies

CFS patients often avoid activity out of fear of exacerbating their symptoms. Complete bed rest should be avoided because of the problems associated with physical deconditioning. Moderate levels of exercise and rest, dictated by common sense, are essential, and physical activity should be gradually increased as tolerated.

Cognitive behavior therapy attempts to alter attitudes, perceptions, and beliefs that can contribute to maladaptive behavior. Cognitive behavior therapy combined with a graded exercise program may be beneficial in improving functioning. In some patients with fibromyalgia, physical therapy may be helpful for morning stiffness and muscle pain.

Antiviral Medications

Acyclovir* (Zovirax) has been well studied and is no better than placebo in treating patients with CFS. Amantadine* (Symmetrel) has been reported to decrease fatigue in patients with multiple sclerosis but only anecdotal information is available regarding its use in CFS patients.

Immunologically Active Drugs

In two well-controlled studies, intravenous immunoglobulin* (Gamimune N) has been given monthly to patients with CFS with conflicting results. At present, this modality of therapy cannot be recommended. Similarly, data do not support the use of transfer factor, interferon alpha,* or high-dose corticosteroids.

Antidepressant Drugs

Depression is common in CFS, and antidepressants are a mainstay in the treatment. If the decision is made to try an antidepressant agent, anecdotal reports suggest that lower doses than are usually prescribed may be effective. Dosing can be increased gradually if the effect with the initial dosage is inadequate. The drug selected should be tried for 4 to 6 weeks before therapeutic failure is considered.

The choice of antidepressant depends, to a great extent, on expected side effects. Although large controlled studies are lacking, tricyclics and serotonin reuptake inhibitors appear to be beneficial. Tricyclic antidepressants are associated with sedative and anticholinergic effects. Anecdotally, patients who have difficulty sleeping sometimes respond well to agents such as amitriptyline HCl* (Elavil) or doxepin HCl* (Adapin) taken once a day at bedtime. In a study of patients who had fibromyalgia, amitriptyline in doses of 25 mg at bedtime, rather than the usual doses of 100 to 150 mg, resulted in less fatigue, improved sleep, and decreased myalgias when compared with placebo. Responses were usually seen in 3 to 4 weeks. Desipramine HCl* (Norpramin), 100 to 200 mg per day, is a less sedating tricyclic drug.

When sedation is not desirable, serotonin reuptake inhibitors, such as fluoxetine HCl* (Prozac), 20 to 40 mg per day; paroxetine HCl* (Paxil), 20 mg per day; or sertraline HCl* (Zoloft), 50 to 150 mg per day, can be helpful. Serotonin reuptake inhibitor agents are usually given in a single dose in the morning or in divided doses in the morning and at noon.

Bupropion HCl* (Wellbutrin), 200 to 300 mg per day, may be effective in patients who are unable to tolerate a tricyclic agent or serotonin reuptake inhibitor. Venlafaxine* (Effexor), 75 to 225 mg per day, is chemically related to bupropion. This new drug inhibits norepinephrine and serotonin reuptake. Adverse effects are similar to those of other serotonin reuptake inhibitors, but dose-related hypertension has also been reported with venlafaxine.

Anxiolytic Agents

Panic disorders and anxiety are common in patients with chronic fatigue syndrome. Although there have been no controlled studies specifically in this patient group, a regimen of alprazolam plus ibuprofen is effective in reducing pain and anxiety in patients with fibromyalgia. Anecdotally, clonazepam* (Klonopin), other benzodiazepines, and buspirone HCl* (BuSpar) also appear beneficial, but controlled studies are lacking. Alprazolam* (Xanax) may be particularly helpful in managing panic attacks.

Analgesics

Headache is treated with analgesics. Acetaminophen, aspirin, and other nonsteroidal anti-inflammatory drugs are often used to treat myalgias and arthralgias associated with chronic fatigue syndrome. In one study of patients with fibromyalgia, a regimen of naproxen sodium (Naprosyn), 500 mg bid, plus amitriptyline, 25 mg at bedtime, was effective in decreasing muscle aches. Response is seen as early as 1 to 2 weeks after starting therapy. The muscle relaxant cyclobenzaprine HCl* (Flexeril), in dosages of 10 to 20 mg at bedtime, results in decreased pain and improved sleep in patients with fibromyalgia.

Sleep Medications

Difficulties in falling and staying asleep, as well as awakening unrefreshed from sleep, are very common in chronic fatigue syndrome. Low doses of amitriptyline,* 25 to 50 mg, or cyclobenzaprine,* 10 to 20 mg,

---

*Not FDA-approved for this indication.

taken at bedtime may be beneficial. Other agents that have been reported anecdotally to help are trazodone HCl* (Desyrel), 25 to 50 mg; doxepin,* 10 to 50 mg; and clonazepam,* 0.5 to 1.0 mg, at bedtime. Zolpidem (Ambien), 5 to 10 mg at bedtime, is a nonbenzodiazepine hypnotic that may be tried for short-term use.

Drugs for Allergies

New allergies or exacerbations of old allergies are commonly reported by patients with chronic fatigue syndrome. Food elimination diets, royal jelly, various herbs, and dietary supplements have not been shown to be helpful in alleviating symptoms. Nonsedating antihistamines, such as astemizole (Hismanal), loratadine (Claritin), or terfenadine (Seldane), can be tried.

SUMMARY

CFS is a chronic waxing and waning illness whose etiology and pathogenesis remain uncertain. There are no specific therapies for CFS. Treatment is symptomatic and supportive. The temptation to try unproved and exotic remedies is strong since anecdotal reports appear promising. However, most of these agents are ineffective and some are potentially harmful and costly. Antidepressants appear particularly beneficial for treating symptoms of CFS. Important nonpharmacologic interventions include the setting of realistic goals, stress reduction, lifestyle modifications, maintaining and increasing activity levels, physical therapy, encouraging participation in counseling and support groups, and using cognitive behavior therapy.

---

*Not FDA-approved for this indication.

MUMPS

method of
BASIM I. ASMAR, M.D.
Wayne State University School of Medicine
Detroit, Michigan

Mumps is an acute, generalized infection caused by a paramyxovirus and characterized by painful enlargement of the parotid glands. Infection is spread by direct contact via the respiratory route. The virus can be demonstrated in the respiratory tract 2 days prior to and up to 7 days following the onset of parotid swelling. Disease incidence is highest during winter and early spring and lowest during summer. Infection occurs throughout childhood, with peak incidence between ages 10 and 14 years. The incidence rates for mumps have declined substantially since the introduction of the vaccine in 1967. However, during 1986 and 1987 outbreaks occurred among susceptible adolescents and young adults in U.S. high schools and colleges, reflecting the underimmunization of individuals born between 1967 and 1977. The incidence peaked in 1987 to

12,848 cases reported to the Centers for Disease Control. Subsequently the incidence gradually decreased among all age groups during 1988–1993 and reached fewer than 2000 reported cases per year in 1993 as a result of improved immunization rates and the initiation of the two-dose vaccination for measles using the mumps-measles-rubella (MMR) vaccine.

CLINICAL MANIFESTATIONS

The incubation period of mumps is 14 to 24 days. The onset of the disease is characterized by pain and swelling in one or both parotid glands. The swollen parotid and the surrounding soft tissue edema push the ear lobe upward and outward. The orifice of Stensen's duct may be red and swollen. Eating or drinking acid food may elicit discomfort. Moderate fever is frequently present and lasts 3 to 4 days, but systemic toxicity is usually absent. Swelling of the submandibular glands may occur along with or in the absence of parotid swelling. Older patients with mumps may complain of headache, caused by involvement of the meninges. Parotid swelling lasts 7 to 10 days. The patient is considered noninfectious 1 week after the onset of parotid swelling.

Complications

Viremia early in the course of infection and the predilection of mumps virus for glandular and nervous tissues account for the widespread complications.

Orchitis is the most feared complication and occurs in about 30% of postpubertal males who develop mumps. Bilateral involvement occurs in one third of these patients. Orchitis usually follows parotitis and causes severe testicular pain, swelling, and tenderness. Atrophy of the testes may follow and result in impairment of fertility; however, absolute sterility is rare because testicular involvement is usually unilateral.

Oophoritis may occasionally occur in females, causing pelvic pain and tenderness, but it does not lead to impairment of fertility.

Meningoencephalitis is the most common complication of mumps in childhood. Neurologic involvement may occur 1 week prior to or 3 weeks following the onset of parotitis. Aseptic meningitis occurs in up to 50% of cases and is usually manifested by mild headache or asymptomatic mononuclear pleocytosis. Mumps virus can be isolated from the cerebrospinal fluid early in the illness. Encephalitic symptoms are rare. Complete recovery in 3 to 10 days is the rule.

Deafness occurs in about 4% of patients with mumps and is usually unilateral; however, bilateral involvement may occur. The hearing loss may be transient or permanent. Development of meningitis does not appear to be related to hearing impairment.

Pancreatitis may manifest as epigastric pain, at times associated with vomiting. Severe pancreatitis is rare. Elevated serum amylase is usually present with or without clinical manifestations of pancreatitis because of involvement of other salivary glands.

Other rare complications of mumps include nephritis, thyroiditis, myocarditis, mastitis, arthritis, transverse myelitis, and thrombocytopenic purpura.

DIAGNOSIS

Diagnosis of mumps parotitis is usually made on the basis of symptoms and physical examination. Elevation of serum amylase is common. Diagnosis can be confirmed by isolating the virus from saliva, blood, or cerebrospinal fluid, or by demonstrating a fourfold rise in mumps antibodies by fluorescent testing or increase in the enzyme-linked immunosorbent assay (ELISA) antibody value during convalescence.

DIFFERENTIAL DIAGNOSIS

Several other viruses, including cytomegalovirus, coxsackievirus A, Epstein-Barr virus, influenza, parainfluenza 1 and 3, and HIV, can cause parotitis. Suppurative parotitis is associated with exquisite tenderness and elevated leukocyte count, and pus can be expressed from the duct. Recurrent parotitis due to salivary calculi or of unknown etiology can result in intermittent gland swelling. Preauricular lymphadenitis and submandibular lymphadenitis can be differentiated from parotitis by their location anterior to the parotid and below the ramus of the mandible, respectively. Parotid tumors and leukemia can also result in parotid enlargement.

THERAPY

Treatment is supportive as mumps is a self-limited disease. Attention should be paid to hydration and nutrition. Analgesics may be needed to relieve discomfort from parotitis or headache. Orchitis may necessitate stronger analgesics. Administration of antiviral agents or gamma globulin is inappropriate. Mumps immune globulin is no longer available.

PREVENTION

Live attenuated mumps virus vaccine is routinely given to children as a combined vaccine containing measles and rubella vaccines (MMR) after the first birthday, usually at 15 months of age. Mumps vaccine induces immunity in more than 95% of recipients and its protective efficacy is long-lasting. It is well tolerated, and adverse reactions attributed to the vaccine are extremely rare and may include rashes, pruritus, and purpura. A second dose of MMR is recommended in late childhood or early adolescence. Mumps revaccination is important because mumps can occur in highly vaccinated populations; a number of cases have occurred in persons with a history of mumps vaccination. Pregnant women and persons with suppressed immunity should not be given the vaccine. However, the vaccine is safe in HIV-infected children who are to be immunized with MMR.

OTITIS EXTERNA

method of
DAVID S. PARSONS, M.D., and
R. NEIL VAN LEEUWEN, M.D.
University of Missouri–Columbia
School of Medicine
Columbia, Missouri

Otitis externa (OE) is a common ailment with up to 10% of the population being affected during their lifetime. During peak season, a typical otolaryngology practice may see several such patients each day. A basic understanding of the external ear canal and the pathophysiology of the disease aids in the treatment and prevention of further episodes of OE. Three types of otitis externa and their treatment will be considered: (1) diffuse otitis externa caused by bacteria, which represents 90% of the infections; (2) fungal otitis externa, or otomycosis, which in some studies represents 9% of otitis externa; and (3) a rare progression to osteomyelitis, which is commonly known as malignant otitis externa.

The external ear canal directs sound to the tympanic membrane and protects the middle ear from injury. The lateral third of the canal is composed of cartilage, with a thin layer of subcutaneous tissue between the cartilage and skin. This portion of the canal contains the glands responsible for the production of cerumen. The medial two thirds of the canal is bony and is covered by a thin layer of skin with almost no subcutaneous tissue. Sloughed skin and cerumen produce an acidic environment. The skin, cerumen, and acidic environment act as barriers to protect the ear from bacterial, fungal, and insect invasion. Any breakdown of this barrier invites local or diffuse bacterial invasion.

Several factors are known to predispose an individual to OE. These include underlying skin conditions such as eczema, humid climate, frequent swimming or ear washing, and localized trauma most often secondary to repeated insertion of a Q-Tip into the ear. Otitis externa begins as localized edema of the canal skin, usually from heat and humidity. This causes a local blockage of the sebaceous glands, with a sensation of fullness and itching in the ear. The natural response to the itching is to scratch, which can lead to injury of the epithelium and open the way for localized pathogen invasion.

Diffuse bacterial OE can present in any age group but is more common in the middle-aged population. The presenting symptoms of otitis externa nearly always include pain and itching. There are also a number of other complaints, including otorrhea, fullness, tinnitus, and hearing loss. On physical examination, findings can range from a very limited erythema or localized pustule to remarkable erythema, canal wall edema which can occlude the canal, or clear to purulent otorrhea. Pain can usually be elicited by palpation of the tragus or manipulation of the pinna. Visualization of the ear canal and tympanic membrane is important to look for granulation tissue, discrete lesions that need biopsy for diagnosis, or tympanic membrane perforations to suggest that middle ear disease might be the predisposing factor for OE. Techniques to examine the tender ear are offered later. The usual pathogens include a predominance of *Pseudomonas* species as well as staphylococci, coliforms, *Proteus* species, and anaerobes.

When the disease is severe, patients often will not allow an examination of the external canal. Four to eight drops of topical 4% lidocaine can be placed into the canal. After several minutes an otowick (Merocel

Sponge Pope Ear Wick) is gently inserted and moistened with additional lidocaine. After 10 to 15 minutes, upon removal of the wick, the ear can either be examined or suctioned or an injectable lidocaine block can be placed to ease the discomfort from the disease or the examination.

The cornerstone of otolaryngologic treatment is aural toilet, sometimes done two to three times weekly if warranted, and topical antibiotics. Treatment includes mopping of debris with a Jobson Horne probe and cotton. In an office equipped with a microscope, suction under direct visualization is the best choice to clean debris. The application of combination topical antibacterial-steroid drops or astringents is important to resolve the OE. When the edema is severe, a wick or antibacterial impregnated gauze must be inserted into the canal to assure adequate penetration of topical medication. This is usually removed in 2 to 3 days. Patients should also be given adequate analgesia, which in severe cases may include narcotics. See Table 1 for expanded treatment regimens.

If treated properly, OE usually resolves in a week. If it is not significantly improved in 1 week, other etiologies must be looked for and debris should be cultured. In addition, topical antibiotic drops containing neomycin may cause a painful localized reaction. If such a reaction occurs, the drops should be switched to a non-neomycin containing antibiotic ear or eye drop.

After OE has resolved, prevention is of utmost importance. Because moisture in the ear canal is a key factor in developing OE, the goal of prevention is to maintain a dry ear canal. Water precautions should be taught, including the use of ear plugs while swimming, showering, and shampooing. Patients should never use Silly Putty to plug their ear. Additionally, patients can be maintained on an acid-alcohol drop (5% boric acid saturated in a solution of 95% alcohol) to dry and clean the ear canal and prevent moisture damage. Hearing aids need to be removed at night to allow drying of the canal.

Etiologies of OE refractory to treatment include progression to malignant otitis externa, underlying immune deficiency, or otomycosis. Otomycosis is found more often in tropical climates. Patients will present with complaints of itching, a foreign body sensation in the ear, discharge, or tinnitus. On physical examination, edema is usually not as pronounced as in diffuse bacterial OE. The most common gross appearance is described as that of a "wet newspaper" and represents mycelium in the ear canal. The most common organisms are *Candida* and *Aspergillus*. If improvement of routine OE is not made after 1 week,

TABLE 1. **Treatment of Otitis Externa**

Clinical Features	Most Likely Organism	Treatment
Diffuse Otitis Externa		
Middle age	*Pseudomonas* sp.	Aural toilet
Severe pain	*Staphylococcus* sp.	TOPICAL
Pruritus	Coliforms	Polymyxin B, neomycin, polysorbate 80, hydrocortisone drops (Cortisporin Otic susp.): 4 drops 3–4 times a day
Fullness	*Proteus* sp.	
Erythema	Anaerobes	
Gross edema		Tobramycin, dexamethasone (TobraDex), 4 drops 3–4 times a day
Debris in canal		
		SYSTEMIC
		Ciprofloxacin (Cipro), 500 mg orally twice a day
Otomycosis		
Tropical climates	*Candida*	TOPICAL
Pruritus	*Aspergillus*	Acid alcohol (5% boric acid saturated in a solution of 95% isopropyl alcohol), 5 drops 4 times daily
Foreign body sensation		
Mild edema		Acetic acid, aluminum acetate (Domeboro), 5 drops 4 times a day
"Wet newspaper" appearance		
		Acetic acid (VōSol), with hydrocortisone (VōSol HC), 5 drops 4 times daily
		Nystatin, triamcinolone ointment (Mycolog II): apply to canal once daily
		SYSTEMIC
		Ketoconazole (Nizoral), 200 mg orally daily
		Fluconazole (Diflucan), 200 mg orally first day, then 100 mg daily
Malignant Otitis Externa		
Elderly diabetic	*Pseudomonas aeruginosa*	TOPICAL
Severe pain, worse at night		Same topical treatment as for Diffuse Otitis Externa
Otorrhea		SYSTEMIC
Granulation tissue		Ciprofloxacin (Cipro), 750 mg orally twice daily OR Aztreonam, 1–2 gram IV every 8–12 hours plus clindamycin (Cleocin), 600 mg IV every 8 hours

then daily application of topical antifungal ointment such as nystatin-triamcinolone (Mycolog-II) should be considered. Debris should be sent for fungal culture. In severe cases, systemic antifungal agents may be necessary.

The most serious form of OE is an osteomyelitis of the temporal bone, described by Chandler as "malignant otitis externa" (MEO). In the past, even with antibiotic treatment, the mortality rate has been reported to be as high as 50%. With the advent of fluoroquinolones, especially ciprofloxacin (Cipro), mortality is rare, therefore, diagnosis and institution of therapy are imperative to recovery. Elderly male diabetics comprise more than 80% of cases. Underlying immunocompromise is the second most common etiology for MEO. Pain, worse at night, and otorrhea are the most common complaints. On physical examination, the hallmark sign is granulation tissue at the bony/cartilaginous junction, which must be biopsied to rule out other granulomatous diseases as well as malignancy. In more advanced cases, cranial nerves may be involved, the most common being CN VII. Diagnosis is confirmed by a technetium 99 scan. The most likely pathogen, in greater than 95% of cases, is *Pseudomonas aeruginosa*.

Treatment of MEO in the past included intravenous synthetic penicillins and aminoglycosides. Surgical débridement was also needed to remove necrotic bone. There was still significant morbidity and mortality using this therapy. The treatment of choice is now fluoroquinolone therapy, most often ciprofloxacin, given either intravenously in the acutely ill or noncompliant patient, or orally on an outpatient basis. Surgery is generally limited to the removal of the granulation tissue. The patient is followed every 6 weeks with a gallium scan. Treatment is continued until the gallium scan is negative. Cure rates have been as high as 96% with ciprofloxacin therapy alone.

PLAGUE

method of
LARRY CROOK, M.D.
Gallup Indian Medical Center
Gallup, New Mexico

Plague is an acute febrile illness caused by a gram-negative bacillus, *Yersinia pestis*. Plague occurs throughout the world, and is enzootic in the small mammal populations, especially squirrels and prairie dogs, in the southwestern United States. Almost all the human cases in the United States have occurred in the western half of the country, with the majority occurring in New Mexico, Arizona, Colorado, or California. Humans are an accidental host in this disease of animals, and human transmission is not a normal part of the natural history of this disease. Human plague is most commonly contracted from the bite of an infected flea, which is also the main method of ani-

mal-to-animal transmission. After a flea feeds on an animal with plague, the bacteria multiply and eventually obstruct the foregut of the flea and are then regurgitated into the open bite wound when the flea attempts to take another blood meal. Direct contamination of open wounds can also occur by handling infected animals or materials, as can direct inhalation of infected droplets from a patient with pneumonic plague. Primary pneumonic plague from human-to-human transmission occurs during epidemics and is the most feared feature of an outbreak of plague. However, in the United States the only primary human pneumonic plague in recent years has occurred in patients exposed to domestic cats with pneumonic plague. Person-to-person spread has not occurred in the United States in over 50 years.

Usually a patient with plague develops an extremely tender, swollen, firm, nonfluctuant lymph node in the region draining the site of the flea bite. The skin overlying the node is usually erythematous, shiny, and edematous. The swollen node, or group of nodes, is called a bubo, and this form of plague is bubonic plague. In a minority of cases a patient will present with an acute febrile illness without a bubo. This form of plague is septicemic plague; it has a much higher fatality rate than bubonic plague, probably related to the atypical presentation that leads physicians away from considering plague in the differential diagnosis, and away from including an antibiotic effective against plague in the initial treatment. Septicemic plague may present with signs and symptoms of a gastrointestinal infection, with nausea, vomiting, diarrhea, and abdominal pain. Other presentations of septicemic plague include signs and symptoms of a urinary tract infection, an upper respiratory tract infection, appendicitis, or a nonspecific viral syndrome. Routine blood cultures are positive in septicemic plague; however, they are positive in most cases of bubonic plague also, and this does not distinguish septicemic from bubonic plague. Both bubonic and septicemic plague can spread by hematogenous dissemination to other organs. Hematogenous spread to the lungs causes secondary pneumonic plague. Patients with pneumonic plague generally have bilateral interstitial infiltrates on radiography and gram-negative rods in their sputum. Hematogenous spread can also cause meningitis, arthritis, ophthalmitis, or infection in almost any other organ. Gram-negative sepsis, septic shock, disseminated intravascular coagulation, adult respiratory distress syndrome, and multiple organ dysfunction have all been associated with plague.

DIAGNOSIS

The physician must maintain a high index of suspicion. Plague can present in patients of any age and frequently occurs in children. In the United States, plague is more common in the summer months. A history of living or traveling in the western half of the United States, especially the southwest, or in other areas of the world where plague is present, is important. Most exposures occur in rural settings, and the presence of dogs or cats at home, or rodents in proximity to the home, increases the risk. A history of a flea bite is seldom obtained.

The incubation period is 2 to 8 days, and the patient usually presents with an acute febrile illness. If a bubo is present, a milliliter of sterile saline should be injected into it and immediately aspirated back into the syringe. This fluid can then be stained by Gram's stain and cultured by routine methods. If necessary, a small amount of lidocaine can be injected into the bubo before the aspiration is per-

---

Disclaimer: The opinions expressed in this article are those of the author and not necessarily those of the Indian Health Service.

formed. Routine blood cultures should also be obtained. The finding of gram-negative bacilli or coccobacilli in a Gram stain of the bubo aspirate increases the probability of plague, but therapy should never be delayed or withheld because of a negative stain. Other appropriate body fluids should likewise be stained and cultured. *Yersinia pestis* has a distinctive "safety pin" appearance when stained with Giemsa, Wayson, or Wright's stain. A specific fluorescent antibody stain is available at reference laboratories. Antibody titers in acute and convalescent serum can also be measured at reference laboratories and are sometimes useful retrospectively. Complete blood counts, routine chemistries, coagulation tests, and arterial blood gases should be obtained. However, the results of these tests are nonspecific and consistent with any gram-negative systemic bacterial infection.

TREATMENT

Survival in plague is directly related to the interval between the onset of symptoms and the onset of a course of appropriate antibiotics. Untreated bubonic plague has a mortality rate of about 40%, untreated pneumonic plague a mortality rate of 100%. However, with appropriate treatment the mortality is less than 10%. Streptomycin is the drug of choice. The usual dose is 15 mg per kg intramuscularly every 12 hours. Chloramphenicol intravenously is the drug of choice for plague meningitis, arthritis, and patients in shock. The dose is 15 mg per kg intravenously every 6 hours. Tetracycline is effective orally and can be given to complete a 10-day course of therapy after an initial good response to parenteral streptomycin or chloramphenicol. The usual dose of tetracycline is 500 mg every 6 hours orally. Gentamicin, doxycycline, and trimethoprim-sulfamethoxazole* (Septra, Bactrim) all appear to be effective, but there is not enough clinical experience with these drugs to recommend them as primary treatment. Disk sensitivities are not reliable in choosing drugs for plague; however, in *Y. pestis* no clinically significant resistance to streptomycin, tetracycline, or chloramphenicol, has been reported. It is important to note that none of the penicillins or cephalosporins have been proved to be effective treatment for plague in humans.

PREVENTION

Patients with plague should be placed in contact isolation, and in strict respiratory isolation if there is any suspicion of pneumonic plague. Family and close contacts of a patient with plague should be identified and followed closely for 8 days. Any such person who develops a fever should be treated for plague as described earlier. Preventive therapy is recommended only for individuals with face-to-face, (within 6 feet) exposure to a case of pneumonic plague. These individuals should receive tetracycline orally for 5 days; children under 12, pregnant women, and others who cannot take tetracycline should be given oral trimethoprim-sulfamethoxazole*

for 5 days. Hospital staff are generally not given preventive therapy. A vaccine is available for people who anticipate exposure, especially in an area of the world where medical care is not readily available.

All cases of plague should be reported to the local public health authorities. The Centers for Disease Control plague center in Fort Collins, Colorado, is also available for help in suspected or proved cases of plague (970-221-6450).

Treatment for plague is highly successful, and virtually all deaths are related to delays in receiving appropriate therapy. The major challenge is to consider the diagnosis and then to treat with appropriate drugs as soon as possible.

PSITTACOSIS

method of
DENNIS E. DURIEX, M.D.
Lubbock, Texas

Psittacosis is a systemic infection of humans caused by *Chlamydia psittaci*. The resultant disease has a very wide spectrum, ranging from a mild, flu-like illness to a severe and often fatal course (if untreated). A typhoidal form of the disease can occur that involves a general febrile state without the respiratory component.

The infection is usually associated with bird exposure (usually to parrots and parakeets, but also turkeys, ducks, and pigeons), through inhalation of dried bird excreta. Persons who work with birds—pet shop employees, zoo workers, veterinarians, and pigeon enthusiasts—are theoretically at risk.

Human disease can also occur after exposure to cows, goats, and sheep. The infection has been implicated as a cause of abortions in sheep and humans. Human-to-human transmission has been reported and is associated with a more severe infection than avian-acquired disease. This occurrence is rare, and isolation of hospitalized cases is not necessary.

C. psittaci is common in birds and domestic animals. A 5% to 8% carriage rate has been found in populations studied. It is likely that all species of birds can be affected. Infected birds can be asymptomatic or be obviously sick, with shivering, anorexia, emaciation, diarrhea, and ruffled feathers. Strains associated with turkeys or psittacine birds seem to be the most virulent for humans.

CLINICAL FINDINGS

Psittacosis has an incubation period of 5 to 15 days. Its onset can be abrupt, with the sudden occurrence of high fever and chills, or more insidious. Symptoms are nonspecific and can resemble a viral syndrome or mononucleosis. Symptoms include severe headache, fever, and chills (>95% of cases), pharyngitis, myalgias (>90%), anorexia, hepatosplenomegaly, adenopathy, and rash. A nonproductive cough can be seen in 50% of cases. Pulse-temperature dissociation can occur. Chest x-ray findings are typically more impressive than physical findings.

Splenomegaly is frequent (70% of cases) and when found in a case of undiagnosed, community-acquired pneumonia, the possibility of psittacosis should be entertained. Cardiac complications include pericarditis, myocarditis, and cul-

---

*Not FDA-approved for this indication.

ture-negative endocarditis. Anemia, pancytopenia, hemolysis and disseminated intravascular coagulation can occur. Poly- and monoarticular as well as icteric hepatitis have been reported. Neurologic complications include cranial nerve palsies, transverse myelitis, and meningoencephalitis. Dermatologic features include Horder's spots, a blanching maculopapular rash that can be confused with the rose spots of typhoid fever.

DIAGNOSIS

The diagnosis is established via clinical acumen, recognizing the clinical features of the disease, and serologic confirmation. Demonstration of a fourfold rise in complement fixing antibodies is considered diagnostic. A single titer of 1:32 or greater is presumptive evidence of infection. Detection of *C. psittaci* using DNA hybridization or polymerase chain reaction (PCR) is also possible, and diagnostic. Isolation of the organism in cultures may be hazardous to laboratory personnel and requires specialized institutions.

TREATMENT

Tetracycline, 2 grams per day, is the treatment of choice. Doxycycline, 100 mg twice daily, is also effective. For allergic or pregnant patients, erythromycin is a reasonable alternative. Treatment should last 10 to 21 days. Clinical improvement is usually seen within 48 to 72 hours.

PREVENTION

Infected avian sources should be treated (tetracycline, chloramphenicol, doxycycline) for at least 45 days. Quarantine is also advisable. Cases of psittacosis should be reported to public health officials. With appropriate treatment, the prognosis is quite good, with a mortality rate of less than 1%.

Q FEVER

method of
DAVID W. STRYKER, M.D.
New Mexico Medical Group
Albuquerque, New Mexico

Q fever (the name is ascribed to either Query or Queensland) is caused by *Coxiella burnettii*. This member of the rickettsial family is a small, intracellular pleomorphic coccobacillus. The organism lives within phagolysosomes at low pH. There is a phase variation characterized by changes in the cell wall. Phase I cells are infectious, while serologic response is largely against phase II. The major mode of transmission is inhalation of dustborne spores. The spores are associated with products of parturition from domestic ungulates as well as other species including cats and rabbits. Spores are quite hardy, surviving for months to years in contaminated surfaces. Outbreaks of disease have been reported in abattoir and agricultural workers and with the birth of kittens. Laboratory outbreaks have occurred, and although isolation of the organism in cell culture is not difficult, it should be attempted only in specially equipped facilities.

Q fever is not a reportable disease, so incidence data are unavailable. In specific exposed populations, serologic positivity may be as high as 59%.

Coxiella burnettii infections in animals usually are asymptomatic, though they may be a cause of abortion in sheep and goats. In humans, the disease is usually mild or subclinical, infrequently requiring hospitalization. Symptomatic illness generally lasts 2 to 40 days (average: 11). Symptoms consist primarily of fever, rigors, malaise, headache, and myalgia. Cough is very common and may be productive with hemoptysis. Other respiratory symptoms include pleurisy and pharyngitis.

Examination usually reveals fever and inspiratory crackles. Neurologic signs, lymphadenopathy, hepatosplenomegaly, jaundice, and *Erythema nodosum* have all been reported. Routine laboratory values show a normal to slightly elevated white count and mildly elevated transaminases. Alkaline phosphatase and bilirubin are minimally elevated.

Although acute mortality is low (0.1 to 0.8%), chronic infection can occur. Q fever is a cause of endocarditis ("culture-negative"), chronic hepatitis, as well as infections of vascular aneurysms, cardiac and other prostheses, and osteomyelitis. Chronically infected patients may have murmur and signs of congestive heart failure. Embolic phenomoma may occur. Chronic infections generally occur in immnosuppresed patients or those with pre-existing endothelial lesions. Specific cellular immune response is lacking in chronic infections, though antibody titers to both phase I and phase II antigens are elevated.

DIAGNOSIS

Since symptoms of Q fever are nonspecific, diagnosis requires a high index of suspicion for patients who are in at risk groups or who have otherwise unexplained compatible illness. Facilities for culturing are not available in most hospitals, so serologic and pathologic methods are used. Testing for serologic response employs complement fixation (CF), immunofluorescent antibody (IFA), and enzyme-linked immunosorbent assay (ELISA). A fourfold increase in CF titers against phase II indicates recent infection. IFA is used to give more specific information about chronicity of disease, or when paired sera are not available. Elevated IgM suggests recent illness, and IgA, particularly that directed against Phase I antigen, suggests chronic disease such as endocarditis. A single IgA titer against phase I of greater than 1:200 is considered diagnostic of endocarditis, as is an elevated ratio of phase I to phase II antibodies. The newer ELISA tests may be more sensitive and can be used for large groups. Biopsy of lung, liver, or bone marrow may show classic "doughnut" granulomas.

THERAPY

Therapy of Q fever requires use of antibiotics that penetrate intracellularly into phagolysosomes. Doxycycline (Vibramycin), 100 mg orally twice daily for 15 to 21 days, is felt to be the standard for acute disease. Trimethoprim-sulfamethoxazole (TMP-SFX) (Bactrim, Septra), DS orally twice daily (sometimes in combination with rifampin (Rifadin), 600 mg once daily), erythromycin* (E-Mycin), 333 mg three times a day), and fluoroquinolones (ciprofloxacin [Cipro],* 500 to 750 mg twice daily, have all been reported to

---

*Not FDA-approved for this indication.

be effective. Chloramphenicol, 50 mg per kg per day, has been used in children and pregnant women. A short course of prednisone, 40 mg per day, may be useful for acute hepatitis.

Chronic infections are difficult to treat, requiring in some cases years of therapy. Combinations of doxycycline, a fluoroquinolone, and rifampin have been recommended. The antiphase I IgA titer should be followed until it is less than 1:200.

PREVENTION

Prevention depends on avoidance of exposure. Screening of potentially infected animals is useful, as is the prompt disposal of products of parturition. Various vaccine preparations have been developed but presently are felt to be too toxic for general use.

RABIES

method of
CATHLEEN A. HANLON, V.M.D., Ph.D.
Albany, New York

and

HILARY KOPROWSKI, M.D.
Philadelphia, Pennsylvania

Rabies is a much dreaded disease of antiquity. It is possible that the disease was already known to inhabitants of India in the 30th century before Christ, since the root of the word "rabies" is a Sanskrit word "rabhas," meaning to do violence. The first factual description of rabies may be found in the Eshuma (pre-Mosaic) Code in the 23rd century before Christ. The Greeks and Romans were apparently familiar with rabies, as was an Italian savant of the 16th century named Fracastoro, who wrote a detailed clinical description of rabies in humans. Despite its antiquity, with successful prevention dating back to Louis Pasteur's postexposure vaccination of Joseph Meister in 1885, there remains no effective cure for clinical rabies. Yet, when postexposure treatment is rendered according to guidelines and without delay, it is unfailingly effective.

In many developing countries, the presence of rabies in domestic dogs continues to be a significant risk to people. It is estimated that approximately 100,000 cases of human rabies may occur worldwide, although the actual magnitude is essentially unknown. Under-reporting of human cases, particularly in developing countries, is widely acknowledged, due to a number of factors relating primarily to a lack of basic resources. Most developed countries have successfully controlled canine rabies with a concomitant significant reduction in human exposures. Overt human mortality due to the disease is held in abeyance in these developed countries, but with significant economic and emotional ramifications from human exposures that still occur, principally from wildlife reservoirs, necessitating post-exposure treatment. Additional burdens related to rabies include appropriate animal management, such as (1) the 6-month quarantine or euthanasia of exposed, unvaccinated domestic animals; and (2) management of an animal (vaccinated or not) that bites a person through either eu-

thanasia and rabies testing, or a 10-day confinement and observation of dogs and cats for the development of clinical signs of rabies to rule in or out the necessity for human treatment. There is neither a reliable antemortem diagnostic test for rabies in animals, nor a definitive diagnostic antemortem technique for the determination of rabies exposure.

EPIDEMIOLOGY

All mammals are thought to be susceptible to rabies, but to varying degrees. Strains of rabies may now be differentiated with modern virologic techniques, such as monoclonal antibody (MAB) typing and the reverse transcriptase-polymerase chain reaction (RT-PCR) assay. This allows for a more precise identification of isolates in relation to principal mammalian hosts, which are responsible for the perpetuation of rabies in discrete geographic regions. All reservoirs belong to the mammalian orders Carnivora or Chiroptera (Table 1).

If rabies can be controlled in a reservoir species, it may be eliminated regionally. One of the first examples of control in a reservoir species was through mandatory dog vaccination and stray dog control, widely implemented in Canada and the United States in the early 1950s. This resulted in the elimination of canine rabies, with the exception of occasional incursions at the Texas–Mexico border. Similarly, the United Kingdom, Scandinavia, Japan, Malaysia, and a few other areas of the Americas have had a history of canine rabies but have achieved secondary eradication. Aggressive control measures, focused on both domestic animals and wildlife, have successfully eliminated rabies, and strict international importation/quarantine regulations have prevented its return. Some geographic regions, particularly islands, including Antarctica, Australia, New Zealand, Hawaii, and Pacific Oceania, have never had known indigenous rabies. Currently, a viral variant of red fox rabies has been largely eliminated over extensive geographic areas of Switzerland, Germany, Belgium, France, and contiguous European countries, as well as in Ontario, Canada, through oral vaccines offered in baits to free-ranging carnivores. In the United States, pilot studies targeting the raccoon and coyote are in progress.

TABLE 1. **Major Global Rabies Reservoirs**

Insectivorous Bats	**Domestic Dogs**
U.S., Canada, and Europe	Major vector of rabies throughout the world, particularly equatorial regions of Asia, Africa, and Latin America
Raccoons	
Southeastern, mid-Atlantic, and northeastern U.S.	
Skunks	**Vampire Bats**
Mid-western U.S. and western Canada	Northern Mexico to Argentina
Foxes	**Yellow Mongooses**
Central and western Europe, the Arctic, eastern Canada, northern New York, and other scattered foci in the U.S.	Asia and Africa
	Indian Mongooses
	Carribbean Islands
Coyotes, and Other Wild Canids	**Raccoon Dogs**
North America, Asia, and Africa	Eastern Europe and Scandinavia

Reprinted with permission from Scientific American SCIENCE & MEDICINE. Copyright © 1995 by Scientific American, Inc. All rights reserved.

Rabies in the United States is geographically widespread in bats and regionally apparent among raccoons, skunks, foxes, and coyotes (Figure 1). Currently, epizootic levels of rabies are occurring among raccoons in the northeastern states and coyotes in Texas. Although domestic dogs are still the most important worldwide reservoir of rabies, cats are now the most common rabid domestic animal in the United States. Rodents, lagomorphs (rabbits and hares), and the opossum (the only North American marsupial) are not important in rabies epizootiology; bites from these animals rarely present a risk of rabies to humans. Infrequently, large-bodied rodents, such as woodchucks (groundhogs), beavers, and domestic rabbits housed in outdoor hutches, have become naturally infected with rabies, and as such, present a risk of infection, should they bite or otherwise expose a human.

Infected animals are the ultimate sources of all known human rabies cases, with the exception of eight human-to-human transmission cases via corneal transplantation. From 1980 through 1995, there have been 30 cases of human rabies diagnosed in the United States; at least 10 cases were apparently acquired abroad in areas with enzootic canine rabies. There was no definite history of an animal bite in 20 of the 30 recent cases, raising the possibility that the event may have been unrecognized as an exposure. Among the 18 cases acquired in the United States since 1980, 15 have been due to rabies variants associated with bats. Further analysis of 13 cases revealed an association with a particular bat genera, as follows: nine with the silver-haired bat, *Lasionycterus noctivagans*; three with the Mexican free-tailed bat, *Tadarida braziliensis*; and one with the genus *Myotis,* or small brown bat. Not much is known about the virus associated with *L. noctivagans,* nor about the bat itself. It is a solitary, migratory species that prefers old growth forest. Encounters with humans are relatively rare, as evidenced by *L. noctivagans* comprising only 1.3% (15 of 1125) of all bats submitted for rabies testing in New York during 1995. While the numbers are small, the trend toward a disproportionate role in human mortality warrants vigilant monitoring.

A bite or possible bite was implicated in only two of the 15 bat-associated cases. A vague history of a bat encounter during a walk was the only significant event in one case. In three cases, the patients had a history (vague in one case) of handling one or more bats. In five cases, no history of animal exposure could be elicited retrospectively. In four recent cases, these was a history of a bat occurring in the house, and in two of these, in the bedroom of the patient, some weeks prior to disease onset, while people were sleeping. In none of these cases did this result in the consideration of the possibility of rabies nor initiate contact with health professionals for rabies testing of the bats. In both a Connecticut and New York case, the patients presented with symptoms initiating focally on an upper extremity, suggesting the possibility of a bite that was insufficient to fully arouse them from sleep. Current recommendations advise that treatment should be considered when rabies cannot be definitively ruled out by laboratory testing of the animal or when a bite or other physical contact with a bat cannot be ruled out.

MOLECULAR VIROLOGY

Rabies viruses are bullet-shaped, membrane-bound, single-stranded, negative-sense RNA viruses that belong to the Rhabdoviridae family, genus *Lyssavirus.* Advanced virologic techniques have demonstrated significant variation within the genus. Besides rabies virus, at least three other so-called rabies-related viruses (Mokola, Duvenhage, and European bat lyssavirus) are known to cause human disease that is clinically indistinguishable from true rabies; these viruses are found only in the Old World. Despite considerable antigenic variation among rabies viruses of major public health significance, there appears to be adequate cross-protection with current vaccines made from relatively homogenous, laboratory-maintained strains of rabies, originating from street isolates of rabies from several decades ago. This may not be true for other lyssaviruses.

Analysis of the molecular structure of the virus has revealed an inner nucleocapsid core of ribonucleoprotein and an outer surface glycoprotein. Glycoprotein is the antigenic determinant of the virus that is responsible for the induction of virus-neutralizing antibodies. In addition to glycoprotein, internal proteins of the virus play a role in the immunogenic response. The outer glycoprotein spikes are implicated in attachment and fusion to nerve cells through attachment to putative receptor molecules, such as gangliosides or the acetylcholine receptor.

PATHOGENESIS

A uniquely diabolical aspect of rabies virus infection is a directed effect upon host behavior that enhances transmis-

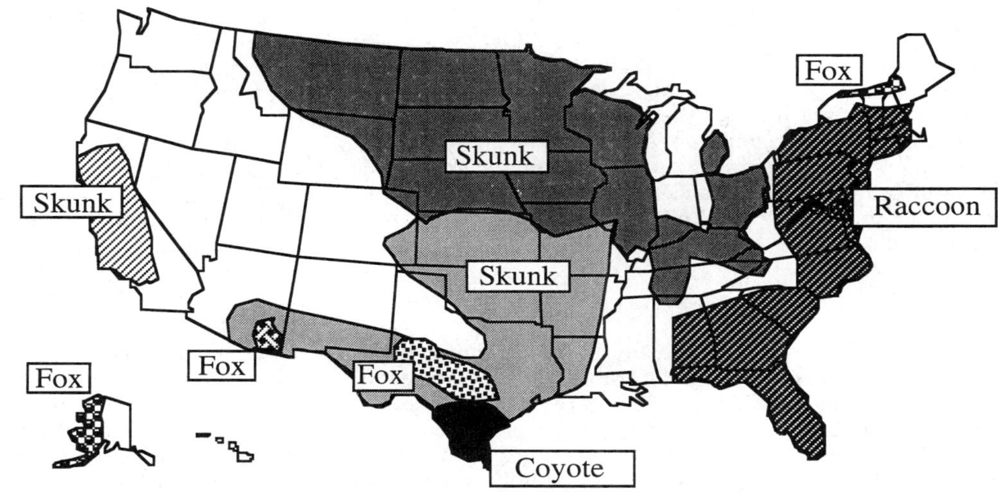

Figure 1. Major terrestrial rabies reservoirs in the United States. Terrestrial animal reservoirs only; multiple strains of rabies occur in bats and are geographically widespread throughout the U.S. (Adapted from Krebs et al. JAVMA, December 1995, pp 1562–1575.)

sion through the induction of unusually irritable and aggressive behavior, including biting. This is most commonly manifested in reservoir hosts to which virus strains have exquisitely adapted. Although maniacal and hallucinatory behavior may occur, biting is uncommon in humans infected with rabies. Virus is typically present in high amounts in saliva as the hosts' behavior reflects an increased propensity to bite, creating an opportunity for virtual inoculation into the next susceptible host. Extremely uncommon routes of human infection may also include contamination of mucous membranes, aerosols (laboratory accidents and bat cave aerosols), corneal transplants, and vaccine-induced cases through inoculation of improperly inactivated rabies vaccine. Environmental contamination of objects or the fur of pets with rabies virus from a rabid animal has not been implicated in transmission to humans.

Following inoculation, infection is virtually undetectable by even the most sophisticated techniques while the virus undergoes a so-called eclipse phase of several hours to days, during which some limited replication may occur locally in muscle cells at the site of entry. Due to the neurotropic nature of the virus, spread within the host does not include a viremic stage, perhaps evidence of an exquisite strategy to avoid host immune defenses. The incubation period is highly variable, ranging in humans from as short as 7 days to well over 1 year, with evidence in one case of over 6 years, although typically averaging several weeks to months. The incubating host is noninfectious until immediately prior to and during the clinical period.

Once within peripheral nerve fibers, virus infection proceeds centripetally via retrograde axoplasmic flow to dorsal root ganglia and into the spinal cord, sometimes manifesting as rapidly progressive, ascending paresis, paralysis, and ultimately with encephalitic signs, once the brain is infected. Ubiquitous infection of the brain parenchyma occurs rapidly, although there is a predilection for the limbic system, the reticular formation, the pontine tegmentum, and nuclei of cranial nerves.

Following infection of the brain, the virus moves to the peripheral nerves and centrifugally invades highly innervated areas, particularly the cornea, skin (especially of the head and neck), salivary glands, and buccal mucous membranes.

Microscopic lesions are nonspecific, although indicative of a viral encephalitis, with perivascular infiltration, neuronophagia, and gliosis. Careful examination may demonstrate spongiform encephalopathy, but inflammatory responses and necrosis may be minimal. Eosinophilic, intracytoplasmic inclusion bodies (Negri bodies) may be identifiable in nerve cells at this stage of infection and are pathognomonic of rabies. Despite profound encephalitic manifestations, there is a relative lack of structural neuronal damage, which raises the issue of functional interference with neurotransmission as one pathogenic mechanism. Moreover, recent investigations implicate higher levels of inducible nitric oxide synthase, which may contribute to increased levels of oxygen radicals leading to neuronal damage.

CLINICAL HUMAN RABIES

Human rabies is rare in the United States. However, at least five of the recent human rabies deaths were not suspected clinically. Rather, they were diagnosed retrospectively, on the basis of histologic findings suggestive of Negri bodies, which spurred further diagnostic investigation. The differential diagnosis of any rapidly progressive

viral encephalitis should include rabies, even in lieu of a history of an animal bite, due to the lengthy incubation period, and consequential poor recall of a possible exposure, particularly with a bat encounter that may have seemed innocuous at the time. The clinical course is acute, usually progressing from initial signs to the need for intensive support within 2 weeks, and death shortly thereafter.

Initial symptoms are often nonspecific, including sore throat, fever, headache, irritability, insomnia, anorexia, dysphagia, cough, nausea, vomiting, and diarrhea. More specific symptoms often include paresthesia, pain, and itching at the presumptive or known site of exposure. The most profound and characteristic clinical manifestations of human rabies are hydrophobia and aerophobia, which are exaggerated respiratory protective reflexes including severe pharyngeal spasms triggered by attempts to swallow, the sight or sound of water, or air currents. Other cranial nerve manifestations include choking, drooling, and diplopia. Along with aerophobia and hydrophobia, there may be central nervous system excitation with anxiety, confusion, hallucinations, disorientation, photophobia, ataxia, and seizures. These periods often present with interluding episodes of normalcy during which the patients may be self-reflective and apologetic for their abnormal behavior. Autonomic excitation may result in labile hypertension, hyperventilation, priapism, palpitations, and a loss of thermoregulatory ability.

A paralytic phase (dumb rabies) may follow the agitated phase, or the patient may progress directly from the prodromal stage to the paralytic phase. Ascending paralysis, either symmetrical or asymmetrical, and brain stem infection ultimately lead to respiratory arrest and the need for mechanical ventilatory support. Hypothalamic and hypophyseal dysfunction may contribute to wasting; rhabdomyolysis and cardiomyopathy have been described. Ultimately, rabies culminates in coma and generalized multi-organ failure that invariably leads to death.

LABORATORY DIAGNOSIS

The most sensitive and definitive diagnostic technique is the fluorescent antibody test for rabies virus antigen in infected tissue, especially fresh brain material. In lieu of a brain biopsy, a nuchal skin biopsy from the nape of the neck (including hair follicles) may test positive during the clinical course; a negative result does not rule out rabies. Saliva may be serially collected for virus isolation and RT-PCR analysis. Cerebrospinal fluid may be cultured for virus and evaluated for the presence of rabies virus neutralizing antibody (VNA) titers. Consecutive serum samples may be evaluated for rising rabies VNA titers in patients with no prior history of either pre- or post-exposure rabies immunization. Light touch impressions of the cornea (avoiding abrasion of the the corneal surface) and scrapings of the buchal mucosa may yield infected epithelium for evaluation with immunofluorescence, as well, although it requires a high level of technical expertise, as epithelium often has some nonspecific fluorescence. In a rapidly fulminating clinical course, all tests may remain negative until death, whereupon only one or more may be positive.

Fresh brain tissue is the optimal diagnostic material. A minimally invasive biopsy approach is through the medial canthus of the eye. Brain material that is formalin fixed may be evaluated histologically for the presence of Negri bodies, which, although not as sensitive as immunofluorescence, is still pathognomonic for rabies. With some additional preparatory steps, the fluorescent antibody test may also be applied to formalin-fixed tissue. Due to recent advances in RNA extraction techniques, rabies genome may often be extracted, amplified with RT-PCR, and genetically sequenced from formalin-fixed tissue, although fresh tissue is optimal, allowing retrospective identification of the animal source.

Routine clinical laboratory tests are nonspecific. Often performed to rule out other diagnoses, computer tomography and magnetic resonance imaging scans are largely unremarkable, and electroencephalographic changes are nonspecific.

CLINICAL MANAGEMENT

In the United States, the predominant responsibility of the clinician is to assess patients presenting for a potential animal source exposure to rabies, rather than management of clinical rabies per se. Clinical rabies remains incurable; extremely rare instances of survival, but with severe sequelae, have been documented, typically with a history of post-exposure with vaccine only. Nonetheless, it is prudent for clinicians to entertain rabies in the differential diagnosis of a rapidly progressive encephalitis, as five recent human rabies deaths in the United States were not suspected ante mortem, despite compatible clinical presentations. Universal precautions and early diagnosis will minimize potential exposure of health care workers and others. Treatment of a rabies-suspect patient is often empirical for other possible etiologies, including antivirals, such as for a herpes encephalitis, and appropriate antibiotics, such as for Lyme borreliosis or other bacterial causes. Specific treatment for rabies is simply supportive and palliative at best, often involving antiseizure medications, sedatives, analgesics, and neuroleptics.

Determination of the necessity for post-exposure treatment requires elicitation of the suspected animal source of exposure. If there is a history of travel and possible exposure abroad, consultation with health authorities familiar with global rabies epizootiology is warranted. If a possible exposure occurred in the community, familiarity with regional rabies epizootiology is essential. Often, local, state, and federal health authorities are trained to provide valuable expertise in these assessments.

If a wild animal has potentially exposed a person and is available for testing, the decision may be based upon test results. If there will be no undue delay in submission for testing, and the circumstances or species of animal suggest a low risk of rabies, treatment may be delayed until test results are available. A negative test result is definitive and reliable in ruling out the necessity for treatment. If the wild animal is a rabies vector species (bat, raccoon, skunk, fox, coyote) that has bitten someone, post-exposure treatment can be initiated immediately but may be discontinued if a negative test result is obtained. In the United States, bites from dogs and cats may be handled with the imposition of a 10-day confinement and observation period, or euthanasia and testing, unless the attack is severe and rabies

is strongly suspected by a veterinarian, whereupon post-exposure treatment should be instituted without a delay for pending test results.

One of the most important aspects of prevention is immediate flushing and cleansing of the animal bite or wound. Ideally, this should occur on site immediately after the encounter but should be instituted upon clinical presentation as well. This will reduce the viral amount that is able to penetrate intracellularly, either in muscle or nerve cells, and enhance success of post-exposure treatment. This is most critical with severe, multiple bites to the head and upper extremities. Management of wounds with surgical repair should be restricted to that which is absolutely essential, as it is theoretically possible to increase exposure through further tissue penetration in the suturing process.

Early intervention with post-exposure treatment consisting of human rabies immune globulin (HRIG) and multiple doses of rabies vaccine is extremely effective in preventing rabies in humans. Post-exposure treatment for rabies-naive patients consists of five vaccine doses of either 1.0 mL human diploid cell vaccine (HDCV; Imovax) or 1.0 mL rabies vaccine adsorbed (RVA), administered on day 0 (day of initiation of treatment; ideally the same as exposure), 3, 7, 14, and 28, and HRIG (Hyperab or Imogam) at 20 IU per kg, administered only once, on day 0. Exogenous HRIG is administered to rabies-naive patients to neutralize residual amounts of extracellular virus, which is why it is important to administer as much as is comfortably possible, up to 50% of the volume, locally around the site of the bite; the remainder should be administered in the gluteal muscle. Rabies vaccine and HRIG should never be mixed in the same syringe or administered at the same anatomic site. If there is a delay in availability of HRIG, it may be administered up to day 7 of post-exposure treatment. It is contraindicated after day 7, as its interference with the patient's endogenous antibody response to vaccination outweighs its utility. If patients have previously received post-exposure with modern cell culture vaccines, or have been pre-immunized with three doses of a cell culture vaccine at any time prior in their lifetime, they are immunologically primed against rabies (even without currently detectable titers) and should respond to post-exposure vaccination with an anamnestic antibody response; hence, HRIG is contraindicated in these patients due to a potential dampening of the endogenous immune response. Post-exposure for pre-immunized patients, and those who may have previously received post-exposure treatment, consists of two vaccinations with either 1.0 mL HDCV or 1.0 mL RVA administered in the deltoid on day 0 and 3.

Pre-exposure rabies prophylaxis is available for persons engaged in high-risk occupations or avocations, such as veterinarians, animal control officers, animal caretakers, rabies researchers, vaccine production technicians, diagnostic laboratory workers, and wildlife rehabilitators. In addition, any person who is likely to come into contact with potentially infected domestic animals or wildlife, such as spelunkers who explore caves where there are bat colonies, and persons spending extended periods (>30 days) in contact with animals in Africa, Asia, or Latin America, should have pre-exposure vaccination. Pre-exposure prophylaxis consists of 1.0 mL of HDCV or RVA given intramuscularly (deltoid area), or a 0.1 mL intradermal administration of HDCV in the deltoid area on days 0, 7, and 21 or 28. When administered intradermally as if for tuberculosis sensitivity testing, inexperienced personnel may have occasionally deposited some vaccinations subcutaneously resulting in markedly inferior serologic responses; current packaging ameliorates this potential problem. A single booster dose is recommended periodically, depending upon the results of serologic testing and the relative risk of continued exposure.

Serologic testing should be conducted every 6 months for persons at constant risk such a laboratory workers, or every 2 years for persons at frequent risk, such as veterinarians, animal control officers, etc., to confirm a titer resulting in complete neutralization at a dilution of 1:5 (or by the World Health Organization standard of a titer of 0.5 International Units). A booster dose is recommended when persons in these categories fall below this predetermined level at the 6-month and 2-year intervals. In lieu of serologic testing, a booster may be empirically administered every 2 years for persons at frequent risk of exposure, although there may be adverse reactions including mild local reactions such as erythema and swelling, mild systemic reactions, such as fever and nausea, immune complex reactions, and even, albeit rarely, a neurologic illness resembling Guillain-Barré syndrome. No serologic testing or periodic booster vaccine administration beyond the primary course is needed for those with an infrequent or episodic risk, such as most law enforcement officers, emergency personnel, etc. (except the day 0 and 3 vaccine administration in response to an exposure).

Pre-immunization against rabies may best be regarded as a priming of the immune response; there is no known "protective" antibody titer. A pre-immunized person remains susceptible to rabies and without appropriate post-exposure booster vaccinations may be still develop rabies, as demonstrated in a pre-immunized Peace Corps worker who was bitten by a puppy with signs of rabies, but did not receive the two dose post-exposure vaccination, and subsequently died of rabies, as well as a pre-immunized rabies researcher who developed clinical rabies following exposure in the laboratory to high concentrations of intentionally aerosolized rabies virus. It is essential that pre-immunized persons remain attentive to episodic rabies exposures and seek appropriate post-exposure treatment with each occurrence.

Outside the United States, several different schedules and routes for use of alternative biologic agents (e.g., purified chick or duck embryo cell vaccine [PCEC, PDEV],* purified Vero cell rabies vaccine [PVRV],* and purified equine rabies sera [ERIG]*)

---

*Not available in the United States.

are commonly employed. In some developing countries, the only available vaccine is prepared from nerve tissue of inoculated animals. Due to the risk of neuroparalytic complications, these should only be used if there will be a significant delay in obtaining access to modern tissue culture vaccines.

Rabies is invariably fatal once clinical signs are present. However, all exposures do not invariably lead to clinical rabies in humans. Without intervention with post-exposure prophylaxis, rabies generally occurs in approximately 60% of persons with a bite exposure from clinically rabid animal and is dependent upon the dose, strain, severity, and location of the injury, as well as other factors.

INFECTION CONTROL

According to American Council of Immunization Practices (ACIP) recommendations, an exposure to rabies is defined as a bite or scratch from a rabid animal, or contamination of open wounds or mucous membranes with infectious material. The most highly infectious material is saliva and nervous tissue. Generally, contact with other body fluids or excreta, such as blood, urine, feces, milk, serous exudate, etc., does not constitute an exposure to rabies. Rabies virus is labile, remaining susceptible to degradation from desiccation, detergents, changes in pH, ultraviolet radiation (i.e., sunlight), etc. The act of simply touching a rabid animal (or human) is not considered an exposure and does not warrant post-exposure treatment. However, extreme caution is warranted with a history involving potential bat contact due to the diminutive size of the animal and the possibility of a nearly imperceptible pinpoint prick from teeth of a millimeter or less.

Blood products do not transmit rabies. Eight cases of corneal transplant–associated rabies are the only documented examples of human-to-human rabies transmission. There has not been any recent documented cases of rabies transmission from a patient to a health care worker, even in developing countries where human rabies is not uncommon and universal precautions are not always practiced. Stringent universal body fluid precautions will virtually eliminate the need for post-exposure treatment in the health care environment.

The control and prevention of animal and human rabies is a great public health challenge for many areas of the world and still of significant concern in the United States, where the occurrence of human rabies is viewed, perhaps appropriately, as a horrible specter. In developing countries, easier access to lower cost prophylaxis remains urgent, along with effective implementation of rabies control at its animal source (i.e., the domestic dog). One of the Healthy People 2000 objectives is to reduce human post-exposure treatments by 50%. This may be unattainable in the face of multiple wildlife rabies epizootics coupled with the ideal of no human rabies cases in the United States. Current approaches include the continuation of aggressive public education about what constitutes an exposure and ways to avoid exposure, and the investigation of novel adjunct control methods, such as oral wildlife rabies vaccination, designed to control rabies at its animal source.

RAT-BITE FEVER

method of
LAWRENCE H. HANAU, M.D., PH.D.
Montefiore Medical Center
Bronx, New York

Rat-bite fever includes disease caused by two different organisms: *Streptobacillus moniliformis* and *Spirillum minus*. Bacillary disease is more common in the United States, while disease caused by *S. minus* predominates in Asia. Infection resulting from a rat bite was first described in India more than 2000 years ago, and in Japan is called *sodoku*, meaning rat poison. The syndrome was first described in the United States in 1839, and by 1916 both organisms had been identified.

The organisms causing rat-bite fever are members of the rat's commensal flora. Fifty to 100% of rats harbor *S. moniliformis* in their oro- or nasopharynx, and 25% are colonized by *S. minus* in their blood or conjunctivae. Infection is acquired through the bite or scratch of an infected animal, though occasionally no bite will have occurred. Infection may also be acquired by the bites of other rodents—for example, mice or squirrels; animals preying on rats, e.g., dogs, cats, or weasels; or in the case of *S. moniliformis*, through the ingestion of food or water contaminated with rat excrement, a syndrome known as Haverhill fever. In the United States today, the largest groups to be infected are laboratory personnel and persons, particularly children under the age of 10, who live in crowded, rat-infested areas.

BACTERIOLOGY

S. moniliformis is a pleomorphic gram-negative rod that may form filaments with bulbous swellings, giving it the appearance of beads on a string. The organism requires enriched media and an atmosphere containing 8 to 10% CO_2 to grow. Of note, growth is inhibited by sodium polyanethol sulfonate, the anticoagulant found in most blood culture bottles today, although the yield may be increased by using resin-containing bottles. In liquid media, *S. moniliformis* forms flocculent puffballs; in solid media, it forms colonies 1 to 2.5 mm in size. The organism may also spontaneously develop penicillin-resistent L forms, whose colonies have a fried-egg appearance. *S. moniliformis* may be definitively identified by its characteristic fatty acid profile in gas-liquid chromatography.

S. minus is a coiled, spiral, gram-negative rod, which is best visualized by dark-field microscopy or in Wright- or Giemsa-stained specimens. It cannot be grown on artificial media.

DISEASE DUE TO *STREPTOBACILLUS MONILIFORMIS*

The manifestations of disease caused by *S. moniliformis* and *S. minus* are summarized in Table 1. Disease due to *S. moniliformis* first manifests itself after an incubation period of 1 to 22 days but most often occurs in less than 10 days. During incubation, the initial bite wound may have healed, and the patient may not remember the bite. The disease is heralded by the abrupt onset of fever, chills, headache, myalgias, arthralgias, and gastrointestinal symptoms. Patients who acquire their disease through oral ingestion will also complain of sore throat and will also note more severe gastrointestinal symptoms, particularly vomiting. Two to 4 days later, the patient will develop a maculopapular or petechial rash that will often involve the palms and soles. In addition, the patient may develop an asymmetrical arthritis involving large joints, such as the knees, ankles, or elbows. The joint effusions, accompanying the arthritis, are generally sterile, though occasionally they may be directly infected, which may result in destruction of cartilage. Notable laboratory findings include an elevated white blood cell count, which may be as high as 30,000, and a false-positive test for syphilis, found in approximately 25% of patients.

Infection may be detected by growing the organism as described previously, or serologically, via the detection of specific agglutinins, which are usually detectable 10 days after the onset of disease. Infection is confirmed by detection of a fourfold rise in titer or an initial titer of 1:80.

Rat-bite fever must be differentiated from other diseases. When a history of exposure to rats has been obtained, a significant alternative is leptospirosis. However, rat-bite fever may also need to be distinguished from Rocky Mountain spotted fever, secondary syphilis, viral infections, meningococcemia, enteric fever, and a drug reaction. In the presence of arthritis, one should also consider disseminated gonococcal infection, Lyme disease, brucellosis, endocarditis, collagen vascular diseases, or acute rheumatic fever.

In the absence of treatment, the fevers will often resolve spontaneously within 3 to 5 days, and most other manifes-

TABLE 1. **Manifestations of Rat-Bite Fever**

Feature	*S. moniliformis*	*S. minus*
Incubation	<10 days	5–30 days
Bite site	Heals well	Inflammation and chancre-like lesion occur at onset of symptoms
Rash	Maculopapular and/or petechial	Macular
Lymphadenitis/lymph node involvement	Minimal to absent	Prominent
Arthritis/arthralgias/myalgias	Prominent	Rare
Relapsing pattern	Irregular	Regular
False-positive test for syphilis	<25%	<50%
Growth in laboratory	On specialized media	Inoculation into laboratory mice/ guinea pigs
Serologic test	Yes	No

tations will resolve within 2 weeks, although joint inflammation may persist for longer periods of time. However, fevers may recur at irregular intervals, and these recurrences may persist for several months. Mortality without treatment is 13%. Other complications include the development of endocarditis, which has a 100% mortality without treatment; purulent joint infections; and there are case reports of myocarditis, pericarditis, meningitis, pneumonia, amnionitis, and a brain abscess being caused by *S. moniliformis*.

DISEASE DUE TO *SPIRILLUM MINUS*

Disease caused by *S. minus* differs from that caused by *S. moniliformis* in a number of ways. The incubation period averages 13 days and may range from 5 to 30 days. Although, the bite wound may heal initially, it later will become painful and swollen and develop a purple color. Eventually it will form a chancre with induration and eschar formation. The changes at the wound site are followed by fevers, chills, headache, and malaise. A rash will also be detected in 50% of patients during the first week of illness. The rash is characterized by blotchy, red-brown to violaceous macules that tend to be larger in size when compared with those caused by *S. moniliformis*; these lesions may coalesce to form large eruptions. In contrast to the bacillary form of the disease, lymphadenitis and lymphangitis are prominent and arthritis and myalgias are usually absent. The white blood cell count will usually be between 10,000 and 20,000, and eosinophilia may be detected. Fifty percent of patients will have a false-positive test for syphilis. As noted, *S. minus* cannot be cultured on artificial media and there are no serologic tests available. *S. minus* occasionally may be visualized in clinical specimens, but detection often requires the inoculation of clinical material into mice or guinea pigs that are free of colonization.

In the absence of treatment, the fevers will resolve after 3 to 5 days but will be followed by relapses at regular intervals; the rash may fade and then recrudesce. Complete clinical resolution usually occurs after 1 to 2 months. Complications of the *S. minus* infection include hepatitis, meningitis, epididymitis, conjunctivitis, nephritis, anemia, myocarditis, and endocarditis, which is rare and usually will occur in patients with pre-existing valvular disease.

TREATMENT AND PREVENTION

The treatment of choice for both forms of the disease is penicillin. The traditional treatment is 600,000 U of procaine penicillin administered intramuscularly every 12 hours, for a week or until a clinical response is achieved. Thereafter, 500 mg of penicillin V should be administered every 6 hours for a total course of 10 to 14 days. Some recommend that the penicillin be administered intravenously, rather than by the intramuscular route. Children may be treated with 200,000 U per kg per day intravenously and then switched to penicillin V, 25 to 50 mg per kg per day in four divided doses. Patients with endocarditis or other serious complications require prolonged treatment with a daily regimen of 15 to 20 million U of penicillin given intravenously in divided doses; endocarditis should be treated for 4 weeks. Some authorities recommend adding streptomycin at 7.5 mg per kg twice daily, to treat the penicillin-resistant

L forms, which develop spontaneously. Treatment of *S. minus* infection may be complicated by development of a Jarisch-Herxheimer reaction.

Alternatives for the penicillin-allergic patient include tetracycline,* 500 mg every 6 hours; streptomycin; or erythromycin,* 500 mg every 6 hours, though some organisms may be resistant. There are reports of treatment with chloramphenicol* and clindamycin (Cleocin).* There are little data regarding the efficacy of these penicillin alternatives for the treatment of disease caused by *S. minus*.

In order to prevent disease, laboratory personnel should wear gloves when working with rodents. Those patients who sustain a bite should wash the wound thoroughly with soap and water and should receive tetanus prophylaxis, if needed. Two grams of penicillin V in divided doses may be given orally for 3 days, though its efficacy is unknown.

---

*Not FDA-approved for this indication.

RELAPSING FEVER

method of
MARK D. LACY, M.D., and
R. WESLEY FARR, M.D.
West Virginia University
Morgantown, West Virginia

Relapsing fevers are arthropod-borne spirochetal infections characterized by recurrent febrile episodes followed by asymptomatic periods. The tick-borne variety is seen worldwide, including the western United States, whereas the louse-borne variety is seen in the developing world but not in the United States unless imported.

ETIOLOGY, EPIDEMIOLOGY, AND PATHOPHYSIOLOGY

Various rodent ticks and the human body louse are the vectors by which humans acquire the spirochetal bacteria causing relapsing fever. These microbes are members of the *Borrelia* spirochete genus and are 8 to 30 μm long with a helix of 3 to 10 loose spirals. They cannot be cultivated in standard media but, unlike other spirochetes causing human disease, they can be readily detected with Giemsa or Wright stains.

Louse-borne disease is caused by *Borrelia recurrentis* and is endemic in the highlands of Africa, South America, and foci in the Far East. It is not observed endemically in the United States. This form of relapsing fever usually occurs in the setting of overcrowding where dissemination of body lice results in epidemics. Untreated, the mortality rate may reach 40% and is related to host factors such as malnutrition and concurrent illnesses.

Over a dozen species of *Borrelia* produce the tick-borne variety of relapsing fever. The vectors are soft ticks of the genus *Ornithodoros*. The natural reservoirs are rodents and other small mammals residing in warm areas throughout the world at elevations of 1500 to 9600 feet. The ticks usually feed at night, have a painless bite, and feed for 5 to 20 minutes; hence, exposures to the vector may go unnoticed. Most cases in North America have occurred in the

Western forests; the number of reported cases there is growing due to increased intrusion of humans into the vectors' environment. Sixty-two visitors lodging in cabins at Grand Canyon National Park in Arizona in 1979 constituted the largest outbreak of the disease in the Western Hemisphere. The characteristic pattern of fevers interspersed with periods of well being are related to the human immune response to the spirochete following inoculation and to this spirochete's ability to reconfigure its outer membrane antigens. A single borrelial spirochete may produce up to 40 different variants or serotype progeny by this multiphasic antigen variation during the same infection. Each surface antigen is encoded by a different gene activated to evade the host's serospecific antibody. Thus, after the first serotype wanes and the fever subsides because of an effective antibody response by the host, another antigen is expressed by a new bacterial variant. Several days later, as this new serotype multiplies, another febrile episode ensues necessitating a retailored antibody response in order to clear the new variant. This cycle of genetic recombination and antigen expression followed by specific antibody response is repeated and is responsible for the periodicity distinctive in this disease.

SYMPTOMS, SIGNS, AND DIAGNOSIS

Tick- and louse-borne relapsing fever have similar manifestations that develop after an approximate 1-week incubation period. Symptoms begin suddenly with high fever, rigors, myalgia and arthralgia, weakness, and a severe headache. Nausea, abdominal pain, diarrhea, vomiting, or nonproductive cough is sometimes reported. During the febrile episodes, patients are acutely ill with lethargy, tachycardia, tachypnea, and occasionally confusion. Nonspecific maculopapular rashes may be seen; petechial rashes are less common. Hepatosplenomegaly is frequent in louse-borne disease but is unusual in the tick-borne variety. Lymphadenopathy usually affecting the cervical chains is not dramatic. Jaundice or mucosal bleeding is an infrequent sign of louse-borne relapsing fever and portends a worse prognosis. Myocarditis is a rare phenomenon. Central nervous system involvement, manifesting as meningitis or cranial nerve deficits, is occasionally seen, particularly in louse-borne disease. Laboratory parameters are nonspecific. Hemograms are usually normal, although thrombocytopenia has been reported. Liver enzymes may be elevated, especially in severe cases of louse-borne relapsing fever. Positive serologic tests for Lyme disease and syphilis occur in less than 5% of patients.

The most useful laboratory study is a thick or thin smear of peripheral blood with a Wright's or Giemsa stain. Organisms may be detected only during febrile episodes. Repeated examinations may be necessary to demonstrate spirochetes. Dark-field and fluorescence microscopy may increase the sensitivity but require more laboratory expertise. Antibody serologic tests are not widely available except in reference laboratories and often lack specificity.

The acute clinical syndrome lasts 1 to 6 days and then terminates as abruptly as it begins. Hypotension and shock have been observed in the primary episode. Subsequent relapses, occurring 7 to 10 days later, are usually less severe. In tick-borne disease, relapses may recur over several weeks; fewer relapses occur in louse-borne disease. The early stages of relapsing fever may simulate other disorders, so geographic and epidemiologic factors are important in the diagnosis. Tick-borne disease may be confused with Colorado tick fever or Rocky Mountain spotted

fever. Early louse-borne relapsing fever may resemble malaria, dengue fever, typhoid fever, or leptospirosis.

TREATMENT

Tetracycline, or erythromycin during pregnancy is the drug of choice and is usually given orally. A single 500-mg dose of either is satisfactory for most episodes of louse-borne disease. A 500-mg oral dose of tetracycline or erythromycin four times daily for 7 to 10 days is given for the tick-borne variety due to a higher rate of treatment failure and relapse. Penicillin and ceftriaxone (Rocephin) are recommended if central nervous system involvement is present. Chloramphenicol is another effective alternative therapy (Table 1).

Hospitalization may be necessary for very ill patients but also as a precaution in anticipation of a Jarisch-Herxheimer type of reaction. Frequently seen within 3 hours after treatment, the reaction elicits fever, increased rigors, and hypotension, persisting for up to 24 hours. Since the exact mechanism of this phenomenon remains unclarified, management consists of supportive care. Corticosteroids and acetaminophen do not modify the Jarisch-Herxheimer reaction. Uncomplicated, adequately treated relapsing fever has a mortality rate of less than 5%.

PREVENTION

Louse-borne relapsing fever is best prevented by minimizing overcrowding and maintaining good hygiene. Malathion-type insecticides may be necessary to successfully delouse crowded housing facilities. Rodent-proofing of lodging facilities and the use of insect repellents may reduce the risk of tick-borne disease if vector habitats cannot be avoided. The Bacterial Zoonoses Branch, Division of Vector-Borne Infectious Diseases, Centers for Disease Control and Prevention, requests that serum samples from patients with documented infections be submitted for its International Borreliosis Reference Collection; telephone 303-221-6400. Cases should also be reported to state and local health departments.

TABLE 1. **Preferred Therapy for Relapsing Fever**

	Drug	Adult Dosage	Duration
Louse-borne relapsing fever	Tetracycline*	500 mg PO	1 dose
	Doxycycline*	100 mg q 12 h PO	2 doses
Tick-borne relapsing fever	Doxycycline	100 mg q 12 h PO/IV	7–14 d
	Erythromycin	500 mg q 6 h PO/IV	7–14 d
Alternative drugs	Chloramphenicol	500 mg q 6 h PO/IV	
	Penicillin V	500 mg q 6 h PO	
	Penicillin G†	5 million units q 6 h IV	
	Ceftriaxone†	2 gm once daily IV	

*Substitute erythromycin, 500 mg PO, for pregnant women. In children less than 8 years old, give 40 mg/kg/day in divided doses q 6–8 h.

†Use in patients with central nervous system manifestations.

RHEUMATIC FEVER

method of
STANFORD T. SHULMAN, M.D., and
JANET A. STOCKHEIM, M.D.
*Northwestern University Medical School and
Children's Memorial Hospital
Chicago, Illinois*

Acute rheumatic fever (ARF) may follow untreated pharyngitis caused by group A beta-hemolytic streptococci. Because ARF can develop after a subclinical or asymptomatic streptococcal pharyngeal infection, primary prevention with antistreptococcal antibiotics is not always possible.

ARF is most common in school-aged children 5 to 15 years of age and is much less common in younger children and adults. Both sexes are affected equally, and the peak season is in the spring. The onset of ARF is 2 to 4 weeks following streptococcal pharyngitis, and ARF is never a complication of streptococcal skin infections.

Once suspected, the diagnosis of ARF is confirmed by fulfilling the Jones Criteria—guidelines first established in 1944 by T. Duckett Jones to aid in the diagnosis and to limit the over-diagnosis of ARF. These guidelines have been revised several times, the last in 1992 by the American Heart Association, and now apply only to the initial attack of ARF. Table 1 outlines the 1992 revised Jones Criteria. Diagnosis of ARF requires two major criteria or one major and two minor criteria, *with supporting evidence of antecedent group A streptococcal infection in either case.*

Migratory polyarthritis is the most frequent finding in ARF, occurring in 75% of patients. It classically involves the larger joints, with pain often preceding the development of hot, red, tender, and swollen joints. Consistent with its migratory nature, a given joint's involvement resolves within 1 to 3 days without treatment, with a new joint becoming involved. Overall, in the absence of therapy, a severe arthritic course may persist for several weeks. Early anti-inflammatory treatment may abort the progression of polyarthritis, and the characteristic dramatic response to salicylates may be useful in establishing the diagnosis of ARF.

Carditis always includes endocarditis. It may be limited to endocarditis alone or may also include myocarditis and/or pericarditis. It occurs in up to 60% of cases, with mitral valve, with or without aortic valve, involvement. Valvar insufficiency is the most characteristic finding in early and convalescent ARF but may progress to valvar stenosis after years or decades. Manifestations of acute rheumatic carditis include tachycardia, murmurs, rhythm disturbances (with myocardial involvement), and signs of pericardial disease (friction rub, muffled heart sounds, tamponade). An echocardiogram will confirm cardiac involvement.

Signs and symptoms of *Sydenham's chorea* include emotional lability, incoordination, poor school performance, uncontrolled movements, and facial grimacing; these occur in 10% to 15% of cases of ARF. Chorea is frequently exacerbated by stress and disappears with sleep. It may not develop until several months after the inciting group A streptococcal infection, when the acute phase reactants are no longer elevated and evidence of the streptococcal pharyngitis is lacking.

Erythema marginatum is the rare but characteristic rash of ARF. It is an erythematous, serpiginous, macular rash with pale centers and is not pruritic. It is distributed over the trunk and extremities, never involving the face.

Subcutaneous nodules are the least frequent major manifestation of ARF, occurring in fewer than 1% of cases. The firm, painless nodules are approximately 1 cm in diameter and are found along extensor surfaces of tendons near bony prominences.

The minor Jones Criteria are divided into clinical and laboratory findings. *Arthralgia* qualifies as a minor criterion only in the absence of polyarthritis as a major manifestation. *Fevers* are typically moderate and occur early in the course of the illness. Note also that the minor manifestation of *prolonged P-R interval* on electrocardiogram does not confirm the presence of the major manifestation of carditis nor predict long-term cardiac disease.

In applying the Jones Criteria, it is mandatory to document evidence of a recent group A streptococcal infection. Throat culture or a rapid streptococcal antigen test performed at the time of presentation of ARF is positive in only 10% to 20% of cases, reflecting spontaneous clearance of the organism. The serum antistreptococcal antibody titers include antistreptolysin O, anti-deoxyribonuclease B, antihyaluronidase, and antistreptokinase. Only 80% to 85% of ARF patients have elevated titers of a specific antibody, but the likelihood of demonstrating at least one elevated titer increases to 95% to 100% if three antibodies are measured.

Once accurately diagnosed, the treatment of ARF is divided into therapy of the acute attack and chronic therapy to prevent recurrences.

TABLE 1. **Jones Criteria for Acute Rheumatic Fever (Revised, 1992)**

Major Criteria	Minor Criteria
1. Migratory polyarthritis	*Clinical*
2. Carditis	1. Arthralgia
3. Chorea	2. Fever
4. Erythema marginatum	*Laboratory*
5. Subcutaneous nodules	3. Elevated acute-phase reactants
	4. Prolonged P-R interval

WITH

Supporting evidence of antecedent group A streptococcal infection:
  Positive throat culture or rapid streptococcal antigen test
    OR
  Elevated or rising streptococcal antibody titer

Adapted from JAMA *268*:2069, 1992. Copyright 1992, American Medical Association.

THERAPY OF ACUTE RHEUMATIC FEVER

Patients with suspected or confirmed ARF should be hospitalized for a full medical evaluation, for observation of their progress before and after the initiation of therapy, and to impress upon them and their families the long-term consequences of rheumatic heart disease and the high risk of recurrence. They should receive treatment for streptococcal pharyngitis (Table 2) even though it is difficult to demonstrate persistent group A streptococci.

Anti-inflammatory agents effectively suppress the inflammatory activity of ARF, and the dramatic clinical response of arthritis to aspirin may be useful in establishing the diagnosis of ARF. There is no consistent evidence that corticosteroids reduce the

TABLE 2. **Treatment of Rheumatic Fever**

Acute Rheumatic Fever

Antistreptococcal Antibiotics

Benzathine penicillin IM, 600,000 U in children weighing less than 60 lbs; 1.2 million U in all others
OR
Oral penicillin, 250 mg 6 h for 10 d
OR
Oral erythromycin, 40 mg/kg/d divided in 4 doses, for 10 days

Anti-inflammatory Agents

Aspirin: 50–75 mg/kg/d in 4 divided doses for patients without cardiac involvement
OR
Aspirin: 75–100 mg/kg/d in 4 divided doses for patients with only mild carditis
OR
Corticosteroids: prednisone, 2 mg/kg/d in 4 doses for 2–4 wk, then taper with addition of salicylates, for patients with moderate or severe carditis

Cardiac Drugs (if needed)

Diuretic therapy as indicated; cautious digitalization as indicated

Antichoreic Drugs (if needed)

Phenobarbital or diazepam (Valium) as indicated

Prevention of Recurrent Acute Rheumatic Fever

Rheumatic Prophylaxis (for all patients)

Monthly benzathine penicillin IM, 600,000 U in children less than 60 lbs; 1.2 million U in all others
OR
Penicillin V PO, 250 mg twice daily
OR
Sulfadiazine PO, 500 mg twice daily (500 mg once daily if less than 30 kg)

Infective Endocarditis Prophylaxis (for patients with cardiac disease)

As recommended by the American Heart Association

Adapted from Shulman ST: Rheumatic fever. *In* Rakel RE (ed): Conn's Current Therapy 1991. Philadelphia, WB Saunders Co, 1991, pp 100–101.

residual cardiac damage caused by ARF. However, administration of corticosteroids does promptly suppress acute inflammation, particularly cardiac inflammation, and on rare occasions can be lifesaving. Anti-inflammatory agents can be withheld in patients who are only mildly to moderately ill and in whom the diagnosis of ARF is not completely clear. This may allow for observation of disease progression, particularly the major manifestation of migratory polyarthritis. Anti-inflammatory therapy should be instituted, however, once the diagnosis is confirmed.

In patients without evidence of cardiac involvement, aspirin should be given at a dose of 50 to 75 mg per kg per day in four divided doses. For those with only mild carditis (i.e., unassociated with cardiomegaly or congestive heart failure), we recommend aspirin at a higher dose of 75 to 100 mg per kg per day in four divided doses. In smaller children, the higher end of the appropriate dose range should be given, with the lower end for larger children. The latter may develop salicylate toxicity at the higher

dosages. In each case, after 2 weeks, the dose may be reduced by half and continued for another 2 to 3 weeks.

Those patients who demonstrate significant cardiac involvement with cardiomegaly and/or congestive failure and/or pericarditis should be treated with prednisone at a dose of 2 mg per kg per day for 2 to 4 weeks. Prednisone should then be tapered over several more weeks, with simultaneous administration of salicylates at a dose of 50 to 70 mg per kg per day in four divided doses to prevent a clinical rebound of inflammatory activity. All anti-inflammatory agents can then be stopped after another 6 to 8 weeks. Bed rest is recommended for patients in congestive cardiac failure. Other supportive therapies include diuretics, fluid and salt restriction, and oxygen therapy. Careful digitalization may be required.

Chorea is a self-limited feature, and many patients benefit significantly from quiet, nonstressful surroundings and the administration of phenobarbital or diazepam (Valium). Chorea follows a much longer latent period than the inflammatory manifestations of arthritis and carditis and tends not to respond to anti-inflammatory therapy alone.

PREVENTION OF RECURRENT ACUTE RHEUMATIC FEVER

Individuals who have had an attack of ARF with or without cardiac disease or who are found to have chronic rheumatic heart disease (RHD) are at risk for recurrent attacks of ARF following streptococcal pharyngitis. Thus, they should receive *continuous* antistreptococcal prophylaxis to prevent recurrences of ARF. Three standard regimens are outlined in Table 2, in order of preference.

The advantage of parenteral penicillin is that one does not depend upon daily patient compliance; however, the injections may be painful. In addition to preventing recurrent attacks of ARF, strict compliance with this regimen has been shown to result in healing of valvar heart disease (as reflected by the disappearance of murmurs) in the majority of patients. Prophylaxis with sulfadiazine has the advantage of avoiding the induction of penicillin-resistant oral flora that could predispose the patient to an episode of bacterial endocarditis due to a penicillin-resistant organism. It should also be noted that sulfadiazine is recommended only for prophylaxis of recurrent ARF and should not be used for treatment of the initial streptococcal infection. Erythromycin has been suggested for the rare patient who is allergic to both penicillin and sulfadiazine.

A subject of considerable controversy is the optimal duration of rheumatic fever prophylaxis. Most recommendations, including those of the American Heart Association and the American Academy of Pediatrics, are to continue lifelong prophylaxis for patients with RHD because the risk of recurrent ARF, while diminishing with time, persists long beyond childhood. In patients without residual cardiac involvement, prophylaxis probably can be discontinued safely at age 21 years if at least 5 years have elapsed since the last attack of ARF.

In addition to rheumatic fever prophylaxis, patients with RHD require infective endocarditis prophylaxis on an episodic basis related to dental or surgical procedures or gastrointestinal or genitourinary tract instrumentation, as recommended by the American Heart Association.

LYME DISEASE

method of
JOSEPH J. BURRASCANO, JR., M.D.
East Hampton, New York

Lyme disease is an extremely complex illness that is still poorly understood. To date, there still is no consensus on many aspects of its management. Despite this, the diagnosis and treatment of Lyme disease is entering a new era, replacing simplistic approaches with more modern ones based on better knowledge, more experience, and the application of common sense. This has resulted in an expansion of syndromes attributable to Lyme disease, thus improving diagnosis, and new treatment recommendations regarding both drug and dose. The existence of seronegativity and chronic persistent infection have been confirmed, as have relapses and treatment failures. With more careful dosing and more prolonged treatment duration, chronic symptoms can be prevented or eliminated in many more patients than ever before.

The diagnosis of Lyme disease is made on clinical grounds, as no currently available test, no matter the source or type, is definitive in confirming whether an infection with *Borrelia burgdorferi* is present, or if so, whether the infection is responsible for the patient's symptoms.

Treatment is also difficult. It is impossible to know how much medication will be necessary to control the infection, because response to therapy is extremely variable. Also, it cannot be determined in advance which of the many complaints will improve with further antibiotics, and which will be permanent. There is no test available that can be used during therapy to indicate how effective the treatment regimen is, and there is no test for cure. That is why the entire clinical picture must be taken into account, including a search for the many subtleties that exist. Patient diaries that succinctly outline symptoms over a course of therapy are vital, and as many objective measures as possible should be followed, such as temperature graphs, notes from physical therapists, and physical findings. This information will help in your assessment of effectiveness of ongoing treatment and guide you in determining optimal duration.

The concept of a "therapeutic alliance" between the caregiver and patient has to be emphasized. This means that the patient has to become part of the medical team and take responsibility for complying with the recommendations given, maintaining the best possible health status, reporting promptly any problems or new symptoms, and especially in realizing that despite all our best efforts, success in diagnosis and treatment is never assured.

GENERAL INFORMATION

Lyme disease is an infectious illness caused by the spirochete *Borrelia burgdorferi* (Bb). Bb is transmitted by the bite of an ixodid tick. Transmission of the organism occurs if the tick has been attached long enough to become engorged (typically more than 24 hours), unless it has been removed improperly, in which case transmission can occur more rapidly. Squeezing the tick's body, irritating it with heat or chemicals in an attempt to get it to back out, and disrupting the tick's integrity, allowing its contents to spill into the wound, all are examples of this. This history is important to elicit when deciding whether to give antibiotic prophylaxis after a tick bite.

DIAGNOSIS

Because of the unreliability of serologic testing for Lyme disease, the diagnosis is a clinical one, based upon the type and pattern of symptoms present and their evolution over time, especially in the setting of a previously healthy patient who has had potential tick exposure. Erythema migrans is the sole absolute indicator of Lyme disease, yet it is observed in fewer than 50% of cases. The other and more common symptoms are nonspecific and protean, but they almost always involve multiple systems and vary over time in both location and intensity, consistent with an active, disseminated infection. A great deal of effort must be made in ruling out similarly presenting illnesses, for often disseminated Lyme becomes a diagnosis of exclusion. Another very important factor is response to treatment: presence or absence of Jarisch-Herxheimer–like reactions, and improvement with therapy. To simplify and clarify diagnosis, a workshop was convened in 1990 and a diagnostic scheme was developed (Table 1). It is important to note that the published reporting criteria of the Centers for Disease Control are for surveillance, not for diagnosis.

Erythema Migrans

Erythema migrans (EM) is a raised, warm, erythematous, centrifugally expanding round or oval lesion with distinct margins. Although usually painless, mild stinging or pruritus can occur. The EM rash can begin 4 days to several weeks after the bite, lasts for several weeks, and may or may not be associated with constitutional symptoms. Multiple lesions are present in 10% to 20% of pa-

TABLE 1. **Lyme Disease Diagnostic Criteria**

	Relative Value
Tick exposure in an endemic region	1
Systemic signs and symptoms consistent with Lyme (other potential diagnoses excluded):	
Single system, e.g., monoarthritis	1
Two or more systems, e.g., monoarthritis and facial palsy	2
Erythema migrans	7
Acrodermatitis chronica atrophicans, biopsy-confirmed	7
Seropositivity	2
Seroconversion on paired sera	3
Tissue microscopy, silver stain	3
Tissue microscopy, monoclonal immunofluorescence	4
Culture positivity	5
B. burgdorferi antigen recovery (when validated)	4
B. burgdorferi DNA/RNA recovery (when validated)	4

Diagnosis	
Lyme borreliosis likely	7 or above
Lyme borreliosis probable	5–6
Lyme borreliosis unlikely	4 or below

tients. A necrotic center may represent a mixed infection, involving other organisms besides *B. burgdorferi*. Atypical lesions may have to be biopsied to aid in diagnosis.

Serologic Testing

Because Lyme serologies often given inconsistent results, you may have to test at more than one laboratory, using different methods if possible. Western blotting is recommended for confirmation. IgM and IgG titers are often reported separately. In Lyme disease, elevated IgM levels do not always indicate an early stage, for these levels may repeatedly peak throughout the course of an active infection. False-negative serologies are common (estimated at 30%) and false-positives occur in up to 10% of patients. Approximately one-third of seronegative patients will become transiently seropositive after completion of successful treatment.

Considerable evidence suggests that in all disseminated Lyme infections, seeding of the central nervous system occurs early (possibly within hours after the bite), yet a recent study has shown that antibodies to Bb can be detected in the cerebrospinal fluid (CSF) in only 20% of such patients. Therefore, spinal taps are not routinely recommended but are performed in patients with pronounced neurologic manifestations, especially if they are seronegative or still significantly symptomatic after completion of treatment. They are done to rule out other neurologic conditions, to determine whether Bb antigens are present, and to determine whether Bb antibodies are being locally produced in the central nervous system. It is especially important to look for pleocytosis and elevated protein, which correlate with the need for more aggressive therapy, as well as the opening pressure, which can be elevated and add to headaches, especially in children.

TREATMENT GUIDELINES

Antibiotic Choices

Because the Lyme spirochete is rapidly distributed to all parts of the body, including the central nervous system, shortly after *B. burgdorferi* enters the bloodstream, all stages of this illness represent disseminated disease. The antibiotic and dose chosen must be able to penetrate all tissues in adequate concentrations to be bactericidal to the organism, even in early infections.

There is no universally effective antibiotic for treating Lyme disease. The antibiotic chosen and dose used will vary based on age, weight, gastrointestinal function, blood levels achieved in light of these factors, and on patient tolerance. For poorly understood reasons, serum antibiotic concentrations vary widely in Lyme patients. Therefore, whenever possible, serum antibiotic levels should be determined to aid in arriving at therapeutic doses.

Four types of antibiotics are in general use for Lyme treatment. The tetracyclines, including doxycycline and minocycline, are bacteriostatic at doses commonly prescribed, and unless high blood levels are attained, treatment failures in early and late disease are common. Tetracycline itself does not penetrate into the CSF as well as doxycycline and minocycline, and its use is not advised. Doxycycline can

be very effective but only if adequate blood levels are achieved either by high oral doses (300 to 600 mg daily) or by parenteral administration.

Penicillins are bactericidal. As would be expected in managing an infection with a gram-negative organism such as *B. burgdorferi*, amoxicillin has been shown to be more effective than oral penicillin V. Because of its short half-life and need for high levels, amoxicillin is usually administered along with probenecid.

Cephalosporins are useful but must be of advanced generation: first-generation drugs are not effective, and second-generation drugs are comparable to amoxicillin and doxycycline both in vitro and in vivo. Third-generation agents are currently the most effective of the cephalosporins because of their very low mean bactericidal concentrations (MBCs) (0.06 for ceftriaxone) and because of excellent tissue penetration. Also, cephalosporins have been shown to be effective in penicillin and tetracycline failures. Cefuroxime axetil (Ceftin), a second-generation agent, is also effective against *Staphylococcus* and thus is useful in treating atypical erythema migrans that may represent a mixed infection, containing some of the more common skin pathogens in addition to Bb. Because it is difficult to tolerate due to gastrointestinal (GI) side effects and is costly, cefuroxime axetil is not used as a first-line drug.

Erythromycin has been shown to be almost ineffective. The advanced macrolides (they are classified as azalides) such as azithromycin (Zithromax) and clarithromycin (Biaxin) have impressively low MBCs, but can be difficult to tolerate due to poor GI tolerance at the high doses needed, and their excessive tendency to promote yeast overgrowth.

When choosing a third-generation cephalosporin, there are several points to remember: cefotaxime (Claforan) and ceftriaxone (Rocephin) both have demonstrated activity in vitro, in vivo, and in clinical studies. Ceftriaxone is administered once daily (an advantage for home therapy) but has 95% biliary excretion and can crystallize in the biliary tree with resultant colic and possible cholecystitis. Gastrointestinal excretion results in a large impact on gut flora. Cefotaxime, which must be given at least every 12, and preferably every 8 hours, is less convenient, but as it has only 5% biliary excretion, it never causes biliary concretions, and may have less impact on gut flora. Biliary complications and gastrointestinal superinfections with ceftriaxone can be lessened if this drug is given in interrupted courses, such as 5 days in a row each week. Table 2 contains a summary of antibiotic choices; other agents with demonstrated in vitro efficacy have been used successfully in treating Lyme patients and are also listed.

Treatment Categories

I have found conclusively that the duration of treatment is just as important as the choice of antibiotic. It is known that *B. burgdorferi* has a very long generation time and may have periods of dormancy.

TABLE 2. Antibiotic Choices

Oral Therapy

(Always check blood levels; goal is peak in midteens; trough [pre-dose] blood level should be greater than 3 μg/mL)

Amoxicillin:
  Adults: 1 gm q 8 h plus probenecid, 500 mg q 8 h
  Pregnancy: 1 gm q 6 h
  Children: 50 mg/kg/day divided into q 8 h doses
Doxycycline:
  Adults: 100 mg tid with food
  Not for children or in pregnancy
Cefuroxime axetil (Ceftin): oral alternative that may be effective in amoxicillin and doxycycline failures; useful in erythema migrans rashes co-infected with common skin pathogens
  Adults and pregnancy: 1 gm q 12 h
  Children: 125 to 500 mg q 12 h based on weight
Tetracycline: Poor response and not recommended
Erythromycin: Poor response and not recommended
Chloramphenicol: Not recommended as not proved and potentially toxic

Poorly Studied but Anecdotally Effective Alternatives

Azithromycin (Zithromax):
  Adults: 500 to 1000 mg/d
  Adolescents: 250 to 500 mg/d
  Cannot be used in pregnancy or in younger children
Clarithromycin (Biaxin):
  Adults: 250 to 500 mg q 6 h
  Cannot be used in pregnancy or in younger children

Parenteral Therapy

Ceftriaxone (Rocephin): Risk of biliary sludging can be minimized with intermittent breaks in therapy (i.e., infuse 5 d in a row per wk)
  Adults and pregnancy: 2 gm q 24 h
  Children: 75 mg/kg/d up to 2 gm/d
Cefotaxime (Claforan): Comparable efficacy to ceftriaxone; no biliary complications
  Adults and pregnancy: 2 gm q 8 h
  Children: 90 to 180 mg/kg/d dosed q 6 h
Doxycycline: Requires central line as it is caustic
  Adults: 300 mg q 24 h, then adjust based upon blood levels
  Cannot be used in pregnancy or in younger children
Penicillin G: IV penicillin G is minimally effective and not recommended
Benzathine penicillin: Useful alternative to oral therapy
  Adults: 1.2 million U once to twice weekly, based upon body weight
  Adolescents: 300,000 to 1.2 million U weekly
  Cannot be used in pregnancy

Poorly Studied but Anecdotally Effective Alternatives

Imipenem: Similar in efficacy to cefotaxime. Must be given q 6 to 8 h
Cefuroxime: Not demonstrably better than ceftriaxone or cefotaxime
Ampicillin: More effective than penicillin G. Must be given q 6 h

---

This has a major effect on the length of treatment needed for the various stages of this illness, for the longer one is infected before adequate treatment is begun, the longer the treatment course will have to be. In humans, Bb seems to regenerate monthly. As antibiotics kill organisms only during their growth phase, therapy is designed to bracket at least one entire 4-week generation cycle. Hence the minimum treatment course is 6 weeks; late, disseminated infections may have to be treated for many months to be controlled. During treatment, symptoms will wax and wane every 4 weeks, reflecting the growth period of this *Borrelia*, similar to what is seen in the relapsing fevers. If the antibiotics are working, over time these monthly flares will lessen in severity and duration. To prevent relapses, treatment has to be continued until all signs of active infection have cleared. The average duration of successful therapy of ad-

vanced cases is 4 months in males, and 6 months in hormonally active females. Treatment failures should alert the clinician to alternative diagnoses, concurrent conditions, and the presence of an otherwise inapparent immune deficiency.

With intravenous antibiotic therapy, a 6-week course is the minimum. If there is a pronounced flare of symptoms during the fourth week, then extend the course to 10 weeks to bracket the next generation cycle. This type of clinical assessment continues, and when these monthly reactions finally lessen in severity, then oral medications can be substituted to the same end point as mentioned earlier. The very occurrence of ongoing monthly cycles indicates that living organisms are still present and that antibiotics should be continued until these cycles no longer occur. Treatment categories are presented in Table 3.

There is more to managing Lyme disease than

TABLE 3. Treatment Categories

Prophylaxis of high-risk groups should consist of education and preventive measures; antibiotics not recommended

Embedded Deer Tick with No Signs or Symptoms of Lyme:

Decide to treat based on the type of tick, whether it came from an endemic area and percent infected, how it was removed, and length of attachment (nymphs: at least 1 day; adults: anecdotally, as little as 4 hours). The risk of transmission is greater if the tick is engorged, or if it was removed improperly, allowing the tick's contents to spill into the bite wound. High-risk bites are treated as follows:

Adults: Oral therapy for 14 days
Pregnancy: Amoxicillin, 1000 mg q 6 h for 6 wk
  Alternative: Cefuroxime axetil, 1000 mg q 12 h for 6 wk
Young children: Oral therapy for 14 days
  Erythromycin: Poor alternative with documented treatment failures

Early Localized: Single erythema migrans with no constitutional symptoms:

Adults and children: Oral therapy for 6 weeks
Pregnancy: 1st and 2nd trimesters: IV for 21 days, then oral for 6 weeks;
  3rd trimester: amoxicillin 1000 mg q 6 h for 6 weeks

Disseminated Disease: Multiple lesions, constitutional symptoms, lymphadenopathy, or any other manifestations of late disease:

Early Disseminated: Present for less than 1 year and not complicated by immune deficiency or prior steroid treatment:

Adults: Oral therapy until no active disease for 4 weeks (4–6 months total)
Pregnancy: As in localized disease, but duration as above. Some experienced clinicians treat throughout pregnancy.
Children: Oral therapy with duration based upon clinical response

Parenteral Alternatives: For sicker patients and those unresponsive to or intolerant of oral medications:

Adults and children: IV therapy for 6 weeks or until clearly improved; follow with oral therapy or IM benzathine penicillin until no active disease for 4 weeks
Pregnancy: IV then oral therapy as above

Late Disseminated: Present greater than 1 year, more severely ill patients, and those with prior significant steroid therapy or any other cause of impaired immunity:

Adults and pregnancy: extended IV therapy (6 to 10 or more weeks), then oral or IM to same end point.
Children: IV therapy for 6 or more weeks

---

simply prescribing antibiotics. It is necessary for the patient to obtain adequate rest and receive any needed physical therapy. Those who have been ill for a prolonged period will also benefit immensely from a careful, thorough, and aggressive graded exercise program when they are well enough to begin. Thrush has to be controlled, and a sensible regimen of adequate nutrition and vitamins, abstinence from smoking and alcohol, and avoidance of caffeine is recommended. Supportive measures cannot be ignored. Table 4 summarizes these points.

Unfortunately, not every Lyme patient will regain his or her former health, and the management of refractory disease is presented in Table 5.

The ever growing number of new cases of this illness underscores the need for better preventive measures, and the many chronically afflicted patients who are resistant to treatment indicate that more research is needed in this area.

TABLE 4. Adjunctive Therapy

Recommended in All Lyme Patients:

Daily yogurt or acidophilus preparations
Multivitamins and B complex, 50 mg daily
Physical therapy and rehabilitation

Prescribe as Needed, Especially in More Severe Cases:

Analgesics and muscle relaxants
NSAIDs and remittive agents
Immune globulins and other immunotherapy if indicated
Antidepressants
Psychosocial evaluation and possibly refer for counseling

Contraindicated:

Alcohol use
Excessive caffeine intake
Any avoidable stresses
Significant sleep deprivation

TABLE 5. Refractory Disease

Persistent Signs and Symptoms That Respond to Antibiotic Therapy

Patients in this group improve on antibiotics, yet relapse repeatedly when medications are discontinued. Persistent infection, somehow resistant to treatment, has been demonstrated in some patients in this category. Recommended: study immune competence, search for concurrent infections, and reconsider the diagnosis

Options for Treatment

Longer duration, including open-ended maintenance therapy
Increased dose
Different drug
Change method of administration (oral to IV)
Supportive therapy as needed

Persistent Signs and Symptoms Not Responsive to Antibiotics

Reconsider the diagnosis
Supportive therapy based on symptoms
NSAIDs and hydroxychloroquine
Antidepressants, analgesics, and muscle relaxants
Synovectomy if the nonjoint symptoms are minimal
Psychiatric/psychometric evaluation
Long-term follow-up
Consider retreatment if condition changes

ROCKY MOUNTAIN SPOTTED FEVER

method of
KATHERINE MINNICK, M.D., and
CHARLES J. SCHLEUPNER, M.S., M.D.
University of Virginia School of Medicine
Salem, Virginia

Rocky Mountain spotted fever (RMSF) is the most common of the spotted fever group of rickettsial diseases. The causative agent, *Rickettsia rickettsii*, is inoculated into the accidental human host by adult ticks near the end of a 6- to 10-hour blood meal. Once in the dermal blood pool, *R. rickettsii* disseminate hematogenously, infecting vascular endothelial cells and thereby setting the stage for multiorgan dysfunction due to vasculitis. Clinical illness follows tick bite by approximately 1 week (range, 3 to 12 days) and is most frequently characterized by fever, headache, myalgias, nausea, vomiting, and anorexia. Rash, if present, may be scant and is delayed until day 3 to 5 of illness. The painless tick bite is often unnoticed and may not be reported. The classic triad of fever, rash, and history of tick bite is rarely encountered in early illness. Unfortunately, severe illness and death are more often associated with delay in treatment rather than delay in seeking medical attention. Therapy must be initiated with a presumptive clinical diagnosis based on understanding the disease and epidemiologic risks of the geographic locale.

EPIDEMIOLOGY

RMSF is associated with factors related to tick activity and human behavior. Incidence is highest among white boys 5 to 9 years of age with a second peak in men over 60 years old. Serving as vector and reservoir, hard-shelled ticks (*Dermacentor* spp., among others) are distributed throughout the United States, Mexico, and Central and South America. Disease prevalence is greater in southeastern states and western south central states; however, RMSF has been reported in every state except Hawaii and Vermont. Most cases are reported from April to October, with wintertime reports occurring in the south during longer warm seasons. Such off-season presentation often delays treatment and is associated with greater mortality. In natural areas, in partially developed suburbs and urban parks, and on unkempt property and roadsides, tall grasses and weeds serve as perches from which ticks await a passing animal. History of exposure to such an environment during the 12 days prior to illness is the key epidemiologic factor.

CLINICAL MANIFESTATIONS

Early signs and symptoms of RMSF—fever, headache, myalgias, gastrointestinal distress—are indistinguishable from more common, benign, self-limiting illnesses. When present, even if palmar or solar, rash is never pathognomonic. Just as the pathogenesis includes inoculation, local replication, spread, endothelial infection, and tissue damage, rash develops in several different stages. Pink macules that blanch with pressure, representing small areas of vasodilation, appear at the ankles and wrists, then the trunk, palms, and soles. With increased vascular permeability, the macules become papular. Advancing vasculitis may be accompanied by hemorrhage into the center of the maculopapule forming a petechia (41 to 59% of cases). Pathogenic events occurring in the skin are reflected in the systemic and pulmonary microvasculature. Altered endothelial function and vascular permeability lead to decreased oncotic pressure and plasma volume, and hypotension. Secondary prerenal azotemia and hyponatremia are common. Edema and hypoalbuminemia correlate with increased severity of illness. Intracardiac pressure monitoring usually reveals a low or normal pulmonary capillary wedge pressure and normal left ventricular function. Extensive infection of the pulmonary endothelium presents as noncardiogenic pulmonary edema, with associated cough and infiltrate on radiography. Severe pulmonary disease may require mechanical ventilation. Pneumonia and acute respiratory distress syndrome (ARDS) are major factors in fatal cases.

Also important in the outcome of RMSF is the involvement of the central nervous system (CNS). Encephalitis occurs in 26 to 28% of cases. Confusion or lethargy with possible progression to delirium, stupor, ataxia, seizures, and coma may appear. Focal deficits may occur. Cerebrospinal fluid reveals pleocytosis (usually 10 to 100 WBC per μl with mononuclear predominance), elevated protein, and normal glucose. Focal hepatic necrosis may lead to enzyme elevations, but hepatic failure does not occur. Jaundice and hyperbilirubinemia occur in some cases as a result of hemolysis. Myalgias reflecting rhabdomyolysis may be associated with striking serum creatinine kinase elevations. Vascular injury activates coagulation and fibrinolytic pathways and platelets; however, thrombotic infarction of tissue is seldom significant. Intravascular coagulation results in platelet consumption leading to thrombocytopenia, but hypofibrinogenemia is exceptional. Cutaneous necrosis and gangrene result from other mechanisms of reduced tissue perfusion. Anemia results primarily from blood loss through damaged vessels. Hemolysis may play a secondary role. Blood may be found in vomitus or stools.

The course of RMSF is slow, with hemorrhagic and severe neurologic signs appearing relatively late. Death occurs at day 8 to 15 of illness if treatment is delayed or absent. Survivors of severe illness may have long-term neurologic sequelae. Fulminant RMSF refers to a rare form with an unusually rapid course; death occurs 5 or fewer days from onset and is strikingly associated with glucose-6-phosphate deficiency in black males.

DIAGNOSIS

A presumptive diagnosis is made on clinical and epidemiologic grounds. Paired acute and convalescent sera should be collected for serologic diagnosis, but results will offer only retrospective confirmation. Skin biopsy of lesions (stained with fluorescent antibodies or immunoenzyme) may be useful in making an earlier diagnosis but should not delay therapy.

TREATMENT

Doxycycline (Vibramycin) is the drug of choice for treatment of RMSF, except when the patient is pregnant, allergic to tetracyclines, or, in the opinion of some, less than 9 years old. In adults and children weighing 45 kg or more, a 200-mg loading dose, followed by 100 mg every 12 hours, is effective. In children weighing less than 45 kg, a 2 mg per kg loading dose, followed by 1 mg per kg every 12 hours, is given. Tetracyclines are avoided in pregnancy because of the effect on fetal bones and teeth. Repetitive administration of tetracycline has been associated with dental staining in children; however, the risk of dental staining after a single short course is minimal. Divalent or trivalent compounds found in antacids, milk, iron, or iron-containing preparations markedly decrease absorption. Chloramphenicol (Chloromycetin) has been used extensively, although not as effectively as doxycycline. Dosing is 50 mg (oral) or 75 mg (intravenous) per kg per day in four divided doses. The most important toxic effects occur in the bone marrow. More common is a dose related and reversible depression of all cell lines. Rare, but generally fatal, is an idiosyncratic aplastic anemia (1 in 50,000 administrations). Monitoring of serum levels and complete blood counts is recommended when this drug must be used. Antimicrobials are given intravenously in severe cases or when nausea and vomiting are present. Response with defervescence may be expected in 48 to 72 hours in milder cases but is delayed in severe illness. Treatment should be continued for 48 hours after defervescence or for a minimum of 7 days. Supportive therapy is given as demanded by the severity of illness. Mild illness treated early may be managed on an outpatient basis. For more severe cases, hospitalization and careful monitoring of vital signs and intravascular volume status are necessary. Intravascular coagulopathy, when present, is best treated by combating its underlying cause. Thrombosis is rare and heparin should be avoided.

PREVENTION

Prevention is best accomplished by avoiding exposure with protective clothing, by careful inspection with prompt tick removal, and by maintenance of tick-free pets. Tick removal requires firm traction with a forceps to include mouth parts. Extracted ticks should be handled carefully, as fluids and tissues may have large quantities of rickettsiae. No vaccine is available for prevention of RMSF. Routine antimicrobial prophylaxis after tick bite is unsound on epidemiologic grounds.

RUBELLA AND CONGENITAL RUBELLA

method of
LAWRENCE R. STANBERRY, M.D., Ph.D., and
SHIRLEY A. FLOYD-REISING, Ph.D.
Children's Hospital Medical Center
Cincinnati, Ohio

Rubella (German measles) is a systemic infectious disease caused by an RNA virus whose only natural reservoir is human beings. Postnatally acquired infection may be subclinical or produce an acute illness with or without rash. Infection during early pregnancy can cause in utero infection resulting in congenital anomalies. This once common infection is now rarely seen in countries where the rubella vaccine is widely used. Rubella, however, should still be considered in the differential diagnosis of exanthematous illnesses and congenital malfunctions.

POSTNATALLY ACQUIRED INFECTION

Approximately 25% of infections are subclinical. For patients with clinically recognized illness, symptoms manifest after a 14 to 21-day incubation period. Malaise and tender lymphadenopathy (usually including suboccipital, postauricular, and cervical nodes) may precede onset of rash by 3 to 4 days. Patients may experience low-grade fever, headache, anorexia, coryza, sore throat, and/or mild conjunctivitis. These symptoms are observed more often in adolescents and adults than in children and generally subside shortly after the rash develops. The exanthem typically begins as pinkish red maculopapules on the face and neck and spreads to the trunk and extremities as the rash fades from the face and neck. Discrete lesions on the trunk may coalesce to form a more uniform red rash. The rash usually fades within 3 to 4 days and uncommonly can cause a mild desquamation. Nontender lymphadenopathy may persist for several weeks after resolution of the acute illness. Complications of childhood rubella are rare and include arthritis, encephalitis, and thrombocytopenia. Joint involvement occurs commonly in adolescents and adults and may persist for 5 to 10 days but resolves spontaneously and without sequelae.

Mild scarlet fever can produce a rubella-like illness, as can infections caused by the enteroviruses, measles, and parvovirus B19.

CONGENITAL RUBELLA

Rubella during pregnancy can result in fetal infection. The extent of fetal damage is influenced by when during gestation the infection occurs. Infection in the first 2 months of pregnancy causes intrauterine death or serious malformations in up to 85% of fetuses. Risk of malformations and significant fetal injury persists through the third month of pregnancy, but evidence of fetal injury is rarely observed after the fourth month. Infection in the first trimester may result in a variety of congenital abnormalities, including growth retardation; ocular, cardiac, and central nervous system defects; deafness; hepatic injury; splenic enlargement; thrombocytopenia; pneumonitis; and bone lesions. Infants who survive the neonatal period are at risk of developing diabetes mellitus, thyroid dysfunction, and psychiatric disorders.

The differential diagnosis of congenital rubella includes perinatal infections due to cytomegalovirus, herpes simplex virus, toxoplasma, and *Treponema pallidum* (syphilis).

EPIDEMIOLOGY

Rubella is spread via the respiratory route. Patients may be contagious from 7 days before to 14 days after the rash develops (typically 5 days before to 6 days after onset of rash). Infants with congenital rubella may shed virus for years, although they are rarely contagious after 1 year of age. Rubella has a worldwide distribution and is endemic in large cities. Before widespread use of the rubella vaccine, epidemics occurred irregularly at 6- to 9-year intervals.

LABORATORY DIAGNOSIS

Virus isolation has limited applicability for routine diagnosis of rubella, and there are few clinical situations for which culture is indicated. Unadapted rubella virus does not produce significant cytopathic effect (CPE) in cell tissue culture, and isolation of this agent may take weeks to complete. In the event that virus isolation is required for situations of rubella cases with severe complications (e.g., encephalitis or thrombocytopenia), specimens should be collected as early as possible after onset of illness. Rubella virus is relatively unstable, and specimens require transport in a protein-containing collection medium.

Serologic techniques for detection of antibodies to rubella virus provide the most reliable method for laboratory diagnosis of acute and congenital infections. There are a number of serologic methods available for the measurement of antibodies to rubella virus. These include hemagglutination inhibition (HI), complement fixation (CF), passive hemagglutination (PHA), enzyme immunoassay (EIA), indirect immunofluorescent assay (IFA), and latex agglutination (LA). IgG antibodies usually persist for the lifetime of the patient, whereas IgM antibodies are present for 5 to 6 weeks after onset of illness. The test that has been used most frequently in the past is the HI test, and it is still the standard by which other methods are compared for sensitivity and specificity. Paired acute- and convalescent-phase sera must be tested together to diagnose infection accurately. The HI test detects both the early IgM and the later-appearing IgG. CF antibodies become detectable a week or more after onset of rash (5 to 7 days after HI antibody appears), but CF antibodies do not persist as long as HI antibodies. The CF test is a useful backup diagnostic test in those cases where acute-phase serum was collected too late to detect an HI antibody rise.

Other tests have increasingly supplanted HI as routine methods for detection of immune status. Both PHA and LA are sensitive and specific and detect rubella antibody, which appears within a few days after acute illness onset and thereafter persists indefinitely. EIA and IFA are equally as accurate and also afford the capability to detect rubella-specific IgM antibody, reflecting recent infection. Detection of specific IgM is considered indicative of recent infection, but all IgM assays may occasionally render false-positive results. IgM serodiagnosis can occur in many other infections, including infectious mononucleosis and parvovirus B19, which may be confused clinically with rubella.

Of the aforementioned tests, the HI, PHA, EIA, and LA methodologies are the most useful to assess an individual's rubella immune status. Accurate diagnosis of rubella infection in the first trimester of pregnancy requires rubella serodiagnosis with acute- and convalescent-phase sera. Traditionally, a fourfold or higher titer rise through testing by HI or CF tests has been used as the criterion for diagnostic significance. The diagnosis can sometimes be established by demonstrating specific rubella IgM antibodies. However, IgM antibodies have a short (5-day) half-life and wane rapidly after the patient recovers from acute illness. A seroconversion is diagnostic and conclusive for recent rubella infection. Patients without clinical symptoms but with diagnostic serology should have their infection confirmed through the absence of late-rising PHA or CF antibodies in the first serum sample. Congenital rubella infection is confirmed serologically by demonstrating the persistence of rubella antibody passively transferred from the mother and, also, by detecting specific rubella IgM antibody in the newborn. Persistence of rubella antibody beyond 6 months of age, after the loss of passively acquired antibody, is highly suggestive of congenital rubella infection.

TREATMENT

Management of the acute illness is supportive. Use of gamma globulin in the exposed pregnant woman does not prevent fetal infection. There are no antiviral drugs effective in the treatment of postnatal or congenital rubella.

RUBELLA VACCINE

The live rubella virus vaccine (RA 27/3 strain) is available as a single vaccine or as a component of the trivalent measles-mumps-rubella (MMR) vaccine. For subjects older than 1 year of age, a single dose of the vaccine induces protective immunity in greater than 95% of recipients. At present, it is recommended that immunocompetent infants at 12 months of age be immunized with the rubella vaccine contained in the trivalent MMR. A second dose of the MMR is recommended at 4 to 5 years of age (Advisory Committee on Immunization Practices) or at 12 years of age (American Academy of Pediatrics). The rubella (MMR) vaccine should be given to asymptomatic HIV-infected children. The vaccine is contraindicated in patients with impaired cell-mediated immunity (excluding HIV-infected subjects) and persons with a history of serious reaction to egg or neomycin. The vaccine is also not given to pregnant women, and it is advised that female recipients not become pregnant for 3 months afterward. Inadvertent immunization during pregnancy occasionally results in infection of the fetus, but no congenital abnormalities have been noted. Immunization should be postponed for 3 months after receiving gamma globulin products. Serious adverse reactions to the vaccine are uncommon. A mild exanthematous illness 2 to 3 weeks after immunization is occasionally noted, and self-limited arthralgias have been reported in 10 to 20% of adult vaccine recipients.

MEASLES
(Rubeola)

method of
PATRICIA A. HUGHES, D.O., and
MARTHA L. LEPOW, M.D.
Albany Medical College
Albany, New York

Measles is one of the most significant causes of childhood mortality in history, and it remains an important cause of death in children in many developing countries. Measles epidemics in developed countries in the 1980s and 1990s and the ongoing problem of disease in developing countries have produced renewed interest in the study and eradication of this virus.

Measles virus is an encapsulated, single-strand 15.9-kilobase RNA morbillivirus in the family of Paramyxoviridae. Humans are the only reservoir for measles. In contrast to many other viruses, measles is relatively genetically stable, which allows for continued protection from both remote infection and vaccination.

Epidemiology. It is estimated that 50 million people worldwide are infected annually with measles, with approximately 1 million resultant deaths. Prior to measles vaccine licensure, everyone except those in certain isolated regions of the world became infected between ages 5 and 9 years. After widespread use of the measles vaccine, it became apparent that epidemics occurred in select populations of school age children and college students. Of particular concern, however, are recent outbreaks among preschool children. In the United States and developing countries, both serologic and epidemiologic data indicate that infants are susceptible to measles at approximately 9 months of age and 6 months of age, respectively. One reason for earlier susceptibility is that mothers who received measles vaccine transfer less antibody to their infants than do mothers who have had natural disease. Urban living, crowding, and limited access to health care are also important factors influencing the trend toward earlier susceptibility. Measles is a winter/spring disease in temperate climates. There is no sexual or racial bias. However, it has been suggested that complications from disease may be greater in male patients.

In nonimmune individuals measles is extremely contagious. It is transmitted by aerosolized respiratory droplets. Small droplets can remain infectious in the air for some time. Larger droplets are acquired by direct contact with either the respiratory epithelium or conjunctiva.

The small number of primary vaccine failures, waning immunity, and most importantly unimmunized individuals explain outbreaks of measles occurring in vaccinated populations.

PATHOGENESIS

Measles attaches to the respiratory epithelium via one of its structural envelope proteins, hemagglutinin. The virus then spreads and multiplies in macrophages in regional lymph nodes. This is followed by a primary viremia with extensive replication of virus at both the initial infection site and endothelial and epithelial cells of many organs, and throughout the reticuloendothelial system (RES). Finally, secondary viremia occurs and is associated with clinical symptoms. The time course from infection to symptoms is approximately 10 days.

The appearance of symptoms also correlates with the onset of the host immune response. By the time the rash appears, specific viral antibody, mononuclear cell infiltration at sites of viral replication, and virus-specific T cells can all be detected. The virus is then efficiently cleared. Individuals with cell-mediated immune defects fail to clear the secondary viremia and often succumb to the disease.

The specific immune response to measles causes a subsequent immunosuppression even in normal hosts. The immunologic abnormality is characterized on the cellular level by a poor response to mitogens, abnormal lymphokine production, and a decrease in T cell number with a normal T cell ratio. In addition, patients fail to respond to delayed-type hypersensitivity antigens, such as tuberculin skin testing, and are susceptible to secondary infection, resulting in most of the significant morbidity and mortality from measles.

Multinucleated giant cells that occur as a result of cell fusion are seen on pathologic examination. They are called Warthin-Finkeldey cells when they appear in the RES.

CLINICAL FINDINGS

Measles is a highly contagious systemic disease. After an asymptomatic incubation period of approximately 10 days, the infected child develops mild respiratory symptoms that can be confused with a cold. One to two days later a cough, coryza, conjunctivitis with severe photophobia, and occasionally nausea appear.

Three to four days after the onset of respiratory symptoms, a fine, bluish-white enanthem called Koplik spots appears on the buccal mucosa. Within 24 hours a generalized, occasionally hemorrhagic, erythematous rash appears at the hairline and in 2 days spreads cephalocaudad over the entire body, including palms and soles. By the third day the rash fades in the same order as it appeared, leaving behind a brownish discoloration. The duration of fever from onset is about 7 days. Infectivity decreases markedly by the second day of full body rash.

Measles can be modified in children who receive a preventive dose of immunoglobulin in an amount insufficient to abort the infection. Infants with waning maternal immunity may also have modified disease. Children who received inactivated measles vaccine in the 1960s and were later exposed to wild or rarely vaccine virus could develop an unusually severe illness with high fever, rash, pneumonia or pleuritis without prodromal respiratory symptoms.

Laboratory examinations that support the diagnosis include virus isolation and antibody testing. IgM antibody can be measured during the first week of illness, while acute and convalescent sera can be obtained to demonstrate a fourfold rise in IgG antibodies. Other tests include hemagglutination inhibition, which correlates well with neutralization. An enzyme-linked immunosorbent assay (ELISA) is the most widely used. Leukopenia, lymphopenia, and thrombocytopenia are characteristic.

Differential diagnosis includes Kawasaki's disease, streptococcal and staphylococcal toxic shock syndrome, and drug eruptions.

COMPLICATIONS

Common complications are otitis media, croup, bacterial tracheitis, and secondary pneumonia due to pneumococcus, staphylococcus, streptococcus, and *Haemophilus influenzae,* as well as herpes simplex virus. Activation of pulmonary tuberculosis has been noted to occur following measles. Children with congenital or acquired immunodeficiencies are at serious risk of pneumonia and death from the natural disease. No teratogenic effects have been described.

There are three types of central nervous complications. Approximately 1 in 1000 children develop acute encephalomyelitis between the second and sixth day after onset of rash, with death occurring within 24 hours in approximately 15%. Subacute sclerosing panencephalitis occurs after a prolonged latent period, with insidious onset of mental deterioration, motor dysfunction, seizures, coma, and death within 2 years. A delayed type, rapidly fatal, acute encephalitis appearing 1 to 7 months after infection occurs in immunocompromised patients. Polymerase chain reaction has been used to diagnose the presence of measles virus in brain tissue in several patients.

Thrombocytopenia commonly occurs but rarely with enough severity to produce serious bleeding. Myocarditis is rare. Diarrheal disease is more common in underdeveloped countries but is often associated with poor outcome. Conditions putatively associated with measles include multiple sclerosis, chronic autoimmune hepatitis, Paget's disease of bone, and otosclerosis.

TREATMENT

No specific treatment exists for measles. Though not approved by the Food and Drug Administration for this indication, ribavirin (Virazole) is effective in vitro. Limited data from underdeveloped countries suggest reduction in severity and duration of disease when ribavirin is given intravenously during the pre-eruptive phase. It has been used in measles-associated delayed acute encephalitis and in immunocompromised children.

Although vitamin A deficiency rarely occurs in the United States, it is associated with poor outcome from measles. The American Academy of Pediatrics recommends that oral vitamin A supplementation of 200,000 IU for children 1 to 2 years of age and 100,000 IU for those 6 months to 1 year of age be given to all infants hospitalized with measles. The dose should be repeated in 24 hours and at 4 weeks in children with ophthalmologic evidence of vitamin A deficiency. These doses are 100 to 200 times the recommended dietary allowance, and patients should be monitored for toxicity.

PREVENTION

Measles vaccine is safe, cost effective, and highly efficacious, with a 95% seroconversion rate. Vaccine strains presently in use are all derived from the original Edmonston strain but are less virulent through serial passage in chicken embryos. It is given as MMR, a trivalent preparation along with mumps and rubella. In 1979 a heat stabilizer was added to the preparation, making reduced efficacy as a result of improper handling less likely.

A two-dose regimen of measles vaccine is currently recommended. The first dose is given at 12 months of age with a second dose at 5 years of age prior to school entry or at 12 years of age. At times of epidemic, measles vaccine may be given as a single preparation at 6 months of age, followed by a booster of MMR at 15 months.

Children with defects in cell-mediated immunity and pregnant women should not receive measles vaccine. However, individuals infected with human immunodeficiency virus (HIV) should receive measles vaccine. Symptomatic HIV-infected individuals exposed to measles should receive postexposure immunoglobulin regardless of immunization status. Contrary to prior beliefs, a recent report in the *New England Journal of Medicine* demonstrated that measles vaccine could safely be given to children with a history of anaphylaxis to eggs. If an individual has received standard-dose immunoglobulin, vaccine should be postponed for 8 months. If a patient has received high-dose immunoglobulin for treatment of Kawasaki's disease or immune thrombocytopenia purpura, immunization should be delayed for 11 months.

In an attempt to achieve antibody responses in infants with circulating maternal antibody to measles, a higher-titer Edmonston Zagreb strain vaccine, attenuated by serial passage in human diploid cells, has been used. Of concern, however, was an increased mortality due to secondary infections in female recipients. In developing countries, when vitamin A supplementation was given orally at the same time as the measles vaccine, there was a reduced seroconversion rate from the vaccine.

POSTEXPOSURE PROPHYLAXIS

Measles vaccine can be given within 72 hours of exposure and may still be protective. Immune globulin given within 6 days of exposure can prevent or modify clinical symptoms. It is given intramuscularly at doses of 0.25 mL per kg in otherwise healthy individuals and 0.5 mL per kg for immunocompromised people. The maximum dose is 15 mL.

TETANUS

method of
JAMES P. RICHARDSON, M.D., M.P.H.
University of Maryland School of Medicine
Baltimore, Maryland

Tetanus, one of the oldest afflictions of humankind, results from infection with the anaerobic gram-positive organism *Clostridium tetani*. The manifestations of the disease are caused by the neurotoxin elaborated by the organism, not by the infection itself. Tetanus usually presents as increased tone of the masseter muscles, or trismus, hence the former name of lockjaw.

ETIOLOGY

The causative organism of tetanus, *C. tetani,* exists as spores that are resistant to heating and disinfectants and hence are nearly ubiquitous. Spores have been found in animal and human feces, and in soil, dust, human dwellings, and hospitals.

EPIDEMIOLOGY

Tetanus is a rare disease in the United States, with an annual incidence of about 0.02 per 100,000. About 50 cases are reported to the Centers for Disease Control and Prevention each year, two thirds of whom are age 50 years and older. Probably many cases of tetanus go unreported, however. There is a slightly higher incidence of tetanus in men. Today the overall case-fatality rate is about 20% to 30%, but this increases with increasing age, reaching 52% in those older than 60 years.

Worldwide, the disease is much more common due to lower levels of immunization. More than one half million infants succumb to neonatal tetanus every year.

PATHOGENESIS

Tetanus spores gain entrance to the body through injuries to the skin. These injuries are often so minor that they do not result in any medical attention (e.g., a prick from a thorn bush, a minor puncture wound). Because *C. tetani* is an obligate anaerobe, the spores will grow only in areas of low oxygen tensions, such as occurs with pressure sores, puncture wounds, or gangrene. Growing, or vegetative, *C. tetani* elaborate tetanospasmin, one of the most potent neurotoxins known, which then spreads via axons to the central nervous system (CNS).

Tetanospasmin becomes bound to gangliosides within the CNS, suppressing inhibitory influences on the motor neurons and inhibiting acetylcholine release at the motor end-plate. This results in reflex irritability, rigidity, and disinhibition of spinal cord reflex arcs. Autonomic hyperactivity is common, resulting from direct stimulation by tetanospasmin. Hypertension and tachycardia, alternating with periods of hypotension and bradycardia, may occur.

CLINICAL PRESENTATION

The incubation period of tetanus is usually from 3 days to 3 weeks, but tetanus can occur several months after an injury. Cases with shorter incubation periods tend to be the most severe.

Generalized disease is the most common presentation of tetanus (Table 1). Common presenting complaints include trismus, neck rigidity, stiffness, dysphagia, restlessness, and reflex spasms. Risus sardonicus is the characteristic grimace that patients with tetanus may display. These patients show raised eyebrows and a wrinkled forehead with the corners of the mouth pulled up. Muscle rigidity usually starts with the jaw and facial muscles and then spreads to the extensor muscles of the limbs. Neonatal tetanus presents as an inability to suck 3 to 10 days after birth. Tetanic seizures, manifested by tonic muscle contractions, may occur in generalized tetanus. Tetanic seizures differ from major motor seizures in that patients with tetanic seizures remain conscious. This activity may be provoked by noise, light, or examination of the patient. These seizures are extremely painful and portend a poor prognosis if frequent.

As the disease progresses, hypoxia may result from involvement of the respiratory muscles. Airway control is very important because laryngospasm may cause further compromise (see later).

Two much less common types of tetanus are localized tetanus and cephalic tetanus. Localized tetanus is characterized by painful spasms of muscles in close proximity to the site of injury. This disorder is usually self-limiting and lasts less than 2 weeks, but progression to generalized disease can occur if untreated. Cephalic tetanus is a frequently severe form of localized tetanus. Minor head trauma or chronic otitis media may be the mode of entry of the organism. Cephalic tetanus may present as single or multiple cranial nerve palsies or trismus and will often progress to generalized tetanus if not treated.

TABLE 1. **Presentations of Tetanus**

Generalized Disease

Trismus
Risus sardonicus
Dysphagia
Opisthotonos
Isolated cranial nerve palsies
Rigidity or stiffness in an extremity
Neck stiffness
Restlessness
Tetanic seizures
Poor sucking (newborns)

Localized Disease

Rigidity or stiffness in an extremity

Cephalic Disease

Single or multiple cranial nerve palsies

DIAGNOSIS

Tetanus is determined by clinical diagnosis; there are no laboratory tests specific for the disease. A history of a predisposing injury and the development of the usual clinical features make the diagnosis clear in most cases. However, as noted earlier, a history of injury is not always present. Laboratory tests such as complete blood counts and routine blood chemistry tests are not helpful. Cultures are positive in only 32 to 50% of patients, and in any event treatment cannot wait for their completion. Absence of any sensory deficits and a clear sensorium support the diagnosis of tetanus. A well-documented history of primary immunization and a booster immunization within the last 10 years makes the diagnosis of tetanus much less likely.

Whereas established generalized tetanus is easily recognized, the diagnosis of early tetanus can present some difficulty. Cranial nerve involvement is common and may confuse the physician. Trismus may result from intraoral disease or an acute reaction to a phenothiazine drug such as chlorpromazine (Thorazine). Muscular stiffness can also be a manifestation of strychnine poisoning, meningitis, hepatic encephalopathy, rabies, and conversion reaction. A delay in the diagnosis of tetanus has occurred in patients presenting with dysphagia. Rigid abdominal muscles may simulate an acute abdomen.

TREATMENT

Whenever possible, patients with suspected tetanus should be transferred to a facility with experience with this disease. Patients should be kept in a quiet, dark environment. Treatment has the following goals: (1) neutralization of circulating toxin, (2) elimination of the source of toxin by careful surgical excision, (3) prevention of respiratory and metabolic complications, and (4) prevention of muscle spasms.

Tetanus antitoxin should be given to prevent further fixation of the toxin to the central nervous system, although it will not reduce manifestations already present. Three thousand to 6000 units of human tetanus immune globulin (TIG) (Hyper-Tet) should be given intramuscularly as soon as possible. Some authorities recommend giving some of this near the site of the wound. Immunization with tetanus-diphtheria toxoid (Td) or diphtheria toxoid–pertussis vaccine–tetanus toxoid (DPT) (DTwP), as appropriate, also should be given, at a site different from that for TIG (Table 2).

Débridement is important for several reasons. Débridement removes existing organisms, creates an aerobic environment unfavorable for further growth, and secures specimens for culture. Débridement should be delayed until several hours after the administration of antitoxin because tetanospasmin may be released into the bloodstream. Antibiotic therapy is essential to sterilize the wound and reduce bacteremia. The antibiotic of choice is now metronidazole (Flagyl), given at a dose of 7.5 mg per kg every 6 hours after a loading dose of 15 mg per kg has been given. Acceptable alternatives are doxycycline (Vibramycin) and imipenem cilistatin (Primaxin). Penicillin, once the drug of choice, should not be used because it may worsen gamma-aminobutyric acid–induced hypertonia.

TABLE 2. **Guide to Tetanus Prophylaxis in Routine Wound Management**

History of Adsorbed Tetanus Toxoid (doses)	Clean, Minor Wounds		All Other Wounds*	
	Td†	TIG	Td†	TIG
Unknown or < three	Yes	No	Yes	Yes
≥ three‡	No§	No	No‖	No

*Such as, but not limited to, wounds contaminated from dirt, feces, soil, saliva, etc.; puncture wounds, avulsions; and wounds resulting from missiles, crushing, burns, and frostbite.

†For children under 7 years old; DPT (DT, if pertussis vaccine is contraindicated) is preferred to tetanus toxoid alone. For persons 7 years old and older, TD is preferred to tetanus toxoid alone.

‡If only three doses of fluid toxoid have been received, a fourth dose of toxoid, preferably an adsorbed toxoid, should be given.

§Yes, if more than 10 years since last dose.

‖Yes, if more than 5 years since last dose. (More frequent boosters are not needed and can accentuate side effects.)

From the Advisory Committee on Immunization Practices (ACIP), The Centers for Disease Control and Prevention: Diphtheria, tetanus, pertussis: Guidelines for vaccine prophylaxis and other preventive measures. MMWR Morb Mortal Wkly Rep *40*:1–28, 1991.

Oxygenation is assured by protecting the airway. In all but the mildest of cases, prophylactic intubation should be initiated early. Intubation will usually require sedation with a benzodiazepine (e.g., lorazepam [Ativan], 2 mg intravenously) and neuromuscular blockade (e.g., vecuronium [Norcuron], 0.08 to 0.1 mg per kg). Patients requiring more than 10 days of intubation or who have generalized seizures should undergo elective tracheostomy. An oropharyngeal airway will allow removal of secretions and prevent biting in mild cases that do not require intubation.

Control of tonic spasms and tetanic seizures is best achieved with the benzodiazepines. Additional benefits are that these drugs produce sedation and amnesia. Diazepam (Valium) can be given at a dose of 0.5 mg per kg to 15 mg per kg per day intravenously. Alternatively, continuous infusions of lorazepam (Ativan) at a dose of 0.1 to 2.0 mg per hour or midazolam (Versed) at a dose of 0.01 to 1.0 mg per kg per hour can be given. The goal is to control muscle rigidity and inhibition of spasm as well as produce the desired level of sedation.

In those patients whose muscle spasms do not respond to sedation, neuromuscular blocking agents, such as vecuronium (Norcuron), are often necessary. These patients will require assisted ventilation, often for several days or weeks. Because neuromuscular blocking agents prevent skeletal muscle movements only and do not reduce pain or provide sedation, it is essential that these patients be monitored very closely for adequate pain relief.

Later in the course of the disease cardiovascular instability may develop through effects on the autonomic nervous system. Both alpha-adrenergic and beta-adrenergic blockade may be necessary with phentolamine (Regitine) and propranolol (Inderal) for treatment of hypertension and tachycardia. Brady-cardia may develop as well, requiring placement of a pacemaker. Hypotension may require monitoring of cardiac output and intravenous fluids or pressor agents.

COMPLICATIONS

Supportive care is critical to the prevention of complications. Most of these complications are those common to immobile patients. Attention to nutritional status and frequent turning of the patient will prevent pressure sores. Low-dose heparin should be administered to prevent deep venous thromboses and pulmonary emboli. Physical therapy should be begun as soon as possible to prevent contractures. Fractures and dislocations may result from tetanic seizures, requiring orthopedic management.

Most patients will eventually make a full recovery, but some patients remain hypertonic. It is important that recovering patients complete a primary series of immunizations because having had the disease does not confer immunity (Table 3).

PREVENTION

Prevention of tetanus through immunization is the key to the elimination of tetanus. It is important to distinguish between primary and booster immunization, however. A never-immunized patient requires two additional doses of tetanus-diphtheria toxoid (Td) beyond the dose given when the wound is treated (see Table 3). Wounded patients who have never been immunized may require tetanus immunoglobulin (TIG) (see Table 2). The elderly population is particularly susceptible, because so many have never been immunized or because their immunity has lapsed.

Physicians should use a case-finding approach to increase tetanus immunization rates. Reminders placed at physicians' desks or computer-generated reminders attached to charts or patients' bills have improved immunization rates. Tetanus-diphtheria toxoid should be given whenever tetanus immunization is necessary, to ensure immunity to diphtheria as well as tetanus.

Td is a safe vaccine. Adverse reactions consist primarily of local edema, tenderness, and fever. Anaphy-

TABLE 3. **Routine Diphtheria and Tetanus Immunization Schedule for Persons 7 Years and Older**

Dose	Age/Interval	Product
Primary 1	First dose	Td
Primary 2	4–8 wk after first dose*	Td
Primary 3	6–12 mon after second dose*	Td
Boosters	Every 10 years after last dose	Td

*Prolonging the interval does not require restarting series.

From the Advisory Committee on Immunization Practices (ACIP), The Centers for Disease Control and Prevention: Diphtheria, tetanus, pertussis: Guidelines for vaccine prophylaxis and other preventive measures. MMWR Morb Mortal Wkly Rep *40*:1–28, 1991.

lactoid reactions are rare. Most adverse reactions occur in persons with evidence of hyperimmunization. The only contraindications to Td toxoid are a history of a neurologic sequela or a severe hypersensitivity reaction following a previous dose.

To reduce neonatal tetanus and protect the mother, pregnant women who are due for a booster should receive Td, preferably during the last two trimesters. TIG should be given to pregnant women only when clearly indicated.

PERTUSSIS

method of
MAUREEN KAYS, M.D.
University of Florida
Gainesville, Florida

and

MICHAEL E. PICHICHERO, M.D.
University of Rochester Medical Center
Rochester, New York

Pertussis, or whooping cough, is a very contagious, acute respiratory tract illness affecting all age groups but with the greatest morbidity in young children. The epidemiology, diagnosis, and prevention of this illness are undergoing rapid reassessment. Pertussis incidence has been on the rise in the United States since 1980. Recognition of high pertussis prevalence in adolescents and adults, the availability of improved molecular diagnostic techniques to detect infection, and the licensure of new acellular, purified pertussis vaccines represent the advances in recent years.

MICROBIOLOGY

Bordetella pertussis is a small, gram-negative coccobacillus with fastidious growth requirements. Recovery is enhanced by direct inoculation of nasopharyngeal secretions, taken with a calcium alginate swab, onto selective media such as Bordet-Gengou, modified Strainer-Scholte, or Regan-Lowe charcoal agar. Colonies appear after 3 to 7 days, making alternative diagnostic methods valuable (see Diagnosis). *Bordetella parapertussis* is an important etiologic agent of a pertussis syndrome in some areas.

Bordetella pertussis expresses multiple antigenic and biologically active proteins that are postulated to play a role in disease. These are listed in Table 1. Fimbriae (FIM), filamentous hemagglutinin (FHA), and pertactin (PRN) are important for attachment of the organism to ciliated respiratory epithelial cells. Pertussis toxin (PT) and adenylate cyclase adversely act on the host immune response, allowing infection to continue after attachment. The toxins heat-labile toxin (HLT), lipopolysaccharides (LPS), and tracheal cytotoxin (TCT) have been implicated in the cytotoxic effects seen in the respiratory tract. Tracheal cytotoxin appears to cause the most epithelial damage.

EPIDEMIOLOGY

Pertussis is highly contagious, with an attack rate of 50% to 100%. Transmission is dependent on aerosolized droplets from an infected case. Environmental survival is limited. Humans are the only host. Females have an increased risk of illness that increases with age. Epidemics occur every 3 to 5 years with a late summer/early fall peak; the cycle has not been affected by immunization. Worldwide there are at least 51 million cases of pertussis with 60,000 deaths a year. The advent of the whole cell vaccine (DTwP) in the United States decreased the incidence of whooping cough from a high of 265,000 cases with 7000 deaths in 1934 to a low of 11,000 cases with 7 deaths in 1976.

Since 1981, there has been an overall increase in the incidence of pertussis in the United States (Figure 1). The largest increase is found predominately in immunized adolescents and adults; however, disease incidence remains highest in children under 1 year of age. Incidence calculations of pertussis do not indicate the true picture owing to underreporting, undue reliance on laboratory diagnosis, and atypical undiagnosed disease. Increased surveillance and improved diagnostic tools such as polymerase chain reaction (PCR) detection methods and serology techniques suggest that approximately 25% of adolescents and adults with cough of 7 or more days have pertussis. Of concern are pertussis epidemics that include children with age-appropriate immunization. In a 1993 outbreak in Cincinnati, 75% of infants diagnosed with whooping cough had received one or more doses of DTwP. Eighty-five percent of the infected 6- to 12-year-old children had received four or more doses of DTwP.

The changing epidemiology of pertussis can be explained by several factors. DTwP vaccine–induced immunity clearly wanes rapidly such that most children beyond 9 to 10 years of age, adolescents, and adults are at risk for infection. DTwP efficacy has wide confidence limits (45% to 95%), and this may reflect the fact that DTwP is more effective at preventing severe pertussis in endemic conditions than in preventing mild-to-moderate disease, especially when disease is widespread.

CLINICAL

The incubation period of pertussis ranges from 6 to 20 days (mean, 7 days). Illness has three phases: catarrhal,

TABLE 1. **Biologically Active Proteins of *Bordetella pertussis* Infection**

Protein	Properties
Pertussis toxin (PT) or lymphocytosis-promoting factor (LPF)	Envelope protein with multiple biologic roles
Filamentous hemagglutinin (FHA)	Cell-surface protein with adhesion properties
Pertactin (PRN), a 69-kD protein	Outer membrane protein with adhesion properties
Fimbriae (FIM) or agglutinogen (AGG)	6 types: type 1 is common to all strains with adhesion properties
Adenylate cyclase	A hemolysin, extracytoplasmic, impairs host phagocytosis
Heat-labile toxin (HLT)	Cytoplasmic toxin
Lipopolysaccharide (LPS)	Envelope-related toxin
Tracheal cytotoxin (TCT)	Cytoplasmic toxin

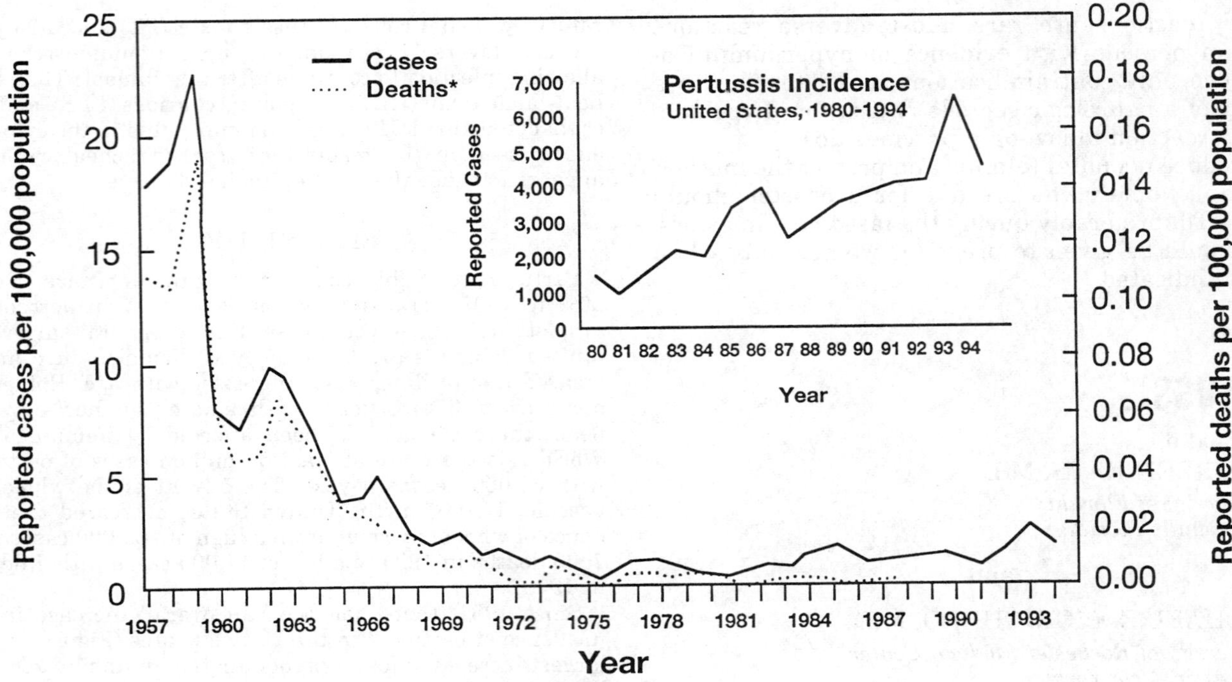

* Data on mortality are not available in all years.

Figure 1. Pertussis incidence and mortality, United States, 1957–1994. (From MMWR *44*:525–529, 1995.)

paroxysmal, and convalescent (Table 2). The total course of illness generally lasts 6 to 8 weeks, although in China pertussis is known as the 100-day cough. The specific clinical manifestations depend on age and immunization status. *Bordetella parapertussis* produces a less severe and shorter clinical illness.

The catarrhal stage is marked by upper respiratory tract symptoms with rhinorrhea, mild cough, low-grade fever and conjunctival injection. These findings are nonspecific and resemble the common cold; therefore the diagnosis of pertussis is not usually considered.

During the paroxysmal stage (2 to 4 weeks), coughing predominates. The characteristic inspiratory whoop occurs after a repetitive spasmodic or paroxysmal cough; post-tussive emesis often follows. Cyanosis and apnea are not uncommon in children less than 1 year of age. Infants are most susceptible to morbidity during this stage. Pneumonia is the most frequent complication and is responsible for 90% of pertussis-associated deaths in children less than 3 years of age. Seizures, encephalopathy, and coma are thought to be either due to cough-related hypoxia or possi-bly due to direct toxin effects. The repetitive coughing attacks are exhausting, leading to lethargy and anorexia.

The final convalescent stage lasts 3 to 4 weeks with decreasing frequency of coughing episodes. However, cough may persist for months to a year. Coughing paroxysms often recur during viral respiratory infections for several years following the initial infection.

Partially immune patients, predominately adolescents and adults, often have a prolonged catarrhal stage without a true paroxysmal stage. The illness may resemble a nonspecific viral or *Mycoplasma* or *Chlamydia* bronchitis.

DIAGNOSIS

During the paroxysmal cough stage, diagnosis can be straightforward clinically. For any patient with cough longer than 7 days, pertussis should be considered in the differential diagnosis. Coughs that patients or parents characterize as severe, spasmodic, or staccato or cough that results in vomiting should raise the diagnosis of pertussis as a significant possibility and prompt laboratory testing.

Leukocytosis (20,000 to 50,000/mm³) with a marked lymphocytosis occurs late in the catarrhal phase and during the paroxysmal phase but is not a consistent finding. Partially immune hosts do not usually respond with a marked leukocytosis. The "gold standard" for diagnosis is culture of *B. pertussis* from the nasopharynx. Culture is best performed with a calcium alginate swab of the nasopharynx left in place until a cough occurs. Suction of deep nasopharyngeal secretions with a No. 5 or 8 French catheter cut to a 3- to 4-inch length connected to a syringe is an excellent alternative method of securing a specimen for culture. Prompt inoculation onto one of several media (Regan-Lowe charcoal with cephalexin is the most commonly used) is essential for optimal bacterial recovery. Cough plates are no longer recommended. During the late cough to early

TABLE 2. **Clinical Manifestations of *Bordetella pertussis* Infection**

Stage	Duration	Contagiousness	Symptoms
Catarrhal	1–2 wk	+ + + +	Rhinorrhea Conjunctival injection Slight cough Low-grade fever
Paroxysmal	2–4 wk	+ + +	Paroxysmal cough Whoop Post-tussive emesis Cyanosis/apnea
Convalescent	3–4 wk	—	Recovery

TABLE 3. Diagnostic Methods for Pertussis

Method	Sensitivity	Specificity	Comments
Culture	+	+ + + +	"Gold standard" requires 3–7 d for growth on selective media; recovery rate affected by antibiotics and late stages of illnesses
Direct fluorescent antibody (DFA)	+	+	Rapid results; recovery rate affected as above
PCR	+ + + +	+ + + +	Rapid results; does not require living organisms
ELISA	+ + +	+ + +	Positive late in paroxysmal or convalescent stage; high antibody with single specimen or demonstration of rise in titer

convalescent stage, culture positivity rates drop to 15%. Antibiotic-treated patients have a much reduced rate of positive cultures.

The low sensitivity of culture during the time when pertussis is often suspected and the lengthy incubation period make other diagnostic methods attractive (Table 3). The direct fluorescein-labeled antibody (DFA) used for detection of *B. pertussis* in nasopharyngeal smears suffers from interobservor variability but can provide a definitive result in just a few hours.

Polymerase chain reaction (PCR) appears to have the best future in the diagnosis of pertussis. PCR assays on nasopharyngeal specimens have a high specificity and a higher sensitivity than culture. This is especially important for the diagnosis in the partially immune or previously treated patient. The speed of the assay is also advantageous. Results can be available in 24 hours. Cost is approximately the same as culture.

New serology methods also show promise. A single serum specimen can be used for diagnosis in many cases. Enzyme-linked immunosorbent assay (ELISA) testing for IgG and/or IgA antibodies to PT, FHA, PRN or FIM is available in some reference laboratories, and high-titered antibody levels can identify a substantial number of patients who are culture negative; specificity can be a problem. Although laboratory diagnosis is often difficult, a clinical case definition can be used (Table 4).

TREATMENT

Antibiotics are effective in aborting the illness completely or decreasing symptomatology if given early in the catarrhal stage. Antibiotics do not markedly change the duration of cough if started beyond 2 weeks into the paroxysmal stage of the illness in most patients. Nevertheless, antibiotics should always be given because after 4 days of appropriate antibiotic therapy, pertussis organisms are eliminated from the nasopharynx. Thus, treatment decreases contagion considerably.

Erythromycin in the estolate formulation (Ilosone) at a dose of 40 mg per kg per day orally for 14 days

TABLE 4. Pertussis Case Definition

Cough lasting ≥14 d with at least one of the following:
  Paroxysms of cough
  Inspiratory whoop
  Post-tussive emesis
  Positive culture or laboratory confirmation with epidemiologic link to a confirmed case

is the drug of choice. Clarithromycin (Biaxin) for 14 days or azithromycin (Zithromax) for 5 days may be reasonable alternatives that produce less gastrointestinal upset but are more expensive. Trimethoprim-sulfamethoxazole (Bactrim, Septra), 8 and 40 mg per kg per day of the trimethoprim and sulfamethoxazole, respectively, for 14 days, is an alternative antimicrobial, although clinical efficacy is lower than that of a macrolide. Antibiotics should be given for a full 14 days (except azithromycin), otherwise relapse is common. Pertussis immune globulin has no efficacy and is not recommended. Supportive care is extremely important. Avoidance of coughing triggers and maintaining hydration and nutrition are all essential. Albuterol and steroids may have an adjunctive role in the treatment of pertussis.

A case of erythromycin-resistant *B. pertussis* has been reported in the United States. Although such resistance is considered rare by the Centers for Disease Control and Prevention, any patient with persistent disease despite compliance with adequate therapy should be recultured and considered a candidate for trimethoprim-sulfamethoxazole treatment.

PREVENTION

Immunization for pertussis was first studied in the 1930s. The DTwP vaccine has been in widespread use for the prevention of pertussis in the United States for 45 years. Although DTwP is efficacious in preventing severe illness, safety concerns exist. Both the medical literature and the popular press have debated the side effects of DTwP. Table 5 lists the relative frequency of common and unusual adverse effects of the DTwP. Concern about these reactions and possible permanent sequelae have led to development of acellular (DTaP) vaccines that are less reactogenic (Figure 2) while remaining highly efficacious.

DTaP vaccines contain one or more purified immunogenic components of *B. pertussis*: PT, FHA, PRN and FIM, rather than a whole cell preparation. All DTaP vaccines contain inactive PT and most contain FHA. The specific quantities, detoxification methods of PT, and the addition of PRN and FIM vary among the products.

In 1995, comparative trials were completed in Italy and Sweden of several DTaP vaccines compared with United States–licensed DTwP. These studies showed

TABLE 5. **Adverse Events Occurring Within 48 Hours of Whole-Cell DTP Immunization**

Event	Frequency* (per Dose)
Local	
Redness	1/3
Swelling	2/5
Pain	1/2
Mild/Moderate Systemic	
Fever ≥38° C (100.4° F)	1/2
Drowsiness	1/3
Fretfulness	1/2
Vomiting	1/15
Anorexia	1/5
More Serious Systemic	
Persistent, inconsolable crying (duration ≥3 h)	1/100
High-pitched, unusual cry	1/900
Fever ≥40.5° C (≥105° F)	1/330
Collapse (hypotonic-hyporesponsive episode)	1/1750
Convulsions (with or without fever)	1/1750
Acute encephalopathy†	1/110,000
Permanent neurologic deficit†	1/310,000

*Number of adverse events per total number of doses regardless of dose number in DTP series.

†Occurring within 7 days of DTP immunization.

From *MMWR 34*:411, 1986; and Cody CL, et al: Pediatrics *68*:650–660, 1981.

TABLE 6. **Efficacy Rates of Acellular Pertussis Vaccines**

Trial	Vaccine Composition	Efficacy Rate (%)
Sweden 1993–1995	PT + FHA + PRN + FIM	85
	PT + FHA	58
	DTwP	48
Italy 1993–1995	PT + FHA + PRN (manufacturer #1)	84
	PT + FHA + PRN (manufacturer #2)	84
	DTwP	36

Abbreviations: PT = pertussis toxin; FHA = filamentous hemagglutinin; PRN = pertactin; FIM = fimbriae.

of age according to the American schedule. The efficacy of the DTwP vaccine was significantly less than what is observed in the United States. However, booster doses of DTwP were not given as recommended in the United States at 15 to 20 months, and both countries had pertussis epidemics during the trial (probably resulting in a higher inoculum and exposure as compared with the United States).

Currently, two DTaP vaccines (Tripedia and Acel-Imune) are approved for use for the fourth and fifth doses (18 months and 4 to 5 years of age, respectively). The Food and Drug Administration is expected to approve one or more DTaP vaccines for infants soon. The routine immunization schedule would not change from current recommendations except for substitution of the DTaP vaccines for the DTwP. Ongoing trials are evaluating the DTaP vaccines in adolescents and adults, since these populations appear to be a continuing reservoir of pertussis infection.

all DTaP vaccines tested to have greater efficacy than DTwP vaccine (Table 6). All DTaP vaccines also had significantly fewer adverse reactions than DTwP. These randomized double-blind trials involved more than 25,000 infants vaccinated at 2, 4, and 6 months

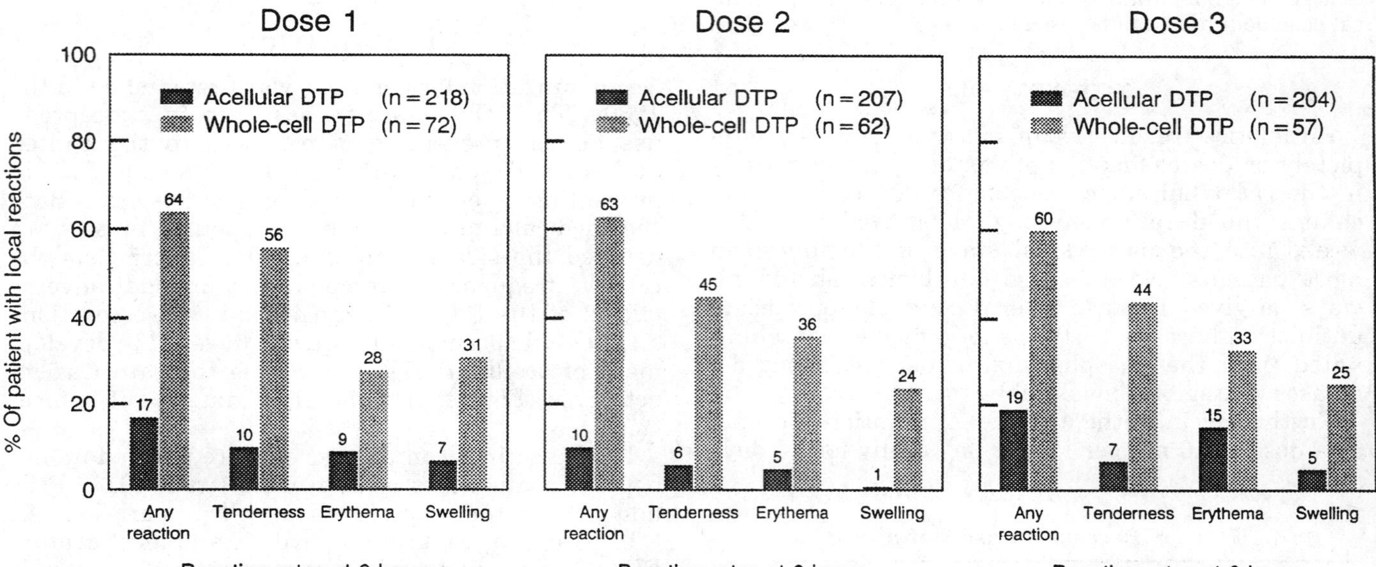

Figure 2. Acellular pertussis vaccine: local adverse effects, USA (2, 4, and 6 months of age). (From Pichichero ME, et al: Acellular pertussis vaccination of 2-month-old infants in the United States. Reproduced by permission of Pediatrics Vol 89, pp 882–887. Copyright 1992.)

IMMUNIZATION PRACTICES

method of
CLIFFORD O. MISHAW, M.D.
Baylor College of Medicine
Houston, Texas

The immunization of children and adults continues as a primary means of preventing disease. However, as epidemics of measles and pertussis in the last decade in the United States demonstrate, many children and adults continue to be susceptible to vaccine-preventable diseases. This is in large part due to a large number children and adults in the U.S. who are inadequately immunized.

Clearly, physicians play an extremely important role in ensuring that their patients are fully immunized on time. This requires prioritizing the administration of immunizations in one's practice. Parents and adults should be educated as to their importance. They should be encouraged to bring their immunization records with them regularly to all patient visits. Every feasible opportunity to immunize should be taken to avoid missed opportunities. Physicians should be encouraged to participate in public health vaccine programs to provide vaccine in their office to those individuals who can't afford it.

This article discusses the pertinent aspects of currently recommended vaccines and certain special circumstances for vaccination.

Table 1 includes the most recently approved immunization schedule for children and adolescents from the Advisory Committee on Immunization Practices for the Centers for Disease Control and Prevention, the American Academy of Pediatrics, and the American Academy of Family Physicians. There are different recommendations for children not immunized according to this schedule.

GENERAL PRINCIPLES

The timely administration of vaccines and immunoprophylaxis with preformed antibody is extremely important. Vaccines are scheduled at a time to induce the best possible immunologic response and when the host is susceptible to the disease. Vaccines may be safely and effectively simultaneously administered. A lapse in time between doses does not require reinstitution of the entire series. The next dose should be given irrespective of the time interval that

TABLE 1. **Recommended Childhood Immunization Schedule: United States, January–June 1996**

Vaccine	Birth	1 mo	2 mo	4 mo	6 mo	12 mo	15 mo	18 mo	4–6 yr	11–12 yr	14–16 yr
Hepatitis B[1, 2]		Hep B-1									
			Hep B-2			Hep B-3				Hep B[2]	
Diphtheria, tetanus, pertussis[3]			DTP	DTP	DTP	DTP[3] (DTaP at 15+ mo)			DTP or DTaP	Td	
H. influenzae type b[4]			Hib	Hib	Hib[4]	Hib[4]					
Polio[5]			OPV[5]	OPV	OPV				OPV		
Measles, mumps, rubella[6]						MMR			MMR[6] or	MMR[6]	
Varicella-zoster virus vaccine[7]						Var				Var[7]	

Vaccines are listed under the routinely recommended ages. Bars indicate range of acceptable ages for vaccination. Shaded bars indicate *catch-up vaccination:* at 11–12 years of age, hepatitis B vaccine should be administered to children not previously vaccinated, and varicella-zoster virus vaccine should be administered to children not previously vaccinated who lack a reliable history of chickenpox.

[1]*Infants born to HBsAg-negative mothers* should receive 2.5 μg of Merck vaccine (Recombivax HB) or 10 μg of SmithKline Beecham (SB) vaccine (Engerix-B). The 2nd dose should be administered ≥1 mo after the 1st dose.

Infants born to HBsAg-positive mothers should receive 0.5 mL hepatitis B immune globulin (HBIG) within 12 hr of birth, and either 5 μg of Merck vaccine (Recombivax HB) or 10 μg of SB vaccine (Engerix-B) at a separate site. The 2nd dose is recommended at 1–2 mos of age and the 3rd dose at 6 mos of age.

Infants born to mothers whose HBsAg status is unknown should receive either 5 μg of Merck vaccine (Recombivax HB) or 10 μg of SB vaccine (Engerix-B) within 12 hr of birth. The 2nd dose of vaccine is recommended at 1 mo of age and the 3rd dose at 6 mos of age.

[2]Adolescents who have not previously received 3 doses of hepatitis B vaccine should initate or complete the series at the 11–12-year-old visit. The 2nd dose should be administered at least 1 mo after the 1st dose, and the 3rd dose should be administered at least 4 mos after the 1st dose and at least 2 mos after the 2nd dose.

[3]DTP4 may be administered at 12 mos of age, if at least 6 mos have elapsed since DTP3. DTaP (diphtheria and tetanus toxoids and acellular pertussis vaccine) is licensed for the 4th and/or 5th vaccine dose(s) for children aged ≥15 mos and may be preferred for these doses in this age group. Td (tetanus and diphtheria toxoids, adsorbed, for adult use) is recommended at 11–12 years of age if at least 5 years have elapsed since the last dose of DTP, DTaP, or DT.

[4]Three *H. influenzae* type b (Hib) conjugate vaccines are licensed for infant use. If PRP-OMP (PedvaxHIB [Merck]) is administered at 2 and 4 mos of age, a dose at 6 mos is not required. After completing the primary series, any Hib conjugate vaccine may be used as a booster.

[5]Oral poliovirus vaccine (OPV) is recommended for routine infant vaccination. Inactivated poliovirus vaccine (IPV) is recommended for persons with a congenital or acquired immune deficiency disease or an altered immune status as a result of disease or immunosuppressive therapy, as well as their household contacts, and is an acceptable alternative for other persons. The primary 3-dose series for IPV should be given with a minimum interval of 4 wks between the 1st and 2nd doses and 6 mos between the 2nd and 3rd doses.

[6]The 2nd dose of MMR vaccine is routinely recommended at 4–6 years of age or at 11–12 years of age, but may be administered at any visit, provided at least 1 mo has elapsed since receipt of the 1st dose.

[7]Varicella-zoster virus vaccine (Var) can be administered to susceptible children any time after 12 months of age. Unvaccinated children who lack a reliable history of chickenpox should be vaccinated at the 11–12-year-old visit.

Approved by the Advisory Committee on Immunization Practices (ACIP), the American Academy of Pediatrics (AAP), and the American Academy of Family Physicians (AAFP).

has elapsed between doses. Recommended doses of vaccines should not be reduced or divided, including those for premature or low-birthweight infants.

Every physician should maintain the immunization history of each patient in a permanent office record that can be easily reviewed and updated and that which will facilitate future timely immunizations. The following data should be documented in the patient's record: (1) month, day, and year of administration; (2) type of vaccine; (3) manufacturer; (4) lot number and its expiration date; (5) site and route of administration; and (6) name and address of the health care provider administering the vaccine. The National Childhood Vaccine Act of 1986 requires that this information be recorded in the patient's personal medical record for mandated vaccines for children.

Parents and patients should be informed about the possible risks and benefits of immunization. They should be questioned about side effects and adverse reactions of previously administered vaccines and conditions that influence the decision to immunize, such as use of immunosuppressive medications, allergies, or an unimmunized household contact.

The National Childhood Vaccine Injury Act of 1986 requires physicians and other health care providers to report certain adverse events to measles, mumps, rubella, polio, pertussis, diphtheria, and tetanus vaccines. The United States Department of Health and Human Services has established a Vaccine Adverse Event Reporting System (VAERS) to accept all reports of any suspected adverse event subsequent to administration of any vaccine. The VAERS toll-free number is 1-800-822-7967.

PRECAUTIONS

Most vaccines are intended for use in healthy individuals or those whose condition is not adversely affected by the immunization. Minor illnesses such as upper respiratory tract and gastrointestinal infections and allergic rhinitis are not a contraindication to immunize. Fever is not a contraindication to immunize. However, if fever or other signs or symptoms suggest a moderate or severe illness, vaccination should be postponed until the individual has recovered.

Routine immunization with measles, mumps, yellow fever, and influenza vaccines of individuals allergic to egg is contraindicated. Skin testing of these individuals with a history of anaphylactic symptoms after egg ingestion is recommended. Mercury hypersensitivity is also a contraindication to administration of vaccines containing mercury compounds such as thiomersal. Neomycin hypersensitivity is a contraindication to administration of inactivated polio vaccine and measles, mumps, and rubella vaccine. Streptomycin hypersensitivity is also a contraindication to administration of inactivated polio vaccine. Any previous hypersensitivity reaction to vaccine administration would also contraindicate further usage.

The concurrent use of antibiotics does not contraindicate vaccination. The appropriate age for immunizing the premature infant is the usual recommended chronologic age.

Immunodeficient and Immunosuppressed Children

Individuals with congenital disorders of their immune function should not be given live vaccines. The use of a short course of systemic corticosteroids or topical corticosteroids in an otherwise healthy child would not contraindicate immunization. However, children receiving larger doses of systemic corticosteroids should not be given live vaccines.

Children with Human Immunodeficiency Virus (HIV) Infection

In general, live virus and bacterial vaccines such as oral polio vaccine (OPV) (Orimune) and bacillus Calmette-Guérin vaccine should not be given to HIV-infected patients who are immunosuppressed. However, since there have been many severe cases and fatalities in measles-infected symptomatic HIV patients, it is recommended to immunize them and asymptomatic HIV patients with measles, mumps, and rubella (MMR) vaccine. Children with asymptomatic or symptomatic HIV infection should also receive diphtheria, tetanus, and pertussis (DTP) vaccine, *Haemophilus influenzae* type b conjugate vaccine, hepatitis B vaccine, and inactivated poliovirus (IPV) vaccine according to the usual recommended immunization schedule. Varicella vaccine should not be given to children with asymptomatic or symptomatic HIV-infection. Pneumococcal vaccine should be given to both asymptomatic and symptomatic HIV-infected children. Symptomatic HIV-infected children should be given yearly influenza vaccine beginning at 6 months of age. Yearly vaccination with influenza vaccine after 6 months of age should be considered in asymptomatic HIV-infected children.

Diphtheria, Tetanus, and Pertussis

Currently, the primary series of diphtheria, tetanus toxoids, and whole-cell pertussis combined (DTP) vaccine is recommended at 2, 4, and 6 months of age. A combination vaccine with an acellular pertussis vaccine component is licensed as an alternative for the fourth and fifth doses, respectively, at 12 to 18 months and 4 to 6 years of age. A combination *H. influenzae* type b conjugate–DTP vaccine may be used for the first 4 doses. However, diphtheria, tetanus, and acellular pertussis (DTaP) (Acel-Imune, Tripedia) vaccine has been preferred for the fourth and fifth doses because of a lower frequency of local and systemic reactions. Universal immunization with pertussis vaccine is recommended only for children less than 7 years of age. In the near future, DTaP may be recommended as an alternative for the entire series including the primary three doses.

A booster with tetanus and diphtheria toxoids (Td)

should first be given at 11 to 12 years of age. Thereafter, adults should be immunized every 10 years with Td. Reactions to the diphtheria toxoid are less in adults because Td contains much less diphtheria toxoid. Adults who have not received a primary series of diphtheria and tetanus toxoids should complete the series with Td. This primary series includes 3 doses of Td with the first 2 doses given at least 4 weeks apart. The third dose may be given 6 to 12 months after the second dose. The combined preparation of Td is preferred for active tetanus immunization for adults, since a large number of adults also lack protective levels of circulating antitoxin against diphtheria. For children less than 7 years of age for whom pertussis vaccine has been contraindicated, tetanus and diphtheria toxoids (DT) may be given.

Common side effects with DTP and DTaP vaccines include erythema, induration and tenderness at the site of the vaccination, crying, and slight to moderate fever. These occur within several hours of administration and resolve without sequelae. These *do not* contraindicate further vaccination. Adverse events after pertussis immunization that would contraindicate further vaccination include (1) anaphylactic reaction and (2) an encephalopathy occurring within 7 days of administration. The following events that were once considered contraindications should now be considered precautions, considering the potential benefits of the vaccine, for instance, during a local outbreak of the disease. These events have not been proven to cause permanent sequelae. They include (1) a convulsion with or without fever occurring within 3 days of DTP or DTaP vaccination; (2) persistent, severe, inconsolable screaming or crying for 3 or more hours within 48 hours of vaccination; (3) collapse or shocklike state (hypotonic-hyporesponsive episode) within 48 hours of vaccination; (4) temperature of 40.5° C or higher, unexplained by another cause, within 48 hours of vaccination. The history of having any of these adverse reactions after previous doses of DTP or DTaP needs to be elicited prior to administering further doses. If the child has had one of these adverse events, the possibility of having another event of equal or greater severity may justify discontinuing pertussis vaccination, although the risks of subsequent adverse events are not known. At each opportunity to vaccinate, the decision to withhold pertussis-containing vaccines should be based on the clinical assessment of the previous adverse event, the risk of exposure to pertussis in the child's community and environment, and the potential risks and benefits of the vaccine.

Any child with abnormal neurologic findings or uncharacterized developmental delay suggesting either a progressive or an undiagnosed neurologic condition should have his or her pertussis vaccine deferred. An adverse event associated with either DTP or DTaP in these individuals may be unwittingly attributed to the vaccine instead of the undiagnosed neurologic condition, such as infantile spasms. Children with unstable or evolving neurologic conditions such as tuberous sclerosis, and certain inherited metabolic and degenerative diseases that predispose to convulsions and neurologic deterioration, should have the pertussis deferred. Once the condition has stabilized or the seizures have been well controlled, the child may receive pertussis vaccine. Similarly, children with uncomplicated developmental delay or cerebral palsy (static encephalopathy) may be vaccinated. These children may be especially at risk for complications of the disease because of their motor and neurologic deficits.

Children who have previously had a seizure are at increased risk of developing a seizure subsequent to a pertussis-containing vaccine. There is no evidence that these vaccine-associated seizures have caused permanent brain damage, epilepsy, or aggravated neurologic disorders or have affected the prognosis in children with underlying disorders. There is also an increased risk of seizures associated with pertussis-containing vaccines in children with a family history of seizures. However, these associated seizures are most probably either benign febrile seizures or seizures in children with a lowered threshold for seizures secondary to fever. A history of a febrile seizure is not an absolute contraindication to administering DTP or DTaP as long as the parents or guardians understand the risks and benefits of the vaccine.

Several studies have indicated that immunization with DTP has not been associated with sudden infant death syndrome (SIDS).

It is currently being investigated whether DTaP may completely replace DTP. Further recommendations regarding this change may be forthcoming in the near future.

Polio

The last known cases of polio secondary to wild virus in the United States and the Western Hemisphere were in 1979 and 1991, respectively. However, wild virus continues to circulate and cause disease in many nations of the world and remains endemic in sub-Saharan Africa and South Asia. The only cases of paralytic poliomyelitis that now occur in the United States are associated with oral polio vaccine (OPV), so-called vaccine-associated paralytic poliomyelitis (VAPP). Approximately 8 to 10 people contract VAPP annually in the United States. The overall risk of VAPP is estimated to be 1 case per 2.5 million doses. These cases have occurred in recent OPV vaccines, mostly infants, direct contacts of recent vaccinees, and immunodeficient children and adults.

Currently, routine immunization of children with trivalent oral polio vaccine is recommended at 2, 4, 6 to 18 months, and 4 to 6 years of age. Inactivated polio vaccine (IPV) should be administered to individuals with congenital or acquired immune deficiency disease such as with HIV infections, immune deficiency states secondary to disease or immunosuppressive therapy, and household contacts of individuals with these conditions.

Routine immunization of previously unvaccinated

adults (≥18 years old) in the United States is not indicated unless they are at increased risk of exposure to the wild virus or to household contacts vaccinated with OPV. This includes travelers to areas of the world where poliomyelitis is endemic. Whenever possible, primary immunization with IPV is recommended. Two doses of IPV should be administered 1 to 2 months apart followed by a third dose 6 to 12 months after the second dose. IPV is preferred in adults, since the risk of VAPP is slightly higher in adults than in children.

In October 1995, the Advisory Committee on Immunization Practices to the Centers for Disease Control and Prevention recommended a new childhood immunization schedule for polio. This would expand the use of IPV with the eventual implementation of an all-IPV schedule that, it is hoped, would decrease the number of VAPP cases in the United States. Further recommendations regarding this issue will probably be forthcoming.

Measles, Mumps, and Rubella

Two doses of the combined vaccine of measles, mumps, and rubella (MMR) are recommended at 12 to 15 months of age and either 4 to 6 or 11 to 12 years of age. Although MMR is a live-virus vaccine, transmission of these vaccine viruses to contacts of vaccinees does not occur.

The risk of complications from measles is highest among infants less than 12 months of age. Monovalent measles vaccine should be given to infants between 6 and 12 months of age during measles outbreaks. Children who were vaccinated before their first birthday will need to receive a second dose between 12 to 15 months of age, and again during their school years.

Adult men and women previously unvaccinated or who have no serologic evidence of immunity to rubella should be immunized. Pregnant females should not be immunized against rubella, and postpubertal females should be warned not to become pregnant for 3 months after receiving rubella vaccine. MMR may be given to adults if they need immunization for measles and/or mumps in addition to rubella.

Pregnancy

Pregnant women should be immunized only when the infection would significantly harm either the mother or the fetus, the risk of exposure to the disease is high, and the vaccine is safe. If otherwise indicated, the only vaccines routinely recommended for administration during pregnancy in the United States are tetanus and diphtheria toxoids. Pregnancy is generally a contraindication to all live-virus vaccines. However, both yellow fever and oral polio vaccines may be given to pregnant women who are at substantial risk of exposure to infection, such as with travel to endemic areas. MMR should not be given to pregnant women. Pregnancy is not a contraindication

to vaccinating women who are otherwise eligible for receiving the vaccine.

Hepatitis B

Universal vaccination for hepatitis B is recommended for all infants born to HBsAg-negative mothers. The first dose is given soon after birth up to 2 months of age. The second dose is given 1 to 2 months later, and the third dose is given between 6 and 18 months of age. There are two licensed recombinant vaccines in the United States, including Recombivax HB (Merck & Co.) and Engerix-B (SmithKline Beecham). Recombivax HB is supplied in four formulations with different concentrations of hepatitis B surface antigen, including a pediatric (5 μg/mL), adolescent/high-risk infant, and adult formulation (10 μg/mL).

Infants born to an HBsAg-positive mother should receive 0.5 mL of hepatitis B immune globulin (HBIG) within 12 hours of birth and the initial dose of hepatitis B vaccine concurrently at a different site within 12 hours of birth. The second and third doses should be respectively given at 1 and 6 months of age. Individuals who have previously not been immunized for hepatitis B should begin the series between 11 and 12 years of age. The second dose should be given at least 1 month after the first dose. The third dose should be given at least 4 months after the first dose and at least 2 months after the second dose.

Children and adults at high risk for exposure to hepatitis B should also be immunized. These include residents of institutions for developmentally disabled persons, homosexual males, users of intravenous drugs, health care workers at risk for exposure to blood or body fluids, and household contacts and sexual partners of hepatitis B carriers.

The only contraindication is an anaphylactic reaction to a previous dose or to common baker's yeast.

Haemophilus influenzae Type b

Four *H. influenzae* type b conjugate vaccines and one combination *H. influenzae* type b conjugate–DTP vaccine are licensed in the United States. One of the conjugate vaccines, ActHIB, may be combined with DTP for injection. These vaccines consist of the *H. influenzae* type b capsular polysaccharide or its oligomers covalently linked to a carrier protein. Recommendations for the different conjugate vaccines vary, since their composition and immunogenicity differ. Whereas three of the conjugate vaccines are recommended beginning at 2 months of age, ProHIBiT (Connaught Laboratories, Inc.) is recommended only for children 12 months and older. Except for PedvaxHIB (Merck & Co.), three doses in the primary series are recommended at 2, 4, and 6 months. A booster of any conjugate vaccine should be given at 12 to 15 months. A dose of PedvaxHIB at 6 months is not required. Children older than 5 years do not need to be routinely immunized. Children not vaccinated on time need to be immunized according to an alternate immunization schedule. Individuals with a history of anaphylaxis to a *H. influenzae* vaccine or a component should avoid vaccination. Children vaccinated with these conjugate vaccines alone should not be considered adequately immunized against the carrier protein.

Meningococcal Vaccine

A serogroup-specific quadrivalent meningococcal polysaccharide vaccine against groups A, C, Y, and W-135 *Neisseria meningitidis* is licensed in the United States and available from Connaught Laboratories, Inc. Routine immunization of children with this vaccine is not recommended. Vaccination of children with either functional or anatomic asplenia and those with terminal complement component deficiencies 2 years of age and older should be considered.

Pneumococcal Vaccine

The 23-valent pneumococcal vaccine is composed of purified capsular polysaccharide antigens. Those children 2 years and older with an increased risk of acquiring systemic pneumococcal infections or with increased risk of developing serious disease if infected should be immunized. These include children with sickle cell disease, functional or anatomic asplenia, nephrotic syndrome, chronic renal failure, conditions associated with immunosuppression, cerebral spinal fluid leaks, and HIV infection.

The following immunocompetent adults who are at increased risk of pneumococcal disease or its complications should be vaccinated: individuals with cardiovascular or pulmonary disease, diabetes mellitus, alcoholism, cirrhosis, or cerebrospinal fluid leaks, or who are 65 years of age and older. Immunocompromised adults at increased risk of pneumococcal disease or its complications should also be vaccinated. These include individuals with splenic dysfunction or anatomic asplenia, Hodgkin's disease, lymphoma, multiple myeloma, chronic renal failure, nephrotic syndrome, and conditions associated with immunosuppression such as organ transplantation. Adults with asymptomatic or symptomatic HIV infection should also be vaccinated.

Revaccination of older children and adults should be strongly considered 6 years or more after the initial dose for those individuals at highest risk of a rapid decline in antibody levels or fatal pneumococcal infection. These include those with chronic renal failure, nephrotic syndrome, transplanted organs, and asplenia. Revaccination of children 10 years old and older 3 to 5 years after the initial vaccination should also be considered in those with similar conditions at high risk of severe pneumococcal infection.

Influenza

The influenza vaccine is immunogenic and safe and has had minimal side effects. The composition is frequently changed in anticipation of the expected prevalent influenza strains. There is both a whole- and split-virus vaccine. The latter should be used in children less than 13 years old. Children less than 9 years of age receiving the influenza vaccine for the first time should receive two doses of the split-virus vaccine administered 1 month apart. It should be annually administered in the autumn before the start of the influenza season to children and adults at least 6 months of age or older.

The use of inactivated influenza vaccine has been the single most significant means of preventing and attenuating influenza infection. Children and adults at risk of influenza-associated complications such as lower respiratory tract complications and death should be immunized. These include the following: (1) persons 65 years old and older; (2) residents of nursing homes and chronic care facilities housing patients of any age with chronic medical conditions; (3) those with disorders of the pulmonary or cardiovascular systems, including children with asthma; (4) children and adults with chronic metabolic diseases including diabetes mellitus, chronic renal disease, hemoglobinopathies including sickle cell disease, or immunosuppression; and (5) children and adolescents receiving chronic aspirin therapy because of their increased risk of developing Reye's syndrome after an influenza infection. This includes individuals with HIV infection. Currently, routine vaccination of all children and adults is not feasible. However, vaccination should be considered if parents or guardians desire that their child's risk of developing the disease be reduced or if any adult wishes to reduce his or her risk of becoming infected.

Unlike the 1976 swine influenza vaccine, subsequent influenza vaccines have not been associated with increased frequency of Guillain-Barré syndrome. Common side effects include erythema and induration for 1 to 2 days at the site of the injection. Although infrequent, malaise, mylagia, and other signs of toxicity may occur, especially in those individuals previously not exposed to the influenza antigens. These symptoms may begin 6 to 12 hours after vaccination and may persist for 1 to 2 days. Allergic reactions may occur and may be due to sensitivity to egg protein. Individuals with a history of anaphylactic reactions after eating eggs should not be given influenza vaccine. Individuals with acute febrile illnesses should not be immunized until their symptoms have abated.

Rabies

Pre-exposure immunization should be considered for animal handlers, veterinarians, certain laboratory workers and field personnel, persons planning to spend more than 1 month in areas of countries where rabies is a constant threat, and persons such as spelunkers whose vocations and avocations bring them into contact with potentially rabid animals such as skunks, raccoons, and bats.

All persons suspected of having been exposed to rabies should be reported to the local health department. The decision to immunize a potentially exposed individual should be made in consultation with the local health department, which can provide information on the risk of rabies in a particular area for each species of animal. In the United States, skunks, raccoons, and bats are more likely to be infected than other animals, but foxes, coyotes, cattle, dogs, and cats have occasionally been infected. Bites from squirrels, hamsters, guinea pigs, gerbils, chipmunks, rats, mice, rabbits, and hares rarely require specific antirabies prophylaxis. An unprovoked attack is also more suggestive of a rabid animal. A suspect dog or cat that has bitten a human should be captured, confined, and observed.

Rabies post-exposure prophylaxis is recommended for all individuals who have been bitten or scratched by wild or domestic animals that may be infected. Human rabies immune globulin (RIG) should initially be given with the first dose of vaccine for post-exposure prophylaxis. One-half of the RIG is used to infiltrate the wound, and the other half is given intramuscularly. A dose of either human diploid cell vaccine (HDCV) or rabies vaccine, adsorbed (RVA) is immediately given intramuscularly in the deltoid area, in a different area than the RIG, with subsequent doses given on days 3, 7, 14, and 28.

Varicella Vaccine

Varicella-zoster virus vaccine (Varivax) is a live attenuated virus vaccine that has now been recommended for susceptible children any time after 12 months of age. Children between the ages of 12 months and 12 years should receive a single dose subcutaneously. Adolescents and adults older than 13 years should receive two doses 4 to 8 weeks apart. Side effects include mild to moderate fever, pain and erythema at the injection site, and a varicella-like rash either at the injection site or generalized. Salicylates should not be used for up to 6 weeks after receiving the vaccine. Becoming pregnant should be deferred for 3 months after receiving this vaccine. Contraindications to use of the vaccine include hypersensitivity to gelatin or neomycin, immunosuppression, active untreated tuberculosis, and an active febrile illness. Vaccinees potentially may transmit the virus to close contacts. Therefore, vaccinees should avoid close contact with susceptible high-risk individuals such as immunocompromised persons. The vaccine should not be given to HIV-infected persons.

Foreign Travel

Travel to foreign countries necessitates consideration of additional immunizations to the routine recommended vaccines. The requisite vaccines vary with the length of stay and the destination. A more detailed reference or the CDC needs to be consulted for specific recommendations for foreign travel.

Hepatitis A

Hepatitis A vaccine (Havrix) is an inactivated virus vaccine and may be given to persons 2 years of age and older. It has been recommended for individuals traveling to countries endemic with the infection, those living in communities with outbreaks, intravenous drug users, males who have sex with other males, people with chronic liver disease, and those at occupational risk of infection.

TOXOPLASMOSIS

method of
BENJAMIN U. SAMUEL, M.D., and
KEITH A. JOINER, M.D.
Yale University School of Medicine
New Haven, Connecticut

Toxoplasma gondii, the causative agent of toxoplasmosis, is an obligate intracellular coccidian parasite with worldwide distribution. Toxoplasmosis refers to the clinical and pathologic disease state caused by *T. gondii*, as opposed to toxoplasma infection which is asymptomatic. *T. gondii* infects all animals and most birds and is one of the most widely distributed of all intracellular parasites. Cats are the definitive primary hosts and maintain an intestinal sexual cycle that results in the production of oocysts; all other animals are secondary hosts and have an extraintestinal asexual cycle with the production of tissue cysts.

Infection with *T. gondii* is acquired by ingestion of cysts or oocysts or by transplacental transmission. Less common modes of acquiring the infection include blood and leukocyte transfusions, organ transplantation, and laboratory accident. Following ingestion of cysts or oocysts, the organisms are released, and they infect the host cells by an active process; dissemination to other parts of the body via the lymph and bloodstream occurs, resulting in acute infection. The tachyzoites, which are the asexual invasive forms of the parasite, can invade and replicate within essentially all nucleated cells. Intracellularly, the tachyzoites reside in a parasitophorous vacuole protected from the host cell-killing mechanisms. After the resolution of the acute phase, chronic (latent) infection ensues in all patients infected with *T. gondii*. In about 7 to 10 days after systemic tachyzoite infection, tissue cysts containing bradyzoites develop virtually in every organ and persist for the life of the host, especially in brain, heart, and skeletal muscles. These persistent, slowly metabolizing forms of *T. gondii* are the most probable source of recrudescent infection in immunocompromised patients.

CLINICAL MANIFESTATIONS

Description of the protean clinical and pathologic manifestations of toxoplasmosis is beyond the scope of this article. Briefly, clinical manifestations of toxoplasmosis fall into four categories: (1) acquired in immunocompetent individuals, (2) acquired or reactivated in immunodeficient hosts, (3) congenital, and (4) ocular. Approximately 10% to 20% of healthy immunocompetent patients with acute toxoplasmosis develop symptomatic illness, usually lymphadenitis or an "infectious mononucleosis"-like syndrome. Rarely, a patient may develop clinically overt illness with myocarditis, pneumonitis, or encephalitis with potentially fatal dissemination.

Acute toxoplasmosis in the immunocompromised patient is usually due to reactivation of the latent infection. The incidence of toxoplasmic encephalitis (TE) in AIDS patients is directly proportional to *Toxoplasma* seroprevalence in the population. In the United States, 10% to 40% of HIV-positive patients are latently infected with *Toxoplasma*, and of these, 30% to 50% develop TE, especially when the CD4 count falls below 100/cmm. In parts of Western Europe and Africa, *Toxoplasma* seroprevalence among HIV-infected persons is much higher. In immunocompromised patients who are seronegative, acute disease may result from exogenous infection.

Focal necrotizing encephalitis is the most common manifestation of toxoplasmosis in patients with AIDS. Other manifestations of toxoplasmosis in AIDS patients include pulmonary disease and chorioretinitis. Pulmonary toxoplasmosis is being increasingly recognized and has a high mortality. The clinical picture may be indistinguishable from that of *Pneumocystis carinii* pneumonia (PCP).

The clinical presentation of TE is varied and may be difficult to differentiate from a number of other HIV-related conditions affecting the central nervous system (CNS). Magnetic resonance imaging (MRI) or computed tomography (CT) scans characteristically show multiple, bilateral cerebral lesions in patients with TE. The lesions on CT scan are typically multiple and contrast enhancing, involving the basal ganglia and corticomedullary junction bilaterally. The findings on MRI/CT scan are not pathognomonic. However, a presumptive diagnosis of TE can be made based on the MRI/CT scan findings and positive toxoplasma serology in symptomatic AIDS patients, and treatment initiated promptly.

Toxoplasmosis in non-AIDS immunocompromised patients, such as transplant recipients and patients with underlying malignancy, is fatal if not recognized early and appropriate treatment given. In transplant recipients, toxoplasmosis may be reactivated or in seronegative patients be acquired via donor organ or blood products, and it causes significant morbidity and mortality. Toxoplasmosis in these patients may present as TE, recurrent attacks of fever, myocardial dysfunction, and pericardial effusions (especially in heart transplant recipients). Other manifestations may be nonspecific or reflect inflammation and necrosis of the organs involved, particularly the heart and lungs.

Transplacental transmission of *T. gondii* occurs in about one third of all women infected during pregnancy. If the infection occurs during the first trimester, the incidence of congenital toxoplasmosis is low (10% to 15%), but the disease is severe. The incidence of fetal infection increases to 30% in the second trimester and 60% in the third trimester, but the disease is less severe. Almost all infected newborn infants of mothers who acquire the disease in the third trimester are asymptomatic at birth, but they have a higher incidence of learning disabilities and chronic neurologic sequelae than uninfected infants. Approximately 85% of subclinically infected infants, if left untreated, develop chorioretinitis that may result in blindness. Otherwise healthy, immunocompetent women who are seropositive for toxoplasma, indicating prior infection (before conception), are not at risk for transmitting the infection to their infants. However, women of childbearing age who are HIV-positive pose unique problems. They are at high risk for acquiring acute toxoplasmosis if they are seronegative, and if they are seropositive for *Toxoplasma* may have reactivation of infection. In either case the fetus is at risk for congenital toxoplasmosis. In infants congenitally infected with HIV and *T. gondii*, toxoplasmosis appears to have a more progressive course, even though at birth most infants co-infected with *T. gondii* and HIV are asymptomatic.

T. gondii infection is one of the major causes of chorioretinitis in the United States and Europe. *Toxoplasma* chorioretinitis is usually congenital but occasionally may be seen in acute toxoplasmosis. In patients with AIDS, ocular toxoplasmosis may occur in conjunction with TE, although this is a less common cause for retinitis than is cytomegalovirus. The lesions, which are usually large and necrotic, progressively destroy retinal tissue. Definitive diagnosis requires either retinal biopsy and demonstration of the organisms in tissue specimens, or isolation of *T. gondii* from vitreous aspirate.

DRUGS ACTIVE AGAINST *T. GONDII*

Drugs with antitoxoplasma activity can be broadly classified into:

1. Drugs interfering with folate metabolism
   a. Pyrimethamine
   b. Trimethoprim*
   c. Sulfonamides, e.g., sulfadiazine
   d. Trimetrexate*
   e. Sulfones—dapsone*
2. Drugs that inhibit protein synthesis
   a. Tetracyclines—chlortetracycline,† doxycycline,* minocycline*
   b. Macrolides—spiramycin,‡ clarithromycin,* azithromycin,* roxithromycin†
   c. Lincosamides, e.g., clindamycin
3. Drugs with an uncertain mechanism of action
   a. Hydroxynaphthoquinone—atovaquone*
4. Miscellaneous

Table 1 gives the dosage and adverse effects of drugs used in toxoplasmosis, and Table 2 gives drug interactions of antitoxoplasma drugs and commonly used drugs.

The first line of therapy is combination drugs that inhibit folate metabolism. Pyrimethamine (a dihydrofolate reductase inhibitor) is combined with sulfadiazine (a dihydrofolate synthetase inhibitor) to block folate synthesis sequentially and produce synergistic activity against *T. gondii*. This combination is the most commonly used regimen. Folinic acid (leucovorin), which is preferentially taken up by mammalian cells and not by *T. gondii*, should be given to prevent pyrimethamine-induced hematologic toxicity. Folinic acid can be given orally, intravenously, or intramuscularly. The optimal dose of folinic acid is not known. A dose of 5 to 10 mg daily is recommended for older children, and 10 to 20 mg daily (up to 50 mg daily) for adults. Although sulfadiazine is the most often used sulfonamide, sulfamethoxazole and trisulfapyrimidines (no longer commercially available in the United States) can be used in conjunction with pyrimethamine. Other sulfon-

---

*Not FDA approved for this indication.
†Not available in the United States.
‡Investigational drug in the United States.

TABLE 1. **Drugs Used in Toxoplasmosis**

	Route of Administration	Major Excretory Route	Dose	Adverse Effects
Pyrimethamine (Daraprim)	PO	Hepatic	200-mg loading dose followed by 75–100 mg qd for acute infection in adults, and 2 mg/kg (up to 100 mg) daily given in 2 equally divided doses as loading dose then 1 mg/kg (max 25 mg) daily, in 2 doses in children Suppressive therapy: 25–75 mg qd	Dose dependent folate deficiency, megaloblastic anemia, pancytopenia, hypersensitivity reactions including SJ syndrome, TEN, dermatitis, pulmonary eosinophilia, serum sickness reactions, hepatitis, GI intolerance and CNS effects such as ataxia, tremors, seizures, and respiratory failure
Sulfonamides Sulfadiazine	PO	Renal	4–8 gm/day q 4–6 h dose adjustment required in renal failure	Allergic reactions—rash, pruritus, SJ syndrome, fever, crystalluria with renal damage, hepatitis, GI intolerance, bone marrow suppression, hemolytic anemia (G6PD deficiency), kernicterus in the neonate, rarely myocarditis and neuropsychiatric disturbances
Trimethoprim-sulfamethoxazole (Bactrim, Septra)	PO IV	Renal	80 mg/kg/day IV of sulfamethoxazole component × 3 wk then 25 mg/kg/d for 3–4 wk	Skin rash, fever, GI upsets, agranulocytosis, aplastic anemia, acute interstitial nephritis, SJ syndrome, TEN, reversible hyperkalemia
Dapsone	PO	Hepatic	100 mg/day	Hemolytic anemia, blood dyscrasias, nephrotic syndrome, allergic reactions, GI intolerance, agranulocytosis, peripheral neuropathy, fever, exfoliative dermatitis
Clindamycin (Cleocin)	PO IV	Hepatic	600–900 mg q 6 h	Diarrhea, *C, difficile* colitis, GI intolerance, skin rash, neutropenia, eosinophilia, blood dyscrasias
Clarithromycin (Biaxin)	PO	Hepatic Renal	1 gm twice daily	GI intolerance, diarrhea, abdominal pain, headache, abnormalities in LFT, dizziness, tinnitus, reversible hearing loss
Azithromycin† (Zithromax)	PO	Hepatic	1 gm loading dose followed by 500 mg to 1.2 gm/d	GI disturbances, nausea, vomiting, diarrhea, abdominal pain, rarely rash, angioedema, cholestatic jaundice, palpitation, chest pain, reversible hearing loss, LFT abnormalities, vaginitis, monilia, blood dyscrasias
Spiramycin*	PO	Hepatic	3 gm/d in adults; 100 mg/kg/day in 2 divided doses in children	Paresthesias, allergic rash, nausea, vomiting, diarrhea
Atovaquone† (Mepron)	PO	GI	750 mg q 6 h	Rash, GI effects such as nausea, diarrhea, vomiting, abdominal pain, headache, anemia, neutropenia, fever, elevated aminotransferases
Trimetrexate† (Neutrexin)	IV		30–280 mg/m²/d	Marrow suppression with neutropenia, thrombocytopenia, hepatitis, altered LFT, rash, GI toxicity

Abbreviations: SJ = Stevens-Johnson; TEN = toxic epidermal necrolysis; GI = gastrointestinal; CNS = central nervous system; PO = orally; IV = intravenous; LFT = liver function tests.
*Investigational drug in the United States.
†Not FDA-approved for this indication.

amides are less active against *T. gondii* and hence should not be used for the treatment of toxoplasmosis. Dapsone is a sulfone with potent activity against *T. gondii*. It acts by inhibiting *T. gondii* dihydropteroate synthesis. Dapsone is well absorbed when given orally and has a long half-life and better toxicity profile than do sulfas, making it a good alternative to sulfadiazine for maintenance therapy. Trimethoprim is markedly less active than pyrimethamine against the dihydrofolate reductase (DHFR) of *T. gondii*. Trimethoprim-sulfamethoxazole has been shown to be active against *T. gondii* in a number of animal models and in a limited number of AIDS patients with TE. Low-dose trimethoprim-sulfameth-

TABLE 2. **Drug Interactions**

Antitoxoplasma Drug	Interacting Agent(s)	Effect of Interaction
Atovaquone*	AZT	Increased AZT levels
	rifampin	Decreased atovaquone levels
	rifabutin	
	trimethoprim-sulfamethoxazole	Decreased TMP-SMX levels
Dapsone	rifampin, didanosine	Reduced levels of dapsone
	pyrimethamine	Increased marrow toxicity
	dideoxycytidine	Peripheral neuropathy
Pyrimethamine	antacids, kaolin	Reduced absorption
	dapsone	Increased marrow toxicity
	phenothiazines	Increased toxicity
	lorazepam	Hepatotoxicity
Sulfonamides	oral anticoagulants	Potentiate effects of coumarin
	cyclosporine	Decreased cyclosporine effect
	digoxin	Decreased absorption of digoxin
	sulfonylurea	Potentiate hypoglycemic effects
	nonsteroidal anti-inflammatory drugs	May have increased effects of sulfonamides
Clindamycin	antimotility drugs	Increased risk and severity of *C. difficile* colitis
	neuromuscular blocking agents	Increased blockage

*Not FDA-approved for this indication.

oxazole given prophylactically for *Pneumocystis carinii* infection was also found to prevent toxoplasmosis in AIDS patients. The optimal dose is not known.

In patients who are allergic to sulfonamides, a combination of pyrimethamine and clindamycin shows efficacy equal to that of pyrimethamine/sulfonamide. The exact mode of action of clindamycin, especially in TE, is not known. Whereas pyrimethamine and sulfadiazine cross the blood-brain barrier well, clindamycin does not. It is not known whether clindamycin accumulates in necrotic areas of the brain, especially when larger doses are used.

Other agents active against *T. gondii* have been less well studied in humans. Newer macrolides—roxithromycin, clarithromycin and azithromycin—have been found to be highly active against *T. gondii* in animal models and have been used successfully in a limited number of patients in combination with pyrimethamine. These macrolide antibiotics have the advantage of greater bioavailability. Higher and more persistent serum and/or intracellular levels can be achieved with these agents. Additional studies are needed to determine the exact role of these drugs. Unlike pyrimethamine and sulfadiazine, which are active in animal models only against the tachyzoite form, azithromycin may have activity against both

tachyzoites and the cyst forms (bradyzoites) of *T. gondii*. The macrolides should not be used as single agent therapy for toxoplasmosis, which is true for all the other agents as well. One exception is spiramycin, which is used to treat toxoplasmosis in pregnant women during the first trimester when pyrimethamine is contraindicated. Although spiramycin alone is less effective than the standard regimen, it remains as a viable option for patients who cannot tolerate pyrimethamine, sulfonamide, and clindamycin. Spiramycin can be obtained in the United States with permission of the United States Food and Drug Administration (FDA) (301-443-9550). Spiramycin does not cross the blood-brain barrier well, and in patients with AIDS, spiramycin, 2 grams daily, has been reported to be ineffective in preventing TE.

Atovaquone,* a hydroxynaphthoquinone, has been shown in a small number of patients to produce a partial or complete clinical and radiologic response. Atovaquone acts by blocking electron transport in parasite mitochondria, which in turn inhibits pyrimidine synthesis in malarial parasites but does not appear to be the mechanism of action in toxoplasma. Atovaquone has activity against both tachyzoites and tissue cysts of *T. gondii*. In vitro and animal studies have shown that atovaquone does not have synergistic effects when used with sulfadiazine, clarithromycin, or minocycline and in fact may even have an antagonistic effect with pyrimethamine. The exact clinical implications of these observations are not clear. Atovaquone is reasonably well tolerated. It is poorly absorbed from the gut, and the bioavailability is improved up to threefold when taken with a fatty meal. It has high protein-binding capacity and a long elimination half-life (50 to 70 hours). Relapse has occurred while on atovaquone maintenance therapy in several patients even after successful induction, thus limiting its use as a single agent in long-term treatment.

Trimetrexate,* a lipid-soluble analogue of methotrexate and a potent inhibitor of *T. gondii* DHFR, has activity against *T. gondii* in animal models. It is cleared both hepatically and renally with up to 41% excreted unchanged in the urine. In a salvage trial of trimetrexate-leucovorin for TE in sulfonamide-intolerant AIDS patients, trimetrexate was given intravenously at a dose of 30 to 280 mg per m² per day with leucovorin. Although the drug was well tolerated and patients had dramatic but transient improvement, relapse was noted while the patients were still receiving the drug, thus limiting the role of trimetrexate as a single agent in the treatment of TE in AIDS patients.

Experimental and anecdotal clinical data suggest that tetracycline/doxycycline has antitoxoplasma activity. In a limited number of patients given doxycycline, relapses occurred while they were still on the drug, raising the possibility of the development of drug resistance.

*Not FDA-approved for this indication.

Piritrexim,* an analogue of methotrexate, is a lipid-soluble folate antagonist active against murine toxoplasmosis when combined with sulfadiazine. Piritrexim has been used in patients with severe psoriasis in place of methotrexate, whose use is limited by the development of hepatic fibrosis and cirrhosis. In initial phase I/II clinical trials, adverse reactions were minimal and dose related. Piritrexim has not been tried in human toxoplasmosis. The nonclassic antifolates such as trimetrexate and piritrexim enter cells via passive diffusion, circumventing the need for the folate transport system(s) (which are absent in *T. gondii*) necessary for the uptake of classic antifolates, such as methotrexate. However, these nonclassic antifolates lack selectivity for parasite DHFR compared with mammalian DHFR, thus necessitating leucovorin rescue when used.

A variety of additional agents from different classes may have activity against *Toxoplasma*. Diclazuril† is an anticoccidial drug used to prevent coccidiosis in poultry in Canada, Europe, and South America. The drug has an excellent safety and toxicity profile in birds and mammals and has been used with some success at 200 mg per day in the treatment of *Isospora belli* infection in AIDS patients. Recently it has been shown to be active in murine toxoplasmosis when used in conjunction with pyrimethamine. The purine analogue arprinocid† is another anticoccidial agent used in veterinary medicine that has been shown to be active in murine toxoplasmosis. Arprinocid competitively inhibits hypoxanthine membrane transport, but it is unlikely that this is the mechanism of action against *T. gondii*. Substituted pyridopyrimidine compounds have been synthesized with more potent and selective activity against parasite DHFR. The clinical usefulness of these novel agents alone or in combination has not yet been established.

Immunomodulators such as gamma interferon‡ (Actimmune) have been shown to be active against toxoplasma both in vitro and in vivo. Interferon gamma appears to act primarily by activating macrophages to kill toxoplasma. The exact role of these immunomodulators either alone or in combination with antitoxoplasma agents has not yet been established.

ISSUES IN THE MANAGEMENT OF TOXOPLASMOSIS

Acute Acquired Toxoplasmosis in Immunocompetent Persons

In the immunocompetent individual, acute toxoplasmosis may go unnoticed because of minimal symptoms. Isolation of *Toxoplasma* from blood and body fluid, or demonstration of tachyzoites in tissue sections or smears of body fluids, establishes the diagnosis of acute toxoplasmosis. A variety of serologic tests are also available, and a diagnosis of recent acquired infection is confirmed if there is seroconversion from a negative to a positive titer. A high IgM titer (measured either by indirect fluorescent antibody test or by ELISA) and a positive Sabin-Feldman dye test are probably diagnostic of recent acute infection, with or without symptoms. Traditionally, treatment is not given for acute acquired toxoplasmosis in immunocompetent patients unless there are severe and persistent symptoms, or clinically overt disease with myocarditis, pneumonitis, or encephalitis, in which case treatment is given for 2 to 4 weeks or longer if warranted. Infection acquired by transfusion or laboratory accident should be treated promptly.

Acute Toxoplasmosis in Pregnancy and Congenital Toxoplasmosis

Treatment of acutely infected pregnant women decreases the incidence of fetal infection. If treatment is to be given during the first trimester, spiramycin* is the current drug of choice. The exact duration of therapy is not known. If the fetus is not infected, it is recommended that spiramycin be given without interruption until delivery. Treatment with sulfadiazine alone (or with an equivalent sulfonamide) is recommended if spiramycin is not available. Fetal infection can be documented by prenatal diagnosis based on detection of the parasites or parasite DNA in the cord blood, amniotic fluid, or placental tissue. Polymerase chain reaction (PCR)–based assays for the detection of *T. gondii* DNA are promising. Detection of specific IgM and IgA in fetal serum must be interpreted with caution because of the possibility of contamination with maternal blood. Fetal ultrasonography should be performed periodically to document evidence of fetal infection. In first and second trimester pregnancies with acute fetal toxoplasmosis, the pregnancy need not be interrupted. Pyrimethamine and sulfadiazine combined with leucovorin rescue can be given in the second and third trimester, and these appear to be superior to spiramycin alone. Pyrimethamine and sulfadiazine can be alternated with spiramycin every 3 weeks until delivery. Both symptomatic and asymptomatic infants with congenital toxoplasmosis can be treated with alternating courses of 4 weeks of pyrimethamine and sulfonamides and 6 weeks of spiramycin through the first year of life. Alternatively, for infants with overt disease, pyrimethamine and sulfonamide should be given for the first 6 months of life, and then this combination can be alternated with spiramycin every 4 weeks through 12 to 18 months of age. Prednisone (1 to 2 mg per kg per day) should be given if there is evidence of inflammation, such as high CSF protein value or chorioretinitis.

HIV-infected pregnant women who are seropositive for toxoplasmosis pose therapeutic problems. Until further data are made available, these women should

---

*Investigational drug in the United States.
†Not available in the United States.
‡Not FDA-approved for this indication.

---

*Investigational drug in the United States.

receive spiramycin during the first trimester of pregnancy if their CD4 lymphocyte counts are less than 200 per mm^3 and pyrimethamine/sulfadiazine or trimethoprim-sulfamethoxazole later on in pregnancy.

Toxoplasmosis in Immunocompromised Patients

Toxoplasmosis has emerged as the single most common opportunistic infection of the central nervous system in patients with AIDS, causing encephalitis or focal cerebral lesions. At present, treatment is usually initiated empirically in AIDS patients with typical findings on CT scan or MRI of the brain and positive toxoplasma serology. In empirically treated patients, clear clinical and radiologic response should be seen within 14 days. Brain biopsy and attempts at definitive diagnosis should be made if empirically treated patients deteriorate clinically by 7 days or do not improve clinically by 10 days. Extracerebral toxoplasmosis (ECT) with dissemination, although rare, is not uncommon in patients with advanced AIDS. Ocular toxoplasmosis is the most common manifestation of ECT, and it is frequently associated with cytomegaloviral (CMV) retinitis, making diagnosis difficult. Cerebral toxoplasmosis could occur before, during, or after ECT diagnosis. Involvement of other organ systems can occur during dissemination, or it may present as isolated, unexplained fevers. Demonstration of parasitemia establishes the diagnosis of ECT in AIDS patients with unexplained fevers.

Primary or induction therapy should be given for 3 to 6 weeks or more, depending on the severity of illness and response to therapy. Although the combination of pyrimethamine and sulfadiazine with leucovorin rescue remains the mainstay of therapy, a substantial number of AIDS patients have severe adverse reactions to this combination (see Table 1), in which case pyrimethamine and intravenous clindamycin becomes the therapy of choice. This latter combination, although efficacious, is associated with a slightly higher rate of failure due to disease progression than with the pyrimethamine-sulfadiazine combination. Use of corticosteroids for reduction of cerebral edema and raised intracranial pressure may complicate interpretation of response to empirical therapy for TE. Seizures occur in up to 35% of patients with TE, necessitating the use of anticonvulsants. However, anticonvulsants should not be used prophylactically.

In a limited number of AIDS patients allergic to sulfonamides and also intolerant of clindamycin, sulfadiazine desensitization has been attempted under close in-hospital supervision. One protocol is to administer gradually increasing amounts of sulfadiazine orally every 3 hours for 4 to 5 days, starting at 10 μg. Sulfadiazine suspensions can be prepared using sulfadiazine and 2% methylcellulose mucilage.

Relapse of toxoplasma encephalitis occurs, even after successful induction, in over 50% of patients if they do not receive subsequent maintenance therapy.

Pyrimethamine (25 to 75 mg per day) plus sulfadiazine (500 mg four times a day) is the recommended suppressive therapy. If sulfonamides cannot be used, then pyrimethamine (75 mg per day) combined with clindamycin (450 mg three times a day) should be given, although retrospective studies indicate a higher rate of relapse with this latter combination. Alternative regimens include pyrimethamine plus either atovaquone* (750 mg q 6 h), dapsone (100 mg per day), or azithromycin (500 mg per day). Folinic acid should be given in conjunction with pyrimethamine.

Ocular Toxoplasmosis

Ocular toxoplasmosis usually occurs as a late sequel of congenital infection. Toxoplasmic chorioretinitis may also be a manifestation of extracerebral toxoplasmosis in AIDS patients. Clindamycin with sulfadiazine (minimum 3 weeks) has been reported to be effective because of rapid resolution of inflammation. Systemic corticosteroids are usually given when lesions involve the macula or optic nerve head, threatening vision. Relapses are common, necessitating retreatment. Photocoagulation may be necessary both for the treatment of active lesions and for prophylaxis.

Prophylaxis

General measures to prevent acquisition of infection are important, especially for pregnant women and immunocompromised patients. Meats should be heated to 60° C or frozen to −20° C or less to kill the cysts. Thorough washing of hands after handling raw meat is a must. Fruits and vegetables may be contaminated with oocysts and hence must be thoroughly washed before eating. Direct contact with cat feces should be avoided.

A single agent that is safe and free of side effects, active against both the cyst form and tachyzoites, which can be used as a prophylactic agent, is not available. AIDS patients with evidence of positive toxoplasma serology have been targeted for primary prophylaxis of toxoplasma encephalitis. Although a number of drugs appear to be useful in prophylaxis against TE, no concrete recommendations can be made since most of the studies were retrospective in design, involving small patient samples. Trimethoprim-sulfamethoxazole (4 to 7 double-strength tablets per week) or dapsone (50 mg per day) combined with pyrimethamine (50 mg per week) or roxithromycin (300 mg three times a week) appears to be effective in the prevention of reactivation of toxoplasmosis. Drug therapy for primary prevention of TE in AIDS patients should be individualized, taking into consideration drug intolerance, adverse effects, and interactions with other drugs commonly used in AIDS patients. Trimethoprim combined with sulfamethoxazole, as a single agent, has the added advan-

---

*Not FDA-approved for this indication.

tage of prevention of *Pneumocystis carinii* infection. The problems associated with this combination are significant side effects and possible reactivation while on the drug.

TRICHINELLOSIS

method of
J. DICK MacLEAN, M.D.

McGill University Centre for Tropical Diseases
Montreal, Quebec, Canada

Trichinellosis is a disease caused by the nematode genus *Trichinella* and is acquired by the ingestion of larvae encysted in the infected muscle of animals. In the past, infected pork was the most common source of human infection, but the frequency of such infections has been greatly diminished with better pig husbandry. At present the most common sources of the infection are animals such as bear, wild boar, and walrus.

After being ingested, infective larvae mature over several days into adults, and the females inhabit the small intestinal mucosa where they begin to produce large numbers of newborn larvae daily for the following 4 to 6 weeks. These larvae enter the systemic circulation, are disseminated, and invade tissues throughout the body. The pathology produced appears to be a combination of a vigorous host inflammatory response and direct damage caused by the 100 by 6 mμ larvae. The larvae have a predilection for striated muscle cells in which they round up in cystlike forms, isolating themselves from the immune response of the host.

The majority of individuals infected with a small number of *Trichinella* will be asymptomatic. In those who become ill, the clinical picture reflects the number of ingested larvae and the evolving life cycle of the parasite. An initial intestinal phase is followed by a visceral phase. The intestinal phase may include abdominal pain, nausea, vomiting, and/or diarrhea lasting several days to weeks. It is superseded by the visceral phase, consisting of pain, tenderness and weakness of muscles, subungual and conjunctival hemorrhages, at times periorbital or peripheral edema, and central evanescent rashes. This phase can persist for up to 4 to 6 weeks. The triad of blood eosinophilia, raised serum creatine phosphokinase, and *Trichinella* antibodies that develop after 3 weeks is highly specific, and it is usually not necessary to confirm the diagnosis with the visualization of larvae in a muscle biopsy. Heavy infections can result in meningo-encephalitis, myocarditis, and pneumonitis. These severe complications are the most frequent causes of death in trichinellosis and reflect the inflammatory response to larvae invading these vital organs.

THERAPY

The goals of treatment for trichinellosis are to decrease the host's inflammatory response and to kill the different stages of the parasite. The advisability of treatment and the nature of the treatment depend on the severity of the infection, the stage of the illness, and the patient's tolerance of medications.

In mild cases without fever, severe symptoms, or involvement of vital organs, treatment may be limited to aspirin or other nonsteroidal anti-inflammatory agents. Mebendazole (Vermox) should be prescribed to eliminate adults and disseminating larvae (200 to 400 mg orally every 8 hours for 3 days, followed by 400 to 500 mg orally, every 8 hours for 10 days). The patient should be followed closely during therapy because the death of worms may lead to an exaggerated inflammatory response and worsening of the illness. Should this occur, corticosteroids may be given (e.g., oral prednisone in declining doses over 4 days, as described later).

In florid disease (high fever, severe pain, extensive edema, or involvement of vital organs), the first line of therapy is corticosteroids. The administration of prednisone, 0.5 to 2.0 mg per kg per day orally in two equal doses every 12 hours, should be started. This daily dosage can be continued for 10 days and then tapered by halving to terminate in 4 to 7 days. This treatment will lead to defervescence, diminution of myalgia, and amelioration of central nervous system dysfunction. After 1 to 2 days of prednisone, mebendazole is added to the therapy (dose as given earlier). Should the mebendazole lead to a deterioration of important clinical functions as a result of the destruction of worms, an increase in prednisone and a decrease in mebendazole is advised. Thiabendazole (Mintezol) has been used as the anthelminthic in the past but appears to have no therapeutic advantage and has more side effects.

Mebendazole has been used successfully as a prophylactic drug during the incubation period in persons known to have ingested infected meat.

TULAREMIA

method of
DAVID A. HAAKE, M.D.

University of California, Los Angeles
Los Angeles, California

Tularemia is a bacterial zoonosis that is usually transmitted to humans by exposure to infected animals or biting arthropods. Both the disease and the causative agent, *Francisella tularensis,* derive their names from Tulare, California, where the bacterium was first isolated in 1912 from ground squirrels. This highly virulent organism is capable of infecting a broad range of animal hosts. Although rabbits and hares are the most important animal reservoirs, hundreds of wild and domestic mammals, birds, amphibians, and fish have been found to be infected. *F. tularensis* is also remarkable for its high infectivity rate and its ability to persist in a wide variety of environmental conditions. Numerous cases of tularemia have been documented in the medical literature involving indirect transmission via water, mud, articles of clothing, or other inanimate objects contaminated by infected animals. Animal-associated cases occur primarily during the rabbit-hunting months of November through February. Transmission by arthropods usually involves ticks, biting flies, and mosquitos that are active during warmer months of May through September. Individuals at increased risk include veterinarians, hunters, trappers, meat handlers and cooks, sheep workers, agricultural workers, campers, and laboratory technicians. Tularemia is found throughout temperate climates of the Northern Hemisphere, except in the United Kingdom. Although the disease is found throughout the United States (except Hawaii), most cases occur in Arkansas, Illinois, Missouri, Texas, Virginia, and Tennessee.

Tularemia can present in a number of different ways, depending upon the localization of the disease process. However, the general features of tularemia are the same regardless of how the disease is manifested. After an incubation period of 3 to 5 days, there is abrupt onset of symptoms, including high fever, chills, headache, cough, and generalized myalgia. Symptoms often subside after 24 to 96 hours only to recur 1 to 3 days later. The illness typically continues for 2 to 3 weeks, associated with fatigue and weight loss. Without appropriate treatment, some patients may develop persistent fatigue lasting for several months.

The classification of tularemia reflects the ability of the organism to enter the body via the skin, mucous membranes, and gastrointestinal or respiratory tracts. The most common presentation is *ulceroglandular tularemia,* which results from cutaneous inoculation. Lymphadenopathy typically begins 1 or 2 days after onset of fever, associated with development of one or more painful, small, red papules at the site of inoculation. The papule progresses to a pustule and then to an ulcer with sharp undermined borders and a flat base. Upper extremity ulcers are usually associated with exposure to infected animals, whereas lesions located on the lower extremities, abdomen, back, or head usually reflect transmission by biting arthropods. Generalized lymphadenopathy may occur, reflecting bacteremic dissemination of the organism. *Glandular tularemia* refers to lymphadenopathy without formation of an ulcerative lesion. Without treatment, the nodes often persist for long periods. Half become fluctuant, leading to drainage and fistula formation. The differential diagnosis of ulceroglandular tularemia includes bubonic plague, ecthyma gangrenosum, sporotrichosis, cat-scratch disease, rat-bite fever, boutonneuse fever, and anthrax.

F. tularensis may also gain access to the body via mucous membranes. When the portal of entry is the conjunctivae, *oculoglandular tularemia* may result. Inflammation and edema of the eyelids and conjunctivitis occur, with regional lymphadenopathy involving the preauricular, submandibular, and cervical nodes. Ingestion of inadequately cooked meat or contaminated food may lead to inoculation via the oropharynx. The resulting condition is referred to as *oropharyngeal (anginose) tularemia.* Exudative pharyngitis and tonsillitis with cervical lymphadenopathy are the usual manifestations. It is important to note that sore throat, with or without physical signs of pharyngitis, may occur in patients with tularemia regardless of whether there is a reason why the oropharynx would be the portal of entry. *Pneumonic tularemia* occurs when there is airborne transmission of the pathogen. Aerosols of *F. tularensis* have resulted in outbreaks of tularemia in occupational, recreational, and laboratory settings. Patients will usually present with fever, nonproductive cough, dyspnea, and substernal and/or pleuritic chest pain. Radiographic studies typically reveal hilar lymphadenopathy and scattered pulmonary infiltrates. Pneumonic involvement also occurs in ulceroglandular or typhoidal illness due to hematogenous dissemination to the lungs.

Typhoidal tularemia presents as disseminated infection with symptoms of sepsis without localizing features or lymphadenopathy. Patients with this form of tularemia typically have underlying medical disorders. Pulmonary infiltrates are frequently present. Severely ill patients may have hyponatremia, meningitis, rhabdomyolysis, myoglobinuria, renal failure, hypotension, adult respiratory distress syndrome, and intravascular coagulopathy. Blood cultures are more likely to be positive due to the high levels of bacteremia. Typhoidal tularemia can mimic typhoid fever, brucellosis, legionellosis, Q fever, rickettsiosis, malaria, endocarditis, and tuberculosis.

The mortality rate for untreated tularemia is 8%. Early diagnosis and treatment reduce the mortality rate to 1% to 2%. Risk factors for an adverse outcome include increased age, serious underlying medical disorders, a delay in initiation of appropriate therapy, significant pulmonary involvement, and typhoidal disease.

LABORATORY DIAGNOSIS

The diagnosis of tularemia is based upon clinical suspicion and confirmed with specific serologic studies. Routine laboratory tests such as white blood cell count, platelet count, and sedimentation rate may or may not be abnormal. Hyponatremia, elevated serum transaminases, increased creatine phosphokinase, and myoglobinuria have been reported. *F. tularensis* is a small, pleomorphic, gram-negative coccobacillus, but it is difficult to identify in infectious material due to its poor staining qualities. Although the organism is fastidious it will occasionally grow in blood culture media. The organism is a serious laboratory hazard due to its virulence and its high infectivity rate. Clinical microbiology laboratory personnel should be alerted if the diagnosis of tularemia is suspected.

Serologic testing for tularemia is widely available. The standard technique involves tube agglutination of a bacterial suspension. This test is usually negative during the first week of illness, becoming positive during the second week, and peaking after 4 to 5 weeks. An acute agglutination titer of 1:160 is supportive of the diagnosis but may also result from infection occurring in the remote past. A fourfold rise in titer between acute and convalescent specimens is definitive evidence of recent infection. More sensitive methods of antibody detection are available in some laboratories, such as the enzyme immunoassay (EIA).

TREATMENT

Tularemia can be challenging to treat due to the toxicity of the recommended antibiotics and the propensity of the disease for relapse. Nevertheless, patients suspected to have tularemia on clinical grounds should be treated empirically even if serologic confirmation is pending. The drug of choice for treatment of tularemia is streptomycin because of the wealth of clinical experience with this agent, the ability of streptomycin to induce a prompt clinical response, and the low incidence of relapse after therapy. The standard regimen is 7.5 to 10 mg per kg intramuscularly every 12 hours for 10 to 14 days. An alternative approach is to give 15 mg per kg intramuscularly every 12 hours the first 3 days, followed by 7.5 mg per kg intramuscularly every 12 hours for the remainder of the course. Eighty percent of patients defervesce within 48 hours. Severely ill patients may require continuation of the 15 mg per kg intramuscularly every 12 hours dosage, although this increases the risk of vestibular and auditory ototoxicity. Doses greater than 2 grams per day are unlikely to provide additional benefit.

Fluctuant nodes should be needle aspirated or surgically drained. However, invasive procedures are not recommended until streptomycin has been administered for 48 hours. Incision and drainage of untreated patients has occasionally resulted in bacteremia and sepsis. Gentamicin is an acceptable alternative to streptomycin, although its efficacy has been less well documented. Gentamicin is administered intravenously at a dose of 3 to 5 mg per kg per day in divided doses for 10 to 14 days. The effectiveness of streptomycin and gentamicin in the treatment of tularemia is related to the fact that aminoglycosides are bactericidal antibiotics. As with all aminoglycosides, the dose of streptomycin and gentamicin should be adjusted in patients with impaired renal function.

Tetracycline and chloramphenicol have occasionally been used in the treatment of tularemia. These agents may be useful as oral therapy in less severely ill patients. However, due to the fact that these drugs are bacteriostatic, there is a much higher incidence of failure or relapse than in patients treated with aminoglycosides. The dosage of tetracycline should be 2.0 grams per day orally in divided doses for at least 14 days. Tetracycline should not be used in children less than 9 years old, during pregnancy, or during lactation. A suggested oral tetracycline regimen in older children is 30 mg per kg per day in divided doses, to a maximum of 2.0 grams per day. Lower doses or shorter courses of tetracycline increase the risk of relapse, which usually occurs within the first 2 weeks after discontinuing therapy. Due to the risk of hematologic toxicity, use of chloramphenicol should be restricted to patients who are not able to receive aminoglycosides or tetracycline. The oral dose of chloramphenicol is 30 to 50 mg per kg per day in three or four divided doses for 14 days. An important role for chloramphenicol is in patients with meningitis. Penetration of the blood-brain barrier by aminoglycosides is poor. If evidence of meningeal infection is present, chloramphenicol, 50 to 100 mg per kg per day intravenously in divided doses, can be added to streptomycin.

A number of alternative drugs have been considered for use in tularemia. Erythromycin,* ciprofloxacin (Cipro)* norfloxacin (Noroxin)* and imipenem/cilastatin (Primaxin)* have been used successfully. However, there are insufficient clinical data to consider these drugs as adequate therapy. In vitro sensitivity testing suggested that the third-generation cephalosporins could be an effective and less toxic substitute for chloramphenicol in the treatment of meningeal infection. However, in vitro data do not necessarily correlate with clinical efficacy. A recent study documented eight failures of outpatient use of ceftriaxone in the treatment of tularemia. These patients were being treated empirically for presumed nontularemia infection and had a clinical deterioration.

---

*Not FDA-approved for this indication.

After the diagnosis of tularemia was made, these patients responded rapidly to standard therapy.

PREVENTION

The risk of tularemia can be reduced significantly through education and simple, common sense measures. Dead or sick animals should be avoided. Hunters and trappers should wear gloves when handling or skinning game, especially rabbits. Game should be cooked thoroughly prior to ingestion. Insect repellents and protective clothing are important in reducing exposure to biting insects. Physical examination for ticks should be performed frequently. Attached ticks should be removed promptly using tweezers or forceps to grasp the tick's mouthparts as close to the skin as possible. *F. tularensis* has a high infectivity rate, so laboratory workers should use caution when working with clinical samples that are potentially contaminated with this organism.

SALMONELLOSIS

method of
ARVID E. UNDERMAN, M.D.
University of Southern California School of
Medicine
Los Angeles, California

Salmonellosis quite obviously is infection caused by members of the genus *Salmonella,* which are gram-negative bacilli belonging to the family Enterobacteriaceae. Classically, four clinical syndromes have been well described to which, I believe, a fifth should be added. The first is acute enterocolitis, which is by far the most common presentation and is usually self-limited. The second is focal extraintestinal infection with either concomitant or antecedent bacteremia (e.g., mycotic aneurysm of the aorta, osteomyelitis, septic arthritis, rarely meningitis). The third is enteric fever that is not caused by *Salmonella typhi,* in about 10% of cases. Fourth, there are chronic asymptomatic carriers. The proposed fifth clinical presentation is that of persistent or recurrent *Salmonella* bacteremia over weeks to months. In the past, this has been seen with hepatosplenic schistosomiasis but now is frequently encountered in human immunodeficiency virus (HIV)–infected individuals, with or without full-blown acquired immunodeficiency syndrome (AIDS).

Microbiologically, salmonellae are motile, gram-negative, nonspore-forming organisms that are differentiated from other Enterobacteriaceae by inability to ferment lactose and sucrose while producing acid, hydrogen sulfide, and, except in the case of *S. typhi,* gas. The taxonomy may delight microbiologists but is a clinician's nightmare, given the existence of 2000 serotypes. The traditional Kauffman-White schema divides the organisms depending upon their somatic lipopolysaccharide (O) antigens, along with their flagellar (H) antigens. The current proper nomenclature divides the salmonellae into three species: *S. typhi, S. choleraesuis,* and *S. enteritidis,* with the latter species containing all but the first two serotypes. For the present, it is expeditious to regard each separately so that all serotypes using their O antigens can be divided into five principal groups, A through E. No more than 10 to 15 serotypes account for most human isolates. It is hoped that new molecular techniques may resolve the confusion. Current techniques, such as plasmid analysis and ribotyping, are tools for epidemiologic tracking. The salmonellae are widely distributed throughout nature and occur both in warm- and cold-blooded vertebrates. Most are adapted to specific hosts, with *S. typhi* and *S. paratyphi* occurring only in humans. The source of human infection is most often related to contaminated food products, especially in the context of improper preparation, cooking, and refrigeration, thereby allowing the organisms to multiply. Novel sources of human salmonellosis include pet turtles, lizards, iguanas, African hedgehogs, rattlesnake meat (as either a delicacy or folk remedy), and even manure-contaminated marijuana.

Clinical infections in immunocompetent humans usually require the ingestion of more than 10^6 organisms. Fewer organisms may cause disease in the following situations: (1) decreased gastric acidity as the result of achlorhydria, surgery, or pharmacologic blockade (cimetidine, ranitidine, omeprazole); (2) impaired cellular immunity as the result of solid tumor, lymphoma, chemotherapy, or HIV infection; (3) chronic hemolytic anemia, most importantly in sickle cell disease; (4) infants less than 6 months of age or the debilitated elderly; (5) splenectomy or cirrhosis with portal hypertension; (6) severe atherosclerosis or endovascular aneurysms, chiefly of the aorta and great vessels. Moreover, concurrent use of antibiotics can markedly reduce the number of salmonellae needed to produce infection by altering or reducing the normal bowel flora.

Human salmonellosis is most often sporadic rather than epidemic. Primary contacts of clinical cases may have positive stool cultures but no illness. The incidence of human salmonellosis is thought to be greatly under-reported, with estimates as high as 1 million cases annually. The majority go undetected because the self-limited nature of the disease obviates either medical attention or the need to perform cultures. Currently there is an ongoing outbreak of salmonellosis caused by *S. enteritidis,* traced to eggs.

The salmonella were among the earliest bacteria to show antibiotic resistance. This has continued on a worldwide basis, facilitated by indiscriminate use of antibiotics, both in medical practice and agriculture. Resistance to ampicillin, a former mainstay of therapy, has approached or surpassed 50%. The small number of effective agents available to us to treat serious infection should mandate their judicious administration.

ENTEROCOLITIS

Clinical Picture

Enterocolitis is by far the most common clinical presentation of salmonellosis. Incubation ranges from 6 to 96 hours, most commonly occurring between 12 and 48 hours. Initial symptoms include nausea and vomiting, followed by headaches, myalgias, malaise, chills, low-grade fever, abdominal cramps, and diarrhea. High temperatures (40° C, or 104° F) should alert the clinician to invasive disease. Stools may be merely loose or profuse and watery. On direct examination, they may or may not contain polymorphonuclear leukocytes or occult blood. The presence of mucus or gross blood in the absence of hemorrhoids or fissures should alert the clinician to organisms causing dysentery. The white count is most often normal or slightly elevated, with a left

shift containing 10 to 15 bands. Low white counts with greater numbers of bands should alert the clinician to possible bacteremia. The diagnosis can be confirmed only by stool or blood culture. Serum serology examinations are not helpful. Most healthy adults have a self-limited, uncomplicated course, with resolution of symptoms without treatment within 48 to 72 hours.

Treatment

Fluid and Electrolyte Replacement

The sine qua non in the treatment of diarrhea is fluid and electrolyte replacement. In most cases, increased oral intake of bland juices coupled with clear broths and temporary elimination of lactose-containing foods will suffice. Commercial electrolyte solutions (Pedialyte) may be useful. Though not readily available in the United States, rehydration salts are widely employed. The World Health Organization recommends and distributes packets containing 90 mmol of sodium, 20 of potassium, 80 of chloride, 30 of bicarbonate, along with 111 mmol of glucose to be dissolved in 1 liter of sterile or boiled water. This mixture should be consumed at a rate sufficient to compensate for diarrheal losses while maintaining a dilute, nonconcentrated-appearing urine output. Within 24 to 48 hours, the diet can be supplemented with bland soft foods given in small, frequent feedings. If the patient has profuse vomiting or severe dehydration as determined by orthostatic changes in blood pressure, parenteral rehydration should be used. Frequently, this can be accomplished in an outpatient infusion room rather than through admission to hospital. When there is persistent emesis, profuse diarrhea, systemic toxicity, or abnormalities in serum electrolytes, parenteral rehydration in hospital is prudent.

Antimotility and Antinausea Agents

The use of agents such as atropine-diphenoxylate (Lomotil) or loperamide (Imodium) should be discouraged. Though they may result in symptomatic improvement in cramps and diarrhea, they have a potential to increase complications and even predispose to bacteremia. In general, if the patient has a fever and the diarrhea contains blood or mucus, their use should be eschewed. Most pediatricians feel they should never be used in children younger than 5 years of age. An alternative is bismuth subsalicylate (Pepto-Bismol). The adult dose is 1 ounce (2 tablespoons) or 2 tablets (262.5 mg) every 30 minutes for 8 hours. The pediatric dose is 1.1 mL per kg at 4-hour intervals for up to 5 days. Although nausea and vomiting are occasional presenting symptoms with enterocolitis, they rarely persist. Prochlorperazine (Compazine) or trimenthobenzamide (Tigan) may be helpful. Both are available in oral, suppository, or parenteral form. Suppositories usually stimulate further diarrhea. Vomiting may preclude oral administration. A singular muscular injection of Compazine, 5 to 10 mg, is often all that is needed. This may be repeated every 4 to 6 hours as needed. Promethazine hydrochloride (Phenergan) is more frequently used in children and may be used orally (0.5 mg per lb or 1.0 mg per kg every 6 hours) or intramuscularly in the same doses. Again, suppositories may stimulate the diarrhea.

Antibiotics

Antibiotics are not needed in the treatment of uncomplicated *Salmonella* enterocolitis in otherwise healthy children or adults. Studies have shown that they neither shorten the course nor improve symptoms. Overuse will contribute to emergence of resistance, as well as increase risk of symptomatic and bacteriologic relapse. Moreover, their use may actually prolong the convalescent excretion or contribute to chronic carriage of the organism. Newer quinolone drugs may be the exception to the latter; however, their frequent use has been paralleled by increasing resistance worldwide. Postponing antibiotic therapy until the return of a stool culture often provides the physician with a way to avert the frequent patient demand for antibiotic therapy. Often patients are better by the time results are available. Nevertheless, high-risk patients, as previously identified, should receive treatment to prevent potential complications of bacteremia. Additionally, if patients are sick enough to require hospitalization, antibiotic therapy should be considered but in no way is mandated.

Appropriate antimicrobial therapy should be guided by susceptibility testing. Initially, trimethoprim-sulfamethoxazole (TMP/SMX) (co-trimoxazole, Bactrim or Septra) may be administered to the non-sulfonamide-sensitive patient. The dose is 5 to 8 mg of trimethoprim per kg every 12 hours for children or 1 double-strength tablet (160 mg trimethoprim/ 800 mg sulfamethoxazole) every 12 hours for adults. Though widely used, trimethoprim-sulfamethoxazole has not yet received FDA approval. If the organism is susceptible, ampicillin, 50 mg per kg orally to 100 mg per kg per day intravenously, each in four divided doses for children, or 2 to 4 grams per day in four divided doses for adults, may be administered. Amoxicillin in equivalent oral dosage may be substituted. The duration of therapy is generally 5 days. If there is complicating bacteremia or systemic infection, the foregoing is modified as outlined next.

Newer quinolone antibiotics, such as ciprofloxacin, ofloxacin, and norfloxacin, are effective. They are, however, contraindicated in prepubertal children and pregnant women. Adult doses are ciprofloxacin (Cipro), 500 mg twice daily, ofloxacin (Floxin), 400 mg twice daily, or norfloxin (Noroxin), 400 mg twice daily. There is definitely a trend in the United States to use these agents empirically for all suspect bacterial diarrhea; however, the clinician should bear in mind that their widespread use is both expensive and contributes to emerging resistance. Therefore, it is recommended that they be reserved for the previously mentioned high-risk groups who have either resistant *Salmonella* or who are intolerant or allergic to sulfonamide or ampicillin.

BACTEREMIA AND FOCAL INFECTION

Bacteremia in acute uncomplicated *Salmonella* enterocolitis is infrequent. Therefore, blood cultures are not routinely necessary except in patients who fall into the previously outlined high-risk categories. Shaking chills or high fever (40° C, 104° F) should alert the clinician to possible bacteremia. Focal suppurative infection subsequent to bacteremia is infrequent but may occur at any site. Thus, *Salmonella* has been associated with bronchopneumonia, empyema, soft tissue infection, aortic mycotic aneurysms, endocarditis, septic arthritis, splenic or hepatic abscesses, meningitis, and osteomyelitis. The clinician should have a high index of suspicion for an endovascular mycotic aneurysm in patients older than 50 years of age. *Salmonella* should always be suspected in individuals with sickle cell disease. Indeed, bone and joint infections are, in general, the most frequent sites of extraintestinal infection with *Salmonella*. Meningitis occurs primarily in infants younger than 5 months of age. In patients with HIV, diagnosis of a *Salmonella* bacteremia will almost always be accompanied by recurrent episodes.

Treatment

Bacteremia and localized suppurative infection require antibiotic therapy. Owing to the problem of resistance, this therapy must be altered according to the results of susceptibility testing. The recovery of the organism is therefore extremely important, and adequate cultures of blood or infected material should be obtained before initiation of therapy. Parenteral ampicillin, 100 to 200 mg per kg per day divided into four doses, or trimethoprim-sulfamethoxazole (TMP/SMX), 8 to 10 mg per kg of trimethoprim per day in three divided doses, may be used. In the case of resistance or sensitivity to the foregoing, third-generation cephalosporins such as cefotaxime (Claforan) or ceftriaxone (Rocephin) have excellent activity, though neither are FDA-approved for this indication. Cefotaxime, 1 to 2 grams every 6 to 8 hours for adults, or 100 to 200 mg per kg per day in three or four divided doses for children, has been found effective in bacteremia, osteomyelitis, septic arthritis, and a variety of other focal *Salmonella* infections. Chloramphenicol's use is superannuated, both by toxicity, availability of other effective agents, and, interestingly, by cost.

Focal infection often requires surgery. Often this is as simple as the drainage of localized suppuration or lavage of a septic joint, but it may require extensive vascular reconstruction, as in the case of infected aortic aneurysms.

The duration of therapy for bacteremia is 10 to 14 days, whereas osteomyelitis and endovascular infections require 6 weeks. Quinolones such as ciprofloxacin, 500 mg twice daily orally, may be helpful in treating osteomyelitis. Trimethoprim-sulfamethoxazole can also be used in this fashion. Both have adequate blood levels after oral administration. I have had to use continuous prophylaxis of either trimethoprim-sulfamethoxazole or ciprofloxacin in several HIV patients to prevent recurrent bacteremia. This was not a problem since prophylactic trimethoprim-sulfamethoxazole is used chronically for *Pneumocystis*.

ENTERIC FEVER

Clinical Picture

The clinical picture of nontyphoidal *Salmonella* enteric fever is indistinguishable from that of typhoid fever, which is discussed elsewhere in this publication.

Treatment

The antibiotic therapy of nontyphoidal enteric fever parallels that of the treatment of typhoid. The reader is referred to that section in this publication. Treatment should be adjusted and altered once the results of susceptibility testing are available. Acceptable regimens include ampicillin, amoxicillin, and trimethoprim-sulfamethoxazole, along with third-generation cephalosporins and quinolone antibiotics. My preference has been to use cefotaxime (Claforan), in the same doses as for bacteremic salmonellosis. The duration is 10 to 14 days. Relapse rates are low; relapse may be seen within 2 to 6 weeks. Relapse requires an equivalent course of therapy in both dose and duration. Comparative studies are ongoing using both third-generation cephalosporins such as ceftriaxone and oral quinolones in short-course therapy of typhoid, as well as nontyphoidal enteric fever. Although these show some promise, they are currently not the standard of practice in the United States. Nevertheless, a strong case can be made for using quinolones inasmuch as intravenous usage can be rapidly converted to oral usage, with obvious cost saving. Otherwise healthy young adults may be treated orally as outpatients. Furthermore, the incidence of relapse may be less, convalescent carriage shortened, and chronic carriage prevented. The foregoing, if for no other reason, should cause the physician not to prescribe quinolones for uncomplicated enterocolitis or other self-limited diarrheas of bacterial origin.

Adjunctive measures are of importance, including attention to fluid and electrolyte balance and nutrition. The use of corticosteroids is controversial and certainly for use only in those patients who are delirious, obtunded, stuporous, comatose, or in shock. It has been my overall impression that nontyphoidal enteric fever is somewhat milder than typhoid itself, and complications such as gastrointestinal bleeding or ileal perforation are exceedingly rare.

CARRIER STATE

Asymptomatic excretion of organisms invariably occurs following clinical *Salmonella* enterocolitis. It exceeds 8 weeks in 5 to 10% of patients. Chronic carriage, either in the stool or urine, is defined as excretion of the organism for greater than 1 year. Its incidence is stated to be 1% in adults and 5% in children less than 5 years of age. This is somewhat less than that seen with *S. typhi*. Convalescent excreters need only maintain strict personal hygiene to prevent transmission of the organism. Those involved in food preparation or health or child care should be maintained off work until three successive cultures are negative at intervals prescribed by the public health department. It goes without saying that all positive cases of salmonellosis are reportable by law to local public health authorities. Recently, oral quinolones have been used (ciprofloxacin, 500 to 750 mg twice daily for 5 to 14 days), to curtail institutional outbreaks, as in nursing homes or psychiatric facilities. While this may be expeditious, eliminating or preventing the source of the outbreak in a prospective fashion is preferable. In the case of food handlers and health or child care workers, some feel that quinolone therapy eliminates the problem of convalescent excretion, hence individuals may return to work without delay. Though data generally support this, the successive negative stool requirement will not be obviated.

As stated, the management of the chronic carriage of nontyphoidal salmonellosis is the same as that of *S. typhi*, which is discussed in detail elsewhere. A 4- to 6-week course of oral antibiotics may be tried when there is no evidence of gallbladder disease; however, if chronic cholecystitis and/or cholelithiasis is present, cholecystectomy is almost always necessary. Despite cholecystectomy, a certain number of individuals will continue to excrete organisms thought to be of hepatobiliary origin. Chronic carriage is seen, albeit rarely, in the United States with either *Schistosoma mansoni* or *Schistosoma haematobium*. When these parasites are treated, subsequent therapy of the *Salmonella* results in termination of the stool or urinary carriage state.

TYPHOID FEVER

method of
THOMAS BUTLER, M.D.
Texas Tech University Health Sciences Center
Lubbock, Texas

Typhoid fever remains a major global infectious disease with an estimated annual world incidence of 12 million cases with 500,000 deaths. In the United States, there are about 300 cases annually, and most of these occur in travelers who have recently returned from countries with high incidences of typhoid fever, such as Mexico, Pakistan, and India.

CLINICAL FEATURES

Infection is transmitted by ingestion of water or food contaminated with *Salmonella typhi*. Unsanitary conditions or unchlorinated water sources, as obtain in developing countries, give rise to infections, or an asymptomatic chronic fecal carrier of *S. typhi* in a household or as a restaurant worker may be identified as a source of infection. Part of the ingested inoculum survives passage through the acid barrier of the stomach to penetrate the intestinal mucosa. Persons with achlorhydria or gastric resection or who are taking antacids are at higher risk for developing infection. The organisms multiply in mononuclear phagocytes of Peyer's patches in the ileum and spread by the bloodstream to the liver, spleen, and bone marrow, where further intracellular multiplication occurs. After an incubation period of about 2 weeks, patients develop the onset of gradually worsening fever, chills, myalgias, headache, and fatigue. Bacteremia permits the diagnosis by blood culture. Most patients will complain of abdominal discomfort or distention, often with diarrhea or constipation. Rose spots develop on the trunks of some patients, and most patients show splenomegaly, hepatomegaly, or abdominal tenderness. Mental confusion or delirium, rectal bleeding, or intestinal perforation occur in a minority of cases, about 2% to 10%, and these patients are at greatest risk of having a fatal outcome after 1 to 3 weeks of untreated disease.

DIAGNOSIS

The diagnosis of typhoid fever is readily made in most patients by blood cultures. Culture of stool or rectal swab will be positive for *S. typhi* in only about 10 to 20% of patients early in their illnesses. Culture of bone marrow will result in an even higher yield of positive cultures than will blood cultures, but this method is not advised for routine clinical situations. Some laboratories employ the Widal anti-Salmonella agglutinin test or use the febrile agglutinins to detect antibodies against O or H antigens of *S. typhi*. Most patients with typhoid fever show elevated titers of these antibodies, but the results are not diagnostically specific because many healthy persons who have lived in endemic areas have elevated titers. Antimicrobial susceptibility to ampicillin, chloramphenicol, and trimethoprim-sulfamethoxazole should be carried out by disk diffusion in agar to guide the use of drugs for therapy.

TREATMENT

Antimicrobial Drugs

Chloramphenicol became the drug of choice in 1948 when it was shown to reduce mortality and to cause defervescence and clinical improvement in most patients in about 5 days. This drug is inexpensive and remains the drug of choice in countries where most *S. typhi* strains remain susceptible: the United States, Mexico, countries of Central and South America, and most countries of southern Europe and the Mediterranean region. In the United States and other industrialized countries, there is a strong reluctance by physicians to employ chloramphenicol because of its association with bone marrow aplasia, a rare idiosyncratic effect that is estimated to occur about once in 30,000 individuals. Accordingly, physicians in the United States have chosen alternative antimicrobial drugs such as ampicillin, amoxicillin, trimethoprim-sulfamethoxazole, and ceftriaxone (Table 1).

In 1989, strains of *S. typhi* showing multidrug resistance (MDR) to chloramphenicol, ampicillin, and trimethoprim-sulfamethoxazole emerged in China, India, and Pakistan. Over the ensuing years these MDR strains became prevalent in these and other Asian countries and some countries of Africa, including Egypt and South Africa. Ciprofloxacin, ofloxacin, and other fluoroquinolones were tested and found to be highly effective in adults. Fluoroquinolones are not advised in children because of the potential of these drugs to injure developing bones. For children, the cephalosporins ceftriaxone, cefotaxime, and cefoperazone (Cefobid), have shown good results. Other drugs that have shown satisfactory results in MDR typhoid fever and may be used are aztreonam (Azactam), cefixime (Suprax), ampicillin-sulbactam (Unasyn), and furazolidone (Furoxone).

The recommended duration of therapy for chloramphenicol was originally set at 14 days. The incidence of relapse, characterized by the return of fever and bacteremia within 6 weeks of stopping therapy, occurred in up to 20% of patients, and, for this reason, shorter courses of therapy have not been attempted. However, clinical trials in the last decade with short courses of 3 to 7 days of ceftriaxone were successful, with rates of relapse of less than 20%. Similarly, ciprofloxacin and ofloxacin have been successful in courses of 5 to 7 days.

Relapses

Following therapy, patients should be advised to return to their physician if fever should recur. Relapses may be expected in about 10% of patients, and most occur within 1 to 6 weeks of stopping therapy. Treatment of the relapse should be the same as for the first episode of illness.

Supportive Therapy

Patients with typhoid fever require attention to fluid and electrolyte balance. Patients with fever and anorexia for several days will be dehydrated, and some with vomiting or diarrhea will have saline depletion and, sometimes, acidosis or hypokalemia. Intravenous fluid support will be required for the severely ill patients. Patients with severe anemia, sometimes caused by intestinal bleeding, will require blood transfusion.

Complications

The most feared complication of intestinal perforation develops in about 4% of hospitalized cases before or during antimicrobial therapy. This should be suspected in patients with severe abdominal pain, distention, or peritonitis and can be diagnosed by an abdominal x-ray film showing free abdominal air. Surgical repair of the ileal or colonic perforation is urgently indicated. Another life-threatening compli-

TABLE 1. **Antimicrobial Therapy for Typhoid Fever**

	Drug of Choice	Alternatives
Chloramphenicol susceptible:	Chloramphenicol 50–60 mg/kg/d PO or IV in 4 divided doses until defervercence, then 30–40 mg/kg/d to complete 14-d course	Trimethoprim-sulfamethoxazole (Bactrim, Septra), one double strength tablet twice daily for 14 d for adults or 8–20 mg trimethoprim/kg/d IV or by oral suspension for children twice daily for 14 d or amoxicillin 1 gm q 8 h for 14 d for adults or 25 mg/kg/d q 8 h for 14 d for children
Multiple drug resistant (MDR) to chloramphenicol, ampicillin, and trimethoprim-sulfamethoxazole:		
Adults	Ciprofloxacin (Cipro), 500 mg PO twice daily for 7 d or ofloxacin (Floxin), 400 mg PO twice daily for 7 d	Ceftriaxone, 2 gm IV once daily for 7 d or cefotaxime, 2–4 gm q 12 h for 7 d
Children	Ceftriaxone (Rocephin), 50–75 mg/kg/d IV once daily for 7 d or cefotaxime (Claforan), 100–200 mg/kg/d IV twice daily for 7 d	Cefixime (Suprax), 20 mg/kg/d q 12 h for 7 d

cation is brisk intestinal hemorrhage from ileal ulcers. This requires transfusions, and, rarely, surgical resection of the ileum.

Pulmonary complications include pneumonia, which is usually a bacterial superinfection that may require additional antimicrobial therapy. Cases of adult respiratory distress syndrome (ARDS) have been described in patients with typhoid fever.

The liver is frequently enlarged with the formation of typhoid nodules and "typhoid hepatitis." In severe cases, there may be jaundice. The liver dysfunction resolves during therapy and does not require special attention. Rare cases of acute cholecystitis requiring surgery have been described.

Patients with severe disease, including delirium or coma or shock, were shown in a study in Indonesia to benefit from corticosteroid therapy in addition to the antibiotic. Dexamethasone was given as 3 mg per kg initially, followed by 1 mg per kg every 6 hours for 48 hours.

Mortality Rate

The mortality rate of typhoid fever is considerably less than 1% in the United States and should approach zero in patients who receive appropriate antimicrobial therapy within a week of onset of illness. In developing countries, the mortality rate is several times higher than this because of delays of starting therapy. Death may be caused by complications, such as intestinal perforation or hemorrhage, and by nutritional deficiencies, especially in young children. Septic shock is a rare fatal complication.

Chronic Fecal Carriers

About 3% of patients treated with antibiotic successfully for typhoid fever will excrete *S. typhi* in their stools during convalescence and will persist in excreting organisms for years although they are asymptomatic. This occurs more often in adult women than in children or men because of a higher likelihood in women of gallstones or other diseases of the biliary tract, where the chronic infection resides. These chronic carriers are important in public health because they are a reservoir for spread to other persons in the home and through food handling. For chloramphenicol-susceptible organisms, carriers should receive amoxicillin or ampicillin, 6 grams a day orally in three to four divided doses, combined with probenecid, 2 grams a day orally in four divided doses, for 6 weeks. For MDR *S. typhi* infection, ciprofloxacin, 500 mg orally twice daily, or norfloxacin, 400 mg orally twice daily, for 4 weeks is effective. Stool cultures need to be repeated at the end of therapy. Failure to eradicate infection is associated with the presence of gallstones. Cholecystectomy, if indicated for symptomatic biliary tract disease, will usually cure the infection.

PREVENTION

Infection can be prevented in many situations by attention to ingesting sanitary drinking water and freshly cooked foods and fresh foods uncontaminated by human sewage. Travelers to Mexico, Central and South America, Africa, and Southern Asia should be advised to drink only bottled beverages or beverages made with recently boiled water and without ice. They should avoid dairy products and cold dishes by choosing freshly cooked foods. Vaccines offer additional protection to travelers who expect to be exposed in endemic areas to uncertain sources of water and food. The live oral Ty21a vaccine (Vivotif) is taken as one capsule orally every other day for 7 days. For continuing exposure, travelers should repeat the vaccination every 5 years. The protection provided by the Ty21a vaccine is equal to that of the parenteral whole cell killed vaccine (Typhoid Vaccine, USP) without the side effects of fever and pain at the injection site.

THE TYPHUS FEVERS

method of
GREGORY A. DASCH, PH.D.
Naval Medical Research Institute
Bethesda, MD

Rickettsiae are small, gram-negative, obligately intracellular bacteria. They cause a large number of arthropod-transmitted diseases, collectively the typhus fevers, which vary somewhat in the details of their clinical presentation. In general, rickettsioses are characterized by a sudden onset of nonspecific symptoms, including high fever, headache, myalgia, arthralgia, and rash. Characteristic necrotic skin lesions, the tache noire or eschar, occur at the site of the tick or mite bites and are highly pathognomonic for boutonneuse fever, African tick bite fever, and scrub typhus. However, their detection requires very thorough examination of the patient, and they may be absent in secondary infections. Similar lesions do not occur in other rickettsioses, notably epidemic or murine typhus, and other tick-transmitted spotted fevers, including Rocky Mountain spotted fever. Elicitation of a history of arthropod exposure is often essential to a correct early diagnosis. Delayed appropriate treatment of rickettsioses is more often associated with a poor therapeutic outcome than is a delay in receiving medical care.

Table 1 lists the principal rickettsial diseases with their respective etiological agents, vectors, reservoirs, and geographic distribution. Activities that bring humans into contact with arthropod vectors and reservoirs are key elements of the epidemiology of these diseases, with the exception of Brill-Zinsser disease (recrudescent epidemic typhus). In that case, a prior history of primary epidemic typhus or immigration from areas with high rates of epidemic typhus must be elicited. The primary rickettsiosis occurring in the United States, Rocky Mountain spotted fever, is described in detail in a separate section. The increasingly large amount of international travel and associated vacations in exotic locations have led to frequent inadvertent exposure to a wide variety of rickettsial agents maintained as zoonoses. The 4- to 14-day delay in onset of illness that occurs after arthropod bites may make diagnosis of imported disease difficult, particularly if any of the usual triad of fever, headache, and rash are absent or slow in manifestation. Confirmation by serology is usually too late to be of clinical value. However, rapid direct methods of diagnosis, such as immunofluorescent or preferably immunoperoxidase staining of rickettsial organisms in skin biopsies, or polymerase chain reaction (PCR) amplification of DNA in biopsies or blood specimens, are reliable diagnostic procedures in 40% to 60% of patients with rickettsioses. Further improvements in these assays, particularly PCR, may be expected, but they are presently done in only a few research laboratories.

Epidemic or louse-borne typhus is presently endemic primarily among populations living at high altitudes or in cold climates where body lice are prevalent, and bathing and laundering of clothing are infrequent. Transmission occurs chiefly by scarification of skin bites contaminated with highly infectious louse feces rather than by the bites themselves. Mortality in untreated epidemic typhus increases in an age-dependent manner to more than 50% at age 50 years. Epidemic typhus has been a scourge of war throughout history. Millions of cases of epidemic typhus occurred in Eastern Europe and the former U.S.S.R. during the two World Wars and created a large latent reservoir of *R. prowazekii*. Factors including stress, other illness, or underlying disease, and immunosuppression may trigger recrudescence of the persistent rickettsial infection as Brill-Zinsser disease. It is often described as milder than primary epidemic typhus, but this is not always the case. In the Eastern United States from Florida to Massachusetts, sylvatic epidemic typhus occurs among people in rural areas, probably by exposure to fleas of flying squirrels living in nearby nests.

Rat flea-borne murine or endemic typhus is maintained worldwide in rat populations. Although often associated with rural populations where it once caused thousands of cases annually in the United States, it now occurs primarily in urban or suburban areas where significant rat populations may exist. Recently, both *R. typhi* and a second typhus-like agent, *R. felis*, have been isolated from cat fleas and opossum tissues, implicating them as novel vectors and hosts in endemic foci of murine typhus-like illness in Texas and Southern California. The agents can be maintained in fleas by transovarial transmission, and infection occurs by both bite and scarification of infected flea feces in bite sites. Although generally milder than epidemic typhus or Rocky Mountain spotted fever, murine typhus requires intensive care in 10% of cases and may be fatal.

Spotted fever group rickettsiae causing human disease are found on every inhabited continent (see Table 1). Pathogenic rickettsiae as well as numerous species of nonpathogenic rickettsiae are maintained by transovarial passage in ticks and in small mammal reservoirs. Transmission to humans occurs by tick bite and by finger contamination of the conjunctiva with fluids from squashed ticks. Spotted fever rickettsioses often occur sporadically but may recur in endemic foci. However, very high attack rates of *R. africae* infections transmitted by highly infected *Amblyomma* ticks occur in southern Africa. *R. akari* infections occur as sporadic focal outbreaks, often in urban settings, when mouse mites bite humans due to a decrease in their normal mouse hosts following rodent control measures or murine disease. Molecular methods have permitted identification of numerous new species of spotted fever group rickettsiae and characterization of their tick vectors, reservoirs, and distribution. Although these spotted fevers are generally milder than Rocky Mountain spotted fever, they can be fulminant and fatal. Glucose-6-phosphate dehydrogenase deficiency is an associated risk factor for severe rickettsial disease. Serologic confirmation of a spotted fever rickettsiosis is facilitated by the extensive cross-reactivity of human sera among species of this group, but identification of the specific agent presently requires acute clinical specimens containing the rickettsiae for PCR characterization or cultivation.

Scrub typhus rickettsiae are transmitted by a variety of trombiculid mites in which they are maintained by transovarial passage. These rickettsiae now belong to the genus *Orientia* in recognition of their numerous antigenic and biologic differences from the closely related typhus and spotted fever rickettsiae. Endemic scrub typhus seroprevalence rates of 30% to 70% are common among humans in many rural areas of Asia, and urban foci of disease are known as humans create disturbed habitats or encroach on infected mite islands containing small mammals and

This investigation was supported by the Naval Medical and Research Development Command, Research Task 61102A.001.01.BJX.1293. The opinions and statements contained herein are the private ones of the author and are not to be construed as official or reflecting the views of the Navy Department or the Naval Service at large.

TABLE 1. **Principal Vectors, Reservoirs, and Distribution of the Typhus Fevers**

Disease	Rickettsial Species	Vector	Reservoir	Distribution
Typhus Group Fevers				
Epidemic (louse-borne) typhus	*R. prowazekii*	Body louse	Humans	S. America, Asia, Africa
Brill-Zinsser disease	*R. prowazekii*	None	Humans	Worldwide
Sylvatic typhus	*R. prowazekii*	Squirrel flea?	Flying squirrels	Eastern U.S.
Murine typhus	*R. typhi*	Rat flea	Rats	Worldwide
Cat flea typhus	*R. felis*	Cat flea	Fleas, opossums	Southwestern U.S.
Spotted Fever (SF) Group				
Rocky Mountain SF	*R. rickettsii*	Tick	Ticks, small mammals	The Americas
Boutonneuse fever	*R. conorii*	Tick	Ticks, small mammals	Europe, Africa to India
Queensland tick typhus	*R. australis*	Tick	Ticks, small mammals	Australia
North Asian tick typhus	*R. sibirica*	Tick	Ticks, small mammals	Central Asia
Astrakhan fever	*R. sp.*	Tick	Ticks, small mammals	Europe
Oriental spotted fever	*R. japonica*	Tick	Ticks, small mammals	Japan
African tick bite fever	*R. africae*	Tick	Ticks, small mammals	Sub-Saharan Africa
Flinders Island SF	*R. honei*	Tick	Ticks, small mammals	Australia
Israeli tick typhus	*R. sharonii*	Tick	Ticks, small mammals	Israel
Rickettsialpox	*R. akari*	Mite	Mites, mice	Worldwide
Scrub Typhus Fever				
Tsutsugamushi disease	*O. tsutsugamushi*	Mite	Mites, small mammals	Siberia to Afghanistan, Pacific Islands, and Australia

their mites. Scrub typhus varies substantially in severity (including fatal illnesses with pneumonia, kidney failure, and jaundice) depending both on host factors and the great biologic variability of *O. tsutsugamushi*. Cases refractory to conventional doxycycline therapy have been described.

Rickettsiae spread hematogenously from the site of inoculation and proliferate in the vascular endothelium and invade distant and contiguous endothelial and vascular smooth muscle cells. Vascular injury leads to increased vascular permeability with resultant edema, hypovolemia, hypoproteinemia, hypotension, and, commonly, hyponatremia. Thrombocytopenia occurs commonly due to the consumption of platelets at the numerous foci of endothelial injury. Rickettsial endotoxins and exotoxins and host immunopathologic or coagulation responses are not considered important pathogenic mechanisms in the majority of cases.

TREATMENT

Antibiotic therapy of rickettsioses (Table 2) must be begun promptly and empirically without laboratory confirmation of disease as there is a greatly increased risk of serious complications in delayed treatment. These include gangrene, cerebral dysfunction, kidney failure, myocarditis, and disseminated intravascular coagulation. Severe or fulminant disease is generally treated with intravenous antibiotics, but generally a course of oral therapy is adequate. Long-lasting doxycycline (Vibramycin), given twice daily in two divided doses, is generally preferred to tetracycline (given in four divided doses in five times larger amount). Prompt defervescence and patient improvement often occurs in 24 to 72 hours. Chloramphenicol has generally been given in pregnancy and early childhood when toxicity and staining of teeth from prolonged tetracycline therapy is a concern. However, treatment failures with chloramphenicol have been reported for murine typhus, scrub typhus, and boutonneuse fever, and the response to tetracycline in Rocky Mountain spotted fever was better than with chloramphenicol. Ciprofloxacin (Cipro)* has been proposed for treatment of murine

*Not FDA-approved for this indication.

TABLE 2. **Drug Treatment of the Typhus Fevers**

Etiologic Agent	Adults	Children
R. prowazekii and *R. typhi*	Doxycycline, 200 mg/d PO for 7–15 d Chloramphenicol, 1.5 gm/d PO for 5 d	Chloramphenicol, 150 mg/kg/d PO for 5 d
R. sibirica and *R. rickettsii*	Doxycycline, 200 mg/d PO for 5 d	Chloramphenicol, 50 mg/kg/d for 5 d
R. conorii	Doxycycline, 200 mg/d PO for 1–5 d Chloramphenicol, 2 gm/d PO for 7–10 d Ciprofloxacin,* 1.5 gm/d PO for 5 d Josamycin,† 3 gm/d PO for 5 d (pregnant women)	Doxycycline, 5 mg/kg PO single dose Chloramphenicol, 50 mg/kg/d PO for 5 d Josamycin, 500 mg/d PO for 5 d
O. tsutsugamushi	Doxycycline, 200 mg/d PO for 7–15 d Chloramphenicol, 2 gm/d PO for 7–15 d	Chloramphenicol, 150 mg/kg/d PO for 5 d

*Not FDA-approved for this indication.
†Not available in the United States.

typhus but appears ineffective for scrub typhus rickettsiae in vitro. Treatment of the newer rickettsioses has not been examined in clinical studies and is based on effective regimens for related agents.

The duration of treatment has varied considerably but has not been subject to critical study. At least 2 days of treatment following defervescence is recommended. Early termination of antibiotic therapy or a single or two-dose doxycycline regimen, particularly in patients treated less than five days after onset of symptoms when full humoral and cellular immunity have not developed, may lead to relapse and febrile recrudescence of disease. Glucocorticosteroids are often given to severely ill patients, but there has been no evaluation of efficacy. Proper fluid and electrolyte maintenance are critical in severely ill patients to maintain organ perfusion.

The Respiratory System

ACUTE RESPIRATORY FAILURE

method of
JOHN W. BRICE, M.D.
W.J.B. Dorn VA Medical Center
Columbia, South Carolina

"In with the good air; out with the bad air." This trite expression gives a succinct representation of normal lung function. Acute respiratory failure can occur from a derangement in either the uptake of oxygen from the atmosphere to the arterial blood or the elimination of carbon dioxide from venous blood back into the atmosphere. While the presence of acute respiratory failure can be suspected from the clinical appearance of the patient, analysis of arterial blood gases (ABGs) is necessary to confirm the diagnosis. An arterial oxygen tension (Pa_{O_2}) of less than 55 torr or an oxygen saturation (Sa_{O_2}) of less than 90% suggests hypoxemic respiratory failure, and an arterial carbon dioxide tension (Pa_{CO_2}) of greater than 50 torr (with an associated drop in pH) indicates hypercapnic respiratory failure. Like many pieces of data, ABGs are best interpreted by comparison with the patient's baseline. A Pa_{CO_2} of 60 torr might be normal for a patient with established chronic obstructive pulmonary disease (COPD). In such a case, the pH should be normal and the plasma bicarbonate elevated, signifying renal compensation for a long-standing respiratory acidosis.

PHYSIOLOGY OF RESPIRATORY FAILURE

Gas Exchange

As ambient air is inhaled, it is saturated with water vapor. Water vapor takes up space and decreases the space available for inspired gases. Upon entering the alveolated lung, the inspired air is further diluted by CO_2 coming in from the pulmonary capillaries. The alveolar oxygen tension (PA_{O_2}) can be estimated using the alveolar gas equation:

$$PA_{O_2} = FI_{O_2}\,(PB - PW) - (Pa_{CO_2}/R)$$

where FI_{O_2} is the fraction of inspired oxygen, PB is barometric pressure, PW is the vapor pressure of water (47 torr at sea level), and R is the respiratory quotient (the ratio of CO_2 production to oxygen consumption).

Several assumptions are made in this equation. One is that Pa_{CO_2} equals alveolar carbon dioxide tension (PA_{CO_2}), which is probably very close to the truth, as CO_2 is a very soluble gas. We also assume that R is 0.8 and while this is an acceptable generalization, it is almost never exactly the case. Therefore, if we were breathing ambient air at sea level ($PB = 760$ torr), then

$$PA_{O_2} = 0.21\,(760 - 47) - (40/0.8) = 100\ \text{torr}$$

Unlike the case with CO_2, there is normally a gradient between PA_{O_2} and Pa_{O_2}. This is due to the relative insolubility of oxygen. This gradient, the $P(A-a)_{O_2}$, is normally less than 10 torr in healthy young adults but rises to around 30 torr in old age. Therefore, the normal patient breathing ambient air at sea level has a PA_{O_2} of around 90 torr. The $P(A-a)_{O_2}$, often called the $A-a$ gradient, is calculated by subtracting the Pa_{O_2} obtained by arterial blood gas measurement (ABG) from the PA_{O_2} calculated by the preceding alveolar gas equation.

Since alveolar hypoventilation will cause PA_{CO_2} to rise, there will be an increase in PA_{CO_2}. This extra CO_2 in the alveolus will occupy additional space, therefore there will be a proportional decrease in PA_{O_2} and thus a decrease in Pa_{O_2}. The calculation of the $A-a$ gradient can help determine whether hypoxemia is due to hypoventilation and increasing CO_2 (normal $A-a$ gradient) or due to an impairment of oxygenation (elevated $A-a$ gradient).

Acute respiratory failure can occur from failure of the lung as ventilatory pump, causing hypercapnea, or from inadequate oxygenation of arterial blood. There are multiple etiologies of both mechanisms, and the clinical scenario of concomitant hypercapnia and hypoxemia is not uncommon. It is imperative to seek out and treat the root causes of both problems.

Hypoxemic Respiratory Failure

Any process that impairs transfer of oxygen from the atmosphere into the capillary blood in the lungs can cause hypoxemia. Hypoxemia is generally defined as a Pa_{O_2} of less than 55 torr and/or a hemoglobin oxygen saturation (Sa_{O_2}) of less than 90%. Hypoxemic respiratory failure is a condition that develops when an acceptable Pa_{O_2} or Sa_{O_2} cannot be maintained despite the provision of supplemental oxygen.

Factors that are external to the patient, such as low partial pressures of inspired oxygen (PI_{O_2}), can be the cause of hypoxemic respiratory failure. Low PI_{O_2} can occur at high altitudes and can be clinically important in management of patients. A person with underlying lung disease and a low, but acceptable, Pa_{O_2} while living on the coastal plain may have problems with hypoxemia if he or she travels to mountainous areas. Air travel can also induce problems in the borderline patient. While newer aircraft are more efficient at maintaining cabin pressure, they also fly at higher altitudes, causing an even lower PI_{O_2}.

In the clinical setting, abnormalities in the ventilation-perfusion ($\dot{V}/\dot{Q}$) equilibrium of the lung are the most common reasons for hypoxemia. If the perfusion and ventilation of lung tissue are not matched, the effectiveness of the lung as a gas transfer device becomes impaired. The causes for abnormal $\dot{V}/\dot{Q}$ relationships are protean. Common causes are COPD, pneumonia, pulmonary embolism, cardiogenic pulmonary edema (e.g., congestive heart failure) and noncardiogenic pulmonary edema (e.g., the adult respiratory distress syndrome).

If an area of lung has no ventilation (a $\dot{V}/\dot{Q}$ ratio of zero), then a shunt is said to exist. This can cause hypoxemia resistant to treatment by supplemental oxygen. Hypoxemia in a patient with shunt is caused by the admixture of venous blood with oxygenated blood from normally functioning areas of the lung. This causes a substantial drop in the final O_2 content of the arterial blood. To understand this, we need to look at the formula for the oxygen content of blood:

$$\text{Oxygen content} = (1.39 \times \text{Hgb} \times \text{Sa}_{O_2}) + (\text{Pa}_{O_2} \times 0.003)$$

where Hgb is hemoglobin concentration in grams per dL. The factor of 1.39 is the amount of O_2 (in mL) that 1 gram of hemoglobin can carry when fully saturated. Multiplying this factor by the hemoglobin concentration and then by the measured oxygen saturation will yield the amount of O_2 bound to hemoglobin. Only a small quantity of O_2 is carried dissolved in plasma, due to the relative insolubility of oxygen (0.003 mL per torr of oxygen tension). Shunted blood does not come into contact with any ventilated lung tissue, therefore an increase in $F_{I_{O_2}}$ will not affect its oxygen content. The blood leaving normal lung is already fully saturated, and an increase in $F_{I_{O_2}}$, while raising the Pa_{O_2}, will not significantly change the oxygen content.

Intrapulmonary shunt is common in patients with the adult respiratory distress syndrome (ARDS) and may rarely be due to pulmonary arteriovenous malformations. Extrapulmonary shunts do occur, as in atrial or ventricular septal defects, but these do not cause hypoxemia until right-sided pressures become so high that the shunt becomes right to left instead of left to right.

The inability of blood to reach equilibrium with the alveolar gases during its trek through the pulmonary vasculature can also cause hypoxemia. Normally the lung is quite efficient in this regard. Equilibration generally occurs in the pulmonary capillary bed with time to spare. Processes that cause thickening of the alveolar capillary membrane can reduce the efficiency of gas exchange. These processes can be inflammatory in nature, such as the interstitial pneumonias, or fibrotic processes, such as asbestosis. Interstitial edema from any cause will also impair diffusion. A reduction in the red cell transit time through the lung may also prevent full equilibration. This reduction must be relatively profound to have a noticeable effect and is generally not clinically important except in patients with widespread destruction of lung tissue and therefore a markedly reduced capillary bed or in cases of dramatically increased cardiac output. Some experts have postulated that a profound reduction in mixed venous oxygen content can be responsible for inadequate diffusion equilibrium.

As discussed earlier, alveolar hypoventilation can cause hypoxemia in the absence of other lung pathology by reducing the Pa_{O_2}, a pattern easily discerned by obtaining ABGs and calculating the $A - a$ gradient, which will be normal if alveolar hypoventilation is the sole cause of hypoxemia. In addition to the aforementioned causes, hypoxemia can also be induced by excessive intrapulmonary oxygen consumption by leukocytes present in lung tissue in cases of severe pulmonary inflammation.

Hypercapnic Respiratory Failure

The level of CO_2 in arterial blood is very strictly maintained at 40 torr in healthy subjects. The hallmark of hypercapnic respiratory failure is an increasing Pa_{CO_2} and a decreasing pH. It is important to remember that patients with a chronic respiratory acidosis (e.g., patients with severe but stable COPD) will have a chronic elevation of Pa_{CO_2}, but the pH will be normal because of renal compensation. If a patient has had an ABG in the past (while stable), it is invaluable in determining what is normal for that patient. Overcorrection of Pa_{CO_2} is a common mistake in the treatment of COPD patients.

Any factor that causes acute CO_2 retention can lead to hypercapneic respiratory failure. Reduced ventilatory drive is one cause of CO_2 retention. Causes of a reduced drive include overdoses (particularly narcotics or sedatives), trauma to or infarction of the mid or lower medulla, profound hypothyroidism, chronic malnutrition, and severe metabolic acidosis. Neuromuscular diseases (such as the muscular dystrophies, Guillain-Barré syndrome, myasthenia gravis, and amyotrophic lateral sclerosis) impair the function of the respiratory musculature even though respiratory drive is normal. Aminoglycosides and calcium channel blockers are weak neuromuscular blockers. This is rarely of clinical importance, but occasionally the failure of a patient to wean from mechanical ventilation is secondary to these drugs. Spinal cord injury in or above the thoracic levels can also lead to ventilatory pump failure.

Electrolyte imbalances, particularly hypophosphatemia, can cause dysfunction of respiratory muscles. Actual muscle atrophy can result from malnutrition and from disuse (as might occur with prolonged ventilatory support). Corticosteroid administration has also been associated with muscle weakness and atrophy.

Increased work loads from mechanical factors, however, are the most common cause of hypercapnic respiratory failure. These loads can be divided into four categories: inertial loads, threshold loads, resistive loads, and elastic loads. Inertial loads are imposed by the inertia of the respired gases themselves. The amount of work required to initiate or stop air flow is not generally of clinical importance. Threshold loads result from the prevention of air movement until a given pressure is obtained. These types of loads are sometimes intentionally applied to patients undergoing pulmonary rehabilitation. Threshold loads are often inadvertently imposed on patients being mechanically ventilated for respiratory failure if modes are used that require the patient to activate demand valves. Outside of such areas, threshold loads are not often significant.

Resistive loads, on the other hand, are quite clinically important and easy to understand. Fatigue from the increased resistive loads associated with obstructive airway diseases, such as COPD and asthma, is a common clinical scenario. Elastic loads are as important clinically as resistive loads. These are the result of abnormal pressure-volume relationships. Increased elastic loads are easy to see in patients with disease processes that cause stiff lungs, such as interstitial fibrosis and pulmonary edema. The work required to expand such stiff lungs is significantly higher than normal. In cases of kyphoscoliosis, the chest wall compliance is reduced, causing similar workload increases. What is less intuitively obvious is that elastic loads can be a problem in the patient with COPD. We are familiar with the idea that, from a pathologic sense, the lungs of a COPD patient are more compliant than normal. That is, a given amount of pressure will distend emphysematous lungs to a greater degree than it will normal lungs. This leads one to believe that elastic loads should be less in this setting. This would be true at low lung volumes; however, because of the loss of elastic recoil in the lung, these patients have hyperinflated lungs and their tidal breathing may be at volumes very near total lung capacity (TLC). Compliance is related to lung volume and at high volumes, the compliance of the lung is actually quite low, and thus, the imposed elastic loads may contribute as much to the development of fatigue and respiratory failure as do resistive loads.

The $\dot{V}/\dot{Q}$ abnormalities discussed earlier cause as much impairment to CO_2 excretion as to O_2 uptake. Despite this, hypercapnia does not often result from $\dot{V}/\dot{Q}$ mismatch alone. This is due to the tight central control of Pa_{CO_2}. Chemoreceptors respond to an increase in Pa_{CO_2} by increasing minute ventilation, which stabilizes Pa_{CO_2} but increases ventilation of nonperfused lung, often referred to as "wasted ventilation." If such compensatory mechanisms are pushed to their limits, fatigue and hypercapnia can occur.

Increased CO_2 production can be another cause of hypercapnia. High loads of carbohydrates will cause elevation of R values. While usually clinically unimportant, this can cause problems in the patient teetering on the verge of respiratory failure.

MANAGEMENT OF ACUTE RESPIRATORY FAILURE

Hypoxemic Respiratory Failure

Correction of the underlying cause is the treatment of choice in dealing with hypoxemia; however, the results of such treatment may take days or even weeks. In this interval, it is imperative that the oxygen content of arterial blood and the delivery of that oxygen to tissues be maintained at adequate levels. Supplemental oxygen can be provided by a variety of methods. Most simply, a nasal cannula can be utilized to deliver oxygen flows of 0.5 to 5 liters per minute; however, FI_{O_2} is not precisely controlled. The minute ventilation of the patient will determine the actual FI_{O_2}. Minute ventilation is defined as the tidal volume multiplied by the respiratory rate. As minute ventilation rises, the supplemental O_2 provided will account for a lesser percentage of the total volume of ventilation, and, therefore, the FI_{O_2} will be less than expected.

Venturi masks produce a more reliable FI_{O_2} (ranging from 0.24 to 0.50); however, the higher FI_{O_2} Venturi systems produce a lower flow of gas, and tachypneic patients may still entrain a significant amount of room air around the mask, diluting the mixture and decreasing the FI_{O_2}. Aerosol units that connect directly to wall oxygen supply can generate an FI_{O_2} of up to 1.0, but such systems also produce lower flows as FI_{O_2} is increased. If a concentration of 50% or higher of oxygen is required, it is best to use two aerosol units and connect them both to the patient with a Y connector in order to produce flow rates that will match the patient's inspiratory flow rate.

Tight-fitting masks with reservoir bags and nonrebreathing valves can be used to approximate an FI_{O_2} of 1.0, but high FI_{O_2} systems such as this should be used only for short-term therapy owing to the risk of oxygen toxicity. With diseases such as pneumonia and ARDS, which are not likely to resolve quickly, oxygen toxicity can develop from exposures to high oxygen concentrations. A patient with hypoxemia that cannot be improved by an FI_{O_2} of less than 0.6 should be considered for intubation and mechanical ventilation, unless she or he has a process that can be easily reversed (e.g., congestive heart failure responsive to diuretics).

Hypercapnic Respiratory Failure

Hypercapnic respiratory failure from overdoses of narcotics and benzodiazepines is easily reversed by naloxone (Narcan) and flumazenil (Romazicon), respectively. Other overdoses may be problematic due to the lack of specific reversal agents. Mechanical ventilatory support may be required until respiratory depression resolves.

Respiratory failure caused by obstructive lung diseases (e.g., asthma and COPD) is a very common problem. In the COPD patient, mechanical ventilation is not required as long as the patient is reasonably oriented, hemodynamically stable, and able to protect his airway. Initial ABGs may look fairly horrendous, but a significant number of these patients can be managed without mechanical ventilation. Aggressive therapy should include (1) aerosolized beta-agonists such as metaproterenol (Alupent) or albuterol (Proventil, Ventolin); (2) aerosolized anticholinergics such as ipratroprium (Atrovent); (3) oxygen therapy as indicated; (4) appropriate antibiotics for any respiratory infection; (5) vigorous pulmonary toilet, including chest physiotherapy if the patient cannot clear sputum.

Oxygen therapy must be applied thoughtfully in these patients but it is mandatory if the patient is hypoxemic. Supplemental O_2 can increase alveolar oxygen tensions in poorly ventilated areas of the lung, reducing autoregulation of blood flow away from these areas. The worsening $\dot{V}/\dot{Q}$ mismatch that results is the most important mechanism of worsening hypercapnia caused by O_2 therapy. The worry over increasing Pa_{CO_2} should never prevent the utilization of oxygen in a hypoxemic patient. If the hypercapnia and acidosis that result from reasonable O_2 therapy is too severe, then intubation and mechanical ventilation are required.

Intravenous aminophylline has fallen out of favor with many physicians; however, it may still be a useful drug in some COPD patients with hypercapnic respiratory failure. Loading doses of aminophylline are no longer recommended. A continuous drip of 0.3 to 0.5 mg per kg per hour is a reasonable starting point. Serum drug levels must be monitored closely. The therapeutic range is considered to be 8 to 12 μg per mL. The mechanism of action of aminophylline is not known, and its bronchodilator action is minimal; however, it may act as a significant diaphragmatic inotrope. The place of corticosteroids in the management of COPD exacerbation is controversial; however, I believe their use is justifiable if there is impending respiratory failure.

The management of refractory asthma leading to respiratory failure (status asthmaticus) is similar to that of COPD with several exceptions. The role of corticosteroids in this area is much clearer. Intravenous methylprednisolone (Solu-Medrol), in a dose of 125 mg (or equivalent) should be given as soon as possible and followed by 40 to 60 mg every 6 hours. Aminophylline is less likely to be of benefit, and beta-agonists should be dosed as frequently as possible without inducing cardiac or other side effects.

In the usual asthma attack, hypocapnia is the rule. If an asthmatic in distress becomes hypercapnic, it may be a sign of impending respiratory failure. While not all such patients will require intubation, the equipment and personnel should be standing by so intubation can be accomplished without delay if it becomes necessary. Once intubated, patients in status asthmaticus can be very difficult to manage due to very high peak inspiratory pressures. Heavy sedation and neuromuscular blockade are sometimes necessary. Recently, a new way of ventilating status asthmaticus patients has been investigated. Permissive hypercapnia uses lower pressures and accepts the hypercapnia and acidosis (which can be quite severe) that result. With vigorous therapy, these patients improve quickly and apparently tolerate the acidosis better than the high peak pressures imposed by more standard therapy.

Respiratory failure from neuromuscular disease can create an ethical quagmire. Patients with the potential for developing irreversible respiratory failure should be queried about their desires for long-term life support measures before such measures become necessary. If the episode of respiratory failure is due to an exacerbation of some other reversible process, then the use of bilevel positive airway pressure (BiPAP) in a timed or synchronized mode can obviate the need for mechanical ventilation in some cases. BiPAP applies a higher pressure to the airway during inspiration and a lower pressure during expiration, creating a gradient and thus, airflow. It can be applied using a nasal mask identical to ones used for nasal continuous positive airway pressure (CPAP).

Mechanical Ventilation

Patients who have hypoxemia or hypercapnia (or both) who fail conservative therapy or who become unstable are candidates for mechanical ventilatory support. The ideal candidate for mechanical ventilation is someone with severe but reversible disease. Patients who develop respiratory failure as the terminal event in the natural history of their disease process should not be automatically intubated and supported. Time spent educating patients and their families on what to expect from any given disease process can prevent a great deal of unnecessary suffering as death approaches.

The goal of mechanical ventilation in acute respiratory failure is to return the patient to a stable condition with the minimum amount of nonphysiologic intervention. Remember, positive pressure ventilation is, by its very nature, nonphysiologic. The Pa_{O_2} should be kept above 60 torr and the Sa_{O_2} above 90%. There is no advantage to raising the Pa_{O_2} to abnormally high levels. The pH should be between 7.35 and 7.45 regardless of what this may do to Pa_{CO_2}.

Ventilator Modes and Settings

When treating acute respiratory failure, it is best to use a mode of ventilation in which all of a patient's attempts to breathe are fully supported. This goal can be accomplished in the majority of cases with assist/control mode ventilation (A/C), a mode that is relatively easy to understand and set. In the emergency situation, the $F_{I_{O_2}}$ should always be set at 1.0 and then adjusted down as quickly as clinically prudent. The short-term goal should be to get the $F_{I_{O_2}}$ below 60%. The tidal volume should be initially set between 5 and 10 mL per kg of ideal body weight and then adjusted based on the results of ABG analysis. In A/C, the respiratory rate set will act as a backup if the patient's spontaneous rate falls. The rate should be set at a level that will assure that the patient receives an adequate minute ventilation. Remember, some acutely ill patients will require a dramatically increased minute ventilation. If a patient becomes suddenly more tachypneic, A/C, if set properly, will be able to keep up with patient demands.

The peak inspiratory flow rate is generally set between 40 and 60 liters per minute, but patients who are very tachypneic may require flow rates as high as 100 liters per minute. If high flow rates are used, they must be reduced as the patient improves and respiratory demands decrease. Dangerously high peak airway pressures can occur from inappropriately high flow rates. Some ventilators are time cycled rather than volume cycled and, because of this, have no independently controllable flow rate. To obtain an increased flow rate on such a machine, the inspiratory time can be decreased (less time for inspiration equals higher inspiratory flow rates).

The addition of a small amount (2 to 4 cm H_2O) of positive end-expiratory pressure (PEEP) has been shown to reduce the work of breathing. It is felt that this prevents microatelectasis and therefore reduces the shear forces caused by reopening collapsed alveoli. Higher levels of PEEP may be needed in patients with diffuse lung disease and refractory hypoxemia (e.g., ARDS). In such instances, PEEP can be increased slowly (in 2- to 3-cm H_2O increments) up to a maximum of 15 to 20 cm H_2O. If a PEEP of above 5 cm H_2O is required, a pulmonary artery catheter is useful to monitor cardiac output and mixed venous blood gases. As PEEP is increased, the intrathoracic pressure increases, and this may impede venous return to the heart. The result may be an improved Pa_{O_2} but decreased O_2 delivery to tissue due to impairment of cardiac output. PEEP should not be used to treat focal processes or obstructive lung diseases because of the risk of hyperinflation of normal lung tissue and iatrogenic lung injury.

If peak inspiratory pressures exceed 50 to 55 cm H_2O or if a PEEP of above 15 to 20 cm H_2O is needed to oxygenate the patient, the risk of barotrauma and iatrogenic lung injury increases. Pressure-controlled ventilation (PC) can be used in this circumstance. PC functions very similarly to A/C, except an inspiratory pressure is set instead of a volume, and the machine cycles off when the inspiratory flow rate slows rather than when a given volume is impaired. Damage from excessive pressures is less likely in this mode of ventilation, but volume becomes a variable. Close attention must be given to any patient on pressure-cycled ventilation. Analysis of pressure-volume waveforms can also help reduce the risk of air trapping and auto-PEEP, a potentially fatal complication. To obtain adequate ventilation in severe ARDS patients, PC can be utilized with the inspiratory to expiratory (I:E) ratio inverted; however, this is very nonphysiologic and requires sedation and usually use of nondepolarizing neuromuscular blockers to paralyze skeletal muscles.

There is a trend to use intermittent mandatory ventilation (IMV) with pressure support (PS) in patients presenting with acute respiratory failure. IMV gives a set number of ventilator-supported breaths per minute and allows all additional breaths to be spontaneous (with no ventilator support). When pressure support is used with IMV, all the spontaneous breaths are then supported by an applied pressure. While this method can certainly be used to ventilate a patient in respiratory failure, the variables that exist are much more complex, and it requires unfailing attention to detail. Many other modes of ventilation exist and have very legitimate uses but are beyond the scope of this text.

Weaning from Mechanical Ventilation

The first question to be answered here is "Does the patient really need to be weaned?" Many patients intubated for respiratory failure can be simply extubated once the underlying pathology has been corrected. If the patient truly needs to be weaned from mechanical ventilation, then the question is more difficult. There is no consensus on how to wean. The medical literature has not been helpful—in fact, it is contradictory. There is no firm evidence that any method is superior to any other. My approach is to place patients on a PS that will deliver a tidal volume of about 7 to 10 mL per kg of ideal body weight. The required PS level must be determined by close bedside observation of the patient. I do not use an IMV back-up. If the patient is not breathing spontaneously, he is not a candidate to be weaned from support. I rest the patient regularly on A/C and slowly extend the time he or she is on PS and also slowly decrease the level of PS. Always rest the patient at night. Stressing a patient at night tends to cause undue agitation. Once the patient can tolerate a PS of 8 to 10 cm H_2O, I attempt extubation.

Best results from weaning can probably be obtained by a consistent, thoughtful approach. If respiratory therapists and ICU nurses know what to expect and what to look for, the success rate will be higher, no matter what method is used.

ATELECTASIS

method of
JOSEPH S. McLAUGHLIN, M.D.
University of Maryland School of Medicine
Baltimore, Maryland

Atelectasis (Gr. *ateles,* imperfect, and *ektasis,* expansion) is the most common morbid state in the 7% of patients who suffer pulmonary complications following surgical procedures. The incidence is doubled in abdominal operations, tripled in smokers, and quadrupled in patients with chronic obstructive pulmonary disease. In large series of patients undergoing thoracotomy and pulmonary resection, the incidence of significant atelectasis approximates 25%. Respiratory insufficiency is the direct cause of death in 25% of surgical mortalities and is a contributory cause in an additional 25%.

In the past, postoperative atelectasis was attributed to the presence of mucous plugs obstructing an airway, but a number of other factors are now recognized that are of equal importance. The most significant are those factors that lead to underventilation and the loss of surfactant. Laplace's law states that the smaller the radius, the greater the surface tension and the greater the tendency to collapse. Surfactant, a wetting agent, reduces surface tension and helps maintain small air sac patency. Normal breathing patterns, which include deep breaths of approximately twice the tidal volume, ventilate small alveoli. Any process that interferes with these normal mechanisms, including pre-existing pulmonary disease, shallow breathing from compression, pain, or inflammation, leads to atelectasis. Gases of higher concentration in the alveoli, including oxygen and anesthetic gases, diffuse into the capillary blood and lead to further collapse. Alveolar collapse leads to fluid accumulation and stagnation, which serves as a prime substrate for bacterial growth and pulmonary infection.

Clinically significant atelectasis presents with fever, tachycardia, and hypoxia. Physical findings may be few and depend upon the amount of lung involved. With lobar collapse, the trachea is shifted toward the involved side, chest excursion is reduced, and the diaphragm is elevated. Rales and tubular breath sounds may be heard. Most commonly, atelectasis is diagnosed by radiographic examination.

Radiographically, atelectasis is loosely classified by its appearance. Platelike atelectasis presents as horizontal densities, usually in the lower lung fields. Segmental atelectasis usually occurs in the basilar segments and refers to partial collapse of a lobe. Lobar atelectasis involves an entire lobe and has a distinctive appearance depending upon the lobe involved. Diffuse atelectasis involves an entire lung and presents as a miliary pattern and decreased lung volume: adult respiratory distress syndrome (ARDS) is the best example.

Prevention is the best treatment, but unfortunately this is not always possible. Cessation of smoking is critical, and a period of 1 month of abstinence is recommended. Treatment of underlying pulmonary disease, especially chronic bronchitis and asthma, is indicated. Patients with reactive airways should be treated with bronchodilators preoperatively and during the postoperative period. Chronic bronchitis should be treated with appropriate antibiotics based on culture results. Pulmonary function studies in the absence of clinical findings have not proved reliable in predicting postoperative pulmonary dysfunction except in patients undergoing pulmonary resection and in elderly people. Performance of these studies should be based on clinical evaluation.

Preoperative training is of value. Patients are instructed to breathe deeply and to cough. Incentive spirometry prior to operation is helpful and is useful in the immediate postoperative period if performed regularly and often. An upright position maintains funtional residual capacity (FRC), which is reduced by as much as 40% when one moves from an upright to a supine position. Thus, patients should be placed in a partially upright position when confined to bed and ambulated in a chair or walking as soon as possible.

Pain produces shallow breathing, splinting, limited diaphragmatic excursion, and ineffective coughing. All these actions lead to atelectasis. Pain control is vital and may be accomplished by a number of means. Oral and parenteral narcotic dosages must be adjusted and balanced to relieve pain but not given to levels at which consciousness is reduced and cooperation and coughing are diminished. The use of patient-controlled pumps (P.C. Narcotic Regulators) is recommended. Epidural anesthesia is particularly useful in reducing pain following thoracotomy and upper abdominal incisions.

Prevention and treatment blend into a continuum of therapy. Coughing and mechanical clearing of secretions can be accomplished by nasal tracheal suctioning and lavage. This technique involves the passage of a catheter through the nasal airway into the trachea. The head is tilted downward and the tongue is grasped with a gauze sponge and pulled forward out of the mouth. The catheter is inserted during a deep breath. The patient must be well-oxygenated during this maneuver, and the use of a finger pulse oximeter is highly recommended. Five to ten ml of saline is injected into the airway, and intermittent suction is carried out for a few seconds at a time. Some expertise is needed to pass a catheter into the trachea and failure is not unusual; however, coughing produced by the attempt is of itself beneficial.

Fiberoptic bronchoscopy has not been shown to prevent atelectasis any more effectively than usual noninvasive preventive measures. The technique is useful in removing secretions and is most valuable when other measures fail. It can be easily and safely carried out with topical anesthesia at the bedside. Lavage is useful, and the addition of 1 to 2 drops of 1/10,000 epinephrine solution to 10 ml of saline may shrink swollen bronchial membranes and help aeration.

If the foregoing measures are ineffective and if the patient is hypoxic, endotracheal intubation and ventilation with positive end-expiratory pressure (PEEP) of 5 to 10 cm of water pressure is indicated. Higher pressures risk the possibility of barotrauma and should be avoided.

CHRONIC OBSTRUCTIVE PULMONARY DISEASE

method of
MORTON SKORODIN, M.D.
Veterans Affairs Medical Center
Muskogee, Oklahoma

Chronic obstructive pulmonary disease (COPD), persistent, largely irreversible airway obstruction, afflicts and ultimately kills millions of people. Nevertheless, the diagnosis is often not made promptly, particularly in milder cases. To facilitate diagnosis, spirometry should be performed in the caregiver's office by all smokers, as well as persons with shortness of breath, to demonstrate whether or not airflow obstruction is present. A forced expiratory volume in the first second (FEV_1) less than or equal to 70% of the forced vital capacity (FVC) and FEV_1 less than 75% of predicted indicate airflow obstruction. A chest x-ray should be obtained initially on all patients with COPD, largely to help diagnose the presence of co-morbidities. Physicians should ask their patients to discontinue smoking. This alone will convince some smokers to quit. Patients may be prescribed nicotine patches (Nicoderm, Habitrol). Dosage is generally 21 mg per day for 2 to 8 weeks, 14 mg per day for 2 to 4 weeks, and finally 7 mg per day for another 2 to 4 weeks. Dosage is reduced for patients weighing less than 45 kg, for persons with known or suspected cardiovascular disease, and for light smokers. Individuals thought to have cardiovascular disorders should be warned about the possibility of myocardial infarction if they continue to smoke while using the transdermal patches. Nicotine prescription is best done in the context of a smoking cessation program. Oral clonidine (Catapres)* 0.1 mg per day to 0.3 mg twice a day, or transdermal clonidine (Catapres-TTS-1, -2, or -3), applied weekly, may be helpful for easing the withdrawal from nicotine.

DRUG THERAPY OF COPD

Bronchodilators are the mainstay of therapy. Ipratropium bromide (Atrovent) by metered-dose inhaler (MDI) or nebulization of aqueous solution is generally effective. This anticholinergic agent only occasionally causes side effects, as it is poorly absorbed.

---

*Not FDA-approved in this indication.

It may be used on a prn basis or on a regular schedule, e.g., up to 4 inhalations by MDI (72 μg) four times a day* if breathlessness is persistent. This is double the generally recommended dose, though safe. Health care providers should instruct patients in the proper use of MDIs. Some patients are too breathless, enfeebled, or demented to use an MDI properly. They may be prescribed motorized nebulizers for use with aqueous solutions (e.g., ipratropium bromide, 0.5 mg as often as every 6 hours). Tidal breathing through a spacer attached to an MDI may also be effective.

Theophylline may be safely used in small to moderate doses for many patients. Serum theophylline levels must be obtained from time to time. The levels should be kept on the low side, e.g. 7 to 10 mg per liter. Side effects, particularly mood changes and supraventricular dysrhythmias, may occur even at these levels. The usual starting dose is 300 mg extended-release capsules twice a day for otherwise healthy individuals weighing 60 to 80 kg. Clinicians must be aware of co-morbidities and medications that alter the clearance of theophylline (Table 1). Side effects include gastroesophageal reflux, diarrhea, insomnia, headache, irritability, tremulousness, and tachycardia. At high levels, serious dysrhythmias (e.g., ventricular tachycardia, seizures, and death) may occur. This underscores the importance of obtaining serum levels. If no benefit is noted, the medication should be discontinued. Beta-adrenergic agents are the author's third choice, occasionally, but not usually, being more effective than ipratropium bromide. The safety of their long-term use is widely questioned, and tolerance to the bronchodilator effect and worsening of the illness may develop during regular therapy. Their use may be important for acute

---

*Exceeds dosage recommended by the manufacturer.

bronchospasm, as in asthma treatment. They are more effective and safer if their use is prn only rather than on a regular schedule. Examples are albuterol (Proventil, Ventolin), terbutaline (Brethaire), and metaproterenol (Alupent, Metaprel), up to 2 inhalations four times a day. Most clinicians prefer to prescribe inhaled beta agonists before going to theophylline. Oral beta agonists are also available. These include terbutaline (Brethine, Bricanyl), 2.5 mg twice per day to 5 mg three times per day, albuterol (Proventil Repetabs, Volmax), 4 to 8 mg twice per day, and metaproterenol (Alupent, Metaprel), 10 to 20 mg three to four times per day. Their use is more likely to result in tremor and cardiovascular effects than is use of the inhaled forms. With all bronchodilators, the clinician must assess whether any clinical benefit is being derived, as these agents are not thought to prolong life in COPD. Spirometry is not adequate to determine this. More important is the patient's subjective assessment, improvement in exercise tolerance and ability to perform activities of daily living, and improvement in gas exchange.

The role of corticosteroids in COPD has not been fully elucidated. Most clinicians prescribe oral steroids such as prednisone if there is spirometrically demonstrated improvement from the medication, e.g., 15% or more increase in FEV_1 after 10 to 14 days of prednisone 40 mg per day. The usual long-term dosage is much lower. It is best not to exceed 10 mg a day or 20 mg every other day, though this is often not possible. One retrospective study indicated that long-term corticosteroid use may prolong life, without regard to whether or not an acute improvement in FEV_1 occurs. Thus the legitimate use of steroids in COPD may go beyond the small proportion of patients with a spirometrically demonstrable improvement.

If steroids are used, the caregiver must be on the lookout for complications caused by these agents. In particular, calcium supplements (calcium carbonate, 650 mg, two tablets twice a day) and vitamin D, 400 to 800 IU per day (1 or 2 multivitamin tablets per day), should be prescribed to help prevent and treat osteoporosis. The role of inhaled steroids in COPD is even less clear. They are widely prescribed in large part because they have a favorable safety profile. It is likely that some patients benefit from these drugs, but it is difficult to tell which ones do. Patients are notoriously nonadherent to treatment with inhaled steroids. This is due, in part, to their delayed onset of action. Patients must be educated about this. They should be prescribed for twice-a-day usage to make adherence easier. Examples are triamcinolone acetonide (Azmacort) and beclomethasone (Beclovent, Vanceril), 4 to 8 inhalations twice a day, and flunisolide (AeroBid), 2 to 4 inhalations twice a day.

REHABILITATION

Unfortunately, bronchodilators are limited in their ability to improve lung function and, even more so, exercise tolerance, because airflow obstruction is

TABLE 1. **Drugs and Conditions that Alter Theophylline Clearance**

Decrease (Higher Serum Levels)	Increase (Lower Serum Levels)
Drugs	
Ciprofloxacin	Phenytoin
Enoxacin	Phenobarbital
Norfloxacin	Carbamazepine
Macrolide antibiotics	Rifampin
Isoniazid	Furosemide
Cimetidine	Tobacco smoking
Propranolol	Cannabis smoking
Calcium channel blockers	
Mexiletine	
Allopurinol	
Oral contraceptives	
Influenza vaccine	
Conditions	
High-carbohydrate, low-protein diet	Hyperthyroidism
Fever	Cystic fibrosis
Viral infection	
Cor pulmonale	
Congestive heart failure	
Liver disease	
Pregnancy	

largely irreversible. Much can be done with a rehabilitation program, either one initiated by the patient or one in an organized setting. Most COPD patients are deconditioned; therefore, exercise is valuable. Swimming is appropriate for many patients, as hyperinflation aids flotation and the rhythm of swimming is compatible with the obligatory prolonged expiratory time along with the short inspiratory time characteristic of COPD. Upper extremity exercise is very difficult for the severely afflicted patient, because the shoulder girdle is recruited to the task of breathing. Consequently, the patient who is too breathless to ambulate may have even more difficulty operating a wheelchair. These patients do best standing behind the wheelchair and bracing their upper extremities and shoulder girdle by using the hand grips while walking and utilizing the seat for their belongings. This is a legitimate use of the wheelchair and it may be prescribed for this purpose. Short bursts of light resistance training may strengthen the shoulder girdle and be well tolerated. Many patients do pursed-lip breathing reflexively. It can also be taught. This maneuver prevents premature airway closure and improves the distribution of ventilation with improvement in gas exchange.

COMPLICATIONS AND CO-MORBIDITIES

Respiratory infections commonly occur, especially in patients who continue to smoke. These are characterized by increased shortness of breath, increased sputum production, and change in the color of the sputum. The presence of two out of three of these symptoms indicates that the patient is likely to respond to antibiotics. Infections are treated empirically. Common organisms are *Streptococcus pneumoniae, Haemophilus influenzae,* and *Moraxella catarrhalis.* The latter two organisms generally produce beta-lactamase. Thus, beta-lactam antibiotics should generally be avoided. Good choices include doxycycline (Vibramycin), 100 mg twice a day, or trimethoprim-sulfamethoxazole (Bactrim, Septra), one double-strength tablet twice a day for 10 to 14 days. Some patients have persistent purulent bronchorrhea and require a course of antibiotics every month or prolonged courses, e.g., 2 months or longer. Pneumococcal vaccination (Pneumovax), 0.5 mL intramuscularly, should be administered. This may be repeated in 6 years.

Viral infections occur frequently. Influenza A vaccine should be administered every fall (0.5 mL intramuscularly). Alternatively, it may be prevented/treated with rimantadine (Flumadine), 100 mg once or twice a day throughout the flu season (prevention) or for 7 days (treatment), or amantadine (Symmetrel), given as 200 mg once a day or 100 mg twice a day for a similiar period. Rimantadine has fewer side effects. Chronic hypoxemia and cor pulmonale are common sequelae of COPD. These are listed together because hypoxemia causes pulmonary hypertension, which, in turn, results in cor pulmonale. Arterial blood gas determinations should be performed on patients when the FEV_1 percent predicted declines to 50% of predicted or below. Pa_{O_2} less than or equal to 55 mmHg ($Sa_{O_2} \leq 88\%$) or 56 to 59 mmHg (Sa_{O_2} 89%) with polycythemia or evidence of cor pulmonale is an accepted criterion for prescription of long-term supplemental oxygen. *Diagnosing chronic hypoxemia and prescribing home O_2 are extremely important, as this treatment has been shown to prolong life in hypoxemic COPD.* It also lowers pulmonary artery pressure. Supplemental O_2 should be titrated to keep Pa_{O_2} at 65 to 80 mmHg or Sa_{O_2} at 91 to 95%. The usual dose is 2 liters per minute. Oximetric testing can be done during exercise, eating, and sleep, states that often require an increased O_2 flow. Often, however, the dose is increased empirically by 1 liter per minute for these times without testing. Whether liquid or gaseous O_2 is used and whether or not O_2 conserving devices are used should be based upon the individual's needs. O_2 should be used as close to 24 hours per day as possible. It should not be prescribed to patients who continue to smoke.

Malnutrition often accompanies COPD. As with cor pulmonale, malnutrition portends a poor prognosis. The etiology of malnutrition in COPD is multifactorial. Aggravating factors include early satiety due to shortness of breath, aerophagia, and abdominal crowding and increased caloric requirements due to excessive work of breathing. Nutritionally compromised patients should be encouraged to eat small meals often. Use of O_2 during meals may be helpful. Fat intake should not be restricted. Attention should be paid to micronutrients of which elderly COPD patients may have marginal intake, such as zinc and folic acid. Zinc deficiency is a concomitant of many chronic debilitating illnesses and may further reduce appetite. Nutritionally depleted patients often gain weight when zinc is supplemented (e.g., zinc sulfate, 220 mg, one capsule three times a day for several months). This relatively high dose should not be continued indefinitely. It is also reasonable to prescribe one multivitamin tablet per day and folic acid, 1 mg per day, for those whose intake of the latter appears marginal. COPD patients with weight loss generally should not be subjected to extensive work-ups for neoplasia, unless the weight loss is out of proportion to the severity of airflow obstruction. There should be some bulk in the diet, or it should be supplemented, e.g., psyllium (Metamucil), 1 tablespoon twice a day in 8 ounces of water or juice, as constipation commonly occurs in COPD due to immobility and medications such as calcium supplements and opiates.

Depression and anxiety commonly occur in COPD. These problems are not always obvious, and the caregiver must conduct an appropriate interview to uncover them. Theophylline and corticosteroids often contribute to mood changes, especially in combination. Depression is commonly successfully treated with counseling and recent-generation antidepressants. As for anxiety, benzodiazepines should generally be avoided. Buspirone (BuSpar) has the advantage of not suppressing ventilatory drive. It also apparently is not habit-forming. Sexual dysfunction is often found in COPD. Patients only occasionally bring up this problem unless questioned. They may be too breathless to engage in sexual intercourse. This may be helped by using an inhaled bronchodilator before and O_2 during sex and assuming a position of comfort.

Many COPD patients lead successful and happy lives despite their disability. This often depends on other factors such as the presence or absence of alcoholism, a successful occupational history, physical conditioning, and, most importantly, a supportive family. These patients should be encouraged to continue to work. For many, this is not possible. Patients should be encouraged to volunteer, develop hobbies, travel, etc. With regard to travel, airlines will allow or supply supplemental O_2 if notified in advance.

All too often, breathlessness is relentless and progressive in COPD despite all efforts. Motivated individuals who have quit smoking may be considered for referral for reduction pneumectomy (removal of surface blebs), either by open thoracotomy or by video-assisted thoracoscopy, recognizing that the role of these procedures has not been fully worked out. Similarly, single-lung transplant may be considered.

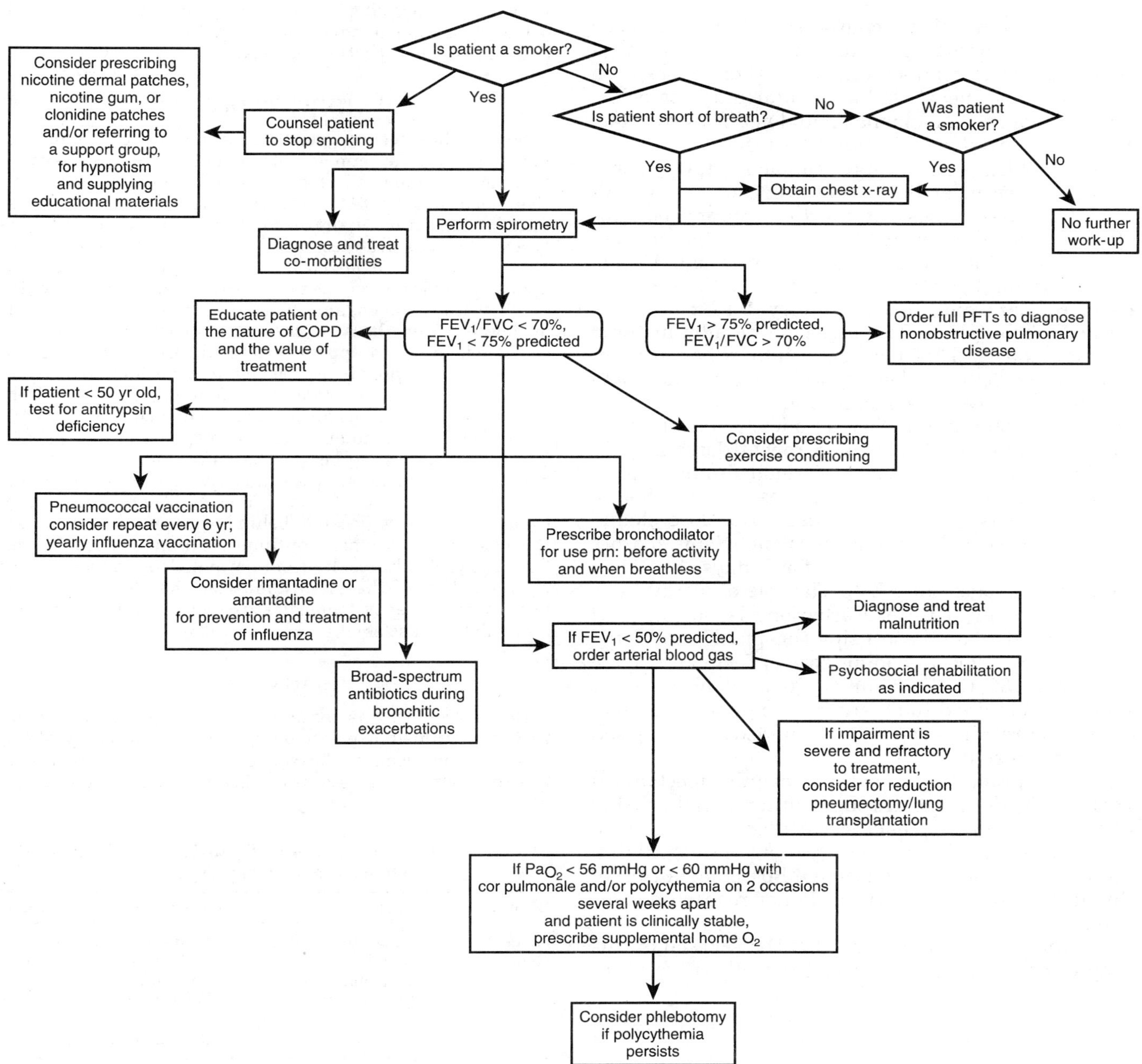

Figure 1. Management of chronic obstructive pulmonary disease (COPD).

Alpha$_1$-antitrypsin deficiency is a special situation. This is a hereditary form of emphysema largely found in persons of Northern European descent. It should be suspected in patients with moderate to severe COPD under the age of 50. Alpha$_1$-proteinase inhibitor (human) (Prolastin), a pooled plasma product rich in alpha$_1$-antitrypsin, may be administered intravenously weekly or monthly. However, this therapy is expensive and not proven efficacious, although it is considered the standard of care for patients with moderate airflow obstruction. Early results with single-lung transplant for this problem are favorable.

ACUTE EXACERBATIONS

Acute exacerbations characterized by increased shortness of breath are common occurrences. Infection is the most common etiology. Other causes such as congestive heart failure, pulmonary embolus, pneumothorax, and anemia should not be overlooked. Exacerbations should initially be treated with low-flow (1 to 2 liters per minute) supplemental O$_2$ and a nebulized bronchodilator or bronchodilators. Although albuterol does not add to the bronchodilator effect of ipratropium at 90 minutes, it has a more rapid onset of action. Doses are ipratropium, 0.5 mg, and albuterol, 2.5 mg. Ipratropium may be repeated every 6 hours and albuterol every 1 to 2 hours, if needed. Terbutaline, 0.25 mg, may be administered subcutaneously. This may be helpful when the patient is "too tight" to benefit well from inhaled beta agonists. Intravenous magnesium sulfate (e.g., 1.2 grams over 20 minutes) has an additive effect and is safe to administer. Higher and repeat doses may be safely given in the absence of renal failure, e.g., 2 to 3 grams over 30 to 60 minutes every 6 hours. Corticosteroids are generally used; the dose should not be excessive. Methylprednisolone (Solu-Medrol), 0.5 mg per kg every 6 hours for 3 days, has been shown to increase the FEV$_1$. The role of intravenous theophylline in acute exacerbations is not clear. If the patient has not been using theophylline or if the serum level is low, a loading dose of 5 mg/kg may be given over 30 to 60 minutes. Arterial blood gases should be obtained to determine whether acute and/or chronic respiratory acidosis and excessive hypoxemia are present.

A small proportion of patients require mechanical ventilation, delivered through either a tight-fitting nasal mask or an endotracheal tube. The vast majority wean relatively easily from the ventilator. Patients and their families should be made aware of this fact to avoid premature "do not resuscitate" orders.

The approach to managing COPD discussed in this chapter can be displayed algorithmically (Figure 1).

SLEEP APNEA SYNDROME

method of
MARY KATHRYN REEVES-HOCHÉ, PH.D.
Respironics, Inc.
Murrysville, Pennsylvania

Sleep apnea syndrome is a common disorder, particularly in middle-aged men. The triad of excessive daytime sleepiness, nightly snoring, and obesity are recognized as characteristics common for this disorder. New data indicate that this disorder is more common in women than previously appreciated. The prevalence of the disease is now thought to occur in 4% to 9% of the middle-aged male workforce and to be as high as 2% in middle-aged women. Previously reported prevalence data indicated a ratio of 4:1 men to women; this has changed to 3:2, with 75% of the women being postmenopausal.

PATHOPHYSIOLOGY

Snoring has been suggested as a marker for the preapneic stage of sleep apnea, with a continuum from asymptomatic continuous snoring to the fully developed obstructive sleep apnea (OSA) syndrome. Apnea is defined as a complete cessation of airflow for 10 or more seconds. Three types of apneas are recognized to occur during sleep: central, obstructive, or mixed in nature (Figure 1). In central apnea, no effort is made to breathe, hence no airflow. In an obstructive apnea, an intact effort to breathe occurs but airflow is absent because the upper airway is completely collapsed. In mixed apneas, a central respiratory pause is followed by an effort to breathe against a collapsed airway. Hypopnea is airflow reduced enough to cause a fall in oxygen saturation, but airflow is not stopped.

All sleeping individuals have some apneas or hypopneas. However, when these become frequent and prolonged, resulting in frequent arousals and hypoxic episodes, OSA can have significant sequelae (Table 1). The etiology of the collapsing airway (located behind the soft palate, or at the base of the tongue) continues to remain speculative. Collapse probably results from normal sleep-induced muscle relaxation of the airway muscles that help maintain pharyngeal patency (genioglossus, genio- and mylohyoid, and palatal muscles).

DIAGNOSIS

Diagnosis of OSA is based on a suggestive history (Table 2), and confirmed by polysomnography. Traditionally, sleep studies have been performed overnight in a laboratory environment. Recent studies indicate that in carefully se-

TABLE 1. **Sequelae and Manifestations of Untreated Obstructive Sleep Apnea**

Event	$\rightarrow$	Sequelae	$\rightarrow$	Clinical Manifestations
Arousal		Fragmented sleep		Daytime sleepiness
Hypoxia		Systemic and pulmonary hypertension		Left ventricular failure
				Cor pulmonale
				Polycythemia
				Arrhythmias
				Sudden death

The clinical sequelae of untreated obstructive sleep apnea are related to the frequent and recurring apneas, hypopneas, and subsequent arousals occurring every time an individual falls asleep.

	Central	**Obstructive**	**Mixed**

Figure 1. The three types of sleep apneas. flow / effort

lected patients, split night studies (diagnostic and therapeutic) may be appropriate. With the emphasis on cost containment, there is a push for screening studies to occur in the home. As portable diagnostic equipment becomes more sophisticated, this option may be more readily available.

TREATMENT

Options for treatment of obstructive sleep apnea include general measures, pharmacology, upper airway appliances, upper airway surgery, and nasal continuous positive airway pressure (NCPAP). General measures for the treatment of OSA aim at modification of risk factors. Accordingly, weight loss is highly recommended in the obese. Smoking cessation has been shown helpful in those with a smoking habit of two or more packs per day. Avoidance of alcohol and other sedatives at least 2 hours before bedtime is essential. Improvement of sleeping hygiene, primarily using the bed to sleep and not as an extension of the living room, is important. In addition, changing sleeping positions might be helpful, since some patients have fewer apnea events while lying on their side.

The pharmacologic therapy for sleep apnea has generally been disappointing. Drugs have been used to reverse hypogonadal conditions and stimulate breathing (medroxyprogesterone [Provera]), treat hypothyroidism (Synthroid), activate muscles of the upper airway (protriptyllin [Vivactil]), and improve depression (fluoxetine [Prozac]).

Upper airway appliances or dental devices have not been scientifically studied for their effectiveness in treating the spectrum of OSA. These devices are designed to hold the mandible forward and thereby increase the posterior oral pharynx space. They also reduce posterior tongue prolapse. Early studies indicate they may be helpful in mild disease. These appliances may offer an alternative to therapy when standard therapy such as NCPAP cannot be tolerated.

Upper airway surgery is another option for treatment. Tracheostomy is generally only used in those who are morbidly ill. Uvulopalatopharyngoplasty (UPPP) may increase airway size by removing the uvula, soft palate, tonsillar pillars, and other redundant pharyngeal tissue. Laser-assisted uvulopalatoplasty (LAUP) is a new methodology for accomplishing the same goal as the UPPP, except that it is an office procedure with no general anesthesia. The current literature is a series of case reports; there are no randomized studies indicating effectiveness.

NCPAP continues to be the standard of therapy for obstructive sleep apnea. NCPAP works by pneumatically splinting the airway open via a nasal or oral/nasal mask connected by a pneumatic circuit to a blower. Side effects generally relate to the interface and are easily corrected with minor adjustments to the mask or headgear. Unfortunately, compliance with NCPAP may be less than desirable in many patients. There are now many long-term, covert, objectively documented studies on NCPAP compliance in typical OSA patients. Self-reported NCPAP use is consistently overestimated by the patient when compared with covert monitoring clocks. Although NCPAP improves objective and subjective sleepiness, patients who are tested in the laboratory following documented use of the device demonstrate daytime sleepiness with shortened multiple sleep latency times. Sleeping without NCPAP for only one night fully reversed any effects of the NCPAP on improving the patient.

TABLE 2. **Signs and Symptoms Characteristic of Obstructive Sleep Apnea**

Physical Examination	Subjective Complaints
Obesity	Morning bloodshot eyes
Short bullneck	Morning headaches
Hypertension (seen in approximately 50% of patients, more prevalent in men than women)	Impotence (reported by spouse)
	Being tired on awakening
	Necessity of daytime naps or having sleep "attacks"
Crowded posterior oral pharynx	Difficulty maintaining vigilance
Large tongue (macroglossia)	Inability to concentrate
Small chin (micrognathia)	Poor memory
Occasional nasal pathologies (polyps, deviated septum)	Poor judgment (reported by employer)
In severe cases (those with daytime hypercapnia): cor pulmonale, severe somnolence, impaired cognition, and mood changes	Irritability and personality changes (reported by spouse)
	Depression
	Witnessed apneas or gasping during sleep (reported by sleeping partner)

CARCINOMA OF THE LUNG

method of
HENRY WAGNER, JR., M.D.

H. Lee Moffitt Cancer Center and Research
Institute, University of South Florida
Tampa, Florida

Lung cancer kills more men and women in the United States than any other malignancy. As the age at which smokers begin their addiction has decreased, so has the age at which lung cancer kills. More than 80% of cases are due to habitual or environmental exposure to the carcinogens present in tobacco smoke, so from one perspective, lung cancer may be considered a disease that is better suited for psychosocial intervention than intervention by surgeons or by radiation or medical oncologists. Indeed, the recent reduction in the death rate from lung cancer in white males in the United States reflects more the decline in the incidence of cigarette smoking that began following the publication of the surgeon general's report in 1965 than great advances in the effectiveness of therapy for this disease.

Disappointment with the results of present therapy must not be confused with nihilism. An overall cure rate of "only" 15% of the 180,000 patients in the United States who present with lung cancer each year still translates to about 27,000 lives saved. Modest improvements in therapy will benefit many individuals, comparable to the modest improvements seen with adjuvant therapy of patients with breast or colon cancer or the striking improvements in the treatment of such uncommon tumors as carcinoma of the testis or Hodgkin's disease. Furthermore, lung cancer is increasingly becoming a disease of healthy former smokers. The previous "typical" lung cancer patient, a male veteran who began smoking during World War II, is being replaced by the man or woman who began smoking in high school during the 1960s, smoked for 20 to 30 years before quitting, and remains at high risk for lung cancer while his or her risk of cardiovascular disease has decreased rapidly following smoking cessation. Several large centers have reported that, in recent years, more than half of their lung cancer patients are former (more than 1 year since cessation) rather than current smokers. This change has key implications in terms of both therapeutic interventions and the possibility of enlisting this population, which has already demonstrated a high degree of motivation by quitting smoking, to participate in studies of early detection and chemoprevention. Although primary prevention by the reduction of tobacco use is likely to be the most effective means of reducing deaths from lung cancer, more than 1 million persons would die of lung cancer during the next decade, even if all smokers were to quit today. An effective strategy aimed at reducing both the mortality and the morbidity of this disease must include efforts at risk reduction (smoking prevention and cessation), screening of asymptomatic individuals at high risk, early detection of lung cancer in those with symptoms, intervention in the process of carcinogenesis, and improvements in the effectiveness of both local and systemic treatment of patients with established lung cancer.

SCREENING AND EARLY DETECTION

The poor overall results of treatment of patients diagnosed with symptomatic lung cancer have spurred efforts to diagnose the disease in asymptomatic individuals. In the United States, the National Cancer Institute sponsored several trials in the 1970s that compared active screening with chest x-ray (CXR) and sputum cytology to "routine" medical care, which, in the populations of male smokers studied, often included annual CXRs. Although these studies showed a shift toward detection of earlier-stage disease in the screened populations, with higher rates of resectability, there was no measurable improvement in overall survival. This led to recommendations to abandon routine screening for lung cancer (warranted by the data) and to pessimism about early diagnosis in general, which is not justified. It remains clear that the patients with lung cancer who are most likely to be cured are those diagnosed with localized disease without spread to regional nodes or distant sites. Although no screening procedures have shown benefit, relegating patients with symptoms suggestive of lung cancer to a policy of watchful waiting, or empirical antibiotic therapy without vigorous follow-up, will only create a self-fulfilling pattern of poor results in treating patients diagnosed with advanced disease. The two groups of patients with lung cancer with the best outcomes are those diagnosed incidentally by CXR obtained for some other indication and those diagnosed by the thorough evaluation of symptoms consistent with lung cancer in a patient at risk (present or former smoker). A high degree of suspicion and vigorous diagnostic work-up are indicated in a patient with symptoms consistent with lung cancer, particularly when there is a past or present history of tobacco exposure, either direct or secondhand.

Molecular technology offers the ability to detect malignant changes in exfoliated cells well before visible morphologic changes appear. Tochman showed that monoclonal antibody staining of cells showing atypia could predict which patients were going to develop frank malignancy with a lead time of about 2 years. Mao reported similar findings using probes for mutations of K-*ras* and *p53* genes. These findings, reported initially in small pilot trials, are currently being validated in large prospective trials seeking to detect second malignancies in patients curatively resected for their first lung cancers.

CHEMOPREVENTION

Patients who have developed one malignancy of the upper aerodigestive tract (head and neck, lung, esophagus) as a result of exposure to the carcinogens in tobacco are at high risk of developing second and subsequent lesions. Careful studies reveal multiple areas of dysplasia and carcinoma in many of these patients at the time of their initial diagnoses, and the risk of a second invasive malignancy is about 3% per year. These individuals require careful follow-up for the early detection and effective treatment of second malignancies, particularly since their initial treatment may have limited the options in treating subsequent malignancies.

The increasing understanding of epithelial carcinogenesis as a process rather than an event has led to the development of strategies aimed at stabilizing or reversing some of these processes, thus delaying or preventing the development of invasive malignancy. Several preliminary trials with *cis*-retinoic acid and retinoyl palmitate have shown promise in reducing the risk of second malignancies in patients with resected head, neck, and lung cancers, and larger confirmatory studies are currently under way. Such chemoprevention strategies do not substitute for smoking cessation in these high-risk individuals. Also, several trials using beta carotene have failed to show any reduction in lung cancer incidence. At present, chemoprevention, at least with retinoids and other specific agents, should be viewed as an area of active research rather than established clinical practice.

PROGNOSTIC FACTORS

As is true for most malignancies, the probable outcome in an individual case of lung cancer is a function of the histology and stage of the disease and the status of the host. Host factors are of major importance in lung cancer, in part due to the advanced age of many patients (median age of diagnosis is in the seventh decade) and the frequency of other illnesses such as chronic obstructive pulmonary disease (COPD) and cardiac disease, which are also tobacco related.

Lung cancer is divided into two major histologic subgroups: small cell lung cancer (SCLC) and the combination of squamous cell carcinoma, adenocarcinoma, and large cell undifferentiated carcinoma, considered collectively as non–small cell lung cancer (NSCLC). Although there are some differences in the behavior of these subtypes of NSCLC, particularly in early-stage disease—with squamous cell carcinoma a bit more likely to remain localized to the chest and adenocarcinoma and large cell carcinoma more likely to disseminate widely, with particular affinity for the central nervous system (CNS)—these distinctions are largely lost with more advanced disease. In the past, SCLC and NSCLC were viewed as quite different diseases, but there is now increasing convergence in modern therapeutic approaches with the understanding that both are usually disseminated diseases that present with substantial bulk disease in the chest, requiring both systemic and locoregional therapies.

The TNM staging system is generally used for patients with NSCLC and is reasonably predictive of outcome (Tables 1 and 2). In patients with SCLC, there is almost always involvement of regional lymph nodes, so the staging is simplified to "limited" disease, in which extrathoracic metastases cannot be demonstrated, and "extensive" disease, in which they can. There are occasional patients with SCLC who do not have nodal involvement, and their prognosis is considerably better than that of other patients with limited disease. The increasing realization of the role of locoregional therapy in achieving long-term survival for patients with limited SCLC may prompt an appropriate return to the use of the TNM staging system, as there is a substantial difference in the prognosis of an individual with small ipsilateral mediastinal nodes and that of a patient with bulky bilateral mediastinal and supraclavicular nodes, both of whom would be considered to have limited disease.

In addition to cell type and anatomic stage, a variety of molecular prognostic factors have been proposed to provide further predictive information in lung cancer (Table 3). These include measures of cell proliferation (e.g., S-phase fraction, PCNA, Ki67, Tpot), mutated or overexpressed oncogenes and/or tumor suppressor genes (K-*ras,* p*53,* HER-2-*neu,* bcl-2), cell surface antigens (ABO blood type antigens and their precursors), and indicators of angiogenesis. Most of these have been proposed on the basis of small series of patients, usually treated in a nonuniform fashion, and often based on univariate rather than multivariate analysis. Their proper validation will require prospective study in large series of patients staged, treated, and followed in a uniform fashion.

RADIOGRAPHIC PROCEDURES IN STAGING

As with any other medical test, radiographic staging procedures should be used primarily when their results

TABLE 1. **International Staging System: TNM Classification**

Stage	Description
T1	A tumor that is 3 cm or less in greatest dimension, surrounded by lung or visceral pleura, and without radiographic or bronchoscopic evidence of invasion proximal to a lobar bronchus.
T2	A tumor more than 3 cm in its greatest dimension or a tumor of any size that invades the visceral pleura or has associated atelectasis or obstructive pneumonitis extending to the hilar region. At bronchoscopy, the proximal extent of demonstrable tumor must be within a lobar bronchus or at least 2 cm distal to the carina. Any associated atelectasis or obstructive pneumonitis must involve less than an entire lung.
T3	A tumor of any size with direct extension into the chest wall (including superior sulcus), diaphragm, or the mediastinal pleura or pericardium without involving the heart, great vessels, trachea, esophagus, or vertebral body, or a tumor in the main bronchus within 2 cm of the carina without involving the carina.
T4	A tumor of any size with invasion of the mediastinum or involving the heart, great vessels, trachea, esophagus, vertebral body, or carina or the presence of a malignant pleural effusion.
N0	No demonstrable metastases to regional lymph nodes.
N1	Metastases to ipsilateral peribronchial or hilar lymph nodes, including direct extension.
N2	Metastases to ipsilateral mediastinal or subcarinal lymph nodes.
N3	Metastases to contralateral mediastinal lymph nodes, contralateral hilar lymph nodes, and ipsilateral or contralateral scalene or supraclavicular lymph nodes.
M0	No distant metastases.
M1	Distant metastasis; specify site(s).
Stage I	T1–2, N0, M0
Stage II	T1–2, N1, M0
Stage IIIA	T1–3, N2, M0
	T3, N0–2, M0
Stage IIIB	T4, N0–3, M0
	T1–4, N3, M0
Stage IV	Any T, any N, M1

Modified from Mountain CF: A new international staging system for lung cancer. Chest *89*:225S, 1986.

will affect the choice of therapy. A second goal is to define very homogeneous groups of patients for clinical research studies. When these tests are so used, the possibility of differences between groups exhaustively staged and the more general population of patients must be kept in mind.

Appropriate radiographic procedures for patients with suspected or newly diagnosed lung cancer depend on the histologic type of cancer and on the therapeutic options. I stage most aggressively those patients with tumors of intermediate aggressiveness and intermediate clinical status. In an otherwise healthy individual who, when presenting for an elective orthopedic procedure, is found to have a 2-cm peripheral lung nodule without any other abnormalities on CXR, chest computed tomography (CT),

TABLE 2. **Rates and Patterns of Relapse Following Resection of NSCLC**

Series	Stage	Histology	No. of Patients	Survival (year)	Chest Only (%)	Distant Only (%)
Feld*	T1, N0	NSCLC	162	ns	9	17
Feld*	T2, N0	NSCLC	196	ns	11	30
Feld*	T1, N1	NSCLC	32	ns	9	22
Pairolero	T1, N0	NSCLC	170	71% (5)	6	15
Pairolero	T2, N0	NSCLC	158	59% (5)	6	23
Pairolero	T1, N1	NSCLC	18	33% (5)	28	39
Thomas*,†	T1, N0	Squamous	226	~85%	5	7
Thomas*,†	T1, N0	Nonsquamous	346	~65%	9	17
Martini†,‡	T1–2, N1	Squamous	93	44%	16	31
Martini†,‡	T1–2, N1	Adenomatous	114	34%	8	54
Martini‡	T2–3, N2	Squamous	46	~30% (5)	13	52
Martini†	T2–3, N2	Nonsquamous	103	~30% (5)	17	61

*First site of relapse only.
†Relapse rates include patients relapsing in multiple sites.
‡Some patients received postoperative radiation and/or chemotherapy.

and routine laboratory studies (complete blood count, chemistry profile including electrolytes, renal and hepatic function), extensive further testing is unlikely to provide any useful information. At the other end of the spectrum, a patient who presents with a history of severe cardiopulmonary disease, substantial recent weight loss, poor performance status, new bone pain, and a large hilar mass requires only an efficient choice of the least invasive means of obtaining a tissue diagnosis and appropriate palliative therapy. Extensive delineation of all sites of metastatic disease in such a setting is expensive and wasteful.

Staging of the Mediastinum

CT scanning is currently the radiographic method of choice for evaluating the mediastinum. Both false-positive and false-negative rates are 20 to 30%, and it is essential to keep this in mind when planning therapy. Diagnostic radiologists are neither uniform nor necessarily precise in their description of the appearance and nature of mediastinal nodes. In some cases, a patient will be said to have "mediastinal adenopathy," with the implication of unresectable N2 disease, when in fact what has been shown by CT is the presence of several 1-cm nodes. The size distribu-

tion of mediastinal nodes in normal individuals easily includes this range, and among nodes 1.5 cm or greater in dimension, about 20% will be histologically benign. The percentage of such false-positives is higher in patients with obstructing endobronchial lesions or extrinsic bronchial obstruction from hilar nodes and postobstructive infection. In a patient who is otherwise a good operative candidate, histologic involvement of such nodes should be confirmed by biopsy before treatment decisions are made. In cases in which normal-size nodes are histologically positive, such involvement is usually intranodal, and the nodes are technically resectable. It is presently unresolved whether these patients are better served by initial resection and postoperative adjuvant therapy or by detection of these N2 nodes by preoperative mediastinoscopy and/or anterior mediastinotomy (Chamberlain procedure) and treatment with neoadjuvant therapy prior to resection.

Although there were initially great hopes that magnetic resonance imaging (MRI) might be superior to CT in distinguishing between benignly enlarged and malignant mediastinal nodes, this has not been the case. CT, with its better spatial resolution and greater freedom from motion artifact, is the superior modality. MRI has a role in the evaluation of lesions that involve the lung apex (and possibly the brachial plexus) as well as medial lesions that abut the vertebrae and may invade the neural foramina. Such involvement would preclude resection and poses a risk of spinal cord compression, and its delineation has important implications for planning radiation therapy.

TABLE 3. **Established and Proposed Prognostic Factors in Resected NSCLC**

Stage
Number of nodal sites
Extranodal extension
Histology
Grade
Ploidy
PCNA staining
Ki67 staining
BRDU labeling
K-*ras* mutation
3p deletion
p53 mutation
p53 overexpression
Angiogenesis
EGFR expression
neu oncogene expression
Blood group A expression
H/Ley/Leb antigen expression
Monoclonal antibody detection of nodal metastases

Evaluation of Distant Metastatic Disease

Most patients with metastatic lung cancer are symptomatic and present with clear indications of the sites of their disease (Table 4). In patients without such symptoms, the question arises when to order "routine" imaging studies. The liver and adrenals are common sites of metastasis for SCLC and NSCLC and are well imaged by CT. I generally order an extended CT of the chest to include the upper abdomen and image all these structures in a single sitting. Although metastases to the adrenals are common, so are adenomas, and the distinction between these may require biopsy in a patient who is otherwise a good candidate for curative resection.

Bone scans are of limited value as routine studies. Many patients have abnormal bone scans due to benign degenerative diseases. The likelihood of detecting occult metastatic

TABLE 4. **Local Expressions of Systemic Metastatic Disease**

Syndrome	Presentation	Management
Brain metastases	Headache; nausea and/or vomiting; altered mental status; focal motor, sensory, or cerebellar deficits; focal or generalized seizures	Corticosteroids; whole brain irradiation; consider resection or radiosurgery for a single metastasis in a patient whose other sites of disease are controlled; avoid prophylactic anticonvulsants
Spinal cord compression	Back pain; motor or sensory deficits; loss of sphincter control	Emergency evaluation by contrast MRI; high-dose corticosteroids; local radiation or surgical decompression
Pleural effusion	Dyspnea; chest pain	Thoracentesis and pleurodesis with doxycycline, bleomycin, or talc, thoracoscopic decortication (?)
Pericardial effusion	Dyspnea; syncope	Emergency evaluation by cardiac ultrasound to exclude atrial collapse; pericardiocentesis or pericardiectomy; avoid diuretics
Superior vena cava obstruction	Dyspnea; facial and neck swelling; distention of superficial chest wall veins	Corticosteroids; mediastinal irradiation
Bone metastases	Pain; may be asymptomatic	Palliative radiation therapy with or without orthopedic stabilization

disease in patients without focal symptoms or elevation in alkaline phosphatase is low, and I do not routinely obtain bone scans except in these settings.

Clinically occult involvement of the CNS, especially in patients with SCLC, adenocarcinoma, and large cell carcinoma, is more common, especially in patients with involvement of mediastinal nodes. Although scanning of the brain is probably not indicated in patients with Stage I or II disease, where the probability of involvement is about 5%, in patients with N2 disease, it is in the range of 15 to 20% as detected with high-resolution gadolinium-enhanced MRI. For patients being considered for aggressive and potentially curative treatment such as chemoradiotherapy with or without surgery, the finding of CNS metastases leads to major changes in therapy, and MRI scanning is warranted. I do not routinely scan patients with known extracranial metastatic disease to look for CNS disease in the absence of symptoms, but instead inquire carefully for early symptoms and scan when they appear.

TNM STAGE GROUPING

The International Staging System as outlined by Mountain in 1986 has been the standard for reporting treatment results during the past decade. The broad outlines of this system are without question. Recently, however, several areas have emerged that indicate a need to modify this system.

Several of the TNM stages have considerable heterogeneity in outcome. This is true to some degree for patients with Stage I disease, where the survival of patients with T1, N0, M0 disease (about 80%) is strikingly better than that of patients with T2, N0, M0 disease (about 60%). It is in Stage III that the problems are greatest, however. These were partially recognized by Mountain, who divided the third stage into IIIA (no invasion of the mediastinum or involvement of contralateral mediastinal or supraclavicular nodes, no pleural effusion), and IIIB (the presence of one or more of the aforementioned characteristics). In retrospect, this has separated a group of patients (IIIA), some of whom can be treated surgically, undergo complete resection, and have a reasonably favorable prognosis (especially T3, N0, M0), from those who are unresectable and are often treated palliatively. If one considers instead those patients with Stage IIIA and IIIB NSCLC who are treated

nonsurgically with radical radiotherapy or chemoradiation, survival differences are much less striking.

It seems reasonable at the present time to consider a restructuring of the subgroups of Stage IIIA NSCLC along the following lines (Table 5):

T3, N0–1, M0: Peripheral T3 lesions or those closer than 2 cm from the carina or involving resectable mediastinal structures, with normal or enlarged hilar nodes but negative mediastinal nodes. These patients are clearly resectable. Current clinical trials are addressing whether they benefit from preoperative chemotherapy.

T1–3, N2a, M0: Involvement of a single mediastinal nodal station, discovered at mediastinoscopy or mediastinotomy or at the time of thoracotomy. In some institutions, these patients are resected and then considered for adjuvant postoperative therapy; in others, they are given preoperative therapy.

T1–3, N2b, M0: Involvement of multiple mediastinal nodal stations with potentially resectable disease. These patients have fared poorly with past therapy. Current trials compare chemoradiotherapy as definitive therapy or followed by resection.

T1–3, N2c, M0: Bulky involvement of mediastinal nodes (e.g., seen on CXR), possibly with superior vena cava compression. Not likely to be resectable even with preoperative therapy and should be considered for definitive chemoradiotherapy.

A distinction in Stage IIIB may also be made between

TABLE 5. **Proposed Substaging of Stage IIIA NSCLC**

Stage	Description
T3, N0, M0	Normal hilum and mediastinum by CT, negative mediastinoscopy
T3, N1, M0	Enlarged hilar nodes on CT, negative mediastinoscopy
T1–3, N2a, M0	Involvement of single mediastinal station at resection
T1–3, N2b, M0	Involvement of multiple mediastinal stations at resection
T1–3, N2c, M0	Multiple station mediastinal node involvement at mediastinoscopy
T1–3, N2d, M0	Bulky mediastinal nodes on CXR, possible superior vena cava compression

those patients with central T4 or N3 disease that can be encompassed within a reasonable radiation therapy portal and those with T4 disease by virtue of malignant pleural effusions in whom all known disease cannot be treated to 60 Gy or more.

CARDIOPULMONARY EVALUATION

Appropriate surgery requires a resectable tumor in an operable patient. In a patient who is quite ill from nonmalignant cardiopulmonary disease, it may be appropriate to determine the physiologic limits to appropriate treatment before embarking on a detailed staging work-up. The determination of operability is also linked to the expected outcome of the operation. One is more willing to consider operating on a patient with marginal cardiopulmonary function for resection of a highly curable T1, N0, M0 tumor than for a doubtfully curable T3, N2, M0 one.

Patients must be able to tolerate loss of the functioning lung that would be removed surgically or ablated by radiation fibrosis. Surgical removal may in some cases improve lung function, both by removing areas currently perfused but unaerated (physiologic shunting) and by improving lung mechanics in patients with severe COPD and overinflation. Radiation fibrosis, on the contrary, does not improve function and may create shunting through volumes of lung unable to perform adequate gas exchange. In addition, irradiation of large volumes of lung may produce an acute inflammatory reaction (acute radiation pneumonitis) characterized by nonproductive cough and dyspnea. Prediction of probable postoperative or postradiation pulmonary function, particularly the forced expiratory volume in 1 second (FEV_1), can be approximated from CT-measured lung volumes and regional ventilation perfusion scans, although these are better at predicting postsurgical effects than postradiation ones. This is due in part to our incomplete knowledge of the complex dose/volume relations involved in late radiation toxicity to the lung. Patients with a predicted post-treatment FEV_1 of less than 800 cc are at high risk for dyspnea at rest, as are those with single breath diffusing capacity of less than 35%.

Patients with a history of myocardial infarction within 6 months prior to planned surgery, unstable angina, poorly controlled ventricular arrhythmias, and uncontrolled congestive failure are all at high operative risk. In these settings, the risks of surgery must be carefully weighed against the loss of treatment effectiveness if nonsurgical therapy is chosen. It is important here to recognize that the patient's preferences regarding immediate risk of operation and long-term effectiveness of cancer treatment may not be that of the physician, and the patient's preference ought to have priority so long as it is based on a clear explanation of the treatment options.

TREATMENT OF NSCLC

Treatment recommendations for operable patients with NSCLC are outlined in Table 6. For patients with resectable disease, the extent of surgical resection depends on both the location of the primary tumor and the extent of hilar or mediastinal adenopathy. Patients with T1–2, N0 disease can usually be resected by lobectomy, whereas those with hilar or mediastinal nodal involvement or central T3 lesions are more likely to require pneumonectomy. Some compromise in the adequacy of the surgical margin may be necessary in patients with marginal pulmonary function who could tolerate lobectomy but not pneumonectomy. In such cases, postoperative radiation to the questionable margin may be indicated. The Lung Cancer Study Group (LCSG) conducted a randomized trial comparing lobectomy with wedge or segmental resection for patients with T1, N0 lesions and found a significantly higher local relapse rate and a marginally inferior survival in patients who had the more conservative resection. Such proce-

TABLE 6. **Recommended Therapy for Good Risk* Patients with NSCLC**

Clinical Stage	Therapy	Comments
T1–2, N0, M0	Resection (usually lobectomy)	If pathologic N0, no adjuvant therapy is indicated; should be considered for trials of early detection and chemoprevention
T1–2, N1, M0	Resection	Consider for postoperative adjuvant therapy
T3, N0–1, M0	Resection	Consider for postoperative adjuvant therapy
T1–3, N2, M0	Resection followed by adjuvant therapy (randomize radiation therapy vs. radiation and chemotherapy)	Single N2 node found at intraoperative mediastinoscopy
T1–3, N2, M0	Induction radiochemotherapy and resection or definitive radiochemotherapy (randomized trial)	Multiple N2 nodes or single node with extranodal extension
T1–3, N3, M0	Definitive radiochemotherapy	Radiochemotherapy clearly superior to "standard" radiation therapy alone; local control remains poor
T4, N1–3, M0	Definitive radiochemotherapy	Consider preoperative radiochemotherapy and resection for patients with T4, N0, M0 lesions, especially those of the superior sulcus
T1–4, N0–3, M1	Symptomatic palliative treatment with radiation and/or chemotherapy	Consider more aggressive therapy, including resection, for patients with T1–3, N0, M1 lesions with a solitary lesion in the brain or adrenal

*Adequate cardiopulmonary function, Eastern Cooperative Oncology Group performance status 0 or 1; weight loss ≤ 5%. Patients not meeting these criteria may still be suitable for therapy but should be evaluated with particular care.

dures should currently be reserved for individuals with very compromised pulmonary status who would not tolerate lobectomy.

Curative Radiotherapy for Medically Inoperable Patients

Despite improvements in surgical technique and perioperative care and the introduction of lung-sparing resection procedures, a small percentage of patients with operable tumors, particularly those with severe cardiac disease, may not be good candidates for resection. Other individuals refuse surgery for personal reasons, even though it is recommended. Radical radiation therapy is curative in a proportion of these patients and should be offered as a reasonable second-line therapy (Table 7). Five-year survival is about 15% overall but rises as high as 70% for good performance status patients with T1, N0 lesions treated to doses of 70 Gy or more. Because of the significant cardiac and pulmonary dysfunction in these individuals, radiation portals should be small, treating only the primary tumor volume without any attempt at elective irradiation of regional lymph nodes.

Adjuvant Postoperative Treatment in Patients with Resected NSCLC

Despite apparently curative surgery, about 30% of patients with resected Stage I and more than 50% of patients with Stage II and III NSCLC have local and/or distant recurrences, and almost all of them die of their recurrent disease. As seen in Table 2, the majority of recurrences are in distant sites, but local failure occurs in about 15 to 20%. Over the past decades, many trials of adjuvant therapy with radiation, chemotherapy, or both have been conducted in the hope of reducing these high relapse rates. To date, the results have been modest at best. For patients with N1 or N2 disease, postoperative mediastinal radiation reduces local recurrence from 20 to 3% (in squamous cell) without measurably changing overall survival. A number of carefully conducted trials of adjuvant chemotherapy in well-staged patients have shown a modest delay in recurrence and death. These trials, conducted primarily in the 1980s, were hampered by the use of drug regimens that were less effective against metastatic disease than those presently available and by poor patient compliance (and low total drug dose received), due in part to the lack of effective antiemetics. Current trials for patients with resected node-positive NSCLC are comparing radiation therapy with radiation therapy plus chemotherapy (cisplatin/etoposide) in the U.S. Lung Intergroup trial and observation with chemotherapy (cisplatin/vinorelbine) in a Canadian National Cancer Institute (NCI) trial. In view of the known toxicities of these regimens and their uncertain efficacy in the adjuvant setting, participation in these studies should be encouraged.

TABLE 7. **Radiation Therapy for Patients with Clinically Resectable NSCLC**

Author	No. of Patients	Stage (Clinical)	Dose (Gy)	Median Survival (mo)	2-Year Survival (%)	5-Year Survival (%)	Local Failure (%)
Morrison	28	Operable	45/4 wks	n/a	14	6 (4 yr)	n/a
Smart*	40	Operable	50–55 (250 kv)	~30	~50	22	n/a
Coy*, †	141	T1–3, Nx	50–57.5	n/a	31	11	45
Cooper	72	T1–3, N0–1	Variable	9	n/a	6	n/a
Haffty	43	T1–2, N0–1	54–59	28	60	21	39
Noordijk	50	T1–2, N0	60	25	56	16	70
Zhang	44	T1–2, N0–2 (80% T1–2, N0)	55–70	>36	~55	32	27 for those with data
Talton	77	T1–3, N0	60	17	36	17	n/a
Sandler	77	T1–2	60	20	30	~10	56†
Ono	38	T1–N0	60–70	~40	68	42	n/a
Dosoretz	152	T1–3, N0–1	50–70	17	40	10	70
	44	T1	50–70	Not reached	~60	~60	30
	63	T2	50–70	~12	~30	~10	80
	41	T3	50–70	~12	~30	~10	86
Hayakawa	17	Stage I	60–80§		75	31	n/a
	47	Stage II	60–80§		44	22	n/a
Rosenthal	62	T1–2, N1	18–65 (median 60)	17.9	33	12	60
Kaskowitz	53	T1–2, N0	50–70 (median 63)	20.9	43	6	55
Graham	103	T1–2, N0–1	18–60 (median 60)	16.1	35	14	
	35‖	T1, N0–1	18–60 (median 60)	n/a	n/a	29	

*Includes some patients with small cell carcinoma.
†Includes some patients with unresectable proximal T3 lesions.
‡Data from autopsies of 31 patients (22% of entire series), of whom 14 had locoregional disease, 17 disseminated disease, and 6 with no evidence of disease.
§Dose received by "majority of patients." Some received lower doses, and 13 patients showing a good response at 70 Gy were boosted to 80 Gy or higher.
‖Subset of entire series of 103.
Abbreviation: n/a = data not available.
Modified from Wagner H: Radiotherapeutic management of Stage I and II lung cancer. *In* Pass HI, Mitchell JB, Johnson DH, Tumsi AT (eds): Lung Cancer: Principles and Practice. Philadelphia, Lippincott-Raven, 1996.

Preoperative Treatment in Patients with Resectable NSCLC

In the 1960s, trials of preoperative radiation therapy for patients with resectable NSCLC showed no benefit but did show increased toxicity, and this treatment cannot be recommended. More recently, three groups reported small randomized trials of immediate surgery or initial chemotherapy followed by surgery (and, in some cases, additional chemotherapy and/or radiotherapy). The two larger trials were halted prior to their planned accrual when interim analysis showed a statistical superiority for the preoperative chemotherapy regimen (Table 8). The third, much smaller trial also suggested a benefit in this approach. Although these results are highly encouraging, one should be cautioned that the overall size of the trials is small, known anatomic prognostic factors were unbalanced, in the study by Rossell there was a known disparity in the frequency of K-*ras* mutations between the two arms (with the status of other molecular markers unknown), not all patients underwent surgical staging, the survival for the patients treated with surgery alone was poorer than expected, and the resectability rates for what were ostensibly similar patients varied considerably between institutions. Confirmation of these results would be desirable, particularly in view of the dramatic nature of the reported improvement in survival.

A current U.S. Intergroup trial is addressing a somewhat different question: whether patients with multiple-level N2 disease are better treated with definitive chemoradiation therapy or lower-dose chemoradiotherapy followed by surgery. This should determine whether such neoadjuvant therapy makes patients more curable or their tumors merely more resectable. Since such multimodality neoadjuvant regimens are toxic, with treatment-related death rates approximately 10%, it is key to demonstrate a survival advantage if such approaches are to become standard practice.

Management of Patients with Unresectable Stage IIIA and IIIB NSCLC

Recent trials in North America, Europe, and Asia have clearly shown improvement in median survival for patients with Stage IIIA and IIIB NSCLC treated with both radiation and chemotherapy compared with either single-modality treatment. Improvements in both median and longer (2- and 3-year) survival are seen, and the Cancer and Leukemia Group B trial of radiotherapy alone (60 Gy over 6 weeks) or preceded by two cycles of cisplatin/vinblastine reported a near doubling in 5-year survival from 10 to 19%. More recent trials employing concurrent as well as sequential chemotherapy suggest even longer median survivals approaching 2 years, albeit at the cost of substantially increased acute esophageal toxicity. Local disease control remains poor, and the use of altered radiation fractionation, dose escalation, and sensitization of radiation-resistant cells remain research priorities.

Palliative Treatment of Local and Metastatic Disease

Most patients with lung cancer will at some time be symptomatic from their intrathoracic disease unless it has been resected. Localized symptoms from brain or bone metastases are also common. Radiation therapy has long been the mainstay of treatment for such patients, with relatively high rates of palliation for irritative and obstructive symptoms and painful bone metastases but poorer results for symptoms of nerve compression such as vocal cord paresis and phrenic paralysis. In the United States, common radiotherapeutic practice has been to treat such patients to doses of 30 to 35 Gy in 10 to 15 fractions over 2 to 3 weeks. In the United Kingdom, several randomized trials conducted by the Medical Research Council have compared such schedules with abbreviated regimens of 17 Gy in two fractions 1 week apart or a single fraction of 10 Gy and have found equally good palliation of symptoms and survival, with toxicity no greater than that for more fractionated treatment (Table 9). Such hypofractionated palliative schedules are particularly attractive for patients who might otherwise have to travel substantial distances or remain hospitalized for the duration of their radiation therapy. Other trials have obtained similar results for bone metastases.

Although most reports of chemotherapy for lung cancer have focused on response and survival rates, several groups recently reported specifically on symptomatic responses (see Table 9). These are in the same range as that reported for radiation therapy.

Treatment of Metastatic NSCLC

With the rare exception of a patient who develops an isolated brain or adrenal metastasis that can be

TABLE 8. **Randomized Trials of Surgery Versus Induction Chemotherapy Followed by Surgery for Patients with Resectable Stage III NSCLC**

Study	No. of Patients	Regimen	% Complete Resection	Median Survival (mo)	p Value
Rossell	30	MIP→S→XRT	85	26	<.001
	30	S→XRT	90	8	
Roth	28	CEP→S→XRT	66	64	<.008
	32	S→XRT	61	11	
Pass	13	EP→S→EP	85	29	0.95
	14	S→XRT	86	16	

Abbreviations: MIP = mitomycin/ifosfamide/cisplatin; CEP = cyclophosphamide/etoposide/cisplatin; EP = etoposide/cisplatin; S = surgery; XRT = radiation therapy.

Rossell R, Gomez-Codina J, Camps C, et al: A randomized trial comparing preoperative chemotherapy plus surgery with surgery alone in patients with non-small cell lung cancer. N Engl J Med 330:153–158, 1994.

Roth JA, Fossella F, Komaki R, et al: A randomized trial comparing perioperative chemotherapy and surgery with surgery alone in resectable Stage IIIA non-small cell lung cancer. J Natl Cancer Inst 86:673–680, 1994.

Pass HI, Progrebnia HW, Steinberg SM, et al: Randomized trial of neoadjuvant therapy for lung cancer: Interim analysis. Ann Thorac Surg 53:992–998, 1992.

TABLE 9. **Percentage of NSCLC Patients Obtaining Palliation of Symptoms with External Beam Irradiation or Chemotherapy**

Symptom	Standard Radiation Therapy (24–30 Gy in 6–10 Fractions)*	17 Gy in 2 Fractions (First Trial/Second Trial)*	Fraction of 11 Gy*	EDAM/MMC/VBL*	DDP/MMC/VBL*
Cough	56	65/48	56	23/10	40
Hemoptysis	86	81/75	72	5/0.3	100
Chest pain	80	75/59	72	21/10	44
Anorexia	64	68/45	55	n/a	n/a
Depression	57	72/na	n/a	n/a	n/a
Anxiety	66	71/na	n/a	n/a	n/a
Breathlessness	57	66/41	43	22/15	66

*From Bleehen NM, Girling DJ, Fayers PM, Aber VR, Stephens RJ: Inoperable non–small cell lung cancer (NSCLC): A Medical Research Council randomised trial of palliative radiotherapy with two fractions or ten fractions. Report to the Medical Research Council by its Lung Cancer Working Party. Br J Cancer, 63:265–270, 1991.

Bleehen NM, Bolger JJ, Hasleton PS, Hopwood P, et al: A Medical Research Council (MRC) randomised trial of palliative radiotherapy with two fractions or a single fraction in patients with inoperable non–small-cell-lung cancer and poor performance status. Br J Cancer 65:934–941, 1992.

†Scores are not percentage of patients improved but rather median symptom severity (0 = least, 100 = most) before and after chemotherapy. From Kris MG, Gralla RJ, Potanovich LM, et al: Assessment of pretreatment symptoms and improvement after EDAM + mitomycin + vinblastine (EMV) in patients with inoperable non–small cell lung cancer (NSCLC). Proc ASCO 9:883A, 1990.

‡From Tumarello D, Graziano F, Isidori P, Cellerino R: Symptomatic, stage IV, non–small-cell lung cancer (NSCLC): Response, toxicity, performance status change and symptom relief in patients treated with cisplatin, vinblastine, and mitomycin-C. Cancer Chemother Pharmacol 35:249–253, 1995.

Abbreviations: n/a = data not available; EDAM = edatrexate; MMC = mitomycin; VBL = vinblastine; DDP = cisplatin.

resected, metastatic NSCLC is not a curable disease. The goals of treatment should be palliation of symptoms and extension of life with a quality that is valuable to the patient. Although economic considerations cannot be forgotten, these cannot dictate therapeutic goals. Recent trials have shown that chemotherapy, when given to patients of good nutritional and performance status, can prolong survival. With the use of serotonin antagonists to reduce nausea, the toxicities of treatment are substantially less than previously. A number of regimens have been developed with response rates in the range of 30 to 50% for patients with Stage IV disease and median survivals of about 1 year (Table 10). These are dramatically superior to prior response rates of 20% and survivals of 24 weeks. Several new agents in development also show significant single-agent activity and are currently being tried in combination regimens (Table 11).

TREATMENT OF SCLC

Staging of SCLC has followed a simpler pattern than that for NSCLC because of the early realization that the vast majority of patients have mediastinal nodal involvement if not extrathoracic metastatic spread readily demonstrable at the time of diagnosis, that the conventional T and N distinctions were not highly prognostic for outcome, and that surgical resection alone for the majority of patients was not a useful treatment strategy. These conclusions were reached at a time antedating the present chemotherapeutic regimens and the use of higher doses of radiation and may be open to reconsideration.

With the exception of the rare patient who presents with a peripheral coin lesion that is resected and found to be SCLC, essentially all patients with this disease have extrathoracic metastatic disease and require systemic chemotherapy as part of their initial

TABLE 10. **Chemotherapeutic Regimens for Metastatic NSCLC**

Regimen	Doses	Comments
EP: etoposide/cisplatin	E 100–125 mg/m^2 P 60–90 mg/m^2	"Standard"
VP: vinblastine/cisplatin	V 4–5 mg/m^2 q wk × 4 P 100 mg/m^2 q 4 wk	Demonstrated survival benefit if used prior to RT
MVP: mitomycin/vinblastine/cisplatin	M 8 mg/m^2 days 1, 29, 71 V 4–5 mg/m^2 q wk × 5, then q 2 wk P 100 mg/m^2 days 1, 29	Limited to brief use before RT or surgery because of cumulative toxicity
TP: Taxol/cisplatin	T 135 mg/m^2 q 4 wk P 75 mg/m^2 q 4 wk	May be used concurrently with chest RT without need for G-CSF
TC: Taxol/carboplatin	T 135–250 mg/m^2 q 4 wk C AUC of 6–7.5 using Calvert formula	Doses of T > 225 mg/m^2 require G-CSF support AUC dosing more physiologically appropriate than mg/m^2
NP: vinorelbine/cisplatin	N 30 mg/m^2 weekly P 120 mg/m^2 days 1, 29, then q 6 wk	Demonstrated survival benefit over vinorelbine as a single agent

Abbreviations: RT = radiation therapy; G-CSF = granulocyte colony-stimulating factor; AUC = area under the curve.

TABLE 11. **Single-Agent Activity of New Chemotherapeutic Agents**

Agent	Mechanism of Action	Response Rate*	Comments
Vinorelbine (Navelbine)	Inhibits microtubule assembly	NSCLC 14–36%	Less neurotoxic than other vincas
Paclitaxel (Taxol)	Prevents microtubule dissociation	NSCLC 21–24% SCLC 34–41%	Toxicities very dependent on rate of infusion
Docetaxel (Taxotere)†	Prevents microtubule dissociation	NSCLC 20–41%	May produce pleural fluid accumulation
Edatrexate (10-EdAM)†	Inhibits dihydrofolate reductase	NSCLC 10–30% SCLC 0%	—
Gemcitabine†	Inhibits ribonucleotide reductase	NSCLC 20–22% SCLC 27%	Modest myelosuppression
CPT-11 (irinotecan)†	Inhibits topoisomerase-1	NSCLC 32% SCLC 47%	Significant myelosuppression; diarrhea
Topotecan†	Inhibits topoisomerase-1	NSCLC 0–18% SCLC 34–35%	Significant myelosuppression

*Complete and partial remissions.
†Investigational drug in the United States.

management. The distinction between what has been termed "limited disease" and "extensive disease" is thus an operational one that is highly dependent on the technology used for staging. Patients with limited disease are those whose detected disease is confined to one hemithorax. Some series have allowed the presence of ipsilateral supraclavicular lymph nodes and pleural effusions, and contralateral paratracheal (but not hilar) nodes have generally been allowed. In some series, the operational nature of this classification has been made explicit, with "limited" disease considered to be that which could be encompassed in a reasonable radiotherapy portal.

The distinction between limited and extensive disease has two important operative features. First, with present therapy, survival is strikingly better for patients with limited than with extensive disease, with a reasonable (e.g., 20%) rather than anecdotal possibility of 5-year survival. As a corollary of this better survival, these patients are at risk from both the long-term sequelae of treatment and the natural history of their disease and other tobacco-associated malignancies, particularly second lung cancers. These considerations are important in designing long-term follow-up and intervention strategies for these patients. Second, at present, the optimal therapy for patients with limited SCLC who have good performance status and reasonable pulmonary function should include thoracic radiation therapy as part of the initial treatment. For patients with extensive SCLC, thoracic irradiation has not been shown to improve survival, and its use is primarily palliative. There may, however, be subgroups of patients with extensive SCLC—particularly those who present with bulky intrathoracic disease and minimal extrathoracic disease and who show a good response to an initial two to three cycles of chemotherapy—in whom the early use of radiation therapy for the thoracic disease and one or two limited metastatic sites (e.g., brain, bone) could be beneficial or even curative.

Patients with peripheral T1–2, N0, M0 SCLC lesions should probably be resected and then considered for adjuvant chemotherapy and radiation therapy. Thus, a patient with a suspicious peripheral coin lesion and normal hilum and mediastinum on CT scan should proceed to thoracotomy without an initial needle biopsy, since the biopsy's failure to diagnose malignancy would be doubted and either a small cell or non–small cell diagnosis would lead to resection.

Radiochemotherapy for Limited Disease

Patients with limited SCLC should be treated with combination chemotherapy and radiation therapy to the primary tumor, ipsilateral hilum, and mediastinal nodes. Larger volumes of prophylactic radiation do not appear to be necessary. The precise timing of radiation and chemotherapy (concurrent vs. alternating vs. sequential; radiation at the start of therapy or after two to three cycles of chemotherapy) remains incompletely defined. A recent intergroup study by ECOG, RTOG, and SWOG gave radiation therapy (45 Gy in either 25 fractions over 5 weeks or 30 fractions over 3 weeks) concurrently with the start of chemotherapy (four cycles of cisplatin/etoposide) and achieved an overall median survival of 20 months, with about 30% of patients alive at 3 years. This cooperative group trial is a reasonable current treatment benchmark. If thoracic radiation is to be delayed, it is probably not wise to do so for more than three cycles of chemotherapy, as a meta-analysis has shown that the survival gains from adding radiation therapy to chemotherapy are achieved only when both modalities are given relatively early.

Chemotherapy of Extensive Disease

Extensive SCLC is responsive to a wide variety of chemotherapeutic agents, but these responses are not durable, and virtually all patients die of their disease. Regimens such as cisplatin/etoposide or cyclophosphamide/doxorubicin/vincristine are widely used and as effective as any reported. Attempts to improve survival by adding other drugs, alternating these two regimens, delivering chemotherapy on a weekly schedule, or increasing drug doses with cytokine and stem cell support have not shown consistent benefit. For patients with poor performance status, simple oral regimens of etoposide or etoposide and cyclophosphamide provide good, albeit temporary, palliation.

Prophylactic Cranial Irradiation

Relapse in the CNS is common in SCLC despite a complete systemic response, and it has been proposed that there are pharmacologic barriers to adequate drug delivery to micrometastatic disease. Radiation therapy given prophylactically to patients in systemic complete remission (CR) has been shown to significantly reduce the incidence of CNS relapse, although a significant improvement in survival has not been demonstrated. Estimates of the frequency with which CNS relapse is truly isolated, as opposed to a component of systemic relapse, suggest that the maximal survival benefit that might be seen with a complete abolition of CNS failure would be 10%—too small to be reliably detected by any of the present randomized trials. Furthermore, prophylactic cranial irradiation (PCI) has been associated with the development of neurologic deterioration in patients with SCLC, although the precise contribution of radiation, chemotherapy, and paraneoplastic syndromes has been difficult to unravel.

At present, we lack consensus on the role of PCI in SCLC. There is agreement that several things should not be done: patients without a CR or near CR should not be given PCI, PCI should avoid large (e.g., 4 Gy) radiation fractions, and PCI should not be given concurrently with induction or consolidation chemotherapy or followed by "maintenance" chemotherapy. Uncertainty arises for a patient who has had a clear-cut CR or excellent partial remission, has a normal brain MRI, and is of good performance status—the sort of patient who has a reasonable shot at long-term survival and stands to lose the most from either CNS relapse or toxicity and to gain the most from their avoidance. For the moment, it seems most honest to explain the pros and cons of both approaches to the patient; be willing to support him or her, whatever the choice; and give, if asked, one's own personal preference (I favor giving PCI in this selected subgroup of patients).

COCCIDIOIDOMYCOSIS

method of
AUGUSTINE D. MUNOZ, M.D., and
JOHN W. CALDWELL, PHARM.D.

Kern Medical Center
Bakersfield, California

Coccidioidomycosis, San Joaquin Valley fever, and in the medical vernacular, "cocci," are all synonyms of the disease caused by the dimorphic fungus *Coccidioides immitis*. The organism grows in the soil from 40 degrees north latitude in California to 40 degrees south latitude in Argentina.

The geography and climate are characteristic of a low-altitude semidesert, with hot summers, moderately wet winters, and infrequent freezes. The mycelial phase matures into arthroconidia, which are infectious to both animals and humans. When detached by a slight breeze they can travel up to 75 miles and survive low moisture and high temperatures. In the mammalian host, inhaled arthroconidia develop into a spherule, which by cytoplasmic cleavage and nuclear division forms endospores (each can produce another spherule). There is no human-to-human nor animal-to-human or animal transmission. Infections are asymptomatic in 60% of individuals and only noted by the conversion to a positive skin test. In the remaining 40%, mild flulike symptoms to acute respiratory failure may ensue. Only 10% to 20% of the total infected population receive a clinical diagnosis. The majority will recover without event; however, when the host's ability to localize the infection through cell-mediated immunity is impaired, significant pulmonary or disseminated disease may occur.

The clinical presentation is divided into three categories: (1) primary pulmonary, (2) disseminated (extrapulmonary), and (3) complicated or protracted pulmonary disease. Symptoms develop 10 to 16 days following exposure and most commonly include fever, chest pain, cough, malaise, anorexia, fatigue, headache, pharyngitis, chills, cutaneous manifestations, and joint pains. The skin manifestations (rash, erythema multiforme, erythema nodosum) and articular symptoms are thought to represent deposition of circulating immune complexes and are not to be confused with dissemination. Clinical outcome is not adversely related to their presence. Pulmonary radiographic manifestations of primary disease include a nonspecific alveolar infiltrate in any lobe, cavitation, nodule formation, and pleural effusion. The exudative pleural effusion can be secondary to direct extension of the pulmonary infection, or an immune complex manifestation. Radiographic findings will clear in 95% of the patients within 6 to 8 weeks.

DIAGNOSIS

The diagnosis of a *C. immitis* infection may be confirmed by having a positive skin test (minimum of 5×5 mm of induration), a positive serology (IgM positivity or complement-fixation titer 1:4 or greater), or the presence of spherules with endospores in the collected specimen (tissue, sputum, pleural fluid). A positive culture can also confirm the diagnosis but will take 3 days to 1 week for results. Skin test results alone are not reliable to diagnose acute illness, especially in the severely ill or immunocompromised host. Serologic testing must be undertaken for confirmation. The antibody response includes the acute-phase development of IgM antibodies (present in 90% of the patients within 4 weeks) measured by enzyme immunoassay or immunodiffusion, and IgG antibodies measured by immunodiffusion or complement fixation. Complement-fixation (CF) titers correlate with disease severity and are strongly associated with dissemination.

Dissemination, which occurs in 5% of clinical cases, can be a serious complication of primary disease. The site of dissemination will generally determine morbidity. Although any organ of the body can be involved, lesions of the skin, soft tissue, bone, and meninges present clinically. A verrucous skin lesion is the most common dermatologic description. Subcutaneous abscesses or masses may also occur. Bones are involved in 10% to 50% of disseminated cases. The frequency in descending order includes vertebral bodies, tibia, skull, metatarsals, and metacarpals.

Joints may also be involved as a direct extension of a bony lesion or from hematogenous spread. The synovial fluid has no characteristic findings. Fluid culture is rarely positive, but biopsy specimens of synovium may be. One third to one half of patients with dissemination will have meningitis. Disease typically involves the basilar meninges, can occur in all age groups, and is uniformly fatal in less than 2 years without treatment.

Residual thin-walled pulmonary cavities or nodules are seen in approximately 5% of cases. Although one third of the cavities may close over a 2-year period, those remaining are at risk for rupture or bleeding or both. Nodules present a diagnostic problem, frequently requiring a biopsy to exclude malignancy when they are discovered incidentally without a prior history of infection. Slowly progressive fibrocavitary changes can also be observed.

TREATMENT

Treatment for mild primary infection with *C. immitis* is not generally required for patients with normal immunity as the illness is self-limited. Those with more significant pulmonary infiltrates, accompanied by shortness of breath, fever, and fatigue, will commonly be treated with oral azoles (ketoconazole [Nizoral], itraconazole [Sporanox], fluconazole [Diflucan]) or amphotericin B (Fungizone). Data from over 500 cases of primary disease were analyzed by our group for factors associated with with serious disease and formed the basis of a treatment algorithm (Figure 1). For patients with severe respiratory distress, hypoxemia, or acute respiratory distress syndrome (ARDS), aggressive treatment with amphotericin B is indicated. We utilize a rapid escalation dosing schedule in such circumstances, beginning at 5 mg and increasing every 8 hours until the dose is 0.75 mg per kg, which is then continued daily thereafter. The minimum total dose is 1 gram, but it may range up to 3 grams in selected cases. Further treatment with amphotericin B or azoles is based upon clinical response, resolution of infiltrates, changes in the CF titer, and response to skin testing. Those with persistent titers greater than 1:16, a negative skin test, and chronic fatigue are treated for longer periods of 3 to 12 months.

In pregnant women, expert advice is needed. Disease presenting in the second and third trimesters or immediately postpartum is associated with increased risk of dissemination and ARDS. Due to the teratogenic potential of all the azoles, amphotericin B is utilized when symptoms are significant. Although many patients will do well without treatment, they require close monitoring for progressive infiltrates, respiratory distress, and rising CF titers. A negative skin test after 1 month will prompt treatment regardless of other positive signs of improvement. Therapy should be continued through the postpartum period as well but may include azoles at this point with careful birth control counseling.

For all other patients with early disease not pre-

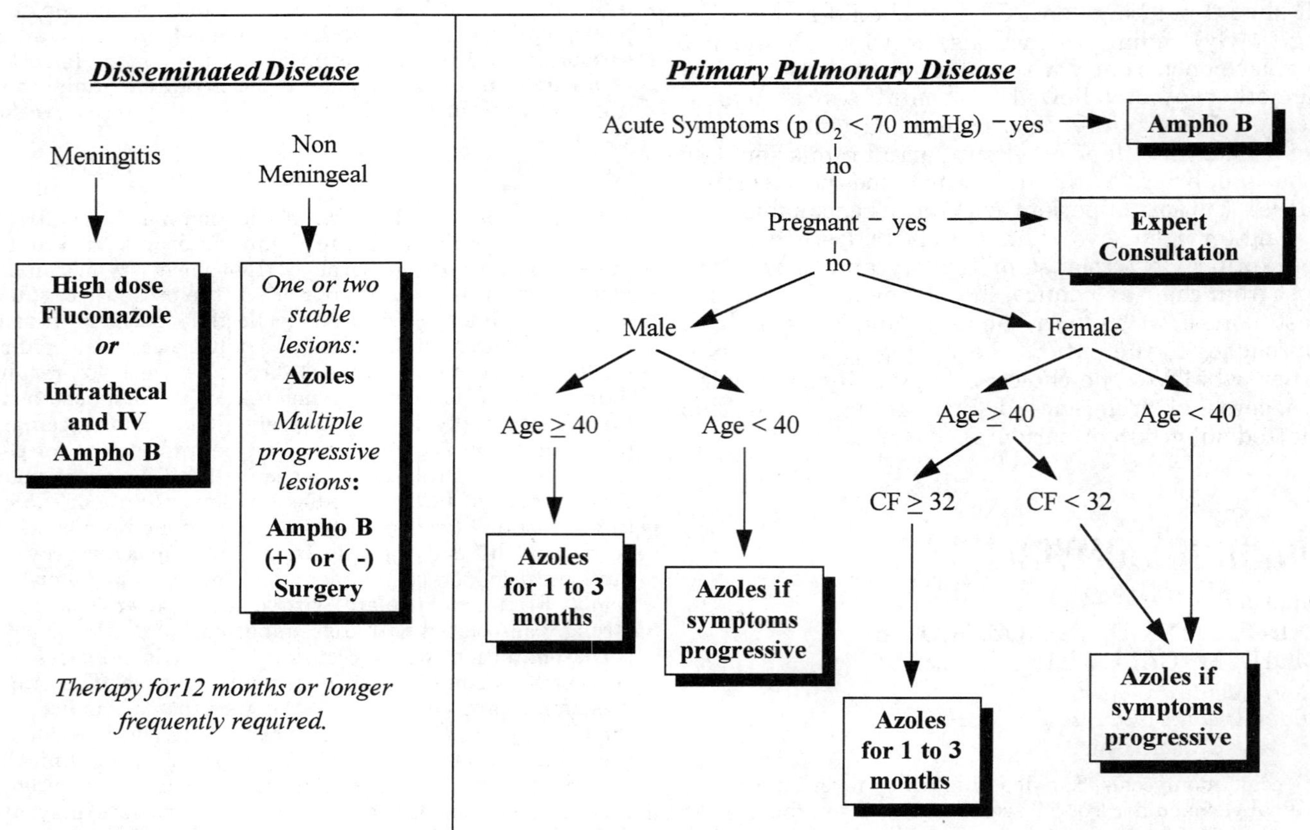

Figure 1. Coccidioidomycosis treatment algorithm. Ampho B = amphotericin B; CF = complement-fixation titer; p O₂ = arterial blood oxygen.

Table 1. Medications for the Treatment of Coccidioidomycosis

	Trade Name	**Indications**	**Dosages**
Amphotericin B	Fungizone	Severe disease Meningitis	1 to 3 gm total dose IV 0.1 to 0.8 mg intrathecally with dose escalation
Ketoconazole	Nizoral	Moderate pulmonary or nonmeningeal dissemination	400 mg/d PO

Fluconazole*	Diflucan	Meningitis
		Moderate pulmonary or
		  nonmeningeal dissemination
			800 to 1200 mg/d† PO
			400 mg/d PO preferred when dosage above 400
			  mg required due to intolerance of other azoles
			  or failure of lower doses

Itraconazole*	Sporanox	Same as ketoconazole	400 mg/d PO

*Currently not approved by the Food and Drug Administration for treatment of *C. immitis*.
†Exceeds dosage recommended by the manufacturer.

senting with dissemination, the algorithm is a useful guide to therapy. The risk of serious disease (late dissemination, death, or chronic pulmonary disease) is associated with male sex, increasing age, CF titers greater than 1:32, and African American race. All men over 40 years of age should receive treatment for 1 to 3 months, depending on response, as well as women over 40 years of age with CF titers greater than 1:32. This represents about 20% of the infected population. In both men and women under this age, and women over 40 years with low titers, treatment should be based on the severity of initial symptoms and clinical course. Over a 1-year period, the risk of serious disease in these lower-risk populations was less than 7% in our retrospective series; however, 36% of them received azoles. In all cases of primary pulmonary disease, the decision to treat or continue previous treatment is based on symptoms and findings. CF titers of 1:16 or greater, a persistently negative skin test, chronic fatigue, and delayed resolution of pulmonary infiltrates are the most common reasons for initiating or continuing oral azoles.

There are no studies in primary cocci with any drug treatment. Research in cases of nonmeningeal dissemination and chronic pulmonary disease does not favor fluconazole* (Diflucan) or itraconazole (Sporanox) over the less expensive ketoconazole (Nizoral). Since side effects with both ketoconazole and itraconazole are increased with doses greater than 400 mg, we prefer fluconazole when dosage ranging above this level is required (Table 1). Although some increase in nausea, alopecia, and arthralgias can occur in fluconazole doses greater than 400 mg, these effects have not led to significant noncompliance. All the azoles have been associated with hepatic toxicity and require liver function test monitoring monthly for the first 3 months of treatment. Enhanced activity of warfarin, phenytoin, and oral hypoglycemics when combined with azoles can lead to significant toxicity and requires careful monitoring.

Patients presenting with a cavitary lesion or fibrocavitary changes on chest radiograph are a unique challenge. A satisfactory treatment regimen is yet to be described that will eliminate the radiographic findings despite a good clinical response. Cavities occur more commonly in patients with diabetes and tend to relapse with cough, fatigue, and positivesputum cultures when treatment is discontinued.Therapy is generally continued for 6 to 12 monthsfollowing symptoms as described for primary disease.

Patients with meningitis have historically been treated with intravenous and intrathecal amphotericin B. In the past few years a choice between amphotericin B or fluconazole has been offered. The excellent bioavailability and penetration of fluconazole in the cerebral spinal fluid has yielded successful treatment responses in 60% to 70% of patients. Although doses of 400 mg per day were initially recommended, we have noted more rapid responses in meningitis scores when patients are started at 800 to 1000 mg* per day. Patients are monitored clinically and with monthly cerebral spinal fluid parameters and CF titers. Relapse after discontinuing fluconazole or amphotericin B is the rule, and treatment may need to be continued indefinitely. Patient quality of life is significantly improved with fluconazole, which avoids the necessity of repeated cisternal amphotericin B injections and the attendant morbidity. Whether the long-term prognosis with fluconazole will equal that of amphotericin B will require more experience.

Nonmeningeal dissemination to skin and soft tissue responds better than disease in the joints or bone. Minimal lesions of skin and soft tissue can be effectively managed with azoles. When sites are multiple or progressive and associated with high CF titers, amphotericin B, total dose of 1 to 3 gms, is preferred, followed by oral azoles. Surgical drainage of abscesses or extraction of the sequestrum in osteomyelitis is commonly required. Local irrigation with amphotericin B (100 mg per liter) for joint involvement failing to respond to systemic treatment can also be effective. Treatment duration is generally for a year or longer until symptoms have resolved and a positive skin test can be demonstrated.

---

*Not FDA-approved for this indication.

*Exceeds dosage recommended by the manufacturer.

HISTOPLASMOSIS

method of
CAROL A. KAUFFMAN, M.D.

*Ann Arbor Veterans Affairs Medical Center and
University of Michigan Medical School
Ann Arbor, Michigan*

Histoplasma capsulatum is the fungus responsible for causing histoplasmosis. This organism flourishes in the soil in areas drained by the Ohio and Mississippi Rivers. It grows exuberantly as a mold when the soil is fertilized by avian nitrogenous waste. Disease is caused when *H. capsulatum* conidia are inhaled into the lower respiratory tract. In the body, at 37°C, the organism is converted to the yeast form. Although the initial infection is almost always pulmonary, histoplasmosis should be viewed as a disease of the reticuloendothelial system (RES), with parasitization of macrophages and subsequent hematogenous spread to all organs of the RES (liver, spleen, lymph nodes, bone marrow).

CLINICAL MANIFESTATIONS

Manifestations of histoplasmosis vary from acute self-limited infection that rarely comes to the attention of a physician and does not require treatment to overwhelming infection with adult respiratory distress syndrome, shock, and disseminated intravascular coagulation. The severity of infection depends upon the number of organisms inhaled as well as the immune response of the host against the organism. Thus, healthy persons who develop acute pulmonary histoplasmosis after exposure to a point source with a large number of organisms may have bilateral alveolar infiltrates and severe systemic symptoms; likewise, patients who are immunosuppressed, such as infants, transplant recipients, and HIV-infected individuals, have a propensity to develop overwhelming pulmonary or disseminated histoplasmosis. The x-ray film often shows a miliary-type infiltrate, but the lesions tend to be more variable in size and nodular than those noted with miliary tuberculosis.

The usual manifestations of acute pulmonary infection in a healthy host are fever, cough, dyspnea, and pleuritic chest pain. Chest radiograph shows involvement of one or more lobes. Other manifestations of pulmonary histoplasmosis include hilar lymphadenopathy, mediastinal lymphadenopathy, and rarely cavitary lesions.

Chronic cavitary pulmonary histoplasmosis occurs almost entirely in patients with pre-existing chronic obstructive pulmonary disease. Lesions are in the apical segments of the lungs, usually bilateral, and often cavitary. Patients present with fever, night sweats, anorexia, weight loss, cough, hemoptysis, and dyspnea. The chest x-ray film is indistinguishable from that seen with reactivation tuberculosis.

Almost all patients have hematogenous dissemination of *H. capsulatum*, but most do not manifest systemic complaints. However, in the immunosuppressed host, acute symptomatic dissemination occurs. This is manifested by fever, night sweats, anorexia, weight loss, mucocutaneous ulcers, hepatosplenomegaly, and pancytopenia. This is the most common manifestation of histoplasmosis in HIV-infected individuals.

Chronic progressive disseminated histoplasmosis usually occurs in middle-aged and elderly men. Widespread involvement of many organ systems occurs, and the disease has a progressive downhill course. Patients generally have fevers, weight loss, night sweats, and mucocutaneous ulcerations and may present with acute adrenal insufficiency secondary to adrenal destruction by *H. capsulatum*.

DIAGNOSIS

H. capsulatum may take 6 to 8 weeks to grow in culture. The organism can be grown from blood in patients with acute dissemination. In an acutely ill patient, it is best to establish a diagnosis by histopathologic examination of tissues. The organism is a small (2 to 4 μm), intracellular budding yeast best seen by silver stains of bone marrow, liver, lymph nodes, or mucocutaneous lesions.

Skin testing should not be performed as it is neither sensitive nor specific. Serology is useful, especially in patients with chronic histoplasmosis. The most commonly used tests are complement fixation and immunodiffusion assays. A radioimmunoassay is currently available for testing urine and serum for *H. capsulatum* antigen; this is most helpful in patients with disseminated infection.

ANTIFUNGAL THERAPY

Prior to the 1980s, the treatment of histoplasmosis was amphotericin B (Fungizone). For chronic cavitary pulmonary histoplasmosis, as well as chronic progressive disseminated histoplasmosis, a total of at least 25 mg per kg was required. The introduction of several new azole antifungal agents has simplified treatment for most patients. Itraconazole (Sporanox) has become the drug of choice for many forms of histoplasmosis; ketoconazole (Nizoral) is also effective. Fluconazole (Diflucan) has not proved to be as efficacious as itraconazole or ketoconazole.

For patients who are seriously ill, especially immunosuppressed patients with overwhelming disseminated histoplasmosis, amphotericin B still remains the drug of choice. Generally, a daily dose of 0.7 to 1.0 mg per kg should be achieved in the first several days and then continued until the patient stabilizes. After several weeks, therapy can be switched to an azole drug.

Patients with pulmonary histoplasmosis can usually be treated with 200 mg of itraconazole per day. The minimum treatment course should probably be 6 months, and patients should be followed for the next year to be certain that relapse does not occur. Ketoconazole, 400 mg daily, is also effective for pulmonary histoplasmosis.

Patients with the chronic cavitary form of pulmonary histoplasmosis usually require therapy for at least 1 year and often for a longer period of time. This form of histoplasmosis is difficult to treat because of the underlying severe chronic obstructive pulmonary disease. A daily dosage of 200 mg of itraconazole can be used; if the patient fails to respond within the first month, this should be increased to 200 mg twice daily. Ketoconazole at a daily dosage of 400 mg can also be used; if the patient fails to respond, then 800 mg daily* should be tried. At this dosage, side effects

---

*Exceeds dosage recommended by the manufacturer.

are common, and treatment is difficult to carry out over the long time required.

Chronic progressive disseminated histoplasmosis responds to treatment with itraconazole or ketoconazole. Usually, 200 mg of itraconazole twice daily is preferred, but 400 to 800 mg of ketoconazole is also effective. Treatment is usually continued for at least 1 year, and some patients require longer treatment. For patients with mild-to-moderate acute disseminated histoplasmosis, 200 mg of itraconazole twice daily can also be used. Those with severe disease should receive amphotericin B initially followed by itraconazole.

It is unclear whether patients with *Histoplasma* meningitis should be treated with amphotericin B or an azole. Little experience exists to recommend using an azole in this situation. On the other hand, meningitis is often chronic, requiring therapy for life, and azoles are better suited to this form of therapy.

In patients with AIDS who have mild-to-moderate histoplasmosis, itraconazole, 200 mg twice daily, has been shown to be effective. For patients with moderately severe or severe disease, an initial course of 1 to 2 weeks of amphotericin B followed by itraconazole is preferred. Lifelong maintenance therapy is required in AIDS patients because relapse is almost a certainty. Itraconazole, 200 mg twice daily, is the drug of choice for maintenance therapy. Ketoconazole is ineffective for treating histoplasmosis in AIDS patients, and fluconazole is less effective than itraconazole.

As noted earlier, itraconazole has become the drug of choice for most forms of histoplasmosis. Two major deterrents to the use of itraconazole are problems with absorption of the drug and drug interactions. An acid environment in the stomach is required for effective absorption, and thus patients should not be treated with concomitant H_2 blockers, omeprazole (Prilosec), or antacids. In elderly patients, many of whom may be achlorhydric, it is appropriate to measure serum itraconazole levels to be certain the patient is absorbing the drug. Itraconazole serum levels increase two- to threefold when given with food.

The other major drawback to the use of itraconazole is the number of drug interactions that occur when this drug is used concomitantly with other drugs metabolized through the P-450 enzyme system. Itraconazole should not be given with rifampin (Rifadin) or rifabutin (Mycobutin), since itraconazole serum levels will decrease dramatically. In addition, phenytoin and carbamazepine have a similar, although less pronounced, effect and should not be used with itraconazole.

Itraconazole increases the serum levels of digoxin and cyclosporine and may lead to serious toxicities. However, the major drug interactions that must be avoided are those with terfenadine (Seldane) and astemizole (Hismanal). Serum levels of these antihistamines are increased when ketoconazole or itraconazole is given; such increases can lead to serious ventricular arrhythmias, such as torsades de pointes.

Loratadine (Claritin) and cisapride (Propulsid) levels also are increased with concomitant ketoconazole use, causing ventricular arrhythmias; presumably this same effect could also occur with itraconazole and thus it too should be avoided when using loratadine and cisapride.

Itraconazole can cause edema, hypertension, and hypokalemia in a small percentage of patients. The mechanism of this side effect is unknown. Other side effects include hepatitis, which is rare, but requires that the drug be stopped, rash, nausea, and vomiting.

BLASTOMYCOSIS

method of
PETER G. PAPPAS, M.D.
University of Alabama at Birmingham School of Medicine
Birmingham, Alabama

Blastomycosis is an unusual but important systemic infection caused by the thermally dimorphic fungus *Blastomyces dermatitidis*. The disease is endemic to most of the eastern United States, excluding Florida and most of New England. The disease also occurs in Canada and has been reported rarely from Central and South America, Western Europe, and Africa. Within the United States and Canada, the disease is concentrated in areas along the Mississippi and Ohio River basins and the Great Lakes. In endemic areas, small point source outbreaks have been associated with recreational and occupational activities occurring in wooded areas along waterways. Current evidence indicates that *B. dermatitidis* exists in warm, moist soil enriched by organic debris including decaying vegetation and wood.

Most infections with *B. dermatitidis* occur through inhalation of aerosolized spores, but there are occasional reports of infection resulting from direct inoculation through the skin. Primary infection is usually asymptomatic or may be associated with a self-limited influenza-like illness. In the minority of patients, chronic pneumonia or extrapulmonary dissemination may occur.

Blastomycosis is usually recognized clinically as a chronic, indolent, systemic fungal infection with a variety of pulmonary and extrapulmonary manifestations. Chronic pulmonary blastomycosis usually presents with chronic productive cough, chest pain, hemoptysis, weight loss, and low-grade fever. Chest roentgenogram may reveal nodular or lobar infiltrates, oftentimes involving multiple lobes. Perihilar mass lesions, with or without cavitation, mimicking other granulomatous diseases or lung neoplasms are often seen. Pleural effusions are uncommon in the normal host. Occasionally, diffuse pulmonary infiltrates consistent with the adult respiratory distress syndrome may occur, and this manifestation is associated with an exceptionally high mortality. Extrapulmonary blastomycosis most commonly involves the skin, bone, male genitourinary tract (especially the prostate and epididymis), and the central nervous system. The skin is involved in 40 to 80% of cases, and multiple system involvement is seen in up to 60% of cases. Blastomycosis involving the central nervous system is relatively uncommon and may present as granulomatous meningitis or an intracerebral mass lesion.

B. dermatitidis is an uncommon opportunistic pathogen, but there are recent data suggesting that blastomycosis may be unusually severe in immunocompromised patients, causing widely disseminated multiple-organ disease. These patients are particularly likely to develop central nervous system involvement. The most common underlying immune disorders among these patients include chronic glucocorticocosteroid use, solid organ transplant recipients, and advanced HIV disease.

A definitive diagnosis of blastomycosis requires a positive culture for *B. dermatitidis* from clinical specimens. A presumptive diagnosis is based on the finding of broad-based budding yeasts with doubly refractile cell walls compatible with *B. dermatitidis* on histopathologic examination of clinical specimens. Ten percent KOH is used to prepare wet specimens such as sputum or skin lesions for examination. Fixed specimens are usually stained with hematoxylin and eosin, periodic acid–Schiff (PAS), or Gomori's methenamine-silver (GMS) reagents. Serologic assays are of very limited value in the diagnosis of blastomycosis. Most of the assays, especially the complement fixation assay, are highly cross-reactive and of little diagnostic value. Among the available tests, immunodiffusion and ELISA assay tests for A antigen of *B. dermatitidis* probably have the best potential as serologic markers of disease. The blastomycin skin test antigen lacks sufficient specificity and sensitivity and should not be used as a diagnostic test.

TREATMENT

At present, there are three drugs approved for the treatment of blastomycosis: amphotericin B (Fungizone), ketoconazole (Nizoral), and itraconazole (Sporanox). Fluconazole (Diflucan),* has also been used successfully to treat milder forms of blastomycosis but is not approved for this purpose. Traditionally, amphotericin B has been the mainstay of therapy for all forms of blastomycosis, but studies over the last few years have proven both ketoconazole and itraconazole to be highly effective alternatives, particularly for patients with more indolent disease that does not involve the CNS. Although there are no comparative trials, itraconazole appears to be more efficacious than ketoconazole and is associated with considerably fewer adverse effects. In a recently published trial, 95% of patients with non–life-threatening, non-CNS blastomycosis were successfully treated with itraconazole, 200 to 400 mg daily for 2 to 6 months. This approximates the observed efficacy of amphotericin B in similar patients; thus itraconazole has become the oral agent of choice. There are similar data concerning the use of ketoconazole, which suggest efficacy in at least 80% of patients receiving 400 to 800 mg daily for 6 months or more. Most patients with blastomycosis can be started on oral therapy with itraconazole, 200 mg daily, and advanced by 100-mg increments at monthly intervals to a maximum of 400 mg daily in patients with persistent or progressive disease. Among patients with more aggressive disease, an initial dose of 400 mg is more appropriate. Ketoconazole is usually begun at 400 mg daily and advanced by 200-mg increments at monthly intervals to a maximum dose of 800 mg daily in patients with persistent or progressive dis-

ease. Therapy with either agent should be given for at least 6 months. Despite its increased cost compared with ketoconazole, itraconazole is generally preferred because it is better tolerated at therapeutic doses, is better absorbed, and is probably more effective than ketoconazole.

The role of fluconazole in the treatment of blastomycosis is probably very limited. The compound appears to be roughly similar to ketoconazole in efficacy but with less toxicity. Fluconazole does not appear to be as efficacious as itraconazole at similar doses; however, at higher doses (400 to 800 mg daily), up to 90% of patients are successfully treated. Because of the excellent penetration of fluconazole into the CNS, this compound may have potential as a therapeutic agent in meningeal or intracerebral blastomycosis. Amphotericin B should be reserved for patients with life-threatening or CNS disease, patients who are immunocompromised, and for those in whom oral therapy has failed. A total dose of 1.5 to 2.5 grams is sufficient therapy for most patients. In selected patients, an induction dose of about 500 mg is given to achieve a rapid fungicidal effect, and this is followed by oral therapy with itraconazole for at least 6 months. Amphotericin B must be given intravenously and can be infused over 2 hours in most settings. Preinfusion saline loading with 500 to 1000 mL and avoidance of other nephrotoxic agents are recommended to avoid amphotericin B–induced nephrotoxicity. Infusion-associated toxicities such as fever, chills, headache, and myalgias can usually be controlled with agents such as ibuprofen, acetaminophen, and diphenhydramine. For more severe cases, intravenous meperidine is given before or during the infusion.

The treatment of acute pulmonary blastomycosis remains controversial. Many investigators choose to observe non-immunocompromised patients without therapy, since available data suggest that most cases resolve spontaneously without therapy. Careful long-term follow-up is essential in these patients to monitor for evidence of active disease.

All patients with chronic blastomycosis should receive antifungal therapy. Itraconazole is generally preferred over ketoconazole because of superior efficacy and less toxicity, although ketoconazole is an acceptable alternative. Higher dose fluconazole may have a role in certain circumstances. All of these agents must be given for at least 6 months. Induction therapy with amphotericin B followed by an azole is indicated in selected patients. Cure rates among non-immunocompromised patients should exceed 90%. Among immunocompromised patients, lifelong chronic suppressive therapy may be necessary to prevent relapsing disease.

---

*Not FDA-approved for this indication.

PLEURAL EFFUSION AND EMPYEMA THORACIS

method of
RICHARD I. WHYTE, M.D.
The University of Michigan Medical Center
Ann Arbor, Michigan

PLEURAL EFFUSION

Pleural effusion is an abnormal collection of fluid within the pleural space; when the fluid becomes infected, the collection is termed an empyema. Normal physiology of the pleural space involves an equilibrium between fluid entering the pleural space and fluid being reabsorbed, with only a small amount (estimated to be between 3 and 10 mL) of fluid being present at any one time. Under normal conditions, fluid is produced by filtration from the parietal pleura; however, under pathologic conditions such as pulmonary edema or visceral pleural inflammation, fluid may originate from other sources. Pleural fluid is generally reabsorbed by the parietal pleural lymphatics. When the normal equilibrium is disturbed and fluid production exceeds reabsorption, an effusion results.

Pleural effusions are categorized as either exudates or transudates—the characteristics of each are listed in Table 1. Most commonly, the distinction is based on protein or lactate dehydrogenase (LDH) concentration. Transudates are typically associated with changes in osmotic and hydrostatic pressure gradients and not with alterations in pleural or capillary permeability. Exudates result from changes in capillary permeability and may be of neoplastic, infectious, or inflammatory origin. Common causes of both exudative and transudative effusions are listed in Table 2.

The symptoms of pleural effusions include dyspnea, cough, and chest discomfort. Other symptoms may also be present, depending on the etiology of the effusion. Small effusions may be asymptomatic. On physical examination, patients may demonstrate decreased breath sounds on the side of the effusion; there may also be egophony and dullness to percussion. The diagnosis of pleural effusion is usually made by a chest radiograph, but it is reported that over 400 mL of fluid must be present before the effusion is apparent on a standard posteroanterior chest radiograph. Lateral decubitus films and computed tomography (CT) are more sensitive. Ultrasonography may be useful in localizing loculated fluid collections but is usually not necessary to make the diagnosis.

Once the diagnosis of pleural effusion has been made, characterization of the fluid is generally indicated. Thoracentesis, or aspiration of fluid from the chest, can usually be performed in a safe fashion using local anesthesia and physical examination for localization. In performing a thoracentesis, care should be taken not to injure the neurovascular bundle that runs adjacent to each rib. Goals of thoracentesis are characterization of the fluid and, if indicated, pleural drainage. Complete evacuation of the pleural space is frequently possible, although removal of over 1 to 1.5 liters of fluid is more likely to result in acute pleuritic chest pain and re-expansion pulmonary edema. Such occurrences can be minimized by slow evacuation of the pleural space, avoiding high-negative intrathoracic pressure, and avoiding removing large amounts of fluid. Pleural fluid samples should be examined for cell count, protein, LDH, glucose and amylase concentrations, culture, pH, and cytology. If a chylothorax is suspected, triglyceride concentration should be determined.

Protein and LDH levels will determine whether

TABLE 2. Causes of Pleural Effusions

Transudates

Congestive heart failure
Cirrhosis
Nephrotic syndrome
Glomerulonephritis
Myxedema
Pulmonary emboli
Peritoneal dialysis
Hypoalbuminemia
Constrictive pericarditis
Malignancy
Atelectasis
Urinothorax

Exudates

Neoplasm—pulmonary, metastatic to pleura, and mesothelioma
Infectious—bacterial, tuberculous, viral, fungal, parasitic
Pulmonary embolism
Gastrointestinal disease—pancreatitis, subphrenic abscess, esophageal perforation
Inflammatory—rheumatoid arthritis, systemic lupus erythematosus, drug-induced lupus, Sjögren's syndrome
Miscellaneous—drug-induced, asbestos exposure, postpericardiotomy syndrome, trapped lung, Meigs' syndrome, uremia, radiation therapy
Chylothorax
Hemothorax

TABLE 1. Characteristics of Transudates and Exudates

	Transudate	Exudate
Protein	<3 gm/dL	>3 gm/dL
Pleural fluid/serum protein ratio	<0.5	>0.5
Pleural fluid/serum LDH	<0.6	>0.6
pH		<7.20 (implies empyema)
Glucose	Same as serum	<60 suggestive of infection
Cytology	Negative	May be positive in malignant effusions
Leukocyte count	<1000/mm³	>1000/mm³
Color	Clear	Cloudy
Specific gravity	<1.016	>1.016
Culture	Negative	May be positive
RBC count	<10,000/mm³	>10,000/mm³
Odor	Odorless	

the fluid represents a transudate or an exudate. A low glucose level is suggestive of empyema, tuberculous infection, neoplasm, or rheumatoid arthritis. An elevated amylase level is suggestive of pancreatitis or esophageal perforation. A triglyceride level of over 100 mg per dL is highly specific for chylothorax. Bloody effusions are associated with neoplasms, tuberculosis, and trauma. Leukocyte count may be helpful in establishing the etiology of a pleural effusion. Transudates typically have leukocyte counts of less than 1000 per mm³; leukocyte counts over 50,000 per mm³ usually denote a parapneumonic effusion or empyema. The color and clarity of the effusion should be noted. Grossly bloody effusions frequently are due to neoplasm or trauma; black fluid may represent an amebic abscess; tube-feed–colored fluid may represent an esophageal perforation or a misplaced feeding tube; cloudy fluid may be either chylous or purulent. Odor is occasionally helpful; a putrid odor indicates that an anaerobic infection is present.

When thoracentesis provides inadequate information, more invasive procedures are necessary. Percutaneous pleural biopsy may be helpful, although findings are frequently nonspecific. Thoracoscopy permits inspection of the entire pleural space, and large biopsy specimens can be obtained from areas visually noted to be abnormal. The diagnostic accuracy of thoracoscopy for the evaluation of undiagnosed pleural effusions is reported to be over 90%.

Treatment of a pleural effusion is directed toward the underlying cause. If the effusion is symptomatic, drainage, either by thoracentesis, tube thoracostomy, or thoracoscopy, may be necessary. Recurrent malignant effusions may be treated by chest tube drainage followed by chemical pleurodesis. Although a number of sclerosing agents are available, video-assisted thoracoscopy (VATS) with talc pleurodesis is over 90% effective in preventing recurrent effusions.

EMPYEMA THORACIS

Empyema thoracis is defined as pus within the pleural space. The condition may arise from a number of conditions; however, most empyemas are secondary to pneumonia. Other causes of empyema include trauma, lung abscess, esophageal perforation, subphrenic abscess, and pulmonary resection or other thoracic surgical procedures. The progression of an empyema has classically been divided into three phases: (1) an acute or exudative phase characterized by thin, purulent fluid, (2) a fibrinopurulent stage characterized by extensive fibrin deposits and turbid cellular fluid, and (3) an organized, or chronic, phase characterized by fibroblast ingrowth and collagen deposition that results in a thick pleural peel that entraps the lung.

Treatment of empyema is based on two premises: (1) drainage of all infected fluid, and (2) obliteration of residual pleural space. Early cases of empyema secondary to bacterial pneumonia have been successfully treated with thoracentesis and appropriate antibiotic administration. This is particularly true with parapneumonic effusions, in which the distinction between it and a true empyema is often unclear. Sometimes repeated aspirations are necessary, but administration of antibiotics alone is rarely adequate treatment. A leukocyte count of over 10,000 per mm³, a pH less than 7.20, a positive Gram's stain, or a glucose concentration less than 40 mg per dL all indicate that thoracentesis is unlikely to provide adequate drainage and that tube thoracostomy will be necessary. Inadequate drainage by thoracentesis, as demonstrated by residual fluid on chest radiograph or CT, is also an indication for tube thoracostomy. When the empyema has reached the fibrinopurulent or organizing stages, tube thoracostomy is generally inadequate and one must resort to surgical drainage. Recently, instillation of fibrinolytic enzymes has been used to break down loculations and improve drainage.

The surgical management of empyemas has traditionally rested on rib resection. In this procedure, effective drainage can be all but guaranteed through a combination of dependent drainage through a large-bore tube and mechanical breakdown of loculations. Initial closed drainage may be converted to open drainage after pleural symphysis; the empyema tube is subsequently slowly withdrawn as the cavity obliterates. Video-assisted thoracic surgery (VATS) may be helpful in the management of patients with empyema—loculations can be broken down, chest tubes can be accurately positioned, and a limited decortication can be performed. A complete decortication can also be performed thoracoscopically although this is tedious and frequently far more time-consuming than an open decortication. The basis of decortication in the management of empyema is removal of the pleural peel, thereby allowing the underlying lung to expand and fill the pleural space. Decortication is typically performed for empyemas in the chronic or organizing phase. When the lung cannot expand to obliterate the pleural space, as may occur following pulmonary resection or radiation, omental or muscle flaps can be rotated to obliterate any residual space. Thoracoplasty is rarely necessary but may be employed when tissue flaps are unavailable.

The management of patients with postpneumonectomy empyema with bronchopleural fistulas merits special mention. Immediate drainage of the infected space is essential, as contralateral pneumonia is frequently fatal. Once the pneumonectomy space is drained, the open bronchial stump should be closed. This can be accomplished by direct suture closure or by reinforcement with intercostal muscle or omental flaps. Long bronchial stumps can be stapled using a transmediastinal approach. Once the source of ongoing sepsis, the bronchial stump, is controlled, the empyema cavity must be addressed. Long-term open drainage—e.g., an Eloesser flap, may be appropriate for patients with limited life expectancy. However, other patients should be managed with either Clagett's procedure or muscle flap obliteration of the pneumonectomy space.

PRIMARY LUNG ABSCESS

method of
NICHOLAS D. D'ESOPO, M.D.
Woodbridge, Connecticut

A primary lung abscess is a localized necrotizing infection that has usually, but not always, liquefied and drained into the bronchial system to form an air-containing cavity.

The offending microorganisms are in at least 90% of cases anaerobic bacteria that have been aspirated from the oral cavity in conditions of depressed cough and/or clouded consciousness. By definition, a primary lung abscess occurs in individuals who have had no antecedent pulmonary or systemic conditions that could have predisposed them to such infections.

The source of the anaerobic bacteria is commonly gingivodental infection, but it is important to appreciate that a primary lung abscess may occur, though infrequently, in edentulous individuals. The foul-smelling sputum characteristic of anaerobic infection is expressed in the term "putrid lung abscess," whereas the primary lung abscess is also, in the older literature, the "nonspecific lung abscess," a term which recognizes that the sputum smear and culture do not disclose a specific bacterial species, such as staphylococci or gram-negative baccilli, which may produce necrotizing pulmonary lesions. The primary pulmonary abscess is distinct from, but related to, anaerobic pneumonia in which necrosis is revealed on the chest radiograph by the presence of multiple small abscesses.

The primary lung abscess contrasts with the secondary lung abscess, which is due to a variety of aerobic microorganisms and occurs in clinically recognizable settings, such as following major surgery, esophageal lesions, head and neck malignancies, prolonged hypotension, abdominal suppuration, steroid therapy, and neutropenia following cancer chemotherapy. In addition, specific infections that may lead to cavitary formation may need to be considered, most of them occurring in clinical circumstances or in geographic areas which suggest them. These include abscesses distal to bronchial obstruction, especially by neoplasms, as well as infections due to *Legionella* spp, *Actinomyces, Nocardia,* and in AIDS patients, organisms such as *Pneumocystis carinii* or *Rhodococcus equi*; also, mycobacteria and fungi, e.g., *Coccidioides immitis, Histoplasma capsulatum, Blastomyces hominis, Cryptococcus neoformans, Aspergillus*; also parasites, such as *Entamoeba histolytica, Paragonimus westermani*; and septic emboli. In addition to these infectious cavitary lesions, certain noninfectious pulmonary space-forming lesions may simulate an abscess. These include cavitating bronchogenic carcinoma; cavitary pulmonary infarction; cysts; bullae and developmental anomalies, such as sequestration; vasculitides, such as Wegener's granulomatosis; and finally, an empyema with an air-fluid level.

In primary lung abscess, the predisposing conditions that lead to the aspiration of anaerobic bacilli are alcoholism, foremost, over-sedation by drugs, neurologic and cardiovascular disease, seizures, and dental problems. In about 10% of patients, no predisposing situation is identified.

The anaerobic bacteria most commonly isolated from patients with primary lung abscess include *Peptostreptococcus* spp, *Fusobacterium nucleatum, F. necrophorum, Bacteroides melaninogenicus* and *intermedius,* and the *Bacteroides fragilis* group. These organisms have been recovered by techniques that bypass the oropharynx, such as percutaneous and transtracheal aspiration or bronchoscopy with protected catheter.

In about half the cases of primary lung abscess, aerobic bacteria have also been recovered, particularly *Streptococcus pneumoniae, Staphylococcus aureus, Escherichia coli, Klebsiella pneumoniae,* and *Pseudomonas aeruginosa.* The role of these aerobic bacteria is uncertain. Their presence or absence does not correlate either with the clinical features of the disease or its response to therapy.

Primary lung abscess frequently pursues an indolent course. It is usually an illness ranging from 2 weeks to 3 months in duration, consisting of cough, occasionally bloody sputum, fever of modest degree (101°F, 102°F), chest pain, malaise, and weight loss. Rigors are very rare. The recall by the patient of the distinct aspiration episode is unusual. Patients who have had a short illness, measured in days, are apt to have suffered an extended period of unconsciousness. Occasionally, the patient can remember the abrupt onset of a large amount of foul sputum, presumably as an abscess breaks into the bronchial tree. Continued respiratory symptoms, pleural pain, and malaise lead the patient to seek medical attention.

Examination of the patient may reveal the stigmata of chronic alcoholism. Clubbing of the fingers and toes occurs in abscesses that have been present for some time. Examination of the chest is not particularly helpful, though cavernous breath sounds may sometimes be elicited. The chest examination is often silent.

No radiographic features distinguish an anaerobic abscess from many of the cavitary pulmonary lesions previously enumerated. The anaerobic abscess is usually a single cavity of varying size. Pneumonic consolidation contiguous with it is generally not extensive and occasionally it is absent, the abscess appearing as a well-circumscribed cavitary mass-lesion. Patchy pneumonia distant from the abscess in the same or other lobes is unusual and suggests an abscess due to organisms found more often in secondary lung abscess. Before the abscess has drained into the bronchial system it may appear as a more or less circumscribed pneumonia. At that time, computed tomography may disclose a lucent center with thick, irregular walls. However, this is an image compatible with several other entities, especially a cavitary bronchogenic carcinoma. The right lung, because of its more vertical main bronchus, is affected more often than the left lung. The most common sites are by far the posterior segment of the upper lobe and the superior segment of the lower lobe. These are regions in which aspirated secretions settle in the recumbent position. Aspiration abscesses also occur in the basal segments of the lower lobes, but these are far more commonly secondary abscesses. The aspiration abscess is almost always contiguous with the pleural surface. Pleural effusion, either sterile or infective, occurs in some cases and should be aspirated and cultured.

Anaerobic bacteria inhabit the normal mouth. Hence, the diagnosis of an anaerobic infection cannot be made by the customary examination of respiratory secretions by smear and culture. The previously mentioned techniques for recovering anaerobic bacteria from the lungs are impractical, unavailable, or expensive for clinical practice. The diagnosis of an anaerobic infection is, in fact, a probable one that is suggested by a chest radiograph consistent with a lung abscess, a patient with an appropriate background for aspiration, and the absence in the respiratory secretions of pathogens that may be responsible for the clinical and radiographic data at hand. The presence of foul sputum, which occurs in about three quarters of the patients, adds immeasurably to the probability that the abscess in question is an anaerobic infection.

TREATMENT

Three drug regimens have been used to treat primary lung abscess: penicillin; clindamycin; and metronidazole in combination with penicillin.

Penicillin, both intravenously and orally, has been used successfully for many years. However, penicillin therapy may fail because anaerobic bacteria have become increasingly resistant to it. It may, however, be employed for patients with mild-to-moderate systemic and local symptoms without extensive disease on the chest radiograph. This is not because penicillin may be sufficient therapy for mild disease but not for severe disease; rather, because the treatment of an illness that does not seem urgent affords an opportunity to assess its efficacy and to turn if necessary to alternative therapy. Penicillin G is administered intravenously in a dose of 10 to 20 million units daily until a definite clinical and radiographic response has been obtained. Therapy may be continued with oral penicillin G, penicillin V, ampicillin, or amoxicillin in dosages of 500 to 750 mg three to four times daily.

In limited clinical trials, clindamycin (Cleocin) was found superior to penicillin in terms of fever, the duration of putrid sputum, and the number of failures. Indeed, clindamycin is considered by many clinicians the drug of choice for primary lung abscess. It is administered intravenously in a dose 600 to 700 mg every 8 hours. It is continued as oral therapy in a dose of 150 to 300 mg three to four times daily, or in more severe cases up to 450 mg every 6 hours. The disadvantage of clindamycin is its high cost, especially since oral therapy often needs to be prolonged.

Metronidazole (Flagyl) is active in many anaerobic infections, but it is not suitable as monotherapy for anaerobic lung abscess. Metronidazole in combination with penicillin may be effective therapy, though this regimen has not been subjected to sufficient clinical trial. Metronidazole may be administered in a dose of 7.5 mg per kg every 6 hours intravenously or orally in the same dosage. This amounts on average to 500 mg every 6 hours. Metronidazole may be used in combination with erythromycin or chloromycetin in patients sensitive to penicillin. Its low cost is attractive. A disulfiram-like reaction should be remembered when dealing with chronic alcoholics.

Other antibiotics to which anaerobes are frequently sensitive are second-generation cephalosporins, such as cefotetan (Cefotan), cefmetazol (Cefmetazon), and cefoxitin (Metoxin). In hospital-acquired lung abscess, aerobic organisms need to be identified and sensitivities determined. Combinations of beta-lactam drugs and beta-lactamase inhibitors, such as ticarcillin plus clavulanic acid, and ampicillin plus sulbactam, are active against all anaerobes.

The response to antibiotic therapy is usually prompt, with improvement in symptoms, a decrease in sputum volume and beginning defervescence. Resolution of the abscess on the chest radiograph lags behind clinical improvement. The abscess, in fact, often progresses during the first several days of therapy. This should not lead to abandoning the first choice of an antibiotic regimen, nor should it prompt investigation for a probable alternative diagnosis. As therapy continues, the abscess cavity progressively diminishes in size, with resolution of the associated pneumonia. Defervescence may be slow, with patients often remaining febrile until the second week of therapy. Bronchoscopy does not have the primary role it once had in the preantibiotic era. Now, it is not routinely performed to enhance drainage of the abscess but should of course be carried out if there is any doubt about the diagnosis. Postural drainage should be conservatively prescribed, if at all.

An antibiotic regimen in the treatment of lung abscess is considered a failure if after 10 to 14 days of treatment symptoms and fever continue, or the cavity fails to progressively decrease in size, or the fluid level persists or recurs, or the pericavitary pneumonia extends locally or in another segment or lobe.

Failure of treatment occurs because of (1) poor selection of an antibiotic regimen, (2) an incorrect diagnosis of primary lung abscess, (3) a very large cavity, i.e., over 6 cm in diameter, (4) a chronic cavity, (5) immunodeficiency in elderly debilitated patients, and finally, (6) an unsuspected and undrained empyema.

The management of the failure will depend on clinical symptoms and the extent and severity of the radiographic disease. The sputum should be examined for predominating aerobic bacteria, as well as organisms such as tubercle bacilli and fungi. Bronchoscopy is now mandatory to rule out an obstructing lesion or other kind of bronchial disease, especially bronchogenic carcinoma. If these measures are unrevealing and if the clinical situation does not seem urgent, additional drug therapy directed toward anaerobes may be employed, such as adding clindamycin to the regimen of a patient who has not responded to penicillin. When all antibiotic therapy appears to have been exhausted, a surgical procedure, usually lobectomy, rarely pneumonectomy, may be considered.

Resection of the abscess is especially indicated in patients for whom the diagnosis of a primary anaerobic abscess has been in doubt, apart from the failure to respond to what was considered a potentially effective regimen. Surgery is also indicated for a chronic lung abscess whose organized cavity wall will render it incapable of responding to any drug therapy. These indolent abscesses often occur in patients who have been afebrile from the beginning and may suggest that the initial diagnosis of an anaerobic lung abscess was in error. Resectional surgery is the therapy-of-choice in some patients who have had a massive hemorrhage, such as 500 mL or more, and, while such a bleeding usually does not recur after rest and sedation, the risk of a second such episode may not be warranted in some patients.

Percutaneous drainage of a lung abscess has been successfully performed in patients who were considered too high a risk for resection. Drainage appears to be especially indicated in patients with a giant cavity, e.g., over 6 cm in diameter. Abscess cavities that attain this very large size do so, in fact, because an inflammatory endobronchitis has led to air trapping. The response to external drainage is usually excellent, with rapid improvement after evacuation of large amounts of pus. Selection of the drainage site is either by CT or ultrasound. Pleural symphysis is assumed to have occurred when the abscess has been present for 2 weeks or more. External drainage has the disadvantage of requiring a drainage tube in place for a number of weeks.

It has been suggested that 2 to 4 months of antibiotic therapy will suffice for most patients with primary anaerobic lung abscess. However, recurrences occur when therapy is too brief. The most conservative practice is to continue therapy until the residual lesion has been stable on repeated chest radiographs. This may require more than 4 months of therapy. It is appreciated that these lesions may shrink in size as they organize for some time after they have been sterilized, but there is no way to recognize this stage. At the point of stability, the residual lesion may consist of one or more thin-walled spaces; these are the healed abscess and/or ectatic bronchi. Sometimes the lung abscess has been converted by therapy into a large cystic space. One is uncertain about what should be done with these. They can bleed extensively, presumably from the bronchial circulation that developed in the healing process. They may be colonized with fungi. It may therefore be justified to resect these spaces as a preventive measure.

Patients with severe symptoms or extensive radiographic disease will be admitted to hospital to receive intravenous therapy in that setting. Those patients with less severe illness, some of who can be afebrile, may justifiably be treated as outpatients from the beginning. Because the diagnosis of an anaerobic abscess is a probable diagnosis supported by the clinical radiographic response to antibiotic therapy, it is critical that these patients be those who are able to make frequent outpatient clinic visits for observation and chest radiographs; and they must be judged to be compliant for prolonged drug therapy.

OTITIS MEDIA

method of
MYLES L. PENSAK, M.D.
University of Cincinnati Medical Center
Cincinnati, Ohio

Otitis media is an inflammation of the middle ear space. Generally associated with bacteriologic infection, it may be provoked by environmental allergens, changes in barometric pressure, viral and fungal contaminants, or systemic pathologies. Because of the frequency with which it is diagnosed (90% of children under age 7 have been diagnosed with at least one episode), this clinical entity raises significant parental concerns, as well as economic issues with both health care providers and payers.

PATHOBIOLOGIC AND ENVIRONMENTAL FACTORS

The tympanic space or middle ear is a mucous membrane–lined, air-filled cavity residing within the temporal bone that houses the ossicular chain. The lateral boundary is defined by the tympanic membrane, while the anterior space (protympanum) contains the introitus of the eustachian tube. The osseous portion of the tube is fixed in size, while the cartilaginous segment varies in diameter with pharyngeal alterations associated with swallowing and respiration. The eustachian tube regulates the flow of air from the nasopharynx to the middle ear space and is found to be at a 10-degree angle directed inferiorly from the horizontal in the infant, maturing to a 45-degree angle in the adult.

Failure to equilibrate air pressure between the middle ear and ambient environment will often lead to negative middle ear pressure, atelectasis, effusion, and chronic changes within the mesotympanum.

A host of extratemporal factors contribute to the development of recurrent otitis media. These include genetic predisposition; craniofacial defects including, but not limited to, cleft palate defects; day care exposure; smoke-filled environments; and infant feeding habits. Other cofactors include concomitant viral infections, allergic and immunologic compromise, and the presence of upper airway obstruction secondary to chronic adenoid infection.

The bacteria most commonly found in most cases of uncomplicated otitis media include *Streptococcus pneumoniae, Haemophilus influenzae,* and *Moraxella catarrhalis.* The frequency of the latter two has been more prevalent as beta-lactamase–producing strains have become prominent. Other organisms, including *Staphylococcus aureus,* group A streptococci, and gram-negative bacilli, are infrequently identified. In contradistinction, *Pseudomonas aeruginosa* is often isolated in cases of chronic otitis media.

CLINICAL PRESENTATION AND MANAGEMENT

Acute otitis media is often heralded by otalgia, fever, and drainage if the tympanic membrane perforates. Examination reveals a red drum with loss of landmarks. As the inflammatory process progresses, the middle ear will contain an effusion of serous, mucoid, or purulent material. Several series have demonstrated that otoscopy may not help to distinguish among these effusions. Recognizing that effusion often accompanies acute infection, it needs to be appreciated that following resolution of an acute infection it can take up to 3 months for the effusion to clear.

Despite the popular employment of antibiotics, recent meta-analysis of data reported from otitis media studies reveals that while antibiotics appear to impact treatment and prevention, they do so in less than dramatic fashion.

While amoxicillin remains the treatment of choice

TABLE 1. **Dosing Schedules of Antibiotics for Pediatric Otitis Media**

Drug	Usual Dosage	Daily Dosage	No. of Days Therapy	Total Dose (mg/kg)	Price 9-kg 20-lb Child	Price 17-kg 32-lb Child
Amoxicillin (Amoxil)	40 mg/kg/day	tid	10	40	$10.50	$11.30
Amoxicillin, clavulanate (Augmentin)	40/10 mg/kg/day	tid	10	400/100	$32.10	$56.20
Azithromycin (Zithromax)	10 mg/kg/day 1	qd	5	30	$27.50	$27.50
Cefaclor (Ceclor)	40 mg/kg/day	bid/tid	10	400	$20.19	$28.59
Cefixime (Suprax)	8 mg/kg/day	qd/bid	10	80	$32.30	$51.20
Cefprozil (Cefzil)	30 mg/kg/day	bid	10	300	$29.60	$49.50
Erythromycin-sulfisoxazole (Pediazole)	50–150 mg/kg/day	tid/bid	10	150	$19.29	$32.29
Loracarbef (Lorabid)	30 mg/kg/day	bid	10	300	$37.40	$62.10
Trimethoprim-sulfamethoxazole (Bactrim)	8–40 mg/kg/day	bid	10	80/400		

for uncomplicated cases, fully 70 to 90% of otitis-prone children will have their otitis resolve without intervention.

In choosing an antibiotic, several factors need to be addressed: cost, tolerance, and efficacy. Since antibiotics seem to help resolve otitis media with effusion only in 14% of patients, compounded by the fact that repetitive courses of antibiotics do not change the overall response rate, the clinician must endeavor to be suspect of all the advertising done related to drugs for otitis media. Table 1 lists commonly employed regimens for uncomplicated acute otitis media. Antihistamines/decongestant therapy has not been shown to effect otitis media outcome. The author and his colleagues reserve the utilization of ventilation tubes for those children who have persistent effusion with conductive hearing loss or those experiencing recurrent episodes of acute otitis media who are refractory to antibiotic management. Most often, these children will have more than five or six acute infections per year.

CONCLUSION

Otitis media is a common, generally uncomplicated disease process affecting millions of children annually. Host, environmental, and therapeutic factors seem to influence the frequency and severity of individual episodes. Complications are uncommon but may be severe.

ACUTE BRONCHITIS

method of
ANTHONY L. ESPOSITO, M.D.,
CHRISTINE J. DEMPSEY, M.D, and
JANE M. DOYLE, M.D.
University of Massachusetts School of Medicine
Worcester, Massachusetts

A diagnosis of bronchitis implies the presence of inflammation of the lower respiratory tract involving the tracheobronchial tree but not the airspaces. Acute bronchitis refers to infections occurring in otherwise normal adults; acute exacerbations of chronic bronchitis applies to patients who have underlying chronic obstructive pulmonary disease. Although they share clinical features, acute bronchitis and acute exacerbations of chronic bronchitis possess distinct microbiologies and therapies and thus, differences exist in the management of patients with these conditions.

ACUTE BRONCHITIS

Most episodes of acute bronchitis are caused by viral pathogens, such as influenza, rhinovirus, adenovirus, and coronavirus; it is not surprising that the incidence of the disease rises during the winter and early spring. Some cases are due to *Mycoplasma pneumoniae, Chlamydia pneumoniae*, and *Bordetella pertussis*, but common bacterial pathogens, such as *Streptococcus pneumoniae* and *Haemophilus influenzae*, play a very minor role in this condition. A cough represents the hallmark complaint, and although some patients will produce purulent pulmonary secretions, most will report a nonproductive cough or the expectoration of clear or mucoid secretions. Substantial variability exists in the magnitude of the associated fever and the severity of accompanying symptoms; because of the spectrum and overlap of symptoms, etiologic diagnoses cannot be reliably established on the basis of clinical manifestations. Nevertheless, the presence of significant chills, fever, headache, malaise, and myalgias in the patient presenting between December and March does suggest a diagnosis of influenza. Similarly, a history of moderate-to-severe symptoms in a young adult who presents in the summer or early fall and whose cough is associated with substernal chest discomfort raises the possibility of mycoplasmal tracheobronchitis.

The exclusion of pneumonia represents a primary goal in the evaluation of the adult with an acute cough syndrome. In general, the likelihood of pneumonia is remote in the fit young or middle-aged adult whose pulmonary and systemic symptoms appear mild, whose vital signs include minimal elevations of the temperature, pulse, and respiratory rate, and whose chest examination reveals normal breath sounds or a few, diffuse rhonchi; these patients do not require a chest radiograph or other laboratory tests. Young adults infected with the human immunodeficiency virus (HIV-1) represent an important exception to this generalization; in particular, adults with documented or undiagnosed HIV-1 disease may seek medical attention because of *Pneumocystis carinii* pneumonia presenting as a subacute illness characterized by fever, a nonproductive cough, and mild shortness of breath on exertion. Similarly, debilitated geriatric patients can experience bacterial pneumonia that is associated with minor complaints and a relatively normal physical examination.

Reassurance that the illness is self-limited and control of disabling symptoms represent the cornerstones of management of the patient with acute bronchitis. Patients should be informed that their cough may persist for 2 to 3 weeks, especially if they smoke cigarettes; patients should also be reminded that since most episodes of bronchitis are viral in origin, antibiotics will not likely alter the course of their disease. Fever and myalgias should be controlled with an antipyretic analgesic, such as acetaminophen. A cough that interferes with sleep or daytime activities can be suppressed with antitussive medications that contain dextromethorphan or with codeine sulfate (15 to 30 mg every 4 to 6 hours). Patients who fail to respond to these conservative measures may require a chest radiograph or antimicrobial drugs. Since influenza can be complicated by bacterial pneumonia, patients should be instructed to contact their practitioner if their illness becomes associated with a deterioration in their sense of well being, a recrudesence of their chills and fever, or the onset of shortness of breath or a cough productive of green or yellow sputum. Finally, an episode of acute bronchitis can trigger bronchospasm that is manifest by frank wheezing or an intractable cough; in the latter case, the presence of bronchospasm can be detected by pulmonary function testing. Patients who experience postinfectious bronchial hyperactivity characteristically respond well to therapy with inhaled beta-agonists or corticosteroids.

The routine use of antimicrobials in treating adults with acute bronchitis remains controversial because of the absence of supportive data from well-designed, placebo-controlled trials. Nevertheless, most practitioners will prescribe an antimicrobial because of the patient's expectation of being treated with such agents and because of the doctor's concern about disease due to potentially susceptible microbes, such as *Mycoplasma pneumoniae, Chlamydia pneumoniae*, or *Bordetella pertussis*. Although antimicrobial therapy is frequently prescribed, this approach ignores the fact that *Mycoplasma, Chlamydia*, and *Bordetella* produce a minority of the episodes and that antibiotics can produce adverse reactions. Further, the liberal use of anti-infective drugs does alter the microbial ecology of the community, facilitating the emergence of antimicrobial resistance.

The role of antibiotics in the treatment of adults with acute bronchitis has been further confounded by the recent description of an entity termed "acute bacterial bronchitis." Occurring in both smoking and nonsmoking adults, this condition is characterized by the presence of purulent pulmonary secretions and the recovery of a potential respiratory tract pathogen, such as *Streptococcus pneumoniae*, from expectorated sputum. Although patients with acute bacterial bronchitis appear to respond well to antibiotics, authorities disagree on the clinical importance of the microbes isolated from the sputa of these patients and thus, on the utility of antimicrobial therapy.

In general, we do not recommend antibiotics for the fit adult with acute bronchitis, unless the epidemiologic history suggests infection due to *M. pneumoniae*; thus, the young adult who presents in the summer or early fall and who reports that a similar illness is moving slowly among family members or close contacts would be a candidate for antimycoplasmal chemotherapy. Some clinicians will also prescribe an anti-infective for possible mycoplasmal or chlamydial disease if the acute cough syndrome persists for more than 5 to 7 days. A macrolide (e.g., erythromycin) or a tetracycline (e.g., doxycycline) would be appropriate therapy; these drugs are active against *M. pneumoniae* and *C. pneumoniae* (Table 1). Patients with "bacterial bronchitis" who appear ill at presentation or who produce purulent secretions for more than 2 to 3 days can be treated with amoxicillin, doxycycline, or erythromycin.

Amantadine (Symmetrel) or rimantadine (Flumadine) will reduce the duration of fever and systemic complaints caused by influenza A if therapy is initiated within 48 hours of the onset of symptoms. In addition, treatment with these drugs will facilitate the resumption of a patient's usual activities. However, at clinically relevant doses, these agents will not alter the course of disease due to influenza B or other viral pathogens. Although the incidence of central nervous system (CNS) side effects is greater with amantadine, both drugs have the potential to produce clinically significant neurologic events, including agitation, an inability to concentrate, toxic psychoses, and seizures; the latter are more likely in patients with a pre-existing epileptic disorder. The risk of an untoward CNS event is enhanced in the setting of advanced age or disease-related renal dysfunction, and, thus, reductions in creatinine clearance require dosage adjustments. The likelihood of an adverse neurologic reaction, such as hallucinations and delirium, is also increased in patients receiving antihistamines, anticholinergics, antidepressants, and perhaps trimethoprim or diuretics. Both antivirals should be avoided in pregnant or breast-feeding patients.

The standard dose of amantadine or rimantadine is 100 mg orally twice daily; in individuals 65 years of age or older, 100 mg daily is sufficient, and in patients with advanced degrees of renal failure, additional dose reductions are necessary. The usual course of therapy is 7 days.

ACUTE EXACERBATIONS OF CHRONIC BRONCHITIS

A diagnosis of chronic bronchitis applies to any person who experiences a cough that is productive of

TABLE 1. **Oral Antimicrobials Useful for Treating Adults with Infectious Bronchitis**

	Daily Dose	Advantages	Disadvantages	Important Drug Interactions
Amoxicillin	500 mg q 8 h	Inexpensive Serious adverse events uncommon	Some *H. influenzae*, most *M. catarrhalis* are resistant	Allopurinol
Amoxicillin-clavulanate (Augmentin)	500 mg q 8 h	Spectrum includes beta-lactamase producing *H. influenzae* and *M. catarrhalis*	Expensive Loose stools common	Allopurinol
Erythromycin	250 mg q 6 h or 500 mg q 12 h	Inexpensive Spectrum includes *M. pneumoniae,* *C. pneumoniae,* *S. pneumoniae,* *M. catarrhalis* Safe for use in patients allergic to penicillins or cephalosporins	GI intolerance common Frequent dosing Most *H. influenzae* are resistant Absorption impaired by food	Theophylline, terfenadine, astemizole, digoxin, Coumadin, cyclosporine, triazolam, carbamazepine
Azithromycin (Zithromax)	500 mg first day, then 250 mg qd for 4 d	Infrequent dosing Short courses of therapy Better tolerated than erythromycin Fewer drug interactions than erythromcyin Spectrum similar to erythromycin but better activity against *H. influenzae* Safe for use in patients allergic to penicillins or cephalosporins	Expensive Absorption impaired by food	—
Clarithromycin (Biaxin)	500 mg q 12 h	Infrequent dosing Better tolerated than erythromycin Spectrum similar to erythromycin but better activity against *H. influenzae* Safe for use in penicillin- or cephalosporin-allergic patients	Costly Caution with use during pregnancy	Theophylline, terfenadine, astemizole, zidovudine, cyclosporine, rifabutin, carbamazepine
Cefaclor (Cefaclor)	250 mg q 8 h	Spectrum includes *S. pneumoniae,* *H. influenzae,* *M. catarrhalis,* including beta-lactamase producing strains Generic less expensive	Not active against *M. pneumoniae,* *C. pneumoniae* Brand expensive	—
Cefixime (Suprax)	400 mg qd	Infrequent dosing Spectrum similar to cefaclor	Expensive Loose stools common	—
Cefpodoxime (Vantin)	200 mg q 12 h	Infrequent dosing Spectrum similar to cefaclor	Expensive Loose stools common Absorption impaired by antacids, H_2 blockers	—

Table continued on opposite page

sputum, that lasts for at least 3 months for 2 or more consecutive years and that cannot be attributed to another disorder, such as bronchiectasis, asthma, sinusitis, gastroesophageal reflux, or cystic fibrosis. In the United States, cigarette smoking represents the most common cause of chronic bronchitis; other potential etiologies include multiple respiratory tract infections during childhood and prolonged exposure to industrial or environmental pollutants.

An exacerbation of chronic bronchitis reflects a deterioration in the patient's pulmonary status. Characteristic symptoms include shortness of breath on exertion, an increase in the volume of sputum produced daily, and a change in the appearance of the secretions from white or clear to yellow or green; many patients will present with all these complaints. Fever of substantial magnitude and extrapulmonary complaints are not common, and their presence should raise concerns about the possibility of pneumonia, a more serious disease. Patients who are well-known to their physicians can often be managed without a trip to the office or clinic; patients who are aged or fragile or who have more severe symptoms or multiple underlying medical conditions should be seen. The primary purpose of the visit is to detect evidence of pneumonia or respiratory decompensa-

TABLE 1. **Oral Antimicrobials Useful for Treating Adults with Infectious Bronchitis** *Continued*

	Daily Dose	Advantages	Disadvantages	Important Drug Interactions
Cefprozil (Cefzil)	500 mg q 12 h	Infrequent dosing Spectrum similar to cefaclor	Expensive	—
Cefuroxime (Ceftin)	250–500 mg q 12 h	Infrequent dosing Spectrum similar to cefaclor	Expensive Loose stools common	—
Loracarbef (Lorabid)	200–400 mg q 12 h	Infrequent dosing Spectrum similar to cefaclor	Expensive	—
Doxycycline	100 mg q 12–24 h	Inexpensive Infrequent dosing Spectrum includes *M. pneumoniae, C. pneumoniae,* and most strains of *S. pneumoniae, H. influenzae, M. catarrhalis* Safe for use in penicillin- or cephalosporin-allergic patients	GI intolerance Photosensitivity Contraindicated in pregnant or nursing women Absorption impaired by antacids, iron, bismuth subsalicylate	Digoxin, Dilantin, barbiturates, carbamazepine
Trimethoprim-sulfamethoxazole (Bactrim, Septra)	1 DS tablet q 12 h	Inexpensive Infrequent dosing Spectrum includes most strains of *S. pneumoniae, H. influenzae, M. catarrhalis* Safe for use in penicillin- or cephalosporin-allergic patients	Potential for serious allergic reactions Increasing prevalence of resistance in *S. pneumoniae* Not active against *M. pneumoniae* or *C. pneumoniae* Caution with use in pregnant patients near term	Dilantin, Coumadin, cyclosporine, azathioprine, methotrexate, sulfonylureas
Ciprofloxacin (Cipro)	500 mg q 12 h	Infrequent dosing Spectrum includes *H. influenzae, M. catarrhalis, M. pneumoniae,* many strains of *S. pneumoniae,* and some strains of *C. pneumoniae* Safe for use in penicillin- or cephalosporin-allergic patients	Expensive Variability in activity against *S. pneumoniae* Absorption impaired by antacids, iron, sucralfate, zinc Should be avoided in pregnant or nursing women	Theophylline, caffeine, cimetidine, Coumadin, cyclosporine, didanosine
Ofloxacin (Floxin)	400 mg q 12 h	Infrequent dosing Spectrum includes *H. influenzae, M. catarrhalis, M. pneumoniae, C. pneumoniae,* and many strains of *S. pneumoniae* Safe for use in penicillin- or cephalosporin-allergic patients	Expensive Variability in activity against *S. pneumoniae* Should be avoided in pregnant or nursing women Absorption impaired by antacids, iron, sucralfate, zinc	Coumadin, didanosine

tion requiring aggressive outpatient interventions or, perhaps, admission to hospital.

Decisions concerning laboratory tests must be made on a case-by-case basis. In the absence of clinical evidence of pneumonia or incipient respiratory failure, a chest radiograph, arterial blood gas (ABG) analysis, complete blood count (CBC), and Gram's stain and culture of sputum are not required, since they rarely provide critical information. Of course, a comprehensive diagnostic assessment would be appropriate for patients who are elderly, who are immunosuppressed by medications (e.g., corticosteroids) or disease (e.g., lymphoma), who have a history of respiratory failure, or who exhibit subtle signs of ventila-tory insufficiency, such as agitation or irritability. Similarly, patients who fail a course of empiric antimicrobial therapy require an evaluation that might include a sputum culture to identify drug-resistant microbes and a chest radiograph to detect the presence of a pneumonia, lung mass, or mild congestive heart failure.

Approximately 50% of all exacerbations of chronic bronchitis are precipitated or perpetuated by bacterial infection; the balance of the flares are attributable to viral infections and environmental insults, including cigarette smoke. The infectious agents most frequently associated with exacerbations include *Haemophilus influenzae, Streptococcus pneu-*

moniae, and *Moraxella (Branhamella) catarrhalis.* Atypical pathogens, such as *Mycoplasma pneumoniae* and *Chlamydia pneumoniae,* represent uncommon agents in this setting. Because of their proclivity to alter pulmonary and systemic host defenses and to predispose to bacterial pneumonia, influenza A and B represent the most important viral agents capable of inducing an exacerbation. Finally, *Staphylococcus aureus, Candida* sp., and aerobic gram-negative bacilli, such as *Escherichia coli,* are occasionally isolated from the expectorated sputa of patients who have received multiple courses of antibiotics; however, these microbes rarely play a significant role in the disease, and their recovery can usually be ignored.

Because many exacerbations are not triggered by bacterial agents and because of the difficulty in distinguishing bacterial from nonbacterial episodes, it is not surprising that investigators have had difficulty in confirming a benefit of antimicrobials in this condition. Nevertheless, contemporary clinical trials have demonstrated that antibiotics decrease the duration of symptoms and reduce the risk that the flare will result in a clinical deterioration requiring additional interventions, such as hospitalization. Most authorities agree that the benefit of antimicrobials is greatest in patients with moderate-to-severe exacerbations characterized by increases in dyspnea and in the volume and purulence of sputum.

A variety of antimicrobials have been employed in the management of patients with acute exacerbations of chronic bronchitis, and these drugs demonstrate comparable clinical efficacies (see Table 1). The standard agents include amoxicillin, doxycycline (or tetracycline), and trimethoprim-sulfamethoxazole. Erythromycin is occasionally prescribed for these patients; however, since the macrolide exhibits very poor activity against *H. influenzae* and since the antibiotic has the potential for inducing a serious drug-drug interaction (see Table 1), we do not recommend erythromycin for patients with flares of their chronic bronchitis.

The newer antimicrobials included in Table 1 offer some advantages over the traditional agents, such as less frequent dosing; however, the more recently introduced anti-infectives are invariably more expensive than the older compounds. The emergence of penicillin-resistant and trimethoprim-sulfamethoxazole–resistant strains of *S. pneumoniae* is worrisome, but the magnitude of the problem in adults with acute exacerbations of chronic bronchitis does not yet require a change in prescribing practices. Thus, we recommend that amoxicillin, doxycycline, or trimethoprim-sulfamethoxazole be employed as first-line agents; these drugs remain active against greater than 90% of the strains of *S. pneumoniae* and *H. influenzae* isolated from adult patients with exacerbations. Of note, *Moraxella (Branhamella) catarrhalis* can produce invasive disease of the lower respiratory tract, and approximately 75% of strains produce a beta-lactamase and thus, are resistant to amoxicillin. Nevertheless, since the prevelance and

virulence of *M. catarrhalis* are relatively low, we continue to utilize amoxicillin in this patient population. A 7- to 14-day course of therapy is usually prescribed.

Patients with acute exacerbations who exhibit wheezing on physical examination or who complain of dyspnea that is associated with a decline in their FEV_1 (forced expiratory volume in 1 second) and FEV_1/FVC (forced vital capacity) are candidates for systemic corticosteroids. Prednisone is often utilized; the initial dose is 0.5 to 1.0 mg per kg per day, and the corticosteroid is usually tapered over a 7- to 14-day period. Finally, systemic corticosteroids should be administered to patients who experience respiratory failure as a consequence of their exacerbation.

Some clinicians who care for patients with chronic bronchitis recommend antibiotic prophylaxis during the winter and early spring months as a mechanism to prevent acute exacerbations and the associated morbidity. In general, antibiotic prophylaxis can be considered for the patient with moderate or severe bronchitis who experiences four or more flares per year. A variety of schemes are employed, including prescribing an antibiotic every day throughout the cold and flu season or daily for 1 week each month during the target period. Amoxicillin, trimethoprim-sulfamethoxazole, and tetracycline are often utilized for prophylaxis. Obviously, in light of the absence of definitive data from controlled studies and because of the potential for widespread antibiotic use to encourage the emergence of drug-resistant bacteria, the practice of prophylaxis remains controversial.

The trivalent influenza vaccine to prevent disease due to the prevalent strains of the A and B viruses and the 23-valent pneumococcal vaccine to reduce the risk of pneumonia represent standard prophylactic interventions in patients with chronic obstructive pulmonary disease. Because the efficacy of these vaccines in this patient population has been confirmed by therapeutic trials or epidemiologic investigations, we strongly recommend their use. The influenza vaccine should be administered annually, preferably between mid-October and mid-November. An allergy to eggs represents the primary contraindication to the use of the influenza vaccine. Optimal protection is not conferred for 10 to 14 days following the administration of the influenza vaccine; thus, in the setting of a confirmed outbreak of influenza A, amantadine or rimantadine can be used for prophylaxis and administered concurrently with the vaccine. High-risk patients should be vaccinated and started on chemoprophylaxis with one of the antiviral agents, which should be given for 14 days following the vaccination. The prophylactic and therapeutic doses of amantadine and rimantadine are identical, and as emphasized previously, dosage adjustments are required in elderly people and in patients with renal dysfunction (see earlier). Finally, the pneumococcal vaccine should be given to all patients with chronic lung disease; although at present controversial, we recommend that a second dose of the pneumococcal vaccine be administered 7 to 10 years after the initial vaccination. The pneumococcal vaccine does not prevent acute exacerbations, but it does reduce the likelihood that a patient with chronic obstructive lung disease will experience pneumonia due to *S. pneumoniae*.

BACTERIAL PNEUMONIA

method of
LAURA C. CAMPBELL, M.D., and
G. DOUGLAS CAMPBELL, JR., M.D.
Louisiana State University School of Medicine–Shreveport
Shreveport, Louisiana

Despite the introduction of broad-spectrum antimicrobial agents, newer diagnostic tests, and improved supportive care, pneumonia remains the sixth leading cause of death in the United States and the most deadly of all infectious diseases. Because pneumonia is not a reportable disease, most available information is derived from vital statistics and clinical studies, and while these studies are inherently limited, certain information is apparent. First, the incidence of pneumonia is greatest at the extremes of life, but pneumonia-associated morbidity and mortality are most common among the elderly (85% of reported mortality occurs in patients ≥65 years of age), those with significant coexisting illness (i.e., chronic obstructive pulmonary disease, congestive heart failure, alcoholism, diabetes mellitus, renal insufficiency, chronic liver disease, etc.) and the immunosuppressed. Second, of the large spectrum of potential infectious etiologies, the likelihood of a specific pathogen causing pneumonia is influenced by a variety of factors, including whether the pneumonia was acquired in the community or hospital, the severity of illness, patient-related factors (age, immune status, presence of coexisting disease), time of the year, and even geographic location. Finally, outcome can be substantially improved by the rapid initiation of appropriate antimicrobial therapy, although antimicrobial choices must be tempered with a knowledge of local antibiotic resistance patterns, a recognition of what constitutes an appropriate clinical response, and an approach to the management of any patient who does not respond clinically.

APPROACH TO DIAGNOSIS

Central to the recognition of any bacterial pneumonia is the presence of a constellation of findings that include chest radiographic evidence of a new or progressive pulmonary infiltrate as well as certain other clinical and laboratory abnormalities that either reflect the broad features of pulmonary inflammation (i.e., fever, leukocytosis, and the production of purulent sputum) or major (i.e., cough, sputum production, fever >37.8°C) and minor (i.e., pleuritic chest pain, dyspnea, altered mental status, evidence of pulmonary consolidation, leucocytosis) characteristics of

pneumonia. Unfortunately, the presence of these findings rely on the ability of the patient's defense mechanisms to respond to infection as well as the virulence of the infecting organism. Not surprisingly, these criteria are less useful among individuals who are elderly, malnourished, immunosuppressed, or have significant coexisting disease or when pneumonia is caused by certain bacterial pathogens (i.e., *Chlamydia pneumoniae, Mycoplasma pneumoniae*). Even when these criteria are present, they are neither capable of identifying a specific pathogen nor are unique to bacterial pneumonia, since tuberculosis, many nonbacterial pathogens (i.e., endemic fungi, respiratory viruses, etc.), and even noninfectious processes (i.e., pulmonary emboli, idiopathic pulmonary fibrosis, broncholitis obliterans organizing pneumonia, etc.) may present with similar findings. Attempts to improve the sensitivity and specificity of diagnosing bacterial pneumonia by looking for specific syndromes (typical versus atypical pneumonia) has yielded similar disappointing results.

Because of the limitations of clinical criteria, additional strategies have been employed in the workup of pneumonia. The approaches taken range from obtaining a large battery of diagnostic tests at the time of presentation to simply initiating empirical therapy.

Diagnostic Procedures

Diagnostic tests are ordered for the following specific reasons: to determine whether the patient has bacterial pneumonia or whether there is another process present; to identify a specific etiology; to identify patients at risk for more complicated illness. There are limitations to diagnostic testing. No single test nor battery of tests is able to identify all potential etiologies in every case of pneumonia; the spectrum of potential infectious agents is simply too large. The diagnostic tests chosen often reflect the physician's biases, regarding both the appropriateness of a specific test or battery of tests and the perceived likely spectrum of potential infectious agents in varying clinical settings. Extensive testing is expensive, often requires special expertise, and, as suggested by the experience from several large clinical studies that employed extensive batteries of tests, identifies a pathogen in only half of the cases. Even when a diagnostic test identifies a pathogen, this often occurs after a delay of hours to days because of the time required for processing and reporting, and precludes the use of these results at the time of initial antimicrobial selection. Therefore, treatment in a majority of patients is, by necessity, empirical.

Despite these limitations, certain tests are of benefit in selected settings. A standard posteroanterior and lateral chest radiograph should be considered in patients presenting with clinical evidence of pneumonia, especially if they have coexisting disease, if the clinical symptoms are severe or unusual, or if the patient is hospitalized or hospitalization is considered. A chest radiograph can be helpful in several ways. Occasionally the radiographic pattern can be suggestive of certain pathogens that are not apparent from the clinical presentation—for example, pneumonia resulting from aspiration, *Mycobacterium tuberculosis*, or *Pneumocystis carinii*. The chest radiograph may identify noninfectious processes that can mimic pneumonia or infectious processes that can complicate the patient's course (e.g., bronchogenic carcinoma, lung abscess, or pleural effusions). Finally, the chest radiograph may help in assessing the severity of illness; for example, the presence of a multilobar infiltrate is associated with more severe illness and is probably best treated with intravenous therapy in the hospital.

Preferably before initiation of antimicrobial therapy, two sets of blood cultures (both aerobic and anaerobic) should be obtained in all hospitalized pneumonia patients. An organism will be isolated from blood cultures in 8 to 20% of cases; however, even a negative blood culture is helpful because it is often associated with less severe illness.

Pleural effusions are common among patients with pneumonia, reported to occur in 40 to 50% of all bacterial pneumonias treated in the hospital, but obtaining a sample of the effusion is not possible or even necessary in most cases. A thoracentesis should be considered in any patient with pneumonia if the effusion is greater than 10 mm on lateral decubitus film or if the patient is severely ill. Once obtained, the pleural fluid should be examined for the presence of gross purulence or putrid smell, which are findings consistent with an empyema. Additionally, certain microbiologic and laboratory tests should be performed, including culture and staining for bacteria, fungi, and *Mycobacterium* spp.; and measurement of pleural fluid glucose, protein, lactic dehydrogenase (LDH), cholesterol, and pH. At the time of the thoracentesis, serum should be obtained for measurement of glucose, protein LDH, and cholesterol, and results should be compared with pleural fluid values. The presence of any of the following findings suggests that the pleural space is infected and closed chest tube drainage of the pleural fluid should be considered: (1) pH<7.2; (2) the presence of gross purulence; (3) pathogenic bacteria on Gram's stain or culture; (4) pleural fluid glucose of <40 mg/dL. If initially there is not an indication for pleural fluid drainage, the physician should continue to monitor the effusion and repeat thoracentesis should be performed if there is concern that pleural space has become infected.

Serum chemistries, CBC, and arterial blood gas determination are not helpful in suggesting a specific etiology but can be useful in identifying coexisting illness, organ dysfunction, or hypoxemia, which are markers of severe illness.

Some physicians continue to believe in the utility of sputum Gram's stain and culture for detecting bacterial pathogens; however, sputum examination is fraught with many difficulties. Collection, processing, and interpretation of sputum Gram's stain requires expertise. The sputum specimen must be relatively free of oropharyngeal contamination, which often contains potentially pathogenic organisms. Results from sputum Gram's stain are unreliable if the patient has recently received antibiotic therapy. The Gram stain does not detect certain pathogens (e.g., *M. pneumoniae, C. pneumoniae,* respiratory viruses), which account for a substantial incidence of pneumonia in certain age populations. Culturing sputum is even less helpful except for pathogens that do not colonize the oropharynx (i.e., *Legionella* spp., *M. tuberculosis,* endemic fungi). Finally, the cost of collection, processing, and interpreting a sputum Gram stain and culture may exceed the cost of oral antimicrobial therapy.

Serology offers the ability of diagnosing many pathogens that are difficult to isolate by culture methods, but its use is limited by time delays resulting from the need for both acute and convalescent sera, and by expense. Serology is useful for epidemiologic purposes and may occasionally be helpful retrospectively in patients who fail to respond to therapy.

Invasive diagnostic testing of the lower respiratory tract has experienced a resurgence in recent years because of improvements in collecting lower respiratory tract specimens using the fiberoptic bronchoscope (FOB). Available invasive diagnostic tests that are commonly employed include FOB with the protected specimen brush (PSB) and bronchoalveolar lavage (BAL), percutaneous needle aspiration (PNA), and, in intubated patients, endotracheal aspiration (ETA).

PNA and FOB with BAL and/or PSB are all highly dependent upon the experience of the operator. Additionally, contamination with upper respiratory tract secretions is common with FOB. Contamination can be minimized if the operator is experienced with all aspects of the procedure, uses BAL and PSB to collect lower respiratory tract specimens, and quantitative culturing of the BAL and PSB specimens is properly performed. These procedures are expensive, and culture results are not available immediately for help in directing therapy. ETA cultures are helpful mainly to exclude potential pathogens, especially among patients receiving mechanical ventilation.

EMPIRICAL THERAPY IN BACTERIAL PNEUMONIA

Because of the limitations of diagnostic testing, the initial therapy chosen is frequently empirical. Recently, the American Thoracic Society developed statements on the treatment of community-acquired pneumonia (Niederman MS, Bass JB Jr, Campbell GD Jr, et al: Guidelines for the initial management of adults with community-acquired pneumonia: Diagnosis, assessment of severity, and initial antimicrobial therapy. Am Rev Respir Dis 148:1418–1426, 1993) and hospital-acquired pneumonia (Campbell GD Jr, Niederman MS, Broughton WA, et al: Hospital-acquired pneumonia in adults: Diagnosis, assessment of severity, initial antimicrobial therapy, and preventative strategies: A consensus statement. Am

J Respir Crit Care Med 1996; 153:1711–1725) in non-immunosuppressed adults. The approach chosen attempted to identify the most likely pathogens in a particular clinical setting based upon easily recognizable factors. Empirical antimicrobial regimens were developed according to the identified spectrum. Both statements stressed the importance of knowing the local antimicrobial resistance patterns, identified factors that might affect the spectrum of pathogens, and developed strategies for patients who do not respond to therapy.

COMMUNITY-ACQUIRED PNEUMONIA

It is estimated that there are 4 million cases of community-acquired pneumonia (CAP) annually in the United States. Approximately 800,000 of these require hospitalization, accounting for 3% of all hospital admissions annually. The reported mortality from CAP ranges from less than 1% to 25%, varying with severity of illness. Mortality in the outpatient setting is uncommon; the rate increases among patients requiring hospitalization, where estimates range from 13 to 25% for patients treated on the ward, and approach 50% in cases of severe CAP requiring admission to the intensive care unit. The spectrum of potential pathogens also varies with certain factors. By separating patient populations into several easily identifiable categories based upon age,

the presence of coexisting disease, and the severity of illness at presentation, it is possible to identify the most likely pathogens present. Using these criteria, CAP can separated into four categories, two outpatient and two inpatient):

CAP Patients Treated in the Outpatient Setting

CAP-1: Patients <60 years old and without co-existing illness

CAP-2: Patients ≥60 years and/or with co-existing illness

CAP Patients Requiring Hospitalization

CAP-3: Patients with mild-moderate pneumonia requiring hospitalization

CAP-4: Patients with severe pneumonia (requiring admission to an ICU)

In this schema, nursing home pneumonia may be included with CAP. While it is appreciated that this population is at greater risk for outbreaks of respiratory viruses and *M. tuberculosis,* and in encountering certain antimicrobial resistance bacteria (methicillin-resistant *S. aureus*), it is felt that the effects of age, coexisting illness, and severity of disease at presentation affect the spectrum of pathogens in a similar manner as with patients with CAP. Displayed in Table 1 are the most frequent or "major" pathogens

TABLE 1. **Etiology and Empirical Treatment of Community-Acquired Pneumonia**

Patient Groups	Pathogens	Antimicrobial Therapy
CAP-1: <60 years, with no coexisting illness	*Major Pathogens:* *S. pneumoniae, M. pneumoniae,* respiratory viruses, *C. pneumoniae, H. influenza* *Miscellaneous Pathogens* Legionella spp., *S. aureus, M. tuberculosis,* endemic fungi, aerobic GNB*	Erythromycin OR Tetracycline *Significant History of Smoking* Azithromycin (Zithromax) OR Clarithromycin (Biaxin)
CAP-2: ≥60 years and/or with co-existing illness	*Major Pathogens:* *S. pneumoniae,* respiratory viruses, *H. influenzae,* aerobic GNB*, *S. aureus* *Miscellaneous Pathogens:* *M. catarrhalis, Legionella* spp., *M. tuberculosis,* endemic fungi	Second-generation cephalosporin Trimethoprim/sulfamethoxazole (Bactrim, Septra) OR Beta-lactam/beta-lactamase inhibitor ± Macrolide
CAP-3: Requiring hospitalization	*Major Pathogens:* *S. pneumoniae, H. influenzae,* polymicrobial, aerobic GNB*, *Legionella* spp., *S. aureus, C. pneumoniae,* respiratory viruses *Miscellaneous:* *M. pneumoniae, M. catarrhalis, M. tuberculosis,* endemic fungi	Second- or third-generation (non-pseudomonal) cephalosporin OR Beta-lactam/beta-lactamase inhibitor ± Macrolide
CAP-4: Requiring admission to the ICU	*Major Pathogens:* *S. pneumoniae, Legionella* spp., aerobic GNB, *P. aeruginosa, M. pneumoniae,* respiratory viruses *Miscellaneous:* *H. influenzae, M. tuberculosis,* endemic fungi	Macrolide PLUS Third-generation (anti-pseudomonal) cephalosporin Imipenem/cilastatin (Primaxin) OR Ciprofloxacin (Cipro)

*Aerobic gram-negative bacilli; does not include *P. aeruginosa.*
Adapted from Niederman MS, et al: Am Rev Respir Dis *148*:1418–1426, 1993.

reported to occur in at least 5% of patients enrolled in most large clinical studies and "miscellaneous" pathogens, which occur less frequently (<1%), along with suggested appropriate antimicrobial therapy for each of the four CAP patient groups.

It is appreciated that certain local or geographic factors could affect both the likelihood of any pathogen and the appropriateness of recommended therapy, especially if antimicrobial resistance (i.e., penicillin-resistant *Streptococcus pneumoniae* or methicillin-resistant *Staphylococcus aureus*) is common. It is also recognized that immunosuppression, especially resulting from HIV infection, may not be clinically apparent and would also affect the spectrum of potential pathogens.

CAP Treated in the Outpatient Setting

The majority of CAP, in excess of 3 million cases annually, is treated in the outpatient setting, where mortality is rare and most patients recover without significant morbidity. Among CAP patients younger than 60 years old and without coexisting illness (CAP-1), mortality is less than 1% and only 8% of patients initially treated in the outpatient setting eventually require hospitalization for CAP. The most likely pathogens are *S. pneumoniae, M. pneumoniae,* respiratory viruses, *C. pneumoniae,* and *Haemophilus influenzae*; and miscellaneous pathogens include *Legionella* spp., *S. aureus, M. tuberculosis, M. tuberculosis,* endemic fungi, and aerobic gram-negative bacilli (excluding *Pseudomonas aeruginosa*). Antimicrobial therapy in this setting should include either a macrolide or tetracycline. If the patient has a substantial smoking history, the likelihood of infection with *H. influenzae* is increased and one of the newer macrolides (azithromycin [Zithromax], or clarithromycin [Biaxin]) should be considered, since erythromycin is minimally effective in this setting.

CAP patients 60 years of age or older and/or with co-existing illness (CAP-2) are also frequently treated in the outpatient setting. Mortality is slightly higher in this group, approximately 3%, but up to 20% of patients initially treated in the outpatient setting eventually require hospitalization for CAP, suggesting the need for close follow-up in this population. The most likely pathogens are *S. pneumoniae,* respiratory viruses, *H. influenzae,* aerobic gram-negative bacilli (excluding *P. aeruginosa*), and *S. aureus.* Miscellaneous pathogens include *Moraxella catarrhalis, Legionella,* spp., *M. tuberculosis,* and endemic fungi. The difference in the spectrum of pathogens and the increased likelihood for the later need of hospitalization are probably a reflection of the increased incidence of coexisting illness, particularly COPD. Antimicrobial therapy in this setting would be a second-generation cephalosporin, trimethoprim/sulfamethoxazole (TMP/SMX), (Bactrim, Septra), or a beta-lactam/beta-lactamase inhibitor. A macrolide should be added if there is concern that the pneumonia may be due to *Legionella* spp.

CAP Requiring Hospitalization

While up to a fifth of CAP patients require hospitalization, the majority of these patients are treated on the wards. CAP morbidity and mortality is higher among patients requiring hospitalization. In CAP-3 patients (patients requiring hospitalization), mortality ranges from 13 to 25%. The most likely pathogens are *S. pneumoniae, H. influenzae,* polymicrobial organisms (including anaerobic organisms), aerobic gram-negative bacilli (excluding *P. aeruginosa*), *Legionella* spp., *S. aureus, C. pneumoniae,* and respiratory viruses. Miscellaneous pathogens include *M. pneumoniae, M. catarrhalis, M. tuberculosis,* and endemic fungi. Therapy in this setting should be delivered intravenously and should include either a second or non-pseudomonal third-generation cephalosporin or a beta-lactam/beta-lactamase inhibitor. If *Legionella* spp. is suspected, a macrolide should be added; if *Legionella* spp. infection is documented, therapy should be further expanded with the addition of rifampin for at least the first few days of therapy.

Mortality in CAP-4 patients, those with severe CAP usually requiring admission to an intensive care unit, frequently approaches 50%. The majority of these patients require ventilatory support. The major pathogens associated with severe CAP include *S. pneumoniae, Legionella* spp., aerobic gram-negative bacilli, *P. aeruginosa, M. pneumoniae,* and respiratory viruses. Miscellaneous pathogens are *H. influenzae, M. tuberculosis,* and endemic fungi. Because of the spectrum of pathogens, therapy should include a macrolide plus either a third-generation cephalosporin with anti-pseudomonal activity or other anti-pseudomonal agents (i.e., imipenem/cilastatin [Primaxin], ciprofloxin [Cipro], aminoglycoside, etc.)

Criteria for Hospital Admission

No single criterion or set of criteria are available that can adequately identify the need for hospitalization. This reflects both the inability to define the exact role of hospitalization and the dynamic nature of pneumonia, which may progress to more severe illness. Even in clinical studies, approximately 20% of CAP patients who are 60 years of age or older and/or have co-existing illness (CAP-2) and are initially treated as outpatients eventually require hospitalization. While admission criteria are lacking, the presence of certain findings may suggest a need for hospitalization. Hospitalization should be considered for patients requiring specialized supportive care (IV therapy, supplemental oxygen, mechanical ventilation), or who may be difficult to manage in an outpatient setting (lack of supportive care, homeless, questionable compliance, chronic mental impairment). The presence of other factors are associated with a more complicated course that may better be treated in a hospital setting. These factors include the presence of coexisting illness, CAP within the last year, suspicion of aspiration, chronic alcohol abuse, malnutrition, extrapulmonary site of infection, sepsis or organ dysfunction, and physiologic abnormalities (i.e., respiratory rate >30 breaths per minute, systolic blood pressure <90 mmHg or a diastolic blood pressure of <60 mmHg, temperature of >38.3°C, Pa_{O2} <60 mmHg or Pa_{CO2} of >50mmHg while breathing room air). If there is doubt as to whether the patient needs hospitalization, admission to an observation area for several hours to monitor early response to therapy might be considered.

Markers of Severity of Infection

Early recognition of severe pneumonia can more rapidly facilitate institution of specific antimicrobial therapy. Again, no universally accepted factors have been identified, but the presence of any of the following suggests that the pneumonia is severe:

1. Respiratory frequency greater than 30 breaths per minute, at initial presentation
2. Respiratory failure with the Pa_{O2}/FI_{O2} ratio less than 250
3. Chest radiograph showing bilateral or multilobar involvement or a 50% increase in the size of the infiltrate within 48 hours of admission
4. Need for mechanical ventilation
5. Presence of shock, defined as a systolic blood pressure less than 90 mmHg or diastolic blood pressure less than 60 mmHg
6. Requirement of vasopressors for more than 4 hours
7. Evidence of organ dysfunction (urine output <20 mL/hour, total urine output <80 mL/4 hours)

HOSPITAL-ACQUIRED PNEUMONIA

Hospital-acquired pneumonia (HAP), defined as pneumonia occurring more than 48 hours after hospitalization, is the second most common nosocomial infection but the most deadly of all nosocomial infections. The overall estimated incidence of HAP is 5 to 10 cases per 1000 hospital discharges, but this incidence varies both with type of hospital and ward service. The incidence of HAP is higher in tertiary referral centers, especially on medical or surgical services, and is increased by an additional 6- to 20-fold in the intensive care unit setting, especially among mechanically ventilated patients. The annual U.S. incidence of HAP is estimated to be between 150,000 and 300,000 cases, with mortality ranging from 20 to 70%.

Most cases of HAP result from microaspiration of oropharyngeal secretions that have previously been colonized with pathogenic bacteria. Certain pathogens are more frequently encountered in the setting of HAP and are referred to as "core pathogens" (Table 2). These include *S. pneumoniae, H. influenzae, S. aureus,* and aerobic gram-negative bacilli (*E. coli, Klebsiella* spp., *Proteus* spp., *Serratia marcescens*). The spectrum of potential pathogens is broadened by

TABLE 2. **Etiology and Empirical Treatment of Hospital-Acquired Pneumonia***

Patient Groups	Pathogens	Antimicrobial Therapy
HAP-1: Mild-moderate, no risk factors OR Severe, early onset (<5 days) no risk factors	Core pathogens: Enteric gram-negative bacilli (*E. coli, Klebsiella* spp., *Proteus* spp., *S. marcescens*) *H. influenzae* Methicillin-sensitive *S. aureus* *S. pneumoniae*	Core antibiotics: Cefazolin (Ancef) and gentamicin Second-generation cephalosporin (Cefuroxime [Zinacef]) Non-pseudomonal third-generation cephalosporin (cefotaxime [Claforan], ceftriaxone [Rocephin]) Beta-lactam/beta-lactamase inhibitor (ampicillin/sulbactam [Unasyn], ticarcillin/clavulanate [Timentin], piperacillin/tazobactam [Zosyn]) Fluoroquinolone (ciprofloxacin [Cipro])
HAP-2 Mild-moderate with risk factors: Gross aspiration, recent abdominal surgery Coma, head trauma, diabetes, renal failure High-dose steroids	Core pathogens—*plus:* Anaerobes *S. aureus* *Legionella* spp.	Beta-lactam/beta-lactamase alone Core antibiotics ± clindamycin (Cleocin) or metronidazole (Flagyl) Core antibiotics *plus:* Vancomycin (Vancomycin) (if MRSA† is likely) Core antibiotics ± macrolide
HAP-3: Severe, with risk factors, OR Severe, no risk factors, late onset (≥5 days)	Core pathogens—*plus:* *P. aeruginosa* *Acinetobacter* spp. Methicillin-resistant *S. aureus*	Aminoglycoside or ciprofloxacin *plus:* Anti-pseudomonal penicillin (Piperacillin [Piperacil], mezlocillin [Mezlin]) Ceftazidime (Fortaz) or cefoperazone (Cefobid) Aztreonam (Azactam) Imipenem/cilastatin (Primaxin) Beta-lactam/beta-lactamase inhibitor

*See algorithm, Figure 1.
†Methicillin-resistant *S. aureus.*
Adapted from Campbell GD Jr, et al: Am J Respir Crit Care Med *153*:1711–1725, 1996.

other factors. It is appreciated that (1) the severity of illness (mild-moderate versus severe), (2) prolonged or repeated exposure to antimicrobial agents and presence of other specific risk factors, and (3) the duration of hospitalization prior to development of HAP (early HAP <5 days, late HAP ≥5 days) all affect oropharyngeal colonization as well as the development and etiology of HAP. By using these factors, a likely spectrum of pathogens can be defined for different clinical settings (Figure 1), and empiric regimens developed.

Mild-Moderate HAP

In patients with mild-moderate HAP, the spectrum of potential infectious agents is primarily affected by the absence or presence of specific risk factors associated with certain pathogens. Essentially all of these patients are appropriately treated on the ward. In patients without risk factors (HAP-1), the core pathogens are the most likely etiology. Duration of hospitalization affects the frequency with which these core pathogens are encountered. *H. influenzae* and *S. pneumoniae* more commonly cause HAP early (<5 days) during hospitalization, while *S. aureus* and aerobic gram-negative bacilli are more common later. Antimicrobial therapy in this setting should include one of the following agents: a beta-lactam/beta-lactamase inhibitor, a second-generation cephalosporin, or a third-generation non-pseudomonal cephalosporin. If the patient is penicillin-allergic, either a fluoroquinolone or a combination of clindamycin (Cleocin) and aztreonam (Azactam) could be used. Since this antimicrobial therapy is directed against core organisms, these agents will be referred to as "core" antibiotics.

In patients with mild-moderate HAP but with specific risk factors for certain pathogens (HAP-2), the most common pathogens include the core pathogens, but other pathogens should be considered according to the presence of specific risk factors. The therapy should be directed against the core organisms as well as pathogens associated with a specific risk factor. Risk factors for the development of anaerobic pneumonia include witnessed gross aspiration and recent thoracoabdominal surgery. In this setting, therapy should include either a single agent such as a beta-lactam/beta-lactamase inhibitor or clindamycin and either a second-generation cephalosporin or a third-generation non-pseudomonal cephalosporin. *S. aureus* is more likely in the presence of coma, head trauma, diabetes mellitus, or renal failure. *S. aureus* is usually methicillin-sensitive, especially if the patient has recently been hospitalized, has not been exposed to antibiotics, and is not an intravenous drug abuser. HAP resulting from *Legionella* spp. infection is more likely if the patient is on high-dose steroids. In patients with multiple risk factors, *P. aeruginosa*, *Acinetobacter* spp., and methicillin-resistant *S. aureus* are more common, and these patients should be treated as if they have severe HAP (HAP-3).

Severe HAP

The spectrum of pathogens encountered in patients with severe HAP is influenced by both the presence of specific risk factors and the duration of hospitalization prior to the development of HAP. If HAP occurs early during hospitalization (<5 days) in patients without specific risk factors, the most likely pathogens are similar to those encountered in HAP-1 and therapy with one of the core antibiotics would suffice. The most common clinical presentation in this setting would be an otherwise healthy individual who experienced a recent medical, traumatic, or surgical event (i.e., myocardial infarction, stroke, car wreck, surgery) and then developed pneumonia.

When HAP occurs 5 days or more after admission and/or specific risk factors are present, the spectrum of potential pathogens broadens to include not only core pathogens but also *P. aeruginosa*, *Acinetobacter* spp., and methicillin-resistant *S. aureus* (HAP-3); therefore, empirical therapy in this setting must be broadened. Since *P. aeruginosa* and *Acinetobacter* spp. are frequently encountered in this setting, the most appropriate therapy should include two agents with known anti-pseudomonal coverage chosen with a consideration of the local antimicrobial resistance

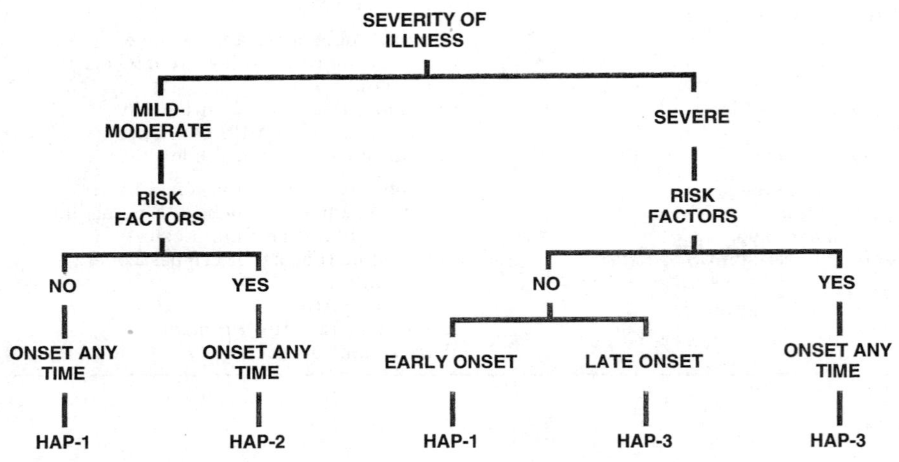

Figure 1. Algorithm for classifying patients with hospital-acquired pneumonia (HAP). (From Campbell GD Jr, et al: Am J Respir Crit Care Med *153*:1711–1725, 1996.)

patterns. The choices include using two beta-lactam agents, or a single beta-lactam agent and either an aminoglycoside or a fluoroquinolone. Because of concern of resistance, two beta-lactam agents have fallen out of favor by many. A beta-lactam agent with a fluoroquinolone, such as ciprofloxacin, or an aminoglycoside is an appropriate alternative. There has been increased interest in prescribing the total daily dosage of aminoglycoside in a single dosage based upon creatinine clearance. A single total dose given once a day ensures high peak levels with good tissue penetration, and a low trough level minimizing toxicity. Need for repeated peak and trough levels is greatly reduced.

PNEUMONIA IN THE IMMUNOSUPPRESSED PATIENT

Immunocompromised patients present special problems for the physician. Not only does the compromised immune system broaden the potential spectrum of both infectious and noninfectious processes (i.e., radiation fibrosis, drug-induced lung disease), but also the clinical findings are often fewer and atypical, requiring the clinician to have a higher index of suspicion. Additionally, if left untreated, an infectious process may rapidly progress, sometimes within hours, to more severe illness and even death. These factors frequently result in the prompt initiation of empirical broad-spectrum antimicrobial therapy and extensive diagnostic testing. Often, an appreciation of the specific immune dysfunction together with a history of the treatment a patient has received may help in limiting the spectrum of potential etiologies, or at least in directing diagnostic studies.

Pulmonary disease is among the most common sequelae of HIV infection, and the majority of severe complications are infectious, but HIV infection is frequently not clinically apparent. Therefore, in any patient presenting with a diffuse, clinically severe, or atypical pneumonic process, the physician should elicit a history of risk factors for HIV infection. *Pneumocystis carinii* pneumonia (PCP) is a frequent presenting infection in HIV-positive individuals. If HIV infection is considered, work-up should be broadened from that discussed previously to include induced sputa, since the sensitivity of this test in some institutions is reported to be up to 90 to 95% for *P. carinii*. Additionally, an HIV test should be obtained and if positive a CD4 count measured, since CD4 count can be helpful in defining the spectrum of likely pulmonary pathogens. The empirical therapy of a pneumonic process in such a patient should include TMP/SMX or pentamidine (Pentam 300), in addition to broad-coverage antimicrobial therapy similar to that used in severe HAP patients. If serial sputa are negative for PCP and the patient is responding to therapy, stopping anti-PCP agents should be considered, since AIDS patients may already have a compromised granulocyte count secondary to their HIV infection and do not need the unnecessary risk of granulocytopenia that may be associated with TMP/SMX or pentamidine.

Pulmonary infection in non-neutropenic cancer patients is similar to that in the general population except in the setting of defective cell-mediated immunity (i.e., Hodgkin's disease), decreased humoral immunity (i.e., multiple myeloma, hypogammaglobulinemic patients), or hematologic malignancies, where qualitative abnormalities of neutrophil function exist in addition to quantitative defects.

Neutropenia, abnormal neutrophil function, and the specific diagnosis-related immune defects increase mortality risk from pneumonia and warrant hospitalization for broad-coverage intravenous antibiotic therapy. The empirical therapy for a pneumonic process in such patients should include two drugs that have broad-spectrum gram-negative bacilli coverage including activity against *P. aeruginosa*. An appropriate choice would be that used for severe pneumonia in non-immunosuppressed patients. Vancomycin should be included in initial empirical therapy only in patients who have been recently hospitalized in an environment in which the methicillin-resistant *S. aureus* rate is high, in patients in whom a central line or indwelling device may be complicated by infection, or in patients with mucositis or skin disruption. In spite of perceived ease or relative cost of a particular regimen, it is prudent to alternate regimens to prevent institutional problems with resistance. Regardless of the initial empirical therapy, modifications in therapy may be required if the patient has not improved or worsens after approximately 4 days of therapy. In that setting, consideration should be given to adding vancomycin. If clinical response is not seen after approximately 7 days of therapy, the addition of antifungal agents should be considered, especially in patients with prolonged neutropenia or who have undergone allogeneic bone marrow transplantation.

In the immunocompromised patient, diagnostic testing may need to be more extensive with a lower threshold for additional testing than in the non-immunocompromised patient, especially in the patient who does not improve with usual therapy.

RESPONSE TO THERAPY

One important aspect in managing patients with pneumonia is to ensure that antimicrobial therapy is effective; but, since an organism is isolated in less than half of all patients and often only after several days of therapy, the antimicrobial resistance pattern for the offending bacteria may not be known. Other parameters should be followed to determine if the expected response is occurring or if antimicrobial agents should be changed. There are a number of different parameters that can be followed; however, these can be affected by both patient and pathogen factors. In mild-moderate pneumonia, the best parameters are fever and white blood cell count, both of which should improve within 2 to 4 days of therapy. Physical examination and chest radiographic findings are slow to improve, especially if pneumonia is due to a virulent organism (i.e., *P. aeruginosa*) or if significant underlying disease is present. In severe pneumonia, especially if it is associated with mechanical ventilation, improvement is frequently delayed. In this setting, the physician can follow physiologic parameters such as oxygenation, organ dysfunction, blood pressure, or can incorporate these findings with more invasive tests (i.e., FOB with PSB and/or BAL). Invasive testing, particularly after 72 hours of therapy, can be used as an indicator of appropriateness of therapy. If pathogenic bacteria are recovered in sufficient numbers (PSB $>10^3$ cfu), the patient is less likely to experience clinical improvement; however, whether changing antimicrobial therapy at this time affects outcome is unknown.

MANAGEMENT OF NONRESPONDING PNEUMONIA

The reasons for antimicrobial failure include bacterial factors (antimicrobial resistance, superinfection, unusual or unexpected pathogens), infection-related complications (lung abscess, empyema, and extrathoracic sites of infection), noninfectious etiologies (pulmonary emboli, cancer, drug-induced lung disease, drug fever, etc.), and development of acute respiratory distress syndrome (ARDS).

In patients who are not responding after several days of therapy or experience rapid deterioration, further investigation is important. Initial work-up should include complete history and physical examination, ECG, and repeat chest radiograph. In addition, different approaches can be taken depending upon on the likelihood of the previously mentioned processes. Serologic testing, for specific pathogens as well as HIV, may be helpful in this setting. In mechanically ventilated patients, ETA is helpful in excluding certain pathogens and antimicrobial resistant organisms. FOB with PSB/BAL to sample lower respiratory tract secretions potentially can identify resistant or unusual bacteria (*M. tuberculosis, Francisella tularensis*) and nonbacterial (endemic fungi, respiratory viruses, *P. carinii*) pathogens, as well as detect endobronchial obstruction that may affect clinical response. CT scanning is helpful in detecting unsuspected empyema, lung abscess, and cancer. V/Q scanning of the lung or pulmonary angiography should be performed when pulmonary emboli are considered. Open lung biopsy can be performed but usually is performed as a last resort and with the realization that the results are often not helpful.

VIRAL RESPIRATORY INFECTIONS

method of
ERIC A. F. SIMOES, M.D., D.C.H.
*University of Colorado Health Sciences Center
and The Children's Hospital
Denver, Colorado*

Viral respiratory infections are the most common acute illnesses of humankind and the leading reason for patient visits to physicians. Viral upper respiratory tract infections are caused by over 100 distinct viruses. The rhinoviruses are the commonest cause; other etiologic agents include coronavirus, parainfluenzavirus, influenzavirus, respiratory syncytial virus, adenovirus, Epstein-Barr virus, and enteroviruses in the summer. In a third of cases no etiologic agent is identified. The majority of these viral respiratory infections result in the common cold. Cold symptoms include nasal obstruction and discharge, sore throat, sneezing, coughing, and fever in young children. Patients with influenza, a less common but a more severe illness, have in addition headache, malaise, myalgias, fever, chills, and occasionally rigors.

TREATMENT OF THE COMMON COLD

The common cold is easily diagnosed clinically, and virologic studies are unnecessary. The mainstays of therapy for this self-limited condition remain reassurance, rest, and fluids. There is no role for antiviral therapy and antibacterial therapy, and combination cold remedies containing compounds for all possible cold symptoms should be avoided.

Topical nasal decongestant preparations, such as 0.1% xylometazoline (Otrivin) or 0.05% oxymetazoline (Afrin), may be administered to adults two to three times a day as intranasal drops or sprays. Sprays (1 or 2 sprays per nostril) are administered with the patient upright, whereas drops (1 or 2 drops per nostril) are administered with the patient in a recumbent position. The patient should be warned about the hazard of rhinitis medicamentosa, which follows prolonged usage of nasal decongestants. Patients being treated with monoamine oxidase (MAO) inhibitors should not use decongestants. A less concentrated solution of xylometazoline (0.05%) may be used for older children, and infants should be given only saline nasal drops.

Oral preparations are available, such as pseudoephedrine hydrochloride (Sudafed), which may be given three to four times daily at a dosage of 15 mg per dose for children aged 2 to 5 years, 30 mg per dose for those 6 to 11 years old, and 60 mg per dose for those over 11 years. Oral preparations are probably less effective than topical preparations. Recent studies have suggested that 1 week's therapy with pseudoephedrine does not cause a significant rise in blood pressure in patients with prior controlled hypertension.

Antihistamines exert a drying effect on the nasal mucosa owing to an anticholinergic side effect, but used alone they do not relieve nasal congestion. The slight possible benefit afforded by adding an antihistamine to a decongestant must be weighed against the antihistamine's prominent side effect of drowsiness, which may impair work performance and automobile driving safety. Newer antihistamines lacking these anticholinergic side effects do not cause drowsiness, but they also do not dry the nasal mucosa because histamine is not involved in the pathogenesis of the common cold.

Sore throat is usually mild and may be relieved by saline gargles, but occasionally an analgesic is required. Aspirin may be given orally every 4 hours (adult dose: 325 to 650 mg, pediatric dose: 10 mg per kg of body weight to a maximum of 650 mg). Acetaminophen (Tylenol, Tempra) may be given orally every 4 hours to patients who are unable to take aspirin. Each dose of acetaminophen is 60 to 120 mg for those 1 to 3 years old, 120 mg for those 3 to 6 years old, 240 mg for those 7 to 11 years old, and 325 to 650 mg for those over 11 years.

Severe sore throat, especially with exudate, cervical adenopathy, and fever, should suggest the possibility of streptococcal pharyngitis, which may be confirmed by throat culture or a streptococcal antigen test. Treatment for this condition is discussed in another article.

Cough does not usually require therapy in patients with the common cold, but moderate-to-severe coughing may require a suppressant after the possibility of pneumonia has been excluded by history, physical examination, and (if necessary) radiography. Effective cough suppressants include codeine and dextromethorphan hydrobromide. Codeine may be given orally every 4 to 6 hours at the following doses: 2.5 to 5 mg per dose for a child 2 to 5 years old, 5 to 10 mg for a child 6 to 11 years old, and 10 to 30 mg for those over 11 years old. Dextromethorphan dosage is the same, not to exceed four doses in 24 hours. Patients taking MAO inhibitors should not receive these cough suppressants. Expectorants have not been proved to provide effective cough therapy.

Constitutional symptoms and headache are usually minimal with a cold but occasionally require treatment with one of the antipyretics or analgesics previously listed.

The most frequent bacterial complication of the common cold is otitis media, which occurs in approximately 2% of colds, involving mostly children. Otalgia, or diminished auditory acuity, indicates the need for pneumatic otoscopy.

Recent studies have shown that about 90% of patients with a common cold have fluid in their sinuses during the first few days of a cold, apparently because of obstruction of the nasal ostiomeatal complex by inflammation due to the viral infection. Acute bacterial sinusitis follows about 1 of 200 colds and tends to occur more frequently in adults. It cannot be distinguished from a cold on the basis of purulent nasal discharge, which may occur in the uncomplicated cold owing to the viral infection itself. Persistent nasal obstruction and facial pain suggest the need for sinus transillumination or radiography or both. These bacterial complications require antibiotic therapy as discussed in other articles in this book.

Patients and their families should be instructed that colds are caused by infectious viruses that spread from person to person. Although the mechanism of spread in the natural setting has not been definitively established, experimental evidence suggests that rhinoviruses are spread by hand contact and also by large-particle aerosols created by sneezing or coughing. Handwashing and conscious avoidance of finger-to-nose or finger-to-eye contact (which

inoculates the virus) after exposure to a cold sufferer may reduce the risk of transmission because large-particle aerosols usually do not travel more than 5 feet. Covering the mouth tightly with a tissue during sneezing and coughing will reduce the number of particles aerosolized.

Ingestion of large doses of vitamin C has been shown to provide ineffective prophylaxis against or therapy for the common cold. Zinc lozenges have also been shown to be ineffective therapy in multiple randomized trials. Prospects for a vaccine are poor because of the multiplicity of viral agents. Interferon has shown activity as a prophylactic agent but has prevented only a minority of colds and has not been considered cost effective.

TREATMENT OF INFLUENZA

The diagnosis of influenza is made on clinical and epidemiologic grounds. As with colds, diagnostic virology is usually unnecessary for management of the patient with influenza, but the practitioner should be aware of reports on influenza activity from the Centers for Disease Control and Prevention or the state health department. During winter these reports give evidence of the predominant type and frequency of influenza virus isolates in sentinel practices.

The systemic symptoms of influenza are the primary target of therapy. Bed rest and increased fluid intake are necessary. During an influenza A epidemic, amantadine (Symmetrel) has been considered the drug of choice because it is more effective than acetaminophen or aspirin and reduces illness duration by half when started within 48 hours of the onset of symptoms.

The oral dosage for adults and children older than 9 years of age is 200 mg initially followed by 100 mg twice daily, and for children 1 to 9 years of age it is 5 mg per kg of body weight twice daily (not to exceed 150 mg per day). The dose for elderly adults is 100 mg once daily because higher doses are associated with a high rate of side effects. Amantadine has not been approved for use in children younger than 1 year. Treatment should continue for 3 to 4 days or until 48 hours after resolution of symptoms. Its use has been associated with minor and reversible side effects on the central nervous system, such as insomnia, difficulty in concentrating, and dizziness. The dose should be reduced in renal failure. Rimantadine (Flumadine) is now available commercially and provides equivalent therapeutic efficacy for influenza A at the same dosage but has a lower incidence of side effects than amantadine. Rimantadine has not been approved for treatment in children. The cost of rimantidine is about twice that of amantadine, however.

When influenza B predominates in the area, acetaminophen may be prescribed (dosage given previously) because amantadine and rimantidine lack activity against this virus. Aspirin should not be prescribed for children in view of recent epidemiologic evidence relating Reye's syndrome to salicylate use for influenza or varicella. Although Reye's syndrome is rare in adults, case reports suggest that aspirin may play a role, and acetaminophen is thus preferred.

Cough is often moderate to severe, requiring prescription of a cough suppressant such as codeine or dextromethorphan (dosage given previously), after the possibility of pneumonia has been excluded. Nasal congestion may warrant a topical decongestant as previously described.

Prevention of influenza is possible by vaccination, which is recommended for those at risk for serious complications and death from influenza. This group includes principally the elderly (over 65 years of age) and those with a chronic disease, especially of heart or lungs. Health care workers in contact with such high-risk patients should also be vaccinated to prevent transmission to their patients. Persons providing essential services to the community should be vaccinated as well. Targeted high-risk children are recommended for vaccination: those with chronic pulmonary diseases, hemodynamically significant cardiac disease, immune-suppressed, hemoglobinopathies, recipients of long-term aspirin therapy, diabetes mellitus, and chronic renal and metabolic diseases. Children under 13 years of age should receive only the split-virus vaccine. Egg allergy is one of the few contraindications to vaccination.

During an epidemic of influenza A, high-risk individuals who are unable to receive the vaccine may be treated prophylactically with amantadine (Symmetrel), 100 mg once daily for adults and for children weighing more than 20 kg. The prophylactic dose for children weighing 20 kg or less remains the same as the therapeutic dose, given in one or two divided doses. If amantadine is begun prophylactically at the time of vaccination, it should be continued for 14 days to allow time for an effective vaccine response. Rimantidine (Flumadine) provides equal protective efficacy against influenza at the same daily dosage as amantadine (100 mg per day for an adult).

MYCOPLASMAL AND VIRAL PNEUMONIAS

method of
WILLIAM SALZER, M.D., and
E. DALE EVERETT, M.D.
University of Missouri-Columbia
Columbia, Missouri

MYCOPLASMAL PNEUMONIA

Lower respiratory tract infection with *Mycoplasma pneumoniae* is a common cause of community-acquired pneumonia in healthy young adults and adolescents but may occur in persons of any age. The clinical presentation is usually a virus-like prodrome followed by symptoms of lower respiratory tract infection. Chest radiographs often reveal multifocal in-

filtrates, which are out of proportion to the clinical appearance of the patient, who usually looks relatively nontoxic with a nonproductive cough and few ausculatory findings. However, severe disease, in some cases leading to respiratory failure, may occur, particularly in persons with sickle cell anemia or immune deficiency.

A definitive diagnosis of mycoplasmal pneumonia requires a diagnostic rise in antibodies or isolation of the organism on special mycoplasma media. These techniques require 2 to 3 weeks. Many patients with mycoplasmal pneumonia develop cold agglutinins after about 7 days of illness, which is supportive but not diagnostic. Since definitive diagnosis is usually not possible early in the illness, therapy must be initiated based on clinical suspicion.

Mycoplasma bacteria are the smallest free-living organisms. They do not have cell walls, so they are not susceptible to beta-lactam antibiotics, nor do they synthesize folate so they are not inhibited by trimethoprim/sulfamethoxazole (Bactrim, Septra). The drugs of choice are erythromycin or tetracycline, 500 mg orally four times daily for 14 days. Doxycycline, 100 mg twice daily orally for 14 days, is effective as well. Therapy for less than 14 days has been associated with relapses. The new macrolides clarithromycin (Biaxin) and azithromycin (Zithromax) probably are effective and may have fewer gastrointestinal side effects than erythromycin but are considerably more expensive. Currently, clarithromycin has an FDA-approved indication for mycoplasmal pneumonia while azithromycin does not. A few small studies support the efficacy of a 5-day course of azithromycin for mycoplasma.

The fluoroquinolones ciprofloxacin* (Cipro) and ofloxacin* (Floxin) have moderate in vitro activity against mycoplasma and achieve good levels in the lung, but there is little published clinical experience in treating mycoplasmal infections with these drugs.

INFLUENZA A

Influenza types A and B are responsible for yearly epidemics of lower respiratory tract infection. The circulating strain can be identified by culture, direct antigen detection on respiratory secretions for type A, or knowledge of the predominant strain from public health authorities. This is important to know since amantadine and rimantadine are effective in treating and preventing influenza A but not B. The dosages used for prevention and treatment are amantadine (Symmetrel) or rimantadine (Flumadine), 100 mg orally twice daily. For patients over 65 years of age, the dosage must be reduced to 100 mg daily, and further reductions are needed for renal insufficiency. Rimantadine is less dependent on renal function and may have fewer side effects but is more expensive. For treatment of acute disease, these drugs are most efficacious when started within 48 hours of the onset of symptoms and are continued until the patient is

---

*Not FDA approved for this indication.

afebrile for 2 days. Strains of influenza resistant to these drugs have developed during therapy and have been transmitted to close contacts. These drugs are also effective in preventing influenza A if given throughout the time of potential exposure or for 2 weeks after influenza vaccination. In the patient with severe influenzal pneumonia and respiratory failure, these drugs may be used, but efficacy in this situation is unproved.

HERPES VIRUSES

Herpes Simplex Virus. HSV may produce a hemorrhagic tracheobronchitis and/or pneumonitis in immunocompromised or critically ill patients, particularly those receiving mechanical ventilation. These patients should be treated with acyclovir (Zovirax), 10 mg per kg intravenously every 8 hours, with dosage reduction for renal impairment.

Varicella. Pneumonitis, often severe, commonly occurs in immunocompromised patients and occasionally in normal adults with chickenpox. These patients should be treated with acyclovir, 10 mg per kg intravenously every 8 hours, which may ameliorate the disease in some patients, particularly if therapy is started within 72 hours of disease onset.

Cytomegalovirus. Pneumonia due to CMV rarely occurs during primary infection in normal adults. Such patients usually improve without antiviral therapy. CMV pneumonia is a significant problem in transplant recipients and other severely immunocompromised patients, in whom it presents as an interstitial pneumonitis often progressing to respiratory failure. Treatment consists of ganciclovir (Cytovene), 5 mg per kg intravenously every 12 hours, and high-dose intravenous immunoglobulin. In bone marrow transplant patients, ganciclovir alone has not reduced mortality. Foscarnet (Foscavir), 60 mg per kg intravenously every 8 hours, is another drug with anti-CMV activity, but there is little experience in treating CMV pneumonia with this agent. Both drugs require dosage reduction for renal insufficiency.

RESPIRATORY SYNCYTIAL VIRUS

RSV is a common cause of bronchiolitis and pneumonia in children under 2 years of age and may cause pneumonia in elderly or immunocompromised adults. Epidemics occur annually during the colder months. RSV infection can lead to respiratory failure in some patients. In this subset of patients with severe disease, aerosolized ribavirin (Virazole) shows some benefit. Ribavirin is nebulized and administered through a mask, into a tent or endotracheal tube. When used in a patient on a mechanical ventilator, in-line filters and close monitoring are required because the drug may occlude tubing and valves in the ventilator circuit. The drug is given for up to 20 hours a day for 2 to 5 days.

LEGIONELLOSIS
(Pontiac Fever and Legionnaires' Disease)

method of
JOYCE A. KORVICK, M.D.*
Center for Drug Evaluation, Food and Drug Administration
Rockville, Maryland

Legionellosis refers to disease caused by bacteria belonging to the family Legionellaceae. *Legionella pneumophila* causes two well-defined clinical syndromes: legionnaires' disease and Pontiac fever.

Since the discovery of *L. pneumophila* in 1977, 17 additional species have been isolated in culture from patients with pneumonia: *L. micdadei, L. bozemanii, L. dumoffii, L. long-beachae, L. jordanis, L. gormanii, L. feeleii, L. hackeliae, L. maceachernii, L. wadsworthii, L. birminghamensis, L. cincinnatiensis,* and *L. oakridgensis.* However, 90% of clinical infection is caused by *L. pneumophila*, serogroups 1, 4, and 6.

CLINICAL SYNDROME

Pneumonia is the most common clinical manifestation of legionnaires' disease. Extrapulmonary manifestations have also been described, including myocarditis, pericarditis, liver abscess, peritonitis, perirectal abscess, cerebral microabscess, hemodialysis fistula infection, pyelonephritis, and prosthetic valvular endocarditis. Symptoms typically include malaise, weakness, chills, dry cough, and fever. Neurologic symptoms range from headache and lethargy to encephalopathy. Watery diarrhea occurs as a prodromal symptom in up to one-half of cases. The degree of illness and severity of pulmonic disease at presentation vary widely. At one extreme, the patient may present with a mild cough and slight fever; at the other extreme, with confusion, multisystem failure, and overwhelming pneumonia. The clinical presentation is nonspecific; thus specialized laboratory tests are needed for definitive diagnosis. However, the following clues should increase the clinician's suspicion of legionnaires' disease: (1) Gram's stain of respiratory secretions containing organisms; (2) hyponatremia (serum sodium level < 130 mEq per liter); (3) failure to respond to beta-lactam or aminoglycoside antibiotics; (4) occurrence in an institution where the potable water is known to be contaminated by *Legionella*. Risk factors include immunosuppression (especially corticosteroids) and cigarette smoking.

Pontiac fever is a nonpneumonic illness. The attack rate is high, and the incubation period is 2 to 4 days. Myalgia, headache, malaise, and fever are presenting symptoms. It is not fatal; recovery usually occurs within 2 days without specific antibiotic therapy. Diagnosis is based on seroconversion to *Legionella* in the context of the clinical syndrome.

DIAGNOSIS

Legionella organisms are faintly staining, gram-negative rods. Direct microscopic evaluation of respiratory secre-

---

**The recommendations expressed herein are those of the author, and do not necessarily represent the position of the FDA.*

tions is accomplished by a fluorescent antibody stain (DFA) specific for *Legionella*.

Since *Legionella* organisms are fastidious, they require specialized media for isolation (buffered charcoal yeast extract agar). Selective agars have been developed that contain antibiotics and suppress the growth of competing bacteria and dyes that color the *Legionella* colonies. Direct fluorescent antibody (DFA) staining is a rapid technique that has a sensitivity of 50 to 70%. Detection of *Legionella* antigen in the urine is also commercially available, with sensitivities comparable with those of other techniques. Urine can be obtained with minimal discomfort to even the most uncooperative or disoriented patient. At present, the urine test identifies only *L. pneumophila* serogroup 1. Serologic testing can be a useful adjunct to direct isolation of the organism. However, in most cases this is a retrospective tool requiring serum from both acute and convalescent stages.

THERAPY

Historically, erythromycin has been the drug of choice for legionnaires' disease (Table 1). Controlled trials have never been performed, and this recommendation is based on the lower case/fatality ratio among patients receiving erythromycin during the 1976 outbreak. The recommended duration of therapy is 14 to 21 days. Therapy for 21 days is recommended for immunocompromised patients and recipients of transplants. Relapses in this population have occurred with shorter courses of erythromycin.

Newer macrolides, including clarithromycin* and azithromycin,* have demonstrated activity against *L. pneumophila* in vitro, in animal models, and in

---

*Not FDA-approved for this indication.

TABLE 1. **Antibiotic Therapy for** *Legionella*
Pneumonia

Antibiotic	Dose and Frequency	Route
Erythromycin (Erythrocin)*	1 gm q 6 h 500 mg q 6 h	Intravenous Oral
Ciprofloxacin (Cipro)	750 mg q 12 h 400 mg q 8 h	Oral† Intravenous
Doxycycline (Vibramycin, Vivox)	100 mg q 12 h	Oral, intravenous
Tetracycline (Achromycin, Sumycin)	0.5–1 gm q 6 h	Oral, intravenous
Trimethoprim-sulfamethoxazole (Septra, Bactrim)	160/800 mg q 8 h 160/800 mg q 12 h	Intravenous Oral
Azithromycin (Zithromax)	500 mg q 24 h	Oral
Clarithromycin (Biaxin)	500 mg q 12 h	Oral

*Clinical experience is limited with agents other than erythromycin, and as such other agents are not currently approved by the FDA for this indication.

†For severe illness, combine with rifampin (Rifadin), 600 mg every 12 hr orally, and/or use intravenous form when available and implement oral therapy after demonstrated clinical improvement.

Adapted from Yu VL: Legionellosis. *In* Mandel GL, et al (eds): Principles and Practice of Infectious Diseases, 4th ed. New York, Churchill Livingstone, 1995, p 2093.

anecdotal reports; however, large clinical trials have not been undertaken with these agents.

Combination therapy (erythromycin and rifampin) is recommended in patients with severe disease. Rifampin (Rifadin) is very active against *Legionella* but should not be administered alone because of the potential for the development of resistance.

Alternative drugs include doxycycline,* trimethoprim-sulfamethoxazole,* and quinolones.* Although no clinical trials have been performed, these antibiotics have been reported to be successful in isolated cases and all have been reported to achieve therapeutic levels in the alveolar macrophage. *Legionella* is an intracellular pathogen, and thus effective anti-*Legionella* agents must penetrate the macrophage to reach their targets.

The majority of patients with *Legionella* prosthetic valvular endocarditis require valve replacement and additional therapy with erythromycin and rifampin. Two months of intravenous therapy with an additional 6 months of oral therapy is recommended.

Side Effects

Gastrointestinal complaints—nausea, vomiting, and diarrhea—are the most common side effects of the macrolides. Erythromycin has been noted to cause nausea, diarrhea, phlebitis, and ototoxicity, which are reversible on cessation of the antibiotic. Intravenous administration requires large fluid volumes, which may complicate the fluid management of severely ill patients.

Rifampin in the oral form may have decreased bioavailability in patients with gastrointestinal dysfunction. In severe cases, the intravenous formulation can be utilized. Rifampin causes nausea, diarrhea, and elevated liver functions, and it interferes with the metabolism of many drugs. Rash, fever, leukopenia, hemolysis, and anemia are rare but have been reported.

Cyclosporine levels must be monitored closely during treatment of legionnaires' disease in recipients of transplants. Erythromycin raises the cyclosporine serum concentration and may lead to nephrotoxicity, whereas rifampin decreases the serum concentration of cyclosporine, which may contribute to rejection of the transplanted organ.

Therapeutic Outcome

The patient should respond with a feeling of well-being and decreasing temperature within 5 days of initiation of therapy. The mortality is 5% in patients receiving appropriate therapy and from 24 to 43% in immunocompromised patients.

---

*Not FDA-approved for this indication.

ACUTE PULMONARY EMBOLISM

method of
C. GREGORY ELLIOTT, M.D.
LDS Hospital
Salt Lake City, Utah

DIAGNOSIS

The diagnosis of acute pulmonary embolism (PE) remains a challenge, in spite of numerous technical advances. The decision to order diagnostic studies and the quantification of the clinician's suspicion that the patient has pulmonary embolism are both critical steps (Figure 1). It is well recognized that patients die from PE that was never suspected by their physicians. Conversely, many patients present with symptoms, signs, and laboratory abnormalities caused by diseases that mimic PE. A low threshold for ordering screening studies is important when the clinical presentation suggests PE in patients who have risk factors (Table 1). Even when risk factors are not present, the common symptoms of sudden dyspnea, unexplained pleuritic chest pain with or without hemoptysis, and hypotension with or without syncope should lead the physician to consider PE. The clinician must also be aware of uncommon presentations of PE, such as abdominal pain, cough, fever, wheezing, sudden unexplained arrhythmia, or oxygen desaturation in the hospitalized patient.

Once the physician suspects acute PE, it is important to estimate how likely this diagnosis is before performing ventilation and perfusion lung scans. This prior probability influences the likelihood that a given lung scan pattern represents acute PE (Table 2). A normal lung perfusion scan excludes clinically important PE and eliminates the need for anticoagulant therapy. However, an abnormal perfusion scan alone is not sufficiently specific to confirm the diagnosis of acute PE. When combined with ventilation scanning and a clinical estimate of prior probability, the likelihood that the patient has PE can be estimated. It is appropriate to treat patients for PE when the ventilation and perfusion scan pattern suggests a high probability for acute PE and the clinical suspicion is high. In general, additional testing is needed if the perfusion and ventilation

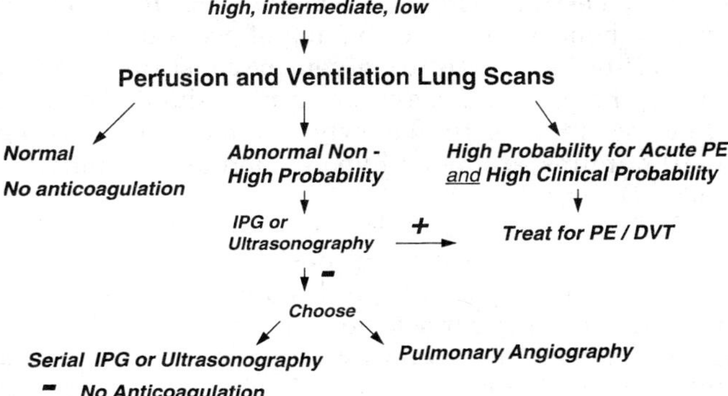

Figure 1. This approach to the diagnosis of acute pulmonary embolism (PE) emphasizes an estimate of the clinical probability for PE and an alternative approach to pulmonary angiography for patients with abnormal ventilation and perfusion scans for which either the scan pattern and/or the estimated clinical probability are not high. The alternative approach to pulmonary angiography does not apply to patients with severe cardiopulmonary compromise.

TABLE 1. Risk Factors for Venous Thromboembolism

Previous venous thromboembolism
Prolonged immobilization
Extensive surgery
Multiple trauma
Major medical illness
Age > 40 years
Underlying prothrombotic disease, e.g., cancer

Modified from Hirsh J: Venous Thromboembolism: Guide to Management. Mississauga, Ontario, Du Pont Pharmaceuticals, 1993.

scans are abnormal, but not high probability; or the physician's estimate of the presence of PE was not high and the scan pattern suggests a high probability for PE. Most patients with abnormal perfusion lung scans will require additional diagnostic tests before a management strategy is chosen.

Pulmonary angiography remains the "gold standard" for the diagnosis of acute PE. However, angiography is invasive, expensive, and not always readily available. These limitations have led to the development of alternative diagnostic strategies. Both serial impedance plethysmography and duplex ultrasonography with compression of the veins rely upon the knowledge that proximal deep venous thrombosis of the lower extremities underlies the majority of PE. Therefore, positive studies confirm the diagnosis of venous thromboembolism, and negative studies of the leg veins over a 2-week period allow the clinician to withhold anticoagulation because the risk for recurrent PE is low (less than 3%). This strategy should not be applied to patients who have serious cardiopulmonary compromise. Whenever possible, these patients should undergo pulmonary angiography, as should patients at increased risk for venous thrombi in other locations—for example, upper extremities, renal veins, or right side of the heart.

TREATMENT

Unfractionated heparin followed by warfarin is highly efficacious therapy for the majority of patients with PE. Rapid achievement of an adequate anticoagulant effect is crucial to prevent recurrent venous thromboembolism. An initial bolus of 5000 units of heparin followed by a constant intravenous infusion should be initiated when the diagnosis is confirmed

TABLE 2. Influence of Prior Probability Upon the Likelihood That Ventilation and Perfusion Lung Scan Patterns Are Due to Acute Pulmonary Embolism*

	Prior Probability for PE		
	High	*Intermediate*	*Low*
Scan Pattern	80–100	20–79	0–19
High	96	88	56
Intermediate	66	28	16
Low	40	16	4

*Prior probability for PE was determined from clinical information by experienced clinicians who estimated the likelihood of PE (high = 80–100%, intermediate = 20–79%, and low = 0–19%). Data express the likelihood (expressed as percent) for identifying acute PE on pulmonary angiograms. Modified from The PIOPED Investigators: JAMA *263*:2753–2759, 1990. Copyright 1990, American Medical Association.

or when clinical suspicion is high and bleeding risk is low (Table 3). An initial heparin infusion of 1000 IU per hour is not sufficient for most patients. The constant infusion should deliver either 1240 IU per hour to patients with a high risk for bleeding complications or 1680 IU per hour for those without identifiable risks for bleeding complications. Alternatively, the initial infusion may be weight-adjusted at 18 IU per kg (actual body weight) per hour. Measurement of the activated partial thromboplastin time (aPTT) approximately 4 to 6 hours later permits adjustment of the heparin dose to achieve aPTT results in the targeted therapeutic range. Emphasis should be placed upon rapidly exceeding the lower threshold of the targeted therapeutic range, since persistently subtherapeutic heparin levels permit recurrent venous thromboembolism. Heparin should be continued for a minimum of 5 days, and it may be continued for 7 to 10 days for more seriously affected patients— e.g., patients with massive PE.

For patients without venous access, subcutaneous low-molecular-weight heparin (enoxaparin, Lovenox) provides an alternative. The initial subcutaneous dose is 1 mg per kg of body weight given every 12 hours. Measurement of the aPTT is not necessary when low-molecular-weight heparin is given. This strategy may also be used for compliant outpatients with deep venous thrombosis, asymptomatic PE, and those at low risk for bleeding complications.

Rarely, therapeutic prolongation of the aPTT cannot be used to guide heparin therapy. When patients with the lupus anticoagulant are seen with pulmonary embolism or when pseudoheparin resistance

caused by increased factor VIII levels leads to persistently "subtherapeutic" aPTT results in spite of large (more than 50,000 IU per 24 hours) heparin doses, heparin levels may be used to guide therapy. The target therapeutic range is 0.2 to 0.4 IU per mL using protamine titration, or an antifactor Xa level of 0.35 to 0.70 IU per mL.

Platelet counts should be monitored daily during initial heparin therapy. When the platelet count falls abruptly, or when the platelet count falls below 100,000 per μL, heparin should be discontinued and alternative treatment should be begun, with heparin-induced thrombocytopenia diagnosed presumptively. Heparin-induced thrombocytopenia is caused by heparin-induced immune complexes, and it may cause life-threatening arterial or venous thrombi. The diagnosis may be confirmed by normalization of the platelet count after discontinuing heparin, exclusion of other causes of thrombocytopenia, and a positive heparin-induced platelet aggregation test. If removal of all heparin is not effective, plasmapheresis may lead to clinical improvement. Anticoagulation can be maintained until warfarin becomes effective by administering Ancrod* (Knoll Laboratories), a defibrinogenating agent, or a heparinoid (Org 10172 or Danaparoid,* Organon, Inc). In the future, specific thrombin inhibitors such as recombinant hirudin* or argatroban* may provide therapeutic alternatives.

Bleeding and heparin-induced thrombocytopenia with or without thrombosis are the major early complications of heparin treatment. Major bleeding complications that require blood transfusion and discontinuation of heparin are more likely to occur in patients who have identifiable risks for bleeding, such as thrombocytopenia, surgery or trauma within the past 2 weeks, or a history of peptic ulcer disease. In the absence of such risks, an excessively prolonged aPTT is not a strong predictor of major bleeding. Most major bleeding episodes can be managed by discontinuing heparin, but when bleeding is life-threatening, the anticoagulant effects of heparin can be reversed more rapidly by protamine. The dose should be estimated (i.e., 1.0 mg of protamine for 100 units of heparin bolus, or 0.5 mg of protamine for the number of heparin units given by constant infusion during the past hour), and protamine should be given (2 mg per ml in saline) slowly—no more than 50 mg in 10 minutes—to avoid hypotension and anaphylactoid reactions.

Warfarin (Coumadin) can be initiated on the first full hospital day. An initial dose of 10 mg is appropriate for most patients. Subsequent doses depend upon the prothrombin time (PT) response. Because there is a delay between warfarin administration and its antithrombotic effect, a prolonged PT during the first 4 days of warfarin therapy does not always indicate that an antithrombotic effect has been achieved. For this reason, heparin and warfarin are overlapped for approximately 4 days, and heparin is discontinued when the anticoagulant effect, as mea-

TABLE 3. **Protocols for Initial Heparin Therapy**

Reference	Initial Bolus	Constant IU Infusion
Hull et al, 1992*	5000 IU	1680 IU/h (low risk to bleed) 1240 IU/h (high risk to bleed†)
Raschke et al, 1993‡	80 IU/kg	18 IU/kg/h

aPTT (sec)§	Dose Change‖ (IU/h)	Additional Action	Next aPTT
≤45	+240	Re-bolus with 5000 IU	4–6 h
46–54	+120	None	4–6 h
55–85	0	None	
86–110	−120	Stop infusion for 1 h	4–6 h after restart
>110	−240	Stop infusion for 1 h	4–6 h after restart

*Hull RD, et al: Optimal therapeutic level of heparin therapy in patients with venous thrombosis. Arch Intern Med *152*:1589–1595, 1992.

†High risk to bleed in the judgment of the attending physician; common criteria include surgery or trauma within 2 weeks, thrombocytopenia, thrombotic stroke, or history of peptic ulcer.

‡Raschke RA, et al: The weight-based heparin dosing nomogram compared with a "standard care" nomogram. Ann Intern Med *119*:874–881, 1993.

§Normal range with Dade-Actin FS reagent is 27–35 sec. Therapeutic range of 55–85 sec corresponds to heparin concentration range of 0.2 to 0.4 IU/mL by protamine titration. The therapeutic range may vary according to thromboplastin reagent and should be determined by each laboratory.

‖Dosage adjustments are made to aPTT measurements during steady state conditions—e.g., 4–6 h after dose adjustments.

Abbreviation: aPPT = activated partial thromboplastin time.

---

*Investigational drug in the United States.

TABLE 4. **Management of High International Normalized Ratio**

INR	Clinical State	Action
< 6.0	No bleeding	Hold warfarin
> 6.0 and < 10.0	No bleeding	Subcutaneous vitamin K_1 (1–2 mg)
> 10.0	No bleeding	Subcutaneous vitamin K_1 (3 mg)

Adapted from Hirsh J, et al: Oral anticoagulants. Chest *108*:231S–246S, 1995.

sured by the international normalized ratio (INR), is between 2.0 and 3.0. More intense anticoagulation (INR = 3.0 to 4.5) with warfarin increases the risk for bleeding but can prevent recurrence for selected patients—e.g., those who have had objectively documented recurrent venous thromboemboli at INR 2.0 to 3.0. Warfarin should be continued for a minimum of 3 months for patients who have had a first episode of PE. Longer courses of warfarin are warranted for patients with continuing risk factors, such as hypercoagulable states. Lifetime treatment is appropriate for patients who have had more than one objectively documented venous thromboembolism. Recurrence is more likely when warfarin dosing is inadequate, and serious bleeding complications are more likely when the anticoagulant effect of warfarin is excessive. Therefore weekly or biweekly measurements of PT are appropriate initially to guide dosage adjustment for most patients. Excessively prolonged PT results can be treated with subcutaneous vitamin K (Table 4). Monthly measurements of PT are appropriate when the PT response to warfarin stabilizes.

Pregnant patients or those who may become pregnant during anticoagulant therapy cannot receive warfarin because of the risk for teratogenicity. In this situation heparin must be continued either as a constant infusion or subcutaneously. Severe osteopenia is a potential complication of prolonged (more than 4 months) heparin administration.

Vena Cava Filter

Vena cava filters offer a therapeutic alternative when anticoagulants are contraindicated or when anticoagulant therapy must be stopped. A vena cava filter also should be placed when massive pulmonary embolism requires surgical embolectomy, or when objectively documented recurrent pulmonary embolism occurs in spite of adequate anticoagulant treatment, or in selected circumstances in which thromboembolism may prove fatal, such as extensive unattached large vein thrombi or smaller thrombi in patients who have had hemodynamically significant pulmonary embolism. In my opinion, anticoagulant therapy should be resumed when possible after vena cava filter insertion in order to prevent further morbidity from deep vein thrombi in the legs.

Massive Pulmonary Embolism

Patients with massive pulmonary embolism—that is, pulmonary embolism that causes hypotension or cardiac arrest—are more likely to die from acute PE. For this reason, more aggressive management options must be considered. These options include insertion of a vena cava filter to prevent recurrence, administration of thrombolytic drugs to dissolve the thrombus more rapidly than endogenous fibrinolysis, use of catheters to fragment the thrombus, and embolectomy performed either with a catheter or surgically. The choice of intervention(s) depends upon available resources and expertise. Furthermore, well-designed clinical trials have not been conducted to prove the efficacy of any of these methods, although the absence of such trials should not preclude judicious use of these therapies.

Thrombolytic therapy accelerates the dissolution of clot when compared with heparin. Thus thrombolysis may be lifesaving for those few patients with acute PE that produces hypotension, cardiac arrest, or profound arterial hypoxemia refractory to supplemental oxygen. Unlike other treatments for massive acute PE, thrombolysis can cause serious bleeding by dissolving hemostatic plugs. For this reason, absolute and relative contraindications to thrombolytic therapy must be considered before administering any thrombolytic drug (Table 5). If available, alternative treatment, such as embolectomy or catheter fragmentation, should be used when relative or absolute contraindications exist. If therapeutic alternatives are not available, thrombolysis may be given in the face of relative contraindications when survival is unlikely without such treatment, such as cardiac arrest or shock refractory to medical management.

A number of thrombolytic agents and dosing regimens are available (Table 6). The selection of the agent and dosing regimen must take into consideration drug availability and cost, as well as the benefits and risks. Shorter infusions of recombinant tissue plasminogen activator (rt-PA) (Activase) or urokinase (Abbokinase) are more rapidly efficacious than FDA-approved regimens for urokinase and streptokinase that are infused over 12 and 24 hours respectively. When cost is not an issue, I prefer a bolus of rt-PA. A constant infusion of heparin should be continued during and after this bolus and titrated to the targeted therapeutic range using the aPTT.

TABLE 5. **Contraindications to Thrombolytic Therapy**

Absolute

Active internal bleeding (gastrointestinal, genitourinary, central nervous system, etc.)

Relative

Major surgery, trauma, or internal bleeding within past 10 days
Cerebrovascular disease
Uncontrolled hypertension (systolic blood pressure > 180 mm Hg and/or diastolic BP > 110 mm Hg
Hemostatic defects (thrombocytopenia, renal failure, liver failure, anticoagulant therapy)
Pregnancy
Pericarditis
Diabetic hemorrhagic retinopathy
Advanced age (> 75 years old)

TABLE 6. Thrombolytic Therapy for Acute Pulmonary Embolism

Discontinue heparin*	
Streptokinase	250,000 IU bolus
(Streptase)	100,000 IU/h infused for 24 h
Urokinase	4400 IU/kg loading dose
(Abbokinase)	4400 IU/kg/h infused for 12 h
	or 3 × 10⁶ IU infused over 2 h
Tissue plasminogen activator (Activase)	100 mg infused over 2 h *or* 0.6 mg/kg bolus infused over 2 min†

*Heparin should be reinstituted approximately 3 to 4 h after the thrombolytic infusion ends and when the thrombin time is less than 2× baseline.

†Heparin infusion can continue during bolus infusion of tissue plasminogen activator.

Pulmonary embolectomy is appropriate for patients who have large, centrally located thromboemboli accompanied by circulatory shock that is unresponsive to medical therapy. In my opinion, surgical embolectomy is also the treatment of choice for patients with intracardiac thrombi. Pulmonary embolectomy can be performed with a suction catheter or surgically with cardiopulmonary bypass. When selected patients undergo this procedure, approximately 80% survive to hospital discharge, and their long-term function is usually excellent. The prognosis is poorer for patients who suffer cardiopulmonary arrest, but reported survival of patients undergoing cardiopulmonary resuscitation makes emergency cardiopulmonary bypass and surgical embolectomy appropriate for selected patients in this situation.

When surgical or catheter embolectomy is not available and thrombolysis is contraindicated, catheter fragmentation can be attempted. Standard cardiac catheters with or without guidewires can be used to make fragments of large proximal PE.

PREVENTION

Ample evidence exists to show that routine prophylaxis of individuals who have well-recognized risks for venous thromboembolism reduces the rate of fatal and nonfatal acute pulmonary emboli. However, despite recognition of the problem and the cost effectiveness of preventive measures, prophylaxis is underutilized.

Prophylactic measures should be applied widely to patients at risk for venous thromboembolism. Risk factors include age (risk increases progressively after 40 years); prolonged immobility or paralysis; prior venous thromboembolism; cancer; major surgery; obesity; congestive heart failure; stroke; and use of high-dose estrogens. Hemostatic abnormalities increase the risk when combined with immobilization or surgery or both. When multiple risk factors coexist, the risks are cumulative.

The choice of preventive strategy depends upon the nature and severity of the risk for venous thromboembolism (Table 7). For example, the risk is high for venous thromboembolism following multiple trauma, but these patients can have a substantial risk for bleeding. Therefore, intermittent pneumatic compression of the lower extremities is the appropriate initial prophylactic measure for such patients. Patients under 40 years of age who undergo short (less than 30 minutes) periods of general anesthesia have a low risk (0.2%) for PE, and they do not require prophylaxis. Patients older than 40 years undergoing major surgery with no other risk factors have a moderate risk (1% to 2%) for PE, and they require less

TABLE 7. Specific Recommendations for Prophylaxis Against Venous Thromboembolism†

Condition	Recommendation
General surgery	
Low risk	No prophylaxis
Moderate risk	Subcutaneous UH, 5000 IU 2 h preop and q 12 h postop
High risk	Subcutaneous UH, 5000 IU 2 h preop and q 8 h postop
Very high risk	(1) Subcutaneous UH, 5000 IU 2 h preop and q 8 h postop, plus IPC applied intraoperatively *or* (2) perioperative W (INR: 2.0–3.0)
Total hip replacement	(1) Subcutaneous E,* 30 mg q 12 h *or* (2) W begun preoperatively and adjusted to INR 2.0–3.0 postop *or* (3) subcutaneous UH dosed to keep the aPTT (6 h post UH injection) normal
Total knee replacement	Postop subcutaneous E, 30 mg q 12 h *or* IPC
Hip fracture surgery	(1) Subcutaneous E, 30 mg begun 2 h preop *or* (2) W adjusted to INR 2.0–3.0
Neurosurgery	(1) IPC *or* (2) subcutaneous UH, 5000 IU q 12 h *and* IPC for high risk patients
Acute spinal cord injury with leg paralysis	(1) Subcutaneous UH in doses adjusted to produce aPTT = 1.5 × control 6 h after dose *or* (2) W adjusted to INR 2.0–3.0 *or* (3) IPC plus subcutaneous UH 5000 IU q 12 h
Multiple trauma	IPC followed by (1) subcutaneous E, 30 mg q 12 h *or* (2) W adjusted to INR 2.0–3.0 when bleeding is unlikely
Myocardial infarction	Subcutaneous UH, 5000 IU q 12 h
Ischemic stroke with paralysis	Subcutaneous UH, 5000 IU q 12 h
General medical patient at bed rest	Subcutaneous UH, 5000 IU q 12 h

*A number of low-molecular-weight heparins will soon be available in addition to enoxaparin.

Abbreviations: UH = unfractionated heparin, IPC = intermittent pneumatic compression, E = enoxaparin (Lovenox), W = warfarin (Coumadin), INR = international normalized ratio.

Modified from Clagett GP, et al: Prevention of venous thromboembolism. Chest *108*:312S–334S, 1995.

intense prophylactic measures than similar patients with multiple risk factors who have a high risk (2% to 4%) for PE. Finally, patients older than 40 years may have a very high risk (4% to 10%) for PE because of the nature of their surgery (hip or knee replacement, hip fracture, extensive cancer resection); the nature of their illness (such as paraplegia); or previous venous thromboembolism. These patients should receive the most intense prophylactic measures.

SARCOIDOSIS

method of
ANDERS G. EKLUND, M.D.
Karolinska Hospital
Stockholm, Sweden

The clinical picture of sarcoidosis differs according to the genetic background of the patient. Thus, Asians have been reported often to present with blurred vision and to have rather limited pulmonary involvement. In contrast, African-Americans seem to get a more aggressive form of disease with pronounced constitutional and respiratory symptoms. In whites, an acute onset is common. This is known as Löfgren's syndrome, with fever, erythema nodosum (predominantly women), ankle arthritis (men), and bilateral hilar lymphadenopathy (BHL). An abrupt onset often indicates a good prognosis, whereas an insidious one may predict an unfavorable outcome, with development of pulmonary fibrosis and lung function impairment.

PATHOGENESIS

Sarcoidosis is characterized by the formation of noncaseating epithelioid cell granuloma in a multiorgan fashion, and about 90% of the patients will have intrathoracic manifestations. During the last two decades, knowledge about the pathogenetic mechanisms has increased considerably, mainly because of the bronchoalveolar lavage (BAL) technique, which has enabled us to study the pattern of the pulmonary inflammatory reaction. In short, there is an accumulation of CD4+ T lymphocytes in the lungs when the disease is active, and often a corresponding inversed ratio of CD4+/CD8+ T cells in the peripheral blood. At the same time noncellular components, e.g., albumin, fibronectin, and procollagen-III-N-terminal peptide, appear in high concentrations in the epithelial lining fluid, reflecting the inflammatory response. Earlier it was believed that the higher the percentage of BAL-fluid lymphocytes, the greater the risk for a poor outcome. However, the accumulation of lymphocytes seems to be highest in patients with Löfgren's syndrome, which is known to have a very good prognosis. Recently it has been shown that HLA-DR3(17)+ DQw2 white patients during active disease get an accumulation in the lungs (but not in the blood) of T cells that express a specific receptor for antigen (Vα2.3). These patients tend to get less advanced radiographic changes and seldom develop chronic disease.

The findings of restricted usage of the T cell receptor at the inflammatory site in the context of a specific HLA type could provide some clues as to the antigenic peptide that may be triggering the inflammation. The causative agent still remains unknown. However, there have been interesting reports—for example, on the increased occurrence of mycobacterial rRNA in spleens from sarcoidosis patients compared with normals, and on a clinical picture compatible with lung sarcoidosis developing in a heart transplant recipient, the donor of which turned out to have sarcoidosis. This could support the notion of a transmissible agent. Also, sarcoidosis patients will develop granuloma in the transplanted organs.

DIAGNOSIS

One should always aim to get histologic confirmation of the diagnosis, which also should be based on a clinical and/or a radiographic picture compatible with sarcoidosis. The biopsy specimens could be obtained from skin lesions, enlarged superficial lymph nodes, the bronchial mucosa, or through transbronchial biopsies of the lung parenchyma. If there is unilateral swelling of hilar lymph nodes, a mediastinoscopy may be advocated to rule out malignant lymphoma. If there is access to Kveim-Siltzbach suspension, the diagnosis, especially in nonfibrotic stages, may be confirmed. The specimens should be thoroughly investigated for possible infectious agents.

CLINICAL DISEASE ACTIVITY

In 1993 there was an international consensus conference on how to define activity in sarcoidosis. It was stated that the disease is active when it undergoes clinical, roentgenographic, or physiologic change indicating ongoing inflammation, granuloma formation, or a fibrosing process. Additionally, it was pointed out that activity does not mean poor prognosis or a need to start treatment. The most useful markers of activity were considered to be the clinical evaluation (fever, uveitis, erythema nodosum, lupus pernio, changing scars, polyarthralgia, dyspnea, cough), and the development of changes in chest x-ray films and lung function (VC, FEV_1, DL_{CO}). In the consensus report (Eur Respir J 7:624–627, 1994), some optional markers of activity were pointed out (serum ACE, [67]gallium scan, computed-tomography, and BAL-fluid cell counts and CD4+/CD8+ ratio). It should be noted that serum angiotensin converting enzyme (ACE) often is normal during the first few months of disease, and that it may be used for monitoring the effect of treatment.

TREATMENT

Although corticosteroids have been the mainstay in the treatment of sarcoidosis since the early 1950s, it still remains to be proved that the patients ultimately benefit from steroid treatment, especially in the long run. Many of our therapeutic modalities are based on empirical findings and not on exact knowledge of the mechanisms behind the effects of the drugs. This has to be kept in mind, together with the fact that the side effects of prolonged treatment cannot simply be ignored. However, the macrophage-lymphocyte interaction appears to be a crucial event in the disease process, and steroids will have a modulating effect on several genes expressed by these cells, thereby influencing their synthesis of cytokines.

Most physicians who are experienced in treating patients with sarcoidosis will be able to recall patients on steroid treatment who seemed to respond to the treatment in a rather dramatic fashion. One reason for the lack of consistent reports may be that at the onset of the disorder it is often difficult to predict the outcome. As this usually is favorable, treatment with steroids will not be started until there are obvious signs of a progressive disorder. When treatment is finally started, possibly the responsiveness to the corticosteroids is reduced. Also, the treatment protocols have mostly been rather rigid and not aimed at giving an optimal effect and maintaining it in the individual patient. It seems that when prolonged treatment is given aiming at optimizing the radiographic improvement, the patients will have a small but significantly better functional outcome in the long run. In recent years, inhaled steroids have been proposed as an alternative or complement to oral steroids.

In 1993 there was an international consensus on the treatment of sarcoidosis (Sarcoidosis *11*:34–40, 1994). It was concluded that most centers seem to prefer daily administration of steroids but may shift to alternate-day long-term maintenance treatment. A common starting dose is 20 to 40 mg of prednisone or prednisolone per day or alternate day. The duration of the treatment should be determined by the results of regular follow-ups of disease activity. Often treatment for 3 to 12 months is advocated. The rationale to start treatment is if an evaluation of the combined findings of symptoms, lung function, chest x-ray changes, and other activity markers indicates deterioration.

Lung Involvement

Stage I. When the patient has bilateral hilar lymphadenopathy (BHL) but is asymptomatic and without lung function impairment, treatment should be avoided. In Löfgren's syndrome, nonsteroidal antiinflammatory drugs administered for some weeks may be helpful in overcoming the arthralgia.

When there are signs from the respiratory tract, such as persistent cough and/or dyspnea, oral steroid treatment may be needed. At least these patients should be closely monitored in order to detect functional deterioration early. If bronchoscopy reveals endobronchial signs of sarcoidosis, perhaps with plaque formation, the indication for starting with oral steroids is increased. If there are simply signs of bronchial hyperreactivity (BHR), inhaled steroids may be an alternative.

Stage II. A considerable number of patients will have stage II (BHL with parenchymal infiltrates) disease at detection. If they are asymptomatic and the lung function is close to normal, there is no obvious need for immediate steroid treatment. However, if during an observation period of 3 to 6 months signs of disease activity and deterioration appear, treatment may be started. The ultimate goal should be that the patient becomes asymptomatic and that there is a normalization of the chest x-ray film, lung function, and other activity parameters. However, this goal may be far from being achieved: when deciding on the doses of steroids as well as the duration of treatment, adverse effects such as weight gain,

hypertension, cataracts, diabetes mellitus, and susceptibility to infections must be taken into account.

Stage III. These patients will not have BHL but instead have parenchymal infiltrates with or without signs of shrinkage of the parenchyma, indicating irreversible fibrotic changes. If there are still indications of active (see earlier) and progressive disease, a trial with steroids is indicated. These patients are more likely not to have radiographic findings compatible with extensive fibrosis. However, if there are no signs of activity, steroid treatment should be avoided, as it may possibly even increase the risk for infections occurring in bronchiectasis or cavitations.

Methotrexate* may be an alternative or additional treatment to steroids in poorly responding active cases. The patients have to be followed closely with regard to the side effects, mainly hepatotoxicity. This treatment should be decided on only by experienced chest physicians, and the same applies to administration of cyclophosphamide* (Cytoxan) and azathioprine* (Imuran). Cyclosporine* (Sandimmune) has so far not proved to be effective in the treatment of pulmonary sarcoidosis.

Inhaled Steroids. An increasing number of reports indicate that inhaled steroids may be beneficial in the treatment of selected cases of patients with pulmonary sarcoidosis. Accumulating data also support the idea that when this treatment is started it should be given in combination with oral steroids in order to achieve a more rapid improvement. The rationales for giving inhaled steroids are to reduce the systemic side effects of oral steroids either by replacing the oral steroids or by supplementing administration of oral steroids in a steroid-sparing manner. Possibly, in some mild cases (e.g., with BHR), inhaled steroids could be the only therapy.

Transplantation. Patients with advanced pulmonary sarcoidosis may undergo transplantation of lungs (single or double). This of course would be considered only when all other therapeutic measurements have failed, and if the clinical picture is still deteriorating. In the transplanted lung(s) there will ultimately be formation of sarcoid granuloma, which also occurs in patients receiving heart and liver transplants due to end-stage sarcoidosis lesions.

Extrapulmonary Involvement

Sarcoidosis may affect almost any organ, and thus some patients will need treatment due to such involvement. Rather often the *eyes* are engaged. Depending on the character and intensity of the changes, corticosteroids may be given as eyedrops or by subconjunctival injection, often in combination with oral treatment in high doses.

Skin lesions can be treated by local and/or systemic administration of steroids. However, the response may be disappointing, and other treatment modalities may have to be considered in advanced cases

---

*Not FDA approved for this indication.

or for esthetic reasons. Hydroxychloroquine* (Plaquenil) could be tried, and alternate-day treatment reduces the ocular toxicity. The dose recommended in the consensus report was 200 mg on alternate days for about 9 months. Eye examinations on a regular basis have to be conducted throughout the treatment. An alternative regimen is administration of methotrexate once weekly (10 mg) for 3 months. Liver function should then be monitored.

Cardiac and neurologic involvement may call for high doses of steroids for prolonged periods of time. Whenever the dose has been reduced and signs of a relapse occur, the dose of steroids has to be increased again. As a general rule, the lowest dose can be chosen at which no sign of relapse was present. In *myocardial* sarcoidosis, additional drugs to compensate for congestive heart failure may be needed, and in some cases a pacemaker has to be inserted. In advanced cases of *neurosarcoidosis*, radiotherapy may be indicated as a final therapeutic approach. Magnetic resonance imaging has proved useful in monitoring the neurologic manifestations of the disease.

Usually modestly raised liver function test levels indicating *hepatic involvement*, or a somewhat *enlarged spleen* or *superficial lymph nodes*, do not call for steroid treatment.

Sarcoidosis may affect the *kidneys* in different ways. If there is hypercalciuria, the patient should be encouraged to avoid food and beverages rich in calcium. In addition, the intake of liquids should be abundant and diuretics may be provided. If there are additional signs of impaired renal function, oral steroids should be given. The consensus panel on treatment of sarcoidosis recommended calcium-chelating agents for hypercalciuria if it becomes necessary to discontinue steroid therapy.

Hypercalcemia

Somewhat less than 10% of all patients with sarcoidosis have hypercalcemia, which is caused by a second hydroxylation of vitamin D by alveolar macrophages and possibly by cells in the sarcoid granuloma. The serum concentrations of the metabolite $1,25\text{-}(OH)_2\text{-}D$ increase, and this metabolite is the major determinant in the intestinal absorption of calcium. Usually treatment with steroids, sometimes in high doses over a prolonged period of time, will be needed.

Pregnancy

Several studies have indicated that pregnancy does not aggravate sarcoidosis. In addition, there does not seem to be any increased risk for the fetus. During the pregnancy, chest radiographic monitoring of the disorder should be avoided if possible. Improvement of the disorder during the pregnancy may occur, either due to spontaneous resolution or due to tempo-

rary hormonal effects caused by the pregnancy. In the latter case, the disorder may return to the previous condition after the child has been delivered.

SILICOSIS

method of
ANDREW J. GHIO, M.D.
National Health and Environmental Effects Research Laboratory, Environmental Protection Agency Research Triangle Park, North Carolina

Silicosis is a fibrotic injury of the lung that follows exposure to respirable silica (silicon dioxide, SiO_2). Silicosis was reported by ancient civilizations. It was the first recognized occupational lung disease. Industrialization greatly increased both the number of workers with a significant exposure to silica and the incidence of silicosis. This pneumoconiosis continues to be associated with a significant morbidity and mortality in this country despite predictions of its pending elimination.

The mechanisms of lung injury after silica exposure have not been defined. Tissue damage after the inhalation of silica is likely to be associated with oxidant generation by the dust. The production of these oxygen-based free radicals results from either the fracture of silica particles or the complexation of a metal cation by surface functional groups. Fracture of the dust directly produces silicon- and oxygen-based free radicals. The accumulation of specific metals by silanol groups at the surface confers a capacity to the silica to transport electrons and catalyze the generation of oxidants via the Fenton reaction. The oxidative stress that results from silica exposure can affect a release of both NF-$\kappa\beta$ and oxidant-sensitive mediators, such as tumor necrosis factor and interleukins. These substances appear to coordinate the lung injury to silica, including the inflammatory and fibrotic responses.

PATHOLOGY AND CLINICAL FEATURES

There are two levels of categorization of silicosis (Table 1). Chronic, accelerated, and acute pneumoconioses are delineated by the relationship of the onset of disease with the initial exposure to silica dust. In addition, chronic and accelerated silicosis, but not acute silicosis, are classified according to the size, shape, extent, and profusion of small opacities and the presence and size of large masses observed on the chest radiograph. Simple silicosis presents as small, rounded opacities (up to 10 mm in diameter) on the chest radiographs. Complicated silicosis results from the coalescence of these small opacities and presents on the radiograph as a large mass (greater than 10 mm in diameter).

Chronic silicosis, both simple and complicated, is the fibrosis of lung tissue after a prolonged (greater than 10 years) exposure to silica. Histologic examination of lung tissue from individuals with chronic silicosis demonstrates silica nodules in the interstitium. These are lesions of concentrically arranged collagen and reticulin fibers surrounded by mononuclear inflammatory cells. By means of polarized light, particles of silica can sometimes be found in the periphery of the nodule. Silica nodules are in highest concentration in the superior regions of the lungs. They

---

*Not FDA approved for this indication.

TABLE 1. **Classification of Silicosis**

	Onset of Disease	Histology	Clinical Features	Chest Radiograph
Chronic silicosis				
Simple	>10 yr	Silicotic nodule, fibrosis	None	Small opacities
Complicated	>10 yr	Silicotic nodule, fibrosis	Dyspnea, cough, phlegm	Large mass
Accelerated silicosis				
Simple	<10 yr	Silicotic nodule, fibrosis	None	Small opacities
Complicated	<10 yr	Silicotic nodule, fibrosis	Dyspnea, cough, phlegm	Large mass
Acute silicosis	<5 yr	Inflammation	Fevers, chills, weight loss, dyspnea, cough, phlegm	Alveolar infiltrates

can also be observed in mediastinal and hilar lymph nodes and in extrathoracic sites.

Silica nodules can grow and coalesce to form a large mass, which, after attaining a size of greater than 10 mm in diameter on the posteroanterior chest film, indicates the onset of complicated silicosis. A large mass of complicated silicosis includes dense hyalinized connective tissue, anthracotic pigment, inflammatory cells, and minimal silica content. These masses are associated with compression and destruction of both airways and vasculature.

Simple silicosis is not usually associated with respiratory symptoms, abnormalities on physical examination, or decrements in pulmonary function. Subsequently, this form of silicosis is most frequently found on a routine chest radiograph that demonstrates a profusion of small, rounded opacities.

Unlike simple silicosis, complicated silicosis can be associated with respiratory symptoms, abnormalities on physical examination, and decrements in pulmonary function. Patients can have a productive cough and are also frequently dyspneic. Pulmonary function tests demonstrate a combination of obstruction and restriction and a decreased diffusing capacity. The alveolar-arterial gradient is increased and widens further with exertion. The chest radiograph will demonstrate both a profusion of small opacities and a large mass with a diameter greater than 10 mm. These large masses can cavitate as a result of avascular necrosis, infection with *Mycobacterium tuberculosis,* or neoplastic transformation (i.e., scar carcinoma). The chest film can also show hilar elevation, tracheal distortion, bullous changes, pleural thickening, pneumothorax, and "eggshell" calcification, which is almost pathognomonic for silicosis. Hypoxemic respiratory failure, pulmonary hypertension, and cor pulmonale develop with progression of the disease and are usually terminal events.

Accelerated silicosis usually is found in workers who have had exposures to higher concentrations of silica relative to those individuals with chronic silicosis. Accelerated silicosis, both simple and complicated, pathologically and clinically resembles chronic silicosis, but the onset of disease is earlier (within 10 years of the initial exposure to silica). Symptoms, findings on physical examination, abnormalities on pulmonary function testing, and radiographic presentation are identical to those of chronic silicosis. As a result of the greater exposure these patients have had, the progression of simple to complicated disease and mycobacterial infection are more common in accelerated silicosis relative to chronic silicosis.

Acute silicosis most frequently follows extremely high exposure to silica. Evidence of lung injury follows a very short exposure time (within 5 years of the initial exposure to silica). Histologically, there are few, if any, silicotic nodules in lung tissue of individuals with acute silicosis. There is significant inflammation and fibrosis diffusely throughout the lung, and this involves the alveolar space as well as the interstitium. In addition, there is an accumulation of an eosinophilic substance, a phospholipid, in the alveolar space, mimicking pulmonary alveolar proteinosis.

Acute silicosis is that form of lung injury after silica exposure that progresses most rapidly. Patients are symptomatic early, with cough, phlegm production, dyspnea, lethargy, fevers, chills, and weight loss. There is restriction and a decreased diffusing capacity on pulmonary function testing, which worsen rapidly. The chest radiograph shows diffuse alveolar filling rather than small, rounded opacities or large masses. Infections with mycobacteria, hypoxemic respiratory failure, and cor pulmonale are more frequently observed with acute silicosis than with either chronic or accelerated silicosis. Death follows in months to a few years.

DIAGNOSIS

A thorough history, with attention to occupation, and a chest radiograph are requisite for the diagnosis of silicosis. Biopsies of tissue are unlikely to contribute to this diagnosis. Other lung diseases that imitate silicosis must be excluded. In chronic and accelerated disease, the diagnosis of simple silicosis demands a history of significant exposure to silica and a chest radiograph demonstrating small (up to 10 mm in diameter), rounded opacities, almost always in the upper lung zones. Verification of dust exposure and the presence of a large mass with a background profusion of small opacities on the chest radiograph make the diagnosis of complicated silicosis. The relationship between the time of onset of exposure and disease will allow the discrimination of chronic from accelerated silicosis.

The diagnosis of acute silicosis requires massive exposure to silica. The chest radiograph shows neither small opacities nor large masses but rather diffuse infiltrates with an alveolar filling pattern (air bronchograms).

PREVENTION AND TREATMENT

There is no effective therapy for silicosis. Consequently, the only reasonable approach is its prevention. The current exposure standard of 100 μg per m³ of respirable silica should prevent the great majority of cases of silicosis. If it is not possible to achieve this standard through ventilation and water suppression, workers should be provided with personal breathing equipment. All individuals with silicosis must be counseled to avoid further exposure to silica. As a result of financial constraints, some patients do not feel they have a choice about their exposure.

Treatment of silicosis is always supportive and directed at the complications of this disease, including obstructive lung disease, bronchitis, mycobacterial disease, hypoxemic respiratory failure, pulmonary hypertension, and cor pulmonale (Table 2). All patients with silicosis should be considered for vaccination against influenza and pneumococcus. Corticosteroids are of little benefit in chronic and accelerated silicosis. In acute silicosis, a role for these medications may exist as a result of the significant inflammation. However, their use will predispose the patient to mycobacterial infection, and they should be employed only with close observation of the patient.

Obstructive lung disease in a patient with silicosis is treated with inhaled beta-2 agonists, such as albuterol (Ventolin and Proventil), 2 puffs every 6 hours when necessary. Inhaled steroids such as beclomethasone (Vanceril and Beclovent), 4 puffs every 6 hours, and theophylline (Theo-Dur) twice a day can also be useful. The dose of aminophylline is determined by blood levels. Corticosteroids can also be given systemically but only in low doses.

Bronchitis in the individual with silicosis warrants hydration and postural drainage for clearance of secretions and antibiotic coverage. Ampicillin, doxycycline, and erythromycin can all be used. If there is little-to-no improvement in the first few days, sputum should be Gram-stained and the antibiotic coverage reassessed.

All forms of silicosis predispose the individual to mycobacterial infection, most commonly *M. tuberculosis*. Patients with silicosis must be evaluated with yearly tuberculin skin tests. Converters are assumed to have active tuberculosis. Cultures are obtained and therapy initiated with isoniazid, 300 mg daily; rifampin (Rifadin), 600 mg daily; pyrazinamide, 1.5 to 2.0 grams daily; and ethambutol (Myambutol), 750 to 1000 mg daily. Testing for sensitivity must be done as a result of an increasing prevalence of drug-resistance in *M. tuberculosis*. If sensitive, isoniazid (INH), rifampin, and pyrazinamide should be continued. If resistant, alternative medications must be considered. The duration of therapy for *M. tuberculosis* with silicosis is controversial but should be at least 6 months. With relapse, lifetime therapy with antimycobacterial agents must be begun. If cultures are negative, prophylactic treatment with INH, 300 mg daily, should be initiated and continued for 1 year. Even after 1 year on INH, a significant proportion of the patients will develop active disease. Isoniazid preventive therapy should also be used whenever the patient with a positive tuberculin skin test is treated with systemic steroids.

In a number of individuals with silicosis, the diagnosis of active tuberculosis can be difficult to achieve. Weight loss, fevers, chills, night sweats, and other systemic symptoms in a patient with silicosis should prompt an evaluation with a chest radiograph, acid-fast stains, and cultures. Active disease and suspected disease should both be treated. If the cultures are negative and clinical suspicion still high, the patient should be evaluated for bronchoscopy.

Hypoxemic respiratory failure, pulmonary hypertension, and cor pulmonale are treated with continuous oxygen therapy and pulmonary rehabilitation. Therapy with continuous oxygen will improve exercise tolerance. In addition, it is hoped that continuous oxygen will either delay or prevent the development of pulmonary hypertension and cor pulmonale. Oxygen delivery should be guided by arterial blood gases. Arterial oxygen tension should be elevated to values greater than 60 mm Hg. Ventilator support is indicated only when respiratory failure results from disease that is reversible. For cor pulmonale, diuretics such as furosemide (Lasix), 20 to 80 mg twice a day, and appropriate cardiac medications should also be considered.

Experimental therapies directed toward silicosis have included immunosuppressive agents, D-penicillamine* (Cuprimine), polyvinyl pyridine-*N*-oxide,† tetrandine,† inhalation of aluminum salts,† and whole lung lavage. Effectiveness of these treatments remains unproved. In addition, the therapeutic use of several of these agents is complicated by significant side effects. Finally, lung and heart-lung transplantation are possible therapeutic choices for a select number of patients with silicosis. This requires early referral and evaluation of these patients.

---

*Not FDA-approved for this indication.
†Investigational drug in the United States.

TABLE 2. Treatment of Complications in Silicosis

Complication	Treatment
Obstructive lung disease	Inhaled β-agonists, inhaled steroids, aminophylline
Bronchitis	Antibiotics (ampicillin, doxycycline, erythromycin)
M. tuberculosis	
Culture positive	Isoniazid (Laniazid), rifampin (Rifadin), pyrazinamide, ethambutol (Myambutol)
Culture negative	Isoniazid
Respiratory failure, pulmonary hypertension, cor pulmonale	Oxygen therapy

HYPERSENSITIVITY PNEUMONITIS
(Extrinsic Allergic Alveolitis)

method of
DEAN A. EMANUEL, M.D.
Marshfield Clinic
Marshfield, Wisconsin

Agricultural workers are exposed to massive amounts of organic dust that may contain large numbers of fungal

TABLE 1. Clinical Features of Organic Dust Toxic Syndrome (ODTS) and Acute Farmer's Lung Disease (FLD)

	ODTS	FLD
Onset	4–8 h	4–12 h
Occurrence	July–October	Winter and spring
Symptoms	Cough, fever, chills, malaise, headache, chest tightness, dyspnea	Cough, fever, chills, dyspnea
Duration	24–48 hours	5 d to weeks
Exposure	Usually massive dust–all exposed develop disease	Minimal—usually individual
X-ray film	Usually normal	Nodular to patchy infiltrate pneumonia
Precipitating antibodies	Usually negative serology	Positive serology
WBC	Leukocytosis to 26,000	Leukocytosis mild

spores and bacterial endotoxins. Dairy farmers, in particular in the upper Midwestern United States and elsewhere in the world, are exposed to large numbers of these products during the winter months while working in closed spaces with poor ventilation. This environment allows inhalation of significant numbers of appropriate-sized (1 to 2 microns) antigenic particles that can be associated with hypersensitivity pneumonitis and/or toxic reactions. Farmer's lung disease and organic dust toxic syndrome are two typical examples. It is important to distinguish between these two illnesses, since their exposures and symptoms are identical but their treatment and eventual outcome are different. Table 1 lists some of these distinguishing characteristics. Table 2 lists rarer examples of hypersensitivity pneumonitis.

Patients who have been exposed to massive amounts of organic dust containing endotoxin will have symptoms similar to those of farmer's lung disease. All individuals so exposed will become ill. Their radiographs, however, are usually normal and they lack precipitins in their blood to the thermophyllic organisms. They will recover in days with no apparent sequelae. The disease is a nonallergic inflammatory systemic response occurring in the airways and alveoli, and it occurs in individuals who have never been exposed to the agent previously. Prior sensitization is not a requirement. The threshold level of endotoxin has been calculated to be 10 to 33 ng/m^3 to induce changes in FEV$_1$.

It should be emphasized that the patient need not be a farmer to develop sensitivity to the thermophyllic group organisms. This type of delayed allergic reaction can also occur in office workers exposed to contaminated air conditioners. The usual victims of exposure to these organisms, however, are dairy farmers who are exposed to moldy forage, whether it be hay or silage. The reaction that is produced is a delayed type of hypersensitivity, often not recognized by patient or physician.

Studies on the long-term effects of exposure to these agents indicate that at least five attacks are necessary before the development of significant pulmonary disease, with pulmonary fibrosis and the consequent pulmonary insufficiency. This is particularly true with farmer's lung disease. At one time it was felt that any patient with this disease should discontinue farming. It has been shown that farmers can continue farming if they are able to change their agricultural practices to avoid further exposure. The use of a disposable mask is advocated, such as the 3-M model 8710 from Minnesota Mining and Manufacturing Company, Minneapolis, Minnesota, which will prevent the inhalation of spores of the 1- to 2-micron size that are a cause of the pulmonary problems.

TREATMENT

Patients who have extensive pulmonary infiltrates as a result of heavy or prolonged exposure may be severely debilitated and require hospitalization, oxygen, fluid therapy, and, on occasion, treatment with corticosteroids. Prednisone, 40 to 60 mg daily for 5 days, then tapering over a 1-month period, will not produce steroid dependence and will result in rapid improvement. Continued use of steroids is to be condemned, since this will not protect the patient from the immunologic response in the lungs and will not prevent the development of progressive disease. Some patients will develop progressive disease with a chronic pulmonary fibrosis, pulmonary insufficiency, and cor pulmonale; the exact reasons for this progressive disease remain undetermined.

The ideal therapy for the patient with hypersensitivity pneumonitis requires removal from the environment to prevent any further inhalation of the offending agent. This requires a detailed history of occupational exposure and, at times, intensive detec-

TABLE 2. Etiology of Hypersensitivity Pneumonitis

Antigen	Antigen Source	Disorders
Micropolyspora faeni	Moldy hay, silage, grain	Farmer's lung
Thermoactinomyces vulgaris	Bagasse (moldy sugar cane), moldy hay	Bagassosis or farmer's lung
Thermoactinomyces vulgaris	Moldy compost	Mushroom worker's lung
Thermoactinomyces candidus	Contaminated humidifier and air conditioning ducts	Humidifier lung and air conditioner lung
Thermoactinomyces viridus	Moldy hay, moldy cocklebur, vineyards, ventilation systems	Vineyard sprayer's lung
Aspergillus fumigatus	Moldy wood chips	Papermill worker's lung
Cryptostroma corticale	Moldy maple logs	Maple bark disease
Animal products		
Pigeon serum protein	Pigeon droppings	Pigeon breeder's lung
Duck protein	Feathers	Duck fever
Turkey protein	Turkey products	Turkey handler's lung
Parrot and budgerigar protein	Bird droppings	Budgerigar fancier's lung
Chicken protein	Chicken products	Feather picker's lung

tive work to determine the etiologic agent. Serologic evidence of the presence of circulating antibodies can often be demonstrated and can usually be obtained in most laboratories, as well as from the Centers for Disease Control in Atlanta. The enzyme-linked immunosorbent assay (ELISA) is one method of providing sensitivity and specificity for the detection of these antibodies.

SINUSITIS

method of
KAY W. CHANG, M.D., and
ANDREW F. INGLIS, JR., M.D.
University of Washington
Seattle, Washington

Sinusitis begins with inflammation of the mucosa of the nasal cavities and paranasal sinuses. Inflammatory edema may produce blockage of the narrow sinus ostia, leading to retained secretions within the sinus cavity. This fluid may or may not become superinfected by bacteria. Therapy is aimed at decreasing inflammation, providing adequate drainage of infected mucus, and sterilizing the sinus cavity. Sinusitis continues to be one of the more common medical problems. In 1993 and 1994, sinus complaints accounted for nearly 25 million office visits to physicians in the United States. The majority of these visits are due to acute sinusitis.

ACUTE BACTERIAL SINUSITIS

It may be difficult to distinguish acute bacterial sinusitis from viral rhinitis. In acute sinusitis, patients present with signs and symptoms of an upper respiratory infection (purulent nasal discharge and congestion) in addition to facial pain or pressure. Fever may be present but is uncommon in bacterial sinusitis. In contrast, viral rhinitis is typically accompanied by systemic symptoms such as fever, generalized aches, and malaise. Viral rhinitis frequently precedes sinusitis, and the two may coexist.

Signs and symptoms often reveal the involved sinus. Toothache or pain over the cheekbone suggests maxillary sinus involvement. Medial canthal pain or pressure and periorbital headache suggest ethmoid involvement. Severe frontal headache and tenderness over the frontal area suggest frontal sinusitis. Severe headache with multiple foci and located at the vertex, retro-orbital, or occipital areas may indicate involvement of the sphenoid sinuses. Acute frontal or sphenoid sinusitis should be viewed as a potential medical emergency and treated aggressively, as severe neurologic complications occur relatively frequently.

Sinusitis is a clinical diagnosis, and routine diagnostic confirmation with radiographs is unnecessary. A clinical diagnosis of sinusitis may be followed up with a fiberoptic intranasal examination. In the hands of a skilled examiner, flexible nasal endoscopy may be used to pinpoint the source of purulence, as well as to identify the condition of the intranasal mucosa. Radiographs should be obtained only when the clinical picture is confusing or when complications are present or suspected. Studies have shown plain sinus x-rays to be unreliable, with both high false-positive and false-negative rates. The most appropriate study is the computed tomography (CT) scan. A screening axial CT scan of the sinuses (which in many centers is similar in price to that of a plain sinus x-ray series) will identify the involved sinuses accurately and is especially appropriate when the presence of frontal or sphenoid sinusitis needs to be confirmed. A full sinus CT with coronal cuts is the technique of choice when delineating anatomy for surgical consideration. Follow-up radiographs to confirm resolution of the sinusitis are generally unnecessary.

The usual bacterial pathogens in acute sinusitis are the same as those causing acute otitis media, namely *Streptococcus pneumoniae*, *Haemophilus influenzae*, *Moraxella catarrhalis*, and *Streptococcus pyogenes*. Appropriate antibiotics for treatment include amoxicillin-clavulanic acid (Augmentin), trimethoprim-sulfamethoxazole (Bactrim, Septra), cefuroxime (Ceftin), loracarbef (Lorabid), clarithromycin (Biaxin), and azithromycin (Zithromax). The widespread prevalence of β-lactamase resistance among these bacteria accounts for the many treatment failures encountered when using amoxicillin and early-generation cephalosporins that do not have activity against many strains of *H. influenzae* and *M. catarrhalis*. Similarly, tetracycline and erythromycin have also been associated with a high rate of treatment failures. New treatment strategies may be necessary as the prevalence of antibiotic-resistant pneumococcus strains increases. A 10-day course of an effective antibiotic will resolve most acute sinus infections. Symptomatic response should occur within 48 to 72 hours. Topical nasal vasoconstrictors such as oxymetazoline (Afrin), and Neosynephrine may aid in shrinking the nasal and sinus mucosa to allow for improved sinus drainage but are not recommended for more than 2 to 3 days because of possible rebound vasodilation. Oral decongestants are of questionable benefit. Nasal saline irrigation may improve mucociliary clearance of inspissated mucopurulent secretions. Antihistamines are generally not recommended because of their drying effect on these secretions.

Patients whose symptoms progress while under treatment may benefit from sinus aspiration (for culture) and lavage, or from surgical drainage.

CHRONIC SINUSITIS

Chronic sinusitis is characterized by persistent, symptomatic mucosal inflammation lasting weeks, months, or years. In general, the symptoms are less severe than those seen in acute sinusitis. The primary complaint is usually nasal discharge or obstruction. Secondary complaints include pain, pressure, headache, and postnasal discharge. Cough may also be present, caused by posterior drainage. Since symptoms are poorly localized and mild, chronic sinusitis may be difficult to recognize. Because the clinical picture may be unclear, and because frequently anatomic anomalies or complications are present, CT scanning is helpful in chronic cases as a diagnostic aid and for guiding therapy.

Initial treatment is similar to that used for acute sinusitis, but usually a more prolonged course (3 weeks or more) of antibiotics is required. Since anaerobic organisms often are implicated in chronic infection, drugs such as clindamycin (Cleocin) or metronidazole (Flagyl) may need to be added to a regimen of one of the antibiotics mentioned earlier. Intranasal cultures are sometimes helpful in this situation to identify the organism and guide antibiotic choice. Because mucosal edema often plays a crucial causative role, therapy aimed at reducing this edema will often be helpful. Intranasal steroids are effective in this setting at reducing mucosal edema, inflammation, and allergic hyperreactivity. Oral steroids are frequently helpful in managing exacerbations.

If aggressive antibiotic therapy fails, a search for underlying causes should be initiated. Any factor impairing the drainage of the sinus may be implicated. Allergies frequently produce mucosal edema and inflammation, which may impair sinus drainage and lead to sinusitis. An allergy evaluation should be considered if symptoms of itchy and runny nose, thin, watery nasal discharge, sneezing, and nasal congestion precede or accompany the symptoms of sinusitis. Anatomic abnormalities such as a deviated nasal septum, a lateralized middle turbinate, polyps, or foreign bodies may also be implicated. The key area that needs to be assessed via CT scan is the ostiomeatal complex, a narrow area in the lateral nasal wall underlying the middle turbinate where the anterior ethmoid, frontal, and maxillary sinuses drain. Minimal anatomic narrowing in this area may lead to sinus obstruction. Rarer diseases such as cystic fibrosis and ciliary dyskinesia impair the normal mucociliary function required to drain the sinus. Immunosuppression from any cause may lead to opportunistic infections.

FUNGAL SINUSITIS

Fungal sinusitis is a special category and can be classified into two types: invasive and noninvasive. Noninvasive fungal sinusitis is an extramucosal, saprophytic colonization that may be further subdivided into allergic and nonallergic or mycetomatous forms.

Allergic fungal sinusitis is usually caused by bipolaris species and produces a clinical picture of nasal obstruction and polyposis, eosinophilia, sinus expansion, and bone erosion. This disease is analogous to allergic bronchopulmonary aspergillosis. Treatment includes surgical drainage and topical and systemic steroids to reduce the inflammatory response.

Noninvasive nonallergic fungal sinusitis may occur in patients who have undergone prolonged adminis-

tration of antibiotics or steroids. These infections are usually caused by *Aspergillus* or *Candida* and result in a fungus ball, or mycetoma, in the sinus cavity without mucosal invasion. Treatment requires drainage of the sinus.

Invasive fungal sinusitis is a much more serious problem that generally occurs in uncontrolled diabetic or immunocompromised patients. *Aspergillus* and *Mucor* are the two most common pathogens. Rapid mucosal invasion occurs and may spread through the bone beyond the sinus into the orbit or cavernous sinus. Intranasal examination reveals necrosis of nasal and sinus mucosa, and CT scan reveals bony invasion. Treatment consists of systemic amphotericin B (Fungizone), with aggressive surgical debridement.

COMPLICATIONS

Complications of sinusitis are caused by the spread of the process beyond the sinus. The most common complication is the spread of infection to orbital structures. This occurs more often in children and usually originates from the ethmoid sinus, which is separated from the orbit by a very thin bone, the lamina papyracea. This infection can progress through several stages. The first is periorbital or preseptal cellulitis, characterized by edema of the eyelids with erythema and fever. There is no proptosis or involvement of the extraocular muscles, and vision is normal. Preseptal cellulitis may progress to orbital cellulitis, with symptoms of proptosis, chemosis, edema, orbital tenderness, and pain. High-dose intravenous antibiotics with careful observation are required. Further progression leads to a subperiosteal or orbital abscess that requires surgical drainage in addition to intravenous antibiotics. A CT scan is almost mandatory to differentiate between these entities.

Mucoceles are mucosa-lined cystic lesions in the paranasal sinuses, which result from chronic inflammation. These lesions expand slowly and can cause bony erosion. Frontal sinus mucoceles present with frontal headache, proptosis, diplopia, and deep periorbital pain. Sphenoethmoidal mucoceles cause subtle symptoms initially. These progress to headache with occipital, vertex, or deep nasal pain; diplopia; visual field abnormalities; and globe displacement. Maxillary sinus mucoceles are usually the asymptomatic cyst or polyp seen in the maxillary sinus on radiographs. Frontal and sphenoethmoidal mucoceles require surgical removal. In contrast, maxillary mucoceles rarely cause symptoms and rarely require therapy.

Occasionally, sinusitis results in osteomyelitis, which generally involves the frontal bone. This requires aggressive treatment, including drainage of the frontal sinus and prolonged high-dose antibiotic therapy.

Rare complications include the orbital apex syndrome, manifested by diminished vision and ophthalmoplegia, and cavernous sinus thrombosis, manifested by bilateral eye findings, high fevers, and meningeal signs. Intracranial extension, including epidural abscess, subdural abscess, brain abscess, and meningitis, requires the appropriate intravenous antibiotics as well as neurosurgical intervention.

STREPTOCOCCAL PHARYNGITIS

method of
LAWRENCE E. SCHWARTZ, M.D., and
ALAN D. TICE, M.D.
Infections Limited
Tacoma, Washington

Sore throat is a common manifestation of many infectious syndromes and a frequent complaint of patients seeking acute medical care. The majority of cases of acute tonsillopharyngitis are caused by viral pathogens, including adenoviruses, enteroviruses, influenza and parainfluenza viruses, and Epstein-Barr virus. Group A beta-hemolytic streptococci (GABHS) are the most common cause of bacterial pharyngitis, with sporadic or epidemic cases due to Groups B, C, and G streptococci. Increasing attention has been given to other bacterial causes of pharyngitis recently, including *Mycoplasma pneumoniae, Chlamydia pneumoniae, Arcanobacterium haemolyticus,* and *Neisseria gonorrhoeae,* but these infections represent only a small percentage of cases of bacterial pharyngitis. A sore throat may also occur in patients with noninfectious illness, such as Behçet's syndrome, Kawasaki disease, or recurrent aphthous stomatitis.

Recommendations vary regarding the evaluation and management of the patient with acute tonsillopharyngitis. The situation is complicated by the fact that a diagnosis of GABHS pharyngitis cannot be made solely based on symptomatology or physical examination. Accurate diagnosis and appropriate treatment of the patient with GABHS infection is important due to the possibility of suppurative sequelae, such as retropharyngeal or peritonsillar abscess, or nonsuppurative sequelae, such as acute rheumatic fever or glomerulonephritis. Indiscriminate treatment of sore throat with antibiotics should be discouraged, particularly in this era of increasingly prevalent drug-resistant bacteria. The following discussion reviews the microbiology and epidemiology of GABHS as well as current diagnostic options and available therapeutic regimens for the patient with acute GABHS tonsillopharyngitis.

THE ORGANISM

Group A streptococci (*Streptococcus pyogenes*) are gram-positive cocci that typically form chains. Most strains form a zone of clear (beta) hemolysis on blood agar around each colony. Differentiation of group A from other hemolytic streptococci is typically done by looking for a zone of inhibition around a bacitracin disk. Group-specific identification of beta-hemolytic streptococci may also be performed, most commonly utilizing a latex agglutination method.

More than 80 types of GABHS have been characterized based on a surface component, the M protein. This protein provokes a serologically distinct immune response and is a major virulence factor, helping the organism evade phagocytosis. Some serotypes are associated with an increased risk of nonsuppurative sequelae following infection with these strains. GABHS have a variety of other surface proteins that enhance virulence, and produce a remarkable number of biologically active extracellular toxins, including streptolysins O and S, erythrogenic toxins A, B, and C, DNAase, and hyaluronidase.

The immune response and host defense against GABHS pharyngitis are not well characterized, but there appears to be an early accumulation of monocytes and neutrophils with subsequent phagocytosis of bacteria. Antibody responses to a type-specific M protein are not detectable for several weeks after an infection and probably serve a protective role against reinfection by the same serotype.

EPIDEMIOLOGY

GABHS are primarily human pathogens and are rarely found in other species. Streptococcal pharyngitis is predominantly a disease of school-age children, with peak incidence occurring between age 5 and 15 years. Infants rarely develop pharyngitis but may develop a purulent rhinitis caused by GABHS known as streptococcosis. Infection is typically more frequent in winter and spring, but sporadic cases occur throughout the year. In cold or temperate climates, approximately one-third of children and 10% of adults who complain of sore throat during the peak winter season are actually infected with GABHS; the remainder of cases are usually viral in origin.

Transmission of GABHS is through close contact and from person to person. The organism is primarily spread through transfer of respiratory secretions or contact with large droplet nuclei containing streptococci. Spread through the air by dust particles or by fomites (environmental objects) does not appear to be involved. Infection among family members or classmates is common. Patients should be considered highly contagious in the acute stage of illness. Treatment with appropriate antibiotics rapidly suppresses growth of GABHS, and the patient may be considered much less contagious after 24 to 48 hours. Carriers of GABHS (to be discussed later) are infectious primarily in the first two weeks after acquisition of the organism. There appears to be little risk of spread after that time.

CLINICAL MANIFESTATIONS

The incubation period is short, with onset of symptoms within 12 hours to 4 days of exposure. Symptoms of GABHS tonsillopharyngitis generally occur suddenly, with the appearance of fever and sore throat. Parents may notice that the child has "bad breath" and that the throat and tonsils are red. The severity of illness may vary from very mild sore throat to severe pharyngitis with toxicity, high fever, nausea, vomiting, and collapse. Headache and abdominal pain are common complaints in children. Many patients will have at least some degree of tender anterior cervical adenopathy. Physical examination will often confirm pharyngitis, with pharyngeal erythema and enlarged tonsils. In 50% to 90% of cases, there is a whitish-yellow exudate over the tonsils or pharynx. It is important to note that unless suppurative sequelae occur, GABHS is a self-limited illness, with symptoms usually subsiding in 3 to 5 days.

DIAGNOSIS

The diagnosis of GABHS pharyngitis has been based on throat culture for many years, and it remains the "gold standard." Attempts to diagnose streptococcal infection based solely on clinical grounds are fraught with error and lead to overtreatment in most cases. Breese and others have developed clinical scoring systems that may be helpful in some cases but generally will have no better than 60% to 70% sensitivity overall. Some clinical features may be helpful in excluding GABHS infection, such as the presence of cough, hoarseness, or conjunctivitis, but these findings are by no means conclusive. The situation is further complicated by the fact that many children are asymptomatic pharyngeal carriers of GABHS, so a positive throat culture result may be seen in a patient with a typical viral pharyngitis. Blood tests are generally not obtained, but leukocytosis is common in GABHS infection, as opposed to many viral etiologies of pharyngitis. The absence of an elevated white blood cell count decreases the likelihood of GABHS as the cause of pharyngitis. C-reactive protein may be elevated in some cases of GABHS but is usually normal with viral infection.

In recent years, rapid diagnostic tests for the detection of group A streptococci have allowed clinicians to make a quick diagnosis of GABHS pharyngitis before the patient leaves the office. While the specificity of most currently available assays is generally better than 90% to 95%, sensitivity is less than optimal. Up to 30% of cases of true GABHS infection will be missed by rapid tests. False-negatives typically occur if the relative numbers of streptococci in the oropharynx are low, or if the throat swab is improperly obtained. False-positives due to chronic carriage of GABHS also present a problem. Whereas these tests facilitate early treatment, this is not clearly a necessary or even desirable approach. Some studies suggest that early antibiotic treatment decreases the development of type-specific immunity and that treatment may be delayed for up to seven to nine days without any increase in risk of nonsuppurative sequelae such as rheumatic fever. The common practice of obtaining a throat culture and withholding treatment until the result is known can be justified early in the course of disease. However, it is also true that early treatment leads to more rapid resolution of symptoms and may limit spread of GABHS to others. A reasonable approach is to treat patients with positive rapid antigen assays and obtain throat cultures on patients with a negative test, deferring treatment until the culture results are known. Routine follow-up throat cultures are no longer recommended.

THERAPY

Treatment of GABHS pharyngitis reduces the duration of symptoms, decreases the risk of suppurative and nonsuppurative sequelae, and limits the spread of illness to others. Although GABHS are susceptible to a variety of antimicrobials, penicillin remains the drug of choice in nonallergic individuals, based both on proven efficacy and low cost. Recent reports suggesting that penicillin has become less effective in eradicating GABHS from the pharynx have appeared, but this has not been substantiated. Speculation that treatment failures occur due to beta-lactamase production by oropharyngeal flora or because penicillin tolerance occurs in some strains of group A streptococci has been difficult to prove; published studies have provided conflicting results. The likely clinical significance of these problems is minor. By far the most common reason for therapeutic failure is noncompliance. Although most patients will improve

symptomatically within 24 to 48 hours of beginning treatment, complete eradication of GABHS from the pharynx is difficult and has led to recommendations for a full 10-day course of therapy. Many patients will discontinue treatment after they feel well, typically within three to four days. Re-exposure to friends or family members who are infected may also explain apparent treatment failures.

A variety of other agents have efficacy in the treatment of GABHS pharyngitis and may be useful when concerns exist about compliance, bacterial copathogenicity (beta-lactamase production by oral flora), penicillin tolerance, or in the face of treatment failure. These will be discussed next and are listed in Table 1. Inappropriate agents for treatment include sulfonamides (including trimethoprim-sulfamethoxazole [Bactrim, Septra]) and tetracyclines, which are not active enough against GABHS.

Penicillins

Oral penicillin V has traditionally been used to treat group A streptococcal infections. Twice-daily dosing is as efficacious as more frequent three or four times a day dosing in eradication of GABHS. Decreased dosing frequency clearly enhances patient compliance. Amoxicillin or ampicillin, while no more active in vitro then penicillin, is an acceptable alternative and may be more palatable than penicillin V for patients receiving an oral suspension. When concern exists about patient compliance or follow-up, a single dose of intramuscular benzathine G is appropriate. This is also the preferred strategy for treatment of epidemic infections due to GABHS. Amoxicillin/clavulanate (Augmentin) is generally not indicated unless concerns about bacterial copathogenicity exist; diarrhea is also a common side effect, making this a less attractive treatment option.

Macrolides

Erythromycin has long been advocated as the best alternative for patients with penicillin allergy or sensitivity who require treatment of GABHS infection. However, it has a higher failure rate than beta-lactam agents, and some strains of GABHS are resistant. Gastrointestinal (GI) side effects also occur frequently and lead to early discontinuation of therapy. Clarithromycin (Biaxin) is a new macrolide with excellent activity against GABHS; it allows the convenience of twice-daily dosing and has a much lower incidence of GI intolerance than erythromycin. Azithromycin (Zithromax) is an azalide drug with a long half-life; this agent may be given once daily for five days with equivalent efficacy to a ten-day treatment course of penicillin for GABHS pharyngitis. Both clarithromycin and azithromycin are available in an oral suspension and should be considered good alternatives to erythromycin in treatment of the penicillin-allergic patient with streptococcal pharyngitis.

TABLE 1. **Antibiotic Dosing for GABHS Pharyngitis***

Antibiotic	Child < 40 Pounds	Adults and Children > 40 Pounds
Penicillin VK	25–50 mg/kg/d divided bid	500 mg bid
Amoxicillin	20–40 mg/kg/d divided tid	500 mg bid
Cephalexin (Keflex)	25–50 mg/kg/d divided bid	250 mg qid
Cefadroxil (Duricef)	30 mg/kg/d qd	1 gm qd
Cefaclor (Ceclor)	20 mg/kg/d divided bid	250 mg tid
Cefuroxime axetil (Ceftin)	20 mg/kg/d divided bid	250 mg bid
Cefprozil (Cefzil)	15 mg/kg/d divided bid	500 mg qd
Cefpodoxime (Vantin)	10 mg/kg/d divided bid	100 mg bid
Loracarbef (Lorabid)	15 mg/kg/d divided bid	200 mg bid
Erythromycin estolate (Ilosone)	40 mg/kg/d divided bid	500 mg bid
Clarithromycin (Biaxin)	15 mg/kg/d divided bid	250 mg bid
Azithromycin (Zithromax)	12 mg/kg/d qd for 5 d	500 mg on day 1, 250 mg qd days 2–5
Clindamycin (Cleocin)	20 mg/kg/d divided tid	150 mg tid

*All treatment courses are 10 days unless otherwise specified.

Cephalosporins

Multiple clinical trials have demonstrated that the majority of currently available oral cephalosporins are at least as effective as penicillin in treatment of GABHS pharyngitis and in many cases have superior rates of clinical and bacteriologic cure. Many of these agents are resistant to a variety of beta-lactamases, eliminating concerns about bacterial copathogenicity. Cephalexin (Keflex) and cefadroxil (Duricef) are commonly prescribed agents; the former has the advantage of low cost, the latter has the advantage of once-daily dosing. Second-generation agents such as cefaclor (Ceclor), and cefuroxime (Ceftin), are also quite effective, but cefaclor may have a greater incidence of adverse side effects such as rash or serum sickness. Recently a variety of novel agents, including loracarbef (Lorabid), cefpodoxime (Vantin), and cefprozil (Cefzil), have been approved by the Food and Drug Administration. These agents are well tolerated and are usually dosed twice daily. Cefprozil has been shown to be efficacious in adults with GABHS pharyngitis when given once a day. Most oral cephalosporins are quite expensive and should generally be considered for use only when a patient has failed treatment with a standard penicillin regimen. A complete list of currently available cephalosporins and dosing regimens is included in Table 1.

RECURRENT STREPTOCOCCAL PHARYNGITIS AND THE CARRIER STATE

Patients who have persistently positive throat cultures for GABHS often provide a dilemma for practicing physicians; if this occurs in the setting of clinical pharyngitis, there is no easy way to determine whether the patient has a refractory group A streptococcus infection or is a chronic carrier of GABHS with a concomitant viral pharyngitis. The carrier state is a puzzling phenomenon in which patients harbor the organism for long periods of time without developing an immune response. Carriers appear to be at low risk for development of rheumatic fever. Fortunately, spread of GABHS from carriers to close contacts is rare.

Patients who fail to improve rapidly on therapy or have a prompt recrudescence of symptoms following completion of a treatment course and have persistently positive throat cultures should be retreated. Retreatment with penicillin is inappropriate. Alternative agents such as cephalosporins or macrolides should be used. Other reasons for treatment failure, such as noncompliance or intrafamilial spread, should be considered. In some cases, culture of family members and treatment of positive results are indicated. If the throat culture remains positive after a second course of therapy, the benefit of more treatment is doubtful. However, if the patient is a persistent carrier and typically has frequent episodes of pharyngitis, interpretation of throat culture results will be difficult. In this setting, attempts at eradication of the carrier state can be considered. Clindamycin (Cleocin) has been demonstrated to be quite effective in this setting, although GI intolerance and concerns about increased risk of antibiotic-associated colitis have limited its use. A combined regimen of penicillin and rifampin (Rifadin), has also been shown to be effective at eradication of the carrier state.

TUBERCULOSIS AND NONTUBERCULOUS MYCOBACTERIAL DISEASES

method of
KEVIN D. MAUPIN, M.D.,
WILLIAM C. BAILEY, M.D., and
NANCY E. DUNLAP, M.D., PH.D.
University of Alabama at Birmingham
Birmingham, Alabama

TUBERCULOSIS

Tuberculosis (TB) remains an important cause of disease in the United States and throughout the world. The persistence of tuberculosis in the United States has been due to four major factors. The first factor is the emergence of human immunodeficiency virus (HIV/AIDS). Individuals who are infected with HIV are more susceptible to both *Mycobacterium tuberculosis* (MTB) infection and progression to MTB disease. Second, the immigration of people from areas where there is a high prevalence of tuberculosis has resulted in increased numbers of cases within the United States. Third, poverty, homelessness, and substance abuse have resulted in increased MTB transmission within these populations. And last, decreased health care funding with deterioration in the health care system has contributed to poor adherence to therapy and development of resistant strains of MTB. Because of these four factors, the transmission of drug-resistant strains of MTB has increased and, therefore, the initial recommendation for chemotherapeutic intervention in the treatment of tuberculosis has changed.

Diagnosis

Correctly diagnosing TB requires understanding of disease presentations and interpretation of diagnostic tests. Along with the medical history and physical examination, Mantoux's tuberculin skin test, chest radiograph, and sputum smear and culture are useful in the evaluation of a person for tuberculosis. It is important to elicit a history of tuberculosis exposure, infection, or disease, and risk factors for disease. Determining whether the patient has an increased opportunity for becoming infected with MTB is important in the exposure history. Close contacts of TB cases, individuals born in areas of the world where tuberculosis is common, persons who live or spend time in certain facilities (nursing homes, correctional institutions, homeless shelters, drug treatment centers), intravenous drug abusers, HIV-infected persons, and elderly people are at increased risk for TB infection. If infected with MTB, certain groups are more likely to progress to TB disease. The most important risk factor for this development is HIV infection. Individuals who have been recently infected with MTB are also at increased risk for progression to TB disease. Certain medical conditions such as diabetes mellitus, cancer of the head and neck, hematologic and reticuloendothelial diseases, immunosuppressive therapy, prolonged corticosteroid therapy, intestinal bypass or gastrectomy, silicosis, and end-stage renal disease are also risk factors for progression to TB disease. Symptoms of TB disease include a prolonged and productive cough, fever, chills, night sweats, chest pain, fatigue, hemoptysis, and weight loss.

The physical examination, although very important, will not confirm or rule out the diagnosis of TB. However, an assessment of the patient's physical condition is necessary in the treatment plan of the patient. Mantoux skin testing, although not diagnostic, is highly indicative of tuberculosis infection. Administration of the test is by an intradermal injection of 0.1 mL containing 5 tuberculin units of purified protein derivative (PPD) with a tuberculin syringe. The test is read at 48 to 72 hours after the PPD injection. The size of the induration, not erythema, is the important variable with this test. Table 1 lists the size of induration suggesting TB infection in different population groups. A negative reaction to the PPD does not rule out disease. Overwhelming miliary or pulmonary TB infection, immunosuppression, HIV infection, overwhelming viral infection, Hodgkin's disease, sarcoidosis, and live-virus vaccination may cause a negative PPD when infection is present. Also, a patient does not convert to a PPD-positive skin test for 10 to 12 weeks after TB infection. Therefore, a PPD may be falsely negative if administered prior to 10 weeks after exposure. False-positive PPD skin tests may also occur since antigens that appear in the PPD preparation are shared with other mycobacteria. These cross-reactions tend to result in smaller areas of induration than with true MTB infections but may cause confusion in interpreting a PPD test in areas of the world where nontuberculous mycobacteria are common. The chest radiograph is never diagnostic of tuberculosis. However, it is useful for ruling out pulmonary tuberculosis in persons with a positive PPD reaction.

Collection and examination of clinical specimens for MTB are very important in diagnosis of tuberculosis. Three sputum specimens in patients with suspected pulmonary tuberculosis should be collected and sent for acid-fast staining and mycobacterial culture. In some instances it may be useful to induce sputum with saline inhalation. Bronchoscopy or gastric lavage may be needed in patients with poor cough. In suspected cases of extrapulmonary tuberculosis, specimens collected directly from the suspected site (biopsy, cerebrospinal fluid, and so on), are necessary for diagnosis. Identification of the species can usually take 2 to 3 weeks, with the isolation taking 6 to 12 weeks.

Management

Report all suspected cases of TB disease to local public health officials as soon as possible. Start ther-

TABLE 1. **Positive PPD Reaction**

Greater than or equal to 5 mm

Confirmed or suspected HIV infection
Intravenous drug user with indeterminate HIV status
Close contacts of TB cases
Chest radiograph suggestive of previous TB disease

Greater than or equal to 10 mm

Intravenous drug user, HIV-negative
Long-term-care facility occupants
Age <4 yr
Groups with high prevalence for TB infection
Medically underserved

Greater than or equal to 15 mm

No known risk factors

apy immediately in a suspected case of TB disease. It is not necessary to await the results of bacteriologic studies. Waiting for results to start treatment will increase the time that the case will be infectious and thus increase the risk of TB transmission to others. Treat suspected cases of tuberculosis with multiple drugs to prevent development of resistant strains of tuberculosis. Directly observed therapy (DOT) is the standard method of administering treatment of all suspected cases of tuberculosis. DOT decreases nonadherence, a major factor in the development of multi-drug resistance tuberculosis. Continued evaluations of the patient's clinical course, difficulties with the medications, and follow-up of the bacteriologic studies and radiographs are necessary components of DOT. A contact investigation should be performed by local health departments on every case of TB. Contacts of a case that are infected with MTB but do not have TB disease can be identified with Mantoux's PPD skin testing. Chest radiographs, to rule out TB disease, should be obtained for all patients with positive PPD skin tests prior to initiation of preventive therapy.

Specific Antituberculosis Agents

Five standard first-line drugs are used in the treatment of tuberculosis: isoniazid (INH), rifampin (RIF), ethambutol (EMB), pyrazinamide (PZA), and streptomycin (SM). It is necessary to know the standard dosage and adverse reactions caused by these drugs (Tables 2 and 3). Patients should be evaluated at least monthly for adverse reactions. It is helpful to have a baseline measurement of hepatic enzymes, bilirubin, complete blood count with platelets, serum creatinine, and uric acid prior to initiating antituberculous drugs. If ethambutol is included in the regimen, visual acuity and red-green color perception should be evaluated. Hearing tests should be performed prior to initiation of streptomycin.

Isoniazid (INH) is metabolized by the liver and is bactericidal. It is an important drug in the management of TB because it can be given orally, is low in cost, and can be used in twice or three times weekly regimens. INH may cause hepatitis and peripheral neuropathy. The risk of hepatitis from INH increases with age and alcohol consumption. Peripheral neuropathy is most prominent in alcoholics and pregnant women and can usually be prevented by the daily administration of pyridoxine (10 mg orally per day). The usual daily dose of INH is 300 mg (or 5 mg per

TABLE 3. First-Line Antituberculosis Drugs

	Adverse Reactions	Monitoring
Isoniazid	Hepatitis, peripheral neuropathy, hypersensitivity, rash	Baseline liver enzymes; repeat if abnormal, high risk, or symptomatic
Rifampin	Hepatitis, thrombocytopenia, rash, febrile reaction, myalgia	Baseline CBC, platelets, and liver enzymes; repeat if abnormal, adverse reaction, or symptomatic
Pyrazinamide	GI upset, hepatitis, rash, arthralgia, gout	Baseline liver enzymes and uric acid; repeat if abnormal, adverse reaction, or symptomatic
Ethambutol	Optic neuritis	Baseline and monthly visual acuity and color vision
Streptomycin	Renal failure, ototoxicity	Baseline hearing and kidney function; repeat if adverse reaction or symptomatic

kg); the twice or three times weekly dosage must be increased to 900 mg (or 15 mg per kg).

Rifampin (RIF) (Rifadin) is bactericidal and metabolized by the liver. RIF is an extremely potent antituberculous agent that is usually well tolerated and can be given orally. It colors the body fluids orange and may permanently discolor soft contact lenses. The principal adverse reactions with RIF are hepatitis and thrombocytopenia. RIF interacts with methadone and oral contraceptives. The usual daily dose of RIF is 600 mg (or 10 mg per kg). Unlike the other first-line agents, RIF requires no adjustment of the dosage when administered twice or three times weekly.

Pyrazinamide (PZA) is a bactericidal agent that can be given orally. It can cause hepatitis, although it is metabolized in the kidneys. The usual daily dose of PZA is approximately 1.5 grams (15 to 30 mg per kg). Dosage is increased to 50 to 70 mg/kg when PZA is given twice or three times weekly. PZA is important early in therapy to decrease the length of chemotherapy.

Ethambutol (EMB) (Myambutol) is the only bacteriostatic agent of the first-line drugs. EMB is excreted through the kidneys and therefore the dosage must be reduced in patients with renal failure. It can cause optic neuritis, and its use is discouraged in children unable to be monitored for changes in vision unless it is needed in the treatment of multidrug-resistant TB. The usual daily dose of EMB is 15 mg per kg. When given two or three times a week, it requires an increased dosage to 50 mg per kg or 30 mg per kg, respectively.

Streptomycin (SM), an aminoglycoside, must be given parenterally. It is metabolized in the kidneys and, like other aminoglycosides, can cause renal toxicity and ototoxicity. The usual daily dose is 0.75 to

TABLE 2. Dosage of First-Line Antituberculosis Drugs

	Daily Therapy	2× Week	3× Week
Isoniazid (mg)	300	900	900
Rifampin (Rifadin) (mg)	600	600	600
Pyrazinamide (mg)	15–30	50–70	50–70
Streptomycin (mg/kg)	10–20	25–30	25–30
Ethambutol (Myambutol) (mg/kg)	15–25	50	25–30

1.0 grams (or 10 to 20 mg per kg). If it is necessary to give SM to elderly patients or those with renal dysfunction, reduce the dose. SM can be given twice or three times weekly.

Preventive Therapy

Preventive therapy for TB infection can prevent progression to TB disease. In patients with a positive PPD skin test, it is vital to rule out TB disease prior to starting preventive therapy.

Unless there is a suspicion of resistance or a contraindication to its use, INH is the drug of choice for preventive therapy. Administer INH, daily or twice or three times weekly, for 6 months in adults, 12 months in HIV-infected persons, and 6 to 9 months in children. If there is a suspicion of INH-resistant tuberculosis, RIF is then the drug of choice. Patients should be followed at least monthly for adverse reactions and nonadherence to therapy.

Treatment of Tuberculosis Disease

TB disease must be treated with multiple drugs to which the organism is susceptible. Administer four drugs—INH, RIF, PZA, and EMB or SM—unless there is little possibility of drug resistance. In circumstances in which resistance to both INH and RIF is possible, a five- or six-drug regimen may be needed until the results of drug susceptibility on the specific MTB organism are available. If the risk of resistance is low, the three-drug regimen with INH, RIF, and PZA can be used. If the patient has not been previously treated for tuberculosis and the MTB organisms are susceptible to all the drugs, a 6-month treatment regimen with INH/RIF/PZA and EMB or SM for the first two months, followed by INH/RIF for the last 4 months, is usually both effective and safe. DOT should be considered in all cases of tuberculosis. Medications can be given daily, or intermittently with twice or three times weekly regimens. Intermittent regimens are administered according to the following schedules:

1. Treat daily with the four drugs for 8 weeks, then, if the TB is susceptible, follow with 16 weeks of INH and RIF at two or three times a week.
2. Treat with four drugs daily for 2 weeks, then twice weekly to complete a full 2 months of therapy with four drugs. Follow with twice-weekly therapy of INH and RIF for 16 weeks.
3. Treat with four drugs three times a week for the entire 6 months.

For those patients who cannot tolerate PZA, a 9-month regimen of INH and RIF is effective. EMB or SM should initially be included in this regimen until the susceptibility of *M. tuberculosis* is known. In the HIV patient, prolong treatment if the clinical or bacteriologic course deems it necessary.

Extrapulmonary tuberculosis should respond to the same regimen as that for pulmonary tuberculosis. Exceptions to the rule are miliary, meningeal, bone, and joint tuberculosis in children. These infections usually require at least 12 months of treatment. Exclude SM from the regimen in pregnant women because of possible ototoxicity in the fetus. A small amount of the drugs passes into breast milk; however, it is not necessary to stop breast-feeding if the mother is taking the standard antituberculous medications.

With MTB disease that is resistant to standard antituberculous drugs or in patients who have intolerance to medication, the treatment of tuberculosis is much more difficult. At least two bactericidal drugs to which the organism is susceptible should be used. Never add a single drug to a failing drug regimen. If a nonstandard drug regimen must be used, consultation with experts in the treatment of tuberculosis should be strongly considered. All treatment of tuberculosis should be given in conjunction with the local health department.

NONTUBERCULOUS MYCOBACTERIAL INFECTIONS

The nontuberculous mycobacterial (NTM) infections have taken on greater importance in human disease in recent years. The HIV population, with its increased susceptibility to infections, is a major reason for an increase in the significance of the NTM infections. These bacteria are present naturally in soil and water. Rarely is infection by human-to-human contact. The NTM infections most commonly causing disease are *Mycobacterium avium* complex (MAC) and *M. kansasii*. HIV-infected persons, persons on immunosuppressive therapy, and immunocompetent persons with pulmonary disease are the groups most susceptible to the NTM infections. Furthermore, there is an increase in the risk of disseminated disease in the HIV-infected population.

Diagnosis of NTM disease is made by culture. However, a positive culture for NTM may represent colonization and not disease. A positive PPD of 5 to 10 mm may occur and is due to weak cross-reactivity between the NTMs and MTB species. Chest radiographs of patients with disease caused by NTMs and MTB may be similar in appearance. Because MTB and NTM organisms are also indistinguishable on acid-fast staining, treatment with multiple antituberculous drugs should be administered until the species identification is reported so that transmission of MTB will be limited. Unfortunately, many of the NTM species are resistant to antituberculous agents as well as to many commonly used antibiotics. Also, it is frequently difficult to determine whether the organism is causing disease or just colonizing the host. Treatment duration varies depending on the site of the infection and the species involved.

Mycobacterium avium Complex Infection

Mycobacterium avium complex (MAC) disease causes disease in the lung, skin, and soft tissues. It may be associated with prosthetic devices or catheters. In immunosuppressed individuals, MAC may result in disseminated disease. MAC infections involving the pulmonary system have been recognized in the patient with chronic lung disease or hematologic malignancy for many years. However, disseminated MAC is now the most common bacterial infection seen in AIDS patients. This infection is seen mainly in patients with CD4+ lymphocyte counts of less than 100 per mm^3. Night sweats, fever, weight loss, fatigue, and gastrointestinal complaints are common in disseminated MAC.

MAC is resistant to many antituberculosis agents. Treatment of MAC infections should include at least two to four drugs for a period of 18 to 24 months. Treatment should continue for 12 months after culture conversion. Ethambutol (Myambutol), clarithromycin (Biaxin), azithromycin (Zithromax), ciprofloxacin* (Cipro), rifabutin (Mycobutin), rifampin (Rifadin), amikacin* (Amikin), and clofazimine* (Lamprene) are possible drug choices. Rifampin, 600 mg per day; ethambutol, 15 mg per kg per day; azithromycin, 500 mg per day, plus clarithromycin, 1000 mg per day, is a reasonable initial regimen. Streptomycin 1 gram two to three times a week for a total of 40 grams, may improve outcome. Surgical excision is the treatment of choice for MAC lymphadenitis. The treatment for a MAC catheter infection is removal of the catheter. Treatment of MAC infection in the HIV patient is lifelong. Prophylaxis for HIV patients with a CD4+ lymphocyte count less than 100 per mm^3 with rifabutin (300 mg per day) may be considered, but only after MTB disease or active MAC infection is excluded.

M. kansasii Infection

M. kansasii is second only to MAC among the NTMs as a cause of disease. *M. kansasii* infections

---

*Not FDA-approved for this indication.

are associated with lymphadenitis, pulmonary, and disseminated disease. Clinically, infection is more closely related to *M. tuberculosis* than to the other NTMs. In the immunocompetent patient, disease usually involves the pulmonary system. However, in the HIV-infected population, it can occur as a disseminated or a pulmonary infection. *M. kansasii* is susceptible to most antituberculosis agents. A reasonable treatment regimen for pulmonary *M. kansasii* is with isoniazid, 300 mg per day; rifampicin, 600 mg per day; and ethambutol, 15 mg per kg per day for at least 18 months. Treatment of lymphadenitis is with surgical excision. Treatment of *M. kansasii* infection is usually successful, and relapse is rare.

Other NTM Infections

M. fortuitum and *M. chelonae* are rapidly growing mycobacteria. Disease is associated with lymphadenitis and with pulmonary, postoperative, skin and soft tissue, disseminated, otologic, foreign body, and catheter-associated infection. Sputum isolation is more commonly due to colonization than to infection. Treatment is variable and depends on the clinical symptoms. Amikacin, tobramycin, erythromycin, clarithromycin, fluoroquinolones, sulfonamides, cefoxitin, imipenem, and doxycycline are agents to be considered in the treatment regimen.

M. xenopi disease is associated with pulmonary infections and with contaminated water supplies. Agents active against *M. xenopi* include rifampin, ethambutol, and streptomycin.

M. malmoense is a rare cause of disease in humans. Unlike most mycobacteria, its incidence of infection is not increased in the HIV population. Disease is associated with lymphadenitis and pulmonary infection. Rifampin, ethambutol, and streptomycin are all active against *M. malmoense*.

ACQUIRED DISEASES OF THE AORTA

method of
D. PRESTON FLANIGAN, M.D.
University of California, Irvine
Irvine, California

There are actually only a few acquired diseases of the aorta. Many diseases affect the aortic branches but they do not involve the aorta itself, and many diseases that do affect the aorta are congenital rather than acquired in nature. The most common acquired diseases of the aorta include occlusive disease, aneurysmal disease, and aortic dissection. Although occlusive disease is caused primarily by atherosclerosis, acute occlusion may occur from thrombosis or embolization from the heart or from the more proximal aorta. Occlusive disease occasionally may be caused by aortitis. Aneurysmal disease also is caused most commonly by atherosclerosis but may follow trauma or aortic infection. Aortic dissection in the absence of congenital disease is usually associated with severe hypertension.

OCCLUSIVE DISEASE OF THE AORTA

Patients with lesser degrees of occlusive disease of the aorta may not be symptomatic, but, as the aorta is further narrowed, intermittent claudication will begin if the patient is sufficiently active. Symptoms more severe than claudication (rest pain, ischemic ulcer, or gangrene) usually do not occur in the absence of concomitant infrainguinal arterial occlusive disease unless embolization or particularly poor collateralization has occurred. Impotence may occasionally accompany claudication as a result of terminal aortic occlusion or severe stenosis (Leriche's syndrome). In most cases the atherosclerotic process also involves the iliac arteries.

Atherosclerosis

Occlusive disease of the aorta is caused almost exclusively by atherosclerosis. The process is generally limited to the infrarenal aorta, where symptoms are usually the direct result of obstruction of blood flow. Occasionally atherosclerosis will affect the suprarenal aorta, but in this situation symptoms are more often due to embolization of thrombus which forms on the atherosclerotic plaque rather than from local obstruction of blood flow. Atherosclerotic aortic plaques also may cause branch artery occlusive problems as the aortic plaque may involve the orifices of aortic branches. This situation is commonly seen in the aortic arch and at the level of the mesenteric and renal arteries. Branch artery occlusion as a result of aortic plaques can cause stroke, mesenteric ischemia, and renovascular hypertension. Most patients with aortic atherosclerosis, however, usually have no symptoms at all and require no therapy other than risk factor modification once the disease is recognized. Physical findings in patients with aortic occlusive disease include decreased or absent femoral pulses, lower extremity hair loss, thin skin, and dystrophic nails.

Many patients with intermittent claudication can be managed without surgery. Medical therapy consists of exercise, if not contraindicated, cessation of smoking, control of serum lipids, weight loss if the patient is overweight, and occasionally pharmacologic therapy. Cessation of smoking has clearly been shown to improve outcome in patients with intermittent claudication. Exercise, if performed regularly, and weight loss have been shown to increase walking distance. Many studies have now shown regression of atherosclerotic plaque in hyperlipemic patients when serum lipids are controlled. In many patients lipids can be controlled by diet alone, but many patients will require lipid-lowering medications selected in accordance with their specific lipid abnormality. Pentoxifylline (Trental) orally, 400 mg three times a day, has been shown to increase walking distance as much as 25%, although in many patients this drug has no effect.

In most patients exercise, medication, and risk factor modification will do more to retard progression than to improve symptoms. Significant symptomatic improvement can currently be achieved only by endovascular or surgical means. The most effective invasive interventions include balloon angioplasty, endarterectomy, and bypass procedures.

In properly selected patients, iliac angioplasty now gives results that approach those achieved by surgical procedures. Screening duplex ultrasound followed by arteriography when appropriate will identify those patients who are good candidates for angioplasty. Good candidates have stenosis rather than occlusion, shorter lesions, and fewer lesions. Angioplasty works best in the iliac arteries: angioplasty of the aorta itself has only been performed on a limited basis and is not yet considered standard treatment.

Surgical means of treating aortic atherosclerosis include endarterectomy and bypass. Endarterectomy is usually employed only when the disease process is truly limited to the aorta and proximal common iliac arteries. Most surgeons, even in this situation, prefer bypass because of similar results and ease of application. Most patients, because of associated iliac artery atherosclerosis, will require an aortic bifurcation graft from the infrarenal aorta to the femoral arteries. When aortic branch occlusion requires intervention, branch vessel endarterectomy or bypass may be combined with aortic endarterectomy or bypass. Currently, endovascular grafts delivered via the femoral arteries are being tested in both patients with occlusive disease and aneurysmal disease of the aorta.

In the absence of infrainguinal arterial occlusive disease, aortoiliac revascularization is usually curative. Even when infrainguinal disease is present, the amount of improvement from aortoiliac revascularization is often sufficient to preclude the need for more distal revascularization.

Some patients are too ill from co-morbid conditions to undergo a major intra-abdominal surgical procedure, or such a procedure may be contraindicated by previous pelvic irradiation, abdominal wall stomas, or multiple previous intra-abdominal procedures. In these situations axillofemoral bypass or axillobifemoral bypass can be utilized. This approach also is used commonly for lower extremity revascularization in the treatment of aortic infection.

Results of invasive procedures for the treatment of aortic occlusive disease are quite good. Aorto-bifemoral bypass and aortoiliac endarterectomy patency rates are usually reported as greater than 90% at 5 years postoperatively. Patency for axillobifemoral bypass is less, at about 50% to 70% at 5 years, and is similar to the results achieved from iliac angioplasty. However, longevity following these procedures is poor (25% to 35% mortality at 5 years) due to underlying coronary artery disease.

Acute Aortic Occlusion

Acute occlusion of the aorta is caused by either aortic thrombosis on top of pre-existing aortic plaque or from embolization. The symptoms include lower extremity pain, weakness, coldness, paralysis, anesthesia, and pallor associated with absent lower extremity pulses to palpation. The legs and lower abdomen may appear mottled. This condition is a true emergency as it is usually fatal if untreated.

If symptoms are mild in the early course of therapy, an attempt at thrombolytic therapy may be justified, especially if the etiology is thought to be thrombotic. Restoration of aortic flow coupled with anticoagulation may allow for a planned elective aortic surgical procedure to correct the underlying aortic problem. In most cases, however, symptoms are acute and severe and usually require immediate surgical intervention. In the case of embolization, transfemoral balloon embolectomy may be curative. When the etiology is thrombosis, emergency aortobifemoral bypass or axillobifemoral bypass is often required. Mortality rates in excess of 50% are not uncommonly reported. Patients with embolic disease often require lifelong anticoagulation to reduce the risk of re-embolization.

Aortitis

The most common form of aortitis is Takayasu's aortoarteritis. This disease is an autoimmune process that primarily affects the branches of the aortic arch but can involve the aorta with both occlusive (coarctation) and, less commonly, aneurysmal disease. The abdominal aorta and its branches are less commonly affected. Most patients are women less than 30 years of age. The symptoms in the acute phase include fever, malaise, and tachycardia usually associated with an elevated erythrocyte sedimentation rate. Late symptoms are those relative to the specific vessels stenosed by the inflammatory process. Steroids are the preferred treatment in the acute phase and can actually lead to improved circulation as the receding inflammatory process allows for a less stenotic arterial lumen. Surgical therapy is more successful if applied during a quiescent phase. Bypass from and to uninvolved areas is the procedure of choice, as endarterectomy generally does not work well in the treatment of this disease.

ANEURYSMAL DISEASE

Ninety to 95% of aortic aneurysms are located below the renal arteries; iliac artery involvement is common. The most common cause of aortic aneurysm is atherosclerosis; a genetic pattern has been identified in some families. Other acquired causes include infection and trauma. Any patient with symptoms arising from aneurysm expansion or rupture requires immediate surgical intervention. Fortunately, most patients have aneurysm repair on an elective basis. The primary indication for surgical repair of an asymptomatic aortic aneurysm is size. For most areas of the aorta it has been shown that aneurysms greater than 5 cm in maximal transverse diameter should be repaired. Below this size, rupture is rare. Longitudinal studies have shown that aneurysms enlarge at an average rate of 4 mm per year. During the course of most of these studies (3 to 5 years), 80% of aneurysms enlarged. When an aneurysm is 4 to 5 cm in diameter and the patient is otherwise healthy, surgical repair is probably indicated. When a patient has numerous co-morbid conditions that increase the surgical risk, it is often preferable to observe aortic aneurysms that are larger, especially when the aneurysm is located in the chest or suprarenal abdominal aorta. Patients selected for observation should have an ultrasound or computed tomography (CT) scan of the aneurysm every 6 to 12 months to monitor size. Patients with aortic aneurysm and/or atherosclerotic occlusive disease have an increased incidence of atherosclerotic disease affecting other crucial arteries, such as the carotid and coronary vessels; thus, risk factor modification is the mainstay of nonsurgical therapy.

Aneurysms of the ascending aorta are not common. In general, surgical repair is indicated for aneurysms of 5.5 to 6 cm in diameter or larger. Cardiopulmonary bypass is required and, for proximal aneurysms, aortic valve replacement and coronary revascularization may be necessary. Operative mortality is approximately 10%.

Repair of aortic arch aneurysms requires cardiac arrest and profound hypothermia. Operative mortality approaches 15%, and stroke occurs in up to 10% of patients.

Descending aortic aneurysm repair does not require cardiopulmonary bypass, but many surgeons have recommended its use despite published data showing equivalent results when it is not used. Repair of descending aortic aneurysms carries an approximate 10% risk of spinal cord ischemia and paralysis.

Thoracoabdominal aneurysms vary in their extent and number of branch vessels involved. The most serious complications include death, paraplegia, hemorrhage, and renal failure. Surgical repair usually involves the inclusion technique in which, after opening the aneurysm, a tube graft is sewn to the aorta at the proximal aneurysm neck. Side holes are cut along the graft, and the orifices of the branch vessels are sewn to the graft. It is probably important to include at least one set of intercostal arteries as well. Finally, the aorta at the distal aneurysm neck is anastomosed to the graft. Numerous new techniques have been developed to try to avoid spinal cord and visceral ischemia, including intercostal/lumbar replantation, spinal cord drainage, and cardiopulmonary bypass through the femoral vessels. Recently the use of prior axillofemoral bypass has been shown to be beneficial. Operative mortality for thoracoabdominal aneurysm repair is approximately 5% to 10%. Repair of aneurysms involving the descending thoracic and visceral abdominal aorta is associated with a 20% paraplegia rate, however.

Infrarenal aortic aneurysms are repaired with either an aortic tube graft or a bifurcation graft, depending on the extent of aneurysmal and occlusive disease involving the iliac vessels. Replantation of branch vessels is rarely required; the risk of paraplegia is extremely rare. When there is concern regarding the circulation to the large bowel, replantation of the inferior mesenteric artery is performed. Elective surgical repair of infrarenal aortic aneurysms can now be accomplished with less than a 3% operative mortality rate. However, operative mortality for ruptured infrarenal aortic aneurysms remains between 40% and 50% in most reports. Overall mortality from rupture is in excess of 90%. These poor results further emphasize the need for early elective repair of aortic aneurysms.

AORTIC DISSECTION

Aortic dissection is a highly lethal condition due to the complications of rupture and branch vessel occlusion. Rupture at the aortic root can cause cardiac tamponade and damage to the aortic valve and coronary arteries. The most common acquired cause is arterial hypertension. Although several classifications have been suggested, the classic classification of DeBakey remains useful. In this classification, Class I dissections start at the aortic root and continue past the aortic arch to the more distal thoracic or abdominal aorta. Class II dissections are limited to the ascending aorta. Class III dissections begin just distal to the left subclavian artery and extend distally variable distances. The dissection begins with an intimal tear that leads to a dissection of blood into the media, causing a false channel. The dissection may tear the orifices of aortic branch vessels such that they may be perfused from either the true lumen, the false lumen, or not at all. Branch vessel occlusion can lead to stroke, extremity ischemia, visceral ischemia, and spinal cord ischemia, causing flaccid paralysis. If the dissection is deep and the adventitia weak, rupture can occur.

The great majority of patients will present with chest or back pain, and about half will have hypertension. The murmur of aortic insufficiency may be heard. Symptoms specific to abdominal organ ischemia may be present. Extremity pulses may be absent. Chest radiograph may show aortic enlargement, and a pulsatile abdominal mass may be palpated. CT scan with contrast is most useful for making the diagnosis.

Initial therapeutic efforts are aimed at the immediate control of hypertension in an intensive care unit setting. Dissections involving the ascending aorta should usually undergo early surgical repair to avoid fatal complications. Indications for emergency surgical repair include severe aortic valvular insufficiency, impending rupture, progression of the dissection, occlusion of major aortic branches, hemothorax, hemopericardium, and unrelieved pain on medical management. Class III dissections are often treated effectively with medical management alone. Surgical therapy may be considered after 1 to 2 months for Class III dissections. Patients with a residual false lumen following repair of any type of dissection should be followed carefully by CT scan for enlargement. Progressive enlargement is an indication for reoperation, as rupture risk is high.

Operative technique varies, depending on the location and type of dissection being repaired; a detailed description is beyond the scope of this chapter. In the repair of all types of dissections, however, the primary goal is re-establishment of the true lumen and perfusion of branch vessels. In ascending aortic dissections, aortic valve repair and coronary bypass may be required.

The natural history of aortic dissection is dismal, with approximately one third of patients dying after 2 days, three fourths dying after 2 weeks, and 90% dying after 1 year. Overall operative mortality for repair of aortic dissection averages 25%. Ascending aortic dissections have both a much worse natural history if untreated and a higher operative mortality rate compared with descending aortic dissections.

MYCOTIC ANEURYSMS

Mycotic aneurysms of the aorta are unusual but carry a high mortality rate. A mycotic aneurysm may occur as a secondary infection of an atherosclerotic aneurysm, or it can be caused by a primary aortic infection resulting in an aneurysm or pseudoaneurysm. The most common organism affecting the aorta is *Salmonella* and the aneurysms are almost exclusively located in the infrarenal portion of the aorta. Treatment requires resection of the infected portion of the aorta. For organisms with low virulence, an in situ aortic reconstruction occasionally may be possible, but aortic ligation with extra-anatomic reconstruction, such as an axillofemoral bypass, is most often required. The rare mycotic aneurysms that involve the visceral aorta must be repaired with an in situ reconstruction. Death for this latter condition is the rule.

AORTIC TRAUMA

Trauma to the abdominal aorta is usually not a diagnostic dilemma. Blunt trauma in this area is rare, and penetrating trauma is usually detected at the time of abdominal exploration. Penetrating abdominal aortic trauma is usually repaired directly or with either in situ or remote bypass; however, mortality remains high. Sudden deceleration, as seen with motor vehicle accidents or falls, can lead to blunt transection of the thoracic aorta, usually just distal to the left subclavian artery. A high index of suspicion is required to make the diagnosis, as the chest radiograph may not be diagnostic. CT scan or aortography is usually required to confirm the diagnosis. The mortality rate is approximately 40% during the first 2 days if the transection is not repaired. A short interpositional graft is usually all that is required to repair the injury. It remains controversial whether shunting is effective in reducing the incidence of spinal cord ischemia associated with the repair.

ANGINA PECTORIS

method of
GEORGE P. HANNA, M.D., and
RICHARD W. SMALLING, M.D., PH.D.
*University of Texas Medical School and
Hermann Hospital*
Houston, Texas

Angina pectoris is a symptom complex that results from an imbalance between myocardial oxygen demand and oxygen supplied by coronary arterial flow. It is usually due to coronary atherosclerotic disease; however, other pathologic conditions may precipitate angina, such as aortic stenosis and hypertrophic obstructive cardiomyopathy, by increasing oxygen demand. Rapid arrhythmias (atrial flutter or fibrillation with rapid ventricular response) may also result in angina. Angina is classically described as substernal pressure, a tightness, squeezing, or heavy sensation over the precordium, and may be associated with dyspnea. The patient may describe it with a clenched fist over the chest, a gesture known as Levine's sign. It may also radiate to the neck, jaw, and left arm, and the patient may describe a numbing sensation along the ulnar distribution of the left arm. Radiation to the same areas on the right side and the epigastrum is not uncommon.

The differential diagnosis of angina pectoris includes pulmonary, gastrointestinal, pleural, musculoskeletal, and vascular pathologies (Table 1).

Angina is usually precipitated by exertion, eating, cold exposure, or emotional upset. It is generally classified as stable or unstable. Stable angina tends to be exertional and is usually predictable in both its frequency and ease of provocation. Unstable angina refers to pain that is of new onset, occurs at night (nocturnal angina) or at rest (angina decubitus) with increasing frequency and duration, and with less predictable provocation and relief. Many consider postinfarction angina unstable as well. Prinzmetal's or variant angina due to coronary spasm often occurs in the early morning hours or following exercise. All types of angina—stable, unstable, or variant (Prinzmetal's)—result in myocardial ischemia; however, they differ in pathophysiology, and the approach to management may differ as well.

UNSTABLE ANGINA

Pathophysiology

Coronary angiography in patients with unstable angina reveals lesions that are often eccentric, with irregular or scalloped margins, and a high incidence of thrombus. Over the past decade, pathologic, experimental, and clinical observations have led to better understanding of the pathophysiologic mechanisms underlying unstable angina. Plaque rupture and fissuring in the atherosclerotic coronary artery, platelet aggregation, and thrombus formation play critical roles. As the plaque ruptures, it exposes several elements that are potent thrombogenic stimuli, one of which is fibrillar collagen type I. Platelet aggregation ensues, and along with activation of the coagulation system a thrombus is generated. Subsequently, fibrinogen and Von Willebrand's factor result in fur-

TABLE 1. **Etiology of Chest Pain**

Potentially Life-Threatening	Non–Life-Threatening

Cardiac
  myocardial infarction
  angina pectoris
  pericarditis
  coronary spasm
	Cardiac
	  mitral valve prolapse
	  aortic stenosis
	  hypertrophic obstructive
	    cardiomyopathy

Mediastinum
  mediastinitis
  esophageal rupture
	Chest wall
	  trauma
	  costochondritis
	  fractures

Great vessels
  dissecting aneurysm
  pulmonary embolus
	Spinal disease
	  cervical/thoracic

Pulmonary
  embolus/infarction
  pneumothorax
  pneumonia/pleurisy
	Infection
	  herpes zoster
	  Bornholm's disease

	Gastrointestinal
	  esophageal/acid reflux
	  esophageal spasm

ther platelet aggregation. Endothelial cell dysfunction over and near the plaque may result in vasoconstriction of the involved coronary segment, thus worsening the coronary luminal diameter. Vasoconstriction is accentuated by many factors produced by platelets, such as serotonin, platelet-derived growth factor, prostanoids, and others that possess vasoconstrictive properties.

Another potential contributing factor in some patients is a low level of nitric oxide (NO). Nitric oxide is a nitrogen-free radical generated by endothelial cells and circulating white blood cells (WBC) through bioconversion of L-arginine into citrulline, which produces vasodilation and platelet inhibition. Dysfunctional endothelium and WBC may lack the ability to produce NO.

Depending on the thrombogenic stimulus and the balance between thrombogenic and vasoconstrictive factors on one hand, and antithrombogenic and vasodilatory factors on the other hand, along with shear rate forces and the severity of the underlying stenosis, plaque rupture may result in thrombus formation that is either transient or permanent. Thrombogenic and vasoconstrictive factors include thromboxane A_2, leukotrienes, histamine, serotonin, and plasminogen activator inhibitor, whereas antithrombogenic and vasodilatory factors include endothelium-dependent relaxing factor (EDRF), prostaglandin I_2, and plasminogen activator. More intriguing is the mechanism underlying the progression of coronary disease in unstable angina. Progression can result from recurrent subclinical cycles of plaque rupture, hemorrhage, and organization.

At the cellular level, the interaction among platelets, monocytes/macrophages, and endothelial cells is critical. These cells express many mitogens, such as platelet-derived growth factor, which is chemotactic for smooth muscle cells and induces proliferation. Other important factors include fibroblast growth factor and interleukin-1, which, along with epidermal growth factor and transforming growth factor produced by platelets and macrophages, may result in plaque progression and neointimal proliferation.

A discussion of the pathophysiology of unstable angina is not complete without mention of the circadian pattern of ischemic events. Many ischemic events, including angina, myocardial infarction, and ischemic strokes, occur in early morning hours. This phenomenon is heterogeneous and involves heart rate, blood pressure, and platelet and coagulation cascade activation, as well as coronary artery tone variation, among others.

In view of the potentially serious ramifications for patients with unstable angina (USA), there has been heavy emphasis in recent years on the importance of early markers to better prognosticate and stratify patients according to risk. Among such markers are tissue-type plasminogen activator, plasminogen activator inhibitor (PAI-1), troponin-T, endothelin-1, C-reactive protein, and serum amyloid A protein. Tissue-type plasminogen activator and PAI-1 levels were found predictive of subsequent cardiovascular events (acute myocardial infarction or severe recurrent angina with or without intervention) at 12-week follow-up in 22 patients. Endothelin-1 was noted to be elevated in USA patients who went on to have acute myocardial infarction or recurrent angina with ECG changes, compared with controls, at 9-week follow-up in a study of 16 consecutive patients. The markers of inflammation, C-reactive protein, and amyloid A protein also have been found predictive of poor outcome in USA and may reflect an important inflammatory component in the pathogenesis of USA. More important still is the recent identification of troponin-T as an early marker for diagnosis of USA as well as a predictive marker of poor outcome in these patients. The role that these markers will play in medical management of patients with USA is rapidly evolving.

Management

As the pathophysiologic mechanisms in unstable angina are elucidated, the approach to management is becoming more and more multifaceted. Future emphasis will be placed on halting the process of accelerated atherosclerosis with an HMG-coenzyme A reductase inhibitor, use of an antiplatelet regimen consisting of serotonin inhibitors and thromboxane synthesis inhibitors, inhibiting platelet aggregation using glycoprotein IIb/IIIa receptor blockers as well as antagonists to the receptor of platelet-derived growth factor (PDGF), along with conventional therapy with aspirin and heparin. Of note is the role of hirudin in USA. Hirudin's mechanism of action has been elucidated by several recent studies; it binds to several key foci of thrombin with high affinity, including the catalytic site and the anion exocite. Figure 1 depicts one scheme for managing unstable angina.

STABLE ANGINA

Pathophysiology

The predisposing pathologic alteration in stable angina is atherosclerosis with or without intimal fibrous proliferation. Narrowing of coronary luminal diameter results in decreased myocardial oxygen delivery, especially when myocardial oxygen demand is increased with conditions that augment heart rate, contractility, and/or myocardial wall tension. Coronary angiographic studies in patients with stable angina frequently reveal smooth, regular plaques with a low incidence of ulceration or thrombi. Moreover, progression of disease in these patients occurs in 40% to 50% (much lower rates in those treated with lipid-lowering agents), but it is generally of small magnitude (10% change in the initial severity of stenosis at 1 year). Also, single vessel disease is more prevalent in patients with stable versus unstable angina.

In addition to the obvious theory of atherosclerosis as the instigator of ischemia in these patients, there

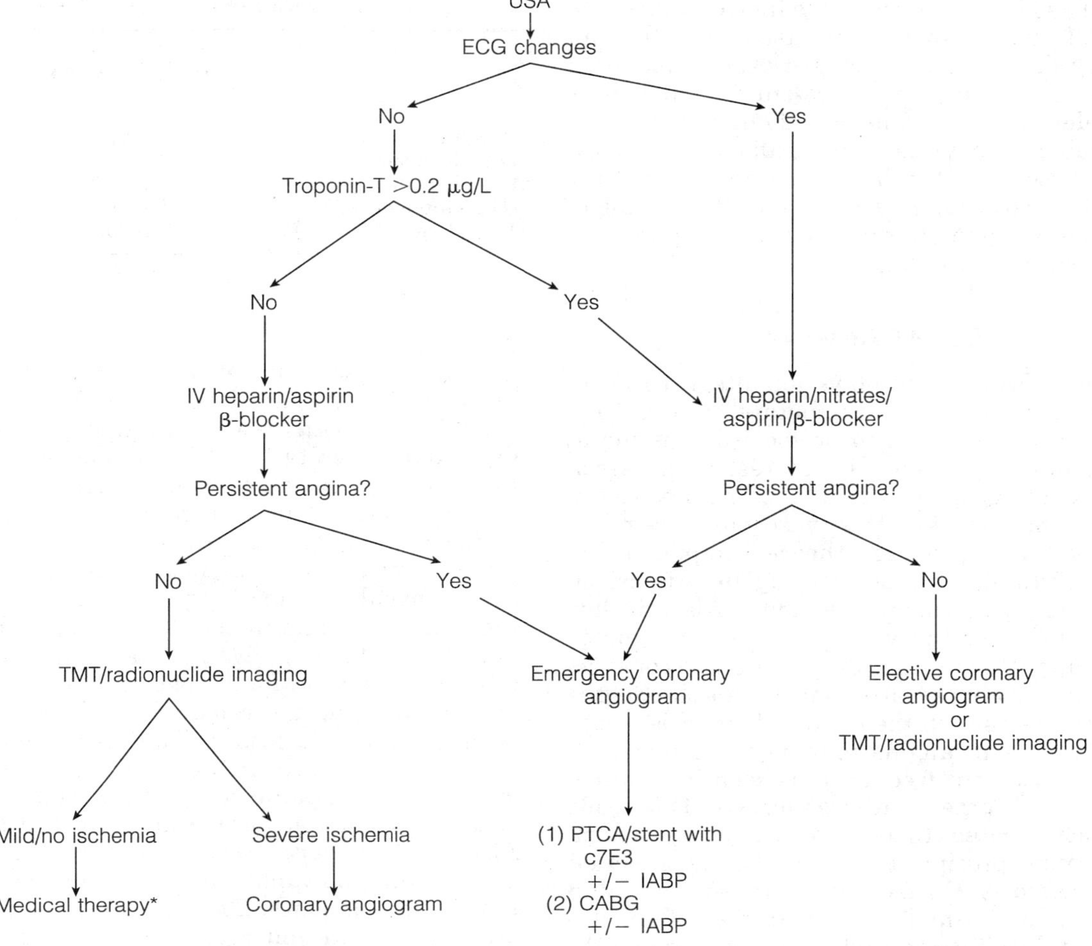

Figure 1. Schematic approach to managing unstable angina. *Medical therapy: antiplatelet agents (aspirin, ticlopidine), beta-blockers, calcium channel blockers, and nitrates. *Abbreviations:* USA = unstable angina; TMT = treadmill testing; PTCA = percutaneous transluminal coronary angioplasty; CABG = coronary artery bypass graft; IABP = intra-aortic balloon pump; IV = intravenous.

are other contributing factors. One is the severity of the lesion; resting blood flow is little affected until stenosis reaches 85% of coronary luminal diameter. Peak hyperemic blood flow, however, is reduced at a 50% occlusion. Another factor is the extent of collateral blood flow bypassing the stenotic segment. A third is the role played by the mediators of vasoconstriction, such as the sympathetic tone, histamine, serotonin, and others as discussed earlier. Fourth is the normal preferential distribution of blood flow to the endocardium at rest, resulting in diminished endocardial coronary flow reserve to respond to stress. Also, as coronary blood flow to the left ventricle occurs in diastole, a shorter diastolic time, as seen with tachycardia, for example, tends to reduce myocardial perfusion, rendering the myocardium more susceptible to ischemia. Therefore, conditions that increase wall stress, elevate left ventricular end-diastolic pressure, shorten diastolic filling time, and diminish coronary perfusion pressure tend to make the subendocardium more ischemic. Based on this pathophysiology, conditions that increase myocardial oxygen demand or decrease myocardial oxygen supply are

likely to precipitate angina in these patients. Therefore, angina may occur with exercise, cold exposure, or after meals. Also, tachycardia, anemia, sepsis, and carbon monoxide poisoning may worsen angina under normally tolerated conditions.

Management

In stable angina, medical management should attempt to alleviate factors that increase myocardial oxygen demand. This includes aggressive control of hypertension and tachycardia, as well as addressing secondary factors such as anemia, hypoxemia, hyperthyroidism, smoking, and drug use (cocaine and other sympathomimetic agents.) Then, pharmacologic therapy with a single agent can be a nitrate, calcium blocker, or beta blocker. All patients should receive an antiplatelet drug unless contraindicated. Beta blockers are probably more effective as initial monotherapy. Nitrates or calcium blockers or both can then be added if symptoms persist. Caution is advised with concomitant use of beta and calcium blockers (verapamil [Calan, Isoptin] and diltiazem

[Cardizem]), as both have negative inotropic and dromotropic effects. In some patients, adequate pain control may be difficult to achieve despite maximal pharmacologic therapy, or persistent ischemia may still be evident on ergonomic or radionuclide testing. It is advisable then to perform cardiac catheterization, and those with "high-risk" coronary anatomy may require revascularization procedures (angioplasty with or without stenting, coronary bypass, and so on) on a case-by-case basis.

VARIANT ANGINA

Coronary vasospasticity plays an integral role in the genesis of variant or Prinzmetal's angina. This coronary vasospasm tends to be focal and is manifested frequently by chest pain at rest with associated electrocardiographic alterations. The precise underlying mechanism for this vasospasm remains undetermined, and proposed theories implicate hypersensitivity to either vasoactive agents (described previously) or parasympathetic tone. Also, it has been suggested that the vasospasm may be due to amplification of the normal physiologic vasoconstriction at sites of coronary atheromas, and the degree of spasm correlates with the degree of stenosis. Angiographically, variant angina may be associated with normal coronaries but frequently is seen in conjunction with some degree of atherosclerosis. This leads to the much-debated theory that coronary spasm may, over time, precipitate endothelial dysfunction and atherosclerosis. (In fact, coronary angioscopy in animals revealed intimal injuries at sites of spontaneous or acetylcholine-induced coronary spasms.) Diagnosis of coronary spasm in symptomatic patients with normal or minimally diseased coronaries (50% diameter stenosis or less) can be achieved angiographically in the cardiac catheterization laboratory using ergonovine maleate. Complications are few, estimated at 0.03% in a Duke University review of 3447 cases of variant angina.

Medical management of variant angina consists of calcium channel blockers, with or without nitrates. Beta blockers should be avoided in patients with variant angina.

ANTIANGINAL MEDICAL THERAPY

Nitrates

Nitrates are widely used in treatment of angina pectoris. Of the various nitrate compounds (Table 2), nitroglycerin is the most widely investigated. The main effect of the drug is decreasing preload by dilating venous capacitance vessels. Dilating coronary arterial vessels, mainly the stenotic segment, is a secondary effect. The effect of nitroglycerin on cardiac metabolism is not well understood, but some studies suggest that it increases the lipid to carbohydrate oxidation ratio, possibly optimizing energy utilization via cardiac unloading.

In the acute setting, nitrates are delivered sublin-

TABLE 2. **Commonly Used Nitrates**

	Recommended Daily Dose (mg)	Duration of Action
Sublingual NTG	0.3–0.8	10–30 min
Oral NTG spray	0.4	10–30 min
Isosorbide mononitrate	40	7–12 h
Isosorbide dinitrate	10–160	2–6 h
NTG ointment (2%)	0.5–2 inches	3–8 h
Transdermal NTG disks	10–50	24 h

Abbreviation: NTG = nitroglycerin.

gually, by spray, or intravenously when available. Transdermal preparations generally should not be used for the acute case owing to slow release of the drug and difficulty in adjusting dosing. When given intravenously in intensive care settings, close monitoring of blood pressure is mandatory. In chronic stable angina, oral or transdermal preparations of nitrates may be used. A nitrate-free period is necessary to avoid tolerance. Typically, relatively long-acting and orally administered nitrates, such as isosorbide dinitrate, are given at 6- to 8-hour intervals during the day, and a nitroglycerin patch or paste is applied at night and removed the following morning after the patient arises. This represents the best available approach to optimize the nitrate effect while avoiding tolerance. Continuous administration of the same nitrate preparation should be avoided. Also, if a transdermal system is to be used alone, the patch should be applied in the morning and removed in the evening hours. The mechanism of nitrate tolerance is not well understood, but there is evidence to suggest depletion of sulfhydryl groups. The nitrate's site of interaction with vascular smooth muscle may play an important role. Side effects of nitrates include hypotension, headache, flushing, and reflex tachycardia.

Beta Blockers

Beta blockers are common and very effective drugs for managing ischemic heart disease. Phasic and tonic increases in the sympathetic outflow to the heart and the circulation have been shown to result in ischemia. They also cause hypertension, tachycardia, and increased contractility, all of which increase myocardial metabolic demand. Beta blockers blunt these effects, thus reducing ischemia and protecting the myocardium postinfarction. Beta blockers with intrinsic sympathomimetic effects, however, are not as useful. Moreover, beta blockers have been shown to reduce free fatty acids (FFA) and shift tissue metabolism to carbohydrate, allowing for greater cardiac energy production. Other beneficial effects of beta blockers include an increase in ventricular fibrillation threshold, a decrease in automatic arrhythmias by reducing phase 4 depolarization, reduced after-depolarizations, and altered refractoriness. Table 3 lists some of the commonly used beta blockers. Shorter-acting beta blockers are useful for titration

TABLE 3. **Commonly Used Beta Blockers**

Name (Formulation)	Recommended Daily Dose	Duration of Action (h)
Cardioselective Preparations		
Acebutolol (Sectral)*	400–1800 mg	24
Atenolol (Tenormin)	50–200 mg	24
Esmolol (Brevibloc) injection	Loading dose, 0.5 mg/kg Infusion, 50–300 μ/kg/min	10–20 min
Metoprolol		
Lopressor	15–240 mg	6–8
Lopressor SR, Toprol XL	50–400 mg	24
Injection	5 mg (may repeat q 5 min × 2–3)	5–8
Noncardioselective Preparations		
Nadolol (Corgard)*	80–240 mg	40
Propranolol		
Inderal	30–60 mg	3–6
Inderal LA	60–160 mg	24
Injection	1 mg (0.1 mg/kg) (may repeat q 4h)	3–4
Pindolol (Visken)*	10–20 mg	8
Sotalol (Betapace)	240–480 mg	24
Timolol (Blocadren)	15–45 mg	6–12

*Significant intrinsic sympathomimetic activity.

of doses in the inpatient setting, whereas longer-acting preparations are desirable for outpatients to improve compliance. Potential side effects include bradycardia, hypotension, bronchospasm, inhibition of insulin release and blunting of metabolic response to hypoglycemia, lethargy, depression, and impotence.

Calcium Channel Blockers

The three major groups of calcium channel blockers are the phenylalkylamines (e.g., verapamil), the benzodiazepines (e.g., diltiazem) and the dihydropyridines (e.g., nifedipine). Their mechanism of action is based mainly on the calcium inward current, which plays an important role in the various physiologic processes of the myocardium and vascular smooth muscle. Therefore, calcium blockers dilate coronary and peripheral arteries; in isolated cardiac tissue, they cause negative inotropic, chronotropic, and dromotropic effects. In the intact animal, however, the peripheral arterial vasodilation results in reflex tachycardia and vasoconstriction, thus counteracting hypotension. Also, calcium blockers have been shown to inhibit myocardial carbohydrate metabolism, increasing the FFA/carbohydrate utilization ratio. Table 4 summarizes the various commonly used preparations.

These drugs differ somewhat in their pharmacokinetics; verapamil results in more potent negative

TABLE 4. **Commonly Used Calcium Channel Blockers**

Name (Formulation)	Recommended Daily Dose	Duration of Action (h)
Diltiazem		
Cardizem	120–360 mg	6–8
Cardizem CD	120–360 mg	24
Cardizem SR	120–360 mg	12
Dilacor XR	60–120 mg	24
Injection	0.25 mg/kg bolus; 10 mg/h infusion	3
Nifedipine		
Adalat, Procardia	30–90 mg	4–8
Procardia XL	30–90 mg	16–24
Verapamil		
Calan, Isoptin	120–360 mg	8
Calan SR, Isoptin SR	120–240 mg	24
Injection	5–10 mg (may repeat in 30 min)	1–6
Nicardipine		
Cardene	60–120 mg	6–8
Cardene SR	60–120 mg	12
Amlodipine (Norvasc)	5–10 mg	24

inotropy and dromotropy than peripheral arterial vasodilation, hence its beneficial effect in left ventricular hypertrophy and diastolic dysfunction. Nifedipine induces potent peripheral vasodilation, resulting in reflex tachycardia, but produces little negative inotropy. The newer dihydropyridines amlodipine (Norvasc), felodipine (Plendil), and nimodipine (Nimotop) have the benefit of inducing coronary vasodilation with little negative inotropy, hence they possess potential benefit in ameliorating angina in patients with mildly depressed left ventricular function when other calcium blockers may be detrimental. However, it is important to keep in mind that all calcium antagonists, to varying degrees, may worsen congestive heart failure in patients with severely depressed left ventricular function. Diltiazem is intermediate with respect to the aforementioned effects. Finally, it is important to adjust dosing of calcium antagonists in elderly people, in patients with renal failure, and when used in conjunction with digoxin, cimetidine, quinidine, and other negative inotropic agents. Side effects may include edema, headache, flushing, bradycardia, hypotension, and, as mentioned earlier, worsening ventricular function.

SILENT ISCHEMIA

Discussion of angina is not complete without mention of silent ischemia. It may be defined as objective evidence of transient myocardial ischemia without symptoms of chest pain or angina equivalent. It has been classified by Cohn into three types:

I. Patients with asymptomatic coronary artery disease with silent ischemia detected by screening exercise testing. In the United States, the prevalence of coronary disease in the asymptomatic population has been estimated at 4% to 5%.

II. Patients with silent ischemia postinfarction. Theroux found 18% of postinfarction patients to have silent ischemia on early exercise testing.

III. Patients with angina who also have episodes of silent ischemia. The latter group encompasses patients with stable, unstable, and variant (Prinzmetal's) angina. In these groups, total ischemic time has been shown to correlate with poor clinical outcome, with increased incidence of infarction, interventions, sudden cardiac death, and hospitalization. It has also been shown to correlate with the severity of coronary artery disease. Moreover, silent ischemia is associated with a high incidence of perioperative complications. Therefore, silent ischemia requires early detection by identifying high-risk patients so that pharmacologic therapy may be provided. The same agents described previously for treatment of angina are good for management of silent ischemia. However, persistent ischemia upon objective stress testing despite maximal medical therapy may require early revascularization. In the Asymptomatic Cardiac Ischemia Pilot Study, silent ischemia and angina were relieved in more patients undergoing revascu-

larization procedures (percutaneous transluminal coronary angioplasty [PTCA] and coronary artery bypass graft [CABG]) than patients receiving medical therapy alone.

CARDIAC ARREST: SUDDEN CARDIAC DEATH

method of
MICHAEL L. MARKEL, M.D., and
TIMOTHY K. KNILANS, M.D.
University of Cincinnati, College of Medicine
Cincinnati, Ohio

Sudden cardiac death can reasonably be defined as natural death due to collapse of circulation, heralded by the abrupt, and often instantaneous, loss of consciousness within 1 hour of the onset of the acute symptoms. It may occur in an individual with or without known pre-existing heart disease but in whom the time and mode of death are unexpected. This is contrasted with a cardiac arrest, in which circulatory collapse caused by a potentially life-threatening cardiac event is appropriately treated and, thus, does not result in death. Farther along this spectrum is an episode of cardiac syncope during which loss of consciousness occurs owing to cerebral hypoperfusion caused by a potentially life-threatening cardiac event that terminates without intervention.

Death from cardiac causes is a major health problem in the United States and all western countries. Approximately one half of cardiac deaths are classified as sudden. It is estimated that between 250,000 and 500,000 people a year experience a cardiac arrest or sudden cardiac death in the United States. Only a small percentage of these individuals are successfully resuscitated or discharged from the hospital alive. It is amazing that this epidemic is largely unrecognized by the medical community and the public at large. The existence of cardiac disease, particularly coronary artery disease, and death from cardiac event seems to be accepted as an inevitable part of the aging process.

ETIOLOGY/PATHOLOGY

Autopsy series performed on victims of sudden death have demonstrated that most of them have cardiac disease (Tables 1 and 2). Approximately 80% have coronary artery disease, 10% to 15% have cardiomyopathy, and 5% have valvular heart disease. The remaining 0 to 5% may have a vascular catastrophe or electrical abnormalities such as Wolff-Parkinson-White (WPW) syndrome or conduction system disease. Atherosclerotic coronary artery disease is by far the major pathologic entity identified. Seventy-five percent of subjects have a prior healed myocardial infarction, and 25% to 30% have evidence of acute myocardial infarction. Approximately 75% of cases will have multivessel disease with at least 75% narrowing in at least two coronary arteries. It is estimated that the initial "symptom" of 20% to 30% of individuals with acute myocardial infarction is sudden death. However, only a distinct

TABLE 1. **Cardiac Disease States Associated with Ventricular Arrhythmias**

Coronary artery disease	Coronary artery spasm	Chagas' disease
Acute myocardial infarction	Hypertrophic cardiomyopathy	Congenital heart disease
Chronic myocardial infarction	Myocarditis	Tetralogy of Fallot
Ischemia	Arrhythmogenic right ventricular dysplasia	Double outlet right ventricle
Left ventricular hypertrophy	Sarcoidosis (also heart block)	Certain coronary anomalies
Dilated cardiomyopathy	Amyloidosis	Transposition of great vessels
Valvular disease		

minority of individuals resuscitated from sudden death have evidence of acute myocardial necrosis. Besides acute and chronic myocardial infarction, ventricular hypertrophy (both primary and secondary) and myocardial fibrosis (as seen in dilated cardiomyopathy) have also been associated with sudden cardiac death. As a general rule, there is evidence of structural cardiac disease in the majority of victims of sudden death. The corollary is that the risk of sudden cardiac death is small in individuals who have a mechanically normal heart.

The arrhythmias responsible for cerebral hypoperfusion, documented at the time of resuscitation of out-of-hospital cardiac arrest, are ventricular fibrillation in 65% to 80% of cases, bradyarrhythmias or asystole in 20% to 30%, and sustained ventricular tachycardia in 5% to 10%. Although these arrhythmias are documented at the time of treatment by the emergency squad, the initial arrhythmia is not necessarily known. Subsequent studies of Holter monitor tracings taken from individuals who were wearing a Holter monitor at the time of cardiac arrest have demonstrated that a majority experienced ventricular tachycardia that degenerated into ventricular fibrillation. The remaining 20% to 30% of episodes occur primarily as bradyarrhythmias, which may then degenerate to ventricular fibrillation

TABLE 2. **Causes of Sudden Death**

	Structurally Abnormal Heart	Either Structurally Normal or Abnormal Heart*	Structurally Normal Heart
Electrical	Venticular tachycardia (VT)†	Heart block/asystole†	Long QT syndrome (VT/VF)
	Ventricular fibrillation (VF)†	Ischemia (VF)	Wolff-Parkinson-White syndrome (VT/VF)
	Electromechanical dissociation (EMD)†	Coronary artery disease	Primary electrical disease (VT/VF)
	Congestive heart failure (VT/VF/ EMD/heart block/asystole)†	Coronary artery spasm	Southeast Asian sudden death syndrome (VT/VF)
		Cocaine/amphetamines (VT/VF)	Right bundle branch block with anterior ST segment elevation (V1–V3) syndrome (VT/VF)
		Drug proarrhythmia (brady or tachy)	
		Digitalis	
		Drugs that increase QT (torsades de pointes)	
		Type IA and Type III antiarrhythmic drugs	
		Terfenadine (Seldane) or astemizole (Hismanal) with ketoconazole (Nizoral) or erythromycin	
		Drugs that markedly slow conduction velocity	
		Type IC antiarrhythmic drugs	
		Metabolic abnormalities (VT/VF/heart block/ EMD/asystole)	
		Hypokalemia/hyperkalemia	
		Hypomagnesemia	
		Acidosis/alkalosis	
		Hypoxia	
		Hypovolemia	
		Anemia	
		Volume overload	
		Hypothermia	
Mechanical	Cardiac tamponade	Massive pulmonary embolism	
	Ball valve thrombus	Tension pneumothorax	
	Cardiac myxoma		
	Massive myocardial infarction (e.g., acute left main coronary artery occlusion)		
Vascular		Rupture of aneurysm of major blood vessel	
		Central nervous system hemorrhage	

*"Structurally normal" refers to mechanical function of the heart: does the substrate exist to support a reentrant tachycardia circuit? Common abnormalities include myocardial infarction, hypertrophy, fibrosis (dilated cardiomyopathy), and valvular disease. Prior to myocardial infarction, the heart may be "normal" mechanically even though coronary artery disease exists. Conversely, the ejection fraction may be normal even in the presence of a (small) previous myocardial infarction, but the heart would be considered abnormal.

†Ventricular tachycardia/ventricular fibrillation/electromechanical dissociation/heartblock/asystole are final common pathways to arrest of the circulation. Sustained monomorphic ventricular tachycardia is extremely unusual if the heart is mechanically normal. Polymorphic ventricular tachycardia and ventricular fibrillation occur in normal or abnormal hearts owing to a variety of factors ("triggers") that can modify the "substrate."

or continue as bradyarrhythmias. These Holter monitor recordings have given us other clues regarding events leading up to cardiac arrest. In some instances, increases in heart rate and decreases in heart rate variability have been documented, implying activation of the sympathetic nervous system. In other instances, ST segment changes have suggested acute ischemia as the initiating event, particularly when ventricular fibrillation occurred as the initial arrhythmia.

PATHOPHYSIOLOGY

This background of information has led to the present conceptual framework. Acute or chronic cardiac structural abnormalities (substrate) exist in conjunction with functional modulation (trigger), which interact to cause the initiation of ventricular tachycardia and ventricular fibrillation (Figure 1). The "PVC theory" states that the majority of episodes of ventricular tachycardia and ventricular fibrillation are initiated by premature ventricular contractions (PVCs). The corollary to this is that abolition of these PVCs would therefore prevent the initiation of ventricular tachycardia and ventricular fibrillation and, thus, decrease the incidence of sudden cardiac death.

This hypothesis was tested in a large multicenter National Institutes of Health (NIH)–sponsored trial, the Cardiac Arrhythmia Suppression Trial (CAST). The somewhat surprising finding was that even though ventricular ectopy was suppressed by the drugs encainide and flecainide, there was an increase in the death rate over placebo therapy. These antiarrhythmic drugs cause profound conduction slowing in the heart. Ischemia also causes conduction slowing. It is thought that the combination of the conduction slowing from the drug, plus that which occurred with ischemia in this postmyocardial infarction population, resulted in the formation of reentrant circuits, allowing ventricular tachycardia and fibrillation to occur. This resulted in the increased death rate seen in the drug treatment group. Therefore, in this instance, drug treatment had a marked effect on the trigger (PVCs), but the effect on the substrate overwhelmed any benefit that may have been seen from the decrease in PVCs. It also points out that PVCs are certainly not the only trigger that can interact with an abnormal cardiac substrate to cause sudden death. Most electrophysiologists now agree that treatment of asymptomatic premature ventricular contractions postmyocardial infarction is unwarranted.

For most diseases, patients will experience some symptoms that they can express to their physician. This results in further evaluation of the symptoms as well as physical examination and possibly ancillary testing, which then results in a diagnosis and treatment. Sudden cardiac death is a different type of problem: patients rarely have any symptoms prior to the episode of sudden death. When they do have a change in the state of their well-being, the symptoms are usually not specific and are referable to the cardiovascular system only 10% to 15% of the time. Also, in contrast to other disease states, once the patient experiences cardiac arrest, the window of opportunity for acute treatment lasts only minutes before irreversible damage and death occur. Ventricular fibrillation that exists untreated for 4 to 6 minutes results in irreversible brain

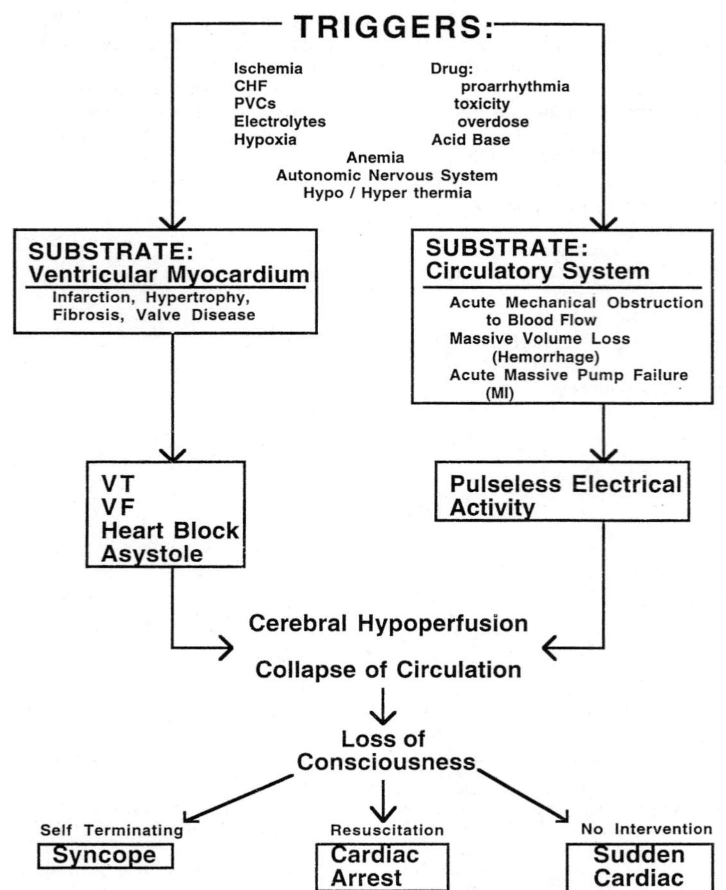

Figure 1. Theory of sudden death. "Triggers" act on (usually) abnormal substrate to cause the sudden arrest of circulation and subsequent loss of consciousness. Self-terminating events result in syncope. If the event is not self-terminating but the patient is resuscitated, then this is a cardiac arrest, but if there is no intervention, the patient will die (sudden cardiac death).

damage. Survival is rare if greater than 8 minutes pass before the onset of basic cardiac life support or if greater than 16 minutes elapse before advanced cardiac life support.

In rare episodes successful resuscitation occurs after longer periods of time. In these instances it is likely that the initial event was a hypotensive ventricular tachycardia or a hypotensive bradycardia that allowed enough blood flow to keep central nervous system cells alive but not enough to maintain consciousness. Even when patients are initially resuscitated, 40% to 60% of out-of-hospital cardiac arrest victims die during the initial hospitalization. Sixty percent of these deaths are due to anoxic central nervous system injury, 30% to congestive heart failure and pump failure, and only 10% to arrhythmias that are unsuccessfully treated once the patient is hospitalized.

The earlier the treatment, the better the chance of survival. Education of the general public about the technique of cardiopulmonary resuscitation (CPR) initially resulted in an improvement in survival. Now, with the awareness and fear of the acquired immune deficiency syndrome (AIDS), bystanders seem to be unwilling to perform CPR on a stranger. Early defibrillation also results in improved survival. The automatic external defibrillator can be operated by an individual not trained in arrhythmia recognition. It is hoped that these devices will become more available to police and firefighters and in public venues. Defibrillation could then be administered earlier and should increase the rate of resuscitation with return to normal function.

RISK STRATIFICATION

Since individuals who experience sudden cardiac death rarely have any preceding symptoms that would indicate they are at risk, it becomes necessary to identify those who are at risk and initiate effective therapy prior to such an event (Table 3). Preventive therapy is generally not well accepted by patients or physicians. Complicating the issue is the fact that "effective therapy" for prevention is still not defined.

The strongest risk factor for sudden death is compromised left ventricular function. The risk of sudden cardiac death begins to increase dramatically as the ejection fraction declines below 40%. The worse the mechanical function of the heart, the more likely it is for electrical instability to exist and thus the propensity for ventricular tachycardia and fibrillation.

Asymptomatic ventricular ectopy is another major independent predictor of sudden cardiac death. The risk of sudden death begins to increase with as few as 3 PVCs per hour and rises steeply between 3 and 10 PVCs per hour. As the frequency of PVCs increases above 10 per hour, the risk of sudden death increases minimally. Also of importance is the presence of complex ventricular ectopy, which includes couplets and nonsustained ventricular tachycardia. The more complex the ectopy, the worse the prognosis.

The presence of late potentials as determined from a signal-averaged electrocardiogram is also an independent predictor of an increased risk of sudden death. The signal-averaged electrocardiogram is obtained by averaging, amplifying, and filtering the ECG to detect low amplitude, high frequency electrical activity in the ST segment. These "late potentials" indicate areas of slow conduction within the ventricular myocardium that are necessary (but not sufficient) for a sustained monomorphic ventricular tachycardia circuit to exist. The presence of late potentials has been associated with the induction of sustained ventricular arrhythmias during electrophysiologic testing and has also been correlated with an increased risk of sudden death after myocardial infarction.

It is necessary to point out that the usefulness of the signal-averaged electrocardiogram is compromised in the presence of a bundle branch block. The delayed activation of one ventricle caused by the bundle branch block results in delayed high frequency, high amplitude signals at the end of the QRS complex that "overwhelm" the low amplitude late potential. Special criteria are being investigated, such as evaluation of the frequency of the components of the signals in the QRS, that may improve the applicability of the technique in patients with bundle branch block.

During sinus rhythm, activation of the inferior and posterior base of the heart normally occurs late, whereas the anterior wall of the heart and septum are activated early during the QRS complex. Therefore, areas of slow conduction in the myocardium due to an inferior myocardial infarction are more likely to result in delayed electrical activity that extends beyond the QRS and into the ST segment and, thus, can be recognized by the signal-averaged ECG as a "late potential." Indeed, it has been shown that late potentials are more common after inferior as compared with anterior myocardial infarction. Even with this caveat, the negative predictive value of a signal-averaged electrocardiogram is quite high, being over 95% in several large studies. The positive predictive value of a late potential in these same studies has ranged from 15% to 30%.

TABLE 3. **Risk Stratification for Sudden Cardiac Death***

	Low Risk		**Moderate Risk**	**High Risk**
Ventricular function (ejection fraction)	Normal	40%–50%	30%–40%	<30%
CHF NYHA Class	I	I–II	II–III	III–IV
Ventricular arrhythmia	≤3 PVCs/h	≤3 PVCs/h	3–10 PVCs/h	≥10 PVCs/h
Complex ectopy	None	Rare	Frequent ectopy, nonsustained VT	Sustained VT/VF
Hemodynamic symptoms with ectopy	None	Minimal	Lightheadedness	Previous syncope Previous cardiac arrest
Signal-averaged ECG	(−) Late potential	(+) Late potential	(+) Late potential	(+) Late potential
Heart rate variability	Normal	Normal	Decreased	Decreased
EP testing	Noninducible	Noninducible	Noninducible	Inducible sustained monomorphic VT

*Categories are not absolute (e.g., even frequent ectopy and nonsustained ventricular tachycardia do not have adverse prognosis if the heart is normal). However, the more high-risk features present, the higher the risk of sudden death.

Abbreviations: CHF = congestive heart failure; NYHA = New York Heart Association; PVC = premature ventricular contraction; VT = ventricular tachycardia; VF = ventricular fibrillation; EP = electrophysiologic.

Heart rate variability is another tool recently evaluated. It is a non-invasive method of assessing autonomic nervous system activity. In conditions with high vagal tone, there tends to be a large amount of sinus arrhythmia, and hence "variability" in the heart rate. When sympathetic tone is increased, the heart rate tends to be more regular and less variable. Factors that increase sympathetic nervous system activity increase the likelihood of ventricular arrhythmias, and those that decrease such activity decrease the chance of ventricular arrhythmias. Conversely, increases in parasympathetic nervous system ("vagal") activity tend to prevent ventricular arrhythmias, and decreases tend to increase them. It has been shown that a decrease in heart rate variability (sympathetic dominance) is associated with an increased mortality rate following myocardial infarction.

Electrophysiologic testing is also utilized for risk stratification. This is a type of right-sided heart catheterization during which multielectrode catheters are placed within the heart. Specific pacing protocols (programmed ventricular stimulation) are performed to determine whether a sustained ventricular arrhythmia can be induced. This usually consists of pacing at a constant rate followed by the introduction of single, double, and triple ventricular extrastimuli (PVCs). This stimulation protocol is usually performed using at least two pacing rates, and pacing is performed from at least two right ventricular sites (usually the right ventricular apex and outflow tract). The induction of a sustained monomorphic ventricular tachycardia carries an adverse prognosis. The induction of polymorphic sustained ventricular tachycardia or ventricular fibrillation is often considered an "artifact" of the testing technique and does not carry an adverse prognostic significance if these arrhythmias are induced with three or more extra stimuli (PVCs).

Programmed ventricular stimulation is often used to guide therapy in survivors of cardiac arrest. If sustained ventricular tachycardia can be induced in the drug-free state but not in the presence of an antiarrhythmic drug, then this implies a favorable outcome. Even if the patient does not respond to antiarrhythmic drug therapy, then other information obtained during electrophysiologic testing, such as the pacing methods by which ventricular tachycardia can be terminated, is useful to select the proper type of implantable cardioverter-defibrillator and to establish proper programming of the device. However, electrophysiologic testing has also been used to determine the risk of sudden death in patients after acute myocardial infarction (without spontaneous sustained ventricular tachycardia) and also in patients with chronic coronary artery disease and nonsustained ventricular tachycardia. In these settings, the induction of a sustained monomorphic ventricular tachycardia also carries an adverse prognosis. In the case of nonsustained ventricular tachycardia, a large NIH-sponsored study is ongoing (the Multicenter Unsustained Tachycardia Trial: MUSTT) to determine whether treatment with antiarrhythmic drugs (which make ventricular tachycardia noninducible) will improve the prognosis in these high-risk individuals.

All these risk-stratifying testing procedures provide different but complementary information. Assessment of the left ventricular ejection fraction is a way of looking at the amount of substrate. In other words, the worse the ejection fraction, the more pathologic left ventricular tissue is present and therefore, the more substrate that is available to support a ventricular tachycardia circuit. The Holter monitor evaluates the presence of ventricular ectopy and ischemia, which may act as potential triggers for the induction

of sustained ventricular arrhythmias. The signal-averaged electrocardiogram assesses the presence of late potentials that indicate areas of slow conduction within the ventricular myocardium. Areas of slow conduction are necessary for the induction of reentrant-sustained monomorphic ventricular tachycardia. However, the presence of such areas of slow conduction is not sufficient to imply that a ventricular tachycardia circuit is present. Heart rate variability assesses autonomic tone, which is known to influence the likelihood of sustained ventricular arrhythmias. Patients with clinical conditions in which high sympathetic tone exists, such as congestive heart failure, or patients after a myocardial infarction may therefore be more likely to sustain a life-threatening ventricular arrhythmia. However, unless a patient has already experienced a sustained ventricular arrhythmia, the only way to determine whether the substrate of a "high-risk" patient will support reentrant-sustained ventricular tachycardia is to perform an electrophysiologic study.

Previously, in subjects who experienced a spontaneous, sustained ventricular arrhythmia, emphasis had been placed on the induction of ventricular tachycardia with the same QRS morphology on 12-lead electrocardiogram as was seen spontaneously ("clinical VT"). However, it has been observed in some patients that "nonclinical" ventricular tachycardia morphologies induced during electrophysiologic testing are eventually seen spontaneously. Now many electrophysiologists consider the induction of any monomorphic ventricular tachycardia to carry adverse prognostic significance since this demonstrates the ability of the substrate to support potentially life-threatening arrhythmias.

DIAGNOSTIC EVALUATION/ TREATMENT

The diagnostic evaluation and treatment for cardiac arrest can be divided into four categories. Group 1 consists of patients in the acute setting of an ongoing cardiac arrest. The evaluation is obviously governed by the electrocardiographic tracings and physical findings obtained during the arrest and follows standard advanced cardiac life support guidelines. Treatment varies depending on whether ventricular fibrillation, ventricular tachycardia, pulseless electrical activity, or asystole is demonstrated. The reader is referred to the American Heart Association's *Textbook of Advanced Cardiac Life Support* for further details of treatment in the acute setting. In group 2 are those individuals who present for treatment of angina, myocardial infarction, or congestive heart failure. Although these individuals may have no signs or symptoms of arrhythmias, their disease state puts them at risk of sudden cardiac death. Consideration should be given to assessing this risk within the limits of our present knowledge and treatment capability in an attempt to alter this prognosis. The third group consists of the individuals with cardiac disease who present with syncope. This should always be considered an aborted sudden death episode and should be aggressively evaluated. The fourth category is the patient who has been resuscitated from a cardiac arrest and is now stable from a cardiac and neurologic standpoint.

Much of the information obtained during the evaluation of patients who present with symptoms of cardiac disease (group 2) is also useful in terms of assessment of the risk of sudden death. Commonly, these individuals' electrocardiograms will demonstrate evidence of prior myocardial infarction, ischemia, conduction system disorder, WPW syndrome, long QT interval, or electrolyte abnormalities that may indicate an increased risk of sudden death. An echocardiogram also provides a large amount of information during a cardiac evaluation. Systolic and diastolic ventricular function are determined, as well as the presence of segmental wall motion abnormalities that would imply coronary artery disease. The presence of primary or secondary ventricular hypertrophy can also be ascertained. The presence of valvular heart disease is easily demonstrated, as well as unusual conditions such as an atrial myxoma, a ball valve thrombus, or pericardial effusion and tamponade. An exercise test is often performed looking for evidence of coronary artery disease and ischemia. Active ischemia, especially in the presence of a previous myocardial infarction, is certainly a predisposing factor to sudden death. Evidence of exercise-induced arrhythmia, such as ventricular tachycardia or heart block, may indicate the propensity to potentially life-threatening tachy- or bradyarrhythmias. A Holter monitor may also look for the presence of silent ischemia and ST segment changes during daily activities. The Holter will also demonstrate the presence, frequency, and complexity of ventricular ectopy that increases the risk of sudden death. Heart rate variability can also be determined from these recordings.

Therefore, with the standard testing that is commonly done for evaluation of a cardiac complaint, most of the information necessary for risk stratification is already available. The signal-averaged electrocardiogram is the only test that is necessary to complete noninvasive risk stratification. Patients with low ejection fractions, congestive heart failure, active ischemia, frequent complex ventricular ectopy, and late potentials on signal-averaged electrocardiogram are at the highest risk of sudden cardiac death. Patients with several of these risk factors may warrant invasive evaluation.

Treatment of patients in group 2 should be directed at the primary problem and in particular to the use of agents that have been shown to prolong life. In the setting of coronary artery disease, chronic treatment with platelet inhibitors such as aspirin should be undertaken. The use of beta blockers (without intrinsic sympathomimetic activity) has been demonstrated to prolong life in patients after myocardial infarction. Unfortunately, the minority of patients are treated with beta blockade after myocardial infarction. The use of beta blockers in individuals with compromised left ventricular function may precipitate congestive heart failure. However, the greatest benefit from beta blockers in the various trials occurred in those patients who had congestive failure and decreased left ventricular function. Also, several early trials have demonstrated that beta-blocker therapy can actually be advantageous in the treatment of congestive heart failure. When administered to patients with active congestive failure, the drugs must be started at very low dose levels and titrated upward. In the context of preventing sudden death, beta blockers should be used in all patients postmyocardial infarction and should be considered as the first line therapy of patients with angina, especially if a previous myocardial infarction is present.

The use of angiotensin-converting enzyme (ACE) inhibitors has been shown to improve longevity in individuals who have congestive heart failure. Thus, these agents should be primary treatment. It is extremely important to maintain potassium and magnesium levels in patients receiving diuretic therapy for congestive heart failure or for hypertension (especially if left ventricular hypertrophy is present).

In the treatment of acute myocardial infarction, it is now apparent that having an "open artery" is better than having a "closed artery." Therefore, consideration should be given to the use of thrombolytic agents early in the course of an acute myocardial infarction if a contraindication is not present. If facilities are available, acute angioplasty of the infarcted vessel may be preferable since prognosis is improved, compared with the use of thrombolytic agents. Several studies have now shown that the incidence of late potentials on the signal-averaged electrocardiogram is markedly decreased when the coronary artery is opened early in the course of the infarct. This implies decreased formation of the appropriate substrate for ventricular arrhythmia and presumably will result in a decreased risk of sudden death in future years.

The second group of patients (who present with symptoms of cardiovascular disease) represent the largest absolute number of patients with the potential to experience sudden death. Therefore the greatest potential impact will be made by effective prophylactic treatment of this group of patients. However, current technology does not allow us to pinpoint with certainty which patients will experience sudden death, and as yet no "silver bullet" is available to prevent sudden death. Although implantable cardioverter-defibrillators (ICDs) are expected to prevent sudden death effectively, the expense and complexity of these devices precludes their use as prophylactic therapy owing to the huge numbers of patients involved. The effectiveness of these devices for prolonging life has not yet been proved with certainty. Therefore, treatment in this second group is aimed primarily at the underlying conditions and treatments that are known to prolong life. A patient whose ischemia and congestive heart failure are effectively treated, who has compromised left ventricular function (left ventricular ejection fraction less than 40%), and who continues to demonstrate complex ventricular ectopy and nonsustained ventricular tachycardia is at an increased risk of sudden death, and consideration should be given to referring this individual for electrophysiologic testing for further risk-stratification. Consideration should then be given to referring the patient to a center that is participating in the MUSTT (Multicenter Unsustained Tachycardia Trial), which seeks to determine the best therapy for these individuals.

Unfortunately, in a cost-conscious environment, it is cheaper for a patient to die without evaluation and thus in some circumstances there is built-in resistance to it. Treatment is costly due to the large numbers of patients involved and the complexity and expense of some therapies. The present risk-stratification procedures do not have a high positive predictive accuracy. However, they do have a very good negative predictive accuracy (greater than 90%). We can reliably identify patients who are not at risk and hence do not require treatment. These individuals live the longest, and they may receive prophylactic therapy for many years with the attendant cost and side effects. Identification of low-risk individuals and elimination of unnecessary treatment will decrease costs and help balance the cost-effectiveness equation.

In the third group is the patient with cardiovascular disease who presents with syncope. Therefore, it is of primary importance to determine whether this patient has cardiovascular disease. If the patient has no history of cardiovascular disease (myocardial infarction, valvular disease, angina, congestive failure symptoms, palpitations, or a heart murmur), an electrocardiogram still should be obtained to look for evidence of conduction system disease, chronic or acute myocardial infarction, a short PR interval and a delta wave consistent with the WPW syndrome, or a long QT interval. An echocardiogram is also useful in this instance. Significant valvular disease should be detected by physical examination, and the presence of coronary artery disease will often be revealed by the electrocardiogram. However, the echocardiogram may demonstrate left ventricular hypertrophy or a cardiomyopathy with a moderate decrease in left ventricular function (with few signs or symptoms of congestive failure) that would still put the patient at risk of sudden death.

If the syncope patient has evidence of cardiovascular disease after this evaluation, he or she should be referred for an electrophysiologic study to assess for arrhythmic causes for syncope and, specifically, to evaluate for inducible, sustained, monomorphic ventricular tachycardia. If the patient presenting with syncope does not have evidence of cardiovascular disease, then the likelihood of death from the process causing syncope is small. If the problem becomes recurrent, referral to an electrophysiologist for tilt table testing (to test for neurocardiogenic syncope) is the most cost-effective route prior to proceeding with a long neurologic evaluation, which is unlikely to be fruitful.

The fourth group consists of those who are resuscitated from a cardiac arrest (Figure 2). As in all areas of medicine, the key to effective therapy is accurate diagnosis, and this is especially true in these patients. Initially (Figure 2A), the patient should receive supportive measures, including pressors and mechanical ventilation as necessary, until it can be established whether the patient has suffered irreversible anoxic central nervous system or cardiac damage. During this time of supportive therapy, serial electrocardiograms and cardiac enzyme testing should be performed to determine whether the patient has suffered an acute myocardial infarction. A drug screen should be performed as part of the initial evaluation, since cocaine may precipitate coronary artery spasm and/or ventricular arrhythmias. An echocardiogram is frequently obtained early in the course after resuscitation to help assess left ventricular function to guide ongoing therapy. It is not uncommon for "postarrest stunning" to be present, and this may improve over the course of several days. Also of note, this stunning may appear as segmental wall motion abnormalities that may resolve with time. Ventricular fibrillation occurring soon after the onset (within 72 hours) of an acute myocardial infarction does not carry adverse long-term prognostic significance. Therefore, further evaluation and treatment are not necessary. Strong consideration should be given to early catheterization and angioplasty to open the "infarct artery." Acute thrombolytic therapy is often relatively contraindicated due to cardiopulmonary resuscitation performed in the cardiac arrest survivor. Chronic beta-blocker therapy as well as aspirin should be given to such an individual, and to any patient after a myocardial infarction.

If there is no evidence of an acute myocardial infarction, and assuming recovery of neurologic status, then the patient should be referred to a cardiovascular center that has the capabilities of performing cardiac catheterization and electrophysiologic testing (Figures 2B and 2C). Even if the patient has no evidence of an acute myocardial infarction, there is a very high incidence (greater than 90%) of advanced atherosclerosis and multivessel coronary artery disease in cardiac arrest survivors. If the patient has normal coronary arteries, then ergonovine should be administered to determine whether or not the patient has coronary artery spasm causing transient ischemia. The patient should undergo a 24-hour Holter monitor to quantify the amount of spontaneous ventricular arrhythmia as well as to document any spontaneous bradyarrhythmias that may not be documented by the standard telemetry system. Ischemia, without infarction, is a well-known cause of polymorphic ventricular tachycardia and ventricular fibrillation. Aggressive treatment of ischemia is necessary and frequently will involve revascularization. It is our custom to proceed with coronary artery bypass grafting (CABG) because of the high (up to 33%) restenosis rate within 6 months of angioplasty. The patient who has silent ischemia and whose only indication of ischemia is ventricular fibrillation runs a very high risk, should restenosis occur. In the days before the transvenous defibrillator, electrophysiologic testing was often performed prior to CABG. If a sustained monomorphic ventricular tachycardia was induced, then epicardial defibrillator patches were placed at the time of surgery, and the patient under-

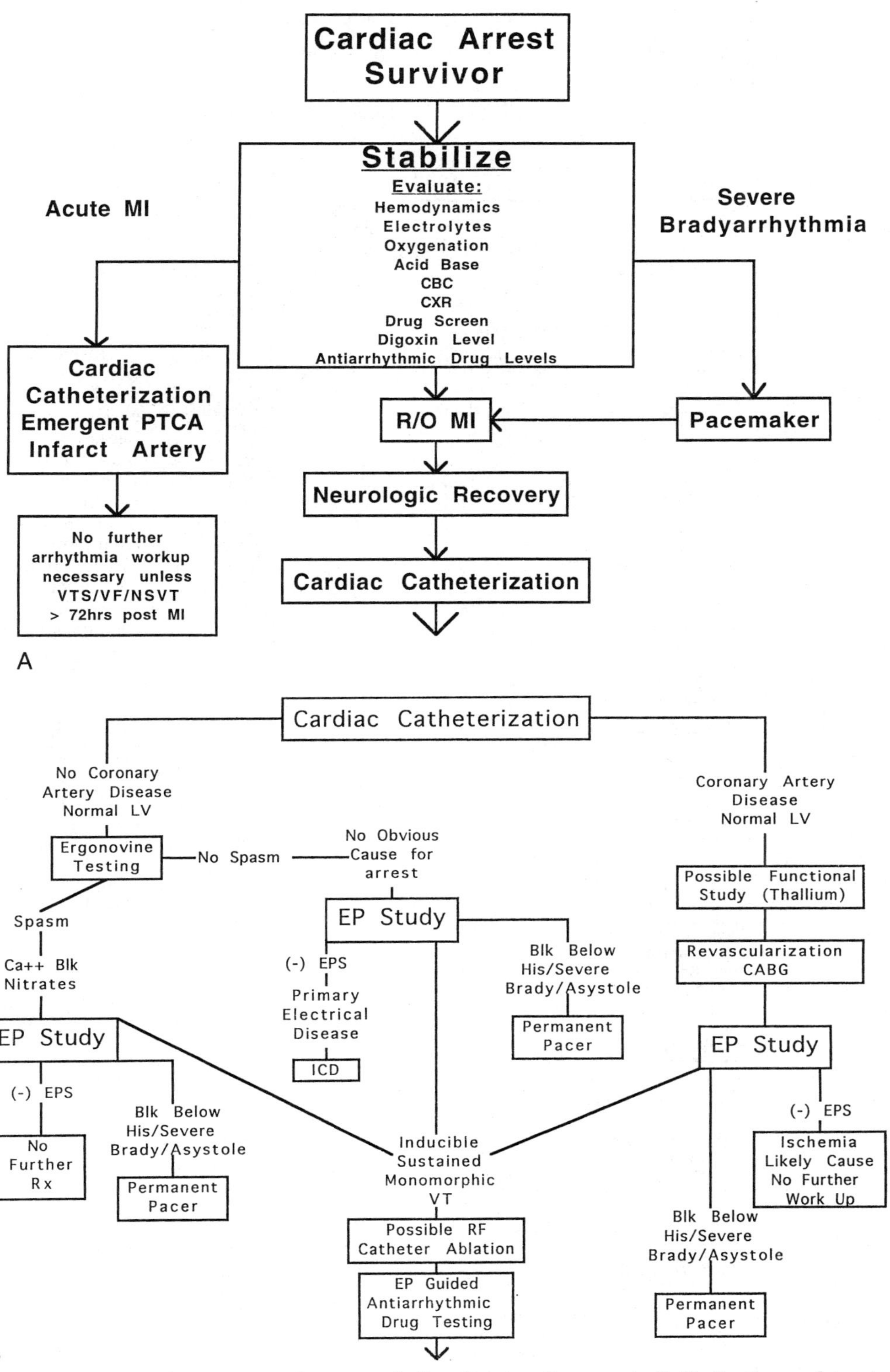

Figure 2. *A*, Initial evaluation and treatment after resuscitation from cardiac arrest. *B*, Evaluation and treatment of the cardiac arrest survivor after initial stabilization. Cardiac catheterization is necessary early to evaluate the "substrate." Schema for patients with normal left ventricular function with and without coronary artery disease.

Illustration continued on following page

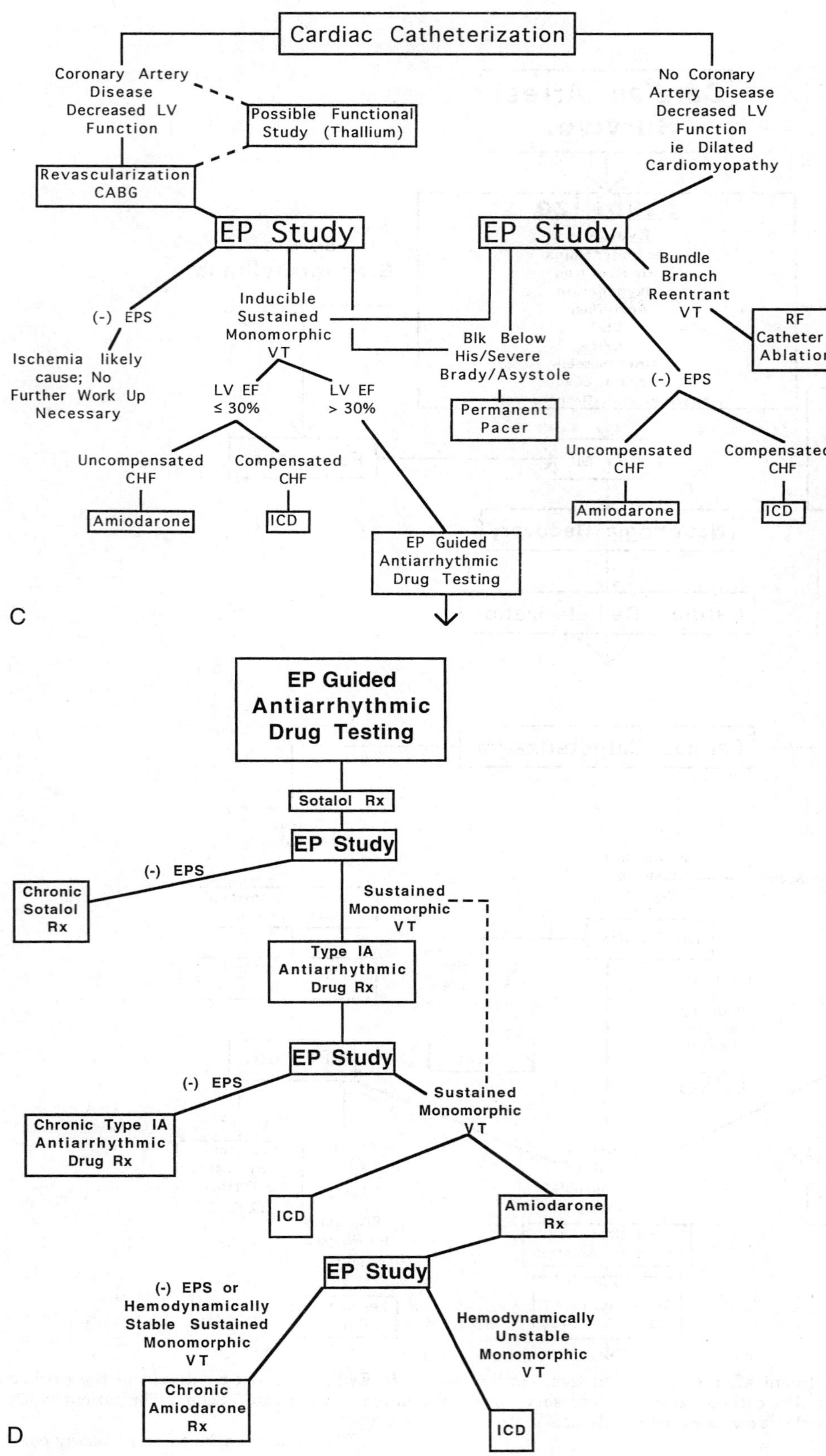

Figure 2. *Continued C*, Evaluation and treatment of the cardiac arrest survivor after initial stabilization. Cardiac catheterization is necessary early to evaluate the "substrate." Schema for patients with compromised left ventricular function with and without coronary artery disease. *D*, Evaluation and treatment of the cardiac arrest survivor after initial stabilization and evaluation. Schema for the use of electrophysiologic testing to assess the efficacy of antiarrhythmic drug therapy for the treatment of inducible sustained ventricular arrhythmias.

BLK = block; Brady = bradycardia; CABG = coronary artery bypass grafting; CBC = complete blood count; CHF = congestive heart failure; CXR = chest radiograph; EF = ejection fraction; EPS = electrophysiologic study; ICD = implantable cardioverter-defibrillator; LV = left ventricle; MI = myocardial infarction; NSVT = nonsustained ventricular tachycardia; PTCA = percutaneous transluminal coronary angioplasty; RF = radiofrequency; R/O = rule out; Rx = treatment; VF = ventricular fibrillation; VT = ventricular tachycardia; VTS = ventricular tachycardia sustained.

went repeat electrophysiologic testing after surgery. With the high success rate of the transvenous defibrillator system, the pre-CABG electrophysiologic test assumes less importance. However, it continues to be our bias to place epicardial defibrillator electrodes at the time of coronary artery bypass grafting in subjects with inducible monomorphic ventricular tachycardia since these epicardial systems are time-tested. In addition, this leaves the possibility for the use of a transvenous lead system in the future should problems with lead failure arise. A failed transvenous lead system may require a potentially risky lead extraction procedure to allow placement of a new system.

After revascularization has been performed and heart failure therapy is maximized, the cardiac arrest survivor should undergo electrophysiologic evaluation. Protocols of treatment differ by institution; this is our general approach (Figures 2*B* and 2*C*): If sustained monomorphic ventricular tachycardia is inducible and the ejection fraction is greater than 30%, then the patient will undergo serial electrophysiologic testing to assess antiarrhythmic drug efficacy (Figure 2*D*). Usually, therapy with two drugs will be attempted: the type III antiarrhythmic drug sotalol (Betapace) and a type IA agent (quinidine [Quinaglute, Quinidex], procainamide [Pronestyl, Procan SR], disopyramide [Norpace]). If the first drug does not prevent the induction of sustained ventricular tachycardia, then the second agent will be tested. If neither of these agents is successful then the patient is "drug refractory," and prolonged trials of more antiarrhythmic drugs are unlikely to be successful. Treatment with an implantable cardioverter-defibrillator would be the usual next step. However, in selected cases, catheter or surgical ablation of ventricular tachycardia or chronic amiodarone therapy is considered.

Less information is available for survivors of cardiac arrest who have a dilated rather than an ischemic cardiomyopathy. It is known that electrophysiologic testing has a lower sensitivity and is less reproducible in patients with a dilated versus an ischemic cardiomyopathy. Reproducibility of the induction of ventricular tachycardia needs to be aggressively verified in these patients, otherwise a drug may be judged to suppress induction of ventricular tachycardia when actually this represents a problem of reproducibility of the testing technique. This has led some electrophysiologists to question the usefulness of serial drug testing in patients with a dilated cardiomyopathy, and they proceed to empiric amiodarone treatment versus an implantable cardioverter-defibrillator. Baseline electrophysiologic testing is still utilized to look for the induction of bundle branch reentrant ventricular tachycardia (curable by catheter ablation) and to determine whether pacing techniques can be used to terminate ventricular tachycardia. This information is used to select and program an implantable cardioverter-defibrillator.

If the patient has inducible sustained monomor-phic ventricular tachycardia during electrophysiologic testing and the ejection fraction is less than 30% (see Figure 2*C*), then the success rate for conventional antiarrhythmic therapy is limited. In this instance, empiric chronic amiodarone therapy or an implantable cardiac defibrillator will be considered as the next step. Patients who have left ventricular dysfunction and severe congestive failure symptoms are unlikely to have any significant improvement in longevity with a defibrillator unless they are considered a cardiac transplant candidate. If the patient has not been limited by heart failure symptoms, then a defibrillator would be expected to prevent sudden death in this individual.

If the patient does not have inducible monomorphic ventricular tachycardia at electrophysiologic testing and an obvious precipitating factor for ventricular fibrillation was identified and has been corrected (e.g., left main coronary artery disease now status post-CABG), then further therapy is not necessary. However, if monomorphic ventricular tachycardia is noninducible, there was no obvious precipitating cause, and the patient continues to have the substrate that puts her or him at risk of sudden death (e.g., dilated cardiomyopathy), then treatment with an implantable cardioverter-defibrillator is usually utilized. However, in some instances, empiric chronic amiodarone therapy may be warranted.

The proper treatment modalities to prevent or treat initial or recurrent cardiac arrest are in a state of flux. Whereas most electrophysiologists believe that the implantable cardioverter-defibrillator markedly improves survival, this has not been proved. Early studies of defibrillator use were retrospective comparisons against historical controls. There were many sources of biases in these studies, especially when cardioverter-defibrillator required a thoracotomy. Many of the "sicker" patients were not felt to be candidates for this therapy, and thus these trials may have been biased to favor the defibrillator. At present several ongoing prospective randomized trials should help determine the effectiveness of the defibrillator. It is possible that the defibrillator simply converts the mode of death in these individuals so that a sudden death is converted to a heart failure death. Although sudden death mortality is improved, total mortality is not affected. Preliminary evidence from the multicenter automatic defibrillator trial (MADIT) has demonstrated a survival benefit in individuals at high risk of sudden death who received an implantable defibrillator compared with those receiving conventional antiarrhythmic therapy. At this time sotalol and amiodarone are thought to be the most effective antiarrhythmic drugs. However, a direct comparison of these therapies with each other and with the defibrillator has never been done and is now ongoing in an attempt to determine the relative benefits of these therapies.

ACKNOWLEDGMENT

The authors thank Venessa A. Bryson for her secretarial assistance in the preparation of this manuscript.

ATRIAL FIBRILLATION

method of
MARSHALL S. STANTON, M.D.
Mayo Clinic
Rochester, Minnesota

Many causes exist for atrial fibrillation (Table 1), but the important causes to exclude in most patients presenting with their first episode are thyrotoxicosis and structural heart disease. The history and physical examination will usually point to the underlying etiology, if one is to be found. Important ancillary tests are thyroid function tests (i.e., sensitive thyroid-stimulating hormone [TSH]) and an echocardiogram. Unless otherwise suspected, it is not necessary to exclude coronary artery disease (CAD) in the patient presenting with new-onset atrial fibrillation, as it is very unusual for CAD by itself, without concomitant left ventricular dysfunction or acute infarction, to be responsible for this arrhythmia.

Beyond diagnosing the cause of atrial fibrillation, the physician must decide (1) how to control the rapid ventricular response that usually accompanies the untreated arrhythmia, (2) whether and how to try to prevent recurrence, and (3) how to minimize the risk of stroke or systemic embolism that exists in these patients.

CONTROL OF VENTRICULAR RESPONSE

Why Control the Ventricular Response in Atrial Fibrillation. Maintaining a well-controlled ventricular response has two goals: (1) improving the patient's symptoms and/or exercise tolerance, and (2) preventing ventricular dysfunction.

During rapid ventricular rates, systolic and diastolic function are impaired. Further, ischemia may occur in patients with coronary artery disease or those with ventricular hypertrophy. Blunting the ventricular response helps maximize cardiac performance. Although many patients with atrial fibrillation and a rapid ventricular response complain of palpitations, fatigue, or dyspnea, a substantial number report no symptoms. The clinician must be wary that although patients claim to be asymptomatic, they may still have reduced exercise tolerance. Studies have shown an increase of about 50% in treadmill exercise time when the ventricular rate is brought under control.

Ventricular dysfunction can arise from a prolonged rapid ventricular rate, a so-called *tachycardia-in-duced cardiomyopathy*. This is a well-studied phenomenon in experimental models in which rapid pacing is used to create a cardiomyopathy. Whenever a patient presents with rapid atrial fibrillation and a dilated cardiomyopathy, the fast rate must be considered as a possible etiology as this is a potentially reversible form of ventricular dysfunction. Of course, it is also possible that the atrial fibrillation is the result rather than the cause of the cardiomyopathy. In either case, controlling the ventricular response is an essential part of the patient's management.

Pharmacologic Control. Three main categories of drugs are used to block the atrioventricular (AV) node in an attempt to slow the ventricular response in atrial fibrillation: digitalis glycosides (predominantly digoxin [Lanoxin]), beta-adrenergic blockers, and calcium channel blockers (Table 2). When using these drugs, it should be remembered that none of them have been shown to be effective in preventing recurrence of atrial fibrillation. The only exception is that meta-analysis has shown that prophylactic use of beta-adrenergic blocking drugs prevents atrial tachyarrhythmias following cardiac surgery. Further, it is probably a misconception that these drugs will convert an acute episode back to sinus rhythm.

Beta-adrenergic blocking drugs are effective in slowing the ventricular response. Acutely, the only ones that are available for intravenous administration are propranolol (Inderal), metoprolol (Lopressor, Toprol), atenolol (Tenormin), and esmolol (Brevibloc). These agents may be particularly useful when atrial fibrillation complicates hyperthyroidism or other hyperadrenergic states (e.g., acute myocardial infarction (MI), postoperatively, sepsis). Intrinsic sympathomimetic activity (ISA) is a characteristic of some beta blockers (e.g., acebutolol [Sectral]) whereby the drug blocks the beta-adrenergic receptor but at the same time provides mild tonic stimulation. This results in a lesser reduction in resting heart rate but still adequately blunts sympathetic effects during exertion or other stress. Beta blockers with ISA may be useful in patients with relative bradycardia at rest in whom beta-adrenoceptor blockade is desired.

TABLE 2. **Treatment of Atrial Fibrillation**

Control of Ventricular Rate
Atrioventricular (AV) nodal blocking drugs
  Beta-adrenergic blocking drugs (e.g., propranolol [Inderal], metoprolol [Lopressor])
  Calcium channel blocking drugs (verapamil [Isoptin, Calan, Verelan], diltiazem [Cardizem])
  Digoxin [Lanoxin]
Catheter ablation/modification of the AV node

Maintenance/Restoration of Sinus Rhythm
Antiarrhythmic drugs
  Class IA: quinidine (Quinaglute, Quinidex), disopyramide (Norpace), procainamide (Procan, Pronestyl)
  Class IC: flecainide (Tambocor), propafenone (Rhythmol)
  Class III: amiodarone (Cordarone), sotalol (Betapace), ibutilide (Corvert)
Maze surgical procedure
Catheter maze procedure?

TABLE 1. **Common Causes of Atrial Fibrillation**

Cardiac	Systemic Diseases
Hypertension	Thyrotoxicosis
Ischemic heart disease	Alcohol (holiday heart syndrome)
Cardiomyopathy	
Valvular disease	Chronic lung disease
Wolff-Parkinson-White syndrome	Electrolyte abnormality
Atrial septal defect	Idiopathic
Tachycardia-bradycardia syndrome (sick sinus syndrome)	

The calcium channel blocking drugs that can control the ventricular rate are verapamil and diltiazem, and they are equally effective. Verapamil and diltiazem are available in intravenous as well as oral preparations. Both of them have negative inotropic effects, with that of verapamil probably being somewhat more potent than that of diltiazem. The dihydropyridines (e.g., nifedipine [Procardia]) are not effective in atrial fibrillation.

Digoxin has two effects on the AV node. The first action, occurring at lower doses, is the indirect effect of increased vagal tone. With higher doses, the more direct action of digoxin on slowing AV nodal conduction occurs. This fact is of more than just academic interest. When observing a patient being monitored at rest, it may appear that an adequate blocking effect on the AV node is present. However when that patient walks, the ventricular rate may increase dramatically if only the vagal effects of digoxin are present. Thus, it is important to note the ventricular response during exercise before concluding that the patient's heart rate is "well controlled."

Digoxin, by itself, is probably not effective in restoring sinus rhythm. In new-onset atrial fibrillation, about 50% of patients will spontaneously revert to sinus rhythm within 24 hours without treatment, and a randomized study has shown no difference in reversion rates between digoxin and placebo. Further, the entire idea of whether digoxin controls the ventricular response at all during recurrences has been called into question. As digoxin shortens action potential duration and refractoriness in the atria, it is conceivable that it may cause *atrial proarrhythmia* and worsen the frequency and duration of a patient's paroxysms of atrial fibrillation.

Most comparative studies between the different types of AV nodal blocking drugs have shown no difference between beta-adrenergic blocking drugs and calcium channel blockers. Digoxin typically does not control the ventricular response as well as the other drugs, particularly during exercise. The best role for digoxin in atrial fibrillation may be in the patient with left ventricular dysfunction or as adjunctive therapy with a beta- or calcium channel blocking drug.

Adenosine (Adenocard) is a potent AV nodal blocker, but its effects dissipate quite rapidly (less than 30 seconds) and thus it has no therapeutic use in atrial fibrillation. Clonidine (Catapres)*, a central alpha-$_2$-receptor agonist that reduces sympathetic nervous outflow, has been shown in one small study to slow the ventricular response but its more routine use in this situation should await further studies.

Atrial fibrillation in patients with the Wolff-Parkinson-White syndrome presents a special case, and acute and chronic management differ from that of atrial fibrillation in other settings. The aforementioned drugs should not be used to control the ventricular response as they all may precipitate an increase in the ventricular rate and possible degener-

*Not FDA-approved for this indication.

ation to ventricular fibrillation. Digoxin enhances conduction over accessory pathways in about one-third of patients, slows conduction in about one-third, and in the other third has no effect. The specific effect of digoxin in any given patient cannot be predicted a priori. The calcium channel blockers can increase the ventricular response by causing hypotension with resultant reflex sympathetic activation. Beta-adrenergic blockers, as well as digoxin and calcium channel blockers, by blocking conduction over the AV node can decrease retrograde concealed conduction into the accessory pathway that may have been helping blunt conduction over the accessory pathway.

Nonpharmacologic Approaches. When the ventricular response during atrial fibrillation cannot be controlled pharmacologically, a procedure can be performed in the electrophysiology laboratory that permanently interrupts conduction from the atria to the ventricles. This procedure, *catheter ablation of the atrioventricular (AV) junction*, is relatively easy to accomplish under local anesthesia by the delivery of radiofrequency energy through a catheter placed near the AV node. Since this results in complete AV block, permanent pacemaker implantation is required afterward. Typically, a rate-responsive ventricular pacemaker (VVIR) is placed. If the patient has paroxysmal atrial fibrillation, a dual-chamber pacemaker with mode-switching capability should be used so that AV synchrony can be maintained when the patient has sinus rhythm. Mode switching is a function available in some newer pacemakers by which atrial fibrillation can be detected and results in the pacemaker automatically changing its pacing mode from dual chamber (atrial and ventricular) to single chamber (ventricular). When sinus rhythm returns, the pacemaker senses this and reverts back to the dual chamber mode, allowing tracking of the patient's native sinus rate. As atrial fibrillation persists after catheter ablation of the AV junction, the risk of thromboembolism is unchanged, and thus aspirin or warfarin therapy still needs to be considered (see later).

Newer approaches using catheter ablation to modify the AV junction so as to slow the ventricular response without creating complete AV block are being attempted. The goal is to attain rate control but avoid a pacemaker. Some investigators have reported success with this technique, but late occurrence of AV block has been reported, and this approach does not have universal acceptance. The irregular ventricular rhythm that remains after AV node modification (as opposed to the regular paced rhythm following AV node ablation) may cause persistent symptoms in some patients.

PREVENTION OF RECURRENCE

A noble goal in the treatment of patients with atrial fibrillation is to prevent recurrence of the arrhythmia. Two important points need to be kept in mind in this regard: (1) treatment of such patients has never been shown to prolong survival or decrease the incidence of stroke or peripheral embolism; (2) the drugs used to prevent recurrence may actually cause new arrhythmias (proarrhythmia).

A meta-analysis of six randomized, controlled trials of quinidine has shown that 1 year after cardioversion 50% of quinidine-treated patients remained in sinus rhythm compared with only 25% of control patients ($p < .001$). However, it was noted that death rates were higher in the quinidine group: total mortality 2.9% vs. 0.8%; sudden death 0.8% vs. 0.0%. Although this study does point out the potential problem of proarrhythmia seen with antiarrhythmic drug therapy, caution must be used so as not to overinterpret the problem, as the total number of patients suffering sudden death was small (3 of 413 patients).

The decision to treat atrial fibrillation is thus made with the intent of reducing symptoms. As with controlling the ventricular response in asymptomatic patients, exercise tolerance also increases once sinus rhythm is restored. Although preventing any recurrence is the best outcome, it is sometimes necessary to settle for a reduction in the frequency of recurrence. It is useful for the patient to be aware of this possible secondary goal of therapy so that any recurrence is not necessarily viewed as a complete failure. Aside from amiodarone, no one antiarrhythmic drug has been shown to be more effective than another in preventing recurrent atrial fibrillation and 1-year recurrence rates are in the range of 50% to 70%. Thus, choice of an antiarrhythmic drug is made based on patient characteristics and side effects of the drugs. Generally, in patients without coronary artery disease and with normal ventricular function, I will choose a Class IC agent (e.g., propafenone [Rythmol]), flecainide [Tambocor]) as first-line therapy. In those patients with coronary artery disease and/or ventricular dysfunction, I begin with a Class IA drug (e.g., quinidine) or sotalol (Betapace). Because of the proarrhythmic potential of all antiarrhythmic drugs, therapy is begun in the hospital while the patient's cardiac rhythm is monitored. Consideration can be given to initiation of Class IC agents as outpatients in those who have no coronary artery disease and normal cardiac anatomy and function. This is because the incidence of serious proarrhythmia in that specific setting is extremely low. However, it is important to involve the patient in this decision. If a Class IC drug is begun as an outpatient, it is best to have the patient return after 3 days of therapy to obtain an electrocardiogram to assess the extent of QRS prolongation (up to 20% beyond baseline is acceptable) and a treadmill exercise test to screen for proarrhythmia. Some arrhythmologists argue that amiodarone can be started on an outpatient basis in individuals without structural heart disease; however, this point is debated.

If neither a Class IA nor IC drug provides the desired control, amiodarone (Cordarone) often prevents recurrent arrhythmia. Additionally, amiodarone is very effective at blocking the AV node and slowing the ventricular response. Although the success of amiodarone is greater than for any other drug, side effects are more prevalent. Some of the most prevalent and/or troublesome are pulmonary fibrosis, hepatitis, and hypo- or hyperthyroidism. During follow-up of patients using amiodarone, it is best to assess them every 3 months during the first year of therapy and every 6 months thereafter. At each visit, in addition to a brief history and physical examination aimed at uncovering side effects, a chest radiograph, liver functions tests, and sensitive TSH should be obtained. I initiate amiodarone therapy in the hospital under continuous ECG monitoring with a loading dose of 800 mg twice a day for 4 days. The patient is then dismissed receiving 400 mg daily with the plan to reduce the maintenance dose to 300 or 200 mg daily within 6 months. Alternatively, some clinicians begin 200 mg daily initially without a loading dose. This latter approach takes longer for the patient to attain maximum antiarrhythmic effect. Ibutilide (Corvert) was recently approved for acute conversion of atrial fibrillation. It is available only as an intravenous preparation.

Nonpharmacologic Approaches. The maze procedure has been developed to prevent recurrences of atrial fibrillation. This operation involves incisions, resuturing, and the placement of cryolesions at different anatomic locations throughout the atrium. The strategic placement of these lesions prevents the occurrence of the reentrant wavefronts needed to support atrial fibrillation. Sinus rhythm is maintained, and atrioventricular conduction is intact in most patients. Long-term prophylaxis against thromboembolism does not appear necessary. Some patients may have early recurrence of atrial fibrillation, but this is likely related to the surgery and due to a different mechanism than the patient's original arrhythmia. This postoperative atrial fibrillation typically resolves within a couple of months. Initial reports are promising, with cure rates greater than 95%. Experience is growing rapidly at some centers, but long-term follow-up is lacking.

Catheter ablation within the atrium to cure atrial fibrillation is being investigated. Analogous to the surgical maze procedure, this technique aims to create multiple lines of block within the atria that prevent atrial fibrillation from occurring. The lines are strategically placed so that the sinus impulse can still traverse the right atrium to the AV node, and AV synchrony is maintained. At present, the catheter maze is early in its investigation. Many more patients and longer follow-ups are needed to determine where this therapy will fit into the treatment of atrial fibrillation. It has the potential to become a major therapeutic advance in the therapy of atrial fibrillation in the next few years.

STROKE PREVENTION

Acute Conversion to Sinus Rhythm. Electrical cardioversion of atrial fibrillation can be associated with embolic events. Whether the same risk exists for medical cardioversion using antiarrhythmic drugs is unknown but should be assumed until data prove otherwise. Exactly how long a person can be in atrial fibrillation before developing a risk of embolism during cardioversion is unclear. If the arrhythmia has been present for more than 24 hours or for an unknown duration, it is safest to proceed as though the risk is increased. In such a situation, oral anticoagulation with warfarin should be accomplished with the International Normalized Ratio (INR) in the 2.0 to 3.5 range for 3 to 4 weeks before attempting reversion to sinus rhythm. Embolic events following cardioversion can occur a week or more following the procedure; thus, anticoagulation should be maintained for an additional 4 weeks and perhaps longer based on the assessment of whether chronic prophylaxis is necessary.

In some instances, there may be a more urgent need to restore sinus rhythm, or there may be a contraindication to long-term anticoagulation. When cardioversion is contemplated in such situations, transesophageal echocardiography (TEE) may be useful in its ability to identify atrial thrombi that would almost always lead to deferral of cardioversion. The ability to detect atrial thrombi is enhanced by using a biplane or multiplane system and by the experience of the operator. A negative TEE reduces but does not exclude the possibility of an embolic event with cardioversion. When a patient is not adequately anticoagulated with warfarin, heparin should be used during the cardioversion as there is suggestive evidence that electrical shocks may be thrombogenic.

Chronic Prophylaxis. Patients with nonrheumatic atrial fibrillation have a risk of stroke or peripheral embolism of 3% to 6% per year, which is about five times that of people in sinus rhythm. Those who have *lone atrial fibrillation*, defined as age less than 60 years and no clinical heart disease or hypertension, appear to be at extremely low risk and probably do not need prophylaxis. Because of the increased incidence of embolism in all other patients, anticoagulant or antiplatelet therapy is strongly encouraged.

Numerous studies have shown that warfarin reduces the incidence of embolism by 64% to 86%. Most of these studies aimed to keep the prothrombin time ratio at 1.2 to 1.5 times control (International Normalized Ratio [INR] 1.5 to 3.0). A meta-analysis of the major anticoagulation trials suggests that an INR of 2.0 to 3.5 provides the greatest protection against embolism with the lowest risk of hemorrhage. The incidence of major bleeding episodes with warfarin was 1.3% to 1.5% per year, and intracranial hemorrhage was seen in 0.5% per year. The results concerning aspirin's efficacy are conflicting. One large study (Stroke Prevention in Atrial Fibrillation I [SPAF I]) showed a benefit to aspirin, 325 mg per day, compared with placebo; another study (AFASAK) reported no improvement with aspirin, 75 mg per day. SPAF II compared warfarin (PT 1.3 to 1.8 times control) with aspirin, 325 mg per day, and found that in patients 75 years old or less, warfarin

tended to have a lower rate of stroke or peripheral embolism (1.3% per year versus 1.9% per year) but not significantly so (p = 0.24). Likewise, in patients over 75 years of age, the primary event rate was nonsignificantly lower in the warfarin group (3.6% per year versus 4.8% per year, p = 0.41). Thus, the results of SPAF II imply that the event rate for patients aged 75 years or less is low enough with aspirin, 325 mg per day, that warfarin does not appear to add any benefit. This is particularly so when these patients have no clinical predictors of thromboembolism: history of hypertension, recent heart failure, or prior thromboembolism (0.5% per year event rate in the absence of those predictors). Diabetes mellitus is a predictor of thromboembolism in some studies. It is noteworthy that the presence of paroxysmal as opposed to chronic atrial fibrillation does not appear to affect the thromboembolic potential.

The results of echocardiography can help stratify for thromboembolic risk. Global left ventricular dysfunction or an enlarged left atrium (more than 2.5 cm per m²) identifies people at increased risk. Recent reports also show that spontaneous echo contrast ("smoke") seen in the left atrium is an independent predictor of thromboembolism in atrial fibrillation, increasing the risk fourfold. This finding can be detected by transesophageal echocardiography (TEE) in 25% to 60% of cases.

Although the use of warfarin versus aspirin must be individualized and the patient should be part of the decision-making process, the following general approach is reasonable. Patients under 75 years old with none of the risk factors just discussed are at low risk for embolism and can be treated with aspirin. Those under 75 years, with any of the risks, should receive warfarin. Patients over 75 years of age are at increased risk of major hemorrhage from warfarin and, although they may be at some increased risk of stroke due to their age, in the absence of other risks may best be treated with aspirin. The elderly patient with risk factors presents a particularly difficult therapeutic problem, and the decision of warfarin versus aspirin must take into consideration the patient's long-term outlook, concomitant medical problems, gait, and overall balance.

PREMATURE BEATS

method of
EZRA A. AMSTERDAM, M.D.
*University of California School of Medicine and
Medical Center*
Sacramento, California

Premature cardiac beats are the most frequent disturbances of cardiac rhythm and one of the most frequent causes of an irregular pulse. They originate from all areas of the heart; in descending order of frequency, they occur in the ventricles, atria, and atrioventricular (AV) junctional tissue. Although premature beats are a frequent manifestation of cardiac disease, they also occur in the absence of structural abnormalities of the heart and can be provoked by numerous cardiac and extracardiac factors. However, the prevalence and complexity of premature beats increase in the presence of cardiac disease, particularly during acute cardiac and noncardiac provoking factors. Although premature beats are frequently an incidental finding in both cardiac patients and healthy individuals, they commonly produce symptoms and can occasionally impair hemodynamic function. Moreover, they may also be harbingers of sustained tachyarrhythmias if not controlled. Their prognostic importance varies from nil to ominous and depends on the setting—a normal or diseased heart—in which they occur. Symptomatic premature beats may be distressing to the patient while asymptomatic premature beats may indicate increased prognostic risk to the physician. The essence of management of these rhythm disturbances is recognition that the patient, rather than the arrhythmia, is the primary consideration. Thus, depending on the circumstances of the individual patient, premature beats may require (1) no specific treatment,(2) correction or elimination of cardiac or extracardiac provoking factors, or (3) pharmacologic therapy.

DEFINITION

A premature beat is defined by its occurrence earlier in the cardiac cycle than the anticipated normal sinus beat, and it is further described by its origin from the atrium (atrial premature beat [APB]), AV junction (junctional premature beat [JPB]), or ventricle (ventricular premature beat [VPB]). A variety of other terms have been applied to premature beats, the most common of which are premature ventricular contraction (PVC), premature ventricular depolarization (PVD), extrasystole, and ventricular ectopic depolarization (VED). This alternative terminology has also been applied to atrial and junctional premature beats. Because an ectopic depolarization may be early (premature) or late (in which case it is an escape beat), and the prefix *extra* provides no information on timing, it is more precise to use the term "premature" to indicate an abnormally early beat.

Documentation of premature beats requires electrocardiograph demonstration to determine their timing and morphology accurately. Morphology reflects their site of origin (atrium, junction, ventricle), as described later under the specific types of premature beats. By common consensus, three or more consecutive premature beats define a tachycardia. For example, three consecutive VPBs, JPBs, or APBs comprise ventricular, junctional, and atrial tachycardia, respectively. Two consecutive premature beats are referred to as coupled premature beats or a couplet (coupled VPBs, JPBs, APBs). Single premature beats that occur after every other normal sinus beat are described as occurring in bigeminy; trigeminy and quadrigeminy indicate occurrence after every third and fourth normal beat, respectively. Only nonrepetitive premature beats will be discussed.

MECHANISMS

Premature beats are caused by the same mechanisms that are primarily responsible for most cardiac arrhythmias: (1) disorders of impulse conduction, represented by reentry, and (2) disorders of impulse generation, comprising abnormal automaticity and triggered activity.

Reentry

This mechanism is generally considered to account for the majority of cardiac arrhythmias. It is considered an abnormality of impulse conduction and involves re-excitation of an area of myocardium by an impulse that returns to the latter focus after traversing a circuitous route. It requires unidirectional block and may include a region of inexcitable tissue, such as a myocardial scar. Reentry accounts for what has been classically termed the "circus movement" that underlies many arrhythmias. If the circus movement results in "endless loop" impulse conduction, a sustained arrhythmia will result. Isolated premature beats occur when the impulse following the reentry pathway dissipates after a single cycle. Reentry is associated with ischemia or fibrosis of the myocardium, as well as drug toxicity and metabolic abnormalities.

Abnormal Automaticity

This mechanism refers to (1) the occurrence of spontaneous depolarization in cardiac tissue such as atrial and ventricular muscle that normally lacks intrinsic automaticity, and (2) increased automaticity in the His-Purkinje system, which is automatic under physiologic conditions. Conditions that can cause abnormal automaticity include ischemia, metabolic abnormalities, and drug toxicity (e.g., digitalis, catecholamine, methylxanthines).

Triggered Activity

This mechanism is defined as the generation of action potentials resulting from afterdepolarizations. Triggered activity differs from automaticity in that it is dependent on the previous action potential rather than representing a spontaneous depolarization. Afterdepolarizations may occur during repolarization (early afterdepolarizations) or after repolarization (delayed afterdepolarizations). Afterdepolarizations may be subthreshold and not result in a premature beat. If individual triggered action potentials reach the threshold for depolarization of the cell, premature beats appear, whereas repetitive triggered activity results in a sustained arrhythmia. Triggered activity can be caused by ischemia, digitalis, and catecholamines.

GENERAL CONCEPTS

Premature beats are detected during evaluation prompted by symptoms or as incidental findings on physical examination or electrocardiogram (ECG). Appropriate management is predicated on a thorough evaluation that includes a careful history, physical examination, and relevant laboratory studies, including a standard 12-lead electrocardiogram, and, in selected patients, special techniques such as ambulatory electrocardiographic monitoring. These methods will provide evidence not only of the presence or absence of premature beats, but also of cardiac and noncardiac conditions that may be etiologic factors for premature beats.

History

Symptoms. Premature beats are frequently suggested by complaints of palpitations, variably described by patients as an irregularity, skipped beats, or pounding. Occasionally, symptoms of dizziness, presyncope, or syncope may be related to premature beats, although they are more likely to indicate a sustained tachy- or bradyarrhythmia.

Palpitation is defined as an unpleasant perception of the heart beat as rapid or forceful. A "skipped beat" suggests an awareness of the compensatory pause frequently associated with premature beats, and a forceful sensation is commonly related to the increased contractility and augmented ejection of the post-extrasystolic beat.

It is noteworthy that there is a frequent discrepancy between palpitations and documented arrhythmia. Thus, in many patients with and without cardiac disease, palpitations do not correlate with premature beats but, rather, represent an unpleasant awareness of the heart beat unassociated with any abnormality. In these cases, the symptom is commonly attributable to anxiety. Moreover, most patients with premature beats, even in relatively high frequency, are not aware of the irregular cardiac activity. By contrast, a much higher proportion of patients with sustained arrhythmias are aware of the abnormality. In this regard, a recent study that evaluated patients with palpitations reported that the symptom was due to a cardiac etiology in less than one half of the group. The next largest category was psychiatric conditions, the majority of which were related to panic disorder.

Arrhythmogenic Factors. Important potential etiologies of premature beats revealed by the clinical evaluation include cardiac disease (ischemic, valvular, hypertensive, primary myocardial, right ventricular dysplasia, mitral valve prolapse), noncardiac disease (pulmonary disease, hyperthyroidism, electrolyte abnormalities), drugs (digitalis, diuretics, psychotropics, sympathomimetics), and habits (caffeine, nicotine, alcohol, cocaine). Optimizing therapy and/or eliminating provoking factors may be sufficient to alleviate premature beats.

Physical Examination

The physical examination provides direct evidence of premature beats by detection of an irregular pulse, and it is thereby important in indicating the need for further, objective evaluation by electrocardiography in selected patients. However, its utility resides in positive findings, since the brevity of the examination renders it insensitive to recognition of even relatively frequent premature beats. Isolated premature beats are distinguished by interruption of a regular rhythm by intermittent, singly occurring premature beats. However, the physical examination is limited beyond this point. It cannot provide the site of origin of the abnormal beat, since all types, by definition, occur early, and each may or may not be associated with a compensatory pause. The latter characteristic is worth emphasizing, since it is a common misconception that a compensatory pause is diagnostic of VPBs. Moreover, frequent premature beats of any site of origin may result in an irregularly irregular rhythm indistinguishable from atrial fibrillation, atrial flutter with variable conduction, and multifocal atrial tachycardia. VPBs may be useful in the clinical diagnosis of hypertrophic obstructive cardiomyopathy (HOCM, previously referred to as idiopathic hypertrophic subaortic stenosis). In this disease, the pulse of the post-VPB sinus beat, assessed by physical examination, is smaller than the pulse associated with sinus rhythm, whereas in normal individuals and those with systolic murmurs not related to HOCM, the post-VPB pulse is greater than that in sinus rhythm. This phenomenon is the result of the increased obstruction to left ventricular outflow caused by the augmented contractility of the post-VPB beat (a result of the force-frequency relation in cardiac muscle). The physical examination can reveal the characteristic click murmur of mitral valve prolapse, a condition commonly associated with VPBs.

Electrocardiogram and Ambulatory Monitoring

The definitive diagnosis of premature beats requires electrocardiographic documentation. The 12-lead electrocardiogram is a simple, relatively inexpensive office method by which abnormal beats can be diagnosed if they are present. If the rhythm is regular and symptoms are intermittent, ambulatory monitoring is the most accurate means of detecting and quantifying abnormal cardiac rhythm and its relation to symptoms and daily activity. However, this is an expensive method and should be reserved for selected patients with significant symptoms or evidence of cardiac disease. In this regard, it has recently been reported that the diagnostic yield and cost-effectiveness of transtelephonic event monitors were superior to those of 48-hour continuous ambulatory monitoring in the assessment of patients with palpitations. The resting electrocardiogram can also provide important evidence of cardiac abnormalities that are potential etiologies of premature beats. Thus, pathologic Q waves indicate prior myocardial infarction or cardiomyopathy. Enlargement of the ventricles or atria can be detected, and ST-T abnormalities may indicate ischemia or fibrosis. Left bundle branch block and combinations of conduction abnormalities are also indicative of structural heart disease. It is essential to search for the short PR interval (<0.12 sec) and delta wave of the Wolff-Parkinson-White syndrome associated with supraventricular arrhythmias and the long QT syndrome associated with ventricular arrhythmias and sudden death.

Exercise Testing

This test is useful in selected patients. It is indicated in patients with symptoms related to exertion in whom it provides objective evidence of exercise capacity; occurrence of symptoms; response of heart rate, rhythm, and blood pressure; and evidence of myocardial ischemia. It thereby can confirm or exclude, in a controlled setting, the presence or absence of cardiac rhythm abnormalities during exertional stress and potential etiologies. Exercise testing is also useful in patients whose symptoms do not occur during exertion to evaluate their threshold for arrhythmias and to detect evidence of cardiac disease. The response of premature beats to exercise testing is of limited use in determining the presence of cardiac disease. Premature beats in most patients, with or without cardiac disease, decrease during exercise and reappear as the heart rate declines postexercise. Exercise-induced reduction in premature beats, therefore, is not evidence of the absence of cardiac disease. However, an increase in the frequency of premature beats during exercise is associated with an increased probability of underlying cardiac disease.

Echocardiography

This method provides noninvasive evaluation of cardiac systolic and diastolic function, chamber dimensions, wall thickness, and valve structure and function. Intracardiac thrombi are also detectable by echocardiography. Abnormalities of all these features of cardiac structure and function may be relevant to the etiology of premature beats. In addition, the single most important factor relative to the prognostic significance of VPBs is left ventricular systolic function. Therefore, this single test provides extensive information on the cardiac status in a patient with premature beats. In selected patients, stress echocardiography provides a noninvasive approach to the detection of inducible myocardial ischemia and thereby to evidence of coronary artery disease.

Summary of General Approach to the Patient

Evaluation should be thorough to confirm or exclude the presence of premature beats in patients with compatible symptoms. The correlation between symptoms and objective evidence of premature beats is frequently weak. Patients with persistent symptoms and no evidence of premature beats on screening studies require further testing by sophisticated methods such as an event recorder or ambulatory electrocardiographic monitoring. Exercise testing and echocardiography provide important information of value in selected patients. The former method is useful in patients with exercise-related symptoms suggestive of premature beats, and the latter provides noninvasive cardiac evaluation that relates to the etiology of premature beats and the prognostic significance of VPBs. Elimination of provoking factors is essential and may obviate the need for further therapy in many patients.

ATRIAL PREMATURE BEATS

Clinical Features

APBs can be detected by prolonged electrocardiographic monitoring in approximately 10% of individuals without evidence of cardiac disease. However, their prevalence rises to 80% or more in patients with disease involving the atria, such as dilatation or fibrosis. The mechanism is usually automatic foci or reentry foci in the atrium, which are promoted by structural disease, but automatic foci may result from excessive adrenergic activity. Provoking factors include most of the etiologies enumerated earlier under History and, in addition, noncardiac conditions such as infection, fever, and emotional stress which involve sympathetic stimulation. APBs may cause symptoms, but the patient is usually not aware of them unless they are of high frequency.

Electrocardiogram

APBs are recognized on the electrocardiogram by the premature appearance and altered morphology of the P wave compared with the sinus P wave. Depending on the site of origin in the atrium and the electrocardiographic lead, alterations may include increased or decreased amplitude, widening, notching, or superimposition on the preceding T wave. APBs may be associated with (1) a compensatory pause before the next sinus P wave, (2) a pause that is greater than compensatory, or (3) no pause. These outcomes depend on the timing of the APB and on whether it penetrates and resets the sinus node. Very early APBs may be nonconducted (blocked) and hidden in the T wave. This can result in significant bradycardia if the APBs are bigeminal. Failure to recognize this abnormality may result in inappropriate therapy, such as a pacemaker, when the proper

approach is an antiarrhythmic agent to abolish the APBs and restore sinus rhythm. APBs may also result in aberrant conduction in the His-Purkinje system, owing to impulse conduction before these fibers are fully recovered. This yields a widened QRS that suggests a VPB if the premature P wave is not identified.

Management

The clinical approach to most patients with APBs consists primarily of identifying and eliminating provoking factors and optimizing treatment of underlying cardiac disease, if present. Specific antiarrhythmic therapy is usually not required unless the APBs precipitate tachycardias, in which case digitalis, a beta blocker, or a calcium channel blocker that inhibits AV node conduction can be utilized.

JUNCTIONAL PREMATURE BEATS

Clinical Features

JPBs are much less frequent than the other two forms of premature beats. They result from abnormal automaticity or reentry mechanisms and are induced by the previously noted provoking factors, most prominent among which are digitalis toxicity, myocardial infarction, and myocarditis. They may also occur in the absence of cardiac disease.

Electrocardiogram

Since the AV junction is located between the atria and ventricles, a JPB depolarizes in both anterograde (to the ventricles) and retrograde (to the atria) directions and can therefore produce both a P wave and a QRS complex. Their sequence on the electrocardiogram depends on both the site of origin of JPB in the junctional tissue and the conductivity of the pathways. If the retrograde impulse reaches the atria before the anterograde impulse reaches the ventricles, the result is a premature, inverted P wave followed by a premature QRS complex; if the atria and ventricles are simultaneously depolarized, the P waves will be lost in the premature QRS complex; and if the ventricles are depolarized initially, a premature QRS complex will precede the premature, inverted P wave. Aberrant conduction within the ventricles may produce a wide QRS that is indistinguishable from a VPB.

Management

Isolated JPBs are managed by correction of the underlying process. Specific antiarrhythmic therapy is usually not warranted unless sustained tachycardia occurs.

VENTRICULAR PREMATURE BEATS

Clinical Features

VPBs are the most frequent form of premature beat. They are associated with increased prognostic risk in patients with left ventricular dysfunction and are, therefore, a continuing therapeutic challenge. Drug therapy to suppress VPBs in order to prevent serious ventricular arrhythmias has been unsuccessful and is associated with increased mortality related to proarrhythmia. Because of these considerations, VPBs are the clinically most important of the premature beats. An encouraging development in this regard is the favorable findings in initial studies with amiodarone, and the results of large trials in progress with this agent are awaited.

The most frequent mechanism of VPBs is reentry, but automaticity and triggered activity are prominent factors in many patients. VPBs encompass the entire spectrum of provoking factors, but significant impairment of left ventricular function is the most important and most difficult to treat. VPBs originate at any site in the His-Purkinje (ventricular) conducting system and depolarize the right and left ventricles consecutively (rather than nearly simultaneously as occurs normally) by abnormal routes, accounting for the altered QRS complex in the electrocardiogram.

Electrocardiogram

A VPB is characterized electrocardiographically by a premature, bizarre, wide ($\geq$ 0.12 sec) QRS complex. The ST segment and T wave are usually directed opposite to the dominant deflection of the QRS, representing a secondary repolarization abnormality. (In the simplest terms, abnormal depolarization results in abnormal repolarization.) A retrograde P wave may be seen but is commonly obscured in the wide QRS complex. Retrograde activation of the atria may also be precluded by their prior depolarization by the normal sinus beat before the arrival of the retrograde impulse. A VPB usually results in a compensatory pause before the next sinus beat, but depending on the timing of the VPB and conduction velocity of the impulses, there may be no pause.

A wide QRS complex may represent a beat of supraventricular origin when *aberrant conduction* is present. This phenomenon occurs when a premature beat arises from a supraventricular focus before the nodal and infranodal conducting pathways (AV node, junctional tissues, and bundle branches) are completely repolarized, so that the impulse traverses an abnormal route. This abnormal conduction is reflected by aberration—distortion and widening—of the QRS complex, which can be difficult to distinguish from a VPB. This is an important distinction because of the different clinical implications of supraventricular and ventricular premature beats. Morphologic criteria have been developed to aid in discrimination of aberrantly conducted beats and VPBs. While these criteria are helpful, they are not definitive.

Descriptors favoring aberration include antecedent P wave, right bundle branch block pattern, triphasic QRS configuration in V1(rsR′), and initial QRS identical to the normally conducted beats. *Descriptors favoring ventricular origin*: fusion beats, capture beats, QRS $\geq$ 140 msec, left axis deviation, AV dissociation, and certain configurational characteristics of the QRS (V1: mono- or biphasic or R>R′; V6: QS or rS; concordance: similar QRS morphology V1–V6).

Management

In patients with and without cardiac disease, symptoms from isolated VPBs are unusual, even when the abnormal beats are frequent. The therapeutic dilemma posed by VPBs is primarily related to their importance as a risk factor for sudden death in patients with left ventricular dysfunction, possibly as triggers for initiating lethal ventricular tachyarrhythmias. Alternatively, they may be markers of electrical instability and high risk without having an initiating role. In studies of survivors of myocardial infarction, it has been established that the presence of high-grade VPBs (>10 per hour) increases the risk of death. Thus, the long-term mortality rate in patients with the combination of left ventricular ejection fraction of less than 40% and greater than 10 VPB per hour was 1.5 to 2.1 times higher than the mortality rate in patients with the same ejection fraction and less than 10 VPB per hour. However, as previously indicated, drug therapy to reduce mortality by eliminating or decreasing the frequency of high-grade VPBs in patients with left ventricular dysfunction, with the goal of preventing lethal arrhythmias, has not only failed to achieve this end but has also been associated with an increase in mortality.

The deleterious outcomes of drug therapy were most recently obtained in the Cardiac Arrhythmia Suppression Trial (CAST), and they have resulted in a general policy of refraining from the use of antiarrhythmic therapy in patients with asymptomatic VPBs. If the early reports of favorable results with amiodarone (Cordarone), are confirmed in current trials with this agent, our approach to antiarrhythmic drug therapy in this high-risk population will be altered. Noninvasive techniques such as the signal-averaged electrocardiogram have been highly accurate in identifying those patients within this population who are at the highest risk and are, therefore, suitable candidates for effective drug therapy. However, until the current trials with amiodarone are completed, the approach to high-grade VPBs in patients with left ventricular dysfunction comprises vigorous management of the underlying disease with the appropriate cardioprotective agents (aspirin, beta-adrenergic blockade, and lipid-lowering therapy for coronary artery disease; angiotensin-converting enzyme inhibitors, a diuretic, and digitalis for left ventricular dysfunction), optimization of anti-ischemic therapy, and correction of metabolic abnormalities.

In patients with acute coronary events (myocardial infarction, unstable angina), asymptomatic VPBs may presage the development of sustained ventricular arrhythmias. Therefore, it is appropriate to use antiarrhythmic drug therapy (lidocaine, procainamide, beta blockade) in this setting if asymptomatic VPBs are frequent (e.g., >10 per hour) or they occur in frequent couplets, and elimination of provoking factors (ischemia, pain, cardiac failure, metabolic abnormalities) does not alleviate the VPBs. VPBs that impair hemodynamic function require therapy.

In patients without evidence of structural heart disease, it is clear that VPBs impose no increase in prognostic risk. Distressing palpitations should be managed by correction of provoking factors and reassurance to the patient. This approach should result in the need for drug therapy in a small minority of this group who have intolerable palpitations associated with anxiety. The most appropriate drug is a beta blocker. This is particularly useful in patients in whom VPBs are related to the adrenergic stimulation associated with exercise or emotional stress.

In summary, specific drug therapy for asymptomatic, isolated VPBs is not currently indicated in patients with or without cardiac disease. In the former, drug therapy has not been beneficial and has been associated with increased mortality. Trials in progress with amiodarone are promising. In the group without cardiac disease, VBPs are not a risk factor for more serious arrhythmias and drug therapy should be avoided in all but exceptional cases.

HEART BLOCK

method of
JAMES H. KAPPLER, M.D., and
BRUCE GENOVESE, M.D.
Michigan Heart and Vascular Institute,
  St. Joseph's Mercy Hospital
Ann Arbor, Michigan

Heart block can broadly be defined as slowing or interruption of a transmitted chemoelectric depolarizing wave from one structure in the heart's specialized conduction system to an adjoining structure. Under normal circumstances, the conducted signal originates in the sinoatrial node (SAN) and propagates through atrial myocardium to the atrioventricular node (AVN). Velocity of conduction slows in this structure, allowing for ventricular diastolic filling. The signal then travels down the bundle of His and along the right and left bundle branches, leading to depolarization and contraction of respective ventricular myocardium. Conduction block can occur in any of the structures mentioned and is commonly categorized based on the resulting electrocardiographic findings. Conduction block can be either physiologic or the result of pathologic processes. The determination of the site of conduction block, as well as symptoms experienced by the patient during heart block, are important pieces of information with respect to prognosis and decisions regarding appropriate therapy.

SINOATRIAL NODE EXIT BLOCK AND SINUS NODE DYSFUNCTION

SAN exit block can be defined as one or more SAN depolarizations that fail to initiate atrial depolariza-

TABLE 1. Drugs Causing Sinus Node Dysfunction

Beta-adrenergic antagonists	Amiodarone
Calcium channel blockers	Sotalol
Verapamil	Digoxin
Diltiazem	Lithium
Quinidine	Phenothiazines
Procainamide	Alpha-methyldopa
Flecainide	Clonidine
Propafenone	

tion in the absence of a competing rhythm. Electrocardiographic manifestation of SAN exit block shows sinus pauses with intervals reproducibly equivalent to an exact multiple of the sinus cycle length or the interval between two normally conducted P waves. Sinus node exit block is one of several bradycardic arrhythmias suggesting sinus node dysfunction or the "sick sinus syndrome."

Sinus node dysfunction can also be diagnosed by evidence of resting sinus bradycardia (heart rate less than 60 beats per minute), sinus arrest, sinus bradycardia following spontaneous or elective termination of various arrhythmias, or inability to mount an appropriate heart rate response during exercise. The prevalence of sinoatrial exit block in the general population appears to become less frequent with age. SAN exit block has been documented in as many as 65% of healthy asymptomatic children, 28% of asymptomatic male medical students, and 1.4% of asymptomatic middle-aged volunteers during ambulatory monitoring. Symptomatic sinus node dysfunction becomes most common in the age group over 50 years old.

Sinus node dysfunction is most commonly caused by drugs (Table 1) but also can be associated with ischemic heart disease, hypervagotonia, dilated cardiomyopathy, cardiac surgery, idiopathic fibrosis of the SAN, hypertension, vasculitis, neoplasms, and infiltrative diseases. Treatment of sinus node dysfunction and SAN exit block should be reserved for those who are symptomatic as a result of the bradyarrhythmia. Care should be taken to ensure that symptoms of fatigue, heart failure, exercise intolerance, syncope, or presyncope are truly a direct effect of the arrhythmia. This can be done with ambulatory monitoring, exercise testing, or a trial of discontinuing potentially offending medications. Treatment for sinus node dysfunction generally involves implantation of a permanent pacemaker. Approximately half of all pacemakers in the United States have been implanted for sinus node dysfunction. Less frequently, anticholinergic medications, such as propantheline (Pro-Banthine)* or disopyramide (Norpace), or phosphodiesterase inhibitors, such as theophylline* preparations, may be used successfully.

ATRIOVENTRICULAR BLOCK

Atrioventricular block can be defined as slowing or disruption of the depolarizing wave front in its nor-

---

*Not FDA-approved for this indication.

mal progression from the atrium to the ventricle (Table 2). This can occur within the atrium, the atrioventricular node, the His bundle, or the bundle branches. The degree of block is based upon electrocardiographic findings and not necessarily on the site of block.

First-Degree Atrioventricular Block. First-degree block can be defined as a PR interval of longer than 200 ms. Because the PR interval prolongs physiologically as heart rate increases, first-degree block should be diagnosed only on electrocardiograms with heart rates less than 100 beats per minute, on which the rhythm is assumed to be originating from the sinus node. First-degree block has been observed among normal adult males with a prevalence of approximately 1%. The PR interval measures the time from initial atrial activation (beginning of the P wave) to earliest ventricular activation (beginning of the QRS complex). Therefore, first-degree block can be caused by intra-atrial conduction delay, atrioventricular node conduction abnormalities, and His-Purkinje conduction abnormalities. First-degree block generally does not cause significant hemodynamic disturbance and has no adverse prognostic implications in the absence of other conduction abnormalities or the diagnosis of coronary artery disease. In general, first-degree block requires no specific therapy. Special considerations will be discussed later.

Second-Degree Atrioventricular Block. Second-degree block can be defined as intermittent failure of the depolarizing wave, originating in the atrium, to reach the ventricle. Prognosis depends on the site of block and the association of symptoms and hemodynamic compromise. Two electrocardiographic types of second degree block have been described.

TYPE I SECOND-DEGREE BLOCK. In general, type I block is characterized by gradual prolongation of the PR interval leading to a P wave that fails to conduct to the ventricle. This may or may not be in association with gradually shortening R-R intervals. Type I second-degree block has been observed in as many as 9% of 24-hour ambulatory monitors among asymptomatic adults. Episodes of type I second-degree block occur more frequently at night and among well-conditioned individuals, suggesting an association with increased vagal tone within the AV node. Invasive electrophysiologic study has confirmed that type I second-degree block most frequently occurs within the AV node but infrequently can occur within the His bundle or bundle branches.

To determine the site of block, both invasive and noninvasive assessment have proved helpful. Atropine, 0.6 to 1.0 mg, can be administered intravenously to enhance AV node conduction and increase the sinus rate. If block is present in the AV node, atropine should decrease vagal tone and 1:1 conduction should be observed. As atropine has little effect on the His-Purkinje system, the increased frequency of conduction through the AV node should result in a higher ratio of block when present below the AV node. Exercise testing may also bring out higher ratios of block in patients with His-Purkinje disease, whereas 1:1 conduction is frequently observed during exercise among patients with block within the AV node. Carotid sinus massage increases vagal tone at the level of the AV node and is likely to result in a higher ratio of block when present at the level of the AV node, whereas patients with block in the His-Purkinje system may show improved conduction ratio during carotid sinus massage as the sinus rate and frequency of conduction through the AV node decrease. Invasive electrophysiologic testing can also assist in the diagnosis of the site of type I block but is rarely necessary.

Morbidity and mortality among patients with type I block depend on association with coronary artery disease, site of block, and symptoms experienced with bradycardia. Symptomatic patients and those with block within the His-Purkinje system have been shown to have reduced mortality with pacemaker implantation. The great majority of patients with type I block are asymptomatic with block located within the AV node and require either no change in therapy or adjustment of medication likely to adversely effect AV node conduction.

TYPE II SECOND-DEGREE ATRIOVENTRICULAR BLOCK. This is characterized by absence of sinus P wave conduction to the ventricle in one or more consecutive beats preceded by at least two conducted sinus P waves with equal PR interval. The first conducted P wave following any series of nonconducted beats will have an equal PR interval. This should be observed in the absence of a competing atrial or ventricular rhythm. Care should be taken to exclude the presence of nonconducted premature atrial beats observed with a shorter P-P interval and different P wave morphology. Type II block is exceedingly rare within the asymptomatic population, and the site of block occurs with relative exclusivity in the His-Purkinje system. Invasive evaluation among patients with type II block shows 30% of block to be within the His bundle and the remainder within the bundle branches and the distal His-Purkinje system. There is a relatively high rate of morbidity and mortality

TABLE 2. **Causes of Atrioventricular Block**

Drug effect
Ischemic heart disease
Intrinsic conduction system disease
  Lev's disease
  Lenegre's disease
Rheumatic heart disease
Myocarditis
Hypoxemia
Electrolyte abnormalities
Trauma/surgery
Chagas' disease
Myxedema
Amyloidosis
Malignancies
Sarcoidosis
Scleroderma (progressive systemic sclerosis)
Muscular dystrophies
Congenital heart disease

among patients left untreated in this group with a high frequency of progression to complete heart block. No medications have been shown to be of benefit. Pacemaker implantation is warranted in all patients with type II atrioventricular block.

Third-Degree Atrioventricular Block. Third-degree block is characterized by the inability of a depolarizing wave originating in the atrium to reach the ventricle. This may be accompanied by a regular escape rhythm from the atrioventricular junction or the ventricle and requires that the supraventricular rate exceed the rate of the escape rhythm when present. Third-degree block can be transient or permanent. The prevalence of third-degree block is rare within the general population both on routine electrocardiography and ambulatory monitoring. The site of block is variable although most frequently in the His-Purkinje system. Third-degree block within the AV node most frequently occurs as a result of drug toxicity or acute inferior wall myocardial infarction and frequently may not require permanent pacemaker implantation. Diagnosis of chronic third-degree block is not difficult and requires pacemaker implantation unless in the setting of acute inferior myocardial infarction, drug toxicity, hyperkalemia, hypercalcemia, hypervagotonia, or recent cardiac surgery.

Transient, symptomatic third-degree block is less easily diagnosed and can be evaluated using ambulatory 24-hour monitoring, patient-activated continuous loop recording, exercise testing, or invasive electrophysiologic assessment. If potentially reversible causes of third-degree block are not present, pacemaker implantation should be performed. Prior to the availability of pacemaker implantation, the mortality of third-degree atrioventricular block was observed to be as high as 78%. The long-term mortality among patients with third-degree block following pacemaker implantation is strictly dependent on age and coexisting illness. Congenital complete heart block should be mentioned in that these patients are frequently young and have a reliable escape rhythm with a high probability of freedom from related morbid events. Pacemaker implantation should be entertained only in those patients with exercise intolerance, syncope, or presyncope, with risk of multiple device implants weighed against potential benefits.

FASCICULAR BLOCK AND BUNDLE BRANCH BLOCK

The conduction system below the His bundle includes the right bundle branch and the left bundle branch, which divides into an array of Purkinje fibers called the anterior and posterior fascicles. Block may occur in any combination of these structures. In general, the morbidity and mortality of isolated right or left bundle branch block and anterior or posterior fascicular block depend on age and co-morbid clinical variables and not on progression of conduction system disease; therefore, prophylactic pacemaker implantation is not indicated in asymptomatic individuals.

Bifascicular block may be defined as left bundle branch block or right bundle branch block (RBBB) in addition to either anterior or posterior fascicular block. Asymptomatic patients require no further evaluation or therapy. For patients with syncope or presyncope, invasive electrophysiologic testing is indicated to assess the potential role of transient high-grade AV block as the cause of syncope as well as that of malignant supraventricular or ventricular rhythms. Patients in whom markedly abnormal resting His-Purkinje conduction intervals have been observed show a high rate of developing third-degree block. However, they have not been shown to have improved survival with pacemaker implantation. Permanent pacemaker implantation is indicated to reduce the risk of syncope and associated morbidity.

Trifascicular block is manifested electrocardiographically by RBBB with alternating anterior and posterior fascicular block. RBBB with either anterior or posterior fascicular block and first-degree block is also sometimes referred to as trifascicular block. Again, prophylactic pacing in asymptomatic patients is not indicated. Symptomatic patients may undergo empirical pacemaker implantation but may benefit from invasive electrophysiologic testing to exclude inducible ventricular arrhythmias as the cause of syncope or presyncope.

TACHYCARDIAS

method of
DAVID J. KESSLER, M.D.,
ROBERT C. CANBY, M.D., and
RICHARD L. PAGE, M.D.
*University of Texas Southwestern Medical
　Center
Dallas, Texas*

The evaluation of patients presenting with tachycardia begins with a careful history. In particular, questions regarding syncope, lightheadedness, chest pain, and congestive heart failure should be addressed. The symptom of palpitations is nonspecific, since it may arise from any change in rhythm or cardiac contractility. Information about regularity, rate, and nature of initiation and termination can provide clues to the diagnosis. In combination with physical findings and 12-lead electrocardiograms obtained during sinus rhythm and tachycardia, the mechanism of tachycardia can be established.

SUPRAVENTRICULAR TACHYCARDIAS

A clinically useful subdivision of supraventricular tachycardias is the distinction between atrial and junctional tachycardias (Table 1). Atrial arrhythmias are defined as arising from atrial tissue, whereas junctional tachycardias require the atrioventricular node as a critical component of the tachycardia mechanism.

TABLE 1. Classifications of Supraventricular Tachycardia

Atrial tachycardias
Sinus tachycardia
Sinus node reentry
Atrial fibrillation
Atrial flutter
Atrial tachycardia
Multifocal atrial tachycardia

Junctional Tachycardias
Atrioventricular nodal reentry
Atrioventricular reentry
Paroxysmal junctional tachycardia

Atrial Arrhythmias

Sinus Tachycardia. Sinus tachycardia may be associated with a variety of physiologic and pathologic processes. Exercise, anxiety, fever, anemia, hypovolemia, heart failure, and hyperthyroidism may cause tachycardia. Typically the rhythm is nonparoxysmal, with onset and termination occurring gradually. Heart rates may exceed 200 beats per minute (bpm). In general, therapy targeted at the underlying state is indicated. Beta-adrenergic blockade can be useful to relieve symptoms when heart failure is not present.

Sinus Node Reentry. This uncommon arrhythmia can mimic sinus tachycardia because the focus occurs in the perinodal tissue, and the P wave morphology is similar or identical to that seen during sinus rhythm. The paroxysmal nature of onset and termination distinguishes it from sinus tachycardia. Heart rates during tachycardia are often less than 130 bpm. Vagal maneuvers may slow the rate or terminate tachycardia. Therapy with calcium antagonists or beta blockers is often successful. Alternatively, catheter ablation has been reported to eliminate this arrhythmia.

Atrial Flutter. Atrial flutter (AFL) is characterized by a regular atrial rhythm typically occurring at approximately 300 bpm. The "flutter waves" on electrocardiogram (ECG) reflect the atrial reentry mechanism and often have a sawtooth pattern in the inferior leads (II, III, aVF). The P wave morphology may be difficult to identify at ventricular rates of 150 bpm when 2:1 atrial to ventricular conduction occurs. Flutter waves are visible at higher degrees of AV block, as often observed with AV nodal blocking drugs or conduction system disease.

The causes of AFL are similar to those responsible for atrial fibrillation (see page 262) and include hypertension, systolic and diastolic heart failure, coronary disease, valvular disease, pulmonary hypertension, pericarditis, and previous atriotomy. The physical examination may reveal flutter waves in the jugular venous waveform. Symptoms are similar to those seen with atrial fibrillation (AF) or rapid atrial tachycardias, although the higher heart rate may precipitate more pronounced hemodynamic compromise. Rarely, AFL will conduct in a 1:1 fashion to the ventricles and cause hemodynamic compromise and syncope.

Management issues for AFL are similar to those of atrial fibrillation and atrial tachycardias: rate control, conversion, maintenance of sinus rhythm, and anticoagulation. Rate control is often more difficult in patients with AFL than in those with atrial fibrillation, and blocking to an atrioventricular ratio of greater than 2:1 may require a combination of AV nodal blocking drugs. The risk of thromboembolic complication of AFL, as compared with that of AF, is undetermined. A prudent approach is to treat atrial fibrillation and AFL in the same way, since patients often have both arrhythmias. Anticoagulation for 3 weeks before and 4 weeks after cardioversion is recommended. Membrane-stabilizing agents may cause pharmacologic cardioversion of AFL and are used to promote and maintain sinus rhythm after electrical cardioversion. They include the Vaughan-Williams class IA (procainamide [Pronestyl], disopyramide [Norpace], quinidine); class IC (flecainide [Tambocor], propafenone [Rythmol]); and class III (sotalol [Betapace], amiodarone [Cordarone]) drugs (Table 2). The efficacy of these agents in maintaining sinus rhythm at 1 year ranges from 30% to 80%, and the use of any specific agent must be balanced against its side effect profile.

Common side effects of type IA agents include nausea and diarrhea (quinidine), anticholinergic symptoms (disopyramide), and a lupus-like syndrome (procainamide). These agents prolong the QT interval and may cause bradycardia-dependent polymorphic ventricular tachycardia (torsades de pointes), so careful monitoring should be maintained during initiation of therapy.

Flecainide and propafenone slow intracardiac con-

TABLE 2. Antiarrhythmic Therapy

Drug	Usual Dose	Elimination
Type IA		
Procainamide (Procan SR)	500–2000 mg q 6 h	Renal, hepatic
Quinidine	300–900 mg mg q 8 h	Hepatic, renal
Disopyramide (Norpace CR)	150–450 mg mg q 12 h	Renal, hepatic
Type IB		
Mexiletine (Mexitil)	150–300 mg g 8 h	Hepatic
Type IC		
Propafenone (Rhythmol)	150–300 mg g 8 h	Hepatic
Flecainide (Tambocor)	50–200 mg g 12 h	Hepatic, renal
Type II		
Beta blockers	See individual drugs	
Type III		
Sotalol (Betapace)	80–240 mg g 12 h	Hepatic, renal
Amiodarone (Cordarone)	200–400 mg daily	Hepatic ?
Type IV		
Diltiazem (Cardizem SR)	120–180 mg g 12 h	Hepatic
Verapamil (Calan SR)	120–180 mg g 12 h	Hepatic
Digoxin	0.125–0.25 mg daily	Renal, hepatic
Adenosine (Adenocard)	6–12 mg IV	

duction, which results in PR and QRS prolongation on the ECG. Their efficacy in atrial fibrillation is similar to that of quinidine and sotalol. These agents are well tolerated, but flecainide increases the risk of sudden death in patients with prior infarction and ventricular ectopy, and both drugs may be proarrhythmic. In general, these agents are not administered as first-line therapy in patients with structural heart disease.

Sotalol has little effect on intracardiac conduction but causes QT interval prolongation and may precipitate torsades de pointes. In addition, sotalol causes bradycardia out of proportion to its beta-blocking effects. Intolerance in patients with lung disease, heart failure, and bradycardia is observed.

Amiodarone has many potential side effects: thyroid and liver abnormalities, skin discoloration, corneal microdeposits, bradycardia, and pulmonary fibrosis. In spite of these side effects, low-dose amiodarone is relatively well tolerated and quite effective in maintaining sinus rhythm.

When an atrial stabilizing agent is administered in therapeutic doses and cardioversion has not occurred, direct current cardioversion can be performed employing low energy (50 to 100 joules). AFL can also be terminated by overdrive pacing of the atrium, either using intracardiac stimulation or noninvasively utilizing a transesophageal electrode. Maintenance therapy with an atrial stabilizing agent is continued after cardioversion has been performed. When sinus rhythm cannot be maintained, chronic rate control with AV nodal blocking drugs or AV junction ablation and pacemaker implantation are indicated. In isolated AFL, catheter-mediated ablation of the flutter circuit is reported to be successful in excess of 80% of selected patients.

Atrial Tachycardia. Atrial tachycardia (AT) is due to spontaneous depolarization of an ectopic focus within the atria. AT accounts for 5% to 10% of supraventricular arrhythmias and occurs also in the setting of structural heart disease. Onset and termination may be sudden or show a "warm-up" phenomenon with gradual onset. Therapy is similar to that of atrial flutter, consisting of AV nodal blocking agents and atrial stabilizing drugs (Table 3). Radiofrequency catheter ablation can offer permanent cure by destroying the ectopic atrial focus. Alternatively, ablation of the AV node with pacemaker placement eliminates symptoms in refractory cases.

Multifocal Atrial Tachycardia. MAT occurs in the setting of lung disease and usually causes minimal or no symptoms. This irregular rhythm is occasionally mistaken for atrial fibrillation. Three or more different P wave morphologies and PR intervals are required to define MAT. The mainstay of therapy is treatment of the underlying lung disease, although verapamil and digoxin have been reported to improve the arrhythmia.

Junctional Tachycardias

AV Nodal Reentry. Atrioventricular nodal reentrant tachycardia (AVNRT) causes approximately 60% of paroxysmal supraventricular tachycardias. These arrhythmias typically have a narrow QRS complex, except in patients with baseline intraventricular conduction delay or bundle branch block, or when there is functional conduction delay with tachycardia. The ventricular rate is typically between 150 and 250 bpm. In the typical form of AVNRT, the electrical impulse travels down the "slow" pathway of the AV node and reenters back up the "fast" pathway. This causes P waves to occur just before, within, or just after the QRS complex. An R′ in ECG lead V1 only during tachycardia represents the superimposed P wave and is diagnostic. In the atypical form of AVNRT (less than 5%), the reentrant circuit is reversed (down the "fast" and reentering the "slow" pathway), causing the P wave to occur substantially after the QRS. AVNRT occurs in structurally normal hearts, with a slight preponderance of women, and increases in incidence with age. Patients present with palpitations, breathlessness, and neck pounding. Presyncope and syncope rarely occur following the onset of tachycardia.

AVNRT may be terminated by transient block within the slow AV nodal pathway; this is accomplished with vagal maneuvers such as carotid massage and Valsalva or with medication. Adenosine, an endogenous nucleoside, is the best drug option and is effective in over 90% of cases. This drug causes transient AV block when administered as an intravenous bolus injection. Mild side effects of breathlessness and anxiety resolve promptly due to the very short half-life of less than 2 seconds. Alternatively, intravenous verapamil or diltiazem is effective. For chronic therapy, calcium channel antagonists, beta blockers, and digoxin usually reduce the frequency of recurrence. In addition, the membrane-stabilizing agents are effective. As an alternative to drug therapy, radiofrequency catheter ablation is offered as first-line therapy in many centers. It is effective in curing AVNRT in over 90% of patients with few complications.

TABLE 3. **Chronic Therapy for Arrhythmias**

Arrhythmia	Target	Drug Class
Inappropriate sinus tachycardia	Sinus node	II, IV, IC
Sinus node reentry	Sinus node	IV, II
Atrial flutter	Atrium	IA, IC, III
	AV node	II, IV
Atrial tachycardia	Atrium	II, IV, IA, IC, III
Nonparoxysmal junctional	AV node	II
AV nodal reentry	AV node	II, IV, IA, IC, III
AV reentry	AV node	II, IV
	Accessory pathway	IA, IC, III
Ventricular tachycardia	Ventricle, HPS	IA, III, IC, II
Ventricular fibrillation	Ventricle, HPS	IA, IC, III, II
Long QT syndrome	Ventricle	II

See Table 2 for drug classes and usual dose; HPS indicates His-Purkinje system.

Atrioventricular Reentry and the Wolff-Parkinson-White Syndrome. AV reentrant tachycardia (AVRT) accounts for 30% of paroxysmal supraventricular tachycardias. The mechanism involves activation of the ventricles using the AV node and reentry to the atria via an accessory atrioventricular pathway. Accessory pathways are congenital and may cross from atrium to ventricle along the mitral annulus, tricuspid annulus, or septum. AVRT most commonly occurs in patients with Wolff-Parkinson-White syndrome (WPW). This syndrome is defined by a short PR interval, QRS prolongation during sinus rhythm (due to a delta wave), and symptoms related to tachycardia. The prolonged QRS in sinus rhythm reflects a fusion between normal ventricular activation and pre-excitation of the ventricle using the accessory pathway. During orthodromic tachycardia, anterograde activation of the ventricles occurs through the AV node, whereas retrograde activation of the atria is via the accessory pathway. In antidromic tachycardia (which is uncommon), the circuit is reversed: ventricular activation occurs through the accessory pathway, with atrial activation occurring retrograde through the AV node. In some patients with AVRT, the accessory pathway is concealed and functions only in the retrograde direction; this allows AVRT, but gives a normal QRS complex during sinus rhythm.

The ECG during AVRT may appear identical to that of AVNRT, although the P wave, if visible, occurs distinctly after the QRS (instead of being fused with the QRS). The rate of tachycardia is similar to that of AVNRT (150 to 250 bpm) but tends to be slightly faster. The prevalence of the WPW pattern in the general population is 1 to 3 per thousand, but less than half of patients with the WPW pattern have tachycardia. WPW occurs primarily in structurally normal hearts, although there is an association with Ebstein's anomaly and mitral valve prolapse.

The tachycardias associated with WPW also may have a wide QRS complex, due to either atrial fibrillation (with anterograde conduction using the accessory pathway) or antidromic AVRT. Pre-excited atrial fibrillation is not uncommon and can cause syncope or even sudden death. Pre-excited AF is recognized by an irregularly irregular wide complex rhythm that may also have occasional narrow beats.

Patients present with symptoms of palpitations, chest discomfort, dyspnea, and lightheadedness, and, rarely, true syncope that may date back to childhood. Rarely, a patient presents with sudden cardiac death due to pre-excited AF and subsequent ventricular fibrillation; for this reason WPW should always be considered in the differential diagnosis of sudden death occurring in a young person.

The acute management of AVRT is similar to that of AVNRT, directed at AV nodal block to terminate the tachycardia. If vagal maneuvers are not successful, then adenosine is the drug of choice. Alternatively, verapamil (Isoptin) can be administered intravenously. If the patient presents with pre-excited atrial fibrillation, AV nodal blocking drugs are con-traindicated since they can accelerate the tachycardia by facilitating conduction down the accessory pathway. In this case, procainamide is the drug of choice since it both blocks conduction in the accessory pathway and may stabilize the atrium.

Medical management for patients with AVRT but no pre-excitation is similar to that for patients with AVNRT, and any AV nodal blocking drug is appropriate. When a delta wave is present, AV nodal blocking drugs are to be avoided, and drugs that impair accessory pathway conduction are indicated (quinidine, procainamide, disopyramide, flecainide, propafenone, sotalol, amiodarone). Alternatively, radiofrequency catheter ablation has become a first-line option. A single procedure confirms the mechanism of the paroxysmal supraventricular tachycardia (PSVT) and allows ablation of the accessory pathway in over 90% of patients.

Nonparoxysmal Junctional Tachycardia. Junctional tachycardia in adults may occur in the clinical settings of acute myocardial infarction, postoperative cardiac surgery, myocarditis, and digitalis toxicity. Nonparoxysmal junctional tachycardia typically accelerates following a premature ventricular or atrial depolarization and may maintain rates between 70 and 130 bpm. AV dissociation is observed, and the rate may be irregular. Therapy is rarely required; however, beta blockade may slow tachycardia until the primary etiology resolves.

VENTRICULAR ARRHYTHMIAS

Monomorphic Ventricular Tachycardia. Ventricular tachycardia (VT) is defined as three or more consecutive QRS complexes of ventricular origin at a rate over 100 bpm; when the VT lasts more than 30 seconds or causes hemodynamic compromise, it is considered sustained. Monomorphic VT (MMVT) is defined by a uniform morphology and cycle length, and polymorphic VT (PMVT) has variable morphology and cycle length.

The majority of MMVT is associated with ischemic heart disease and is secondary to reentry in the area of a previous myocardial infarction. MMVT also occurs in patients with dilated cardiomyopathy, hypertrophic cardiomyopathy, infiltrative diseases (sarcoid or RV dysplasia), and occasionally in patients with structurally normal hearts.

The patient with a sustained, regular, wide complex tachycardia may present with minimal symptoms, chest pain, dyspnea, presyncope, syncope, or sudden death. It is necessary to distinguish MMVT from supraventricular tachycardia in order to direct acute and chronic therapy. A history of prior infarction, coronary disease, or coronary risk factors are all suggestive that a wide complex tachycardia is VT. Although patients with VT are usually hypotensive, a normal blood pressure does not exclude the diagnosis. Intermittent cannon a waves of the jugular venous waveform and variability of the first heart sound suggest dissociation of atrial and ventricular contraction and imply the diagnosis of VT.

A number of complex schemes have been published for evaluation of the 12-lead ECG, but a few simple guidelines will help establish the diagnosis of VT (as opposed to aberrant supraventricular tachycardia). Atrioventricular dissociation is the only truly diagnostic finding. This is demonstrated by P waves on the ECG that march through the wide complex tachycardia at a slower rate, or the presence of capture or fusion beats. A capture beat is an early, narrow, complex beat caused by atrial activation conducting to the ventricle without interrupting tachycardia. Fusion beats are caused by the combination of a sinus beat and a VT complex; capture beats are similar, although the ventricle is completely activated by the narrow complex QRS. Several criteria suggestive of VT are listed in Table 4.

The unstable patient with a wide complex tachycardia (or any unstable tachycardia) should undergo immediate DC cardioversion. If the patient is hemodynamically stable and without angina, pharmacologic management is warranted. The first drug of choice for suspected VT is lidocaine, although recent data suggest that procainamide is preferable for VT that is unrelated to acute ischemia. If the diagnosis is in doubt (VT vs. supraventricular tachycardia), and especially if pre-excited AF is considered, intravenous procainamide is the drug of choice. Direct current cardioversion (with as low as 50 joules) should be performed if drug therapy is unsuccessful or if the patient becomes unstable.

Inspection of the ECG during sinus rhythm can assist in diagnosis of wide complex tachycardia. For example, a delta wave or fixed bundle branch block would suggest a supraventricular origin of the tachycardia. Following cardioversion, the patient is observed in a monitored setting, and myocardial infarction is ruled out. Continued therapy with lidocaine or procainamide should be considered if the patient was unstable with the VT.

After myocardial infarction has been ruled out, evaluation for etiology is undertaken. Echocardiography is used to assess for the presence of structural heart disease: wall motion abnormalities consistent with ischemia, hypertrophy, congenital anomalies, or valvular abnormalities causing ventricular dilatation. Most patients should undergo cardiac catheterization to assess coronary anatomy. In patients with structurally normal hearts and MMVT with a left bundle branch block pattern, cardiac magnetic resonance imaging (MRI) is useful to assess for RV dysplasia. Exercise testing may demonstrate exercise-related VT. A 24-hour ambulatory (Holter) monitor will quantify the amount of spontaneous ventricular arrhythmias and may help evaluate further therapy. Clinical electrophysiology (EP) study will confirm the diagnosis and help guide therapy.

Ventricular tachycardia occurring in the setting of coronary disease will be reproduced at EP study in 95% of cases. This is useful to determine whether the VT may be terminated by overdrive pacing. If so, the patient may be a candidate for an implantable cardioverter-defibrillator (ICD) with antitachycardia pacing. Additionally, the response to intravenous procainamide may be assessed in the laboratory. Traditional management of VT included serial EP studies that evaluated the response to one or more antiarrhythmic drugs. Today, only one or two drugs are evaluated, if drug testing is undertaken at all. As an alternative to invasive EP testing, Holter-guided therapy can be considered. Antiarrhythmic agents used for the chronic treatment of VT include quinidine, procainamide, disopyramide, flecainide, propafenone, moricizine, sotalol, and amiodarone. In selected cases, if the VT is tolerated hemodynamically and is unifocal in origin, radiofrequency ablation may be effective.

The implantable cardioverter-defibrillator (ICD) has become a mainstay of therapy for patients with hemodynamically significant VT or sudden cardiac death. ICD implantation has become a relatively minor procedure since the electrodes are placed via the subclavian vein and the generator can be placed in the pectoral region. Third-generation devices offer both low-output cardioversion shocks and antitachycardia pacing to terminate VT along with bradycardia pacing.

In patients with nonischemic cardiomyopathy and sustained VT, the clinical arrhythmia can be induced only about 60% of the time at EP study. EP study is still recommended, since it allows assessment of pace-terminability of the rhythm and may assist in the choice of therapy. Additionally, about 5% to 10% of patients with a dilated cardiomyopathy and sustained VT will have a bundle branch re-entrant VT that can be cured with radiofrequency ablation.

As mentioned, ventricular tachycardias can occur in structurally normal hearts. The most common, known as repetitive MMVT, originates in the right ventricular outflow tract and typically has a left bundle branch morphology and inferior axis (negative QRS in lead V1 and positive in leads II, III, and aVF). It is often exercise-related and suppressed by beta blockers or calcium channel blockers. Another normal heart VT, known as idiopathic left ventricular tachycardia, originates at the base of the posterior papillary muscle and demonstrates a right bun-

---

TABLE 4. **12-Lead ECG Discrimination of Supraventricular and Ventricular Tachycardias**

Wide Complex Tachycardia: Criteria for VT

AV dissociation
  P waves marching through tachycardia
  Fusion complexes
  Capture beats
  Absence of RS in all chest leads (V1–V6)
QRS morphology
  LBBB pattern (monophasic downward in V1): greater than
    0.16 sec
  RBBB pattern (monophasic upward in V1): greater than
    0.14 sec
  R/S ratio in V6 less than 1 (mostly negative QRS complex in
    V6)

Abbreviations: LBBB = left bundle branch block; RBBB = right bundle branch block.

dle branch, left axis pattern (positive in V1, I, and aVL; negative in aVF). It is responsive to verapamil and most antiarrhythmic agents. Both tachycardias are also amenable to radiofrequency ablation for permanent cure.

Patients with ventricular tachycardia occurring in the setting of arrhythmogenic right ventricular dysplasia may at first appear to have a structurally normal heart, although there is often substantial fatty infiltration of the right ventricle. These changes are best visualized with MRI, but echocardiogram and right ventriculogram may also show abnormalities. There may be several different VT morphologies, all originating from the right ventricle, and tachycardia may be precipitated by exercise. Due to the risk of sudden cardiac death and the difficulty of suppression or ablation, ICD therapy is often recommended.

Polymorphic Ventricular Tachycardia. Like MMVT, this occurs in the setting of ischemic and nonischemic cardiomyopathy. At times, an MMVT will degenerate to polymorphic ventricular tachycardia (PMVT). Likewise, PMVT may degenerate to ventricular fibrillation. The diagnosis is usually straightforward, although pre-excited AF in the setting of two or more accessory AV pathways may resemble PMVT.

The mechanism responsible for PMVT is suggested by the presence or absence of QT prolongation during sinus rhythm. In the absence of QT prolongation, PMVT is treated in a similar fashion to poorly tolerated MMVT or ventricular fibrillation. In the presence of QT prolongation and bradycardia, PMVT is called torsades de pointes. Afterdepolarizations that occur during the prolonged plateau phase of the cardiac action potential (which is the intracellular equivalent of a prolonged QT interval) are believed to be responsible for torsades. It is recognized in two distinct situations. First, torsades occurs with an "acquired long QT." Prolongation is due to medication toxicity and/or electrolyte abnormalities (such as quinidine or sotalol and hypokalemia and hypomagnesemia). Treatment is directed at correcting the precipitating factor and increasing the heart rate with isoproterenol or pacing.

The second cause for torsades is congenital. Two inherited forms have been recognized: the Jervell–Lange-Nielsen syndrome is an autosomal recessive trait associated with deafness; the Romano-Ward syndrome is an autosomal dominant trait associated with normal hearing. Patients may present with syncope, sudden cardiac death, or, simply, a family history of sudden cardiac death. They commonly develop arrhythmias during periods of increased adrenergic tone such as fright, exertion, and stress. Management of these patients includes beta blockers, pacemaker therapy, stellate ganglion blockade or resection, and implantation of an ICD.

Ventricular Fibrillation and Sudden Cardiac Death. Ventricular fibrillation (VF) is recognized on the ECG by a coarse, undulating baseline without other electrical activity. VF often occurs in the same setting as VT (other than for "normal heart" VT); in fact, VF can be a result of degeneration of VT. VF may also be a consequence of acute ischemia.

The patient who experiences VF loses consciousness within seconds. If cardiopulmonary resuscitation is not initiated, irreversible neurologic injury will result within minutes. The first treatment is immediate DC defibrillation. If the first three shocks do not result in conversion, countershock is repeated following epinephrine, then lidocaine, then beryllium.

In spite of improved life support training and paramedic availability, at best only one patient in three survives out-of-hospital arrest. VF resulting from a reversible cause, such as ischemia, does not require further evaluation or therapy. In the absence of a reversible cause, survivors of cardiac arrest are at high risk of recurrence. VF is typically evaluated by invasive EP study. The finding of MMVT implies that VT may have caused VF. The provocation of VF is a nonspecific response, but it is significant if the pacing protocol to induce the rhythm was not aggressive. In the past, drug therapy was guided by the serial EP studies. Recently the use of the ICD (with or without EP study) has replaced drug therapy in most cases. In addition, empirical amiodarone therapy appears to improve survival in patients with VF. Studies are underway to determine which treatment option is superior.

CONGENITAL HEART DISEASE

method of
SCOTT E. FLETCHER, M.D.
*Creighton University and University of Nebraska Childrens Hospital
Omaha, Nebraska*

Congenital heart disease is relatively uncommon, with an incidence of approximately 8 cases per 1000 live births. Over the past several decades, with improvement in surgical or catheter intervention, most children with congenital heart disease lead healthy lives long after their intervention. The most common presentations are (1) an infant or child with a murmur, (2) a cyanotic newborn infant, and (3) an infant with congestive heart failure.

MURMUR EVALUATION

Most murmurs in pediatric patients are innocent and unrelated to any cardiac abnormality. Innocent murmurs can be made louder by conditions that increase cardiac output, such as fever, exercise, or anemia. The most common innocent, or functional, systolic murmurs are (1) the branch pulmonary artery flow murmur in the neonate, (2) pulmonary outflow murmur, (3) Still's murmur, (4) supraclavicular bruit, and (5) cardiorespiratory murmur. A venous hum is a continuous murmur that can be made to disappear by supine positioning or jugular compression.

Pathologic murmurs are often but not always present with congenital heart disease. Pathologic murmurs cannot be made to disappear by position changes; however, they may change in intensity. Diastolic murmurs are always pathologic.

CYANOSIS

Cyanosis occurs when more than 5 gm per dL of deoxygenated hemoglobin is present in blood. Cyanosis is usually respiratory in origin, with intrapulmonary right-to-left shunting due to ventilation-perfusion mismatch, but intracardiac right-to-left shunting due to heart disease must be considered. Cyanosis may be more apparent in the polycythemic child or the patient with poor cardiac output and increased oxygen extraction at the tissue level.

CONGESTIVE FAILURE

Major manifestations of congestive heart failure include tachypnea, tachycardia, excessive sweatiness, poor feeding, and failure to thrive. Rales and peripheral edema typically appreciated in adult patients with congestive heart failure are rare in infants and children. Hepatomegaly from passive congestion of a distensible liver capsule is a common but late finding in congestive heart failure. Cardiomegaly by chest radiograph is the rule. Infants and children are usually given a diuretic (furosemide) with or without digoxin therapy. Some patients may benefit from afterload reduction with angiotensin-converting enzyme (ACE) inhibitors.

VENTRICULAR SEPTAL DEFECT

By far, the most common congenital heart defect is ventricular septal defect (VSD). The typical presentation of a VSD is a murmur with or without signs of congestive heart failure. The manifestations, as well as management decisions, of a VSD are dictated by the relative pulmonary and systemic vascular resistances and the size and location of the septal defect. The systolic murmur of VSD is usually harsh and can be best heard at the mid to lower left sternal border. When significant left-to-right shunting occurs, a diastolic flow rumble can also be heard across the mitral valve.

Four general types of VSD are encountered. Perimembranous VSD is the most common. These defects account for nearly 80% of all significant communications within the ventricular septum. Infants with a large perimembranous VSD usually present between 2 weeks and 2 months of age with evidence of pulmonary overcirculation. Infants with large VSDs and normal pulmonary vascular resistance may minimally benefit from increased caloric-density formulas for improved weight gain. In a subgroup of patients with large VSD, pulmonary vascular resistance remains high and the patient does not manifest signs of overt congestive heart failure. With recent advances in neonatal cardiac surgery, most infants with large perimembranous ventricular septal defects are

operated within the first 6 months of life for closure of the defect. Moderate-sized perimembranous VSDs may present with signs and symptoms of congestive heart failure; however, not all defects will require surgical closure. Some perimembranous VSDs may close spontaneously or decrease in size over the first several years of life to a point of being hemodynamically insignificant. Spontaneous closure tends to occur by incorporation of tissue of the septal leaflet of the tricuspid valve into the defect. Some moderate-sized ventricular septal defects do not close or decrease in size spontaneously, and surgical intervention is warranted. This surgery is usually performed prior to 2 years of age. Small perimembranous VSDs can close spontaneously. This generally occurs in the first year of life; however, late closure has been documented.

All perimembranous VSDs place patients at risk of bacterial endocarditis, and patients should receive prophylaxis at times of risk. Perimembranous VSDs are occasionally associated with the development of progressive aortic insufficiency owing to prolapse of the aortic valve into the septal defect. Reports of left ventricular (LV) to right atrial (RA) shunts have been described, with spontaneous closure by septal tricuspid leaflet tissue ingrowth. Most cardiologists recommend surgical repair at time of recognition of LV to RA shunts, as well as of progressive aortic insufficiency that may occur with valve tissue prolapse into VSDs.

The second most common location for VSD is in the trabecular muscular septum. In early infancy, they are as common as perimembranous VSD. Muscular VSDs tend to close spontaneously in the first months of life with growth and thickening of the ventricular septum. Muscular VSDs may be associated with other forms of congenital heart disease. Rarely an isolated muscular VSD is large enough to require surgical intervention. Surgical closure can be difficult because of the heavy trabeculations within the right ventricle.

A third location of VSD is in the inlet septum. Inlet VSDs, also known as AV canal-type VSDs, tend to be large and do not close spontaneously. This subtype of VSD is commonly associated with Down's syndrome. Usually a cleft in the anterior mitral valve leaflet is associated. Surgical closure with or without repair of the mitral valve is generally required.

The fourth location of VSD is in the juxta-arterial position. These defects are also termed supracristal. Supracristal VSDs are most frequently seen in Asian populations and are relatively rare in other ethnic groups. Supracristal VSDs do not close spontaneously and are often complicated by significant aortic valve insufficiency. The mechanism of aortic valve insufficiency is prolapse of a valve cusp into the septal defect. Surgical therapy is probably warranted upon discovery of this rare VSD.

ATRIAL SEPTAL DEFECT

Atrial septal defect (ASD) is the second most common congenital heart lesion. It is by far the most common defect to be diagnosed after infancy. A systolic murmur may be heard over the pulmonary listening area secondary to increased flow. A fixed split-second heart sound is classic. When significant left-to-right shunting occurs, a diastolic flow rumble across the tricuspid valve can be heard.

Except for mild growth deficiency, symptoms are unusual in the first decade of life. By the fifth decade of life, significant ASDs usually result in some exercise intolerance. Pulmonary vascular congestion, arrhythmias, and right ventricular failure are typical late symptoms.

The outcome of atrial septal communications discovered during the neonatal period depends on the size of the defect. Defects less than 3 mm will universally undergo spontaneous closure or result in a probe patent foramen ovale. Defects between 3 and 8 mm in size have a 75% chance of decrease in size to a hemodynamically insignificant level. Generally, defects larger than 8 mm will need surgical or transcatheter intervention.

Secundum ASDs account for over 80% of ASDs, are located in the region of the fossa ovalis, and usually present with an asymptomatic heart murmur or cardiomegaly on screening radiograph. If ASD closure is performed prior to 5 years of age, most patients do well. Atrial arrhythmias occur with increased frequency in patients with unrepaired ASD or those undergoing late closure. Surgical closure of secundum ASDs is accomplished with an extremely low morbidity and mortality. Transcatheter therapy with several types of ASD devices has been successfully used in small to medium-sized atrial communications. Even small atrial septal communications pose a theoretical risk of paradoxical systemic emboli. In patients suffering a stroke, management of such defects is controversial.

The second most common location of ASD is in the ostium primum region. Often associated with VSD of the AV septal type, ostium primum ASDs do not close spontaneously. Ostium primum defects may be part of a complete AV septal complex. Primum ASDs are always associated with clefts in the mitral valve, so mitral insufficiency may result. Because of associated mitral insufficiency, all primum ASDs will require bacterial endocarditis prophylaxis when patients are placed at risk. Transcatheter closure techniques are not considered appropriate to close primum ASDs because of the proximity of the defect to the atrioventricular valves. Surgical repair before the age of 5 years is usually recommended.

Less common, sinus venosus ASDs occur near the junction of the superior vena cava and the right atrium. This type of defect is almost always associated with anomalous connection of right-sided pulmonary veins. Physical findings and natural history are similar to secundum atrial septal defect with the addition of significant sinus node disease following surgical closure and baffling of the pulmonary veins to the left atrium. The rarest atrial septal communication is in the coronary sinus. Coronary sinus ASDs occur in the region of the coronary sinus ostia via unroofing the sinus such that left atrial blood has easy access to the coronary sinus. Closure of the atrial septum (sinus os), leaving the coronary sinus unroofed, results in a small residual right-to-left shunt, but eliminates the right-sided volume load.

PULMONARY STENOSIS

Pulmonary stenosis (PS) may occur as an isolated defect and is a common component in complex congenital heart defects. A systolic murmur of variable intensity is heard at the upper left sternal border. A systolic ejection click is common. Isolated PS usually occurs at the level of the pulmonary valve. Typical stenotic pulmonary valves are thin and form a dome in systole. A subgroup of stenotic pulmonary valves are truly dysplastic. These valves have characteristic supravalve narrowing and thickened cauliflower-like leaflets. Transcatheter therapy in the form of balloon valvuloplasty has become the treatment of choice for pulmonary valve stenosis. Dysplastic pulmonary valves are less amenable to standard valvuloplasty techniques.

Severity of PS is graded into four categories: A right ventricular-to-pulmonary artery gradient of less than 30 mmHg is considered mild. Mild PS rarely progresses and may actually improve with time. Most patients are asymptomatic, and the course is benign. PS is termed moderate when the right to left ventricular pressure ratio is between 50% and 100% and right ventricular to pulmonary artery pressure gradient is less than 80 mmHg. Most patients will have electrocardiographic evidence of right ventricular hypertrophy, which can lead to endocardial fibrosis and right ventricular dysfunction. If noninvasive evaluation with electrocardiogram, physical examination, or echocardiogram suggests moderate pulmonary valve stenosis, cardiac catheterization is warranted, and pulmonary balloon valvuloplasty is usually performed.

PS is considered severe when right ventricular pressure is equal to left ventricular pressure or the right ventricular to pulmonary artery gradient is greater than 80 mmHg. The majority of children with severe PS have symptoms of exercise intolerance. An attempt at pulmonary balloon valvuloplasty in the catheterization laboratory is warranted and usually successful. When the pulmonary valve is dysplastic or severe subvalve narrowing is present, surgical therapy may be necessary. If balloon valvuloplasty or surgical therapy is successful in achieving mild PS or better, the long-term course of PS is usually benign. Critical PS occurs in a small subgroup of pulmonary valves that present in infancy with ductal dependent pulmonary blood flow. Some infants require palliative systemic to pulmonary artery shunts whereas other patients may be treated with balloon valvuloplasty alone. A combination of a palliative shunt and an outflow procedure is used in some patients. The size and function of the heavily hypertrophied right ventricle will ultimately determine whether a complete two-ventricular repair is feasible.

AORTIC STENOSIS

Aortic valve stenosis (AS) is the most common left heart obstructive lesion. One to two percent of the general population have a bicuspid aortic valve that may become dysfunctional to the point of requiring surgical attention in middle to late adulthood. A smaller number of functionally bicuspid aortic valves cause significant obstruction to LV outflow and require intervention during childhood years. Intervention in the form of balloon valvuloplasty or surgical valvuloplasty is usually performed in an effort to relieve left ventricular hypertrophy that may result in fibrosis and ischemic changes. The natural history of severe aortic valve stenosis suggests that sudden death in untreated AS is relatively common, as is endocarditis. With current management and antibiotic prophylaxis, these risks have significantly decreased. The typical presentation of AS is a murmur in an asymptomatic patient. The murmur of AS is systolic, usually with a click, and heard best at the upper right sternal border.

In addition to auscultatory findings, chest radiograph may show cardiomegaly, and the patient with poor left ventricular function may have pulmonary vascular congestion. In the older child, the electrocardiogram may demonstrate left ventricular hypertrophy; however, the neonate with critical AS demonstrates right ventricular hypertrophy. Echocardiography is a reliable noninvasive method of assessing the severity of aortic stenosis in children. Doppler-derived mean transvalvular gradients appear to correlate best with peak-to-peak LV to aortic gradients measured in the cardiac catheterization laboratory. Significant ST-T wave changes during performance of a maximal exercise test may indicate a need for intervention in the patient with AS. These exercise results, however, can be somewhat confounding in the patient with mild AS, as judged by echocardiographic evaluation.

We define mild aortic stenosis as a peak-to-peak pressure gradient of 40 mmHg or less in an asymptomatic patient. In general, no therapy is required except for the use of subacute bacterial endocarditis (SBE) prophylaxis when placed at times of risk; however, these patients require diligent follow-up to investigate for worsening ventricular hypertrophy, ischemic symptoms, or progressive stenosis by noninvasive means.

Moderate AS, defined as a gradient less than 40 mmHg with symptoms or between 40 and 70 mmHg peak-to-peak gradient without symptoms is generally treated. These catheter-measured gradients usually correlate with a mean transvalvar gradient of 25 mmHg or more by Doppler echocardiography. Palliative therapy consists of balloon valvuloplasty in the catheterization laboratory or surgical valvotomy. Either can be associated with recurrence of stenosis as well as new aortic insufficiency (AI).

In severe AS, there may be T wave changes in the lateral precordial leads, suggesting ventricular strain or ischemia. Dilatation of the ascending aorta is common. Balloon valvuloplasty is our procedure of choice, with a target result of 60% reduction in gradient. Greater relief of gradient may be associated with more severe AI. Critical aortic stenosis is seen exclusively in the neonatal period. Systemic cardiac output is dependent on right ventricular output through the patent ductus arteriosus. Critical AS is associated with unicommissural aortic valves. Critical AS can be treated with balloon dilatation via umbilical, femoral, or carotid artery approaches. Careful attention to balloon size (i.e., 90% annular diameter or less) should be observed because AI is poorly tolerated in this age group. Repeat valvuloplasty may be required at a later date.

Valve replacement is sometimes necessary in children with moderate-to-severe AS or AI. More recently, the Ross procedure with placement of a pulmonary autograft in the aortic position and a cadaveric homograft in the pulmonary position has been used with gratifying results. This procedure alleviates the need for long-term anticoagulation.

COARCTATION OF THE AORTA

Coarctation of the aorta (COA) is due to medial thickening of the proximal descending aorta. The clinical presentation of COA depends on the severity of obstruction and the age of the patient. Neonates may present with congestive heart failure or even shock. Associated cardiac defects such as VSD are frequent. Neonatal coarctation is associated with hypoplasia of the transverse aortic arch and aortic isthmus. Although balloon angioplasty may be successful in relieving symptoms of congestive heart failure, recurrence of obstruction is common. We prefer an aggressive surgical approach with augmentation of the transverse aortic arch.

Children with COA of the aorta outside the neonatal period generally present with upper extremity hypertension, decreased lower extremity pulsation, and possibly continuous murmurs from collateral blood flow around the COA. A systolic ejection click as a manifestation of frequently associated bicuspid aortic valve can often be appreciated. Without intervention, greater than 90% of patients with COA will die by age 50 years. Causes of death are aortic rupture, dissection, endocarditis, congestive heart failure, or intracranial hemorrhage. Successful repair reduces the risk of morbidity and mortality from all these causes. Intervention for COA should be undertaken when there is an upper to lower extremity resting blood pressure gradient of 15 to 20 mmHg or greater in the face of normal cardiac output. This degree of obstruction is generally associated with left ventricular hypertrophy by electrocardiogram.

Presently, surgical repair of COA using either an end-to-end anastomosis, subclavian flap, patch repair, or extended end-to-end anastomosis is done. Rarely, aneurysm formation at the site of repair has been described for all techniques; however, it is more frequent when the patch repair is performed. Residual transverse arch hypoplasia may predispose to aneurysm formation. Balloon arterioplasty of discrete coarctation has been well described and is gaining acceptance. To avoid rare aortic aneurysm, the balloon size should not exceed the diameter of the aorta at the level of the diaphragm.

Balloon arterioplasty is regarded as the treatment of choice for recurrence of COA after initial successful balloon angioplasty surgical repair. In a small number of patients, balloon arterioplasty with placement of endovascular stents has been used. The long-term results of aortic endovascular stents and the interventionalists' ability to redilate them with patient growth are under investigation.

TRANSPOSITION OF THE GREAT ARTERIES

Transposition of the great arteries (TGA) presents in the first several weeks of life with moderate-to-severe cyanosis. The pulmonary artery arises from the left ventricle and the aorta from the right ventricle, giving rise to parallel circulations. To sustain life, a significant mixing lesion must be present at the level of the atrial septum, ventricular septum, or patent ductus arteriosus. Auscultation alone may be unimpressive except for a single second heart sound from the anteriorly malpositioned aorta. ECG may show right axis deviation and right ventricular hypertrophy. In neonates with an inadequate site of mixing, prostaglandin E_1 (Prostin VR Pediatric) infusion may be used to open the ductus arteriosus in order to stabilize the patient.

In simple TGA, most infants are currently managed with an arterial switch procedure. This surgical procedure involves transection above the level of the semilunar valves and moving the great vessels to their appropriate ventricle with transfer of the coronary arteries. The arterial switch is generally performed in the first several weeks of life. Intermediate term follow-up of patients repaired via the arterial switch procedure is encouraging and supports continued use of this approach. In some patients with TGA, associated cardiac anomalies such as valvar or subvalvar pulmonary stenosis or complicated coronary artery anatomy may necessitate an alternative surgical approach.

In the past, patients with TGA were managed with an atrial repair known as the Mustard or Senning procedure. Both consist of redirecting systemic venous return to the mitral valve so that deoxygenated blood may be pumped to the pulmonary arteries by a morphologic left ventricle and oxygenated blood pumped to the systemic circulation by a morphologic right ventricle. Although many patients having undergone the atrial baffle procedure continue to do extremely well, problems with the right ventricle serving as a systemic ventricular pump are increasingly encountered. Other postoperative problems include baffle obstruction, atrial and ventricular arrhythmias, and rarely, sudden death.

PATENT DUCTUS ARTERIOSUS

Patent ductus arteriosus (PDA) is a normal vascular structure in fetal life. The ductus arteriosus generally closes within the first 24 to 72 hours of extra-uterine life. Persistent patency of the ductus is more common in premature infants and may impose a significant volume load on a relatively noncompliant left ventricle in these small neonates. Because of significant respiratory distress, some premature infants will require pharmacologic ductus closure with prostaglandin inhibitors or surgical ligation.

In older children, a patent ductus arteriosus is diagnosed by the presence of an asymptomatic heart murmur in an infant or child. Typically, the murmur is continuous and heard best in the left infraclavicular area. In large PDA, left ventricular hypertrophy and left atrial enlargement may be present on ECG. Chest radiograph may show increased pulmonary vascular markings and cardiomegaly. Untreated, the natural history of patent ductus arteriosus includes congestive heart failure, endocarditis, and rarely, pulmonary vascular disease. PDA closure is recommended at any age. In the asymptomatic patient, closure should be delayed until 1 year of age, as spontaneous resolution of the left-to-right shunt has been reported. In the past, surgical ligation and division has been the treatment of choice. A national PDA coil registry provides evidence that transcatheter occlusion of small to medium-sized ductuses with Gianturco embolization coils has now become a suitable alternative. Rashkind transcatheter PDA devices (not presently available in the United States) have also been demonstrated effective in achieving ductal closure.

TETRALOGY OF FALLOT

Malalignment ventricular septal defect, pulmonary stenosis, overriding aorta, and right ventricular hypertrophy make up the tetralogy of Fallot (TOF). In the extreme case, deviation of the outlet ventricular septum may be so significant as to result in pulmonary atresia. The degree of cyanosis depends on the amount of obstruction to pulmonary blood flow. Cyanosis is very severe in TOF with pulmonary atresia and absent in the so-called pink tetralogy with mild pulmonary stenosis. Typically the patient is suspected of having heart disease based on the systolic murmur of blood flow across the right ventricular outflow obstruction. The murmur is harsh and loudest at the left upper sternal border, with radiation into both lung fields. ECG shows right ventricular hypertrophy, and the classic chest radiograph demonstrates a boot-shaped heart caused by right ventricular enlargement and hypoplasia of the main pulmonary artery segment.

The approach to TOF has undergone significant evolution since 1945 when Drs. Blalock and Taussig treated a TOF patient with a subclavian artery-to-pulmonary artery anastomosis. Presently palliative shunts to augment pulmonary blood flow are used only when associated anomalies preclude complete repair. Generally closure of the ventricular septal defect and relief of the right ventricular obstruction can be performed with minimal morbidity and mortality in patients greater than several months of age. In younger patients with marked cyanosis, patients with anomalous coronary arteries requiring cadaveric homograft placement, or patients with severe pulmonary artery hypoplasia, palliative shunts such as the modified Blalock-Taussig shunt to the central pulmonary arteries or palliative balloon valvuloplasty is used. In this selected group of patients, definitive repair is performed at a later date. The postoperative course in patients with tetralogy of Fallot is frequently benign but may be complicated by residual pulmonary stenosis, pulmonary regurgitation, residual ventricular septal defect, right ventricular dysfunction, arrhythmias, and on rare occasions, sudden death.

ATRIOVENTRICULAR SEPTAL DEFECT

Atrioventricular septal defect (AVSD), also known as endocardial cushion defect or AV canal defect, is common among children with Down syndrome. In a complete AVSD, there is a large-inlet muscular ventricular septal defect as well as an ostium primum atrial septal defect and a cleft in the anterior leaflet of the mitral valve. Symptoms are similar to those of a large ventricular septal defect. Unrepaired, these patients may have accelerated development of pulmonary vascular obstructive disease. In patients with persistent elevation of pulmonary vascular resistance, growth may be near normal; however; more commonly failure to thrive is seen. Repair of AV septal defect by the one- or two-patch technique should be performed in infancy.

In some patients, the AVSD may be incomplete with only a VSD or a primum ASD. In fact, some patients may have isolated cleft of the mitral valve apparatus. In this particular scenario, surgical repair may be recommended at a later date. In a minority of patients with AVSD, right or left ventricular hypoplasia is present and may preclude a biventricular repair. Surgery for AVSD is more difficult than for isolated ASD or VSD, and success is often determined by postoperative mitral valve function.

HYPOPLASTIC LEFT HEART SYNDROME

Hypoplastic left heart syndrome (HLHS) is a severe congenital heart defect that is characterized by hypoplasia of left-sided cardiac structures. The mitral valve is critically stenotic or atretic, as is the aortic valve. The left ventricle is of inadequate size to perform systemic work. With spontaneous constriction and ultimate closure of the patent ductus arteriosus in the first several days of life, the left ventricle is asked to provide systemic cardiac output that was previously provided by the morphologic right ventricle. The left ventricle is inadequate for

this purpose, and severe metabolic acidosis and shock will occur. In patients diagnosed prenatally by fetal echocardiography or postnatally because of mildly decreased peripheral pulses, hepatomegaly, and mild respiratory distress, this insult of acidosis may be avoided by the use of prostaglandin E_1 to maintain ductal patency.

Without intervention, more than 95% of infants die in the first several months of life, with only rare survivors beyond 1 year. If the family pursues medical treatment, two palliations are possible. The first is heart transplantation, which requires lifelong immunosuppression and is limited by donor organ availability. A second option is a staged reconstructive palliation. The first stage "Norwood procedure" is a high risk operation that prepares the morphologic right ventricle to perform as the systemic ventricular pump. This operation requires a great deal of expertise, but recent advances suggest a greater than 80% survival for stage I Norwood. The second and third stage operations are described in the following section.

FUNCTIONAL UNIVENTRICULAR HEARTS

A host of congenital cardiac lesions associated with hypoplasia of either the right or left ventricular chambers now receive palliation with a univentricular repair. The Fontan procedure, initially described for tricuspid atresia, is used for double-inlet left ventricle, hypoplastic left heart, hypoplastic right heart, unbalanced AV canal, and other congenital cardiac defects in which two functional ventricles are not present. The Fontan procedure routes systemic venous return from the inferior and superior caval systems to the pulmonary arteries without a ventricular pump in this circulation. This procedure can be staged such that only superior caval flow is directed to the pulmonary arteries at first (hemi-Fontan or bidirectional Glenn). Following a period of adaptation, inferior caval flow is directed to the pulmonary arteries. Success of the Fontan procedure depends on adequate systolic function of the systemic ventricle, undistorted pulmonary artery anatomy, low pulmonary vascular resistance, normal diastolic relaxation of the systemic ventricle, and absence of significant atrioventricular valve regurgitation.

HYPERTROPHIC CARDIOMYOPATHY

method of
LAWRENCE S. COHEN, M.D.
Yale University School of Medicine
New Haven, Connecticut

Isolated descriptions of patients with probable hypertrophic cardiomyopathy appeared in the European medical literature in the mid-nineteenth century. But it was in 1907 that Schmincke definitively described severe diffuse hypertrophy in the hearts of two women, considering the disorder to be congenital in origin and responsible for left ventricular outflow tract obstruction. As is often the case with scientific discoveries, interest in this syndrome did not ignite until almost 50 years later when the ability to define the hemodynamics in patients with this entity in the cardiac catheterization laboratory became a reality. These latter investigations initiated a series of studies into the nature of the disease, its patterns of inheritance, the presence or absence of true obstruction, its medical and surgical treatments, and its natural history. Controversies surrounding the nature of the syndrome spawned a variety of terms to describe hypertrophic cardiomyopathy— idiopathic hypertrophic subaortic stenosis (IHSS), hypertrophic obstructive cardiomyopathy (HOCM), muscular subaortic stenosis (MSS), and asymmetric septal hypertrophy (ASH), to name a few. Most early investigators stressed the dual concepts of left ventricular hypertrophy and dynamic subaortic stenosis. Careful analysis of left ventricular angiograms identified that the basis for the subaortic obstruction was systolic apposition of the anterior leaflet of the mitral valve against the hypertrophied interventricular septum.

As further understanding of the disease developed, it became clear that some symptomatic patients with hypertrophied ventricles might not evidence any features of left ventricular outflow tract obstruction. These observations led to the thesis that abnormalities in left ventricular compliance might also contribute to the abnormal pathophysiology of these patients. The concept of diastolic dysfunction contributing to left heart failure became an increasingly attractive explanation in certain patients. The introduction of M-mode echocardiography opened a new era in the diagnosis and understanding of hypertrophic cardiomyopathy. Asymmetric septal hypertrophy was a consistent feature of the disease whether or not patients were symptomatic and whether or not outflow tract obstruction was present. Systolic anterior motion of the mitral valve was seen most frequently in the subset of patients who had outflow tract obstruction. The echocardiogram allowed for extensive screening of family members and helped demonstrate that the disease is transmitted as an autosomal dominant trait with a high degree of penetrance. The preceding introduction to this disease entity can be summarized as follows: Hypertrophic cardiomyopathy should be thought of as a primary myocardial disease resulting in a nondilated, hypertrophied ventricle (usually asymmetrical), with or without dynamic outflow tract obstruction, and usually of a familial nature, manifesting typical clinical signs and symptoms with a characteristic clinical course and response to treatment modalities.

Patients with hypertrophic cardiomyopathy most often present with dyspnea, angina, or dizziness (presyncope). Other symptoms such as edema or palpitations are less frequent. In greater than two thirds of patients, dyspnea is the predominant symptom, and in the majority of patients it is the presenting symptom. Dyspnea and paroxysmal nocturnal dyspnea are a consequence of decreased compliance of the left ventricle with consequent increase in left ventricular filling pressure. This leads to elevation of left atrial and pulmonary venous pressures. Chest pain is a frequent symptom and is likely due to a mismatch between coronary artery supply and the excessive demands of a hypertrophied myocardium. The chest pain may be more prolonged than the usual angina due to ischemic heart disease. It may worsen after administration of sublingual nitroglycerin. The pain may not be associated with physical or emotional stress but may come on after the

cessation of physical activity. It may be made worse by standing and be improved by lying down. Syncope or presyncope is the third most common symptom. This symptom may have a variety of pathophysiologic determinants. It may be secondary to cardiac arrhythmias or to a low cardiac output due to a sudden increase in subvalvular gradient or low cardiac output due to decreased cardiac compliance.

In patients with left ventricular outflow tract obstruction, the use of either physiologic maneuvers or pharmacologic agents at the bedside can be very useful. Any intervention that decreases left ventricular volume (preload) or decreases systemic arterial pressure (afterload) or increases left ventricular ejection velocity (contractility) will augment the resting outflow tract gradient. Conversely, any intervention that increases left ventricular volume, increases systemic arterial pressure, or diminishes left ventricular contractility will decrease the resting outflow tract gradient. An understanding of the foregoing makes interpretation of the physical examination more rational.

The heart is generally enlarged on physical examination. The precordial impulse is often displaced laterally. A presystolic impulse is often present, corresponding to atrial systole with an augmentation of blood flow into a poorly compliant ventricle. In some patients there is a late systolic impulse leading to a triple apical impulse. A systolic thrill is present frequently and is felt most regularly at the cardiac apex. A thrill is present in many patients with obstruction but is not present in patients without an obstructive component to their disease.

Examination of the jugular venous pulse may reveal a prominent "a" wave that augments with inspiration. This reflects the diminished compliance of the right ventricle. The arterial pulses are brisk, and the carotid pulse may have a double impulse in patients with obstruction. An atrial gallop (fourth heart sound) is extremely common in patients with and without obstruction. A diastolic filling gallop (third heart sound) is appreciated somewhat less frequently. The second heart sound is at times paradoxically split.

A systolic murmur is present in all patients with obstruction and may vary in intensity, depending upon the magnitude of the subvalvular gradient. The murmur is most prominent at either the lower sternal border or at the cardiac apex. For reasons stated earlier related to the pathophysiology of the disease, the murmur often increases with standing, the Valsalva maneuver, tachycardia, and a postextrasystolic beat. Conversely, squatting, isometric handgrip, and bradycardia will decrease the intensity of the murmur. In a minority of patients a diastolic rumble may be present, probably related to abnormalities in flow across the mitral valve secondary to a poorly compliant left ventricle.

Most patients will have an abnormal resting 12-lead electrocardiogram, even if they are asymptomatic. The most common electrocardiographic abnormalities are left ventricular hypertrophy and ST and T wave abnormalities. Because of asymmetric hypertrophy of the left ventricle, patients may have large Q waves in the anterior, lateral, or inferior leads. This finding, especially in young patients, is a distinct clue to the diagnosis of the disease. Other frequent electrocardiographic abnormalities are left atrial or right atrial enlargement, left axis deviation, or PR prolongation. Sudden death is uncommon in patients with ventricular arrhythmias other than sustained ventricular tachycardia. The presence of sustained ventricular tachycardia on Holter monitor identifies a subgroup of patients with as high as an 8% annual mortality rate. There are no specific radiologic findings, but the chest roentgenogram may mimic mitral stenosis, mitral regurgitation, or congestive cardiomyopathy. Most patients have an enlarged left ventricle and left atrium, and about half have evidence of right ventricular enlargement as well. On left ventricular cineangiography, the shape of the left ventricle may be quite variable but is always abnormal. In end-diastole, there is frequently the typical banana-shaped ventricle (ballerina shape), with end-systolic cavity obliteration. Systolic anterior motion (SAM) of the mitral valve may be seen in the left anterior oblique projection. Mitral regurgitation is seen in between half and all patients in reported series.

The hemodynamic findings in this disease are quite unique. Systolic pressure gradients in the right ventricular outflow tract may be present in approximately 15% of patients with hypertrophic cardiomyopathy. The degree of right-sided obstruction is usually less than 30 mmHg and does not contribute to clinical symptoms.

Considerable controversy surrounded the question of whether left ventricular pressure gradients were real or spurious, caused by catheter entrapment in the left ventricle. The result of numerous investigations clarified the issue. It is now clear that there are patients with hypertrophic cardiomyopathy who have true obstruction caused by apposition of the anterior leaflet of the mitral valve and the hypertrophied interventricular septum. Other patients have generalized cardiac hypertrophy but do not develop obstruction. Further understanding of the natural history of this disease has demonstrated that some patients who have normal or supranormal systolic function early in their disease may develop impaired systolic function late in their disease. The impaired systolic function may be due to myocardial fibrosis and/or myocardial ischemia. The clinical picture in these patients mimics that of patients with a dilated cardiomyopathy. There is left ventricular dilatation, cardiac output is low, and filling pressures are elevated.

Mitral regurgitation is commonly present in obstructive cardiomyopathy and less commonly present in the nonobstructive variety. There is a direct relationship between the severity of the outflow tract gradient and the degree of mitral regurgitation. The gradient is initiated by the anterior mitral-leaflet–septal coaptation. This anterior movement leads to faulty midsystolic coaptation of the two mitral leaflets and consequent mitral regurgitation.

Abnormalities in diastolic function are often present in this disease and at times may dominate the hemodynamic picture. The thickened left ventricle has decreased compliance, and myocardial fibrosis leads to an increase in muscle stiffness.

In patients with a subvalvular gradient, there is a marked variability of outflow tract obstruction that can be demonstrated during cardiac catheterization and after physiologic or pharmacologic interventions. Interventions that (1) increase cardiac contractility, (2) decrease preload (smaller diastolic chamber size), or (3) decrease afterload (lower aortic diastolic pressure) will augment the left ventricular–aortic gradient. Conversely, interventions that (1) decrease contractility, (2) increase left ventricular size, or (3) increase aortic diastolic pressures will lessen the gradient. Therefore, digitalis, sympathomimetic amines, nitroglycerin, Valsalva maneuver, and standing will augment the gradient. Conversely, beta-adrenergic receptor blockade, calcium channel blockers (verapamil), phenylephrine, squatting, and isometric handgrip will all lessen obstruction.

The echocardiogram has been the most useful laboratory examination in the detection and tracking of patients with this entity. The finding of anterior motion of the anterior mitral leaflet, beginning with the onset of ejection and reaching its peak upon contacting the interventricular septum in midsystole, was one of the first echo abnormalities described. The finding of asymmetrical septal hypertrophy became synonymous with hypertrophy cardiomyopathy. The ratio of the thickness of the interventricular septum to the thickness of the posterior free wall is greater than or equal to 1:3. Furthermore, most patients have a septal thickness greater than or equal to 15 mm. In addition to its thickness, the interventricular septum has decreased systolic excursion. In patients with systolic obstruction, there is premature closure of the aortic valve. Further, there is a prolonged relaxation time index, the time from end-systolic dimension to mitral valve opening. Transesophageal studies are valuable in defining further abnormalities of the mitral valve and in guiding intraoperative procedures.

The natural history of patients with this entity is quite variable. The rate of progression of the disease may be more rapid in children and young adults. The discovery of a heart murmur usually antedates the onset of symptoms by years. The natural history at any stage may be punctuated by the occurrence of sudden death. The risk factors for sudden death are considered to be a "malignant" family history, young age, syncope, evidence of myocardial ischemia, increased septal thickness, sustained ventricular tachycardia on electrophysiologic testing, and ventricular tachycardia on ambulatory monitoring if associated with altered consciousness. The appearance of atrial fibrillation will often initiate symptoms in a previously asymptomatic individual. Infective endocarditis may occur, especially on the mitral valve. Transmural myocardial infarction or pulmonary or systemic embolization may have a negative impact on the clinical course. Sudden death may be due to atrial or ventricular tachyarrhythmias, bradyarrhythmias, heart block, obstruction to left ventricular outflow, diastolic dysfunction, and myocardial ischemia. This last factor is achieving greater significance in most studies. Early studies placed the annual mortality at 3% to 4%, but with wider use of echocardiography to establish the diagnosis, the annual mortality is probably somewhat lower at 1% to 2%.

Recent studies have identified a genetic abnormality in this disease. There is strong evidence that mutations in the β-MHC (major histocompatibility complex) gene are responsible for many of the familial forms of the entity. Multiple families have been shown to be genetically linked to the β-MHC locus on chromosome 14. Affected members of a family have the same mutation and unaffected members do not. This β-MHC mutation is not present in the general population. Hypertrophic cardiomyopathy is an autosomal dominant disease, so that half of the offspring of an affected individual will inherit the disease. The other half will be normal.

TREATMENT

Treatment of patients with hypertrophic cardiomyopathy is aimed at alleviation of cardiac symptoms and prevention of sudden death. For the past 30 years, the mainstay of therapy has been the use of beta-adrenergic blocking agents. These drugs decrease cardiac contractility, slow the heart rate and, therefore, allow for increased ventricular filling and end-diastolic size. Although strictly controlled randomized trials have not been carried out, it is generally acknowledged that beta-blocking drugs are the mainstay of therapy for patients with this disorder. Calcium channel blocking agents, particularly verapamil (Isoptin, Calan), have been used to good advantage in patients with this disorder. Drugs in this class inhibit the inward transmembrane flow of calcium ions in cardiac muscle, in smooth muscle of the coronary and systemic arteries, and in cells of the intracardiac conduction system. There is some enthusiasm for the use of verapamil because of its negative inotropic, chronotropic, and muscular relaxant qualities. In patients with diastolic dysfunction, verapamil may have unique qualities. The negative inotropic effect of disopyramide (Norpace), a type 1A antiarrhythmic agent, has led to its use in patients with systolic obstruction.

Dual-chamber pacing has recently been extensively studied and used in patients with hypertrophic cardiomyopathy. The exact mechanics by which the obstructive gradient is decreased is unknown but may be related to decreased or paradoxical septal motion. The long-term efficacy of this therapy is still unknown. A cornerstone of its success is complete ventricular capture. Therefore, in patients with normal or prolonged PR intervals, it is more successful. In patients with short PR intervals, the hemodynamic benefits are more difficult to achieve.

For the past 30 years, surgical intervention has offered help to symptomatic patients. It is now generally agreed that a transaortic ventriculomyotomy and myectomy is the operation of choice. The operation reduces resting and provoked peak systolic gradients. Relief of obstruction is associated with improvement in mitral regurgitation and improvement in all the echocardiographic indices of obstruction. Although prolongation of life has not been proved, most clinicians feel that in the symptomatic patient, operation has improved the prognosis.

MITRAL VALVE PROLAPSE

method of
ROBERT A. LEVINE, M.D.
*Harvard University and Massachusetts General
   Hospital
Boston, Massachusetts*

The most critical element in the management of mitral valve prolapse (MVP) is correct diagnosis: most of the confusion surrounding MVP has reflected nonspecific diagnosis. A variety of criteria based on the history, physical examination, and echocardiogram have produced an apparent epidemic of MVP involving up to 10% to 15% of the general population. The great majority of these individuals, however, are in good health, and few develop complications; management is therefore uncertain. To resolve this confusion requires a return to the fundamental definition of the condition.

Prolapse is the slipping or displacement of a body part from its usual or normal position with respect to surrounding structures. Mitral valve prolapse, therefore, is displacement of the mitral leaflets from their normal or usual position with respect to their surrounding structures and can simply be defined as superior billowing of the leaflets into the left atrium. There are two prerequisites for implementing this definition in practice: first, we need a technique that can display the relation of the mitral leaflets to surrounding structures, and second, we need to know the normal range of these relations, because prolapse is by definition an abnormality, not a variant of normal. Failure to satisfy these conditions has led to the widespread diagnosis of MVP through the use of nonspecific techniques that do not display the fundamental relations of the valve to other structures, and extrapolation of findings such as systolic clicks from small groups of symptomatic individuals without establishing a normal range. Recent progress has moved to satisfy these prerequisites using the noninvasive technique of cardiac ultrasound to display the fundamental relations defining prolapse, combined with improved ability to distinguish normal from abnormal patterns through increased understanding of the normal three-dimensional shape of the mitral valve, as discussed later under Diagnosis.

MECHANISMS

Mitral valve prolapse, defined as superior protrusion or billowing of portions of the mitral valve into the left atrium, has several mechanisms:

1. Leaflet and chordal elongation, with floppy leaflets characterized by myxomatous degeneration of the fibrous backbone of the valve, as in idiopathic MVP and Marfan's syndrome; in idiopathic MVP, the posterior mitral leaflet bulges most severely, and symptomatic mitral regurgitation occurs most commonly in men over 50 years old.
2. Loss or diminution of chordal support from trauma, endocarditis, and occasionally, papillary muscle stretching in chronic ischemic heart disease; the extreme of chordal rupture produces flail, with the leaflet everting into the left atrium and a visible gap in coaptation.
3. Geometric or secondary prolapse related to decreased left ventricular cavity size, with leaflet extrusion toward the left atrium (occasionally seen in patients with ostium secundum atrial septal defects and other forms of right ventricular volume overload).
4. A combination of the foregoing (hypertrophic cardiomyopathy, for example, with nonmyxomatous leaflet elongation and a small ventricular cavity). Acute rheumatic valvular involvement causes dysjunction of the leaflets by posterior annular dilatation, which stretches the posterior leaflet away from the anterior, combined with stretching of the chords to the anterior mitral leaflet, causing failure of coaptation but without prominent superior leaflet billowing.

DIAGNOSIS

Most patients evaluated for MVP present with auscultatory findings or symptoms referred to as the "MVP syndrome," including nonspecific chest pain, dyspnea, fatigue, palpitations, and anxiety. The mid- to late systolic click, variably associated with a subsequent murmur, relates to prolapse that occurs as left ventricular pressure rises, the left ventricular cavity shrinks, and the papillary muscles yield to imposed stresses. These findings are widely used to screen for the possibility of MVP but have diagnostic limitations. A holosystolic murmur may be the only finding in patients with fully developed disease and important mitral regurgitation. These findings are also *nonspecific* and insufficient to make the diagnosis of prolapse based on the relations of the leaflets to surrounding structures. Although the specificity of these findings is felt to be improved by their response to maneuvers (for example, respiratory variation, and earlier occurrence with decreased left ventricular cavity size upon standing), many patients referred for clicks and apical systolic murmurs have completely normal valves by cardiac ultrasound. In such cases, the findings may relate to chordal systolic anterior motion, reflecting normal chordal laxity, and trivial amounts of physiologic regurgitation, as seen in structurally normal hearts. Symptoms short of true heart failure are likewise nonspecific, occurring commonly in unselected populations without relation to mitral valve abnormalities.

Diagnosis must therefore be based on a technique that displays the relations of the leaflets to surrounding structures and assesses the effectiveness of mitral coaptation; two-dimensional and Doppler echocardiography is ideal for providing such an assessment noninvasively. The echocardiographic diagnosis has traditionally been made on the basis of superior protrusion of the leaflets from the left ventricle into the left atrium, beyond a line connecting their annular hinge points (see later for broader definition). Because of the difficulties created by nonspecific diagnosis, it is worthwhile reviewing the rationale for current criteria. This information can be of value to the clinician in deciding whether a previously made diagnosis needs to be reassessed in view of current understanding.

Initial criteria assumed the mitral annulus was planar and that leaflet displacement could be assessed in any two-dimensional view cutting across the left atrium, annulus, and left ventricle. Three-dimensional reconstruction of the normal mitral valve and annulus, however, has revealed that the entire structure has a saddle-like shape, with its low points (closest to the apex) located medially and laterally and its high points located anteriorly and posteriorly near the aortic root and posterior left ventricular wall. This shape can produce *apparent* leaflet displacement superior to the annulus in a two-dimensional view containing the low points of the saddle, because the leaflets must connect the low points and the high points of the annulus and are located in between. This realization has allowed us to reduce the frequency of MVP diagnosis by roughly 75% by eliminating the diagnosis based on apparent superior displacement of the anterior leaflet in the mediolateral four-chamber view, which shows that leaflet attaching to the medial central fibrous body of the heart, which is most apically located. The diagnosis of prolapse is then made in long-axis views that contain the high points of the annulus, with the ultrasound beam scanned systematically through the medial, central, and lateral segments of the leaflets to look for prolapse. It should be noted that the saddle shape primarily eliminates the nonspecific diagnosis of *anterior* leaflet bowing in the four-chamber or mediolateral view; in contrast, localized protrusion of the *posterior* leaflet relative to the anterior, particularly its lateral scallop, can be diagnosed in that view and reflects deficient chordal support or localized leaflet elongation.

Based on clinical correlations, superior leaflet displacement that is less than 2 mm relative to the line connecting the annular hinge points is not regarded as abnormal prolapse but as superior systolic leaflet displacement within the range of normal leaflet motion, given the physiologic variation in mitral leaflet position relative to the annulus that occurs with changing left ventricular volume. (The previous single-dimensional M-mode technique that displays valve motion versus time fails to provide the full spatial appreciation of the two-dimensional technique, and displays a *posterior* component of leaflet motion as opposed to the *superior* billowing that is used in the definition and corresponds to surgical observations.)

Several other features of the mitral valve are noted during interpretation of the echocardiogram: (1) Presence of abnormal and typically diffuse leaflet thickening characteristic of myxomatous degeneration and associated with valve-related complications (significant mitral regurgitation and endocarditis) in follow-up studies. (2) Assessment of the presence and degree of mitral regurgitation by Doppler color-flow mapping, using the area of the regurgitant jet within the left atrium, the size of the proximal jet origin (reflecting the regurgitant orifice), and Doppler measures of regurgitant flow rate, volume, and effective orifice area. (3) Superior traction or tug of the papillary muscles in parallel with leaflet motion, with an associated hyperdynamic inward motion of the intervening posterobasal myocardial segment (see later section on arrhythmias).

The fundamental concept of MVP as an abnormal relation of the mitral leaflets to their surrounding structures can be broadened to include leaflet billowing not only relative to the annulus, but also relative to *each other*, at the site where regurgitation actually occurs. Such leaflet dysjunction, with superior protrusion of one leaflet (typically the posterior) relative to the other, produces *malcoaptation* and the most severe degrees of mitral regurgitation, leading to the need for surgery.

It is important to note that the correlation between altered leaflet *geometry* and abnormal valve *function*, with clinical complications and progressive valvular changes, remains to be refined by prospective clinical studies. The evolution of idiopathic MVP remains to be determined: it does not appear to be present at birth; mild displacement of thin leaflets does not appear to progress over 10 years; the clinical course of classic myxomatous disease is typically slow (over 10 years) but may be accelerated by chordal rupture or supervening infection.

MANAGEMENT

Diagnosis

In presenting the diagnosis to the patient, great care must be taken to avoid what Aubrey Leatham referred to as the "MVP fiasco": the anxiety resulting from a diagnosis despite trivial or inapparent hemodynamic or clinical consequences. This explains the technical focus in the prior discussion, with new criteria aiming to minimize diagnosis in otherwise normal individuals. Increased insurance premiums based on the diagnosis and exclusion from activities at critical risk from arrhythmias, such as piloting aircraft, have been unfortunate consequences of nonspecific diagnosis.

Valve-Related Complications

Patients with important (moderate-to-severe) mitral regurgitation are followed noninvasively by two-dimensional and Doppler echocardiography at annual intervals for increasing prolapse, progressive regurgitation, and deteriorating left ventricular systolic function. Left ventricular *unloading* by the regurgitant orifice tends to mask declining contractile function; increasing end-systolic volume is a useful

TABLE 1. **Recommended Standard Prophylactic Regimen for Dental, Oral, or Upper Respiratory Tract Procedures in Patients Who Are at Risk***

Drug	Dosing Regimen†
Standard Regimen	
Amoxicillin	3.0 gm PO 1 h before procedure; then 1.5 gm 6 h after initial dose
Amoxicillin/Penicillin–Allergic Patients	
Erythromycin	Erythromycin ethylsuccinate, 800 mg, or erythromycin stearate, 1.0 gm PO 2 h before procedure; then half the dose 6 h after initial dose
or	
Clindamycin (Cleocin)	300 mg PO 1 h before procedure and 150 mg 6 h after initial dose

*Includes those with prosthetic heart valves and other high-risk patients.

†Initial pediatric doses are as follows: amoxicillin, 50 mg/kg; erythromycin ethylsuccinate or erythromycin stearate, 20 mg/kg; and clindamycin, 10 mg/kg. Follow-up doses should be one half the initial dose. *Total pediatric dose should not exceed total adult dose.* The following weight ranges may also be used for the initial pediatric dose of amoxicillin: <15 kg, 750 mg; 15–30 kg, 1500 mg; and >30 kg, 3000 mg (full adult dose).

Reproduced with permission from the American Medical Association from Dajani AS, et al: Prevention of bacterial endocarditis. Recommendations by the American Heart Association. JAMA *264*(22):2919–2922, 1990. Copyright 1990, American Medical Association.

index of incipient failure. Current practice advocates an earlier move to surgery, even in patients with relatively mild symptoms, to avoid irreversible left ventricular dysfunction; this is possible because of the increased availability and success of mitral valve *repair*, which generally combines resection of elongated leaflet portions with annuloplasty to increase leaflet apposition. Preoperative evaluation of the mitral valve scallops by transesophageal echocardiography is routinely used to guide surgical planning; real-time three-dimensional reconstruction is currently practical and provides animated images of the valve from a surgical perspective (left atrial view) that dramatically enhances communication of findings to the surgeon. Postoperative development of systolic anterior motion (SAM) of the mitral valve with dynamic left ventricular outflow tract obstruction can be reduced by shortening excessively long posterior leaflets, which otherwise shift the coaptation point anteriorly toward the left ventricular outflow tract and favor the development of SAM.

Antibiotic Prophylaxis for Bacterial Endocarditis

Prophylaxis is provided based on American Heart Association guidelines for patients with important mitral regurgitation—that is, more than the trace amounts seen in structurally normal hearts (see Tables 1, 2 and 3). Prophylaxis is also prudent for patients with abnormal leaflet thickening because of the frequent association between that finding and mitral regurgitation, and the evidence it provides of intrinsic leaflet abnormality.

Arrhythmias, Syncope, and Sudden Death*

Ventricular and supraventricular tachycardias are most frequently associated with hemodynamically

*Method of Drs. Michael Roberts and Brian McGovern.

significant mitral regurgitation. The true frequency of sudden death in MVP is unknown, although case reports and postmortem series suggest that it actually occurs, perhaps because of traction on the papillary muscles, which experimentally lowers the threshold for lethal ventricular arrhythmias. Risk factors for sudden death are, unfortunately, difficult to determine but include leaflet elongation, a definite history of syncope, survival following aborted sudden cardiac death, QT prolongation, and ventricular ectopic activity with exercise, as well as significant mitral regurgitation with left ventricular dilatation. Given the rarity of this event, it is important not to burden the great majority of patients with the anxiety related to it. Patients with MVP and ventricular ectopy, even when frequent, do not require evaluation or therapy. Patients with a definite history of nonvasovagal or orthostatic syncope are evaluated with echocardiography, ambulatory ECG monitoring, and exercise stress testing to determine whether nonsustained ventricular tachycardia occurs. Electrophysiologic testing is best reserved for patients with symptomatic supraventricular tachycardia, and those with syncope, presyncope, aborted sudden death, and symptomatic runs of ventricular tachycardia on am-

TABLE 2. **Alternate Prophylactic Regimens for Dental, Oral, or Upper Respiratory Tract Procedures in Patients Who Are at Risk**

Drug	Dosing Regimen*
Patients Unable to Take Oral Medications	
Ampicillin	IV or IM administration of ampicillin, 2.0 gm, 30 min before procedure; then IV or IM administration of ampicillin, 1.0 gm, or PO amoxicillin, 1.5 gm, 6 h after initial dose
Ampicillin/Amoxicillin/Penicillin–Allergic Patients Unable to Take Oral Medications	
Clindamycin (Cleocin)	IV administration of 300 mg 30 min before procedure and an IV or PO dose of 150 mg 6 h after initial dose
Patients Considered High Risk and Not Candidates for Standard Regimen	
Ampicillin, gentamicin, and amoxicillin	IV or IM administration of ampicillin, 2.0 gm, plus gentamicin, 1.5 mg/kg (not to exceed 80 mg), 30 min before procedure; followed by amoxicillin, 1.5 gm PO 6 h after initial dose; alternatively, the parenteral regimen may be repeated 8 h after initial dose
Ampicillin/Amoxicillin/Penicillin–Allergic Patients Considered High Risk	
Vancomycin (Vancocin)	IV administration of 1.0 gm over 1 h, starting 1 h before procedure; no repeated dose necessary

*Initial pediatric doses are as follows: ampicillin, 50 mg/kg; clindamycin, 10 mg/kg; gentamicin, 2.0 mg/kg; and vancomycin, 20 mg/kg. Follow-up doses should be one half the intial dose. *Total pediatric dose should not exceed total adult dose.* No initial dose is recommended in this table for amoxicillin (25 mg/kg is the follow-up dose).

Reproduced with permission from the American Medical Association from Dajani AS, et al: Prevention of bacterial endocarditis. Recommendations by the American Heart Association. JAMA *264*(22):2919–2922, 1990. Copyright 1990, American Medical Association.

TABLE 3. **Regimens for Genitourinary/Gastrointestinal Procedures**

Drug	Dosage Regimen*
Standard Regimen	
Ampicillin, gentamicin, and amoxicillin	IV or IM administration of ampicillin, 2.0 gm, plus gentamicin, 1.5 mg/kg (not to exceed 80 mg), 30 min before procedure; followed by amoxicillin, 1.5 gm PO 6 h after initial dose; alternatively, the parenteral regimen may be repeated once 8 h after initital dose
Ampicillin/Amoxicillin/Penicillin–Allergic Patient Regimen	
Vancomycin and gentamicin	IV administration of vancomycin, 1.0 gm, over 1 h plus IV or IM administration of gentamicin, 1.5 mg/kg (not to exceed 80 mg), 1 h before procedure; may be repeated once 8 h after initial dose
Alternative Low-Risk Patient Regimen	
Amoxicillin	3.0 gm PO 1 h before procedure; then 1.5 gm 6 h after initial dose

*Initial pediatric doses are as follows: ampicillin, 50 mg/kg; amoxicillin, 50 mg/kg; gentamicin, 2.0 mg/kg; and vancomycin, 20 mg/kg. Follow-up doses should be half the initial dose. *Total pediatric dose should not exceed total adult dose.*

Reproduced with permission from the American Medical Association from Dajani AS, et al: Prevention of bacterial endocarditis. Recommendations by the American Heart Association. JAMA *264*(22):2919–2922, 1990. Copyright 1990, American Medical Association.

bulatory monitoring. However, the utility of programmed ventricular stimulation is limited in patients with ventricular arrhythmia and MVP, as the findings are frequently limited to nonsustained polymorphic ventricular tachycardia.

Those symptomatic with frequent ventricular ectopy or runs of nonsustained ventricular tachycardia will usually benefit from beta-blocker therapy, in addition to refraining from the use of aggravating agents (caffeine, alcohol, and sympathomimetics). In the case of syncope or sudden cardiac death, serial electrophysiology-guided drug testing with Class III agents (sotalol [Betapace], 80 mg twice daily, or amiodarone [Cordarone], 200 to 400 mg daily, after a loading dose) may be appropriate for life-threatening ventricular arrhythmias. Mexiletine (Mexitil), 100 to 200 mg three times a day, may also be used. The use of an implantable cardioverter-defibrillator is indicated in patients with failed drug suppression or unacceptable side effects, or those resuscitated from cardiac arrest, particularly those who remain noninducible at an electrophysiologic study. The implantable defibrillator affords the most secure insurance against sudden death. Although mitral valve repair has been advocated as a prophylactic measure, it cannot provide the same confidence.

Systemic Emboli

In the absence of endocarditis, recent results show no positive evidence for an association between MVP and acute ischemic stroke in any age group. Evalua-

tion should therefore focus on other causes, with appropriate therapy, including aspirin and dipyridamole, as indicated.

Genetic Counseling

This should be provided to patients with Marfan's syndrome as appropriate for that condition. The true inheritance pattern of idiopathic MVP based on the above criteria has yet to be defined.

Acute Rheumatic Fever with Mitral Valve Prolapse

Physical rest and, in the case of significant mitral regurgitation, valve repair to arrest the cycle of active carditis are indicated.

CONGESTIVE HEART FAILURE

method of
URI ELKAYAM, M.D.
University of Southern California School of Medicine
Los Angeles, California

Congestive heart failure is a complex syndrome that involves myocardial dysfunction, hemodynamic abnormalities, and changes in the neurohormonal, autocrine, and paracrine functions. It is associated with typical signs and symptoms such as shortness of breath, orthopnea, paroxysmal nocturnal dyspnea, decreased exercise capacity, weakness, peripheral edema, and cardiac cachexia. This condition is also associated with reduced longevity due to malignant arrhythmias, thromboembolic events, or progression of heart failure.

The most common causes of congestive heart failure are coronary artery disease, hypertension, idiopathic dilated cardiomyopathy, myocarditis, valvular heart disease, excessive alcohol consumption, hypertrophic cardiomyopathy, and congenital heart disease. Factors that precipitate or exacerbate congestive heart failure include infection, increased fluid and dietary salt intake, uncontrolled hypertension, cardiac arrhythmias, poor compliance with therapy, myocardial ischemia, renal failure and thyrotoxicosis, anemia, high environmental temperature, emotional stress, pregnancy, obesity, ethanol ingestion, thiamine deficiency, and drugs that suppress myocardial contractility, promote sodium and fluid retention, or reduce renal function.

The incidence of congestive heart failure has been increasing despite a decline in mortality rates secondary to cardiovascular disease and stroke. The reasons for this phenomenon are multifactorial and include aging of the population and improved survival of patients with coronary artery disease, myocardial infarction, valvular heart disease, hypertension, and diabetes mellitus, owing to improved pharmacologic and surgical management. Approximately three million individuals in the United States are diagnosed with heart failure, with 400,000 new cases diagnosed annually. The incidence of this condition doubles in the general population with each decade of life over 45 years, and at the present time, heart failure is the third leading cause for hospitalization in all age groups and the principal cause of hospitalizations in patients over the age of 65 years. Approximately 35% of diagnosed heart failure patients require hospitalization every year, and multiple hospitalizations are common (over 40% of hospitalized patients are readmitted to the hospital within three months after their discharge). The common causes for the high rate of hospitalizations include inadequate management, lack of patient compliance to prescribed therapy and diet, use of drugs that cause a detrimental effect, and progression of underlying disease.

COMMON SYMPTOMS AND SIGNS OF CONGESTIVE HEART FAILURE

The two most common symptoms occurring in patients with heart failure are dyspnea and fatigue. Exertional dyspnea is one of the earliest symptoms; patients with a more severe form of the disease also experience orthopnea and bouts of paroxysmal nocturnal dyspnea that usually occur several hours after falling asleep. Other symptoms include oliguria, nocturia, and epigastric fullness and discomfort. The clinical signs of congestive heart failure can include tachycardia, borderline low blood pressure, tachypnea, leg edema and in more advanced cases presacral edema, increased central venous pressure, diffuse and forceful left ventricular heave with point of maximal impulse displaced both downward and laterally, hepatomegaly, ascites, jaundice or cyanosis, and Cheyne-Stokes respiration. The auscultatory findings often include an increased intensity of P2 and the presence of S3 and/or S4, murmurs of mitral and tricuspid regurgitation, and inspiratory rales. The common laboratory findings in patients with severe heart failure may include cardiomegaly on chest radiograph, plus interstitial edema (Kerley's B lines), vascular flow redistribution, bronchial cuffing, and pleural effusion.

The electrocardiographic findings are related to the etiology and can show evidence of old myocardial infarction, left ventricular hypertrophy, left atrial enlargement with or without right atrial enlargement, tachycardia, frequent premature beats, nonsustained ventricular tachycardia, atrial fibrillation, and nonspecific abnormalities of the ST segment and T waves. In patients with idiopathic cardiomyopathy, one often finds low voltage in the limb leads concomitant to high voltage in the chest leads. The echocardiographic findings depend on the underlying disease and usually demonstrate dilatation of all cardiac chambers; mitral and/or tricuspid valve regurgitation is commonly seen. The echocardiogram is helpful in diagnosing and estimating the severity of valvular abnormalities in patients with valvular heart disease, and abnormal cardiac anatomy and function in patients with congenital heart disease. It is likely to demonstrate segmental wall motion abnormalities in patients with ischemic heart disease and a history of myocardial infarction. Thallium scintigraphy increases sensitivity for diagnosing myocardial ischemia and can help in the assessment of myocardial viability. Myocardial viability can also be assessed with PAT (paroxysmal atrial tachycardia) scanning and dobutamine echocardiography. Exercise testing will reveal reduced exercise tolerance and oxygen consumption and lack of normal increase of blood pressure with exercise. It may be useful in the diagnosis of myocardial ischemia in patients with coronary artery disease.

LABORATORY TESTS

Abnormalities of renal function with elevated serum creatinine and urea levels are commonly seen in patients with heart failure. In more severe forms of the disease, hyponatremia and abnormalities of liver function with elevated transaminase and bilirubin levels are also commonly seen. In patients receiving diuretic therapy, hypokalemia, hypomagnesemia, and hyperuricemia are not uncommon.

NEW YORK HEART ASSOCIATION FUNCTIONAL CLASSIFICATION

The New York Heart Association classification is the most commonly used method for the assessment of functional capacity, grading the severity of heart failure and assessing efficacy of therapy. Class I indicates no undue symptoms on ordinary activity and no limitations of physical activity. Class II—slight to moderate limitations of activity, without symptoms at rest. Class III—marked limitations of activity, without symptoms at rest. Class IV—severe failure as evidenced by discomfort with any physical activity and symptoms at rest.

PATHOPHYSIOLOGY

The first phase in the development of congestive heart failure is an insult to the myocardium resulting in impairment of ventricular function. The disease process that is responsible for heart failure can be ongoing for an extended period of time before symptoms occur. Ventricular dysfunction eventually leads to hemodynamic abnormalities, activation of neurohormonal as well as cardiovascular and paracrine-autocrine systems, and changes in endothelial function, which produce symptoms and physical findings of congestive heart failure.

Neurohormonal Change. Heart failure is associated with an increase in plasma norepinephrine, renin, atrial natriuretic factor, and arginine vasopressin. These neurohormonal changes are proportional to the severity of the condition. The major consequences of neurohormonal activation are vasoconstriction and retention of sodium and water. Neurohormonal systems have, therefore, become important therapeutic targets in the treatment of heart failure. Other factors that may play a role in the development and progression of this clinical syndrome are elevated levels of tumor necrosis factor, which may lead to a worsening of myocardial damage and abnormality in endothelial function that may result in impairment of vasodilatory capacity and decreased regional perfusion.

DIAGNOSIS

The common symptoms of congestive heart failure are dyspnea, orthopnea, weakness and easy fatigability, paroxysmal nocturnal dyspnea, nocturia, swelling of the feet and ankles, and epigastric fullness and discomfort. The physical examination often reveals tachycardia, borderline decreased blood pressure with narrow pulse pressure, and distended neck veins with prominent a and v wave either unprovoked or induced by applying pressure to the abdominal area (hepatojugular reflux). Point of maximum left ventricular impulse is diffuse and displaced both laterally and downward; right ventricular heave is prominent, and closure of the pulmonic valve may be palpable. Auscultation of the heart often reveals augmented P2 and the presence of S3 and holosystolic murmurs of mitral regurgitation and/or tricuspid regurgitation. Auscultation of the lungs may reveal inspiratory rales and, at times, decrease in breath sounds and dullness to percussion because of pleural effusion. Inspection of the patients often reveals tachypnea, Cheyne-Stokes respiration, and peripheral edema.

Electrocardiographic changes vary according to the etiology of heart failure and often will demonstrate signs of acute or previous myocardial infarction, left ventricular hypertrophy, left and right atrial enlargement, conduction abnormalities, and arrhythmias. In patients with heart failure caused by myocardial infarctions, Q waves and reduction in QRS voltage are commonly seen. In patients with idiopathic cardiomyopathy, low voltage QRS complexes in the limb leads and high voltage QRS complexes in the chest leads are commonly found. The chest radiograph usually shows cardiomegaly, left and right atrial enlargement, a prominent main pulmonary artery, and enlarged right pulmonary artery (left pulmonary artery is less well visualized because of overlap with the cardiac silhouette). Right ventricular enlargement can be reflected by the large anterior mediastinal silhouette noted on lateral x-ray projection. When left atrial pressure is elevated, there is redistribution of blood flow from the base of the lungs to the apices and linear densities, reflecting interstitial edema in the base of the chest (Kerley's lines), and pleural effusion can be seen.

Echocardiography often demonstrates enlargement of all four cardiac chambers, with decrease in wall motion and decreased fractional shortening and ejection fraction. Segmental wall motion abnormalities are commonly seen in patients with ischemic heart disease but can be seen also in patients with other etiologies. Doppler studies will often demonstrate regurgitation of the tricuspid, mitral, and less frequently the pulmonic and aortic valves. Pericardial and pleural effusion are often seen on echocardiography in patients with congestive heart failure. The echocardiogram is of great use in evaluation of the anatomy and the integrity of the various valves and the presence of congenital heart disease. The presence and extent of ischemic heart disease can be evaluated by a thallium scintigraphy. Further analysis of wall motion as well as ejection fraction can be studied by nuclide angiography. Cardiac catheterization and coronary angiography are especially useful in evaluation of the presence and severity of coronary artery disease and assessment of cardiac as well as pulmonary pressures and left ventricular systolic function and wall motion abnormalities. Transesophageal echocardiography is advantageous in some cases with valvular heart disease, especially those with prosthetic valves in whom endocarditis is suspected to be the cause of deterioration of congestive heart failure symptoms.

ACUTE CONGESTIVE HEART FAILURE

Management

In the treatment of acute congestive heart failure, the clinician should attempt a rapid improvement of hemodynamic abnormalities and concomitantly look for precipitating or exacerbating factors that need to be corrected. Since the immediate problem in patients with acute congestive heart failure is an elevated left ventricular end-diastolic pressure and pulmonary edema, these should be given the highest priority. Nitroglycerin either sublingually (0.4 mg repeated every 5 to 10 minutes to achieve the desired effect) or intravenously (initial dose, 20 μg per min increased by 10 to 20 μg per min every 5 to 10 minutes) is the drug of choice. Titration should be done carefully to avoid excessive reduction in systemic blood pressure. Sodium nitroprusside can be used as an alternative to nitroglycerin (initial dose,

0.1 mg per kg per min). Administration of oxygen is important to improve blood oxygenation. Intravenous diuretics (furosemide [Lasix], 20 to 80 mg intravenously) are useful to lower blood volume. However, it is important to remember that in patients with ischemic heart disease, pulmonary congestion is often due to left ventricular compliance and mitral regurgitation rather than fluid overload. Correction of ischemia and the use of vasodilators should, therefore, be effective, and excessive diuresis should be avoided to prevent hypovolemia and thus hypotension and tachycardia.

Morphine sulfate (3 to 5 mg intravenously) is useful for alleviation of pain and anxiety and can contribute to reduction of venous return and improvement of pulmonary edema. The use of bronchodilators is not indicated in the majority of the cases, especially since the tachycardic effect of most of these agents can be detrimental in patients with coronary artery disease or tachyarrhythmias. Intubation and mechanical ventilation are effective and needed in patients with severe hypoxemia in spite of oxygen administration. Hemodynamic monitoring with the aid of indwelling pulmonary catheters can provide important information and guide in the selection of therapy. The possibility of an acute ischemic event should be considered in every patient with acute heart failure. When evidence for ischemia or myocardial infarction exists, early cardiac catheterization and reperfusion with either angioplasty or bypass surgery will provide the best results. The early use of two-dimensional echocardiography and Doppler studies can be extremely useful in the diagnosis of correctable mechanical problems such as acute mitral regurgitation due to ruptured chordae tendineae or endocarditis, rupture of the ventricular septum, acute aortic regurgitation due to endocarditis and proximal aortic dissection, and acute mechanical valve thrombosis. For evaluation of valves, a transesophageal echocardiogram often provides better information.

In patients with cardiogenic shock, intra-aortic balloon counterpulsation can provide stabilization and be used as a bridge for coronary angioplasty or bypass surgery. In patients with cardiogenic shock and severe hypotension (systolic pressure 80 mmHg or less), use of a vasoconstrictive dose of dopamine (greater than 5 μg per kg per min) may be required. It should be noted, however, that medical therapy for cardiogenic shock is doomed to fail in the great majority of the cases.

The treatment of patients with acute exacerbation of chronic congestive heart failure is similar to the treatment described above; however, diuresis should play the predominant role since this condition is almost always associated with increased body water. Massive diuresis is often required to correct edema, ascites, and pleural effusion. Patients may also be resistant to the usual dose of diuretics and may require a more aggressive regimen, including repeated doses of intravenous boluses of loop diuretics (furosemide, 40 to 80 mg) and the addition of a non-loop diuretic such as hydrochlorothiazide or metolazone (Zaroxolyn). Some patients may require a continuous infusion of high-dose diuretics (10 to 100 mg of furosemide per hour) to achieve diuresis. The use of renal-dose dopamine (1 to 5 μg per kg per min) is useful in increasing renal blood flow and urine output.

Inotropic support may be useful to optimize the hemodynamic profile of the patients. Drugs such as dobutamine (5 to 10 μg per kg per min) and milrinone (Primacor) (initial bolus of 50 mg per kg over 10 minutes followed by continuous infusion of 0.5 μg per kg per min) may result in a significant reduction in left ventricular filling pressure and increase in cardiac output. Use of these medications, however, may be associated with reduction of blood pressure, acceleration of heart rate, and an increase in the incidence of cardiac arrhythmias. Because of their positive inotropic effect, these drugs can lead to an increase in myocardial oxygen consumption and to myocardial ischemia in some patients with coronary artery disease. In patients who do not respond to aggressive diuretic therapy, hemofiltration or dialysis should be considered for removal of excess fluid. Frequent blood samples for measurement of serum potassium should be obtained during massive diuresis to prevent hypokalemia and cardiac arrhythmias. The usefulness of magnesium administration has not been clearly established; however, many patients with chronic congestive heart failure have been demonstrated to be magnesium-depleted, and magnesium replacement seems to make good clinical sense. Repletion should be done with caution in patients with impaired renal function.

CHRONIC CONGESTIVE HEART FAILURE

Management

Patients with chronic heart failure should be treated with medications regardless of the presence or the degree of their symptoms. Left ventricular systolic function should be assessed in every patient at high risk for either coronary artery disease or myocardial disease. The presence of left ventricular systolic dysfunction is a strong indication for a thorough evaluation for the etiology. Reperfusion by either coronary angioplasty or coronary artery bypass surgery is indicated in patients with myocardial ischemia or evidence for hibernating myocardium. Persistence of left ventricular dysfunction in such cases and the presence of left ventricular dysfunction in patients with other conditions is an indication for drug therapy. Multiple studies have uniformly demonstrated the usefulness of angiotensin-converting enzyme (ACE) inhibitors in the prevention of left ventricular remodeling and dilatation, worsening of systolic dysfunction, development of symptoms, hospitalizations, myocardial ischemia, and death. The protective effect of ACE inhibitors seems to be a class effect and is not drug-specific. Experimental and clinical information has also demonstrated the protective effect of organic nitrates for the prevention and even regression of remodeling. These drugs, therefore, can substitute for ACE inhibitors in patients who cannot tolerate the latter.

SYMPTOMATIC HEART FAILURE

Patients with symptomatic heart failure should be treated with diuretics and digoxin in addition to ACE inhibitors. The use of diuretics alone in patients with mild symptoms of congestive heart failure is not justified for the following reasons: Combination therapy of diuretics plus either an ACE inhibitor or digoxin has been shown to be more effective than diuretics alone in relieving symptoms and in the prevention of hospitalization for worsening of heart failure. Since the use of diuretics alone is associated with activation of neurohormones, this may lead to diuretics resistance.

Digitalis should be added to the therapeutic regimen in patients with systolic function who remain symptomatic on ACE inhibitors and diuretics. Hydralazine, 75 mg four times daily, and isosorbide dinitrate (Isordil), 40 to 80 mg three times a day, can be used as an alternative to ACE inhibitors in patients who cannot tolerate these drugs. Preliminary reports have demonstrated that the angiotensin II receptor antagonist losartan (Cozaar),* 50 mg daily, may be an adequate alternative to ACE inhibitors in patients with heart failure. In more severely symptomatic patients with heart failure who continue to be symptomatic on triple therapy (ACE inhibitors, diuretics, and digitalis), additional drugs should be considered after optimization of the dose of each of these medications. A high dose of furosemide may be needed to prevent fluid retention in patients with chronic heart failure (80 to 120 mg two or three times daily).

Close follow-up and education of the patient and family regarding compliance in taking medications, appropriate nutrition with emphasis on a low-salt intake, and the importance of daily monitoring of the patient's body weight are critical in the attempt to prevent worsening of heart failure and hospitalizations. Body weight should be measured on a daily basis; a weight gain of three or more pounds should be promptly treated by increasing the dose of furosemide given orally or intravenously. The addition of hydrochlorothiazide, 25 to 50 mg daily, or metolazone, 5 to 10 mg daily, for 2 to 3 days will be effective in increasing diuresis and return of body weight to its baseline.

A number of drugs may improve symptoms and outcome in patients on triple therapy who continue to be symptomatic. Isosorbide dinitrate, in a dose of 40 to 80 mg three times a day, may be useful mostly by reduction of right and left ventricular filling pressures. Because of the rapid development of tolerance, this drug should be given on a three-times-daily ba-

---

*Not FDA-approved for this indication.

sis, allowing the patient at least 12 hours of washout interval after the third dose. Since the benefit of nitrates for cardiac function, exercise tolerance, and survival has been demonstrated only in combination with hydralazine and because of recent information indicating prevention of nitrate tolerance with hydralazine, the use of this drug combination makes good clinical sense. A recent large study has demonstrated a substantial improvement of survival in patients with nonischemic cardiomyopathy and severe symptoms of heart failure due to severe left ventricular systolic dysfunction (ejection fraction 30%) who receive the calcium antagonist amlodipine (Norvasc), 10 mg daily. However, there was no effect from amlodipine on quality of life or symptoms in this patient population. Amlodipine, therefore, should be considered in addition to triple therapy in patients with nonischemic cardiomyopathy for further protection and prolongation of life.

Several studies have demonstrated a beneficial effect of beta-blocking agents on left ventricular function, exercise tolerance, morbidity, and mortality in patients with symptomatic heart failure. Metoprolol (Lopressor) has reduced the need for heart transplantation in patients with idiopathic dilated cardiomyopathy. Bisoprolol and carvedilol reduced hospital admissions for heart failure, and carvedilol reduced mortality in a preliminary study. Although the use of beta blockers for the treatment of chronic heart failure needs to be further established, it may be considered in selected patients. Because of potential worsening of cardiac function and symptoms with commencement of therapy, the initial dose should be very small, and titration should be gradual and continuous.

Intermittent infusion of inotropic drugs has been used for improvement of symptoms in end-stage patients with heart failure. Although the benefit of this therapy has not been evaluated by adequate prospective and randomized studies, it is being used in patients in whom maximal conventional therapy fails to provide adequate compensation. Dobutamine or milrinone are the drugs most used for this indication; they are administered with a pump through a central venous access catheter. Infusions of several hours once or twice weekly have been mostly utilized. The recommended doses are 5 to 10 μg per kg per min for dobutamine and an initial bolus of 50 μg per kg over 10 minutes, followed by a continuous infusion rate of 0.5 μg per kg per min for milrinone. This therapy is mostly used at the present time as a bridge to heart transplantation.

An implantable left ventricular assist device (LVAD) is another option for a bridge for transplantation in patients with end-stage heart disease. Under the current FDA guidelines, the pump is indicated for patients with severe heart failure awaiting a heart transplantation who remain unresponsive to maximum medical therapy, including inotropic drugs and intra-aortic balloon pump. The most widely used device is connected to the left ventricular apex, and blood is ejected into the ascending aorta. This device allows most morbidly ill patients to regain physical activity and to undergo pretransplant rehabilitation, which allows a smoother post-transplant recovery. Due to "textured lining" inside the device, thromboembolic events are rare and there is no need for anticoagulation.

Dynamic cardiomyoplasty has also been used in various centers for cardiac support in patients with severe heart failure. Because of high mortality associated with this procedure in New York Heart Association class IV patients, this procedure does not seem to be an alternative to cardiac transplantation at the present time. Although symptomatic and functional improvements have been reported in less sick patients (Class III), the yield of the procedure has not been proved in an appropriate randomized trial against medical therapy. To place cardiomyoplasty definitively into the perspective of heart failure management schemes, a randomized clinical trial has been instituted for comparison of outcome with this operative intervention and aggressive medical management of patients with less than New York Heart Association class IV heart failure.

Cardiac transplantation is now a well-accepted surgical therapy for end-stage heart failure. The procedure has been performed in over 30,000 patients around the world. According to the registry of the International Society of Heart and Lung Transplantation, the survival postcardiac transplantation has been 76% after 12 years, with an approximate 4% mortality rate per year. Recent information indicates survival of 93% at one month and 84% at 12 months postcardiac transplantation. The maximum hazard for death is seen early after heart transplantation and falls rapidly over the next six months, with a gradually declining risk thereafter. The two most common causes of death are infections and early graft failure; these account for 45% of total deaths. Predictors for death include, in adult patients, advanced age, need for mechanical ventilation at the time of transplantation, abnormal renal function, low pretransplantation cardiac output, high pulmonary vascular resistance, longer donor ischemic time, older donor age, and donor and recipient not both blood type O.

ANTIARRHYTHMIC TREATMENT IN PATIENTS WITH HEART FAILURE

There is an increased incidence of atrial as well as ventricular arrhythmias in congestive heart failure, and at least 50% of these patients die of an arrhythmic death. The most common atrial arrhythmia in patients with chronic heart failure is atrial fibrillation. Heart rate control is challenging in patients with atrial fibrillation with rapid ventricular response who have a severe depression of left ventricular systolic function. The use of verapamil is contraindicated because of its strong negative inotropic effect and the potential for further depression of left ventricular systolic function and hypotension. Digoxin has been traditionally used for heart rate control in this patient population. However, it should be noted that digoxin is less effective in controlling heart rate in these patients when sympathetic activity is markedly elevated. The use of intravenous diltiazem (Cardizem), has been demonstrated to be both effective and safe for acute heart rate control in patients with heart failure. Chronic use of diltiazem, however, is not recommended because of its potential deleterious effect.

Since heart failure is a strong predictor for thromboembolic events in patients with atrial fibrillation, every effort should be made to convert atrial fibrillation to sinus rhythm. Electrical cardioversion is the procedure of choice because of the potential side effects of available medications. Cardioversion should be performed 3 to 4 weeks after initiation of anticoagulation or within one or two days of admission in patients in whom left atrial thrombi have been ruled out by transesophageal echocardiogram and after at least 12 to 24 hours of intravenous heparin administration. Anticoagulation should be continued for at least a month postcardioversion, even in patients who maintain sinus rhythm, to allow recovery of left atrial function.

In patients who fail to convert to sinus rhythm or fail to maintain sinus rhythm, a second attempt should be made after a loading dose of amiodarone (Cordarone). Chronic heart rate control in patients who remain in atrial fibrillation is best achieved with amiodarone, digoxin, and beta blockers. As previously indicated, initiation and titration of beta blockers in patients with left ventricular systolic dysfunction should be extremely cautious to prevent worsening of left ventricular dysfunction. Use of the nondihydropyridine calcium antagonists for chronic heart rate control is not recommended because of their deleterious long-term effects in patients with congestive heart failure.

The value of the treatment of premature ventricular beats and even short runs of nonsustained ventricular tachycardia has never been proved in patients with congestive heart failure. Such arrhythmias, therefore, should be treated if they are symptomatic. The use of class I antiarrhythmic drugs has been clearly demonstrated to be deleterious in recent years. The majority of these drugs have negative inotropic and proarrhythmic effects and may result in life-threatening arrhythmias. For this reason, amiodarone has been the drug of choice for the treatment of ventricular arrhythmias in most cases. Chronic use of amiodarone has been shown to improve left ventricular function. One large-scale study has recently demonstrated improved survival in patients with severe heart failure regardless of the presence of arrhythmias. In patients with sustained ventricular tachycardia, or an episode of near sudden death, the use of an automatic implantable cardioverter defibrillator should be seriously considered. Amiodarone is usually used in patients with automatic defibrillators to reduce recurrent arrhythmias and the need for electrical discharge by the device. It should be noted that the treatment of congestive heart failure, especially the use of ACE inhibitors, has been demonstrated to have an antiarrhythmic effect and reduce the incidence of sudden death.

ANTICOAGULATION

The incidence of clinically apparent arterial thromboembolism has been reported to be low in patients with chronic heart failure who are not in atrial fibrillation, ranging between 0.9 to 5.5 events per 100 patients per year. At the same time, however, postmortem studies have demonstrated a higher incidence of peripheral and pulmonary thromboembolism. For this reason, many physicians administer anticoagulation to patients with severe left ventricular systolic dysfunction (ejection fraction 20%) or patients with echocardiographic evidence for intracardiac thrombus. The efficacy of this practice, however, has not been tested by controlled trials. Since heart failure has been shown to be a predictor for thromboembolic events in patients with atrial fibrillation, anticoagulation to achieve the target of an international normalized ratio (INR) of 2.0 to 3.0 is indicated for these patients.

DIASTOLIC DYSFUNCTION

Approximately 30% to 40% of all patients presenting with symptoms and signs of congestive heart failure have normal or near-normal left ventricular systolic function. They have left ventricular diastolic dysfunction, which leads to elevated left ventricular end-diastolic pressure, pulmonary pressures, and symptoms of heart failure. The most common causes for left ventricular diastolic dysfunction are myocardial ischemia, hypertension, aging, diabetes mellitus, hypertrophic cardiomyopathy, and pressure overload due to aortic stenosis or coarctation of the aorta. There is no simple diagnostic test for diastolic properties of the left ventricle at the bedside. This condition should be suspected in a patient with symptoms and signs of heart failure without left ventricular systolic dysfunction. The presence of left ventricular hypertrophy, either on the electrocardiogram or on the echocardiogram, supports the diagnosis of diastolic dysfunction. Change in the pattern of mitral valve diastolic flow obtained by the Doppler technique, may be helpful in demonstrating an augmentation of the A-wave reflecting increased contribution of the atrial contraction to left ventricular filling. This sign, however, is not highly sensitive and specific.

Since ischemic heart disease is a common cause of diastolic dysfunction, patients should be evaluated for underlying coronary artery disease using noninvasive and, if indicated, invasive diagnostic methods. A finding of elevated left ventricular filling pressure during cardiac catheterization in an euvolemic patient with normal left ventricular systolic function is diagnostic for diastolic dysfunction. The differential diagnosis of constrictive pericarditis should be considered in patients with left ventricular diastolic dysfunction, especially in those with elevated central venous pressure, peripheral edema, and a history of tuberculous pericarditis, cardiac surgery, and radiation to the chest. Echocardiography, computed tomography, or magnetic resonance imaging may be helpful in the diagnosis of this condition.

In patients in whom myocardial ischemia is the cause of diastolic dysfunction, ischemia should be corrected either with medications or with a reperfusion procedure, including coronary angioplasty or coronary artery bypass surgery. In the patients without a surgically and mechanically correctable cause for left ventricular diastolic dysfunction, the use of beta-blocking agents is of primary importance. Reduction in ventricular rate and prolongation of diastolic time allow a better filling of the left ventricle, reduction in left ventricular end-diastolic pressure, and augmentation of cardiac output. Use of calcium antagonists may be helpful because of their direct effect on augmentation of myocardial relaxation, which leads to improvement of diastolic properties. Since elevation of left ventricular end-diastolic pressure is an important contributor to the symptoms of patients with this syndrome, reduction in venous return to the heart by the use of diuretics, organic nitrates, or ACE inhibitors may be beneficial. However, since maintenance of adequate cardiac output may depend on elevated filling pressure in these patients, the use of diuretics and venodilators should be done cautiously to prevent hypotension.

INFECTIVE ENDOCARDITIS

method of
JAYASEELAN AMBROSE, M.B., M.R.C.P., and
BARRY H. GREENBERG, M.D.
UCSD Medical Center
San Diego, California

"Acute and subacute bacterial endocarditis" are classic clinical syndromes of infected heart valves, and these distinctions remain useful in making empirical management decisions. However, most authorities use the broader term "infective endocarditis" (IE). IE often presents with protean symptoms and signs that may result in a missed or delayed diagnosis. Before the antibiotic era, IE was a uniformly fatal disease. This outcome suggests that host defense mechanisms play a relatively minor role in the eradication of this infectious process and highlights the importance of effective antimicrobial therapy and/or timely surgical intervention. Despite significant advances, the overall mortality remains significant at approximately 10 to 20%. Basic principles of management remain important in all forms of IE; they include recognition of the clinical syndrome, isolation of the organisms from blood or tissue samples, appropriate antimicrobial therapy, prompt recognition and treatment of complications, and antibiotic prophylaxis for individuals at risk.

PATHOGENESIS

Animal models have been used to study the mechanisms leading to the formation of bacterial vegetations, the patho-

logic hallmark of IE. This infectious process is thought to begin with endothelial damage resulting from immune complex deposition or hemodynamic changes such as regurgitant blood flow, high pressure gradients, or turbulent flow through narrow orifices. This results in the accumulation of platelets, red blood cells, and fibrin strands, termed "nonbacterial thrombotic endocarditis," which adhere to the endothelial surface of the valve. These microthrombi appear to be a prerequisite for IE and form the nidus for bacterial growth as a result of seeding during transient bacteremia. Bacterial adherence is an important component of this process, and it appears that elaboration of dextran by the organisms and binding to fibronectin are important pathogenic mechanisms. Subsequently, additional platelet and fibrin deposition and further bacterial deposition occur, creating a series of layers that ultimately forms a vegetation. This allows both rapid unrestricted growth of bacterial colonies within the vegetation and protection from normal host defense mechanisms. Depending on the host factors and the virulence of the microorganism, the presentation may be acute, subacute, or chronic. The understanding of the pathogenic mechanisms leading to IE has established the principle of using high-dose bactericidal antimicrobials for effective treatment.

EPIDEMIOLOGY

With the caveat that published data reflect the referral bias of tertiary care institutions, the estimated incidence of IE is approximately 1 per 1000 hospital admissions, or 3 to 4 cases per 100,000 person-years. Although the incidence has remained relatively unchanged, there has been an evolution in the epidemiology as well as in the clinical and microbiologic spectrum. As in other illnesses, the mean age of affected individuals has increased.

Previously, chronic rheumatic valvular heart disease was the most common predisposing cardiac lesion. This has been supplanted by mitral valve prolapse, along with degenerative aortic and mitral valve disease and hypertrophic cardiomyopathy. There is also an increasing proportion of patients over the age of 65 with IE who have minimal or no identifiable underlying structural heart disease. A relatively new group of affected individuals are the intravenous drug users. Another population that continues to grow are individuals with prosthetic valve endocarditis. Among children, congenital heart disease is the most common predisposing cause, with cyanotic heart disease associated with shunts and stenotic valves being particularly high risk.

The microbiologic spectrum has been altered by the aging population, the increase in the number of intravenous drug users, and the aggressive use of medical interventions, in particular intravascular prostheses and monitoring equipment. Further apparent microbiologic diversity has been brought about by improved microbiologic techniques that have demonstrated a slightly increased prevalence of nutritionally variant streptococci, *Chlamydia, Legionella, Coxiella burnetii* (Q fever), and other fastidious organisms.

ETIOLOGY

Streptococci and staphylococci continue to be the most prevalent isolates, affecting at least 75% of patients who are not intravenous drug users (Table 1). Intravenous drug use (IVDU) associated IE is most often caused by *Staphylococcus aureus, Staph. epidermidis,* gram-negative bacilli, or *Candida.* Prosthetic valve endocarditis (PVE) can be

TABLE 1. **Etiologic Agents of Infective Endocarditis**

Organism	Native Valve	Prosthetic Valve
	Approximate Percentage	
Streptococci		
Alpha-hemolytic	60	10–30
Enterococci	10	5–10
Pneumococci	1–2	<1
Beta-hemolytic	<1	<1
Others	<1	<1
Staphylococci		
Staphylococcus aureus	25	15–20
Coagulase-negative	<1	25–30
Gram-Negative Organisms		
Enterics	<5	<5
Pseudomonas spp	<5	<5
HACEK	<5	<1
Neisseria spp	<1	<1
Fungi		
Candida spp	<1	5–10
Others	<1	<1

Abbreviations: HACEK = *Haemophilus* spp, *Actinobacillus actinomycetemcomitans*, *Cardiobacterium hominis*, *Eikenella* spp, and *Kingella kingae*.
From Dajani AS: Infective endocarditis. *In* Rakel RE (ed): Conn's Current Therapy 1994. Philadelphia, WB Saunders, 1994.

divided into "early-onset," less than 60 days postoperatively, or "late-onset," greater than 60 days postoperatively. Early PVE is most commonly due to *Staph. epidermidis* and *Staph. aureus*. Other organisms include aerobic gram-negative bacilli and fungi (usually *Candida* or *Aspergillus*). On the other hand, the organisms responsible for late PVE are similar to those that cause "native valve endocarditis."

"Culture-negative endocarditis" occurs in less than 5% of cases of IE and is usually due to the effects of prior antibiotic therapy. Other causes include failure to grow fastidious organisms, such as the HACEK group (*Haemophilus* spp, *Actinobacillus actinomycetemcomitans*, *Cardiobacterium hominis*, *Eikenella* spp, and *Kingella kingae*), nutritionally variant streptococci, *Corynebacterium*, *Legionella*, and fungi, such as *Aspergillus*. These organisms may require specialized culture techniques for isolation. Rare causes of sterile blood cultures include IE with *Coxiella burnetii* (Q fever) and *Chlamydia*. Systemic illnesses such as systemic lupus erythematosus and malignancies may also give rise to a syndrome of noninfective endocarditis.

Polymicrobial IE is a relatively recent problem that has predominantly affected intravenous drug users and patients with indwelling central venous catheters. These patients have an overall mortality of 30%, and prognosis is worse with infections involving *Candida*, *Pseudomonas*, and enterococci.

CLINICAL FEATURES

The presentation of IE is quite variable. The virulence of the organism and the host response in large part determine the presentation of the illness. Previously used diagnostic criteria were too strict, and therefore IE was uniformly underdiagnosed. Recently, D. T. Durack and colleagues of the Duke University Endocarditis Service have proposed new diagnostic criteria that more closely reflect the changing epidemiology of IE and also take into account advances in echocardiographic diagnosis. These are modeled after the Jones criteria for rheumatic fever (Tables 2 and 3). Several different investigators have dem

onstrated the validity of these criteria when compared with the "gold standard" of IE diagnosis, namely, pathologic confirmation of valvular vegetations at surgery or autopsy. However, further evaluation of these criteria are required, especially in situations such as PVE and IE in children.

Clinical features of IE are a reflection of systemic toxicity, localized intracardiac infection and their related complications, bland or septic embolic phenomena, and immune complex disease.

Systemic features almost always include fever, and in subacute forms there may be complaints of malaise, weight loss, myalgias, and arthralgias.

Intracardiac infection primarily involves the valvular apparatus and usually results in a regurgitant murmur. The sensitivity of this finding in defining the presence of endocarditis increases significantly if the murmur is new-onset or has changed in character. Rupture of chordae tendineae or papillary muscle and perforation of the valve leaflet usually results in hemodynamically significant regurgitation and can lead to the abrupt onset of congestive heart failure (CHF).

The presentation of acute aortic insufficiency (AI) differs from chronic AI in that the diastolic murmur tends to be short, and it may decrease in intensity as the degree of regurgitation worsens. This is explained by rapid elevation in left ventricular (LV) end-diastolic pressure with consequent reduction in the gradient between the aortic root and the left ventricle. LV dilatation is also not marked since there has been insufficient time for the ventricle to adapt to the acute volume load. However, a drop in the diastolic blood pressure, a soft S1 and loud S3 along with pulmonary congestion remain consistent findings in hemodynamically significant acute AI.

Acute mitral insufficiency may result from destruction of the chordae, the papillary muscle, or the valve leaflet itself. Examination reveals a hyperdynamic precordium

TABLE 2. **Proposed New Criteria for Diagnosis of Infective Endocarditis**

Definite Infective Endocarditis

Pathologic Criteria
  Microorganisms: Demonstrated by culture or histologic appearance in a vegetation, *or* in a vegetation that has embolized, *or* in an intracardiac abscess, *or*
  Pathologic Lesions: Vegetation or intracardiac abscess present, confirmed by histologic examination showing active endocarditis

Clinical Criteria, Using Specific Definitions Listed in Table 3
  2 major criteria, *or*
  1 major and 3 minor criteria, *or*
  5 minor criteria

Possible Infective Endocarditis

  Findings consistent with infective endocarditis that fall short of "definite," but not "rejected"

Rejected

  Firm alternative diagnosis for manifestations of endocarditis, *or*
  Resolution of manifestations of endocarditis, with antibiotic therapy for ≤ 4 days, *or*
  No pathologic evidence of infective endocarditis at surgery or autopsy, after antibiotic therapy for ≥ 4 days

Reprinted by permission of the publisher from Durack DT, Lukes AS, Bright DK: New criteria for diagnosis of infective endocarditis: Utilization of specific echocardiographic findings. Reprinted from American Journal of Medicine: Vol. 96; 1994 (pp 200–209). Copyright 1994 by Excerpta Medica Inc.

TABLE 3. **Definitions of Terminology Used in the Proposed New Criteria**

Major Criteria

1. *Positive blood culture for infective endocarditis*
   Typical microorganism for infective endocarditis from two separate blood cultures
   Viridans *streptococci,* Streptococcus bovis,* HACEK group, *or*
   Community-acquired *Staphylococcus aureus* or enterococci, in absence of primary focus, *or*
   Persistently positive blood culture, defined as recovery of microorganism consistent with infective endocarditis from
   (a) Blood cultures drawn more than 12 h apart, *or*
   (b) All of three sets, or majority of four or more separate sets of blood cultures, with first and last drawn at least 1 h apart
2. *Evidence of endocardial involvement*
   Positive echocardiogram for infective endocarditis
   (a) Oscillating intracardiac mass, on valve or supporting structures, *or* in path of regurgitant jets, *or* on implanted material, in absence of alternative anatomic explanation, *or*
   (b) Abscess, *or*
   (c) New partial dehiscence of prosthetic valve, *or*
   (c) New valvular regurgitation (increase or change in preexisting murmur not sufficient)

Minor Criteria

1. *Predisposition:* Predisposing heart condition *or* intravenous drug use
2. *Fever:* ≥38.0° C (100.4° F)
3. *Vascular phenomena:* Major arterial emboli, septic pulmonary infarcts, mycotic aneurysm, intracranial hemorrhage, conjunctival hemorrhages, Janeway lesions
4. *Immunologic phenomena:* Glomerulonephritis, Osler's nodes, Roth's spots, rheumatoid factor
5. *Microbiologic evidence:* Positive blood culture but not meeting major criteria as noted previously† *or* serologic evidence of active infection with organism consistent with infective endocarditis
6. *Echocardiogram:* Consistent with infective endocarditis but not meeting major criteria as noted previously

---

*Including nutritional variant strains.

†Excluding single positive cultures for coagulase-negative staphylococci and organisms that do not cause endocarditis.

Reprinted by permission of the publisher from Durack DT, Lukes AS, Bright DK: New criteria for diagnosis of infective endocarditis: Utilization of specific echocardiographic findings. Reprinted from *American Journal of Medicine:* Vol. 96; 1994 (pp 200–209). Copyright 1994 by Excerpta Medica Inc.

---

with evidence of pulmonary congestion and a systolic murmur of variable quality.

Tricuspid valve endocarditis with regurgitation is almost entirely a disease associated with IVDU. Quite often there is no discernible murmur. However, the peripheral manifestations of tricuspid regurgitation are usually obvious. These include a large V wave in the jugular venous pulse, an enlarged pulsatile liver, and peripheral edema in the absence of pulmonary congestion.

Prosthetic valve dysfunction may manifest with a new regurgitant murmur and/or loss of appropriate opening and closing sounds.

Occasionally intramyocardial abscesses may form and rupture, resulting in a variety of intracardiac shunts. Rarely, valvular stenosis may result from an obstructing vegetation or thrombus.

Clinically evident emboli occur in approximately 25% of patients. The classic embolic findings consist of Osler's nodes (painful nodules on the pads of the fingers and toes), Janeway's lesions (nontender hemorrhagic lesions on the palms and soles), Roth's spots (white-centered hemor-

rhages in the fundus), splinter hemorrhages (linear red streaks in the nail beds), and petechiae (conjunctiva, palate, buccal mucosa, and skin above the clavicle). These classic findings are more often seen in the subacute form of IE. It should be noted that although these are considered classic "embolic phenomena," they may in fact be related to immune complex formation. In addition, emboli may occur to the cerebral circulation, resulting in stroke or mycotic aneurysm formation. Mycotic aneurysms may form in any part of the arterial tree and are due to bacterial seeding of the endothelial surface, which results in structural damage to the arterial wall with subsequent aneurysm formation. These aneurysms can rupture and bleed and cause clinical syndromes based on their location. Other organs such as the spleen and rarely the kidney may be sites for systemic emboli. A common feature among IVDU-associated IE is septic pulmonary emboli that appear as nodules, infiltrates, and cavitary lesions on chest x-ray films.

The immune system is activated in IE with the formation of circulating immune complexes, which may be responsible for Osler's nodes and also for the glomerulonephritis that sometimes accompanies IE.

Splenomegaly is present in approximately 30% of affected individuals and may be related to activation of the immune system or as a result of splenic infarcts. Clubbing is a chronic manifestation of IE and is seen typically in illnesses lasting greater than 6 weeks.

Acute IE may present rapidly with fever, metastatic abscesses, valvular destruction, and CHF.

LABORATORY EVALUATION

The presence of continuous bacteremia with an organism known to cause endocarditis in the appropriate clinical setting confirms the diagnosis of IE. Therefore, the most important diagnostic test is properly obtained blood cultures.

Since the number of colony-forming units per mL of blood is relatively low, it has been shown that at least 10 mL of blood is necessary per culture. In order to demonstrate continuous bacteremia, three sets should be collected at 1-hour intervals or longer. At least two of the three sets should be positive. If antibiotics have been used previously, it may be more beneficial to wait 48 hours before drawing blood in order to improve the chances of isolating the infecting organism. However, if the clinical course is fulminant, three blood samples for culture should be obtained at 30-minute intervals and empirical antibiotic therapy initiated.

It is extremely important to alert the microbiology laboratory that the diagnosis of IE is being considered. This enables the laboratory to hold cultures for longer periods of time and also to initiate any specialized techniques that may be necessary to isolate fastidious organisms.

Other laboratory parameters may be abnormal but are not diagnostic. Normochromic, normocytic anemia is usually present, and the white blood cell count may be normal or elevated depending on the acuity of the illness. Thrombocytopenia may occur, and the erythrocyte sedimentation rate is usually elevated. Up to 50% of patients with IE develop a positive rheumatoid factor. The urinalysis may be abnormal, with the presence of microscopic hematuria and/or proteinuria. This may indicate immune complex–mediated glomerulonephritis or renal emboli. A reduction in serum complement levels usually parallels abnormal renal function.

An electrocardiogram (ECG) is an important tool in the assessment of conduction system disease that may result from extension of the infection into the septum, particularly from the aortic valve. Abnormalities in conduction typically manifest as atrioventricular (AV) block, hemiblock, or bundle branch block. Conduction system disease may be transient or permanent, reflecting either edema or complete destruction of the conduction system, respectively. Higher degrees of AV block and bundle branch block are more specific for the detection of septal extension of the infective process. The sensitivity of ECG abnormalities for this condition, however, remains low and should not be relied on to rule out intramyocardial involvement secondary to IE.

The chest roentgenogram is valuable in the assessment of the hemodynamic status and complements the physical examination findings of left heart failure. In tricuspid valve endocarditis, the x-ray film is an extremely important diagnostic tool and usually demonstrates the presence of infiltrates and cavitary lesions consistent with septic pulmonary emboli.

ECHOCARDIOGRAPHY

Because of significant advances in echocardiographic technology and the relative ease and noninvasiveness of this technique, it has become a frequently used test in the evaluation of patients with suspected IE. The recent introduction of the Duke University criteria for IE (see Table 2) recognizes the diagnostic importance of echocardiographically defined abnormalities; however, the definitive diagnosis of IE must be made in conjunction with clinical and microbiologic findings. The existing echocardiographic technology includes two-dimensional color flow and Doppler evaluation. Imaging can be performed using either transthoracic echocardiography (TTE) or transesophageal echocardiography (TEE).

The issue of vegetation size and its prognostic significance has been the subject of much debate. The overall consensus suggests that larger vegetations (particularly greater than 10 mm) are associated with a higher embolic rate. However, whether this embolic potential predicts progression to heart failure, the development of perivalvular extension of infection, the need for valve surgery, or death remains controversial. What remains clear is that the decision to proceed with valve surgery should not be based exclusively on vegetation size. Furthermore, follow-up studies to document the resolution of vegetations have not provided any greater prognostic information than can be obtained clinically.

In cases of CHF, echocardiography becomes an indispensable tool that can evaluate the degree of valvular abnormality, define underlying structural heart disease, and assess left ventricular function. With the addition of color mapping and Doppler flow techniques, it is possible to define in a semiquantitative fashion the degree and nature of the valvular regurgitation. In addition, these modalities can be helpful in the diagnosis of fistulous tracts and intracardiac shunts, which can develop as complications of IE. An absolute indication for either TEE or TTE would be persistent bacteremia despite adequate antibiotic therapy, suggesting perivalvular extension of infection.

Some debate still exists in the choice of TTE versus TEE. In general, TTE and TEE are complementary in the assessment of LV function. Furthermore, the relative ease of performing a TTE tends to favor this technique as the initial approach followed by the TEE if there is inadequate visualization or further information is required.

Screening for IE by echocardiography remains a complex issue, and several factors need to be considered. Since a missed diagnosis and delayed therapy can be fatal, echocardiography by itself, even by the transesophageal approach, cannot entirely rule out the diagnosis of IE. This is true for several reasons, which include the inability to resolve structures less than 2 mm and impaired visualization in the presence of heavily calcified leaflets or prosthetic valves. On one hand, in the specific case of nosocomial *S. aureus* bacteremia, it appears fairly clear that screening for IE is not cost-effective unless there is a new regurgitant murmur, underlying structural heart disease, or persistent bacteremia despite removal of the presumed primary focus. On the other hand, community-acquired *S. aureus* bacteremias with no clinical stigmata of IE are associated with a 20% likelihood of having occult vegetations or predisposing structural heart disease. Finally, not all cases of endocarditis are associated with vegetations, particularly early in the course of the disease. For all these reasons, echocardiography is a tool that should be used thoughtfully, and, more importantly, the findings must be integrated with the existing clinical and microbiologic information.

CARDIAC CATHETERIZATION

The primary role of cardiac catherization is the preoperative evaluation of patients who require surgery for complications related to IE. Most clinical cardiologists would agree that preoperative catheterization is a useful step to assess hemodynamics, assess LV function, define aortic root anatomy, and evaluate for the presence or absence of coronary artery disease. In addition, when there are uncertainties regarding the echocardiographic assessment of valvular insufficiency and LV function, cardiac catheterization remains a useful tool for clarifying the diagnosis and severity of disease. Prosthetic valves can also be evaluated visually under fluoroscopy, and if the characteristic rocking motion is seen, this suggests valve dehiscence.

TREATMENT

The cornerstones of the management of IE are identification of the organism, initiation of appropriate antimicrobial therapy (Table 4), recognition of complications, and prompt surgical intervention when indicated. The principles of antimicrobial therapy are to use bactericidal agents, ensure adequate blood levels of these agents, utilize synergistic combinations when possible, and maintain therapy for an appropriate duration. In general, all forms of IE should be treated for a period of not less than 4 weeks. The two notable exceptions are IE caused by "penicillin-susceptible" *Streptococcus viridans* and selected cases of right-sided endocarditis due to *Staph. aureus*.

Acute IE is usually quite fulminant and is accompanied by some degree of sepsis syndrome, and therefore therapy should not be delayed. In the subacute form, therapy may be initiated after identification of the organism. In the case of previous antibiotic therapy, organism recovery is extremely low for approximately 2 weeks, and therefore the risk of delayed therapy must be weighed against the benefit of organism isolation. Despite these uncertainties in diag-

TABLE 4. **Antimicrobial Therapy for Endocarditis***

Microorganism	Regimen	Duration (Weeks)
Penicillin-Susceptible Streptococci (Viridans streptococci)		
Native valve	Aqueous penicillin G 10–20 × 10^6 U IV q 24 h +	2
(Relatively resistant viridans streptococci and *Streptococcus bovis* should be treated with 4 weeks of penicillin G and 2 weeks of gentamicin.)	Gentamicin 1 mg/kg IM or IV q 8 h	2
	or	
	Aqueous penicillin G 10–20 × 10^6 U IV q 24 h	4
	or	
	Ceftriaxone (Rocephin) 2 g IV or IM single daily dose	4
	or	
	Vancomycin 15 mg/kg IV q 12 h	4
Prosthetic valve	Aqueous penicillin G *or* vancomycin in same dose as above	4–6
	+	
	Gentamicin 1 mg/kg IM or IV q 8 h	2
Enterococci (Streptococcus faecalis, Strep. faecium, Strep. durans) *and resistant viridans streptococci*		
Native valve and infections of <3 months' duration	Aqueous penicillin 20–30 × 10^6 U IV q 24 h +	4
(For prosthetic valves and infections of >3 months' duration, 6 weeks of therapy is recommended.)	Gentamicin 1 mg/kg IV q 8 h	4
	or	
	Vancomycin 15 mg/kg IV q 12 h +	4
	Gentamicin 1 mg/kg IV or IM q 8 h	4
Coagulase-Positive Staphylococci		
Native valve		
Staphylococcus aureus, methicillin-susceptible	Nafcillin (Unipen) *or* oxacillin (Bactocill) 2 g IV q 4 h	6
	or	
	Cefazolin (Ancef) 2 g IV q 8 h	6
	or	
	Vancomycin 15 mg/kg IV q 12 h	6
Staph. aureus, right-sided, methicillin-susceptible	Nafcillin *or* oxacillin 2 g IV q 4 h	2
(If extrapulmonary infection exists, nafcillin should be continued for 4–6 weeks.)	+	
	Tobramycin (Nebcin) *or* gentamicin 1 mg/kg IV q 12 h	2
Staph. aureus, methicillin resistant	Vancomycin 15 mg/kg IV q 12 h	6
Prosthetic valve		
Staph. aureus, methicillin-susceptible	Vancomycin 15 mg/kg IV q 12 h	≥6
(The use of rifampin in this setting is controversial.)	+	
	Rifampin (Rifadin) 300 mg PO q 8 h	≥6
	+	
	Gentamicin 1 mg/kg IV or IM q 8 h	2
Coagulase-Negative Staphylococci (*Staph. epidermidis,* methicillin-resistant)†		
Native valve	Vancomycin 15 mg/kg IV q 12 h	6
Prosthetic valve	Vancomycin 15 mg/kg IV q 12 h	≥6
	+	
	Rifampin 300 mg PO q 8 h	≥6
	+	
	Gentamicin 1 mg/kg IV or IM q 8 h	2
Diphtheroids	Vancomycin 15 mg/kg IV q 12 h	6
HACEK organisms	Ceftriaxone 2 g IV *or* IM q 24 h single dose	4
	or	
	Ampicillin 2 g IV q 4 h +	3
	Gentamicin 1.0 mg/kg IV q 8 h	
Gram-Negative Organisms (Should be treated according to antibiotic susceptibility; suggested regimes are listed.)		
Pseudomonas aeruginosa	Piperacillin (Pipracil) 3 g IV q 4 h *or* ceftazidime (Fortaz, Tazicef) 2 g IV q 8 h *or* Aztreonam (Azactam) 2 g IV q 6 h *or* imipenem 0.5–1 g IV q 6 h	6
	+	
	Tobramycin 1.7 mg/kg IV q 6 h	6
Enterobacteriaceae	Cefotaxime 2 g IV q 6 h *or* imipenem 0.5–1 g q 6 h *or* aztreonam 2 g IV q 6 h	4–6
	+	
	Tobramycin 1.7 mg/kg IV q 8 h	6
Q-Fever Bacteria and Chlamydia	Doxycycline 100 mg PO q 12 h *or* Tetracycline 500 mg PO q 6 h	
	+	1–2 years or longer
	Co-trimoxazole (160 mg trimethoprim and 800 mg sulfamethoxazole) PO q 8 h	
Fungi	Amphotericin B (Fungizone) IV 1 mg/kg/24 h	6–8
	+	
	Flucytosine (Ancobon) 37.5 mg/kg PO q 6 h	
Culture-Negative (empirical therapy)	Vancomycin 15 mg/kg IV q 12 h	6
	+	
	Gentamicin 1 mg/kg IV or IM q 8 h	6

*Dosages recommended are for patients with normal renal and hepatic function.
†Antimicrobial therapy for methicillin-susceptible strains is identical to that for methicillin-susceptible *Staph. aureus.*
From Wilson WR, Thandroyen FT: Infective endocarditis. *In* Willerson JT, Cohn JN (eds): Cardiovascular Medicine. Churchill Livingstone, New York, 1995.

nosis, fairly reliable empirical judgments can be made based on the acuity of the clinical presentation and also the site and type of valvular involvement. The major categories of IE are native valve endocarditis (NVE), PVE, and right-sided endocarditis, which is usually associated with IVDU.

The vast majority of NVE cases are caused by viridans streptococci, enterococci, and staphylococci. A combination of penicillin G, gentamicin (Garamycin), and nafcillin (Unipen) is a reasonable choice if one cannot wait for the results of microbiologic cultures. In the setting of early PVE, there is a greater concern for *Staph. epidermidis* infections, and therefore vancomycin should be used in place of nafcillin. Late-onset PVE has organisms similar to those of NVE, and therefore a similar empirical regimen may be used. Infective endocarditis related to IVDU is predominantly *Staph. aureus* infection, and a combination of nafcillin and gentamicin would be a reasonable choice. It should be emphasized that these are short-term empirical regimens that should be modified as soon as culture and susceptibility testing are available.

"Susceptible" viridans streptococci are defined by the minimal inhibitory concentration (MIC), which is the minimal concentration of antibiotic that inhibits the growth of the organism in a test tube. Organisms with MICs of 0.1 µg per mL or less can be effectively treated with a 2-week course of penicillin G and gentamicin. The concentrations of gentamicin required to act synergistically with penicillin G are quite low (peak of 3 µg per mL or less; trough of 1 µg per mL or less) and minimize the risk of nephrotoxicity and eighth cranial nerve damage. Recent studies have demonstrated efficacy with a 4-week regime of ceftriaxone (Rocephin) two grams per day intravenously or intramuscularly. This antibiotic course offers the possibility of a home-based form of therapy that could significantly reduce health care costs and at the same time be safe, effective, and convenient. However, only patients with uncomplicated IE who are hemodynamically stable and have documented clearance of bacteremia would qualify for this treatment option. For relatively resistant strains of viridans streptococci (MIC 0.1 to 0.5 µg per mL), e.g., nutritionally variant streptococci, *Strep. bovis,* a 4-week course of penicillin G along with gentamicin in the first 2 weeks is recommended. Resistant viridans streptococci (MIC of 0.5 µg per mL or more) are treated with a 4- to 6-week course of penicillin G and gentamicin.

Enterococci (*Strep. faecalis, Strep. faecium, Strep. durans*) are the third most common cause of NVE and occur more commonly in elderly men. Such NVE is best treated with a 4-week course of both penicillin G and gentamicin, or ampicillin and gentamicin. The likelihood of cure using antibiotics alone improves if the infection has been less than 3 months in duration. Highly gentamicin-resistant strains may require surgical removal of the infected valve for a complete cure. Enterococci causing PVE should be treated with the same regimen as above for a period of 6 weeks.

Staphylococcal IE is treated on the basis of methicillin susceptibility or resistance, left- versus right-sided valvular involvement, and the presence or absence of prosthetic material. Methicillin-susceptible staphylococcal left-sided NVE or PVE (right- or left-sided) can be treated with 6 weeks of nafcillin alone or it can be combined with low-dose gentamicin for 3 to 5 days. The addition of gentamicin decreases the duration of bacteremia but does not improve survival or reduce complications. Methicillin-susceptible right-sided staphylococcus NVE (typically IVDU-related) not associated with an extrapulmonary foci of infection can be treated successfully with a 2-week course of nafcillin and tobramycin, or nafcillin and gentamicin. Those with extrapulmonary involvement should receive a 4- to 6-week course of nafcillin, combined in the initial 2 weeks with tobramycin or gentamicin. *Staphylococcus aureus* (methicillin-resistant) NVE should be treated with vancomycin for 6 weeks. Methicillin-resistant strains of *Staph. epidermidis* are typically associated with early-onset PVE and are best treated with a combination of vancomycin and rifampin for 6 weeks with gentamicin added in the first 2 weeks.

Endocarditis associated with the HACEK group of organisms accounts for approximately 9% of non-IVDU-associated cases. These can be effectively treated with 3 weeks of ampicillin. In penicillinase-producing strains, ceftriaxone may be substituted.

Gram-negative infections with other than the HACEK group account for 5% of NVE, 13% of PVE, and 30% of IVDU-associated IE. According to their in vitro susceptibility, these infections should be treated for 4 to 6 weeks utilizing cefotaxime, imipenem, or aztreonam in combination with high-dose gentamicin. There is some evidence to suggest that intravenous ciprofloxacin may now be the preferred therapy in Enterobacteriaceae and *Pseudomonas aeruginosa* infections. A combination of an extended-spectrum penicillin (piperacillin or azlocillin) combined with high-dose tobramycin also appears to be an effective regimen for *P. aeruginosa* IE. This combination therapy may be effective in right-sided NVE; however, the cure rate for left-sided infections is quite dismal, and early valve replacement is recommended.

COMPLICATIONS

The vast majority of deaths related to IE result from congestive heart failure. The major complications can be broadly divided into (1) local valvular destruction, (2) perivalvular extension of infection, (3) embolic complications, (4) systemic sepsis, and (5) intractable infection (Table 5).

Local valvular destruction caused by bacterial vegetations constitutes the most common cause of valvular regurgitation; however, infection of the chordal apparatus or perivalvular abscesses formation may also give rise to insufficiency of the affected valve. In the case of acute aortic insufficiency or mitral

TABLE 5. Complications of Infective Endocarditis

Local valvular destruction, which often accounts for congestive
  heart failure
  Aortic insufficiency
  Mitral regurgitation
  Tricuspid regurgitation (right-sided heart failure, particularly
    in the presence of pulmonary hypertension)
Perivalvular extension of infection, may be associated with
  Persistent, uncontrolled infection
  Valvular insufficiency
  Cardiac conduction defects
  Left-to-right shunts
  Arrhythmias
Embolic phenomena
  Systemic: cerebrovascular accidents, splenic or renal infarcts,
    myocardial infarction, mesenteric/limb ischemia, or
    metastatic abscesses
  Pulmonary: cavitary lesions or pneumonia
Other
  Systemic sepsis (usually secondary to staphylococcal or gram-
    negative infections)
  Mycotic aneurysms
  Valve obstruction by vegetation (rare, but may occur with
    exuberant growth of large, bulky vegetations, particularly on
    prosthetic valves)

From Larsen G, Greenberg B: Infective endocarditis. *In* Rakel RE (ed):
Conn's Current Therapy 1988. Philadelphia, WB Saunders, 1988.

regurgitation, rapid evaluation of the hemodynamic
status and prompt intervention form the basis for
effective therapy. Right heart catheterization can be
invaluable in making this important assessment. If
CHF is suspected by clinical examination, the patient
should be transferred to the coronary care unit and
a pulmonary artery (PA) catheter placed. If normal
pulmonary capillary wedge pressures (PCWPs) are
found, the PA catheter can be removed and medical
therapy for IE may be continued. In the case of mild
elevations in the PCWP, medical treatment for CHF
should be initiated with diuretics and aggressive intravenous vasodilator therapy. We prefer using intravenous nitroprusside as a first-line agent. If the CHF
can be easily controlled, continued medical management would be appropriate and the patient may be
followed sequentially to determine the need for valve
replacement. If, however, there is a failure of medical
therapy for CHF or initial catheterization reveals
severe elevation in the PCWP, urgent surgical evaluation should be planned with concomitant aggressive
treatment of CHF. Failure to proceed with surgical
therapy within 24 to 48 hours after the diagnosis of
severe unresponsive heart failure usually results in
cardiogenic shock and death.

Right-sided endocarditis differs in that the effects
of tricuspid valvular regurgitation with right ventricular volume overload can often be controlled with
diuretic therapy. However, if right-sided heart failure
becomes intractable, a number of surgical procedures
may be considered. These include replacement with
a prosthetic valve and valvuloplasty. Since most
cases of right-sided IE are found in intravenous drug
users, there are significant implications when considering the placement of prosthetic valves in these
patients. Unfortunately, a large percentage of these
individuals continue to use intravenous drugs and
therefore put themselves at significant risk for PVE,
which carries a higher mortality and almost always
requires surgical intervention. This has led several
groups to consider valvuloplasty as a possible alternative. Initial reports have been encouraging; however, these were at fairly specialized centers and
therefore their wider application must await larger
clinical experience.

The incidence of perivalvular extension of infection
(PVEI) varies considerably depending on the series
that is studied. The incidence among NVE patients
is in the order of 10%, and the incidence among PVE
patients is approximately 50 to 60%. Aortic valve
infections are the most common source of PVEI. Typically, PVEI comes to the attention of the clinician
as persistent bacteremia despite adequate antibiotic
therapy, or as worsening CHF. In both these situations TTE and TEE become invaluable for appropriate management. The manifestations of PVEI may
reflect both its extent and its location. PVEI secondary to prosthetic valve endocarditis may result in
paravalvular regurgitation as well as valve dehiscence. From 5 to 10% of patients may develop
arrhythmias and heart block as a result of PVEI,
and therefore the ECG remains a valuable although
somewhat insensitive tool for diagnosis. Occasionally,
infection may spread outside into the pericardium,
resulting in purulent pericarditis, which requires
prompt surgical drainage. Infection may also involve
the papillary muscles, causing disruption of the subvalvular apparatus and resulting in mitral regurgitation. Destruction of intracardiac septae may result in
shunt formation with consequent volume overload.
All these conditions may be associated with myocardial abscess formation. Usually surgery is indicated;
however, with the increasing use of TEE earlier in
the course of IE, smaller myocardial abscesses are
likely to be detected and may not necessarily require
immediate surgical intervention.

Clinically evident embolic phenomena occur in 22
to 43% of patients with IE. There are also likely to
be a large number of clinically silent events, particularly to the spleen or kidney. They may also present
dramatically with an acute arterial occlusion in the
limb or mesentery. Rarely, vegetations may embolize
to the coronary arteries, resulting in myocardial infarction. However, cerebral emboli remain the most
profound embolic complication because of their potential for death and long-term disability. The embolic risks appear to be related to the size of the
vegetation, the duration of antimicrobial therapy,
and the type of organism. Despite the advances in
echocardiographic technique, valvular surgery cannot be recommended strictly on the basis of vegetation size. If, however, there are recurrent embolic
events despite adequate antimicrobial therapy, especially in the presence of organisms such as group B
streptococci, nutritionally variant streptococci, HA-
CEK organisms, or fungi, a stronger consideration
could be given for surgical intervention. Currently
the most effective treatment for reduction of embolic

risk is prompt antimicrobial therapy, which results in a significant reduction in embolic rates in the second and third week of treatment.

Septic embolization can result in metastatic abscesses and also mycotic aneurysms. Metastatic abscesses are most often caused by *Staph. aureus* and in general require surgical drainage. There are, however, clinical situations in which they may resolve with antibiotic therapy, in particular septic emboli to the lung from right-sided IE. Mycotic aneurysms are caused by weakening of the vascular wall as a result of local endovascular bacterial seeding. They can occur in any vascular structure and in most cases result in catastrophic hemorrhage. They are relatively rare complications and are usually diagnosed by their pressure effects. Cerebral mycotic aneurysms typically present with unremitting headache and homonymous hemianopsia, and this symptom complex should alert the physician to the possibility of a serious intracranial complication. In general, if mycotic aneurysms are detected, the therapy of choice is surgical excision.

Systemic complications include systemic inflammatory response syndrome (SIRS), particularly with *Staph. aureus* and aerobic gram-negative infections. These complications may not reverse immediately with prompt antibiotic therapy and may therefore require supportive care in an intensive care setting. In addition, meningitis and encephalopathy may result secondary to the bacteremia and systemic sepsis.

Intractable infection may occur in the setting of fungal, gram-negative, or staphylococcal infection of prosthetic valves. Consequently these infections are associated with a greater incidence of complications including valve dysfunction and PVEI. In addition native valve infections due to aminoglycoside-resistant enterococcus and *P. aeruginosa* have a very poor response to antimicrobial therapy, and therefore

TABLE 6. Indications for Surgery in Infective Endocarditis

Generally Accepted Indications
Congestive heart failure refractory to routine management
Uncontrolled infection despite appropriate antimicrobial therapy
Fungal endocarditis
Suppurative pericarditis
Unstable prosthetic valve
Recurrent disabling systemic emboli after 1–2 weeks of adequate antimicrobial therapy
Mycotic aneurysms

Relative Indications
Infection with gram-negative organism
Staphylococcus aureus infection of left-sided valve (particularly aortic)
Recurrent relapse after apparent cure
Evidence of perivalvular extension of infection
Rupture of sinus of Valsalva or of ventricular septum
Early prosthetic valve endocarditis
New periprosthetic leak
Metastatic abscesses not responding to antimicrobial therapy

From Larsen G, Greenberg B: Infective endocarditis. *In* Rakel RE (ed): Conn's Current Therapy 1988. Philadelphia, WB Saunders, 1988.

TABLE 7. Cardiac Conditions

Endocarditis Prophylaxis Recommended
Prosthetic cardiac valves, including bioprosthetic and homograft valves
Previous bacterial endocarditis, even in absence of heart disease
Most congenital cardiac malformations
Rheumatic and other acquired valvular dysfunction, even after valvular surgery
Hypertrophic cardiomyopathy
Mitral valve prolapse with valvular regurgitation

Endocarditis Prophylaxis Not Recommended
Isolated secundum atrial septal defect
Surgical repair without residua beyond 6 months of secundum atrial defect, ventricular septal defect, or patent ductus arteriosus
Previous coronary artery bypass graft surgery
Mitral valve prolapse without valvular regurgitation*
Physiologic, functional, or innocent heart murmurs
Previous Kawasaki disease without valvular dysfunction
Previous rheumatic fever without valvular dysfunction
Cardiac pacemakers and implanted defibrillators

*Individuals who have mitral valve prolapse associated with thickening and/or redundancy of the valve leaflets may be at increased risk for bacterial endocarditis, particularly men 45 years of age or older.

From Dajani AS, Bisno AL, Chung KJ, et al: Prevention of bacterial endocarditis. Recommendations by the American Heart Association. JAMA 264:2919–2922, 1990. Copyright 1990, American Medical Association.

early valve replacement may be the only viable option.

In general most IE relapses occur between 4 and 8 weeks of stopping antimicrobial therapy. Though there are no clear guidelines, most authorities agree that IE relapse caused by antibiotic-sensitive viridans streptococci and enterococci can be successfully treated with a repeat course of antibiotics. In cases of recurrent relapses and in first-time infections involving Q fever or other resistant organisms, cardiac valve replacement is the appropriate approach.

A summary of the absolute and relative indications for surgery are listed in Table 6. However, the decision to proceed to surgical intervention and valve replacement must be made carefully after assessing all the available clinical, laboratory, echocardiographic, and hemodynamic information.

PREVENTION

Despite the lack of data from controlled trials, there does seem to be a strong association between medical and surgical instrumentation and IE in individuals with underlying structural heart disease. Antibiotic prophylaxis has assumed an important role in the prevention of IE in such individuals. These guidelines were last revised by the American Heart Association (AHA) in 1990 and are summarized in Tables 7, 8, and 9. They represent an attempt to simplify the antibiotic regimen previously used before dental procedures. Specifically, patients with prosthetic valves no longer require parenteral prophylaxis. It is important to remember that general measures are also important. These include the maintenance of excellent oral hygiene and also the use of chlorhexidine (Peridex) mouthwash before dental procedures. These general measures can significantly decrease the amount of subsequent bacteremia. As a corollary to these preventive measures, there is a need to improve awareness among physicians, dentists, and patients regarding the need for antibiotic prophylaxis and the maintenance of good

TABLE 8. Endocarditis Prophylaxis

Procedures for Which Endocarditis Prophylaxis Is Recommended

Dental Procedures
  Dental extraction
  Professional dental cleaning
  Periodontal surgery

Oropharyngeal and Respiratory Tract Procedures
  Tonsillectomy
  Adenoidectomy
  Surgical procedures involving respiratory mucosa
  Bronchoscopy with a rigid bronchoscope

Genitourinary Procedures
  Cystoscopy
  Prostatic surgery
  Urethral dilation
  Urethral catheterization if urinary tract infection is present*
  Urinary tract surgery if urinary tract infection is present*

Gastrointestinal Procedures
  Gallbladder surgery
  Esophageal dilation
  Sclerotherapy for esophageal varices
  Intestinal surgery

Gynecologic and Obstetric Procedures
  Vaginal hysterectomy
  Vaginal delivery in the presence of infection*

Incision and Drainage of Infected Tissue

Procedures for Which Endocarditis Prophylaxis Is Not Recommended†

Dental or Oral Procedures
  Filling of cavities above the gum line
  Simple adjustment of orthodontic appliances
  Shedding of primary teeth
  Injection of local intraoral anesthetic (except intraligamentary injections)

Lower Respiratory Tract Procedures‡
  Endotracheal intubation
  Bronchoscopy with a flexible bronchoscope, with or without biopsy

Genitourinary Procedures‡
  Gastrointestinal endoscopy with or without biopsy

Gynecologic and Obstetric Procedures (in the absence of infection)‡
  Cesarean section
  Uncomplicated vaginal delivery
  Dilation and curettage
  Therapeutic abortion
  Sterilization procedures
  Insertion or removal of intrauterine devices

Cardiac Catheterization

---

*In addition to prophylaxis for genitourinary procedures, antibiotic therapy should be directed against the most likely pathogen.

†Not intended to be all-inclusive.

‡In patients who have prosthetic heart valves, a previous history of endocarditis, or surgically constructed systemic-pulmonary shunts or conduits, physicians may choose to administer prophylactic antibiotics.

From Dajani AS, Bisno AL, Chung KJ, et al: Prevention of bacterial endocarditis. Recommendations by the American Heart Association. JAMA *264*:2919–2922, 1990. Copyright 1990, American Medical Association.

TABLE 9. Recommended Regimens for Various Procedures

Recommended Prophylactic Regimen for Dental, Oral, or Upper Respiratory Tract Procedures in Patients Who Are at Risk

Standard Regimen

PATIENTS NOT ALLERGIC TO PENICILLINS
  Amoxicillin 3.0 g PO 1 h before procedure, then 1.5 g 6 h after initial dose

PENICILLIN-ALLERGIC PATIENTS
  Erythromycin ethylsuccinate 800 mg or *erythromycin stearate* 1.0 g PO 2 h before procedure, then half the dose 6 h after initial dose
            or
  Clindamycin 300 mg PO 1 h before procedure, then 150 mg 6 h after initial dose

Parenteral Regimen for Patients Unable to Take Oral Medications

PATIENTS NOT ALLERGIC TO PENICILLINS
  Ampicillin 2.0 g IV or IM 30 min before procedure, followed by ampicillin, 1.0 g IV or IM, or amoxicillin 1.5 g PO, 6 h after initial dose

PENICILLIN-ALLERGIC PATIENTS
  Clindamycin 300 mg IV 30 min before procedure, followed by 150 mg IV or PO 6 h after initial dose

Regimens for Genitourinary or Gastrointestinal Procedures

Standard Regimen

PATIENTS NOT ALLERGIC TO PENICILLINS
  Ampicillin 2 g IM or IV plus *gentamicin* 1.5 mg/kg (not to exceed 80 mg) IM or IV 30 min before procedure; followed by *amoxicillin* 1.5 g orally 6 h after initial dose; alternatively, parenteral regimen may be repeated once, 8 h after initial dose

PENICILLIN-ALLERGIC PATIENTS
  Vancomycin 1.0 g IV slowly over 1 h plus *gentamicin* 1.5 mg/kg (not to exceed 80 mg) IM or IV, 1 h before procedure, may be repeated once, 8 h after initial dose

Alternative Low-Risk Patient Regimen
  Amoxicillin 3.0 g orally 1 h before procedure; then 1.5 g 6 h after initial dose

Pediatric Doses

  Initial pediatric doses are as follows: amoxicillin, 50 mg/kg; erythromycin ethylsuccinate or erythromycin stearate, 20 mg/kg; clindamycin, 10 mg/kg; gentamicin 2 mg/kg; and vancomycin 20 mg/kg. Follow-up doses should be half the initial dose. *Total pediatric dose should not exceed total adult dose.* Following weight ranges also may be used for initial pediatric dose of amoxicillin; <15 kg, 750 mg; 15–30 kg, 1500 mg; and >30 kg, 3000 mg (full adult dose).

From Dajani AS, Bisno AL, Chung KJ, et al: Prevention of bacterial endocarditis. Recommendations by the American Heart Association. JAMA *264*:2919–2922, 1990. Copyright 1990, American Medical Association.

oral health. The AHA has IE-prevention patient cards that can alert both physicians and dentists to the need for antimicrobial prophylaxis. Using this type of system can significantly improve patient and doctor compliance with the AHA guidelines.

HYPERTENSION

method of
M. A. SIDDIQUI, M.D., and
J. R. SOWERS, M.D.
Wayne State University School of Medicine
Detroit, Michigan

The incidence of nonfatal and fatal cardiovascular disease, renal disease, and all causes of mortality increases progressively with higher levels of both systolic and diastolic blood pressure. These associations are strong, continuous, independent, and predictive. More than 50 million Americans have hypertension, which is defined as systolic blood pressure of 140 mmHg or more and/or diastolic blood pressure of 90 mmHg or more. Despite tremendous advances in drug therapy, hypertension still remains a major cause of morbidity and mortality. The prevalence of hypertension increases with age and is greater in African Americans and those of lower socioeconomic status. In young adults and middle age groups, hypertension is more prevalent in males; thereafter, the reverse is true.

Important advances in understanding the pathophysiology of hypertension have been made over the last several years. It is now regarded more as a disease of the vascular system, associated with a variety of metabolic derangements that increase the risk for cardiovascular and cerebrovascular accidents. A large number of antihypertensive agents are available, which are often synergistic in their antihypertensive properties, and thus they can be chosen to maximize antihypertensive properties and minimize side effects.

PATHOPHYSIOLOGY

Hypertension can be classified into two groups: primary or essential hypertension and secondary hypertension. In the majority of hypertensives with the essential type, no obvious etiology is evident, whereas secondary hypertension is usually a manifestation of some underlying potentially correctable disease process. In essential hypertension, the multiple interactions of neural, hormonal, autocrine, paracrine, rheologic, geometric, and intracellular factors determining the blood pressure obscure the role of any single effector system in development of elevated blood pressure. Several abnormalities have been described in patients with essential hypertension, often with a claim that one or more of these are primarily responsible for the hypertension. While it is not clear at present whether these individual abnormalities are primary or secondary, varying expressions of a single disease process or indicative of separate disease processes, the accumulating data support the latter hypothesis. Therefore, just as fever can be due to a number of different causes and is considered an abnormal physical sign, so also can essential hypertension have a number of causes.

Autonomic Dysfunction

Many antihypertensive medications act by regulating sympathetic neurotransmission, either by blocking the cardiac or vascular adrenergic receptors or by stimulating central adrenergic receptors. The occurrence of these findings has led to suggestions that an adrenergic mechanism is the cause of elevated blood pressure. It has been proposed that in essential hypertension, there are four factors that interact and produce an increase in sympathetic outflow, which in turn leads to an increase in total peripheral vascular resistance. These factors include (1) stress, (2) baroreflex resetting, (3) genetic constitution, and (4) renin-angiotensin-aldosterone system in brain and periphery.

Contributions to hypertension may include alterations in circulating levels of humoral factors such as the endothelins, vasopressin, angiotensin II, endogenous digoxin-like substances, insulin/insulin-like growth factors, steroids, and catecholamines. The other etiologic factors include maladaptive changes in the vascular wall and rheologic factors such as blood viscosity as well as an imbalance between endothelium-derived contracting and relaxing factors. Changes in the cell membrane include lipid changes, alteration in vasoactive hormone receptor numbers and type, intracellular mechanisms such as second messengers, ion channels, and protein phosphorylation. These changes all interact with the sympathetic nervous system to produce abnormal vascular tone and renal sodium handling. Indeed, there is often an association between increases in vascular tone and renal sodium retention early in the development of hypertension.

The unanswered issue about the etiology of essential hypertension is not the individual components in the constellation of the systems but rather the interaction of the entire constellation of maladaptive factors to maintain elevated blood pressure. It has been proposed that the central nervous system adapts to these factors to maintain an elevated blood pressure by increasing vascular responsiveness through adjustments in cardiovascular reflexes and enhanced sympathetic drive.

Evidence of Autonomic Imbalance. The presence of a reduced baroreceptor sensitivity, elevated mean heart rate, and increased vascular contractile responses in young borderline hypertensive individuals lends credence to the view that increased sympathoneural and decreased parasympathetic outflow plays an important role in early elevations of blood pressure. Studies have shown that distributions of antecubital venous plasma norepinephrine levels in hypertensive patients are wider and shifted significantly toward a higher range than the order of distribution observed in normotensive controls. Abnormalities in norepinephrine kinetics are also apparent in young hypertensive patients, which is generally characterized by increased spillover of norepinephrine in cardiac, renal, and brain tissue, suggesting that spillover in certain circulations causes development of hypertension. Although there is substantial overlap in the distribution curves, combined assessment of plasma norepinephrine levels and hemodynamic responses to adrenergic agents can augment the accuracy of identifying the patients with increased sympathoneural contribution to essential hypertension. For example, hypernoradrenergic subjects have larger depressor responses to clonidine and larger pressor responses to yohimbine than the pressure-matched subjects with normal levels of plasma norepinephrine. Furthermore, these subjects also tend to have elevated renin activity and enhanced vasodepressor responses to beta blockers. The combination of high baseline levels of norepinephrine, plasma renin activity, a large depressor response to clonidine, and an accentuated pressor response to yohimbine may help in identifying subjects with increased sympathoneural contribution to blood pressure.

Central Vasomotor Control and Baroreflexes

The central nervous system has a very important role in both long- and short-term regulation of arterial blood pressure and development of hypertension. The short-term regulation of blood pressure is exerted by second-to-second modulation in the activity of sympathetic postganglionic and cardiovagal neurons, while the long-term effects are mediated by humoral and neural mechanisms. The brain can regulate blood pressure by contributing to the control mechanisms that define this relationship: **Blood pressure (BP) = TPR × CO** (total peripheral vascular resistance times cardiac output). The sympathetic postganglionic neurons control blood pressure by selective and differential actions on splanchnic beds and cardiac output. Cardiac output can be modified by changes in the volume of large veins, thereby altering cardiac filling and/or regulating the cardiac contractility. The neural regulation is the result of actions caused by discharges from the postganglionic neurons, which are in turn controlled by signals from preganglionic neurons, which represent the principal effector limbs of the high- and low-pressure cardiovascular reflex systems. The preganglionic neurons are spontaneously active and normally generate a background of sympathetic nerve activity, which is then transmitted to spinal postganglionic neurons, thus contributing to the resting vascular tone. The medulla is the principal target site of the action of centrally acting antihypertensive agents. It is also important in integrating and coupling myriad signals generated in higher brain areas with appropriate cardiovascular reflexogenic responses. The neurogenic theory for development of hypertension postulates that excessive centrally mediated adrenergic vasoconstriction leads to elevation in blood pressure.

Cardiopulmonary or low-pressure baroreceptors are located predominantly in ventricles, atria, and venoatrial junctions. They discharge during systole, and their discharge rate is directly related to intensity of contraction and filling pressures of the heart. The afferent signals from the receptors converge on to the nucleus of the tractus solitarius (NTS) situated in the brain stem. Generally, excitation of these receptors causes inhibition of efferent sympathetic neural outflow to the heart and vasculature leading to decrease in heart rate and blood pressure, along with a concomitant increase in the efferent parasympathetic neural outflow resulting in sinus node slowing and prolongation of atrioventricular conduction. Although abnormalities of cardiopulmonary baroreflexes cause hypertension, by itself hypertension can cause secondary abnormalities in cardiopulmonary baroreflexes controlling the blood pressure. Studies conducted in different phases of hypertension show that baroreflexes are progressively blunted as the duration of untreated hypertension increases. Once the appropriate antihypertensive regimen is instituted and regression of left ventricular hypertrophy (LVH) occurs, there is gradual restoration of low-pressure cardiopulmonary as well as high-pressure sinoaortic baroreflex sensitivity.

Hemodynamics in Hypertensive Patients. Mean arterial pressure is the product of cardiac output and total peripheral vascular resistance. The normal population as it ages tends to develop a decrease in cardiac output and heart rate, while the systolic blood pressure tends to increase slightly due to loss of elasticity of large vessels and decrease in baroreflexes. These changes are associated with an increase in total peripheral vascular resistance. In contrast, younger individuals with Stage I and II hypertension have elevated cardiac index, elevated heart rate, and relatively normal total peripheral vascular resistance. However, the total peripheral vascular resistance is elevated when it is extrapolated to the amount of blood flow. When exercised, these patients show a decrease in cardiac index and total peripheral resistance index, but the decrease is not as prominent as in normal subjects. Studies performed on offsprings of hypertensive patients revealed that resting heart rate and total peripheral vascular index are slightly elevated with a normal cardiac index.

Patients with class III and IV hypertension have an elevated basal total peripheral resistance and heart rate and left ventricular thickness along with a decrease in stroke volume and left ventricular compliance. When exercised, these individuals show a steeper increase in vascular resistance and blood pressure. Vascular resistance increases in all circulatory beds, including pulmonary, which can decrease the right ventricular ejection fraction, leading to functional disturbances in both left and right ventricles.

Neurohumoral Circulatory Control. Although an increase in total peripheral vascular resistance is the hallmark of established hypertension, it is a very infrequent finding in patients with borderline hypertension. A hyperkinetic circulation is an established finding in young, borderline hypertensive patients. Many of these patients have hemodynamic features suggestive of sympathetic overactivity, which includes increased heart rate, cardiac output, and stroke volume, while the total peripheral vascular resistance is normal to slightly elevated. The presence of increased sympathetic tone can be confirmed by various techniques, including direct microneurographic recording of the activity in sympathetic nerve fibers of peroneal and tibial nerves and plasma norepinephrine and norepinephrine spillover rates, all of which are increased in patients with borderline hypertension.

It is unclear as to how the initial cardiac hyperactivity leads to an increase in total peripheral vascular resistance and development of sustained hypertension. It has been speculated that arterioles undergo morphologic changes, in response to either increased flow and pressure or higher circulating levels of catecholamines. The changes in the vasculature include an increase in media/lumen ratio and an enhanced responsiveness to vasoconstrictive stimuli. This increased vascular responsiveness is indicative of the presence of a generalized hyperreactive state in the vasculature. The renin-angiotensin-aldosterone system may also interact with the sympathetic nervous system in causing increased vascular reactivity. The increased vascular reactivity in response to sympathetic stimulation and angiotensin II appears to result because of early abnormalities of vascular smooth muscle cells (VSMC).

It has been suggested that alterations in humoral and local vasomotor control mechanisms lead to establishment of sustained hypertension with significant structural changes in the vasculature.

Autoregulatory Theory of Hypertension. This hypothesis is based on evidence that the kidney is the primary long-term controller of blood pressure, which is closely adjusted to mediate pressure natriuresis. Thus a primary defect in renal sodium handling leads to water retention, an increase in cardiac preload and cardiac output, and an increase in total peripheral vascular resistance. Thus, normal tissue perfusion is maintained at the expense of an elevated resistance and arterial pressure. The increase in pressure is associated with natriuresis, so as to return the blood pressure to normal, but very frequently in hypertensive individuals there is resetting of the pressure natriuresis relationship leading to further salt and water retention.

Neurogenic Theory. This hypothesis suggests that excessive centrally mediated sympathetic vasoconstriction causes centralization of blood volume, an increase in cardiac preload, and a tendency to have an inappropriately high cardiac output for a given level of arterial resistance. In this setting, an imbalance between cardiac output and resistance contributes to the development of hypertension.

Functional and Structural Mechanisms

A number of functional factors can lead to an increase in vascular resistance in hypertension. These are classified as extrinsic and intrinsic, based on their relationship to VSMC. Examples of the intrinsic factors include abnormalities in membrane transport of sodium, calcium, and potassium; increase in vasoagonist receptor sensitivity; and decreased production of vasodilatory substances such as nitric oxide (NO)/cyclic guanosine monophosphate (cGMP), prostacyclin, and natriuretic peptides by vascular cells. Abnormalities in the VSMC signal transduction system leading to increased calcium-mediated VSMC contractility have also been described.

The extrinsic factors influencing VSMC contractility include an imbalance in endothelium-derived vasodilatory and vasoconstrictive agents; increased levels of angiotensin, serotonin, vasoactive prostaglandins, endothelins, and various other vasoactive agents; and/or reduced levels of NO, vasodilatory prostaglandins, and natriuretic peptides. The modulating effect of endothelium on VSMC tone has garnered increasing attention. The abnormalities of the endothelium-dependent vasodilatation present in hypertensive patients appear to include a defect in production of endothelium-derived NO as well as other vasodilatory factors.

Nitric Oxide (NO). This endothelium-derived relaxing factor is a free radical that can act as a neurotransmitter or as an autacoid or paracrine substance. NO can regulate diverse physiologic effects, including vascular relaxation, and studies have shown that cGMP mediates the effects of NO on VSMC. NO is formed from endogenous arginine or from exogenous sources such as nitroglycerin. The enzyme catalyzing the formation is called nitric oxide synthase (NOS), and multiple isomers (i.e., endothelial, inducible, and neuronal NOS) of this enzyme have been described. A variety of drugs and hormones can alter NOS. For example, estrogen, insulin, and insulin-like growth factors can increase endothelial NOS, mediating their vasodilation in part through stimulation of NO production. In contrast, hyperglycemia inhibits endothelial NOS, leading to decreased NO production and related vasoconstriction. The endotoxins and a variety of cytokines can stimulate inducible NO in a number of tissues, including VSMC, leading to vasodilatation and low blood pressure in conditions such as septic shock. The NO/cGMP transduction system can also affect platelet function (decreased platelet aggregation) and inhibit vascular growth and remodeling and thus the atherogenic process.

Endothelins. These are very potent vasoconstrictor polypeptides produced by endothelium. The family consists of the three isoforms ET1, ET2, and ET3 plus snake venom toxin sarafotoxin and vasoactive intestinal polypeptide (VIP). All three active isopeptides contain 21 amino acid residues with two internal disulfide bridges. The actions of endothelins include the following:

1. Contraction of vascular smooth muscle cells; the contraction is remarkably long-lasting and resistant to vasodilators.

2. Mitogenic responses are elicited through activation of protein kinase C and subsequent expression of early genes such as C-*fos* and C-*myc*.

3. Protein kinase C activation also activates the sodium hydrogen transport system, resulting in intracellular alkalization and subsequent vascular growth.

Endothelin production may be elevated under certain pathophysiologic conditions, such as drastic reductions in glomerular filtration rate caused by cyclosporine or prolonged spasm of cerebral vessels post hemorrhage.

Heredity

The children of hypertensive parents have an increased risk of developing elevated blood pressure. Most studies support the concept that the inheritance is probably multifactorial and polygenic. Although the specific genes contributing significantly to the development of hypertension are unknown, a number of candidate genes are currently being investigated.

Environment

A number of environmental factors, including occupation, alcohol intake, family size, stress, obesity, and dietary intake of cations, fat, and sugar, have been implicated in the development of hypertension. These factors are assumed to be important in the increase in blood pressure with age in Western and industrialized civilizations.

Salt. The response to salt illustrates the heterogeneous nature of essential hypertension, with less than 60% of patients with elevated blood pressure being salt sensitive. The elderly, African Americans, diabetic individuals, and obese persons appear to be relatively salt sensitive. Salt loading in the salt-sensitive individual may cause an increase in digoxin-like natriuretic factor, which causes inhibition of ouabain-sensitive Na,K-ATPase, which leads to an increase in intracellular sodium and thus calcium. The other theories of salt sensitivity include a salt-induced renal loss of calcium and/or potassium, lack of appropriate salt modulation of renal blood flow, and aldosterone production. The INTERSALT study demonstrated a linear relationship between salt intake and the development of hypertension. It is unclear at this time whether increasing potassium, calcium, and magnesium in the diet will modulate this small but significant salt-related increase in blood pressure in large populations.

Renin-Angiotensin System

Low-Renin Essential Hypertension. About 20% of patients with essential hypertension have a low-renin state, which is more frequent in African Americans and the elderly. These patients have expanded extracellular volume and increased vascular resistance. There may be increased sensitivity of the adrenal cortex to angiotensin II in many of these individuals, implying that they may have mild adrenal hyperplasia.

High-Renin Essential Hypertension. Approximately 15% of patients with essential hypertension have elevated plasma renin activity, suggesting that elevated levels of angiotensin II may play a role in the pathogenesis of elevated blood pressure in these patients. Studies performed on these patients showed a decrease in blood pressure in 50% of the population with the use of saralasin, and these patients have excellent blood pressure–lowering effects from angiotensin-converting enzyme inhibitors.

Nonmodulating Essential Hypertension. These individuals may compose 25 to 30% of the hypertensive patients. They are called nonmodulators due to the absence of the sodium-mediated modulation of the target tissue (i.e., kidney and adrenal) responses to angiotensin. These individuals have normal to high levels of renin and have a salt-sensitive form of hypertension due to a defect in the kidneys' ability to excrete sodium appropriately. This abnormality appears to be genetically determined and can also be corrected by use of an angiotensin-converting enzyme inhibitor.

Insulin Resistance

Hyperinsulinemia associated with insulin resistance in the obese may contribute to hypertension by many mechanisms. Insulin causes sodium reabsorption from both proximal and distal tubules, and obese individuals are particularly sensitive to the salt-retaining action of insulin. This salt retention is attenuated by weight reduction and an accompanying decrease in insulin levels. Insulin may also contribute to hypertension by inducing vascular growth and remodeling, a process mediated through vascular insulin-like growth factor–mediated mechanisms. Insulin normally exerts vasodilatory effects on vessels, in part, through stimulation of NO production. It attenuates VSMC calcium influx by means of both voltage- and receptor-mediated effects. These observations have led to the concept that decreased effect of insulin on vascular tissues may lead to increased vascular contractility.

Insulin is known to regulate the two vascular smooth muscle pumps, namely Na,K-ATPase and Ca-ATPase. Decreased activity of both pumps and an associated increase in intracellular calcium have been reported in insulin-resistant obese states of hypertension. Thus, decreased cellular insulin actions may lead directly to abnormal cellular cation metabolism and enhanced peripheral vascular resistance. Furthermore, chronic hyperinsulinemia may lead to accelerated atherosclerosis and vascular remodeling. These observations may explain why patients with insulin resistance, such as those with non–insulin dependent diabetes and/or obesity have a high prevalence of hypertension.

CLASSIFICATION OF HYPERTENSION

The fifth report of the Joint National Committee on the Detection, Evaluation and Treatment of Hypertension (JNC-V) has provided a new classification of adult blood pressure based on its impact on the risk (Table 1). The traditional terms "mild hypertension" and "moderate hypertension" have been abandoned, as they failed to convey the impact of elevated blood pressure on the risk of developing a cardiovascular disease. The new classification includes high-normal blood pressure as a category because persons having systolic and diastolic blood pressure ranging from 130 to 139 and 85 to 89 mmHg, respectively, are at an increased risk of developing definitive high blood pressure and of experiencing nonfatal and fatal cardiovascular events compared with similar persons having lower blood pressure.

TABLE 1. **JNC-V Classification of Blood Pressure for Adults Age 18 Years and Older**

Category	Systolic (mmHg)	Diastolic (mmHg)
Normal	<130	<85
High-normal	130–139	85–89
Hypertension		
Stage 1 (mild)	140–159	90–99
Stage 2 (moderate)	140–159	100–109
Stage 3 (severe)	180–209	110–119
Stage 4 (very severe)	>210	>120

DIAGNOSIS

Detection and Confirmation

Hypertension control begins with detection of high blood pressure and requires continued surveillance. It has been suggested that hypertension should not be diagnosed on the basis of a single measurement. The initial elevated reading needs to be reconfirmed on at least two subsequent visits one to several weeks apart, with the average systolic blood pressure 140 mmHg and above and/or the average diastolic blood pressure 90 mmHg and above being required for the diagnosis of high blood pressure.

The following are some of the techniques to be used for measuring the blood pressure so that the values obtained reflect the patient's usual levels:

1. Measurement should begin after 5 minutes of rest.
2. Patient should be seated with arm bared, supported, and at heart level.
3. The patient should not have smoked or ingested caffeine within the past 30 minutes prior to measurement.
4. The appropriate cuff size should be used for ensuring accurate measurement. The bladder should nearly or completely encircle the arm.
5. Measurements should be taken with a mercury sphygmomanometer, a recently calibrated aneroid manometer, or a calibrated electronic device.
6. Both systolic and diastolic pressures should be recorded. The disappearance of the Korotkoff sound (phase V) should be used for the diastolic reading.
7. Two or more readings separated by 2 minutes should be averaged. If the first two readings differ by more than 5 mmHg, additional readings should be obtained.

It is of paramount importance that patients be informed and taught the meaning of their elevated blood pressure readings and advised regarding the need for periodic remeasurement.

Medical History

As our understanding of the epidemiology, pathophysiology, and molecular biology of hypertensive disorders improves, the heterogeneity of hypertensive disorders becomes evident, and from a clinician's point of view this is apparent in several ways:

1. A blood pressure reading may be an unreliable indicator of the type, severity, and prognosis of hypertension.
2. Blood pressure readings may not accurately reflect the efficacy of the antihypertensive therapy.
3. Only 73% of the hypertensive population undergo therapy with medications, and only 21% of those are adequately controlled.

In view of the fact that cardiovascular disease accounts for most of the morbid and mortal events associated with hypertension, the goal of antihypertensive therapy should be to prevent stroke, myocardial infarction, congestive heart failure, and sudden death.

The rapidity of the diagnostic evaluation and initiation of treatment will depend upon several features: the patient's age, duration of hypertension, coexisting diseases, associated symptoms, and magnitude of the blood pressure elevation. Normally, the evaluation is accomplished over several visits spaced at weekly or biweekly intervals.

The following points should be carefully considered in the evaluation of the patient: Was the blood pressure elevation discovered merely on routine examination? Has there been loss of well-being, or a decline in vigor? What, if any, antihypertensive medications has the patient been given? Has the patient been taking any medications that are known to elevate the blood pressure? These include oral contraceptives, steroids, nonsteroidal anti-inflammatory drugs (NSAIDs), nasal decongestants and other cold remedies, appetite suppressants, cyclosporine, erythropoietin, tricyclic antidepressants, and monoamine oxidase inhibitors.

Variant hypertensive patterns can be recognized. A positive family history of elevated blood pressure suggests a hereditary basis for the patient's elevated blood pressure. A history of renal disease in patient and family should be considered; symptoms of nocturia or polyuria and a history of hematuria, recurrent urinary tract infections, renal colic, renal trauma, glomerulonephritis, proteinuria, or microalbuminuria are suggestive of a renal basis of hypertension. Polycystic kidney disease is among the most common primary renal parenchymal diseases associated with hypertension. The patient should be asked whether any family member required dialysis or has died prematurely from stroke, heart attack, or renal failure.

Questions about the patient's lifestyle and environment, which include alcohol intake, smoking, lack of physical activity, and diet, may uncover the presence of associated risk factors. Review of systems focusing on primary target organ damage—brain, cardiovascular, and kidney—is central to clinical history. Headaches can be a symptom of hypertension, particularly if they are occipital, pulsatile in nature, and most prominent on awakening. This complaint is characteristic of patients with pheochromocytoma, hypertensive encephalopathy, and with renovascular hypertension. It is a less specific symptom in patients with uncomplicated essential hypertension and is not a reliable indicator of the magnitude or degree of blood pressure control.

The presence of lethargy and proximal muscle weakness is often associated with metabolic disturbances such as primary and secondary hyperaldosteronism and hyperparathyroidism, when accompanied with weight gain; it is a feature of Cushing's disease and hypothyroidism. Focal sensory and motor changes are of immediate concern, as they are usually an indication of a stroke or a transient ischemic attack (TIA). Symptoms of autonomic instability are common in hypertensive patients, manifesting as light-headedness, syncope, and nocturia that reflect orthostatic changes in blood pressure. Autonomic instability may also manifest as tremors, abnormal sweating, blurred vision, depression, and decrease in libido. Early or uncomplicated hypertension is usually free of symptoms, although young patients with labile hypertension may have symptoms of hyperdynamic circulation including tachycardia and palpitations.

Hypertension is a common manifestation of systemic diseases associated with renal insufficiency, notable among which are diabetes mellitus and connective tissue disorders. A renal biopsy may be required to ascertain the diagnosis and guide treatment. A common curable cause of hypertension is renovascular disease. This diagnosis is suggested by a history of abrupt onset of severe hypertension, particularly at the extremes of age, and a poor response to antihypertensive medications. The other commonly associated features include a history of cigarette smoking and high plasma renin levels with or without hypokalemia; when both kidneys are involved, an elevated level of serum creatinine is generally observed. The renal function worsens on initiation of therapy with angiotensin-converting enzyme inhibitors in patients with bilateral renal artery stenoses.

Physical Examination

The general appearance is often unremarkable except for central obesity in most patients with uncomplicated hypertension. The presence of florid facies is indicative of vasomotor instability, possibly due to an underlying metabolic disorder. Ruddy complexion with a bluish tinge characterizes some patients with essential hypertension, obesity, and polycythemia (Gaisböck's syndrome). Scleroderma crises, associated with high-renin hypertension, are associated with dusky appearance and acrocyanosis. Marked truncal obesity with moon facies, frontal baldness, atrophic extremities, abdominal striae, skin atrophy, and spontaneous ecchymoses suggests Cushing's syndrome. Multiple neurofibromas, mucosal neuromas, and café au lait skin discoloration suggest a familial disorder with associated pheochromocytoma. Hypertension can be related to hypothyroidism characterized by lethargy, dry skin, coarse speech, and delayed reflexes. Renal failure may be manifest as pallor of mucosa and skin, periorbital as well as peripheral edema, and uremic breath.

Blood pressure is measured as discussed previously, and it is good practice to check blood pressure in both arms. A disparity of more than 10 mmHg should be confirmed by repeat measurements, and a consistent disparity is suggestive of the presence of an occlusive disease in the subclavian artery. The most likely cause is atherosclerotic plaque in elderly individuals, while in the younger population it may be due to aortic coarctation or vasculitis. Blood pressure should also be measured in the thigh to rule out the possibility of the presence of coarctation of the aorta. Normally the systolic blood pressure is higher and diastolic blood pressure is lower in the popliteal artery compared with the brachial artery. During the initial visit, blood pressure should be measured in all the three positions: sitting, supine, and standing. Postural changes in the blood pressure are especially prominent in the elderly and in patients with autonomic neuropathy (e.g., with long-standing diabetes).

Funduscopic Examination. This is a very important part of the physical examination; it provides assessment of the target organ damage, severity of hypertension, and urgency for treatment. The Keith-Wagener-Barker system of classification is employed for grading the retinal changes:

Grade I: Minimal disease manifests as spasm, copper wire, or silver wire appearance of the arterioles with tortuosity and segmental constriction.

Grade II: Grade I changes accompanied by evidence of arteriolar sclerosis. Heightened light reflex and presence of arteriovenous nicking are suggestive that disease has been present for years.

Grade III: In addition to the preceding changes, overt retinal hemorrhages and exudates are present. Hemorrhages are flame shaped and radiate from the optic disk, along the vascular tree. Exudates can be either hard or soft; the former are shinier and circumscribed, while the latter ones are like cotton wool spots. Hard exudates indicate an older healing process, while soft exudates and hemorrhages suggest an ongoing severe or accelerated hypertension requiring urgent treatment.

Grade IV: These changes are usually the hallmark of malignant hypertension, characterized by edema of disk margins accompanied by hemorrhages and soft exudates.

Examination of the Heart. The mechanical effects on the heart due to sustained increase of pressure work are reflected in the physical findings. Forceful left ventricular apex manifests early in the disease period and is especially exaggerated in variant hyperdynamic states. Sustained left ventricular thrust indicates substantial left ventricular hypertrophy. The presence of an S_4 gallop is an indication of reduced left ventricular compliance and occurs during atrial systole. The S_3 gallop may occur in young patients with rapid left ventricular filling but in older patients is a late manifestation of hypertension as a result of reduced left ventricular diastolic compliance.

Hypertension is usually systolic in nature in patients with aortic regurgitation; physical findings include diastolic murmurs and wide pulse pressure. The physical findings in patients with aortic stenosis are systolic murmur, ventricular heave, narrow pulse pressure, and pulsus parvus. A harsh systolic murmur over the precordium or the midscapular space in young patients may be due to coarctation of the aorta; this physical finding should be corroborated by measuring the blood pressure in all four extremities. An echogram of the heart should also be obtained to rule out the presence of bicuspid aortic valve, which commonly occurs in patients with coarctation of the aorta.

Examination of the Vascular System. Hypertension leads to accelerated atherosclerosis that causes vaso-occlusive disease. Evaluation includes auscultation of peripheral arteries, including carotids, subclavian, abdominal aorta, renal, and femoral arteries. The presence of the diastolic component to a bruit or thrill suggests a tighter stenosis. All the distal pulses should be palpated and the extremities inspected for evidence of vascular insufficiency.

Neck. The neck should be palpated for the presence of thyromegaly, and the carotid pulses should be carefully examined.

Abdominal Examination. The aorta should be carefully palpated due to the increased prevalence of the risk of aortic rupture in hypertensive patients. The presence of enlargement of one or both kidneys suggests hydronephrosis, tumor, or polycystic renal disease. Occasionally pheochromocytoma can be large enough to be palpated; this urge should be curbed, as the cardiovascular responses can be potentially catastrophic. Careful auscultation in the paraumbilical area will elicit the presence of renal artery bruit, which usually has a to-and-fro component.

Neurologic Examination. Strokes, hypertensive encephalopathy, or an underlying metabolic abnormality related to the primary disturbance should be excluded.

Laboratory Tests and Diagnostic Procedures

Diagnostic tests that should be routinely performed before initiating therapy include urine analysis, complete blood count, blood glucose, serum potassium, calcium, creatinine, uric acid, cholesterol (total and HDL), triglycerides, and an ECG. Additional optionable tests include urinary microalbumin determination, assessment of cardiac anatomy and function by means of echocardiography, and estimation of plasma renin/urinary sodium.

Complete Blood Count. This is a measure of the patient's general health. Anemia may be a concomitant finding in a variety of chronic diseases, including renal failure. Polycythemia may identify hypertension in certain settings—e.g., excessive erythropoietin administration. Eosinophilia in the setting of atherosclerosis may signal spontaneous or iatrogenic atheroembolic renal or peripheral vascular disease.

Serum Potassium. Low serum potassium (<3.6 mg/L) when associated with urinary potassium wasting points toward disorders of aldosterone. Spontaneous hypokalemia may also be the consequence of renal tubular acidosis,

gastrointestinal losses, or diuretic therapy. If the serum potassium is borderline or low (i.e., ≤3.6 mEq/L), it should be repeated on two or three separate occasions. Hyperkalemia is the result of renal failure, especially during treatment with ACE inhibitors.

BUN, Creatinine, Urinalysis, Microalbuminuria. Blood urea nitrogen (BUN) and serum creatinine provide an important longitudinal marker of progressive decline of renal function in patients with hypertension. Routine urinalysis including microscopic examination of sediment is an important screening test of renal parenchymal disease. An abnormally increased excretion of albumin in a 24-hour urine collection is a sensitive indicator of impaired renal function. In diabetics microalbuminuria suggests possible incipient renal insufficiency, and in nondiabetics it is associated with increased risk of cardiovascular morbidity/mortality.

Fasting Blood Glucose. This test is generally performed to identify the presence of diabetes, which is commonly associated with hypertension. Diabetes is a strong independent risk factor for cardiovascular disease.

Serum Uric Acid. Diuretics stimulate urate absorption in the proximal renal tubules and may promote acute gouty arthritis in predisposed individuals. A markedly elevated serum uric acid level may reflect an underlying lead nephropathy; in addition, it is an important marker of preeclampsia in hypertensive pregnant patients.

Serum Cholesterol. An elevated level of serum cholesterol, especially the LDL fraction, is an important risk factor for the development of cardiovascular disease. Treatment of hypertension with a certain group of medications like high-dose diuretics and beta blockers is associated with an increase in LDL cholesterol levels and an increase in triglycerides and reduction in HDL (beta blockers). Thus, it is important to establish the baseline fasting lipid profile before starting the antihypertensive therapy. Studies have shown a decrease in cardiovascular morbidity and mortality in patients who are treated for elevated serum cholesterol levels.

12-Lead ECG. Performing a 12-lead ECG helps in identifying the presence of LVH and ischemic heart disease. A number of studies, including the Framingham study, have shown that left ventricular hypertrophy (LVH) is a strong predictor of myocardial infarction, stroke, and death. It is important to note that electrocardiography is not a sensitive but a very cost-effective method of identifying the previously mentioned abnormalities.

Echogram of Heart. This is a very sensitive method for detecting the presence of LVH; it also helps in quantifying the ventricular function and identifying the presence of wall motion abnormalities.

LVH can regress with therapy, but there are insufficient data to suggest a preferential response to certain pharmacologic classes of antihypertensive agents. The persistence of LVH during therapy suggests a higher cardiovascular risk when compared with individuals in whom it regresses. However, echocardiograms should not be routinely obtained in patients with essential hypertension.

Plasma Renin Activity. This is usually performed when either renovascular hypertension or hyperaldosteronism is suspected as a cause of elevated blood pressure. Low plasma renin activity in face of normal sodium intake is suggestive of hyperaldosteronism, whereas an elevated activity is strongly suggestive of renovascular hypertension. An exaggerated renin activity response to captopril is strongly suggestive of renal artery stenosis.

End-Organ Damage

The Heart in Hypertension. Left ventricular hypertrophy (LVH) is defined as an increase in left ventricular mass that is abnormal when adjusted for age, sex, and race. It is said to be present if echocardiographically determined left ventricular mass exceeds 130 gm/m² body surface area in males and 110 gm/m² in females.

The pathophysiologic abnormalities commonly associated with LVH are (1) impaired left ventricular filling, (2) ventricular dysrhythmias, (3) myocardial ischemia, and (4) decreased left ventricular contractility. The increase in left ventricular mass can be quantitated by chest x-ray, ECG, two-dimensional echocardiography, CT scan, and MRI. The chest x-ray is a very semiquantitative method and is not recommended. Even though ECG is a very specific test, it is not very sensitive in detecting LVH, as 20 to 30% of patients with normal ECGs will have LVH as detected by two-dimensional echocardiography. The most sensitive and specific method of confirming the presence of LVH is echocardiography.

The Kidney in Hypertension. Hypertension is both a cause and consequence of renal failure. The presence of hypertension accelerates deterioration in renal function by causing worsening of intrinsic renal failure and hastening age-related nephron loss. The incidence of hypertensive nephropathy, which is defined as renal insufficiency in which hypertension is the only known cause, is difficult to quantify, as hypertension develops as a consequence of renal failure and many patients labeled to have hypertensive nephropathy very frequently have other causes of renal failure.

The clinical features suggestive of hypertensive nephrosclerosis as proposed by Luke and Curtis are as follows:

1. African Americans.
2. Positive family history; onset of hypertension between ages 25 and 45 years.
3. Long-standing or very severe hypertension.
4. Evidence of hypertensive retinal damage and left ventricular hypertrophy.
5. Onset of hypertension before development of proteinuria.
6. Absence of any cause for primary renal disease.
7. Biopsy evidence: degree of glomerular ischemia and fibrosis compatible with degree of arteriolar and small arterial vascular disease.

Classically, the kidneys in hypertensive nephrosclerosis are shrunken, scarred, and granular in appearance. There are pathologic changes in the vasculature, including intimal thickening, fibrosis, and reduplication of internal elastic lamina in the arcuate and interlobular arteries, as well as hyalinization of arterioles. The glomerular injury is generally focal in nature and consists of tuft shrinkage along with loss of cellularity and eventual sclerosis. The tubules are very frequently atrophic.

The mechanisms of injury include hemodynamic changes as well as destruction caused by elevated levels of cholesterol and endothelial dysfunction.

Hemodynamic Injury. Hypertension causes damage to kidneys in various ways; one such mechanism is ischemia with glomerular hypoperfusion causing glomerulosclerosis, which is most evident in patients with renovascular hypertension and to a certain extent in patients with essential hypertension. In contrast to the setting of hypertension secondary to intrinsic renal disease, glomerular capillary hyperfiltration and hypertension rather than ischemia are important pathogenetic mechanisms. Furthermore, increase in capillary pressure leads to enhanced traffic of macromolecule into the mesangium. This may stimulate synthesis of matrix components by the mesangial cells. Peristent proteinuria may accelerate disease by contributing to tubulointerstitial injury and rapid glomerulosclerosis.

Cholesterol and Endothelial Dysfunction. This is based on experimental evidence that hypertension and dyslipidemia accelerate glomerular injury, while therapy with lipid-lowering agents slows the disease progression. In studies examining the potential additive effects of systemic hypertension and hyperlipidemia, the combination induces more glomerular injury than either risk factor alone. It is speculated that oxidation of LDL lipoprotein may be a critical injury-promoting step among all other mechanisms. The presence of fibrinoid materials in the glomerulus in many forms of renal injury is suggestive of endothelial cell dysfunction. Abnormalities in capillary hemodynamics and hemostasis occur, which are triggered by endothelial dysfunction.

Cerebral Circulation. Chronic hypertension is associated with adaptive and degenerative structural changes in the cerebral resistance vessels. In the large conduit arteries, hypertension accelerates atherosclerosis and contributes to the development as well as rupture of saccular aneurysms. In smaller arteries and arterioles, hypertension causes structural remodeling, which consists of wall thickening and luminal narrowing. In patients with long-standing hypertension, degenerative changes in the form of lipohyalinosis may prevail, sometimes associated with a tendency to develop Charcot-Bouchard microaneurysms. These degenerative changes may be the source of smaller lacunar infarcts and hemorrhages. Binswanger's encephalopathy, also known as leukocraniosis or subcortical arteriosclerotic demyelination with progressive dementia, may also be associated with hypertension.

Follow-Up

The blood pressure measurement needs to be repeated to confirm the persistence of initial elevated levels or to determine whether they have returned to normal and need only periodic reassessment. The initial blood pressure readings that are markedly elevated (i.e., diastolic 120 mmHg or greater, or systolic 210 mmHg or more) or are associated with evidence of target organ damage may require immediate drug therapy. Follow-up recommendations by JNC-V based on initial blood pressure measurements for adults aged 18 years and older are as follows: systolic pressure 130 and diastolic pressure 85 mmHg, blood pressure needs to be rechecked in 2 years. For systolic 130 to 139 and diastolic 85 to 89 mmHg follow-up in 1 year and advice about lifestyle modifications, including weight loss, moderation in alcohol and sodium intake, and increased physical activity, are needed. If systolic blood pressure is 140 to 159 and diastolic is 90 to 99 mmHg, these readings need to be reconfirmed within the next 2 months. Immediate evaluation needs to be performed for systolic pressures 160 to 179 and diastolic 100 to 109. A systolic blood pressure of more than 210 and diastolic blood pressure of more than 120 need immediate referral to the source of care, in comparison with a systolic pressure of 180 to 209 and a diastolic of 110 to 119, in which the patient can be referred to the source of care in 1 week. It is also important to note that if the systolic and diastolic categories are different, recommendation for shorter follow-up should be employed (e.g., 160/85 mmHg should be evaluated or referred to source of care within 1 month). The scheduling of follow-up should be modified by reliable information about past blood pressure measurements, other cardiovascular risk factors, or target organ damage.

Ambulatory BP Monitoring (ABPM)

There is increasing evidence that target organ damage correlates better with out-of-office measurements, including those with ABPM. Studies conducted at the authors' center have shown that ABPM offers useful insight into physiologic blood pressure variations and may alter the decision to treat elevated blood pressure readings measured in the office. The authors have also shown that ABPM is cost effective in an outpatient setting in preventing unwarranted drug therapy and the inappropriate diagnosis of hypertension.

Clinical situations in which ambulatory blood pressure monitoring are helpful include the following:

1. White coat hypertension.
2. Evaluation of drug resistance.
3. Evaluation of nocturnal blood pressure changes.
4. Episodic hypertension.
5. Hypotensive symptoms associated with antihypertensive medications or autonomic dysfunction.
6. Carotid sinus syncope and pacemaker syndromes (along with electrocardiographic monitoring).

Ambulatory blood pressure can be recorded either by noninvasive or invasive equipment. The former is a more practical way of measuring the blood pressure, as it eliminates the need for an indwelling arterial catheter and the associated risk of infection. Noninvasive blood pressure monitoring can be performed either intermittently or continuously; an example of the instruments is the Spacelabs 90207. Current monitoring devices are fully automatic, lightweight, and portable, and can measure and store blood pressure and heart rate data for more than 24 hours. Each device needs to be calibrated initially and then at least yearly afterward against standard methods of checking the blood pressure. The two protocols that have been published for evaluating the noninvasive discontinuous blood pressure monitors are those of the British Hypertension Society and the Association for the Advancement of Medical Instrumentation. While ABPM is a unique tool for research and for extended assessment of particular hypertensive patients with special clinical problems, it is not recommended for routine diagnosis and management of most patients.

PRIMARY PREVENTION OF HIGH BLOOD PRESSURE

Primary prevention of high blood pressure can be accomplished by population-based and targeted strategies. The former include application of interventions to the general population with the objective of achieving a downward drift in the distribution of blood pressure. The targeted strategies include attempts at decreasing the blood pressure in persons with high-normal blood pressure, family history of elevated blood pressure, and those with one or more of the various lifestyle factors that contribute to the development of hypertension. These lifestyle factors include high-sodium diet, excessive calorie consumption, low levels of physical activity, and low content of dietary potassium. They form the basis of intervention strategies that have shown promise in prevention of high blood pressure. The data are less convincing for stress management; supplementation with calcium, potassium, magnesium, and fish oil; a high-fiber diet; and an alteration of macronutrient consumption.

However, achievement of the intervention goals is severely constrained by various societal barriers, including lack of satisfactory food substitutes and the absence of a national campaign to advocate adoption of the population-based and targeted intervention strategies necessary to prevent development of hypertension.

TREATMENT

Approach to Management

The goal of treating hypertensive patients is to prevent morbidity and mortality associated with elevated blood pressure and to control hypertension with the least intrusive means. This is generally achieved by lowering and maintaining the arterial blood pressure below systolic blood pressure 140 mmHg and diastolic pressure less than 90 mmHg, while simultaneously modifying other cardiovascular risk factors. A further reduction of blood pressure to 130/35 mmHg, especially in those with diabetes, can be pursued with due regard to cardiovascular function. At this point, it is unclear as to how far the diastolic blood pressure should be reduced below 85 mmHg, especially in the elderly population. The results of the HOT trial (Hypertension Optimal Treatment) are eagerly awaited.

Lifestyle Modifications

Modifications in lifestyle include weight reduction; increase in physical activity; and moderation in dietary alcohol, fat, and salt intake. They offer hope of disease prevention, are effective in lowering the blood pressure, and reduce the risk of premature cardiovascular disease. Even when they do not adequately decrease the blood pressure alone, they do often decrease the number and doses of antihypertensive medications. Lifestyle modifications are particularly helpful in a large proportion of patients with additional risk factors for premature cardiovascular disease (CVD) such as dyslipidemia or diabetes mellitus.

Stage I and II Hypertension

JNC-V recommends that if the blood pressure remains at or above 140/90 mmHg during a 3- to 6-month period despite lifestyle modifications, antihypertensive medications should be initiated, especially in individuals with evidence of target organ disease and or other known risk factors for cardiovascular disease. Data from clinical trials strongly indicate that drug therapy should be initiated before development of target organ damage.

Drug Therapy. The recommended initial drug therapy for stage I and II hypertension is monotherapy—that is, start with a single drug. Low-dose diuretics and perhaps beta blockers may be preferable for monotherapy, as they have been shown to decrease cardiovascular morbidity and mortality in controlled clinical trials. The demographic characteristics of the patient, presence of concomitant diseases, quality of life, and economic considerations should be carefully considered while choosing the antihypertensive therapy.

In general, African Americans and the elderly are somewhat more responsive to diuretics and calcium channel blockers than angiotensin-converting enzyme (ACE) inhibitors. ACE inhibitors are generally recognized as the initial antihypertensive agent of choice in diabetic hypertensive persons because of their salutary renal effects. Antihypertensive agents may worsen some clinical problems while improving others; for example, beta blockers may worsen asthma, diabetes, and peripheral vascular disease while improving angina pectoris, cardiac dysrhythmias, and migrainous headache. Drugs chosen to treat elevated blood pressure may affect the quality of life; many of these agents cause impairment in sexual functioning and decrease the mental acuity and exercise tolerance.

The lowest dosage of the medication chosen is generally used to initiate therapy and is continued for several weeks, even if the blood pressure is not well controlled, before increasing to the next dosage level. It is important to note that adherence to medications improves substantially as the prescribed dose frequency decreases. Because of better compliance and increased safety (especially with calcium antagonists), sustained slow-release preparations are preferable.

After 1 to 3 months of follow-up, if the response to initial therapy is still inadequate and the patient has not experienced significant side effects, the physician must make sure that the patient is compliant with the prescribed therapy before considering the following three options:

1. Increase the dose of the first drug to or toward maximal levels.
2. Substitute an agent from another class.
3. Add a second drug from another class.

The method of combining the medications with different mechanisms of action will very frequently allow smaller doses of the drugs to be used in achieving blood pressure control and also minimizes the potential for dose-dependent side effects. If a diuretic is not chosen as the first drug, it will be helpful as a second agent because its addition enhances the effects of the other agents. If the addition of the second antihypertensive agent leads to satisfactory blood pressure control, an attempt should be made to withdraw the first agent, as blood pressure is adequately controlled with one agent alone in nearly 50% of patients. If the response is inadequate, consider adding a third agent and/or a diuretic if it is not already prescribed. At each step, the physician must carefully consider the causes for lack of responsiveness to therapy (Table 2).

Once the blood pressure is controlled to an optimal level and the maintenance doses of the antihypertensive agent have been established, substituting comparable combination tablets may simplify the

TABLE 2. **Causes for Lack of Responsiveness to Antihypertensive Therapy**

Nonadherence to Therapy
Cost of medication
Lack of clear instruction/inadequate patient education
Side effects of medications/inconvenient dosing
Organic brain syndrome
Drug-Related Causes
Doses too low
Rapid inactivation
Drug interactions, e.g., NSAIDs, antidepressants, nasal decongestants, cocaine, cyclosporine, erythropoietin
Associated Conditions
Increasing obesity
Alcohol abuse
Increasing stress
Secondary Hypertension
Renal failure
Renovascular hypertension
Primary hyperaldosteronism
Pheochromocytoma
Pseudohypertension

patient's regimen and promote adherence to the treatment program.

Stage III and IV Hypertension

The general principles of management are similar to those described as previously but certain modifications may be appropriate for patients presenting with a systolic pressure of 180 mmHg or more and/or a diastolic pressure of 110 mmHg or more. These include the following:

1. Decreased interval between changes in medication.
2. Initial multidrug therapy.
3. More frequent follow-ups.
4. The maximum dosage of some medications may be increased.

It is recommended that patients presenting with a diastolic blood pressure of 120 mmHg or more be given immediate drug therapy, and if significant target organ damage is present, they may require hospitalization and management by a specialist.

Drugs

Diuretics

The thiazides and related compounds comprise the most frequently used antihypertensive agents in the United States. These drugs have a similar pattern of pharmacologic effects and are generally interchangeable with appropriate adjustment of dosage. The blood pressure–lowering effect is seen at lower doses that produce a small natriuretic effect; increasing the dosage will not increase the antihypertensive effect unless the patient is on a high-salt diet, in which case the lower dose may not produce a net loss of sodium ion. The use of higher doses is associated with a marked increase in the side effects and symptoms that lead to poor patient compliance. Lower doses of diuretics are particularly preferable in the elderly and in patients with diabetes.

The exact mechanism by which diuretics reduce blood pressure is uncertain. These drugs first decrease the extracellular volume and the cardiac output. However, the hypotensive effect is maintained during long-term therapy due to decreased vascular resistance, even though the cardiac output returns to the pretreatment level and the extracellular volume remains somewhat reduced, leading to decreased blood pressure. This effect is not observed in anephric patients and is reversed by high salt intake or infusion of saline. Postulated mechanisms of action include a decrease in interstitial fluid volume and a fall in smooth muscle sodium concentration that secondarily reduces intracellular calcium concentration, such that the cells are more resistant to the contractile stimuli. It is possible that there may be a change in the affinity and response of the cell surface receptors to vasoconstrictive hormones.

Side Effects. Use of high-dose diuretics (i.e., 50 mg or greater of hydrochlorothiazide) may be associated with hypokalemia, hypomagnesemia, hyperuricemia, hypercalcemia, and possibly hyperglycemia and hypercholesterolemia. The associated metabolic abnormalities may be associated with cardiac arrhythmias and muscle weakness. Much has been written about the worsening of the metabolic profile, particularly in patients with diabetes mellitus and hypertension, but careful analysis of the clinical studies reveal a comparable benefit in overall mortality and morbidity in these subgroups of patients being treated with diuretics. Data from the Systolic Hypertension Elderly Program (SHEP) trial as well as studies performed in Europe suggest that low-dose diuretic therapy decreases the cardiovascular mortality and slows the progression of renal disease. Thus, low-dose diuretics are firmly established as having an important role in the therapy of most patients with essential hypertension.

Drug Interactions. NSAIDs, cholestyramine, and colestipol may decrease the antihypertensive effectiveness of diuretics, the former by antagonizing diuretic effectiveness and the latter by decreasing its absorption. Loop diuretics such as furosemide (Lasix) are not effective antihypertensives and should be reserved for patients with severe renal impairment.

Diuretics can raise the levels of lithium leading to increased toxicity and can make management of dyslipidemias and diabetes difficult.

Potassium-Sparing Diuretics. These include amiloride (Midamor), spironolactone (Aldactone), and triamterene (Dyrenium). These agents generally act by competitive inhibition of aldosterone action at the distal convoluted tubules, thus decreasing the potassium loss. Amiloride is the drug of choice in the management of primary hyperaldosteronism. As a class, potassium-sparing diuretics are weak diuretics and are generally used in combination with other diuretics to avoid or reverse hypokalemia from other agents. Potassium-sparing agents should be used with caution in patients with renal impairment, and their hyperkalemic effect may be exaggerated in patients being treated with ACE inhibitors. Use of spironolactone is associated with development of gynecomastia and a decrease in libido in males. Triamterene usage can cause formation of renal calculi.

Adrenergic Inhibitors

Adrenergic inhibitors include beta blockers, beta blockers with intrinsic sympathomimetic activity (ISA), alpha and beta blockers, and alpha$_1$-receptor blockers.

Beta blockers: Atenolol (Tenormin), betaxolol (Kerlone), metoprolol (Lopressor), and propranolol (Inderal).

Beta blockers with ISA: Includes acebutolol (Sectral), pindolol (Visken), and carteolol (Cartrol).

Alpha-beta blockers: Labetalol (Normodyne, Trandate) is the prototype.

Alpha$_1$-receptor blockers: Examples are doxazosin (Cardura) and terazosin (Hytrin).

The antihypertensive action of beta blockers is mediated through effects on cardiac output, renin secretion, and adrenergic neuronal function, and possibly through increases in baroreceptor sensitivity. The beta blockers without ISA cause an initial decrease in cardiac output and a rise in peripheral vascular resistance with no net change in arterial pressure. In subjects who respond with a reduction in blood pressure, peripheral vascular resistance returns to pretreatment values in a few hours or a few days. It is this recovery of vascular resistance in the face of persistently reduced cardiac output that accounts for the decrease in arterial blood pressure. Plasma renin activity is generally reduced due to decrease in renal renin production.

Drugs with ISA produce less effect on resting heart rate and cardiac output and a fall in vascular resistance below pretreatment levels, probably because of stimulation of vascular beta$_2$-adrenergic receptors that mediate vasodilatation.

The usage of beta blockers may cause exacerbation of asthma in predisposed individuals, worsening of peripheral vascular disease, fatigue, insomnia, impotence, decrease in left ventricular function, lipid abnormalities (decrease in HDL and increase in LDL and triglycerides), and reduced exercise tolerance. These medications can mask symptoms of hypoglycemia. The use of these agents is generally contraindicated in patients with asthma, chronic obstructive pulmonary disease, congestive heart failure, and conduction disturbances of the heart. Caution should be exercised when beta blockers are used in patients with peripheral vascular disease and insulin-treated diabetes. Alpha blockers block the postsynaptic alpha$_1$ receptors and cause vasodilatation. They work by reducing the vascular constrictor response to sympathetic nerve discharge. They have potential beneficial effects on lipids and may improve the activity of the fibrinolytic system, regress left ventricular hypertrophy, and decrease symptoms associated with prostate enlargement. They are the agents of choice in the management of pheochromocytoma and are also useful agents in the treatment of patients with renovascular hypertension, asthma, peripheral vascular disease, and diabetes. Alpha blockers may be associated with development of orthostatic changes, syncope, palpitations, headache, priapism, nasal decongestion, vomiting, diarrhea, and rash.

Drug Interaction. Rifampin (Rifadin), smoking, and phenobarbital decrease the serum levels of beta blockers by induction of liver enzymes, thus decreasing the antihypertensive effects. Cimetidine and quinidine may enhance the antihypertensive actions. The use of beta blockers along with calcium channel blockers or reserpine can worsen conduction defects.

While beta blockers do cause masking of hypoglycemic symptoms and worsening of dyslipidemias, it is important to note that they are the only medications that are known to decrease mortality in the post–myocardial infarction period, and diabetics benefited the most in subgroup analysis. Therefore, clinicians should not hesitate to use beta blockers as antihypertensive agents in appropriate settings.

ACE Inhibitors

Angiotensin-converting enzyme (ACE) inhibitors are serum protease inhibitors and block the formation of angiotensin II; in addition, they decrease the degradation of various kinins including bradykinin. A number of experiments have shown a direct relationship between serum bradykinin level and formation of nitric oxide (NO) by endothelium. Thus elevated bradykinin levels increase the levels of NO, which is a potent vasodilator; in addition, it is speculated that kinins may decrease the formation of fetal myocardial proteins, which is generally observed in patients with congestive heart failure.

The use of ACE inhibitors results in decrease in blood pressure, improvement in cardiac output, and decrease in heart size, all of which manifest as increase in exercise tolerance and decreased hospitalization in patients with heart failure. The ACE inhibitors have made a remarkable impact on the management of patients with cardiac failure, as evidenced by the results of several large clinical trials.

ACE inhibitors cause a decrease in the tone of efferent arterioles that results in a decrease in intraglomerular pressure and hyperfiltration; this manifests clinically as a decrease in proteinuria. The results of recently published trials have shown ACE inhibitors to be beneficial in preventing the progression of renal failure in patients with diabetes.

Side Effects. Side effects of ACE inhibitors include cough, rash, angioneurotic edema, hyperkalemia, and rarely neutropenia and proteinuria. These medications can cause irreversible and acute renal failure in patients with bilateral renal artery stenosis or unilateral renal artery stenosis, in patients with a solitary kidney, or in volume-depleted states, particularly in the elderly. These medications are absolutely contraindicated in pregnancy, as use of agents that alter the renin-angiotensin-aldosterone system may be associated with development of renal failure, craniofacial hypoplasia, intrauterine growth retardation, hydramnios, and patent ductus arteriosus.

Drug Interactions. The concomitant use of diuretics leads to excessive hypotensive effects. The hyperkalemic effect of ACE inhibitors becomes more prominent with the use of potassium supplements, potassium-sparing diuretics, and NSAIDs. The dosage of lithium needs to be adjusted in patients being managed with ACE inhibitors.

Calcium Channel Blockers

The clinical effects of this chemically, pharmacologically, and therapeutically heterogeneous group of agents is related to blocking the L class of voltage-gated calcium channels in vascular smooth muscle and cardiac tissue. The calcium channel blockers have attracted interest as blood pressure–lowering agents, as they reduce vascular resistance without a significant effect on cardiac output. The ability of these agents to decrease the cytosolic calcium concentration within the VSMC probably explains most of their vasodilatory properties. Experimental data suggest that calcium channel blockers interfere with both angiotensin II and alpha$_2$ adrenoreceptor–mediated vasoconstriction, and the maximal vasodilatory response may be inversely related to the patient's plasma renin activity and angiotensin levels. These agents are more effective in dilating constricted as opposed to nonconstricted vascular beds, and greater vasodepressor responses occur in patients with higher levels of blood pressure. The use of these agents is associated with natriuresis, which most likely results from improvement in blood supply, decreased renal tubular sodium reabsorption, and a reduction in aldosterone secretion.

Calcium channel blockers have a differential effect on heart rate; while the nondihydropyridines induce a 10% reduction in heart rate, mainly during exercise, the dihydropyridines acutely tend to cause reflex tachycardia, which is especially pronounced with shorter-acting preparations. This factor might be the cause of higher cardiovascular death rate recently observed in patients being treated with calcium channel blockers. These observations make short-acting dihydropyridines unsuitable for antihypertensive therapy under most clinical conditions.

Centrally Acting Alpha$_2$ Agonists

Examples of this subgroup include clonidine (Catapres), guanabenz (Wytensin), and methyldopa (Aldomet). These agents act by stimulating the central alpha$_2$ receptors that inhibit the efferent sympathetic activity leading to decreased total peripheral vascular resistance. They are generally effective in hyperdynamic, high-renin states of hypertension and are generally safe and effective in most patients with renal disease. They are also very effective in regressing left ventricular hypertrophy (LVH).

Side Effects. These agents can cause rebound hypertension if discontinued abruptly, especially with prior administration of high doses or with continuation of concomitant beta-adrenergic therapy. The other side effects include drowsiness, sedation, dry mouth, fatigue, and orthostatic dizziness. Methyldopa can cause liver damage, fever, and Coombs-positive hemolytic anemia. However, these agents generally do not have adverse effects on carbohydrate or lipid function.

Drug Interactions. Tricyclic antidepressants decrease the effects of centrally acting medications. The concomitant antihypertensive therapy, especially with diuretics, increases the chances of developing postural hypotension.

Peripheral-Acting Adrenergic Antagonists

The agents generally used in clinical practice are guanadrel (Hylorel), guanethidine (Ismelin), rauwolfia root, and reserpine. While the first two medications inhibit the catecholamine release from neuronal storage sites, reserpine and rauwolfia root cause depletion of tissue stores of catecholamines. Although these agents are used sparingly, reserpine in low doses is a safe and effective antihypertensive agent.

Side Effects. These include orthostatic and exercise-induced hypotension, diarrhea, lethargy, nasal congestion, and depression. These drugs are contraindicated in patients with a history of mental depression or with active peptic ulcer disease, as they may accentuate these problems.

Direct Vasodilators

Hydralazine (Apresoline) and minoxidil (Loniten) are commonly used vasodilators; they act by direct (primarily arteriolar) smooth muscle dilatation. These agents can cause reflex tachycardia and salt and water retention, which can be of such severity that diuretic treatment might be required.

Side Effects. These agents generally do not regress LVH and may even worsen this condition. The use of hydralazine may be associated with the development of lupus-like syndrome, with a positive antinuclear antibody and antihistone antibody test, but the anti–double-stranded DNA antibodies will be absent. The use of minoxidil can cause hypertrichosis and aggravation of pre-existing pleural and pericardial effusions.

Angiotensin II Receptor Blockers

Losartan (Cozaar), an angiotensin receptor blocker, was recently approved for management of hypertension. It is an angiotensin II type I receptor blocker in various tissues, including adrenals, brain, kidneys, liver, lung, heart, and VSMC. It has no agonist activity and inhibits most of the physiologic responses to angiotensin II. This agent is metabolized to an active compound, and the inhibitory effects of losartan to the pressor responses to angiotensin are closely correlated to the plasma concentration of its active derivative. Clinical trials have suggested that the antihypertensive potency of these newer agents is similar to that of ACE inhibitors.

The adverse effects noted with use of these agents are dyspepsia, muscle cramps, dizziness, insomnia, nasal stuffiness, and cough. They are contraindicated for use in pregnant females and in individuals with impaired renal functioning. In controlled clinical studies, of the total number of patients tried on losartan, approximately 20% were 65 years and older. There was no overall difference in effectiveness or safety noted in these individuals, when comparisons were made with younger individuals. The use of losartan is associated with uricosuria; this property has been utilized in making combination pills with a diuretic for management of patients who become symptomatically hyperuricemic when treated with diuretics.

Effects of antihypertensive therapy on liquid and lipoprotein levels are summarized in Table 3.

Impact of Drug Therapy on Survival

The results of two major randomized trials, namely the Hypertension Detection and Follow-up Program (HDFP) and the study of the Medical Research Council (MRC), along with meta-analysis of several small randomized trials, suggest that the use of antihypertensive therapy is associated with a decrease in the incidence of stroke, total mortality, and coronary heart disease. The reduction in stroke is quite close to the estimate derived from the association of blood pressure with event rates in epidemiologic studies. For coronary heart disease, the reduction in incidence is generally less than predicted from the epidemiologic studies.

J Curve. It has been a long-held view that decreasing the blood pressure beyond a certain point in hypertensive patients will increase the risk of strokes and cardiac events. Studies conducted on hypertensive patients have not shown a consistent J-shaped relationship between treated blood pressure and strokes, but some of the studies did show a consistent J-shaped relationship for cardiac events and treated diastolic blood pressure. These observations have led to the speculation that decreasing the diastolic blood pressure beyond 85 mmHg will be deleterious for patients.

The postulated mechanisms by which lowered blood pressure leads to increased cardiovascular morbidity and mortality were as follows:

1. Fifty percent of hypertensive patients have left ventricular hypertrophy. A hypertrophied left ventricle has increased myocardial oxygen consumption compared with normal-sized left ventricles. If a decrease in coronary blood flow occurs as a result of a decrease in diastolic blood pressure, a hypertrophied left ventricle may be more prone to ischemic events.

2. In hypertensive patients, oxygen extraction in the coronary circulation at baseline is near maximum; in low-flow situations, the heart may not be able to compensate by increasing the oxygen extraction.

3. Autoregulation, which is the primary defense mechanism in patients with coronary artery disease, is adversely affected in hypertensive individuals.

TABLE 3. Effects of Antihypertensive Therapy on Lipid and Lipoprotein Levels

Drug Class	Total Cholesterol	LDL Level	Triglyceride Level	HDL Level
Thiazide diuretics	Increases	Increases	Increases	No effect
Beta blockers	No effect	No effect	Increases	Decreases
Beta blockers (ISA)	No effect	No effect	No effect	No effect
Alpha and beta blockers	No effect	No effect	No effect	No effect
Alpha$_1$ blockers	Decreases	Decreases	No effect	No effect
Central adrenergic blockers	Decreases	Decreases	No effect	No effect
ACE inhibitors	No effect	No effect	No effect	No effect
Calcium blockers	—	—	—	—
Angiotension II blockers	—	—	—	—

ISA = intrinsic sympathomimetic activity; LDL = low-density lipoprotein; HDL = high-density lipoprotein.

4. Excessive lowering of the diastolic blood pressure gives rise to decreased coronary blood flow, which can lead to increased blood viscosity and platelet adhesiveness. All these changes could lead to thrombus formation, a key event in the development of myocardial infarction.

5. The areas of well-perfused myocardium adjacent to the ischemic areas precipitated by low diastolic blood pressure may cause a build-up of metabolic gradients giving rise to ventricular arrhythmias.

Careful analysis of the studies on which these assumptions are based has revealed that these studies were not designed to establish optimal treatment goals; accordingly, conclusions are invalid. Furthermore, these studies did not control for metabolic side effects of the therapy such as hypokalemia, hyperlipidemia, hyperglycemia, and thus for risk factors or for associated co-interventions. All these factors could very well account for the observed J-shaped relationship and thus serve as confounders in using these study findings to determine treatment goals. If the J curve does exist, it appears to have little bearing in the management of hypertensive patients. In the SHEP study (in which as high as 60% of patients had abnormal electrocardiograms, suggestive of cardiovascular dysfunction), diastolic blood pressure was reduced as low as 70 mmHg in a significant number of patients and was associated with a significant reduction in cardiovascular events. It is recommended that in patients with pre-existing cardiac disease, blood pressure should be lowered carefully using appropriate antihypertensive medications. These patients should be followed up at regular intervals, with careful attention to symptoms such as weakness, dizziness, palpitations, etc., onset of which warrants alteration in therapy.

Management of Hypertensive Crises

Hypertensive crises can be classified as hypertensive emergencies and hypertensive urgencies. *Hypertensive emergencies* are usually associated with the presence of progressive target organ damage, and immediate reduction in blood pressure is required. Ancillary measures such as intubation, ensuring adequate urine output, seizure control, and hemodynamic monitoring form an important part of patient management. Examples of hypertensive emergencies include hypertensive encephalopathy, hypertension with left ventricular failure, hypertension with subarachnoid or intracerebral bleed, unstable angina, and aortic dissection. Accelerated or malignant hypertension is considered an emergency if target organ damage is present. Clinical findings consistent with malignant hypertension include papilledema and altered mental states.

Hypertensive urgency is elevated blood pressure without any evidence of target organ damage. It is the presence of target organ damage, not the height of blood pressure reading, that determines whether intensive care unit, regular hospital bed, emergency room, or the physician's office be the site of treatment.

The patient with hypertensive crises needs to be carefully evaluated for selecting the appropriate antihypertensive medication. The duration of the hypertension, complaints at time of presentation, and the medications that the patient is at present using need to be ascertained. Evidence of the target organ damage should be sought by performing a very careful and thorough history and physical examination with particular attention to optic fundi, central nervous system, heart, lungs, abdomen, and peripheral arterial pulsations.

Treatment of Hypertensive Emergencies

In true hypertensive emergencies, antihypertensive medications should be started soon after obtaining an ECG. There is no need to withhold treatment waiting for the results of investigative tests, which should include chemical analysis of blood; complete blood picture; x-ray of the chest; and CT scan of the head if the patient is confused, disoriented, comatose, or has focal neurologic deficits. The most important thing to understand in the management of patients with hypertensive emergencies is the mechanism of autoregulation. It is a phenomenon that protects organs from damage when there are variations in blood pressure levels. When blood pressure rises, blood vessels supplying the organs undergo vasoconstriction; whereas when blood pressure falls, vessels dilate, increasing the blood supply. The heart, kidneys, and brain all have the mechanism of autoregulation but the brain has been the most extensively studied and is hence described here. An increase in blood pressure is associated with cerebral vasoconstriction, whereas vasodilatation occurs when blood pressure falls so that the blood flow remains constant during fluctuations of the mean arterial pressure (MAP) from the normal of 60 to 70 mmHg to well over 150 mmHg. When the MAP drops below the lower limit of the autoregulation, the brain extracts more oxygen to compensate for the decreased flow, and symptoms of ischemia do not occur until this protective mechanism fails. While normal individuals can tolerate changes in blood pressure, this is often not the case in patients with chronic hypertension, cerebral vascular disease, and aging.

Chronic hypertension causes an increase in the tone as well as hyperplasia of vascular smooth muscle cells, which tends to shift the autoregulation curve to the right. The end result of these changes causes the brain to have low blood supply at higher blood pressure. It is very important to note that the lower limit of cerebral autoregulation is roughly 25% below the MAP; hence it is suggested that the goal in hypertensive emergencies should be to lower the MAP by 20 to 25% over a period of minutes to hours depending on the nature of the emergency. For example, patients with pulmonary edema secondary to left ventricular failure or patients with aortic dissection need to have their blood pressure lowered very aggressively within 15 to 30 minutes to very low levels compared with those with other emergencies. However, in patients presenting with hypertensive encephalopathy, the reduction in blood pressure should be effected in 2 to 3 hours.

Hypertensive Encephalopathy. Patients presenting with hypertensive encephalopathy often have a history of untreated or poorly treated hypertension. The symptoms include headache, nausea, vomiting, and visual disturbances; patients have varying degree of obtundation, and blood pressure is elevated (systolic blood pressure usually above 240 mmHg; diastolic blood pressure above 140 mmHg). Hypertensive encephalopathy is the result of hyperperfusion of the brain. It occurs when the upper limit of cerebral autoregulation capacity is exceeded, leading to cerebral edema, petechial hemorrhage, and microinfarcts. This phenomenon can also occur with acute elevations of blood pressure even though the upper limit of cerebral autoregulation is not exceeded in these scenarios; examples include preeclampsia and acute glomerulonephritis. The drug of choice for treating hypertensive encephalopathy is sodium nitroprusside (Nipride). Blood pressure should be lowered gradually to a systolic pressure of 140 to 160 mmHg and diastolic pressure of 90 to 110 mmHg. If the decrease in blood pressure does not improve the sensorium, the diagnosis of hypertensive encephalopathy needs to be reconsidered.

Subarachnoid Hemorrhage. This clinical condition is usually the result of rupture of a berry aneurysm or an arteriovenous malformation. Cerebral angiography in these patients reveals an area of intense

vasospasm adjacent to the area of hemorrhage. This finding has led to reluctance in treating hypertension in these patients, as lowering the blood pressure might precipitate an infarction in the borderline ischemic zone. The cooperative study of aneurysmal subarachnoid hemorrhage showed that the risk of death and rebleeding has a U-shaped relationship to systolic blood pressure. The chances of an adverse event (death or rebleed) are higher when the systolic blood pressure is less than 127 mmHg or more than 159 mmHg compared with blood pressure between 127 and 158 mmHg. This study further revealed that treatment with antifibrinolytic agents reduces mortality more than treatment with antihypertensive agents. Although mortality and incidence of rebleeding are reported to be higher in patients with systolic blood pressure greater than 159 mmHg, the benefit of using antihypertensive agents in this scenario is unclear; some studies report a decrease in mortality, while others do not.

It is appropriate to treat acutely and severely elevated blood pressure in the setting of subarachnoid hemorrhage; however, the benefits of reducing mildly elevated blood pressure are unproven. Nitroprusside should be used in this setting because of its rapid onset of action and easy titration, even though sodium nitroprusside can elevate the intracranial pressure. The increase in intracranial pressure can be treated with mannitol infusion, intubation, intravenous dexamethasone, and/or hyperventilation.

There are reports suggesting that the use of nimodipine, a calcium channel blocker, improves the neurologic outcome in patients with subarachnoid hemorrhage. The postulated mechanism for this improved outcome is prevention of calcium influx into the ischemic neurons, thus preserving neuronal function. There are some studies that suggest that use of propranolol might also improve the outcome in this setting. Nevertheless, the current treatment of choice is nitroprusside.

Hypertension Associated with Intraparenchymal Bleed. The presence of intracranial bleeding is usually associated with cerebral edema and vasospasm, but the degree of vasospasm is not as intense as that associated with subarachnoid hemorrhage. The development of cerebral edema leads to increased intracranial pressure, requiring higher arterial pressure to perfuse the brain adequately.

Those experienced in treating patients with ischemic strokes and intracranial bleeds recommend the following: no antihypertensive treatment for blood pressure readings less than 180/105 mmHg, and oral labetalol, captopril (Capoten), or nifedipine (Procardia), for blood pressure levels ranging between 180/105 and 230/120 mmHg that persist for greater than 60 minutes. In case of inability to administer medications orally due to the presence of altered mental status, intravenous labetalol is recommended. If the systolic blood pressure is more than 230 mmHg and diastolic blood pressure is more than 120 mmHg and these values persist for more than 20 minutes, intravenously administered labetalol is recommended; for diastolic blood pressure more than 140 mmHg, intravenous sodium nitroprusside is recommended.

The suggested target blood pressure levels are 160 to 170 mmHg (systolic) and 95 to 100 mmHg (diastolic) for patients who were previously normotensive, whereas the target blood pressure levels in patients with a prior history of hypertension are 180 to 185 mmHg (systolic) and 105 to 110 mmHg (diastolic). If heparin sodium is to be administered, the target levels should be lower to prevent intracranial bleeding. It is very important to note that if reduction of blood pressure makes obtundation worse or coma deeper or causes progression of neurologic deficit, the antihypertensive medication should be modulated accordingly. Prognosis is so poor in hypertensive intraparenchymal hematoma that it is difficult to evaluate the effectiveness of blood pressure reduction, and no controlled trials have been undertaken.

Acute Ischemic Stroke. Sodium nitroprusside is the agent of choice to acutely lower elevated blood pressure in patients with ischemic stroke. Nimodipine (Nimotop) has been used with equivocal results. One group reported improved survival in males but not in females; the improvement was greatest in patients with moderate to severe deficit at baseline, whereas others reported no benefit in survival or neurologic outcome except for those patients who had mild deficit at the outset, who seemed to achieve greater recovery when treated with nimodipine.

Acute Left Ventricular Failure. Left ventricular failure is associated with increases in levels of physiologically occurring vasoconstrictor hormones, including catecholamines and angiotensin II. In patients who are hypertensive, these changes combined with enhanced peripheral vasoconstrictor responses can severely impair left ventricular performance. Reduction in blood pressure is associated with a decrease in the workload of a failing left ventricle and takes precedence over other measures such as administration of digoxin when pulmonary edema occurs in patients with uncontrolled hypertension. The agent of choice for lowering the elevated blood pressure is sodium nitroprusside. Other agents that have been tried include intravenously administered nitroglycerin, nifedipine, and alpha-adrenergic blockers. Many reports recommend concurrent use of a rapidly acting diuretic along with nitroprusside or nitroglycerin. ACE inhibitors should be prescribed once the patient is able to take oral medications. In situations that are not as emergent, ACE inhibitors along with diuretics can provide effective vasodilation for patients with significant left ventricular dysfunction.

Hypertension in Presence of Myocardial Ischemia or Infarction. Acute ischemia of the left ventricle with or without actual infarction is at times accompanied by severe hypertension, for which emergency treatment is required. Presumably, the increase in blood pressure is secondary to reflex initiated in the ischemic left ventricle. The goal of antihypertensive therapy in this setting is to reduce the myocardial oxygen consumption and to increase the myocardial blood supply.

Based on studies utilizing scintigraphic techniques to study the infarct size, it was concluded that infarct size was limited and left ventricular function was better in patients treated with intravenously administered nitroglycerin. However, follow-up studies performed on these patients show no statistical difference in mortality at 3 months.

Nitroglycerin acts by venodilatation, thus decreasing the preload and the amount of work being done by the heart; it also increases regional blood flow distal to a severe arterial stenosis and is at present the drug of choice in this condition. Reduction in blood pressure in this clinical situation is ancillary to emergency measures to improve or restore coronary patency, which include intravenously administered heparin or thrombolytics, coronary angioplasty, and coronary artery bypass grafting (CABG).

Dissecting Aortic Aneurysm. Dissecting aortic aneurysms can be classified as type I, II, or III, depending on the location of the tear. The first two types generally involve the arch of the aorta, while the third one begins distal to the left subclavian artery. Surgical intervention is routinely required for type I and II, while type III is generally managed medically. Acute blood pressure reduction is needed to decrease shear forces on the damaged aorta. Since reflex sympathetic activation that accompanies administration of arterial vasodilators increases both the rate and the velocity of the left ventricular ejection, leading to further damage of injured aorta, agents like hydralazine and diazoxide are contraindicated.

The drug of choice is a beta blocker followed by administration of intravenous nitroprusside. It is generally recommended to decrease and maintain systolic blood pressure and MAP at 100 mmHg and 80 mmHg, respectively. When pain persists or increases and there is difficulty in controlling the blood pressure, it generally portends an ominous prognosis. Parenteral therapy can be discontinued as soon as the oral regimen becomes effective. A variety of medications can be tried orally, the list of which includes beta blockers, guanethidine, guanadrel, and reserpine.

Emergencies Associated with Hypercatecholaminemia. The situations in which this occurs include pheochromocytoma, drug and food interactions, clonidine withdrawal, and ingestion of sympathomimetic agents including cocaine. These situations can be mostly handled as hypertensive urgencies and treated with oral medications. Prazosin (Minipress), a peripheral alpha-adrenergic blocker, is generally the medication of choice. If need arises to treat the patient with intravenous medications, either phentolamine or nitroprusside can be used.

Perioperative Hypertension. This is not considered an emergency in the usual sense, but parenteral medications are needed to control elevated blood pressure. CABG and other procedures requiring cross-clamping of aorta, such as resection of aortic aneurysm, renal revascularization, and surgeries performed on carotid arteries, are associated with elevated blood pressure. Even a small increase in blood pressure may be fraught with chances of bleeding at suture sites. The medications that can be used include intravenous nitroglycerin and nitroprusside, both of which are equally efficacious and are not associated with a decrease in cardiac output. The disadvantages are that both require close monitoring, and prolonged use of nitroglycerin is associated with development of resistance and tachyphylaxis. If nitroprusside is used for more than 24 hours, the chances of developing cyanide toxicity increases markedly and this must be monitored.

There are reports of patients treated with other medications, such as isradipine (DynaCirc), nicardipine (Cardene), labetalol, and methyldopa with good results. While treating elevated blood pressure, particular care must be taken to avoid hypotension, as these patients can develop thrombosis at suture lines.

Accelerated or Malignant Hypertension. Malignant hypertension constitutes a syndrome of severe elevation of blood pressure associated with vascular damage, which manifests on physical examination as papilledema and often retinal hemorrhages and exudates as well as a change in mentation. The term accelerated hypertension is often used when this syndrome presents without papilledema. Malignant hypertension usually occurs as an accelerated phase of pre-existing hypertension but can occur in the absence of prior hypertension. In the latter instance (e.g., hypertension associated with acute glomerulonephritis), the vessel wall lacks the protective structural thickening seen with chronic hypertension. In severe hypertension of recent onset, the upper limit of cerebral autoregulation is still relatively low and consequently the risk of encephalopathy or hemorrhage is greatly increased. Generally immediate treatment is warranted in this setting, if there is papilledema and/or a change in mental status.

In malignant hypertension, the vascular lesions consist predominantly of myointimal proliferation and fibrinoid necrosis, and the severity of these lesions parallels the severity and duration of hypertension. These patients also have medial thickening due to vascular smooth muscle hypertrophy and collagen deposition. This can be accompanied by cellular intimal proliferation that gives rise to characteristic onion skin appearance of small blood vessels in patients with severe hypertension. Collectively, these changes cause reduced luminal diameter and decreased luminal to wall diameter ratio. The medial thickening is variably reversible after blood pressure control, but intimal thickening contributes to irreversible luminal narrowing. It is believed that this vascular damage is initiated by chronic or extreme elevations of blood pressure and interaction of elevated blood pressure with hormonal changes that lead to progression of benign hypertension to an accelerated phase. Accelerated hypertension is characterized by the appearance of fibrinoid necrosis in the vessel wall and is associated with spasm and overdilatation of segments in the vessel wall.

The vascular damage associated with chronic and extreme elevation of blood pressure leads to an increase in levels of renin and aldosterone. The elevated levels of renin set in motion a vicious cycle in which elevated angiotensin levels enhance vasoconstriction, leading to further worsening of renal ischemia and increase in blood pressure. At this point, pressure natriuresis results in intravascular volume depletion, which further increases renin secretion and sympathetic activity. The complications associated with malignant hypertension are hypertensive encephalopathy, renal failure, and microangiopathic hemolytic anemia. Again, the treatment of choice for accelerated hypertension is intravenous nitroprusside.

Isolated Systolic Hypertension. Isolated systolic hypertension is defined as systolic blood pressure consistently above 160 mmHg associated with simultaneous diastolic blood pressure of less than 90 mmHg. It is estimated that the prevalence rate of systolic hypertension in individuals above 75 years of age is 25 to 30%, and it is more common in females. Elevations in systolic blood pressure are associated with increase in mortality from stroke, congestive heart failure, coronary artery disease, and peripheral vascular disease. In fact, epidemiologic studies suggest that systolic blood pressure is a greater, independent, and important predictor of morbidity and mortality than diastolic blood pressure. When isolated systolic hypertension occurs in young adults, it often indicates a hyperdynamic circulation as exists in hyperthyroidism or diabetes mellitus. As stated previously, it portends significant cardiovascular morbidity and mortality, and the impact of not treating these patients can be enormous. Lifestyle modifications should be initially tried to lower the blood pressure; if these are not successful, antihypertensive therapy with low doses of diuretics should be instituted irrespective of the age of the patient.

White Coat Hypertension. This phenomenon can be defined as persistently elevated blood pressure in the clinic and a normal blood pressure reading at other times. It cannot be diagnosed on the basis of a single elevated office reading, as many individuals have a relatively high blood pressure when first seen, which generally regresses to mean with repeated office visits. The prevalence is predicted to be 21% in patients with borderline hypertension and 5% in patients with advanced blood pressure and is more common in children and patients above age 65 years, including those with isolated systolic hypertension.

The mechanisms implicated in development of this condition are as follows:

1. Exaggerated alerting or orienting responses and thus generalized hyperreactivity to novel stimuli.
2. A learned or conditioned response.
3. A precursor of sustained hypertension.

When white coat hypertension is suspected, either a 24-hour ambulatory blood pressure measurement should be performed or the patient should be advised to check his or her blood pressure at home and carefully document readings for review with the physician.

SECONDARY HYPERTENSION (Table 4)

Renovascular Hypertension

The sustained elevations in arterial pressure caused by stenoses, constrictions, or lesions in the renal vasculature are characterized as renovascular hypertension. The importance of identifying this curable form of hypertension has been magnified by recent advances in management modalities, which include percutaneous transluminal renal angioplasty (PTRA). The development of the captopril suppression test has led to an increase in the office diagnosis of patients identified as having renovascular hypertension. This potentially curable form of hypertension is suggested by sustained, significantly elevated blood pressure in extremes of age, particularly if accompanied by normal serum potassium, creatinine, and blood sugars.

The two main categories of renovascular hypertension are unilateral and bilateral renovascular hypertension; this classification includes conditions of one remaining kidney as in renal transplant patients with stenoses of a transplanted kidney. The resulting hypertension is in large part mediated by an increased activity of the renin-angiotensin system.

TABLE 4. **Important Causes of Secondary Hypertension**

Renal

Acute and chronic glomerulonephritis
Chronic pyelonephritis
Renovascular stenosis or renal infarction
Polycystic disease
Other severe renal disease
Renin-producing tumors

Endocrine

Oral contraceptives
Adrenocortical hyperfunction
   Cushing's disease and syndrome
   Primary hyperaldosteronism
   17-Alpha-hydroxylase and 11-beta-hydroxylase defects
    (adrenogenital syndromes)
Pheochromocytoma
Myxedema
Acromegaly

Neurogenic

Raised intracranial pressure
Spinal cord transection
Diencephalic syndrome

Miscellaneous

Coarctation of aorta
Increased intravascular volume
Polyarteritis nodosa
Hypercalcemia
Medications (cyclosporines, epoetin [Epogen],
   glucocorticoids)

Bilateral Renal Artery Stenoses

Bilateral renal artery stenoses involve stenoses or lesions in the vasculature of both kidneys, which reduce glomerular perfusion pressure and compromise renal blood flow. The stenoses can be caused by arteriosclerotic vascular disease, fibromuscular dysplasia, external compression by tumor, or stenoses at the suture site in transplanted kidneys.

The critical initiating event in the development of sustained hypertension is a decrease in renal perfusion pressure even if there is not a sustained reduction in renal blood flow or glomerular filtration rate. The reduction in perfusion pressure to kidneys prevents adequate sodium excretion and also serves as a stimulus to enhance renin secretion. The initial phase in bilateral renal artery hypertension is associated with angiotensin-induced vasoconstriction; with the passage of time, angiotensin dependency is attenuated because of progressive retention of salt and water and consequent volume expansion. The functional renal mass is subjected to decreased perfusion pressure, which causes sodium conservation (related to pressure natriuresis phenomenon) and activation of the renin-angiotensin-aldosterone system, both of which cause sodium and water retention. The resultant volume expansion slowly transforms this condition into the second phase in which hypertension is predominantly volume dependent. While the net salt and water balance is eventually restored, it requires sustained systemic hypertension to maintain an adequate perfusion pressure beyond the stenoses. Treatment with ACE inhibitors may exert deleterious renal effects in the face of bilateral renal artery stenoses because renal perfusion is either at or below the lower limit of autoregulatory range. When angiotensin blockade lowers renal perfusion pressure below the autoregulatory range, the glomerolar filtration rate decreases. There will be more vasodilatation of efferent arterioles than of the already vasodilated afferent arterioles, which may further contribute to a precipitous decrease in renal function.

The pathophysiology of hypertension in the setting of unilateral renal artery stenoses depends on how the normal kidney responds and adapts to progressive changes in hormonal, neuronal, and hemodynamic influences resulting from stenoses of the opposite kidney. In response to a decrease in perfusion of a single kidney, the hypoperfused tissue increases renin production and elevates systemic levels of angiotensin II and systemic blood pressure. However, the resultant hypertension can cause the nonstenotic kidney to increase sodium excretion; this effect is blunted because the nonstenotic kidney is also subjected to high angiotensin II levels. The unique difference between hypertension caused by unilateral renal artery stenoses and bilateral involvement is angiotensin dependency, which remains even during the steady-state phases associated with unilateral stenoses. The pressure distal to the stenoses is usually not completely restored, so that there is always a continuous stimulus for renin release from the stenotic kidney. In addition, the nonstenotic kidney does not completely escape the effects of inappropriately elevated angiotensin II levels. Recent studies have suggested an increase in renin production by the normal kidney in response to an increase in circulating levels of angiotensin II. This amplification mechanism is sustained as long as there is even a small excess of renin production from the stenotic kidney. The sustained elevations of arterial pressure eventually elicit hypertension-induced glomerular injury in the nonstenotic kidney. This may lead to progressive renal dysfunction. Once this is established, vascular repair will not restore arterial pressure to normal and there is progressive renal insufficiency. Thus it is very important to detect and correct hypertension arising from renal vascular lesions before the irreversible damage sets in.

Management. Medical therapy may be used only in the short term, while patients are being prepared for interventional therapy. Alternatively, long-term medical therapy may be utilized in medically unstable patients or older patients with easily controlled hypertension and well-maintained renal function. Generally, hypertension is difficult to control and frequently requires multiple medications. In unilateral stenoses, ACE inhibitors alone or in combination with other agents generally control blood pressure adequately. In bilateral renal artery stenoses, ACE inhibitors are contraindicated, as they often cause progressive worsening in renal function. Calcium channel blockers alone or in combination with other agents are generally preferred in this scenario. The definitive therapy includes percutaneous angioplasty or surgical revascularization, and in some cases nephrectomy may be necessary.

Method for Performing the Captopril Suppression Test

1. The patient should maintain normal salt intake and receive no diuretics.
2. If possible, all antihypertensive medications should be withdrawn 3 weeks prior to the test.
3. The patient should be seated for at least 30 minutes, and blood pressure measured at 20, 25, and 30 minutes (average the three readings for baseline).
4. Captopril (50 mg diluted in 10 mL of water immediately prior to the test) is administered orally.
5. Blood pressure is measured 15, 30, 40, 45, 50, 55, and 60 minutes after administration of captopril; at 60 minutes, a venous blood sample is drawn for measurement of stimulated plasma renin activity.

Renin Criteria for Captopril Suppression Test

Three renin criteria for the captopril suppression test that together distinguish patients with renovascular hypertension from those with essential hypertension are as follows:

1. Stimulated plasma renin activity of 12 ng/mL or more.
2. Absolute increase in plasma renin activity of 10 ng/mL/hour or more.

3. Percent increase in plasma renin activity of 150% or more, or 400% or more if baseline plasma renin activity is less than 3 ng/mL/hour.

Primary Hyperaldosteronism

Primary hyperaldosteronism accounts for approximately 1% of the hypertensive population and is especially prevalent in women aged 30 to 50 years. The blood pressure levels are variable, and accelerated hypertension is rare. Patients generally complain of weakness, loss of stamina, nocturia, and paresthesias. The orthostatic fall in blood pressure without reflex tachycardia and absence of hypertensive overshoot and bradycardia after Valsalva's maneuver are highly suggestive of aldosterone excess. The presence of hypokalemia, which has a reliability of 75 to 90%, along with low plasma renin activity (PRA) is strongly suggestive of aldosterone excess in hypertensive patients. Elevated 24-hour urine aldosterone excretion rate, along with hypokalemia secondary to renal potassium wasting and suppressed plasma renin activity, is very suggestive of primary hyperaldosteronism.

The subsets of primary hyperaldosteronism include aldosterone-producing adenoma (Conn's syndrome) and idiopathic hyperaldosteronism (bilateral hyperplasia). Adenomas account for approximately 75% of cases of primary hyperaldosteronism. In this syndrome, a diurnal pattern of aldosterone secretion is maintained, which suggests that aldosterone production is under control of adrenocorticotropic hormone. In such patients, aldosterone secretion does not increase normally in response to assumption of an upright posture because of marked suppression of the renin-angiotensin-aldosterone system and insensitivity of adenoma to angiotensin II. In idiopathic hyperaldosteronism, which accounts for at least 25% of cases of primary aldosteronism, there is frequently bilateral micro- or macronodular adrenal hyperplasia. Furthermore, these patients have a two- to threefold increase in aldosterone concentration during assumption of an upright posture, suggesting persisting adrenal sensitivity to angiotensin II. This response, along with iodocholesterol scanning, helps in differentiating between these two disorders.

Other causes of mineralocorticoid hypertension include glucocorticoid-remediable hyperaldosteronism, enzymatic deficiencies, and Liddle's syndrome. Even though inherited syndromes are relatively rare, they should be entertained in differential diagnoses and work-up for mineralocorticoid-related hypertension.

Medical therapy that is indicated in bilateral adrenal hyperplasia or adrenal adenoma in patients who are poor surgical risks generally consists of a potassium-sparing diuretic, either amiloride or spironolactone. In bilateral hyperplasia, this therapy usually results in correction of hypokalemia and may normalize blood pressure. Definitive management of adrenal adenomas consists of surgical removal of the adenoma; this usually results in decreased blood pressure and reversal of biochemical defects.

HYPERTENSION IN SELECTED SUBGROUPS

African Americans

The frequency of hypertension is relatively high in this population and is generally associated with a relatively high morbidity and mortality. Epidemiologic studies suggest that the prevalence of hypertension in African Americans is about 38.2% and that approximately 25% have uncontrolled hypertension. This population appears to develop hypertension at an earlier age, and at any decade of life hypertension is generally more severe in African Americans than in whites. It has been suggested that as much as 30% of all deaths in hypertensive male African Americans and 20% of women may be related to elevated blood pressure. This earlier onset, higher frequency, and greater severity of hypertension in this segment of population results in a 1.3-fold greater rate of nonfatal stroke and a 1.8-fold greater rate of fatal stroke. The cardiovascular death rate and progression to end-stage renal diseases increase by 1.5- and 5.0-fold, respectively.

The prevalence of hypertension among blacks is considerably different in various parts of the world. For example, the prevalence of high blood pressure in rural Africans is considerably less than in African Americans in the United States and the Caribbean. These observations suggest that environmental factors have a large role in determining the prevalence of hypertension in this population.

Hypertension in this group is generally characterized by low plasma renin, increased intravascular volume, and salt sensitivity. This tendency for low-renin state in blacks becomes apparent in childhood and is present even in normal and volume-contracted states. Expanded plasma volume is not secondary to increased dietary intake of salt, although studies have suggested that decreased intake of potassium and calcium may contribute indirectly to salt retention and resultant increased volume. This notion is based on the observation that increasing the dietary potassium and calcium is associated with natriuresis and a negative sodium balance. Investigations of salt sensitivity have revealed blacks to have greater variability in blood pressure associated with changes in salt content of diet and also decreased ability to generate renal natriuretic factors such as dopamine, prostaglandins, and kinins.

Racial differences in cellular cation metabolism may also contribute to the increased prevalence of salt-sensitive hypertension in blacks. There may be racial differences in the membrane transport as well, which account for increased intracellular sodium and calcium. There is also a higher incidence of obesity and insulin resistance in blacks, which may contribute to the abnormal cation metabolism.

Indeed, studies performed at the authors' center have shown higher incidence of hyperinsulinemia and insulin resistance in the first trimester of pregnancy as a predictor of development of hypertension in urban black nulliparous women. Currently, it is unclear whether insulin resistance is acquired or inherited in conjunction with hypertension secondary to environmental influences.

Management

Data from controlled trials have shown diuretics to be very effective in decreasing the morbidity and mortality associated with hypertension. They are effective in lowering blood pressure in the African American population, and hence should be the first line of therapy. ACE inhibitors, calcium channel blockers, alpha$_1$ blockers, and alpha and beta blockers are as effective in blacks as in the white hypertensives. Higher doses of ACE inhibitors may be necessary in African Americans, but even low doses of ACE inhibitors in conjunction with diuretics are a very effective combination in this population. African American hypertensive patients generally require multidrug therapy due to the greater severity and often duration of hypertension.

Hypertension in Diabetic Patients

Individuals with diabetes mellitus have twice the prevalence of hypertension as those without diabetes, as evidenced by the presence of three million people in the United States with both hypertension and diabetes. Hypertension occurs more frequently in patients with type I diabetes than those with type II diabetes after adjustments have been made for age. The most significant effect of this combination is that they confer a greater than additive risk of macrovascular disease in the affected individuals. Therefore, it is crucial to treat both the diseases aggressively to prevent end-organ damage in affected individuals. The decision regarding the choice of the antihypertensive agent is generally dictated by the presence of dyslipidemia, renal disease, micro- and macrovascular disease, and autonomic neuropathy. While essential hypertension accounts for majority of the cases of hypertension in patients with diabetes, diabetic nephropathy also contributes to development of hypertension in both type I and type II diabetes.

Diabetic Nephropathy

Diabetic nephropathy is associated with hypertension and is characterized by sodium and fluid retention, increased peripheral vascular resistance, and abnormally high cardiac output, which is especially pronounced in patients with anemia. Isolated systolic hypertension can occur at any age group but is generally more frequent and pronounced in patients with diabetes because of accelerated atherosclerotic vascular changes. There is substantial difference in the causes of hypertension in type I and type II diabetes; while nephropathy appears to be a more common cause of hypertension in the former group, obesity and insulin resistance play a significant role in the development of hypertension in the latter group. A strong family history of hypertension identifies those patients with type I diabetes who are likely to develop elevated blood pressure. The mechanisms through which insulin resistance and uncontrolled hyperglycemia lead to elevated blood pressure and accelerated atherosclerosis are multiple and currently under study by a number of investigative groups.

The clinical evaluation of patients with diabetes and hypertension should take into consideration the following:

1. Is the patient taking any medication, prescribed or over the counter, which is known to alter the blood sugars or blood pressure? For example, oral contraceptives, steroids, NSAIDs, nasal decongestants, appetite suppressants, and tricyclic antidepressants can cause an elevation of blood pressure.

2. Presence of cardiovascular risk factors, other than hypertension and diabetes, examples of which include dyslipidemias, smoking, and family history of coronary artery disease.

3. The presence of target organ damage due to diabetes and hypertension.

4. The degree of hypertension and diabetes control.

Physical Examination

The blood pressure in the hypertensive diabetic should be checked in all three positions—i.e., lying down, sitting, and standing—after giving enough time for the patient to relax because of an increased prevalence of autonomic dysfunction in this group of patients. In addition, a careful funduscopic, neck, cardiac, extremities, and neurologic examination should be performed to look for evidence suggestive of target organ damage, which includes diabetic/hypertensive funduscopic changes, carotid artery bruit, pedal or sacral edema, and loss of sensory and vibratory sensation. Laboratory evaluation should include a urinalysis, spot urine protein, serum potassium, creatinine, glycosylated hemoglobin, fasting blood sugars, and lipoprotein profile.

Therapy in the Diabetic Hypertensive

Only a few large-scale clinical trials have enrolled patients with diabetes in appreciable numbers. Ten percent of the participants in the HDFP (High Blood Pressure Detection and Follow Up) had a fasting blood pressure of 140 mg/dL or more at baseline or were reported to have been taking medications for diabetes. The effect of diuretic-based stepped care (SC) on the total mortality in this subset did not differ significantly from that in the overall cohort compared with those receiving referred care (RC). In the SHEP trial, 10% of participants had diabetes; in this trial, chlorthalidone was the first-step medication. However, the doses used were much lower than in the HDFP trial. The relative risk reductions in the subgroup with diabetes for all major end points—fatal and nonfatal stroke, cardiovascular disease, and total mortality—were very similar to the results in the total cohort. This beneficial effect was seen despite a slight rise in fasting plasma blood sugar with active treatment.

The goal of treating hypertension in patients with diabetes is to prevent associated morbidity and mortality. The lifestyle modifications are very important in these patients and form the cornerstone of therapy. Changes in lifestyle can enable individuals on drug therapy to reduce the number and dosages of medications needed for the control of hypertension and diabetes. The lifestyle modifications consist of weight reduction, moderation in alcohol intake, regular physical activity, and cessation of smoking. Studies have shown a beneficial effect on blood pressure and glycemic control with modest reduction in weight. Furthermore, weight loss is associated with decrease in LDL cholesterol and increase in HDL cholesterol levels that decrease progression of coronary atherosclerosis.

Even though the general approach to using pharmacologic agents in patients with diabetes and hypertension is very similar to that used with hypertension only there are several qualifications:

1. The goal blood pressure in patients with diabetes has been set at 130/85 mmHg. If this goal is not achieved with hygienic measures, pharmacologic therapy should be instituted.

2. Diabetic renal disease is an important complication that must be taken into consideration. Thus, therapeutic decisions need to consider effects of specific antihypertensive therapy on renal function and the progression of diabetic nephropathy.

3. Special concerns need to be directed at adverse effects of antihypertensive medications on lipid and glucose metabolism.

4. Autonomic dysfunction, which can result in postural hypotension, is common in diabetes and must be considered in therapeutic decisions. Thus, blood pressure should be measured in all three positions and if needed home monitoring of blood pressure should be performed.

ACE inhibitors are good first-line antihypertensive agents in these patients, as they do not cause any adverse effects on the patients' metabolic state and reduce proteinuria associated with diabetes nephropathy. The major risks of using ACE inhibitors is the potential acceleration of renal insufficiency, particularly in patients with bilateral renal artery stenosis and hyperkalemia, because of the high prevalence of type IV renal tubular acidosis (hyporeninemic hypoaldosteronism). Thus, close monitoring of renal function as well as serum potassium is needed.

The other agents that are useful in management of the hypertensive diabetic include low-dose thiazide diuretics, alpha$_1$ blockers, and calcium antagonists. In patients with supine hypertension and orthostatic hypotension due to autonomic neuropathy, short-acting vasodilators can be tried just before bedtime to reduce the nocturnal supine blood pressures. However, because of the increased cardiovascular morbidity and mortality with short-acting dihydropyridines, these drugs should be avoided in a high-risk population such as those with coexisting hypertension and diabetes.

Elderly Patients

The most rapidly increasing fraction of the U.S. population is that group over 65 years of age. At present, there are 31 million Americans older than 65 years, and it is projected that this number will double in the next three decades. Hypertension is an important risk factor for cardiovascular disease in the elderly population. In the Framingham study, borderline hypertension (blood pressure 140/90 to 160/95 mmHg) was associated with an increase in mortality from stroke and coronary artery disease, and this increase in mortality was more evident with advancing years. Data from the Multiple Risk Factors Intervention Trial indicate that elevated systolic blood pressure is a more potent risk factor than diastolic blood pressure in development of end-organ damage, mortality, and morbidity. Indeed, systolic blood pressure of more than 160 mmHg presents a greater risk than diastolic blood pressure of 95 mmHg. An age-related increase in blood pressure, especially systolic hypertension, occurs in industrial, westernized societies, to a much greater extent than in non-industrialized nations. This indicates that the age-related rise in blood pressure may be secondary to environmental factors such as sedentary lifestyle, obesity, and diet.

Aging is associated with increased rigidity and a markedly decreased elasticity of the large blood vessels. This is due to fracturing and uncoiling of elastic fibers and deposition of calcium along with collagenous material in the vessel wall. These changes result in reduced compliance of vessel walls, which leads to transmission of pulse generated during systole to the aorta and its tributaries, resulting in further degeneration and senescent changes in these large vessels. There is damage to the endothelium that causes a decrease in the release of NO and prostacyclin, which are important relaxing factors, while the actions of vasoconstrictors continue unopposed, leading to increased vascular tone. The reduction in compliance of the vessel wall is associated with decreased distensibility of the juxtaglomerular apparatus and renin release. Thus hypertension in the elderly is generally characterized as low-renin hypertension.

There is an age-related decrease in the ability of the body to excrete salt load, which is due to a decrease in glomerular filtration rate, renal blood flow, renal concentrating ability, and the ability of the kidney to produce natriuretic substances. Despite the salt sensitivity, intravascular volumes are usually decreased in the elderly hypertensive. Salt sensitivity in the elderly thus manifests itself as increased vascular reactivity, perhaps related to abnormal VSMC sodium and calcium metabolism. There is also a decrease in baroreceptor sensitivity, which most likely predisposes elderly patients to postural hypotension, especially in response to vasodilators or volume depletion.

Alterations in cardiopulmonary low-pressure baroreceptor function may relate to the increasing prevalence of left ventricular hypertrophy with aging. Age-related increases in insulin resistance and abnormalities in carbohydrate metabolism also likely contribute to the increasing prevalence of hypertension.

Evaluation and Treatment

The diagnosis of hypertension is established if blood pressure readings are elevated on three consequent office visits. Hypertension in the elderly should be treated at any age unless the patient has severe co-morbid diseases that severely limit their lifespan, or the toxicity from therapy is so severe that it potentially outweighs the benefits. Lifestyle modifications also play an important role in management of elevated blood pressure in this population, as weight reduction and salt restriction can have significant antihypertensive effects. The initial target of blood pressure control is to decrease the systolic blood pressure to less than 160 mmHg for patients with systolic blood pressure more than 180 mmHg; for patients with systolic blood pressure between 160 and 179 mmHg, the goal is to lower the systolic blood pressure by 20 mmHg. If this well tolerated, it may be appropriate to decrease the blood pressure even further. The targeted diastolic blood pressue should be less than 90 mmHg.

Low-dose diuretics have been shown in several large clinical trials to reduce stroke and cardiac morbidity and mortality in the elderly and form the cornerstone of therapy in this population. A cardinal rule is that therapy should be started at lower doses and increase in dosages should be spaced at longer intervals in elderly patients. The clinical trials have proved that elderly patients tolerate antihypertensive therapy well if the medications are administered cautiously.

Hypertension in Pregnancy

This includes chronic essential hypertension, pregnancy-induced hypertension, and preeclampsia. In the first condition, the onset of hypertension usually antedates pregnancy or starts with conception. Pregnancy-induced hypertension develops during pregnancy but is not associated with significant proteinuria. Preeclampsia is a clinical disorder of pregnancy characterized by hypertension; significant proteinuria; and, on occasion, liver function, coagulation, and platelet abnormalities. There are no data to suggest that treating hypertension in pregnancy prevents preeclampsia and its associated complications. Patients developing hypertension during pregnancy require close monitoring, physical rest, and institution of antihypertensive medications if diastolic blood pressure is more than 105 mmHg. The onset of significant proteinuria that characterizes preeclampsia usually warrants patient hospitalization, with strict bed rest and close monitoring of liver function as well as platelet count. The definitive therapy is termination of pregnancy if the fetus is mature; if this is not feasible secondary to fetal immaturity, patient treatment with antihypertensive medications is justified. Blood pressure should not be decreased too rapidly, as this will have a deleterious effect on fetoplacental circulation. There is considerable experience with use of methyldopa and hydralazine, which are generally recommended as the first-line agents. There is an emerging body of data suggesting that calcium channel blockers are also useful. The onset of eclampsia warrants parenteral therapy, and usually either hydralazine or methyldopa is used in combination with magnesium sulfate; it is important to note that nitroprusside is contraindicated because its use is associated with development of cyanide toxicity in the fetus. The other agents that are contraindicated in these patients are ACE inhibitors, which can cause renal failure in the newborns. There are studies that suggest the use of aspirin and a diet rich in calcium prevents development of pregnancy-induced hypertension, but further large-scale randomized trials are needed to confirm the benefit of these measures before universal recommendation.

Hypertension and Heart Disease

While treating patients with hypertension and ischemic heart disease, the benefits of lowering the blood pressure must be weighed carefully against the requirements of coronary circulation for an adequate perfusion pressure to maintain the required myocardial blood flow. Though it makes sound clinical sense to lower blood pressure gradually in patients with hypertension and angina pectoris, it is unclear at present as to how much the blood pressure can be reduced safely.

Therapy should utilize agents that reduce myocardial oxygen requirements and/or increase coronary blood flow. These include beta blockers, calcium channel blockers, and nitrates. Concern has been generated recently about increase in mortality with the use of calcium channel blockers in these patients; it is important to note that only short-acting dihydropyridines were used in these studies, which are associated with intense reflex tachycardia and rapid swings in blood pressure and are generally not recommended for management of hypertension. For similar reasons, other vasodilators such as hydralazine are also contraindicated.

Antihypertensive agents of choice in this setting are beta-adrenergic blockers. These agents, except those with intrinsic sympathomimetic properties, have been found to decrease mortality after acute myocardial infarction, presumably partly by a reduction of cardiac arrhythmias. Nitrates also lower the blood pressure as well as alleviate the symptoms of myocardial ischemia. The mechanism of action includes dilatation of veins leading to a decrease in preload and at higher doses a reduction in afterload secondary to arterial vasodilatation. These two actions reduce myocardial oxygen demand. Nitrates may also increase coronary blood flow by dilating the large epicardial coronary vessels, block coronary spasm, and increase the collateral blood flow in the coronary tree, thus improving perfusion distal to coronary stenoses. Lifestyle modification, including cessation of smoking, management of dyslipidemia, and weight reduction, play a very important role in improving survival in these patients.

Hypertension and Coexistent Renal Disease

Renal disease is a relatively common cause of secondary hypertension, which occurs in more than 80% of patients with chronic renal failure and contributes to the progression of renal disease. Hypertension is the most important predictor of coronary artery disease, which is a leading cause of death in patients with renal disease. The nocturnal dipping of blood pressure is significantly blunted in patients with renal failure, due to autonomic dysfunction or alteration of sleeping patterns, and this nondipping phenomenon has also been associated with an increase in cardiovascular morbidity. A number of factors, including sodium retention, activation of the renin-angiotensin-aldosterone system, abnormalities of the adrenergic system, and an imbalance between endothelium-derived vasoconstrictor and vasodepressor agents, have been implicated in the development of hypertension in patients with renal failure.

A good control of blood pressure is of paramount importance in preventing or slowing the progression of renal disease. Nonpharmacologic therapy includes dietary reduction of salt and fat. Treatment medications include diuretics (may require loop agents), given the central role of volume expansion in renal parenchymal hypertension. Other useful agents used include adrenergic blockers, ACE inhibitors, and calcium channel blockers. Potent direct-acting vasodilators like minoxidil may be required, but salt retention often occurs, requiring additional diuretic use. When the glomerular filtration rate falls below 30 mL/minute, a rapid and marked reduction of sodium intake or vigorous therapy with diuretics may result in significant volume contraction, since the failing kidney cannot conserve sodium normally. There are a number of studies that suggest ACE inhibitors may attenuate the development of progressive renal impairment when used early in renal disease, but caution must be exercised because worsening of renal failure or hyperkalemia can occur. Indeed, these agents must be used with extreme care when the creatinine level is more than 3 mg/dL.

ACUTE MYOCARDIAL INFARCTION

method of
STEPHEN T. SMITH, M.D.
Henry Ford Hospital
Detroit, Michigan

Each year there are approximately 1.5 million myocardial infarctions in the United States, with approximately twice that number of hospital admissions for unstable angina pectoris, known myocardial infarction, or to "rule out" myocardial infarction. Despite the declining incidence of coronary heart disease over the last several decades, it remains the major cause of death in North America, with great economic burden to health care. In addition to the declining incidence, however, therapeutic advances in early and late management have contributed to a substantial decline in acute myocardial infarction mortality. In 1995, a first myocardial infarction may still carry up to a 25% mortality at 1 year in North Americans.

PATHOPHYSIOLOGY

The commonest reason for an acute myocardial infarction (AMI) is an unstable or ruptured atherosclerotic plaque and subsequent thrombosis in an epicardial coronary artery, with transmural infarction presenting most often due to a totally thrombosed artery. The sequence of events includes the long-term development of the intramural atherosclerotic plaque, disruption of the endothelial cellular monolayer with exposure of the thrombogenic plaque matrix, and thrombus formation within the plaque, extending into the vascular lumen. Platelets are recruited with enlargement of the thrombus and plaque volume, release of vasoactive substances, arterial spasm with further reduction in coronary blood flow, and, finally, infarction. Acute myocardial infarction may also occur less commonly without atheromatous disease via embolization (endocarditis, myxoma), in congenital coronary anomalies, with acute prolonged hypoxia and/or hypotension (carbon monoxide poisoning, cardiac arrest), vasculitis, trauma (coronary dissection, intravascular manipulation), or other more obscure mechanisms (coronary spasm, syndrome X, cocaine ingestion).

Coronary occlusion may be complete and may result in permanent, extensive damage to the myocardium, or it may be incomplete with more limited injury due to protective coronary collateral circulation, spontaneous thrombolysis, or through pharmacologic treatment (thrombolysis) or mechanical treatment (percutaneous transluminal coronary angioplasty [PTCA]). The prior definitions of Q wave myocardial infarction equaling transmural infarction and non–Q wave myocardial infarction equaling nontransmural injury are no longer as applicable in the current era of rapid, effective treatment and more sophisticated technology for the detection of residual viable myocardium.

Identifiable precipitators of AMI are not found in the majority of patients. Some circadian periodicity is present, with the peak incidence occurring in the first few hours after awakening, though AMI may occur at any time of the day. Other factors implicated as precipitators include sudden, strenuous physical exertion, emotional trauma or duress, direct trauma (myocardial contusion), indirect trauma (acute neurologic injury), or other types of physiologic stress (noncardiac surgery).

DIAGNOSIS

Acute prolonged thoracic discomfort is the predominant *symptom* in the majority of patients, although the specific location of the discomfort and the individual description of the symptom may vary. The pain is usually present from one-half hour to several hours; often is described as crushing, squeezing, or burning; and may be accompanied by diaphoresis, nausea, and dyspnea. Important components of the differential diagnosis of patients with severe prolonged thoracic or epigastric discomfort include acute pulmonary embolus with or without infarction, pneumothorax, pneumonia, aortic dissection, pericarditis, esophagitis, and peptic ulcer disease.

The *physical examination* is often nonspecific but may show a pale, anxious, diaphoretic individual complaining of thoracic pain. Specific findings may include ventricular gallop tones, murmurs of mitral insufficiency or ventricular septal defect, hypotension, arrhythmias, elevated central venous pressures, or pulmonary vascular congestion.

The 12-lead *electrocardiogram* will be diagnostic or at least abnormal in the majority of patients and is most sensitive for anterior and inferior infarctions. Classically, ST segment elevation of 0.1 mV or greater in two or more contiguous leads is considered acceptable for the diagnosis. Q waves may be present at initial evaluation or may evolve as the infarction progresses. New bundle branch block or anterior precordial ST segment depression with an increase in R wave amplitude suggestive of a true posterior infarction may be the initial electrocardiographic findings. One should recall that other conditions may mimic the ECG findings of AMI, including pericarditis, acute pulmonary disease, abnormal repolarization as with pre-excitation syndromes, and possibly electrolyte disturbances such as hyperkalemia.

Enzyme analysis is focused on the isoenzyme MB of creatine kinase (CK), which begins to rise 4 to 8 hours following the initiation of cellular damage, declining to normal after several days. Other enzyme tests such as lactate dehydrogenase (LDH), LDH ratio, and aspartate transaminase are not as helpful and are best used when the CK-MB is nondiagnostic. Serial CK-MB measurements are required to exclude AMI. The level of CK correlates roughly with the size of infarction and survival and may be affected by reperfusion, with earlier peaking and reduction in total value. In the future, troponin T, which peaks late and is more specific, and/or myoglobin levels that peak early in AMI, though are less specific for myocardial damage, may be used; however, these are not routine at present.

TREATMENT

Once the patient is identified with possible myocardial infarction in the emergency facility, rapid assessment of the diagnostic criteria for myocardial infarction, as well as indications and contraindications for thrombolytic therapy, should begin. Experimental and clinical observational data show that the longer myocardial ischemia persists, the more complete is the damage. Also, it is estimated that we treat about 25% to 30% of total AMI patients and 60% to 70% of eligible AMI patients with thrombolytics as per the GUSTO (Global Utilization of Streptokinase or TPA for Occluded Arteries) data, although in clinical practice these numbers may be much lower. In the United States, the average time for presentation following symptom onset is 4 to 5 hours, and the time to treatment is 1 to 2 hours. An attractive goal would be to increase the public awareness so that prehospital delays in seeking treatment could be reduced and to enhance the identification and initiation of treatment on arrival so that the "door to needle" time could be shortened to 30 minutes, when the most benefit can be gained. Any patient with prolonged thoracic discomfort presenting within 12 hours and having ECG criteria consistent with myocardial infarction should be considered for such therapy (Table 1).

TABLE 1. **Patient Eligibility for Thrombolysis**

Male or female of any age
Presentation with chest pain
Presentation within 12 h of onset of symptoms or ongoing
   ischemic pain up to 24 h following presentation
Lack of major contraindications to thrombolysis
Suitable ECG criteria, including 0.1 mV ST segment elevation in
   two or more contiguous ECG leads, new or presumed new
   RBBB or LBBB, anterior precordial ST segment depression
   with enlarging R wave consistent with a posterior myocardial
   infarction
Specific patients for TPA include those with administration of
   SK or APSAC within the last 12 months, persistently
   hypotensive patients, or patients <75 yr old presenting within
   4 h of symptom onset, especially with large anterior infarctions

Abbreviations: ECG = electrocardiographic; RBBB = right bundle
branch block; LBBB = left bundle branch block; TPA = tissue plasminogen
activator; SK = streptokinase; APSAC = anisoylated plasminogen streptokinase activator complex.

Aspirin

Oral antiplatelet agents in the form of aspirin at
160 to 325 mg, either chewed or swallowed, should
be given. The Second International Study of Infarct
Survival (ISIS-II) demonstrated a substantial reduction of 24% in mortality with immediate therapy.
With the addition of aspirin to thrombolytic therapy,
a synergistic effect on survival is seen, with a resultant 8% absolute mortality as opposed to 13.2% untreated mortality.

Thrombolytics

Thrombolytic therapy has been shown in virtually
all trials as being most effective when given immediately, with benefit declining steadily as time elapses
from the onset of symptoms. This mandates that
therapy be initiated without delay as soon as the
diagnosis is reasonably suspected in the emergency
room. Criteria for patient eligibility for thrombolysis
are given in Table 1. After 12 hours have elapsed,
benefit in mortality has declined markedly although
benefit may still be seen, especially in those patients
who have ongoing symptoms. The first major study
that popularized the intravenous use of thrombolysis
was GISSI I (Gruppo Italiano per lo Studio della
Streptochinasi nell'Infarto Miocardio), which demonstrated the ease of administration, efficacy in promoting survival, and safety in the intravenous use of
streptokinase. Subsequent studies, including ISIS
III, showed the equal benefit of streptokinase (SK),
anistreplase, and tissue plasminogen activator (TPA)
on survival (see Table 2 for dosing schedules). Other
trials, such as GISSI III, have demonstrated the lack
of additional benefit to thrombolysis with nitrates
and magnesium. The GUSTO trial was an international trial of 41,021 patients comparing treatment
with streptokinase with front-loaded TPA. The results suggested that both agents were nearly equal
in efficacy; however, front-loaded TPA appeared to
provide additional mortality reduction of 0.9% over

SK, especially in patients under the age of 75 years
with anterior infarctions.

Potential problems with thrombolysis are primarily related to bleeding. The risk of major bleeding
ranges from 1% to 5%, and the most feared hemorrhagic complication, intracranial hemorrhage (ICH),
occurs in 0.5% to 1.5%. Elderly people appear to
have a higher risk for ICH; however, AMI deaths
are higher as well, with the benefit of thrombolysis
generally outweighing the risk. In many studies, TPA
had a slightly higher risk of intracranial hemorrhage, which may offset its mortality benefit. Other
risk factors for stroke include older age, higher blood
pressure, history of hypertension, and prior stroke.
Stroke is a complication of the disease and the therapy, with most hemorrhagic strokes occurring within
the first 24 hours and most ischemic strokes occurring after 48 hours. Any new focal neurologic abnormality should be promptly investigated by clinical
examination and computed tomography (CT) or magnetic resonance imaging (MRI). It has been suggested
that in the future, very fibrin-specific thrombolytic
agents such as staphylokinase may help resolve the
stroke issue with thrombolytic therapy. Hypotension
may be a risk with SK and anistreplase. These
agents should be used cautiously in patients presenting with hypotension that is prolonged and not
responsive to fluid resuscitation. Anaphylaxis is a
rare, usually unpredictable event with SK and anistreplase but not with TPA. Neutralizing antibodies
may develop with SK and anistreplase that may preclude a second dose of either of these agents unless
resolution of antibody resistance has been shown
—rTPA being the preferred agent in this circumstance. Contraindications to thrombolysis as per the
Fourth American College of Chest Physicians Consensus Conference on Antithrombotic Therapy are
given in Table 3.

Beta-Adrenergic Receptor Antagonists (Beta Blockers)

Beta-blocking medications are currently recommended for routine use in most patients following
AMI. Their benefit is seen both in the short- and
long-term reduction in mortality. Long-term oral
therapy in the Beta-Blocker Heart Attack Trial
(BHAT) and acute and oral therapy in ISIS I demon-

TABLE 2. **Thrombolytic Agents Available for
Intravenous Use**

Agent	Available Forms	Dose
Streptokinase (SK)	Kabikinase	1.5 million U/60 min
Tissue plasminogen activator (TPA, alteplase)	Activase	15 mg bolus followed by 0.75 mg/kg over 30 min (up to 50 mg), followed by 0.5 mg/kg over 60 min (up to 35 mg)
Anistreplase	Eminase	30 U IV bolus over 5 min

TABLE 3. Contraindications to Thrombolysis

Absolute Contraindications

Aortic dissection
Acute pericarditis
Active bleeding
Any history of intracranial hemorrhage, intracerebral
    vascular disease (aneurysm, arteriovenous malformation),
    or cerebral neoplasm

Relative Contraindications

Within 6 mo: GI hemorrhage, GU hemorrhage, or ischemic
    stroke
Within 2–4 wk: major surgery, organ biopsy, puncture of
    noncompressible vessel, prolonged CPR, major trauma, head
    trauma
Diabetic proliferative retinopathy
Severe, uncontrolled hypertension (SBP >200 mmHg and/or
    DBP >120 mmHg)
History of bleeding diathesis, hepatic dysfunction, cancer
Pregnancy

Abbreviations: CPR = cardiopulmonary resuscitation; SBP = systolic blood pressure; DBP = diastolic blood pressure.

strated this benefit with beta blockers in the prethrombolytic era. The TIMI 2 trial in the thrombolytic era did not show a mortality benefit, although a reduction in recurrent ischemia and infarction was shown. Theoretical mechanisms for benefit include reduction in oxygen consumption, lowering of heart rate and blood pressure, shifting of myocardial blood flow from the epicardial areas to the subendocardium, and "electrical stabilization" with a reduction in the propensity toward ventricular fibrillation. Clinical benefit is seen with survival benefit, reduction in ischemia and AMI, reduction in episodes of ventricular fibrillation, and possibly reduction in cardiac rupture following AMI. Contraindications to beta blockers include severe congestive heart failure, severe obstructive pulmonary disease, and heart block. See Table 4 for recommended immediate therapy.

Anticoagulants

Heparin

The indirect antithrombin agent heparin is routinely used in ischemic heart disease of a variety of subtypes, including AMI, though it is not FDA-approved for this use. Several major thrombolytic trials, including ISIS III and GUSTO have shown that subcutaneous heparin is not effective in reduc-

ing mortality when routinely given following thrombolytics and aspirin in AMI, and that intravenous use following streptokinase and aspirin is unhelpful. When used following TPA and aspirin, heparin improves patency with some increased risk of bleeding. It is administered as a bolus followed by continuous infusion for the first 24 to 48 hours, keeping the activated partial thromboplastin time 1.5 to 2.5 times normal.

Complications of heparin therapy are primarily related to hemorrhage, although less commonly thrombocytopenia may develop. Other antithrombins, including low-molecular-weight heparin and compounds based on hirudin, are not well studied as yet and are not currently recommended.

Coumadin

Coumadin (warfarin) has been used in a number of small clinical trials since the 1940s and is in a large clinical trial now with the Coumadin-Aspirin Reinfarction Study (CARS) for secondary prevention following a first AMI. Preliminary data analysis does not suggest additional benefit with Coumadin at this level of anticoagulation. While effective at standard levels of anticoagulation, this therapy is limited by patient compliance and the necessity of monitoring the anticoagulant effect. Thus anticoagulant therapy with Coumadin is not routinely recommended following AMI, for aspirin is more easily applied and is clearly effective. Coumadin does have a role in large anterior infarctions for the prevention of thrombotic embolization within the first 3 to 6 months and possibly longer in patients with severely impaired left ventricular function. The proper range is an International Normalized Ratio (INR) of 2.0 to 3.0. When specifically used for the prevention of reinfarction, the target INR is 2.5 to 3.5.

Angiotensin-Converting Enzyme Inhibitors

In addition to their known use in patients with heart failure due to systolic dysfunction, a number of trials have investigated the use of angiotensin-converting enzyme (ACE) inhibitors following AMI with measurable or symptomatic LV dysfunction. A recent consensus paper coordinated by the GISSI group with participation by the investigators of the CONSENSUS, AIRE, SAVE, SOLVD, ISIS, GISSI III, and V-HeFT trials suggested that any patient with signs or symptoms of LV dysfunction at any time following AMI should be treated with an individually dosed ACE inhibitor in the absence of contraindications and that such therapy could be started on the first day following standard therapy with aspirin, thrombolytics, and beta blockers. This is suggested not because of known efficacy but rather because this is the most highly mortal period of AMI. Such therapy need not be continued indefinitely without symptoms or measurable LV dysfunction following 4 to 6 weeks of therapy.

TABLE 4. Available Beta-Blocking Medications for Usage in Acute Myocardial Infarction

Agent	Dose
Metoprolol (Lopressor)	5 mg IV q 5 min for 3 doses, followed by 50 mg PO q 6 h for 8 doses, followed by 100 mg PO q 12 h indefinitely
Atenolol (Tenormin)	5 mg IV for 2 doses separated by 10 min, followed by 50 mg PO for 2 doses, followed by 100 mg daily as a single or divided dose

Nitrates

Nitrates may be administered in a variety of oral, sublingual, transcutaneous, and intravenous forms, although intravenous nitroglycerin is most commonly used for AMI. Pharmacologic effects include redistribution of coronary blood flow to the subendocardial regions, dilatation of coronary arteries, reduction of preload through dilatation of venous capacitance vessels with reduction in myocardial oxygen consumption, and systemic arterial dilatation with a reduction in blood pressure and afterload. Clinically this may give relief of ischemic pain, control of hypertension, and a reduction in symptoms of pulmonary vascular congestion, although hypotension is a risk, especially with volume depletion and right ventricular infarction. It is surprising that large clinical trials, such as ISIS IV and GISSI III with nitroglycerin therapy in acute myocardial infarction, have not demonstrated any important benefit in survival following standard care. When given, intravenous nitroglycerin should be begun at 5 to 10 µg per minute, with titration to clinical effect or to unacceptable reduction in systemic blood pressure or to achievement of 200 µg per minute at which the maximal effect is present.

Antiarrhythmics (Lidocaine)

Lidocaine is a Vaughan-Williams class 1B antiarrhythmic agent that inhibits the fast sodium channel without prolonging the QT interval and is a first choice in ischemic ventricular arrhythmias. Routinely used in the past, lidocaine is no longer a prophylactic agent for ventricular fibrillation in AMI, partly due to the low incidence of ventricular fibrillation and a possible increase in asystolic arrest with its use. It is indicated now for the prevention of second events in patients who have experienced ventricular tachycardia or ventricular fibrillation. One should begin with a 100-mg or 1.0- to 1.5-mg per kg intravenous bolus, a second intravenous half-dose bolus 20 minutes later, followed by a continuous infusion of 1 to 4 mg per minute for 24 to 48 hours. After this time, intravenous antiarrhythmic therapy is usually stopped and the patient is observed and monitored for a recurrence. Chronic oral antiarrhythmic therapy is not indicated in the absence of recurrent complex, symptomatic ventricular arrhythmias.

Nonroutine Limited Medical Therapy

Other therapies have been tried in large clinical trials. They are routine in clinical use but have not been shown to be beneficial in a majority of patients or have been shown to be detrimental. *Magnesium* therapy was thought to promote survival primarily through the prevention of lethal arrhythmias following a meta-analysis of a number of small published trials. The ISIS IV trial, however, showed no benefit over standard care. Magnesium may have some role in electrolyte-provoked arrhythmias.

Calcium channel blockers are also routinely used without much support in large clinical trials. Most trials have suggested minimal or no benefit in survival following AMI. 1-Dihydropyridine was shown in the Holland InterUniversity Nifedipine Trial (HINT) to increase mortality following AMI. In general, calcium channel blockers should not be used unless another clinical reason exists, such as hypertension or recurrent angina, and dihydropyridines should not be used unless with beta-blocking drugs.

Table 5 summarizes the current medical therapy recommendations.

Interventional Therapy

Primary angioplasty has been used as an acute treatment for AMI in place of or in the absence of thrombolysis. Some centers have achieved good success with this method, but most hospitals in the United States do not have cardiac catheterization laboratories or provide interventional techniques. In addition, such therapy requires a large commitment of resources and personnel, 24-hour staffing of the catheterization laboratory, and the experienced operator capability to do quality angioplasty within the initial several hours of the myocardial infarction. In most centers, primary angioplasty even when available probably does not provide a major benefit over medical thrombolytic therapy.

Another possible use of interventional therapy may be as an adjunct to thrombolysis. The Thrombolysis in Myocardial Ischemia 2A (TIMI 2A) study was the first to demonstrate the lack of benefit from immedi-

TABLE 5. **Medical Priorities in Acute Myocardial Infarction**

Agent	Timing of Administration	Recommended
Aspirin	Immediate	All patients
Thrombolytics	Immediate	All eligible patients
Beta blocker	Immediate if no contraindication	Most patients without severe COPD, CHF
Heparin	Immediate after TPA or if no thrombolysis	Some patients
Coumadin	First week after heparin	Patients with large anterior infarctions
ACE inhibitors	First week or later	Patients with subjective or objective LV dysfunction
Nitrates	Variable, usually not mandatory	Some patients with angina or CHF
Lidocaine	Immediate if specifically indicated	Specific patients for prevention of recurrent VT/VF
Magnesium	Generally not indicated	Rare patients
Calcium channel blockers	Generally not indicated	Occasional patients with hypertension or angina

Abbreviations: COPD = chronic obstructive pulmonary disease; CHF = congestive heart failure; TPA = tissue plasminogen activator; LV = left ventricle; VT/VF = ventricular tachycardia/ventricular fibrillation.

ate versus delayed catheterization and angioplasty. Most subsequent clinical trials, including TIMI 2B, European Cooperative Study Group (ECSG), and the Thrombolysis in Acute Myocardial Infarction (TAMI 1) study, did not support routine catheterization and angioplasty following thrombolysis. No mortality benefit and an increase in procedure-related complications were seen in several patient groups. Patients with uncomplicated, completed infarctions may safely undergo stress testing without catheterization for risk stratification after AMI. In patients with recurrent spontaneous or demonstrable ischemia, catheterization and angioplasty or bypass surgery is indicated owing to the significantly higher morbidity and mortality in this group.

One group in which both primary and adjunctive angioplasty may be indicated is composed of patients presenting in shock or developing shock within the first 24 hours. In these patients, deaths may be reduced from 90+% to 50% with successful reperfusion. Given the dismal prognosis in cardiogenic shock due to AMI with medical therapy alone, careful consideration of revascularization should be given in clinically indicated patients.

Intra-Aortic Counterpulsation

Intra-aortic counterpulsation therapy or "balloon pumping" (IABP) is an invasive therapy used as an adjunct to other therapy for acute myocardial infarction. It involves the percutaneous placement of a balloon in the descending aorta, which inflates with cardiac diastole and deflates with cardiac systole. This gives an increase in diastolic perfusion pressure of the coronary arteries while decreasing cardiac afterload, an effect that cannot be duplicated pharmacologically. The role of this therapy has been debated extensively as it does not appear to change survival; however, it may be empirically useful as a bridge to other procedures such as percutaneous transluminal coronary angioplasty (PTCA), coronary artery bypass graft (CABG), mitral valve replacement, or ventricular septal repair or for hemodynamic support following revascularization. Complications include intra-arterial thrombosis and embolization, vascular occlusion, vascular damage or perforation, and bleeding.

Initial General Care

Initial care in the intensive care unit involves bed rest with bedside commode, supplemental oxygen, intravenous access, and cardiac arrhythmia monitoring. Ischemic pain control using morphine sulfate or meperidine hydrochloride (Demerol) should be given. Anxiolytics, sleep sedation, and stool softeners may be empirically beneficial. Blood work should be monitored for electrolyte disturbances, blood cell loss, coagulation profile, and return to baseline of cardiac enzymes. Daily ECGs are useful but daily routine chest radiographs are not, in the absence of clinical indication. Uncomplicated infarctions may be transferred to step-down units after 24 to 48 hours of observation. Patients with uncomplicated infarctions may be discharged from the hospital in less than 1 week.

Complications

Arrhythmias constitute the commonest early complication of AMI. Early *ventricular arrhythmias* are responsible for the majority of first-day deaths, although the incidence of ventricular fibrillation has declined to less than 2%. Ventricular tachycardia and ventricular fibrillation should be promptly treated with defibrillation, followed by lidocaine bolus and infusion for 24 to 48 hours. Electrolyte abnormalities, hypoxia, and recurrent ischemia should be looked for and corrected if present. VT or VF following this period should be thoroughly investigated for correctable causes, and because of a much higher late mortality, such patients should be considered for empirical or electrophysiologically directed antiarrhythmic therapy. Routine prophylactic antiarrhythmic therapy for ventricular arrhythmias is not indicated owing to clear lack of benefit, as seen in the Cardiac Arrhythmia Suppression Trial (CAST).

Supraventricular arrhythmias are even more common and range from benign to serious. Sinus tachycardia generally requires no specific treatment. Sinus bradycardia is usually transient and responsive to atropine, although occasionally pacing may be required if hemodynamic compromise exists. Atrial fibrillation and other supraventricular tachycardias are usually easily controlled with digoxin, calcium channel blockers (intravenous diltiazem [Cardizem]), or beta blockers (intravenous esmolol [Brevibloc]), with cardioversion being reserved for arrhythmias that provoke ischemia, hemodynamic compromise, or persist. Long-term treatment is usually not necessary.

Symptomatic bradyarrhythmias and *conduction disorders* should be considered for temporary transcutaneous or transvenous pacing. Sinus, junctional, or idioventricular bradycardia unresponsive to medical therapy, with hypotension, hypoperfusion, or ischemia related to the rhythm, should be paced. Other indications for pacing include complete AV block, Mobitz 2, Mobitz 1 with symptoms, and "new" bifascicular block. Most conduction disorders are transient. Permanent pacing may be required for persistent conduction disorders, and electrophysiologic testing should be considered when the need for pacing is in doubt.

Congestive heart failure may be present in the initial stages of infarction, with symptoms of pulmonary vascular congestion, hypoxia, or radiographic congestion. This should be promptly treated with diuretics in the absence of hypotension. ACE inhibitors and nitrates should be used to reduce afterload and preload in the absence of contraindications. Arterial vasodilators may also be useful if systemic pressures are high. Invasive hemodynamic monitoring may be helpful if the proper pharmacologic approach is in doubt or if a mechanical complication is suspected.

Venous thrombosis and *pulmonary embolus* contributed significantly to the morbidity and mortality of myocardial infarction in the past; with declining inpatient times and with routine subcutaneous heparin prophylaxis, their risk has waned.

Recurrent ischemia and infarction may occur at any time following myocardial infarction, is heralded by recurrence of symptoms and further electrocardiographic changes, and carries a clearly worse short- and long-term prognosis. Following identification, these patients should be promptly treated with heparin and nitroglycerin and referred for catheterization and potential revascularization. This may be seen more commonly in non–Q wave infarctions, patients with diabetes, and possibly following thrombolysis but should be watched for in all patients.

Mechanical complications of AMI include shock due to pump failure, ventricular septal defect, papillary muscle rupture with acute mitral regurgitation, and cardiac rupture. All may manifest as hypotension, hypoperfusion, low cardiac output, and pulmonary vascular congestion, and all carry a dismal prognosis without treatment. Following the clinical appearance of shock in a patient with AMI, prompt identification of the etiology by echocardiography with or without invasive hemodynamic monitoring and catheterization should be done. IABP, inotropes, pressors, and diuretics may be immediately required. Directed interventions including PTCA for cardiogenic shock due to extensive infarction, valve repair or replacement for acute mitral regurgitation, and ventricular repair for ventricular septal defect or free wall rupture may be lifesaving.

A *right ventricular infarction*, while not strictly a mechanical complication, warrants mention because of its potential to simulate shock due to other causes. The typical patient has an inferior myocardial infarction with a proximal right coronary artery occlusion, elevated central venous pressure, clear lungs, and low cardiac output. The diagnosis can often be confirmed by right-sided precordial ECG, especially with V3R, but also by echocardiography. Such patients usually respond promptly to volume expansion and may not require other interventions. Dobutamine (Dobutrex) may be used for temporary inotropic support.

Systemic embolization is a late complication usually seen in patients with extensive anterior infarction. Patients with these infarctions demonstrated by ECG or patients with identifiable large anterior wall motion abnormalities on echocardiography or ventriculography may benefit from anticoagulation with Coumadin for 3 to 6 months following infarction and may be switched to aspirin after this period as the risk of embolization is low after 6 months.

Risk Stratification

Following initial management but prior to release from the hospital, it is routine to evaluate patients for evidence of recurrent ischemia, a significant negative prognosticator in the short and long term. Early low-level standard stress testing can be safely used if the ECG is relatively normal or exercise testing with echocardiographic or nuclear imaging if it is not. Exercise with echocardiography may provide an additional estimation of ventricular function, another factor important in long-term prognosis. Patients with "positive" exercise testing, indicating low-level ischemia, should be referred for catheterization and appropriate revascularization by PTCA or CABG. Patients with "negative" low-level exercise testing should undergo maximal exercise testing within 4 to 6 weeks following infarction.

Secondary Prevention

Secondary prevention refers to the long-term prevention of morbid and mortal events following AMI, especially recurrent infarction and sudden cardiac death. Although some patients with depressed ventricular function and multivessel coronary disease will have clear survival benefit from definitive treatment of ischemia via revascularization, virtually all patients will benefit in a prognostic sense from medical therapy. Aspirin at a daily dose of 160 to 325 mg and an oral beta blocker (without intrinsic sympathomimetic activity) individually dosed should be considered for all patients unless clear contraindications exist. Coumadin should be considered for patients who cannot take aspirin. Cholesterol-lowering therapy with simvastatin has recently been shown in the Scandinavian Simvastatin Survival Study (4S) to improve long-term survival following AMI, with the benefit extending to at least 5 years, and is indicated in hypercholesterolemic patients. Cardiac rehabilitation, with attention to risk factor modification and prudent exercise, is advisable for all patients.

CARDIAC REHABILITATION

method of
HENRY S. MILLER, JR., M.D.
Bowman Gray School of Medicine, Wake Forest University
Winston-Salem, North Carolina

Cardiac rehabilitation should begin as soon as the patient is stabilized in the hospital. After early assessment and therapy, be it thrombolytic or interventional or both, the patient should begin early activity and self-care. After transfer from the Coronary Care Unit, progressive ambulation should begin. During the next 4 days in the hospital, individual and group discussions include a description of the pathophysiology of the disease and the patient's specific problem, dietary methods of lipid control, and behavioral modifications related to smoking, obesity, and stress by the cardiac rehabilitation staff, nurses, and dietitian.

The patient may or may not have a predischarge exercise test. The uncomplicated patients are discharged with information concerning symptoms that may occur, i.e., angina, dyspnea, weakness, and arrhythmias; progressive physical activity as to duration, frequency, and intensity, with an exercise heart rate range; and dietary instructions.

The availability of coronary arteriograms and left ventriculograms for most patients allows the physician to determine the likelihood of residual myocardial ischemia and left ventricular function. Risk stratification of the patient allows modification of hospital therapy, as well as medication decisions and instructions at discharge.

The patients are brought into the outpatient rehabilitation program at approximately 2 weeks after the myocardial infarction, coronary artery bypass surgery, or valvular surgery; 4 to 5 days following coronary interventional procedures such as percutaneous transluminal coronary angioplasty (PTCA), atherectomy, and so on; 3 to 4 weeks after heart transplant; and when angina is stable.

PATIENT ASSESSMENT

1. Resting electrocardiogram and symptom-limited graded exercise test.
2. Laboratory tests, including lipid profile, SMAC, complete blood count, and drug levels.
3. Height, weight and body fat measurement.
4. Seven-day food record plus food preference and frequency questions.
5. Psychological testing designed to evaluate depression, anxiety, Type A behavior of aggression, rage, anger, and so on.
6. Vocational assessment when appropriate.

Exercise tests and laboratory studies are not repeated if done within 1 month and reports are available.

After evaluation of the psychological test, all patients are seen by the clinical rehabilitation nurse specialist or psychologist or both for discussion of the test results. Appropriate referrals are made for therapy if needed. Utilizing the lipid and glucose laboratory results, height, weight and body fat measurements, and food records, the dietitian discusses the good points of the diet and those that need correction with the patient, spouse, or others. Outlines of an appropriate diet with instructions in food purchasing and preparation are given. The vocational counselor reviews the records on each patient and discusses any employment modification or special circumstances with the patient and employer. A safe and effective exercise prescription is developed from the graded exercise test results, observations of the patient's ability to walk, information related to peripheral vascular disease, and musculoskeletal problems.

After evaluation, the patients discuss what they wish to accomplish in the rehabilitation program with the nurse specialist or program director. These are considered in light of the goals the staff feels are the top rehabilitative needs. These goals are then established with the patients and serve as a benchmark for them to work toward in physical conditioning and risk factor control when they are re-evaluated at 3-, 6-, and 12-month intervals.

The rehabilitation participants meet three times a week in three separate areas in the university gymnasium, with the patients divided into beginners (first 2 to 3 months), advanced (3 to 9 months), and cardiac fitness programs (for patients who wish to continue after the rehabilitation program and those with risk factors). Moving from beginners to advanced is usually at 3 months but varies depending on the patients' physical condition and risk stratification. The exercise consists of walking and jogging, with upper and lower extremity bike exercise and free-weight exercises. The warm-up and cool-down exercise routines include games with balls, including volleyball. The intensity of the individual physical activity program gradually increases with physical conditioning and requires the patients to exercise more vigorously to reach their prescribed heart rate range.

After 7 to 10 minutes of stretching and warm-up, the patients exercise for 40 minutes in their heart rate range. After the first 1 to 2 months, use of free-weights during the last 10 minutes of exercise is added. Varied routines are used to condition different muscle groups. Under supervision, patients assume the role as leaders in the stretching, calisthenics, and free-weight exercises to stimulate interest and add to the enjoyment.

Except for a rare patient who exercises with a Holter monitor, none of the patients have continuous ECG monitoring. In the beginners program, each patient has blood pressure and pulse rate recorded using "Quick-Look" defibrillator paddles before exercise and one to two times during exercise to evaluate the rhythm and rate. They are taught to count their pulse rate at 5 minutes and 15 to 20 minutes of exercises, with free-weight training, and during cooldown. Each patient has counters to record the number of laps walked and to record the distance ridden during bike exercise. The heart rates, laps walked, blood pressure, and weight are recorded on a daily log, with any signs and symptoms and a rhythm strip. All the rhythm strips are carefully re-examined by the exercise coordinator, nurse, or physician after each session to check for abnormalities. The patient's personal physician is informed of any abnormalities.

Once each week during the first 3 months, the patients have a 10- to 12-minute lecture on the reason for and importance of all phases of rehabilitation and secondary prevention, i.e., exercise, lipid control, weight control, smoking, stress management, and others. These topics plus an update of the medical and surgical therapy in more detail are given on a monthly basis. In addition, the patients are taught relaxation techniques and have special weight reduction classes weekly. Smoke Stopper Programs are held as needed. Emergency drills are held monthly in each exercise area and the locker rooms. Test and evaluation information, progress reports, and any status change are sent to the referring physician, who remains in control of the therapeutic decisions.

NEED FOR CONTINUOUS MONITORING

The question of continuous electrocardiographic monitoring has been debated over many years, but to date, there is no evidence that this reduces the incidence of sudden death or cardiac events. Close observation by trained personnel after careful initial evaluation seems to provide better monitoring and allows the patients to become more accustomed to monitoring themselves and more comfortable with exercising outside the program. In the absence of adequate personnel, continuous monitoring may improve the recognition of potential problems and alert the staff about the high-risk patients and those with significant arrhythmias. These patients probably represent 5% to 10% of the total patient population referred to cardiac rehabilitation. The monitoring can be limited to 10 to 12 sessions and used intermittently thereafter. Of interest, cardiac arrest, ventricular fibrillation, and other events that have occurred in our patients have been after 1 year in the program in all but two patients. One was 6 months after infarction and the other was at his initial visit.

Safety. In 1996, the safety of exercising patients with cardiovascular disease in a rehabilitation program should not be a concern to physicians. Van-Camp and Peterson surveyed 167 rehabilitation programs that included about 51,000 patients exercising for 2,350,000 hours. Cardiac arrests occurred in 1 per 112,000 patient hours of exercise, of which 86% were successfully resuscitated with no cardiovascular complication. There was one fatality every 784,000 patient hours of exercise, and nonfatal myocardial infarction occurred every 300,000 patient hours of exercise. Considering the fact that all these patients had coronary artery disease and most had had myocardial infarction or coronary artery bypass grafting or both, this seems to be extremely low. Careful planning maximizes the safety of any cardiac rehabilitation program. Emergency cardiac drugs, defibrillators, and methods of ventilatory support should be on the scene. As a minimum, all personnel should be certified in basic life support, and emergency drills should be carried out in all locations, including exercise areas, dressing rooms, and testing laboratories. In a carefully planned emergency system, the time from a patient arrest to the ability to administer electroshock in the rehabilitation programs with equipment immediately available is less than 1 minute in the exercise areas, and slightly longer in the dressing rooms. This is significantly better than in most hospitals with patients outside Intensive Care or the catheterization laboratories.

PATIENTS WITH SPECIAL PROBLEMS

Patients with poor left ventricular function, with and without congestive heart failure, and those with arrhythmias present some special problems, but almost all do surprisingly well and show improvement in the rehabilitation programs. It is surprising that the 30 patients in our program with left ventricular ejection fractions of under 40% have an exercise capacity that does not correlate with their ejection fraction. Many of them have measured exercise capacities of 35 to 38 mL O_2 per kg without significant dyspnea or angina. Care should be given to the level at which these individuals begin their exercise program; and progression may be a bit slower. However, the results are extremely encouraging, particularly to the patients. In a current research study, patients with symptomatic congestive failure have improved functional capacity with no untoward events.

Exercise testing has proved to be an excellent way to determine the effect of various levels of physical activity on arrhythmias. With this test, one can usually determine the need for electrophysiologic or other studies and specific therapy before beginning exercise training. Careful evaluation to determine a safe, effective training heart rate at a level that does not produce the arrhythmias is very important. Again, the ability of the patients to improve their physical capacity and enter into more vigorous exercise activities is quite gratifying. More frequent monitoring with "Quick-Look" paddles and Holter monitors is performed on these patients.

The number of patients above 65 years of age and even above 75 years who are referred to cardiac rehabilitation has increased dramatically. Many more retired individuals are taking part in cardiac rehabilitation to assure them of their ability to maintain an active lifestyle. In elderly people, one must consider the changes in the musculoskeletal system with increasing arthritis, the decrease in ventilatory capacity, and the changes in the ability of the myocardium to relax. These factors not only cause some difficulty in their ability to walk or exercise in other ways but also in increasing shortness of breath and inability to increase stroke volume with exercise. However, in spite of these changes, the training exercise markedly improves their functional capacity. It takes more time than in younger people, but the improvement is significant and the ability to return to or maintain a functional lifestyle is gratifying. It is interesting that many patients over age 75 years who have been physically active most of their life have a good physical capacity and no significant symptoms of shortness of breath or cardiac symptoms. Because of the change in pulse rate and blood pressure response to activity, which is more pronounced as the patient gets older, it is frequently better to try to obtain metabolic parameters such as oxygen uptake to determine their exercise capacity. However, if this is not available, the pulse and blood pressure response can be used to establish a safe, effective training heart rate.

As with all patients in cardiac rehabilitation, exercise tests are done to determine functional capacity and not for diagnoses. Therefore, patients should be tested using all the medications that they will take during training. Never use heart rate tables to determine training heart rates in patients with cardiac disease who are on medications. At best, they will be only a rough estimate. Most heart rate tables were established on normal individuals and should not be applied directly to the medicated patients with cardiovascular disease.

Approximately 35% of the patients with coronary disease have peripheral vascular disease, and in our patient population, 80% of patients with documented peripheral vascular disease have significant obstructive coronary disease (less than 70% in one artery). Also, 25% of those with myocardial infarctions in our rehabilitation program had asymptomatic carotid artery disease by ultrasound, with only 2% being significantly obstructed (less than 85%). Peripheral vascular disease can present a problem because of the inability to exercise; but studies have shown that prolonged walking (1 hour four times weekly for 9+ months) produces a good increase in the distance walked and decrease in claudication pain. Our subjects with peripheral vascular disease exercise the upper and lower extremities on a bicycle primarily, plus walking, and accomplish a significant increase in overall functional capacity. Swimming has proved to be good exercise for these patients, but, unfortunately, it does not improve their ability to walk or decrease their claudication significantly even with good increase in physical capacity. Subjects with asymptomatic carotid disease are exercised in a similar fashion to other patients. It has been shown in good longevity studies that surgical correction of obstructive carotid stenosis, even when asymptomatic, is beneficial and reduces cerebrovascular events. Examination of the carotids should always be part of the evaluation.

With the high frequency of diabetes in the cardiovascular disease population, each patient should be carefully screened for glucose abnormalities. In insulin-dependent diabetics, it is best to evaluate the blood sugar before exercise and establish minimal and maximal levels within which they may be allowed to participate in the physical activity. Symptomatic hypoglycemia may occur at different levels with blood sugars in different individuals, but those with a blood sugar below 70 are asked to take their glucose supplementation before walking and to recheck the blood sugar after 10 to 20 minutes. It is best if one of the staff members walks with them initially and observes them for hypoglycemic symptoms and other problems. A blood sugar of 360 has been used as the upper limit. The time that the patients have eaten and had their insulin injections will change the results. If the patients have no ketones and are asymptomatic, they are allowed to exercise for 10 minutes, and then the glucose is rechecked. If there is an increase, they are stopped and told to follow the instructions given to them by their physicians. If they are symptomatic or problems are recurrent, they are referred or taken to their physicians.

PROBLEM OF UNDERUTILIZATION

Cardiac rehabilitation centers are becoming more available. Some centers now have satellite operations in small surrounding towns. But with 53 major cardiac rehabilitation centers in North Carolina, only 15% of the patients that are candidates enter the programs. Several factors play a part, such as the patients' unwillingness to attend, distance to the programs, physician disinterest, or delay in referring the patients. Feelings that low-risk patients do not need the rehabilitation and secondary prevention services and that high-risk patients are too ill or too risky to participate or that the interventional or surgical procedure has corrected the problem are often implied by physicians and other medical personnel. In fact, all patients need some aspect of the rehabilitation program, whether it be conditioning, risk factor control, education, or lifestyle changes, to prolong the remainder of their lives.

To reach the goal that all patients with cardiovascular events and procedures participate in cardiac rehabilitation programs, home programs are being established in many areas. Some home rehabilitation programs have been in operation since the mid-1980s in a few locations. Tele-electronic monitoring has been used in several programs. Currently, a five-city study of home rehabilitation programs using this technique is underway. The preliminary results are encouraging, showing good compliance. In these centers, the nurse or rehabilitation specialists can monitor the heart rate and talk with the patients by telephone to discuss their symptoms and encourage them. This personal contact helps what may be lost in not participating in group exercise.

Prior to starting the home program, patients are best evaluated and their rehabilitative and preventive needs determined. In some centers, patients attend 3 to 12 exercise sessions following evaluation, during which the exercise routine, ability to count the pulse, and psychological, dietary, and risk factor therapy are established. Patients are asked to perform their exercise routines to the training heart rate and rate of perceived exertion three to four times per week for 30 to 40 minutes per session. A warm-up of 5 minutes before the exercise and a 5-minute cool-down period afterward is included. In our home program, two of our staff visit the patients at home initially to design and discuss the exercise routine and observe the first exercise session. The patients record their pulse at rest, after 5 to 20 minutes of exercise and 5 minutes of cool down, plus the distances walked or ridden on a bicycle. The patients are called by the staff three times the first few weeks and one to two times every week thereafter, as required, to evaluate and motivate the patients. They return to our center every 3 months for testing and risk factor evaluation. Results from preliminary information seem very encouraging as to their increase in physical capacity and lipid control and compare favorably with those exercising in the rehabilitation center.

An increasing number of universities have graduate programs that are providing us with well-trained and dedicated rehabilitation and prevention specialists in the field of exercise physiology, nursing, physical therapy, and others. With the ability to evaluate and treat patients with coronary artery disease more accurately and completely, risk stratification and determining the rehabilitative and preventive needs can be established early. With the availability of better trained and more experienced personnel, cardiovascular rehabilitative exercise can be safely held in many areas such as malls, high school and college gyms, and recreational centers. Again, careful rules and safety guidelines have to be established and the intensity of exercise and training heart rate determined by a careful and well-monitored graded exercise test. Patients should be tested in the mode in which they will be exercising, i.e., bike test for biking and treadmill test for walking and jogging. The patients should be referred by their physicians, as would be true of the center and home-based programs. Here especially it would be beneficial for the participants to exercise at a rehabilitation center for a few sessions to become familiar with the exercise routine, become comfortable with their ability to count their pulse rate, and be observed for any arrhythmias or undue exercise problems. This will make the participant more secure when exercising in the local exercise facility.

Cardiac rehabilitation participants who now lead some of our exercise routines could also lead exercise sessions in these locations under the direction of trained rehabilitation personnel. In part, this is being carried out in many locations in "mall walker's groups." They are designed primarily for well patients, but many cardiac patients participate because of the convenience, and the supervising personnel are frequently not as well trained. Adding physician referral to get appropriate information, careful evaluation, and early education of these patients should make this a much safer and more effective mechanism of rehabilitation. Exercising in groups adds to the enjoyment and safety, as there is always someone to provide or call for assistance.

BENEFITS

The effect of exercise rehabilitation programs on all-cause and cardiovascular mortality has been determined by examining the data from programs that had matched controls. With approximately 2200 patients in both the control and rehabilitative groups, there was an average 25% decrease in the cardiovascular and overall mortality through a 3-year period in the exercise group. Equally beneficial results have been noted in studies in which patients with documented cardiovascular disease have lipid control that approximates the new lipid guidelines for patients with coronary disease: total cholesterol less than 180, LDL less than 100, and HDL more than 40. When the patients were restudied by coronary arteriography after 2 years, there was a significant decrease in plaque progression, and in some segments regression of the plaques was noted. In further follow-up in several of the studies, there was a decrease in the rate of cardiovascular events.

All these studies point to the fact that rigid control of the major risk factors of *inactivity, hyperlipidemia,* and *smoking* over time will reduce deaths and cardiac events and improve the quality of an active, useful life. As we enter the era of capitated medical care, primary and secondary prevention will become more important. There is a strong suggestion in more recent studies that tight control of risk factors in patients who have known coronary disease is reducing the frequency of interventional procedures, coronary artery bypass graft surgery, and thus the hospitalizations for those procedures and other problems. The money saved from a 1- to 2-day hospitalization for interventional therapy will currently pay for two to three patients in ours and most other rehabilitation programs for 6 months, including all the testing. We in the medical field need to continue to work toward 100% participation of all patients with cardiovascular disease in cardiac rehabilitation and prevention programs. The same systems serve equally well for risk factor screening and primary prevention. Food for thought for the future!

PERICARDITIS

method of
J. SOLER-SOLER, M.D., and
J. SAGRISTÀ-SAULEDA, M.D.
Hospital General Universitari Vall d'Hebron
Barcelona, Spain

MANAGEMENT OF ACUTE EPISODE

Most patients with acute pericarditis complain of chest pain and fever. Frequently, some degree of pericardial effusion is present, and some patients may suffer cardiac compression because of tense fluid (tamponade). Therefore, treatment of acute pericarditis is to relieve the symptoms and to remove pericardial effusion when needed. In addition, some specific etiologies, such as tuberculous and bacterial pericarditis, require the administration of adequate antimicrobial therapy.

Relief of Symptoms

Pain and fever are usually satisfactorily managed by using common analgesic-antipyretic drugs, alone or in combination. For patients with no contraindications, the first choice is aspirin, 250 to 500 mg orally every 4 to 6 hours. In patients with contraindications or intolerance to aspirin, other types of nonsteroidal anti-inflammatory drugs (NSAIDs) should be used. Acetaminophen (Tylenol), 500 to 750 mg every 4 to 6 hours, can be succesful in patients with mild or moderate symptoms. In patients with severe symptoms, the most effective drugs are indomethacin (25 to 50 mg every 6 to 8 hours) and ibuprofen (800 mg every 6 to 8 hours). For patients with severe refractory symptoms, different combinations of these drugs can be attempted (aspirin plus acetaminophen, indomethacin plus acetaminophen, ibuprofen plus acetaminophen). Drug therapy should be maintained up to 1 week after the relief of symptoms.

Very rarely (in our experience less than 2% of patients), symptoms are considered to be refractory and the choice of corticosteroid administration may arise. Corticosteroids are very effective drugs that quickly control pain and pericardial effusion. However, they must be considered the last resort, because some patients become "hooked" on a drug and symptoms reappear every time the dose is diminished, leading to the unpleasant situation of recurrent pericarditis. Therefore, an effort should be made to avoid these drugs; it is probably much better for the patient to put up with the symptoms some additional days than to begin prematurely with the easy resource of corticosteroid administration. Only patients with surgically induced pericarditis, especially those needing concomitant anticoagulant therapy, should be given corticosteroids as first-choice therapy.

In our opinion, most patients with acute pericarditis can be managed at home. Only those patients with severe or persistent symptoms, those with evidence of more than mild pericardial effusion, and those with tamponade should be hospitalized in a center equipped to perform drainage of pericardial fluid or any other adequate clinical investigation.

Treatment of Cardiac Tamponade

First, it should be stated that cardiac tamponade is not an "all or nothing" condition but a continuum that ranges from mild venous distention and a small degree of pulsus paradoxus with good clinical tolerance to a very acute, severe, and life-threatening hemodynamic compromise. In fact, not all patients with cardiac tamponade require drainage of pericardial fluid. Some patients with mild tamponade, especially the young ones in whom idiopathic or viral pericarditis is the most probable etiology, can be successfully managed with bed rest and anti-inflammatory drugs. Of course, these patients should be carefully monitored, with prompt removal of pericardial fluid if the clinical situation deteriorates. In patients with moderate-to-severe tamponade, drainage of pericardial fluid is mandatory; additionally, important etiologic information may be obtained in some patients.

The choice between pericardiocentesis and surgical drainage depends highly on hospital resources and the personal experience of the operator. Pericardiocentesis should be avoided if there is less than 5 mm of anterior echo-free space. Pericardiocentesis should be performed by a skilled cardiologist. Surgical drainage is usually performed through a subxiphoid approach under local or general anesthesia. The procedure is safe and, furthermore, it allows resection of pericardial tissue for laboratory examination. However, surgical drainage is, in some way, more aggressive, and in most patients (about 70%) tamponade is successfully resolved by pericardiocentesis. Our choice is to begin with pericardiocentesis and reserve surgical drainage for the patients in whom tamponade persists or recurs.

Management of Pericardial Effusion in Patients with Acute Pericarditis but Without Tamponade

Pericardial effusion occurs frequently (40% to 60%) in acute pericarditis, including the idiopathic/viral form. If tamponade is not present, routine pericardiocentesis is not indicated because its diagnostic yield is very low and pericardial effusion will disappear spontaneously. Pericardiocentesis should be performed only in patients with a strong suspicion of purulent pericarditis, for diagnostic purposes.

Management of Acute Pericarditis with a Prolonged Clinical Course

The possibility of specific etiologies would arise in these patients. We advocate subxiphoid pericardial biopsy and drainage in patients with persisting clinical activity (pain, fever, pericardial effusion) only after 3 weeks of hospitalization. The diagnostic yield of this procedure depends largely on the relative incidence of specific etiologies (especially tuberculosis), so its indication and timing should be individualized in each clinical and geographic context. Blind antituberculous treatment should be avoided.

TREATMENT OF SPECIFIC ETIOLOGIC FORMS OF PERICARDITIS
Idiopathic/Viral Pericarditis

Idiopathic/viral pericarditis usually resolves in a few days with bed rest and NSAID. However, occasionally the disease may last a few weeks longer. Pericardial effusion is frequent, and tamponade is not exceptional. As stated, an effort should be made to avoid corticosteroid therapy.

A special form is the so-called *recurrent idiopathic benign pericarditis*. Each recurrence should be managed as an acute episode of pericarditis. In about 50% of patients, colchicine* (1 to 2 mg per day) controls the recurrences. Wide-open pericardiectomy is not indicated for two reasons: recurrences are not prevented in most patients, and the disease will finally heal after some recurrences.

Tuberculous Pericarditis

In patients with demonstrated tuberculous pericarditis (isolation of tubercle bacilli or demonstration of granulomas in pericardium or other tissues), antituberculous therapy should be given with isoniazid, 300 mg once daily (450 mg in patients weighing more than 90 kg) for 6 months, rifampin (Rifadin), 600 mg once daily (450 mg in patients weighing less than 50

---

*Not FDA-approved for this indication.

kg, 750 mg in patients weighing more than 90 kg) for 6 months, and pyrazinamide, 30 mg per kg per day for 2 months. Corticosteroids can be given during the inflammatory-effusive phase, but their usefulness has not been proved and the indication remains controversial. In the first weeks or months in the evolution of the illness, attention should be paid to the possibility of constriction, which may happen in about 50% of patients, requiring pericardiectomy.

Nontuberculous Bacterial Pericarditis

In this form of pericarditis, surgical drainage is mandatory. Appropriate antibiotic treatment matched to the causative microorganism is also necessary. If the microorganism cannot be identified, antibiotic selection should be made depending on the surrounding infection. Instillation of antibiotics into the pericardial sac is not necessary since antibiotic diffusion to the pericardial space is very good. Progression to constrictive pericarditis occurs in one third of patients.

Postmyocardial Infarction Pericarditis

This form of pericarditis, which is present in 20% to 30% of patients suffering acute myocardial infarction, should be managed like acute idiopathic pericarditis. Anticoagulant therapy is not absolutely contraindicated but probably should be avoided in patients with strong inflammatory signs and severe pericardial effusion.

Postpericardiotomy Pericarditis

Cardiac surgery is now a common cause of pericarditis. The need for anticoagulant treatment in many of these patients complicates the management of pericarditis. Because of this, the probable best therapeutic approach is administration of corticosteroids.

Radiation-Related Pericarditis

Radiation of the chest for Hodgkin's lymphoma or breast neoplasia may cause different forms of pericardial disease, including acute and chronic pericarditis and pericardial effusion. Acute symptoms should be managed like acute idiopathic pericarditis. Massive effusion and tamponade are initially managed by pericardiocentesis, but if massive effusion recurs, wide-open pericardiectomy is indicated.

Metabolic Pericarditis

Classic uremic pericarditis in nondialyzed patients improves after the onset of dialysis; occasionally, pericardiocentesis may be necessary because of tamponade due to rapid hemorrhage or induced by dialysis if fluid is removed too rapidly from the intravascular compartment. Pericarditis in patients on chronic hemodialysis should be managed by increasing the frequency and duration of the hemodialysis sessions and using local instead of general heparinization. Switching from hemodialysis to peritoneal dialysis may solve the problem in some patients. If the patient does not get better and, especially, if tamponade appears (frequently during hemodialysis), pericardiocentesis with instillation of a nonabsorbable corticosteroid in the pericardial sac may be useful. If tamponade recurs, wide-open pericardiectomy may be necessary.

Pericarditis in Vasculitis–Connective Tissue Disease

Pericarditis in systemic lupus erythematosus and related syndromes usually responds to corticosteroid therapy, although an additional dose of aspirin or NSAID may be necessary. Tamponade is very infrequent.

Neoplastic Pericarditis

Except in cases of leukemia or lymphoma, there is no efficacious treatment for neoplastic pericarditis. Pericardial effusion should be drained only if tamponade is present, and the simplest procedure (including repeated pericardiocentesis with instillation of tetracycline* or bleomycin [Blenoxane] in the pericardial sac) should be used.

Pericarditis in AIDS Patients

Although some specific forms of pericardial involvement, such as bacterial and tuberculous pericarditis and Kaposi's sarcoma, have been said to be more frequent in patients with AIDS, pericarditis is actually idiopathic in origin in most patients. Therefore, aspirin or NSAIDs should be used, and pericardiocentesis or biopsy should be reserved for patients with tamponade or persisting active disease.

TREATMENT OF PERICARDIAL EFFUSION IN PATIENTS WITHOUT CLINICAL SYMPTOMS OF ACUTE PERICARDITIS

Pericardial effusion is not an uncommon finding in patients with congestive heart failure and during pregnancy. Sometimes pericardial effusion is found in individuals with no evidence of heart or general disease. In these cases, hypothyroidism should be ruled out. In most of these instances pericardial effusion is mild or moderate, and pericardial fluid drainage is not indicated. A special condition is chronic massive pericardial effusion (pericardial effusion with echo-free spaces in the anterior and posterior sac larger than 20 mm lasting over 3 months). Although this condition can be well tolerated or even absolutely asymptomatic, these patients are at risk of tamponade, so pericardial fluid removal seems advisable.

---

*Not FDA-approved for this indication.

TREATMENT OF CONSTRICTIVE PERICARDITIS

Chronic constrictive pericarditis with clinical symptoms of congestive heart failure is a clear indication for pericardiectomy. However, in older patients, especially those with important calcifications, mortality is quite high. Therefore, if symptoms are satisfactorily controlled with diuretics and sodium restriction, medical treatment seems the most appropriate. Another special situation is postirradiation constrictive pericarditis. In such cases, the myocardial damage caused by the irradiation increases the risk of surgery and its outcome. The syndrome of effusive-constrictive pericarditis is amenable to wide-open pericardiectomy, as cardiac compression by the thick pericardium persists after resolution of tamponade by pericardiocentesis.

One special form of constrictive pericarditis is acute-subacute constriction that can appear in the evolution of tuberculous and bacterial pericarditis. Particularly in the latter case, constriction may evolve very quickly so that urgent pericardiectomy may be needed. Mild constriction (frequently subclinical) is very common in the phase of resolution of pericardial effusion in acute benign pericarditis, and in almost all the patients constriction resolves spontaneously (transient constriction). In these patients, a conservative approach is indicated.

PERIPHERAL ARTERIAL DISEASE

method of
KENNETH E. McINTYRE, JR.
University of Texas Medical Branch
Galveston, Texas

Vascular occlusive disease of the lower extremities commonly occurs in humans as they age. Atherosclerotic plaques, which begin to form earlier in life, continue to progress with age and produce symptoms when major blood vessels become narrowed. Elderly patients are commonly unaware that they have circulatory impairment and often attribute difficulty in walking to the aging process. At least 10% of the U.S. population over the age of 70 has symptoms of vasculogenic claudication. Atherosclerosis can also occur in patients less than 40 years of age, but rarely. When patients develop symptoms of vascular impairment at a young age, other uncommon causes of arterial disease should be sought.

SYMPTOMS CAUSED BY CHRONIC VASCULAR OCCLUSIVE LESIONS

The most common symptom experienced by patients with chronic occlusive disease of the lower extremity is pain. When the pain is brought on by exercise and relieved by resting, the symptoms are referred to as claudication (from the Latin *claudicatio,* to limp). The pain is often referred to as a muscle cramp and most commonly occurs in the calf muscle. Undoubtedly, the gastrocnemius-soleus muscle complex in the calf requires the most energy during walking and therefore develops ischemia when oxygen supply cannot meet demand. Foot claudication rarely occurs, because the few small muscle groups in the foot are not required for ambulation. Thigh or buttocks claudication occurs less commonly, generally when there is significant occlusive disease at the level of the aorta and iliac arteries. Older patients may not walk fast enough to induce cramps but notice early fatigue or weakness of their legs. Patients may attribute difficulty with walking to arthritis or to the aging process itself. As occlusive disease progresses, the ability to walk decreases. In a small percentage of patients, claudication progresses to ischemic rest pain. This pain involves the feet and usually occurs at night when the legs are elevated. Since the pain is caused by nerve ischemia, it is not surprising that patients describe the pain as burning. The pain is severe and is seldom relieved by narcotic medication, but at least initially, some relief may be obtained by placing the foot in a dependent position.

RISK FACTORS FOR ATHEROSCLEROTIC OCCLUSIVE DISEASE

Every patient who undergoes an examination for vascular complaints should be questioned about risk factors. There are three major risk factors for the development of occlusive plaques: cigarette smoking, hypertension, and hypercholesterolemia. Secondary risk factors, including diabetes mellitus and family history, are also important. When these risk factors are present occlusive plaques tend to occur in several areas, including the aorta and the coronary, carotid, renal, mesenteric, iliac, femoral, popliteal, and tibial arteries. Therefore, an adequate history in a patient with claudication includes questions about angina pectoris, myocardial infarction, stroke, and transient ischemic attack (TIA).

PHYSICAL EXAMINATION

It is extremely important to have the patient remove his or her clothes prior to beginning the examination. Undergarments may be worn, and the examining room should be warmed. The physical examination should begin with the vital signs, including a measurement of the blood pressure in both arms. In addition, a careful cardiorespiratory examination is imperative, since it is common for patients with vascular occlusive disease to have hypertensive and/or ischemic heart disease as well as chronic obstructive pulmonary disease. Although upper extremity arterial occlusive disease seldom produces symptoms, a decrease in upper extremity blood pressure is often the first sign of subclavian artery stenosis.

The examination of the end organ (foot) is as important as the examination of the pulses. A foot with chronic ischemia may be cool to the touch and demonstrate pallor on elevation to 30 degrees, hair loss on the toes and dorsum of the foot, and thickened toenails. In more advanced cases, the skin develops subcutaneous tissue atrophy and may ulcerate. Ischemic ulcerations occur primarily on the dorsum of the toes and are necrotic or gangrenous. In addition, ischemic ulcers are quite painful. In the dependent position, a severely ischemic foot may demonstrate rubor, a purplish-red hue that involves the toes. Sensation is usually intact except in those patients with severe ischemia or diabetic patients with neuropathy.

It is important to palpate pulses, because absence of a pulse generally indicates an obstruction in the arterial segment at or proximal to that pulse. The character of the pulse is recorded as normal, diminished, or absent. The abdominal aortic pulse should always be palpated, since abdominal aortic aneurysms are most commonly detected by physical examination. Next, the groin pulses (common femoral artery) are palpated. The femoral pulse is quite important, because any reduction in it is usually caused by more proximal (aortoiliac) occlusive lesions. It is also important to palpate the popliteal pulse, since femoropopliteal occlusive disease is quite common among those with claudication. Finally, both pedal pulses (dorsalis pedis and posterior tibial) should be palpated. These pulses may be difficult to palpate if the patient is cold or if more proximal tibial occlusive disease (as seen in diabetes mellitus) is present. The upper extremity pulses (brachial and radial) as well as the common carotid pulse in the neck should also be recorded.

Bruit is the audible equivalent of a palpable thrill. Both are signs of turbulent blood flow, and although they may be present in patients with normal vessels (e.g., those with anemia, hyperdynamic state), they usually occur as a consequence of an occlusive plaque. The best places to detect bruits are over the common carotid artery in the neck and over the common femoral artery in the groin. Unfortunately, the presence of a neck bruit does not often correlate with stenosis of the carotid artery. Abdominal bruits may also be detected but can occur from a number of sources, including the mesenteric, renal, and iliac arteries, as well as the aorta.

NONINVASIVE VASCULAR LABORATORY STUDIES

The noninvasive vascular laboratory is a tremendous resource in evaluating patients with suspected vascular occlusive disease. The laboratory helps diagnose vascular disease; determine the location, severity, and progression of atherosclerotic occlusive lesions; and monitor the results of surgical revascularization. The tests are noninvasive and inexpensive and are performed in the outpatient setting.

The most important test is the Doppler-derived ankle-brachial index (ABI). The ABI is determined by measuring the pedal pressure and dividing it by the brachial artery pressure. Normally, the value should be 1.0 or greater. Values greater than 0.9 are usually not associated with symptoms. Patients with claudication have ABIs in the range of 0.5 to 0.8. When the ABI falls to below 0.5, disabling claudication usually occurs. Ischemic rest pain is associated with ABI values of 0.2 to 0.5, and tissue loss (nonhealing ischemic ulcers and/or gangrene) with values less than 0.2. Care should be taken when using the ABI to evaluate leg ischemia in a patient with end-stage renal disease and/or diabetes mellitus. Due to calcification of the blood vessels in these patients, the ABI is supranormal and should be disregarded. In this circumstance, measurement of the toe pressures using photoplethysmography (PPG) is often of benefit and can identify those patients whose ischemic ulcers will heal spontaneously without surgical revascularization. In general, a toe pressure greater than 60 mmHg is associated with spontaneous healing.

In patients with claudication, exercise testing on a treadmill is an important part of the noninvasive laboratory examination. Treadmill walking helps increase blood flow across stenotic arterial segments in the lower extremities. When flow is increased, any pressure drop across a stenosis is augmented, thereby enhancing the sensitivity of the ABI. An example is a patient with only a mildly decreased ABI at rest. Treadmill exercise is performed until claudication symptoms occur. A decrease in ABI greater than 20% establishes the hemodynamic significance of the occlusive lesion. The treadmill should not be used in patients with severe disabling claudication or ischemic rest pain. In addition, cardiac monitoring should always be performed during treadmill exercise, since exercise may initiate an attack of angina pectoris and/or arrhythmia.

NATURAL HISTORY AND NONOPERATIVE THERAPY

The greatest concern among patients with symptomatic vascular occlusive disease of the lower extremities is loss of a limb. Fortunately, the risk of amputation is reasonably low, about 1 to 2% per year. Of greater concern is the documented risk of myocardial ischemia or stroke. Twenty to 25% of patients with claudication may experience myocardial infarction, and 15% may suffer stroke during 5 years of follow-up. Moreover, the mortality rate among those with claudication is significantly higher than that among age-matched controls. The mortality rate is 30 and 50% at 5 and 10 years, respectively, and is directly related to the degree of leg ischemia. It is no surprise that the leading cause of death among claudicants is ischemic heart disease. Since the risk of progressive leg ischemia is low, conservative therapy should almost always be recommended prior to any consideration of operative therapy. In patients who present with mild claudication and can walk several blocks before developing symptoms, the risk of developing progressive limb-threatening ischemia is quite low. In this group, modification of risk factors and walking exercise are the cornerstones of treatment.

Complete cessation of smoking is mandatory. Patient education and support from nonsmokers are beneficial in the treatment of cigarette addiction. In some cases, the use of transdermal nicotine patches may also be of benefit. Hypercholesterolemia should also be treated aggressively. If the low-density lipoprotein (LDL) cholesterol fraction is greater than 130 mg per dL, therapy should be instituted with an HMG CoA reductase inhibitor such as lovastatin (Mevacor) or simvastatin (Zocor). These agents are well tolerated and effectively lower the level of LDL as well as raise the level of high-density lipoprotein (HDL). Finally, hypertension and diabetes should be carefully controlled. Today, there is no controversy that careful monitoring and control of blood sugar lead to fewer long-term complications in patients with diabetes mellitus. Daily walking exercise is as important as risk reduction in a patient with claudication. Walking helps the claudicant by causing adaptation in the muscle enzymes of the leg so that ischemic muscle can extract oxygen more efficiently without requiring anaerobic metabolism for energy production. Patients are instructed to walk until they develop symptoms. They should continue to walk for another 10 to 15 yards *with the pain* before resting for a full 5 to 7 minutes. This process should be repeated several times during 1 hour each day. If walking is terminated with the onset of pain, the positive effect of exercise is lost. Within weeks, the beneficial effects of walking exercise become apparent. If patients are compliant and participate actively, one can anticipate an increase in walking distance of 200 to 300%.

Although many agents to improve claudication are currently being studied, only one drug has received Food and Drug Administration (FDA) approval for the treatment of claudication. Pentoxifylline (Trental), has been tested extensively and has been shown to be of benefit in about 30 to 50% of patients. Unfortunately, when it does have an effect, walking distance is only modestly improved by 30 to 40%. Pentoxifylline should be given for a minimum of 6 to 8 weeks to achieve maximum benefit. There is universal agreement that pentoxifylline is of no benefit in patients with limb-threatening ischemia (rest pain and/or tissue loss). Other agents are often used by clinicians to treat claudication, but there are no good scientific data to support their use. These agents include aspirin,* carnitine,* naftidrofuryl,† and niacin.* Aspirin has been shown to reduce the incidence of stroke following TIA, enhance the patency of infrainguinal and coronary bypass grafts, and reduce the incidence of myocardial infarction and death. For these reasons, aspirin therapy is commonly used in patients with vascular occlusive lesions in the lower extremities. Chelation therapy has been shown to be of no value in the treatment of patients with atherosclerotic occlusive lesions as the cause of claudication.

OPERATIVE THERAPY FOR INTERMITTENT CLAUDICATION

Operative therapy for patients with atherosclerotic occlusive lesions of the lower extremities should be reserved for those with either limb-threatening ischemia (rest pain and/or tissue loss) or disabling claudication. Moreover, the indications should not be altered if a patient is considered a candidate for percutaneous angioplasty to treat occlusive lesions. Patients should not be considered candidates for elective vascular reconstructive operations unless their operative risks (cardiopulmonary) and expected longevity have been carefully scrutinized by the surgeon. For example, it would not be reasonable to propose a vascular operation to treat claudication in a patient whose walking was limited by severe congestive heart failure or whose life was limited because of metastatic carcinoma.

Operations for claudication are grouped by the location of the obstructing atherosclerotic lesions to be treated: aortoiliac (suprainguinal, proximal, inflow), femoropopliteal, and tibial/pedal (distal, outflow). In general, proximal lesions causing a hemodynamic reduction in blood flow should be repaired prior to considering bypass of more distal lesions. In those patients with both proximal and distal occlusive disease, a combination of percutaneous angioplasty and traditional vascular reconstructive operation may be of benefit. In this circumstance, angioplasty can be performed prior to or in conjunction with the vascular bypass operation. For example, a segmental common iliac artery stenosis may be dilated by angioplasty before an ipsilateral femoropopliteal bypass is performed.

Aortoiliac Occlusive Disease

The conventional treatment for patients with proximal occlusive disease has been aorto-bifemoral bypass. The durability (5-year patency rate of 85 to 90%) and the low 30-day mortality rate (less than 3%) have made this operation the standard by which other forms of therapy are measured. Bypass to the external iliac arteries is generally not performed, because progressive occlusive lesions distal to the anastomosis will invariably require extension of the bypass to the femoral arteries. Unilateral aortofemoral bypass is also not commonly done, because patients with iliac disease confined to a single side invariably develop occlusive lesions on the contralateral side. Because an abdominal incision is required, patients with multiple prior abdominal operations, intestinal or urinary stomas, or severe cardiac and/or respiratory insufficiency are not considered good candidates for this procedure, and alternative procedures such as angioplasty or extra-anatomic bypass should be considered. Since the aorta and femoral arteries are much larger than the saphenous vein (commonly used for infrainguinal bypass), prosthetic bypasses constructed of either Dacron or expanded polytetrafluoroethylene (e-PTFE) are commonly used.

If the occlusive process is confined to the aorta and common iliac arteries alone, aortoiliac thromboendarterectomy (TEA) may be performed as an alternative to conventional aorto-bifemoral bypass. The patency and mortality rates for this procedure are similar to those for aorto-bifemoral bypass, and an added advantage of aortoiliac TEA is that no prosthetic graft material is required.

The newest technique for the treatment of aortoiliac occlusive disease is percutaneous angioplasty with or without stent placement. Angioplasty is ideally suited for those patients with localized segmental occlusive plaques in the common iliac arteries. When angioplasty is utilized for these lesions, success rates parallel those of surgical treatment. Although the use of stents appears to offer some advantages over angioplasty alone, long-term follow-up data are not available. The early data on patency rates after iliac stent placement are promising, but only continued follow-up will document whether these intraluminal devices are beneficial in the treatment of aortoiliac occlusive disease over the course of time.

Femoropopliteal Occlusive Disease

The femoropopliteal portion of the arterial tree is the most likely to be affected by atherosclerotic

---

*Not FDA-approved for this indication.
†Not available in the United States.

plaques among patients with claudication. Often, the occlusive lesions begin in the adductor canal of Hunter, a tightly bound fascial compartment where the superficial femoral artery becomes the popliteal artery. Occlusion of this arterial segment alone commonly causes claudication, but symptoms seldom progress to limb-threatening ischemia. For this reason, a conservative approach to patients with isolated superficial femoral artery occlusions is warranted. If surgical therapy is considered, above-knee or below-knee femoropopliteal bypass is the standard procedure. Although this procedure can be performed with prosthetic conduits, the best bypass patency results are achieved with the use of saphenous vein. The mortality rate from femoropopliteal bypass is 1 to 3%, and the 5-year graft patency rate is 63 to 75% when saphenous vein is used, compared with 22 to 59% when PTFE is used.

The results of angioplasty for femoropopliteal occlusive lesions in selected patients with segmental stenoses or occlusions may be similar to surgical results. Unfortunately, occlusive disease in the superficial femoral artery is seldom isolated, requiring several balloon inflations to effectively treat multiple lesions. Early re-stenosis following angioplasty for femoropopliteal occlusive disease continues to be a problem. The role of stent placement to augment angioplasty for femoropopliteal occlusive lesions remains unknown.

In summary, femoropopliteal occlusive disease occurs commonly among patients with leg ischemia. Most patients can be treated conservatively, but if an intervention is required for limb salvage, femoropopliteal bypass with saphenous vein continues to be the standard.

Tibial/Pedal Occlusive Disease

Occlusive lesions at the tibial/pedal level pose the greatest challenge to physicians. Disease of the proximal tibial arteries is usually the cause of ischemic leg symptoms in patients with diabetes mellitus. These arteries are small and require bypass using saphenous vein for successful revascularization. Severe disease at this level usually causes limb-threatening ischemia, and operative procedures are reserved for this indication. These procedures are technically demanding but produce excellent limb salvage results that are comparable in diabetic and nondiabetic patients. Although the proximal tibial arteries are severely diseased in patients with both insulin dependent and non–insulin dependent diabetes, the distal tibial and pedal arteries are often normal, facilitating bypass to these levels. The mortality rate of tibial/pedal bypass is 1 to 2%, with a 3-year patency rate of 56 to 88%. Although prosthetic bypasses can be used in the absence of saphenous vein, the results for tibial/pedal bypass are poor. Angioplasty has been used to treat arterial stenoses at this level, but the results have not been encouraging.

ACUTE EXTREMITY ISCHEMIA

Few clinical presentations are as impressive as that of a patient with acute extremity ischemia. The symptoms occur suddenly, and without emergent treatment, there is a significant risk to both life and limb. The universal symptom that occurs shortly after the acute event that produces ischemia is severe pain in the foot and calf. The pain is so severe that even narcotic medication seldom totally relieves it. Acute ischemia can be caused by either thrombosis or embolism, and the etiology is often difficult to prove. Patients with embolism as the cause of acute ischemia are generally older, have a history of heart disease (chronic arrhythmia such as atrial fibrillation, mitral and/or aortic valve stenosis or insufficiency, ventricular aneurysm, or acute myocardial infarction), and usually have no history of vascular occlusive disease of the lower extremities. Acute ischemia caused by thrombosis occurs more commonly in younger patients with a prior history of claudication or vascular bypass or angioplasty for vascular occlusive disease.

The physical examination may also help differentiate between embolism and thrombosis as the etiology of acute ischemia. Patients with embolism may have signs of acute or chronic heart ailments (arrhythmia, murmur) and often totally normal pulses in the unaffected extremity. Patients with thrombosis as the cause of acute ischemia often demonstrate signs of chronic arterial insufficiency, such as loss of hair over the toes and feet or thickened toenails. In addition, scars from prior bypass operations may be present, and there may be an abnormal pulse examination in the contralateral extremity.

The classic description of the history and physical findings in a patient with acute extremity ischemia includes the five P's: pain, pallor, pulselessness, paresthesia, and paralysis. Pain, pallor, and pulselessness occur soon after acute ischemia begins, but neurologic deficits are usually not present immediately after the onset of pain. Depending on the severity of ischemia, the nerves soon manifest dysfunction, with the development of paresthesia and finally paralysis. The leg is termed "viable" until the onset of paresthesia and paralysis. If restoration of blood flow can be accomplished before the development of neurologic symptoms, the outcome for both patient and extremity is improved. The window of opportunity for treatment is narrow, because untreated acute ischemia ultimately leads to limb loss. The sooner blood flow is restored, the better the outcome will be. If blood flow can be re-established within 4 to 6 hours after the onset of ischemia, there are usually few if any complications. Unfortunately, even if therapy is undertaken in a timely fashion, the complications from acute muscle ischemia (myoglobinuric renal failure, hyperkalemia, acidemia, and compartment syndrome) may still occur and influence the eventual outcome.

As soon as the diagnosis of acute extremity ischemia is made, intravenous heparin must be given.

Usually a bolus dose of 5000 to 10,000 U is followed by an intravenous infusion of 1000 U per hour. Heparin anticoagulation helps prevent propagation of thrombus. In addition, it is critical that patients receive adequate intravenous hydration as quickly as possible. Adequate hydration helps lower blood viscosity, thereby improving ischemia. Moreover, high urinary output helps reduce the risk of acute renal failure from myoglobin pigment precipitating in the tubules.

If there are no neurologic signs (paresthesia, paralysis) present, arteriography should be performed if it can be accomplished in a timely fashion. Arteriography helps identify the pathologic process (thrombosis or embolism) and offers the option of treatment with thrombolytic therapy. Urokinase (Abbokinase) is a direct activator of plasminogen, converting it to plasmin. Catheter-directed urokinase infusion directly into the thrombus may effectively treat the ischemia without the need for surgical intervention. The usual dose of urokinase is 250,000 to 400,000 U given as a bolus within the thrombus, followed by 2000 to 4000 U per minute as an infusion. Continuous monitoring of the patient is necessary to ensure that ischemia does not worsen during the infusion. As the thrombus or embolus lyses, ischemia may worsen transiently before improvement occurs. This occurs as small fragments of clot break loose and embolize distally. Continued infusion usually results in symptomatic improvement. An arteriogram should be repeated in 4 hours to evaluate the effect of thrombolysis. Urokinase is usually continued until lysis is complete or no further lysis occurs. The infusion should not be continued longer than 48 hours, because bleeding complications become more common. Fibrinogen concentrations are monitored every 6 to 8 hours during the infusion. If the fibrinogen level falls to below 100 mg per dL, the infusion should be stopped, because spontaneous bleeding may occur. Overall, the risk of major hemorrhage (requiring surgery and/or transfusion) is 5 to 15%, and the risk of intracranial hemorrhage is less than 1%. Thrombolytic therapy should not be used in patients who have active gastrointestinal bleeding, recent stroke, or other intracranial pathology.

Arteriography and/or thrombolytic therapy should not be employed if the patient presents with advanced ischemia (i.e., neurologic deficits). Under these circumstances, surgical intervention is necessary. Operative thrombectomy or embolectomy carries an operative mortality of 10 to 25% that is due largely to ischemic heart disease and the metabolic disturbances created by muscle ischemia. In addition, there is a similar incidence of major amputation following surgical intervention for acute leg ischemia.

DEEP VENOUS THROMBOSIS OF THE EXTREMITIES

method of
FELIPE NAVARRO, M.D., and
J. MICHAEL BACHARACH, M.D.
Cleveland Clinic Foundation
Cleveland, Ohio

Deep vein thrombosis (DVT) is an underdiagnosed entity in hospitalized patients, yet it is common and leads to considerable morbidity and mortality. DVT also occurs in ambulatory patients who have been exposed to certain risk factors within the preceding 90 days (see Table 1). Once DVTs are recognized, appropriate treatment can be instituted to avoid their major complications: chronic venous insufficiency, acute pulmonary embolism, or phlegmasia cerulea dolens.

PATHOGENESIS

The pathogenesis of DVT is based on Virchow's triad: venous stasis, vessel endothelial damage, and hypercoagulable state. Any one of these often potentiates the other. Conditions that produce venous stasis prevent the dilution of activated coagulation factors by nonactivated blood, prevent activated coagulation factors from being cleared, and prevent activated coagulation factors from mixing with their inhibitors. Venous stasis is caused by clinical conditions that cause immobility and raised venous pressure, such as perioperative immobility, congestive heart failure, and pregnancy. Venous stasis and hyperviscosity are closely linked together; polycythemia, erythrocytosis, and dysproteinemias are risk factors for DVT.

Damage to the endothelial wall has been postulated to expose subendothelial collagen, which in turn activates the intrinsic pathway through activation of factor XII by collagen, and the activation of factors XII and XI by activated platelets. The endothelial wall may sustain damage by conditions that cause extrinsic trauma, such as in orthopedic and gynecologic operations, as well as the thoracic outlet syndrome. Direct trauma such as thrombectomy, endovascular procedures, and even complete lysis of a venous thrombus leaves the endothelial wall traumatized.

The list of hypercoagulable states continues to grow. Some conditions lead to production of hypercoagulable substances, such as in malignancies. Malignancies also increase the risk of developing phlegmasia cerulea dolens as a sequela of iliofemoral DVT. The acquisition of certain antibodies, such as a circulating anticoagulant or an anticardiolipin antibody, can increase the susceptibility of spontaneous thrombosis. Congenital deficiencies, such as protein-C and protein-S deficiencies and antithrombin III deficiency, also increase the risk of spontaneous thrombosis. Table 1 summarizes risk factors for DVT.

DIAGNOSIS

The diagnostic dilemma of DVT is reflected by the fact that as many as 50% of patients with DVT are asymptomatic, and as many as 70% of patients with clinically suspected DVT have negative results from objective testing. The time-honored Homans' sign is insensitive and nonspecific; other "classic" signs are often eponymized but are more of historic than diagnostic value. Patients with venous thrombosis usually do not develop signs or symp-

TABLE 1. **Risk Factors for DVT**

Venous Stasis

Immobilization
Anesthesia induction/surgery
Varicose veins
Advanced age
Congestive heart failure
Myocardial infarction
Stroke
Pregnancy

Endothelial Wall Injury

Hip/long bone fractures
Orthopedic surgery
Trauma
Mechanical thrombectomy
Thrombolytic therapy
Previous DVT

Hypercoagulable States

Congenital
  Protein-C deficiency
  Protein-S deficiency
  Antithrombin III deficiency
  Activated protein-C resistance
  Paroxysmal nocturnal hemoglobinuria
  Hyperviscosity
Acquired
  Circulating anticoagulant (lupus anticoagulant)
  Anticardiolipin antibody
  Malignancy
  Inflammatory bowel disease
  Oral contraceptives

toms until the thrombus is large and occlusive. Approximately 80% of venous thrombi in symptomatic patients are in or have extended into the popliteal and more proximal veins.

The most common clinical symptoms are pain, tenderness, and swelling. Night cramps, erythrocyanosis, dilated veins, and elevated skin temperature also occur but are not specific to venous thrombosis. Moreover, the differential diagnosis of DVT is extensive and may include a ruptured Baker's cyst, ruptured medial head of the gastrocnemius, cellulitis, lymphedema, congestive heart failure, hematoma, and tumors. These conditions should be excluded by history, physical examination, and objective testing since their treatment differs from that of an acute venous thrombosis. For example, anticoagulating a patient who complains of an acutely painful and swollen leg may have dire consequences if the patient had in fact sustained a ruptured medial head of the gastrocnemius instead of an acute DVT.

Ascending contrast venography is the "gold standard" for the objective diagnosis of deep vein thrombosis. It has a higher sensitivity than duplex ultrasound for calf vein thrombus and is often used for inadequate or equivocal duplex examinations. The most reliable criterion for confirming an acute venous thrombosis is an intraluminal filling defect visualized in multiple views. Nonfilling of venous segments cannot be reliably used to diagnose acute venous thrombosis. Venography is invasive and not free of complications. Complications may include hypersensitivity reactions, renal impairment, local skin and tissue necrosis secondary to extravasation, and, ironically, venous thrombosis in as many as 1% to 2% of patients with negative venograms.

Duplex ultrasonography has emerged as the diagnostic tool of choice of upper and lower extremity DVT. It is noninvasive and has a sensitivity and specificity approaching 95% for proximal DVT. However, the sensitivity falls in the assessment of the calf veins, and results are often operator dependent.

TREATMENT

The treatment of choice for DVT is anticoagulation. Anticoagulation therapy, with heparin and warfarin, is prophylactic against immediate and long-term complications. In the acute setting, anticoagulation therapy has been proved to prevent thrombus extension, pulmonary embolism, and, subacutely, phlegmasia cerulea dolens. Therefore, unless contraindications exist, a bolus of heparin should be administered once the diagnosis of DVT is entertained until objective testing is completed. The long-term goal of anticoagulation is the prevention of recurrent DVT and chronic venous insufficiency.

Intravenously administered unfractionated heparin is the drug of choice for DVT. It binds to antithrombin III, or heparin cofactor II, enhancing the ability of antithrombin III to inactivate factors XIIa, XIa, IXa, and thrombin. This in turn effectively and rapidly prevents extension of the thrombin. Recurrence rates of venous thromboembolism can be reduced by maintaining the activated partial thromboplastin time (aPTT) at 60 to 80 seconds, particularly during the first 24 hours. A weight-based heparin nomogram consisting of an intravenous bolus of 80 U per kg, followed by 18 U per kg per hour infusion, has been shown to attain this target more effectively and safely than the traditional 5000 U bolus and 1000 U per hour infusion. An aPTT should be checked 6 hours after the infusion is started and 6 hours following any adjustment of the infusion rate. In addition to the aPTT, a complete blood count (CBC) should be obtained every 48 hours to monitor for platelet-associated thrombocytopenia as well as to guard against occult bleeding.

Oral anticoagulation with warfarin (Coumadin) should be started on the same day as heparin. The anticoagulation effect of warfarin is monitored by the International Normalized Ratio (INR), which should be kept between 2.0 and 3.0. Warfarin is a vitamin K antagonist that depletes the vitamin K–dependent factors II, VII, IX, X, protein-C and protein-S. The half-lives of factors II, IX, and X range between 72 and 96 hours, whereas that of factor VII is between 8 and 12 hours. Therefore, heparin and warfarin should overlap between 4 and 5 days even if a therapeutic INR is reached sooner. The early rise in the INR represents depletion of factor VII, which has the shortest half-life. In addition, protein-C and protein-S, which are natural anticoagulants, are also depleted in the early stages of warfarin treatment. Therefore, premature discontinuation of heparin may result in a net thrombogenic state since the other vitamin K–dependent coagulation factors have not been depleted.

After a loading dose of 10 mg, subsequent doses of warfarin are regulated according to the INR (between 2.0 and 3.0). The first documented, unexplained episode of DVT or pulmonary embolism requires 3 to 6 months of anticoagulation. The second episode requires 6 to 12 months, and the third unexplained episode generally commits the patient to lifelong Coumadin.

Low-molecular-weight heparins (LMWHs) are fractionated heparins of about 4000 to 6500 daltons (compared with 12,000 to 15,000 daltons for unfractionated heparin). LMWHs have a longer plasma half-life, have a predictable response based on a weight-adjusted dosing, and, therefore, make laboratory monitoring of aPTT unnecessary. LMWHs' higher ratio of antifactor Xa to antifactor IIa activity (4 to 1) results in optimal antithrombotic activity coupled with a lower bleeding tendency compared with unfractionated heparin, which has a lower antifactor Xa to antifactor IIa activity (1 to 1). In the United States, the LMWH enoxaparin (Lovenox) has been approved by the Food and Drug Administration for DVT prophylaxis in orthopedic surgery. Studies have also shown LMWHs to be at least as effective as intravenous unfractionated heparin in the treatment of acute DVT. LMWHs can be used when a patient develops unfractionated heparin-induced platelet antibodies. There is approximately a 25% to 50% cross-reactivity with LMWHs for heparin-induced platelet antibodies. Therefore, when a patient develops unfractionated heparin-induced platelet antibodies, LMWH-induced antibodies should also be checked before instituting LMWH. Thus, the use of LMWH should still be accompanied by monitoring of platelet counts. The cost of LMWH is higher than that of conventional intravenous heparin, but since the use of LMWHs does not require the frequent laboratory monitoring of aPTT or hospitalization, the cost is offset by these savings.

The use of thrombolytic therapy for the treatment of deep venous thrombosis is controversial. The premise of its use in the treatment of DVT is that complete lysis of the thrombus will preserve valvular function and, therefore, prevent the postphlebitic syndrome. Thrombolytic therapy has been shown to be more effective than heparin in achieving complete resolution of acute DVT. However, although many studies *suggest* that thrombolytic therapy reduces the frequency of postphlebitic syndrome, there is no firm evidence for this. Moreover, thrombolytic therapy is not better than standard anticoagulation in the prevention of acute pulmonary embolism.

We do use thrombolytic therapy in patients with acute iliofemoral DVT and "effort thrombosis" of the subclavian-axillary veins. In the former condition, resolution of the thrombus burden via thrombolysis has the potential of being of most benefit in preventing the postphlebitic syndrome. With Paget-Schroetter syndrome or so-called effort thrombosis of the subclavian-axillary veins, significant morbidity and mortality can be reduced with thrombolysis.

To achieve the best results, the fibrinolytic agent should be delivered via an infusion catheter that is embedded directly into the thrombus. In this way, the fibrinolytic agent, which activates the fibrin-bound plasminogen within the thrombus, is not only locally concentrated but also protected from plasminogen activator inhibitors. The directed delivery of the thrombolytic agent improves the likelihood of clot lysis and allows lysis to be achieved with shorter-duration infusions. In this fashion, an acute DVT may be completely lysed within 24 to 48 hours.

The standard dose of urokinase (Abbokinase)* is a 4400 U per kg infusion followed by a 4400 U per kg per hour infusion through the infusion catheter. If recombinant tissue plasminogen activator (rt-PA) (Activase)* is used, an infusion rate of 0.05 mg per kg per hour is administered via the infusion catheter. Intravenous heparin at 1000 U per hour should be given concomitantly to prevent pericatheter thrombus formation. Following complete thrombolytic therapy, a standard anticoagulation course with heparin and warfarin is initiated as the intima has been damaged and, therefore, prone to recurrent thrombosis.

In the case of effort thrombosis of the subclavian-axillary veins, identifying any underlying stenotic lesion is extremely important. A number of options now exist to treat the stenotic lesion, including balloon angioplasty with or without endovascular stenting. Surgical correction of an extrinsic source of thoracic outlet compression is an important therapeutic alternative. In the case of a patient who has undergone lytic therapy to open the vein, there is usually a 4- to 6-week period of treatment with anticoagulation prior to surgical intervention.

ALTERNATIVES WHEN ANTICOAGULATION IS CONTRAINDICATED

Prior to the initiation of either anticoagulation or thrombolytic therapy, the patient should be screened for relative and absolute contraindications. Relative contraindications must be determined for the individual patient; they are considered in relation to available alternatives and the risks of the procedure. Absolute contraindications include active bleeding, recent stroke, recent head trauma, and bleeding diathesis, including the development of heparin-induced thrombocytopenia with thrombosis (HITT).

Inferior vena cava interruption, introduced in 1983 as an inferior vena cava ligation, is now done via percutaneous placement of a caval filter. There are a variety of caval filters, with the most commonly used being Greenfield's filter. Its cone-shaped geometry allows most of the cone to be filled with thrombus without significant reduction in caval blood flow. The preservation of caval blood flow coupled with renal vein blood flow allows gradual resolution of the thrombi caught in the filter. For this reason, long-term filter patency rates independent of anticoagulation reach 98%. Long-term caval patency is also 98%. Indications for placement of a caval filter include (1)

---

*Not FDA-approved for this indication.

propagation or embolism of acute thrombus despite adequate anticoagulation; (2) bleeding on anticoagulation requiring transfusion, (3) the presence of other contraindications to anticoagulation, (4) diminished cardiopulmonary reserves or massive pulmonary embolism, which predispose the patient to severe hemodynamic instability in the event of a subsequent pulmonary embolism of any size, and (5) patients undergoing surgery while on anticoagulation for acute DVT.

SPECIAL CLINICAL CIRCUMSTANCES

Free-Floating Thrombi. When diagnosed by ascending venography or ultrasonography, a free-floating thrombus raises serious concern in the clinician regarding its implication. The intuitive concern is that these thrombi would be more likely to embolize to the lung than thrombi that are adherent to the vein wall. The literature has many studies assessing the risk of embolization of free-floating thrombi compared with non–free-floating thrombi. There is no consensus in the literature on how best to treat free-floating thrombi or whether to treat them any differently, i.e., the placement of an inferior vena cava filter. The main question to be answered is what proportion of free-floating thrombi represents the remnants subsequent to pulmonary emboli or the actual source of the embolization. In our practice, we treat free-floating thrombi the same way we treat any acute DVT.

Pregnancy. Gravid patients with DVT pose a challenge to the clinician. Warfarin, unlike heparin, crosses the placenta. Warfarin should not be used during pregnancy due to its potential teratogenic and hemorrhagic effects on the fetus. Gravid patients should be treated with intravenous heparin and then converted to full-dose subcutaneous heparin. As with intravenous heparin, the aPTT should be kept between 60 and 80 seconds. The daily dose of subcutaneous heparin will be higher than that of intravenous heparin. Alternatively, LMWH may be used during pregnancy. In pregnant patients who develop heparin-induced platelet antibodies from both unfractionated and LMWH, the heparinoid danaparoid (Org 10172) may be used. Anticoagulation should be continued until term. Postpartum, anticoagulation is reinstated with heparin and warfarin until a therapeutic INR is reached. Thereafter, warfarin is continued for an additional 4 to 6 weeks.

Calf Vein Thrombosis. There is a great deal of controversy in the literature about the indications to treat as well as to the treatment of calf vein thrombosis. However, because calf vein thrombosis is reported to be the source of fatal pulmonary emboli in 15% to 25% of patients, we treat calf vein thrombosis by one of two approaches. For calf vein thrombi that are extensive, are symptomatic, or occur in patients with significant risk factors, full anticoagulation with warfarin for 6 to 8 weeks is recommended. This may be done without heparinization in the outpatient setting. For calf vein thrombi that occur in asymptomatic, ambulatory patients with minimal risk factors, or in patients who have absolute contraindications to anticoagulation, serial duplex ultrasound twice weekly for 2 to 3 weeks is acceptable. If the thrombus propagates proximally into any part of the popliteal vein, then either immediate anticoagulation with heparin and warfarin is initiated, or a caval filter is inserted.

Prophylaxis. Every patient should be considered for DVT prophylaxis at the time of admission. The patients should be categorized according to risk factors for DVT. Table 2 summarizes recommendations for prophylaxis.

Recurrence. This is a very challenging aspect in the treatment of venous thrombosis. The symptoms of recurrent DVT resemble those of the postphlebitic syndrome. The diagnosis of recurrent acute DVT requires documentation with a venogram or duplex ultrasound. The patient is treated with anticoagulation with heparin and warfarin and an underlying cause is sought. In the patient who develops a recurrent acute DVT despite *adequate* anticoagulation, an

TABLE 2. **Recommended Prophylaxis Regimens**

Low Risk	
(Minor surgery in patients <40 yr with no risk factors; general medical patients with CHF, MI, stroke)	Heparin 5000 U every 12 h or intermittent compression stockings
Moderate Risk	
(Major surgery in patients >40 yr with no other risk factors)	Heparin 5000 U 2 h before and q 12 h after surgery or Low-molecular-weight heparin, or Intermittent pneumatic compression stockings
High Risk	
(Major surgery in patient > 40 yr with other risk factors)	Heparin 5000 U 2 h before and every 8 h after surgery or Low-molecular-weight heparin, or Intermittent pneumatic compression stockings
Very High Risk	
(Major surgery in patients >40 yr plus previous DVT or malignant disease or orthopedic surgery or hip fracture or stroke or spinal cord injury)	Heparin 5000 U 2 h before surgery followed by therapeutic heparin or Low-molecular-weight heparin or Warfarin (INR 2–3) or Intermittent pneumatic compression stockings (+one of the above)
Patients with indwelling venous catheters	Add warfarin 1 mg daily
Patients at risk for intracranial bleed (Hemorrhagic stroke, CNS/eye surgery)	Intermittent pneumatic compression stockings

Modified from Clagett G: Prevention of venous thromboembolism. *CHEST 108*:316S, 1995.

aggressive search for underlying causes is mandatory. Solid malignancies should be ruled out, as Trousseau's syndrome may result in thrombosis resistant to warfarin. Antiphospholipid antibody syndrome, consisting of the lupus anticoagulant and anticardiolipin antibody syndrome, carries a high risk of recurrent thrombosis. In these patients, the INR is to be kept above 3.0. Other conditions, such as resistance to activated protein-C, protein-C and protein-S deficiencies, and other hematologic hypercoagulable states, should be excluded. In patients with recurrence while on Coumadin, levels of factors II and X should be checked to make sure they are adequately suppressed despite a therapeutic INR.

APLASTIC ANEMIA

method of
LYLE L. SENSENBRENNER, M.D.
University of Maryland School of Medicine
Baltimore, Maryland

Aplastic anemia is a clinical syndrome characterized by pancytopenia of varying degree. In addition, hypoplastic marrow with no evidence of infiltrating disease present must be demonstrated. What hematopoietic cells remain usually show no evidence of dysplastic changes. Although macrocytosis may be seen in the erythroid lines in some patients, no dyserythropoiesis or dysplastic changes of the granulocytic or megakaryocytic lines should be seen. Chromosomal analysis of those hematopoietic cells in the marrow must show no clonal abnormalities such as chromosomal deletions or translocations. Occasionally a clone of cells demonstrating an abnormality of the X chromosome's gene for a protein involved in the biosynthesis of glycosyl phosphatidylinositol anchors (PIG-A gene), resulting in paroxysmal nocturnal hemoglobinuria (PNH), will be present in patients with aplastic anemia. This will result in markedly increased susceptibility to complement lysis of all blood cells derived from the PNH clone.

Aplastic anemia is classified in several ways. The two most commonly used classifications are according to the severity of the pancytopenia (severe, supersevere, and not severe or moderate) and etiologically—that is, whether or not there is an inherited condition predisposing to the disorder or whether the disease is acquired in the absence of a recognized underlying predisposition (inherited versus acquired aplastic anemia). These classifications are shown in Table 1.

The end result of the pathogenic process is the failure of the marrow to produce an adequate number of precursors and mature cells. Toxins and other marrow-damaging agents may clearly be acting through a direct destruction of the earliest stem cells in the marrow. However, it appears that in addition to total destruction of the stem cell, nonlethal damage to some marrow cells, presumably early progenitors, exposes antigens, which sets off processes that induce an autoimmune destruction or suppression of early stem and progenitor cells. This autoimmune process may play a major role in the ablation of the marrow. Whatever the pathogenesis or etiology, replacement of the stem cells and immune system from an allogeneic donor appears able to correct the defect, since allogeneic marrow transplantation has been reported to be successful in restoring normal hematopoiesis in all forms of aplastic anemia thus far identified.

CLINICAL PRESENTATION

Since pancytopenia is the major manifestation of aplastic anemia, a complication of one of the cytopenias usually results in symptoms forcing the patient to seek medical attention. The most common presenting feature is bleeding secondary to thrombocytopenia. This is usually first manifested by petechiae, especially of the dependent portions of the body, or minor bleeding from other sources, such as the gums when brushing one's teeth. The petechiae frequently will progress to ecchymosis for which the patient has no history of trauma to explain their presence. The second most common presenting symptom is frequent or severe infections with no clear explanation. These infections are frequently at the site of minor trauma such as a small cut or skin break or in the mouth, throat, nasal passages, and sinuses. Anemia with its symptoms of fatigue, shortness of breath on exertion, and weakness is occasionally the factor initiating the patient's visit to the physician's office.

LABORATORY STUDIES

The diagnosis of aplastic anemia is made by a careful, complete blood count performed on at least two occasions in order to determine the degree of pancytopenia. In addition, a careful inspection of the peripheral blood smear and marrow aspirate is essential to rule out any dysplastic changes in any of the cell lineages or their precursors. A bone marrow biopsy is essential to accurately assess the

TABLE 1. **Classification of Aplastic Anemia**

Severity

Supersevere	Neutrophils $< 200/mm^3$
	Platelets $< 20,000/mm^3$
	Reticulocytes $< 40,000/mm^3$
Severe (2 of 3)	Neutrophils $< 500/mm^3$
	Platelets $< 20,000/mm^3$
	Reticulocytes $< 40,000/mm^3$
Moderate	Pancytopenia less than severe

Etiologic Classification

Acquired aplastic anemia
  Idiopathic
  Secondary to a recognized etiologic agent
    Toxins and chemicals—benzene, trinitrotoluene, chlorophenol pesticides
    Drugs—chloramphenicol, hydantoins, gold, carbamazepine, phenylbutazone, sulfonamides, penicillamine, cancer chemotherapeutics
    Viruses—Epstein-Barr virus, hepatitis (not A, B, C, or D, possibly G)
    Autoimmune disorders
    Radiation
    Pregnancy
Inherited aplastic anemia
  Fanconi's anemia
  Dyskeratosis congenita
  Shwachman-Diamond syndrome
  Amegakaryocytic thrombocytopenia
  Familial aplastic anemia

cellularity of the marrow and to determine the presence of any infiltrating diseases, such as metastatic cancer or lymphoma. Chromosomal analysis of the marrow aspirate cells should also be done to rule out any clonal dysplastic disorder. In patients under the age of 35 years, careful attention to the physical examination is essential to be sure whether Fanconi's anemia is or is not present. If there is any suspicion that Fanconi's anemia might be the underlying etiology (short stature, history or presence of extra or missing digits on the hands, numerous café au lait spots, or congenital renal abnormalities) a clastogen-induced chromosomal breakage study of peripheral blood lymphocytes should be done to rule in or out the disorder. A careful history attempting to determine any underlying etiology or familial incidence is of value for determining the type of aplastic anemia the patient might have. The approach to therapy in some cases such as Fanconi's anemia varies significantly from that used in acquired forms of the disorder.

THERAPY

Bone Marrow Transplantation

Specific therapeutic approaches are determined to a great extent by the severity and etiology of the aplasia, as well as the age of the patient. For patients who have severe acquired aplastic anemia, the therapy of choice is marrow transplantation if the patient is less than 55 to 60 years of age. However, for such a procedure to be successful it is necessary for the patient to have an HLA identical donor. A sibling donor is preferred. If none is available, one can occasionally find a perfectly matched donor in the unrelated donor registry. Since the earlier in the course of the disease one attempts transplant the more successful the procedure is, one should refer all potential transplant patients to a transplant center immediately upon making the diagnosis of severe aplastic anemia. With allogeneic marrow transplantation utilizing an HLA-matched sibling donor, one expects a long-term disease-free survival of greater than 75%, and if there is no radiation in the regimen used to prepare the patient for transplant, a very low incidence of late neoplastic complications (less than 5%).

Patients with inherited forms of aplastic anemia are also candidates for marrow transplantation if a suitable donor can be found. However, it is essential to determine the underlying disease process such as Fanconi's anemia, since those patients are exceedingly sensitive to both radiation and alkylating agents and must be prepared for transplant with a much milder regimen. Patients with Fanconi's anemia who have no donor readily available do frequently respond to androgen therapy, but their response to immunosuppressive therapy has been very poor.

Immunosuppressive Therapy

If the patient is over 55 to 60 years of age, or no donor can be readily identified, immune suppressive therapy should be attempted. The most commonly used regimen is antithymocyte globulin (ATG) (At-

gam), and a successful regimen is 40 mg per kg per day for 4 consecutive days intravenously, followed by 3 to 4 months of cyclosporine (Sandimmune),* starting at 5 mg per kg per day as a continuous infusion, and after 5 days gradually tapering the dose to maintain a blood level of between 150 and 450 ng per mL of whole blood. If the patient can tolerate the drug orally, it may be given in doses of 10 to 20 mg per kg per day in divided doses every 12 hours. Careful attention to blood levels of cyclosporine and creatinine are necessary, with adjustments in the cyclosporine dose should toxicity occur.

Serum sickness is a common complication of ATG therapy. It is treated with a steroid such as methylprednisolone (Solu-Medrol) at a dose of 0.5 to 1.0 mg per kg per day. This dose should be tapered and then discontinued as soon as the process subsides.

If patients have not responded to the therapy by 4 months after starting the cyclosporine, it should be stopped. However, if the patient has responded, the cyclosporine is tapered slowly at no more than 5% a week, watching the blood counts carefully and reinstituting higher doses should the counts begin to fall. Most patients can be tapered off the drug entirely.

Another immune suppressive regimen recently reported by us to be very effective in a small series of patients with severe acquired aplastic anemia is the use of cyclophosphamide (Cytoxan),* 45 mg per kg per day for 4 days given as an intravenous infusion over 1 to 2 hours. Unlike patients who respond to ATG-based immune suppressive regimens, the patients in this small series who responded to cyclophosphamide had no episodes of relapse of their disease and no late clonal disorders.

Androgens

Androgens either alone or in combination with immunosuppressive therapy have had some degree of efficacy, but the results have been extremely variable. Reported studies vary from no responders to greater than 30% of patients responding. There is no doubt that some people with aplastic anemia respond to androgens. The most commonly used agent has been oxymetholone (Anadrol-50),† at a dose of 3 to 5 mg per kg per day orally. However, at the present time this compound is no longer available in the United States. Nandrolone decanoate (Deca-Durabolin), a compound that is as effective as oxymetholone, is available and possibly has less hepatotoxicity. However, it must be given intramuscularly, a potential problem in patients with low platelets and neutrophils. The dosage is 3 to 5 mg per kg weekly for up to 12 weeks. The drug is given deep intramuscularly in the buttocks. We have also used danazol (Danocrine),* 400 to 800 mg per day orally, with some success.

---

*Not FDA approved for this indication.
†Investigational drug in the United States.

Blood Product Support

Since pancytopenia is the major manifestation of aplastic anemia, life-saving emergency supportive measures must be directed to correcting the complications of bleeding, infections, and anemia. Thrombocytopenic bleeding can be a serious and even lethal complication of aplastic anemia and is corrected primarily by the use of platelets to support the patient. Major bleeding almost never occurs in patients with aplastic anemia when the platelets are greater than 20,000 per µL of blood. Significant bleeding usually occurs only when the platelet count has fallen to 5000 per µL of blood or less. Since platelet transfusions can and often do lead to severe alloimmunization, resulting in refractoriness to further platelet infusions, the fewer transfusions given the patient the less likely alloimmunization will result. Therefore our guidelines are to transfuse only if one of the following is present: (1) the platelet count is 5000 or less, (2) the patient is bleeding, (3) the patient is febrile, with a platelet count of 10,000 or less, (4) the patient has clearly demonstrated bleeding at a count greater than 5000 per µL of blood, and the count is now that low, or (5) the patient is to undergo a procedure that could cause bleeding, such as a surgical operation, a diagnostic scoping procedure, or tooth extraction.

Since alloimmunization is a major problem and is contributed to by the leukocytes contaminating a platelet transfusion, the use of leukocyte-depleted platelet products should be standard practice whenever transfusing aplastic anemia patients. Filters are now available that will adequately remove the leukocytes present. If platelet support is required, 10-minute post-transfusion platelet counts are done in order to determine whether or not an adequate increment rise in platelet count was obtained with each transfusion. If a poor response to the transfused platelets is detected, studies of lymphocytotoxic antibody should be carried out. If evidence of severe alloimmunization is detected, either the use of platelet cross-matching or obtaining platelets matched for the class 1 HLA antigens of the patient may be required to identify a platelet product for obtaining an adequate increment in the platelet count with transfusion. Alloimmunization becomes a very severe problem for patients who might be candidates for allogeneic bone marrow transplantation. White blood cell antigens are also responsible for the rejection of an allogeneic marrow graft. It has been clearly shown that the fewer the number of transfusions a patient with aplastic anemia has received, the more likely the patient is to accept an allograft. Thus it is vitally important that patients who might be candidates for a transplant receive as few transfusions as possible and that the transfusions they receive be leukocyte depleted.

As the disease progresses, anemia becomes a severe problem, and red blood cell transfusions are required. Most patients can tolerate a slowly developing anemia as long as the hemoglobin level remains at 7 grams per dL or higher. If the patient is symptomatic from his or her anemia at a level greater than 7 and unable to carry out normal functions, transfusions of red blood cells are indicated. If bleeding is a problem, or patients are to undergo a procedure that could result in bleeding, the hemoglobin level should be maintained at least 2 grams higher—that is, above 9 grams per dL, or 2 grams above the symptomatic level if the symptomatic level is greater than 7 grams per dL. As with platelets, all red blood cell products should be administered leukocyte-depleted to prevent alloimmunization.

Each unit of red blood cells contains about 250 mg of iron, an element the body has no mechanism for removing. If iron stores develop to a high level, damage to pancreas, liver, and heart can result, with lethal consequences. To prevent such complications, chelation therapy should be instituted early in the course of the disease. At the present time, the only chelating agent available is deferoxamine mesylate (Desferal Mesylate), which must be administered either very slowly intravenously or by subcutaneous infusion. The usual dose of deferoxamine is 1.5 to 2.5 grams per day subcutaneously, using a portable pump. Chelation therapy should begin after 20 to 50 units of red blood cells have been administered or the serum ferritin level is greater than 600 ng per mL.

Neutropenia results in increased susceptibility to bacterial and fungal infections. For the severely neutropenic patient, meticulous care should be taken to prevent such infections. This includes careful cleansing and prevention of breaks in the skin. Finger or earlobe sticks to obtain blood should be avoided. Careful handwashing is essential, as is good oral hygiene and dental care to prevent infectious sites from developing. The use of prophylactic antibiotics is to be avoided except to cover the patient during an invasive procedure such as tooth extraction or colonoscopy. The routine use of antibiotic prophylaxis with an agent such as fluconazol (Diflucan) can and often does lead to overgrowth of resistant fungi. Infections that do occur in neutropenic patients must be treated promptly with empiric broad-spectrum antibiotics while awaiting the results of cultures of blood, urine, throat, sputum and any potentially infected site.

Imipenem (Primaxin), 500 to 1000 mg intravenously every 6 hours, or ceftazidime (Fortaz, Tazicef, Tazidime), 1.0 to 2.0 grams every 8 hours intravenously, is an effective empirical antibiotic regimen that can be used in febrile, neutropenic patients while one is attempting to isolate and identify the causative organism. If after 48 to 72 hours the patient remains febrile with little in the way of signs of improvement, vancomycin (Vancocin or Vancoled), 1 gram every 12 hours intravenously, is added to cover possible gram-positive organisms. If fever continues more than another 72 hours on the double antibiotic regimen and a source and organism have not been determined, or if the patient appears to be deteriorating, antifungal coverage with amphotericin B (Fungizone, Amphozone), 0.75 to 1 mg per kg per day intravenously, should be added. If the patient demonstrates a serious infection with an organism shown to be resistant to antibiotics, granulocyte transfusions may be considered but are fraught with severe reactions in addition to alloimmunization. In addition, in patients with no defined neutropenia, granulocytes are frequently ineffective in the long run.

The injudicious use of blood products in patients who are possible candidates for allogeneic transplant could jeopardize a later transplant. Many viruses can be transmitted with transfusions. One that is particularly important is the cytomegalovirus (CMV). Patients who are CMV serologically negative and who have a donor who is serologically negative have the best chance of not developing problems with the virus during the transplant. Therefore all blood products given to a patient with aplastic anemia who is a potential transplant candidate should be from a CMV-negative donor until the CMV serologic status of the patient has been established. If the patient or the donor is CMV serology–positive, the CMV status of the blood product is not important. However if the patient is CMV-negative, all blood products should be from CMV-negative donors only. Since alloimmunization is a major problem for the patient with aplastic anemia, as few transfusions as possible from as few donors as possible should be given. Since family members could share minor antigens with the donor, antigens the patient may not have, one should never use family members as donors of blood products for a patient who might be a candidate for a family member transplant.

Hematopoietic Growth Factors

If the granulocyte count is less than 500 per μL, granulocyte colony-stimulating factor (G-CSF) (Neupogen) or granulocyte-macrophage colony-stimulating factor (GM-CSF) (Leukine) may be used temporarily to raise the granulocyte counts. The usual dosage is 250 μg per m^2 per day given subcutaneously. However, this rarely causes a rise in the hemoglobin level or the platelet count, and the granulocyte count drops back to the pretreatment level shortly after stopping the drug. Thus far the utility of growth factors in patients with aplastic anemia has been very limited and appears to work best in those with higher granulocyte counts to start with.

IRON DEFICIENCY ANEMIA

method of
JONATHAN GLASS, M.D.
Louisiana State University Medical Center
Shreveport, Louisiana

Iron deficiency remains a worldwide problem. In the developed countries, the problem arises from specific problems in individual patients—for example, the increased blood loss that might ensue from gastritis in a patient using nonsteroidal anti-inflammatory agents (NSAIDs). In the developing world, the problem is one of public health and improving the nutritional status of populations at risk. Although yeoman efforts in many countries have addressed endemic iron deficiency, intensive nutritional education and programs of nutritional supplementation are still required. The ease of sampling blood and measuring hematologic parameters makes it easy to forget that iron deficiency is a systemic disease of which the anemia is but one manifestation. The effects of iron deficiency on work performance and exercise tolerance may have significant negative economic impact by impeding work productivity. Iron deficiency occurring during early childhood growth and development may adversely affect psychomotor development and cognitive function that may not correct despite repletion of iron stores. Finally, because of the unique limits on iron stores and the ability to increase iron absorption, iron deficiency may serve as a herald of underlying pathology. Hence, prevention of the onset of the iron deficiency state and early recognition of iron deficiency is extremely important and requires that the physician be attuned to a variety of aspects of iron nutrition. In particular, the clinician needs to be cognizant of distribution of iron in foodstuffs; the mechanisms of intestinal iron absorption, including the site of absorption and factors influencing absorption; and the mechanisms of iron transport within the body. The clinician needs to be able to recognize those illnesses that arise from lack of the nutrient and distinguish the disorders of iron deficiency from disorders of malutilization of the nutrient. Most importantly, the clinician must remember that iron deficiency anemia is a signal for underlying pathology and that ferreting out the abnormality is as much a part of the treatment of iron deficiency as is replacing the iron.

IRON STATUS

There are multiple means for evaluation of the iron stores in an individual. Iron deficiency anemia, as with all anemias, is not a disease but a sign of the disease. Hence, patients may present with the manifestation of the underlying disease as well as symptoms of the anemia. The majority of patients will seek medical attention because of the symptoms that arise from the iron deficiency anemia; a minority of patients present because of the disease causing the anemia. The recognition of iron deficiency as a cause for an anemia is aided by understanding the various conditions that may lead to iron deficiency. Table 1 lists the more common causes for iron deficiency anemia.

Pregnancy imposes a serious drain on iron stores. Iron

TABLE 1. **Causes of Iron Deficiency**

Increased Requirements and/or Decreased Intake
Pregnancy
Growth spurts
Infancy and prematurity
Decreased Absorption
Gastric surgery
Achlorhydria
Malabsorption
Increased Loss
Menses
Gastritis
Colon cancer

is required for the increased maternal blood volume and for transfer to the fetus. In addition there is blood loss in the placenta and cord and blood loss in delivery. The average requirement for iron during pregnancy is about 2.5 mg per day in comparison to the normal female daily requirement of 1.0 to 1.5 mg per day. At birth, the total body iron is about 250 mg, of which about 25% is in iron stores, 70% is in hemoglobin, and the remainder in myoglobin and various iron-containing enzymes such as the cytochromes. During the first 4 to 6 months, the total body iron is relatively stable, and iron is shifted from stores to hemoglobin to allow for the increased red blood cell mass and myoglobin and enzymes. Hence, unless the infants were premature and had not developed sufficient iron stores or unless there was perinatal blood loss, iron deficiency anemia is uncommon in the first few months of life. Subsequently, from about 4 months to 12 months of age, there is a substantial growth spurt requiring an increase of total body iron to about 420 mg to accommodate both the rapid growth and the concomitant increase in blood volume. Iron supplementation of infant diets, especially for the preterm infant, is required to prevent iron deficiency.

The growth spurt of adolescence is another period when iron stores may be marginal. Iron deficiency occurs with similar frequency in males and females, the former having a larger increase of blood volume, the latter having the additional loss above basal amounts from the onset of menses.

The absorption of iron depends on many factors, including gastric acid production, the acid required to maintain iron solubility, and an intact duodenum, the site of iron absorption. Hence, after total or partial gastrectomy, iron deficiency may occur both from loss of acid production and, in the case of a Billroth II procedure, from bypassing the duodenum. Many patients with pernicious anemia will also develop iron deficiency anemia because of the achlorhydria, although the use of H_2 blockers results in no clinical iron deficiency. Patients with celiac sprue and tropical sprue frequently have an iron deficiency anemia. Both pica and pagophagia may be engaged in because of iron deficiency. The ingestion of certain substances, including ice, soothes the irritation that results from a thinned, iron-deficient mucosa. However, certain substances, especially clay (geophagia) and laundry starch (amylophagia), can impede iron absorption. Hence, pica resulting from custom or culture can result in iron deficiency anemia.

While there is regulation of iron absorption, there is no regulatory mechanism for iron excretion. Normally, approximately 1 mg per day, primarily from shed intestinal mucosa and blood loss, is lost. Menses impose another approximate 0.5 to 1.0 mg per day loss as there is about 0.5 mg of iron per milliliter of blood. A normal Western diet contains about 6 mg of iron per 1000 calories, and, although the intestine can increase absorption in response to low iron stores, maximum absorption is about 1.5 to 2 mg of iron per day. Hence, as little as 3 to 4 mL per day of blood loss can result in negative iron balance.

There are multiple causes for increased blood loss. In the gastrointestinal tract, drugs are a major offender, especially aspirin and the other NSAIDs. Benign conditions include reflux esophagitis, gastric and peptic ulcers, colonic diverticuli, ulcerative colitis, and inflammatory bowel disease. In addition, various infestations such as hookworm, *Necator americanus*, and *Ancylostoma duodenale* can be important causes of gastrointestinal blood loss in the tropics. Increased menstrual losses, especially if coupled to multiple pregnancies, are a major cause of iron deficiency anemia in women of childbearing age.

TABLE 2. **Evaluation of Iron Stores**

Hematologic observations: microcytosis, hypochromia, anisocytosis
Serum iron and iron-binding capacity
Serum ferritin
Serum transferrin receptors
Bone marrow iron stores

EVALUATION OF IRON STORES

Having recognized the condition that leads to the anemia, the physician can look for signs that indicate iron deficiency. These may include koilonychia, papillary atrophy of the tongue, and angular stomatitis. In addition, it may be possible to demonstrate achlorhydria or occult blood in the stools. Shortly, however, the iron stores will need to be assessed through a variety of laboratory tests as outlined in Table 2.

The size of the red blood cell is controlled in part by the concentration of hemoglobin, the differentiating red blood cell undergoing an additional division within the bone marrow to achieve as normal a corpuscular hemoglobin concentration as possible. Hence, any disorder that impedes hemoglobin synthesis will result in a microcytic, hypochromic anemia. Decreased hemoglobin synthesis may result either from decreased heme or decreased globin production. Decreased heme synthesis will occur with iron deficiency (too little iron to be placed into protoporphyrin); the anemia of chronic disease (iron is prevented from leaving storage sites and from entering the red cell); lead poisoning (lead inhibits heme synthesis); and sideroblastic anemias (an intrinsic defect in mitochrondrial synthesis of protoporphyrin). Decreased globin synthesis may be the result of one of the thalassemias. The red blood cell size may be assessed from the peripheral smear. The red blood cell is normally the size of the nucleus of a mature lymphocyte. The hemoglobin concentration may be judged from the central pallor that is normally about one third the diameter of the cell. With the automated laboratory equipment available, the size or mean corpuscular volume (MCV) in femtoliters (fL) and the mean corpuscular hemoglobin concentration (MCHC) in grams per deciliter (gm/dL) is readily available and more reliable than one's eye. In addition, anisocytosis or differing sizes of red blood cells is also quantified as the red cell distribution width (RDW) and is frequently elevated in iron deficiency.

As will be discussed, the five disorders leading to microcytic, hypochromic anemias can be distinguished by the history, the physical examination, and the judicious application of the other tests noted in Table 2. One common problem, especially in children, is to distinguish the hypochromic anemia of iron deficiency from that of thalassemia minor. Various discriminant functions have been devised. One easily applied calculation is the MCV/RBC, which in iron deficiency is greater than 13 and in thalassemia minor is less than 13.

Serum iron and iron-binding capacity are a reasonable next step for evaluating iron stores. The major limitations of these tests are the variability in the values, especially between laboratories. The limitations of the variability may be overcome by determining the transferrin saturation with the following formula:

$$\text{Transferrin saturation (\%)} = \frac{\text{Serum iron} \times 100}{\text{Total iron-binding capacity (TIBC)}}$$

In iron deficiency, the transferrin saturation is frequently less than 10%. The low saturation is the result of decreased iron entering the plasma, increased plasma iron turnover, and increased transferrin synthesis by the liver in response to decreased stores. In the anemia of chronic disease, iron is inhibited from leaving storage sites and therefore serum iron is often low. However, the saturation is usually not as severe as in iron deficiency and is in the range of 10% to 15%. In the other conditions, the transferrin saturation is frequently elevated: In the thalassemias, the hemolytic anemia increases intestinal iron absorption; in lead toxicity and the sideroblastic anemias, the incorporation of iron into heme is blocked by decreased heme synthesis and iron cannot be unloaded from transferrin.

Serum ferritin concentrations have been widely used as a measure of iron stores. Ferritin synthesis is proportional to iron stores, and as a certain proportion of ferritin is exported into the plasma, serum ferritin levels reflect iron stores, with 1 μg per liter being the equivalent of about 8 to 12 mg of storage iron. In a normal population serum ferritin concentrations range from 12 to 300 μg per liter. The proportionality of serum ferritin to tissue stores of iron is lost under certain circumstances, in particular when tissue damage results in release of more ferritin. Hence, with inflammatory diseases, infections, liver disease, and malignancies, serum ferritins may not be of diagnostic value. Nonetheless, serum ferritin concentrations can often discriminate between iron deficiency and the other causes of a microcytic, hypochromic anemia.

More recently the serum transferrin receptor has been used as a sensitive and early predictor of iron deficiency. The transferrin receptor is highly expressed on plasma membrane of differentiating erythroid cells. The expression is inversely proportional to the iron stores of the cells. Fortuitously, a proportion of the receptor is proteolytically cleaved and released to the plasma where the receptor can be readily assayed. The synthesis of the transferrin receptor is not affected by inflammation, infection, or malignancies. Serum concentrations of the receptor increase as stores are depleted, and the transferrin receptor concentration is an early indicator of depleted iron stores.

The definitive measurement of iron stores is by Prussian blue staining of bone marrow spicules obtained by aspiration of the marrow. Provided that there are sufficient spicules on the smear, the blue granules of iron in tissue histiocytes can be graded from 0 to 6+ and correlate well with iron stores. In addition, the hematologist can assess whether granules are present in erythroid precursors and macrophages. In the anemia of chronic disease, hemosiderin will be present only in macrophages. In the sideroblastic anemias, iron granules will ring the nuclei of the erythroid cells, giving the characteristic ringed sideroblast. Bone marrow biopsies are not adequate for evaluating stores. The sections through a biopsy do not include an entire cell and therefore may underestimate iron stores.

The net result of the hematologic observations and the various laboratory studies is summarized in Table 3 as used to distinguish among the various microcytic, hypochromic anemias.

TREATMENT

The first principle in the treatment of iron deficiency anemia is to know the etiology of the iron deficiency and to correct the underlying disease. In general in most patients, the onset of the disease is insidious and the progression of the symptoms is gradual. Therefore, one is not frequently pressed to correct the anemia urgently unless there are signs of cardiac failure. The principle of correcting the iron deficiency is to replenish the iron stores with the simplest, least expensive preparation possible.

Iron can be administered orally, intramuscularly, or intravenously. The oral route is the safest and is usually well tolerated. For those individuals who cannot tolerate oral iron preparations, or if prior gastric surgery has bypassed the duodenum, it may be necessary to administer iron intravenously. The standard oral preparation is ferrous sulfate, ferrous gluconate, or ferrous fumarate. Ferrous sulfate is the most commonly used form, and the 300-mg tablet contains 60 mg of elemental iron.

Iron absorption is greatest when the stomach is empty. Maximal iron absorption occurs when ferrous sulfate is taken 1 to 2 hours before meals. An additional ferrous sulfate tablet at bedtime will further maximize the daily absorption. With this regimen in a severely iron-deficient patient, about 40 to 50 mg of iron can be absorbed daily; however, as the anemia abates the rate of absorption will decrease. Since a deficit of 1 gram of hemoglobin corresponds to about 150 mg of iron in an average-sized adult, about 500 to 1000 mg of iron will have to be absorbed to correct

TABLE 3. **Findings in Hypochromic Anemias**

| | | | Serum | | | | Marrow Iron | | |
Disease	Hct (%)	Morphology	Fe	TIBC	Fe/TIBC	Ferritin	Tf Receptor	Siderocytes	Macrophages
Iron deficiency	20–30	Microchromic, microcytic, pencil shapes	↓	↑ ↑	<10%	↓	↑ ↑	Absent	Absent
Anemia of chronic disease	28–32	Microchromic, rarely hypochromic	↓	↓	10–15%	N, ↑	N	Absent	Present
Lead intoxication	26–30	Microcytic, basophilic stippling	N, ↑	N	N, ↑	N, ↑	N, ↓	Present	Present
Sideroblastic anemias	15–30	Dimorphic	N, ↑	N	N, ↑	N, ↑	N, ↓	Rings	Present
Thalassemias	15–30	Microcytic, hypochromic, targets, teardrops, nucleated RBC	N, ↑	N	N, ↑	N, ↑	N, ↓	Present	Present

Abbreviations: Hct = hematocrit; Fe = iron; TIBC = total iron-binding capacity; Tf = transferrin.

the anemia and an equal amount to replenish iron stores. Because the rate of iron absorption will decrease with iron repletion, the anemia will be corrected in 1 to 2 months, and a total of about 3 to 4 months of iron supplementation will be needed to replete stores fully.

The response to iron can be observed by measuring the reticulocyte count that should rise to about 5% to 10% at about 10 days after therapy is initiated. Failure to respond to therapy can result from many causes: noncompliance of the patient in taking the medication; incorrect iron preparation or instructions for taking the prescribed iron; incorrect diagnosis; a concurrent illness that prevents erythropoiesis; malabsorption of iron; and/or continuing iron loss in excess of iron repletion. In reviewing these causes, it is important to remember situations in which concurrent causes for anemia can occur. For example, iron deficiency can occur in rheumatoid arthritis from the use of anti-inflammatory drugs, but the anemia of chronic disease is also common in rheumatoid arthritis. Likewise, pernicious anemia and iron deficiency can coexist, leading to a so-called dimorphic anemia.

There is no evidence that more expensive preparations have a therapeutic advantage. Iron with ascorbic acid increases the side effects of iron therapy, and the increase in iron absorption can be achieved by increasing the dose of ferrous sulfate. Enteric-coated tablets are designed to delay the dissolution of the tablet. As a consequence, the iron preparation may pass by the duodenum and not be absorbed.

The major side effect of iron therapy is gastrointestinal intolerance, with symptoms including heartburn, nausea, abdominal cramps, and diarrhea. In many patients, the symptoms can be relieved by taking the iron with meals although this maneuver will decrease the amount of iron absorbed. The symptoms can be minimized also by decreasing the dose. In some patients, ferrous sulfate elixir, 125 mg per mL of ferrous sulfate, or 25 mg per mL of elemental iron, is better tolerated.

The indications for parental iron are for individuals who (1) cannot tolerate oral iron; (2) are not compliant with medication; (3) malabsorb iron because of gastric resection and/or Bilroth II operation; or (4) continue to lose blood at a rate that is too rapid for oral absorption to compensate. Iron is given intravenously as the iron-dextran complex with 50 mg of iron per milliliter. The amount of iron to be given is calculated from the formula:

Iron to be injected (mg) =
Patient's hemoglobin (g/dL) × body weight (kg) × 3

After a test dose is administered, the entire dose of iron-dextran, diluted into 100 mL of normal saline, can be given over several hours. Immediate side effects include hypotension, urticaria, headache, nausea, and anaphylactic reactions. Delayed reactions include fever, arthralgia, lymphadenopathy, and myalgia.

AUTOIMMUNE HEMOLYTIC ANEMIA

method of
KAUSHIK A. SHASTRI, M.D., and
GERALD L. LOGUE, M.D.
*State University of New York at Buffalo and
Veterans Administration Medical Center*
Buffalo, New York

Autoimmune hemolytic anemia occurs when autoantibodies against one's own red cells are produced that lead to shortened red cell survival. When the bone marrow compensation can keep up with the shortened red cell survival, the patient does not become anemic and is said to be in a compensated hemolytic state. When the bone marrow cannot adequately compensate for the degree of hemolysis, either because of severity of hemolysis or reduced bone marrow compensation, as with folate deficiency or parvovirus infection, the patient becomes overtly anemic.

Table 1 shows the broad classification of autoimmune hemolytic anemias. In the most common type, the autoantibodies that are usually IgG react as well at body temperature as at lower temperatures and are called warm-reacting autoantibodies. The warm-reacting autoantibodies can occur in the presence of underlying connective disorders such as systemic lupus erythematosus, lymphoproliferative disorders like chronic lymphocytic leukemia, and miscellaneous disorders such as ulcerative colitis and solid tumors. About half the cases occur without an underlying cause and comprise the idiopathic warm-reacting hemolytic anemias.

The cold-reactive antibodies (cold agglutinins) are generally IgM autoantibodies that react with I or i antigens on the erythrocytes and bind optimally in cold temperatures, usually below 31°C. They can be seen in adolescents and young adults secondary to *Mycoplasma pneumoniae* infection or infectious mononucleosis and produce a self-limited disease. Chronic cold agglutinins, often in very high titers, occur in older patients with malignant lymphoproliferative disorders. Idiopathic chronic cold agglutinin disease also occurs in elderly people and is due to monoclonal IgM antibodies. Some of these patients go on to develop B cell lymphoproliferative disorders. Paroxysmal cold hemoglobinuria is a very uncommon form of autoimmune hemolytic anemia in adults. Previously associated with syphilis, it

TABLE 1. **Autoimmune Hemolytic Anemias**

Hemolytic Anemia Due to Warm-Reacting Antibodies

Idiopathic (primary)
Secondary to
  Other autoimmune diseases
  Lymphoproliferative diseases
  Miscellaneous diseases

Hemolytic Anemia Due to Cold-Reacting Antibodies

Idiopathic (primary)
Secondary to
  Lymphoproliferative diseases
  Infections (infectious mononucleosis, *Mycoplasma*)
Paroxysmal cold hemoglobinuria

Drug-Induced Hemolytic Anemias

Hapten (e.g., penicillin G)
Immune complex (e.g., quinine, quinidine)
Autoantibody (e.g., alpha-methyldopa, procainamide)

now occurs in chronic idiopathic form in about 1% of adult hemolytic anemias. It is caused by a cold-reactive IgG antibody that has a P antigen specificity. It is characterized by recurrent bouts of massive intravascular hemolysis. A related but self-limiting form occurs in children after a variety of viral infections and accounts for as many as 30% of childhood hemolytic anemias.

In drug-induced hemolytic anemias, which may account for 12% to 24% of immune hemolytic anemias, it may be difficult to prove that the hemolysis is drug induced. Patients are often on several drugs, and in some cases the metabolites and not the parent drug may produce immune hemolysis. The assays to document drug-induced hemolysis depend on the mechanism of hemolysis and are not well standardized. Many drugs can occasionally produce hemolytic anemia, and the drugs belong to a wide range of chemical classes. The three mechanisms that can cause a positive direct Coombs' test (direct antiglobulin test) and possible hemolysis are drug absorption (hapten), immune complex formation, and autoimmune induction.

Nonimmunologic adsorption of proteins to red cells may cause a positive Coombs' test but does not produce hemolysis. With the hapten mechanism, the patient develops antidrug antibodies that react with the drug bound to erythrocyte membrane, leading to extravascular destruction of erythrocytes. Penicillin is the classic example.

In the immune complex mechanism, the offending drug or drug metabolite binds to the antidrug antibody in the serum and then adheres to red cells. The immune complexes activate complement that may lead to intravascular hemolysis with resultant hemoglobinemia, hemoglobinuria, and renal failure. Only small concentrations of drug are required to initiate hemolysis once an individual has been sensitized and had antidrug antibodies. Quinine and quinidine are classic examples for immune complex formation.

In the third mechanism, the drug induces autoantibody production that reacts with red cell antigens and not the drug. Alpha-methyldopa (Aldomet) is one of the drugs that represents this group. It produces a positive direct Coombs' test in about 20% of people but produces hemolysis in about 0.5%.

CLINICAL AND LABORATORY FEATURES

The clinical presentation in warm autoimmune hemolytic anemia is variable and relates to symptoms of anemia itself or the underlying disorder. A point to consider in deciding upon transfusion is that many times the onset of anemia is so gradual that patients can tolerate severe anemia with minimal symptoms. Rapid, severe hemolysis can produce dyspnea, palpitations, and congestive heart failure. Jaundice and pallor are evident. Splenomegaly is frequently present.

Most patients with cold agglutinin hemolytic anemia have mild-to-moderate anemia with or without jaundice. Significant chilling in the microvasculature upon cold exposure gives rise to cyanosis in the fingers, toes, ears, and nose. An occasional patient can have episodic severe hemolysis with hemoglobinuria upon exposure to cold. Other physical findings depend on the underlying disorder, but splenomegaly may also be observed in idiopathic form. Hemolysis following *M. pneumoniae* infection is usually acute and self-limited, lasting for 1 to 3 weeks. Hemolysis in infectious mononucleosis occurs either at the onset or within 3 weeks. During a paroxysm of paroxysmal cold hemoglobinuria, constitutional symptoms are common. After cold exposure, the patient develops body ache, chills,

and fever. The first urine passed contains hemoglobin. Raynaud's phenomenon and cold urticaria sometimes occur.

Laboratory findings in autoimmune hemolytic anemias vary, depending on the severity of hemolysis. Reticulocytosis is usually present, but about a third of patients may not have corresponding elevation of reticulocytes. Peripheral smears may show polychromasia, microspherocytes, and nucleated red cells. Red cell agglutination may be seen on blood smear in cold agglutinin diseases. Other features include elevated lactic dehydrogenase enzyme and indirect bilirubin, and low haptoglobin.

The hallmark of autoimmune hemolytic anemias is the positive direct antiglobulin test (Coombs' test). In the majority of warm reactive autoimmune hemolytic anemias, this test is positive for IgG autoantibody with or without complement. In less than 5% of cases, the Coombs' test can be negative if there are fewer molecules of antibody on the cells and below the threshold of detection (less than 100 to 500 molecules), or the autoantibodies are of the IgA class. In the cold agglutinin diseases, the Coombs' test is positive for complement alone since the IgM antibodies dissociate at the testing temperatures, and the reagents used in the Coombs' test detect only IgG and complement. The IgG antibody of paroxysmal cold hemoglobinuria also detaches at warmer temperatures and remains undetected. It can be detected by the Donath-Landsteiner test, in which the patient's fresh serum is incubated with red cells in cold; upon warming at 37°C, intense hemolysis ensues.

In judging the clinical significance of cold agglutinins, the thermal amplitude and the titer of antibodies must be considered. Most cold agglutinins of low titers (less than 1:64) have no pathologic significance. Thermal amplitude is the highest temperature at which the antibody causes agglutination. The closer the thermal amplitude is to body temperature, the greater the potential for hemolysis.

TREATMENT

The treatment of autoimmune hemolytic anemia depends on the degree and acuity of anemia and the underlying etiology, when identified. It also differs based on the cold or warm reactive nature of the antibody, and hence these two entities are considered separately.

All patients with hemolytic anemia should receive 1 mg of folic acid orally every day because their folate requirements are increased due to compensatory erythroid hyperplasia, and folate deficiency under these circumstances can lead to profound anemia.

The need for blood transfusions in patients with autoimmune hemolytic anemia should be assessed on the basis of important symptoms of anemia. The presence of autoantibody presents problems in cross-matching, and alloantibodies may be missed. When blood transfusion is indicated on clinical grounds, appropriate serologic methods, such as absorption of a patient's serum with the patient's own red cells prior to cross-matching, should be used.

In drug-induced hemolytic anemias, discontinuing the offending drug alone may be sufficient. This is particularly important and potentially lifesaving for drugs that induce hemolysis by the immune complex mechanism. It is important to remember that when autoantibodies are induced by drugs such as alpha-methyldopa, the Coombs' test may remain positive for months after discontinuation of the drug.

Warm-Reacting Autoimmune Hemolytic Anemia

Corticosteroids are usually the first line of treatment in a patient with warm reactive autoimmune hemolytic anemia. The exact mechanism of the action of corticosteroids is not entirely clear. Potential mechanisms of action include reticuloendothelial blockade and decreased antibody production. Approximately two-thirds of patients respond to steroid treatment with stoppage or slowing of the hemolytic process. Response is usually seen within 1 to 2 weeks. Treatment is started at 60 to 100 mg of oral prednisone per day in adults. If a response is seen, the dose is tapered after 2 weeks by 20 mg every week to a baseline daily dose of 20 mg of prednisone. This dose is continued for 6 to 8 weeks after the acute hemolytic episode has subsided. The prednisone dose is further reduced over the next 4 to 8 weeks, while the hemoglobin and reticulocyte counts are closely monitored. Patients requiring continued corticosteroid treatment are best managed on alternate-day steroids because of lesser side effects, but this should be attempted only after the patient has a stable hemoglobin with a daily prednisone dose of 15 to 20 mg per day. Patients achieving complete remission of hemolysis should be followed for several years for possible relapse.

An alternative but not universally accepted strategy is the use of danazol (Danocrine)* with corticosteroids as the first-line treatment of warm-reacting autoimmune hemolytic anemia. Danazol is a synthetic derivative of ethinyl-testosterone with mild androgenic properties. Because of its potential synergistic effect with corticosteroids, fewer relapses, longer remissions, reduction in the dose of steroids, and less frequent need for splenectomy may occur. For severe hemolytic anemia, corticosteroids at the previously indicated doses can be started initially, with danazol in doses of 600 to 800 mg per day. Once the hemolysis has subsided, corticosteroids can be reduced gradually and then discontinued. If improvement is maintained, the dose of danazol can be lowered to 200 to 400 mg per day. The duration of maintenance therapy with danazol is not known, but it should be continued for a year. In one study, prednisone was able to be completely stopped in six of ten patients and reduced to 5 to 7.5 mg daily in two other patients.

Potential adverse effects of danazol include acne, hirsutism, deepening of the voice, weight gain, and altered libido. Microscopic hematuria, headaches, myalgia, muscle cramps, and elevated liver and muscle enzymes have also been reported.

Splenectomy is generally performed in patients who do not respond to corticosteroids after an adequate trial for 6 to 8 weeks, with or without danazol, or who require continued corticosteroids (prednisone in excess of 15 mg daily). About two-thirds of patients have partial or complete response to splenectomy, but relapses are frequent. Patients who relapse after splenectomy or who have suboptimal response to splenectomy may then respond to corticosteroids, frequently at lesser doses. The rationale for splenectomy is to remove the principal site of cell destruction. Splenectomy is more likely to be successful when the antibody does not fix complement, since for complement-coated erythrocytes the liver also becomes an important site of destruction. Pneumococcal vaccination should be given to all patients prior to splenectomy.

Immunosuppressive agents should be given only to patients who do not respond to corticosteroids, danazol, and splenectomy, or who have failed corticosteroids and danazol and are poor surgical candidates. Cyclophosphamide (Cytoxan),* in doses of 1 to 2 mg per kg of body weight orally, or azathioprine (Imuran),* 1 to 2 mg per kg of body weight orally, is used. Either drug may be continued for several months awaiting a response. If a response does ensue, the drugs are gradually reduced. The side effects of these agents are primarily bone marrow suppression. Cyclophosphamide can also induce hemorrhagic cystitis.

Other treatment modalities that may be used in refractory patients to induce at least a transient response after all others have been exhausted include intravenous gammaglobulin and plasmapheresis. The success of intravenous gammaglobulin has been much less compared with its use in immune thrombocytopenia. Higher doses are required (0.5 to 1 gram per kg of body weight) because of the up-regulation of the reticuloendothelial system in autoimmune hemolytic anemia. Only about a third of patients achieve transient benefit. Plasmapheresis has likewise been transiently successful in occasional case reports. In contrast to the mainly intravascular nature of IgM antibodies, the IgG antibodies are mainly extravascular, making removal by plasmapheresis difficult. There are also anecdotal reports of responses to oral cyclosporine in steroid-resistant autoimmune hemolytic anemia.

Cold-Reacting Autoimmune Hemolytic Anemia

In cold-reacting autoimmune hemolytic anemia, avoidance of cold exposure is required, and the patient should be kept warm, particularly in the extremities. Steps such as the wearing of gloves when opening the refrigerator may have to be taken. In refractory and severe chronic idiopathic cold agglutinin disease, this may involve encouraging the patient to move from the colder climate to a warmer climate.

The postinfectious causes of cold-reacting autoimmune hemolytic anemia are self-limited, and avoidance of cold may be all that is needed. In the lympho-

---

*Not FDA-approved for this indication.

*Not FDA-approved for this indication.

proliferative disease–associated cold agglutinin syndromes, treatment of the underlying neoplasm has beneficial effects on the cold antibody titers. In fact, the titer of cold agglutinins can be used to determine the success of therapy of underlying lymphoma.

In idiopathic cold agglutinin disease, cold avoidance may be all that is needed in a patient with mild hemolysis. With severe hemolysis, treatment with immunosuppressive agents as described for warm-reacting autoimmune hemolytic anemia may be attempted. Anecdotally, alpha-interferon has been used with good response. In critically ill patients, plasmapheresis may reduce the antibody transiently and reduce the hemolysis. Glucocorticoids and splenectomy are generally not helpful. When associated with syphilis, treatment of the underlying syphilis may bring about remission.

Cold agglutinins potentially can present significant problems when hypothermia is used during cardiopulmonary bypass. When the presence of cold agglutinins is known beforehand, the thermal amplitude of the antibodies should be elucidated, and the patient's temperature kept above that temperature. A variety of management strategies have been used by cardiothoracic surgeons in such cases, including crystalloid cardioplegia, normothermic ischemic arrest, and warm blood-potassium cardioplegia. In a patient with high titer and high thermal amplitude antibodies, plasmapheresis may temporarily reduce the levels of antibodies, since IgM antibodies are mainly intravascular.

NONIMMUNE HEMOLYTIC ANEMIA

method of
KENZABURO TANI, M.D., PH.D.
Institute of Medical Science, University of Tokyo
Tokyo, Japan

Hemolytic anemia is caused by increased red cell destruction and is characterized by an actual or potential shortening of red cell life span. Patients with typical hemolytic anemia are characterized clinically by anemia, jaundice, and splenomegaly. However, in some cases, marrow compensatory efforts may prevent any clinical manifestation other than a slight reduction in oxygen-carrying capacity, or exposure to a drug or an infection may result in clinical symptoms in those with minimum defects.

The pathogenesis can be subdivided into intrinsic abnormalities and extrinsic abnormalities. The intrinsic abnormalities include abnormalities in membranes, red cell enzymes, globins, and heme; the extrinsic abnormal environment causes injury and destruction by means of mechanical forces, chemicals or microorganisms, antibodies, and sequestration in the monocyte-macrophage system. Table 1 shows the classification of hemolytic anemia. This section focuses on non–antibody-mediated hemolytic anemia—namely, nonimmune hemolytic anemia. A disease caused mainly by so-called intramedullary hemolysis due to ineffective erythropoiesis is excluded from the discussion.

TABLE 1. **Classification of Hemolytic Anemia**

Intrinsic Abnormality

Membrane defect
  Hereditary spherocytosis, elliptocytosis, and pyropoikilocytosis
  Hereditary acanthocytosis and stomatocytosis
Enzyme deficiency
  Glucose-6-phosphate dehydrogenase deficiency
  Pyruvate kinase and other enzyme deficiencies
  Porphyria (congenital erythropoietic porphyria, erythropoietic protoporphyria)
Globin abnormality (hemoglobinopathy)
  Sickle cell disease and related disorders
  Unstable hemoglobins
Paroxysmal nocturnal hemoglobinuria

Extrinsic Abnormality

Mechanical
  March hemoglobinuria and sports anemia
  Traumatic cardiac hemolytic anemia
  Microangiopathic hemolytic anemia
Chemical or physical agents
Infection with microorganisms
Antibody-mediated
  Acquired hemolytic anemia due to warm-reacting autoantibodies
  Cryopathic hemolytic syndrome
  Drug reaction involving antibodies reacting with erythrocytes
  Alloimmune hemolytic disease of newborns
Hyperactivity of the monocyte-macrophage system
  Hypersplenism

DIAGNOSIS

General Approach

The first step in the diagnostic approach to anemia is to obtain hematologic values, including hemoglobin and hematocrit levels, red blood cell and reticulocyte counts, and white cell and platelet counts, and a peripheral blood film examination. In this initial screening procedure, the mean corpuscular volume (MCV) of red blood cells is calculated. Usually, MCV is normal or decreased in hemolytic anemia. A high reticulocyte count is often encountered in hemolytic anemia, and in some cases, a certain type of red cell morphologic abnormality is diagnostically important.

When hemolytic anemia is suspected, biochemical tests, including serum levels of bilirubin, haptoglobin, lactate dehydrogenase (LDH), and free hemoglobin; urinalysis for hemoglobin or hemosiderin; bone marrow examination; red cell life span; ferrokinetics; and abdominal echogram are all helpful in making a definitive diagnosis. In hemolytic anemia the hemoglobin level ranges from normal to very low, the reticulocyte index [% reticulocytes (decimal) × red blood cell count (in millions/mm^3)/50,000 (normal reticulocyte count)] is 2 or greater, and the serum (indirect) bilirubin level is increased. Increased serum LDH levels and decreased serum haptoglobin levels are also common. Bone marrow examination, red cell life span, and ferrokinetics reveal the picture of increased red cell production as well as destruction. The abdominal echogram frequently shows gallstones. It is often advisable to do the same studies on family members in cases of a possible hereditary hemolytic anemia.

Specific Plan

To establish the mechanism of hemolysis, specific laboratory tests are used for each type of hemolytic anemia. As shown in Table 2, each type of hemolytic anemia has its

TABLE 2. **Diagnostic Tests for Hemolytic Anemia**

Mechanism	Diagnostic Test
Intrinsic Abnormality	
Membrane defect	
Hereditary spherocytosis, elliptocytosis, pyropoikilocytosis	Spherocytosis, elliptocytosis, poikilocytosis, increased osmotic fragility, membrane protein deficiency, family cases, DNA diagnosis
Hereditary acanthocytosis	Acanthocytosis, abetalipoproteinemia, family cases
Hereditary stomatocytosis	Stomatocytosis, increased osmotic fragility, family cases
Enzyme deficiency	
G6PD deficiency	Drug related, sex-linked heredity, enzyme assay, Heinz bodies, DNA diagnosis
Pyruvate kinase and other enzyme deficiencies	Enzyme assay, family cases, DNA diagnosis
Congenital erythropoietic porphyria	Abnormal red cell morphology (e.g., anisocytosis), enzyme assay, accumulated uroporphyrin I in red cells, autosomal recessive, DNA diagnosis
Globin abnormality	
Thalassemia	Hypochromic and microcytic, hemoglobin electrophoresis, family cases, DNA diagnosis
Sickle cell disease	Sickling, hemoglobin electrophoresis, isoelectric focusing, solubility test, DNA diagnosis, family cases
Unstable hemoglobins	Heat or isopropanol instability test, hemoglobin electrophoresis, family cases, DNA diagnosis
Paroxysmal nocturnal hemoglobinuria	Ham test, sugar water test, flow cytometric analysis using monoclonal antibodies to CD59 or CD55
Extrinsic Abnormality	
Mechanical	
March hemoglobinuria and sports anemia	Schistocytes and spherocytes, increased plasma hemoglobin, history
Traumatic cardiac hemolytic anemia	
Microangiopathic hemolytic anemia	
Chemical or physical agents	History
Infection with microorganisms	Identification of cause of infection
Hyperactivity of the monocyte-macrophage system	
Hypersplenism	Ultrasound, computed tomography, diagnosis of underlying disease

own established methods for definitive diagnosis. One method is biochemical analysis, including enzyme activity and characterization, and protein structural analysis using electrophoresis or purification for amino acid sequencing. Recent progress in DNA cloning technology has contributed enormously to this molecular diagnosis. It is now relatively easy to identify the pathognomonic gene for each disorder from the partial amino acid sequence of purified protein or the so-called positional cloning method using a genetic linkage map. Compared with the genomic structure of a normal gene, the abnormal counterpart cDNA or genome can be cloned with relative ease from the patient's somatic cells. It is also worth mentioning that recent progress in flow cytometric analysis enables us to diagnose paroxysmal nocturnal hemoglobinuria more sensitively using monoclonal antibodies of CD55 and CD59. The combination of these new technologies allows us to diagnose nonimmune hemolytic anemia more efficiently, as well as to diagnose hemolytic anemia of unknown etiology.

TREATMENT

Treatment depends on the cause of hemolysis. Hemolytic anemia due to extrinsic abnormalities can be treated only by avoiding the causative factors and is discussed elsewhere. Here I focus on hemolytic anemia caused by intrinsic abnormalities. General therapy for hemoglobinuria and hypotension is most important in patients with hemolysis, particularly in the case of hemolytic crisis. Management in this situation includes preservation of intravascular volume and protection of renal function. Urine output should be maintained at 100 mL per hour or greater with the use of intraveneous (IV) fluids, diuretics, or mannitol, if necessary. The excretion of free hemoglobin may be improved by alkalization of the urine. Sodium bicarbonate may be added to IV fluids to increase the urinary pH to 7.5 or greater.

Education

For chronic hemolytic anemia, education on the nature of the disease, psychosocial assessments of patients and their families, and genetic counseling in cases of hereditary hemolytic anemia are important. Patients should be instructed how to prevent acute crisis, for example, avoiding offensive agents for patients with glucose-6-phosphate dehydrogenase (G6PD) deficiency, other enzyme deficiencies, or unstable hemoglobins. G6PD-deficient individuals should avoid most antimalarial agents, some sulfa drugs, some urinary antibiotics (e.g., nalidixic acid [NegGram], nitrofurantoin [Macrodantin]), mothballs, some dyes, and fava beans. Quinacrine (Atabrine), quinine, sulfoxone, sulfadiazine, sulfisoxazole (Gantrisin), aminopyrine, acetaminophen, phenacetin, para-aminosalicylic acid, L-dopa, doxorubicin (Adriamycin), probenecid (Benemid), and dimercaprol (BAL in Oil), are not considered to be associated with significant hemolysis in G6PD-deficient individuals. Some patients with unstable hemoglobins can exhibit episodic hemolysis in response to the same oxidative stressors that exacerbate the clinical phenotype of G6PD-deficient patients, because of these molecules' propensity to be hypersensitive to oxidation. Avoidance of surgical stress, infections, and pregnancy is helpful in preventing acute exacerbation of chronic hemolytic anemia due to pyruvate kinase deficiency. In cases of sickle cell anemia, detailed instructions concerning daily life activities are necessary to protect the patient from unnecessary stress and achieve a better quality of life. Other precautions include the preparation of individualized blood bank files; early detection of infection and an enlarging spleen; immunization against *Streptococcus pneumoniae, Haemophilus influenzae,* hepatitis B, and influenza in childhood; and prophylactic use of penicillin and folic acid. Retinal evaluation in school-age patients and birth control for sexually active women are also recommended. In cases of paroxysmal nocturnal hemoglobinuria (PNH), the most common causes of death are thrombosis or bone marrow failure. All patients should be educated about these complications and be instructed to seek medical assistance as soon as possible if they experience abdominal pain, backache, headache, neurologic abnormalities, or skin pain. They should also be informed of the necessity of taking thrombolytic agents in this situation.

Transfusion

Transfusion is not usually required for patients with red cell enzymopathies or membrane defects, except for some cases of severe hemolytic crisis or aplastic crisis due to parvovirus B19 infection or some other cause. Chronic transfusion is associated with alloimmunization, iron overload, and transmission of viral illness. Chelation therapy with deferoxamine is recommended when the total body iron is elevated. Usually, serum ferritin levels should not exceed 2000 µg per mL. Leukocyte-depleted red cell transfusions may be of value in reducing alloimmunization and the transmission of viral illness. The use of group- and type-specific red cells is recommended to prevent isoimmunization. In cases of sickle cell anemia, simple transfusion is sufficient to supply oxygen carrying capacity and blood volume, but partial exchange transfusion is recommended because of the improved viscosity effects and reduced iron burden of this approach. In thalassemia major, therapy consists of regular red cell transfusions to maintain a baseline hemoglobin level of greater than 9 to 10 grams per dL (hypertransfusion program), coupled with intensive parenteral chelation therapy with deferoxamine. Supertransfusion programs are used to suppress erythropoiesis further by keeping hemoglobin levels at greater than 12 grams per dL, but the long-term effects on quality of life and prognosis have not been determined. Some patients with severe PNH require transfusion. Washed red blood cells were recommended because the infusion of packed cells was thought to aggravate hemolysis by simultaneously infused complements, but transfusion of packed red cells is now considered safe.

Drug Therapy

As mentioned earlier, transfusional hemosiderosis is the major cause of late morbidity and mortality in patients with chronic hemolytic anemia who require regular transfusion. Establishment of a more favorable iron balance should lead to improved survival. Although several drugs have been developed, only deferoxamine mesylate (Desferal), a siderophore iso-

lated from cultures of *Streptomyces pilosus* and introduced in 1960, is currently used because of its nearly specific iron-chelating properties and low toxicity. To obtain good patient compliance, it would be desirable to use oral drugs rather than the current chronic parenteral administration of deferoxamine mesylate. Although several possibilities have been reported, no oral chelators have proved to be effective. For thalassemia and sickle cell anemia, 5-azacytidine,* hydroxyurea (Hydrea) with or without erythropoietin (Epogen), and butyrate have been used mainly for the purpose of augmenting red cell hemoglobin F production. The significance of these drugs in the clinical setting is still undetermined. For sickle cell anemia, besides inducing hemoglobin F synthesis, various kinds of drugs have been tried to decrease hemoglobin S polymerization, increase membrane activity, decrease membrane deformability, or counter the detrimental effects of oxidation. No cure has been reported yet. In PNH, glucocorticoid (0.3 to 0.5 mg per kg per day) is the only drug that can ameliorate hemolysis due to the activation of complement. During an acute episode of hemoglobinuria, the dose may be increased to 1 mg per kg per day and be administered every day until the bout is over. Antithymocyte globulin (Atgam) is one choice for a PNH patient with deficient hematopoiesis. Although both androgens and erythropoietin can stimulate erythropoiesis, these have only limited effectiveness.

Splenectomy

Splenectomy is considered curative therapy for hereditary spherocytosis (HS) and may also be indicated for other membrane defects accompanied by severe anemia. Splenectomy corrects hemolytic anemia, although red cell survival may remain slightly shortened in some patients. Spherocytosis becomes less prominent, and the osmotic fragility improves. In patients with severe autosomal recessive HS associated with spectrin deficiency, in those with combined spectrin and ankyrin deficiency, and in others with unknown molecular defects, hemolytic anemia is only partially improved by splenectomy. Unequivocal indications for splenectomy in HS include either growth retardation and a symptomatic hemolytic disease or mild HS associated with gallstones or a history of gallstones in other relatives with a similar severity of hemolytic disease. Because of the increased frequency of postsplenectomy infection in young children, splenectomy should not be performed in patients younger than 3 to 5 years of age. Children with severe hemolysis, growth retardation, or skeletal deformities may require partial splenectomy, which maintains the splenic phagocytic function and improves the hemolytic anemia. Several weeks prior to splenectomy, patients should be immunized with polyvalent vaccine against pneumococcus, *H. influenzae,* and meningococcus.

In enzymopathies, particularly in severe cases of

---

*Investigational drug in the United States.

pyruvate kinase deficiency, splenectomy results in increased erythrocyte and reticulocyte counts and hemoglobin concentrations and frequently reduces or eliminates transfusion requirements. In other severe cases of red cell enzymopathies, except for triosephosphate isomerase deficiency, splenectomy may also be beneficial to reduce transfusion dependence and elevate peripheral hemoglobin concentration and red cell counts.

In thalassemia, splenectomy is indicated if there is progressive shortening of the survival rate of transfused blood cells, as evidenced by an increased transfusion requirement of more than 180 to 200 mL per kg per year of packed red blood cells. The transfusion requirements of splenectomized patients are considerably less than those of patients with intact spleens. In the case of sickle cell anemia, splenic sequestration is characterized by acute exacerbation of anemia; persistent reticulocytosis; a tender, enlarging spleen; and sometimes hypovolemia. After the event has abated, splenectomy is recommended. Again, it may be better to withhold splenectomy until a patient is at least 5 years old, if chronic transfusion can control the anemia. When early symptoms of splenic sequestration are evident, parents are instructed how to prevent the toxic state.

In other hemoglobinopathies of unstable hemoglobin disorders, splenectomy is indicated if hypersplenism has developed. In congenital erythropoietic porphyria or erythropoietic protoporphyria, splenectomy may be beneficial if the hemolytic anemia is accompanied by splenomegaly. Splenectomy is usually not indicated for PNH. In PNH patients, thromboembolic complications of the surgical procedure can be expected, and this approach should be avoided.

Bone Marrow Transplantation

Bone marrow transplantation (BMT) should be considered in young thalassemia major patients, particularly those less than 5 years old who have an HLA-compatible donor. The currently reported mortality is 10 to 20%, and disease-free survival after 3 to 5 years is 75 to 90%, depending on age and iron status at the time of BMT. Usually older children and adults have significant hepatic hemosiderosis and fibrosis. Factors that predict poor survival are hepatomegaly, portal fibrosis on liver biopsy prior to transplant, and a need for iron chelation therapy to prevent the complication of hemosiderosis. Disease-free survival was reported to be 49% in patients with all three factors, and 94% for patients with none. Patients with some of these factors should be informed of the low success rate before they give their consent for BMT.

Patients suffering from sickle cell anemia with severe symptoms are now also considered candidates for BMT. A recent experience with matched-sibling BMT showed that more than 90% of patients were free of disease at 36 months median follow-up. The obstacle is the lack of HLA-identical donors because of the existence of the same disorder in family members. Broadening the ethnic composition of the registry donor pool and improved supportive care at the time of BMT from unrelated donors may contribute to the treatment for severe forms of sickle cell anemia. Both the aplastic and nonaplastic forms of PNH are curable with BMT. As PNH is a clonal disorder of pluripotent stem cells, conditioning regimens consisting of myeloablation and immune suppression are required. Allogeneic BMT may be considered for patients with a poor prognosis if donors are available. BMT for red cell enzymopathy may also be considered for patients with a poor prognosis.

Gene Therapy

Gene therapy is one of the most promising treatments for chronic nonimmune hemolytic anemia. Single nucleotide substitution of the responsible gene in cases of sickle cell anemia, red cell enzymopathy, unstable hemoglobin disorders, and PNH can be the first target and may provide a cure with the further development of homologous recombination techniques. To attain this end point, specific targeting of red cell lineage is required. There are still technical difficulties in the development of these two techniques, but gene transfer into pluripotent stem cells with retroviral vector, where the responsible gene is under the control of erythroid-specific promoter, can be used for the time being. In cases of thalassemia, it may be more difficult to develop this kind of therapy, because the well-balanced production of both alpha-globin and beta-globin is required. Further investigation is required to develop safe, specific, and effective gene transfer techniques.

PERNICIOUS ANEMIA AND OTHER MEGALOBLASTIC ANEMIAS

method of
ROBERT J. JACOBSON, M.D.
Good Samaritan Medical Center
West Palm Beach, Florida

With few exceptions, megaloblastic anemias are produced by a deficiency of either vitamin B_{12} (cobalamin) or folic acid. Pernicious anemia (PA) ranks as the commonest cause of cobalamin deficiency. The megaloblastic anemias develop as a consequence of impaired DNA synthesis since cobalamin and folic acid are essential for thymidylate formation, an essential component of DNA. Tissues with rapid cell turnover, such as the hematopoietic marrow cells and the epithelial surface cells of the gastrointestinal and genitourinary tracts, all manifest megaloblastic changes when cobalamin or folate is deficient. The impaired DNA synthesis results in characteristic morphologic changes in the blood and marrow. Oval macrocytes causing an elevated mean corpuscular volume (MCV) and hypersegmented neutrophils (a single cell with six or more lobes is diagnostic) may be observed in the peripheral blood smear. Indeed, a hypersegmented neutrophil may be one of the earliest findings before an elevated MCV is present. Bone marrow erythroid precursors are enlarged, with relatively primitive nuclei seen within a mature-appearing cytoplasm. These enlarged or megaloblastic erythroblasts are abundant, and bi- and multinucleated cells may be present as well. Large myelocytes and giant metamyelocytes with horseshoe- or doughnut-shaped nuclei are present; they are usually the first marrow abnormalities to appear and often the last to disappear after initiation of replacement therapy. Severely anemic patients may also manifest with leukopenia and thrombocytopenia, and hypernucleated megakaryocytes may be present in the bone marrow.

In addition to the blood and bone marrow morphologic findings, patients with megaloblastic anemia have an elevated lactic dehydrogenase (LDH) level due to intramedullary cell death. Some of the highest levels of LDH have been recorded in these anemias. For the same reason, there may be an elevated serum bilirubin (mostly unconjugated) and a low or absent serum haptoglobin. Hypogammaglobulinemia and a decrease in serum cholesterol and triglycerides may also be found. Serum iron and percent saturation of transferrin may be increased since iron is not utilized.

Although the blood and bone marrow examination cannot be used to distinguish vitamin B_{12} deficiency from folic acid deficiency, a number of important clinical and laboratory features help distinguish the two. A history of alcoholism or poor dietary habits and pregnancy all indicate that megaloblastic anemia is most likely due to a dietary lack of folic acid. Neurologic abnormalities, particularly of the posterior and lateral columns, point to cobalamin deficiency. Patients who are symptomatic with pernicious anemia may complain of paresthesias and have a decreased sense of vibration in the lower extremities.

The most frequently encountered neurologic defect is diminished vibration sense and next, the loss of proprioception. It has been reported that up to 40% of patients with cobalamin deficiency exhibit neurologic symptoms or signs. More severe neurologic abnormalities include loss of touch and pain sensation, ataxia, limb weakness, visual loss, spasticity, and altered mental status. Fortunately, subacute combined degeneration of the cord is uncommon. The mental changes of impaired memory, dementia, and depression may be overlooked, particularly in elderly patients in whom they may mimic Alzheimer's disease. It is important to remember that neurologic abnormalities may exist in the absence of anemia and macrocytosis.

Determination of serum vitamin B_{12} and serum and erythrocyte folate levels are reliable screening laboratory studies to detect the etiology of megaloblastic anemia. Deficient states can be documented when serum vitamin B_{12} is less than 200 pg per mL, serum folate below 3 ng per mL and red cell folate less than 160 ng per mL. There are several points to consider when ordering these studies: First, a substantial number of patients with clinical and laboratory evidence of cobalamin deficiency may have serum values within the normal range. This may be due to R proteins (rapid electrophoretic proteins) in the commercial kits competing with the purified intrinsic factor for the radiolabeled cobalamin and allowing more of the patient test serum cobalamin to bind to intrinsic factor (this assay is based on a competitive inhibition method). Second, serum folate levels fluctuate widely and reflect recent folate absorption from the bowel. The level will readily increase after a meal containing folate-rich foods. Red cell folate reflects total body stores and provides information about the patient's nutritional status over the preceding 3 months. Third, patients with folate deficiency may also have low levels of serum cobalamin even in the range of

deficiency. The exact cause of this is unknown and may reflect redistribution of cobalamin between cells and plasma. Conversely, patients with severe pernicious anemia may have low serum folate levels owing to malabsorption of folate from megaloblastic small bowel epithelium.

Schilling's test, which reveals correction of vitamin B_{12} malabsorption when intrinsic factor is added (Part II), and serum intrinsic factor antibody are diagnostic of pernicious anemia. Other etiologies of cobalamin deficiency may reveal an abnormal Part II Schilling's test—for example, when there is malabsorption due to celiac disease or tropical sprue. Serum and urinary levels of methylmalonic acid (MMA) are increased in cobalamin deficiency and are very reliable and practical studies to confirm the diagnosis of pernicious anemia. Because cobalamin is essential in the folate-dependent conversion of homocysteine to methionine and the folate-independent conversion of methylmalonyl CoA to succinyl CoA, cobalamin deficiency will result in the accumulation of both homocysteine and MMA, whereas folate deficiency results in the accumulation of homocysteine only.

THERAPY OF PERNICIOUS ANEMIA

Patients with pernicious anemia are treated with parenteral vitamin B_{12}, given by intramuscular or subcutaneous injection. Once the diagnosis of cobalamin deficiency has been made, treatment is initiated. It is not advisable, when faced with a patient with megaloblastic anemia, to administer one of these vitamins blindly or to use large doses of both vitamins before establishing the etiology of the anemia. Not only does it diagnostically mislead the physician, but in patients with cobalamin deficiency, small doses (100 µg) or more of folic acid may improve the hematologic parameters but cause neurologic manifestations to progress and even become irreversible.

My approach is to treat patients initially with intramuscular injections of 1000 µg of cyanocobalamin daily for 5 days. I continue, thereafter, with once-a-week injections for the next 4 weeks to ensure replenishment of the vitamin stores. Patients or family member(s) should be taught to inject the cobalamin themselves, and the opportunity to learn this skill should be offered. It is most important to educate the patient fully about the disease and the need for lifelong treatment with vitamin B_{12}. Patients can be maintained in remission with 1000 µg of cyanocobalamin given every month by intramuscular injection. Unfortunately, relapse in pernicious anemia is not uncommon. For a variety of reasons, patients may discontinue the monthly maintenance injections and, in periods varying from 1 to 10 years, present again with overt megaloblastic anemia. Physicians must stress to their patients the need for lifelong therapy.

The patient's response to vitamin B_{12} replacement is often dramatic and predictable. Within 1 to 2 days of the first injection, patients describe a general feeling of well-being. Appetite returns, glossitis resolves, and mood brightens within a week. A reticulocyte response is first noted after 3 days, and the hematocrit and red cell count begin to rise 5 to 7 days after treatment. Macrocytic red cells take up to 3 weeks to disappear from the peripheral blood, although megaloblastic changes in the bone marrow disappear within 48 hours after treatment. The serum iron will also begin to fall in this short time period. By the fourth week after treatment, the hypersegmented neutrophils have disappeared from the peripheral blood. All the hematologic parameters should return to normal by the second month after the initiation of therapy. Neurologic abnormalities may take longer to resolve, and the degree and likelihood of complete response depends on the pretreatment severity and duration of neurologic symptoms and deficiencies. Most patients respond completely or partially by 6 months of treatment. It is not known whether larger doses of cobalamin are needed to correct neurologic deficiencies than are needed to correct hematologic abnormalities. But, it is prudent to treat patients with neurologic manifestations of pernicious anemia more intensely with cobalamin in the initial 4- to 6-week period.

The two forms of vitamin B_{12} available for therapy are cyanocobalamin and the physiologic form, hydroxocobalamin. Cyanocobalamin is the most widely used form of vitamin B_{12} in the United States. It is inexpensive and in the body is converted to the physiologic form of cobalamin. Hydroxocobalamin is retained longer in the tissues than cyanocobalamin, and maintenance injections can be reduced to 1000 μg every 3 months. It is more expensive and is used more frequently in the United Kingdom and Europe. A small proportion of patients develop antibodies when given hydroxocobalamin, and the antibody is directed against the cobalamin and binding protein complex (transcobalamin II). Injections of cyanocobalamin and hydroxocobalamin are well tolerated and are associated with virtually no toxicity. Rare patients may have local allergic reactions to the injections, and this appears to be directed against the preservative rather than the actual vitamin.

It has been known, but not widely appreciated, that pernicious anemia can also be treated with oral cobalamin. About 1% to 2% of orally ingested cobalamin is absorbed without the need for intrinsic factor. In Sweden, patients have been maintained with oral cobalamin, 1000 μg daily, for many years. The initial treatment to replenish the stores requires a larger oral dose—2000 μg twice daily—or intramuscular injections. Patient compliance is an issue when presenting an oral medication for a prolonged period, but for patients who have a problem with monthly injections, oral cobalamin offers an acceptable alternative.

Patients who are in remission are followed annually with a clinical examination and complete blood count. There is an increased risk of gastric carcinoma in patients with pernicious anemia. The risk estimates have varied from ten times that of control subjects to minimal risk. I do not recommend performing routine endoscopic or radiologic evaluations in asymptomatic individuals but confine gastrointestinal examinations to patients who have suggestive symptoms and signs such as abdominal pain, persistent dyspepsia, weight loss, and occult blood in the stool. There is also evidence indicating that gastric carcinoid and argentaffin tumors are more common in patients with pernicious anemia than gastric carcinomas and may be encountered on endoscopy. Patients with pernicious anemia also manifest other autoimmune diseases, particularly of the thyroid and adrenal glands, and vitiligo of the skin.

THERAPY OF OTHER CAUSES OF VITAMIN B_{12} DEFICIENCY

Patients who have had a total gastrectomy or ileal resection require parenteral cobalamin for the rest of their lives. I give these patients monthly injections of 1000 μg of cyanocobalamin or injections of hydroxocobalamin every 3 months. After surgery, these patients usually have adequate vitamin B_{12} stores, but I check the serum cobalamin level to ensure that daily loading doses of vitamin B_{12} are not required. Patients with blind loop syndrome, ileal inflammatory bowel disease, tropical sprue, and celiac disease require continuing monthly vitamin B_{12} injections until the underlying disease is medically or surgically corrected. Vegetarians who have cobalamin deficiency can be treated after replenishing the stores with oral cyanocobalamin, 25 μg daily, or they can be given 1000 μg of intramuscular vitamin B_{12} every 3 months. It is most important to educate vegetarian mothers of the need for cobalamin supplementation during pregnancy and when breast-feeding infants. Children born of strict vegetarian mothers have been reported at birth to manifest severe neurologic abnormalities.

There is a group of individuals who are asymptomatic and yet have a low level of serum cobalamin. Some of these individuals are physiologically normal yet their serum values are below the low range of normal and must be distinguished from truly deficient subjects. To further complicate the issue, absorption of cobalamin as determined by Schilling's test may also be normal. In the deficient individuals, two findings are particularly helpful. The peripheral blood smear reveals multilobed neutrophils, and elevated levels of homocysteine and MMA are present in the serum and urine. These cobalamin-deficient individuals should be treated with oral cobalamin, 25 μg, and if normal levels of cobalamin are not achieved in 1 to 2 months, then monthly injections of cyanocobalamin are indicated.

THERAPY OF FOLIC ACID DEFICIENCY

The daily requirements of folic acid are 100 to 200 μg; since body stores (8 to 12 mg) are sufficient for only about 4 months, deficiency can readily occur. Dietary deficiency is the commonest cause of folic acid deficiency, and this is particularly prevalent in alcoholics and in individuals who subsist on a "tea and toast" diet. I treat patients with megaloblastic anemia due to dietary folate deficiency with 1 mg of folic acid by mouth daily for 3 months (100 tablets). Thereafter, if most patients have been instructed about the need for folate-rich foods—fresh vegetables and fruit—the deficiency does not recur. In alcoholic patients, folic acid deficiency often accompanies the overall poor nutritional state. Lack of compliance and interest makes these patients susceptible to recurrent deficiency. I treat them initially with large doses of folic acid, 5 mg daily, because maintenance therapy is often difficult and unpredictable. Since folic acid is a heat-labile vitamin, boiling, steaming, or even canning these foods greatly reduces the amount of vitamin. Adolescents or young adults who mainly eat in fast food restaurants or who have unusual diets or food faddism may have little or no folate in their diets. From puberty on, the growth spurt in teenagers is accompanied by a greater need for folate, and their diet may be insufficient in folic acid to meet this need. Educating them about their physiology and correct dietary practice goes a long way in resolving this and other dietary deficiencies.

Pregnancy is another physiologic condition in which there is an increased utilization and requirement of folic acid. To prevent and treat megaloblastic anemia in pregnancy, 1 mg of oral folic acid daily is administered throughout the pregnant state and period of lactation. Furthermore, there is now strong evidence to indicate that folate deficiency during pregnancy is associated with neural tube defects in the child. In women who supplement their diets with folic acid before pregnancy at a low dose of 0.4 mg per day, there is also a significant reduction in the likelihood of infant neural tube defects. It is cautionary to obtain a serum cobalamin level before embarking on long-term folate supplementation.

An increased need for folic acid occurs in patients with chronic hemolytic anemias (sickle cell anemia and thalassemia) and patients requiring long-term hemodialysis. Folic acid, 1 mg daily by mouth, is sufficient to prevent deficiency. Patients who have developed folate deficiency while taking anticonvulsants (particularly phenytoin) or oral contraceptives can be continued on these drugs if they take 1 mg of folic acid daily. In patients with malabsorption (sprue) syndromes, folic acid in daily doses of 2 to 5 mg should be administered. Megaloblastic anemia in patients with tropical sprue is treated with both folic acid and vitamin B_{12}. If the malabsorption syndrome is uncorrectable, then the patients are maintained indefinitely on folic acid, 2 mg per day, and intramuscular cyanocobalamin, 1000 µg every 3 months.

Intravenous folic acid is indicated in patients with folic acid deficiency who are unconscious or unable to take oral medication or poorly absorbing folic acid, as with severe malabsorption. Five milligrams administered intravenously twice weekly is sufficient to correct megaloblastic anemia. Oral folic acid is begun when the patient's clinical condition allows. Folinic acid (citrovorum factor) is a metabolically active form of folic acid that is also administered by intravenous or intramuscular injection. Folinic acid is used in preventing the toxicity from the drug methotrexate, which blocks the folic acid reducing enzyme dihydrofolate reductase.

THERAPY OF COEXISTING IRON DEFICIENCY

Iron deficiency may be combined with the vitamin B_{12} lack in patients with pernicious anemia or after gastrectomy and may be associated with folic acid deficiency in pregnancy and in alcoholics. The absence of bone marrow iron may mask the development of macrocytes, but the white cell precursors will show megaloblastic features and the neutrophils will have hypersegmentation. Patients with combined deficiency respond to oral iron (325 mg of ferrous sulfate three times a day) and vitamin B_{12} or folic acid, depending on which vitamin is lacking. Iron deficiency should also be suspected in patients who do not fully respond to cobalamin or folate therapy. These patients have marginal iron stores that become depleted when hematopoiesis increases with the specific vitamin therapy. One of the values of performing a bone marrow aspirate in megaloblastic anemia is the assessment of the iron stores.

THERAPY OF SEVERELY ANEMIC OR ACUTELY ILL PATIENTS

In most patients with megaloblastic anemia, the gradual decrease in red blood cell count has enabled them to compensate and not manifest circulatory disturbances. If they are severely anemic, with hematocrit counts under 20%, and have no signs of cardiac failure or other distress, I confine the patients to bed and obtain the appropriate diagnostic studies. It is *not* necessary immediately to start these patients on both vitamin B_{12} and folic acid or to consider transfusion therapy. Within a few days the specific deficiency is identified and the therapy begun.

Patients with deteriorating neurologic manifestations or altered mental status should be immediately started on vitamin B_{12} therapy. If there is a history of alcoholism or poor dietary intake, I also administer folic acid, 5 mg intravenously. It is stressed that in emergency situations in which megaloblastic anemia and neurologic dysfunction are found, folic acid should *not* be administered alone but together with vitamin B_{12}.

There are a few indications for transfusion therapy, such as patients with megaloblastic anemia and signs of circulatory distress. Elderly patients particularly may have angina pectoris, cardiac failure, or cerebral dysfunction with even moderate degrees of anemia (hematocrit counts about 25%) and require a more rapid rise of their blood count than that provided by vitamin therapy alone. After obtaining a blood sample for the vitamin measurement, I transfuse such patients *slowly* with 1 or 2 units of packed red cells and also administer a diuretic and replacement potassium as indicated. Patients with a megaloblastic anemia coexisting with another disease (such as hepatic or renal failure, gastrointestinal bleeding, or respiratory insufficiency) that requires immediate treatment with blood transfusion are managed the same way. Serum potassium should be measured in patients during the initial week of therapy. Hypokalemia may occur as a result of plasma potassium entering the proliferating hematopoietic cells that are responding to vitamin B_{12}. I administer oral potassium to those patients with hypokalemia, to patients with heart failure, and to those receiving diuretic therapy. Plasma volume overload is a problem in patients with megaloblastic anemia; careful monitoring, especially for pulmonary edema, is necessary when transfusing patients. In my experience, when megaloblastosis is associated with leukopenia and thrombocytopenia, the administration of either vitamin B_{12} or folic acid is sufficient to correct these abnormalities, and no other therapeutic agent or transfusion is necessary.

THALASSEMIA

method of
GRIFFIN P. RODGERS, M.D., M.M.Sc.
*National Institute of Diabetes, Digestive and
    Kidney Diseases, National Institutes of Health
Bethesda, Maryland*

The *thalassemia syndromes*, which may be the most common single gene disorders in the world, constitute a very diverse group of genetic defects of hemoglobin synthesis, characterized by diminished or absent production of the alpha- or beta-globin chains of adult hemoglobin (hemoglobin A). Thus, in patients with beta-thalassemia there is a decrease in beta-chain production relative to alpha-chain, and the converse is true for alpha-thalassemia. The resultant imbalance in globin chains leads to globin chain precipitating in erythrocytes, ineffective erythropoiesis, and accelerated red cell destruction, with hypochromic, microcytic anemia of varying severities (Figure 1). These disorders are to be distinguished from the *hemoglobinopathies*, which result from mutations in the coding sequences of the alpha- or beta-globin genes that alter the protein structure, resulting in disease manifestations (e.g., HbS in sickle cell disease). These two disorders are not mutually exclusive, in that some mutations (i.e., HbE and Hb Constant Spring) alter both the structure of a globin chain and the rate that it is produced.

A number of structural genes encode for the globin polypeptides in maturing human erythroid cells. Normal functional hemoglobins consist of a tetramer of two alpha-like and two beta-like globin polypeptide chains. The globin chains are encoded by two clusters of closely linked genes. The nonalpha (beta-like) genes reside on chromosome 11 and include the two adult genes, delta (δ) and beta (β); the two very similar fetal genes, gamma-A ($^A\gamma$) and gamma-G ($^G\gamma$); and the single embryonic epsilon (ϵ) gene. On chromosome 16 is found the alpha-like genes, including the duplicated and almost identically functional two alpha-genes (alpha$_2$ and alpha$_1$) that are present in the fetal and adult stages of erythropoiesis, and the embryonic zeta (ζ)-gene. A theta (θ)-gene exists downstream from the alpha$_1$-gene, although its functional significance is still uncertain. As the descriptors of these genes imply, several distinct hemo-

globin species are present during the transitions from intrauterine to adult life. Although the process by which there is a developmental change in the type of globin gene expression—"hemoglobin switching"—has not been fully defined on a molecular level, mutation or deletions of critical elements in the alpha- and beta-globin genes may lead to disease manifestations ranging from inconsequential laboratory findings (microcytosis and hypochromia in alpha- and beta-thalassemia trait) to events incompatible with normal intrauterine growth and development (hydrops fetalis) (Table 1). This summary will briefly examine the clinical features, laboratory diagnosis, and current and experimental approaches to the clinically significant thalassemia syndromes.

CLINICAL FEATURES

Alpha-Thalassemias. The alpha-globin gene cluster is a dynamic locus in which tandemly duplicated long blocks of nucleotide sequences promote nonhomologous recombination between chromosomes during meioses. Thus, the alpha-thalassemia syndromes are predominately due to deletions of one or more of the four genes coding for the alpha-chain, although nondeletional forms have been described. These disorders have their highest prevalence among African American (up to 25%) and Southeast Asian (up to 30%) populations.

The clinical spectrum of the alpha-thalassemia syndromes is directly related to the number of functioning alpha-globin genes. Accordingly, deletions of one ($\alpha\alpha/-\alpha$) or two (($-\alpha/-\alpha$), ($--/\alpha\alpha$)) alpha-globin genes, which occur very frequently in many parts of the world, are virtually asymptomatic. Hemoglobin H disease, due to deletions of three genes ($--/-\alpha$), presents as a moderately severe anemia with splenomegaly and a hypochromic, microcytic blood film appearance (see Table 1). Hemoglobin H ($\beta4$) is demonstrable by special staining of the red cell and by hemoglobin electrophoresis. Generally, however, the anemia in hemoglobin H disease is partially compensated, with an average hemoglobin value of 8 to 10 grams per dL, and therefore chronic transfusion therapy may not be required. Folic acid, 1 mg orally, should be administered daily to compensate for folate loss due to accelerated red cell turnover. Splenectomy may be indicated for progressive anemia. Finally, in its most severe form, in which all four genes are deleted, alpha-thalassemia is incompatible with life, and the fetus is stillborn or critically ill with hydrops fetalis. According to recent reports, mothers carrying affected infants have a high incidence of pregnancy-induced hypertension, seizures, and other peripartum complications. Accordingly, every effort should be made to identify these women (especially Asian American women who are statistically the most affected) early during the course of their pregnancy for appropriate referral. These facts notwithstanding, discussions of thalassemia, and treatment thereof, generally refer to the beta-thalassemia syndromes.

Beta-Thalassemia. The beta-thalassemia syndromes represent the classic molecular paradigm in which disparate defects in a eukaryotic structural gene can culminate in a decreased-to-absent polypeptide chain production. This diverse group of disorders for the most part is due to single nucleotide changes in or around either or both of the two beta-globin genes. Some of the molecular mechanisms accounting for the thalassemic phenotype include nonsense, frame shift, splicing, and polyadenylation mutations, as well as insertions and deletions. In addition, long deletions lead to more complex forms of beta-thalassemia syndromes, such as delta beta-thalassemia or hereditary

All material in this article is in the public domain, with the exception of any borrowed figures or tables.

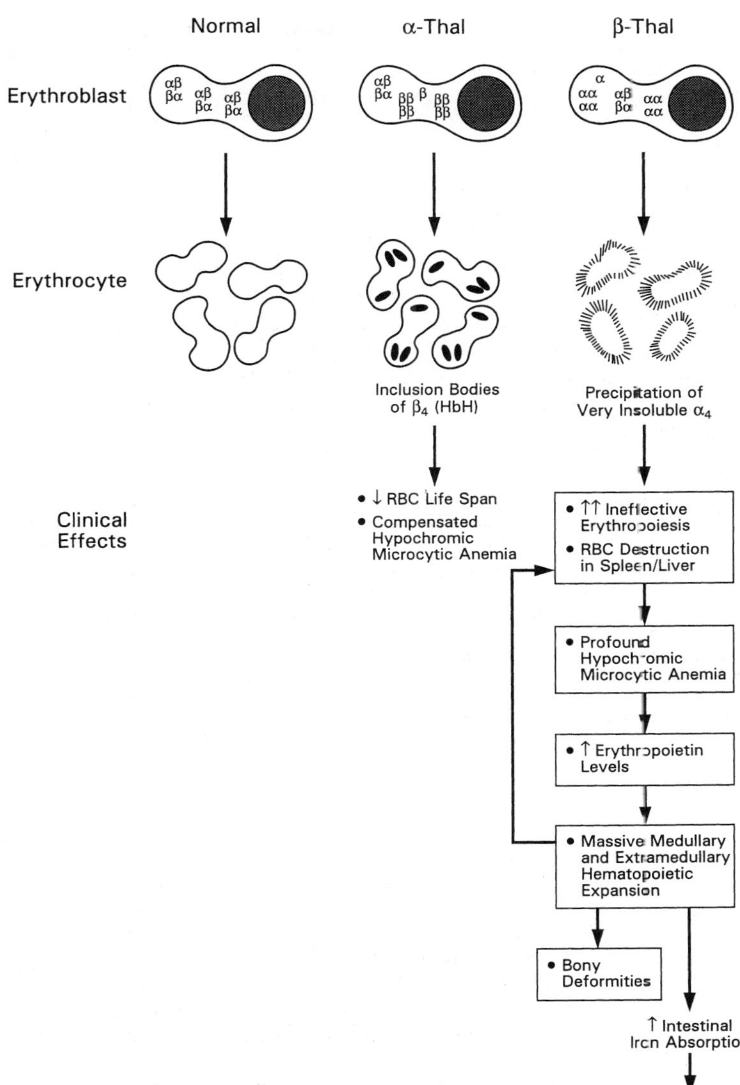

Figure 1. A schematic representation of the pathophysiology of the clinically significant α- and β-thalassemia syndromes (see text).

persistence of fetal hemoglobin (HPFH), but such deletions in the beta-globin cluster occur less commonly than in the alpha-globin cluster. These alterations give rise to significant changes in the level of gene transcription, leading to absent (β^0) or markedly diminished (β^+) amounts of beta-mRNA (see Table 1).

The condition is ubiquitous, but especially common in Mediterranean, Asian, and African populations (and their American descendants) in whom the high gene frequency has been thought to reflect geographic areas with a high malaria prevalence. Within a given ethnic group, relatively few genotypes account for the majority of the cases, each of which now has been defined by DNA sequencing analysis. At a lower level of resolution, the pattern of DNA resolved on gel electrophoresis following restriction enzyme digestion has been used to define certain haplotypes. Specific beta-globin cluster haplotypes are genetically linked to certain of these thalassemic mutations, and hence haplotype analysis has been used to define mutation prevalence in various populations.

The clinical spectrum of disease severity in the beta-thalassemia syndromes is directly related to the quantitative effect of individual mutations of beta-globin synthesis. Reduced or absent beta-globin synthesis results in free alpha-globin accumulations, which precipitate during early erythroblast development because of the relative insolubility of alpha-chains. These inclusions lead to ineffective erythropoiesis in the bone marrow and enhanced peripheral destruction of those erythrocytes that emerge from the bone marrow. The associated pathophysiologic changes resulting from the subsequent anemia include splenomegaly with hypersplenism, osteoporosis, and other skeletal and soft tissue changes associated with an expanded bone marrow, and iron overload resulting from enhanced gastrointestinal absorption and iatrogenic delivery with each red cell transfusion. The liver, heart, pancreas, pituitary, and other endocrine tissues serve as the major sites of excessive iron deposits, leading to their ultimate damage and failure. Figure 1 summarizes the major pathophysiologic processes occurring in the beta-thalassemia syndromes.

LABORATORY DETECTION

Traditional detection of beta-thalassemia relies heavily on the hematologic features. With the more generalized

TABLE 1. **Classification of the Thalassemias**

α-Thalassemia Syndromes

"Silent carrier"	(-α/αα)*
α-Thalassemia trait	(-α/-α; --/αα)
HbH disease	(-α/--)
Hydrops fetalis	(--/--)
Hb Constant Spring genotypes	(αα^{CS}/αα)
Co-inherited α-thalassemia + β-thalassemia	

β-Thalassemia Syndromes

β-Thalassemia minor [trait]	(β/β$^+$)†
β-Thalassemia intermedia	(β/β^0; β$^+$/β$^+$; β$^+$/β^0) = β$^+$
β-Thalassemia major	(β^0/β^0) = β^0

Complex β-Thalassemia syndromes

Hereditary persistence of fetal hemoglobin (HPFH)	(HbF → 25%–100%)
γ-Thalassemia	(HbF → ~ 0%)
δ-Thalassemia	(HbA$_2$ → ~ 0%)
γδβ-Thalassemia	(HbF + HbA$_2$ → ~ 0%)

*Normally one inherits 2 alpha-globin genes from each parent, resulting in a full complement of 4 alpha-globin genes, designated (αα/αα). The alpha-thalassemia syndromes usually result from deletions in one or more alpha-genes, indicated by the dash (-), or from mutations in the coding sequence (e.g., α-Constant Spring, α^{CS}).

†A single beta-globin gene is inherited from each parent; the full complement is thus normally designated as β/β. The β-thalassemia syndromes typically are derived from mutations that lead to a *decreased* level of normal β-chain production (β$^+$), or *absence* of β-chain production (β^0). Various combinations of these mutations give rise to syndromes of increasing severity.

use of electronic cell counters, the diagnosis is first suspected by the discovery of a low mean corpuscular volume (MCV) and mean corpuscular hemoglobin concentration (MCH) on routine complete blood counts. Increased levels of HbA$_2$ (to 4% to 6%) and/or increased HbF (to 5% to 20%), demonstrated by quantitative hemoglobin electrophoresis, support the diagnosis. Unfortunately, the differentiation between iron deficiency anemia and beta-thalassemia trait can be difficult in practice, if there are no reciprocal increases in HbA$_2$ levels and/or HbF. Moreover, in the presence of concomitant iron deficiency, HbA$_2$ levels in beta-thalassemic individuals may fall into the normal range. Occasionally, the diagnosis of iron deficiency cannot be made on the basis of measurements of serum iron, iron-binding capacity, or the absence of stainable iron in the bone marrow. In these instances, the demonstration of a reduced beta-globin synthetic rate or chain ratios (compared with alpha-globin), generally employing ^{3}H-leucine to analyze globin chain production in reticulocytes, will be required for a conclusive diagnosis.

Within the last decade, with improvements in techniques in molecular biology and with the cloning of the human globin genes, one is now able to clone and sequence the β-globin genes directly from a suspected patient. More recently, it has been appreciated that a number of these point mutations that result in the thalassemic phenotype are genetically linked to specific restriction fragment length polymorphisms or haplotypes. Thus, by isolating DNA from peripheral white blood cells, one can perform restriction enzyme digestion of genomic DNA and Southern blotting to examine for the presence of specific haplotypes from which one can infer the particular thalassemic mutation. These traditional DNA diagnostic tests are increasingly being supplanted by the use of the polymerase chain reaction (PCR) directed against specific sequences or the entire structural beta (or alpha-)-globin gene. The advantage of this approach results from contemporary knowledge of the entire alpha and beta sequence (and many thalassemic variants), the requirement for only minuscule quantities of starting DNA to be amplified, and the ability to devise highly sensitive and specific assay conditions.

One additional strategy for the diagnosis of thalassemia is the demonstration of decreased or absent amounts of a specific globin mRNA from early erythroid cells. This approach exploits the common denominator that all forms of thalassemia, despite the heterogeneity of molecular mutations and deletions, have a reduction of either the amounts or functional capacity of the mRNA that encodes for globin chains. A recent report using reverse transcriptase followed by quantitative PCR of RNA isolated from peripheral blood erythroid cells to determine the alpha/beta-globin mRNA ratio present therein demonstrates the feasibility of the approach. Figure 2 offers a diagnostic algorithm for the approach to evaluating hypochromic, microcytic red cell disorders in the presence or absence of anemia. Important (and remedial) differential diagnostic possibilities include iron deficiency, in which the cause for blood loss must be identified, and lead poisoning, especially if basophilic stippling of red cells is prominent.

THERAPY OF BETA-THALASSEMIA

As treatment of severe beta-thalassemia has improved, so have morbidity and median survival. Thus, while untransfused patients in the 1920s had a median survival of 2 years, transfusion therapy aimed at maintenance of a hemoglobin concentration of 11 to 13 grams per dL (pre-transfusion level greater than 10 grams per dL) has been shown to extend the average survival into the second decade, as well as minimizing the bony abnormalities and improving the sexual development. Transfusion support is generally initiated once the hemoglobin drops below 7 grams per dL, and remains there in the absence of infection, blood loss, and so on. To minimize febrile reactions, and not to prejudice the potential future application of bone marrow transplantation (see later), leukocyte-poor RBCs should be administered. An accurate record of the date and amount of blood administered, along with pre- and post-transfusion hemoglobin levels and the occurrence of any transfusion reactions, facilitates optimal therapy of patients. Patients should be tested for the presence of hepatitis B antibodies; those testing negative should be immunized. Splenectomy is usually recommended in children or adolescents (more than 6 to 7 years of age) when their transfusion requirements exceed 1.5 times normal (e.g., over 200 mL per kg per year). Prior to elective splenectomy, all patients should receive polyvalent pneumococcal vaccine, and pediatric patients should also be given *Haemophilus influenzae* type b vaccine.

Though intensive transfusion programs have led to this markedly improved survival, patients will die from iron overload unless chelation therapy is appropriately instituted and maintained. Currently, this involves the use of subcutaneous deferoxamine, although a search for an effective oral chelator is currently underway. Many patients can be placed in iron balance by taking a 12- to 24-hour infusion of

Diagnostic Evaluation of Hypochromic/Microcytic Indices

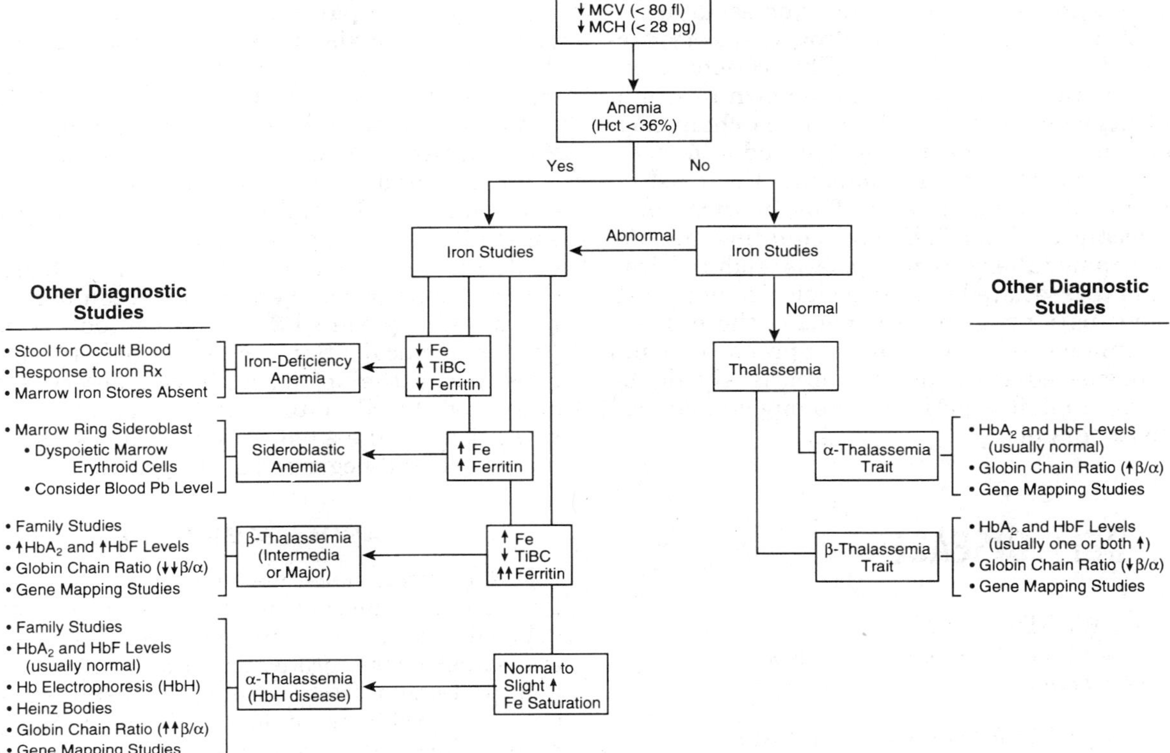

Figure 2. Diagnostic algorithm for the evaluation of red cell hypochromia and microcytosis in the presence (or absence) of anemia (see text).

deferoxamine, 5 or 6 days a week. Chelation therapy should be individualized based on age, risks, compliance history, and other factors. For younger patients who are not yet at risk for the complications of iron overload, 1.5 to 2.0 grams per day, 5 to 6 days per week, should be administered. Individuals aged 13 years or older should receive 2.0 to 2.5 grams per day depending on their ability to tolerate subcutaneous infusions. Patients with high liver iron concentrations (over 6000 μg per gram of dry tissue) or those with evidence of cardiac involvement (e.g., congestive heart failure, dysrhythmias) require more intensive intravenous therapy or should be managed at specialized medical centers caring for large numbers of patients requiring chronic transfusion support.

Periodic assessment of the effectiveness of chelation therapy should include an estimate of iron burden (e.g., serum iron, total iron-binding capacity, ferritin) and an estimate of liver iron concentration by the judicious use of percutaneous liver biopsy or, more ideally, by validated noninvasive testing. A yearly cardiac evaluation should be performed in an effort to detect clinical evidence of cardiac disease, which should include a complete history and physical examination, electrocardiogram, echocardiogram, and chest radiograph. A Holter monitor should be obtained for any patient who complains of palpitations or who is noted on physical examination to have an irregular heart beat. Potential iron-induced damage of endocrine glands should be evaluated by a glucose tolerance test, thyroid function, and cortisol determinations. Hormone replacement therapy is dictated by the results of basal and/or provocative endocrine function studies.

Various complications associated with the use of deferoxamine include visual disturbances, tinnitus, and renal dysfunction (azotemia and proteinuria). All these are reversible on discontinuation of the drug and generally do not recur when the drug is subsequently given at lower doses. For these reasons, annual ophthalmologic and audiologic evaluation is strongly recommended for patients receiving chronic deferoxamine therapy.

Allogeneic bone marrow transplantation (ABMT) is increasingly effective for patients with homozygous beta-thalassemia. Since the initial report in 1982, over 600 patients have undergone ABMT in a single center in Italy. Among good-risk children (as defined by good compliance with chelation and the absence of hepatomegaly and portal fibrosis), the 3-year event-free survival is 93%. Older patients, or those exhibiting one or more risk factors, have rejection-free survivals of less than 75%. Thus, at the moment, ABMT can be recommended only as a reasonable option for selected good-risk candidates with suitable donors.

One alternative form of therapy currently being investigated deserves special mention. This involves the manipulation of globin gene expression using agents such as 5-azacytidine, hydroxyurea, erythropoietin, or butyrate analogues. The rationale for these trials is that these agents are known to stimulate fetal hemoglobin synthesis. Gamma-chain augmentation may compensate for the reduced beta-chain synthesis, thereby normalizing the existing alpha- to nonalpha-chain ratio. This in turn could lead to decreased transfusional requirements, decreased extramedullary hematopoiesis, reduced iron overload, and associated pathophysiologic effects. Although some patients have responded to these therapies very impressively, this general approach should still be considered experimental; efforts should be made to enroll eligible patients into ongoing clinical trials where possible.

SICKLE CELL DISEASE

method of
PAUL S. SWERDLOW, M.D.
Wayne State University School of Medicine
Detroit, Michigan

TYPES OF SICKLE CELL DISEASE

Sickle hemoglobin (HbS) is caused by a point mutation changing a single amino acid residue in the beta-globin chain of hemoglobin. Once deoxygenated, HbS polymerizes, wreaking havoc on first the red cells, then the body. Clinically, the disorders are inherited hemolytic anemias accompanied by pain and organ damage. In sickle cell anemia, both beta-globin genes have the mutation. Patients with one sickle gene and either an HbC or a thalassemic beta-globin mutation are also at risk for sickling (sickle—C disease or sickle—beta-thalassemia). Patients with one sickle beta-globin gene and one normal gene (sickle trait) are essentially normal, without hemolysis or anemia. They may have complications with extreme altitude (2500 meters) or dehydration. They occasionally have hematuria. Hyphema requires ophthalmic intervention, since even trait cells in the anterior chamber sickle and can elevate optic pressures to dangerous levels.

DIAGNOSIS

The diagnosis can be made at birth by screening programs. Unscreened children who are at risk should be tested by age 4 months to allow timely institution of prophylactic penicillin. Definitive diagnosis requires hemoglobin electrophoresis or other direct techniques, not a sickle preparation or Sickledex test. Referral to a specialized center provides confirmation and facilitates consultation, should complications develop.

PEDIATRIC CARE

Follow-up every 2 months the first year and every 3 months the second year is needed, as mortality is high in untreated patients. A routine diet should be supplemented with folic acid. Iron supplements after the first year require evidence of low iron stores.

Routine immunizations are encouraged. Pneumococcal vaccine, *Haemophilus influenzae* B conjugate, and hepatitis B are particularly important. A key intervention is prophylactic penicillin, 125 mg orally twice daily to age 3 years, and 250 mg orally twice daily from ages 3 to 5 years. Children who are allergic to penicillin can be given erythromycin ethyl succinate, 20 mg/kg/day divided into two daily doses.

Parents and children must work to ensure adequate fluid intake and avoid extreme temperatures, especially swimming in cold water. Bed wetting may be due to hyposthenuria. Parents must learn to recognize symptoms of anemia, take a temperature, and palpate the spleen so that they can determine when prompt medical attention is needed. In splenic sequestration, the spleen massively enlarges with sequestered blood, often leading to shock. Prompt transfusion is life-saving. Routine ophthalmic examinations should begin at age 10 years.

ADOLESCENT CARE

Frank discussions are needed regarding limitations owing to disease, issues of retarded growth and delayed sexual development, avoidance of tobacco and street drugs, protection of ankles, contraception and protection from sexually transmitted disease, and any problems of low self-esteem and missed school. Discussion of role models may be helpful, as are support groups and academic and vocational counseling. Ideal jobs allow for intermittent absences and avoid severe physical effort. The difficult transition to adult medicine is eased by communication among pediatrician, internist, family, and patient.

ADULT CARE

Many adults benefit from discussing disease complications and preventive measures, such as drinking adequate fluids and avoiding prolonged cold. Vaccinations and routine health screens should be up to date, including visits with the dentist and ophthalmologist. Patients must know to present immediately when they have fever, cough, dyspnea, orthostasis, or neurologic symptoms. The physician should be supportive in the patient's dealings with prospective employers or with disability forms.

Many patients can control most pain at home. Some respond to nonsteroidal agents. Others require short-acting narcotics such as codeine or oxycodone. For many patients, small supplies last for months. Others who have daily pain need significant supplies of medication to avoid frequent visits to emergency rooms. To optimize care, it is important that one physician or group prescribe all pain medication. The patient must schedule an appointment for medication renewal before running out. Emergency requests for medication are discouraged. More severely affected patients have a poorer prognosis and a shortened survival. They need to be seen frequently and their pain taken seriously. Many qualify for hydroxyurea therapy.

TABLE 1. **Hydroxyurea for Sickle Cell Anemia According to the Multicenter Study of Hydroxyurea (MSH) in Sickle Cell Anemia**

Eligibility

Age at least 18 years
More than three painful crises per year requiring hospital or emergency treatment
Reliable enough to take medication properly and follow up every 2 weeks
Not currently attempting to have children (male or female) or breast-feeding
Informed of long-term potential risks

Dosing

Start at 15 mg/kg/day as a single daily oral dose
Increase at 12 week intervals by 5 mg/kg/day to maximum of 35 mg/kg
If toxic:
   Stop hydroxyurea until counts normal (generally by next visit)
   Restart at a dose 2.5 mg/kg/day lower
   If after 12 weeks no toxicity, increase by 2.5 mg/kg/day

Toxicity

Check for toxicity every 2 weeks until MTD,* then every 4 weeks
Any one of the following counts as toxicity:
   ANC† less than 2,000/mm³
   Platelets less than 80,000/mm³
   Hb less than 4.5/mm³
   Hb less than 5.0 with ARC‡ less than 320,000/mm³ if pretreatment Hb was more than 7.0
   Hb less than 9.0 if ARC is less than 80,000/mm³

*MTD (maximal tolerated dose) is the highest dose that does not produce toxicity.

†ANC (absolute neutrophil count) is the number of neutrophils per mm³ of blood. It is reported directly by some laboratories. It is calculated as the total white count multiplied by (% polys + % bands)/100.

‡ARC (absolute reticulocyte count) is the number of reticulocytes per mm³ of blood. It is reported directly by some laboratories. It is calculated as the total red cell count per mm³ (not hemoglobin or hematocrit) multiplied by the % reticulocytes/100.

Abbreviation: Hb = hemoglobin in gm/dL.

Hydroxyurea, when used according to Table 1, reduces emergent pain by 44% and decreases acute chest syndrome and the necessity for transfusion. Patients whose dosage falls in between the 500-mg capsules can take the medication on alternating days. The physician and patient must carefully weigh the risks and benefits. Short-term toxicity is due to marrow suppression. It is strongly recommended that only 2-week supplies be prescribed and that toxicity criteria be strictly followed. Long-term safety remains unknown. A small increased risk of leukemia is suggested by some but not all studies in cancer patients. Hydroxyurea causes birth defects in animals, so neither men nor women attempting to have children should be on therapy. Use in children awaits controlled clinical trials, since pediatric toxicity is unknown.

EMERGENT PAIN EPISODES

Patients frequently present emergently with pain. A careful evaluation is imperative, since nearly a third of patients who die initially present with pain, acute chest syndrome, or stroke. A focused history and physical examination should ensure that there is no intercurrent infection and no other cause for pain and that the patient is not dehydrated, hypoxic, or having a stroke. Patients can often tell whether the pain is "sickle" pain or not. Hydration either orally or intravenously (5% dextrose at 3 to 5 mL per kg per hour) and oxygen are often begun routinely. Oxygen should be stopped if there is no hypoxia, since it can suppress erythropoiesis. Overhydration is of no benefit. Given the risks of infection, one should have a low threshold for ordering chest x-rays, urinalyses, and cultures. As early as feasible, the pain should be controlled.

Pain is poorly treated by most practitioners owing to a fear of narcotics and a lack of trust in the patient's perception of pain. There are no clinical or laboratory tests to indicate that a patient is having a pain episode. A patient's report of pain is the most accurate indicator. Initial doses for emergent treatment of severe sickle cell pain are presented in Table 2. Intravenous doses can be repeated every 10 minutes if needed. Subcutaneous and intramuscular doses can be repeated every 30 minutes or so. Avoiding intramuscular injections prevents sterile abscesses and preserves the patient's limited muscle mass. Patients who are narcotic-naive or elderly or who have liver disease or limited respiratory drive may need smaller doses. Tranquilizers should be avoided. Where available, patient-controlled analgesia (PCA) is useful both in an inpatient setting and emergently, as long as an adequate bolus is given.

Patients who regularly experience pain learn to use distraction (watching TV, talking on the phone) to avoid focusing on the pain. If interrupted, they

TABLE 2. **Initial Doses of Narcotics Recommended for Acute Emergent Pain***

Medication	Adult Dose (Pediatric Dose in mg/kg)	Routes	Interval	PO Equivalent (mg/kg)	Comments
Morphine	10 mg (0.15)	IV, SC, IM	q 3–4 h	40 mg (0.6)	Drug of choice
Hydromorphone (Dilaudid)	1.5 mg (0.02)	IV, SC, IM	q 3–4 h	6 mg (0.04)	Expensive
Methadone	10 mg	IV, SC	q 6–8 h	20 mg	Mild withdrawal
Meperidine (Demerol)†	75 mg (1.1)	IV, IM	q 2–3 h	300 mg	Seizure risk‡

*If adequate relief is not obtained, doses can be repeated every 10 min for IV and every 30 min for IM or SC, with the patient being carefully monitored. Intervals shown maintain the pain relief achieved with the first dose. The elderly or those with liver disease or decreased respiratory drive may need lower doses.

†Included for comparison only. Not recommended for pain in sickle cell patients.

‡Normeperidine levels increase for many days with repeated use and can cause seizures. Normeperidine is contraindicated in those with a history of central nervous system disease or those on monoamine oxidase inhibitors.

again focus on the pain. This may be misinterpreted as "faking"—for example, an active patient who complains of pain when staff arrives. Few sickle patients are truly addicted to pain medication. Such a determination is best made on an outpatient basis by skilled personnel, not in an emergency room. The use of placebos is of no help, since they often work for known pain. The few patients who become addicted should be detoxified. Such patients may still receive narcotics in the hospital for pain, provided they are tapered off before discharge.

Nonaddicted patients who are tapered too rapidly may go through withdrawal and return with acute pain. The pain should be treated and the medication tapered more slowly. Transferring such patients to long-acting oral medications, such as methadone or a controlled-release narcotic, before discharge minimizes withdrawal symptoms. The medication is then tapered up to 20% per day as an outpatient. Although the government restricts the use of methadone for substance abuse treatment to approved programs, the use of methadone for pain control is not limited. Breaking cycles of withdrawal pain can dramatically improve a patient's well-being and decrease medication utilization.

TRANSFUSION

Transfusions are greatly overused in sickle cell disease, resulting in acute volume overload, chronic iron overload, and sensitization to blood group antigens. The need for each transfusion must be carefully considered, since sensitization may limit later transfusions. Careful matching of blood can delay sensitization but requires prior red cell typing. In life-threatening anemia, transfusion should always be performed with the most compatible blood available, even if it cannot be fully cleared by the blood bank.

Simple and exchange transfusions have different indications. Simple transfusion is indicated for *symptomatic* anemia. Patients with chronic anemia are not benefited by transfusions at arbitrary hemoglobin cutoffs. Patients who tolerate hemoglobin levels of 4 g per dL without ill effect should be allowed to do so. Angina, orthostasis, dyspnea, or neurologic symptoms attributable to anemia are good indications for transfusion. Despite popular wisdom, transfusions do not decrease pain or shorten established pain episodes. Generalized weakness, malaise, or a longer than usual hospital stay is *not* a sufficient indication for transfusion. Simple transfusion may be needed in patients with rapidly falling hemoglobins due to bleeding, splenic sequestration, or aplastic or hemolytic crises.

For stroke and uncontrollable hypoxia—and, less certainly, for persistent priapism and before certain surgeries—it is important to decrease the sicklable cells to less than 30% of the circulating pool while keeping the total hemoglobin around 10 grams per dL. Exchange transfusion via pheresis machine is an elegant way to achieve these goals. Instructions for manual exchange are found in an excellent mono-

graph, "Management and Therapy of Sickle Cell Disease," NIH publication no. 92-2117.

CONTRACEPTION AND PREGNANCY

There are no contraindications to contraception in patients with sickle cell disease. Many patients find that medroxyprogesterone (Depo-Provera) or levonorgestrel (Norplant) helps minimize cyclical menstrual sickle pains. Pregnancy carries increased risk for mother and fetus, but the increase is modest, and positive outcomes are the rule. Nondirective genetic counseling should be offered, with hemoglobin typing of the partner. Prenatal diagnosis is feasible early in pregnancy. Ideally, folic acid, 1 mg per day, is begun before pregnancy. Frequent visits with an obstetrician or clinic specializing in high-risk pregnancy are recommended. Patients should be screened for blood alloantibodies, and the pregnancy should be followed carefully for possible hemolytic disease in the fetus. Because of the frequency of iron overload, iron supplements should be withheld unless iron stores are low.

Pregnancy generally results in increased pain. Fortunately, there is no contraindication to narcotics. Unfortunately, transfusion is commonly performed for uncomplicated pain crises despite a randomized trial of transfusion in sickle cell disease, which found no difference in maternal or fetal outcome. Women with a repeated history of miscarriage may benefit from repeated exchange transfusions, but the risks must be weighed against the possible benefits.

INFECTION

Infection tends to occur in tissues damaged by sickling, such as lung, urinary tract, and bone. Infections must be treated rapidly to avert sickling complications and because patients are functionally asplenic. Temperatures above 101°F should be assumed to be due to infection and treated empirically. Urinary tract infections tend to recur. Repeating urine cultures 2 weeks and then several months after infection ensures complete eradication. Aplastic crises are often due to parvovirus B19, the causative agent of fifth disease. Owing to hemolysis, the hemoglobin falls dramatically when the reticulocyte count is suppressed. Transfusions are usually required. Folate deficiency is another cause of aplastic crisis.

LUNG PROBLEMS

Acute chest syndrome is a new segmental or larger pulmonary infiltrate accompanied by cough, wheezing, tachypnea, new chest pain, or a temperature above 38.5°C (101.3°F). This dangerous syndrome includes both pneumonia and pulmonary infarction, and elements of both may be present. Marrow fat embolism may contribute in many cases. Management includes antibiotics to cover common organisms (pneumococcus and mycoplasma) and careful attention to oxygenation. If there is doubt that the P_{O_2}

can be maintained above 60 mmHg (70 mmHg in a child), exchange transfusion must be performed. Repeated episodes of acute chest syndrome can result in pulmonary hypertension with cor pulmonale. Chronic transfusions or night-time oxygen may help. A related syndrome of multiorgan failure involves some combination of the pulmonary, renal, central nervous, and hepatic systems. Patients who are exchange transfused often make a full recovery.

Splinting due to chest wall pain is a frequent cause of atelectasis, which may lead to acute chest syndrome. Patients with splinting need adequate pain relief to allow full and deep respiration, preferably with an incentive spirometer, to minimize atelectasis. Dyspnea due to chest wall pain is not a contraindication to narcotic use. Indeed, respiration increases as the pain is relieved.

STROKE

One in 15 sickle cell patients will suffer a stroke, the majority before age 18 years. Rapid exchange transfusion to less than 30% sicklable cells may prevent progression and should take precedence over imaging studies. For thrombotic strokes, the high risk of recurrence mandates transfusion for 5 or more years, at least in children. Exchange transfusion can minimize iron overload and may obviate the need for later chelation. Patients who have suffered two strokes are likely to need transfusions for life. Hemorrhagic stroke requires angiography, after exchange, to rule out surgically correctable lesions.

GALLBLADDER AND LIVER

Pigment gallstones affect most patients before age 30 years and many by age 10 years. Cholecystectomy should be performed in those with symptoms attributable to gallstones or with frequent abdominal pain. Some recommend that simple transfusion to a hemoglobin of 10 g per dL be performed before even laparoscopic cholecystectomy.

Acute sickle liver disease usually resolves within 2 weeks. It may be characterized by bilirubin values in the teens and elevated liver enzymes. Care must be exercised in evaluating lactate dehydrogenase (LDH), which may be due to red cell hemolysis, and alkaline phosphatase, which may be due to bony sickling. Rarely, liver disease is severe, with bilirubin values approaching 100 or evidence of hepatic failure. Exchange transfusions are then indicated. Chronic liver disease may be due to viral hepatitis, hemosiderosis, pulmonary hypertension, or repeated sickle infarcts. Liver biopsy may clarify the diagnosis.

LEG ULCERS

Leg ulcers commonly cause morbidity. Patients should be advised that wounds near the malleoli heal poorly, so they should keep these areas clean and well moisturized. Once an ulcer develops, local care

is key. The wound must be kept clean and well débrided with regular dressing changes, such as wet-to-dry saline solution with fine mesh gauze, enzyme-based ointments (e.g., Elase), or whirlpool therapy. Moisturizing the surrounding skin with baby oil or Eucerin cream is helpful. Systemic antibiotics are indicated only for accompanying cellulitis. Edema is treated with elevation and compression stockings. Zinc supplements or hydroxyurea may help. As a last resort, hypertransfusion for 6 months with or without skin grafting may be tried.

BONY DISEASE

Many pain episodes focus on bones, but permanent damage does not usually result. Sickling of growth plates can cause uneven growth of bones. Osteomyelitis is not common, but when it occurs, it is often with salmonella or staphylococcus. Nuclear medicine scans do not easily differentiate osteomyelitis from bony infarcts, and plain films may prove more useful. It is important to obtain a biopsy of any affected bone to determine the appropriate antibiotics to use.

Both hips and shoulders are subject to avascular necrosis, which can lead to chronic arthritis and the need for joint replacement. Early diagnosis is often better with magnetic resonance imaging (MRI). Avoidance of weight bearing for several months may prevent collapse of the femoral head. Some advocate core decompression, but data on efficacy are lacking. Vertebrae are subject to central collapse, causing "fish mouth" or "Lincoln log" deformities, which can result in chronic arthritis.

Gout should be suspected if a joint is swollen, warm, red, and exquisitely tender. Aspiration is essential to document gout crystals and rule out septic arthritis. Acute therapy is with indomethacin (Indocin), 50 mg every 8 hours. Allopurinol (Zyloprim), 300 mg per day, is used for prevention only after repeated episodes.

RENAL COMPLICATIONS

Hyposthenuria is nearly universal. To avoid dehydration, adults should drink at least 4 liters of fluid daily (150 mL per kg for children). Defects in secretion of acid and potassium may result in metabolic acidosis and hyperkalemia, but in severe cases, alternative causes should be sought.

Hematuria, usually painless, is common in sickle cell disease and trait. Evaluation should consider tumor, stones, glomerulonephritis, infection, and bleeding disorders, but papillary necrosis is most common. Most episodes clear spontaneously with good hydration. If hematuria persists, epsilon-aminocaproic acid, 5 grams every 8 hours for four doses, may be helpful, but the risk of clot formation in the renal pelvis and ureter requires careful monitoring. DDAVP (1-deamino-8-D-arginine vasopressin) and cauterization of bleeding sites in the renal pelvis have also been reported to help. Transfusions may be needed, including exchange if hematuria remains refractory. Iron supplementation should be given only if stores are low. Nephrectomy should be avoided, as bleeding may occur in the remaining kidney.

Proteinuria greater than 2 grams per 24 hours may need biopsy for evaluation. Hypertension should be treated with nondiuretic medications. Neither dialysis nor transplantation is contraindicated in chronic renal failure, but those patients undergoing transplant should expect an increase in pain.

PRIAPISM

Priapism is a prolonged, painful erection that can be caused by sickling. There is no established effective therapy. Avoidance of prolonged sexual activity, alcohol, and dehydration may reduce the incidence. Home therapies include hot baths, exercise, or prostatic massage, which, although awkward, can be performed by most patients after brief instruction. Prolonged episodes require emergent evaluation. One must ensure adequate hydration, oxygenation, and pain control; the absence of infection; and the ability to urinate. A Foley catheter may be needed. Nifedipine (Procardia),* 10 mg, or hydralazine (Apresoline),* 10 mg, can be tried acutely. Irrigation of the corpora is a low-risk procedure that is easily performed by a urologist in the emergency room. After 12 to 24 hours, exchange transfusion is usually considered, but there are few data indicating that it helps. Shunt procedures are considered if this fails, but there remains an overall 25% risk of impotence. Those who develop impotence should be referred to a urologist. For patients with repeated episodes, nightly therapy with a nitroglycerin patch* (0.2 to 0.4 mg per hour) or hydralazine, 10 mg before bedtime, may help. Luteinizing hormone–releasing hormone (LHRH) agonists such as luprolide (Lupron)* may help by decreasing testosterone to castration levels.

SURGERY AND ANESTHESIA

A randomized multi-institutional study found that preoperative exchange transfusion was no better than simple transfusion to a hemoglobin of 10 g per dL in decreasing surgical complications. It is critical that good oxygenation be maintained throughout surgery and especially in the postoperative period. Aggressive pulmonary toilet with incentive spirometry helps minimize pulmonary complications. Surgery that is unlikely to cause respiratory splinting, such as hip replacement, may not require any transfusion pre-operatively. Dental procedures should be performed with nitrous oxide only if no good alternatives exist and the nitrous oxide is given with pure oxygen.

FUTURE THERAPY

Related bone marrow transplant can result in cure, but at the risk of substantial morbidity and mortal-

---

*Not FDA-approved for this indication.

ity. Newer agents that increase fetal hemoglobin, block polymerization, alter oxygen affinity, or increase cellular water are being tested. Before any new drugs can be recommended, appropriate randomized trials must be performed. There is a great temptation to try anything in sickle cell disease because of the frustrations encountered in dealing with the disease or the patients. Outside of controlled clinical trials, such temptations must be resisted in the best interests of the patient.

NEUTROPENIA

method of
PETER E. NEWBURGER, M.D.
University of Massachusetts Medical School
Worcester, Massachusetts

Neutropenia, a below-normal number of peripheral blood neutrophils, is determined by calculation of the absolute neutrophil count (ANC) from the total white blood cell count multiplied by the proportion of neutrophils (including both segmented and band forms) on the differential count. The clinical significance of the neutropenia depends upon the level of depression of the ANC, as indicated in Table 1. Severe neutropenia, with ANC less than 200, is also termed *agranulocytosis*, even though eosinophils and basophils (which are also granulocytes) generally remain normal in number.

Fever in the setting of an ANC of less than 500 is a medical emergency that compels immediate evaluation and antibiotic treatment.

CLINICAL PRESENTATION

Neutropenia causes no clinical symptoms or signs per se, so the clinical presentation derives only from secondary infections. Some patients are asymptomatic, but most eventually present with fever, with or without localizing signs of infection. Stomatitis, often with thrush, also occurs commonly; regular periodic stomatitis every 21 days is a hallmark of cyclic neutropenia. Predictable but often

TABLE 1. **Clinical Significance of Absolute Neutrophil Counts**

ANC (neutrophils/mm³)	Clinical Significance
> 1500	Normal
1000–1500	Statistically abnormal but not clinically significant
500–1000	Very slight predisposition to infection; outpatient antibiotic treatment for febrile illness
200–500	Significant predisposition to infection; usually inpatient IV antibiotic treatment; antibiotic treatment for febrile illness
<200 (agranulocytosis)	Very high risk of infection, often with decreased local signs of inflammation; aggressive inpatient IV antibiotic treatment for febrile illness

asymptomatic neutropenia follows 10 to 14 days after administration of intensive cancer chemotherapy.

Neutropenic patients can develop infection in virtually any organ system. The most common forms are cellulitis, particularly perirectal; pneumonia and lung abscess; enteritis, which can progress rapidly to peritonitis; lymphadenitis; and sepsis, which is particularly likely in patients with indwelling central venous catheters. With agranulocytosis, clinical signs may be limited to fever and limited local inflammation; pus is formed slowly or not at all. Common pathogens include *Staphylococcus aureus* and enteric gram-negative bacilli, including *Escherichia coli* and *Pseudomonas* species. Fungi and unusual, opportunistic, or multiple-antibiotic-resistant bacteria generally cause infection only after prolonged neutropenia and broad-spectrum antibiotic therapy but need to be considered even at initial presentation.

EVALUATION

Table 2 presents a differential diagnosis of neutropenia, which can serve as a guide for diagnostic evaluation. In an acutely ill patient, the initial evaluation needs to be completed rapidly (within hours at the most) and should include assessment of potential sites and causes of infection, but with minimal or no manipulation of the rectum or genitourinary tract.

Acquired neutropenia often accompanies viral infection and requires only monitoring of blood counts until recovery. However, depletion of bone marrow reserves can also reduce the ANC in bacterial sepsis in the neonate or in overwhelming bacteremia, as with meningococcus. Drug-induced neutropenia can be associated with a large number of agents, including, but by no means limited to, antibiotics, anticonvulsants, anti-inflammatories, antithyroid drugs, diuretics, and phenothiazines. Antineutrophil antibodies may be detected by flow cytometry or agglutination assays, but false-negative and borderline-positive results may obscure the diagnosis of immune neutropenia. Careful review of the peripheral blood smear may reveal blasts or nucleated erythrocytes indicative of bone marrow involvement by malignancy or may demonstrate abnormal neutrophil morphology associated with a congenital form of neutropenia.

Bone marrow examination (including cytogenetics) is indicated in cases of severe neutropenia or when other bone marrow lineages are abnormal. In some of the less severe forms of congenital neutropenia, such as chronic benign neutropenia, adequate bone marrow reserves of mature neutrophils can be demonstrated by steroid stimulation of their release into the peripheral blood, evaluated by white blood cell and differential counts before and 6 hours after prednisone, 1 to 2 mg per kg orally (or methyl prednisolone intravenously). Serial blood counts, twice weekly over 6 to 9 weeks, are necessary to make the diagnosis of cyclic neutropenia and to document the period and the duration and depth of the nadir. The syndromes listed in Table 2 include unique phenotypic features that aid in the diagnosis; most pediatric hematology texts provide detailed descriptions. Evaluation of the immunoglobulins and cellular immunity not only contributes to the diagnosis of neutropenia associated with immunologic abnormalities but may also indicate a need for more aggressive management if other arms of host defense are impaired. Organic acidurias, detectable by urine screening tests, may produce neutropenia accompanying severe neurologic dysfunction in neonates. Excessive neutrophil margination in benign "pseudoneutropenia" may be demonstrated by epinephrine administration.

TREATMENT

Supportive Care

Fever (greater than 38.5°C peak or 38°C sustained) or other signs of infection require immediate, aggressive antibiotic therapy in the neutropenic patient with an ANC of under 500. Antibiotics specific to the sensitivities of identified organisms provide ideal treatment for infections with positive cultures. In the absence of neutrophils, synergistic combinations of antibiotics may be preferable to single agents to assure eradication of persistent organisms such as *Pseudomonas* species. However, the initial treatment of most febrile illnesses and the entire therapy of many with negative cultures will rely on an empirical choice of antibiotics. The best data for this clinical setting come from studies of fever and neutropenia in patients treated with chemotherapy for malignancy. Most studies recommend a combination of broad-spectrum antibiotics, such as an aminoglycoside (e.g., gentamicin [Garamycin], tobramycin [Nebcin]) and either a third-generation cephalosporin (e.g., ceftazidime [Fortaz]) or a semisynthetic penicillin with anti-*Pseudomonas* activity (e.g., piperacillin [Pipracil], ticarcillin [Ticar]). Patients with indwelling central venous catheters may require substitution of an agent with better gram-positive coverage (e.g., nafcillin [Unipen] or vancomycin [Vancocin]) for the aminoglycoside. Each institution needs to base its empirical antibiotic usage upon the identity and antibiotic sensitivities of bacteria in the local community or hospital (depending upon the likely site of acquisition of infection), with the final choices made in consultation with the local microbiology or infectious disease division. Fever persisting for more than 2 days generally

---

TABLE 2. **Differential Diagnosis of Neutropenia**

Acquired

Viral bone marrow suppression
Overwhelming bacterial sepsis
Drug-induced
Immune (iso- and autoimmune)
Bone marrow replacement; preleukemia
Splenomegaly
Nutritional

Congenital

Congenital neutropenia
  Severe congenital agranulocytosis (Kostmann's)
  Intermediate forms of congenital neutropenia
  Cyclic neutropenia
Syndromes including neutropenia
  Shwachman-Diamond syndrome
  Cartilage-hair hypoplasia
  Fanconi's anemia
  Chédiak-Higashi syndrome
  Reticular dysgenesis
  Dyskeratosis congenita
  Myelokathexis
Neutropenia associated with immunologic abnormalities
Neutropenia associated with metabolic disorders
Pseudoneutropenia

indicates the need for empirical modification of antibiotic coverage; prolonged fever (more than 1 week) requires addition of empirical antifungal therapy such as amphotericin B (Fungizone), usually in consultation with an infectious disease specialist.

For hospitalized patients, handwashing needs to be strictly enforced, but more aggressive "reverse precautions" do little to prevent the majority of infections, which derive from the patient's own skin, mucosa, and gastrointestinal flora. Careful oral, perianal, and skin hygiene may help reduce the prevalence of infection in patients with acute or chronic neutropenia.

Prophylactic antibiotics are useful in severe chronic neutropenia, particularly for the prevention of *Staphylococcus* colonization and infection. First- or second-generation cephalosporins are appropriate for this indication, as is trimethoprim/sulfamethoxazole (Bactrim, Septra). The latter provides broader spectrum coverage with very little toxicity but may itself cause neutropenia and so must be used with caution.

Specific Therapy

For patients with autoimmune neutropenia, high-dose intravenous gamma globulin (2 grams per kg, as a single dose or divided daily over 3 to 4 days) may provide a transient elevation of ANC. The limited response may be sufficient to help clear an infection or aid postoperative wound healing but usually does not last long enough for prophylactic use.

Patients with systemic rheumatologic disorders, including Felty's syndrome, may benefit from therapy with glucocorticosteroids (e.g., prednisone), but there is rarely any indication for their use in other forms of neutropenia. Administration of steroids to a patient with neutropenia may do more harm than good, particularly if there is little or no response. Steroids add immunosuppression to an already compromised host defense system and predispose to fungal infection. However, brief use is safe as a diagnostic test for mobilization of bone marrow neutrophils.

The most important recent advance in the treatment of neutropenia has been the advent of recombinant human colony–stimulating factors: granulocyte colony–stimulating factor (G-CSF), marketed as filgrastim (Neupogen), and granulocyte-macrophage colony–stimulating factor (GM-CSF) marketed as sargramostim (Leukine). Food and Drug Administration (FDA)–approved indications for G-CSF include neutropenia associated with cancer chemotherapy and severe congenital neutropenia. G-CSF accelerates the recovery of peripheral blood neutrophil numbers following chemotherapy, resulting in significantly shorter and often less severe periods of neutropenia and hence lower morbidity and decreased hospitalization. Administration of 5 μg per kg per day, subcutaneously or intravenously, should begin 24 hours after the completion of each course and continue until the ANC has reached its nadir and risen again to 5000 to 10,000/mm^3. The ANC

briefly falls again after discontinuation of G-CSF. If administered by the intravenous route, G-CSF should be diluted to no less than 5 μg per mL and protected from adsorption to plastic tubing by addition of albumin (human) to a final concentration of 2 mg per mL.

Treatment with G-CSF can also correct the ANC to the normal range in most patients with severe congenital neutropenia, including Kostmann's agranulocytosis and cyclic neutropenia. Successful correction of the peripheral blood count also normalizes the prevalence of fever, stomatitis, and infection-related symptoms and risks. At the initiation of therapy, or if the ANC rises far above normal, expansion of myelopoiesis may cause bone pain or splenomegaly. The major concern about long-term use of G-CSF in these patients is the risk of accelerating the conversion to myelodysplasia or leukemia. Most reported cases of myelodysplasia or secondary myeloid leukemia in severe congenital neutropenia patients, both treated and untreated, have been associated with acquired chromosome 7 deletion or abnormality. Therefore, bone marrow cytogenetics need to be examined prior to initiation of G-CSF and periodically during its chronic administration. An international registry is now accumulating data to determine the actual versus the relative risk of myelodysplasia and leukemia associated with G-CSF therapy in severe congenital neutropenias. Because the risk is still uncertain, the drug should be used only for those patients who are frequently symptomatic or most severely affected. Sensitivity to G-CSF varies considerably in severe congenital neutropenia, so dosage needs to be titrated for each patient, usually within a range of 1 to 20 μg per kg per day, subcutaneously.

The use of G-CSF for acquired neutropenia is more controversial. Although it has been demonstrated to hasten recovery in drug-induced neutropenia, discontinuation of the myelosuppressive drug is usually sufficient, and the advantage of a few days' diminution of neutropenia does not justify the major expense, except in patients with severe infection. An empirical trial of G-CSF in acquired forms of severe chronic neutropenia may be warranted for symptomatic patients.

The primary indication for GM-CSF is the acceleration of bone marrow recovery after hematopoietic stem cell transplantation. It may also be effective in some cases of bone marrow failure, but GM-CSF is not indicated for severe congenital neutropenia due to clinically significant eosinophilia.

Granulocyte transfusion, although rarely indicated, may provide additional therapeutic support for newborn infants with sepsis and bone marrow neutrophil storage pool depletion, as well as for some agranulocytic patients with persistent sepsis or fungal infection after an adequate trial of aggressive antibiotic therapy. However, the risks of transfusion reaction, pulmonary sequestration, and graft-versus-host disease are high, and the actual survival advantage conferred by granulocyte transfusion remains uncertain.

HEMOLYTIC DISEASE OF THE FETUS AND NEWBORN

method of
CARL WEINER, M.D.

*Maryland Center for Advanced Fetal Care,
School of Medicine, University of Maryland
at Baltimore
Baltimore, Maryland*

Hydrops fetalis, jaundice, and anemia of the neonate were recognized in 1932 as a single disease characterized by perinatal hepatosplenomegaly, extramedullary hematopoiesis, and nucleated red blood cells on peripheral smear. Multiple investigators have since contributed to the vast body of knowledge demonstrating that IgG antibodies (principally anti-D) bound to the red blood cells (RBCs) of affected neonates lead to their destruction and that transplacental fetal-to-maternal hemorrhage is the main cause of maternal isoimmunization. This work stimulated the development of immunoprophylaxis with anti-Rh-D immunoglobulin, now standard in the industrialized world. Despite these advances, fetal hemolytic disease remains a serious and common cause of perinatal morbidity and, in some countries, perinatal mortality.

INCIDENCE

Anti-D remains the prototype for maternal red cell alloimmunization, though immunoprophylaxis has diminished its relative importance while enhancing that of the other antigen groups (Table 1). The prevalence of RBC alloimmunization approximates 0.5%. The incidence of Rh − individuals varies by race. Fifteen percent of North American whites are Rh −.

PATHOPHYSIOLOGY

Fetal RBCs are seen on a Kleihauer-stained peripheral smear at some time either during pregnancy or at delivery in 75% of women. The frequency and size of the bleed increase from 3% and 0.03 mL respectively in the first trimester to 45% and up to 25 mL in the third trimester. Spontaneous abortion is also associated with fetal-to-maternal hemorrhage, but the incidence is less than 1% and the volume usually less than 0.1 mL. In contrast, surgically

TABLE 1. **Antigens Causing Fetal Hemolytic Disease and Requiring Treatment**

Common

rhesus family: D, C, E, c, e
Kell

Uncommon

JK[a] (Kidd)
Fy[a] (Duffy)
Kp[a or b]
k
S

Rare

Do[a], Di[a or b], Fy[b], Hutch, Jk[b], Lu[a], M, N, s, U, Yt[a]

Never

Le[a or b], P

---

induced abortion has a 20% to 25% risk of transplacental hemorrhage, and the volume is greater. The overall risk of immunization during pregnancy is close to 20% independent of ABO compatibility if the fetus is Rh+, immune prophylaxis is not given, and the woman conceives again. The risk of immunization approximates 4% after therapeutic abortion of an at-risk pregnancy.

The initial immune response to the D antigen appears over 6 weeks to 12 months. Thus, the first sensitized pregnancy is not usually at great risk. A second antigen challenge generates an amnestic response that is both rapid and almost exclusively IgG. The longer the duration between challenges, the greater the increase in both the amount and strength of antibody.

The Rh antigens are well developed by the 30th day of gestation. The antibody-coated RBCs are destroyed within the reticuloendothelial system. The response of the affected fetus is quite variable and reflects the quantity and possibly the subclass of IgG antibody, the efficiency of placental passage, the avidity with which the antibody binds the antigen site, and the maturity of the reticuloendothelial system. Anemia may develop slowly in association with a low reticulocyte count and a normal bilirubin, or within a week in association with a reticulocytosis and hyperbilirubinemia. Both the fetal liver and spleen are enlarged secondary to extramedullary hematopoiesis and congestion.

All fetal sequelae of hemolytic disease stem directly or indirectly from the anemia. Though the fetus tolerates mild-to-moderate anemia well, other metabolic alterations such as metabolic acidemia and hyperlactatemia develop as the anemia worsens. The precise mechanism underlying the development of hydrops is uncertain, but it likely is a combination of hematologic and cardiac events. Cardiac dysfunction, probably mediated by hypoxemia, occurs in most hydropic fetuses. It manifests immediately prior to the appearance of hydrops as an elevated umbilical venous pressure. The umbilical venous pressure declines into the normal range within days following the first RBC transfusion but before hydrops has resolved.

Hyperbilirubinemia is an important part of alloimmune hemolytic disease. Both the fetus and neonate have reduced levels of glucuronyl transferase, the enzyme necessary for the production of the water-soluble diglucuronide. Indirect bilirubin not bound to albumin can penetrate the lipid neuronal membrane, causing cell death. During normal pregnancy, both the fetal serum albumin and bilirubin rise linearly with advancing gestation. Since placental bilirubin transport is limited, the normal fetal total bilirubin is 5 to 10 times above normal adult levels. The levels rise progressively as the severity of the hemolysis increases. The neonate with severe hyperbilirubinemia is at risk for an encephalopathy (kernicterus), which has a high mortality rate. The concentration of bilirubin necessary for kernicterus rises with advancing gestational age. All complications of fetal hemolytic anemia are potentially preventable by treatment.

DETECTION OF ALLOIMMUNIZATION
ANTIBODY DETECTION

The identification and management of fetal hemolytic disease employs several methods for the detection of antibodies either in the maternal sera or bound to the fetal red blood cell:

1. Agglutination tests:
Saline. Rh-positive red blood cells suspended in saline agglutinate if the patient's serum contains IgM but not IgG. IgM does not cross the placenta.

Colloid. Rh-positive red blood cells suspended in a colloid media (such as bovine albumin) agglutinate when the patient's serum contains either IgM or IgG. Thus, if both saline and colloid tests are positive, the antibody may be *either* an IgM or an IgG. The IgM can be eliminated by pretreating the serum to disrupt the sulfhydryl bonds of IgM. The IgG is unaffected.

2. Antiglobulin or Coombs' test:

Indirect. Red blood cells of specific or mixed antigen type are incubated with the patient's serum. Antihuman antiglobulin causes the red cells to clump if they have adsorbed antibody from the serum. The titer is the reciprocal of the highest dilution of serum that causes agglutination.

Direct. Antihuman antiglobulin is added directly to the patient's red blood cells. Clumping indicates antibody bound to the red blood cell. The antibody may be eluted and identified by performing an indirect test using type-specific antigen-type cells.

MANAGEMENT OF PREGNANT RH– WOMEN

All pregnant women should have blood drawn at first visit for the determination of ABO and Rh blood type unless they have previously been tested twice by the same laboratory. An indirect Coombs' test should also be performed. Laboratory error remains a frequent cause of anti-D prophylaxis failure. In addition, almost 50% of patients managed in our unit since 1983 have an RBC antibody directed against an antigen other than D. There is controversy as to how women who are Rh+ should be managed after the initial screen. The most complete approach is to repeat the screen at 32 weeks in search of newly developed non-anti-D antibodies, but this approach is not cost effective. The indirect Coombs' test should be repeated in Rh– women without evidence of sensitization at monthly intervals beginning at 18 to 20 weeks. In some societies, it may be reasonable to test the father's Rh status. Unfortunately, paternity is occasionally other than claimed or simply unknown. The decision whether to consider paternity in management is best left to the physician's discretion.

Routine antenatal anti-D immunoglobulin therapy is cost effective and should be administered to all nonsensitized Rh– women at 28 weeks' gestation. Women with vaginal bleeding of unknown origin should also receive anti-D immunoprophylaxis. Amniocentesis carries a 2% risk of maternal sensitization even if performed under ultrasound guidance; anti-D immunoglobulin should be administered routinely after amniocentesis. At delivery, cord blood is obtained to determine the neonatal ABO and Rh blood type and the detection of red blood cell–bound antibodies. Three hundred micrograms of anti-D immunoglobulin prevents maternal sensitization if the volume of fetal-to-maternal hemorrhage was less than 30 mL of fetal Rh+ blood. About 1 in 400 puerperal women experience a bleed of at least this magnitude. Larger bleeds should be routinely sought in all Rh– women delivering Rh+ children. Cesarean section and manual removal of the placenta each increase fetal-to-maternal hemorrhage and thus the risk of Rh sensitization.

Management of Alloimmunized Women

Noninvasive Evaluation

The prediction of fetal risk by a combination of the maternal obstetric history and serologic examination is at best an imprecise art. The risk of hydrops in the undiagnosed and untested situation approximates 10% in the first sensitized pregnancy. If maternal indirect Coombs' antibody titer determinations are performed in the same hospital using constant techniques, the results are reproducible and of some value in predicting the risk of severe fetal disease *especially during the first sensitized pregnancy.* However, the actual correlation of the titer and course of disease is so low that some argue against its use. When the maternal titer is below the critical threshold (variously 8, 16, or 32), it should be repeated at monthly intervals. Once the critical threshold is crossed, titer and history are inadequate measures upon which solely to base management.

High-resolution ultrasound aids the monitoring of fetuses at risk for hemolytic anemia. Relevant findings include amniotic fluid volume, liver length or thickness, splenic circumference, placental thickness, increased bowel echogenicity, and the cardiac biventricular diameter. Unfortunately, both the utility and the reproducibility of these findings have been low. Ultrasound is not a replacement for an invasive evaluation.

Fetal Testing

A number of approaches now permit identification of at-risk fetuses. Amniocytes obtained at the time of early second-trimester amniocentesis can be tested directly for a number of RBC antigens, including c, d, e, C, D, E, and Kell. Depending upon the population, a third to a half of fetuses will be found to be antigen-negative. Spectrophotometry (ΔOD450) uses a specimen of amniotic fluid obtained by ultrasound-guided amniocentesis after 20 weeks' gestation to measure and semiquantify bilirubinoid products for the prediction of hydrops. Finally, a blood sample obtained by cordocentesis can be tested directly. Each approach has potential advantages and disadvantages. Ultimately, the method selected should reflect the facilities available and the physician's experience. As the incidence of maternal alloimmunization is declining, any individual physician's experience with the management will be less than in the past. This makes consultation or referral to a more experienced individual an increasingly important consideration. *Once maternal alloimmunization has been confirmed, the patient should be referred to a Fetal Diagnosis and Treatment Unit.*

Amniotic Fluid Spectrophotometry. The fetus with hemolytic anemia typically has an elevated serum bilirubin, which enters the amniotic fluid via the urine and tracheal/pulmonary effluent. Liley standardized an approach based on this fact that has remained unchanged since its initial report. While the ΔOD450 can satisfactorily predict the relative fetal hematocrit, it is better at predicting hydrops. The principal advantage of amniocentesis in the 1990s is that most obstetricians are familiar with the technique. Amniotic fluid is obtained and transported to the laboratory in a light-resistant container to prevent degradation of bilirubin. The optical density is measured and the result plotted on semilogarithmic paper, with gestational age on the X axis and the ΔOD450 on the Y axis. Based on the study of 101 single amniotic fluid specimens obtained between 28 and 35 weeks' gestation, Liley observed that the ΔOD450 normally declines with advancing gestation. He divided the graph into three ascending zones:

Zone 1 represents mild or no fetal disease.
Zone 2 is intermediate, with the severity increasing as Zone 3 is approached.
Zone 3 indicates severe disease, with the chance of hydrops occurring within 7 days.

Amniocentesis is repeated at 1- to 2-week intervals, depending upon gestational age, the zone, and the change from the preceding sample. Management is dictated by the trend. Fetal transfusion (or delivery) is considered when either the ΔOD450 is in Zone 3 or serial amniotic fluid specimens reveal a progressive and rapid rise of the ΔOD450 into the upper 80% of Zone 2.

Amniotic fluid spectrophotometry has several major disadvantages. *First*, its application requires the performance of serial invasive procedures over the space of several weeks, a mean of three procedures per patient in experienced hands. Each procedure is associated with a risk of enhanced maternal sensitization as well as a risk of either amnionitis or premature rupture of the membranes. *Second*, amniotic fluid spectrophotometry is an indirect test for fetal anemia. It is not surprising that there is a wide range in disease severity for a single ΔOD450 between 28 and 34 weeks. This is true for both Zone 2 and Zone 3 measurements. Bowman opined that "the experience and judgment of the individual assessing the amniotic fluid findings are more important than the method used." Yet, in their almost unparalleled experience, 9% of the predictions made based on a Zone 2 ΔOD450 (which comprised almost 50% of their measurements) were erroneous. Few clinicians in this era of anti-D immunoglobulin prophylaxis have their experience and none likely will in the future. The *third* disadvantage of amniocentesis is that there is no clinically useful correlation between the ΔOD450 reading and the fetal hemoglobin prior to 28 weeks. The normal ΔOD450 in the second trimester is mid-Zone 2 of the Liley curve. Yet, amniocentesis is often initiated weeks before since the advent of high-resolution ultrasound. The *fourth* disadvantage of the ΔOD450 measurement is that it is subject to a variety of extrinsic errors that can interfere with its laboratory measurement.

Fetal Blood Sampling. The pregnancy loss rate for cordocentesis reflects the indication, the presence of hypoxemia, the vessel actually punctured, and the technique used (needle guide versus freehand). The use of a needle guide to eliminate lateral movement of the needle significantly decreases the complication rate. Cordocentesis for this indication is safe ($<\frac{1}{400}$ risk of a loss) in experienced hands. The placenta is avoided, as would be the practice for amniocentesis, by targeting the umbilical vein in a free loop of cord. When placental puncture is avoided, the magnitude of the fetal-maternal bleed after cordocentesis, as reflected by the percent rise in the maternal serum alpha-fetoprotein concentration, is similar to that after amniocentesis.

The first cordocentesis is performed when the maternal indirect Coombs' titer exceeds the critical threshold between 24 and 28 weeks, unless there is a history of a severely affected fetus earlier in gestation, or the initial indirect Coombs' titer is very high or increasing rapidly. Laboratory tests performed on the first and on any subsequent fetal blood samples are listed in Table 2. Either a strongly positive direct Coombs' test or a *manual* reticulocyte count outside the 95% confidence interval is a high risk factor for the development of antenatal anemia. It is essential that the norms for the reticulocyte count be based on the raw data and not a mathematical derivation, since the actual correlation of the reticulocyte count with gestational age, though significant, is quite low.

The protocol for risk assessment and the timing of any repeat cordocenteses are shown in Table 3. There is a significant direct correlation between the reticulocyte count, the strength of the direct Coombs' test, the risk of fetal anemia, and the trimester in gestation it will occur. Using direct fetal hematologic and serologic tests, a sensitive and specific assessment of the risk for developing pathologic levels of fetal anemia can be made. Approximately 50% of alloimmunized women require only one cordocentesis, as opposed to serial amniocentesis. By employing ultrasound as a backup, delivery may be safely deferred until 37 to 38 weeks, with only a 2% risk of unexpected anemia. Eighty percent of pregnancies requiring more than one cordocentesis ultimately require a fetal transfusion for a hematocrit less than 30%. This protocol for assessment is predictive of antenatal anemia only, not postnatal hyperbilirubinemia. Untreated neonates remain at significant risk for postnatal hyperbilirubinemia. Delivery of the nontransfused fetus should occur between 37 and 38 weeks' gestation in a center capable of dealing with a potentially ill neonate.

The direct testing of the fetus at risk for hemolytic

TABLE 2. **Fetal Blood Tests**

Hematocrit, reticulocyte count (manual), total bilirubin*
ABO type, Rh phenotype, specific other antigen testing, direct
 Coombs' titer

*It is essential that age-adjusted norms be used for the interpretation of these parameters.

TABLE 3. **Criteria for Repeat Cordocentesis if Fetus Is Affected**

Pattern	Hematocrit	Reticulocytes	± Direct Coombs' Test Result	Interval for Cordocentesis (wk)	Interval for Scan (wk)	Comments
1	Normal	Normal	−/trace	—	4	Repeat if initial maternal indirect Coombs' test result <128 and twofold increase documented
2	Normal	Normal or <2.5th percentile	1+/2+	5–6	2	Do not repeat after 32 wk if unchanged; deliver at term
3	Normal	>97.5th percentile	3+/4+	2	1	Continue through 34 wk; if hematocrit stable, deliver at 37–38 wk if not transfused
4	<2.5th percentile but >30%	Any	Any	1–2	1	Repeat as long as hematocrit criteria fulfilled; deliver with pulmonary maturity if not transfused

From Weiner C, et al: Am J Obstet Gynecol, *165*:546–553, 1991.

anemia offers several advantages over amniotic fluid ΔOD450 testing. Both sensitivity and specificity for the diagnosis and the prediction of fetal anemia are much greater than with the ΔOD450. Direct testing of the fetus for anemia has a zero false-positive rate and a 2% false-negative rate. As a result, fewer invasive procedures are necessary, reducing the overall risk of premature rupture of the membranes, amnionitis, and worsening of sensitization.

TREATMENT OF THE ANEMIC FETUS

Suppression of Maternal Antierythrocyte Antibodies

Several methods have been used to suppress or ameliorate either the maternal antibody concentration or its effect on the fetus. None are of documented efficacy, and only two appear to have limited potential: plasmapheresis and immune globulin therapy.

Fetal Transfusion

Anemia must be confirmed directly before initiating transfusion therapy. We define anemia as a hematocrit less than 30% since it is below the 2.5 centile for all gestational ages greater than 20 weeks. These procedures should be performed by individuals in units with considerable and regular experience, at least 8 to 10 transfusions per year.

Blood injected into the intraperitoneal cavity is absorbed via the lymphatics. Approximately 10% of the transfused cells are absorbed per day. Absorption is less efficient in hydropic fetuses. The volume infused is limited by fetal size. Bowman recommends that the volume be based on gestational age:

$$volume = (weeks' gestation - 20) \times 10\ mL$$

The second transfusion is performed when the first has been completely absorbed and thereafter at 3- to 4-week intervals. If the fetus is hydropic and survives the first intraperitoneal transfusion, the fetal abdomen is drained as completely as possible at the sec-

ond transfusion to minimize pressure and maximize the amount of fresh packed cells infused.

Intraperitoneal transfusion places the fetus at risk for abdominal trauma and the obstruction of cardiac return if intra-abdominal pressure rises too high. Thus, the last intraperitoneal transfusion is performed no later than 32 weeks' gestation. Although there have been no randomized trials comparing the intraperitoneal and intravenous routes, a historical comparison from the team in Winnipeg, Canada, indicates that the rate of death per intraperitoneal transfusion is six times greater than that of intravascular transfusion in their experienced hands. Intravenous transfusion is the preferred route unless percutaneous access to the fetal vasculature is extremely difficult, as it might be prior to 18 weeks.

The goal of *intravascular* transfusion therapy is the *term* delivery of a healthy, nonanemic neonate. Transfusions are begun when the fetal hematocrit declines below 30%. This is a pragmatic selection, since the fetus can tolerate a hematocrit of 25% or lower without clinical sequelae. However, it is reasonable since:

1. 30% is less than the 2.5 centile after 20 weeks' gestation.
2. Many patients referred to a Fetal Diagnosis and Treatment Unit come from a great distance away and cannot visit on a semiweekly or even weekly basis without great hardship.
3. It is difficult to predict how fast the fetal hematocrit will decline.
4. Treatment of anemia prevents the development of hydrops, which greatly increases the likelihood of an adverse, poor outcome.

Blood for transfusion should be fresh when possible and compatible with both mother and fetus. It is filtered, rendered leukocyte-poor, washed several times in saline to remove particles associated with transmission of viral infection, resuspended in saline to a hematocrit between 70% and 80%, and irradiated to eliminate the small risk of fetal graft-versus-host disease. Infectious agents usually tested for include cytomegalovirus, hepatitis A, B, C, and human immune deficiency virus. Prostaglandin synthetase inhibitors to minimize uterine activity are contraindicated since an increase in fetal prostacyclin and prostaglandin E_2 is part of the normal adaptive response to the abrupt increase in intravascular volume.

The goal is a post-transfusion hematocrit of 48% to 55%, except for the first transfusion of a hydropic fetus. The volume needed depends upon gestational age, the initial hematocrit, and the presence of hydrops. Assuming similar opening and closing hematocrit measurements, the volume is strongly dependent on gestational age and frequently equals or exceeds the calculated total fetal-placental intravascular volume. Because most hydropic fetuses have myocardial dysfunction that prevents them from tolerating significant volume expansion, the target hematocrit for their first transfusion is only 25%. Since pump dysfunction corrects rapidly as the oxygen-carrying capacity increases, the hematocrit can typically be brought safely to 50% 24 hours later. The decline in umbilical vein pH that normally occurs during transfusion appears especially important in severely anemic fetuses. The red blood cell is the principal fetal buffer, and the pH of the banked blood preserved in citrate is approximately 6.98 to 7.01. We believe the acidemia aggravates the pump failure and now infuse bicarbonate in 1-mEq increments to maintain the pH greater than 7.30. Since that practice was initiated, there have been no further losses of hydropic fetuses. We transfuse half the estimated total volume and check the incremental increase in the hematocrit. Based on the increase achieved with the first aliquot, the remaining volume necessary can be accurately and rapidly calculated.

Except for the hydropic fetus, the second transfusion is performed two weeks after the first. Subsequently, the decline in hematocrit per week is quite predictable for any given fetus. The rate at which the hematocrit drops also decreases with advancing gestation, so that by 34 to 35 weeks, delivery may be safely delayed 4 to 5 weeks without another transfusion.

It is advantageous to perform at least two transfusions 3 weeks apart prior to delivery since postnatal complications of hyperbilirubinemia are significantly less likely after two or more antenatal transfusions. In experienced hands, fetal losses are uncommon and confined to the previable fetus. *There is no justification for routine preterm delivery.* The last transfusion is performed at 34 to 35 weeks' gestation and labor induced at 37 to 38 weeks.

The obstetric philosophy for delivery need not be altered for the nonanemic, transfused fetus. There is no reason to deny either a vaginal birth after cesarean section or the vaginal delivery of the appropriately selected breech just because of an antenatal transfusion. If the final hematocrit at the end of the last transfusion was 50%, it will be in the mid-30s in the umbilical cord at delivery. Typically, the neonatal hematocrit increases 5 to 15% within 8 hours of delivery, reflecting a massive shift of extracellular and intravascular fluid. Over the next few days to weeks, the hematocrit will decline to or below the delivery level.

Postnatally, infants who received *in utero* transfusion therapy do remarkably well, with an average hospitalization time of less than 7 days, much of which is simply observation. Their hyperbilirubinemia is managed with phototherapy. Because they deliver at term, a higher neonatal bilirubin concentration can be tolerated. Double-volume exchange transfusion is rarely needed when there have been at least two antenatal transfusions. However, small, simple transfusions are often necessary beginning at several weeks of age. The neonatal hematocrit and reticulocyte count should be monitored weekly. When this is not done, we have seen severe anemia with resulting high-output failure and failure to thrive occur. The pediatric goal is to keep the neonate asymptomatic but with a modest anemia (16%) so the erythropoietic stimulus is maintained. The use of erythropoietin (Epogen) postnatally is under study. Though the period of neonatal anemia is transient, neonates may go 16 weeks before reticulocytes appear on a peripheral smear. Once reticulocytosis is noted, further transfusion therapy is generally unneeded.

HEMOPHILIA AND RELATED CONDITIONS

method of
W. KEITH HOOTS, M.D.
University of Texas M. D. Anderson Cancer Center
Houston, Texas

Hemophilia A (Factor VIII deficiency) and hemophilia B (Factor IX deficiency) are X-linked inherited hereditary bleeding disorders. By contrast, von Willebrand's disease (vWD) is autosomally inherited, so that males and females are affected equally. Hemophilias A and B present as clinically identical conditions; the primary morbid manifestations are joint bleeding (hemarthrosis) and joint destruction. The reason that the clinical findings are indistinguishable is that Factor VIIIc (hemophilia A) and Factor IX (hemophilia B) are essential cofactors for activating Factor Xa in the intrinsic clotting pathway. Each of these factors is primarily produced in the liver. Factor IX is a serine protease, and Factor VIIIc is a large glycoprotein essential for configuring the clotting enzymes on the platelet surface so that enzyme-substrate reactions occur at optimal maximal kinetics.

Both hemophilias A and B exhibit a range of clinical severities that correlates fairly well with assayed factor levels. Specifically, severe disease is defined as less than 1% assayed clotting factor in plasma, whereas approximately 1 to 5% and greater than 5% of normal are defined as moderate and mild disease, respectively. Males within a family almost always have the same degree of impairment since they share the same defect in the DNA coding for the clotting protein.

Both hemophilia A and hemophilia B are coded for by DNA on the long arm (q) of the X chromosome. The Factor VIII gene, coding for a glycoprotein that is substantially larger than the Factor IX protein (approximately 340,000 vs. approximately 70,000 daltons), has been demonstrated to be highly susceptible to mutation events including delegations and missense and nonsense mutations. Though significantly smaller than the Factor VIII gene, the Factor IX gene has also been shown to be prone to new mutation events, particularly of the missense and nonsense type. In practical terms, this results in approximately 25 to 30% of newly diagnosed cases of either hemophilia A or hemophilia B representing a *new* mutation event within a family previously unaffected by hemophilia. This also accounts for the exceptional consistency of prevalence and incidence of both hemophilia A and hemophilia B across all racial and ethnic groups.

The incidence of hemophilias A and B together is between 1 in 5000 and 1 in 10,000 live male births. Approximately 80 to 85% of these affected neonates have hemophilia A. Approximately two-thirds of those with hemophilia A have severe or moderately severe (≤1% Factor VIII) disease. By contrast almost half of hemophilia B patients have greater than 1% Factor IX levels. Hemophilias A and B of comparable severities bleed with similar frequency.

vWD results when there is a defect in the gene for von Willebrand factor (vWf), which is located on chromosome 12. The disease is among the most prevalent of genetic diseases. As high as 1% of certain cohort studies using molecular biologic analyses for gene mutation have shown abnormalities. The glycoprotein coded for by the vWf gene is a large subunit of approximately 226,000 daltons that multimerizes into large cell-adhesive molecules that are essential both for platelet aggregation via cross-linking of glycoprotein IB receptors between platelets and for platelet adhesion at the site of blood vessel endothelial cell injury. In addition, these vWf multimers that are secreted from both endothelial cells and platelets are essential for stabilizing Factor VIIIc from proteolysis in the circulating plasma. This explains the low level of Factor VIIIc seen in several types of vWD (see later) despite the fact that both the Factor VIIIc gene and its coded protein are entirely normal.

Unlike the pattern in hemophilias A and B, the clinical bleeding pattern of vWD is primarily localized to mucous membrane surface. Hence, epistaxis, menorrhagia, post-dental surgical, and gastrointestinal bleeding are common manifestations in individuals with vWD. Postsurgical bleeding or hemorrhage secondary to significant trauma occurs to differing degrees, depending on the qualitative or quantitative defect or deficiency in the circulating vWf molecule.

Despite the heterogeneity of the molecular defects of vWf, the categorization of clinical vWD is based on the amount and the functional capacity of the vWf protein in the plasma. Abnormalities have been divided into three major types based on the specific laboratory tests that assess both the quantity and the function of vWf in the plasma of an affected individual.

Type I (Type 1) vWD is a heterozygous state in which the genetic defect inherited from one parent (or representing a new mutation) is partially compensated for by normal vWf production directed by the normal gene from the other parent. This Type I, or classic, vWD is the clinical state most commonly diagnosed. *Quantitative* laboratory studies that measure vWf protein immunologically (Factor VIII–related antigen) are abnormal. The results of vWf (Factor VIII vWf: ristocetin cofactor activity [FVIII vWf:RCoF]) *functional* studies that measure qualitative function in the plasma are proportionally reduced. Further, as noted previously, the Factor VIIIc level in the plasma is frequently abnormal as well, since the diminished FVIII vWf:RCoF level results in a decreased plasma half-life of the Factor VIIIc molecules produced by the hepatocyte.

Type II (Type 2) vWD consists of multiple genetic defects sharing one common defining characteristic: there is normal production of vWf protein that is measured by protein antigen assays in the plasma; however, these vWf molecules are functionally defective to differing degrees. A comprehensive discussion of all the Type II variants of vWD is beyond the scope of this article. Nonetheless, several distinct categories that illustrate the heterogeneity can be listed: abnormalities in the multimerization of the vWf subunits, a defective Factor VIIIc binding site, and a defective secretion of vWf from platelets despite normal plasma vWf structure and function. Any and all may produce clinical bleeding syndromes. Further, as with vWD in general, there is often substantial clinical heterogeneity between individuals of the same Type II variant.

Persons with Type III (Type 3) vWD have a defect in the vWf genes of both chromosomes 12. In many cases, neither parent has a clinically significant bleeding history since subclinical disease among Type I heterozygotes is common. By contrast, the individual with Type III homozygous vWD has severe clinical bleeding since he or she has little if any vWf protein or circulating Factor VIIIc. The latter is deficient since a paucity of vWf in plasma results in rapid proteolysis of Factor VIIIc even though its production is normal. Hence, individuals with Type III vWD may experience both the mucous membrane hemorrhage pattern seen with vWD and bleeding into deep tissue or organs (e.g., hemarthroses) seen more commonly in hemophilic persons. Further, chronic morbidity is much more commonly observed in these individuals.

Inherited bleeding diatheses secondary to abnormalities of other plasma proteins, platelets, or blood vessels are much less common than either hemophilia or vWD. Genetic defects in Factors XI, prekallikrein, and high-molecular-weight kininogen result in prolongation of the activated partial thromboplastin time (aPTT) and may cause clinical bleeding syndromes, although usually less severe than in hemophilia A or B. By contrast, inherited Factor XII deficiency, although prolonging the aPTT, produces no clinical bleeding.

Autosomally inherited Factors V, VII, and X and prothrombin deficiencies are quite rare. When diagnosed they may produce a significant hemorrhagic state, the severity of which correlates inversely with the circulating plasma concentration of the deficient protease (Factors II [prothrombin], VII, and X) or glycoprotein (Factor V).

Factor VII deficiency is suggested when the prothrombin time (PT) is prolonged but the aPTT is normal. Homozygous autosomal afibrinogenemia, the clinical incidence of which is approximately 1 in 1 million live births, may present in the neonatal period with life-threatening hemorrhage necessitating emergent and aggressive replacement therapy with cryoprecipitate. Abnormalities in Factors II, V, and X and fibrinogen prolong both the PT and the aPTT.

Two inherited protein deficiencies are notable for their likelihood of producing hemorrhagic syndromes despite normal PT and aPTT screening tests. The first, Factor XIII deficiency, frequently presents with an indicative clinical history: delayed bleeding after initial adequate hemostasis. This occurs because Factor XIII is required for clot stabilization. The second, homozygous deficiency of the inhibitor alpha$_2$-antiplasmin, also produces a bleeding diathesis, since a dearth of this natural inhibitor of the fibrinolytic protein plasmin permits exaggerated clot lysis by plasmin, thus producing clinical bleeding after tissue injury. Inherited disorders of platelet and endothelial cell function do, in a number of circumstances, cause clinical bleeding.

TREATMENT

Hemostatic Abnormalities

Replacement Therapy

For the majority of inherited coagulation disorders, primary therapy consists of infusing a protein product that replenishes the deficient clotting component. Historically the source of these replacement clotting proteins has been human plasma. The majority of these clotting proteins have their hemostatic activity defined as units of clotting activity per milliliter of pooled normal human plasma. Hence, the blood bank and pharmaceutical strategy for improving the replacement capacity for the specific deficient factor has been to concentrate the specific protein. In some cases, similar proteins co-purify in the concentration process from the source plasma. The first successful strategy for concentrating such clotting proteins from source plasma was cryoprecipitate, which results from the slow thawing of freshly frozen plasma and results in a severalfold concentration of the following clotting proteins: Factor VIIIc, Factor VIII vWf, fibrinogen, Factor XIII, and fibronectin.

Commercial fractionation of cryoprecipitate yielded the first generation of lyophilized Factor VIII concentrates, which resulted in an approximate 100-fold increase in the concentration of Factor VIII per milliliter of infusate. This commercial scale-up resulted when source plasma from 5 to 25,000 donors was converted into lyophilized vials of Factor VIII. These vials ranged in potency from 200 to 1500 U (20 to 35 U per mg of protein) per vial. For the first time, convenient home infusion for hemophilia-associated hemorrhage was feasible. Unfortunately, because of the number of donors contributing to the commercial plasma pool, transfusion-transmitted viral disease (particularly transfusion-associated hepatitis and human immunodeficiency virus [HIV] infection) became a common complication in the hemophilia A population. Purification strategies to alleviate or ultimately eliminate this viral risk awaited advances in technology.

Similar viral transmission risk existed for the fractionated therapeutic clotting factor produced for hemophilia B. Since cryoprecipitation does not enrich the product with Factor IX, the initial step in the fractionation of Factor IX clotting factor products has traditionally been barium or aluminum sulfate adsorption followed by further column fractionation. For therapies used in the 1970s and 1980s, this resulted in co-purification of all the molecularly similar vitamin K–dependent factors (II, VII, IX, and X), yielding a final product called prothrombin complex concentrates (PCCs). Like the production of Factor VIII products, the production of PCCs yielded a final

vial concentration of 200 to 1500 U (20 to 40 U per mg of protein) per vial. Like the factor VIII products, these commercially produced factor concentrates were, in the years before more effective viral-attenuation techniques, almost invariably virally contaminated, notably with several species of hepatitis and with HIV (after 1979).

The co-purification of Factors II, VII, and X in the preparation of Factor IX concentrates sometimes resulted in the selective conversion of one or more of these protease zymogens to its active enzyme (e.g., Factor VII is converted in trace amounts to Factor VIIa). This trace contamination with active proteases means that PCCs have a thrombogenic potential. Indeed, PCCs given therapeutically in high and recurrent dosing schedules have produced significant and sometimes fatal clotting events in patients with hemophilia B—particularly in individuals receiving the PCCs to provide hemostasis in association with orthopedic surgery. Other clinical situations in which thrombogenesis may be associated with the infusion of PCCs include (1) sustained crush injuries, (2) large intramuscular bleeds (e.g., psoas or thigh), (3) the treatment of neonates with hemophilia B who have immature natural anticoagulation, and (4) hemostatic therapy given to individuals with severe chronic hepatitis (since this may adversely affect their ability to make antithrombin III and the vitamin K-dependent inhibitors protein-C and protein-S in their hepatocytes). In its most severe manifestations, dosing with PCCs has produced acute myocardial infarction and disseminated intravascular coagulation. The latter risk may be mitigated by not infusing more than 75 U per kg per dose daily when recurrent dosing is required (e.g., after surgery or to treat life-threatening hemorrhage) and by adding small amounts of heparin to each infusion. Fortunately, more advanced purification technologies have resulted in the production of single-component Factor IX products that are free of any significant trace-activated proteases. These now provide the mainstay for therapy of hemophilia B patients when high-dose, recurrent infusion therapy is required.

Later-Generation Clotting Factor Concentrates

Therapeutic Options for Treatment of Hemophilias A and B in the mid-1990s

FACTOR VIII PRODUCTS

Because of the high frequency and profound impact of transfusion-associated transmission of hepatitis and HIV infection in the hemophilic population during the 1970s and 1980s, there were rapid and profound advances in the attenuation (and even elimination) of these and other viral contaminants. The first step in this evolution was heat treatment of Factor VIII products first licensed for use in 1983. Subsequent advances included pasteurization; solvent-detergent treatment to eliminate lipid-envelope viruses; advanced sepharose chromatography; affinity chromatography with monoclonal antibodies directed against the Factor VIIIc–Factor VIII vWf complex or against Factor IX; and most recently, the commercial production of a recombinant Factor VIIIc product in transfected mammalian cell systems. Each non-recombinant clotting factor concentrate presently produced in the United States is made from a donor pool screened for HIV, hepatitis B virus, and hepatitis C virus. In addition, each of the currently marketed products undergoes either heating to high temperatures for a long time or solvent-detergent treatment. Both processes appear sufficient to remove the risk of HIV transmission but not necessarily the hepatitis risk particularly when concomitant donor screening is employed.

This degree of confidence that the product is safe in terms of HIV infection does not exist for cryoprecipitate and fresh-frozen plasma (FFP), which typically undergo no viral attenuation other than donor screening (an exception is the investigational pasteurized FFP product made by the New York Blood Center). Efficient donor screening has reduced the relative risk of infection from either of these single-donor products to between 1 in 40,000 and 1 in 100,000 per donor unit for HIV and to 1 in 3000 or less per donor unit for hepatitis C virus. Even though the risk of hepatitis B infection from single-donor cryoprecipitate or FFP is similarly low, anyone likely to be treated with *any* plasma-derived product (whether single-donor or pooled, attenuated product) *should* receive a full three-inoculation course of the hepatitis B vaccine.

Each one of the Factor VIII concentrates available at this time is considered safe in terms of transmission of HIV and similar retroviruses. However, they are not all free of hepatitis C transmission risk. Fortunately the relative risk that any single lot of any of the products will transmit hepatitis C appears low. Nonetheless, documentation of transmissions of hepatitis C virus, hepatitis A virus, and human parvovirus B19 from some existing Factor VIII products has been documented. Current products can be classified by relative product purity, although any comparisons may quickly become outdated as technology advances.

The intermediate-purity factor concentrates are so designated because even though they undergo aggressive viral inactivation with heat (even pasteurization) and/or solvent detergent, the final concentration of Factor VIII in the end product represents a small percentage of the total heterogeneous plasma proteins present (6 to 10 U of Factor VIIIc per mg of total protein excluding albumin).

High-purity products are factor concentrates that have at least 50 U (range: 50 to 150) of Factor VIIIc per mg of protein (excluding albumin for stabilization). In the majority of cases, specialized column chromatographic techniques (e.g., heparin sepharose) result in the significantly higher purity, although there still is trace contamination with immunoglobulins or other plasma proteins. The chromatographic technique provides some viral attenuation, but enhanced viral safety is dependent on postchromatographic pasteurization or solvent-detergent treatment. The end products are considered safe in terms of HIV and relatively but not absolutely safe in terms of hepatitis C virus.

Ultrahigh-purity products are the monoclonal antibody affinity-purified plasma-derived factor concentrates and the recombinant Factor VIII products. For the former the affinity chromatography step is not only efficient at removing all non-Factor VIIIc protein but is a very efficient viral attenuation process as well. Nonetheless, effective elimination of hepatitis C virus from the monoclonal products has required subsequent pasteurization or treatment with solvent detergent. The specific activity of the monoclonal preparations (before the addition of human serum albumin) is 3000 U of Factor VIIIc per mg of protein. This is essentially identical to the effective purity of the licensed recombinant products, which also require comparable dilution with albumin to maintain stability after lyophilization.

With regard to theoretical viral safety, a notable distinction must be made between the monoclonal and the recombinant products. Since the recombinant Factor VIII products are affinity-purified from the cell culture of transfected hamster-derived cell lines, there is no requirement for any further viral attenuation. The addition of human serum albumin constitutes the sole theoretical source of human viral contamination. A theoretical risk of contamination by other nonhuman mammalian viruses or other infective species remains.

Frequent infusions of ultrapure products (specifically the monoclonal products) have been shown to produce a stabilization of the CD4 count in HIV-infected hemophilic patients when compared with chronic infusion of similar amounts of intermediate-purity clotting factor concentrates. It is suspected that in these ultrapure products this results from the absence of other protein contamination rather than from greater purity in terms of viral contamination. Nonetheless, most physicians treating hemophilia have opted to use one of these ultrapure products to treat their HIV-infected patients. Many have also chosen to treat their previously untreated hemophilia A patients (particularly the young children) with these products because of a perceived theoretical viral safety. This safety margin is inferred from (1) studies showing an enhanced capacity to remove surrogate viruses during the monoclonal processing, and (2) the bypassing of a human plasma source (with the exception of the added human serum albumin) from the recombinant products.

It should be noted that there are ongoing clinical trials of a recombinant Factor VIIIc preparation from which the B domain of the gene has been removed before transfection of the hamster cell lines. The protein portion of Factor VIII coded for by the B domain of the gene is not required for efficient clotting function; further, its deletion confers greater stability on the resultant smaller Factor VIIIc molecule. Hence there is no requirement for human serum albumin to stabilize the final lyophilized product. This may provide a higher level of confidence that the product is safe from any future microbiologic contamination. It is not yet apparent when this product will be available for clinical use.

FACTOR IX PRODUCTS

The clotting factor products available for treating hemophilia B must be assessed for two potential factors: (1) theoretical viral safety and factor purity (activity per milligram of protein), and (2) thrombogenicity. The Factor IX products determined to be free of thrombogenic potential are those preparations that have effectively purified the Factor IX protein from the other prothrombin complex proteins (Factors II, VII, and X). Two technical strategies have been employed to purify Factor IX from the other vitamin K factors and thereby to remove the thrombogenic risk: (1) chromatographic partitioning followed by solvent-detergent treatment, *and* (2) monoclonal affinity purification of Factor IX. The product produced by the former process contains some residual nonclotting plasma proteins. By contrast the monoclonal product is free of other plasma proteins. Viral attenuation to remove HIV appears effective in both processes. The hepatitis virus risk is significantly reduced by both processes. However, studies using surrogate viruses imply greater safety from hepatitis C or similar viruses with the monoclonal Factor IX concentrate.

The other clotting factor concentrates available for treating hemophilia B patients are PCCs. They can produce thrombotic complications when given in high doses or after repeated or sequential dosing. Viral-attenuation strategies for PCCs are either solvent-detergent treatment or heating to 80° C for more than 10 hours. PCCs made by using the heat process may provide a greater viral attenuation for some viruses, although this has not been proved. Either of these PCCs may prove efficacious for treating moderate bleeding (e.g., hemarthrosis) in individuals with highly responsive Factor VIII inhibitors for whom Factor VIIIc concentrates are nonhemostatic because of the Factor VIII antibody.

ANTI–INHIBITOR CLOTTING PREPARATIONS

Since PCCs are thrombogenic because of their trace contamination with the active proteases (e.g., Factor VIIa or Factor Xa), they have been used for nearly 2 decades to treat bleeding in Factor VIII–deficient patients with high responsive (i.e., anamnestic) Factor VIII antibodies. Later manufacturers of PCCs increased the trace amounts of these active proteases to produce activated PCCs (aPCCs). There is no in vitro assay for either of the two licensed aPCC products that correlates with in vivo hemostatic efficacy. Hence, it is often difficult to predict the hemostatic efficacy of aPCCs. Both the individual response and the therapeutic efficacy for specific hemorrhagic episodes vary widely. Stated another way, it is problematic, if not impossible, to predict a priori whether a given dose (units per kilogram of body weight) will provide the necessary hemostasis after a single infusion in a patient with no prior use of aPCC. This is true even though the aPCCs are supplied according to units of hemostatic activity (Factor VIIIc "bypassing" activity) per vial and are dosed accordingly (typical dosing for hemarthroses is 100 U per kg per dose.) To further complicate the issue, there are two aPCC preparations. One may be ineffective in a patient whereas the other may produce effective hemostasis for acute bleeding for that patient. Conversely, the alternative aPCC may prove superior in a second patient with a similar bleeding episode. Because of this capriciousness of aPCC therapy in patients with inhibitors, an individualized therapeutic plan must be established empirically. However, certain principles generally apply: (1) effective dosing of aPCCs is minimally 75 to 100 U per kg; (2) dosing frequency more often than every 6 hours predisposes to significant thrombogenicity, particularly after the third to fourth consecutive dose (hence monitoring for markers of disseminated intravascular coagulation is warranted when sequential dosing over several days is required), and (3) since the activated proteases that account for the procoagulant activity of aPCCs are short-lived, initial hemostasis may be followed by breakthrough bleeding between doses that may create difficulty for maintenance hemostatic therapy. Therapy with aPCCs is expensive, is less than reliable, and carries a risk of significant complications. Experience and expertise in their use help to mitigate these risks and to differentiate the appropriate use of aPCCs from the other alternatives for inhibitor therapy cited later.

One alternative therapy for treating patients with inhibitors is porcine Factor VIII. This product is produced from porcine plasma using a polyelectrolyte resin separation technology. The residual nonhuman protein is relatively low, although this does not completely eliminate the anaphylactoid potential of this product. Another characteristic of porcine Factor VIII often limits its efficacy in many individuals with inhibitors. In many cases, the specific anamnestic antibody directed against the human Factor VIIIc glycoprotein cross-reacts with shared epitopes on the porcine molecule. Therefore, before the therapeutic efficacy of the product of porcine Factor VIII can be assessed in a patient, it is necessary to quantitate the neutralizing capacity of the antibody against both the porcine and the human Factor VIII product using the Bethesda assay. In those instances in which the anti-porcine product Bethesda unit titer is significantly lower (10 Bethesda U) than the corresponding anti-human product Bethesda titer, therapy with porcine Factor VIII may be the therapy of choice. Before infusing the first dose of porcine Factor VIII (at a starting dose of approximately 100 U per kg), there is need to infuse a test dose of approximately 100 U to ensure that there is no immediate hypersensitivity reaction. If none occurs, a slow infusion over 20 to 30 minutes with careful monitoring for allergic symptoms can proceed. Further, since the porcine

Bethesda unit inhibitor assay provides an in vitro estimate of the neutralizing capacity of the anti–Factor VIII antibody against porcine Factor VIII, it is essential to monitor Factor VIII levels in these patients. As with most therapies for Hemophilia A patients with inhibitors, therapy with porcine Factor VIII is quite costly.

The indications for the use of other more esoteric and experimental therapies for Factor VIII inhibitors (e.g., Factor VIIa, immune tolerance induction, or antibody depletion using a staphylococcal protein A sepharose chromatographic column) are beyond the scope of this discussion. Comprehensive hemophilia treatment centers provide expertise for these specialized therapeutic procedures. Further, since optimal methodologies are still to be determined by collaborative research protocols, discussion with physician-scientists at these centers offers the best prospect for providing clinicians with up-to-date information about therapeutic options for treating complex inhibitor patients.

THERAPIES FOR VON WILLEBRAND'S DISEASE

Patients with Type I and most with Type II vWD may often be treated with desmopressin acetate (DDAVP), a synthetic analogue of the antidiuretic hormone 1-deamino-8-D-arginine vasopressin. Because of its efficacy in inducing the release of vWf multimers from endothelial cells, it results in a concomitant rise in Factor VIIIc levels (because vWf spares the latter molecule from rapid proteolysis in plasma). DDAVP at a dose of 0.3 µg per kg by slow intravenous infusion increases circulating vWf by approximately 250% in the average individual and increases Factor VIIIc approximately 300%. Therefore it becomes the treatment of choice for mild-to-moderate bleeding in most individuals with both mild hemophilia A (e.g., 5% Factor VIII activity) and Types I and II vWD. (Note: In Type IIb vWD, in which the largest vWf multimers are missing from plasma but are released in excess following DDAVP use, there is a theoretical risk of thrombocytopenia from excessive platelet aggregation. Hence its use in this subgroup must be evaluated on an individual case basis.) Since a two and one-half to threefold increase in both Factor VIIIc and Factor VII vWf is often sufficient to raise both to normal ranges in vWD patients, many such individuals may never require any other type of therapy for either acute hemorrhage or prophylaxis for surgical or dental procedures. Tachyphylaxis after repeated dosing with DDAVP can occur because of depletion of the vWf stores in the endothelial cells. Therefore, monitoring of in vivo clotting factor activity levels in those individuals requiring frequent dosing (i.e., daily or more often) is indicated.

Recently, a highly concentrated (1500 µg per mL) intranasal form of DDAVP (stimate) has been licensed in the United States. Two inhalations in a single nostril acutely in adults and one inhalation in children typically achieve approximately two-thirds of the therapeutic effect of the intravenous dosing. As with the intravenous preparation, facial flushing, mild to moderate blood pressure elevation, and antidiuresis are expected side effects.

For individuals with Type III vWD, for those with Types I and II who either fail to respond to DDAVP or do so to a degree inadequate to achieve complete and predictable hemostasis, and for those vWD patients who experience tachyphylaxis precluding required repeated therapy, other therapeutic options are needed. Traditionally, cryoprecipitate administered in a dose calculated to elevate either the Factor VIIIc, or the Factor VIII:vWf level or both to the normal range has been the most effective means for achieving hemostasis in such patients. However, as noted previously, single-donor cryoprecipitate has a very small but finite risk of causing hepatitis virus and even HIV infection.

Hence, many hematologists have chosen to employ one of three intermediate- or high-purity Factor VIII concentrates that have been demonstrated to have most sizes of vWf multimers present after reconstitution. Unlike cryoprecipitate, these concentrates may not have the ideal ratio of vWf multimers when compared with the physiologic state. Nonetheless, the theoretical viral safety conferred by the attenuation they undergo in preparation more than compensates for this theoretical hemostatic deficit. Several studies have shown clinical efficacy to be good even when individuals with severe disease (Type III) have experienced potential or actual life-threatening hemorrhage.

ANTI–FIBRINOLYTIC AGENTS

Tranexamic acid (Cyklokapron) and epsilon-aminocaproic acid (EACA) (Amicar) act by inhibiting plasminogen activation, thereby enhancing clot stability. These two agents are useful therapeutic adjuncts to stabilize clots that have formed after therapy in patients with underlying hemostatic defects. For patients with inherited clotting disorders, they have proved particularly efficacious for bleeding in the oral cavity (e.g., after dental or oral surgical procedures or trauma to the mouth) and for epistaxis. Dosing for oral tranexamic acid is 25 mg per kg per dose every 6 to 8 hours; for EACA it is 75 to 100 mg per kg per dose every 6 hours (maximal dose is 3 to 4 grams every 6 hours). For patients with hemophilia and vWD, treatment may be required for 7 to 14 days, depending on the amount of tissue injury. In hemophilia B, it is prudent to use a purified Factor IX preparation rather than PCC when concomitant antifibrinolytic therapy is contemplated because of the added thrombotic risks of the two latter agents together.

PREVENTIVE CARE

Male infants born to known or suspected hemophilic carrier mothers should not be circumcised until hemophilia in the infant has been excluded by laboratory testing. Blood for assay for aPTT and Factor VIII or Factor IX assay (or both if the family history is uncertain) should be obtained from cord blood.

When a cord blood sample is not available, venipuncture should be performed in a superficial limb vein in order to lessen the likelihood of producing a hematoma that might then require the patient to have replacement therapy. Femoral and jugular sites must be avoided.

Routine immunizations requiring injection such as diphtheria-pertussis-tetanus (DPT) or measles-mumps-rubella (MMR) may be given in the deep subcutaneous tissue (rather than deep intramuscular as is the usual practice), using the smallest gauge needle that is feasible. Hepatitis B vaccine should be given as soon after birth as possible to all infants with confirmed diagnosis of hemophilia. The oral polio live attenuated viral vaccine should not be given to an infant whose hemophilic older brother (or grandfather in the household) is known to be HIV immune-suppressed; Salk vaccine may be substituted.

Early infant dental examination is recommended to teach proper teeth brushing and to ensure adequate household water fluoridation. In addition to education about hemophilia, both genetic and psychosocial counseling are important for the mother of a newborn with hemophilia. This is particularly true for the approximately 30% for whom the hemophilia represents a new mutation and for whom there is no previous family experience with the disease. Reluctance to clean the teeth routinely should be dispelled early, and anticipated problem areas for causing bleeding should be discussed.

Both parents should be encouraged to participate intensively in every part of the infant's care. Further, normal socialization opportunities must not be limited because of the hemophilia. Experienced personnel should discuss specifically what minimal limitations are reasonable versus what constitutes overprotection and therefore may jeopardize the child's normal development.

An appropriate exercise regimen that excludes "contact" sports (e.g., tackle football) should be encouraged as a daily routine. Further, the role of such a program for the child and adult following episodes of hemarthrosis is best discussed before the child has a joint bleed.

SPECIAL CONSIDERATION FOR HEMOPHILIC BLEEDING

It should be emphasized that early treatment improves the quality of life. It is not only necessary but in many cases diminishes the ultimate duration of therapy. For example, infusion for an acute hemarthrosis with an appropriate dose of factor concentrate (generally 15 to 25 U per kg of body weight) immediately on recognition of pain may obviate the need for a second infusion by forestalling the inflammatory response in the joint. This may curtail the predisposition for rebleeding in the same joint. Appropriate dosage is chosen to ensure some circulating factor level for at least 48 hours. The strategy for always maintaining such a minimal level is known as

"prophylaxis" and has been demonstrated to be efficacious in preventing essentially all joint bleeding in patients with both hemophilia A and hemophilia B. A decision to undertake primary prophylaxis requires extensive prospective evaluation and is best done in close consultation between the parent of the hemophilic child and professionals in the comprehensive hemophilia treatment center.

For life-threatening bleeding in a hemophilic patient, the exigency for immediate infusion is superseded only by resuscitative requirements. Every effort should be made to keep the factor level in the normal range (i.e., 50%) until this bleeding emergency has passed. Further, an acutely hemorrhaging hemophilic patient should be transported, if at all possible, to an emergency center that stocks appropriate plasma products. All head injuries must be considered nontrivial unless proved otherwise by observation and computed tomography or magnetic resonance imaging scan. Late bleeding after head trauma can occur as long as 3 to 4 weeks after the injury. Hence, patients with head and neck injuries should be infused immediately unless one is totally convinced that the injury is insignificant. Additionally, if the patient is not hospitalized, the patient and his or her family should be instructed in the neurologic signs and symptoms of central nervous system bleeding so that the patient will return for reinfusion, clinical and radiologic reassessment, and hospitalization at the earliest manifestation of bleeding.

Bleeding from the floor of the mouth or the pharynx or epiglottic region frequently results in partial or complete airway obstruction. Therefore, such bleeding should be treated with an aggressive infusion program with extended clinical follow-up to ensure resolution. Such bleeding may be precipitated by coughing, tonsillitis, oral or otolaryngologic surgery (e.g., extraction of wisdom teeth, tonsillectomy, adenoidectomy), or regional block anesthesia. For surgery and anesthesia, prophylaxis with appropriate infusion therapy before the procedure usually obviates the need for further treatment.

Patients with hemophilia who have gastrointestinal lesions, such as ulcer, varices, or hemorrhoids, must be managed with an appropriate continuous infusion regimen that maintains nearly normal circulating levels of Factor VIIIc or IX until some healing has been achieved. Concomitant transfusions with packed red blood cells may also be required.

Selected types of hemarthroses may be particularly problematic. Hip joint or acetabular hemorrhages can be dangerous because increased intra-articular pressure from bleeding and the associated inflammation may lead to aseptic necrosis of the femoral head. Twice-daily infusion therapy designed to sustain a factor level above 10 U per dL for at least 3 days should be given, along with enforced bed rest that includes Buck's traction for immobilization.

A hemarthrosis of the hip may, at first appearance, be difficult to differentiate from a bleed in the iliopsoas muscle. The latter limits primary hip extension, whereas a bleed in the joint makes any motion of the hip excruciatingly painful. Further, an iliopsoas bleed may decrease sensation over the ipsilateral thigh because of compression of the sacral plexus root of the femoral nerve. Ultrasonography may demonstrate a hematoma in the iliopsoas region. Treatment of the two is similar, although rehabilitation from the hip bleed is more protracted. Both benefit from a physical therapy regimen that strengthens the supporting musculature while slowly mobilizing the affected area. Closed compartment muscle and soft tissue hemorrhages are dangerous because they frequently impinge on the neurovascular bundle. These can occur in the upper arm, forearm, wrist, and volar aspect of the hand as well as the anterior or posterior filial compartments. Swelling and pain precede tingling, numbness, and loss of distal arterial pulses. Infusion must maintain an adequate hemostatic level of Factor VIIIc or IX. Other possible therapeutic maneuvers include elevation to enhance venous return and, as a last resort, surgical decompression if medical therapy fails to forestall progression.

COMPREHENSIVE CARE

Special treatment centers have been established in the United States and many other countries to provide multidisciplinary care for patients with hemophilia and related disorders. Many patients infused with plasma-derived factor concentrates before 1984 to 1985 were infected with the HIV and/or one of the hepatitis viruses. The comprehensive hemophilia centers provide voluntary testing for these viruses, counseling of patients found seropositive for previous infection, and access to appropriate care and therapy. Risk reduction counseling and education are as essential elements of comprehensive treatment centers as is repeated testing for evidence of hepatitis infection.

Comprehensive hemophilia treatment centers are also the mainstay for ongoing education of patients and families about the management of their bleeding disorder. The centers coordinate home therapy and preventive services and work closely with hemophilia consumer organizations to advocate advances in therapy and care.

Further information about hemophiliac care, hemophilia centers, and HIV risk reduction and counseling is available through the National Hemophilia Foundation, The Soho Building, 110 Greene Street, Suite 303, New York, New York 10012 (telephone, 212-219-8180 or 800-424-2634) or from its local chapters.

PLATELET–MEDIATED BLEEDING DISORDERS

method of
SHANNON M. BATES, M.D., and
JOHN G. KELTON, M.D.
Chedoke-McMaster Hospital and McMaster University
Hamilton, Ontario, Canada

Thrombocytopenia is a very common laboratory abnormality. Thrombocytopenia, like any other cytopenia, signifies an underlying disorder that has caused the cytopenia. Indeed, it is our opinion that thrombocytopenia is much more likely to cause greater morbidity because of the nature of its underlying cause (for example, septicemia) than is bleeding from the thrombocytopenia itself. The majority of patients with thrombocytopenia do not bleed (Figure 1). A greater morbidity (and mortality) is associated with those uncommon intravascular acute platelet-mediated thrombotic disorders, heparin-induced thrombocytopenia, and thrombotic thrombocytopenia purpura than is associated with isolated thrombocytopenia by itself. Recognizing these caveats, when faced with a thrombocytopenic patient, the physician must simultaneously determine the cause of the thrombocytopenia and also the risk (usually bleeding, but occasionally thrombotic) that the thrombocytopenia itself poses to the patient. We briefly review the steps taken in assessing the bleeding risk, the approach used to diagnose thrombocytopenic disorders, and a brief description of common thrombocytopenic disorders that are seen both in inpatients and outpatients.

ASSESSMENT OF THE BLEEDING RISK IN A THROMBOCYTOPENIC PATIENT

Some thrombocytopenic patients present with bleeding. However, for an increasing number of patients, particularly those in the hospital, the thrombocytopenia is first identified as a laboratory abnormality, and it is the thrombocytopenia that initiates additional investigation. As in any unexpected laboratory abnormality, the first step is to repeat the abnormal test (the complete blood count), and also the blood film should be carefully reviewed by a knowledgeable physician. The reason to examine the blood film is twofold: first, a small but important percentage of apparently thrombocytopenic patients have a laboratory abnormality in

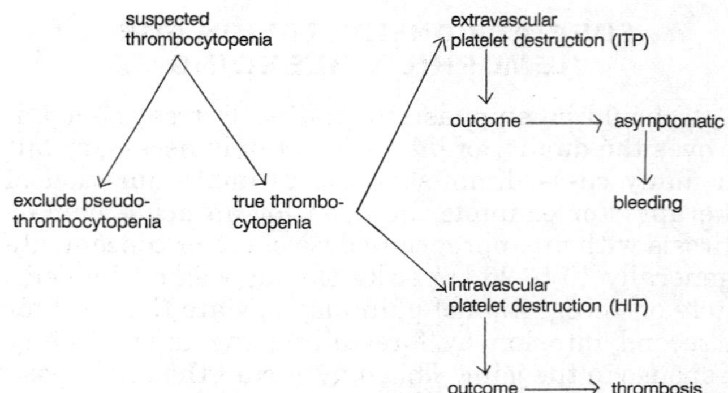

Figure 1. Examples of thrombocytopenia caused by extravascular platelet destruction (e.g., immune thrombocytopenia, ITP) or intravascular platelet destruction, as illustrated by heparin-induced thrombocytopenia (HIT).

which platelet clumping is initiated by the anticoagulant used to reverse clotting (EDTA, ethylenediaminetetraacetic acid). The diagnosis is confirmed by examining the stained blood film and looking for platelet clumps. This is an important laboratory artifact that does not require further investigation or treatment. The second reason why the blood film should be examined before the patient is assessed is that it can provide important information concerning the cause of the thrombocytopenia. For example, the presence of an elevated white count and immature white cells could indicate that an infective process is causing the thrombocytopenia. Red cell fragmentation could indicate a fragmentation syndrome such as disseminated intravascular coagulation (DIC).

The platelet count can provide some information about the relative bleeding risk. However, it must be emphasized that there is not a direct relationship between the platelet count and the risk of bleeding. There are two reasons for this. First, platelets are only one contributor to the hemostatic system (the others being coagulation factors and the integrity of the blood vessel itself). Hence, the patient with a mild coagulation defect (a hemophilia carrier) or impaired vascular integrity (postoperative) will be at greater risk of bleeding at the same platelet count than a patient whose other components of the hemostatic system are intact. The second reason for the relatively poor correlation between the platelet count and the risk of bleeding is the considerable variability in platelet function. Platelets can vary dramatically in their hemostatic ability, depending upon intrinsic and extrinsic factors. Disorders that are characterized by increased platelet turnover result in stimulation of the megakaryocytes to produce more platelets, which in turn leads to the release of larger and more granular platelets that have an elevated mean platelet volume (MPV). Hence, patients with a preponderance of these types of platelets (who typically have disorders of enhanced platelet destruction) will have enhanced platelet function and lower bleeding risk at the same platelet counts compared with those with smaller, less granular platelets. This latter group of patients, who typically have a normal or reduced MPV, typically have thrombocytopenia caused by impaired platelet production.

Extrinsic factors also influence platelet function. Patients with uremia have impaired platelet function as do patients who have an inherited abnormality of von Willebrand factor, a protein important in platelet function. There are also a number of uncommon but important platelet disorders, characterized by abnormal platelet membrane or granular content and a lifelong bleeding tendency.

In general, and unless there is an intrinsic or extrinsic cause for platelet dysfunction, patients with thrombocytopenia tend not to bleed when their platelet count is above 50,000 per µL. Disorders of increased platelet turnover, which are characterized by an elevated MPV, seldom have serious bleeding unless the platelet count falls below 10,000 to 20,000 per µL. Indeed, some patients can be asymptomatic even at extremely low platelet counts. The patients with thrombocytopenia caused by reduced platelet production (for example, those receiving chemotherapy to treat leukemia) begin to show physical signs of hemostatic impairment when their platelet count falls below 20,000 per µL and can suffer from serious bleeding when the platelets are less than 5000 to 10,000 per µL.

The cardinal sign of thrombocytopenic bleeding is petechiae. These are tiny subcutaneous collections of red cells that appear on dependent regions of the body. Minor trauma in these patients produces larger ecchymotic lesions that may or may not be painful, depending on their size and the secondary inflammatory response they trigger. The presence of petechiae and purpura means that the patient requires treatment to raise the platelet count to safe levels. We also carefully examine the patient for evidence of mucous membrane bleeding, which most frequently manifests as blood blisters in the mouth and less commonly as gastrointestinal (GI) or genitourinary (GU) bleeding. These "wet purpura" are an indication for urgent intervention to raise the platelet count to safe levels.

The rest of the physical examination should be directed at determining the cause of the thrombocytopenia. For example, patients with the most common cause of isolated thrombocytopenia, idiopathic thrombocytopenic purpura (ITP), will have a normal physical examination and will not have lymphadenopathy or splenomegaly. Hepatosplenomegaly is consistent with a lymphoproliferative cause. Splenomegaly may also be caused by portal hypertension secondary to hepatic cirrhosis. Lymphadenopathy is seen in patients with lymphoproliferative and infectious causes of thrombocytopenia, such as infectious mononucleosis or human immunodeficiency virus (HIV).

GENERAL GUIDELINES FOR SUPPORTING A THROMBOCYTOPENIC PATIENT

Depending upon the clinical situation, which is defined by both the platelet count and the physical evidence of hemostatic impairment, the physician can determine the urgency of intervention. Unfortunately, some physicians treat all thrombocytopenic patients with platelet transfusions. For many patients this will not result in hemostatic improvement and may put the patient at risk for a transfusion-acquired infection. For a few patients, particularly those with intravascular platelet-mediated thrombotic disorders such as heparin-induced thrombocytopenia, thrombotic thrombocytopenic purpura, and hemolytic uremic syndrome, platelet transfusions worsen the disorder. The decision to give a thrombocytopenic patient a platelet transfusion depends upon the presence or absence of active bleeding and the cause of the thrombocytopenia. In general, any patient with potentially life-threatening bleeding caused by thrombocytopenia should receive platelet transfusions. Even if the patient's platelets are rapidly destroyed by the underlying disorder (septicemia, drug-induced thrombocytopenia, immune thrombocytopenia), platelets may exert some hemostatic benefit before being destroyed themselves.

For those patients who have physical evidence of hemostatic impairment (petechiae and bruising) but do not have life-threatening bleeding, we administer platelet transfusions depending upon the cause and chronicity of the thrombocytopenia. For example, if the thrombocytopenia is caused by a disorder of increased platelet destruction (Table 1), the transfused platelets themselves will rapidly be destroyed and benefit will be limited. At the same time, for those patients who have a potential long-term thrombocytopenic risk (aplastic anemia) and in whom there is considerable risk of sensitization to the transfused platelets, platelet transfusions should be given only after carefully weighing the risks and benefits.

TABLE 1. **A General Classification of the Mechanism of Thrombocytopenia**

Cause of the Thrombocytopenia	Isolated Thrombocytopenia	Risk of Bleeding	Example
Underproduction	Very rare	Moderate	Chemotherapy, aplastic anemia
Hypersplenism	Uncommon	Rare	Hypersplenism due to cirrhosis
Destruction	Typical	Moderate	Immune DIC, immune ITP

Abbreviations: DIC = disseminated intravascular coagulation; ITP = idiopathic thrombocytopenic purpura.

Currently, the largest use of platelet transfusions is in the prevention *(prophylactic transfusions)* of bleeding in patients who have a short-term episode of thrombocytopenia caused by impaired platelet production. Typically these are leukemic patients who have recently received chemotherapy. Currently, there is debate about the "transfusion trigger" used to give platelet transfusions to these patients. Until recently, most physicians transfused these patients if their platelet count fell below 20,000 per μL. It is now apparent that serious bleeding does not occur unless the platelet count is below 5000 to 10,000 per μL and, increasingly, physicians are comfortable with this as the indication for platelet transfusion therapy.

Depending upon the platelet count and the clinical situation, other nonblood product interventions can be used, particularly in patients in whom the bleeding is caused by or contributed to by platelet dysfunction rather than severe thrombocytopenia. These include DDAVP (desmopressin), which stimulates the release of von Willebrand factor (vWF) from endothelial cells, and antifibrinolytic agents such as epsilon-aminocaproic acid. Care should be taken to avoid hemostatic challenges (surgery, intramuscular injections) and the use of medications (aspirin, many nonsteroidal anti-inflammatory agents) that impair platelet function. Alcohol inhibits platelet function and can cause bleeding in an otherwise hemostatically intact but thrombocytopenic patient.

Investigation of a Thrombocytopenic Patient

As noted previously, the first step is confirmation, by repeat testing and examination of the film, that the patient is thrombocytopenic. Many thrombocytopenic patients are not bleeding and have no physical signs of hemostatic impairment.

The focus of the laboratory investigation of the thrombocytopenic patient depends upon the situation. We find it convenient to differentiate between thrombocytopenia identified in the hospitalized patient and unexpected thrombocytopenia found in an outpatient who may or may not be symptomatic. The inpatient most frequently has thrombocytopenia caused by increased platelet destruction and can have infection-induced thrombocytopenia; drug-induced thrombocytopenia, which may be caused by virtually any pharmacologic agent, but with heparin being the most common; dilutional coagulopathy; DIC in pregnant, infected, and cancer patients; post-transfusional purpura in patients at risk, and so

on. Isolated thrombocytopenia in the outpatient most frequently is caused by immune platelet destruction with the most common cause being idiopathic thrombocytopenia purpura. There are many causes of thrombocytopenia, and specific investigations (for example, blood cultures, antinuclear antibodies, HIV testing) depend upon the setting. The relevant investigations and physical findings will be briefly commented upon subsequently (Table 2).

Classification of Thrombocytopenic Disorders

Thrombocytopenia, like any hematologic cytopenia, can be divided into disorders of underproduction, disorders of increased destruction, and disorders caused by sequestration of the platelets within a body organ, almost always the spleen (see Table 1). The circulating blood cells originate from a common stem cell precursor; disorders of impaired platelet production usually, therefore, are characterized by leukopenia and anemia. Depending upon the relative acuteness of the marrow insult, the thrombocytopenia and neutropenia can precede the anemia. Rarely, amegakaryocytic thrombocytopenia (bone marrow failure at the level of the megakaryocyte) can present with isolated thrombocytopenia. Splenic sequestration causing thrombocytopenia also can usually be easily diagnosed. The patient has a dramatically enlarged

TABLE 2. **Classification of Immune Thrombocytopenic Disorders**

Primary immune thrombocytopenia—idiopathic
  thrombocytopenia purpura (ITP), also known as AITP or ATP
Secondary immune thrombocytopenia disorders
  Lymphoproliferative disorders:
    Chronic lymphocytic leukemia
    Non-Hodgkin's lymphoma
    Hodgkin's disease
  Certain carcinomas
  Miscellaneous immune disorders:
    Immunologic joint disease—rheumatoid arthritis
    Systemic lupus erythematosus
    Other immunologic joint diseases (ankylosing spondylitis,
      and so on)
    Immunologic bowel disease (Crohn's disease, ulcerative
      colitis)
    Immunologic liver diseases (chronic active hepatitis)
Infectious diseases
  Bacterial infections
  Certain viral infections
  Chronic and persisting viral infections
  HIV infections
  Epstein-Barr virus

spleen, and often there is depression in one of the other cell lines (most frequently the white cells.) Thrombocytopenia caused by hypersplenism is only mild to moderate in severity, and seldom do these patients have serious bleeding problems caused by the thrombocytopenia itself.

The usual cause of isolated thrombocytopenia in inpatients and outpatients is an increased rate of platelet destruction that overwhelms the ability of the bone marrow to produce new platelets. The destruction can be from immune (ITP, viral infections) and nonimmune (DIC, thrombotic thrombocytopenic purpura [TTP]) causes.

Based upon a careful history, targeted physical examination, and review of the complete blood count, it is usually possible to categorize the general mechanism responsible for the thrombocytopenia. Most physicians will perform bone marrow examinations in a thrombocytopenic patient, but often these tests are uninformative. Typically, the bone marrow examination will be normal in patients with thrombocytopenia caused by an increased rate of destruction or hypersplenism. We perform a bone marrow aspiration in those patients in whom it is suspected that they have thrombocytopenia caused by underproduction, if the patient has an atypical disorder such as an otherwise apparent ITP that resists therapy, ITP with positive physical findings such as lymphadenopathy, and so on. Seldom are "blind" bone marrow aspirations informative. Indeed, it is important to have considered the possible diagnosis at the time of the performance of the bone marrow aspiration to ensure that appropriate investigations are performed. For example, patients with aplastic anemia, amegakaryocytic thrombocytopenia, and other disorders of production need cytogenetic analysis. Patients with pancytopenia and mild splenomegaly require specific investigations for hairy cell leukemia (tartrate-resistant acid phosphatase and immunophenotyping).

Thrombocytopenia in a Hospitalized Patient

Thrombocytopenia in a hospitalized patient is defined as new thrombocytopenia in a patient who was admitted with a normal platelet count. For this group of patients, the thrombocytopenia is also unexpected; not included in this group are those patients in whom the thrombocytopenia is a predictable consequence of treatment such as chemotherapy. The relative frequency depends upon the population under study. For example, thrombocytopenia from DIC would be more likely to be seen in patients with malignancy and septicemia. Thrombocytopenia due to dilution is seen in patients who have major surgery. In the intensive care unit and on the medical wards, thrombocytopenia is most frequently observed in patients with septicemia and with drug-induced thrombocytopenia.

IDIOPATHIC THROMBOCYTOPENIC PURPURA

Idiopathic thrombocytopenic purpura (ITP) is a very common autoimmune disease that targets the platelets for destruction by the cells of the reticuloendothelial system, with the destruction mediated by antiplatelet autoantibodies. ITP can be thought of as the inverse between adults and children. In children, 80% of the patients will have an acute episode of ITP that resolves spontaneously and never recurs. The opposite is true in adults. About 80% of adults who develop ITP will have a chronic disease that will persist unless more definitive treatment is taken. The children who develop ITP in late childhood or early adolescence fall between these two groups and, although they may not necessarily develop chronic ITP (like adults), are much less likely than young children to have spontaneous remissions of their illness.

Acute Idiopathic Thrombocytopenic Purpura in Children

Acute ITP of children is a common illness that develops in young children (often under age 5 years), affecting both girls and boys. Typically, it follows a recent viral infection or vaccination by several weeks. The illness is characterized by the acute development of severe thrombocytopenia (platelet counts typically less than 20,000 per µL), with evidence of hemostatic impairment that can range in severity from easy bruising and petechiae to mucous membrane bleeding. Untreated, the illness typically resolves within several weeks. The use of corticosteroids (prednisone or the equivalent at a dose of 1 mg per kg per day) will shorten the thrombocytopenic interval. High-dose intravenous IgG (IVIgG) (1 gram/kg per day for 2 days) will raise the platelet count to a safe level in the majority of children within a few days. Because of the safety of this preparation, it is the treatment of choice of most physicians managing these patients. Because the diagnosis is readily apparent in most children, extensive laboratory investigation, including bone marrow examination, is seldom required.

Idiopathic Thrombocytopenic Purpura in Adults

ITP in adults typically occurs from age 20 to 50 years and has a female predominance of 2 to 3:1. The illness can present in one of three ways. Most frequently, the patient gives a history of several years of easy bruising and occasional episodes of epistaxis, with medical attention being sought because of an acute episode of thrombocytopenic bleeding that can follow a flu or the ingestion of an antiplatelet agent such as aspirin. Less commonly, patients first present with an acute episode of severe thrombocytopenia with generalized mucous membrane bleeding. Increasingly, patients are identified who have a mild-to-moderate thrombocytopenia and may or may not have easy bruising. These patients have a laboratory abnormality and, as will be discussed, in our opinion frequently do not require specific therapy.

Investigation of the Patient with Idiopathic Thrombocytic Purpura

With the exception of physical evidence of hemostatic impairment (petechiae, bruising, and oral wet purpura), the physical examination of a patient with ITP is entirely normal. In particular, there should be no evidence of lymphadenopathy or splenomegaly. Either of these findings would indicate a secondary cause of immune thrombocytopenia, such as a lymphoproliferative disorder or a viral infection such as HIV or infectious mononucleosis (see Table 2).

The laboratory investigation of a patient with suspected ITP is directed at looking for disorders that can be associated with ITP and excluding other conditions that can be confused with ITP. ITP has a strong association with immunologic hyper- and hypothyroidism; consequently, all patients with ITP should have regular thyroid-stimulating hormone (TSH) monitoring. A small proportion will have evidence of a more systemic autoimmune disorder, and antinuclear antibodies (ANA) should be measured at presentation and periodically during the patient's illness. Seldom does a patient present with ITP and then progress to a more generalized autoimmune condition such as systemic lupus erythematosus. ITP remains a diagnosis of exclusion, and currently there is no definitive test to confirm its presence. Platelet-associated IgG (PAIgG) is frequently measured, but this test has too low a specificity to be useful in the diagnosis of ITP. Currently, the assays measuring the direct interaction with an autoantibody with platelet-specific glycoproteins are being evaluated for their diagnostic usefulness in ITP. Many patients with ITP have autoantibodies against platelet glycoprotein IIb/IIIa. Additionally, patients with autoantibodies to certain platelet glycoproteins (particularly platelet glycoprotein Ib/IX) may be at risk for having more severe and refractory disease. Depending upon the patient presentation, age, and associated findings, other investigations may be appropriate. Young people should be investigated for possible infectious mononucleosis. Infectious mononucleosis can produce severe immune thrombocytopenia that can persist for several months.

Immune thrombocytopenia can be the first manifestation of HIV infection, and although mild thrombocytopenia characterizes every patient with HIV, a small proportion will have an illness indistinguishable from ITP. Patients with Hodgkin's disease and certain lymphoproliferative disorders also have an ITP-like illness that can be independent of the activity of the underlying disease. Many patients with ITP will have a bone marrow examination performed, although as stated previously, the yield on this test is very low in a patient with isolated thrombocytopenia. For patients with obscure thrombocytopenia, we have found that a platelet survival test is very useful and often diagnostic. [111]Indium is the optimum radiolabel and can determine whether the patient has thrombocytopenia associated with hypersplenism, thrombocytopenia due to reduced platelet production, or thrombocytopenia caused by increased platelet destruction (consistent with ITP).

Treatment of the Patient with Idiopathic Thrombocytopenic Purpura

Perhaps the most important issue is to determine whether a patient with ITP requires any treatment. Patients who have severe thrombocytopenia (platelet count of less than 10,000 per μL) and clinical evidence of hemostatic impairment require treatment to raise their platelet count. Although it is important to increase the platelets as quickly as possible, seldom is it extremely urgent (unless the patient has a potential life-threatening bleed). We use one of three treatments. The least expensive treatment is oral prednisone at a dose of 1 mg per kg administered on a daily basis. This will raise the platelet count within 1 to 2 weeks in at least 75% of patients, and as the platelet count rises, the prednisone dosage can be decreased, first to alternate-day therapy and then progressively over several weeks. The platelet count should be monitored. As the prednisone is tapered, most patients will have a decline in platelet count that will necessitate increasing the prednisone dosage. The least dose of prednisone required to raise the patient's platelet count to safe levels, but not necessarily to normal levels, is the ideal dose.

The second treatment is high-dose IVIgG delivered at a dose of 1 gram per kg over 6 to 8 hours. This treatment can be repeated the following day. High-dose IVIgG will raise the platelet count in at least 75% of patients within several days. However, this is not a permanent treatment, and the platelet count will begin to decline within several weeks of completing treatment. The high cost of this treatment limits it widespread usage.

The third treatment that is being used increasingly in Canada and Europe is small doses (25 μg per kg per day for 2 days) of an intravenous preparation of anti-D in Rh-positive individuals (85% of the population). The anti-D coats the patient's own red cells and induces a mild compensated hemolytic state. Presumably, this produces blockage of the reticuloendothelial system and produces a rise in platelet count. Anti-D results in a rise in the platelet count in about the same proportion of ITP patients as does IVIgG, but it has the advantage of being much less expensive and capable of being given over a much shorter interval (minutes instead of hours).

None of these treatments cure ITP patients, and most patients will require more definitive treatment such as splenectomy.

DISSEMINATED INTRAVASCULAR COAGULATION

method of
SUSAN SOLYMOSS, M.D., and
JACQUES R. LECLERC, M.D.
The Montreal General Hospital and McGill University
Montreal, Quebec, Canada

Disseminated intravascular coagulation (DIC) is a dysregulated consumptive coagulopathy giving rise to a wide spectrum of clinical presentations ranging from thrombosis in Trousseau's syndrome to life-threatening bleeding or tissue necrosis in purpura fulminans. The diagnosis relies on both the appropriate clinical context and corroborating laboratory studies, as no single clinical or laboratory abnormality is unique to DIC.

PATHOGENESIS

Consumptive coagulopathy results from a severe imbalance in activation of the procoagulant and fibrinolytic pathways, thus escaping the control and feedback mechanisms that maintain normal hemostasis as a self-limiting process. Activation most typically starts with increased tissue factor expression, which triggers activity of the extrinsic pathway of coagulation. Through the common pathway, amplified by the intrinsic pathway and concurrent with platelet activation, thrombin is produced. Cleavage of fibrinogen yields soluble fibrin and thrombus deposition. Secondary activation of fibrinolysis initiates fibrin and fibrinogen degradation. Ongoing activation of coagulation leads to the depletion of some coagulation factors and their inhibitors. With simultaneous fibrin formation and depletion of factors, clinical manifestations of DIC range from large vessel thrombosis to tissue necrosis due to microvascular thrombosis to severe, uncontrolled bleeding.

Etiologic factors commonly encountered as triggers of DIC are listed in Table 1. Massive release of tissue factor accompanies tissue injury, trauma, and gunshot wounds, as well as obstetric accidents such as abruptio placentae. Widespread endothelial injury and increased tissue factor expression are also seminal in sepsis-associated DIC. Bacterial proteases, endotoxin, and inflammatory mediators such as tumor necrosis factor (TNF) and interleukin-1 (IL-1) modulate significantly the severity of the consumptive process. Although both gram-positive and gram-negative sepsis, as well as viral, parasitic and rickettsial infections, can be associated with DIC, gram-negative organisms are the most common infectious cause of DIC. Meningococcal sepsis is classically associated with purpura fulminans and rapidly progressive skin necrosis, and also is seen with acquired or congenital protein-C deficiency. Localized endothelial injury stimulates DIC in association with aortic aneurysms and in Kasabach-Merritt syndrome. Cellular procoagulants released from various cancer cells and from acute promyelocytic leukemia (APL) cells also induce a consumptive coagulopathy. DIC can occur if proteases not normally found in circulation are released. These include tumor cell protease, leukocyte elastase, trypsin, and certain snake venoms.

Although abnormal activation of clotting is invariable in DIC, many other factors influence its clinical severity. Slow activation, typical of a malignancy or retained dead fetus, yields chronic low-grade DIC, at times only a laboratory abnormality. In contrast, amniotic fluid embolus with rapid massive activation of clotting results in immediate circulatory and respiratory collapse, severe bleeding and up to 80% mortality. Inflammatory cytokines, formation of immune complexes, activation of the complement cascade, and participation of leukocytes all fuel the consumptive process. Compensatory steps that attenuate DIC include synthesis of coagulant proteins by the liver and release of platelets by the bone marrow.

DIAGNOSIS

Accurate and prompt diagnosis of DIC requires the astute clinician to have an index of suspicion and to confirm the diagnosis by laboratory testing. Bleeding or thrombosis in a patient at clinical risk for DIC should trigger evaluation of laboratory parameters, including a complete blood count, prothrombin time (PT), partial thromboplastin time (aPTT), fibrinogen level, thrombin time (TT), and cross-linked fibrin degradation products (FDP or D-dimer). Typical laboratory findings are shown in Table 2. Decreased platelet count and red cell fragmentation may accompany DIC; however, these may also be found in many other conditions, notably hemolytic uremic syndrome (HUS) and thrombotic thrombocytopenic purpura (TTP). If the consumption is severe, both the PT and aPTT will be abnormally prolonged, a finding not typical for HUS or TTP. Prolongation of these screening tests reflects the combined effect of a decrease in fibrinogen concentration and in other factor levels.

Fibrinogen should be quantified directly and assessed qualitatively by the TT. Fibrinogen concentrations need to be interpreted in the clinical context, as an absolute de-

TABLE 1. **Common Etiologic Causes of Disseminated Intravascular Coagulation**

Infectious	Obstetric
Meningococcus	Retained dead fetus
All gram-negatives	Septic abortion
Gram-positives; some	Amniotic fluid embolism
viruses; some	Abruptio placentae
septic shock	**Vascular**
Malignant	Aortic aneurysm
Adenocarcinomas	Kasabach-Merritt syndrome
Leukemias	Vasculitis
Promyelocytic leukemia	**Other**
Tissue Damage	Acute hemolytic transfusion
Crush injury	reaction
Brain injury	Some snake bites
Ischemia	Peritoneovenous shunt
Severe burn injury	

TABLE 2. **Laboratory Abnormalities in Disseminated Intravascular Coagulation**

	Platelet Count	PT	aPTT	Fibrinogen	TT	FDP
Low-grade DIC	N/low	N	N	N/low	N/P	+ +
Severe DIC	low	P	P	low	P	+ + +

Abbreviations: N, normal; P, prolonged; PT, prothrombin time; aPTT, activated partial thromboplastin time; TT, thrombin time; FDP, fibrin degradation products.

crease will not always be found. In the setting of a malignancy or pregnancy, for example, in which high fibrinogen levels are not unusual, the finding of low-normal fibrinogen concentration would corroborate a consumptive process. One of the most sensitive tests for DIC is the presence of FDPs, and this may be the earliest abnormality found. The usefulness of this test, however, is limited by its relative nonspecificity. FDPs are commonly found in the postoperative state or other conditions in which fibrin is generated, such as thrombosis. Decreased clearance of FDPs is a typical hallmark of liver disease. In fact, the coagulopathy of liver cirrhosis versus DIC may be a difficult distinction to make. Both conditions can present with thrombocytopenia, positive FDPs, and a decrease in factor levels. Factor VIII tends to be relatively spared in liver disease, and tests for liver function can also be useful. Specific factor assays help gauge the severity of DIC but are not routinely required for the diagnosis. Measurement of protein-C in purpura fulminans can guide replacement therapy. Novel assays of the activation of coagulation, such as fibrinopeptide A (FPA) and thrombin-antithrombin (TAT), are not yet in clinical use but may provide additional information in the future.

TREATMENT

The essential element of the treatment plan for DIC is to control the underlying illness that has given rise to the consumptive process. By eliminating the stimulus for DIC, the coagulopathy is attenuated and compensatory responses allow laboratory parameters to return to normal. Supportive measures should be provided as necessary to resuscitate patients from vascular collapse and respiratory or other major organ damage. Prompt use of antibiotics for sepsis and quick evacuation of the uterus in case of an obstetric problem are important. Replacement with folate and vitamin K should be considered.

Blood product use needs to be tailored, based on the severity of bleeding and evaluation of laboratory results. Transfusion of packed red blood cells should be given as necessary to maintain hemoglobin. Brisk bleeding, when accompanied by a fibrinogen level of less than 100 mg per dL, warrants replacement of fibrinogen in the form of cryoprecipitate. Transfusion of 10 to 15 units should be followed by laboratory monitoring to assess response. Fresh-frozen plasma is a source of coagulation factors and their inhibitors for those patients with severe factor deficiencies and bleeding. A starting dose of 10 to 20 mL per kg should be given and assessed by looking for improvement in the PT and aPTT. Platelet transfusions are indicated if the platelet count has fallen to less than 20,000 per μL with ongoing bleeding. In case of a major bleed, platelet support may be required at platelet counts of less than 40,000. Antithrombin III and protein-C concentrates, not in routine use, have shown benefit in animal models of DIC and in selected clinical studies.

Anticoagulation with full-dose heparin is indicated for the treatment of venous thrombosis in Trousseau's syndrome. Low-dose heparin can provide clinical and laboratory benefit in the presence of microvascular thrombosis, as in purpura fulminans. The use of low-dose heparin in DIC and acute promyelocytic leukemia may provide no additional benefit over and above prompt blood product support. If low-dose heparin therapy is instituted in patients with evidence of thrombosis, improvement in fibrinogen and FDPs would indicate a beneficial response.

THROMBOTIC THROMBOCYTOPENIC PURPURA

method of
LINDA LACROIX, M.D., and
JACQUES R. LECLERC, M.D.
The Montreal General Hospital and McGill University
Montreal, Quebec, Canada

Thrombotic thrombocytopenic purpura (TTP) is an uncommon disorder characterized by a classic triad of severe thrombocytopenia, microangiopathic hemolytic anemia, and fluctuating neurologic signs. At times, fever and renal impairment can be seen completing the traditional pentad of symptoms. A related disorder, the hemolytic uremic syndrome (HUS), is seen mainly in children. TTP and HUS likely represent overlapping syndromes with similar pathologic processes. In both disorders, the hallmark pathologic lesion is that of microvascular thrombotic occlusions caused by platelet aggregation. With the advent of plasma exchange as the treatment of choice, TTP can now be successfully treated in over 80% of all cases seen.

ETIOLOGY AND PATHOGENESIS

Although most cases of adult TTP are idiopathic and sporadic, a number of known clinical entities may be associated with the development of the syndrome. A list of associated clinical syndromes and etiologies is given in Table 1. It may occur in both sexes although a female preponderance has been noted.

TTP was first recognized in 1924 as a disorder characterized by the presence of hyaline thrombi in the terminal arterioles and capillaries. Since that time, multiple theories as to the exact nature of the pathogenesis have been studied in detail. Early vascular lesions consist of intraluminal platelet thrombi resulting from platelet aggregation in the microcirculation. An abundance of abnormally large von Willebrand factor has been found in the plasma of patients with TTP/HUS. These von Willebrand multimers may function as bridges promoting platelet-platelet adhesion and aggregation. In addition, immune or toxin-mediated endothelial cell injury is thought to play a pathophysiologic role.

In keeping with the theory that there is abnormal interaction between endothelium and platelets, one of the more recently proposed pathologic mechanisms for classic TTP is the lack of a plasma factor leading to decreased synthesis of prostaglandin I_2 (PGI_2) by the endothelium. As PGI_2 is a vasodilator and inhibitor of platelet aggregation, this lack of prostaglandin I_2 may result in widespread microthrombi. Restoration of the normal antithrombogenic endothelium may occur after plasma therapy supplies the putative deficient factor.

TABLE 1. **Clinical Presentations of Thrombotic Thrombocytopenia Purpura**

Presentation	Precipitating Factors
Idiopathic TTP/ hemolytic uremic syndrome	Postviral illness
Epidemic childhood HUS	Postdiarrheal prodrome secondary to verotoxin *Escherichia coli* 0157.H7 *Shigella dysenteriae* 1
Pregnancy	
Drugs	Mitomycin C Cyclosporine Marrow transplant (total body irradiation—chemotherapy) Quinine Oral contraceptive pill
Metastatic cancer	
Human immunodeficiency disease	
Miscellaneous	Bee sting venom Carbon monoxide poisoning Vasculitides (systemic lupus erythematosus)

DIFFERENTIAL DIAGNOSIS

The presence of both severe thrombocytopenia and microangiopathic hemolysis should alert the clinician to several different clinical scenarios as outlined in Table 2. The most frequent diagnostic dilemma is between TTP and disseminated intravascular coagulation (DIC). One should note that the clinical features and peripheral blood abnormalities seen in TTP are usually more extreme and are associated with normal coagulation parameters, unlike those seen in DIC.

CLINICAL AND LABORATORY FEATURES

Intravascular platelet aggregation results in organ damage and severe thrombocytopenia, often less than 20,000 mm^3. Bleeding complications may occur, with particular affinity for the skin. Hemolysis is usually severe, with elevated serum lactate dehydrogenase (LDH) levels and polychromasia seen on the smear due to red cell destruction. Neurologic signs remain extremely variable, ranging from abnormal mentation, headache, transient pareses, to coma. Renal dysfunction is seen in 50% to 75% of patients with TTP and includes cases of hematuria, proteinuria, or severe renal failure. Less frequently, retinal ischemia with visual defects, cardiac dysfunction with conduction anomalies, and mesenteric ischemia with abdominal pain accompany the TTP syndrome.

TABLE 2. **Differential Diagnosis of Thrombocytopenia and Microangiopathic Hemolysis**

Disseminated intravascular coagulation (DIC)
Preeclampsia/eclampsia
HELLP (hemolysis, elevated liver function, low platelets)
Malignant hypertension
Gastric carcinoma
Severe vasculitides (systemic lupus erythematosus)
Evans' syndrome
Idiopathic thrombocytopenic purpura (ITP)

TABLE 3. **Laboratory Features of Thrombotic Thrombocytopenic Purpura**

Feature	Expected Result
Complete blood count	Anemia, thrombocytopenia, reticulocytosis
Peripheral smear	Red cell fragmentation
Serum LDH	Increased
BUN/creatinine	Normal or increased
Coagulation studies	
Prothrombin time/aPTT/thrombin time	Normal
Fibrinogen	Normal
Fibrin degradation products	Increased

Abbreviations: LDH, lactate dehydrogenase; BUN, blood urea nitrogen; aPPT, activated partial thromboplastin time.

TTP remains a clinical diagnosis. The defining features of TTP—low platelets and red cell fragmentation—are readily available by examination of the peripheral blood smear. Tissue biopsies are often not required to establish the diagnosis. The typical laboratory features of TTP are listed in Table 3.

TREATMENT AND PROGNOSIS

With the advent of plasma exchange and plasma therapy as the treatment of choice in TTP, current survival figures are often over 80%. This is in stark contrast to a 90% mortality seen prior to the 1970s. Although treatment remains empirical, it is presumed that either platelet-aggregating substances are being removed or normal plasma is replacing a deficient protective factor. The most effective initial treatment is plasma exchange of 1 to 1.5 volumes per day. Treatment should be initiated as soon as there is adequate clinical suspicion, as most mortality from TTP is seen during the first week of the illness.

Fresh-frozen plasma is the traditional replacement product, although recent data from the Canadian Apheresis Group suggest that cryosupernatant, lacking the large von Willebrand molecules, may be superior to plasma. If plasma exchange is not readily available, the infusion of fresh-frozen plasma can be initiated with up to 8 to 10 units per day to be infused. Less-proven therapies include the use of glucocorticoids, intravenous weekly vincristine (Oncovin),* splenectomy, azathioprine (Imuran),* intravenous gamma globulin* and cyclosporine (Sandimmune).* The use of antiplatelet agents such as aspirin* and dipyridamole (Persantine)* remains controversial because of the possible potentiation of a hemorrhagic tendency. Transfusion of platelets should be avoided unless life-threatening bleeding occurs, as temporary exacerbation of the thrombotic process may occur.

As a rule, prompt exchange should be initiated daily and continued until platelet counts and serum LDH levels normalize, usually 1 to 2 weeks following diagnosis. Approximately 40% of patients will have recurrence of symptoms when exchange is inter-

*Not FDA-approved for this indication.

rupted. Of these patients, 15% to 20% will demonstrate a chronic course with intermittent relapses at variable intervals of months to years. It is important to note that in recovering patients renal and neurologic symptoms may persist despite complete hematologic recovery.

TTP in pregnancy may be indistinguishable from preeclampsia. Delivery should be induced in these patients, and patients should be informed of the risk of recurrence of TTP in subsequent pregnancies.

HEMOCHROMATOSIS

method of
CLAUS NIEDERAU, M.D., and
GEORG STROHMEYER, M.D.
Heinrich Heine Universität
Düsseldorf, Germany

The term *hemochromatosis* refers to diseases in which a progressive increase in total body iron stores leads to deposition of iron in parenchymal cells of liver, heart, pituitary, gonads, pancreas, and other organs, and to subsequent morphologic and functional damage to these organs. Primary, idiopathic, hereditary hemochromatosis is an autosomal recessive disorder. The gene frequency may be as high as 1:20, but the exact gene product is still unknown. Secondary hemochromatosis (previously often classified as hemosiderosis) is most often associated with chronic hemolytic anemias (e.g., thalassemia major, spherocytosis, sideroblastic anemia). The factors in these forms of secondary hemochromatosis that lead to iron overload include iron released from breakdown of hemoglobin and exogenous iron from blood transfusions. Prolonged parenteral and, rarely, enteral iron administration can also lead to secondary hemochromatosis.

Laboratory diagnosis of hemochromatosis includes measurements of serum iron, transferrin saturation, and serum ferritin, as well as tests of liver function and enzymes. The diagnosis is confirmed by liver biopsy with histochemical or biochemical quantification of iron. Alternatively, semiquantitative determination of liver iron concentration may be performed by magnetic resonance or biomagnetometry techniques. Human leukocyte antigen (HLA) typing is useful only for screening in families with an already diagnosed case of primary hemochromatosis. Results from several recent studies suggest that screening of nonselected subjects in the general population may be cost effective to identify patients with hemochromatosis at an early stage in which prophylactic iron removal may prevent most of the complications associated with iron overload.

TREATMENT

Genetic Hemochromatosis

The most effective method for removing excessive iron is by repeated phlebotomies. There is strong evidence that rigorous and complete removal of iron by phlebotomies markedly improves the prognosis. Patients who are diagnosed in an early stage without hepatic cirrhosis and in whom the excessive iron is completely removed by phlebotomy therapy have a normal life expectancy. Therapy starts with a rigorous schedule of phlebotomies until the complete removal of iron can be documented by a liver biopsy or, alternatively, by magnetic resonance or biomagnetometry techniques; therapy has to be maintained by less frequent phlebotomies for the rest of the patient's life (Table 1).

The number of phlebotomies necessary to remove iron during the initial treatment period directly depends on the amount of excessive iron and varies from 50 to 150 phlebotomies during a period of 9 to 24 months. Phlebotomy treatment often markedly improves liver disease and in many cases also cardiac abnormalities. In patients with severe decompensated cardiomyopathy, heart transplantation is, however, usually the only way to save the patient's life. Therapy has no major beneficial effect on arthropathy, insulin-dependent diabetes mellitus, or endocrine abnormalities. Early treatment in the noncirrhotic stage almost completely prevents further complications, including the development of liver cancer. In cirrhotic patients, however, liver cancer is a frequent complication, which often occurs many years after complete removal of excessive iron.

Secondary Hemochromatosis

In most forms of secondary hemochromatosis, excessive iron cannot be removed by phlebotomies because of an underlying anemia that often requires blood transfusions. Therefore, iron-chelating agents are used to remove excessive iron and to prevent or at least to slow down the consequences of iron overload. Deferoxamine (Desferal) is the most widely used agent. After parenteral administration, it chelates iron by building a water-soluble complex, which is subsequently excreted in urine and bile. In adults, a daily dose of approximately 2 grams of deferoxamine is recommended. Because of severe neurotoxic side effects, the daily dose should not exceed 50 to 60 mg per kg.

The most effective form of treatment is a continuous subcutaneous infusion via a portable pump over 24 hours per day, but subcutaneous infusion for 8 to 12 hours overnight is the most widely used form of treatment; it can achieve 80 to 90% of the maximal

TABLE 1. **Phlebotomy Treatment in Genetic Hemochromatosis**

To remove excessive iron
  One or two phlebotomies of 500 mL of blood every wk
    (500 mL of blood contains 250 mg of iron)
  Hemoglobin controlled weekly
  Plasma protein, transferrin saturation, and ferritin
    controlled every 1 to 2 months
  Liver biopsy (or alternatively a magnetic resonance or
    biomagnetometry technique) recommended to
    document complete removal of iron

To prevent reaccumulation of iron
  Phlebotomy 4–8 times/yr (to keep serum ferritin in the
    lower-normal range)
  Therapy should never be discontinued for a longer time!

---

effect. The maximal effect of iron-chelating agents is less than that of phlebotomy therapy. In patients with a form of thalassemia major that requires regular blood transfusions, iron chelation therapy should start early, before complications of iron overload have developed.

Because of the need for parenteral administration of deferoxamine, its limited effects, the neurotoxic side effects, and the high costs, research is currently under way to develop nontoxic, effective, and cheap iron-chelating agents that can be given orally. Currently available oral chelators such as deferiprone are associated with a risk of agranulocytosis and therefore are restricted to patients who are unable or unwilling to use deferoxamine.

HODGKIN'S DISEASE: CHEMOTHERAPY

method of
SANDRA SCHNALL, M.D.
Temple University Cancer Center
Philadelphia, Pennsylvania

Hodgkin's disease is a neoplasm of lymphoid tissue initially described by Thomas Hodgkin in 1832. The etiology and pathogenesis of Hodgkin's disease have been the source of controversy since that time. Despite this, the treatment outcomes have generally been favorable.

INCIDENCE AND ETIOLOGY

In the United States, Hodgkin's disease is diagnosed in 7 of every 100,000 people annually. The incidence has been relatively stable, with a bimodal curve. Rates rise through early life and peak in the third decade. A second peak occurs at age 55 to 75 years. There is a male predominance at all ages. Interestingly, there has been an association between the young adult subtype and high socioeconomic status. There is also a well-defined geographic variation that occurs in young children in underdeveloped countries.

The potential infectious etiology of Hodgkin's disease has long been a topic of discussion. Considerable epidemiologic evidence supports the association of the Epstein-Barr virus (EBV) in Hodgkin's disease. This is based on the increased incidence in young adults with infectious mononucleosis as well as the demonstration of clonal episomal EBV genome in Reed-Sternberg (RS) cells.

There has also been some evidence to support a genetic basis or inherited susceptibility to Hodgkin's disease. There are reports of Hodgkin's disease in monozygotic twins as well as an increased incidence in siblings (in the same sex, a ninefold increase; in the opposite sex, a fivefold increase). Other poorly understood associations have been reported in woodworkers, in patients after tonsillectomy or appendectomy, and in patients with certain human leukocyte antigens (HLAs). There is also a questionable association with human immunodeficiency virus (HIV) infection (see the later discussion).

PATHOLOGY

The diagnosis of Hodgkin's disease is typically based on the recognition of the RS cell. The classic RS cell is a bilobed nucleus with prominent eosinophilic nucleoli. RS cells, however, are not pathognomonic for Hodgkin's disease, and variants may be seen in other reactive and neoplastic conditions. The precise cellular origin of Hodgkin's disease and the RS cell is not firmly established, but theories include an origin in the B lymphocyte series or possibly a macrophage cell line. The antigen markers CD15 and CD30 are commonly seen in the RS cell, along with the absence of CD45. However, this antigenic marking pattern is not absolutely specific.

Cytogenetic studies may reveal hyperdiploid karyotypes but no other pathognomonic chromosome changes or defects.

There are four histologic subtypes of Hodgkin's disease: mixed cellularity (MC), lymphocyte depleted (LD), nodular sclerosis (NS), and lymphocyte predominant (LP). MC occurs in 30 to 50% of patients and is commonly associated with advanced disease. LD occurs in less than 10% of patients and predominates in the older population. NS is noted for its distinct histologic appearance and clinical presentation. It most commonly occurs in the cervical or supraclavicular nodes in adolescents, particularly females, and accounts for 40 to 70% of cases. LP is considered to be a variant of or possibly related to B cell lymphomas. Ten percent of patients present with this subtype, often with early-stage disease.

CLINICAL PRESENTATION

The clinical presentation of Hodgkin's disease is often accompanied by constitutional symptoms such as fever, night sweats, and weight loss exceeding 10% of the baseline body weight. These have been designated the "B symptoms" in the staging classification and imply a poorer prognosis. Other manifestations of probably little prognostic significance include pruritus and pain in lymph nodes after the ingestion of alcohol.

Approximately 68% of patients present with enlarged cervical nodes, 6 to 20% in the axillary area, and 6 to 10% in the inguinal region. A minority of patients present with exclusively subdiaphragmatic disease. Liver involvement is rarely seen without spleen involvement and is often related to cell subtype.

DIAGNOSIS AND STAGING

The classic staging system was established by the Ann Arbor workshop in 1971. In 1989, a new classification was proposed and designated the Cotswold system (Table 1). Table 2 outlines the current recommended staging studies needed to evaluate patients with Hodgkin's disease.

CHEMOTHERAPY

The treatment for Hodgkin's disease is dependent on the stage of the disease (Table 3). It is often curable with radiation and/or chemotherapy. Single-agent chemotherapy rarely plays a role in the initial treatment of Hodgkin's disease. Although remissions are attainable, they are rarely sustained.

In 1970, DeVita and colleagues published the four-drug regimen that included nitrogen mustard, vincristine (Oncovin), procarbazine (Matulane), and prednisone (MOPP) as primary treatment for Hodgkin's disease (Table 4). In an attempt to modify toxicity, several regimens were designed as alterna-

TABLE 1. **Cotswold Staging Classification of Hodgkin's Disease (Modified Ann Arbor)**

Stage	Description
I	Involvement of a single lymph node region (I) or of a single extralymphatic organ or site (IE)
II	Involvement of two or more lymph node regions on the same side of the diaphragm (II) or localized involvement of an extralymphatic organ or site and of one or more lymph node regions on the same side of the diaphragm (IIE)
III	Involvement of lymph node regions on both sides of the diaphragm (III)
	III$_1$—spleen, splenic, celiac, or porta hepatis nodal involvement
	III$_2$—para-aortic, iliac, or mesenteric nodal involvement
IV	Diffuse or disseminated involvement of one or more extralymphatic organs or tissues with or without associated lymph node enlargement

Subcategories

A	No systemic symptoms
B	Unexplained weight loss greater than 10% of body weight in the previous 6 months and/or unexplained fever with temperatures above 38°C and/or night sweats
E	Involvement of single extranodal site that is contiguous to a known nodal site
X	Bulky disease, a mass >10 cm, or mediastinal mass larger than one-third the thoracic diameter

tives to MOPP. In MVPP, the vincristine has been replaced by vinblastine, to decrease neurotoxicity. In ChlVPP, the nitrogen mustard has been replaced with another alkylating agent, chlorambucil (Leukeran), to decrease nausea and vomiting. Other regimens include LOPP and BVCPP (see Table 4).

In the 1970s, Bonadonna and colleagues in Milan designed an alternative regimen for patients who had failed MOPP, using non–cross-resistant agents. This regimen included doxorubicin (Adriamycin), bleomycin (Blenoxane), vinblastine (Velban), and dacarbazine (ABVD). Due to its excellent response rate in MOPP-resistant patients, ABVD was introduced as initial therapy for patients with advanced Hodgkin's disease. Comparison studies of MOPP versus ABVD as first-line treatment in advanced disease showed no notable differences in remission rates,

TABLE 2. **Recommended Staging Procedure for Hodgkin's Disease**

Required

Adequate surgical biopsy
Detailed history with emphasis on absence/presence of B symptoms
Complete physical examination
Chest x-ray (posteroanterior and lateral)
Computed tomography scan of chest, abdomen, pelvis
Lab studies: complete blood count, liver and renal functions, alkaline phosphatase, lactate dehydrogenase, calcium

Recommended

Bone marrow aspirate and biopsy
Bipedal lymphangiogram (dependent on institution)
Staging laparotomy and splenectomy (if it will change therapy)
Gallium scan

TABLE 3. **Treatment by Stage**

Stage	Therapy
I/IIA (nonbulky)	Radiation
I/IIA (bulky)	Chemotherapy → radiation
IIB (clinical)	Chemotherapy
IIB (pathologic)	Radiation
IIIA (minimal upper abdomen)	Radiation
IIIA (other)	Chemotherapy
IIIB/IV	Chemotherapy

disease-free survival, or overall survival. However, secondary leukemias and infertility occur less commonly with ABVD than with MOPP (see later).

Overall, the reasons for the failure of primary treatment for Hodgkin's disease are not clear but may be due to drug resistance or lack of dose intensity. In 1979, Golde and Coldman suggested that the best approach to avoiding drug resistance would be to administer rapidly alternating cycles of chemotherapy that did not produce cross-resistance. The National Cancer Institute (NCI) of Milan piloted the first trial comparing ABVD with alternating cycles of MOPP and ABVD. Although there was no substantial difference in complete remission rates, disease-free survival and overall survival favored the combined arm rather than MOPP alone (73 versus 50%, 84 versus 64%, respectively). However, the doses of MOPP in this study were reduced from the original NCI–U.S. trial, perhaps influencing the outcome. The Cancer and Leukemia Group B (CALGB) reported the results of its important study comparing MOPP alone, ABVD alone, and MOPP plus ABVD. Again, dose reductions in the MOPP arm were noted. The data suggested that MOPP plus ABVD was better at preventing early relapse compared with MOPP alone, but there was no overall advantage compared with ABVD alone.

Another variant was designed by Conners and Klimo in Vancouver and designated the MOPP/ABVD hybrid program (see Table 4). In this regimen, the dacarbazine is omitted, and the use of doxorubicin is increased. All other drugs, except prednisone, are given in 8-day cycles. When long-term results were compared with those of standard MOPP plus ABVD in a randomized trial in Canada, the two programs appeared to be equal. However, the hybrid regimen is probably easier to tolerate. An intergroup trial in the United States is now under way comparing the MOPP/ABV hybrid with ABVD, in an attempt to confirm the initial excellent results in the ABVD arm alone.

As mentioned earlier, dose intensity may be an important factor in remission rate outcomes. It is thought that treatment failure in Hodgkin's disease may be secondary to underdosing rather than resistance alone. To test this hypothesis, a trial is under way giving dose-intensive courses of MOPP with growth factor (granulocyte colony-stimulating factor) support in patients with Stage III and IV Hodgkin's disease.

TABLE 4. **Combination Chemotherapy Programs Effective in the Treatment of Hodgkin's Disease**

Drugs	Recommended Dose (mg/m²)	Route	Days*
MOPP regimen			
Nitrogen mustard	6	IV	1, 8
Vincristine (Oncovin)	1.4	IV	1, 8
Procarbazine	100	PO	1–14
Prednisone	40	PO	1–14
MVPP regimen			
Nitrogen mustard	6	IV	1, 8
Vinblastine	6	IV	1, 8
Procarbazine	100	PO	1–14
Prednisone	40	PO	1–14
ChlVPP regimen			
Chlorambucil	6	PO	1–14
Vinblastine	6	IV	1, 8
Procarbazine	100	PO	1–14
Prednisone	40	PO	1–14
LOPP regimen			
Chlorambucil	6	PO	1–14
Vincristine	1.4	IV	1, 8
Procarbazine	100	PO	1–14
Prednisone	40	PO	1–14
BVCPP regimen			
BCNU (carmustine [BiCNU])	100	IV	1
Vinblastine	5	IV	1
Cyclophosphamide	600	IV	1
Procarbazine†	100	PO	2–10
Prednisone	600	PO	1–10
ABVD regimen			
Doxorubicin (Adriamycin)	25	IV	1, 15
Bleomycin (Blenoxane)	10	IV	1, 15
Vinblastine	6	IV	1, 15
Dacarbazine	375	IV	1, 15
MOPP/ABVD alternating regimen			
(alternating months of MOPP and ABVD)			
MOPP/ABV hybrid regimen			
Nitrogen mustard	6	IV	1
Vincristine	1.4	IV	1
Procarbazine	100	PO	1–7
Prednisone	40	PO	1–14
Doxorubicin	35	IV	8
Bleomycin	10	IV	8
Vinblastine	6	IV	8

*Each cycle lasts 28 days.
†Procarbazine is also given 50 mg orally on day 1.

LIMITED EARLY-STAGE HODGKIN'S DISEASE

Favorable or limited-stage Hodgkin's disease is defined as Stage I or II supradiaphragmatic disease without bulky sites and no or one extranodal site. A decision to proceed with a staging laparotomy should be based on the ability to determine the risk of finding occult subdiaphragmatic tumor. In general, extended field (subtotal nodal) radiation therapy is the treatment of choice. This is thought to be superior to involved field radiation alone due to the significant improvement in freedom from relapse (32% for involved field vs. 80% for extended field). Recent studies demonstrated that chemotherapy can substitute for extended field radiation in Stage I and II tumors. Regimens studied included MOPP and ChlVPP. Excellent results have been achieved, with cure rates greater than 70 to 80%. The advantage of chemotherapy over radiation is limited. However, the long-term effects of radiation (i.e., second solid tumors) are likely diminished. Radiation therapy may also cause developmental growth delay in children, possibly making chemotherapy more advantageous in this subgroup.

Combination therapy with radiation and chemotherapy in limited disease has also been explored. It may improve remission rates and freedom from relapse rates, but to date it has not demonstrated an improvement in survival over chemotherapy given as salvage therapy for radiation failure. A trial from the NCI–U.S. is now in progress, randomizing patients to receive ABVD chemotherapy with or without radiation therapy in the hope of addressing these questions.

BULKY OR EXTENSIVE EARLY-STAGE HODGKIN'S DISEASE

Special mention must be made of early-stage tumors with extensive or bulky involvement (i.e., extending into the lung, pericardium, or chest wall or with a pleural effusion or a mass greater than one-third of the chest diameter). These patients, when treated with radiation alone, have a failure or relapse rate of up to 50%. Therefore, combined-modality therapy is often recommended as initial treatment in these patients. The timing, dose, and regimen of therapy are variable. Currently, most patients receive standard chemotherapy at full dose (i.e., MOPP, ABVD, or combination) and subsequent radiation therapy. This sequence of chemotherapy followed by radiation therapy often reduces the volume of radiation given and allows full-dose chemotherapy to be given. Patients often receive a lower dose of radiation than that given for curative intent in limited-stage disease.

Subdiaphragmatic disease also deserves special attention. Patients often undergo pathologic staging with a laparotomy. Patients with Stage I and II disease may be treated with an inverted Y field of radiation therapy (para-aortic and pelvic nodes). Extensive Stage II patients often require total nodal radiation. Therefore, chemotherapy may be considered a more attractive option in this subset.

ADVANCED DISEASE

The optimal therapy for Stage IIIA Hodgkin's disease is a topic of debate. Several authors have demonstrated that patients with Stage IIIA$_2$ may have a poor outcome with radiation alone. Patients with Stage IIIA and more than five splenic nodules may also have a poorer outcome with single-modality radiation therapy. Therefore, several trials have shown that patients with Stage IIIA$_2$ or bulky Stage IIIA$_1$ may benefit from chemotherapy, with a disease-free survival of over 90%. However, patients with Stage IIIA and fewer than five splenic nodules may be treated with radiation alone.

Chemotherapy is the primary treatment of choice, with curative intent for patients with Stage IIIB and IV Hodgkin's disease and for those patients whose disease has recurred after radiation therapy alone. The different treatment sequences and regimens have been discussed earlier (see Table 4). Consideration must be given to the long- and short-term side effects, and treatment should be individualized for each patient outside of a protocol setting.

RELAPSED OR RECURRENT TUMOR

Unfortunately, patients do relapse after radiation therapy, but they may have an excellent chance at survival with salvage chemotherapy. Most data to date have employed MOPP chemotherapy. The outlook is less optimistic for patients who fail chemotherapy or combined-modality regimens. The length of time since the last chemotherapy (i.e., greater or less than 1 year) has a significant effect on the response to subsequent therapies. Patients relapsing after either MOPP or ABVD can be offered the alternative regimen. Patients failing the MOPP/ABVD

alternating or hybrid regimen may be rechallenged with the same regimen, be given a different regimen, or consider newer agents and/or transplant options.

The availability of autologous bone marrow transplantation or peripheral stem cell support has expanded treatment modalities as well as remission and cure rates. Disease-free survivals of 50 to 60% have been reported in patients undergoing bone marrow transplant/stem cell support after a first or second relapse. The data are influenced by initial remission duration, documented response to standard chemotherapy while in relapse prior to transplantation, performance status, and number of prior relapses.

HODGKIN'S DISEASE IN HIV PATIENTS

Although controversy exists whether there is an increased risk of Hodgkin's disease in HIV-infected patients, most studies show an increased incidence compared with that expected in age-matched controls. Unfortunately, HIV-positive patients often present with advanced disease, advanced histology, B symptoms, or an atypical pattern of involvement. Response to chemotherapy is often poor due to decreased tolerance to chemotherapy and an increased risk of opportunistic infections. However, standard full-dose regimens are generally offered to these patients.

COMPLICATIONS OF THERAPY

Treatment of Hodgkin's disease with chemotherapy and/or radiation therapy has been associated with many acute and chronic side effects (Table 5). Acute toxicity of chemotherapy may include nausea, vomiting, and immune dysfunction.

Secondary malignancies are devastating complications of therapy. Acute leukemia and myelodysplastic syndromes are seen in 1 to 10% of patients after treatment with MOPP; the alkylating agent nitrogen mustard is the most implicated agent. Several studies have demonstrated that splenectomy prior to MOPP increases this risk. There is likely no further risk of developing hematologic malignancies in patients treated with combined-modality therapies (i.e., radiation therapy and chemotherapy). The risk of acute leukemia is significantly less, but not absent, for patients treated with ABVD alone.

There is also an increased risk of B cell lymphomas after treatment with chemotherapy for Hodgkin's dis-

TABLE 5. **Complications of Therapy**

Acute	Chronic/Late
Nausea/vomiting	Second malignancies
Alopecia	Infertility/sterility
Immunologic dysfunction	Cardiac dysfunction
Cytopenias	Pulmonary fibrosis
Neuropathy	

ease. There is no clear association with any specific chemotherapy regimen.

Solid tumors are also known to occur after therapy for Hodgkin's disease. The risk is related to radiation exposure, with tumors occurring in the field or at the edges of the radiation port. In a review from Stanford University, the risk at 15 years was approximately 18%. Tumors that occur include cancers of the lung, stomach, bone, soft tissue, breast, and thyroid.

Radiation therapy has also been associated with premature coronary artery disease as well as constrictive pericarditis and cardiomyopathy.

Sterility is an unfortunate complication of chemotherapy for Hodgkin's disease, as many patients are young adults. About 90% of males are sterilized by MOPP chemotherapy, likely secondary to the alkylating agent nitrogen mustard. Female fertility after MOPP is somewhat dependent upon age at therapy. ABVD is associated more commonly with temporary amenorrhea and azospermia. The option of sperm banking should be offered to male patients. There have been no reported increases in birth defects or complications of pregnancy in those patients who do conceive after chemotherapy.

NEW DRUGS AND AGENTS

Evaluating new agents in Hodgkin's disease is challenging, as the current treatment options and salvage regimens are so successful. However, ongoing trials are in progress for patients who have refractory or relapsed disease. Treatment with biologic response modifiers, including interferon and interleukin-2, has been evaluated in Hodgkin's disease. Due to the different side effects, toxicities, and modalities of action, biologic response modifiers are now being used in conjunction with standard chemotherapy regimens in the protocol setting.

HODGKIN'S DISEASE: RADIATION THERAPY

method of
NANCY PRICE MENDENHALL, M.D.
University of Florida College of Medicine
Gainesville, Florida

Radiation is the single most effective agent available in the treatment of Hodgkin's disease. It may be used as the sole treatment in early-stage patients, in combined modality treatment regimens in patients in all stages, as the sole salvage therapy in patients with nodal recurrence after chemotherapy, as part of salvage regimens that include standard or high-dose chemotherapy, and for palliation or in situations requiring rapid tumor response. Successful radiation treatment requires appropriate equipment, an experienced radiation oncologist, and adequate imaging to define the limits of disease.

RADIOTHERAPY TECHNIQUE

Treatment Volume

Involved-field irradiation (IF) refers to treatment of only the site(s) of clinical involvement. *Extended-field irradiation* (EF) refers to treatment of site(s) of clinical involvement plus elective treatment of contiguous, clinically uninvolved lymph node areas at risk for subclinical disease. *Total nodal irradiation* (TNI) refers to treatment of all nodal and extranodal areas commonly involved in Hodgkin's disease, including the mantle, spleen, para-aortic, and pelvic nodal fields; in some clinical settings, the liver is also treated. *Subtotal nodal irradiation* (STNI) differs from TNI in that the pelvis is not irradiated.

The *mantle* is an irregularly shaped volume that includes the cervical, supraclavicular, infraclavicular, axillary, mediastinal, and hilar lymph nodes. When indicated (because of large mediastinal adenopathy, hilar or subcarinal disease, pleural effusion or involvement, pericardial effusion or involvement), treatment of the whole lung, hemilung, or heart may be incorporated into treatment of the mantle. Opposed anterior and posterior fields are used. The lower border of the mantle is approximately at the bottom of T10 when there is either minimal or no mediastinal disease. The upper border is at midtragus. Custom blocks made of Lipowitz's metal shield the lung parenchyma, larynx, humeral heads, and portions of the mandible and parotid glands. In patients with mid or upper cervical lymph nodes, the preauricular nodes are treated with separate preauricular fields. In patients with bulky upper neck adenopathy, it may be necessary to treat a *Waldeyer's ring* field, which includes not only the preauricular nodes but also the deep upper cervical, occipital, and submental nodes as well as the lymphoid tissue in Waldeyer's ring. The mantle field may be combined with the spleen and para-aortic fields. The advantages of the combined field are shorter treatment time and better dose distribution in the area of field junction. The disadvantage is increased acute toxicity.

The *spleen* field includes the spleen and the splenic hilar nodes. If the spleen has been removed, the splenic hilar nodes may be treated through a small field if the splenic pedicle is clipped by the surgeon at the time of splenectomy. If there is extensive splenic involvement, consideration is given to elective irradiation of the liver because of the high risk for subclinical involvement.

The *para-aortic* field includes all para-aortic and paracaval lymph nodes between the aortic bifurcation and the bottom of the mantle field. The celiac axis nodes are incidentally covered. The para-aortic volume is treated through opposed anterior and posterior fields, matched (with an appropriate gap) to the mantle fields superiorly, the pelvic fields at the bottom of L4 inferiorly, and the spleen field laterally. The spleen and para-aortic fields may be treated in a single combined field.

The *pelvic* field includes the femoral nodes and the

common, external, and internal iliac nodes. The pelvic volume is treated through opposed anterior and posterior fields. The superior border is at the bottom of L4, matched, with an appropriate gap, to the bottom of the para-aortic fields. A customized block made of Lipowitz's metal shields the iliac wings and the midline structures not at risk, including the ovaries after transposition at laparotomy or laparoscopy. In males, special testicular shielding is required to decrease indirect exposure by radiation scattered from the pelvic field, which otherwise could cause azoospermia. An *inverted Y* field combines the pelvic and para-aortic fields. A *spade* field is similar to the inverted Y but does not include the femoral or pelvic lymphatics below the level of the common iliac nodes.

Time-Dose Factors

The doses used at the University of Florida for treatment of adults with radiotherapy alone are 35 Gy for clinically involved sites and 30 Gy for sites suspected of harboring subclinical disease. The dose for elective treatment of the lung or liver is 10 to 15 Gy. After a complete response to six cycles of chemotherapy, doses are reduced to 30 Gy for previously involved sites and 25 to 30 Gy for sites suspected of harboring subclinical disease. Dose reductions are not typically made after only two to three cycles of chemotherapy or in patients whose response to chemotherapy is poor. In children, after four or more cycles of chemotherapy, the dose to clinically involved sites is 25 Gy. In sites of nodal disease, the dose per fraction is 1.5 to 1.8 Gy. The dose per fraction is limited to 1.5 Gy or less when the entire cardiac silhouette is included in the field. When hemilung or whole lung is treated, the dose per fraction must be limited to 1 Gy per day or less through the use of thin lung transmission blocks.

Patients are treated once a day 5 days a week. In the rare patient with rapidly progressive disease, it may be necessary to treat twice a day. Occasionally, the treatment course may be split, with a 2-week break to allow for tumor shrinkage and field reduction for the high-dose area. This schema of split-course radiotherapy in Hodgkin's disease (in contrast to split-course radiotherapy for carcinomas) has no detrimental effect on control rate.

Sequencing in Combined Modality Therapy

In combined modality therapy, chemotherapy is delivered first. Chemotherapy treats all sites of clinical and subclinical disease in nodal and extranodal sites at once, whereas typically only one region may be treated at a time with radiotherapy. In addition, the response to chemotherapy typically results in tumor shrinkage that permits reduction in the radiation field size and consequently less exposure to normal tissue.

TREATMENT RECOMMENDATIONS

Cure is achieved in approximately three quarters of patients treated for Hodgkin's disease, and atten-

tion must be paid to sequelae of successful treatment. Treatment goals are not only relapse-free survival and survival but also survival without complications of treatment. Treatment alternatives include radiation therapy alone, chemotherapy alone, and a combination of the two modalities. Treatment selection depends on stratification of patients into prognostic groups and consideration of the late sequelae of available treatment options. Patients may be grouped into low-, intermediate-, and high-risk groups based on Ann Arbor stage and other prognostic factors such as tumor bulk (more than 6 cm or mediastinal mass greater than one third the maximum intrathoracic diameter), number of sites involved (greater than three or four), and presence and extent of splenic disease. Because of the possibility of salvage after the first treatment failure, it is occasionally appropriate to select an initial management approach that results in a lower probability of freedom from relapse but a higher probability of freedom from treatment sequelae. The results achieved with the approach used at the University of Florida are shown in Table 1.

Adults

Low Risk. Patients with stage IA and IIA disease with less than three or four sites of involvement and no bulky disease are at low risk for treatment failure with radiotherapy alone. If the patient is clinically staged, the radiotherapy volume should be STNI or TNI. Ten-year relapse-free, cause-specific, and absolute survival rates approach 85%, 95%, and 85%, respectively. If the patient has undergone staging laparotomy and has lymphocyte predominant or nodular sclerosis histology and a normal erythrocyte sedimentation rate, mantle irradiation alone may be considered. Relapse-free and absolute survival rates approach 75% and 85%.

TABLE 1. **Treatment Recommendations and Results at the University of Florida**

| | | 10-Year Survival Rates (%) | | |
| | | *Relapse-Free* | *Overall* | *Cause-Specific* |
Stage	**Treatment**			
Low Risk				
IA, IIA with small volume disease and <4 sites involved	STNI or TNI	84	85	95
Intermediate Risk				
IB, IIB; IA, IIA with bulky disease or ≥4 sites involved	Chemo × 2–3 and STNI	81	69	78
IIIA	Chemo × 2–3 and STNI	91	80	88
High Risk				
IIIB	Chemo × 6 and IF RT*	60	40	43
IVA, B	Chemo × 6 and IF RT*	53	64	64

*Usually STNI or TNI.

Abbreviations: STNI = subtotal nodal irradiation; TNI = total nodal irradiation; chemo = chemotherapy; IF = involved field; RT = radiation therapy.

Intermediate Risk. Patients with stage IA and IIA disease with more than three or four sites of involvement or bulky disease, or stage IIIA, IB, and IIB disease, are at intermediate risk of treatment failure and may be treated with radiotherapy alone or with combined modality therapy. With radiotherapy alone, the relapse-free and overall survival rates are approximately 50% and 80% at 10 years. Two basic combined modality approaches are commonly used in patients with intermediate risk disease: two to three cycles of chemotherapy followed by standard irradiation (usually STNI) and four to six cycles of chemotherapy followed by IF irradiation. Our institutional preference is two cycles of chemotherapy followed by radiotherapy, except in the patient with extensive subcarinal involvement that would require more cardiac irradiation. With combined modality therapy, the relapse-free, cause-specific, and overall survival rates are approximately 80%, 80%, and 70%, respectively.

High Risk. Patients with stage IIIB and IV disease are usually treated with combined modality therapy or chemotherapy alone. If combined modality therapy is used, the role of radiation may be to treat all areas of clinical involvement, only areas of bulky involvement, or only areas of incomplete response to chemotherapy. The radiation volume and dose will vary with the role of radiotherapy in a particular combined modality approach. There is a low probability of salvage after initial treatment with chemotherapy. Freedom from relapse, cause-specific, and absolute survival rates have been 60%, 40%, and 43%, respectively, for stage IIIB and 53%, 64%, and 64%, respectively, for stage IV at 10 years.

Children

Because of the musculoskeletal hypoplasia after radiation doses of greater than 25 Gy, chemotherapy is used more extensively in children, even in the early stages of disease. When radiation is used in children who have not reached growth potential, doses are generally limited to 25 Gy or less. Children may be treated with chemotherapy alone, but the doses required are six or more cycles, even in early-stage disease; alternatively, they may be treated with combined modality therapy using low-dose irradiation to involved fields as a means of limiting the chemotherapy dose. In early-stage disease, a common approach is three to four cycles of chemotherapy followed by irradiation with 25 Gy to involved fields. In intermediate and advanced disease, a common approach is four to six cycles of chemotherapy followed by involved field radiotherapy with 20 to 25 Gy.

POTENTIAL SIDE EFFECTS AND COMPLICATIONS

Acute Side Effects

Acute side effects occur during therapy and are usually resolved within 2 to 3 weeks after treatment. Expected side effects of mantle and Waldeyer's ring irradiation include transient hair loss, xerostomia, and an erythematous skin reaction. Hair loss is particularly noticeable in the occipital and preauricular regions in all patients and in the beard and anterior chest of men. Partial regrowth is usually observed within 2 to 4 months of treatment. Transient xerostomia occurs in many patients because of incidental parotid irradiation. Recovery of normal salivary function is related to the patient's pretherapy salivary output and age; young patients usually recover full salivary function, and older patients occasionally retain some mild xerostomia. The skin reaction is usually most prominent on the neck and over the shoulders and may be tender or pruritic. Lotions based on petrolatum (Aquaphor), lanolin, vitamin E, or aloe provide symptomatic relief and promote skin healing.

Nausea is frequently associated with splenic and para-aortic irradiation and may be controlled with standard antiemetics such as prochlorperazine maleate (Compazine), promethazine HCl (Phenergan), metoclopramide HCl (Reglan), chlorpromazine HCl (Thorazine), or ondansetron HCl (Zofran).

Bone marrow suppression may occur with TNI or irradiation preceded by chemotherapy. Thrombocytopenia is usually the first and most significant cytopenia resulting from irradiation. Treatment interruption may be required to allow for bone marrow recovery. Generally, radiation therapy is withheld until the platelet count is greater than 50,000 and the white blood cell count is greater than 2000.

Subacute Side Effects

Fatigue and loss of energy are common complaints during and after irradiation. Although most patients continue their routine activities during treatment, it may be 4 to 6 months after completion of treatment before the patient is back to a normal baseline energy level.

Within 1 to 4 months after completion of mantle irradiation, some patients experience Lhermitte's syndrome, usually characterized by an electric shock sensation associated with neck flexion; this may last from several weeks up to 9 months and is not associated with late or permanent neurologic sequelae of treatment.

Patients with Hodgkin's disease have a propensity to develop herpes zoster. The outbreak usually occurs within 2 years of treatment; later recurrences may be associated with recurrence of Hodgkin's disease. Typically, the outbreak is restricted to a single dermatomal distribution and is self-limited. The pain may be excruciating and the pruritus may be unrelenting. The symptoms and course may be ameliorated by acyclovir (Zovirax). Disseminated disease should be treated in the hospital.

Radiation pneumonitis occurs in less than 5% of patients, primarily in patients with extensive mediastinal disease, 2 to 4 months after mantle irradiation. The syndrome is characterized by a dry, hacking cough with an infiltrate confined to the radiation portals on chest roentgenogram. Symptoms may also include dyspnea, chest tightness, and fever. Occasionally the radiographic changes may extend outside the radiation portals. Although the condition is usually self-limited, severe cases may be fatal if not managed aggressively and expeditiously. If the patient has a cough without dyspnea, close observation is appropriate. If dyspnea is present, pulmonary function studies are helpful in assessment. If there is significant clinical pulmonary dysfunction or evidence of compromise on pulmonary function testing, patients are treated with prednisone (40 to 100 mg a day). With mild compromise, outpatient treatment is adequate with close surveillance, but if there is significant compromise, patients are hospitalized. It is important to rule out other processes such as *Pneumocystis* pneumonia. Steroid initiation should not be delayed for biopsy, however, in the compromised patient. Once steroids are initiated, the treatment is continued until the patient is asymptomatic, and then steroids are tapered slowly, usually over 1 to 2 months.

Acute pericarditis occurs in 1% to 2% of patients (usually those who had extensive mediastinal and pericardial disease) 2 to 6 months after mantle irradiation. Most patients are asymptomatic, and the diagnosis is made from plain chest roentgenograms. The amount of effusion present can be assessed with echocardiogram. Symptomatic patients report fatigue, dyspnea, and chest pain or tightness and may show signs of pericardial friction rub or paradoxical pulse and electrocardiogram changes. Nonsteroidal anti-inflammatory medications such as indomethacin (Indocin) or ibuprofen are usually effective at relieving symptoms. The patient should be observed for increasing pericardial effusion and possible tamponade, in which case emergency pericardiocentesis may be indicated.

Late Complications

Potential late complications include hypothyroidism, sterility, pulmonary fibrosis, cardiac damage, transverse myelitis, nephritis, growth abnormalities, and second malignancies.

Because thyroid dysfunction develops in 25% to 50% of patients, symptoms are routinely assessed, and annual thyroid function tests are obtained in asymptomatic patients. Estrogen replacement is instituted in women if ovarian ablation occurs as a result of radiotherapy or chemotherapy. No effective treatment is known for mediastinal or pulmonary fibrosis, but pericardiectomy can be performed for symptomatic constrictive pericarditis. Hyperbaric oxygen is used but is of limited value in transverse myelitis.

The use of doses greater than 25 Gy in preadolescent children results in hypoplastic development of the irradiated tissues. Musculoskeletal deformities detract from the child's sense of well-being and may contribute to psychosocial dysfunction. The younger the child and the higher the dose of radiation, the more significant the subsequent growth abnormality will be. Common sequelae include a "skinny neck" and shortened interclavicular distance secondary to mantle irradiation, a posterior left abdominal wall deficit from the spleen field, and shortened sitting height secondary to irradiation of the mantle and para-aortic fields.

Survivors of Hodgkin's disease have an increased risk of second malignancy. In particular, excesses of leukemia, non-Hodgkin's lymphoma, and breast, lung, and thyroid cancer have been observed. Some of the increased risk is related to the use of alkylating-agent chemotherapy, some to radiation, and some to host factors. Although the leukemias usually appear between 2 and 8 years after treatment, the solid malignancies may occur 20 or more years after treatment. In addition, an excess of cardiac disease, particularly coronary artery disease, has been noted in Hodgkin's disease survivors. Patients should be advised of the risk of late effects and counseled with respect to other risk factors, such as smoking, high blood cholesterol levels, obesity, and stress. Women should be advised to do breast self-examinations and receive routine mammography.

NEW DIRECTIONS

With the high survival rates currently achieved in Hodgkin's disease and the variety of effective treatment approaches, attention is focused on reducing the late effects of treatment. As most serious late effects from both chemotherapy and radiation are dose related, combined modality therapy is being used as a means not only of reducing the risk of relapse associated with single modality therapy, but also of limiting the doses of each modality. In children, the use of chemotherapy has permitted a lowering of the radiation dose so that little if any hypoplasia is expected. In adults, combined modality therapy has been used with only two to three cycles of chemotherapy producing a lower relapse rate than single modality therapy, as well as a lower risk of leukemia, sterility, and cardiac and lung problems than expected with six cycles of chemotherapy.

ACUTE LEUKEMIA IN ADULTS

method of
STEVEN D. GORE, M.D.
Johns Hopkins Oncology Center
Baltimore, Maryland

The acute leukemias comprise a group of clinically and biologically diverse diseases of the lymphohematopoietic system. In all cases of acute leukemia, clonal expansion of a hematopoietic progenitor cell eventually results in severe anemia, thrombocytopenia, and neutropenia. Clinical remission (restoration of normal hematopoiesis with less than 5% bone marrow blasts) can be achieved in the majority of patients using aggressive induction chemotherapy. Without further therapy, essentially all patients will relapse.

In the past decade, better postremission management of patients with acute leukemias has dramatically improved long-term outcomes and cure rates. Improved supportive care enabling aggressive postremission therapy has provided practitioners and patients with a sometimes bewildering number of choices for management. The appropriate use of clinical prognostic variables can help guide the choice of postremission therapy. New techniques for monitoring the amounts of minimal residual leukemia during clinical complete remission are being evaluated as adjuncts for assessing the success of a treatment course, enabling an early change in management when appropriate.

The optimal treatment for any subtype of acute leukemia has not been determined. Certain subsets of acute leukemia can be cured in 50% to 70% of cases using intensive chemotherapy. However, the treatment of patients with acute leukemia is extremely complicated, even when standard treatments are used to treat patients in good-risk subsets. Patients with acute leukemia receive optimal therapy from practitioners with particular expertise in this area in centers that treat a significant volume of such patients. Because treatments for acute leukemia are by no means optimized, patients should be entered on clinical trials whenever possible. The responsibility of a primary care practitioner who identifies acute leukemia is to make a rapid referral and transfer to a leukemia specialist, stabilizing the patient while preparing the transfer.

CLINICAL PRESENTATION

The clinical presentation of acute myeloid leukemia (AML) and acute lymphoblastic leukemia (ALL) can be similar. Fatigue and exertional dyspnea due to severe anemia are common presenting symptoms and have often been present for several weeks. Thrombocytopenia can lead to gingival bleeding, petechiae, and epistaxis. Unresponsive infection may lead to a complete blood count indicating the more serious underlying disorder.

The white blood cells (WBC) can be elevated, normal, or depressed in patients with AML and ALL; neutropenia is present in most patients. While hyperleukocytosis is commonly recognized as a potential problem when the WBC exceeds 100,000 per μL, some patients with AML will develop this syndrome at WBC counts of significantly less than 100,000 per μL. Hyperleukocytosis leads to abnormal blood viscosity owing to the circulating white cell mass, as well as specific vaso-occlusive phenomena arising from the adhesive properties of myeloid blast cells. Because lymphoblasts are smaller and less adherent, patients with ALL rarely develop hyperleukocytosis even at WBC counts of greater than 100,000 per μL. Hyperleukocytosis leads to pulmonary insufficiency and altered mental status. Patchy or diffuse infiltrates are found on chest radiograph or CT scan. Specific cranial neuropathies are more common with leptomeningeal leukemia, whereas frank quadri- or hemiparesis usually indicates a localized central nervous system (CNS) event such as hemorrhage or a CNS tumor of myeloid blasts (granulocytic sarcoma or chloroma). Hyperleukocytosis can also lead to dermal nodules, priapism, retinal hemorrhage, and Roth spots. Hyperleukocytosis should be treated as a hematologic emergency.

Patients with untreated leukemia may present with acute tumor lysis syndrome. Such patients have hyperuricemia, hyperphosphatemia, and renal insufficiency. In addition, patients may have subclinical or clinical evidence of disseminated intravascular coagulation (DIC) resulting from procoagulant activity released by dying leukemic cells. Significant DIC is most common in acute promyelocytic leukemia (AML M3), but it can also be seen in leukemias with monocytic differentiation (M4 and M5) and even ALL. Whereas all patients with leukemia should be evaluated for coagulopathy, any patient who presents with bleeding should be evaluated on an emergency basis for DIC, even if the bleeding may be explained by thrombocytopenia. As with DIC caused by other disorders, leukemia-induced DIC can occasionally be clinically manifest as thrombosis rather than bleeding.

Other abnormalities are less common in acute leukemia. Infiltrative symptoms include splenomegaly, hepatomegaly, lymphadenopathy, gingival hypertrophy, and leukemia cutis (skin infiltration by blasts). Acute leukemia can also be associated with Sweet's syndrome (neutrophilic dermatosis). In such cases, skin biopsy reveals infiltration with granulocytes rather than blast cells. Rare patients present with isolated granulocytic sarcomas without evidence of leukemia in their blood or bone marrow. Such patients must be treated as if they had acute leukemia, since most will relapse with systemic leukemia if treated with only local measures (surgery and/or radiotherapy).

INITIAL EVALUATION AND MANAGEMENT

The initial clinical determinations when evaluating a patient with possible acute leukemia focus on whether a leukemic emergency exists. The presence of hyperleukocytosis and/or DIC must be rapidly identified. The initial emergency laboratory determinations obtained on all patients suspected of acute leukemia include a complete blood count (CBC) with differential and platelet count, prothrombin time, partial thromboplastin time, quantitative fibrinogen, fibrin degradation products, electrolytes, BUN, serum creatinine, uric acid, phosphorus, and calcium. Patients without hyperleukocytosis, DIC, or tumor lysis syndrome most likely do not present an oncologic emergency and can be evaluated in a controlled but urgent manner. However, the WBC count can double rapidly in patients with acute leukemia, and arrangements for urgent transfer to a specialist in leukemia management should begin with the initial recognition of leukemia, even for patients with a WBC of less than 50,000 per μL.

The diagnosis of acute leukemia should be confirmed as soon as possible through a bone marrow aspirate and biopsy. It is important that when acute leukemia is suspected, sufficient marrow samples be aspirated to obtain studies that allow subclassification of the leukemia and critical prognostic information. Histochemistry and flow cytometry can establish a specific lineage diagnosis in 95% of cases of acute leukemia; morphologic classification of acute leukemia is inadequate. In addition to myeloperoxidase and granulocyte- and monocyte-associated esterases, AML usually expresses myeloid antigens such as CD13 and/or CD33 and HLA-DR. Acute promyelocytic leukemia is the important exception, which routinely is negative for HLA-DR. B lineage ALL can be recognized by the presence of the μ chain of immunoglobulin in the cytoplasm; HLA-DR and B lineage antigens such as CD19 and CD20 are identified by flow cytometry. In contrast, T-ALL lacks HLA-DR expression in at least 90% of cases but is positive for T cell antigens such as CD7, CD5, and CD2. Terminal deoxynucleotidyl transferase (TdT) is expressed in 90% to 95% of cases of ALL but is not specific. Recent additions to the FAB classification make flow cytometry an essential component of leukemia diagnosis. M0 AML denotes cases of AML that are negative for myeloperoxidase but bear myeloid surface antigens detected by flow cytometry. Megakaryoblastic AML (M7) blasts also lack myeloperoxidase but demonstrate megakaryocyte-specific antigens such as CD61 by flow cytometry or platelet-specific peroxidase by electron microscopy.

Flow cytometric analysis of leukemia should always include assessment of expression of the hematopoietic progenitor cell antigen CD34, which has important prognostic significance in AML (see later). All marrow aspirates obtained for the diagnosis of leukemia should be sent for cytogenetic analysis. Clonal chromosomal abnormalities constitute some of the most powerful prognostic information in leukemia (discussed later). In addition, samples should be obtained and stored for possible future use in molecular diagnostic studies.

In patients presenting with fever and granulocytopenia, blood and urine cultures should be rapidly obtained, empiric antibiotics initiated urgently, and a thorough investigation for sites of infection rapidly commenced. Antibiotic management must include adequate coverage for enteric gram-negative organism, including *Pseudomonas aeruginosa*. Leukemic patients may have less common sites of infection, such as sinusitis and perirectal infections. Although every effort should be made to document such infections, thrombocytopenia and neutropenia diminish the ability of leukemic patients to recover from invasive procedures. Surgical débridement is usually ineffective and inappropriate; however, diagnostic aspirations are often tolerated sufficiently well. If a specific source of infection is identified, appropriate specific antibiotics should be added to the gram-negative coverage.

In preparation for chemotherapy, all patients should be started on allopurinol (Zyloprim), and aggressive saline hydration (200 to 250 mL per h), with forced diuresis once the patient is clinically euvolemic to prevent the complications of tumor lysis (the common practice of urine alkalinization may decrease the solubility of phosphate). The efficacy of phosphate binders has never been definitively demonstrated, but they are used at many centers. Renal-dose dopamine can help maintain urine flow through the initial period of cytoreduction.

The multiple intravenous medications, blood products, and phlebotomies required during acute leukemia therapy necessitate long-term venous access. This can be accomplished using permanent or temporary multilumen central venous catheters. Once placed, a carefully maintained multiple lumen central venous access device can be used for all phlebotomy, medication, and blood product administration.

The use of prophylactic antibiotics in neutropenic patients undergoing prolonged bone marrow aplasia remains controversial. Orally administered quinolones are superior to placebo in delaying first neutro-

penic fever and in reducing gram-negative bacteremia. Prophylactic vancomycin (Vancocin) has been shown to decrease the incidence of gram-positive infections in granulocytopenic patients with indwelling catheters; however, the emergence of vancomycin-resistant enterococcus and the cost of vancomycin has brought this practice into question. Nonetheless, highly virulent alpha-hemolytic streptococci can lead to fulminant demise in patients not treated rapidly with vancomycin. Acyclovir (Zovirax) has been demonstrated to reduce the incidence of herpes simplex infections, which can significantly contribute to the development of mucositis as well as febrile viremia.

Hyperleukocytosis represents a leukemic emergency. Therapy directed at lowering the WBC must be instituted. When available, leukopheresis can serve as a useful temporizing measure. Aggressive administration of hydroxyurea (Hydrea), 3 gm per m², orally can lower the WBC count, although its effect is less rapid than that of leukopheresis. Hydroxyurea is therefore often used in conjunction with leukopheresis, particularly when transfer to another center is anticipated. High doses of cyclophosphamide (Cytoxan), 60 mg per kg, administered over 30 minutes following institution of aggressive hydration, prevent further increase in the WBC, and lead to a gradual decline in the WBC over 3 to 7 days. Administration of cyclophosphamide, while technically fairly simple in an emergency situation, may delay definitive cytosine arabinoside (ara-C, cytarabine [Cytosar-U])–based therapy (in the case of AML) and may cause hemorrhagic cystitis. Institution of definitive ara-C-based remission induction therapy for AML with hyperleukocytosis may be effective; however, this may be complicated by "tumor lysis pneumopathy" with development of adult respiratory distress syndrome. Thus, emergency reduction of the tumor mass before institution of ara-C-based chemotherapy represents prudent "pretreatment" stabilization.

The transfusion of red cells in the setting of hyperleukocytosis must be avoided. Despite a low hematocrit, patients with hyperleukocytosis will have a normal or elevated total blood cell volume, due to the increased "leukocrit." Transfusion of red cells to such a patient may cause hyperviscosity with acute difficulties in cranial and pulmonary perfusion. If red cells need to be replaced emergently (for example, because of cardiac ischemia), this can be done using leukopheresis to reduce the white cell mass simultaneously, with careful monitoring of the total packed cell volume. Pulse oximetry provides a more reliable measure of oxygenation in the patient with hyperleukocytosis than conventional arterial blood oxygen tension, owing to in vitro oxygen consumption by the blasts (serum glucose determination may be similarly artifactually decreased).

A screening lumbar puncture is reasonable in all patients with acute leukemia, and certainly in patients with neurologic changes. Although CNS involvement is less common in AML than in ALL, patients with higher WBC and patients with monocytic differentiation are at risk of leukemic meningitis. Lumbar puncture should be delayed until the WBC count is brought under control to minimize the risk of introducing leukemia into the spinal fluid. Some investigators advocate instilling intrathecal chemotherapy at the time of screening lumbar puncture (usually methotrexate, 12 mg, or ara-C, 100 mg). Treatment of established meningeal leukemia requires ongoing intrathecal therapy twice weekly until two lumbar punctures are clear. Cranial irradiation is often added if the patient is symptomatic. All patients with ALL should receive prophylactic intrathecal therapy. For patients with no evidence of CNS leukemia, CNS prophylaxis most often consists of five intrathecal injections of methotrexate, ara-C, or "triple therapy" (methotrexate, ara-C, and hydrocortisone). In some regimens, high systemic doses of methotrexate or ara-C that provide therapeutic CSF levels replace some or all intrathecal therapy.

HLA typing of the patient and siblings should be performed as early as possible. Apart from potential future marrow donation for allogeneic bone marrow transplantation, HLA-matched siblings can serve as platelet donors for alloimmunized patients who achieve inadequate increments in platelet counts following transfusions from random donors.

SUPPORTIVE CARE

All successful induction and postremission therapies of acute leukemia require meticulous attention to details of supportive care. Successful management includes strict attention to prophylaxis and management of tumor lysis syndrome (see earlier) and DIC, aggressive and appropriate management of hyperleukocytosis, and excellent support during the period of marrow aplasia, which can last from 2 to 4 weeks, depending on the type of leukemia and induction regimen used. Support during aplasia requires adequate replacement of red cells and platelets and empiric use of antibiotics for febrile neutropenia. Red cells are generally transfused to maintain the hematocrit greater than 23% (or greater in older patients or patients with ischemic symptoms). Platelets are transfused to maintain the platelet count above 10,000 to 20,000 per μL. If patients are actively bleeding, more frequent transfusions to maintain platelets at 50,000 per μL or greater may be helpful. Premenopausal female patients should have menses suppressed through administration of exogenous estrogens or progestational agents.

Ideal management of febrile neutropenia should be tailored to the microbiologic flora of the center at which the patient is treated. In most centers, otherwise stable febrile patients are observed for 3 days following institution of a new antibiotic change before determining antibiotic failure and initiating another antibiotic change. The first neutropenic fever is usually treated with broad-spectrum antibiotics directed against gram-negative organisms, including *Pseudomonas* species. Many centers will add vancomycin at that time (if not used prophylactically, see

earlier); others withhold specific gram-positive coverage until second fever. At Johns Hopkins, our most common microbiologic isolates during second fever have been fungal (primarily *Candida* species) since the institution of routine norfloxacin and vancomycin prophylaxis. We therefore routinely utilize amphotericin (Fungizone), as empiric therapy for second fever (0.5 mg per kg per day). Antibiotic changes for subsequent fevers can include broadened antibacterial coverage or empiric increase of amphotericin dosage (usually to 1.0 mg per kg per day) to cover potential resistant fungal organisms. With each new fever, a thorough search for the source of fever should be attempted, with careful attention to the sinuses, lungs, and perianal area. In neutropenic patients, chest computed tomography (CT) may be more sensitive than chest radiograph for detection of early fungal lesions; sinus CT may also be more sensitive than plain sinus films. Radiographic demonstration of fungal pneumonitis or sinusitis mandates empiric coverage for potential infections with *Aspergillus* species. This requires therapy with high-dose amphotericin (1.25 to 1.5 mg per kg per day). 5-Flucytosine has in vitro synergy with amphotericin against *Aspergillus* and serves as a useful adjunct in such patients. Lipid formulations of amphotericin may have less renal toxicity than standard amphotericin; such formulations are significantly more expensive. Renal toxicity of amphotericin is usually reversible upon completion of the course.

Abdominal CT scan can reveal the diagnosis of typhlitis (neutropenic enterocolitis), which requires anaerobic coverage in addition to the usual gram-negative coverage. Surgical treatment of such complications during prolonged aplasia is rarely successful because of the difficulty in subsequent patient support; all attempts at aggressive conservative therapy should be made. It is imperative that the microbiologic and mycologic laboratories involved in the care of leukemic patients detect and report organisms that might be considered commensal in patients with normal defense mechanisms but may be pathogenic in neutropenic patients. Antibiotics are generally withdrawn in afebrile patients once the neutrophil count is greater than 500 per μL. If bacteremia has been documented, appropriate antibiotics should be continued for at least 1 week following recovery of neutrophils. Fungal pneumonitis or sinusitis requires prolonged courses of amphotericin, particularly if further cytotoxic therapy is planned. In the case of fungal sinusitis, surgical débridement may be required following bone marrow recovery.

Several of the drugs used in the induction therapy of acute leukemia can cause severe oropharyngeal, esophageal, and intestinal mucositis. Supportive care includes adequate fluid replacement and local measures to provide pain relief. Continuous infusions of narcotics may be required; patient-controlled anesthesia pumps may be useful. Diarrhea that arises in the context of mucositis should be screened carefully for infectious causes, including *Clostridium difficile*. If diarrhea is noninfectious, bulk-forming agents such as psyllium hydrophilic mucilloid may decrease the frequency and fluidity of bowel movements. If this is not successful, loperamide or other anti-motility agents may be helpful.

In both ALL and AML, myeloid growth factors have been successfully used to decrease the time to marrow recovery during induction chemotherapy. Although decreased days of neutropenia have been demonstrated, significant decreases in serious infections, days in the hospital, and cost effectiveness have not been shown. An increase in primary resistance or early relapse of leukemia due to administration of myeloid growth factors has not been demonstrated. However, the long-term effects of growth factor administration are not yet known, and studies will need to continue to mature to ensure that the rate of relapse and incidence of secondary leukemia are not increased. Many investigators advocate reserving growth factor administration for patients with prolonged aplasia (and hypoplastic bone marrows) or patients with life-threatening infections who will not survive without WBC recovery. However, the efficacy of growth factors administered in this fashion has not been well studied.

Interest in the use of myeloid growth factors to sensitize leukemic blasts to the effects of chemotherapy comes from the recognition that the most active agents in the treatment of leukemia, in particular ara-C, are highly dependent on cells traversing the cell cycle. A variety of trials of growth factor augmentation of induction chemotherapy have been performed, with no overall benefit yet demonstrated. The biologic impact of growth factor administration on leukemic blasts appears markedly heterogeneous, with similar numbers of bone marrow samples showing increased and decreased ara-C sensitivity following cytokine infusion. It is therefore unlikely that randomized trials will demonstrate a marked advantage to the administration of growth factors. Further elucidation of the biologic heterogeneity of AML response to growth factors may enable selective administration of these compounds to patients likely to benefit from this approach. At this time, the administration of growth factors to augment the effects of chemotherapy should be limited to clinical trials.

CLASSIFICATION OF AND PROGNOSTIC FACTORS IN ACUTE MYELOID LEUKEMIA

Whereas the French-American-British (FAB) system remains the standard classification system in AML, cytogenetics provides the most important prognostic information. Good-risk subsets of AML include myelomonocyctic leukemia with abnormal eosinophils (M4 Eo), and M2 with significant differentiation (characterized by t[8;21]). Most authorities consider M3 AML a good- or average-risk subset of AML. Erythroleukemia (M6) and megakaryoblastic leukemia (M7) are poor-risk subsets; M0 AML may also carry a poor prognosis. Karyotyping has rapidly eclipsed morphology as a critical source of prognostic

information. Evaluation of a new case of AML is not complete without cytogenetic studies, preferably performed on bone marrow cells. Certain cytogenetically defined subsets have cure rates greater than 50% with nonmyeloablative chemotherapy. The two subsets of AML with the best overall prognoses are those characterized by abnormalities of chromosome 16 involving band q22, and those with t(8;21). Some equally good-risk leukemias may have these cytogenetic abnormalities without the classic associated morphology. Hybrid mRNA resulting from these translocations can be detected through reverse transcriptase–polymerase chain reaction (rt-PCR), which is likely to become a standard diagnostic test for newly diagnosed AML with "normal" karyotype. The great majority of cases of M3 AML have t(15;17). In most cases that do not demonstrate this translocation, the resulting fusion gene, involving the α-subunit of the retinoic acid receptor (RARα), can be detected by Southern blot analysis or rt-PCR. Cases that do not have this fusion gene are unlikely to respond to induction therapy with retinoic acid (see later).

Other cytogenetic abnormalities mark cases of AML as prognostically inferior and unlikely to be cured with nonmyeloablative doses of chemotherapy. These include cases characterized by deletions of the long arms of chromosome 5 or 7, cases with abnormalities of chromosome 11, band q23 (site of the MLL gene), and cases with t(6;9). Trisomy 8, a common abnormality in AML, has been found in some series to identify a subset with poor prognosis; however, in other series trisomy 8 represents "average" risk, with some long-term cures. Normal cytogenetics are considered "average" risk in AML and are likely to represent a biologically heterogeneous group of diseases.

Expression of the progenitor cell antigen CD34 on leukemic blasts portends an unfavorable prognosis; however, some good-risk subsets can express CD34 (such as t[8;21]). Expression of the multidrug resistance glycoprotein (mdr1, P-glycoprotein) is also of negative prognostic significance. Although the biologic significance of mdr1 expression is not certain, clinical trials that aim to overcome the drug efflux function of mdr1 are ongoing in AML.

Leukemias that arise from antecedent hematologic disorders (AHD) are inferior prognostically. However, in the Hopkins experience, history of AHD is not an independent prognostic factor when cytogenetics are included as variables; patients with AHD with normal cytogenetics have survivals similar to those of patients with normal cytogenetics and no history of AHD. AML that arises as a result of prior exposure to cytotoxic therapy (therapy-related AML, or secondary AML) tends to be resistant to induction chemotherapy (especially with "conventionally dosed" ara-C-based regimens) and is rarely if ever cured with nonmyeloablative chemotherapy. AML induced by exposure to alkylating agents is frequently characterized by deletions of chromosomes 5 and 7, often arises from a context of myelodysplastic syndrome (MDS), and may have other poor-risk features such as CD34 expression and M6 or M7 phenotype. In contrast, AML induced by exposure to topoisomerase II inhibitors has a short latency period of 1 to 2 years, monocytic phenotype, and a rapidly progressive course. Such leukemias manifest abnormalities of chromosome 11q23 with rearrangements of the MLL gene. Such leukemias may enter remission easily but often relapse rapidly.

Advanced age persists as an independent prognostic factor in most series in AML. The prognostic significance of age likely represents both decreased tolerance for intensive chemotherapy and increased incidence of innate chemoresistance. High WBC increases the risk of failure to achieve remission; it may also have independent prognostic significance for remission duration, but this is likely to be treatment-dependent.

Acute Myeloid Leukemia Induction Chemotherapy

Cytosine arabinoside (ara-C) is the single most active agent in AML. Effective strategies of ara-C administration aim at maintaining an adequate steady-state concentration for several days. Ara-C is commonly administered as a 7-day continuous infusion at doses of either 100 or 200 mg per m^2 per day, usually in conjunction with 3 days of anthracycline (so-called "3 plus 7" or "7 and 3" schedule). More recent strategies aim at achieving more pharmacodynamically optimal steady state plasma concentrations: these include high doses administered twice daily (so-called "high-dose ara-C," or HiDAc), as well as intensive 3- to 4-day infusional schedules (total dose, 2 to 6 grams per m^2). Both methods are reported to have high response rates. HiDAc has a significant incidence of cerebellar toxicity that can be severe and irreversible; incidence is highest among elderly patients and patients with abnormal renal function. Intensive infusional schedules have almost no significant cerebellar toxicity but may be more likely to cause fluid retention and capillary leak syndrome, including adult respiratory distress syndrome.

In large series, complete remission (CR) rates from administration of conventionally dosed "3 and 7" regimens average approximately 60%. Idarubicin (Idamycin) may have a modest benefit when compared with daunorubicin (Cerubidine) in "3 and 7" induction therapy. Response rates using "3 and 7" induction are considerably lower in elderly patients and in patients with antecedent hematologic disorders (AHD) who are often excluded from clinical trials. Higher CR rates, in the 70% to 90% range, have been reported in Phase II studies of regimens with greater dose intensity of ara-C. Several series include additional drugs, such as topoisomerase-II inhibitors. At Hopkins, ara-C is administered during induction as a 3-day infusion (total dose of 2 grams per m^2) in conjunction with daunorubicin (45 mg per m^2 per day daily for 3 days), followed by VP-16 (etoposide [VePesid]) (400 mg per m^2 per day as a 6-hour intravenous infusion) on days 8, 9, and 10. This regimen has a 70% CR rate, with an approximate 50% CR rate in elderly patients and patients with AHD. It is not yet clear whether there is a single optimal schedule of ara-C for remission induction. The results of ongoing studies that randomize between various induction regimens are awaited to determine whether dose intensity of ara-C during induction is important for any or all patients, or whether it is beneficial in particular subsets, such as CD34+ cases of AML, or AML with a history of AHD.

Special consideration must be given to induction therapy for acute promyelocytic leukemia. It is now well recognized that oral administration of all-*trans*-retinoic acid (ATRA [Vesanoid]) 45 mg per m^2 per day) can induce remission in 70% to 90% of patients with M3 AML (ATRA is not effective in patients with AML which resembles M3 morphologically but does not demonstrate the t(15;17) or RARα-PML gene rearrangement). ATRA induces terminal differentiation of the leukemic cells, followed by restoration of nonclonal hematopoiesis. Administration of ATRA leads to rapid resolution of coagulopathy in the majority of patients, and heparin administration is not required in patients receiving ATRA. However, randomized trials have not shown a reduction in morbidity and mortality during ATRA induction when compared with chemotherapy. Administration of ATRA can lead to hyperleukocytosis, as well as a syndrome of respiratory distress now known as the "ATRA syndrome." Prompt recognition of the ATRA syndrome and aggressive administration of steroids can prevent severe respiratory distress. The optimal management of ATRA-induced hyperleukocytosis has not been established; neither has the optimal postremission management of patients who receive ATRA induction. However, two large cooperative group trials have demonstrated a significant relapse-free and overall survival advantage to patients with M3 AML who receive ATRA at some point during their antileukemic management.

Postremission Management of Acute Myeloid Leukemia

Although individual patients have been reported to have long disease-free survival or cure with a single cycle of chemotherapy, intensive postremission therapy is always indicated in therapy planned with curative intent. There is no convincing evidence in AML that low-dose "maintenance" chemotherapy prolongs disease-free survival, and it is rarely included in current protocols. Non-myeloablative consolidation therapy using ara-C–containing regimens has treatment-related death rates under 10% and yields disease-free survivals ranging from 20% to 50%. A recent large randomized trial performed by the Cancer and Leukemia Group B (CALGB), which compared three different ara-C–containing consolidation regimens, showed a clear benefit in survival to patients under age 60 years who received high-dose ara-C (HiDAc). In a subsequent analysis presented in abstract form, the benefit of receiving HiDAc consolidation was not extended to patients with poor-risk cytogenetics. The optimal number of cycles of HiDAc consolidation has not been determined (the CALGB trial planned four cycles of HiDAc, but few patients received more than two cycles).

We have reported similar results using only one cycle of infusional ara-C–based chemotherapy. In the Hopkins consolidation regimen, a total dose of 6 grams per m² of infusional ara-C is administered over the first 3 days, in conjunction with three doses of daunorubicin (Cerubidine), (45 mg per m² per day). This is followed by 3 additional days of infusional ara-C (total dose, 2 grams per m²) on days 10 to 12 (Ac-D-Ac). This highly ara-C–intensive regimen led to a 40% disease-free survival in patients who received it during remission, but it has a long duration of aplasia and a significant incidence of capillary leak syndrome. Because the optimal doses, schedules, and duration of consolidation chemotherapy have not been determined, patients with AML should be included in clinical trials at institutions treating large numbers of such patients in order to answer these questions. However, in 1996 it is clear that ongoing cycles of "3 and 7" consolidation chemotherapy do not cure adequate numbers of the most curable leukemias.

In bone marrow transplantation (BMT), high doses of "marrow ablative" chemotherapy or chemoradiotherapy are administered to eradicate residual leukemia cells. A source of stem cells is then infused that subsequently repopulates the lymphohematopoietic organs. Allogeneic BMT (alloBMT) results in the lowest incidence of leukemic relapse of all postremission management strategies, even when compared with BMT from an identical twin (syngeneic BMT). This has led to the concept of an immunologic graft-versus-leukemia effect, similar and related to graft-versus-host disease (GVHD). The improvement in freedom from relapse using alloBMT as primary post-remission therapy is offset, at least in part, by increased morbidity and mortality due to GVHD, veno-occlusive disease of the liver, and interstitial pneumonitis. In GVHD, donor T cells recognize minor histocompatibility antigens on the host cells, causing an immune process that can lead to dermatitis, bone marrow and hepatic failure, immune compromise, and severe enteritis.

Disease-free survival using allogeneic transplant in first remission has ranged from 45% to 60%. The use of alloBMT as primary postremission therapy is limited by the need for an HLA-matched sibling donor and the increased mortality of alloBMT in patients in the fifth or sixth decade. The mortality from alloBMT using an HLA-matched sibling donor ranges from 20% to 40%, depending on the series. However, ongoing improvements in alloBMT, such as T cell depletion, are leading to decreased mortality from this treatment modality. Ongoing studies will determine whether such improvements will decrease the mortality of alloBMT without increasing the relapse rate. The use of matched, unrelated donors for alloBMT is being investigated at many centers but currently has a very substantial rate of treatment-related mortality, with disease-free survival less than 35% due to an increased incidence of graft failure and a high incidence of severe GVHD.

In autologous BMT (autoBMT), bone marrow is harvested from patients in remission. Such marrow is cryopreserved and subsequently used as a source of stem cells following the administration of myeloablative therapy similar to that used in alloBMT. When compared with alloBMT, autoBMT has two potential problems: the infusion of viable residual leukemia cells that have been harvested, and the lack of an immunologic antileukemia effect. Despite these potential drawbacks, autoBMT provides disease-free survival reported between 35% and 50%. Because of the lack of GVHD, treatment-related mortality of autologous BMT ranges from 10% to 20%. Substantial issues about the optimal use of autoBMT remain. It is currently unclear whether autoBMT can cure significant subsets of patients who are not cured with ara-C intensive consolidation regimens. Ongoing controversies include the timing of autoBMT and whether autoBMT should be preceded by consolidation therapy. The role of ex vivo treatment (purging) of the bone marrow graft with chemotherapy, such as 4-hydroperoxycyclophosphamide (4-HC)* or mafosphamide,* or monoclonal antibodies such as anti-CD33,* is a critical question. A recent randomized trial compared the use of autologous BMT in first remission to consolidation chemotherapy, with the latter group eligible for autoBMT in second remission. The two arms had equivalent survival. Autologous BMT using 4-HC–purged bone marrow is currently being compared with high-dose ara-C consolidation therapy in a randomized trial.

Because BMT can cure many patients who relapse following chemotherapy, some have suggested that alloBMT can be reserved for second complete remission or early relapse without compromising the numbers of patients ultimately cured. However, clinical and cytogenetic information can define certain subsets with predictable better and worse outcomes using consolidation chemotherapy. Patients with good-risk AML, including t(8;21), inv(16), and t(15;17), have a reasonable chance at cure with intensive consolidation, so transplantation should probably be deferred in this group. Patients with poor-risk factors, including deletions of 5q and 7q, trisomy 8, t(6;9), and t(9;22), are unlikely to be cured with consolidation chemotherapy, and alloBMT in the first CR is a reasonable option for patients with available sibling donors. The efficacy of autoBMT in the poor-risk group is the subject of active clinical trials. Patients with normal cytogenetics comprise an intermediate-risk group, and postremission management should be individualized, or ideally managed according to a clinical trial. Patients with chemotherapy-induced

---

*Investigational drug in the United States.

secondary AML are probably never cured with chemotherapy and should be considered for allogeneic BMT; the efficacy of autologous BMT in this group is under investigation.

PROGNOSTIC FACTORS IN ACUTE LYMPHOBLASTIC LEUKEMIA

Advances in the cure rate in adult ALL have followed adaptation of treatments pioneered in pediatric ALL; however, adult ALL is cured far less often than pediatric ALL. The higher failure rate in adults cannot be completely explained by an increased incidence of leukemias with poor prognostic features. Nonetheless, the overall cure rate in adult ALL ranges from 35% to 40%, which is significantly better than the overall cure rate in AML.

High WBC count is a generally accepted risk factor for failure to achieve CR as well as remission duration. Inferior remission durations have been demonstrated using WBC cutoffs ranging from 5000 to 30,000 per μL. WBC may not impact on survival of patients with a T cell phenotype (see later). CD10-negative B-lineage ALL (so-called "null cell ALL") has been shown by several groups to be high risk for failure to achieve remission and for poor remission duration. This may be due to the high number of patients with this phenotype who have poor-risk cytogenetic abnormalities. Prognosis is extremely poor in patients with ALL over age 60 years. However, some studies suggest increased risk of treatment failure in patients over age 25 or 35 years. L3 ALL (mature B cell phenotype) fares poorly with most current ALL regimens and should be treated with other approaches (discussed later).

As with AML, cytogenetics and molecular diagnostic testing provide critical prognostic information. In pediatric ALL, hyperdiploidy (greater than 52 chromosomes per cell) indicates good risk. Insufficient adult cases are available to verify this as a positive prognostic factor. Several cytogenetic abnormalities have important negative prognostic import in adult ALL. Foremost among these is the Philadelphia chromosome (Ph 1+; t[9;22]). As in CML, the Ph1 chromosome in ALL encodes for a fusion gene combining portions of the *c-abl* oncogene and a second gene known as *bcr*. The fusion gene is known as *bcr/abl*. Essentially no cases of Ph1+ ALL are cured with nonmyeloablative doses of chemotherapy. Some cases of ALL that appear karyotypically normal have *bcr/abl* detectable by rt-PCR or by pulsed field gel electrophoresis. Because of the significant negative prognostic import of this genetic abnormality, it is reasonable to screen all cases of B-lineage ALL with normal karyotype by rt-PCR or pulsed field gel electrophoresis. A second major group of cytogenetic abnormalities with negative prognostic import involves chromosome 11q23 and the MLL gene (such as t[4;11]). Such cases relapse early and are rarely cured without bone marrow transplantation. As noted earlier, cases of L3 leukemia do poorly with ALL therapy. Such cases have translocations that place the *c-myc* oncogene,

located on chromosome 8, under the influence of regulators of the immunoglobulin gene ([t(2;8), t(8;12), and t(8;22)]). Patients with these cytogenetic abnormalities should be on treatment protocols designed particularly for L3 ALL.

In several series, T cell ALL has long-term disease-free survival with nonmyeloablative chemotherapy of 60% to 70%. In contrast, B-lineage ALL is cured in only approximately 35% to 40% of patients. The cure rate in B-lineage ALL is clearly higher if patients with t(9;22), t(4;11), and L3 leukemias are excluded from analysis.

Acute Lymphoblastic Leukemia Chemotherapy

Current induction regimens in ALL combine prednisone, vincristine, and an anthracycline. Some regimens add additional drugs such as cyclophosphamide (Cytoxan) and/or asparaginase (Elspar). Complete remission should be achieved in 70% to 90% of adults with ALL. Successful strategies for postremission chemotherapy often include complicated intensive multiagent sequences of chemotherapeutic drugs. These include alkylating agents, vinca alkaloids, steroids, cytosine arabinoside, anthracyclines, methotrexate, 6-mercaptopurine, and L-asparaginase. Newer dose-intensive chemotherapeutic schedules can be difficult and should be administered by physicians experienced in these regimens at centers equipped to deal with potential complications. In general, several cycles of intensive consolidation are followed by ongoing maintenance therapy. Although the mechanism behind the efficacy of maintenance is largely unknown, the need for ongoing maintenance therapy has been demonstrated in randomized trials. Most ALL chemotherapeutic regimens continue maintenance for 18 to 24 months.

Bone Marrow Transplantation in Acute Lymphoblastic Leukemia

As with AML, alloBMT is the postremission management resulting in the lowest incidence of leukemic relapse. In a retrospective study comparing the outcome of alloBMT in first remission to aggressive chemotherapy, the outcome of the two treatments in first remission appeared identical (40% cure). A more recent prospective trial led to similar conclusions. In the latter trial, alloBMT led to significant survival benefit for patients with high-risk ALL (CD10−; B-lineage ALL with WBC greater than 30,000; Ph1+ ALL), confirming previous single institution experience suggesting the utility of alloBMT for the cure of high-risk ALL. Because of this and similar data, it seems reasonable to reserve alloBMT in first remission for patients with poor-risk cytogenetics or other high-risk features.

AutoBMT has been less successful in the management of ALL in first remission. Long-term disease-free survival estimates range from 20% to 40% with autoBMT. There are no data demonstrating efficacy of autoBMT in high-risk ALL. The long-term survival of patients who received chemotherapy and autoBMT was identical in a randomized trial. It is possible that the efficacy of autoBMT in ALL may be improved by the use of maintenance chemotherapy or immune modulation following transplantation. Because the optimal postremission therapy for patients with ALL is still unclear, patients should be entered in clinical trials whenever possible.

The outlook for patients with L3 leukemia appears to be improving. Newer regimens that resemble treatment for non-Hodgkin's lymphoma combine cyclophosphamide, doxorubicin, vincristine, teniposide, steroids, and high-dose methotrexate. Intrathecal prophylaxis is commenced early in the treatment course. Treatment is aggressive and completed within 5 months, compared with 2 years for most ALL regimens. Using this approach in patients with well-documented L3 leukemia (surface immunoglobulin positive), complete response rates of 60% to 70% are now reported, with at least 50% long-term disease-free survival.

PRIMARY REFRACTORY AND RELAPSED LEUKEMIA

Cases of AML that have failed to go into remission after two cycles of "3 and 7" induction have been considered to be primarily refractory to treatment. In 1996, it may be reasonable to consider retreatment of patients who do not go into remission with a single cycle of "3 and 7" with a more ara-C–intensive regimen rather than proceeding with a second cycle of less dose-intensive therapy. Patients who fail to go into remission with a single course of HiDAc or an intensive infusional ara-C–containing regimen may be considered primarily refractory to treatment. Similarly, patients with ALL who fail to achieve remission with two aggressive induction regimens can be considered to have primarily refractory leukemia. Approximately 20% of such patients can achieve long-term disease control with allogeneic BMT. There is no evidence that continuing induction attempts on such patients prior to allogeneic BMT from an HLA-matched sibling improve outcome; rather the attempts may compromise the chances of success of allogeneic BMT by increasing end-organ toxicity and promoting development of fungal infections. Patients with primary refractory leukemia who do not have an HLA-matched sibling (or unrelated donor if one can be identified in an appropriate time frame) are excellent candidates for Phase I and Phase II investigations of new treatment modalities, including investigational drugs, monoclonal antibodies, and biologic response modifiers.

Patients who relapse after receiving nonmarrow ablative chemotherapy are unlikely to be cured without bone marrow transplantation. Ideally, the availability of potential HLA-matched siblings will have been determined during the first course of chemotherapy. With careful surveillance, some patients will be identified in early relapse, with excellent performance status and minimal hematopoietic compromise. Such patients may do well with allogeneic BMT without reinduction therapy. Retrospective data from The Fred Hutchison Cancer Center suggest that there is no advantage to reinduction before alloBMT in first relapse; however, this type of data is likely to be highly biased toward patients thought to be in first remission but who were found to be in early relapse at the time of arrival in Seattle for BMT. Certainly, such data do not include patients who have an aggressive relapse with declining performance status. Such patients are likely to benefit from reinduction therapy before alloBMT. The choice of reinduction therapy depends on the previous chemotherapy administered. If patients went into remission easily and remission lasted longer than 2 years, reinduction with a similar regimen is reasonable. More intensive regimens, including additional drugs such as topoisomerase II inhibitors, may be beneficial, especially if patients received less intensive chemotherapy initially. Whenever possible, such patients should be entered on clinical trials.

Patients who achieve a second remission but do not have an HLA-matched sibling may receive curative therapy in the form of autologous BMT or allogeneic BMT from a matched unrelated sibling. Autologous BMT, performed with ex vivo purging with 4-HC, can cure approximately 30% to 40% of patients with AML in second complete remission; the cure rate is less for patients with ALL. Successful matched unrelated transplant depends on the ability to identify and mobilize a donor in a rapid time frame. The high incidence of severe GVHD and graft failure continues to make this form of BMT a difficult, but rapidly evolving, treatment modality. Patients who fail to go into second remission are candidates for Phase I and Phase II investigations if alloBMT is not an option.

SURVEILLANCE DURING REMISSION AND MONITORING OF MINIMAL RESIDUAL DISEASE

Patients with acute leukemia in first remission should be monitored carefully so that relapse can be detected and potentially curative salvage therapy instituted early. Routine bone marrow aspirations, even with cytogenetic monitoring, do not appear to detect relapse more than several weeks before peripheral blood counts manifest changes. For this reason, patients whose complete blood counts with differential are normal probably do not need routine bone marrow surveillance outside the context of clinical trials. In addition to monthly blood counts, patients with ALL should be monitored with intermittent lumbar punctures to screen for early evidence of CNS relapse. Any patient with a history of extramedullary disease or primary granulocytic sarcoma should have intermittent radiographic studies performed to monitor relapse at the extramedullary site.

In recent years, a number of more sensitive techniques for the detection of minimal residual disease have been developed. Multiparameter flow cytometry can detect rare numbers of cells with the properties of blasts with leukemia-specific antigen combinations. The specificity and predictive value of such monitoring for relapse are currently being investigated. Leukemias with specific chromosomal translocations and leukemia-specific fusion genes can have exquisitely small amounts of residual leukemia monitored in the bone marrow or peripheral blood using PCR-based techniques. The significance of PCR-detectable disease varies among diseases. Patients with a history of M2 AML with t(8;21) have been found by PCR to have residual cells with this translocation greater than one decade after primary therapy, at a time when they are highly unlikely to relapse. In contrast, persistent or recurrent PCR-detectable RARα-PML several months following consolidation chemotherapy for M3 AML appears to have strong positive predictive power for relapse. If detection of an upward trend in the percentage of such cells has strong positive predictive value for subsequent relapse, such monitoring may enable very early decision about salvage BMT, or change in chemotherapy management if treatment is ongoing as in ALL. Ongoing studies of the use of these techniques to monitor minimal residual disease prospectively will identify which subsets of patients should be screened and when therapeutic intervention is warranted.

PALLIATIVE AND HOSPICE CARE OF PATIENTS WITH REFRACTORY ACUTE LEUKEMIA

Despite superb management, some patients will never achieve remission, and many other patients will relapse and subsequently die of leukemia. The palliation and management of terminal care of such patients is an important part of the job of the treating hematologic oncologist. Hydroxyurea can be used to keep the WBC from rising in patients who are not prepared to die of hyperleukocytosis. Ongoing transfusion support is important palliative care for patients and is consistent with a hospice approach. The administration of red cells to anemic patients improves quality of life and prevents air hunger. Platelet administration can avoid epistaxis and hemoptysis. Many patients with chronic thrombocytopenia tolerate a lower platelet level than patients whose platelet count drops precipitously. Thus attempts may be made to restrict platelet transfusions to patients with platelet counts less than 10,000 per µL or who are actively bleeding. The administration of quinolone antibiotics such as norfloxacin (Noroxin) can avert infections in chronically neutropenic patients whose bone marrows are not going to improve. Whether intravenous antibiotics are administered to such patients when febrile should be decided jointly by the physician and patient. Although patients who have refractory leukemia will never recover their neutrophil count, occasionally short courses of antibiotics will effectively control infection. Long-term antibiotic administration is clearly neither feasible nor appropriate. Pain is not usually a major feature of late-stage acute leukemia unless the disease is infiltrative, causing painful splenomegaly or gingival hypertrophy. Hydroxyurea can provide palliation in some patients; splenic irradiation can also be beneficial. However, patients with significant pain should be provided with appropriate access to narcotic analgesics and be instructed to use them at regular intervals to maintain pain control. Most patients will eventually succumb to infection or to hyperleukocytosis. With appropriate supportive care, many patients with refractory leukemia can survive several months or a year with significant quality of life.

ACUTE LEUKEMIA IN CHILDREN

method of
FAITH H. KUNG, M.D.
UCSD Medical Center
San Diego, California

Each year in the United States, approximately 3000 children under 15 years of age are diagnosed as having acute leukemia. The acute leukemias are the most common childhood malignancy and represent about 30% of all childhood cancers. Like most if not all cancers, leukemias begin in a single cell, in this case a precursor hematopoietic cell. In a manner that is incompletely understood, accidents occur during cell division, mutating the DNA. If the cell survives and the genetic lesion impairs that cell's ability to respond to the milieu of control signals that regulate cell division, it may evolve into a clone of cancer cells. Inexorable cell division and disorderly tissue formation result. Descendants of the original leukemic cell crowd out normal marrow cells, causing bone marrow failure. Leukemic cells may spill into the peripheral blood and are seen as "blasts" in the background of anemia, thrombocytopenia, and a paucity of normal white cells. These cells may accumulate in lymphoid tissues, producing organomegaly and adenopathy. In the usual case, the peripheral blood count is low, but massive leukocytosis may also occur.

Approximately 80% of the childhood acute leukemias are derived from the lymphoid lineage and are classified as acute lymphoblastic leukemia (ALL), 15% are acute nonlymphoblastic (myelogenous, monomyelogenous, or monoblastic) leukemia, and a small portion are not easily classifiable as belonging to either the lymphoid or the myeloid lineage. Indeed, some seem to have attributes of both lineages. Marker studies and genetic evidence indicate that there may be many subgroups of each leukemia. The peak incidence for ALL is between 3 and 5 years, but no such peak is found in the acute nonlymphoblastic leukemias. The incidence of ALL is higher in white children than in black, and higher in males than in females.

There is no convincing evidence that environmental factors such as electromagnetic fields or geography predispose to cancer in children. Leukemias seldom run in families. Factors that may predispose children to acute leukemias are cited in Table 1.

DIAGNOSIS

Children with ALL may present with fever, fatigue, anorexia, irritability, easy bruising, bleeding, respiratory distress from an enlarged thymus, or pain in the abdomen,

TABLE 1. **Risk Factors for Acute Leukemia in Children**

Increased maternal age
Maternal history of fetal loss
Larger birth weight
Fathers exposed to medical x-rays involving the lower
    gastrointestinal tract and lower abdomen prior to conception
Trisomy 21
IgA deficiency
Ataxia telangiectasia
Bloom syndrome
Fanconi's anemia
Shwachman syndrome
Klinefelter's syndrome
Poland's syndrome
Neurofibromatosis

bone, or joint. Rarely is there joint swelling. Often the family relates that the child "never got over a cold." There may be lymph node, liver, and splenic enlargement. See Table 2 for the differential diagnosis. In addition to a complete history and physical examination, the diagnostic work-up for acute leukemia should include the items listed in Table 3.

ACUTE LYMPHOBLASTIC LEUKEMIA

Initially, pathologists classified the leukemias on morphologic criteria. Recently, using monoclonal antibodies specific to B cell or T cell antigens, ALL was divided into B-ALL and T-ALL. Immunophenotyping and cytogenetic studies further classified ALL into early pre-B-ALL, pre-B-ALL, B-ALL, and T-ALL. Children with the following characteristics generally have a poor outcome and are considered as high risk:

1. High initial white blood cell count greater than 50,000 per μL
2. Age at diagnosis 1 year or less or greater than 10 years
3. Hypoploidy or pseudodiploidy
4. Chromosomal abnormalities: t(1;19), t(8;14), t(5;11), t(9;22)
5. DNA index 1.16 or less
6. p53 or Philadelphia expression on leukemic cells

TABLE 2. **Acute Leukemia in Children: Differential Diagnosis**

Marrow infiltrative process from other malignant diseases
    (neuroblastoma, non-Hodgkin's lymphoma, Ewing's sarcoma,
    retinoblastoma, rhabdomyosarcoma)
Epstein-Barr virus or other viral infections
Pertussis
Acute infectious lymphocytosis
Cat-scratch disease
Henoch-Schönlein purpura
Idiopathic or immune thrombocytopenic purpura
Neutropenia
Congenital or acquired aplastic anemia
Juvenile rheumatoid arthritis

TABLE 3. **Diagnostic Work-Up for Acute Leukemia in Children**

Complete blood counts with differential and reticulocyte count
Coagulation studies for evidence of disseminated intravascular
    coagulation
Urinalysis
Chemistry panel, including serum electrolytes, creatinine,
    alanine aminotransferase calcium, phosphorus, uric acid, and
    lactate dehydrogenase
IgG, IgA, and IgM determinations
Chest x-ray for hilar adenopathy and mediastinal mass
Bone marrow aspiration for histochemistry and other specialized
    studies, as noted below:
    Immunophenotype using a standardized panel of monoclonal
        antibodies for classification
    Karyotype for chromosomal abnormalities
    Flow cytometry for DNA index
Lumbar puncture for identification of blasts
HLA typing for possible identification of a bone marrow donor

Treatment

Newly Diagnosed Patients

Induction. Nearly all children with cancer are treated on protocols in conjunction with one of the programs approved by the Pediatric Oncology Group (POG) or Children's Cancer Group (CCG). As the work-up continues, the patient is observed for metabolic complications of leukemic cell breakdown and renal impairment secondary to hyperuricemia. Prophylaxis with allopurinol (Xyloprim) and hydration with intravenous bicarbonate are administered. After the diagnosis is established, vincristine (Oncovin), prednisone, and L-asparaginase (Elspar) are given by a standard protocol over 4 weeks. Daunorubicin (Cerubidine) may be added for patients considered to be at higher risk for relapse. This combination produces a complete remission in over 90% of patients. Patients who require more than 4 weeks to achieve remission or fail to show significant response to therapy by the end of 1 or 2 weeks of induction are at higher risk for relapse and may require a change in therapy.

Consolidation. Even though normal hematopoiesis is re-established and leukemic cells are not evident to even the most sensitive techniques for detecting blasts in the peripheral blood or bone marrow, experience has shown that more therapy is needed to prevent relapse in the bone marrow or in other so-called sanctuary sites within the brain, testicles, or lymphoid tissues. The best method for eliminating the last few logs of leukemic cells is not known but is under intense study. Following are some of the approaches used:

STANDARD-RISK ALL. For children who appear to be at a lower risk for relapse (standard risk), one approach is to give methotrexate (MTX) in moderately large doses intravenously, followed by 6-mercaptopurine (6-MP; Purinethol) intravenously,* alternating every other week with daily oral 6-MP, plus

____

*Intravenous form available only from the National Cancer Institute for patients on clinical protocols.

weekly intramuscular injections of MTX for 6 months.

HIGH-RISK ALL. Several groups of patients have a risk for relapse exceeding 50% (see the earlier list). They are best treated with more aggressive chemotherapy during this period, but the best approach is not known. Using a rationale based on previous experience, one approach is to give intense pulses of drugs that may include teniposide (Vumon), doxorubicin (Rubex), cytosine arabinoside (cytarabine), and cyclophosphamide (Cytoxan) for 6 to 8 months.

Maintenance. Most treatment programs employ the combination of daily oral 6-MP and weekly intramuscular injection of MTX with or without pulses of vincristine and prednisone for about 3 years.

Central Nervous System Prophylaxis. Without preventive measures, 60 to 70% of children with ALL eventually develop central nervous system (CNS) leukemia. Intrathecal MTX alone or in combination with cytosine arabinoside and hydrocortisone is administered to children with standard-risk ALL during induction and consolidation phases and periodically throughout the maintenance phase. Cranial irradiation may be added in children with high-risk ALL. To eliminate the neurotoxicity that is associated with cranial irradiation, high-dose systemic MTX and cytosine arabinoside plus intrathecal therapy without cranial irradiation is currently under clinical evaluation.

Relapsed Patients

Bone Marrow Relapse. After achieving complete remission, 70% of children enjoy long-term disease-free survival. Most appear to be cured of their disease, and over the last 30 years, many have grown up with no evident residua of their disease, married, and had children of their own. But for the 30% of children who relapse in the first years of therapy, much work remains to find an effective cure. Some features have emerged. Those children who have a long first remission and relapse more than a year after discontinuation of therapy appear to have a long second remission as well. Some appear to be cured with chemotherapy alone. However, if the relapse occurs either during therapy or within a year of discontinuation of initial therapy, the prognosis for long-term survival is poor, with less than a 5% chance for survival. An aggressive approach such as allogeneic bone marrow transplantation for those with a human leukocyte antigen (HLA)–matched donor raises the probability of long-term remission compared with chemotherapy alone.

CNS Relapse. On current treatment programs, the incidence of isolated CNS relapse in children with ALL is probably less than 10%. The treatment for CNS relapse usually involves repeated courses of intrathecal medications and more systemic chemotherapy to prevent seeding of leukemic cells to marrow and other sanctuary sites, with or without cranial irradiation. Unfavorable prognostic factors for survival after isolated CNS relapse include high white blood cell count at diagnosis, short duration of first remission, male sex, and prior cranial irradiation. For standard-risk children who have not received cranial irradiation as part of their CNS prophylaxis, more than half can be salvaged with intensified chemotherapy and cranial irradiation.

Testicular Relapse. The testes are sanctuary sites for leukemic cells. Isolated testicular relapse occurs in 7 to 33% of boys. Monthly pulses of vincristine and prednisone reduce the frequency of testicular relapse and confer some advantage in long-term disease-free survival. The treatment for testicular relapse includes systemic chemotherapy and CNS prophylaxis plus testicular irradiation.

ACUTE MYELOGENOUS LEUKEMIA

The presenting symptoms and diagnostic work-up for children with acute myelogenous leukemia (AML) are similar to those for children with ALL. However, treatment strategies that cure children with ALL are ineffective in AML, and overall cure rates using chemotherapy alone are low.

Treatment

Newly Diagnosed Patients

Induction. Complete remissions can be induced in 70 to 80% of patients with combinations that include an anthracycline such as doxorubicin and high doses of cytosine arabinoside. Vincristine and prednisone and other drugs such as epipodophyllotoxins may be added to these agents. Unlike the initial therapy in ALL, induction in AML is usually associated with protracted periods of severe bone marrow hypoplasia, and the risk for complications is very high.

Intensification. Employing the same drugs as in the induction therapy, but in a slightly different dosage and schedule, for up to a year may be useful. Long-term remission rates of 40 to 50% appear to be realistic for some types of AML. Many treatment programs now transplant patients who have an HLA-compatible sibling.

Maintenance. There is no evidence that maintenance approaches such as those used for ALL improve survival.

Relapsed Patients

Bone Marrow Relapse. Those children who have HLA-compatible siblings but have not received bone marrow transplants are often transplanted at this stage. A cure rate of 50 to 60% can be expected. Children without HLA-compatible donors can be treated with autologous bone marrow transplantation. The cure rate may be as high as 35%. There is still considerable controversy over whether autologous bone marrow transplantation is superior to aggressive chemotherapy. Several large, prospective, randomized trials are under way to resolve this issue.

CNS Relapse. Although it was not initially obvious because of the short survival of children with AML, it is now evident that 10 to 30% of children with AML who do not receive CNS prophylaxis develop CNS relapse. However, it has not been demonstrated that CNS prophylaxis improves disease-free survival.

LONG-TERM SEQUELAE

Some therapies used in the treatment of childhood leukemia may result in complications years later. Depending on the age at which it was administered, children who received cranial or craniospinal irradiation may suffer lower IQ, reduced height, and primary germ cell dysfunction. Second neoplasms (CNS tumors in those who have received cranial radiation, or AML and lymphomas) may occur, and in some instances, these are attributed to the mutagenicity of the therapy itself. The cumulative incidence of second cancers appears to be no more than 10% and is probably a good deal less. Higher stress reaction scores, lower well-being scores, and emotional deficit may also become evident in these young adults. Other treatment-related complications include cardiac dysfunction caused by anthracyclines and pituitary dysfunction caused by cranial irradiation.

In an attempt to minimize the treatment-related late effects, the treatments for childhood ALL are now risk based, so that standard-risk patients will be spared the intensive and potentially more toxic therapy, and high-risk patients will receive more aggressive treatment to improve their chances for cure. It is important to emphasize, however, that any evaluation of the late effects of therapy for a potentially life-threatening disease must be balanced by an understanding of the consequences of inadequate treatment.

FUTURE CONSIDERATIONS

Despite enormous advances in the treatment of childhood leukemias, there is room for improvement in the following areas:

1. Greater biologic understanding of the disease, with further delineation of the genetic lesions that cause uncontrolled growth.
2. More effective therapy for high-risk and relapsed patients.
3. Better understanding of why treatment can fail even in low-risk patients.
4. Sensitive methods for detecting residual disease.
5. Better strategies to minimize adverse sequelae without compromising therapeutic efficacy. Hematopoietic growth factors such as granulocyte colony-stimulating factor (filgrastim [Neupogen]), is an example of an agent that appears to shorten the period of severe neutropenia in some patients undergoing intensive chemotherapy.

CHRONIC LEUKEMIAS

method of
VICKI A. MORRISON, M.D.
University of Minnesota and Veterans Affairs
  Medical Center
Minneapolis, Minnesota

The chronic leukemias are a spectrum of diseases with diverse clinical manifestations and approaches to therapy. Significant advances have recently been made in the biology of these disorders. In addition, the therapeutic role of biologic response modifiers, nucleoside analogues, monoclonal antibodies, and bone marrow transplantation (BMT) is being defined. The pathologic features, clinical characteristics, and therapy of chronic lymphocytic leukemia, chronic myeloid leukemia, hairy cell leukemia, prolymphocytic leukemia, and large granular lymphocytic leukemia will be summarized.

CHRONIC LYMPHOCYTIC LEUKEMIA

Chronic lymphocytic leukemia (CLL) accounts for 30% of leukemias diagnosed in the United States, but less than 5% in the Eastern Hemisphere. Although T-CLL predominates in Asia, over 95% of American cases are B-CLL. The incidence of CLL is age dependent, being greatest in patients over 60 years of age. The cause of CLL is unknown.

Pathologic Features

The surface immunoglobulin (Ig) most commonly expressed in B-CLL is IgM; either kappa or lambda light chains may be present. By definition the cells are CD5 positive, but they also express such other B cell antigens as CD19, CD20, CD21, CD23, and CD24; T cell associated antigens are not expressed. Rearrangements of Ig heavy and light chains are present. Approximately 50% of patients will have chromosomal abnormalities, of which trisomy 12 is the most common.

Clinical Characteristics

Clinical Presentation. The median age at diagnosis is 65 years; the disease is twice as common in men as in women. The diagnosis may be incidental, with up to 60% of patients having no systemic complaints. The remainder have nonspecific symptoms like fatigue and malaise. Physical examination may be normal or reveal varying degrees of lymphadenopathy, hepatomegaly, and splenomegaly. Even if initially absent, lymphadenopathy and splenomegaly will later occur in most patients. Patients with advanced-stage disease may present with symptoms and signs referable to anemia, lymphadenopathy, and infection.

Diagnosis and Staging. The present diagnostic criteria for CLL were established in the late 1980s

(Table 1). Both the Rai and Binet staging systems have been used. Problems with these systems are that intermediate-risk patients are heterogeneous, immune thrombocytopenia is not distinguished from thrombocytopenia related to bone marrow infiltration, and low-risk patients are not differentiated into those with stable (versus progressive) disease.

Complications. A variety of complications may occur in the disease course, caused by associated immune problems and disease evolution. Hypogammaglobulinemia occurs in over 50% of patients, is more common in advanced-stage disease, and is not reversed by therapy. Whereas an acquired autoimmune hemolytic anemia occurs in 10% to 25% of patients, immune thrombocytopenia or granulocytopenia occurs in less than 10%. Pure red cell aplasia is rare.

Infections complicate the course of more than 75% of patients. The majority are caused by such common bacteria as *Streptococcus pneumoniae, Staphylococcus aureus*, and various gram-negative organisms. The respiratory tract is the most frequent site of involvement. A new spectrum of infections emerging in patients treated with fludarabine, pentostatin, or 2-chlorodeoxyadenosine includes *Pneumocystis, Listeria,* and *Nocardia* infections, in addition to disseminated *Candida, Aspergillus*, herpesvirus, and cytomegalovirus infections. Intravenous Ig (400 mg per kg every 3 weeks) has been used in patients with a low IgG or a history of at least one major bacterial infection. Although this decreases moderately severe bacterial infections by 50%, the incidence of minor infections is unchanged, therapy is costly, and, importantly, survival is not prolonged. Lower doses (250 mg per kg) may be as effective as higher doses.

Several forms of disease transformation may occur. The evolution of CLL to a large cell lymphoma, or Richter's syndrome, occurs in 3% to 10% of patients. Patients present with fever, weight loss, bulky disease, and extranodal involvement. Response to cytotoxic therapy is uncommon, and mean survival after transformation is 4 months. A clonal transformation of CLL to prolymphocytic leukemia is less common, occurring in 5% to 10% of cases. This transformation is gradual, manifested by progressive anemia, thrombocytopenia, lymphadenopathy, splenomegaly, and resistance to therapy. Lastly, acute leukemia occurs in less than 2% of patients; most cases are acute lymphoblastic leukemia.

Prognosis. The most important prognostic factors are the lymphocyte doubling time (LDT) and the pattern of bone marrow infiltration. Patients with a short LDT (less than 12 months) have a significantly shorter survival than those with an LDT of greater than 12 months. Likewise, patients with a diffuse pattern of bone marrow involvement tend to have a shorter survival than those with nondiffuse (nodular, interstitial, or mixed) patterns of involvement. Response to therapy is also associated with prolonged survival.

Therapy and Outcome

Despite treatment advances, there is no curative therapy for CLL. Median survival is 4 to 6 years, with death due to disease progression with infectious or hemorrhagic complications.

Approach to Patients with Low-Risk Disease (Rai Stage 0, Binet Stage A). As the median survival of these patients is more than 10 years, no cytotoxic therapy is recommended unless they have a progressive clinical course with a short LDT or diffuse bone marrow infiltration.

Approach to Patients with Intermediate-Risk Disease (Rai Stages I/II, Binet Stage B). Median survival of these patients is 8 years. Although progressive systemic symptoms, anemia and/or thrombocytopenia, autoimmune cytopenia(s), massive splenomegaly, bulky lymphadenopathy, and increased frequency of infections have been used as indications for therapy, no clear data support this.

Chlorambucil (Leukeran) is commonly used in two-dose schedules. An initial daily dose of 3 to 4 mg per m^2 orally until a response is seen, followed by 1 to 2 mg per m^2 daily may be used. An alternative scheme is 30 mg per m^2 orally every 2 weeks. The most common toxicity is myelosuppression, which may be dose-limiting and prolonged. Although the duration of therapy is not well defined, treatment is usually continued for as long as the patient responds. Responses are common, but most are partial responses. This therapy delays disease progression but does not prolong survival. The addition of prednisone to chlorambucil results in a higher response rate but no significant increase in survival. Results with multiagent chemotherapy, such as CVP (cyclophosphamide [Cytoxan], vincristine [Oncovin], prednisone) or CHOP (cyclophosphamide, doxorubicin [Adriamycin], vincristine, prednisone), are not better than the single agent chlorambucil.

Prednisone, in a daily oral dose of 30 to 100 mg, is

TABLE 1. **Minimum Requirements for the Diagnosis of Chronic Lymphocytic Leukemia**

Absolute peripheral blood lymphocytosis with mature lymphocytes, sustained for ≥ 4 wk, with no other identifiable cause
    Absolute lymphocyte count (ALC) > 10 × 10^9/L with either marrow involvement or a B cell phenotype

    OR

    ALC > 5.0 × 10^9/L with *both* marrow involvement and a B cell phenotype
Hypercellular or normocellular bone marrow with ≥ 30% mature lymphocytes
Peripheral blood lymphocyte phenotype:
    B cell lineage with expression of low-density surface Ig with either κ or λ light chain
    CD5+, CD2−, CD3−
    Rosette formation with mouse RBCs
Mature lymphocytes with < 55% atypical mature or immature lymphoid cells

Criteria devised by the National Cancer Institute–Sponsored Working Group for CLL and the International Workshop on CLL. CA Cancer J Clin 44:353–377, 1994.

used for autoimmune complications such as hemolytic anemia. This will also lead to a rapid decrease in bulky lymphadenopathy and hepatosplenomegaly. If no response is seen after 1 to 2 weeks, cyclophosphamide, high-dose Ig, cyclosporine, splenectomy, or splenic radiation are other treatment options.

Approach to Therapy of High-Risk Patients (Rai Stage III/IV, Binet Stage C). As the median survival of these patients is 1.5 years, therapy is commonly instituted. In a multicenter study, treatment with monthly chlorambucil and prednisone resulted in the highest response rate (47%), compared with daily chlorambucil and prednisone (38%), or prednisone alone (11%). However, no survival differences were seen. The CVP regimen offers no advantage over chlorambucil and prednisone with regard to response and survival.

A variety of approaches may be used for second-line therapy, including multidrug regimens, such as CVP and CHOP, or the new adenosine analogues (see later). Splenic or involved field radiation may palliate splenomegaly or bulky lymphadenopathy. Splenectomy is reserved for patients with massive splenomegaly or immune cytopenias.

Newer Approaches to Therapy

Fludarabine (Fludara). This adenine nucleoside analogue is the preferred second-line treatment for CLL; ongoing trials will determine whether it will supplant present first-line therapy. The most commonly used dose is 25 mg per m² intravenously daily for 5 days, with cycles repeated every 4 weeks. Response rates are up to 60% in previously treated patients, with a median remission duration of 21 months. In previously untreated patients, response rates are up to 80%, with a median remission duration of 33 months. Myelosuppression is the dose-limiting toxicity. Other complications include infection, especially pneumonia and fever of unclear origin, minor neurologic toxicities, a decline in lymphocyte subpopulations, and, rarely, tumor lysis.

Fludarabine has been used in combination with such agents as cyclophosphamide, doxorubicin, cytosine arabinoside, chlorambucil, and cisplatin; no improvement in the response rate over single-agent fludarabine has been seen. Longer follow-up will be needed to evaluate survival. The addition of prednisone does not alter the response rate but increases the risk of infectious complications.

2-Chlorodeoxyadenosine (2-CdA). This agent (cladribine [Leustatin]), used in an every-4-week dose of 0.1 mg per kg per day for 7 days by continuous infusion, has resulted in response rates of up to 55% in patients with relapsed or refractory disease and up to 85% in previously untreated patients. However, in preliminary results from fludarabine-refractory patients, the response rate is lower, and thrombocytopenia and anemia are rarely corrected. The combination of 2-CdA and chlorambucil is being studied. Myelosuppression, with fever and/or infection, is

a common toxicity. Tumor lysis has also been reported.

Pentostatin (Nipent). Pentostatin (2′-deoxycoformycin [DCF]), an adenosine deaminase inhibitor, when given in a dose of 4 mg per m² intravenously every 2 to 3 weeks in previously treated patients, has resulted in response rates of 20 to 30%. Toxicities include myelosuppression, nausea, rash, and stomatitis. An increased incidence of opportunistic infections, especially with herpesvirus, *Candida*, and *Pneumocystis*, has been seen.

Biologic Response Modifiers. Interferon-alfa* (2a or 2b) is not effective in advanced-stage patients; however, a decrease in the lymphocyte count, splenomegaly, and lymphadenopathy may occur in previously untreated patients with early-stage disease, when used in a dose of 1.5 to 3 million U per m² subcutaneously, three times per week. This agent and interleukin-2 may have a role as a component of combination regimens.

Monoclonal Antibodies. Anti-CD5 monoclonal† and anti-idiotype antibodies,† along with CAM-PATH-1H,† an antibody to a lymphocyte antigen, have been studied in CLL patients. Their use for minimal residual disease after primary therapy may warrant further study.

Bone Marrow Transplantation. Both allogeneic and autologous BMT have been utilized for highly selected young patients who have advanced-stage disease or poor risk factors at diagnosis. Although engraftment generally occurs, the durability of the response and the impact on survival need further evaluation with longer periods of follow-up.

PROLYMPHOCYTIC LEUKEMIA

Prolymphocytic leukemia (PLL) may occur de novo or as a terminal transformation of CLL. The incidence of PLL is 10% that of CLL.

Pathologic Features

Prolymphocytes are large cells (10 to 15 μm) having a round nucleus with condensed chromatin, a large vesicular nucleolus, and abundant pale blue cytoplasm. The majority (80%) of cases are B cell, with high-density surface Ig (usually IgM). Heavy and light chain Ig gene rearrangements are present. The cells are CD10, CD20, CD21, CD22, and HLA-DR positive; terminal deoxynucleotidyl transferase (TdT) is negative. The remaining 20% of cases are T cell, with 75% CD4 positive and 25% CD8 positive. No surface Ig is present. The cells are CD2, CD3, CD5, and CD7 positive; TdT and HLA-DR are negative. Reticuloendothelial organs typically involved include the spleen and the bone marrow (in a nodular or diffuse pattern).

Cytogenetic abnormalities include abnormalities of chromosome 14 and translocations involving chromo-

---

*Not FDA-approved for this indication.
†Investigational drug in the United States.

somes 6 and 12 in B-PLL, and inv(14)(q11;q32) in T-PLL. The presence of trisomy 12 with either 14q+ or t(6;12) suggests a case of CLL with prolymphocytic transformation.

Clinical Characteristics

The median age at diagnosis is 70 years, with a slight male predominance. Patients present with weakness, fatigue, weight loss, fever, and splenic pain. Splenomegaly, often massive, is present in 70% of cases; hepatomegaly is minimal. Lymphadenopathy is minimal to absent in B-PLL but present in 67% of T-PLL patients. Although uncommon in B-PLL, cutaneous involvement occurs in 30% of T-PLL patients. Hyperleukocytosis (white blood cell count greater than 100×10^9/L) occurs in 75% or more of cases; mean WBC is 355×10^9/L, and most circulating cells are prolymphocytes. Anemia and thrombocytopenia are common.

Three subgroups of prolymphocytic transformation of CLL have been described. Patients with a stable count of 10% or less prolymphocytes are classified as CLL. In the second group, classified as CLL/PLL, prolymphocytes range from 11% to 55%. The presence of more than 55% prolymphocytes defines a case as PLL.

Therapy and Outcome

Patients with PLL are typically refractory to therapy and have progressive disease with short survival. Median survival is 3 years; it is shorter in T-PLL than in B-PLL patients.

Combination chemotherapy should be considered in younger patients with a good performance status. Alkylators, with or without vincristine and prednisone, result in response rates of 20%; occasional responses may occur with CHOP. L-Asparaginase (Elspar), interferon-alfa, and CAMPATH-1H* (a monoclonal antibody) have also been used. Response rates with fludarabine are up to 35%. A 48% response rate, with a median remission duration of 9 months, was seen in a series of T-PLL patients treated with pentostatin. In older patients with a poor performance status, one may consider splenic radiation, splenectomy, or leukapheresis.

LARGE GRANULAR LYMPHOCYTIC LEUKEMIA

Large granular lymphocytic leukemia (LGLL) was first described in 1977. This T cell disorder has also been called T suppressor cell CLL, T cell lymphocytosis with neutropenia, chronic T γ lymphocytosis syndrome, T8 hyperlymphocytosis, and granular lymphocyte proliferative disorder.

Pathologic Features

Large granular lymphocytes, which comprise 10% to 15% of normal circulating mononuclear cells, ac-

*Investigational drug in the United States.

count for most natural killer (NK) cell activity. These large cells have a high nuclear to cytoplasmic ratio, condensed nuclear chromatin, and coarse azurophilic cytoplasmic granules. They are negative for esterase, TdT, and myeloperoxidase. The cells express pan-T cell antigens; CD2 is positive in 50% of cases, and CD3 in 80%. The cells are commonly CD8 and CD56 (NK-associated antigen) positive, but usually CD4 and CD5 negative. A classification scheme with four subtypes has been recently proposed. Two subtypes are CD3 positive and are separated by CD16 expression and whether a rearranged or germ-line configuration in the T cell receptor beta-gene is present. The other two subtypes are CD3 negative and are divided by CD57 expression; those who are CD57 positive have indolent disease, whereas CD57 negative patients have aggressive disease.

Clinical Characteristics

The median age of patients is 60 years; sex distribution is equal. The majority of cases occur in whites. Presenting complaints include fever and fatigue; 25% are asymptomatic at diagnosis. Mild-to-moderate splenomegaly is present in 50% or greater of patients. Only 20% will have hepatomegaly; lymphadenopathy occurs in less than 10%. In contrast to other T cell disorders, skin infiltration is rare. The clinical course is commonly complicated by recurrent bacterial infections, especially of the skin, sinuses, and perirectal area, and autoimmune phenomena.

This diagnosis should be suspected in any patient with a T cell lymphocytosis over 5.0×10^9/L of several months' duration with no apparent cause. Median lymphocyte count is 5.0×10^9/L, with most being large granular lymphocytes. Neutropenia, which can be cyclic, is present in most cases. Although anemia is common, thrombocytopenia occurs in less than 10%. Marrow lymphocytosis ranges from 30% to 75%, with nonparatrabecular lymphoid infiltrates in a nodular, diffuse, or interstitial pattern.

Therapy and Outcome

In contrast to most chronic lymphoproliferative disorders, therapy is usually not necessary for patients with LGLL, as the majority of patients have a benign clinical course with long survival and do not require cytotoxic therapy. Indications for treatment include severe neutropenia or anemia, tissue infiltration, marked organomegaly, or marked lymphocytosis. Various therapeutic approaches utilized for patients with disease progression include chemotherapy with single-agent alkylators, steroids, pentostatin, and such regimens as CVP, splenectomy, splenic irradiation, and cyclosporine (Sandimmune).

HAIRY CELL LEUKEMIA

Hairy cell leukemia (HCL), which was first described in 1958, accounts for 1% to 2% of adult leukemias. There are no known predisposing toxic or occupational exposures; rare cases are associated with human T cell lymphotropic virus (HTLV)-II infection.

Pathologic Features

The hairy cell has an indented, eccentric nucleus with characteristic cytoplasmic projections. These cells are usually tartrate-resistant, acid phosphatase (TRAP) positive, and negative for peroxidase and chloracetate esterase. Hairy cells must be present in the bone marrow for diagnosis. The marrow, which cannot be aspirated in over 50% of cases, is normo- to hypercellular, with hairy cells and increased reticulin present. Other sites of involvement are the spleen, liver, and lymph nodes.

The hairy cell is a B cell in mid- to late-stage differentiation. It is usually positive for CD19, CD20, HLA-DR, CD22, CD25, CD45 RA, and PCA-1, and negative for CD21 and pan-T cell markers. The most common cytogenetic abnormalities involve chromosome 14.

Clinical Characteristics

The median age of HCL patients is the early 50s; a male predominance (3 to 5:1) exists. Presenting symptoms include fatigue and splenic pain; weight loss, fever, and night sweats are uncommon. A minority of patients are asymptomatic. Splenomegaly, often massive, is present in 70% to 90%; hepatomegaly and shotty lymphadenopathy are less common.

Pancytopenia, present in 50% of cases at diagnosis, is multifactorial, related to hypersplenism, marrow insufficiency, growth factor deficiency, circulating hematopoietic inhibitors, and abnormal hematopoietic stem cells. From 15% to 20% of patients will be leukemic, with a WBC count of greater than 10.0×10^9/L and more than 50% hairy cells.

Infection, related to defects in cell-mediated immunity, monocytopenia, and granulocytopenia, occurs in more than 67% of patients and is the major cause of death. Bacteremia and pneumonia are most common, often caused by enteric gram-negative organisms or atypical mycobacteria. Less common complications include an autoimmune syndrome, lytic bone lesions, and splenic rupture. An increased incidence of second malignancies, both hematopoietic and solid tumor, has been reported.

Therapy and Outcome

Hairy cell leukemia is a chronic disease for which there is no curative treatment. Median survival in untreated patients is more than 5 years. The majority of patients will require therapy at some time in their disease course. Indications for therapy include a hemoglobin level of 10 grams per dL or less, a neutrophil count of 1.0×10^9/L or less, a platelet count of 100×10^9/L or less, leukemic phase, symptomatic splenomegaly, bulky lymphadenopathy, recurrent or serious infections, bone involvement, autoimmune syndrome, and tissue infiltration.

Splenectomy. Splenectomy will lead to improvement in at least one cell line in 90% of patients. The platelet count can normalize within days, whereas anemia and neutropenia resolve in weeks to months. Patients with bone marrow cellularity of less than 85% and platelet counts greater than 60×10^9/L derive the greatest benefit from splenectomy. However, 50% of patients will relapse at a median of 1.5 years postsplenectomy, whereas the remaining 50% develop bone marrow failure.

Interferon. The mechanism of action of interferon in HCL is not clear, but it may have a direct antiproliferative effect or an immunomodulatory effect, or it may promote differentiation of pluripotent stem cells. The two regimens most commonly used are recombinant interferon-alfa-2b (Intron A), 2 million U per m² subcutaneously three times per week for 12 months, or recombinant interferon-alfa-2a (Roferon-A), 3 million U per day subcutaneously for 6 months, followed by three times per week for 6 months. Although most patients will have normalization of peripheral blood counts, less than 5% will have a complete bone marrow remission. Blood counts commonly decline in the first month of therapy, then improve. The platelet count will normalize over 2 months and the red cells and granulocytes over 3 to 5 months. Circulating hairy cells decrease within a month. Improvement in the bone marrow occurs over 6 to 9 months, with a decrease in hairy cells but no impact on reticulin fibrosis. Splenomegaly improves over 2 months. Approximately 5% of patients will develop neutralizing antibodies to interferon.

Treatment for longer than a year does not improve outcome, nor does subsequent splenectomy affect progression-free survival. Once interferon is stopped, bone marrow involvement progresses more rapidly than do peripheral blood findings. The median time to failure is 18 to 25 months. However, reinstitution of interferon results in responses in up to 77% of patients.

Common toxicities include mild-to-moderate, reversible myelosuppression. A self-limited flulike syndrome is common early in therapy. Fatigue, anorexia, nausea, and paresthesias may also occur.

Pentostatin (Nipent). Pentostatin (2'-deoxycoformycin, DCF), an adenosine deaminase inhibitor, is most commonly used in a dose of 2 to 4 mg per m² per day intravenously over 1 to 2 minutes, given every 2 weeks. Prehydration is necessary to ensure adequate urine output. The average duration of therapy is 6 months; treatment is usually continued for one to two cycles after a complete remission (CR) is attained. The response rate is more than 95% (60% to 90% CR). Circulating hairy cells will decrease in 1 to 2 days, with improvement in the platelet count in 1 to 2 weeks, the neutrophil count and hemoglobin over 2 to 8 weeks, and the bone marrow in 2 to 6 months. However, by molecular diagnostic techniques, patients in a morphologic complete remission may have residual bone marrow hairy cells. A more rapid hematologic response is seen than with interferon, with a median time to CR of 4 to 5 months.

Relapses are infrequent and usually manifest solely in the bone marrow.

In a recent randomized comparison of DCF and interferon-alfa in previously untreated HCL patients, response rates were significantly higher with DCF than with interferon-alfa (79% versus 38%). In addition, relapse-free survival was significantly longer with DCF therapy. However, myelosuppression was more common with DCF.

Pentostatin is also effective in patients who have failed interferon therapy, with response rates of up to 84%. In splenectomized patients, DCF and interferon result in similar response rates, but remissions occur more quickly and last longer in patients receiving DCF.

Fever and infection, related to drug-induced lymphopenia that may persist for over a year after treatment, occur in 15% to 40% of patients. Other toxicities include nausea, vomiting, diarrhea, lethargy, conjunctivitis, and hepatitis; a reversible renal insufficiency is rare.

2-Chlorodeoxyadenosine (2-CdA) (Cladribine [Leustatin]). This nucleoside analogue, when administered in a dose of 2 to 8 mg per m^2 per day by continuous infusion over a 7-day period, has resulted in CR rates of 78% to 92% with a prolonged remission duration, with only one to two cycles of therapy. In several reports, subcutaneous 2-CdA (3.4 mg per m^2 daily for 7 days) has resulted in similar response rates. Prior therapy with interferon, DCF, or splenectomy has no impact on outcome, implying a lack of cross-resistance between the two adenosine analogues (2-CdA and DCF). Toxicities include myalgias, nausea, rash, headache, and weakness. Culture-negative fever occurs in 40%, and documented infections in 20% of patients, related to persistent drug-induced lymphopenia.

Summary. With results of the recent trial comparing interferon with DCF as initial therapy, it appears that DCF has supplanted interferon as the treatment of choice in previously untreated HCL patients. Whereas a rapid response and high CR rate result from DCF, the long-term complications of lymphopenia need to be considered. Alternatively, interferon results in a high response rate, and in initial reports 2-CdA has significant activity with prolonged responses; however, prospective comparative trials will be needed to assess its efficacy and toxicities in comparison with DCF and interferon. Although splenectomy will transiently improve cytopenias and alleviate symptoms, it should be reserved for select patients, such as those with significant splenomegaly and minimal bone marrow involvement.

CHRONIC MYELOGENOUS LEUKEMIA

Chronic myelogenous leukemia (CML), a clonal disorder involving the pluripotent hematopoietic stem cell, accounts for 15% of all leukemias. Although its etiology is unknown, the disease has an increased incidence in people with radiation exposure.

Pathologic Features

The Philadelphia (Ph[1]) chromosome, present in more than 95% of CML cases, is found in cells of granulocytic, monocytic/macrophage, erythroid, megakaryocytic, eosinophilic, and basophilic lineage but is not in somatic cells, bone marrow fibroblasts, or T lymphocytes. It arises from a reciprocal translocation between the abl proto-oncogene located on chromosome 9 and the bcr gene on chromosome 22, resulting in a shortening of the long arm of chromosome 22, or t(9;22)(q34.1;q11.21). This translocation, detectable by fluorescent in situ hybridization, Southern blot, and polymerase chain reaction techniques, results in a chimeric bcr-abl gene that leads to the production of a protein with tyrosine kinase activity. The presence of this fusion gene may be a better diagnostic criterion for CML than the presence of the Ph[1] chromosome; it is present in some patients lacking the Ph[1] chromosome. Additional chromosome abnormalities appear in 80% of patients, evolving to the accelerated or blast phase. The Ph[1] chromosome is also found in cases of acute lymphoblastic (25% in adults, 10% in children) and adult acute myeloid (5%) leukemia.

Clinical Characteristics

The median age of patients is 50 years with a slight male predominance. The disease is divided into chronic, accelerated, and acute (blastic) phases. Median survival is 60 to 65 months, with a 3-year survival of 75% to 85% and a 5-year survival of 50% to 60%.

Chronic Phase. Most patients present with fatigue, headache, weight loss, splenic discomfort, and early satiety; 20% to 30% will be asymptomatic. Splenomegaly is common; hepatomegaly and lymphadenopathy are unusual. The duration of this phase is 3 years.

By definition, patients in the chronic phase have 20% or less immature myeloid cells in the peripheral blood and 30% or less in the bone marrow. The mean WBC count is 225×10^9/L, with less than 5% myeloblasts and an absolute basophilia. The platelet count is over 450×10^9/L in 50%, and over 1.0×10^{10}/L in 25% of patients; 10% will be thrombocytopenic. The bone marrow is hypercellular, with granulocytic and megakaryocytic hyperplasia; myeloblasts are normal to slightly increased in number; reticulin may be increased. Serum lactic dehydrogenase, uric acid, vitamin B_{12} and B_{12}-binding capacity are often elevated. Leukocyte alkaline phosphatase (LAP) is absent to low.

Patients lacking the Ph[1] chromosome may have slightly different clinical characteristics. The median age is 60 years, and splenomegaly is less prominent. The WBC count is 50 to 75 $\times 10^9$/L, and the median platelet count is 170 $\times 10^9$/L. Anemia and monocytosis are more common, whereas basophilia is uncommon. Extensive bone marrow fibrosis with increased myeloblasts may be present. In contrast to

Ph[1]-positive CML, the LAP is normal or increased. Median survival ranges only from 10 to 19 months. However, patients with the bcr-abl rearrangement have clinical features and a response to therapy similar to those of Ph[1]-positive patients.

Accelerated Phase. In most patients there is a gradual transition from the chronic to the acute phase called the accelerated phase, which is characterized by progressive systemic complaints, anemia, basophilia, quantitative platelet abnormalities, circulating myeloblasts (bone marrow or peripheral blasts 10% or greater), increased bone marrow reticulin fibrosis, splenomegaly, and resistance to therapy. This phase lasts from less than 1 to 1.5 years.

Acute or Blastic Phase. Although most patients undergo a gradual transition of their disease process over a median of 4 years, 20% to 25% will evolve directly from the chronic to blastic phase without an accelerated phase. There is a 25% likelihood of blastic conversion for each year of the chronic phase. This phase is defined as the presence of 30% or more circulating or bone marrow myeloblasts or extramedullary blastic infiltrates. Patients present with fever, night sweats, weight loss, splenic pain, bone pain, fatigue, easy bruisability, and hepatosplenomegaly. The WBC count is usually greater than 50×10^9/L, with anemia and thrombocytopenia. In contrast to the chronic phase, the LAP is normal to increased. The blast crisis is myeloid in 60% of cases and lymphoid in 20%. An undifferentiated acute leukemia occurs in 15%, while the remaining 5% have either a megakaryoblastic, erythroid, or progranulocytic blast crisis. Patients with extramedullary blastic transformation may manifest with lymphadenopathy, lytic bone lesions, cutaneous or soft tissue infiltrates, or epidural tumors with cord compression; these findings may precede bone marrow transformation by several months. Median survival in this phase is 2 to 4 months.

Therapy and Outcome

Therapy of Patients in the Chronic Phase. Busulfan and hydroxyurea may be used for chronic phase therapy, with response rates of 70% to 80% and median survival of 30 to 45 months, compared with 19 months in untreated patients. However, cytogenetic remissions are uncommon. The usual dose of busulfan (Myleran) for remission induction is 3 to 4 mg per m² per day orally until the WBC count decreases by 50%, followed by a daily oral dose of 1 to 2 mg per m². The drug should be discontinued when the WBC count is less than 20×10^9/L, as it has a protracted effect. This alkylator has its greatest effect on stem cells. Toxicities include severe myelosuppression (fatal in 5% to 10%), organ fibrosis (lung, heart, and bone marrow), hyperpigmentation, hypogonadism, and an addisonian-like wasting syndrome.

Hydroxyurea (Hydrea), an inhibitor of DNA synthesis that acts on late progenitor cells, is used more often than busulfan because of its better toxicity profile. An initial daily dose of 1 to 2 grams per m² orally will result in a fall in the WBC count within 2 days. For each 50% decline in WBC, the dose should be reduced by 50%, aiming for a target WBC count of 20 to 30×10^9/L. Side effects include a reversible myelosuppression and minor dermatologic changes.

Alternative therapeutic approaches have been utilized in these patients. Intensive combination chemotherapy does not significantly increase survival. Splenectomy or splenic radiation is reserved for patients with symptomatic splenomegaly unresponsive to chemotherapy, or anemia/thrombocytopenia related to hypersplenism. Leukapheresis is used for emergency leukostatic complications, or in pregnant females who are symptomatic.

INTERFERON-ALFA IN CHRONIC PHASE DISEASE. Interferon-alfa has a direct antiproliferative effect on the leukemic clone. Two recombinant products used are interferon-alfa-2a (Roferon-A) or interferon-alfa-2b (Intron A), in a daily subcutaneous or intramuscular dose of 5 million U per m². The dose should be reduced if the WBC count is less than 2×10^9/L or the platelet count is less than 60×10^9/L. A hematologic response occurs in 70% of patients at a median of 3.4 months; a complete or partial cytogenetic response occurs in 40%. A higher response rate is seen when therapy is started within a year of diagnosis. The duration of hematologic response may be up to 41 months, and is longer in patients who achieve a cytogenetic response. A significant survival benefit, with a median survival of 60 to 65 months, is seen with interferon, owing to prolongation of the chronic phase. Although interferon has been used concomitantly or sequentially with agents such as hydroxyurea, busulfan, cytosine arabinoside, 6-mercaptopurine, and interleukin-2,* the addition of these agents does not have a significant impact on the natural history of the disease.

In a recent trial, patients received induction therapy with cytotoxic agents and were then randomized to maintenance therapy with either interferon-alfa or chemotherapy (hydroxyurea or busulfan). The cytogenetic response was 30% in the interferon arm, compared with 5% in those treated with conventional agents. The time to progression to an accelerated/blastic phase and median survival were significantly prolonged in the interferon arm, whether or not a concomitant cytogenetic response occurred.

Early toxicities of interferon, such as fever, chills, malaise, myalgias, arthralgias, anorexia, fatigue, and headache, are common but usually resolve after 1 to 2 weeks of therapy. Toxicities with prolonged therapy include nausea, diarrhea, weight loss, insomnia, persistent fatigue, hair thinning, proteinuria, hepatitis, immune hemolysis, and hypothyroidism. Neurologic toxicities include a frontal lobe syndrome of apathy, memory and concentration problems, a parkinsonian syndrome, depression, and psychosis. These late side effects are dose-limiting in 10% to 25% of patients. Elderly patients tolerate therapy more poorly than younger patients.

---

*Investigational drug in the United States.

Interferon gamma-1b (Actimmune)* has modest activity in CML, with a hematologic response rate of 20% to 30%. Several trials examining the concomitant or sequential use of alfa and gamma interferon have yielded disappointing results.

BONE MARROW TRANSPLANTATION (BMT) IN CHRONIC PHASE DISEASE. Allogeneic BMT is the sole curative therapy for CML. The best outcome occurs in patients transplanted in the chronic (versus accelerated, second chronic, or acute/blastic) phase. The 5-year disease-free survival (DFS) for patients transplanted in the chronic phase is 50% to 60%, compared with 30% for those in accelerated phase, and 10% to 20% for those in acute phase. The corresponding relapse rates are less than 20%, 40%, and 60%, respectively. The most favorable outcome of BMT in chronic phase occurs in patients less than 30 years old who are transplanted within a year of diagnosis. Unrelated donor BMT and allogeneic BMT with mismatch at one locus are other options, but they have an increased risk of acute and chronic graft-versus-host disease (GVHD), graft failure, and early mortality, with a 2-year DFS of 30%. The best outcome is in young, chronic phase recipients in whom the donor and recipient are identical at the HLA-A, -B, and -DR loci. Graft-versus-leukemia effect, which is associated with the presence of chronic GVHD, is important in the prevention of relapse following BMT. With the use of T cell depletion, there is a decreased incidence of GVHD but an increased risk of graft failure and leukemic relapse.

Autologous BMT results in a high engraftment rate, low mortality, and a high rate of re-establishment of a second chronic phase of brief duration. Special treatment of the bone marrow, as in in vivo or in vitro purging with gamma interferon or chemotherapeutic agents, may be done prior to BMT. Other autologous BMT approaches involve the use of peripheral blood stem cells and CD34+/Dr− stem cells.

The optimal approach for patients relapsing after BMT is not clear. A second BMT is successful in 50% of patients but with a significant risk of peritransplant toxicities. Interferon may be used following BMT to reverse early cytogenetic relapse and results in responses in up to 30% of patients. Hydroxyurea may be used to palliate symptoms. Buffy coat infusions can result in a cytogenetic remission in some patients.

SUMMARY. Allogeneic BMT should be considered for patients with chronic phase disease who are less than 50 to 55 years old and have a matched sibling donor; the role of unrelated donor BMT is more controversial. For patients in whom BMT is not an option, interferon is tolerable, effective therapy, with the potential for cytogenetic remission and prolonged survival. Hydroxyurea and busulfan, while not resulting in cytogenetic remission, will control the blood counts, and they remain alternative therapeutic options.

---

*Not FDA-approved for this indication.

Therapy of Patients in the Acute (Blastic) Phase. The outcome for patients with acute phase disease is poor. Patients with a myeloid blast crisis can be treated with cytarabine (cytosine arabinoside, ara-C), either high dose or in combination with an anthracycline, resulting in a 20% to 30% response rate; however, responses are of short duration, and median survival is 2 to 12 months. Patients with a lymphoid blast crisis may be treated with vincristine and prednisone, with or without an anthracycline and cytarabine. Response rates are 40% to 70%, with a remission duration of 6 to 10 months and a median survival of 9 to 12 months. Lastly, hydroxyurea (Hydrea), in a dose of 2 to 4 grams per day, may be used for palliative management, with reduction in the WBC, platelet count, and spleen size. Interferon has minimal activity in the acute phase.

NON-HODGKIN'S LYMPHOMA

method of
PAULA MARLTON, M.B., B.S., and
FERNANDO CABANILLAS, M.D.
*University of Texas M. D. Anderson Cancer
Center*
Houston, Texas

Improvements in the therapy for non-Hodgkin's lymphoma (NHL) made over the last 20 years now promise cure for a substantial percentage of lymphoma patients and improved length and quality of life for others. Associated advances in our understanding of the biology of lymphoma afford further optimism for future therapeutic developments.

The lymphomas constitute a heterogeneous group of disorders: the incidence has been increasing for 2 decades. A large and sometimes confusing array of therapeutic approaches has evolved. Treatment decisions for individual patients are based on a number of criteria, the most fundamental of which are tumor histology and extent or stage of disease.

The importance of histology underlies the absolute necessity to perform an adequate diagnostic lymph node biopsy in all cases. Fine-needle aspiration is of value in establishing relapse and in occasional urgent cases when establishing a rapid diagnosis would require major surgery. Histologic classification attempts to identify separate entities with distinct prognoses and natural histories. It remains an imperfect and difficult science, often requiring the assistance of additional special studies on biopsy material, which may include immunophenotypic analysis, molecular studies, and cytogenetics. Several systems of classification have been devised, the most recent of which is the very comprehensive Revised European-American Classification of Lymphoid Neoplasms (REAL classification). This represents a significant advance over the Working Formulation (WF), the classification currently in use in America (Table 1). However, it awaits widespread acceptance and clinical validation. The WF has replaced the formerly popular Rappaport classification, which first identified two important favorable prognostic features: follicular architecture and predominance of small lymphocytes. In Europe, the Kiel classification has been widely accepted. It is based

TABLE 1. **Abbreviated Working Formulation in Lymphoma**

Low-Grade Lymphoma

Small lymphocytic (consistent with CLL)
Follicular small cleaved cell
Follicular mixed small cleaved and large cell

Intermediate-Grade Lymphoma

Follicular large cell
Diffuse small cleaved cell
Diffuse mixed small cleaved and large cell
Diffuse large cell

High-Grade Lymphoma

Immunoblastic
Lymphoblastic
Small noncleaved cell (Burkitt's and non-Burkitt's)

on the morphologic identification of the lymphoma cell of origin now updated to incorporate immunophenotypic data. The WF identifies low-, intermediate-, and high-grade lymphomas based on the correlation between histology and survival data. This provides a convenient clinical template on which to consider further the therapy of lymphoma and will be used here.

Staging is the process by which extent of disease is evaluated and is used to stratify patients to appropriate treatments. The most widely used staging system is the Ann Arbor system, which was originally developed for Hodgkin's disease (Table 2, *A*). The system is imperfect for NHL, providing, for example, little prognostic discrimination between stage III and stage IV diffuse large cell lymphoma. Attempts have been made to enhance this system by evaluating other patient parameters known to correlate with prognosis. At our hospital, the tumor score system has been developed that incorporates serum lactate dehydrogenase (LDH), beta$_2$ microglobulin (β_2M), tumor bulk, presence of B symptoms (fever, sweats, or weight

TABLE 2. **Staging of Lymphoma**

A.	**Ann Arbor Staging System**
I	One lymph node (LN) region
IE	One extranodal organ or site
II	Two or more LN regions on the same side of the diaphragm
IIE	Stage II plus one extranodal organ or site
III	LN regions on both sides of the diaphragm
IIIE	Stage III plus one extranodal organ or site
IIIS	Stage III plus spleen
IIISE	Stage IIIS plus one extranodal organ or site
IV	One or more extranodal organs with or without associated LN involvement (diffuse or disseminated) (H = liver, P = lung, M = bone marrow)

B.	**Tumor Score System**	
Parameter	*Adverse Feature*	
Ann Arbor stage	III-IV	
Symptoms	Presence of B symptoms	
Tumor bulk	Mass >7 cm or CXR-detectable mediastinal mass	
β_2M	>3.0	
LDH	>685	

Each adverse feature scores 1 point. Totals of 3 or greater define poor-risk patients.

Abbreviations: LN = lymph node; β_2M = beta$_2$ microglobulin; LDH = lactate dehydrogenase; CXR = chest radiograph.

loss), and Ann Arbor stage to define good and poor risk patients (Table 2, *B*). Other efforts to identify patient risk groups according to prognostic factors have culminated in the development of the International Index, which similarly examines five pretreatment parameters to stratify patients with clearly separable outcomes.

An initial staging work-up should be performed in all patients at diagnosis, which generally includes the procedures listed in Table 3. Restaging is required to assess disease response to therapy after two or three courses. Simple tests should be checked after every course. Other assessments specifically addressing potential drug toxicities may include nuclear cardiac scan, electrocardiogram, and lung diffusion capacity.

LOW-GRADE LYMPHOMA

Low-grade lymphoma (LGL) constitutes 30% to 40% of all lymphomas and includes small lymphocytic, follicular small cleaved cell (the most common subset), and follicular mixed small cleaved and large cell lymphomas. Newer entities recognized separately in the REAL classification include marginal zone lymphoma (encompassing the MALT [mucosa-associated lymphoid tissue] lymphomas). Biologically, the majority of these tumors are characterized by an indolent protracted course, recurrent late relapse, and a long median survival of 5 to 8 years.

Early stage disease, although uncommon, is potentially curable. For stage I and stage II patients, radiation therapy has been the mainstay. Involved field (IF) radiation in relatively small doses of 30 to 40 Gy will achieve long-term disease-free survival in at least 50% of patients with laparotomy-proved stages I and II low-bulk disease. Chemotherapy has more recently been evaluated in combination with IF radiation. CVP- and CHOP-based regimens (Table 4) similar to those employed in more advanced disease have been utilized with favorable results and are our recommended approach.

The therapy of advanced-stage disease has been greatly influenced by its apparent incurability coupled with its long natural history and median survival. Conservative approaches, including watchful waiting for asymptomatic patients or single-agent chemotherapy (Table 4), have been advocated in the past and are still useful in elderly patients. However,

TABLE 3. **Staging Work-up**

History of B symptoms: fever, sweats, weight loss
Detailed physical examination
Adequate node biopsy
Blood work: CBC, biochemical profile including LDH & β_2M, serum protein electrophoresis, ESR, HIV serology
Bone marrow aspirate & biopsy (bilateral in LGL)
Chest radiograph
CT chest, abdomen, and pelvis
Lymphangiogram (in some cases might be indicated)
Gallium scan
±Bone scan, GI work-up, CSF examination (when indicated)

Abbreviations: CBC = complete blood count; LDH = lactate dehydrogenase; β_2M = beta$_2$ microglobulin; ESR = erythrocyte sedimentation rate; HIV = human immunodeficiency virus; LGL = low-grade lymphoma; CT = computed tomography; GI = gastrointestinal; CSF = cerebrospinal fluid.

TABLE 4. **Chemotherapy in Low-Grade Lymphoma**

Single Agent

Chlorambucil (Leukeran)	10–15 mg/m²/d × 5 d PO q 21–28 d
	OR
	0.1–0.2 mg/kg/d for 4–6 wk
Cyclophosphamide (Cytoxan)	500–1000 mg/m² IV q 21–28 d
	OR
	60–100 mg/m² PO qd

Combinations

CVP:	
Cyclophosphamide (Cytoxan)	400 mg/m² PO d 1–5
Vincristine (Oncovin)	1.4 mg/m² IV d 1
Prednisone	100 mg PO d 1–5 (21-d cycle)
CHOP:	
Cyclophosphamide	750 mg/m² IV d 1
Doxorubicin (hydroxydaunomycin) (Adriamycin)	50 mg/m² IV d 1
Vincristine (Oncovin)	1.4 mg/m² IV d 1
Prednisone	100 mg PO d 1–5 (21–28 d cycle)

Salvage Regimen

NOPP:	
Mitoxantrone (Novantrone)	10 mg/m² IV d 1
Vincristine (Oncovin)	2 mg IV d 1
Procarbazine	100 mg/m² PO d 1–14
Prednisone	100 mg PO d 1–5

with the realization that most patients eventually die from their disease, and that a substantial percentage will transform to higher-grade histology and manifest therapy resistance, more aggressive treatments are justifiably being explored. These include chemotherapy combinations utilized in intermediate-grade disease (Table 4), which achieve complete remission in a shorter time, are less leukemogenic than long-term single agents, and may confer improved survival. Doxorubicin (Adriamycin)-containing regimens appear superior to non-doxorubicin-containing regimens, particularly for the follicular mixed-cell types. Other investigational approaches to LGL therapy include high-dose chemotherapy with autologous bone marrow transplant (ABMT) or peripheral blood stem cell transplant (PBSCT) and allogeneic bone marrow transplant (BMT) in young patients. This swing toward intensive therapy represents a major change in the philosophy of treating advanced-stage LGL, stimulated by the search for a curative strategy in a clearly chemotherapy-sensitive disorder. Current survival curves for low-grade and the more aggressive lymphomas ultimately cross as the slow but inexorable attrition of patients with LGL meets the plateau of cured patients with higher-grade disease. This is the justification for the ongoing investigation of high-risk approaches.

Biologic response modifiers are also under study in LGL. Alpha-interferon* (IFN-α) has activity in follicular small cleaved cell lymphoma, and we have

---

*Not FDA-approved for this indication.

found it prolongs remission duration when used as maintenance after standard chemotherapy. Patients with divergent histologies (intermediate grade in one site and low grade in another) may also benefit from IFN-α maintenance. Newer agents, including fludarabine (Fludara) and 2-chlorodeoxyadenosine (cladribine), show promising activity and will likely find a role in standard therapy. Experimental approaches utilizing targeted monoclonal antibodies conjugated with toxins or radioisotopes are also being studied.

Once undertaken, the treatment goal in LGL should be attainment of complete remission (CR) since patients with a lesser response have inferior survival. Watchful waiting prior to treatment may forfeit the best chance of achieving a durable CR and, although not yet proven to worsen survival, has been associated with poorer quality of life.

Relapsed LGL that has not transformed histologically may respond again to initially successful treatment. Active salvage regimens include cytarabine (Cytosar-U) and cisplatin (Platinol) combinations (e.g., ASAP: Table 5) and mitoxantrone (Novantrone)-based therapy (e.g., NOPP: see Table 4).

INTERMEDIATE-GRADE LYMPHOMA

Intermediate-grade lymphoma (IGL) includes follicular large cell, diffuse small cleaved cell, diffuse mixed, diffuse large cell lymphoma (the commonest subtype), and immunoblastic lymphoma (classified as high grade in the Working Formulation, but biologically intermediate-grade). Entities recognized separately in the REAL classification include large cell anaplastic lymphoma (Ki-1-positive) and mantle cell lymphoma, some variants of which share more characteristics with LGL. Achievement of cure for at least 50% of patients with the common subtypes of IGL (with the exception of mantle cell) is one of the great triumphs of modern chemotherapy.

Stage of disease again dictates appropriate therapy. True stage I disease is uncommon but when laparotomy-proved and of very low tumor bulk can be cured with extended field radiotherapy alone (70% 10-year disease-free survival). Stage II disease, however, requires systemic chemotherapy (30% 10-year disease-free survival with radiotherapy alone). Because of the limitations of clinical staging and the morbidity of definitive pathologic staging, it is therefore recommended that clinical stage I patients be treated with combination chemotherapy, knowing that many will have early dissemination of disease. We have found that three courses of CHOP (see Table 4) plus IF radiotherapy produce excellent results in stages I and II patients with very low tumor bulk. The cure rate achievable is as high as 80% to 90%. However, other prognostic indicators must be taken into consideration when planning treatment. For example, stage II patients with high levels of LDH and β_2M with large tumor bulk are poor candidates for this regimen and require more aggressive therapy.

Advanced-stage disease requires full-dose combination chemotherapy. Since the development of the

TABLE 5. **Chemotherapy for Intermediate-Grade Lymphomas**

First-Generation Regimens

CHOP (see Table 4)	
CHOP-Bleo:	
CHOP plus	
Bleomycin (Blenoxane)	10 U/m² IV d 1
OPEN:	
Etoposide (VePesid)	100 mg/m² IV d 1–3
Mitoxantrone (Novantrone)	10 mg/m² IV d 1
Vincristine (Oncovin)	1.4 mg/m² IV d 1
Prednisone	100 mg PO d 1–5

Second-Generation Regimens

M-BACOD: (Cycle: 21 d)	
Bleomycin	4 U/m² IV d 1
Doxorubicin (Adriamycin)	45 mg/m² IV d 1
Cyclophosphamide (Cytoxan)	600 mg/m² IV d 1
Vincristine (Oncovin)	1 mg/m² d 1
Dexamethasone (Decadron)	6 mg/m² PO d 1–5
Methotrexate	3 gm/m² IV d 14
Leucovorin (Wellcovorin)	10 mg/m² IV 24 h after methotrexate infusion, then 10 mg/m² PO q 6 h for 72 h

Third-Generation Regimens

MACOP-B:	
Methotrexate (MTX)	400 mg/m² IV wk 2, 6, and 10
Leucovorin	15 mg/m² PO q 6 h × 6 doses commencing 24 h after start of MTX
Doxorubicin	50 mg/m² IV wk 1, 3, 5, 7, 9, 11
Cyclophosphamide	350 mg/m² IV wk 1, 3, 5, 7, 9, 11
Vincristine	1.4 mg/m² IV wk 2, 4, 6, 8, 10, 12
Bleomycin	10 U/m² IV wk 4, 8, 12
Prednisone	75 mg/m²/d PO taper wk 11 and 12
ASAP—M-BACOS—MINE:	
ASAP [IdSHAP]*	
Doxorubicin	50 mg/m² over 48 h d 1–2
Methylprednisolone (Solu-Medrol)	500 mg/d IV d 1–5
Cytarabine (Cytosar-U)	1.5 gm/m² over 2 h after Platinol d 5
Cisplatin (Platinol)	100 mg/m² over 96 h d 1–4
M-BACOS [MBIdCOS]*	
Methotrexate	1 gm/m² IV d 2
Leucovorin rescue	
Bleomycin	10 U/m² d 1
Doxorubicin	50 mg/m² d 1 over 48 h
Cyclophosphamide	750 mg/m² IV d 1
Vincristine	1.4 mg/m² IV d 1
Methylprednisolone	500 mg/m² IV d 1–3
MINE	
Mesna (Mesnex)	500 mg/m²/d PO d 1–3
	PLUS
	1.5 gm/m²/d IV d 1–3
Ifosfamide (Ifex)	1.5 gm/m²/d d 1–3 IV
Mitoxantrone (Novantrone)	10 mg/m² IV d 1
Etoposide	80 mg/m²/d IV d 1–3

*Idarubicin 2 mg/m²/d IV d 1–3 is substituted for doxorubicin in a randomized fashion in the alternatives IdSHAP and MBIdCOS to compare directly the efficacy of these two agents.

CHOP regimen, the first definitively curative lymphoma therapy, a multitude of combinations have been investigated. Table 5 outlines representative examples of these so-called first-, second-, and third-generation regimens that have evolved from CHOP by including additional active agents and modifying delivery schedules and strategies. Initial data from the trials of third-generation combinations reported much higher CR rates than the early South West Oncology Group (SWOG) experience with CHOP (75% to 85% versus 58%). When compared directly, however, in a multicenter randomized SWOG study, these differences did not hold even when patients were stratified according to prognostic index. Thus current evidence reinstates CHOP as standard therapy for IGL. Ongoing, however, is the search for an improvement.

Our current emphasis is on the stratification of patients according to prognosis. Those with high-risk disease receive intensive chemotherapy (see Table 5: ASAP or IdSHAP alternating with M-BACOS or MBIdCOS for four courses, consolidated with MINE for three courses). Those with favorable pretreatment characteristics receive curtailed therapy (three courses of CHOP-Bleo chemotherapy plus IF radiation or CHOP-Bleo alternating with OPEN for a total of six courses, depending on extent of disease). Strict restaging after two and four courses with planned cross-over to high-dose therapy with autologous bone marrow transplant (ABMT) or peripheral blood stem cell transplant (PBSCT) for inadequate responses is another important aspect of the current studies.

Relapsed disease after multiagent front-line therapy carries a poor prognosis. Salvage therapy utilizes known active agents. High-dose cytarabine and cisplatin–based regimens exploiting the synergism between these agents are useful in this setting. Ifosfamide (Ifex),* mitoxantrone (Novantrone),* and etoposide (VePesid)* are other active agents used successfully in combination. For patients with chemotherapy-sensitive relapse, current data indicate that consolidation with high-dose chemotherapy followed by ABMT or PBSCT produces better survival than chemotherapy alone.

HIGH-GRADE LYMPHOMA

High-grade lymphoma (HGL) includes lymphoblastic and small noncleaved cell (SNCC) (Burkitt's and non-Burkitt's) lymphomas. Burkitt's lymphoma is the prototypical high-grade disorder with a rapid growth rate paralleling a high S-phase fraction on flow cytometric cell kinetic analysis. This unique disorder is more common in children and AIDS patients, and has a characteristic karyotypic abnormality (t(8;14)) in the majority of cases. Although baseline staging information is still required, therapeutic decisions are little influenced since all cases are presumed to be disseminated at presentation. Different clinical staging systems, such as the Ziegler system, have been applied to Burkitt's lymphomas. Tumor lysis frequently complicates therapy, thus hydration, allopurinol, sodium bicarbonate, and meticulous monitoring are mandatory. Again, identification of poor prognostic features such as central nervous system

---

*Not FDA-approved for this indication.

(CNS) or bone marrow disease has been used to target high-risk patients prospectively.

Specific treatment programs have evolved for HGL. The early National Cancer Institute regimens in the 1970s demonstrated curative potential for this previously lethal disorder. In general, treatment consists of dose-intense systemic chemotherapy with emphasis on multiagent alternating non–cross-resistant regimens and CNS prophylaxis or therapy, since this is a frequent site of relapse or dissemination. The use of growth factors has enhanced our ability to administer aggressive therapy in rapid cycles. Hyperfractionated delivery of cyclophosphamide (Cytoxan) in an attempt to overcome the very rapid cycling of cells is also being explored in high-grade disease. High-dose chemotherapy and BMT is often part of planned therapy in the highest-risk patients. Overall, approximately 50% of patients are cured. Relapsed patients are difficult to salvage and almost always die from disease.

Lymphoblastic lymphoma is generally a T cell disorder and frequently presents with a large mediastinal mass. This disorder bears a relationship to acute lymphoblastic leukemia (ALL) analogous to that which small lymphocytic lymphoma and chronic lymphocytic leukemia (CLL) share. Treatment approach is in general similar to ALL therapy, utilizing multiagent combinations in induction, consolidation/intensification, CNS prophylaxis, and long-term maintenance phases. Again, cure is possible in approximately 50% of patients, with alternative strategies needed for the remainder. High-dose chemotherapy and autologous or allogeneic BMT is again utilized in the poorest-risk patients.

AIDS-RELATED LYMPHOMA

AIDS-related lymphoma (ARL) is worthy of separate discussion since NHL occurring in the setting of HIV infection manifests differences in both natural history and therapeutic outcome. The probability of AIDS patients developing NHL has been variously predicted at 46% and 29%. The distribution of histologic subtypes differs from the non-AIDS population and appears to vary with the stage of HIV-related disease. Almost 75% of tumors are high-grade lesions of immunoblastic or small noncleaved cell type. The remaining 25% are IGLs. Widely disseminated extranodal disease is present in the majority at presentation. Chemotherapy for ARL patients is often compromised by poor bone marrow reserve exacerbated by antiretroviral therapy and the development of intercurrent opportunistic infections. Consequently, the high complete response rates expected of second- and third-generation regimens are diminished significantly. The CD4 count, pre-existing opportunistic infections, and performance status are all important prognostic indicators. Overall median survival has been reported as less than 6 months. Attempts to improve therapeutic outcome have been made utilizing lower doses of standard regimens and hematopoietic growth factors. Reduced dose M-BACOD (see Table 5) has been used with no reduction in median survival but less toxicity. CHOP has been used with GM-CSF* (sargramostim) (Leukine) with effective reduction in febrile neutropenic episodes. Use of CNS prophylaxis, as well as prophylaxis against *Pneumocystis* and antiretroviral maintenance, is also recognized as important.

Our own approach has been to utilize a novel experimental, minimally myelosuppressive regimen for patients with CD4 counts below 200. This incorporates continuous infusion of 5-fluorouracil (5-FU), leucovorin (Wellcovorin), and cisplatin (Platinol), with provision for use of G-CSF† (filgrastim) (Neupogen). For patients whose counts are over 200 and who have no prior history of opportunistic infections, standard intensity regimens are used. Patients with localized nonbulky disease and histology other than small noncleaved cell lymphoma are treated with abbreviated chemotherapy (CHOP-Bleo × 3) and local radiotherapy. CNS lymphoma accounts for 10% to 50% of lymphoma in AIDS patients but only 1% to 2% in nonimmunocompromised patients. The majority of patients have low CD4 counts and prior AIDS-defining opportunistic infections. Distinction of CNS lymphoma from toxoplasmosis often requires brain biopsy. Standard therapy has been whole brain radiation and steroids. This has improved median survival from 42 days in untreated cases to 136 days in one series. Chemotherapy has proved extremely difficult to deliver effectively to this group, and no good results have been achieved. Intercurrent infection rather than tumor is the usual cause of death. Non-HIV-positive patients with CNS lymphoma receive cytarabine and methotrexate-based chemotherapy following brain radiation.

GASTROINTESTINAL LYMPHOMA

As many as 25% of non-Hodgkin's lymphomas are extranodal in origin. The majority of these are diffuse large cell type. The specific organ of involvement is of importance in determining appropriate therapy. The majority of extranodal lymphomas arise in the GI tract, and the majority of these are gastric. Recently, a strong association between the presence of *Helicobacter pylori* and the development of gastric lymphoma has been shown. Dramatic responses can occur when this is treated with antibiotics. Optimal management of GI lymphoma is somewhat debated, although the role of surgery is declining in favor of front-line chemotherapy. Surgical resection of gastric lymphoma may cure up to a third of cases but remains a morbid procedure following which many patients will still require adjuvant therapy. Stomach conservation with primary chemotherapy has been studied extensively at our institution. It has proved a favorable alternative with few patients requiring subsequent operative intervention. Perforation is an infrequent complication. GI bleeding, while more

---

*GM-CSF = granulocyte-macrophage colony-stimulating factor.
†G-CSF = granulocyte colony-stimulating factor.

common, usually occurs in the setting of extensive gastric involvement and is generally self-limited after the first course of chemotherapy.

Drug regimens employed are those applicable to intermediate-grade lymphomas (see Table 5). Radiation therapy has historically been a very important adjuvant modality for stage I and stage II patients. It remains a useful alternative in chemotherapy-intolerant patients or as an adjunct for bulky, intraabdominal disease.

MULTIPLE MYELOMA

method of
JAMES R. BERENSON, M.D.,
ROBERT A. VESCIO, M.D., and
GARY SCHILLER, M.D.
*West Los Angeles Veterans Affairs Medical
   Center and UCLA School of Medicine
Los Angeles, California*

Multiple myeloma is a bone marrow–based malignancy of terminally differentiated cells of the B-lymphocyte lineage, the plasma cells. Recent evidence suggests that small numbers of cells also circulate in the blood of these patients. Although no common genetic or chromosomal changes have been observed in the malignant cells in these patients, abnormalities of the N-*ras, Rb, p53,* and *c-myc* genes may be found in a minority of patients. The role of cytokines in the pathogenesis of myeloma is not clearly understood, but interleukin-6 and to a lesser extent interleukin-1 and tumor necrosis factor play important roles in the growth as well as the clinical manifestations of the disease.

There are approximately 13,000 new cases of myeloma each year in the United States. There is controversy regarding whether there is an increasing incidence of this malignancy. The median age at diagnosis is approximately 65 years, and the disease is more frequent in men than women. This cancer is twice as frequent in blacks as in whites. The etiology is unknown, although genetic and perhaps environmental factors both probably play a role.

The most frequent clinical manifestations of the disease are related to its bony complications, although generalized weakness, anemia, recurrent infections, renal failure, hypercalcemia, and hyperviscosity are also important features. The median survival is approximately 3 years but varies tremendously depending upon the amount of disease at the time of presentation.

DIAGNOSIS

All patients suspected of having multiple myeloma should have both a serum and urine electrophoresis. The latter evaluation is important since nearly one quarter of myeloma patients will have tumors that secrete only the light chain portion of the Ig molecule. This small Ig fragment is rapidly cleared by the kidney and, therefore, may not be detectable in the serum. In addition, in patients with elevated globulin fractions on routine blood chemistry examinations, a serum protein electrophoresis should be performed. If a monoclonal protein is identified in the serum or urine of any patient, an immunoelectrophoresis should be performed to characterize the Ig subtype, which

will help in classifying the disease type associated with the paraprotein. Once a paraprotein has been identified, it should be determined whether the paraprotein results from a monoclonal plasma cell proliferation that is malignant—usually multiple myeloma, or the nonmalignant condition—monoclonal gammopathy of undetermined significance (MGUS). This differentiation is based on the amount of paraprotein present in the serum and/or urine, bone marrow histology, presence or absence of skeletal disease, hypercalcemia, anemia, or renal dysfunction. In addition to a 24-hour urine collection to measure the urinary excretion of the monoclonal proteins, laboratory tests should include a complete blood count and serum levels of creatinine and calcium. A radiographic bone survey, including long bones, spine, pelvis, and skull, should be performed on all patients. A nuclear medicine bone scan should not be requested, since most myelomatous bony lesions are purely lytic in nature and will be missed by this procedure. Magnetic resonance imaging (MRI) may be helpful in identifying lesions not obvious on plain radiographs. A bone marrow aspirate and biopsy complete the general work-up by assessing plasma cell morphology and infiltration. A marrow plasma cell percentage above 30% coupled with a paraprotein abnormality is sufficient for a neoplastic classification even in asymptomatic patients. Many of these latter patients will have a more slowly progressive form of the disease, appropriately termed "indolent myeloma," and should be followed without treatment until symptoms develop. Rare patients have a nonsecretory form of the disease, which can be diagnosed by finding a pathogenic plasma cell proliferation on biopsy. Patients with only a solitary plasmacytoma lesion should be managed differently, as outlined later.

TUMOR STAGING AND PROGNOSIS

The most common and widely accepted form of staging for multiple myeloma was developed by Durie and Salmon and is based upon tumor bulk and renal function. This relatively complicated staging system is divided into stages I, II, or III based upon the amount of monoclonal protein, hemoglobin level, number of lytic lesions, and serum calcium. In addition, renal function as assessed by serum creatinine is used to subclassify patients into A or B. Patients with stage I disease have median survivals of 48 to 80 months, in comparison to 6 to 33 months for patients with more advanced stage III disease. Because of its complexity, a simpler staging system using simply serum beta$_2$-microglobulin levels has been used. This value is the most important predictor of outcome in myeloma patients. Its level is higher in patients with poor renal function, but it has been shown to be an independent prognostic variable in studies using multivariate analysis. Moreover, rises in beta$_2$-microglobulin levels during the course of the disease predict a poor outcome. In addition, serum C-reactive protein (CRP) has been shown to be a prognostic factor, although a small minority of patients will have the elevated CRP levels associated with poor prognosis. A high plasma cell labeling index has also been shown to be associated with poor outcome. High serum lactic dehydrogenase (LDH) levels and plasmablastic morphology also portend a shortened survival.

TREATMENT

Assessing the Response to Therapy

To determine whether treatment for multiple myeloma is effective, one must first review the clinical and biologic factors that may influence response and the course of disease. As indicated, specific laboratory indicators (hemoglobin and serum levels of calcium, creatinine, and beta$_2$-microglobulin) and clinical features (the amount of bone disease) provide important prognostic information with respect to response and progression-free and overall survival. In addition, the duration of disease not requiring systemic therapy and response to prior therapy determine the likelihood and duration of response and survival. It is important to note that clinical trials reporting improved progression-free survival in myeloma may be biased by the inclusion of patients with less aggressive disease biology. Thus, new therapeutic developments must be evaluated in the light of disease biology and patient selection.

Response assessment is also difficult since there are no uniform criteria by which treatment may be judged. The Southwest Oncology Group (SWOG) defines partial remission as a 75% or greater reduction from diagnosis of bone marrow plasmacytosis and serum or urine paraprotein levels, without progressive bony lesions. Complete remission is defined as normal bone marrow cellularity with less than 5% plasma cells, absence of paraprotein in the serum and urine by immunoelectrophoresis or immunofixation, and no evidence of progressive bony lesions. Some studies have shown that patients with no change in their M-protein after initial treatment may have a similar survival to patients achieving a partial or complete response. However, recent results show that achievement of a reduction in M-protein on chemotherapy is associated with an improved survival, but the amount of protein decrease is not necessarily related to outcome. Disease progression is typically defined as an increase in the amount of serum or urinary M-protein (more than 25% increase) or development of new lytic bone lesions. Disease that fails to respond to initial therapy is typically referred to as refractory myeloma. Patients whose disease demonstrates an initial response but who have subsequent progression despite continued therapy are referred to as secondarily unresponsive. Patients with secondarily unresponsive disease have a better prognosis than patients with refractory disease, who typically do very poorly.

Initial Treatment

The treatment against which all other therapy for multiple myeloma must be compared consists of alkylating agents and glucocorticosteroids. As a single agent, melphalan (Alkeran) produces responses in 25% of patients. The addition of glucocorticosteroids improves the response rate to 40%. In fact, the response rate and overall survival with glucocorticosteroid therapy alone (dexamethasone) may be similar to the combined treatment with melphalan and prednisone (MP). The addition of infusional vincristine and doxorubicin to oral dexamethasone (VAD) leads to a more rapid and higher response rate, although its impact on overall survival is unclear. Potential

disadvantages of VAD include a requirement for central venous access to deliver the vesicant drugs and a higher risk of infections from neutropenia and high-dose dexamethasone. Other therapeutic combinations of alkylating agents have also been employed based on the hypothesis that nonoverlapping toxicities would permit the use of noncross-resistant drugs. Several trials of combined alkylating agents and/or anthracyclines have suggested higher response rates than those achieved with MP. However, most randomized trials and meta-analyses have suggested little impact on overall survival with the added toxicity of these more aggressive combination chemotherapy regimens.

In determining what type of therapy to initiate in the newly diagnosed patient, it is important to consider the extent of disease and associated clinical problems as well as whether the patient is a candidate for myeloablative chemotherapy, followed by hematopoietic transplant support. In patients undergoing autologous transplants, regimens without alkylating agents are preferable because of the permanent damage done to hematopoietic stem cells by these drugs. In patients requiring a rapid response because of severe bone disease, hypercalcemia, or renal disease, VAD is the treatment of choice. By contrast, in elderly patients or in those individuals unable to tolerate aggressive chemotherapy, oral dexamethasone alone or MP is an appropriate form of treatment.

Interferon

The antineoplastic activity of human leukocyte interferon (IFN) has been demonstrated in a variety of malignancies, including hairy cell leukemia and renal cell cancer. Early studies in multiple myeloma used purified IFN-alfa at a dose of 3 million (M) U daily. Higher doses have been associated with minimal antitumor activity at the expense of considerable toxicity, including asthenia, fevers, transient granulocytopenia, anemia, and thrombocytopenia. Furthermore, the efficacy of this agent when used alone seems to be greatest in untreated or chemotherapy-sensitive myeloma, but safer and less toxic chemotherapeutic regimens are better choices for these patients. In refractory disease, the drug has little activity. This biologic agent has been more frequently combined with multiagent chemotherapy or given following a response to the patient's chemotherapy (see Maintenance Therapy, next).

Maintenance Therapy

Whereas conventional doses of chemotherapy frequently lead to reductions in tumor mass and circulating paraprotein, few patients will achieve a complete response. Most patients enter a "plateau phase," at which point the monoclonal protein level remains constant despite continued chemotherapy. It is believed that the remaining tumor cells within the patient at this timepoint are relatively quiescent and resistant to chemotherapy. Continuation of chemotherapy once the paraprotein level stabilizes does not improve overall survival and leads to a permanent reduction in bone marrow reserve and increases the risk of secondary leukemia. Therefore, chemotherapy should be stopped for most patients who enter plateau phase, defined as a stable M-protein level for 3 months on treatment. This will limit the patient's exposure to myelotoxic and leukemogenic drugs. Patients who obtain a complete remission or who had an initial low tumor mass are the most likely to exhibit long, unmaintained remissions.

Maintenance therapy with IFN-alfa has been assessed in numerous randomized studies with conflicting results. Most studies demonstrate a prolongation of progression-free but not overall survival for patients randomized to IFN-alfa therapy. Patients with stable disease during induction chemotherapy do not appear to benefit from treatment. More promising results have been demonstrated for patients with initially responsive disease, particularly if higher doses of drug (3 to 5 MU per m^2 thrice weekly) are used. Even for this latter subgroup of patients, the overall prolongation of survival is minimal (3 to 4 months). As a result, one must weigh the considerable toxicity and expense against the minimal benefit of this agent before considering its use in myeloma patients.

Bone Marrow Transplant

Based on the higher response rates achieved with more aggressive combinations of alkylating agents, high-dose chemotherapy with or without hematopoietic support has been studied. Initial trials involved patients with resistant multiple myeloma who were treated with melphalan (Alkeran) in doses of 70 to 140 mg per m^2. Although dramatic responses were noted, these responses were short-lived and associated with significant morbidity related to protracted myelosuppression. Hematopoietic support using autologous bone marrow was added to shorten the duration of granulocytopenia, allowing for more intensive preparative conditioning with higher doses of melphalan (200 mg per m^2) alone or lower doses (140 mg per m^2) combined with total body irradiation (TBI) or busulfan (Myleran) and cyclophosphamide (Cytoxan). In these early studies, despite treatment eligibility based on resistance to conventional chemotherapy, impressive cytoreduction was achieved, but progression-free survival was brief. Several favorable prognostic factors for sustained response were identified and included chemotherapy-sensitive myeloma and a shorter duration of primary treatment. Based on these results, autologous bone marrow transplantation was used on recently diagnosed patients with chemotherapy-responsive disease. These studies showed very high response rates and suggested improved long-term myeloma-free survival compared with patients treated with conventional chemotherapy alone.

In a recent randomized French study of untreated intermediate- to high-stage multiple myeloma, patients assigned to high-dose chemotherapy and autologous bone marrow transplantation achieved higher overall response rates and better progression-free survival than that achieved by patients continued on conventional chemotherapy. However, a potential problem unresolved by the use of autologous bone marrow support is the presence of clonogenic plasma cells in the autologous bone marrow product. One approach to overcome this problem has been to change the source of hematopoietic support from bone marrow to autologous peripheral blood progenitor cells obtained by leukaphereses. This latter product contains much less tumor contamination than found in bone marrow harvests. A further possible way to reduce the risk of tumor cell contamination in the autograft is through purification of the leukapheresis material by negatively purging with a battery of anti-B-cell antibodies, or by positive selection for hematopoietic progenitor cells.

The lack of uniform expression of B-cell antigens on malignant plasma cells reduces the efficacy of the former technique. On the other hand, in a recent study of positive hematopoietic progenitor cells selected by their expression of the early hematopoietic CD34 antigen, residual clonogenic tumor cell contamination was markedly reduced. Using a PCR-based assay, it was shown that the CD34-selected product showed a greater than 2.7 to greater than 4.5 log reduction in contaminating tumor cells compared with the unselected leukaphereses. Furthermore, the CD34-selected progenitor cells produced rapid hematologic recovery after a myeloablative preparative regimen of busulfan and cyclophosphamide. The median time to both neutrophil and platelet recovery was 12 days, and the median numbers of erythrocyte and platelet transfusions were 7 and 3, respectively. Complete and partial remissions were achieved in 33 of 43 evaluable patients, and the actuarial progression-free and overall survival 1 year after transplantation was 67% plus or minus 19% and 68% plus or minus 21%, respectively.

Given the high response rate and likelihood of prolonged progression-free survival with relatively low treatment-related mortality (5%) in patients undergoing high-dose chemotherapy with autologous progenitor cell support, this treatment modality should be considered for patients aged 70 years or less with intermediate- to advanced-stage multiple myeloma responsive or stable following conventional chemotherapy.

Allogeneic bone marrow transplantation has also been used in myeloma. Its potential advantage includes the complete absence of malignant cells in the infused product as well as a possible therapeutic form of adoptive immunotherapy or graft-versus-tumor effect mediated by the allogeneic bone marrow. Occasionally patients relapsing after autologous transplantation have been treated with this procedure, but the outcome has been generally poor. Due to age restrictions and lack of available donors, very few studies have been published, and most contain small numbers of patients. The results have been disappointing, with a high risk of treatment-related mortality attributable to early transplant-related organ toxicity and graft-versus-host disease. Although early results from the largest study of allogeneic transplants from the European Bone Marrow Transplant Registry were encouraging, a recently published update showed that many patients have relapsed, with very few patients alive and disease-free. Thus, there has been no demonstrated clinical advantage of allogeneic transplantation as hematopoietic support following myeloablative chemotherapy in multiple myeloma.

Therapy of Refractory and Relapsing Myeloma

Thirty percent to 50% of multiple myeloma patients will have progressive disease despite conventional therapy. Of patients who do achieve an initial response, nearly all will ultimately relapse and develop disease unresponsive to initial therapy. The former group whose disease progresses or fails to respond to initial treatment has a particularly poor prognosis. Numerous studies of standard-dose alkylating agents, anthracyclines, spindle toxins, and other drugs have failed to produce results in refractory patients. Likewise, nucleoside antagonists, taxanes, and nitrosoureas have been tried without therapeutic effect. However, high-dose glucocorticosteroids such as prednisone, in a dose of 200 mg every other day or given in a pulse fashion (60 mg per m^2 daily for 5 days every 8 days), or dexamethasone, 40 mg daily for 4 days repeated every 8 to 14 days, may produce excellent responses even in refractory patients. Toxicities include insomnia, hyperglycemia, mental status changes, and increased risk of infections. VAD may be used in patients who initially failed MP, but its efficacy in patients who previously failed high-dose dexamethasone therapy alone is less impressive. This salvage regimen remains one of the most active treatments and is very well tolerated by most patients. Etoposide-containing regimens such as EDAP or ICE have demonstrated some activity in refractory myeloma. Intensive treatment with high-dose alkylating agents and radiation may produce dramatic response in patients with refractory disease. However, these responses are short-lived and cannot be considered a standard form of salvage treatment.

Complications

Hypercalcemia

Hypercalcemia results from the overproduction of specific cytokines (IL-1beta, tumor necrosis factor (TNF), and IL-6) in the myeloma bone marrow environment. Although early studies suggested hypercalcemia occurred in nearly one third of patients at diagnosis, most recent series suggest that only approximately 10% of myeloma patients present with hypercalcemia requiring specific treatment. This complication may also develop during the course of the patient's disease. The symptoms may be nonspecific, including fatigue, generalized motor weakness, anorexia, nausea, constipation, polyuria, dehydration, or confusion. Rehydration with saline should be initiated immediately, which will both correct the calciuresis-induced dehydration and lead to renal excretion of calcium. However, rehydration alone is often not sufficient to maintain normocalcemia. Control of the tumor using chemotherapy should be the primary goal for most patients, since a good tumor response will be the most important factor in the long-term maintenance of normal calcium levels. Glucocorticosteroids are frequently effective in treating this complication because of their combined antitumor properties and suppressive effect upon hypercalcemia-inducing cytokines. Since the hypocalcemic response to both glucocorticosteroids and chemotherapy may be delayed, other agents should be used for a more immediate effect. Calcitonin (Calcimar), has a rapid onset of action that can be important for patients with severe hypercalcemia, but patients rapidly become resistant to its efficacy. Finally, bisphosphonates such as pamidronate (Aredia), are extremely effective, with a single infusion of 90 mg over 4 hours leading to normocalcemia in the great majority of patients after 4 to 5 days.

Renal Failure

Renal dysfunction (creatinine greater than 2.0 mg per mL) occurs in 15% to 30% of patients at diagnosis but will develop in half of patients during the course of their disease. The nephropathy has multiple causes but most commonly results from effects of the Bence Jones proteins, leading to cast nephropathy or monoclonal Ig deposition disease, and/or hypercalcemia. Patients with κ light chain only–secreting tumors have the highest risk for developing the less common Ig deposition disease. Particular structural features of κ light chains resulting from usage of the VκIV subgroup of variable genes may be responsible for this abnormality by promoting tissue deposition. In contrast, the majority of patients with "myeloma kidney" have λ light chain–secreting tumors. Bence Jones proteins precipitate within the distal tubule and combine with Tamm-Horsfall glycoprotein, leading to intraluminal obstruction and eventually renal failure. The primary factors influencing this cast formation are the type and amount of Bence Jones proteins and tubule fluid flow rate. Consequently, exposure to exacerbating factors such as hypercalcemia-inducing diuretics or radiocontrast agents should be minimized. Dehydration should be avoided, and patients with active disease should be advised to drink 2 to 3 liters of fluid per day. Fortunately, successful treatment of the myeloma tumor burden by chemotherapy is often capable of reversing renal dysfunction. Regimens with a rapid response rate such as VAD are preferable. Plasmapheresis has been used successfully during initial management of some patients with renal failure and may be warranted as a therapeutic trial. It is important to note that the reversal of renal dysfunction often takes several months.

Infections

Myeloma patients have been shown in vitro to have defects in B as well as T cell immunity. The older literature suggested that these patients' myelomas were at very high risk of infection, particularly with encapsulated organisms, because of the associated hypogammoglobulinemia. However, recent reports show the higher infectious risk mainly occurs during chemotherapy-induced neutropenia or in the terminal stages of the disease. In fact, myeloma patients develop types of infections similar to other types of cancer patients, in whom infections are associated with neutropenia. Commonly, these involve gram-negative bacterial infections in patients without central venous catheters, and staphylococcal or candidal infections in patients with these lines. In patients receiving intermittent glucocorticosteroid therapy, Pneumocystis carinii must be considered in any patient with a pulmonary infection. In addition, viral infections with herpes simplex or more commonly, herpes zoster, may occur, and require immediate treatment with acyclovir (Zovirax). The use of intravenous immunoglobulins may somewhat reduce the risk of infection but is very costly and probably not justified on a routine basis.

Bone Disease

Bone disease is the major cause of morbidity in multiple myeloma, resulting from stimulation of osteoclasts by bone-resorbing cytokines (TNF, IL-1beta and IL-6), which are overabundant in the myeloma bone marrow. Osteolytic lesions and generalized osteoporosis may lead to severe pain, pathologic fractures, and spinal cord compression and collapse. These complications often require radiation therapy to relieve pain or to treat actual or impending pathologic fractures or spinal cord compression. Plasma cell tumors are relatively responsive to radiation treatment. Responses typically occur rapidly, with most lesions treated with approximately 3000 cGy. However, it is important to avoid unnecessary radiotherapy since its myelosuppressive effect may limit the ability to deliver cytotoxic doses of systemic chemotherapy. Often the latter treatment alone will be effective for relieving skeletal pain. High doses of analgesics may be necessary until pain control is achieved with radiation treatment or chemotherapy. Surgery may be necessary to treat actual fractures or prevent large lytic lesions from developing fractures. The placement of intramedullary rods is usually the surgical procedure of choice. Spinal disease may require surgical decompression or stabilization of the spine. Previous attempts to reduce the development of these skeletal complications with calcium, sodium fluoride, and/or androgenic steroids have been unsuccessful. Bisphosphonates inhibit osteoclastic activity and are effective in the treatment of hypercalcemia associated with myeloma (see previous discussion of Hypercalcemia). Previous attempts to use relatively weak first-generation bisphosphonates (etidronate or clodronate) orally as an adjunct to chemotherapy had no significant effect on the skeletal complications.

A recent large randomized trial compared the effect of the more potent second-generation agent pamidronate, given as a monthly 90-mg 4-hour infusion, with placebo on the development of bony complications in patients on chemotherapy. Pamidronate was successful in both reducing the percentage of patients developing at least one skeletal event as well as reducing the number of events experienced by the patient. In addition, patients experienced less pain after beginning pamidronate therapy, their requirement for analgesic usage was less than that of placebo-treated patients, and individuals treated with the bisphosphonate showed a better Eastern Cooperative Oncology Group (ECOG) performance status. Although this trial involved patients with Durie-Salmon stage III myeloma, it is likely that this drug will also be efficacious in reducing these complications in patients at earlier stages of the disease.

Anemia

The high incidence of anemia in multiple myeloma results from multiple factors, including renal failure, hyperviscosity, chemotherapy-induced marrow suppression, and suppression of erythropoiesis by cytokines (TNF, IL-1beta and IL-6) overproduced in the myeloma bone marrow. Many myeloma patients have inappropriately low levels of erythropoietin (EPO) (Epogen) levels for their degree of anemia. Treatment of the tumor burden with antimyeloma chemotherapy will increase hemoglobin levels in many patients. However, in patients resistant to this form of treatment, subcutaneously administered EPO at 10,000 U thrice weekly may be highly effective. Most responses occur within 2 months of initiation of this form of therapy. Some patients may require higher doses of EPO to raise their hemoglobin. This treatment is more effective in patients whose endogenous EPO levels are inappropriately low for their hemoglobin level. The dose may be reduced once an adequate response has been achieved.

Hyperviscosity

Features suggestive of hyperviscosity include high-output cardiac failure, hearing loss, visual changes, purpura, epistaxis, headache, and a decreased level of consciousness. Although the hyperviscosity syndrome more commonly occurs in patients with Waldenström's macroglobulinemia, patients with advanced stages of myeloma may also present with these symptoms, especially if the circulating paraprotein is of the IgA or rare IgM phenotype. Serum viscosity levels are commonly three to four times normal in symptomatic patients, but this laboratory test does not always correlate well with symptomatology. An irregular dilation of retinal veins (sausage-link appearance) with hemorrhages and exudates is pathognomonic for the condition. Treatment should include plasmapheresis and the reduction of tumor burden with chemotherapy.

Special Clinical Presentations

Monoclonal Gammopathy of Undetermined Significance

Most patients presenting with a monoclonal gammopathy, in fact, do not have a malignant B cell disorder. Monoclonal gammopathies occur at a higher frequency in the elderly population, with approximately 3% of individuals over age 70 years possessing a paraprotein. In a minority (15% to 25%) of cases, MGUS may eventually progress after many years to a malignant disorder. When malignant transformation occurs, most patients develop myeloma, although lymphomas and Waldenström's macroglobulinemia may occur in patients with IgM paraproteins. No factors predict if and when patients will transform to malignant disease. Patients with MGUS should be seen periodically (every 6 to 12 months) and undergo measurement of paraprotein levels, complete blood count, and routine chemistries. However, more extensive re-evaluation of bone marrow and skeletal disease is unwarranted unless it is clinically indicated.

Solitary Plasmacytoma of Bone or Soft Tissue (Extramedullary Plasmacytoma)

Five percent of patients with a plasmacytoma of bone are found to have it at only a single site. By definition, these patients should not have systemic signs of disease such as anemia, hypercalcemia, or more than 30% marrow plasmacytosis. Approximately half these patients will have a monoclonal Ig protein detectable in the serum or urine, which may resolve after successful treatment of the local disease. Radiotherapy with doses of 4000 to 5000 cGy is recommended. Radiation fields should encompass the entire medullary cavity to treat potential intramedullary spread of disease. Although occasional patients can be cured, most eventually relapse with systemic disease within 10 years. Patients developing recurrent myeloma tend to have a more indolent course, with median survivals comparable to those with stage I disease. MRIs of the spine have proved useful to identify patients more likely to develop systemic disease eventually, although it is not clear that the identification of additional abnormalities using this modality should influence treatment decisions.

Localized extramedullary plasmacytomas typically present as a submucosal mass in the tissues of the upper airway passages. Conversion to systemic disease is less common than is observed in solitary plasmacytoma of bone, and in one series 71% of patients remained progression-free at 10 years. Radiation therapy, with doses of at least 4000 cGy, is the treatment of choice. If the disease does relapse, soft tissue spread is more common.

Plasma Cell Leukemia

Plasma cell leukemia is diagnosed when the number of circulating plasma cells reaches 2000 per μL; it occurs in a small minority (3% to 4%) of myeloma patients at diagnosis. These patients have complex cytogenetic abnormalities and higher frequencies of *ras* and *p53* abnormalities than do other myeloma cases. They respond poorly to conventional chemotherapy, especially MP, with brief remission duration and shortened survival compared with other myeloma patients. Plasma cell leukemia also occurs in a similar percentage of patients during the course of the disease termed "secondary plasma cell leukemia," and when it occurs in this setting portends a very short life expectancy.

Plasma Cell Dyscrasia with Polyneuropathy

Occasional patients with myeloma present with multiple sclerotic instead of lytic bony lesions. Many of these patients will also have symptoms of organomegaly (hepatosplenomegaly, lymphadenopathy), endocrinopathies (diabetes mellitus, gonadal dysfunction, hypothyroidism), skin changes (hypertrichosis or hyperpigmentation), and sensorimotor polyneuropathy. Typically, the patients are young men, and the symptom complex has been attributed to increased serum levels of IL-1beta and IL-6. Since these features are part of a paraneoplastic syndrome, effective therapy of the malignant plasma cell proliferation with either chemotherapy or radiation can alleviate most of the symptoms. Steroids may be particularly useful by reducing cytokine production in addition to their direct cytotoxic effect. Experimental treatment with anti-IL-6 and potentially anti-IL-1beta antibodies may also be of benefit, as has been shown for the related Castleman's disease.

POLYCYTHEMIA VERA

method of
ANGELA OGDEN, M.D.
Texas Children's Hospital
Houston, Texas

Polycythemia vera (PV) is a myeloproliferative disorder of the pluripotent stem cell manifest by extreme erythrocytosis and variable thrombocytosis and leukocytosis. The clonal nature of the disease has been demonstrated in affected female patients heterozygous for glucose-6-phosphate dehydrogenase (G6PD) deficiency in which a single G6PD isoenzyme is found in multilineage hematopoietic cells. Clonality from an abnormal stem cell is also demonstrated by the presence of chromosomal abnormalities in multilineage hematopoietic cells that are not present in other tissues. PV is typically a disease of elderly people, with a median age at presentation of 60 years. Less than 0.1% of cases occur in persons less than 20 years of age. The overall incidence of PV is 1.0 to 2.7 cases per 100,000 per year. The incidence rate appears to be increasing over the past decade, but this is most likely due to improved recognition. The highest age-specific incidence rates are in men over 80 years of age (18.3 cases per 100,000 per year) and in women between 70 and 79 years of age (14.6 cases per 100,000 per year).

The median survival from diagnosis is 9 to 14 years, similar to age-matched controls. The most common disease-related cause of death is thrombosis, followed by acute leukemia, other cancers, hemorrhage, and the spent phase.

PV progresses through three fairly distinct stages. Clinical symptomatology relates to the degree of erythrocytosis and thrombocytosis during these periods. Most patients present in the proliferative stage. Many are plethoric and may complain of headache, tinnitus, vertigo, pruritus, bone pain, and weakness. There may be evidence of a hypermetabolic state, manifest by fever, night sweats, and weight loss. Splenomegaly is present at the time of diagnosis in 40% to 70% of cases. A subset of patients present with thrombotic or hemorrhagic events. Erythromelalgia, characterized by paroxysmal burning and throbbing pain in the extremities associated with mottling of the skin, has been well described in PV as well as in other myeloproliferative syndromes.

Patients will proceed from the proliferative stage to the stable phase. This period is characterized by relatively normal peripheral blood counts requiring the discontinuation of specific therapy. During this time, the patient is asymptomatic. Normalization of the red cell mass and platelet count is due to a decrease in the proliferative rate of the marrow, fibrosis of the marrow cavity, or a combination of both. Gradually, 20% to 30% of patients will enter the spent phase of the disease, with pancytopenia due to progressive marrow fibrosis. Patients exhibit marked hepatosplenomegaly from myeloid metaplasia. Overall, 7% to 12% of patients will develop acute leukemia (AL). There is considerable debate whether there is a natural progression of the abnormal clone to acute myelogenous leukemia (AML) or whether leukemic transformation occurs because of cytotoxic therapy. It appears to be a combination of both: 2% of patients treated with phlebotomy develop AL compared with 15% to 20% of patients treated with myelosuppressive agents.

THROMBOTIC AND HEMORRHAGIC EVENTS

Thrombotic events occur in one third of patients with PV, most within the first 2 years of diagnosis. These include deep vein thrombosis, cerebral infarction/ischemia, myocardial infarction, pulmonary embolism, splenic infarction, peripheral gangrene, and arterial embolism. Repeat episodes are common. During the proliferative stage, thrombosis is the most common cause of death. Hemorrhagic episodes, including gastrointestinal bleeding, skin and mucosal bleeds, intracerebral hemorrhage, postoperative bleeding, and retinal hemorrhage, occur in one quarter of PV patients. Less than 10% of patients will demonstrate both hemorrhagic and thrombotic complications. The risk of thrombosis is highest in elderly patients, those patients treated by phlebotomy alone, and patients with a prior history of thrombotic events. In those patients treated with phlebotomy alone, the risk of thrombosis is highest in those patients with a high venesection requirement. It is suggested that patients less than 40 years of age may also have an unusually high incidence of thrombotic complications. The degree of erythrocytosis and thrombocytosis is not associated with the risk of thrombotic or hemorrhagic complications.

DIAGNOSIS

The diagnosis of PV can be made only after the exclusion of other causes of polycythemia. Relative polycythemia

due to vascular contraction, such as dehydration, diuretic therapy, or uncontrolled hypertension, must be excluded. Absolute polycythemia can then be divided into primary polycythemia and secondary polycythemia. Secondary polycythemia can be due to an appropriate response to erythropoietin production, as in chronic lung disease, chronic hypoventilation (pickwickian syndrome), cyanotic heart disease, high altitude, hemoglobinopathy with high oxygen affinity, and carboxyhemoglobinemia. Inappropriate erythropoietin production can result from malignant tumors (renal cell carcinoma, hepatoma, lung cancer, ovarian carcinoma) or benign tumors (pheochromocytoma, adrenal adenoma, uterine fibroids). Renal cysts, renal transplantation, hydronephrosis, and Bartter's syndrome are also associated with increased erythropoietin levels. Anabolic steroid abuse should be sought. Polycythemia due to cigarette smoking is multifactorial, so the determination of polycythemia in smokers may be difficult. There is an element of vascular contraction that can be corrected by abstinence for several days. Several months may be required, however, to reduce the red cell mass resulting from the carboxyhemoglobin from cigarette smoke.

The classic diagnostic criteria for PV were established by the Polycythemia Vera Study Group (PVSG) in 1967. Patients must exhibit an elevated red cell mass, normal arterial oxygen saturation, and splenomegaly (major criteria). In the presence of only two of the major criteria, patients must also exhibit two of the minor criteria: thrombocytosis, leukocytosis, elevated leukocyte alkaline phosphatase, or elevated serum vitamin B_{12} or unbound B_{12} binding protein. Patients early in the course of the disease and patients with erythrocytosis concurrent with other chronic diseases may be excluded by the criteria. Prolonged observation of such patients will reveal whether they indeed have PV.

Bone marrow aspirates in PV are hypercellular, with increased myeloid, erythroid, and megakaryocytic progenitors. The megakaryocytes in particular may be markedly increased, forming sheets of cells. In contrast, the marrow of patients with secondary polycythemia demonstrates erythroid hyperplasia only. Although marrow fibrosis occurs late in the course of the PV, increased reticulin fibers are noted at the time of diagnosis in 10% to 20% of all cases. Marrow and serum iron stores are decreased due to increased iron utilization in the polycythemic state. Serum erythropoietin levels are decreased or undetectable. The increased cell turnover results in increased uric acid levels in 40% to 50% of patients. Erythroid progenitors (CFU-E) in PV proliferate in soft agar culture in the absence of serum or erythropoietin, in contrast to normal erythroid progenitors that require one of these additional factors for growth.

Cytogenetic studies performed at the time of diagnosis of PV are abnormal in 15% to 20% of cases. The most common abnormalities noted in untreated patients and in those who are treated with phlebotomy are +8, +9, and 20q−. Late in the course of PV, cytogenetic abnormalities are much more common, occurring in 70% to 87%. These patients are more likely to have been treated with myelosuppressive therapy. There is no clear correlation between the presence or evolution of abnormal clones and progression of the disease to myeloid metaplasia and myelofibrosis. The finding of monosomy 5, monosomy 7, 5q−, 7q−, and t(1;7) suggests that myelosuppressive therapy has induced secondary AML.

TREATMENT

The primary goal of therapy in the proliferative stage of the disease is to decrease the red cell mass.

This can be accomplished with phlebotomy, alkylating agents, radioactive phosphorus (^{32}P), or interferon. The choice of therapy must be modified according to the risk factors of the particular patient: leukemic transformation is a greater risk in the younger patient treated with myelosuppressive therapy, and thrombotic events occur more frequently in elderly patients.

Patients Below 50 Years of Age

The initial treatment of newly diagnosed PV without prior thrombotic events is simple phlebotomy. Initially, removal of 500-mL aliquots of blood every 2 to 3 days till the hematocrit is below 45 will reduce the blood viscosity. Subsequent phlebotomy every 1 to 2 months is performed to maintain the hematocrit between 42 and 45. It is expected that chronic phlebotomy will result in iron deficiency. The resultant low mean corpuscular volume (MCV) will help maintain a low hematocrit. Patients may become symptomatic from iron deficiency, however, with anorexia, weakness, lethargy, and glossitis. A trial of iron could be attempted, but brisk reticulocytosis and exacerbation of the disease will result. Myelosuppression should be initiated.

Hydroxyurea (Hydrea),* 15 mg per kg per day, with adjuvant phlebotomy as needed, is the myelosuppressive agent of choice. The dose may be increased or decreased by 5 mg per kg per day every 2 weeks to maintain platelets between 150,000 and 600,000 and WBC greater than 3500 per mm³. The usual dose is between 500 and 1000 mg per day. Response is noted in the majority of patients within 3 weeks. No response by 12 weeks indicates treatment failure. Due to the significant myelotoxicity that can occur with hydroxyurea, blood counts should be obtained biweekly for the first several months of therapy. Discontinuation results in rapid rebound thrombocytosis within 7 to 10 days. Due to these factors, scrupulous patient compliance with therapy is necessary. Hydroxyurea has not been demonstrated to be mutagenic to date, although long-term follow-up is necessary to quantify the risk of malignancy in PV.

Since thrombotic events occur more frequently in patients with very high venesection requirements and in patients with a prior thrombotic event, hydroxyurea therapy should be initiated early in young patients with these risk factors.

Patients Above 70 Years of Age

Since elderly patients are at higher risk for thrombotic events, myelosuppression is the primary mode of therapy after acute symptomatology is relieved by phlebotomy. Elderly patients may not tolerate rapid changes in their blood volume, so venesection aliquots of 250 mL are preferable. Intravenous ^{32}P, 2.7 mCi per m² (maximum, 5 mCi per dose) results in a smooth reduction in the red cell mass within 10 weeks in 75% to 85% of treated patients. Complications such as thrombocytopenia and severe anemia are rare and can be managed by the judicious use of blood products. Occasional patients require a second dose at a 25% dose increase if there has not been sufficient reduction in splenomegaly or thrombocytosis within 12 weeks. Therapy should be changed if adequate control cannot be achieved after three doses. Remissions are maintained up to 24 months. Adjuvant phlebotomy to maintain the hematocrit below 45% may be required. The risk of AL after ^{32}P therapy is highest 6 to 10 years after therapy, but the risk is acceptable in this population.

Patients Between 50 and 70 Years of Age

There are no clear-cut guidelines for the treatment of patients in this age group. In the physiologically young patient, phlebotomy is the treatment of choice. Those patients with risk factors for thrombotic complications should be treated with hydroxyurea therapy. Radioactive phosphorus may be the treatment of choice for those patients who cannot tolerate other therapies. The risk of leukemic progression should be weighed against the patient's expected life span.

Other Therapies

Alkylating Agents

Chlorambucil (Leukeran)* is associated with a high rate of secondary malignancy within 5 years of therapy. Use of this agent is no longer recommended for PV. Busulfan (Myleran)* therapy has not been adequately studied in the United States to recommend its use.

Interferon

The use of alfa-interferon in chronic myeloproliferative diseases such as chronic myelogenous leukemia is well documented. The use of alfa-interferon in patients with previously treated PV has now been reported. Dosage is 3×10^6 IU subcutaneously three times per week, which is then tapered to a minimal effective dose, individualized for each patient. More intensive therapy of 3×10^6 IU subcutaneously daily for 6 months has been used. Most patients have normalization of peripheral blood counts, decreased splenomegaly, and resolution of pruritus, bone pain, and hypermetabolic symptoms. Phlebotomy requirements are reduced in most patients and may be eliminated in some. Side effects of myalgia, lethargy, and fever are minimal, with elderly patients most affected. Symptoms resolve with 50% dosage reduction. In those patients followed for more than 1 year who had repeat bone marrow examination, there was no increase in marrow fibrosis over the period of observation. Large trials comparing alfa-interferon with standard therapy to verify the efficacy of this agent have not been reported to date, but the preliminary reports are encouraging.

---

*Not FDA-approved for this indication.

Antiplatelet/Antiaggregating Agents

Addition of aspirin (ASA),* 300 mg three times a day, and dipyridamole (Persantine),* 75 mg three times a day to phlebotomy therapy in a PVSG-sponsored trial did not reduce the incidence of thrombosis. There was an unacceptably high complication rate in the ASA arm, primarily gastrointestinal hemorrhage. Lower-dose aspirin (300 to 325 mg) when the hematocrit is kept below 45% by phlebotomy has been advocated to attempt to decrease the thrombotic complications without increasing the hemorrhagic episodes. There is no consensus at this point, however, whether low-dose aspirin therapy is beneficial in PV.

Ticlopidine (Ticlid),* an antithrombotic agent that primarily affects platelet function, has been evaluated to determine whether it will decrease the thrombotic complications of patients with PV without severe thrombocytosis (platelet count less than 600,000) who have additional thrombotic risk factors such as hyperfibrinogenemia, diabetes mellitus, hypertension, or overt vascular disease. Although the agent decreases the fibrinogen level, blood viscosity was unchanged. The use of this agent is not recommended at this point without further clinical investigation.

Anagrelide† is a compound not yet commercially available that has an antiaggregating effect on platelets and induces thrombocytopenia. Reduction in thrombocytosis has been demonstrated in patients with PV, essential thrombocythemia, and chronic granulocytic leukemia at doses of 1.5 to 4.0 mg per day. The role of this agent in the long-term treatment of PV, however, has not yet been defined.

Pruritus and Gout

One half of patients with PV suffer from intense pruritus exacerbated by bathing and by rough towel drying. Standard antihistamines such as diphenhydramine are of little benefit. Cimetidine (Tagamet),* 300 mg three or four times per day, or cyproheptadine hydrochloride (Periactin), 4 to 16 mg per day, may be beneficial. Cholestyramine (Questran)* is of questionable value to decrease pruritus. The pruritus in PV is not affected by phlebotomy therapy but may be ameliorated by myelosuppressive therapy. Exacerbations occur with relapse of the disease. Interferon therapy may ameliorate or eliminate pruritus in affected patients.

The rapid turnover of hematopoietic cells results in increased urate production. Five percent to 10% of PV patients will develop gout. Presentation is usually atypical, with elbows and ankles affected in a chronic, noninflammatory manner. Therapy with allopurinol (Zyloprim), 100 to 300 mg daily, should then be initiated until remission is attained.

Pregnancy

There is a high incidence of spontaneous abortion and fetal wastage in women with PV, but successful pregnancy can occur. The incidence of preeclampsia is increased, however. Phlebotomy requirements decrease during the course of gestation as blood counts gradually normalize. Delivery is not associated with thrombotic or hemorrhagic complications. Post partum, the hemoglobin will gradually rise, and phlebotomy requirements will resume.

Surgery

Surgical and dental procedures are associated with a high complication rate, primarily hemorrhage and thromboembolism. Hematocrit greater or equal to 52% conveys the highest risk. It is recommended that elective surgery be performed when the patient has been in good hematologic control for at least 4 months. Postoperatively, thrombotic complications can be further reduced by early ambulation.

Spent Phase

There is no recognized curative therapy for the spent myelofibrotic phase of the disease. Postpolycythemic myelofibrosis appears to be more lethal than idiopathic myelofibrosis, with a median survival of 3 years. Treatment guidelines, however, are the same. Asymptomatic patients should be observed. When the patient becomes symptomatic, therapy should be directed to alleviate the specific complaint. If bone marrow failure is the primary problem, androgen therapy with fluoxymesterone (Halotestin), 10 mg three times per day orally, may improve erythropoiesis in those patients with residual ineffective erythropoiesis. Therapy is limited by hepatic dysfunction, congestive heart failure, and virilization.

Pain from splenic enlargement, hypersplenism, or overt hemolytic anemia secondary to splenic enlargement may be the most prominent complaint. Temporary relief may be obtained from low-dose splenic irradiation, 600 to 1000 cGy per fraction. Since the spleen is a site of extramedullary hematopoiesis, pancytopenia may be exacerbated. Peripheral blood counts should be monitored two to three times weekly during therapy. Interferon and hydroxyurea therapy have been beneficial in decreasing the splenomegaly in myelofibrosis. Addition of these agents is beneficial in some patients. Splenectomy is a controversial procedure in these patients. Although the patient may have an improved quality of life postoperatively, the procedure has a substantial surgical risk, with up to 25% mortality. When splenectomy is performed early in the course of myelofibrosis, there has been no appreciable prolongation of life span compared with supportive care. Therefore, splenectomy should be performed when the risk of hypersplenism or hemolysis outweighs the benefit of the spleen as a site of extramedullary hematopoiesis.

Leukemic Transformation

Acute leukemia in PV is usually of myeloid lineage. There may be a period of myelodysplasia, primarily

---

*Not FDA-approved for this indication.

†Investigational drug in the United States.

refractory anemia with excessive blasts, or the spent phase of PV prior to the development to overt leukemia. In general, acute leukemia following PV is unresponsive to chemotherapy, similar to leukemia secondary to chemotherapy or radiotherapy. Current therapeutic regimens using high-dose cytosine arabinoside have induced remission in some patients.

THE PORPHYRIAS

method of
KARL E. ANDERSON, M.D.
*The University of Texas Medical Branch at
    Galveston
Galveston, Texas*

and

ATTALLAH KAPPAS, M.D.
*The Rockefeller University Hospital
New York, New York*

Porphyrias result from deficiencies of enzymes in the heme biosynthetic pathway. This pathway consists of eight enzymes and is most active in bone marrow and liver. Pathway intermediates include the porphyrin precursors δ-aminolevulinic acid and porphobilinogen, and porphyrins (mostly in their reduced forms known as porphyrinogens). These intermediates do not have important physiologic functions or normally accumulate in the body in significant amounts. Heme, on the other hand, is a vital substance for a variety of hemoproteins. The enzyme deficiencies underlying each of the porphyrias are indicated in Table 1. Most porphyrias are inherited, but other factors are important in determining their severity. When porphyrias are clinically expressed, there are striking accumulations of heme pathway intermediates. All inherited porphyrias that have been studied at the molecular level are genetically heterogeneous, and they occur in all races.

Two major types of clinical manifestations occur in porphyrias. *Cutaneous photosensitivity* results from accumulation of porphyrins, which are activated by long-wave ultraviolet light (UV-B) and generate oxygen radicals that damage the skin. *Neurologic effects* occur when the porphyrin precursors δ-aminolevulinic acid and porphobilinogen accumulate. The mechanism of neuron damage is poorly understood. The four types of porphyria in which neurologic manifestations occur are often termed acute porphyrias. Heme pathway intermediates accumulate in some disorders other than porphyria. For example, lead inhibits δ-aminolevulinic acid dehydratase, the second enzyme in the pathway. Succinylacetone, which accumulates in hereditary tyrosinemia, also inhibits this enzyme. Therefore, δ-aminolevulinic acid accumulates in both lead poisoning and tyrosinemia, and both can cause symptoms that resemble acute porphyrias.

This report emphasizes therapies for acute intermittent porphyria, porphyria cutanea tarda, and erythropoietic protoporphyria, the three most common porphyrias. These are likely to be encountered from time to time by any physician. Because these three conditions differ markedly from each other in their major clinical manifestations, exacerbating factors, laboratory testing important for diagnosis, and effective therapies (Table 2), a feature learned about one of them will not apply to the others. For example, there is virtually no similarity in the major therapies for these three conditions. Acute intermittent porphyria and porphyria cutanea tarda do have features in common with some of the other less common porphyrias. Therapy of congenital erythropoietic porphyria, which is very rare, is discussed only briefly.

DIAGNOSIS

Appropriate treatment of the acute porphyrias requires an accurate diagnosis. It is important to maintain a high

TABLE 1. **Enzymes of Heme Biosynthetic Pathway and Classification and Inheritance of Porphyrias**

			Classifications of Porphyrias*			
Enzyme	**Disease**	**Inheritance**	*Hepatic*	*Erythropoietic*	*Acute*	*Cutaneous*
δ-Aminolevulinic acid dehydratase	δ-Aminolevulinic acid dehydratase-deficient porphyria (ADP)	Autosomal recessive	?X		X	
Porphobilinogen deaminase†	Acute intermittent porphyria (AIP)	Autosomal dominant	X		X	
Uroporphyrinogen III cosynthase	Congenital erythropoietic porphyria (CEP)	Autosomal recessive		X		X
Uroporphyrinogen decarboxylase	Porphyria cutanea tarda (PCT)‡	Autosomal dominant	X			X
	Hepatoerythropoietic porphyria (HEP)	Autosomal recessive	X	X		X
Coproporphyrinogen oxidase	Hereditary coproporphyria (HCP)	Autosomal dominant	X		X	X
Protoporphyrinogen oxidase	Variegate porphyria (VP)	Autosomal dominant	X		X	X
Ferrochelatase	Erythropoietic protoporphyria (EPP)	Autosomal dominant		X		X

*The preferred classification is based on the specific enzyme deficiencies. Other classifications refer to the major tissue site of overproduction of heme pathway intermediates (hepatic vs. erythropoietic) or the type of major symptoms (acute neurovisceral or cutaneous).

†This enzyme is also known as hydroxymethylbilane synthase, and formerly was called uroporphyrinogen I synthase.

‡Porphyria cutanea tarda is primarily acquired and is due to one or more factors, such as iron, hepatitis C, excess alcohol, and estrogens. An inherited deficiency of uroporphyrinogen decarboxylase sometimes contributes. In such cases, the disease is termed as familial.

TABLE 2. **The Three Most Common Human Porphyrias and Their Distinctive Major Features**

	Presenting Symptoms	Exacerbating Factors	Test for Screening	Treatment
Acute intermittent porphyria	Neurovisceral (acute)	Drugs (mostly P450-inducers); progesterone; dietary restriction	Urinary porphobilinogen	Heme, glucose
Porphyria cutanea tarda	Blistering skin lesions (chronic)	Iron; alcohol; estrogens; hepatitis C virus; halogenated hydrocarbons	Plasma (or urine) porphyrins	Phlebotomy, low-dose chloroquine
Erythropoietic protoporphyria	Painful skin and swelling (mostly acute)		Plasma (or erythrocyte) porphyrins	β-Carotene

index of suspicion so that the diagnosis is not delayed. A diagnosis of acute porphyria should be *suggested* by neurovisceral signs and symptoms. But the signs and symptoms of these conditions are nonspecific; a diagnosis of acute porphyria must be *established* (or excluded) by laboratory testing. Porphyrin precursor excretion is strikingly increased in all types of acute porphyria during attacks. Skin lesions due to porphyria are also not specific. Plasma porphyrins are increased in patients with concurrent skin lesions due to porphyria, and this laboratory finding is highly specific. Therefore, although the symptoms and signs are nonspecific, it is usually not difficult to establish or exclude a diagnosis of porphyria if urinary porphyrin precursors or plasma porphyrins are measured.

Many laboratory tests are available for diagnosis of porphyria but are frequently overused. Unfortunately, misdiagnosis of porphyria in patients with suggestive symptoms and minimal laboratory abnormalities has become a common problem, and this may lead to inappropriate therapy. For example, heme therapy is much too commonly administered to patients who eventually prove not to have porphyria. Both the misdiagnosis of porphyria and overuse of tests can be avoided using the approach shown in Table 3, which for screening of patients with symptoms emphasizes a few first-line tests that are both specific and sensitive. Second-line tests should be reserved for patients with positive screening tests or with clinically latent porphyria, preferably in consultation with a center with clinical and laboratory expertise in porphyrias. Misinterpretation of second-line tests, including assays for erythrocyte porphobilinogen deaminase and other enzymes and fractionation

of urinary and fecal porphyrins, accounts for many of the mistaken diagnoses of porphyria.

For screening patients with symptoms, the preferred approach is to rely on measurement of *urinary porphyrin precursors (δ-aminolevulinic acid and porphobilinogen)* for patients with neurovisceral symptoms, and a fluorometric measurement of *total plasma porphyrins* when it is suspected that skin photosensitivity might be due to porphyria. Urinary porphobilinogen is always increased during attacks of acute intermittent porphyria, hereditary coproporphyria, and variegate porphyria. Therefore, a normal level effectively excludes these disorders as a cause of current symptoms. Urinary δ-aminolevulinic acid (and coproporphyrin) but not porphobilinogen is increased in δ-aminolevulinic acid dehydratase-deficient porphyria, a very rare form of acute porphyria due to an inherited deficiency of δ-aminolevulinic acid dehydratase. A plasma porphyrin assay is the most sensitive screening test for variegate porphyria, even in latent stages.

TREATMENT OF THE ACUTE ATTACK

Most of the following treatment recommendations apply to acute intermittent porphyria, hereditary coproporphyria, and variegate porphyria. Because very few cases of porphyria due to δ-aminolevulinic acid dehydratase deficiency have been reported, there is little experience with its treatment. Glucose and heme therapy are not uniformly effective in this condition. And although avoidance of drugs that are

TABLE 3. **Laboratory Tests Appropriate for Screening for Porphyria***

Symptoms Suggesting Porphyria	First-Line Test†	Second-Line Tests‡
Acute neurovisceral symptoms	Urinary δ-aminolevulinic acid and porphobilinogen (quantitative; random or 24-hour urine)	Urinary δ-aminolevulinic acid, porphobilinogen and total porphyrins (quantitative; 24 hour urine) Urinary porphyrin fractionation (if total is increased) Total fecal porphyrins (fractionation if total is increased) Erythrocyte porphobilinogen deaminase§ Total porphyrins in plasma (if increased, record wavelength of fluorescence maximum at neutral pH)
Cutaneous photosensitivity	Plasma porphyrins (if increased, record wavelength of fluorescence maximum at neutral pH)	Erythrocyte porphyrins Urinary δ-aminolevulinic acid, porphobilinogen and total porphyrins (quantitative, 24 hour urine) Urinary porphyrin fractionation (if total is increased) Total fecal porphyrins (fractionation if total is increased)

*Depending upon the type of symptoms that suggest the diagnosis.

†Sensitivity and specificity of these tests are high when symptoms suggesting porphyria are present.

‡In patients with acute symptoms, these tests are seldom necessary if the appropriate first-line testing is normal. Most lack sensitivity and/or specificity and are problematic for screening but are useful after a first-line test is positive.

§This enzyme is also known as hydroxymethylbilane synthase. It was formerly known as uroporphyrinogen I synthase, a term still used by many commercial clinical laboratories.

harmful in other acute porphyrias is prudent, it is not known whether this is helpful.

General and Supportive Treatment Measures. Attacks of porphyria are often severe and require hospitalization. Adequate doses of narcotic analgesics are given for pain, which is characteristically severe and is most commonly in the abdomen and extremities but also occurs in the back, chest, and other areas. Chlorpromazine (Thorazine) or another phenothiazine is administered, usually in small doses and for short periods of time, for nausea, vomiting, anxiety, and restlessness. Large doses of phenothiazines (as used for treating acute psychiatric conditions) may produce unpleasant side effects in acute porphyria patients. Acute intermittent porphyria is listed as a specific treatment indication for chlorpromazine in United States labeling, at a suggested dosage of 25 to 50 mg by mouth (or 25 mg intramuscularly) three or four times a day for several weeks, with maintenance therapy required for some patients. But in our experience, considerably smaller dosages are effective for acute attacks, and maintenance therapy is rarely indicated unless there are continuing psychiatric symptoms. Phenothiazines do not specifically address the underlying pathophysiology or reduce the overproduction of porphyrin precursors in acute porphyria.

Chloral hydrate can be given for insomnia. Diazepam and other commonly used benzodiazepines in low doses are probably safe if a minor tranquilizer is required. Observation for neurologic complications and electrolyte imbalances is important. Hyponatremia is sometimes due to inappropriate antidiuretic hormone (ADH) secretion, but gastrointestinal or renal fluid and electrolyte losses are sometimes the major cause.

Glucose loading is considered a specific form of therapy for an acute attack, as discussed next, but if nausea, vomiting, or ileus precludes oral intake for a prolonged period, a more complete nutritional regimen, including intravenous vitamins, lipids, and amino acids should be considered. The safety and efficacy of different parenteral nutrition regimens have not been studied in porphyria. High dietary fat intakes may increase porphyrin precursor excretion in acute porphyria, and high-protein diets can induce hepatic cytochrome P450 enzymes and thereby stimulate porphyrin-heme synthesis. Therefore, it may be prudent to limit the amounts of fat and protein in the intravenous regimen to basic requirements.

Response to treatment is facilitated by identifying and removing inciting factors, such as harmful drugs, and by correcting nutritional deficiencies. Cyclic attacks in women during the luteal phase of the menstrual cycle usually resolve with the onset of menses.

Specific Therapies. Heme therapy and carbohydrate loading are considered specific therapies for acute attacks of porphyria because they repress hepatic δ-aminolevulinic acid synthase, the rate-limiting enzyme of the heme biosynthetic pathway, and thereby reduce the overproduction of excess amounts of porphyrin precursors. Heme therapy is much more effective in this regard than glucose. Intravenous glucose (at least 400 grams daily) is recommended for patients hospitalized with attacks of porphyria. Neither intravenous glucose nor heme therapy has been studied adequately with regard to clinical efficacy in controlled trials. However, extensive clinical experience strongly supports their efficacy.

Mild attacks may respond to glucose alone. It was previously recommended that heme therapy be started only after there was no response to intravenous glucose for several days. However, heme therapy is now often started without an initial trial of glucose alone, especially for a severe attack. Delaying heme therapy favors progression of neuronal damage and slows recovery. Advanced neurologic damage and subacute or chronic symptoms of porphyria often show no clear response to heme therapy.

Heme Preparations for Treatment of Porphyria. Heme (iron protoporphyrin IX) is insoluble at neutral pH but can be prepared as hematin (heme hydroxide) for intravenous infusion at pH 8. A lyophilized hematin preparation is marketed in the United States for treatment of porphyria (Panhematin, Abbott).* Hematin solutions are unstable. Degradation products form rapidly when hematin is reconstituted with sterile water as recommended in the product labeling, and these bind to endothelial cells, platelets, and clotting factors and cause transient anticoagulant effects and phlebitis at the site of infusion. These occur commonly even when hematin is infused promptly. Loss of venous access is common in patients who develop phlebitis from repeated courses of hematin. Particularly if hematin is infused into a peripheral vein, we recommend that it be reconstituted with human albumin,† even though this adds intravascular volume-expanding effects and increases the cost. This procedure stabilizes the heme as heme albumin, harmful degradation products do not form, and anticoagulant effects and phlebitis are prevented. Uncommonly reported side effects of hematin, some of which may also be prevented with albumin, include fever, aching, malaise, hemolysis, and circulatory collapse. Excretion of hematin in urine and acute renal tubular damage occur only with excessive doses.

Heme arginate‡ (an incompletely characterized preparation of heme and arginine) is available in some countries other than the United States and is the preferred heme preparation for intravenous administration. Heme arginate is an investigational drug for treatment and prevention of acute porphyric

---

*This product has a shelf life of 3 months and is usually special-ordered from the manufacturer by phone (1-800-255-5162) and shipped overnight to the treatment site for each treatment course.

†Hematin for injection can be reconstituted with albumin as described by Bonkovsky (Bonkovsky HL, Healey BS, Lourie AN, Gerron GG: Am J Gastroenterol 1991;*86*:1050–1056). To do this, add 132 mL of 25% human serum albumin to a vial of Panhematin (instead of 43 mL of sterile water). The volume required to deliver the desired dose should then be calculated based on this volume.

‡Investigational drug in the United States.

attacks at any location in the United States.* It may eventually become the most widely used preparation for heme therapy. The considerably longer shelf life of heme arginate (2 years, versus 3 months for lyophilized hematin) should greatly enhance the availability of heme therapy for prompt treatment of acute porphyric attacks. Phlebitis is reported much less often with heme arginate than with hematin. When heme arginate is infused intravenously, the heme becomes bound to circulating hemopexin and albumin. Therefore, hematin, heme albumin, and heme arginate do not differ in regard to distribution in vivo or apparent efficacy. Another investigational approach is to combine heme therapy with an inhibitor of heme breakdown, such as Sn-protoporphyrin, to prolong the efficacy of the administered heme.

Heme is effective for treatment of acute porphyric attacks when infused as a single dose of 3 mg per kg daily for 4 days, if treatment is initiated early. There is no definite evidence that continuing beyond 4 days is beneficial, even when the start of treatment was delayed. However, for severe or prolonged attacks, it is reasonable to continue heme infusion for up to 7 days and sometimes at 2- to 3-day intervals thereafter until there are clear signs of recovery. Porphobilinogen levels in urine or serum are generally reduced to normal levels within 2 to 3 days of starting heme therapy and may be monitored to document biochemical response during more prolonged treatment. However a biochemical response to heme therapy is not necessarily predictive of clinical response. For example, if heme therapy is delayed, there may be a good biochemical response, but rapid recovery is less likely because nerve damage is more advanced.

Heme therapy is not effective for conditions other than acute porphyrias and perhaps a few other closely related conditions. Unfortunately, it has become increasingly common for patients to be misdiagnosed as having porphyria and treated unnecessarily with heme. Therefore, it is appropriate to begin heme therapy only when the diagnosis of an acute porphyria is established by demonstrating a marked increase in urinary porphobilinogen. This can be accomplished promptly by qualitative or preferably quantitative measurement of porphobilinogen, such that heme therapy can be initiated within 24 hours. Because porphyrin precursors in plasma and urine fall promptly and dramatically after heme administration, the diagnosis of acute porphyria is more difficult during and for several days after heme therapy.

Other Therapies. Those sometimes used for acute attacks include β-adrenergic blocking agents to control tachycardia and hypertension. Nonspecific membrane effects rather than β-adrenergic blockade account for the effects of propranolol in reducing experimentally induced porphyrias in animals. Propranolol (Inderal)† probably does not hasten recovery from acute attacks in humans. Propranolol may even be hazardous in patients with hypovolemia and incipient cardiac failure, because it may interfere with the effects of increased catecholamines that can represent an important compensatory mechanism. Numerous other therapies, including zinc,* EDTA (Endrate),* adenosine monophosphate (Adenocard), vitamin E,* folic acid,* hemodialysis, and hemoperfusion, have been tried in this disease but are not generally regarded as effective. EDTA may have unwanted effects on the heme biosynthetic pathway. Sorbents have been shown to bind porphyrin precursors in vitro but have been little studied in vivo.

Treatment of seizures in patients with acute porphyria is problematic, because virtually all antiseizure drugs (except bromides) have at least some potential for exacerbating acute porphyria. Some patients with both idiopathic epilepsy and porphyria sometimes must be treated with antiseizure medications that can worsen porphyria. Clonazepam may be less harmful than phenytoin or barbiturates.

PREVENTION OF ACUTE ATTACKS

Prevention measures are highly effective in most patients who have had acute attacks. Because multiple harmful factors usually have contributed to exacerbations of porphyria in a given patient, a broad approach to prevention is important. These include avoiding harmful drugs. Lists of safe and harmful drugs are available.† However, the effects of many drugs on porphyria are not known. Because dietary indiscretions may be inapparent unless a careful dietary history is taken, consultation with a dietitian may be useful. If body weight is near normal, patients should be advised to follow a well-balanced diet with sufficient calories to maintain weight. The diet can be somewhat high in carbohydrate (60% to 70% of total calories). There is little evidence that if such a diet is followed, consumption of additional dietary carbohydrate helps further in preventing attacks. Patients who wish to lose excess weight should do so gradually and when they are clinically stable. They can be instructed on a diet that provides about 10% fewer calories than what is required to maintain weight and should understand that this will result in gradual weight loss over a period of months. Iron deficiency should be corrected because it might impair hepatic heme synthesis.

Attacks of acute porphyria that are clearly related to the menstrual cycle are usually premenstrual and due to high circulating levels of progesterone during the luteal phase of the cycle. If these are occurring frequently, they can be prevented by administration of a gonadotropin-releasing hormone (GnRH) ana-

---

*Contact Karl E. Anderson, M.D., at the University of Texas Medical Branch, Galveston, Texas (409-772-4661) for information about enrollment in these studies.

†Not FDA-approved for this indication.

---

*Not FDA-approved for this indication.

†Drug lists and information regarding drugs not on current lists can be obtained through the American Porphyria Foundation, PO Box 22712, Houston, Texas 77227 (713-266-9617). The Foundation has brochures about porphyrias, publishes a newsletter, and may refer specific inquiries regarding drug safety and methods for diagnosis and treatment to academic medical centers that specialize in clinical porphyrias.

logue. This is not immediately effective if ovulation has already occurred or if a premenstrual attack is already in progress. Attacks partially associated with the menstrual cycle are less effectively prevented. If there is a good response to a GnRH analogue for several months, low oral or transdermal doses of estradiol can be added to control adverse effects of low endogenous estrogens, without exacerbating porphyria. A GnRH analogue is seldom needed for longer than 1 to 3 years, which suggests that cyclic attacks do not occur throughout the reproductive period of life in women with porphyria. Because this and other treatment options are available, oophorectomy is not an acceptable option for preventing cyclic attacks.

Exogenous estrogens, progestins, and androgens given alone or in combination have prevented cyclical attacks in some women with porphyria. However, such steroids sometimes worsen the disease. Synthetic steroids with an ethynyl substituent are potentially harmful in porphyria on theoretical grounds and should probably be avoided. Danazol is definitely contraindicated.

Limited experience suggests that cyclic attacks can also be prevented by heme therapy given at weekly intervals, or at intervals of several days during the luteal phase of the cycle. Hematin is approved in the United States for prevention as well as treatment of acute attacks of porphyria, but no particular regimen is widely recommended. Studies of heme arginate to prevent attacks are underway using once- or twice-weekly infusions.

Congenital Erythropoietic Porphyria

This very rare autosomal recessive disorder is due to a deficiency of uroporphyrinogen III cosynthase. Intramedullary hemolysis and shortened survival of circulating erythrocytes are caused by porphyrins that are produced and accumulate in bone marrow erythroid cells that are actively synthesizing hemoglobin. Splenomegaly can contribute to anemia and cause leukopenia and thrombocytopenia. In most cases, reddish urine and severe cutaneous photosensitivity are noted in early infancy, but the disease may present before birth as nonimmune hydrops. In some cases symptoms began in adult life. Blistering skin lesions resemble those in porphyria cutanea tarda but are usually more severe and are prone to rupture and infection. Loss of digits and facial features can then result. Porphyrins are deposited in the teeth (producing a reddish-brown color termed "erythrodontia") and in bone. Life expectancy is often shortened by infections or hematologic complications.

Protection of the skin from sunlight and minor trauma and prompt treatment of secondary bacterial infections help prevent scarring and mutilation. Blood transfusions sufficient to suppress erythropoiesis may be the most effective treatment. Improvement may occur after splenectomy. Oral charcoal may be helpful by increasing fecal excretion of porphyrins. In affected families, heterozygotes with intermediate deficiencies of the cosynthase can be detected. The disease can be diagnosed in utero. Therefore, there are options for preventing genetic transmission.

Porphyria Cutanea Tarda

Porphyria cutanea tarda is the most common porphyria and also the most readily treated. It is fundamentally an acquired disorder and is due to a deficiency of uroporphyrinogen decarboxylase in the liver. In some cases an inherited deficiency of this enzyme is a predisposing factor. Blistering lesions develop on sun-exposed skin and are the major clinical feature. Chronic liver disease and hepatocellular carcinoma are more long-term complications.

Acquired factors lead to inactivation of hepatic uroporphyrinogen decarboxylase by an oxidative mechanism that requires hepatic iron. Cytochrome P450 enzymes may be involved in the oxidation of the porphyrinogen substrates for the enzyme. Alcohol intake may promote iron absorption, stimulate hepatic heme and porphyrin synthesis, or generate free radicals that damage the decarboxylase. Estrogens, but apparently not other steroids, can exacerbate this condition, perhaps by an unknown oxidative mechanism. A recently described strong association with chronic hepatitis C virus infection suggests that hepatocellular damage induced by this virus, which appears to be accentuated by iron, can involve specific cellular proteins including uroporphyrinogen decarboxylase.

A course of phlebotomies is the preferred treatment and almost always produces a remission. Patients are also advised to discontinue alcohol, estrogens, iron supplements, or other contributing factors. Because iron stores in porphyria cutanea tarda are seldom markedly increased and may be normal, removal of a total of only 5 to 6 units of blood, each at 1- to 2-week intervals, is usually sufficient. Plasma (or serum) ferritin and porphyrin levels should be followed. Ferritin decreases more rapidly than porphyrin levels. Phlebotomies should be stopped when the serum ferritin concentration is near the lower limit of normal. Further iron depletion is of no additional benefit and may cause anemia and associated symptoms. Remission occurs after plasma porphyrin levels return to normal and may be prolonged even if the ferritin level increases at a later time. In some cases a relapse occurs and responds to another course of phlebotomy. Deferoxamine, an iron chelator, may be effective but is much less efficient than phlebotomy.

A course of low-dose chloroquine (Aralen)* (e.g., 125 mg twice weekly for several months or as needed) or hydroxychloroquine (Plaquenil)* is usually effective when repeated phlebotomies are contraindicated. The mechanism of their effects in this condition is not established. One hypothesis is that chloroquine forms complexes with porphyrins and

---

*Not FDA-approved for this indication.

promotes their removal from the liver. Chloroquine given in usual doses to porphyria cutanea tarda patients can cause nausea, malaise, fever, and hepatocellular damage, as well as marked increases in photosensitivity and in porphyrin levels in plasma and urine. Although these adverse effects are generally transient and are followed by complete remission, it is prudent to avoid them by employing a low-dose regimen.

Therapy is more difficult when porphyria cutanea tarda occurs with advanced renal disease because phlebotomy is usually contraindicated by anemia (usually due to erythropoietin deficiency). Recent studies indicate that genetic recombinant erythropoietin can mobilize excess iron, support phlebotomy, and lead to remission of porphyria cutanea tarda in these patients.

Phlebotomy and low-dose chloroquine are specific therapies for porphyria cutanea tarda and are not effective for other types of porphyria. For example, even though the skin lesions that develop in some patients with variegate porphyria and hereditary coproporphyria are identical to those seen in porphyria cutanea tarda, patients do not improve with these therapies.

Erythropoietic Protoporphyria

This autosomal dominant condition is due to a deficiency of ferrochelatase, the final enzyme in the heme biosynthetic pathway. Ferrochelatase is deficient in all tissues in this disease but becomes rate-limiting for protoporphyrin metabolism primarily in bone marrow. Some obligate carriers have little or no increase in red cell protoporphyrin. Individuals with clinically expressed disease accumulate excess protoporphyrin in erythroid cells, plasma, bile, and feces. Bone marrow reticulocytes are the primary source of the excess protoporphyrin. The cutaneous manifestations usually begin in childhood and are distinctly different from those of other porphyrias. Burning, itching, erythema, and swelling can occur within minutes of sun exposure. Diffuse edema of sun-exposed areas may resemble angioneurotic edema. Vesicles, scarring, and skin findings characteristic of other cutaneous porphyrias seldom occur in protoporphyria. There also are no neuropathic manifestations except in some patients with severe hepatic complications. The diagnosis is established by finding excess protoporphyrin in erythrocytes, plasma, bile, and feces; urinary porphyrins and porphyrin precursors are normal. A minority of patients with protoporphyria develop liver disease, which is often preceded by increasing levels of erythrocyte and plasma protoporphyrin, abnormal liver function tests, marked deposition of protoporphyrin in liver cells and bile canaliculi, and increased photosensitivity. Hepatic complications can progress rapidly to death from liver failure. Excess protoporphyrin itself may have cholestatic effects and damage hepatocytes. Intercurrent factors such as viral hepatitis, alcohol, iron deficiency, fasting, and oral contraceptive steroids have played a role in some patients.

Treatment with β-carotene is beneficial to many patients with erythropoietic protoporphyria. Improvement is usually maximal 1 to 3 months after initiation of treatment. β-Carotene doses of 120 to 180 mg daily in adults will usually achieve serum carotene levels in the recommended range of 600 to 800 μg/dL, but sometimes doses up to 300 mg daily are needed. Suntanning resulting from better tolerance of sunlight may lead to further protection. Mild, dose-related skin discoloration due to carotenemia may occur. The mechanism of action of β-carotene is not fully established but may involve quenching of singlet oxygen or free radicals. The drug appears less effective in other forms of porphyria associated with photosensitivity, such as congenital erythropoietic porphyria and porphyria cutanea tarda. Oral cysteine,* which may also quench excited oxygen species, is currently being investigated for treatment of this disease. Topical dihydroxyacetone and lawsone (napthoquinone)* can darken the skin and thereby partially block exposure of the dermis to light and be of some benefit in erythropoietic protoporphyria. Cholestyramine may reduce protoporphyrin levels by interrupting its enterohepatic circulation. Iron deficiency, caloric restriction, and drugs or hormone preparations that impair hepatic excretory function should be avoided.

Hepatic complications may be life-threatening but can resolve spontaneously if a reversible cause of liver dysfunction, such as viral hepatitis or alcohol, is contributing. Transfusions or heme therapy may suppress erythroid and hepatic protoporphyrin production and contribute to improvement. Splenectomy, correction of iron deficiency, and cholestyramine or activated charcoal may be beneficial. Liver transplantation is sometimes required to prevent death from progressive hepatic failure.

ACKNOWLEDGMENTS

Preparation of this chapter was supported in part by grants from the United States Food and Drug Administration Office of Orphan Product Development (FD-R-000710), the American Porphyria Foundation, and the National Center for Research Resources, National Institutes of Health (MO1 RR-00073).

---

*Investigational drug in the United States.

THERAPEUTIC USE OF BLOOD COMPONENTS

method of
PAULA LUTZ, M.D., and
WALTER DZIK, M.D.
Deaconess Hospital
Boston, Massachusetts

Effective component therapy is the successful blend of art and science. General criteria have been established for the transfusion of packed red blood cells (RBCs), fresh-frozen plasma (FFP), platelets (PLTs), and cryoprecipitate (CRY). However, decisions to transfuse must be evaluated individually. Laboratory values, such as hematocrit (Hct), platelet count, prothrombin time (PT), and partial thromboplastin time (PTT), should not be interpreted in isolation. Various questions must be asked to determine the appropriate transfusion trigger for each patient. The questions include (1) *Is the patient actively bleeding?* If so, is the bleeding diffuse (suggestive of a coagulopathy) or localized (suggestive of a fixed lesion)? A local measure may be the sole therapy needed to treat local bleeding. For example, a well-placed suture could halt oozing from a central line site in a patient with fulminant hepatic failure without the need for FFP transfusion. However, the transfusion of FFP would be appropriate if the same patient had diffuse gastrointestinal bleeding or oozing from a well-sutured central line site.

(2) *Is the patient awaiting a procedure?* Preprocedure transfusions of PLTs, FFP, or CRY should be evaluated by the potential bleeding risk per procedure. A vascular procedure (such as a major surgical procedure or the placement of a central line) may warrant the transfusion of FFP to increase coagulation factors to an acceptable level in a patient with a markedly prolonged PT. A nonvascular procedure (such as a paracentesis) should not require pretreatment. Preprocedure transfusions given to patients with mild prolongation of the PT or moderate depression of the platelet count are of little or no value and should be avoided. Certain surgical procedures require a more stringent degree of hemostasis. A platelet count of $50,000/\mu L$ in a patient with multiple myeloma would be acceptable for an appendectomy but inadequate for a neurosurgical procedure.

(3) *Does the patient have a coexisting medical illness that would affect the transfusion trigger?* For example, the presence of severe coronary artery disease in an anemic man might warrant the early transfusion of RBCs as a means to avoid cardiac ischemia.

(4) *Are there alternatives to transfusion?* A minimally symptomatic patient with a chronic megaloblastic anemia from vitamin B_{12} deficiency could be safely treated with vitamin B_{12} injections alone without the need for RBC transfusion.

(5) *Has the patient given informed consent to the transfusion?* As discussed later, the patient must be informed of and agree to the treatment plan using transfusions. The following pages should provide a framework to aid in the decision analysis on the appropriate transfusion of RBCs, PLTs, FFP, and CRY. Additionally, general or patient-specific questions should be directed to the blood bank staff (medical technologists and transfusion medicine physicians) who serve as a valuable resource on patient component therapy.

RBC transfusion is indicated to increase RBC mass and therefore improve tissue oxygenation in a symptomatic anemic patient (Table 1). The patient may manifest signs and symptoms of anemia such as tachycardia, hypotension, breathlessness, or dyspnea on exertion. Additionally, the anemic patient may show symptoms of impending organ ischemia, such as the onset of angina. The transfusion trigger for RBC transfusion should take into account the aforementioned signs and symptoms of the anemia, along with the tempo (acute versus chronic) of the anemia. For example, patients with chronic anemia may be acceptable candidates for the use of RBC transfusion alternatives, such as erythropoietin to treat the anemia of chronic renal failure. In the acute setting, patients who have lost less than 20% of their blood volume from active bleeding usually do not require RBC support. Moreover, RBC transfusions are not indicated as a source of volume replacement in patients with adequate oxygen delivery. Preoperative autologous blood donation may be an option for some patients, particularly those awaiting orthopedic or cardiovascular surgery. Intraoperative alternatives to allogeneic RBC transfusion include the use of intraoperative blood salvage, or isovolemic hemodilution.

PLT transfusions are indicated to increase the functional platelet mass as a treatment of active bleeding from thrombocytopenia or a qualitative platelet defect (Table 2). In these settings, increased surgical bleeding may be seen or "platelet-type bleeding" such as the development of petechiae or bleeding from the mucosal surfaces of the oral pharynx, nose, and gastrointestinal or urinary tract. Great care should be used in determining the appropriateness of PLT transfusions. PLT transfusions are beneficial to treat bleeding from the dilutional thrombocytopenia of massive transfusion. Also, the qualitative platelet defect that develops during cardiopulmonary bypass may improve with PLT transfusion. PLT transfusions should not be given to patients who fail to respond. To evaluate responsiveness, a platelet count can be obtained as quickly as 15 to 30 minutes post-transfu-

---

TABLE 1. Red Blood Cell Transfusion

Effect	Increase RBC mass and O_2-carrying capacity	
ABO requirements	*Recipient*	*Donor*
	A	A or O
	B	B or O
	AB	A, B, AB, O
	O	O
	Unknown (emergency)	O (non–cross-matched)
Time to prepare	Type and screen:	60 minutes
	Cross-match:	5–60 minutes
Typical orders	1. Type and screen and cross-match 'x' units	
	2. Transfuse 'x' RBCs each over 2 h	
	3. Check Hct 30 min post-transfusion (expect 3-point Hct rise per unit in adult)	
Modifications	Leukodepleted	
	CMV-seronegative	
	Irradiated	
	Washed	
	Frozen-deglycerolized	
	Antigen-negative	

TABLE 2. **Platelet Transfusion**

Effect	Increase functional platelet mass
Volume	250–330 mL per 6-unit pool; 300 mL per apheresis bag (= 6–8 units)
ABO requirements	Recipient's RBCs ideally ABO-compatible with donor plasma (not required)
	Rh-negative recipients ideally receive Rh-negative PLTs (not required)
Time to prepare	Pooling: 15 minutes
Typical orders	1. Type and screen
	2. Transfuse 6 units PLTs over 30 min
	3. Check platelet count 30 min post-transfusion (expect 5000–10,000 platelet rise per unit)
Modifications	Leukodepleted
	CMV-seronegative
	Irradiated
	HLA-matched
	Cross-match compatible
	Antigen-negative

sion to determine whether there has been an adequate platelet increment (each unit of platelets should increase the platelet count by 5000 to 10,000/μL).

Consumptive states such as disseminated intravascular coagulation (DIC), immune thrombocytopenic purpura (ITP), and thrombocytopenia from hypersplenism often have a poor post-transfusion platelet increment. Transfused platelets also will not correct the qualitative platelet defect of uremia. PLT transfusions are considered to fuel the thrombotic state of thrombotic thrombocytopenic purpura (TTP) and heparin-associated thrombocytopenia with thrombosis, and therefore their use is absolutely contraindicated in these diseases. Caution should also be used when deciding to give prophylactic PLT transfusions to prevent spontaneous bleeding. Previously, PLT transfusions were given to stable patients with leukemia to maintain a platelet count of more than 20,000/μL. This practice was based on few scientific data and is no longer warranted. The decision to transfuse PLTs before a procedure should be evaluated by the type of procedure (vascular versus nonvascular) planned. A poor post-transfusion platelet increment is also seen in women who have become HLA-alloimmunized through previous pregnancies. The presence of HLA alloimmunization may require the transfusion of HLA-matched or cross-match-compatible PLTs. Many platelet disorders are best treated by the use of alternatives to PLT transfusions. For example, qualitative platelet defects (such as mild type I von Willebrand's disease or the defect of uremia) may respond well to the use of DDAVP with its release of Factor VIII and von Willebrand's factor (vWF) from endothelial cells. TTP is best treated with plasma exchange. Patients with quantitative platelet defects (such as postchemotherapy or in ITP) have been found to have decreased bleeding when treated with antifibrinolytics. Intravenous immunoglobulin, intravenous Rh$_0$(D) immune globulin, steroids, and splenectomy are acceptable alternatives for the treatment of immune thrombocytopenic purpura (ITP).

FFP transfusion is indicated to treat a variety of factor deficiencies, particularly in the setting of active bleeding (Table 3). By definition, 1 mL of plasma from a normal donor contains 1 unit of any coagulation factor. As a result of the volume of distribution of coagulation factors, each unit of FFP should raise coagulation factor levels by 5% to 10% in an adult. Most isolated factor deficiencies (involving Factors II, V, VII, IX, X, and XI) are treated with FFP transfusion. Hemophilia A is best treated with Factor VIII concentrate. FFP transfusion is also used to treat multiple factor deficiencies, such as seen in hepatic failure, DIC, and the dilution of massive transfusion. Caution should be exercised in the use of FFP simply to correct prolonged coagulation times. The PT and PTT are often mildly prolonged by factor deficiencies that are not associated with impaired in vivo hemostasis. Patients with more extreme coagulation factor deficiencies, such as seen with a PT greater than two times control, may be suitable candidates for FFP transfusion prior to a vascular procedure. A factor activity of 50% is usually the aim for major surgery. FFP transfusion will rapidly reverse the effects of warfarin. However, vitamin K will reverse the effects of warfarin within 8 hours and is an acceptable alternative if time permits. Antithrombin deficiency, whether congenital or resulting from hepatic failure or heparin use, may be treated with FFP transfusion. Antithrombin concentrate is also available as an alternative. FFP transfusion is not indicated for volume expansion, nutritional source of protein, or source of gammaglobulin.

CRY is a concentrate of high-molecular-weight proteins (Factor VIII, Factor XIII, vWF, fibrinogen) that precipitate when FFP is thawed at 4° C (Table 4). There are limited indications for the use of CRY. CRY transfusion is indicated for the correction of Factor VIII and XIII deficiencies, although specific Factor VIII concentrate remains the treatment of choice for hemophilia A. The high levels of vWF in CRY make it an excellent treatment for von Willebrand's disease and to treat the bleeding associated with the uremic

TABLE 3. **Fresh-Frozen Plasma Transfusion**

Effect	Source of clotting Factors I–XIII, antithrombin	
Volume	225 mL	
ABO requirements	*Recipient*	*Donor*
	A	A or AB
	B	B or AB
	AB	AB
	O	AB, AB, O
Time to prepare	Thawing: 30 minutes	
Typical orders	1. Type and screen	
	2. Transfuse 'x' units FFP each over 30 min	
	3. Check labs as indicated 30 min post-transfusion; consider PT, PTT, factor levels, antithrombin	
Modifications	Solvent detergent–treated FFP (virally inactivated)	

TABLE 4. **Cryoprecipitate Transfusion**

Effect	Source of Factors VIII and XIII, vWF, fibrinogen
Volume	250 mL per 10 units pooled
ABO requirements	Recipient's RBCs ideally ABO-compatible with donor plasma (not required)
Time to prepare	Thawing and pooling: 45 min
Typical orders	1. Type and screen 2. Transfuse 10 units CRY over 30 min 3. Check labs as indicated 30 min post-transfusion; consider Factor VIII, vWF, fibrinogen
Modifications	None

platelet disorder. As a source of fibrinogen, CRY is useful to treat congenital fibrinogen deficiencies or the acquired deficiency associated with hepatic failure and fibrinolysis. CRY is also used with thrombin as a topical hemostatic agent known as fibrin glue. A fibrin mesh is formed when thrombin converts the CRY fibrinogen to fibrin. Fibrin glue is used in dental surgery to control gum bleeding, during cardiothoracic surgery to control serosal bleeding, and as an aid to close enterocutaneous fistulas.

Informed consent is required prior to transfusion, and the discussion should be documented in the patient's chart. The patient-physician discussion should include the *indications* for transfusion and the potential *benefits* and *risks*. *Alternatives* to transfusion should also be discussed, such as the use of erythropoietin for the anemia of renal failure. Generally, competent adults have the right to refuse transfusion. Special circumstances may apply to pregnant women or to a parent of a minor child, however. *Directed donor* blood donations (from donors selected by the patient) have been found to be no safer than blood from regular community donors, and the use of directed donors is generally discouraged unless medically indicated (such as the use of a sibling's blood for a patient with a rare blood type).

Numerous steps are necessary to ensure a successful transfusion. It is paramount that blood bank samples be drawn by qualified individuals who correctly identify the intended recipient and the blood sample. Two common physician orders are *"type and screen"* or *"type and cross-match."* A *type* determines the patient's blood group via a front type (antigens on the RBC) and a back type (antibodies in the serum). For example, a patient's samples with no A or B antigens on the RBC but with anti-A and anti-B in the serum is classified as group O. A *screen* looks for RBC alloantibodies or autoantibodies in the patient's serum over various incubations. A type and screen order is the appropriate way to request that blood be generally available for a patient. If the patient has no history of RBC alloantibodies and has a current negative screen, an abbreviated *cross-match* may be performed using a serum sample that is less than 3 days old. If the patient has a current or past history of a clinically significant RBC alloantibody, a longer cross-match using Coombs' reagent (anti-IgG) must be performed.

A "type and cross-match" should be ordered when a specific number of RBCs are expected to be transfused. For surgical cases, the number of RBCs cross-matched is usually based on the blood usage per procedure as listed in the maximum surgical blood ordering schedule (MSBOS). For example, in many programs 10 units of RBCs are cross-matched automatically for patients requiring mitral valve replacement. A type and screen is performed for operative cases in which blood usage is unlikely, such as a cholecystectomy. Follow-up *laboratory tests* should be performed after the transfusion of RBCs, FFP, PLTs, or CRY to determine the adequacy of treatment. For example, a lack of an increment to platelet transfusion may indicate HLA alloimmunization that would require the use of HLA-matched apheresis PLTs or cross-matched apheresis PLTs.

Modern day transfusion relies on *component therapy*. Whole blood is separated into components (RBCs, FFP, PLTs) within 8 hours of being drawn from volunteer donors. Each component has different storage requirements and expiration dates. RBCs are best stored at 4° C for 35 to 42 days (as determined by the anticoagulant-preservative solution), FFP and CRY at −18° C for 1 year, and PLTs at 24° C for 5 days. Glycerolized frozen RBCs may be stored at −65° to −120°C for up to 10 years. Rare antigen-negative RBCs are often stored frozen as a ready supply for patients with RBC alloantibodies. The expiration date of a component may change as the component is prepared for transfusion. FFP has an expiration date of 24 hours once thawed, and PLTs have an expiration date of 4 hours once pooled. *Time* is required to prepare components for transfusion and varies according to whether a cross-match (abbreviated or full) is needed or the component is to be thawed or pooled. If RBCs are needed emergently, *non–cross-matched group O RBCs* may be released from the blood bank while the type and screen or cross-match is ongoing.

Premedication with acetaminophen and diphenhydramine hydrochloride prior to transfusion was previously the standard to modify various transfusion reactions. Currently, many transfusion reactions can be prevented through *component modification* without the need for pretreatment. The *washing* of RBCs and PLTs removes plasma and may be indicated for patients with IgA deficiency and anti-IgA antibodies or for patients with recurrent severe allergic reactions to transfusion. RBCs and PLTs may also be rendered *leukodepleted* by filtration to prevent febrile transfusion reactions or primary HLA alloimmunization. Patients requiring prolonged platelet support, such as those with leukemia, often receive leukodepleted components. The prevention of transfusion-transmitted cytomegalovirus (CMV) infection may be done with the use of leukodepleted cellular components or components from CMV-seronegative donors. Transfusion-transmitted CMV infection is a concern for transfusions given in utero or to very-low-birthweight neonates, to CMV-negative HIV-positive patients, and to CMV-negative recipients of CMV-negative transplants (bone marrow, liver, heart and/or lung, and kidney). Transfusion-related graft-versus-host disease (TR-GVHD) may be prevented by the gamma *irradiation* of RBCs and PLTs. Immunocompromised patients at risk for TR-GVHD include those receiving intrauterine transfusions or who carry the diagnosis of congenital immunodeficiencies, aggressive non-Hodgkin's lymphoma, Hodgkin's disease (or history of), acute leukemia, or those receiving a bone marrow transplant. Patients who are HIV positive do not routinely receive irradiated components. Cellular components transfused to an immunocompetent blood relative should also be irradiated due to the risk of TR-GVHD in HLA-related kindreds.

ADVERSE REACTIONS TO BLOOD TRANSFUSION

method of
ROBERT G. WESTPHAL, M.D.,
MARK A. POPOVSKY, M.D., and
E. MARY O'NEILL, M.D.

American Red Cross Blood Services
Dedham, Massachusetts

Adverse reactions to blood occur in 1% to 3% of transfusions, more frequently in hematology and oncology patients. The transmission of infectious diseases will not be discussed except to note that:

1. Bacterial contamination of room temperature–stored platelets is currently the greatest infectious risk from transfusion; although fatal reactions have been documented, the incidence, though unknown, is estimated at 1:4000 to 12,000.
2. The risk of acquisition of human immunodeficiency virus, hepatitis B, or hepatitis C from a blood component is currently estimated to be 1:425,000, 1:200,000, and 1:2000–6000 respectively:
3. Transmission of malaria, Chagas' disease, or babesiosis is unusual in North America, but measurable.

Transfusion reactions may be caused by immunologic, chemical, allergic, mechanical, physical, or infectious means and may be further divided into acute or delayed categories (Table 1).

IMMUNOLOGIC MECHANISMS

Acute Hemolytic Transfusion Reaction. Acute hemolytic transfusion reactions (AHTRs) are almost always due to ABO incompatibility, although there have been reports implicating acquired alloantibodies, such as Rhesus (Rh) or Kidd (Jk[a]). Almost all of these are due to preventable clerical errors and typically occur when a group O patient receives non-group O red cells. These reactions are often severe and life threatening, due to rapid hemolysis of red blood cells. Complement-fixing antibodies and cytokine release cause acute intravascular hemolysis,

TABLE 1. **Adverse Effects of Transfusion of Blood Components**

	Acute	Delayed
Immune	Acute hemolysis	Delayed hemolysis
	Anaphylactic reaction	Alloimmunization
	Urticarial reaction	Post-transfusion purpura
	Acute lung injury	Graft-vs.-host disease
	Febrile, nonhemolytic	Immune suppression
Infectious	Bacterial contamination	Parasitic disease
	Hepatitis and other viral infections	
Chemical	Hyper(hypo)kalemia	Iron overload
	Citrate toxicity	
	Acidosis/alkalosis	
Physical	Hypothermia	
	Volume overload	
	Osmotic hemolysis	
	Thermal hemolysis	
	Coagulation defects	

disseminated intravascular coagulation (DIC), hypotension, shock, and acute renal failure (ARF).

The "classic" presentation includes fever, flank pain, and red urine, but this is uncommonly seen; fever ($\geq 1°$ C rise) and chills are almost invariably present. In comatose or anesthetized patients, oozing from venipuncture sites and hemoglobinuria may be the earliest signs. Because fever is the most common sign of a "benign" febrile, nonhemolytic transfusion reaction (see later), fever must be assumed to be due to hemolysis until proved otherwise.

Thus, the onset of fever in a red cell–containing transfusion recipient requires:

1. Immediate cessation of the infusion (leave intravenous line attached);
2. Begin infusion of normal saline (not Ringer's lactate or dextrose);
3. Draw a blood sample for direct antiglobulin test and plasma-free hemoglobin from a site other than the transfusion line; and
4. Check for clerical error.

The plasma of a patient with an acute hemolytic reaction will be pink (plasma-free hemoglobin ≥ 25 to 40 mg/dL), and a direct antiglobulin test (DAT) will be positive. The DAT may show only a partial or mixed-field reaction, or it may be negative if all transfused cells have been destroyed. In the presence of the sudden onset of fever and hypotension, with or without flank pain and red urine, generous fluid replacement with saline and forced diuresis should be initiated even before the laboratory testing is complete. Supportive care should be vigorous and may include the use of vasoactive drugs such as dopamine and heparin.

Delayed Hemolytic Transfusion Reaction. Delayed hemolytic transfusion reactions (DHTRs) are due to an anamnestic antibody response caused by previous sensitization (pregnancy or transfusion) and when the antibody has fallen below levels detectable by pretransfusion testing. Antibodies of the Jk[a] system, as well as the Rh system, particularly C, c and E, and e, are commonly implicated.

Generally, these antibodies are not complement fixing, and extravascular hemolysis over a period of days is the norm. Occasionally, rapid hemolysis can occur. The diagnosis is often made by the blood bank staff, who find a positive antiglobulin test or antibody screen when more blood is ordered. These reactions generally occur 7 to 10 days after transfusion and lead to a mild elevation in unconjugated bilirubin, decreasing hematocrit, microspherocytosis, and, occasionally, clinically detectable jaundice.

In the absence of brisk hemolysis, no treatment is necessary; however, it is important to make the diagnosis and identify the antibody so that appropriate records are maintained to prevent future occurrences. Future transfusions must lack the antigens of the implicated antibodies.

Febrile, Nonhemolytic Transfusion Reaction. Febrile, nonhemolytic transfusion reactions (FNHTRs) are the most common of the adverse reactions, with an incidence of 1% to 10%. They manifest with fever and shaking chills and sometimes mild dyspnea, within 1 to 6 hours of transfusion. They are benign in that they cause no lasting sequelae; however, they can be very uncomfortable, sometimes alarming, for patients. Because fever may be the first, or only, sign of an AHTR, cessation of the transfusion (see section on Acute Hemolytic Transfusion Reaction) is necessary until hemolysis is ruled out.

Only 15% of people who have a FNHTR will have a second. It has been thought that FNHTRs were caused by antibodies (HLA or granulocyte-specific) directed against contaminating leukocytes in red cell and platelet components. Credence was lent to this since if one removes leukocytes by filtration, washing, or freezing/deglycerolizing/washing, such reactions are usually diminished or prevented.

Recent work indicates that although leukocyte-specific antibodies of recipients may play an etiologic role, more often the FNHTR is caused by cytokines (such as interleukin-6 and tumor necrosis factor) from leukocyte metabolism that accumulate in the supernatant plasma during blood storage.

Leukocyte removal by filtration prior to storage of red cells and platelets is effective in preventing these reactions. Prestorage leukoreduction is expensive, adding $25 to $40 to the cost of such a component. Whether the benefits of leukocyte reduction outweigh these costs is currently under study.

For FNHTRs that are not prevented by such leukoreduction, management consists of:

1. Ensuring that AHTR is not occurring;
2. Administration of antipyretics (avoid aspirin in thrombocytopenic patients); and
3. Modest doses of Demerol for severe chills and rigors.

Anaphylactic Transfusion Reaction. The sudden onset of anaphylaxis—shock, hypotension, angioedema, respiratory distress—in a transfusion recipient is a potentially lethal event and generally occurs within seconds to a few minutes of receiving any blood component that contains plasma. It is usually due to the presence of class-specific IgG, anti-IgA antibodies in patients who are IgA deficient. Significant IgA deficiency is not rare; it occurs in about 1:500 people, but not all who are deficient develop the offending antibody. Diagnosis is usually made after the fact.

Treatment consists of:

1. Discontinuing the transfusion, but keeping the IV open;
2. Administration of epinephrine, 0.3 mL, 1:1000, intramuscularly;
3. Possible administration of an epinephrine drip, 1 mL, 1:1000, diluted to 10 mL in normal saline, intravenously, over 5 to 10 minutes;
4. Consider dopamine, 1 μg per kg per minute;
5. Maintain oxygenation/airway; and
6. Maintain volume with crystalloids.

Prevention consists of making a diagnosis and using IgA-deficient blood products, which may consist of frozen deglycerolized or "ultra" washed red cells, or components from IgA-deficient donors. IgA-deficient blood products may be obtained through the regional blood centers of the American Red Cross, the American Association of Blood Banks, or the Canadian Red Cross.

Urticarial Transfusion Reaction. These reactions are thought to be due to soluble substances in the plasma of the donated unit which react with recipient IgE antibodies, causing histamine release from mast cells and basophils, leading to hives, pruritus, and, occasionally, mild dyspnea. The transfusion should be temporarily interrupted and 50 mg of diphenhydramine (Benadryl) given intravenously through a saline line. The transfusion may be resumed when the urticaria wanes, but the patient should be closely observed to make sure anaphylaxis or angioedema does not occur.

Transfusion-Related Acute Lung Injury. Transfusion-related acute lung injury (TRALI) is a life-threatening complication of transfusion characterized by acute respiratory distress, hypoxemia, hypotension, fever, and bilateral pulmonary edema. The symptoms usually begin within 2 to 4 hours of transfusion. It is indistinguishable from the adult respiratory distress syndrome related to etiologies such as sepsis, but it has a much more favorable prognosis. Death occurs in less than 10% of cases. Recovery is otherwise complete and generally occurs within 96 hours. In 80% to 85% of cases, donor lymphocytotoxic, HLA-specific, or granulocyte antibodies are found in the donor plasma. In 5% of cases the patient is found to have such antibodies. The mechanism is not clearly understood; it is thought to be related to complement activation and granulocyte aggregation in the pulmonary vasculature, leading to the release of superoxide radicals with consequent damage to the pulmonary interstitium. Prompt treatment consists of respiratory support (supplementary oxygen/mechanical ventilation) and pressor agents to treat the vascular collapse. Although infrequently reported, recent evidence suggests that TRALI may be one of the most common causes of death from transfusion.

Post-Transfusion Purpura. Post-transfusion purpura (PTP) is rare and occurs predominantly in women (male-to-female ratio is 1:26). It is characterized by the rapid development of thrombocytopenia 5 to 10 days following transfusion of a platelet-containing blood product. The thrombocytopenia is severe and lasts days to weeks.

PTP patients are usually PL[A1] negative, but through prior exposure (pregnancy/transfusion) they become sensitized to PL[A1]. The immune destruction of platelets includes not only the transfused PL[A1]-positive platelets but also the patient's own PL[A1]-negative platelets. The mechanism for this auto-destruction is unknown but may be related to immune complexes, autoantibodies, or attachment of soluble PL[A1] antigen to PL[A1]-negative platelets.

Treatment options include plasma exchange, high-dose steroids, and/or intravenous immune globulin. Transfusion of PL[A1]-negative platelets may be beneficial, but these may undergo destruction as just noted.

CHEMICAL MECHANISMS

Citrate Toxicity. Citrate toxicity is rare. In general, more than 1 unit of citrated whole blood every 5 minutes is required to cause significant calcium chelation and subsequent hypocalcemia. The manifestations include carpopedal spasm, arrhythmias, and tetany. Red cells prepared with additive solutions contain very little residual citrate. In the setting of exchange transfusions in neonates or massive transfusion of citrated blood in patients with severe liver disease, citrate toxicity may occur. The intravenous administration of calcium salts can also cause severe arrhythmia; thus, it is better to simply monitor such cases and give slow infusions of calcium bicarbonate if electrocardiographic evidence of severe hypocalcemia is noted.

Hyperkalemia and Metabolic Acidosis. Despite moderately increased levels of extracellular potassium seen in red cells approaching the end of their storage time, hyperkalemia is rarely seen in adult patients. Hyperkalemia may occur in some exchange transfusions in newborn infants using "old" blood (more than 7 days old). The same is true of acidosis.

Citrate is rapidly metabolized to bicarbonate, the latter "driving" potassium into the cells and causing alkalosis. Thus, when large volumes of citrated blood are transfused rapidly (1 to 2 blood volumes in 24 hours), it is often necessary to *give* potassium salts; i.e., hypokalemia is very common after massive transfusion whereas hyperkalemia is rare.

Iron Overload (Hemosiderosis). Each unit of whole blood or red cells contains 250 mg of iron. In chronically transfused patients, this may pose problems when reticuloendothelial sites for iron storage become saturated. Iron is then deposited in other tissues, particularly the liver, heart, skin, and pancreas and other endocrine organs, resulting in hepatic fibrosis/cirrhosis, cardiomyopathy, arrhythmias, and endocrine dysfunction, so-called "bronze diabetes."

Hemosiderosis occurs in chronically transfused patients, e.g., congenital hemolytic anemia. Iron deposits can be reduced by the administration of deferoxamine (Desferal).

Osmotic and Thermal Hemolysis. Only 0.9% saline is acceptable as a blood infusion additive. No drugs should ever be added to a blood component or given through an intravenous line through which blood is flowing since osmotic hemolysis may result. Mixing blood with 5% dextrose and water, or having an excess of anticoagulant/preservative, leads to rapid uptake of glucose by the red cells, which in turn take up H_2O and lyse. Lysis also occurs if red cells are frozen without cryoprotectants or are excessively heated. Only carefully monitored blood warming units or refrigerators for blood storage should be used. Transport of blood in extreme temperatures also requires careful monitoring.

Coagulation Defects Due to Massive Transfusions. Dilution of coagulation factors, including platelets, can occur with massive transfusions but is much less common than expected. Such dilution does not occur, even for platelets, based on a simple "wash-out" calculation, since there are significant extravascular reserves of all factors, including platelets. In individuals with normal baseline coagulation, coagulation defects due to transfusion are not detectable until more than 1 blood volume has been transfused. Since massive transfusion generally occurs in the presence of shock and severe blood loss, it is useful to monitor coagulation factors that are large in size, such as platelets, fibrinogen, Factor V, Factor VIII, and von Willebrand's Factor, since they are most commonly affected and do not have large extravascular reserves.

To accomplish this, monitor the platelet count, prothrombin time (PT), and activated partial thromboplastin time (PTT) during massive transfusions. In general, the PT and PTT will remain normal as long as 20% to 25% of normal plasma clotting factors are present. No intervention is needed unless the PT and/or PTT is 1.5 times or greater than the control value in the presence of abnormal bleeding. In nonsurgical, nonbleeding situations, platelet counts (unaspirinated) as low as 10,000 to 20,000/μL can be tolerated.

Circulatory Overload. Transfusion-associated circulatory overload (TACO) is pulmonary edema secondary to congestive heart failure. TACO occurs in the very young or old, usually in the setting of rapid or massive infusion of blood. Symptoms include dyspnea, tachycardia, and hypertension and begin within 6 hours of transfusion. Headache and seizures have also been reported. Recent data suggest that TACO may complicate 1% of transfusion episodes, at least in older surgical patients. Treatment consists of fluid mobilization (e.g., diuretics) and supplementary oxygen; if symptoms persist, phlebotomy in 250-mL increments may be necessary.

Summary. The preceding remarks are necessarily brief, but a common message remains throughout: Never transfuse unless it is necessary. Volume replacement is more important than red cell replacement. The heart cares less what it pumps around, but cares greatly that there is enough of it.

If a patient has an acute transfusion reaction the following guidelines apply:

1. Stop the transfusion;
2. Keep the intravenous line open with saline;
3. Identify and treat the cause; and
4. Transfuse only if necessary.

CHOLELITHIASIS AND CHOLECYSTITIS

method of
ATTILA NAKEEB, M.D., and
KEITH D. LILLEMOE, M.D.
The Johns Hopkins Medical Institutions
Baltimore, Maryland

The management of calculous disease of the biliary tract has undergone dramatic changes in the decade of the 1990s. Yet cholelithiasis and its complications remain significant health problems in the United States and throughout the world. The prevalence of cholelithiasis in the United States is between 10% and 15%, with an additional 1 million Americans diagnosed with gallstones each year. More than 700,000 cholecystectomies will be performed this year, with the overall treatment costs for gallstones exceeding 5 billion dollars.

Gallstones are traditionally classified into three types: cholesterol, pigment, and mixed cholesterol and pigment stones. In reality, pure cholesterol stones are rare (approximately 10%) with most stones in Western countries, approximately 65%, being of mixed composition. Pigment stones, which account for approximately 25% of stones in the United States, can be subdivided into black pigment (20%) and brown pigment (5%). Cholesterol gallstones form as the result of a complex interaction of factors, including the supersaturation of bile with cholesterol, the promotion and inhibition of cholesterol monohydrate crystal growth by pro- and antinucleating proteins present in bile, and stasis of bile in the gallbladder. Female gender, advanced age, obesity, and rapid weight loss all predispose patients to the development of cholesterol gallstones.

Pigment gallstones form when bilirubin and inorganic salts precipitate out of bile because of altered solubilization of unconjugated bilirubin. Black pigment stones contain more inorganic components and mucin than brown pigment stones and are associated with hemolytic disorders, cirrhosis, long-term parenteral nutrition, and ileal resection. Brown pigment stones typically have bacteria in their matrix and are associated with biliary stasis and bacterial or parasitic biliary tract infection.

NATURAL HISTORY OF GALLSTONES

An understanding of the natural history of gallstone disease is necessary for the appropriate management of patients with cholelithiasis. The presence or absence of symptoms remains the most important factor in the determination of the natural history of gallstones. Several studies have shown that only 10% to 20% of patients with asymptomatic gallstone disease will ultimately develop symptoms if followed for 5 to 10 years. Furthermore, the majority of patients developing symptoms will present with uncompli-

cated biliary colic. Therefore, most patients with asymptomatic gallstones should be managed expectantly without cholecystectomy.

In select groups of patients, however, prophylactic cholecystectomy should be considered (Table 1). *Children* with gallstones almost always develop symptoms and should be considered for early cholecystectomy. In patients with *sickle cell disease*, cholecystitis can precipitate a crisis with substantial operative risks. Therefore, these patients are best treated with elective cholecystectomy. A *nonfunctioning gallbladder* usually indicates advanced disease, with over 25% of these patients developing symptoms that require cholecystectomy. *Large gallstones (>2.5 cm)* are more frequently associated with acute cholecystitis, and prophylactic cholecystectomy may also be indicated in these patients. Patients with a *calcified gallbladder* should also undergo prophylactic cholecystectomy because of the high incidence of associated gallbladder cancer in this setting. Finally, acute cholecystitis is a potentially life-threatening condition in immunosuppressed patients. For this reason, prophylactic cholecystectomy has been recommended *prior to major organ transplantation*.

Prophylactic cholecystectomy is no longer indicated in patients with diabetes and asymptomatic gallstones. Although diabetic patients have an increased risk with emergency cholecystectomy, recent studies have shown that they also have an increased risk with elective cholecystectomy. This increased risk is related to co-morbid conditions, not to the diabetes itself. Furthermore, there is no evidence to suggest that asymptomatic diabetic patients are at increased risk of developing complications of gallstone disease.

In contrast to patients with asymptomatic gallstones, patients with symptomatic gallstones do not do well with expectant management. In large series of patients with symptomatic gallstones, the majority have increased or persistent symptoms. Symptomatic patients are also more likely to develop complications than asymptomatic patients, further supporting the

TABLE 1. **Indications for Cholecystectomy in Asymptomatic Patients with Gallstones**

Children
Sickle cell disease
Nonfunctioning gallbladder
Stones > 2.5 cm
Calcification of the gallbladder
Prior to major organ transplantation

role of routine cholecystectomy for symptomatic patients.

BILIARY COLIC AND CHRONIC CHOLECYSTITIS

Biliary colic is the most common symptom of cholelithiasis. It results from the impaction of a stone at the gallbladder–cystic duct junction. This obstruction is generally transient, as the stone either falls back into the gallbladder or passes through the cystic duct. Classically, biliary colic has been associated with the ingestion of fatty foods; however, attacks may be precipitated by any food. Biliary colic is characterized by the sudden onset of right upper quadrant pain. The pain characteristically increases in intensity over 30 minutes to an hour, persists for 4 to 6 hours, and then gradually resolves over 2 to 3 hours. Whereas the pain is typically in the right upper quadrant, it can be epigastric and may radiate to the back or the tip of the right scapula. Associated symptoms include dyspepsia, nausea, and occasionally emesis. On physical examination, patients with biliary colic are usually afebrile, in mild distress secondary to pain, and have mild right upper quadrant tenderness. These findings usually resolve with the resolution of their symptoms and physical examination is usually normal in the interval between attacks. Recurrent episodes of biliary colic lead to a chronic inflammatory response and pathologic changes of chronic cholecystitis. Ultimately, the gallbladder will become contracted and scarred and often becomes nonfunctional.

In addition to typical biliary colic, a number of more vague, nonspecific symptoms may be seen in patients with gallstones. These symptoms include dyspepsia, vague epigastric discomfort, or increased flatulence. Patients with nonspecific dyspeptic symptoms without biliary colic are less likely to benefit from cholecystectomy; however, up to 70% of such patients will still derive significant benefit from the operation.

Diagnostic Evaluation

The diagnosis of symptomatic cholelithiasis is made by the combination of clinical presentation and the documentation of gallstones in the gallbladder. Plain abdominal radiographs demonstrate gallstones in only 20% of patients. Therefore, use of radiographs is limited to the exclusion of other intra-abdominal conditions such as intestinal obstruction or perforation. On the other hand, ultrasonography can demonstrate gallstones in more than 95% of patients with cholelithiasis. Ultrasonography can also provide valuable information on common bile duct size, pericholecystic fluid collections, gallbladder wall thickness, and other abdominal masses. These factors make ultrasonography the preferred test for the evaluation of patients with gallbladder disease. Oral cholecystography, once the "gold standard" for diagnosis of gallbladder disease, is seldom currently used.

Surgical Therapy

The treatment for symptomatic gallstone disease is cholecystectomy. Cholecystectomy effectively treats the symptoms of pain (95%) and dyspepsia (75%) in patients with gallstones. The options for cholecystectomy include the open and laparoscopic techniques. Open cholecystectomy has been performed since 1882, and until 1990 was the standard for treatment of symptomatic cholelithiasis. A recent review of 42,000 open cholecystectomies has documented an operative mortality rate of 0.17%. The mortality rate in patients less than 65 years of age was 0.03%, compared with 0.5% in patients over 65 years.

Since its introduction in 1989, laparoscopic cholecystectomy has rapidly become the preferred treatment for the majority of patients with symptomatic gallstone disease. Laparoscopic cholecystectomy offers several advantages to open cholecystectomy, including less postoperative pain, shortened hospital stay, rapid return to full activity, and decreased cost. Although in early reports several absolute and relative contraindications existed for laparoscopic cholecystectomy, currently over 90% of patients will be candidates for the procedure performed by experienced surgeons. Previous upper abdominal surgery, obesity, cirrhosis, portal hypertension, pregnancy, and acute cholecystitis increase the technical difficulty but do not preclude the laparoscopic approach.

The operative mortality rate for laparoscopic cholecystectomy is 0.01%, and the morbidity rate is similar to that of open cholecystectomy. The incidence of bile duct injury with laparoscopic cholecystectomy is slightly higher than with open cholecystectomy (0.2% to 0.5% versus 0.1% to 0.2%), but the incidence is low enough to justify laparoscopic cholecystectomy as effective therapy for almost all patients with symptomatic gallstone disease. In most series, the conversion rate from laparoscopic to open cholecystectomy is between 2% and 5%.

Common bile duct stones are found in approximately 10% of all patients who undergo cholecystectomy for symptomatic gallstone disease. Factors suggesting common bile duct stones include a history of jaundice or pancreatitis, dilated biliary tree on ultrasound or computed tomography (CT) scan, and elevations in serum bilirubin, liver function tests, or amylase. If common bile duct stones are strongly suspected, preoperative endoscopic retrograde cholangiopancreatography (ERCP) and endoscopic sphincterotomy may be indicated to clear any common duct stones. Intraoperative cholangiography can be used either routinely or selectively to evaluate the biliary tree for stones, as well as to define the biliary anatomy. Either laparoscopic common bile duct exploration, conversion to an open procedure with common duct exploration, or postoperative ERCP and sphincterotomy are appropriate options, depending on local expertise, if stones are detected at laparoscopic cholecystectomy.

Nonsurgical Therapy

The nonsurgical options for the treatment of gallstone disease include oral dissolution therapy with the bile acid ursodeoxycholic acid (Actigall) or contact dissolution therapy with the organic solvent methyl tert-butyl ether (MTBE). Oral dissolution therapy is indicated in symptomatic patients with cholesterol gallstones and functioning gallbladders. These agents are effective in the dissolution of cholesterol gallstones only and therefore are not indicated if stones are radiopaque or if calcifications can be detected on CT scan. In carefully selected series, complete stone dissolution can be achieved in 40% of patients; however, the recurrence rate is 50% within 5 years if therapy is stopped. Contact dissolution with organic solvents requires cannulation of the gallbladder with direct infusion of the agent into the gallbladder. Again, only cholesterol gallstones are amenable to contact dissolution, and the recurrence rate is similar to that of oral dissolution therapy.

Extracorporeal shock wave lithotripsy was originally thought to be a promising nonoperative alternative for the management of symptomatic gallstones. The widespread application of laparoscopic cholecystectomy has greatly limited the role of all nonoperative techniques to a very select group of patients.

ACUTE CHOLECYSTITIS

Acute cholecystitis is the most common complication of gallstones, occurring in 20% to 30% of patients with symptomatic disease. As in biliary colic, acute cholecystitis results from a stone impacting at the gallbladder–cystic duct junction. The extent of inflammation and the progression to acute cholecystitis are likely related to the duration and degree of obstruction. Acute cholecystitis is primarily an inflammatory and not an infectious process, with bacterial infection appearing as a secondary event. Approximately 50% of patients with acute cholecystitis will have positive bile cultures, with *Escherichia coli* being the most common organism noted.

Patients with acute cholecystitis typically present with right upper quadrant pain that is similar to that of biliary colic. However, in acute cholecystitis the pain is usually unremitting, may last several days, and is often associated with nausea, emesis, and anorexia. On physical examination, patients with acute cholecystitis usually have a low-grade fever and exhibit localized right upper quadrant tenderness with or without rebound. The presence of Murphy's sign, an inspiratory arrest during deep palpation of the right upper quadrant, is the classic physical finding of acute cholecystitis. A palpable right upper quadrant mass is appreciated in one-third of patients and usually represents omentum that has migrated to the area in response to the inflammation. Laboratory evaluation can show a mild leukocytosis (WBC, 12,000 to 15,000) and mild jaundice (bilirubin < 4.0 mg per dL) in up to 20% of patients.

Diagnostic Evaluation

Ultrasound and radionuclide scanning are the primary imaging modalities for the diagnosis of acute cholecystitis. Ultrasound documents the presence of gallstones and can demonstrate gallbladder wall thickening, pericholecystic fluid, and gallbladder enlargement. Radionuclide imaging involves the intravenous injection of ^{99m}technetium-labeled iminodiacetic acid derivatives that are taken up by hepatocytes and then rapidly excreted into bile. Nonvisualization of the gallbladder indicates cystic duct obstruction, which is diagnostic of acute cholecystitis in the appropriate clinical setting.

Treatment

The treatment of choice for acute cholecystitis is cholecystectomy. In the past, delayed cholecystectomy was preferred. Patients were initially managed nonoperatively and discharged home after their symptoms resolved. Elective cholecystectomy was then performed 6 weeks later after the acute inflammation had resolved. Prospective trials have shown that early open cholecystectomy (within 3 days of symptom onset) can be accomplished with a morbidity and mortality rate similar to that of delayed cholecystectomy, and it has the advantage of a reduced total hospital stay. In addition, 20% of patients treated with delayed cholecystectomy develop recurrent symptoms requiring hospitalization within 6 weeks. Initially, acute cholecystitis was felt to be a contraindication to laparoscopic cholecystectomy. As experience has increased, however, it has become clear that laparoscopic cholecystectomy can be performed safely in the setting of acute cholecystitis. Of note, the rate of conversion from laparoscopic to open cholecystectomy in the setting of acute cholecystitis approaches 30%.

The current practice for the management of acute cholecystitis involves nothing by mouth and intravenous hydration. A nasogastric tube is placed if there is persistent nausea and vomiting or abdominal distention. In almost all cases, broad-spectrum antibiotics, such as a second-generation cephalosporin, should be started and maintained into the immediate postoperative period. Laparoscopic cholecystectomy should be performed within 24 to 72 hours of diagnosis. Early conversion to an open procedure should be considered if dissection is difficult or clear progress cannot be made by the laparoscopic technique.

In certain high-risk patients whose medical conditions preclude cholecystectomy, a cholecystostomy can be performed for acute cholecystitis. Although previously performed operatively and under local anesthesia, percutaneous drainage techniques can now accomplish the procedure in most patients. In most cases, prompt improvement is seen after gallbladder drainage and appropriate antibiotics. Elective cholecystectomy can then be performed at a later date.

Complications

Several complications of acute cholecystitis are recognized in clinical practice: empyema of the gallbladder, emphysematous cholecystitis, perforation, and cholecystoenteric fistula. All these complications can be associated with significant morbidity and mortality and, therefore, require prompt surgical intervention.

Empyema. Gallbladder empyema represents an advanced stage of cholecystitis, with bacterial invasion of the gallbladder and actual pus in the lumen. Patients present with severe right upper quadrant pain, high-grade fever, rigors, and significant leukocytosis. Sepsis, including cardiovascular collapse, may be seen. Treatment consists of broad-spectrum antibiotics and emergency cholecystectomy or cholecystostomy.

Emphysematous Cholecystitis. The potentially lethal complication of acute emphysematous cholecystitis is characterized by radiographic demonstration of gas within the gallbladder wall or lumen. The condition is more common in elderly and diabetic patients and is the result of infection with a gas-forming bacteria, usually *Clostridium perfringens.* Appropriate antibiotics and prompt cholecystectomy are necessary.

Perforation. Gallbladder perforation can be categorized as being either localized or free. The incidence of perforation in acute cholecystitis is approximately 10%. Localized perforation generally results in the formation of a pericholecystic abscess as the omentum walls off the perforation and limits it to the right upper quadrant. Free perforation is less frequent (1% of cases) and occurs if the omentum is unable to wall off the inflammatory process. Free perforation results in the spillage of bile into the peritoneal cavity and generalized peritonitis. Evidence for perforation includes an increase in pain and tenderness, fever and chills, elevation in white blood cell count, and hypotension. These patients require aggressive fluid resuscitation, antibiotics, and emergency operative exploration.

Cholecystoenteric Fistula. In 1% to 2% of patients with acute cholecystitis, the gallbladder will perforate into an adjacent hollow viscus. The duodenum (79%) and the hepatic flexure of the colon (17%) are the most common sites. Generally, after the fistula forms, the episode of acute cholecystitis resolves as the gallbladder spontaneously decompresses. If a large gallstone passes from the gallbladder into the small intestine, a mechanical bowel obstruction may result, termed *gallstone ileus.* Gallstone ileus occurs in 10% to 15% of patients with a cholecystoenteric fistula. These patients should be treated like those having a mechanical small bowel obstruction: aggressive fluid resuscitation, nasogastric suction, and surgical exploration. Operative management consists of treating only the bowel obstruction by enterostomy and removal of the obstructing stone. Cholecystectomy and closure of the fistula should be deferred until later, if done at all.

Acalculous Cholecystitis

Acalculous cholecystitis is found in approximately 5% of patients operated on for acute cholecystitis. It is usually seen in hospitalized patients suffering from major trauma, significant burns, sepsis, or prolonged illness. The underlying illness often leads to delayed diagnosis. The diagnosis can be confirmed by ultrasound, which shows an enlarged tender gallbladder, thickened gallbladder wall, and pericholecystic fluid collections. Treatment of acalculous cholecystitis includes broad-spectrum antibiotics and urgent cholecystectomy or cholecystostomy.

CIRRHOSIS

method of
VELIMIR A. LUKETIC, M.D., and
MITCHELL L. SHIFFMAN, M.D.
Medical College of Virginia
Richmond, Virginia

As the final stage in the progression of almost all chronic liver disorders, cirrhosis remains one of the most common serious medical conditions seen by practicing physicians. Historically, alcohol and hepatitis B have been responsible for the vast majority of cases of cirrhosis worldwide. However, recent improvements in our ability to detect hepatitis C have dramatically changed this picture. Today, hepatitis C is the most frequent cause of chronic liver disease and the most common indication for hepatic transplantation in the United States. A comprehensive list of etiologies of cirrhosis is given in Table 1.

Cirrhosis is best defined morphologically. A cirrhotic liver is usually small and nodular, reflecting both a loss in cell mass and an increase in connective tissue. Histologically, structurally abnormal nodules are surrounded by fibrous tissue. The pattern is diffuse and results in disorganization of the hepatic lobular and vascular architecture. These structural changes are responsible for both the hemodynamic and the functional disturbances associated with cirrhosis. Once established, cirrhosis is irreversible.

TABLE 1. **Etiologies of Cirrhosis**

Drugs and Toxins	**Metabolic Disorders**
Alcohol	Hemochromatosis
Methotrexate	Wilson's disease
Isoniazid	Alpha$_1$-antitrypsin deficiency
Nitrofurantoin	Glycogen storage diseases
Methyldopa	Galactosemia
Amiodarone	Tyrosinemia
Trichloroethylene	Abetalipoproteinemia
Hypervitaminosis A	**Venous Outflow Obstruction**
Infections	Budd-Chiari syndrome
Viral hepatitis (B, C, D)	Veno-occlusive disease
Syphilis	Cardiac failure
Brucellosis	**Other**
Schistosomiasis	Autoimmune hepatitis
Cholestasis	Nonalcoholic steatohepatitis
Primary biliary cirrhosis	Sarcoidosis
Chronic biliary obstruction	Indian childhood cirrhosis
Primary sclerosing	Jejunoileal bypass for obesity
cholangitis	Cryptogenic cirrhosis
Biliary atresia	
Graft-versus-host disease	
Cystic fibrosis	

However, it is not uniformly fatal. Up to 40% of cases are first discovered at autopsy, and a substantial proportion of affected patients remain asymptomatic.

The prognosis of a patient with cirrhosis depends on the activity of the underlying liver disease, the extent of hepatic dysfunction, and the development of complications of cirrhosis. The Child-Turcotte classification was originally developed to predict the risk of shunt surgery in patients with cirrhosis and portal hypertension. As modified by Pugh, the scale divides patients into three groups (A, B, and C) on the basis of easily available clinical (ascites, hepatic encephalopathy) and laboratory (bilirubin, albumin, and prothrombin time) features. The Child-Pugh scoring system is presented in Table 2. Mean survival for patients with Class A, B, and C cirrhosis is only 40, 32, and 8 months, respectively. It is particularly important to recognize that even patients with stable Child's Class A cirrhosis (i.e., normal hepatic function) have limited survival. This is because most patients with nonalcoholic liver disease have continued progression in the underlying liver disorder and develop complications of cirrhosis, with worsening of the Child-Pugh score. Child's class remains useful for estimating survival for cirrhotics undergoing elective surgery. This ranges from 90% for patients with Child's Class A to 24% for Child's Class C disease. Abdominal surgery for biliary tract, peptic ulcer, or colonic disease is associated with an increased mortality compared with surgery outside the abdominal cavity.

Recently, metabolic liver function tests have increasingly been utilized to predict mortality in patients with cirrhosis. This is particularly important for identifying patients with Child's Class A cirrhosis who would benefit from hepatic transplantation. The simplest of the metabolic liver function tests assesses the liver's ability to convert lidocaine to its primary metabolite, monoethylglycinexylidide (MEGX). Lidocaine is administered intravenously at a dose of 1 mg per kg (maximum dose 100 mg) over 1 to 2 minutes. A serum sample is drawn 15 to 20 minutes later and assayed for MEGX production. There is uniform agreement that MEGX values below 10 ng per mL identify patients with a 50% mortality over the ensuing 1 to 2 years.

EVALUATION AND TREATMENT OF LIVER DISORDERS

Effective therapy is now available for many forms of chronic liver disease. It is therefore imperative that all patients with liver disease, even known alcohol abusers, undergo a complete evaluation to define disease etiology. A list of serologic screening tests for various liver disorders and their treatment is provided in Table 3. The best response to these treatments is achieved in patients prior to the development of cirrhosis or in stable Child's Class A patients. Those with advanced cirrhosis (Child's Class B and C) should be referred for hepatic transplantation.

TABLE 2. Child-Pugh Classification

Parameter	Points		
	1	*2*	*3*
Encephalopathy (stage)	None	1–2	3–4
Ascites	Absent	Slight	Poorly controlled
Bilirubin (mg/dL)	<2.0	2.0–3.0	>3.0
Albumin (gm/dL)	>3.5	2.8–3.5	<2.8
Prothrombin time (seconds prolonged)	1.0–4.0	4.0–6.0	>6.0

Class A: 5–6 points; Class B: 7–9 points; Class C: 10–15 points

TABLE 3. Screening Tests and Treatment for Chronic Hepatitis

Etiology	Screening Test	Treatment
Hepatitis C	Anti–hepatitis C virus	Interferon Liver transplant
Hepatitis B	Hepatitis B surface antigen Hepatitis B e antigen	Interferon Liver transplant
Autoimmune hepatitis	Antinuclear antibodies Anti–smooth muscle	Prednisone Liver transplant
Hemochromatosis	Iron saturation >50%	Phlebotomy Liver transplant
Wilson's disease	Ceruloplasmin	D-penicillamine Liver transplant
Alpha₁-antitrypsin deficiency	Alpha₁-antitrypsin level	Liver transplant

Liver Biopsy

Percutaneous liver biopsy is one of the most important and helpful tests to perform in patients with chronic liver disease. Liver histology can confirm the diagnosis suspected by screening tests and provides valuable information regarding the severity of the underlying liver disorder. In most cases, cirrhosis can be confirmed only by liver biopsy. This is especially true in patients with normal hepatic synthetic function and no complications of liver disease (Child's Class A). In patients with several possible etiologies for their liver disease (e.g., viral hepatitis in a patient with modest alcohol consumption), liver biopsy can be invaluable to help dissect the contributions of these various etiologic factors. Liver biopsy is also helpful in assessing the effectiveness of treatment of chronic liver disease. The procedure is performed in an outpatient setting; in patients with normal platelet counts and normal prothrombin and bleeding times, the complication rate is less than 0.1%.

Alcoholic Liver Disease

The best evidence that elimination of a toxic agent can markedly influence prognosis is provided by patients with alcoholic cirrhosis. The 5-year survival for those patients who stop drinking before they develop complications of cirrhosis (jaundice, variceal hemorrhage, ascites, and/or encephalopathy) approaches 90%. Even when these complications are present, abstinence improves 5-year survival from 34 to over 60%. Thus, the most effective treatment for alcoholic cirrhosis is abstinence. In fact, since regular alcohol consumption also hastens disease progression in patients with nonalcoholic liver disease, all patients with cirrhosis, regardless of its etiology, should avoid alcohol. Patients who develop complications of cirrhosis despite abstinence from alcohol should be considered candidates for hepatic transplantation.

Patients with severe alcoholic hepatitis (with or without cirrhosis) who have either hepatic encephalopathy or a discriminant factor greater than 32 (4.6 × [patient prothrombin time − control prothrombin time] + total bilirubin in mg/dL) have an extremely high in-hospital short-term mortality. Corticosteroids can dramatically improve survival in these patients from 20 to 30% to 70 to 80%. The dose is 40 mg of prednisone or its equivalent per day for 28 days, at which point the dose can be tapered and discontinued. Treatment is contraindicated in patients with pancreatitis, infection, gastrointestinal bleeding, or renal failure.

Colchicine* has been advocated by some studies to prevent the progression of cirrhosis in patients with alcoholic liver disease. This agent acts by disrupting microtubule function and inhibiting procollagen secretion. Although colchicine is both inexpensive and well tolerated, the data to support its effectiveness are both limited and controversial. We do not routinely recommend colchicine for the treatment of patients with cirrhosis. However, for physicians who wish to utilize this agent, the dose is 1 mg per day.

Chronic Hepatitis

Chronic hepatitis is defined as persistent elevation in serum liver transaminases for more than 6 months' duration. The ratio of aspartate aminotransferase (AST) to alanine aminotransferase (ALT) is always less than 1.0 unless cirrhosis is present. Viral hepatitis B and C are the most common etiologies for chronic hepatitis worldwide. Their diagnosis is based on appropriate serologic testing (see Table 3). Patients with an elevated serum ALT generally have active hepatitis when assessed by liver biopsy. However, ALT can fluctuate widely in patients with hepatitis C and from time to time may fall within the normal range. The treatment for viral hepatitis is interferon-alfa-2b (Intron A). The dose for patients with hepatitis C is 3 to 5 million U administered subcutaneously three times weekly for 6 to 18 months. The dose for chronic hepatitis B is 5 million U daily for 16 weeks. Approximately 50% of patients with chronic viral hepatitis respond to this treatment, with normalization in serum liver transaminases. Liver histology should always be evaluated prior to the start of interferon therapy, if possible. In addition, since interferon can exacerbate autoimmune processes, autoimmune hepatitis must be excluded prior to embarking on therapy. Treatment of many patients is limited by side effects: severe flulike symptoms (myalgia, arthralgia, headache, and fever), leukopenia, and thrombocytopenia.

Autoimmune hepatitis is commonly observed in young to middle-aged women who test positive for antinuclear antibodies (ANA). The treatment is immune suppression. Prednisone is utilized in patients with elevated serum liver transaminases and active hepatitis on liver biopsy. The starting dose is 40 to 60 mg daily for the first 1 to 2 weeks. This is reduced to 20 mg daily for an additional 4 weeks and then to 10 mg daily for an additional 6 to 9 months. Unfortunately, most patients relapse once prednisone is discontinued and require long-term maintenance therapy. Azathioprine (Imuran)* at a dose of 50 to 100 mg per day can be added to reduce the dose of steroids necessary to maintain biochemical remission. In patients with mild disease, as assessed by liver biopsy, the side effects of corticosteroid therapy (infections, protein catabolism, osteoporosis, aseptic necrosis of the hips, cataract formation, and diabetes mellitus) may outweigh any potential treatment benefit.

Hemochromatosis is one of the most common genetic disorders in the Western world. The therapy for hemochromatosis is phlebotomy. This should initially be performed weekly until the patient's hemoglobin falls to 10 mg per dL. The frequency of phlebotomy can then be reduced stepwise. Iron saturation and ferritin do not typically decline until patients become mildly anemic. In most patients, phlebotomy needs to continue for 6 months or longer to achieve complete iron reduction from vital organs. Iron chelation therapy may also be performed with deferoxamine (Desferal). If hemochromatosis is recognized early, iron depletion can prevent the development of cirrhosis and other end-organ complications of this disease. It can also improve overall well-being, hyperpigmentation, liver function, congestive heart failure, and diabetes mellitus, even in patients who have developed cirrhosis. Although hepatic transplantation is an option for patients with decompensated cirrhosis, survival is reduced for patients with hemochromatosis compared with those having other liver disorders.

Wilson's disease and alpha₁-antitrypsin deficiency are uncommon autosomal recessive disorders. In Wilson's disease, the copper-binding protein ceruloplasmin cannot be excreted from the liver. Copper accumulates within the liver and other tissues, and this is responsible for the neuropsychiatric abnormalities, hemolytic anemia, and renal tubular acidosis commonly observed in this disorder. The diagnosis is confirmed by low serum ceruloplasmin and elevated urinary copper excretion. The treatment of Wilson's disease is copper chelation with D-penicillamine (Cuprimine). For patients who develop hypersensitivity to this agent, trientine hydrochloride (Syprine) is utilized. In alpha₁-antitrypsin deficiency, a point mutation prevents the secretion of this protein from the liver. Large amounts of alpha₁-antitrypsin accumulate within hepatocytes, and this can be visualized on liver biopsy. The diagnosis is confirmed by a low serum alpha₁-antitrypsin level. No treatment is currently available. Hepatic transplantation is performed when patients develop complications of cirrhosis.

---

*Not FDA-approved for this indication.

*Not FDA-approved for this indication.

Cholestatic Liver Disease

There are two major cholestatic liver disorders that lead to cirrhosis, primary biliary cirrhosis (PBC) and primary sclerosing cholangitis (PSC). Both disorders are manifested by destruction of bile ducts and a persistent elevation in serum alkaline phosphatase. Serum bilirubin is usually normal until end-stage disease. Bile ducts are not dilated on imaging studies. Patients with PBC test positive for antimitochondrial antibody (AMA). Patients with PSC may test positive for ANA and/or anticytoplasmic neutrophil antibody (p-ANCA). Up to 90% of patients with PSC also have inflammatory bowel disease, either ulcerative colitis or Crohn's disease. In PBC, the small intrahepatic bile ducts are destroyed by an as yet undefined immunologic process. In PSC, there is stricture formation and sclerosis of large bile ducts. Such bile duct abnormalities cause reduction in bile flow and accumulation of bile salts within the liver. Since bile salts are hydrophobic molecules with detergent-like properties, they destroy hepatocytes, which leads to cirrhosis. The treatment of these disorders is ursodiol (Actigall). This agent is a hydrophilic bile acid that counteracts the toxic effects of native bile salts. The dose is 10 to 15 mg per kg per day administered as a single dose or in divided doses.

SYSTEMIC MANIFESTATIONS OF CIRRHOSIS

Malnutrition

Malnutrition is a common finding in patients with advanced liver disease. Clinically, it manifests itself as weight loss, decrease in muscle mass, and decrease in fat stores as measured by triceps skinfold thickness. The pathogenesis is multifactorial, and several causes can be operative in an individual patient. Anorexia, nausea, and vomiting often lead to poor dietary intake. The problem is made worse by unpalatable low-sodium and low-protein diets and early satiety attributable to tense ascites. Prolonged fasting leads to consumption of fat stores, an increase in gluconeogenesis, and thus a depletion of structural and functional proteins. Protein catabolism can be aggravated by repeated episodes of sepsis, bleeding, and spontaneous bacterial peritonitis. Finally, malabsorption can develop because of both chronic use of lactulose and neomycin for hepatic encephalopathy and a decrease in intraluminal concentrations of bile salts by cholestasis and cholestyramine. Moderate steatorrhea is found in up to 50% of cirrhotics and contributes to inadequate levels of fat-soluble vitamins (A, D, E, K).

In well-compensated Child's Class A cirrhotics, a normal balanced diet and a daily intake of 1 gram of protein per kg body weight are generally adequate to maintain nitrogen balance. In patients with more advanced liver disease (Child's Class B and C), additional protein and calories are required to achieve positive nitrogen balance and prevent further tissue catabolism. In patients with ascites or infection, caloric needs may be as much as 150 to 175% of the basal daily energy requirement (35 to 45 kcal per kg per day). Supplemental feedings should therefore be considered early, even in patients who appear to have an adequate oral intake. In hospitalized patients, tube feedings are a convenient way to deliver adequate calories to those with anorexia, and this has been shown to improve nutritional indices, Child's class, and short-term survival. In patients with hepatic encephalopathy, protein should be limited to 40 to 60 grams per day. Vegetable proteins are better tolerated and limit the degree of encephalopathy in such patients. Encephalopathy can also be avoided by central or peripheral administration of standard amino acid solutions. Frequent small meals can prevent episodes of hypoglycemia. Cirrhotics, especially those still abusing alcohol, should also receive vitamin and mineral supplements, including vitamin A, thiamine, pyridoxine, vitamin B, folic acid, zinc, magnesium, calcium, and phosphorus. Vitamin D and K supplementation is discussed later.

Fatigue

Fatigue is one of the most common symptoms reported by patients with chronic liver disease and cirrhosis. The underlying mechanism is unknown but may be due to reduced muscle mass and/or altered hepatic gluconeogenesis. Typically, the patient feels well in the morning and tires as the day progresses. Midday rest usually allows the patient to continue to be active for the remainder of the day. Persistent activity in spite of fatigue often leads to prolonged generalized malaise. There is no effective treatment for fatigue, and patients should simply learn how to pace themselves. Within these parameters, cirrhotics should remain as active as possible. Regular exercise promotes general well-being, minimizes osteoporosis, and reduces the risk associated with transplant surgery.

Hepatic Osteodystrophy

Bone disease, both osteoporosis and osteomalacia, occurs in patients with cirrhosis. This is most commonly observed in patients with chronic cholestatic liver disease and those receiving long-term corticosteroids. Affected patients have a decrease in bone density, a loss of trabeculae, and thinning of the bone cortex. Bone pain is the most common symptom and can be present even in the absence of fractures. All patients at risk should therefore receive calcium and vitamin D 50,000 U orally per week. Although this dose should be sufficient to maintain normal serum levels, the potential for toxicity exists, and periodic monitoring of serum vitamin D levels is recommended. There are no data regarding the use of estrogens in preventing bone disease in persons with chronic cholestasis. In postmenopausal women with stable Child's Class A cirrhosis, estrogen supplementation can be safely utilized.

Coagulopathy

The liver is the source of all coagulation proteins except Factor VIII and von Willebrand factor. Since the synthesis of Factors II, VII, IX, and X is dependent on adequate vitamin K, a coagulopathy can develop in any patient with liver disease and malabsorption of fat-soluble vitamin K. In patients with cirrhosis, several abnormalities in the coagulation system have been described. These include a prolongation in prothrombin time, decline in fibrinogen, and increase in fibrin split products. The later effect is secondary to reduced hepatic clearance of activated clotting factors and should not be attributed to disseminated intravascular coagulation. Thrombocytopenia develops with worsening portal hypertension and hypersplenism but may also be secondary to marrow suppression, particularly in patients who consume alcohol. Platelet aggregation is also impaired in cirrhosis. These abnormalities cause the development of spontaneous ecchymoses, petechiae, and gingival bleeding and increase the severity of gastrointestinal hemorrhage.

All patients with a prolonged prothrombin time should receive subcutaneous vitamin K (AquaMEPHYTON). The dose is 10 mg and is administered subcutaneously for 3 consecutive days. This corrects the coagulopathy in patients with vitamin K deficiency from either fat malabsorption or malnutrition but cannot correct a prolonged prothrombin time due to severe parenchymal liver disease. Fresh-frozen plasma can replace all missing clotting factors and is indicated in patients with active bleeding and prior to performing invasive procedures. It is usually administered at a rate of 1 U per hour by continous infusion until bleeding stops or the prothrombin time has been adequately corrected. Plasmapheresis using fresh-frozen plasma replacement can be utilized to rapidly correct severe coagulation abnormalities before performing invasive procedures. Platelet infusions are also indicated in cirrhotics with active bleeding or prior to invasive procedures when the platelet count is less than 75,000 per mL. Desmopressin (DDAVP), a vasopressin analogue, can improve bleeding time and partial thromboplastin time by transiently increasing the levels of Factor VIII and von Willebrand factor. The dose is 0.3 μg per kg diluted in 50 mL saline and infused over 30 minutes.

Pruritus

Pruritus is an often overlooked manifestation of chronic liver disease and cirrhosis. It is most frequently observed in patients with cholestasis. The substance responsible for pruritus is not known; proposed agents have included bile acids and other retained constituents of bile and, more recently, endogenous opiods. The therapy is therefore empirical. The initial drug of choice for mild intermittent pruritus is hydroxyzine (Vistaril, Atarax) 25 to 50 mg as needed. Since pruritus is most troublesome at bedtime, the sedative properties of antihistamines often help pa-

tients sleep. Cholestyramine (Questran)* is utilized for patients with more frequent complaints or in those patients who cannot tolerate antihistamines. This is an anion exchange resin that binds bile acids and other complex molecules thought to contribute to pruritus and increases their fecal excretion. The dose is 8 to 12 grams per day in divided doses. The major side effects are bloating and constipation. Colestipol (Colestid) can be utilized in place of cholestyramine at a dose of 5 grams three times per day. Since ion exchange resins bind most medications, these agents must be taken at least 2 hours apart from other medications. For patients with pruritus refractory to these treatments, enzyme-inducing agents such as phenobarbital* (2 to 4 mg per kg per day, adjusted to maintain a plasma concentration of 10 μg per mL) and rifampin* (300 to 600 mg per day in divided doses) can be utilized. In emergency situations, naloxone (Narcan)* can be administered intravenously in doses of 0.2 μg per kg per minute over 24 hours to provide temporary relief until liver transplantation can be performed.

Prevention of Infection

Bacterial infections are common in patients with cirrhosis. As many as half either have an infection upon admission or develop one during the course of a hospitalization. Urinary tract infections are the most frequent, followed by peritonitis, respiratory infections, and bacteremia. Alcoholics are especially predisposed to community-acquired pneumonia due to *Streptococcus pneumoniae* and *Haemophilus influenzae*. Factors that predispose cirrhotics to infection include malnutrition, which alters cell-mediated and humoral immunity, and impaired phagocytic activity of the hepatic reticuloendothelial system and spleen from portal hypertension. Patients with cirrhosis should therefore be vaccinated with the polyvalent pneumococcal (Pneumovax) and the *Haemophilus* (ProHIBiT) vaccines. In addition, all cirrhotics should receive yearly influenza vaccines. Since an episode of acute viral hepatitis can precipitate liver failure in a patient with cirrhosis, those patients who are seronegative for hepatitis A and B should receive hepatitis A (Havrix) and B (Recombivax-HB, Engerix-B) vaccines.

COMPLICATIONS OF CIRRHOSIS

Once patients with chronic liver disease progress to cirrhosis, they are at risk of developing major life-threatening complications (Table 4). These, in turn, cause decompensation in hepatic function and worsening of the Child-Pugh score. Both the risk of developing complications and the mortality associated with these events increase with worsening Child's class. Since many patients with cirrhosis are awaiting hepatic transplantation, prevention and ag-

---

*Not FDA-approved for this indication.

TABLE 4. **Complications of Cirrhosis**

Hepatocellular dysfunction
  Malnutrition
  Fatigue
  Hepatic osteodystrophy
  Coagulopathy
  Pruritus
  Impaired reticuloendothelial system function
Portal hypertension and gastrointestinal bleeding
  Esophageal varices
  Gastric varices
  Congestive gastropathy
  Intestinal and rectal varices
  Hypersplenism with thrombocytopenia
Hepatic encephalopathy
Ascites and renal insufficiency
  Ascites
  Cirrhotic hydrothorax
  Spontaneous bacterial peritonitis
  Umbilical hernia (spontaneous rupture)
  Prerenal azotemia
Cholelithiasis
Hepatocellular carcinoma

gressive management of these complications are vital for long-term survival.

Variceal Hemorrhage

Bleeding from esophageal and gastric varices is one of the most common complications contributing to morbidity and mortality in patients with cirrhosis. The subject is thoroughly discussed in the article "Bleeding Esophageal Varices."

Hepatic Encephalopathy

Hepatic encephalopathy (HE) is a neuropsychiatric syndrome whose manifestations range from subtle personality changes to coma (Table 5). Although the hallmark for this process is an elevation in serum ammonia, other small metabolic products (i.e., mer-

captans, aromatic amino acids, false neurotransmitters, gamma-aminobutyric acid, and endogenous benzodiazepine-like substances) produced when colonic bacteria degrade protein are thought to be responsible for this syndrome. Normally, these substances enter the portal circulation and are rapidly metabolized by the liver. In cirrhotics, however, hepatic insufficiency, portal hypertension, and venous shunting allow these substances to reach the systemic circulation and cross the blood-brain barrier. Several factors may precipitate hepatic encephalopathy, including excess dietary protein, infection, gastrointestinal bleeding, and the use of sedatives. A comprehensive list is provided in Table 6. We consider hepatic encephalopathy of Stage II or greater a major life-threatening complication of cirrhosis. The alteration in mental status experienced by these patients affects the gag reflex and increases the risk for aspiration pneumonia.

The initial step in the management of hepatic encephalopathy is to exclude other causes for the alteration in mental status, such as subdural hematoma, cerebrovascular accident, drug overdose, delirium tremens, Wernicke's syndrome, hypoglycemia, or organic brain syndrome. The second is to identify and treat precipitating factors. All other interventions are directed at reducing the absorption of products of protein degradation. In patients with severe Grade III or IV encephalopathy, gut-cleansing enemas should be administered, and oral protein should be eliminated. Calories can be supplied as glucose, either enterally or parenterally. As the grade of encephalopathy improves, protein can be slowly added to the diet in 10- to 20-gram increments every other day until normal protein intake is achieved. Patients requiring more than 2 days without protein should receive parenteral protein supplementation. Standard amino acid solutions are adequate. The use of branched chain amino acids or special hepatic diets is rarely necessary. For patients with milder Grade I or II encephalopathy, the protein content of the diet should be limited to 40 to 60 grams.

Lactulose (Cephulac) is utilized for the treatment

TABLE 5. **Clinical Stages of Hepatic Encephalopathy**

Stage	Impairment	Symptom	Signs
I	Mild	Subtle personality changes	± Asterixis
			Impaired handwriting
		Disordered sleep	
		Subtly impaired computations	Poor coordination
II	Moderate	Inappropriate behavior	Asterixis
		Drowsiness, lethargy	Hypoactive reflexes
		Disorientation (time)	Slurred speech
III	Severe	Somnolent but arousable	Asterixis
		Marked confusion	Hyperactive reflexes
		Incoherent speech	Ataxia
IV	Coma	Unconscious	Decerebrate or decorticate posturing

TABLE 6. **Common Events Precipitating Hepatic Encephalopathy**

Dehydration
  Diuretics
  Diarrhea (lactulose induced)
  Vomiting
Electrolyte imbalance
  Hypokalemia
  Alkalosis
  Hyponatremia
Sedative or hypnotic drugs
Gastrointestinal hemorrhage
Excess dietary protein
Infection
  Spontaneous bacterial peritonitis
  Urinary tract infection
  Pneumonia
Constipation
Worsening liver disease

of all grades of hepatic encephalopathy. This synthetic disaccharide is metabolized by colonic bacteria to nonabsorbable short chain fatty acids, which acidify the colonic luminal contents and thereby prevent the absorption of ammonia and other nitrogenous waste products. This nonabsorbable sugar also produces an osmotic diarrhea that helps flush protein, nitrogenous wastes, and bacteria from the colon. The usual dose of lactulose is 15 to 30 mL orally two to four times daily, and this is titrated to produce two to four semisoft stools per day. In patients with high-grade encephalopathy or those who cannot take oral feedings, this agent can be administered via nasogastric tube or as a retention enema (300 mL lactulose in 700 mL water three to four times per day). Side effects of lactulose include profuse diarrhea, cramps, and flatulence. Patients need to be monitored carefully for electrolyte disturbances and volume contraction.

Oral neomycin is a poorly absorbed aminoglycoside that reduces intestinal ammonia-producing flora. The dosage is 2 to 4 grams per day in divided doses. It can be administered in combination with lactulose for patients with severe refractory hepatic encephalopathy. As an aminoglycoside, neomycin can cause oto- and nephrotoxicity. Since bowel edema in patients with portal hypertension allows neomycin to be absorbed, we do not advocate its use in patients with renal dysfunction. When lactulose is not sufficient treatment for hepatic encephalopathy, metronidazole (Flagyl)* can be given at a dose of 250 mg orally three times daily.

Ascites

Ascites is a frequent problem encountered by patients with cirrhosis. This is caused by portal hypertension, a decline in plasma oncotic pressure, and specific changes in the renin-angiotensin axis that strongly favor sodium retention. The development of ascites decreases both survival and the quality of life in patients with cirrhosis. Reported 1- and 5-year survival rates after the appearance of ascites are approximately 50 and 20%, respectively. The most common problems faced by patients with ascites are abdominal discomfort, early satiety, and anorexia. These exacerbate the malnutrition observed in patients with cirrhosis, as discussed previously. As the volume of ascites increases, inguinal and umbilical hernias may develop. Rupture of an umbilical hernia is a life-threatening emergency. Massive ascites may lead to intravascular volume depletion and renal insufficiency. Pulmonary insufficiency may develop, because tense ascites limits diaphragmatic excursion.

Diagnostic paracentesis should be performed in any patient with a new onset of ascites or in a known cirrhotic with ascites and evidence of clinical deterioration, fever, alteration in mental status, or abdominal tenderness. The procedure can be safely performed with a 21-gauge needle, even in the presence of a coagulopathy and thrombocytopenia. In patients with only small amounts of ascites, this procedure can be performed under ultrasound guidance. The fluid can be analyzed for total protein, albumin, triglycerides, amylase, cell count with differential, culture, and cytology. In patients with cirrhosis, the ascitic fluid is typically transudative (total protein less than 2.5 gram per dL). An albumin gradient (serum albumin − ascites albumin) of 1.1 or greater is highly specific for cirrhosis and portal hypertension as the etiology for ascites.

All patients with ascites should decrease their sodium intake. Restriction to 40 to 60 mEq per day results in complete resolution of ascites in up to 20% of patients and reduces the diuretic requirement in the rest. Because it counteracts the effects of aldosterone in the distal tubule, spironolactone (Aldactone) is usually the first diuretic tried. Because of its long half-life, the single dose of 100 mg per day is adjusted only after 3 to 4 days of monitoring. The maximum dose is 400 mg per day. Patients who develop significant painful gynecomastia can be changed to triamterene (Dyrenium) 50 mg twice daily (up to 300 mg per day) or amiloride (Midamor) 5 mg twice daily (up to 20 mg per day). For patients who fail to respond, a loop diuretic such as furosemide (Lasix) 40 mg daily (up to 160 mg per day) or bumetanide (Bumex) 2 mg daily (up to 8 mg per day) can be added. The goal of diuretic therapy is to produce a weight loss of no more than 1 kg per day. The limiting factor is the rate at which ascitic fluid can be resorbed (<900 mL per day). Larger losses, especially in patients without peripheral edema, are at the expense of the intravascular volume and can result in renal insufficiency. Mental status and electrolytes should be followed closely for evidence of complications.

Large-volume paracentesis—removal of 6 or more liters of fluid—has been shown to be effective and safe in patients who present with tense ascites or whose ascites is refractory to sodium restriction and diuretics. To prevent fluid shifts and hypovolemia, albumin should be infused at a rate of 6 to 8 grams for each liter of ascites removed. Diuretics should be continued between paracenteses sessions. Large-volume paracentesis can be particularly useful in patients who have developed respiratory difficulties because of tense ascites.

Patients who fail large-volume paracentesis should be considered candidates for a surgically placed peritoneovenous shunt (LaVeen or Denver shunts). This device, placed between the peritoneal cavity and the superior vena cava, decompresses ascites directly into the vascular system. Contraindications to shunt placement include peritonitis, recent variceal hemorrhage, hepatic encephalopathy, and congestive heart failure. Unfortunately, these shunts are associated with numerous complications, including infection, disseminated intravascular coagulation, and thrombosis. The patency of these devices is rarely greater than several months. More recently, the transjugular intrahepatic portal systemic shunt (TIPS) has shown great promise for the treatment of refractory ascites.

---

*Not FDA-approved for this indication.

Hepatic Hydrothorax

Approximately 10% of patients with cirrhosis develop hepatic hydrothorax. Such patients typically present with large right-sided pleural effusions without ascites. This process occurs in patients who have small congenital defects in the diaphragm that permit movement of ascites into the pleural space in response to negative intrathoracic pressure. Adequate treatment of ascites usually controls mild cases of cirrhotic hydrothorax. Patients with large pleural effusions and respiratory distress have a grave prognosis and limited life expectancy without hepatic transplantation. Serial thoracenteses and aggressive diuretic therapy is the only treatment. Placement of a chest tube is absolutely contraindicated: it only accentuates the negative intrathoracic pressure responsible for the movement of ascites into the pleural cavity. Pleuradesis utilizing talc or tetracycline is rarely successful. Recent case reports have suggested that TIPS may be effective in selected cases.

Renal Failure

All patients with ascites are at high risk for developing renal dysfunction. The hepatorenal syndrome (HRS) carries the gravest prognosis. HRS is characterized by progressive oliguria, increasing blood urea nitrogen and creatinine, urine sodium excretion of less than 10 mEq per liter, a fractional excretion of sodium less than 1%, and a normal urinalysis. The kidneys are histologically normal and function well if transplanted into another individual. HRS is thought to be secondary to a massive elevation in circulating endothelin, severe vasoconstriction of the afferent arteriole, and shunting of blood from the renal cortex. It is most commonly observed in patients with severe Child's Class C cirrhosis who develop variceal hemorrhage and spontaneous bacterial peritonitis. HRS is not responsive to volume expansion, dopamine infusion, or dialysis and is associated with a mortality of over 90%. Hepatic transplantation may result in restoration of renal function.

More frequently, renal impairment in patients with cirrhosis is secondary to either prerenal azotemia or nephropathy. The former is the result of intravascular volume depletion from overaggressive diuresis, paracentesis, lactulose-induced diarrhea, and gastrointestinal hemorrhage. Nephropathy is most commonly caused by intravenous contrast agents, aminoglycosides, and nonsteroidal anti-inflammatory agents. In patients with cirrhosis, and especially those with ascites, the kidney is much more sensitive to toxic injury from these agents. Since adequate renal function is one of the most important factors affecting survival following hepatic transplantation, every attempt should be made to avoid nephrotoxic agents in patients awaiting this procedure. Whenever these agents are utilized, renal function should be closely monitored.

Spontaneous Bacterial Peritonitis

Spontaneous bacterial peritonitis (SBP) is a bacterial infection of the ascitic fluid without evidence of a source. The route of colonization is thought to be hematogenous. The infection is usually monomicrobial. Gram-negative aerobic bacteria are much more common than gram-positive cocci. Most patients with SBP present with fever and diffuse abdominal tenderness. Many, however, can be identified only by deterioration in clinical status with the onset of encephalopathy or worsening liver and kidney function. It is important to make the diagnosis, because SBP carries a mortality rate of 30 to 50%. The presence of 250 polymorphonuclear leukocytes (PMNs) per μL of ascitic fluid is sufficient to make the diagnosis and start therapy. Approximately 30% of cases are culture negative. Culture yield is significantly increased if 10 mL of ascitic fluid is inoculated into a culture bottle as soon as possible after paracentesis.

The treatment is the third-generation cephalosporin cefotaxime (Claforan) administered as a single agent. The dose is 2 grams intravenously two to three times daily for 5 days. Repeat paracentesis should be performed in patients who have not had significant clinical improvement within 48 hours. If the PMN count of the ascitic fluid has not decreased by 50%, antibiotic coverage should be broadened, and other possible etiologies for peritonitis should be considered. Once a patient has an index episode of SBP, there is a 50% risk of recurrent infection within the next 12 months. Prophylactic treatment with norfloxacin (Noroxin) 400 mg per day can substantially decrease this risk and should be considered in patients following an episode of gastrointestinal hemorrhage, in patients with more than one episode of SBP, and in patients awaiting hepatic transplantation.

LIVER TRANSPLANTATION

Hepatic transplantation is the only effective long-term treatment for patients experiencing complications of cirrhosis and should be considered for all such patients. Overall long-term survival following hepatic transplantation is related to Child's class. For patients with Child's Class A or B cirrhosis, survival is excellent and exceeds 80% at most centers. In contrast, the survival for patients with decompensated Child Class C disease is only 60%. This is reduced even further in patients with tense refractory ascites, renal insufficiency, severe malnutrition, and muscle wasting.

Over the past decade, the number of patients referred to liver transplant centers and placed on the active waiting list has continued to rise and now far exceeds the donor population. As a result, the waiting time to obtain a liver transplant for any given patient continues to increase. During this waiting period, patients are at risk of developing additional complications of cirrhosis, and an increasing number die before undergoing transplantation. Other patients simply have a worsening in their Child's class, which reduces post-transplant survival. Early referral to a liver transplant center is the single most important intervention that a primary care physician can provide a patient with cirrhosis to increase his or her chance for long-term survival. The referral should be prompted by the first major complication of cirrhosis (e.g., variceal hemorrhage, refractory ascites or hydrothorax, spontaneous bacterial peritonitis, hepatic encephalopathy, hypoalbuminemia, or coagulopathy).

It is the role of the transplant center to select candidates with the greatest chance for long-term survival. Factors important in this decision include not only the etiology of the liver disease and it severity but also psychosocial factors. Patients with a history of alcoholism and/or drug use should demonstrate abstinence from these activities for a significant period of time prior to undergoing transplantation. All transplant candidates are assessed for hepatocellular carcinoma, which is considered a relative contraindication to transplantation at most centers because of the high rate of post-transplant recurrence and poor survival. Recurrence of chronic hepatitis B had been frequent following hepatic transplantation, but most cases can now be prevented by the use of long-term human hepatitis B immune globulin (HBIG). Chronic hepatitis C recurs in nearly all patients following hepatic transplantation, but this process appears to be relatively mild and nonprogressive and does not affect long-term survival.

BLEEDING ESOPHAGEAL VARICES

method of
KAJ JOHANSEN, M.D., PH.D.
University of Washington School of Medicine
Seattle, Washington

Cirrhosis of the liver is a ubiquitous health care problem, ranking ninth among all causes of death in the United States. Although manifold acute and chronic clinical problems may result from hepatic cirrhosis, none is so dramatic nor so immediately lethal as bleeding esophageal varices (BEV). The mortality rate approaches 50% for each episode of BEV; worldwide, it is the leading cause of lethal gastrointestinal hemorrhage.

ANATOMY AND PATHOPHYSIOLOGY

The parenchymal fibrosis and remodeling that characterize hepatic cirrhosis result inexorably in obstruction of the intrahepatic portal venous system. The resulting portal hypertension leads to the dilatation of multiple portosystemic collaterals, the most important of which are those connecting the portal and azygous systems via the coronary vein and the esophagogastric venous plexus. Others of clinical relevance include the hemorrhoidal venous plexus and the portosystemic collaterals that may form around abdominal wall stomas or intraperitoneal adhesions. Because the portal venous system is devoid of valves,

pressure is constant throughout the entire portal system, usually exceeding 25 mmHg and occasionally reaching values in excess of 40 mmHg.

Most bleeding secondary to portal hypertension arises from esophageal varices. A smaller percentage results from varices in the mucosa of the upper stomach or from a diffuse abnormality of the gastric mucosa termed portal hypertensive gastropathy. Cirrhotic patients' bleeding tendencies result not only from the high venous pressure in their thin-walled gastroesophageal varices but also from thrombocytopenia and various coagulopathies secondary to acute and chronic hepatocellular dysfunction.

CLINICAL PRESENTATION AND DIAGNOSIS

Bleeding from esophagogastric varices most commonly presents as massive painless hematemesis; rarely, melena or hematochezia occurs and nasogastric aspiration demonstrates dark blood in the stomach. Patients with BEV commonly exhibit signs of their underlying chronic hepatic disease; in North America and Western Europe, approximately 90% of such patients are alcoholic, with the remainder suffering the consequences of postnecrotic or other less common forms of cirrhosis.

As for all forms of significant upper gastrointestinal hemorrhage, hallmarks of early management include protection of the airway, volume resuscitation, and early fiberoptic endoscopy. This last diagnostic intervention is crucial not only for diagnosis (up to one-fifth of patients with portal hypertension may be bleeding from some other source, such as peptic ulcer disease, Mallory-Weiss tear, or erosive gastritis) but also to permit endoscopic variceal injection sclerotherapy or banding. In experienced hands, such endoscopic therapy can provide acute control of variceal bleeding in 90% of patients. Intravenous vasopressin (Pituitrin) or octreotide (Sandostatin) is frequently administered in patients with variceal hemorrhage because of these agents' demonstrable effect in diminishing total splanchnic blood flow and thereby portal pressure; whether such treatment significantly reduces early mortality from BEV is unclear.

In the occasional patient with persistent or early recurrent BEV following endoscopic sclerotherapy or banding, temporary balloon tamponade of the varices using the Sengstaken-Blakemore device or one of its analogues may be considered. Substantial mortality rates are associated with the use of emergency balloon tamponade, primarily because its use indicates failure of primary endoscopic therapy. Use of tamponade devices is frequently accompanied by pulmonary or esophageal complications.

DEFINITIVE THERAPY

Because BEV almost always occur in a context of far-advanced liver failure, all such patients should theoretically be considered candidates for orthotopic liver transplantation (OLT). Indeed, liver transplant recipients who had BEV prior to liver replacement enjoy immediate and long-term outcomes no different from those of other types of patients undergoing OLT. Those transplant recipients with alcoholic cirrhosis as a cause of their BEV demonstrate an acceptably low alcohol recidivism rate.

Ever-lengthening waiting lists and the fact that a majority of patients with BEV either have enough residual hepatic function (Child's Class A or B, see Table 1) not to require OLT or are demonstrably noncompliant and would be unable or unwilling to maintain the follow-up and medication schedule required of OLT recipients make liver replacement an uncommon solution for patients with BEV. Because the likelihood of rebleeding within 1 year after the first episode of BEV approaches 90%, some other definitive therapy to prevent further bleeding must be chosen. At various stages in the natural history of a patient with BEV, one or another therapy may be appropriate for consideration, including drugs, chronic endoscopic therapy, or some form of surgical or angiographic decompressive shunt.

Medications that have been useful in patients with portal hypertension and BEV include primarily beta blockers, such as propranolol (Inderal). Several randomized controlled trials demonstrated significant reductions in portal pressure and in variceal rebleeding among patients treated with beta blockade; data are conflicting whether the overall survival of patients so treated is significantly improved.

Whereas acute endoscopic sclerotherapy is designed to halt bleeding by thrombosing the offending varix, chronic endoscopic therapy—by either injection sclerotherapy or banding—is designed to obliterate esophagogastric variceal channels during repeated endoscopic sessions. The approach has the virtue of avoiding operation and general anesthesia, and it can be quite effective when a complete course of esophagogastric variceal obliteration can be carried out, but patients must be willing and able to return for repeat surveillance endoscopic sessions. This approach is not useful in patients who are unwilling to undergo repeated endoscopy, and it carries a cumulative risk of esophageal complications (stenosis, ulceration, perforation).

Endoscopic therapy, either acute or chronic, is ineffective for bleeding from gastric varices or from portal hypertensive gastropathy. Most important, in large series of patients treated with recurrent endoscopic therapy in an attempt to obliterate the esophagogastric variceal plexus, the overall rebleeding rate is approximately 50%; the data are once again unconvincing that chronic endoscopic therapy for BEV significantly improves survival.

Numerous operative approaches to the definitive management of BEV have been attempted. Some, such as transesophageal variceal ligation and most forms of surgical devascularization, have been discarded because of unacceptably high rates of variceal rebleeding. A possible exception is the radical two-stage esophagogastric devascularization procedure of Sugiura; this procedure has demonstrated, in its developer's hands, a remarkably low rate of operative mortality and variceal rebleeding, but these results have not been confirmed outside Japan.

Much more durable has been the record, both positive and negative, for various surgical shunts. Developed experimentally almost a century ago, the portacaval shunt, which anastomoses the portal vein and inferior vena cava directly (or, more recently, by means of an interposed prosthetic graft), is extremely effective at permanently controlling bleeding from esophagogastric varices. The method is technically straightforward and is contraindicated only in the uncommon circumstances of portal vein thrombosis. Results are poor in high-risk (Child's Class C) patients.

The major complication of the standard portacaval shunt is an unacceptably high risk of postshunt portosystemic encephalopathy (PSE), an incompletely understood neuropsychiatric disorder that occurs in the presence of concurrent hepatocellular dysfunction and portosystemic shunting. PSE rates of 25 to 100% have been reported in large series of patients undergoing standard portacaval shunting; this is the primary reason that several randomized controlled trials comparing shunting with maximal medical therapy have shown at best only trends toward improved survival in surgical patients. Recent clinical experiments suggest that the use of limited-size shunts to produce "partial" portal decompression may mitigate this well-documented risk of postshunt neurologic deterioration.

Other shunt constructions have been developed, primarily to attempt to diminish the risk of PSE while providing effective and durable portal decompression. The mesocaval shunt acts physiologically like a portacaval shunt but is burdened by a much higher risk of shunt thrombosis; it is rarely indicated except when the portal vein is occluded. The distal splenorenal shunt attempts to preserve portal perfusion of the liver while decompressing the esophagogastric variceal complex via the spleen and the splenic vein into the left renal vein. This procedure is quite effective at preventing further variceal rebleeding; its relatively low rate of postshunt PSE probably relates mostly to the selection of good-risk patients for operation, since portal perfusion of the liver is lost in a majority of patients by 1 year (especially in those with alcoholic liver disease). The procedure is technically challenging and is rarely indicated except in large academic referral centers that perform it frequently.

Operative shunts may complicate future liver transplantation by virtue of substantial scarring and anatomic distortion at the site of the original opera-

TABLE 1. **Child's Classification of Hepatic Function**

Parameter	Class A	Class B	Class C
Bilirubin (mg/dL)	<2.0	2.0–3.0	>3.0
Albumin (mg/dL)	>3.5	3.0–3.5	<3.0
Ascites	None	Reversible	Refractory
Encephalopathy	None	Minimal	Spontaneous
Nutritional status	Normal	Fair	Poor

tion. This complication is especially marked following shunt procedures in the right upper quadrant. Mesocaval or distal splenorenal shunts cause much less interference with future OLT and are preferred in patients with a high likelihood of undergoing later liver replacement.

The newest therapeutic innovation in the management of BEV is the transjugular intrahepatic portosystemic shunt (TIPS), an interventional radiologic procedure involving transcatheter dilatation of a channel through the liver substance, usually between the right hepatic vein and the right portal vein, with stenting of this channel to prevent immediate reocclusion. The early technical success of TIPS is approximately 95%, and the procedure has been confirmed as an effective, relatively low-risk "bridge" in patients who develop BEV while awaiting liver transplantation.

Unfortunately, an exuberant neointimal proliferative response leads to stenosis or occlusion of the TIPS channel in up to 50% of patients within 1 year, rendering this approach ineffective as a definitive therapy for BEV. Serial ultrasound surveillance of the TIPS channel can detect impending stenosis or occlusion in time to permit repeat dilatation or stenting or placement of a new TIPS channel. As is true for several other therapies for BEV, this approach requires patient compliance with serial evaluation.

DYSPHAGIA AND ESOPHAGEAL OBSTRUCTION

method of
JOSEPH A. TRUSZKOWSKI, M.D., and
KONRAD S. SCHULZE-DELRIEU, M.D.
University of Iowa Hospitals and Clinics
Iowa City, Iowa

Dysphagia is a malfunction of swallowing that most patients experience as the sensation of a bolus not passing smoothly from the mouth to the stomach. Typical descriptions of "trouble swallowing" include "sticking," "hanging up," or "choking" when attempting to swallow. Other symptoms of the underlying disorder, such as heartburn, cough, dyspnea, and chest pain, may be present and, importantly, may constitute the primary complaint. In fact, difficulty swallowing may not be spontaneously reported at all. A history must establish the relative importance and the temporal sequence of dysphagia and associated symptoms.

NORMAL SWALLOWING

Swallowing involves a complex sequence of events for effective bolus transport and airway protection. In the oral phase, food is chewed, mixed with saliva, and compacted into a bolus that is centered in the oral cavity between the tongue and the palate. With the voluntary initiation of a swallow, the mouth closes, sealing the lips and fixing the mandible, and the anterior tongue compresses against the hard palate. A progressive contraction wave in the mid to posterior tongue then pushes the bolus into the orophar-

ynx. The pharyngeal phase involves a rapid series of involuntary reflex-mediated motions in which the bolus is further pushed into the hypopharynx. The soft palate elevates, closing the nasopharynx and preventing nasal regurgitation. The pharynx and larynx are displaced anterosuperiorly as the epiglottis closes over the airway, temporarily halting respiration and preventing tracheal aspiration. The upper esophageal sphincter (UES) relaxes and is also pulled open, as a wave of peristaltic contractions in the hypopharynx delivers the bolus to the proximal esophagus. The esophageal phase begins after the bolus traverses the UES and involves the continuation of pharyngeal peristaltic contractions into the cervical esophagus and esophageal body. The lower esophageal sphincter (LES) relaxes as the bolus reaches the mid esophagus and remains relaxed until after the bolus is propelled into the stomach. Altogether, it usually takes 6 to 8 seconds to deliver a food bolus from the oral cavity to the stomach.

The oral phase requires intact function of both cranial nerves and striated muscles of the face, mouth, and neck. The pharyngeal phase involves reflexes mediated by the swallowing center in the brain stem, where the motor nuclei of cranial nerves V, VII, IX, X, XI, and XII reside. The esophageal phase requires intact esophageal muscle and nerve plexuses within its wall. Each phase of swallowing can be disrupted by many pathologic processes. In approaching patients with dysphagia, one should search for not only disorders that most commonly affect each phase but also those for which specific therapies exist or from which important prognostic information might be gained.

OROPHARYNGEAL DYSPHAGIA

Oropharyngeal dysphagia refers to problems with bolus formation, bolus transfer from the mouth into the esophagus, and protection of the airway. Oropharyngeal dysphagia is typically described as difficulty initiating a swallow, sticking of material in the throat, or incomplete clearance of the mouth or throat, requiring repeated swallowing attempts or expectoration. It may also present with hoarseness or cough due to impaired protective function and aspiration. In silent aspiration, loss of protective reflexes results from the inability to sense aspirated material and to clear the airway by cough. Silent aspiration should be suspected in cases of lobar pneumonia involving the dependent basilar and posterior segments. Aspiration of saliva is at least as significant as aspiration of food in the etiology of bronchopulmonary infections. Esophageal disorders may present with oropharyngeal symptoms; therefore, assessment should include a complete evaluation of the esophagus as well.

Oropharyngeal dysphagia is often caused by structural abnormalities (Table 1). Direct visualization of the oral, pharyngeal, and laryngeal mucosa is necessary to rule out treatable inflammatory and infectious processes and resectable neoplasms. Vocal cord paralysis contributing to aspiration may respond to Teflon injection or a medialization procedure. A barium study may show a Zenker's diverticulum or a prominent obstructing cricopharyngeal bar. If symptomatic, the former is best treated by cricopharyngeal myotomy with diverticular resection or suspen-

TABLE 1. **Causes of Oropharyngeal Dysphagia**

Neurologic Diseases

Cerebrovascular disease
　Cerebral hemispheric stroke or transient ischemic
　　attack
　Brain stem stroke or transient ischemic attack
Amyotrophic lateral sclerosis
Multiple sclerosis
Cranial nerve disease
　Seventh nerve
　Vagus nerve
　Recurrent laryngeal nerve
Central nervous system neoplasm
Central nervous system trauma
Miscellaneous
　Parkinson's disease
　Spinocerebellar degeneration
　Huntington's disease
　Poliomyelitis
　Neurosyphilis
　Wilson's disease
　Diphtheria
　Botulism
　Tetanus

Neuromuscular and Myopathic Diseases

Myasthenia gravis
Polymyositis/dermatomyositis
Myotonic dystrophy
Oculopharyngeal dystrophy
Hypothyroidism
Inclusion body myositis

Mucosal and Structural Abnormalities

Mucosal inflammation
　Bacterial, fungal, viral pharyngitis
　Vincent's angina
　Radiation injury
Xerostomia
　Dehydration
　Anticholinergic drugs
　Sicca syndrome
Benign structural lesions
　Zenker's diverticulum
　Cricopharyngeal bar
　Cricopharyngeal web
Local malignancy
Resective surgery
Extrinsic compression
　Cervical vertebral hyperostosis
　Cervical lymphadenopathy
　Thyromegaly

Underlying Esophageal Disease

sion, and the latter by myotomy alone. Esophageal problems commonly cause oropharyngeal symptoms, so a complete mucosal and functional evaluation is indicated. Webs and strictures in the pharynx and proximal esophagus are treatable with dilatation procedures described in the section "Benign Esophageal Obstruction."

Permanent deficits with persistent oropharyngeal dysphagia can result from stroke, brain tumor, intracranial hemorrhage, and head and neck surgery. Symptoms range from oral retention alone to severe and recurrent aspiration. Tumor resections involving extensive neck dissection pose particular problems. Glossectomy severely impairs food bolus compaction and propulsion, as does pharyngeal muscle resection.

Laryngectomy results in impaired UES opening, and vocal cord removal eliminates a crucial barrier to aspiration. Videofluoroscopy utilizing varying consistencies of barium allows evaluation of the swallowing mechanism and of responses to compensatory measures aimed at optimizing transport, clearance, and protective functions. Examples include reducing bolus size, thickening bolus consistency, flexing the head forward, and rotating the head toward the weak side with swallows. Patients with ineffective pharyngeal peristalsis, hypopharyngeal stasis, and aspiration after swallowing can be shown by videofluoroscopy how to elevate the larynx during and after swallowing, which holds the UES open and facilitates bolus transfer into the esophagus. Patients who aspirate during swallows can learn the supraglottic swallow, in which the breath is held and released as a forceful cough after swallowing, in order to clear the airway.

If compensatory measures fail, other interventions become necessary. Impairment of mucosal and muscular integrity from resective and reconstructive neck surgery is a particular problem. Patients unable to maintain weight with oral feeding alone should receive supplemental nutrition through a percutaneous endoscopic gastrostomy (PEG) feeding tube. If they have become malnourished, they may benefit from temporary nasoenteric feeding to optimize wound healing. Patients who aspirate only liquids may continue to eat solids and receive supplemental fluid through a PEG tube. Those who aspirate all consistencies should abandon the oral feeding route and receive all nutrition through a PEG tube. This particularly applies to patients who have undergone extensive neck dissection, glossectomy, and laryngectomy for cancer. Individuals with gastroesophageal reflux and aspiration should follow postprandial and nocturnal reflux precautions and may benefit from a modified PEG in which a feeding tube is passed into the jejunum (PEJ). In patients with progressive neurologic disorders, particularly amyotrophic lateral sclerosis, in which oropharyngeal dysphagia inevitably leads to aspiration, early intervention is extremely important, and PEG feeding tubes should be placed before patients lose the ability to cough effectively. Although PEG and PEJ tubes help prevent the aspiration of food material, they do not prevent the aspiration of saliva, and this remains a significant source of morbidity. In severe cases of recurrent aspiration, laryngeal closure and tracheostomy may be performed.

Most cases of oropharyngeal dysphagia are caused by neuromuscular diseases. Although many of these cannot be cured, some may respond to disease-specific treatment. Oral and pharyngeal muscle fatigability from myasthenia gravis is preventable with pyridostigmine. Oropharyngeal and esophageal dysmotility caused by hypothyroidism should improve with levothyroxine. Pharyngeal muscle weakness due to polymyositis or dermatomyositis may respond to corticosteroids or immune suppressive drugs. With Parkinson's disease, however, levodopa and anticholinergics can actually worsen associated oropharyngeal and esophageal dysfunction, even though other symptoms improve. Brain stem and cerebral hemispheric strokes can acutely impair cranial nerve and swallowing center reflux function. In these settings, the risk of aspiration is high, and barium studies to assess dysphagia can be dangerous. Swallowing often improves after short periods of time with supportive care involving nasoenteric feeding and aspiration precautions. In cases of stroke, antiplatelet or anticoagulant therapy is indicated to prevent further cerebral infarcts.

ESOPHAGEAL DYSPHAGIA

Esophageal dysphagia refers to incomplete bolus transport from the proximal esophagus to the stomach. Esophageal dysphagia is sensed more than 1 to 2 seconds after initiating a swallow. A sticking or fullness perceived in the lower chest suggests a distal esophageal problem, but symptoms in the upper chest or neck do not necessarily indicate a proximal process, as the sensation may be referred or material may back up. Similarly, oropharyngeal symptoms may represent esophageal disorders, even distal lesions, so complete esophageal assessment is indicated. Dysphagia to solids alone, especially meat and bread, suggests a mechanical obstruction. Intermittency and slow progression imply a benign process, such as a ring, web, or peptic stricture (Table 2).

TABLE 2. **Causes of Esophageal Dysphagia**

Mucosal and Structural Lesions

Schatzki and muscular rings
Webs
Esophagitis/mucosal injury
   Gastroesophageal reflux
   Infection
   Caustic ingestion
   Radiation injury
   Pill-induced injury
Benign strictures
   Reflux-induced
   Corrosive/caustic
   Radiation-induced
   Pill-induced
Malignant strictures
   Adenocarcinoma
   Squamous cell carcinoma
Extrinsic compression

Motor Abnormalities

Achalasia
Progressive systemic sclerosis/CREST syndrome
Spastic motor disorders
   Diffuse esophageal spasm
   Nutcracker esophagus
   Hypertensive lower esophageal sphincter
Nonspecific esophageal motility disorders
   Metabolic
      Diabetes mellitus
      Hypothyroidism
      Electrolyte abnormalities
   Esophagitis/mucosal injury
   Miscellaneous
      Medications

Rapid progression to involve both solids and liquids implies a malignant process, as do anorexia, weight loss, and continuous chest pain. Dysphagia to both solids and liquids, especially if intermittent and nonprogressive, suggests a motor disorder. Associated heartburn suggests a peptic stricture or motor disorder rather than a cancer. Odynophagia, or pain with swallowing, usually represents infectious or corrosive esophagitis or cancer.

Achalasia

Achalasia is a disorder in which the number of ganglion cells in the smooth muscle portion of the esophagus and the LES is reduced. This results in aperistalsis of the mid and distal esophagus and functional obstruction by an LES that fails to adequately relax. Dysphagia occurs with both solids and liquids. Patients may use compensatory maneuvers to improve bolus passage, such as arm raising, erect posturing, and slow, deliberate swallowing. Eventually the esophageal body dilates, and patients experience retrosternal fullness or pain and regurgitation of nonacidified, undigested food. Nocturnal regurgitation may produce coughing spells and aspiration. Significant weight loss is common. On physical examination, a supine test swallow with auscultation over the subxiphoid area may suggest aperistalsis by the absence of sound within 6 to 8 seconds of initiating a swallow of water. A chest x-ray may demonstrate absence of a gastric air bubble, mediastinal widening with a double density, an air-fluid level within the esophagus, and aspiration pneumonia.

A barium swallow with videofluoroscopy shows an aperistaltic, usually dilated esophageal body, with distal tapering to a "bird's beak" configuration. In the upright position, gravity may force barium through the LES into the stomach, independent of swallowing. There may be large amounts of retained food. A study in the prone position shows failure of esophageal clearing. Esophageal manometry demonstrates absent distal esophageal peristalsis and an LES with elevated resting pressure and incomplete relaxation with swallows. Endoscopy is mandatory to rule out cancer at the gastroesophageal junction, especially gastric adenocarcinoma, which can cause an achalasia-like syndrome through invasion of the nerve plexus, with or without mechanical obstruction. In some cases of chronic retention of food, endoscopy may reveal bezoars, pressure ulceration, or even *Candida* esophagitis.

Therapy of achalasia aims to reduce the functional obstruction at the LES to improve esophageal clearance. In order to prevent complications such as weight loss and aspiration pneumonia, it is essential to treat early, before massive esophageal dilatation occurs. Pneumatic dilatation forcefully disrupts the circular muscle layer of the LES. It involves passing a balloon dilator over a guidewire that has been placed in the stomach. Under fluoroscopic guidance, the dilator is centered within the gastroesophageal junction and inflated to its maximum diameter of

3.0, 3.5, or 4.0 cm with a pressure of 9 to 12 psi for 30 to 60 seconds. With inflation there should be a gradual disappearance of the LES indentation on the balloon; if not, the procedure should be repeated with a larger dilator. The risk of perforation is up to 5%, and clinical signs may be lacking, particularly if the dissection is intramural only, so an immediate post-procedure esophagram with water-soluble contrast should be obtained. Half or more of such cases respond to conservative measures, including esophageal suction and antibiotics, without requiring surgery. Although pneumatic dilatation is initially successful in over 75% of cases, recurrent symptoms develop in up to one-third of patients, especially younger adults and children, and the success rate of subsequent dilatations is only 50%.

The modified Heller myotomy involves the surgical division of the anterior circular muscle fibers of the LES, with extension 1 cm or less onto the stomach and several centimeters up the esophagus. It is successful in up to 90% of cases, with only rare relapses. With improvements in technique, the occurrence of postsurgical gastroesophageal reflux and peptic stricture formation has been reduced to less than 10% without requiring an antireflux procedure at the time of myotomy. Although the operative mortality may be low, morbidity and cost are high relative to pneumatic dilatation, and myotomy should be considered second-line therapy for patients in whom dilatation fails after one or two attempts. Thoracoscopic myotomy studies report short-term success rates similar to those of open procedures, but shorter recovery times and lower cost.

Drugs that may be used in the treatment of achalasia include isosorbide dinitrate (Isordil)* 5 to 10 mg or nifedipine (Procardia)* 10 to 30 mg sublingually before meals. Studies have shown inconsistent symptomatic improvement, and it is unknown whether medical therapy alone can prevent or halt esophageal dilatation. As initial therapy, drugs are a poor substitute for pneumatic dilatation or myotomy and should be reserved for patients who refuse or are unsuitable candidates for the procedures. Temporary medical therapy may allow some patients to regain weight and improve their nutritional status while awaiting either procedure. Favorable results have been reported with injection of botulinum toxin† into the LES. This and drug treatment should be reserved for patients who are unwilling to undergo pneumatic dilatation or who are poor operative risks for myotomy.

Esophageal Dysmotility Syndromes

The spastic disorders of the esophagus consist of diffuse esophageal spasm (DES), nutcracker esophagus, hypertensive LES, and the nonspecific motility disorders. They are often described separately, but there is significant overlap of features, and they may be variants of the same disease. They manifest as dysfunction of the distal smooth muscle segment of the esophagus 5 to 10 cm above the LES, frequently including the LES. They present by early to mid adulthood with intermittent, nonprogressive dysphagia to both solids and liquids of varying severity. Intermittent, retrosternal chest pain lasting from minutes to hours is more common than dysphagia, and they seldom occur together. Severe pain episodes are characteristically followed by residual prolonged aching that may be indistinguishable from angina. Regurgitation and weight loss are less common than with achalasia. Physical findings are typically lacking.

Esophageal manometry defines the spastic disorders. DES is characterized by high-amplitude contractions that are simultaneous in onset. Other abnormalities include spontaneous or prolonged contractions and an LES with high resting pressure and incomplete relaxation. Nutcracker esophagus is defined by propagating contractions with above-normal amplitudes and sometimes with prolonged durations. Hypertensive LES occurs as an isolated phenomenon or in association with another spastic disorder, especially DES. Manometry shows elevated resting LES pressure but normal relaxation and peristalsis. Nonspecific esophageal motility disorders are those with manometric abnormalities that do not allow classification within the other three entities. With all these disorders, there is poor correlation of dysphagia with manometric findings. Since they all can be caused by esophagitis, strictures, tumors, and esophageal adhesions, however, evaluation of esophageal structural and mucosal integrity with endoscopy and biopsies is indicated. If unrevealing, barium videofluoroscopy or 24-hour pH monitoring may be helpful.

Therapy for the spastic disorders is most likely to be effective if an underlying cause is identified. Esophageal dysmotility is most commonly due to gastroesophageal reflux disease (GERD), so a therapeutic trial of standard antireflux measures as outlined in the article on GERD may be useful. If endoscopy is grossly unrevealing, empirical esophageal dilatation with a 21-mm bougie dilator may be helpful, as minor strictures, subtle adhesions, and reduced compliance may be missed. Surgical myotomy has been used with some reported success in isolated severe, refractory cases. Nonspecific therapy may include isosorbide dinitrate* 5 to 10 mg or nifedipine* 10 to 30 mg sublingually or orally before eating, diltiazem (Cardizem)* 30 to 60 mg orally before eating, or trazodone (Desyrel) 100 to 150 mg orally each day. Either hyoscyamine sulfate (Levsin) 0.125 to 0.250 mg or dicyclomine hydrochloride (Bentyl) 10 to 20 mg orally four times daily may also be tried.

Esophageal dysmotility, with weak peristalsis and LES incompetence seen on manometry, is common in patients with progressive systemic sclerosis (PSS), CREST syndrome, and diabetes mellitus. PSS and

---

*Not FDA-approved for this indication.
†Investigational drug in the United States.

*Not FDA-approved for this indication.

CREST involve replacement of esophageal smooth muscle with fibrotic tissue, and diabetes causes neuropathy. All may be complicated by delayed gastric emptying, reflux esophagitis, *Candida* esophagitis, and recurrent peptic strictures, which can be quite severe in PSS and CREST. Aggressive antireflux therapy is indicated. Prokinetic drugs, such as metoclopramide (Reglan) 10 to 30 mg, cisapride (Propulsid) 10 to 20 mg, and erythromycin* 250 mg orally before meals and at bedtime, tend to be more useful in diabetics.

Other forms of mucosal disease commonly result in esophageal dysmotility. Infectious esophagitis due to *Candida*, herpes simplex, or cytomegalovirus necessitates systemic antifungal or antiviral therapy and further evaluation for immunodeficiency, if not already known. Pill-induced esophagitis should be suspected in individuals with sudden odynophagia and mid-esophageal lesions who take tetracycline, doxycycline, potassium chloride, quinidine, iron preparations, or nonsteroidal anti-inflammatory drugs; therapy involves stopping the offending drug and temporary antireflux measures. If the medications are necessary, patients should be given suitable alternative formulations. Small, smooth, oval pills are better than large tablets with squared edges. Patients should sit upright during and after swallows and should take plenty of liquid. Semiliquids such as applesauce may provide better propulsion. Radiation therapy to the chest causes both acute and chronic mucosal injury, with odynophagia and dysphagia from secondary dysmotility. Ingestion of strongly acidic or alkaline substances causes acute mucosal injury to the entire esophagus and, in severe cases, esophageal perforation. Emesis results in further damage and should be avoided. Dilution of acids immediately with milk or water may be helpful but should be avoided with alkali. Careful laryngoscopic and endoscopic examination when patients are stable allows staging of injury. Severe cases may require nasoenteric feeding, antibiotics, and endotracheal intubation.

Benign Esophageal Obstruction

Severe inflammation or repetitive mucosal injury can result in an esophageal stricture. Patients report dysphagia primarily to solids that slowly progresses. Peptic strictures due to reflux are the most common type and are suggested by a history of heartburn and regurgitation. They usually form in the distal esophagus but can occur at any level. Proximal strictures can present with oropharyngeal symptoms. Mid-esophageal stricturing may complicate severe pill-induced esophagitis. Radiation-induced strictures tend to occur several months after doses of 6000 cGy or more and after a period of acute injury. Corrosive strictures due to the ingestion of caustic substances can involve long segments of the esophagus.

---

*Not FDA-approved for this indication.

Barium studies show smooth, tapered stenoses, but active esophagitis can cause ulcers and mucosal irregularity. Endoscopy with biopsies and brushings is necessary to rule out Barrett's metaplasia and cancers. Treatment consists of forceful dilatation to a luminal diameter of more than 13 mm, and several options exist. Mercury-filled dilators are passed at the time of endoscopy, with the patient in the sitting or left lateral decubitus position and mildly sedated with a benzodiazepine and narcotic analgesic. Dilators are passed by having the patient swallow increasingly large ones in sequence, such that resistance is met with the last three. If necessary, the procedure can be repeated at 1- to 2-week intervals. In cases of high-grade stenosis, esophageal tortuosity, or hiatal herniation, a guidewire system is preferred. Stiffer, tapered polyvinyl dilators are passed over an endoscopically placed guidewire in a similar sequential fashion. Aggressive antireflux therapy is essential to prevent recurrences.

A Schatzki ring represents a circumferential mucosal protrusion into the distal esophageal lumen. It consists of squamous epithelium superiorly, columnar epithelium inferiorly, and a thin layer of lamina propria in between. It often forms the superior margin of a hiatal hernia sac. Most are asymptomatic unless the lumen measures 13 mm or less, at which point patients experience intermittent dysphagia to solids, classically to meat or bread during a rushed meal. A muscular "A" ring presents similarly but includes a layer of muscle and usually occurs above the squamocolumnar junction. A web is a very thin, noncircumferential membrane of squamous epithelium in the proximal or mid esophagus, usually on the anterior wall. Rings and webs are not caused by esophageal inflammation and do not progress over time. They are best appreciated on barium studies. Endoscopy is less sensitive diagnostically but allows definitive therapy with the single passage of a bougie dilator 17 mm or larger in diameter, preferably over a guidewire if there is a hiatal hernia. Balloon dilatation, as with achalasia, is also an option.

Esophageal Cancer

Esophageal adenocarcinoma usually presents in older individuals with rapidly progressive dysphagia to solids, anorexia, and weight loss out of proportion to the degree of dysphagia. Patients often have long-standing reflux symptoms, but their absence is common in the setting of Barrett's metaplasia, the premalignant lesion associated with chronic reflux. Squamous cell carcinoma presents similarly, but reflux and Barrett's metaplasia are not associated, and it occurs more proximally within the esophagus, sometimes presenting with oropharyngeal symptoms. Barium studies suggest the diagnosis, but endoscopy with biopsies and brushings is required for confirmation. Cure is realistic only with complete surgical resection, but many adenocarcinomas have metastasized and most squamous cell cancers have infiltrated adjacent tissue too extensively at the time of diagnosis. Staging is important, and assessment of resectability may be enhanced by endoscopic ultrasonography.

Palliative therapy for esophageal cancers aims at relieving dysphagia so patients can achieve and maintain adequate oral intake. Dilatation procedures are indicated early to establish luminal patency and are the same as for benign strictures. Methods of maintaining patency with progressive tumors include follow-up dilatations, endoscopic Nd:YAG laser thermal ablation, and peroral esophageal stents. Surgical debulking procedures in unresectable cases can be helpful. Palliative radiation has more of a role with squamous cell cancers than with adenocarcinomas. If oral intake is limited to liquids, nutritional supplements should be given.

Acute Foreign Body Obstruction

Acute esophageal obstruction usually results from impaction of a food bolus at the site of a structural lesion, particularly a stricture, ring, or web. Patients often describe sudden chest fullness or pain after swallowing a large piece of meat. There is poor correlation between the perceived and the actual location of the obstruction. Regurgitation and choking suggest a proximal lesion or a completely filled esophagus from a distal lesion and require immediate attention. Odynophagia and sharp pain may occur if a sharp object such as a bone fragment or toothpick has been swallowed and may also signify laceration or perforation. Other commonly ingested foreign bodies include coins, disk batteries, and safety pins. Initial evaluation with plain x-rays should include anteroposterior and lateral views of both the neck and the chest, with soft tissue technique to try to localize the object. If it is impacted in the UES or cervical esophagus, or if a sharp object is lodged at any site, rigid esophagoscopy by an otolaryngologist using general anesthesia and airway protection is indicated. For suspected food bolus impactions within the esophagus, glucagon 0.5 to 1.0 mg intravenously may allow esophageal and LES relaxation, with subsequent bolus passage into the stomach. If an obstructed esophagus is filled with fluid, an orogastric tube may allow careful lavage to prevent aspiration and facilitate therapeutic endoscopy. Instillation of meat tenderizer with proteolytic enzymes should be avoided because of the risk of perforation. Endoscopy may allow an impacted bolus to be pushed into the stomach, and if this is not possible with gentle pressure, one may try to fragment the bolus first. If retrieval is necessary because the material is undigestible, an overtube is required for airway protection and, in the case of a sharp object, protection of the esophageal mucosa. Alkaline batteries can cause severe corrosive injury and must always be retrieved. Endoscopic reassessment and dilatation of webs, strictures, and rings is indicated as an elective procedure in all patients with bolus impaction of food. Repeat examination is also indicated when persistent

esophageal injury from a foreign body must be ruled out.

DIVERTICULA OF THE ALIMENTARY TRACT

method of
WILLIAM S. HAUBRICH, M.D.
The Scripps Clinic and Research Foundation
La Jolla, California

Diverticula are outpouchings that can occur anywhere along the wall of the alimentary tract from the proximal esophagus to the distal colon. Traditionally, diverticula have been classified as "true" (containing all layers of the wall) or "pseudo" (only the mucosa and submucosa penetrating the otherwise intact muscular wall); in clinical practice, this distinction serves little purpose. Some diverticula are congenital, i.e., developmental defects present at birth; most are acquired during life as a consequence of motility disorder abetted by a focal weakness in the wall.

Diverticula are usually asymptomatic and discovered incidentally in the course of a diagnostic procedure, such as contrast radiography or endoscopy, performed for another purpose. However, occasionally patients present with symptoms and signs sufficient to arouse suspicion of diverticular disease, thereby prompting objective confirmation and requiring consideration of treatment.

ESOPHAGEAL DIVERTICULA

Hypopharyngeal Diverticulum. A fairly common and frequently symptomatic mucosal protrusion is from the posterior wall of the hypopharynx, in a gap between the oblique fibers of the inferior constrictor muscle above and the transverse fibers of the cricopharyngeus muscle (the upper esophageal sphincter) below. This is the familiar Zenker's diverticulum, which is situated in the hypopharynx and not in the esophagus proper. Less frequent are diverticula that protrude laterally in this segment. Presumably, the cause of protrusion is excessive hypopharyngeal pressure generated by swallowing and impeded by an unduly tight and unrelaxing upper esophageal sphincter. Such diverticula typically become evident in persons older than 60 years.

Often the earliest symptom is repeated coughlike attempts to clear the throat, sometimes magnified as paroxysms of choking. Telltale is an occasional and annoying bubbling sensation felt at the back of the throat. Actual dysphagia in the course of eating or drinking is relatively infrequent and transient. Brief periods of spasm in the upper esophageal sphincter, with or without swallowing, can be felt as aching pain deep in the throat. Coughing, sometimes with regurgitation of trapped food particles or a previously swallowed pill or capsule, is particularly troublesome for recumbent patients at night. In some way, a hypopharyngeal diverticulum tends to stimulate salivation, and nocturnal drooling is an occasional symptom. The most serious complication, fortunately rare, is aspiration of regurgitated diverticular content.

Patients with an incidentally discovered or minimally symptomatic hypopharyngeal diverticulum can often be managed by explanation, reassurance, and simple dietary advice: to eat slowly, take small bites of food, chew thoroughly. When symptoms become unduly burdensome, the treatment of choice is surgical excision of the diverticulum, usually accompanied by myotomy of the upper esophageal sphincter. The operation can be performed under local anesthesia, if necessary, and seldom requires more than an overnight stay in the hospital. After several days limited to liquid oral intake, a normal diet can gradually be resumed. The result is almost always satisfactory, and the rate of complication or recurrence is nearly nil.

Mid-Esophageal Diverticulum. Mucosal diverticular protrusion from the lumen of the mid-esophagus is distinctly unusual and almost always an incidental finding. Seldom do mid-esophageal diverticula give rise to symptoms; if esophageal symptoms have prompted their discovery, evidence of an underlying motility disorder should be sought. The old concept that a mid-esophageal defect might be caused by traction on the wall by adjacent inflammation or neoplasia is rarely borne out. The discovery of a mid-esophageal diverticulum alone requires no treatment, unless the diverticulum is egregiously large.

Epiphrenic Diverticulum. Such a mucosal protrusion appears, typically as an incidental finding, in the distal esophagus within 10 cm of the esophagogastric junction. Symptoms, if present, are almost always of an underlying motor disorder, e.g., hypertensive lower esophageal sphincter or an unyielding distal stricture. Treatment, when called for, should be aimed at correcting the underlying disturbance. Only rarely does an epiphrenic diverticulum itself require excision.

Diffuse Intramural Diverticulosis. This unusual condition is marked by clusters of small mucosal outpouchings in segments of varying length, typically in areas of luminal constriction or stasis. The picture, by contrast radiography or endoscopy, is unmistakable. The diverticulosis itself is asymptomatic, except when attended by infection, e.g., candidiasis. Treatment, when indicated, is directed to the associated infection, luminal stenosis, or gastroesophageal reflux.

DIVERTICULA OF THE STOMACH

The vast majority of diverticula of the stomach are stereotypical mucosal protrusions from the posterior wall at the cardial neck of the stomach, averaging about 3 cm in greatest dimension. Most are probably congenital. The cause of symptoms should always be sought elsewhere in the stomach, particularly at or near the cardioesophageal junction. Any temptation to excise a cardiogastric diverticulum should be suppressed.

Occasionally, what appears to be a diverticulum may be seen in the body or antrum of the stomach; more often than not, such a lesion is found, on closer inspection, to be a burrowing neoplasm, a penetrating peptic ulcer, or a scarred deformity produced by previous ulceration or inflammation.

DIVERTICULA OF THE SMALL INTESTINE

Duodenal Diverticulum. Extramural globular protrusions from the supra- or periampullary duodenum are fairly common incidental findings during contrast radiography or endoscopy. Most are thought to be congenital. Only rarely do they give rise to symptoms, and their discovery merits little more than mention. Periampullary diverticula may be associated with a higher than expected frequency of gallstones. If symptoms are present, their cause should be sought in a source other than the diverticula. Almost never do duodenal diverticula, in themselves, justify the considerable risk of attempted excision.

Diverticulum of the Mesenteric Small Bowel. A single outpouching from the small bowel wall is exceedingly difficult to discern on contrast radiographs, which may be just as well, since a lone diverticulum is usually insignificant (with the important exception of a Meckel's diverticulum, noted later). Jejunal and ileal diverticula are often multiple, vary in size from a few millimeters to several centimeters, and typically protrude between the leaves of the mesentery. They are best demonstrated radiographically in progressive films taken after administration of a contrast meal. Their significance is threefold:

1. They may be associated with motility disorders, such as those seen with certain diseases marked by degenerative fibrosis (e.g., scleroderma), with chronic inflammation (e.g., Crohn's disease), or with various visceral myopathies and neuropathies.

2. Stasis within diverticular cavities, especially in the jejunum, is conducive to bacterial overgrowth and consequently to diarrhea, steatorrhea, and nutritional deficiency; recent evidence emphasizes the added role of impaired mucosal function incident to stasis.

3. Rarely, small bowel diverticula may be the cause of spontaneous pneumoperitoneum, which is often asymptomatic and discovered incidentally.

In cases of small bowel diverticulosis, bacterial overgrowth is difficult to demonstrate directly by aspiration and quantitative culture of intestinal contents, especially when diverticula are situated in the ileum. For this reason, indirect tests of bacterial overgrowth are employed; currently, the most reliable is the ^{14}C-D-xylose breath test.

If symptoms cannot be allayed by conservative measures and small bowel diverticula are sufficiently clustered, consideration may be given to surgical resection of the affected segment. However, this is seldom the case, and treatment is best aimed at suppressing bacterial overgrowth. This can be accomplished by administration of an antibiotic agent (or combination of agents) effective against *both* aerobic and anaerobic enteric bacteria. An example is amoxicillin/clavulanate potassium (Augmentin) 250 to 500 mg three times daily. Sometimes a course of 7 to 10 days is rewarded by remission of symptoms for several months; more often, an intermittent course of therapy (e.g., 1 week in every 4) is required for sustained remission. Useful as an adjunct is restriction of dietary fat, as well as substitution of long chain fats by medium chain triglycerides. Supplements of calcium carbonate, fat-soluble vitamins, and parenteral cobalamin may be required. Because lactase deficiency often attends small bowel bacterial overgrowth, elimination of dietary lactose or the use of lactase supplements can be beneficial. Another more recently available approach is the subcutaneous administration of *small* doses of octreotide (Sandostatin), 25 to 50 μg at bedtime, to stimulate intestinal motility and thus help clear bacterial stasis; larger doses tend to aggravate stasis.

Meckel's Diverticulum. This singular congenital anomaly (a remnant of the embryonic vitelline duct) is evident as an elongated protrusion from the anti-mesenteric border of the ileum, usually within 100 cm of the ileocecal junction. Such an anomaly, said to be present in 2% of the general population, may never give rise to symptoms. However, because heterotopic gastric mucosa, capable of acid-peptic secretion, occurs within the lining of most Meckel's diverticula, complication by ulceration, bleeding, or intussusception is a potential hazard. In cases of otherwise occult intestinal bleeding, the presence of a suspected Meckel's diverticulum is best confirmed by a technetium-99m pertechnetate scintiscan. The proper management of any Meckel's diverticulum, whether symptomatically complicated or discovered incidental to exploratory abdominal laparotomy, is surgical resection.

DIVERTICULA OF THE COLON

Mucosal outpouchings from the wall of the large intestine represent acquired defects that occur in more than half the elderly population of the Western world; curiously, the prevalence is far less among people of the same age in Asia and Africa. The commonly accepted explanation is the low-fiber diet favored by Westerners, in contrast to the high-fiber diet on which Eastern and Southern people subsist. This may be an oversimplification; other factors, perhaps genetic, probably play a role. Among Western people, diverticula may be found in any segment of the colon or occur diffusely throughout the colon, but typically they cluster in the sigmoid segment. Among Asian people, diverticula in the proximal colon are more common.

The frequency of colonic diverticula in populations of Europe and North America raises a question: is the presence of large bowel diverticula a disease, or is it a natural consequence of aging? One approach to an answer lies in a definition of terms. The mere presence of diverticula is properly referred to as "diverticulosis" and is not, in itself, a disease; "diverticular disease" is a term that should be reserved for complicating conditions, namely (1) infection leading to inflammation ("diverticulitis") and potentially to perforation or fistula or sometimes to stenotic scarring, and (2) hemorrhage. Diverticulosis is common; diverticular disease is not.

Inflammation and hemorrhage are seldom concurrent; inflamed diverticula tend not to bleed, and bleeding typically occurs in the absence of signs of diverticulitis.

The presence of colonic diverticula is usually demonstrated by barium enema radiography but is often evident at colonoscopy; however, neither the radiographic configuration nor the colonoscopic appearance can be relied on to confirm the presence or absence of active diverticulitis. An exception is when a fistula is clearly demonstrated by barium enema. Computed tomography (CT) scanning, with or without contrast, gives a much more informative picture of the presence and extent of diverticulitis and is being increasingly used for this purpose. Neither contrast radiography nor CT scanning can tell when a diverticulum has bled.

Diverticulosis. Asymptomatic and uncomplicated colonic diverticulosis requires no specific treatment. Patients found to harbor colonic diverticula should be so informed and warned of the possibility of future complications; at the same time, they can be reassured that complications ensue in a fairly small fraction of cases. A patient with known diverticulosis is well advised to adopt a relatively high-fiber diet; the regular use of a supplemental hydrophilic colloid (e.g., a natural psyllium derivative or synthetic substitute, such as methylcellulose) can be beneficial in allaying symptoms of irritable bowel that may attend diverticulosis. The old admonition that patients with diverticulosis must scrupulously avoid foods containing vegetable seeds has little or no validity.

Diverticular Bleeding. Bleeding from a colonic diverticulum (usually only a single diverticulum bleeds at any given time) typically occurs in otherwise asymptomatic patients. Bleeding tends to be brisk and is evident as hematochezia rather than melena. It is important to bear in mind that a source of occult gastrointestinal bleeding or iron-deficiency anemia is rarely, if ever, properly attributable to the mere presence of colonic diverticula.

An acute episode of diverticular bleeding can be expected to subside naturally in the majority of cases. Rare is the threat of exsanguination. The risk of a second episode of diverticular bleeding is about 25%; that of a third or fourth episode is about 50%. Even when an initial episode of intestinal bleeding has been attributed to diverticular disease, one can never be sure that a subsequent appearance of blood in the stool is from the same source; any recurrence requires repeated search for a cause.

Precise location of the diverticulum that is the origin of blood loss is often difficult. Neither contrast radiography nor CT scanning can tell whether a diverticulum is bleeding or has bled. The best that one can do by means of endoscopy, scintigraphy, or selective angiography is to direct attention to the miscreant segment of the colon. Identifying an actively bleeding site by selective arteriography—a procedure that is not always necessary—has the advantage of providing the possibility of control by embolization or injection of a vasoconstricting agent.

The threat of exsanguinating hemorrhage, a rare occurrence, can be countered by exigent surgical resection of that portion of the colon known to be or strongly suspected of being the site of bleeding. More often, surgical intervention is considered as an elective means of stopping repeated episodes of diverticular bleeding. So-called blind colectomy—i.e., operation undertaken when the source of hemorrhage is unknown or only supposed—in the case of either acute or repeated bleeding is not generally recommended. Recent anecdotal reports suggest that active bleeding can be stopped by colonoscopic instillation of absolute alcohol or diluted solutions of epinephrine.

Diverticulitis. The clinical symptoms and signs of acute diverticulitis (pain, typically in the right lower quadrant; marked tenderness over the involved segment, with or without a palpable mass; usually fever; and leukocytosis) are essential to the diagnosis. Most authorities deny the existence of a syndrome of "chronic" diverticulitis, except as represented by scarring that results from acute inflammation.

Whether a given episode of acute diverticulitis can be treated safely and with a reasonable chance of success in an outpatient setting or requires admission to the hospital for more closely supervised care is a matter of judgment by the attending physician. Such judgment must rely largely on clinical assessment, because patients suspected of active, acute diverticulitis are properly spared the risk of invasive investigation, such as barium enema or colonoscopy. In this situation, CT scans can be helpful.

Patients with only mild-to-moderate symptoms and no signs of sepsis can often be managed satisfactorily without resorting to hospital confinement. Such patients are advised to remain at rest and to consume clear liquids in small volumes at frequent intervals. Oral antibiotics effective against both aerobic and anaerobic bacteria should be prescribed, such as amoxicillin/clavulanate (Augmentin) 250 mg/125 mg every 8 hours or ciprofloxacin (Cipro) 500 mg every 12 hours. It is important to keep in mind that infection and inflammation incident to colonic diverticula are actually pericolitis, not a disease of the bowel lumen. No benefit can be expected from the administration of antibacterial agents that are active only within the lumen of the colon.

Patients admitted to the hospital are treated in much the same manner, with the use of intravenously administered fluids and antibiotics (often as "triple therapy," e.g., combining ampicillin, gentamicin, and metronidazole), when necessary. The chief advantage of hospitalization is strict supervision of treatment and closer vigilance to guard against additional or progressive complications. In a considerable majority of patients, acute diverticulitis so treated shows signs of abating within several days and may completely resolve within a week or two. Failure to abate and resolve indicates a complication, notably perforation and abscess formation; sepsis can be lethal. Other complications that pose a hazard include acute free perforation and enteroenteric or enterovesical fistula formation. Percutaneous CT-guided drainage of a diverticular abscess frequently hastens resolution, lessens the risk of further complications, and shortens hospital stay.

Surgical consultation should be sought early in the course of the disease whenever there is suspicion of extensive involvement or threatening progression. Fortunately, the colon is naturally adept at walling off leaks in its wall, but does not always succeed. Exigent surgical intervention is mandated in cases of unconfined perforation attended by spreading peritonitis. This entails a series of staged operations: abdominal drainage, temporary colostomy, then later resection of the affected segment and closure of the colostomy. This sequence—now seldom called for—should be avoided insofar as the patient's safety permits. Much more satisfactory to all concerned is controlling the acute disease by properly intensive, conservative means, thereby allowing reasoned consideration of safer, less complex surgical intervention.

More often, when the acute reaction has subsided, the surgeon may be recalled to provide a definitive "cure" by resecting the affected segment and establishing a primary anastomosis. This is the treatment of choice following an initial episode of unusually severe diverticulitis or repeated episodes of less threatening disease. One episode of mild-to-moderate diverticulitis, favorably resolved, does not call for serious consideration of surgical intervention. A substantial majority of patients—upward of two-thirds—who fully recover from an initial bout of diverticulitis do not suffer a recurrence, especially when they are attentive to their condition. Elective surgical resection is usually reserved for those who have sustained two or more acute attacks or for those whose disease has been complicated by fistula formation or bowel obstruction. In some cases, surgical exploration is required to resolve the differential diagnosis of diverticulitis versus carcinoma. The two conditions may coexist.

Fortunately, resection of the involved segment is almost always curative. Even when diverticula abound throughout the colon, resection of the affected portion, typically the sigmoid segment, yields a favorable prognosis. Subtotal colectomy is rarely required.

Diverticular disease of the colon provides one of the more gratifying patient-physician encounters. Diagnosis is relatively straightforward, effective treatment is available, and the outcome is almost always satisfying to all concerned.

ULCERATIVE COLITIS

method of
ANDREW T. MARSHALL, M.D., and
MARK A. PEPPERCORN, M.D.
Beth Israel Hospital
Boston, Massachusetts

Ulcerative colitis is a diffuse, superficial inflammation of the colonic mucosa and submucosa that almost always involves the rectum and may extend in a contiguous fashion throughout the entire colon. Different terms are used to describe the extent of disease. "Ulcerative proctitis" refers to disease limited to the rectum. "Distal ulcerative colitis" and "proctosigmoiditis" describe disease within the reach of the flexible sigmoidoscope. "Left-sided colitis" refers to the inflammatory process extending to, but not beyond, the splenic flexure. Disease beyond the splenic flexure is termed "pancolitis." It is a chronic disease with remissions and exacerbations. Ulcerative colitis is seen throughout the world with varying incidences. It is more common in developed countries, especially the United States and Western Europe. Ulcerative colitis has been diagnosed in all decades of life, with a peak occurrence between the ages of 15 and 40 years. A second peak occurs in the sixth or seventh decade of life. The etiology of ulcerative colitis remains unknown. The disease causes morbidity secondary to its disabling features of bloody diarrhea, tenesmus, fecal incontinence, abdominal pain, and weight loss; from the adverse effects of surgery; and from possible malignancy. Patients with extensive ulcerative colitis of long duration are at risk for colorectal cancer. Colonoscopic surveillance has been suggested for such patients.

The differential diagnosis of ulcerative colitis includes both acute disorders and several chronic diseases. These include colitis caused by infectious agents, ischemia, radiation, drugs, and Crohn's disease.

The management of ulcerative colitis relies on many different therapeutic agents. The choice of therapy depends on the extent of disease and the severity of the clinical presentation. Truelove and Witts' criteria classify the severity of disease in ulcerative colitis. Mild disease refers to presentations with fewer than four stools daily, with or without blood, and no systemic features. Moderate disease is characterized by more than four stools per day associated with minimal systemic features; patients with severe disease have more than six stools daily with blood and systemic manifestations such as fever, tachycardia, or anemia. For many years, the treatment for ulcerative colitis focused on the use of sulfasalazine and corticosteroids. Over the past several years, the aminosalicylates derived from sulfasalazine and the immunomodulator agents have added greatly to the management of ulcerative colitis. We begin with a brief review of the available agents and then discuss the management of specific clinical presentations.

AMINOSALICYLATES

Sulfasalazine (Azulfidine)

Sulfasalazine was first described in 1942 for the treatment of rheumatoid arthritis but was then found to be effective in the management of ulcerative colitis. Sulfasalazine is composed of 5-aminosalicylic acid (5-ASA) linked to sulfapyridine by an azo bond that is cleaved by the bacterial flora of the colon. The sulfapyridine moiety is rapidly absorbed and excreted in the urine, never reaching distal disease sites. The salicylate component is only minimally absorbed from the colon and thus remains in contact with the colonic mucosa. These observations suggested that the 5-ASA moiety might be the active portion of the drug.

Several placebo-controlled trials established the efficacy of sulfasalazine in the treatment of active ulcerative colitis regardless of disease extent. In addition, sulfasalazine has proven efficacy in the maintenance of remission. Seventy percent of patients in remission on sulfasalazine remained disease free for 1 year, whereas only 24% of control patients did so.

Unfortunately, side effects of sulfasalazine are common and are reported to occur in up to 20% of patients. Gastrointestinal side effects include nausea, anorexia, and dyspepsia. Other common adverse reactions include headache, rash, and fever. Hematologic side effects include leukopenia, agranulocytosis, and hemolytic anemia. Hepatitis, pancreatitis, pericarditis, fibrosing alveolitis, and exacerbation of the underlying colitis also have been reported. Sulfasalazine has been shown to cause male infertility by decreasing sperm counts and affecting sperm morphology and motility. Infertility is reversible after discontinuation of the drug.

Since most of the adverse effects associated with sulfasalazine could be attributed to its sulfa portion, and since the pharmacologic studies suggested that 5-ASA was its active moiety, alternative ways of delivering 5-ASA to the colon were developed.

Topical and Oral 5-Aminosalicylates

Azad Kahn and coworkers first showed that enemas of 5-ASA were just as effective as sulfasalazine enemas in inducing remission in patients with ulcerative proctosigmoiditis. Subsequent studies have confirmed the efficacy of 5-ASA enemas (Rowasa) in active proctosigmoiditis and of 5-ASA suppositories in active ulcerative proctitis. Moreover, both forms of 5-ASA, known generically as mesalamine in the United States and as mesalazine in Europe, have proved effective at maintaining remission for proctosigmoiditis and proctitis, respectively. Since topical forms of 5-ASA are usually not effective for disease beyond the reach of the flexible sigmoidoscope, it was important to develop orally delivered forms for more proximal disease.

The oral preparations of 5-ASA include two mesalamine preparations (Asacol and Pentasa) and olsalazine (Dipentum). Asacol contains the 5-ASA moiety coated with an acrylic resin (Eudragit S) and is released at a pH greater than 7. In the Pentasa formulation, 5-ASA is contained in ethyl cellulose microspheres and releases into the colonic lumen in both a time- and a pH-dependent manner. Dipentum is composed of two 5-ASA molecules linked by an azobond that, like sulfasalazine, requires bacterial action for release of the active free 5-ASA moieties.

Controlled clinical trials have shown the oral 5-ASA preparations to be more effective than placebo in active ulcerative colitis; they are as effective as sulfasalazine and more effective than placebo in maintaining remission. These agents appear to exert their effects in a dose-dependent fashion.

Side effects of the 5-ASA drugs have been reported in less than 5% of patients. Eighty to 90% of patients who are allergic to or intolerant of sulfasalazine are able to tolerate either topical or oral 5-ASA preparations. Caution must be taken when treating patients who are allergic to sulfasalazine, however, as 10 to 20% may exhibit similar adverse reactions to the 5-ASA agents. Adverse effects of the 5-ASA products include anal irritation (enemas), watery diarrhea (especially with olsalazine), nephritis, pericarditis, pancreatitis, pneumonitis, and an exacerbation of existing colitis. The 5-ASA preparations do not cause male infertility.

CORTICOSTEROIDS

Truelove and Witts in 1955 showed that corticosteroids are effective in the management of active ulcerative colitis. A cortisone dosage of 100 mg per day achieved a clinical remission in 40% of patients, compared with 15% of control patients. Since that time, corticosteroids have been the mainstay of treatment for active ulcerative colitis. Prednisone, prednisolone, and methylprednisolone are the oral forms most frequently used for moderate degrees of illness. However, low doses of oral steroids are no more effective than placebo in the maintenance of clinical remission. Furthermore, the long-term use of oral steroids has been associated with significant morbidity. Topical corticosteroids (enemas, suppositories, foams) have also been shown to be effective in patients with active ulcerative proctitis or proctosigmoiditis. Steroid suppositories and foams are effective in up to 75% of patients with active ulcerative proctitis. As with oral forms, topical steroids are not useful in maintaining remission.

Although there is agreement that parenteral corticosteroids are necessary for the treatment of severe active ulcerative colitis, the form of corticosteroid to use is still debated. Studies revealed that hydrocortisone was more effective than corticotropin (ACTH) in patients who had recently been treated with oral corticosteroids. Patients who had not been treated with corticosteroids for at least 30 days fared better with ACTH than with hydrocortisone.

The well-known adverse effects of corticosteroid therapy include electrolyte abnormalities, fluid re-

tention, emotional lability, hypertension, glucose intolerance, and avascular necrosis.

IMMUNOMODULATORS

Azathioprine and 6-Mercaptopurine (6-MP)

The immune suppressive agents azathioprine (Imuran)* and 6-mercaptopurine (Purinethol)* are increasingly being used in the treatment of corticosteroid-refractory or corticosteroid-dependent ulcerative colitis in the attempt to avoid colectomy. Their use in ulcerative colitis is less well established than in Crohn's disease, but studies have supported their efficacy in both treating active ulcerative colitis and maintaining remission in the disorder.

Adverse effects occur in less than 10% of patients and include rash, fever, hepatitis, and pancreatitis; these reverse upon discontinuation of the drugs. Frequent monitoring of cell counts usually avoids neutropenia, pancytopenia, and agranulocytosis in patients treated with these agents. A recent retrospective study suggested that patients on these drugs are at no increased risk for cancer, but cerebral lymphoma has been rarely associated with their use.

Cyclosporine

Cyclosporine (Sandimmune)* has revolutionized the transplant field and the therapy for several autoimmune disorders. Recently, literature has emerged on cyclosporine treatment for active ulcerative colitis. A randomized, double-blind, controlled study of cyclosporine in the management of severe steroid-refractory disease showed a response rate of 82%, compared with no responders in the placebo group. The long-term response of these patients has been questioned, however, as many eventually require colectomy or are hampered by the adverse effects of this agent. Potential toxicities include hirsutism, paresthesias, tremors, seizures, hypertension, irreversible renal damage, and the acquisition of opportunistic infections.

Methotrexate

The reported experience with methotrexate* in the treatment of active ulcerative colitis is limited to open trials. These trials suggested its efficacy for patients with steroid-dependent active ulcerative colitis. However, the long-term remission rates for patients on maintenance methotrexate therapy have been somewhat disappointing. A recent study showed efficacy for this agent in the management of chronic ulcerative colitis. In this study, patients improved symptomatically and were able to significantly decrease or discontinue steroid therapy, but they tended to have incomplete remissions. Side effects of the drug include leukopenia, pneumonitis, and hepatotoxicity.

---

*Not FDA-approved for this indication.

MISCELLANEOUS AGENTS

Nicotine

Recently, a small controlled trial using transdermal nicotine* patches suggested the efficacy of this agent in the management of patients with active ulcerative colitis. However, a recent study showed no role for nicotine in the maintenance of remission in patients with ulcerative colitis.

Fish Oil

Several small clinical trials investigated the role of fish oil (eicosapentaenoic acid)* in patients with mild to moderate active ulcerative colitis and suggested that this agent is effective as a steroid-lowering agent. There is no role for fish oil in the management of patients in clinical remission.

ANTIDIARRHEAL, ANTICHOLINERGIC, AND PSYCHOTROPIC AGENTS

The use of antidiarrheal agents is contraindicated in severe active ulcerative colitis, because of the possible risk of developing toxic megacolon. However, in patients with stable disease and mild symptoms, these agents may be useful in decreasing the frequency of diarrhea and in promoting stool formation. Anticholinergic agents (dicyclomine [Bentyl], hyoscyamine [Levsin]) may be beneficial in patients who have symptoms suggestive of an associated functional bowel component. Mild tranquilizers, such as lorazepam (Ativan) and diazepam (Valium), may be useful for patients troubled by the psychosocial stresses of their chronic disease. On occasion, the addition of antidepressant agents can be considered. Lithium can be of use in those who develop severe psychic reactions while on steroids.

NUTRITIONAL SUPPLEMENTATION

Although complete bowel rest is usually indicated in acute fulminant disease, there is no evidence that feeding is harmful in lesser degrees of active disease. Moreover, neither total enteral nor parenteral nutrition is useful as primary therapy to induce a remission, but both can serve as adjuncts to drug therapy. In general, patients with active symptoms feel better on a decreased-residue diet. Lactose intolerance should be excluded in these patients.

FUTURE MEDICAL THERAPY

In addition to the agents commonly used in clinical practice, potential new therapeutic approaches to the management of ulcerative colitis are currently under active investigation and include the following.

Rapidly Metabolized Steroids

Recent advances have included the development of potent steroid agents with minimal systemic bio-

availability. Budesonide* has been shown to have a higher affinity for the steroid receptor than hydrocortisone and has reduced systemic adverse effects. This agent has been beneficial in the treatment of Crohn's disease, and an enema preparation of budesonide has been effective for distal ulcerative colitis.

FK-506

The immunomodulator *FK-506* (tacrolimus [Prograf]),* approved for organ transplantation, is currently undergoing a randomized clinical trial to study its efficacy in ulcerative colitis. Although the results of clinical trials are not currently available, FK-506 may be useful in the treatment of pyoderma gangrenosum and in fistulous disease.

Immune Globulins

Intravenous gamma globulin has been administered in an open trial to a small number of patients with refractory ulcerative colitis. A subgroup of patients in this study showed an objective positive response, with improvement in disease activity and lowering of steroid dosage.

Anti-CD4 Antibodies

Administration of a monoclonal antibody directed against CD4 cells to patients with refractory ulcerative colitis has been shown in open trials to possibly be effective. Larger controlled trials are needed before this technique can be applied to standard clinical practice.

Short Chain Fatty Acids

Short chain fatty acids (SCFAs) have been studied in patients with refractory ulcerative colitis. Stool frequency, rectal bleeding, histologic inflammation, and endoscopic appearance improved on SCFA enemas in open trials, but placebo-controlled trials gave conflicting results.

Antioxidants

The hypothesis that reactive oxygen metabolites cause mucosal damage in colitis and amplify the inflammatory cascade has led to the investigation of antioxidants in the management of ulcerative colitis. A recent controlled trial assessed the use of allopurinol in the treatment of ulcerative colitis and suggested a possible future role for this group of agents in the management of ulcerative colitis.

Antibiotics

Initially developed for the treatment of *Trichomonas* infection, metronidazole (Flagyl) has been beneficial in patients with inflammatory bowel disease.

---

*Not FDA-approved for this indication.

Although much of the experience has been with Crohn's disease, metronidazole may be of benefit in the management of ulcerative colitis in remission. Ciprofloxacin (Cipro)* appears to be beneficial in certain patients with steroid-dependent ulcerative colitis. Further studies are awaited, however, before the routine use of antibiotics in ulcerative colitis can be recommended.

MEDICAL MANAGEMENT OF SPECIFIC CLINICAL PRESENTATIONS

Proctitis

Ulcerative proctitis is limited to the rectum and can present with rectal bleeding, urgency, tenesmus, diarrhea, or constipation. Approximately 30% of patients with ulcerative colitis present with disease limited to the rectum. There are many different approaches to the management of proctitis. Initial therapy for patients with ulcerative proctitis is usually topical, with 5-ASA suppositories, steroid foams, or steroid enemas. We favor initiating treatment with 5-ASA suppositories at a dose of 500 mg two times per day. Most patients have a prompt clinical response, and the majority are in complete remission within 6 weeks. The partial responders or the nonresponders should be continued on 5-ASA treatment, but the dose can be increased to three times per day and continued for an additional 4 to 6 weeks. Once the disease is in clinical remission, the dose can be gradually decreased to as little as one suppository every third night. Long-term therapy should be considered for patients who do not respond promptly to treatment, do not respond to conventional therapy, or suffer a relapse shortly after discontinuing initial treatment. Hydrocortisone foams (Cortifoam, 90 mg) or enemas (Cortenema, 100 mg) can be used as an alternative initial therapy or in patients who have an inadequate response to the 5-ASA suppositories. On occasion, patients with active proctitis seem to do better with combined therapy (5-ASA suppositories in the morning and afternoon in conjunction with topical steroids in the evening). Disease extent should be reassessed in patients who appear to be refractory to conventional therapy.

Proctosigmoiditis

Proctosigmoiditis can be managed with topical therapy. Initial therapy for mild to moderate proctosigmoiditis may be either a nightly 4-gram 5-ASA enema or a hydrocortisone enema. 5-ASA enemas are our preferred therapy, given their efficacy in maintaining long-term remission. Response should be noticed within 2 to 6 weeks. If symptoms persist, a morning 5-ASA or steroid enema can be added to the medical regimen. Once remission is established, therapy can be tapered gradually to a single 5-ASA enema every third night. For those patients who

*Not FDA-approved for this indication.

either do not respond adequately to topical therapy or cannot tolerate topical therapy, oral 5-ASA preparations can be implemented. A recent trial suggested that the combination of an oral 5-ASA agent and a 5-ASA enema is more effective than either alone. Treatment can be initiated with oral mesalamine 1 to 1.2 grams per day, olsalazine 500 mg per day, or sulfasalazine starting at 1 gram per day. These medications can be increased to a maximum dosage of 4.8 grams per day, 3 grams per day, and 4 to 6 grams per day, respectively. A common error in clinical practice is to assume a therapeutic failure when there is no response with the starting doses and to fail to increase the doses to maximum levels. Once the patient enters a clinical remission, doses can be reduced gradually to maintenance levels of 2 to 2.4 grams per day for mesalamine, 1 gram per day for olsalazine, and 2 grams per day for sulfasalazine. It is not clear whether the combination of an oral 5-ASA drug and topical 5-ASA therapy is better than either alone for long-term maintenance.

Prednisone is indicated for a patient with severe proctosigmoiditis or with moderate colitis who has not responded to 5-ASA and topical steroid therapy. Prednisone can be started at 40 to 60 mg per day and continued for 10 to 14 days before gradual tapering at a rate of about 5 mg per week, with the hope of complete withdrawal of the oral steroid.

Mild to Moderate Left-Sided Colitis and Pancolitis

Therapy for a mildly to moderately ill patient is usually initiated with a combination of oral aminosalicylates and either 5-ASA or steroid enemas. The topical agents are used to relieve symptoms of rectal involvement such as tenesmus and urgency. Oral 5-ASA preparations and sulfasalazine are used in a similar fashion to their use in the management of proctosigmoiditis. Once a clinical remission is established, the dose of the oral aminosalicylate, 5-ASA enema, or both can be tapered to maintenance levels.

For patients not responding to the above measures or for those too ill to wait the several weeks that may be required for these agents to show efficacy but not sick enough to require hospitalization, therapy with prednisone should be initiated, as detailed above.

Severe Colitis

Patients with severe disease require prompt hospitalization and are at an increased risk of progressing to toxic megacolon and subsequent perforation. Thus, a flat plate of the abdomen should be obtained in addition to surgical consultation. Therapy initially includes fluid and electrolyte resuscitation, bowel rest, and intravenous steroids. Hydrocortisone (300 mg per 24 hours), methylprednisolone (48 mg per 24 hours), or prednisolone (60 mg per 24 hours) is given as a continuous infusion. The latter two agents are favored, since they are less salt retaining and potassium wasting than hydrocortisone. Although we favor continuous infusion, there are no data to support this route of administration over bolus infusion. Topical 5-ASA, steroids, or both may be added and oral aminosalicylate agents initiated or continued. There are no data, however, investigating the role of these agents in severely ill patients. Moreover, since the 5-ASA agents may exacerbate ulcerative colitis, consideration should be given to stopping them if disease exacerbation corresponds to their use. For patients who have not been on any steroids within the previous 30 days, ACTH 120 units per 24 hours as a continuous infusion may be considered.

For severely ill patients who appear toxic with or without a dilated colon, in addition to the prompt correction of fluid and electrolyte abnormalities and the initiation of intravenous corticosteroids, broad-spectrum antibiotics such as metronidazole plus a third-generation cephalosporin should be initiated. A nasogastric tube should be inserted for decompression in those with a dilated colon, and parenteral nutrition should be started. Patients with megacolon should be turned from the supine to the prone position for 20 minutes every 2 hours in an attempt to redistribute gas from the transverse to the left colon. Roughly 50% of cases of acute dilatation resolve with medical therapy.

The role of antibiotics in a patient with severe ulcerative colitis who is not toxic appearing and who does not have colonic dilatation is not clear. Although controlled trials have failed to show an efficacy for broad-spectrum antibiotics in such patients, a subgroup that is refractory to steroids with persistent low-grade fevers and leukocytosis with bands may improve with antibiotic treatment. Whether such patients have an undetected pathogen, a *Clostridium difficile* infection despite a negative stool for toxin, or a bacterial flora contributing to the inflammatory process is not clear.

Toxic patients with or without megacolon should respond to treatment within 72 hours; if they do not, a colectomy is indicated. Patients with severe colitis who are not toxic should demonstrate a response within 7 to 10 days of treatment. If a response is not evident within this period, the physician and patient must consider the options of colectomy or treatment with cyclosporine. Cyclosporine* is administered at a dose of 4 mg per kg per day by continuous infusion. A positive response is usually seen within 1 week. If patients respond to intravenous cyclosporine, they are changed to oral cyclosporine at a dose of 8 mg per kg per day, and parenteral steroids are changed to prednisone at an initial dose of 60 mg per day. For those who continue to do well on oral cyclosporine as the prednisone is tapered, 6-MP is added for its steroid-sparing effects and efficacy in maintaining remissions. Because surgery is curative in ulcerative colitis, eliminates the future risk of colorectal carcinoma, and can now be performed with continent-sparing procedures, the surgical option should be strongly considered for patients with disease intractable to 2 or 3 weeks of above therapies.

Steroid-Refractory Ulcerative Colitis

A subgroup of patients, regardless of the extent of their disease, will not respond to corticosteroid therapy and will remain symptomatic. Options for this group of patients with chronic steroid-refractory disease include colectomy or further medical treatment with fish oil, nicotine, or immunomodulator agents. Before attempting therapy with these agents, the physician must make sure that the patient has received maximal doses of standard therapy. In patients who choose further medical therapy, a trial of 15 to 18 fish oil capsules per day containing 2.7 to 3.2 grams of eicosapentaenoic acid may be effective in inducing remission. Similarly, transdermal nicotine patches beginning at a dose of 7 mg daily may be effective in patients with mild to moderately active disease. This therapy is especially attractive for recently stopped smokers or for smokers wishing to stop cigarettes. For most such patients, however, azathioprine or 6-MP becomes the primary consideration. Azathioprine or 6-MP is initiated at a dose of 50 mg per day and is increased gradually to a maximum dose of 2.5 mg per kg per day or 2 mg per kg per day, respectively. It may take 3 to 6 months before a clinical response to these drugs is evident; thus, steroids are continued and gradually tapered during this period. If no clear response is noticed after 6 months of therapy, methotrexate should be considered. Therapy with methotrexate is initiated at a dose of 2.5 mg per week orally and increased over 4 weeks to a maximum dose of 25 mg per week. Methotrexate can also be given intramuscularly to ensure complete bioavailability.

Steroid-Dependent Ulcerative Colitis

Many patients with ulcerative colitis remain well on moderate doses of oral steroids (15 to 30 mg per day) but become symptomatic when the steroid dosage is tapered below these levels. These patients are at risk for significant steroid-related morbidity. Fish oil, nicotine, azathioprine, and 6-MP are used for the management of patients who are steroid-dependent in a manner similar to those who are steroid-resistant. For patients who are ultimately treated successfully with azathioprine or 6-MP, it is unclear how long to continue such therapy. Although studies report a significant relapse of disease for patients who discontinue immunomodulator therapy after a prolonged remission, we favor an attempt to stop these medications in patients with ulcerative colitis after approximately 2 years of remission.

PREGNANCY

Medications are an integral component of the management of a pregnant patient with ulcerative colitis, and certain aspects should be clarified with a patient

---

*Not FDA-approved for this indication.

who is either planning a pregnancy or currently pregnant. There is no evidence that sulfasalazine causes birth defects or adversely influences the course of pregnancy. Experience with topical and oral 5-ASA derivatives is much more limited, but it appears that these agents are just as safe as sulfasalazine in pregnancy. Although corticosteroids cross the placenta and levels of these substances can be detected in fetal blood, they do not adversely affect pregnancy or the fetus. Sulfasalazine, the newer topical and oral 5-ASA drugs, and corticosteroids can be used in pregnant patients in a similar manner to their use in nonpregnant patients.

Recent interest has focused on the use of azathioprine or 6-MP in pregnancy. Published series of patients with inflammatory bowel disease (IBD) taking these agents have not shown any teratogenic effects. In a recent report of pregnant women with IBD taking azathioprine, no adverse effects on the pregnancy or fetus were reported. However, congenital abnormalities have been reported in infants exposed to azathioprine. Our recommendation is that women or men trying to conceive stop either azathioprine or 6-MP 2 to 3 months before attempting conception. For those patients whose disease does not allow cessation of this therapy, we suggest stopping the drug at the time of conception. Neither methotrexate nor cyclosporine should be used in a patient who wants to become pregnant.

Similar recommendations apply with regard to breast-feeding newborn infants. Sulfasalazine, the 5-ASA agents, and prednisone can be continued during the postpartum period and have no adverse effect on the newborn. The effects of 6-MP and azathioprine on nursing newborns are not currently known, so breast-feeding should be avoided if the mother is taking these immune suppressive agents.

COLON CANCER AND SURVEILLANCE

Numerous studies have firmly established that there is an increased risk of developing colorectal cancer in patients with extensive, long-standing ulcerative colitis. Many of these studies were retrospective reviews from large, tertiary referral centers and suggested a higher incidence of colorectal cancer than is currently believed to exist. The cumulative risk of colon cancer is likely on the order of 5 to 10% for patients with pancolitis and disease duration of 20 years. This risk increases with increasing disease duration. The risk rises to 15% at 25 years and may reach as high as 30% at 35 years of disease duration.

Risk factors for cancer development in patients with ulcerative colitis include total duration of colitis and the extent of disease. The increased risk of colorectal cancer appears to start about 8 years after the onset of disease. However, patients with shorter disease durations should not assume that they are risk free, as the diagnosis of ulcerative colitis may have been delayed from its initial onset. Patients with proctitis or proctosigmoiditis are not believed to be at an increased risk for cancer development.

Although the efficacy of surveillance programs is debated, we suggest that patients with pancolitis for 8 years and patients with left-sided colitis for 12 years be enrolled in a surveillance program in an attempt to decrease the incidence of colorectal cancer. Colonoscopy of the entire colon should be performed every year or every other year, with multiple random biopsies taken at 10-cm intervals throughout the length of the colon. Prophylactic colectomy in patients with long-standing ulcerative colitis has also been proposed as an alternative cancer preventive strategy but is rarely practiced in the United States.

Morson in 1967 showed that dysplasia on rectal biopsy is a specific marker to identify patients with ulcerative colitis who are at high risk for developing colon cancer. Since that time, many studies have confirmed this finding. Unfortunately, certain limitations also exist with the use of dysplasia as a premalignant marker. Newer modalities are currently being evaluated to be used in conjunction with dysplasia in identifying premalignant lesions, and other methods that are more sensitive than dysplasia are being investigated. These include DNA flow cytometric analysis, lectins, and specific antibodies directed against tumor-associated antigens. One of these antigens, sialosyl-Tn, has shown promise in conjunction with the use of dysplasia in detecting premalignant lesions in patients with long-standing ulcerative colitis. Currently, although problems exist, dysplasia is still the best available marker for premalignant lesions. There is general agreement that the finding of high-grade dysplasia confirmed by two experienced pathologists should lead to a recommendation for colectomy. Although there is less general agreement about a similar recommendation for the finding of low-grade dysplasia, many gastroenterologists, including the authors, believe that confirmed low-grade dysplasia is an indication for colectomy.

CROHN'S DISEASE

method of
ARVEY I. ROGERS, M.D.
Miami VA Medical Center
Miami, Florida

and

BRETT R. NEUSTATER, M.D.
University of Miami School of Medicine
Miami, Florida

Crohn's disease (CD) is a chronic inflammatory condition of the gastrointestinal tract. Although significant advances have been made over the past 20 years, its origin and pathogenesis remain unclear. Consequently, therapy is directed at reducing inflammation and providing symptomatic relief. The approach to a patient with CD depends on the location, severity, and duration of that patient's disease, as well as the presence of any complicating factors or sequelae. Although it may seem self-evident, the first step in the approach to treatment of a patient with CD is to establish the presence of active disease, given that the adverse effects of therapy can occasionally be worse than the disease itself. This is not always easy, as there are a number of conditions that can imitate CD, and endoscopic and clinical correlation of disease activity does not always exist. Table 1 lists some possible causes of diarrhea in a patient with CD that are not directly attributable to disease reactivation and consequently require alternative therapies. The difficulty of specifically defining the presence and activity of CD is emphasized by the existence of several detailed indices, such as the Crohn's disease activity index; because of their complexity, these indices are used mainly to judge disease activity in the setting of a study protocol.

Once the presence of active disease necessitating treatment is established, we believe that it is useful to view the medical treatment of CD in a stepwise fashion, with each step up in therapy representing another "rung" in the therapeutic armamentarium. At the bottom of the ladder are the approximately 75% of patients with relatively mild disease who respond well to "conventional" therapy, including 5-ASA agents, antibiotics, and nutritional support. From there, the therapeutic options expand to include steroids, immunomodulators, surgery, and less conventional modalities as the patient's disease becomes more complicated and refractory to therapy.

The effective medical management of CD should also focus on considerations other than the clinical application of traditional and newer pharmacotherapies. Equally important are considerations of which patients require therapy, when it should be instituted, what form should be utilized and in what dosage, what duration of therapy is appropriate, and when maintenance therapy should be utilized. It is not always possible to find a successful recipe, but patient-individualized clinical judgment should be a constant ingredient.

FIRST-LINE THERAPY

Initial treatment includes sulfasalazine (Azulfidine), mesalamine (Asacol, Pentasa, Rowasa), antibiotics, nutritional support, and symptomatic therapy. Sulfasalazine and 5-aminosalicylic acid (mesalamine [5-ASA]) are first-line drugs for patients with active mild to moderate disease. The active component of sulfasalazine is 5-ASA, which is linked by an azo bond to sulfapyridine. The sulfasalazine compound is largely unabsorbed in the small intestines and is delivered to the colon, where bacteria split the bond, releasing the topically active 5-ASA. Because of its distal site of action, it is most effective in colonic and ileocolonic Crohn's. Anecdotal evidence suggests that either stricture-associated or fistula-induced bacterial overgrowth in the small bowel or the reflux of released 5-ASA from the colon into the distal small intestine through a bypassed or incompetent ileocecal valve may be responsible for its efficacy in ileal disease.

We initiate therapy with sulfasalazine 500 mg orally twice daily and gradually increase the dose over 1 week to a treatment dose of 1 to 1.5 grams four times daily. As sulfasalazine inhibits folate absorption, we routinely prescribe daily folate supplementation (1 mg orally per day). Unfortunately, up to half of patients experience some mild side effects of sulfasalazine therapy, including anorexia, nausea, vomiting, headache, and reversible oligospermia in men. Although there is an approximately 10% cross-reactivity, mesalamine preparations are generally much better tolerated, because they do not contain the sulfa group, which is responsible for the large majority of adverse effects. Despite its higher cost, mesalamine has become the preferred agent of many.

Various preparations of mesalamine have been formulated, with most demonstrating equal or better efficacy when compared with sulfasalazine either as initial therapy or for relapses. Asacol is an orally administered, resin-coated mesalamine product that is released at a high luminal pH, thus enabling delivery of the active drug to the more distal small bowel and colon. The usual dose for treatment and maintenance of remission is 2.4 grams per day, although we and others commonly increase the dosage up to 4.8 grams per day if needed. Another coated preparation is Pentasa, which releases microgranules of mesalamine throughout the gastrointestinal tract, including the small intestine; this is our 5-ASA of choice for small bowel CD. The major drawback to its use, however, is the need to take three to four 250-mg capsules four times daily. Olsalazine (Dipentum) consists of two 5-ASA molecules linked together by an azo bond, which, like sulfasalazine, is cleaved by colonic bacteria to release the active 5-ASA; its utility in CD has not been well studied, and it can cause worsening diarrhea as a result of increased small intestinal bicarbonate secretion. Topically acting formulations of mesalamine (Rowasa) are available in enema and suppository form and may occasionally be helpful in a patient with distal (rectal or anorectal) Crohn's colitis. We usually prescribe an initial dose of one enema or suppository twice daily or at bedtime.

Antimicrobial agents are utilized frequently in patients with mild to moderate CD with or without

TABLE 1. **Causes of Diarrhea in Crohn's Patients Other Than Disease Flare**

Cause	Treatment
Enteroenteric fistula	Antibiotics, surgery
Bile acid malabsorption	Cholestyramine
Lactase deficiency	Low-lactose diet
Short bowel syndrome	Low-fat diet, elemental diet, total parenteral nutrition
Bacterial overgrowth	Antibiotics
Antibiotic related	Stop antibiotics, treat *Clostridium difficile* if present
Coexistent irritable bowel syndrome	Fiber, antispasmodics
Drugs used to treat Crohn's disease	Exclude other causes, stop drugs

perianal disease, fistulization, intra-abdominal abscess, or secondary bacterial overgrowth. Metronidazole (Flagyl)* is most commonly used and likely functions by reducing bacterial endotoxin and granuloma formation by suppressing cell-mediated immunity. At a dose of 10 to 20 mg per kg per day (750 to 1500 mg per day), metronidazole may be theoretically equivalent to sulfasalazine in patients with ileal or colonic CD, but it is associated with a high rate of recurrence after its withdrawal. In addition, a host of side effects, including a variably reversible neuropathy manifested by paresthesias, limits its long-term utility as maintenance therapy. Various other antibiotics have shown some efficacy, most notably ciprofloxacin (Cipro),* although none has been demonstrated to be as effective as metronidazole. Speculation that *Mycobacterium paratuberculosis* may play an etiologic role in CD prompted several studies using antituberculous drugs that yielded mixed results. At this time, antituberculous therapy cannot be recommended outside of clinical trials.

Nutritional therapy may also be of benefit in patients with CD. Seventy to 80% of patients with CD have weight loss, 25 to 80% have hypoalbuminemia, and many also have vitamin and trace element deficiencies. Patients who have had prior small bowel resection are at even greater risk of nutritional deficiencies. We place all patients with small intestinal disease on a low-lactose diet, and those with strictures on a low-fiber diet. Elemental diets have been shown to be as effective as 5-ASA or steroid therapy acutely in several trials in children, but their unpalatability and poor patient compliance limit their utility. Furthermore, these results have come under scrutiny because a high dropout rate precludes accurate assessment of the data. The combination of bowel rest and total parenteral nutrition (TPN) has also demonstrated short-lived effectiveness in nonrandomized studies, but its role in acute therapy remains largely adjunctive. Fish oil* has been proposed as a possible effective treatment in CD, but poor patient tolerance has been a problem. More recently, a newer coated fish oil preparation (Purepa, Tillots Pharma AG), with which we have had no personal experience and for which there is limited overall experience, was shown to be well tolerated and reduce the risk of relapse in a population of Crohn's patients in remission. We await the results of larger, comparative trials in order to better assess the efficacy of this potentially promising treatment. At this point, however, we have not found much value in nutritional therapy as the *primary* therapy for patients with CD.

The role of adjunctive therapies in CD should not be ignored. As irritable bowel syndrome often coexists in Crohn's patients, we have found regularly scheduled or as-needed antispasmodics and antidiarrheals to be helpful in patients with mild to moderate disease. In patients with ileal resections of less than 100 cm, cholestyramine (Questran)* can improve bile salt–induced choleretic diarrhea but should be used cautiously in patients with small bowel strictures. It should be stressed that symptomatic improvement and not necessarily mucosal healing is the goal of therapy, as the two often do not correlate.

SECOND-LINE THERAPY

Corticosteroids are the mainstay of second-line therapy. We initiate treatment with corticosteroids in CD patients who are very ill and are responding poorly to more conservative management. Oral or parenteral steroids induce remission in 76 to 92% of patients, but unfortunately, relapse after their withdrawal is common, and long-term therapy is associated with significant morbidity, including agitation, insomnia, cataracts, metabolic bone disease, osteonecrosis, diabetes, skin striae, a cushingoid appearance, acne, and possibly peptic ulcer disease. We use a starting dose of prednisone 40 to 60 mg orally per day (or its equivalent) until significant clinical improvement is noted (usually less than 14 days), followed by a gradual taper that is dependent on the duration and severity of symptoms but is usually no greater than 5-mg-per-week decrements. Doses greater than 60 mg per day administered for several months have been associated with increased side effects but not improved efficacy. Patients with severe disease should be admitted to the hospital and placed on an equivalent dose of intravenous steroids (methylprednisolone, hydrocortisone, or corticotropin [ACTH]) as well as antibiotics and possibly enteral (elemental or formula) or parenteral nutrition. Some physicians advocate treatment with a continuous intravenous steroid infusion, although this is likely no better than single- or divided-dose therapy. Others advocate the use of ACTH in patients who have not previously received steroids, but no benefit over corticosteroids has been demonstrated conclusively. A recent abstract suggested that prior steroid use did not adversely affect the efficacy of ACTH, which was again shown to be comparable to steroid therapy. Budesonide† is a very potent, topically active steroid with a high first-pass hepatic metabolism that is not currently available in the United States. Early trials have demonstrated good efficacy with somewhat less pituitary-adrenal axis suppression than prednisone but no greater overall effectiveness than conventional steroids. We believe that any future role for budesonide will likely be as maintenance therapy. Further studies are needed, however, before its use becomes more widespread. The small subset of patients who do not respond to first- and second-line therapies, cannot be tapered off steroids, or have fistulizing CD are candidates for third-line therapy with immunomodulating drugs.

---

*Not FDA-approved for this indication.

*Not FDA-approved for this indication.
†Not available in the United States.

IMMUNOMODULATOR THERAPY

Immunomodulating drugs include azathioprine (Imuran),* 6-mercaptopurine (Purinethol),* cyclosporine (Sandimmune),* and methotrexate.* Azathioprine and its metabolite 6-mercaptopurine (6-MP) are purine analogues that competitively inhibit the biosynthesis of purine ribonucleotides, with subsequent selective T cell and anti-inflammatory effects. Although no comparative trials of the two have been conducted, both agents have been clearly demonstrated to have beneficial effects in patients with CD. These effects include the induction of remission, maintenance of remission, reduction in the dosage of steroids required to maintain remission, and fistula healing in approximately two-thirds of patients. Although therapy is effective regardless of disease location, those with colitis and ileocolitis may benefit the most. The major downside of therapy is its slow onset of action, which averages 3 months but can be 4 months or longer in up to 20%. Concurrent therapy with steroids, antibiotics, nutritional support, and possibly other immunomodulating drugs such as cyclosporine is necessary while awaiting a therapeutic response. Toxicity has been a concern, as has the risk of malignancy. Concerns over the development of neoplasms, in particular lymphoma, were based on data from transplant patients receiving higher-dose therapy; the development of malignancy has not been observed in patients with CD to date. Since long-term prospective trials have not demonstrated an increased risk of malignancy with the use of purine analogues in patients with inflammatory bowel disease, we now believe that there is enough evidence to justify their use in patients who may benefit from them. The most significant adverse reactions include leukopenia, hepatitis, and pancreatitis. Although the pancreatitis is usually not severe, reinstitution of therapy with either 6-MP or azathioprine should not be attempted, as a recurrence is sure to follow. The same applies for other idiosyncratic allergic reactions, such as the *early* development of leukopenia and hepatitis. We generally initiate therapy with 25 to 50 mg per day orally for the first 1 to 2 weeks, followed by a gradual increase to a goal of 1.1 to 1.5 mg per kg per day for 6-MP and 2 mg per kg per day for azathioprine. The exact dosage should be decided on a case-by-case basis, as some patients require significantly higher doses. A complete blood count, liver function tests, and amylase should be monitored every 2 weeks for the first month and then monthly if blood counts and liver function tests remain stable. It can be useful to follow the decline in the white blood cell count (with a goal of 3500 to 5000 mm^3) as an index of effective dosing. The dose of 6-MP or azathioprine should be reduced by 50% in patients taking allopurinol (Zyloprim), a xanthine oxidase inhibitor, as xanthine oxidase is required for 6-MP and azathioprine degradation.

Cyclosporine selectively inhibits cell-mediated immunity by decreasing T helper cell production of various cytokines, including interleukin-2. Its current role in CD is as "salvage" therapy for patients with refractory disease and in the treatment of fistulizing disease. In patients with refractory disease, a response is seen in approximately two-thirds, independent of the site of disease. Unfortunately, withdrawal of therapy is associated with a very high relapse rate, and maintenance therapy with low-dose oral cyclosporine has not been efficacious. Cyclosporine's advantage over 6-MP and azathioprine lies in its more rapid onset of action (weeks vs. months). This has prompted some to use both drugs concurrently and continue the 6-MP after discontinuing the cyclosporine. The toxicity of cyclosporine can be significant, and side effects include hypertension, nephrotoxicity, seizures, hepatotoxicity, hypertrichosis, paresthesias, headache, and, rarely, tumor neogenesis. The usual starting dose is 2 to 4 mg per kg per day intravenously, followed by 4 to 8 mg per kg per day orally. Because of variable, slow intestinal absorption, close monitoring of serum levels is important, with a therapeutic goal of 500 to 700 ng per mL (polyclonal TDX assay). In addition, as cyclosporine is metabolized by the cytochrome P-450 system, many other medications that interact with the cytochrome P-450 system can raise or lower serum concentrations.

Weekly intramuscular injections of 25 mg of methotrexate have been shown to produce a clinical remission in 39% of patients with refractory CD. Toxicity includes leukopenia, nausea, vomiting, diarrhea, hepatotoxicity, and hypersensitivity pneumonitis. Its role in CD is likely in the treatment of patients with refractory disease who either do not respond to or cannot tolerate 6-MP.

Patients with CD may also have a number of complicating presentations that deserve special mention.

FISTULIZING OR PERIANAL DISEASE

Fistulas in CD may be enterocutaneous, enteroenteric, rectovaginal, or enterovesicular. So-called innocent enteroenteric fistulas that are largely asymptomatic do not require any specific therapy. However, more symptomatic fistulous disease or that associated with secondary complications, including local abscess formation, requires intensive therapy. Patients with rectovaginal and enteroenteric fistulas and severe diarrhea benefit from therapy aimed at reducing the volume of diarrhea. Those with severe proctitis and perineal or perianal disease should receive intensive treatment for the proctitis. Steroids have not been demonstrated to have any beneficial effect in fistulizing CD, and antibiotics should be the drugs of first choice. Metronidazole with or without the addition of another antibiotic such as ciprofloxacin may be effective, although it is generally poorly tolerated on a long-term basis. 6-MP and cyclosporine (intravenously or orally) have a high initial response rate in controlling fistulous drainage but achieve long-term fistula closure in less than half of

---

*Not FDA-approved for this indication.

patients. TPN and bowel rest are most useful in the treatment of postsurgical fistulas without a focus of active inflammation and are also occasionally employed to speed the healing process while awaiting the effects of immunomodulatory therapy. Alone, however, the use of TPN and bowel rest is associated with a high incidence of fistula reopening upon resumption of oral feeding. Some centers also advocate perioperative hyperalimentation, although supportive data are lacking. Severe perianal disease can be extremely distressing and refractory to therapy. Newer modalities, including hyperbaric oxygen therapy, may prove useful if other therapies fail.

The association of an abscess warrants immediate drainage and antibiotics. There is no consensus regarding the use of surgical resection or percutaneous drainage and antibiotics; each patient's therapy must be decided on a case-by-case basis. Persistent complications of fistulas typically require surgical resection of the originating, usually inflamed or obstructed, bowel segment.

FIBROSTENOTIC DISEASE

After fibrostenosis is distinguished from severe inflammatory or fistulizing disease, surgery remains the only effective treatment for recurrent obstructive symptoms. Usually, the obstruction occurs in the small intestine but can present in the colon as well. The goal of surgery should be to limit the bowel resection to only the obstructed segment or segments. Strictureplasty is a safe, effective option available to a relatively small number of patients with short, not actively inflamed, fibrous strictures. Because approximately one-third of patients with CD require additional surgeries for recurrent disease, the concept of limiting the amount of resected bowel is important.

MAINTENANCE THERAPY

The two goals of maintenance therapy in CD are to prevent the recurrence of disease after resection of a diseased segment of bowel and to maintain remission after its successful induction with medical therapy. Despite the inference from some earlier trials, therapy with mesalamine has been shown to be effective in both scenarios. As opposed to ulcerative colitis, however, higher doses of 5-ASA appear to be required. The best 5-ASA preparation for maintenance therapy is not clear, as no direct comparative studies are available. Azathioprine and 6-MP have demonstrated efficacy and are used in patients with refractory disease or frequent flares. Cyclosporine does not appear to have any role in maintenance therapy.

NEW THERAPIES

Several new therapies are currently being evaluated for CD. These include potent immune suppressants such as FK-506 (tacrolimus [Prograf],* anti-

---

*Not FDA-approved for this indication.

tumor necrosis factor antibodies,* fusidic acid,* allopurinol,† various cytokine antagonists,* leukotrienes,* anti-CD4 monoclonal antibodies,* interferons,† T cell apheresis,* and immune globulin infusions.* Nutritional therapy with glutamine and butyrate also appears promising.

The therapeutic arena is constantly in flux. Concerned clinicians must maintain a critical awareness of effective new therapies and discard ineffective therapies if they are to provide optimal care to patients afflicted with Crohn's disease.

---

*Investigational drug in the United States.
†Not FDA-approved for this indication.

IRRITABLE BOWEL SYNDROME

method of
JOHN R. MATHIAS, M.D., and
MARY H. CLENCH, PH.D.
The University of Texas Medical Branch
Galveston, Texas

In the past, irritable bowel syndrome (IBS) was the universal diagnosis used to describe patients with a broad spectrum of gastrointestinal (GI) symptoms, including chronic abdominal pain, alternating or persistent diarrhea and constipation, and abdominal distention. In short, IBS was a term, not a disease; it was useful for labeling these symptoms in the many patients whose conventional studies (e.g., complete blood count, biochemical profile, upper GI x-ray series, barium enema, colonoscopy, esophagogastroduodenoscopy, or computed tomography of the abdomen) showed no objective changes. IBS was considered "functional" (GI symptoms in the absence of objective findings). In 1992, an international group of experts in gastroenterology met in Rome, Italy, and agreed on symptom-based criteria to define IBS (Table 1). Thus, for the practicing clinician, IBS is now a disease based on specific criteria that should lead to a more meaningful diagnosis and avoid costly clinical evaluation. In addition to the Rome criteria, symptoms not related to lower-tract disease occur commonly in patients with IBS and include a high prevalence of heartburn and gastroesophageal reflux.

TABLE 1. 1992 Rome Criteria for Irritable Bowel Syndrome

At least 3 months' continuous or intermittent symptoms of:
Abdominal pain or discomfort that is relieved by defecation and/or associated with a change in stool frequency or consistency

Plus

Two or more of the following occurring on at least 25% of occasions or days:
Altered stool frequency
Altered stool form (lumpy, hard or loose, watery)
Altered stool passage (straining, urgency, or feeling of incomplete evacuation)
Passage of mucus
Bloating or feeling of abdominal distention

Adapted from Drossman DA, et al: Identification of sub-groups of functional bowel disorders. Gastroenterol Int 3:159–172, 1990; and Thompson WG, et al: Working team report: Functional bowel disease and functional abdominal pain. Gastroenterol Int 5:75–91, 1992.

PREVALENCE

The true prevalence of IBS is unknown, but current epidemiologic studies suggest that 10 to 26% of adults have IBS symptoms. In Western countries, typical patients with IBS are young white women between the ages of 20 and 35 years; the disease is two to six times more common in women than in men, and up to five times more common in white than in black patients. In contrast, in India and other less-developed countries, IBS seems to be more prevalent in men, possibly because they seek medical care more often than women do. IBS also occurs in the elderly and in young adults, and it is more common than is generally appreciated. In an office-based GI practice, patients with IBS symptoms may account for 25 to 50% of referrals. Interestingly, most people with mild IBS symptoms do not seek medical care; they either treat themselves with over-the-counter medications or ignore the problem altogether. Another reasonable explanation why women may not consult physicians is that the symptoms of IBS often correlate with their menstrual cycles, occurring or worsening just before or during the onset of menses. Many women recognize that GI symptoms may be part of the normal physiologic changes associated with the cycling of reproductive hormones.

Studies have shown that approximately 20% of people with IBS seek medical care. Although it has been suggested that psychological factors are responsible for "health-seeking" behavior, the patients in these studies were obtained from a clinical setting where they *were* actively seeking health care. In contrast, Heitkemper and colleagues reported a prospective study of GI function in 1995, in which the women had been recruited by advertising in a large university setting. These investigations found no difference in psychological profiles in patients with IBS compared with those with GI symptoms that did not meet the Rome criteria. The differences in results in the two types of study may be explained by the sampling techniques—volunteers with GI tract symptoms who were "psychologically" healthier than patients seeking health care in a clinical setting. This issue remains unclear.

PATHOGENESIS

The enteric nervous system (ENS) consists of two intrinsic nerve plexuses with individual neurons, ganglia, neurotransmitters, hormones, and neurocircuits that form a highly organized neural tube. The ENS regulates and controls absorption, secretion, and muscle contraction (of both the muscularis mucosa and the circular smooth muscle) and interacts with the immune system of the GI tract. The two plexuses have different functions: the submucosal (Meissner's) plexus is largely sensory, receiving information from ongoing events in the lumen of the bowel; the myenteric (Auerbach's) plexus receives information from the submucosal plexus, sympathetic and parasympathetic innervation from the spinal cord, and vagal input from the central nervous system (CNS). Although the complex ENS intestinal "brain" is considered autonomous and regulates the ongoing events of the GI tract, it may be overridden by the CNS during times of flight or fright. The complex interactions between the ENS and CNS account for much of our confusion regarding the pathogenesis of IBS. Current information suggests that IBS is a motility disorder involving dysfunction of the sensory-perception pathways that results in disordered responses of GI smooth muscle contraction or neurotransmitter release. Several studies using a balloon catheter or barostat have shown hypersensitivity of the nociceptive neural pathways. Richie compared the volume of air necessary to distend a balloon catheter and cause pain in the rectum in patients who had IBS and in control subjects; the IBS patients experienced pain with less pressure. Since that study, others have shown similar results in the esophagus, stomach, small intestine, and colon. It is now appreciated that many stimuli to the GI tract, such as eating, intestinal distention, emotional stress, physical stress, drugs, infection, environmental toxins, and hormones released from the hypothalamic-pituitary axis or gonads (especially the ovaries), may result in a hyper-response by the intestine and an amplified signal in the perception centers in the CNS. The cause of this resetting of the sensitivity scale remains unknown, but a reasonable hypothesis is that infections, especially viral, set the stage for chronic and ongoing IBS symptoms. In addition, certain areas of the CNS are affected in this disease. It is not uncommon for patients with IBS to relate a history of sensitivities to their environment. They become ill on exposure to certain types of light, especially the flickering of fluorescents or the strobe effect of light (as in a dance hall, in motion pictures, or from a ceiling fan). They are sensitive to noise, especially in a room full of people all chattering at the same time. They are sensitive to odors, particularly perfumes, cigar or cigarette smoke, organic solvents, or cleaning materials such as chlorine bleach. Some patients may actually display symptoms of recognized panic disorder, which is a documented neurotransmitter problem in the limbic system. This sensitivity to the environment suggests dysfunction of the neurons in the limbic system of the CNS and may help explain the relationship between GI tract complaints and emotional factors in some patients.

Several recent studies have shown that sexual or physical abuse during childhood or later in life may be a significant risk factor for the development of IBS symptoms. The prevalence of this condition remains unknown, but if this information is obtained in the history, counseling should begin as soon as possible. The family environment may also influence the behavior of a growing child, such as during bowel training, or the attitude of the family toward GI complaints. Drossman and associates noted that, in general, patients who seek medical care have higher scores on tests that assess psychoneurotic behavior and psychological stress than do nonpatients (subjects with IBS-like symptoms who do not seek health care). As the study by Heitkemper and colleagues suggested, however, protocol and sampling conditions can significantly alter results regarding a correlation between stress factors and symptoms. An alternative explanation is that whatever causes IBS may also affect both the ENS and specific areas in the CNS such as the limbic system, associated with emotion and autonomic function. For example, extraintestinal manifestations of IBS may include back pain, lethargy and malaise, palpitations, headache, and urinary frequency, urgency, and nocturia; it may also include dysmenorrhea and dyspareunia in women. This conglomeration of symptoms suggests an increased sensitivity of systemic nerves or smooth muscle or both. A patient with IBS may be seeing several specialists for individual symptoms when, in fact, an empathetic and informed primary care physician may be all that is necessary for good medical care. It is clear that in moderate to severe disease, only the combination of medication, psychological counseling, and behavior modification is effective in controlling the symptoms of these patients.

DIAGNOSIS

The diagnosis of IBS can be made with a careful history and physical examination. It is no longer a wastebasket

TABLE 2. **Disorders Constituting Idiopathic Neuromuscular Disease***

Gastrointestinal motor dysfunction (nonulcer dyspepsia)
  Symptoms: unexplained abdominal pain, chronic nausea, intermittent intractable vomiting
Sphincter of Oddi dysfunction
  Symptoms: right upper quadrant (RUQ) pain radiating to the back
Ampulla of Vater–duodenal wall spasm
  Symptoms: epigastric-to-RUQ pain that radiates to the back in the absence of stones or a dilated common bile duct
Recurrent abdominal pain in children
  Symptoms: unexplained abdominal pain, chronic nausea, intermittent intractable vomiting
Acute colonic pseudo-obstruction (Ogilvie's syndrome)
  Symptoms: abdominal distention, pain often absent, no stooling
Chronic intestinal pseudo-obstruction
  Symptoms: unexplained abdominal pain, chronic nausea, intermittent intractable vomiting
Chronic intermittent pseudo-obstruction
  Symptoms: intermittent unexplained abdominal pain, distention, chronic nausea, intractable vomiting
Idiopathic intestinal hollow visceral neuropathy
  Symptoms: bowel, bladder, and biliary complaints
Idiopathic intestinal hollow visceral myopathy
  Symptoms: bowel and bladder complaints associated with ocular palsy
Severe intestinal constipation
  Symptoms: chronic obstipation (subtype of pseudo-obstruction)
Roux-en-Y syndrome
  Symptoms: unexplained abdominal pain, chronic nausea, intermittent intractable vomiting worsened by eating

*Most of these disorders require a motility recording for a definitive diagnosis.

Adapted from Mathias JR, Clench MH: Neuromuscular diseases of the gastrointestinal tract. Postgrad Med 97:95–108, 1995.

term but one that is clearly defined by the Rome criteria (see Table 1). The Rome definition helps distinguish subjects with IBS from patients with other functional disorders involving enteric nerves, intestinal smooth muscle, or organic disease (Tables 2 and 3). Complaints of weight loss, fever, bleeding from the GI tract, arthralgia or arthritis, or more systemic symptoms such as progressive deterioration, sudden onset of symptoms, nocturnal symptoms, or fat or blood in the stool should indicate to the physician other types of GI disease (Table 4). In addition, any laboratory findings that are abnormal and suggest underlying organic disease should be investigated and defined.

EXAMINATION OF THE PATIENT

Recognition of the IBS symptom complex allows the physician to approach a patient with minimum testing and a cost-effective evaluation. Exhaustive testing in pursuit of

TABLE 3. **Known Causes of Neuromuscular Disease**

Collagen-vascular disease
Muscular dystrophies
Endocrine disorders
Neurologic disorders
Pharmacologic disorders

Adapted from Mathias JR, Clench MH: Neuromuscular diseases of the gastrointestinal tract. Postgrad Med 97:95–108, 1995.

TABLE 4. **Differential Diagnosis of Organic Diseases That May Mimic Irritable Bowel Syndrome**

Endometriosis
Diverticulosis, diverticulitis
Pelvic inflammatory disease
Neoplasm of the gastrointestinal tract
Malabsorption states
Peptic ulcer disease (*Helicobacter pylori* infection)
Biliary tract disease
Inflammatory bowel disease (Crohn's disease, ulcerative colitis)

a "rule-out diagnosis" should be avoided. A careful dietary and medication history is vital. Many foods cause IBS-like symptoms (Table 5). These include lactose-containing milk or milk products and some medications (lactose is used as a filler in many drugs). Yogurt also contains significant amounts of lactose but is usually tolerated by patients because of its continued fermentation process. Other foods can provoke or exacerbate IBS-like symptoms—fruits that contain sorbitol, as well as many sugarless candies, mints, and chewing gums; cola beverages and fruit juices that contain fructose; some vegetables and legumes; and bran and branlike products. A careful dietary history should identify foods that are contributing factors. Obtaining a history of the drugs, especially over-the-counter medications, used by the patient is also important. When asked for a list of their medications, most patients focus only on prescribed drugs, but antacids that contain magnesium, fiber supplements with senna, analgesics such as narcotics or aspirin, antispasmodics, and antidiarrheal drugs may all cause IBS-like symptoms.

The physician may also ask the patient to keep a daily diary for 4 to 6 weeks, recording both symptoms and foods or medications ingested, to specifically identify unrecognized offending substances. Limiting the amount of space in the diary, such as three or four lines per day, emphasizes to the patient that the diary is to be used as a tool and should not become a part of the patient's "disease."

Tests that should be considered in evaluating IBS include a complete blood count to assess for anemia. A biochemical profile provides general information about the patient's well-being and helps reassure the patient and provides confidence to the physician regarding the patient's management. A routine urinalysis should also be done to complete the general evaluation. The practice of "taking a look" with either air-contrast barium enema and flexible sigmoidoscopy or a complete colonoscopy should be avoided if possible. Use of these tests depends to a large extent on the patient's age and whether there is a family history of colon polyps, cancer, or inflammatory bowel disease. The sudden onset of symptoms in someone over 35 years of age is a clear indication for this type of assessment, and it reassures both the patient and the physician if no serious

TABLE 5. **Foods That May Cause Symptoms Like Those of Irritable Bowel Syndrome**

Lactose: milk and milk products (cream, ice cream, ice milk), some medications
Sorbitol: apples, peaches, pears, cherries, prunes, sugar-free chewing gum and candy
Fructose: cola beverages, fruit juices
Vegetables: broccoli, Brussels sprouts, cabbage, eggplant, zucchini, some legumes
Grains: bran, branlike products

problem is present. These costly procedures should be avoided, however, if they are not clearly indicated. Investigation of stool samples for bacteria and parasites is costly, but assessing for white blood cells in the stool can be done quickly in the office; it requires only a drop of stool mixed with a drop of methylene blue and examination under a microscope. The presence of white blood cells in a stool sample indicates a break in the mucosal integrity, and the patient should then be evaluated with appropriate tests (stool samples and x-ray or endoscopy). Certain key factors in the history may also provide important clues for appropriate testing. Development of symptoms after recent travel, either within or outside the United States, may suggest a pathogenic bacterium or parasite; for instance, certain areas have a high prevalence of *Giardia lamblia*.

Because it is not uncommon for symptoms of lower abdominal pain to be mistaken for dysfunction of the pelvic organs, there should be a close working relationship between the gastroenterologist and a female patient's gynecologist. Our understanding of endometriosis and its relationship to GI symptoms is not clear-cut by any means. Symptoms often attributed to endometriosis are actually those of IBS, and therapy should be focused on controlling the bowel problem.

Recurrent or chronic urinary tract infections are also not uncommon in patients with IBS. Urinary tract evaluation, other than a urinalysis, should be done only when a patient has repeated urinary tract infections, urinary infrequency (once or twice a day), or urinary frequency (more than eight to 10 times per day); the normal mean for urine passage is four to five times a day. The presence of urinary tract disease as determined by an intravenous pyelogram, a cystometrogram, or both, associated with GI tract symptoms, is part of a more serious nerve disease—hollow visceral neuropathy. Interaction between the gastroenterologist, urologist, and gynecologist is imperative in caring for patients with this disorder.

Other tests such as computed tomography, magnetic resonance imaging of the abdomen, or laparoscopy are expensive and almost always unnecessary. These tests should be avoided in a patient with IBS because they only add to the patient's underlying concern about a serious problem. A diagnosis of IBS can be made with confidence based on the aforementioned specific criteria (see Table 1), and therapy should be directed at correcting diet, reducing stress factors, and providing a sound physician-patient relationship.

THERAPY

A strong physician-patient relationship is the focal point of IBS therapy. The primary care physician needs to be well informed about this disease and have the confidence to deal with a patient who has a chronic medical disorder in which the symptoms can fluctuate from day to day. The stress in a patient's life clearly has a strong effect on symptoms, and getting the patient to become a problem solver should be the physician's primary aim. First, it should be recognized that the patient's symptoms are *real* (this is a real disease, even if the pathophysiology is not fully understood). Second, the physician needs to provide reassurance and care to allay the patient's fear of an underlying serious organic disease. Third, objective goals must be established for both short-term (control of the immediate symptoms) and long-term therapy (developing a plan for lifestyle changes). In our experience, most patients can recognize factors that trigger or worsen their symptoms and modify their behavior by keeping a limited daily diary. We ask them to record what they have eaten, their activities, and any unusual events. If the patient cannot accomplish this effectively, referral to a psychologist trained in behavior modification should be considered. Fourth, patients must be involved in treatment decisions—after all, this is their disease, and they must be involved if successful gains are to be made. And fifth, it is the physician's duty as caregiver to teach patients about their disease; understanding is the beginning of successful short-term as well as long-term therapy.

After the initial visit, it is important to reach a confident and positive diagnosis of IBS as quickly as possible. Tests should be completed rapidly so that patients can be assured that they do not have a serious organic disease (cancer is usually what they suspect). Studies have shown that if physicians spend time with their patients as soon as possible after diagnosis and take the time to explain what is wrong and what must be done to control chronic and changing symptoms, people get well sooner and stay well. We have found that sitting down with patients and discussing the following treatment plan in detail is highly effective.

TREATMENT PLAN

Diet. Patients are put on a caffeine-free diet; decaffeinated coffees, teas, and colas are also excluded, because these beverages all contain excitatory transmitters that are not necessarily caffeine. A tyramine-free diet is prescribed as well. Tyramine is an amino acid that binds to the same receptors as do catecholamines or amphetamines. Foods that contain tyramine are listed in Table 6. Patients should also restrict the amount of fat in their diet. Studies have shown that fat stimulates the gastrocolic response and cannot be blocked by anticholinergic medication. Using a spray cooking oil such as Pam (canola oil and lecithin) or small amounts of olive oil is recommended; frying food in the usual animal fats or vegetable oils is strongly discouraged.

Diary. The daily diary should help identify other things that cause patients to have symptoms: foods, drinks, or snacks that may contain sorbitol or fructose (see Table 5). The diary should be used as a tool and not become a part of the disease.

Fiber. The patient should try to consume a high-fiber diet, but it is often difficult to consume enough dietary fiber or raw bran to achieve effective therapeutic control. In addition, some patients ingesting high-bran diets may have worsening symptoms and gas production. Effective products that provide adequate dietary fiber include psyllium, methylcellulose, or polycarbophil taken with adequate amounts of water. Psyllium (Metamucil) can be given initially in small amounts (1 to 2 tablespoons per day) and gradually increased to 3 to 5 tablespoons daily, usually taken in the morning. If patients cannot tolerate

TABLE 6. **Tyramine-Restricted Diet**

Food Group	Unrestricted Foods	Foods Allowed in Moderation	Foods to Avoid
Cheese	Cottage cheese, ricotta, cream cheese	Processed American cheese, Gouda	Aged cheeses—brick, blue, cheddar, Camembert, Swiss, Romano, Roquefort, Stilton, mozzarella, Parmesan, provolone, Emmentaler, boursin, Brie; sour cream, yogurt
Beverages	Milk	White wine (not aged in wood), vodka	Ale, beer, sherry, brandy, liqueurs, liquor (scotch, bourbon, etc.), red wine, white wine aged in wood, bouillon, coffee, tea, hot chocolate, cola drinks
Meats	White meat of fresh or frozen poultry, eggs	—	All red meat, canned meats, liver, fermented (hard) sausage or salami, pepperoni, summer sausage, bologna, Genoa salami
Fish	Fresh or fresh-frozen fish or shellfish	—	Salt herring, dried fish, caviar, pickled herring
Vegetables	Most	—	Flat beans, Chinese pea pods, broad (fava) beans, mixed Chinese vegetables, eggplant
Fruit	Most	—	Figs, avocados, bananas
Miscellaneous	Garlic, herbs, spices	—	Chocolate, soy sauce, protein extracts, yeast concentrates or products made with them, any sauces with unknown ingredients

psyllium, products with methylcellulose (Citrucel) are good substitutes. Patients should be instructed that these fiber products can initially make them feel bloated and full but that this discomfort subsides in a short time.

Exercise. Some form of exercise is beneficial to everyone. Brisk walking in moderation is recommended.

Sleep. An adequate amount of sleep is necessary to reduce stress. Both quantity and quality of sleep are important. Medications may be necessary to provide appropriate sleep. It is important that the patient go to sleep at the same time each night and get up at the same time each morning, thus helping the body to establish its rhythm.

Stress. Psychosocial factors are often involved in patients with IBS; these factors are not the cause of the disease, but they can contribute strongly to the symptoms. Identifying specific stresses and discussing ways to reduce or eliminate them may accelerate a patient's improvement. Other psychosocial factors may be identified that require immediate professional counseling.

Patients should be seen in a follow-up visit at about 8 weeks. If there is significant improvement, they should be encouraged to continue the plan outlined above. However, 8 weeks may not be enough time for bulking agents to become effective; it often takes 3 to 5 months to produce the full effect. Patients should also be forewarned that symptoms may recur periodically and not to be alarmed if they do. After 8 weeks, if there is little or no improvement in the patient's symptoms and condition, the case should be reassessed and referral to a gastroenterologist considered. Further testing should be avoided unless there are new complaints or changing conditions. Additional medication may provide effective control of symptoms, as outlined in Table 7. Reassurance should be provided, and the physician-patient relationship should continue to be nurtured.

UNRESPONSIVE OR COMPLICATED PATIENTS

Patients with IBS who do not respond to the aforementioned plan are few, but they are difficult to manage. Referral to a gastroenterologist is clearly indicated for patients with intractable symptoms of diarrhea, constipation, pain, gas, or bloating. The gastroenterologist should review the patient's history carefully, perform a thorough physical examination, and review the laboratory tests. If the diagnosis of IBS seems appropriate, further testing should be avoided and the patient should be counseled once

TABLE 7. **Drugs for Specific Gastrointestinal Complaints**

Indication	Drug
Diarrhea predominant, incontinence	Loperamide (Imodium) 1–2 tablets tid (antidiarrheal and tightens anal sphincter); cholestyramine 4 grams tid PO (Questran) (binds bile salts)
Constipation predominant	Psyllium, adjust dose, or wheat bran 1/2 cup to one bowl, or calcium polycarbophil 2 tablets qid; lactulose (Chronulac), osmotic sugar; polyethylene glycol and electrolytes (GoLYTELY, Colyte)
Gas, bloating, flatus	Simethicone (Maalox, Mylanta, Riopan); alpha-D-galactosidase (Beano) at beginning of meal
Pain predominant	
Pain after meals	Dicyclomine (Bentyl) 10–20 mg before each meal (antispasmodic, anticholinergic)
Chronic pain syndrome	Amitriptyline (Elavil)* in individual doses

*Not FDA-approved for this indication.

Reproduced with permission, from Drossman DA, Thompson WG: Irritable bowel syndrome: A graduated multicomponent treatment approach. Ann Intern Med *116*:1009–1016, 1992.

again about IBS. The consultant gastroenterologist should be as supportive as possible of the primary care physician, who will most likely provide long-term care for the patient. Emphasis should be placed on control of chronic disease rather than on a "cure." Once again, the patient should be reassured that there is no serious underlying organic disease.

The psychosocial factors in the patient's life need to be readdressed; behavior modification by a psychologist trained in this area may be necessary and is our approach of choice. Other treatments—relaxation therapy, hypnosis, biofeedback, some form of meditation, and group discussion (support groups)—are also acceptable; a patient who needs psychotherapy is unusual. A number of the available psychotropic drugs should also be avoided, especially the serotonin uptake inhibitors such as fluoxetine (Prozac), paroxetine (Paxil), and sertraline (Zoloft). These drugs block the presynaptic receptors for and up-modulate serotonin. They may actually worsen symptoms by making the gut more excitable. One of the therapy combinations useful in treating difficult patients is the benzodiazepine clonazepam (Klonopin)* and cyproheptadine (Periactin).* Klonopin is a gamma-aminobutyric acid (GABA$_A$) receptor agonist, stabilizing nerve cells by opening chloride channels, causing the cell interior to become more negatively charged. Myenteric neurons have been shown to have abundant GABA$_A$ receptors. Cyproheptadine is an old drug that is classified as an antihistamine but also has potent postsynaptic serotonin-blocking action. It down-modulates serotonin and makes the gut less excitable. Only very small doses of these medications are needed for therapeutic effect. We usually begin with Klonopin 0.25 mg three times a day. Two weeks later, Periactin syrup is added at a dosage of 10 drops in the morning and 5 drops at night.

We have also had excellent success in treating more difficult or refractory cases with the gonadotropin-releasing hormone (GnRH) analogue leuprolide acetate (Lupron).* We have identified GnRH receptors on cultured mammalian myenteric plexus neurons. A phase-II, randomized, double-blind, placebo-controlled study of 30 patients using three monthly intramuscular injections of Lupron Depot 3.75 mg showed significant symptomatic improvement in 93% of patients who were on the drug. A 1-year follow-up of 28 of these study patients, but using daily subcutaneous injections, showed even more striking and significant improvement. We now primarily use the daily subcutaneous form. For women with ovaries, daily doses gradually titrated from 0.5 mg to reach 1.0 to 1.25 mg are effective; postmenopausal women and men require 2.0 mg for effective therapy. Because GnRH analogues suppress all gonadotropins, we add estrogen supplements to prevent osteoporosis. It is important to remember that drugs such as Klonopin, Periactin, and Lupron should be used only in difficult patients who have failed conventional approaches to therapy.

*Not FDA-approved for this indication.

HEMORRHOIDS, ANAL FISSURE, AND ANORECTAL ABSCESS AND FISTULA

method of
DAVID E. BECK, M.D.
Ochsner Clinic
New Orleans, Louisiana

An understanding of anatomy is essential to properly diagnose and treat anorectal problems. The area of discussion encompasses the distal rectum, the anal canal, and the perianal spaces. The dentate line divides the rectal mucosa above (generally insensate and lined with columnar mucosa) and the anoderm below (highly sensitive due to somatic enervation provided by the inferior hemorrhoidal nerve and lined with modified squamous mucosa). The anal canal is surrounded by two muscles. The internal sphincter, innervated by the autonomic nervous system, maintains the resting anal tone and is under involuntary control. The external sphincter, innervated by somatic nerve fibers, generates the voluntary anal squeeze and is most important in maintaining anal continence.

The area surrounding the anorectum is divided into four spaces. Knowledge of these spaces is particularly important when evaluating perirectal abscesses and fistulas. The *perianal* space is a subcutaneous space between the dentate line and the most superficial fibers of the external sphincter. The *ischiorectal* space surrounds the perianal space and extends into the fat of the buttock. The *supralevator* space is adjacent to the rectum and proximal to the levator ani, the muscle that serves as the pelvic floor. Finally, the *intersphincteric* space is the area between the internal and external sphincters within the anal canal. All these spaces may be sites for perirectal abscesses.

HISTORY AND PHYSICAL EXAMINATION

In diagnosing and treating anorectal disorders, a dedicated history and physical examination are essential. In most instances, the diagnosis can be predicted by the patient's responses and need only be confirmed by physical examination. Four areas must be investigated:

1. Pain—the character of the pain (e.g., knifelike or achy) and its relationship to bowel movements, its duration, and any causative factors.
2. Bleeding—the character (i.e., dark red, bright red), quantity, and timing of bleeding (i.e., mixed with stool, dripping into the toilet with bowel movements, or occurring between bowel movements).
3. Bowel habits—constipation, diarrhea, incontinence, straining at stool, or change in bowel habits.
4. Masses—prolapsing masses with bowel movements, tender perianal masses, or nontender perianal masses.

Most patients with anal problems dread visiting their physicians, not only because of the embarrassing nature of their problem but mostly because of fear of the examination. Reassurance and gentleness are required to overcome the patient's concern. Explaining the details of the examination in advance helps alleviate the patient's anxiety.

The examination starts with a visual inspection. Spreading the buttocks reveals anal pathology (e.g., perianal abscess, thrombosed external hemorrhoid, prolapsing internal hemorrhoid), and gently everting the anal verge in the posterior midline often allows an anal fissure to be identified. This procedure is followed by careful palpation of the perianal area, looking especially for masses, tenderness, or fluctuance (abscess). A digital examination with a well-lubricated finger is performed next. Following this, anoscopy (a side-viewing anoscope is best) is used to evaluate internal hemorrhoids and other anal pathology. A rigid or flexible sigmoidoscopy can also be performed to examine the mucosa of the distal rectum to rule out inflammatory bowel disease, infectious proctitis, polyps, or rectal cancers.

It is important to remember that not every patient requires every aspect of the anorectal examination just described. For example, a patient with an acute anal fissure may require only visual inspection with gentle eversion of the anoderm; in this case, a digital examination and anoscopy do not add information and only cause the patient discomfort. These examinations should be performed after the acute pathology (e.g., anal fissure) has healed.

HEMORRHOIDS

Hemorrhoids are fibrovascular cushions that line the anal canal and are classically found in three locations: right anterior, right posterior, and left lateral. Contrary to popular belief, hemorrhoidal location in the anal canal has no relationship to the terminal branches of the superior hemorrhoidal artery and vein, and pathologic hemorrhoids are not engorged perianal varices. Hemorrhoids are part of normal anal anatomy and become engorged during straining or performance of the Valsalva maneuver as a component of the normal mechanism of fecal continence. Hemorrhoidal engorgement most likely completes the occlusion of the anal canal and prevents stool loss associated with nondefecatory straining. However, when the term "hemorrhoid" is used in medical literature, it almost exclusively refers to pathologic hemorrhoids, and it will be used as such in the following paragraphs.

Hemorrhoids are divided into internal and external components. Internal hemorrhoids are found proximal to the dentate line, whereas external hemorrhoids occur distally. External hemorrhoids are redundant folds of perianal skin generally related to prior perianal swelling; they remain asymptomatic unless they are thrombosed and are treated entirely differently from internal hemorrhoids.

Internal Hemorrhoids

Internal hemorrhoidal disease is demonstrated by two main symptoms—painless bleeding and protrusion. Pain is rarely associated with internal hemorrhoids because they originate above the dentate line in insensate rectal mucosa. The most popular etiologic theory states that hemorrhoids result from chronic straining at defecation (upright posture and heavy lifting may also contribute). This straining not only causes hemorrhoidal engorgement but also creates forces that decrease the fixation between the hemorrhoids and the rectal muscular wall. Continued straining causes further engorgement and bleeding, as well as hemorrhoidal prolapse. Internal hemorrhoids are categorized into four grades based on symptoms: I, bleeding without prolapse; II, prolapse that spontaneously reduces; III, prolapse requiring manual reduction; and IV, irreducible prolapse.

Questioning often reveals a long history of constipation and straining at defecation. Patients with internal hemorrhoids are commonly extensive bathroom readers, spending many hours in the bathroom each week. Symptoms start with painless bleeding and may progress to anal protrusion. Hemorrhoidal prolapse must be distinguished from true full-thickness rectal prolapse. The physical examination again begins with visual inspection and may reveal prolapsing hemorrhoidal tissue as a rosette of three distinct pink-purple hemorrhoidal groups. If prolapse is not present, anoscopy reveals redundant anorectal mucosa just proximal to the dentate line in the classic locations.

The majority of patients with internal hemorrhoids can be treated without surgical intervention. All patients with Grade I or II hemorrhoids and most patients with Grade III hemorrhoids should be treated initially with efforts to correct their constipation. Recommendations should include a high-fiber diet, liberal water intake (six to eight 8-ounce glasses of water daily), and fiber supplements such as Metamucil, Konsyl, or Citrucel. Sitz baths are recommended for their soothing effect. Hemorrhoidal creams may be added but have never been proved effective. Suppositories should be avoided because they deliver medication to the rectum and not the anus. Patients should be instructed to avoid prolonged trips to the bathroom, and all reading materials should be removed.

If these measures are not effective, a number of nonoperative therapies are available, such as rubber band ligation, infrared coagulation, sclerotherapy, and others. These methods are equally effective and are most successful when applied to Grade I and II hemorrhoids, but they also cure some patients with Grade III hemorrhoids. All may be performed with excellent results in the office setting. Patients with Grade II and III internal hemorrhoids that are refractory to nonoperative measures, patients with Grade IV hemorrhoids, and patients with combined internal and external hemorrhoids are candidates for operative hemorrhoidectomy. Hemorrhoidectomy can be performed under local, regional, or general anesthesia, and it can be either an inpatient or an outpatient procedure. Recurrence following hemorrhoidectomy varies from 2 to 5%.

Hemorrhoids commonly flare during pregnancy, related to constipation and local effects of the gravid uterus. The majority of these patients improve dramatically following delivery. Therefore, efforts to control constipation are usually all that is required.

External Hemorrhoids

External hemorrhoids are asymptomatic except when secondary thrombosis occurs. Thrombosis may be the result of defecatory straining, or it may be a random event. Patients present with acute onset of constant anal pain and often report a sensation of sitting on a tender marble. The physical examination identifies the external thrombosis as a purple mass at the anal verge. The treatment is dependent on the patient's symptoms. In the first 48 hours following the onset of thrombosis, the pain generally increases and excision is warranted. After 48 hours, the pain is generally diminishing and expectant treatment is all that is necessary. Patients should be advised that some drainage should occur. If operative treatment is chosen, the entire thrombosed hemorrhoid should be excised under local anesthesia. Incision and drainage of the clot are avoided, as this results in rethrombosis and worsening symptoms.

ANAL FISSURE

An anal fissure is a tear or split in the anoderm just distal to the dentate line. Fissures are characterized as acute or chronic. An acute fissure is generally caused by the mechanical force of a large, hard bowel movement being passed through an anal canal too small to accommodate safe, easy passage (although diarrhea can also cause anal fissures). These forces usually cause a split to occur in the posterior midline (90% of the fissures in females and 99% of fissures in males are located posteriorly). Decreased local blood flow or increased mechanical stress may account for these fissures' propensity to occur posteriorly. Repeated injury (e.g., from hard or watery bowel movements) can result in development of a chronic fissure.

Symptoms associated with anal fissures include anal pain and bright red rectal bleeding associated with bowel movements. The pain is usually described as a knifelike pain or tearing sensation, and the associated anal sphincter spasm may persist for several hours following each bowel movement. The bleeding is usually minor, red in color, and seen mainly on the toilet tissue. Physical examination is difficult, because the patient has an extremely tender anus and is fearful. Often, visual inspection with gentle eversion of the anoderm in the posterior midline is all that is required. Physical findings include an approximately 1-cm split in the anoderm in the posterior midline just distal to the dentate line. In chronic fissures, the classic triad may be present: hypertrophy of the anal papilla, anal fissure, and sentinel skin tag. Once an anal fissure has been diagnosed, further examination is very painful, unrewarding, and unnecessary. More extensive investigation can be performed after the fissure has healed.

Multiple fissures, or fissures occurring away from the anterior or posterior midline, are unusual and should raise suspicion for other problems such as inflammatory bowel disease, sexually transmitted disease (e.g., syphilis), acquired immune deficiency syndrome (AIDS), tuberculosis, or malignancies.

Acute fissures are arbitrarily defined as those present for less than 6 weeks and are treated nonoperatively. Fiber supplements, stool softeners, and generous intake of water, along with sitz baths and local anesthetic ointments, improve symptoms rapidly and usually result in complete healing. Anal suppositories are to be avoided because they are painful, and once inserted, they rest in the rectum rather than the anal canal.

Chronic fissures are fissures that have been present for more than 6 weeks and are more likely to have an associated hypertrophied papilla and skin tag. They respond poorly to nonoperative treatment, although in some cases a short course of therapy similar to that for an acute fissure may be indicated. The most common surgical treatment for fissures is a lateral internal sphincterotomy. In this procedure, the internal sphincter distal to the dentate line is cut in a lateral aspect of the anal canal. This allows for relaxation of the forces keeping the fissure from healing and results in cure in 90 to 95% of patients.

ANORECTAL ABSCESS

Anorectal abscesses, like abscesses elsewhere in the body, are the result of local, walled-off infections. Most perirectal abscesses have a cryptogenic origin. That is, they begin as infections in the anal glands that surround the anal canal and empty into the anal crypts at the dentate line. The ducts leading to and from these glands become obstructed due to feces or trauma, and a secondary infection develops that follows the path of least resistance, resulting in an anorectal abscess.

Abscesses are characterized as perianal, ischiorectal, supralevator, or intersphincteric. Perianal abscesses are the most common; together with ischiorectal abscesses, they account for more than 90% of all perianal infections. Perianal abscesses occur in the perianal space immediately adjacent to the anal verge. Ischiorectal abscesses are larger and often more complex than their perianal counterparts, and they usually present as a tender buttock mass. Supralevator abscesses occur above the levator ani muscles, present with poorly localized pain, and are exceedingly rare. Intersphincteric, or intermuscular abscesses occur in the plane between the internal and external sphincters, high within the anal canal. The location of these abscesses is important because it dictates subsequent therapy.

Regardless of their location, anorectal abscesses are associated with constant perianal pain. Accompanying symptoms may include fever, chills, and malaise. In rare cases, systemic toxicity may be evident. History reveals a gradual onset of rectal pain that has progressively increased until the time of presentation. Occasionally, spontaneous drainage decompresses the abscess and the patient presents with a purulent discharge.

Again, visual inspection of the perineum often clinches the diagnosis. A fluctuant, erythematous, tender area identifies the abscess. In the rare case of a supralevator or intersphincteric abscess, there may be no external manifestations, and a tender mass on digital examination above the anal canal, adjacent to the rectal ampulla (supralevator abscess), or within the anal canal (intersphincteric abscess) provides the only clue to diagnosis.

Treatment for anorectal abscesses, similar to abscesses elsewhere, is adequate drainage. These abscesses may be drained either in the office (or emergency room) or in the operating room. In general, simple perianal and small ischiorectal abscesses can be drained safely in the office setting. However, recurrent or complex abscesses, abscesses in immunocompromised hosts (including diabetics), and intersphincteric and supralevator abscesses are more appropriately drained in the operating room.

When draining an abscess in the outpatient setting, there are several important points to remember. Local anesthetic works poorly in the presence of infection (because of acidity within the tissues), and the addition of one part sodium bicarbonate to 10 parts local anesthetic may improve its effectiveness. Adequate drainage is essential. Drainage can be established in several ways. One method is to place a catheter (such as a 10 to 16 French Pezzar catheter) through a small stab incision. This allows the pus to drain through the catheter as the cavity closes down. After the cavity closes down, the catheter is removed and the small remaining cavity heals. The incision should be placed over the fluctuant area, as close to the anal canal as possible. This results in a shorter fistula if the abscess does not heal completely. A second drainage option involves creating a larger elliptical incision. Unroofing the abscess allows it to heal without the need for packing. A small incision should be avoided, as it requires painful packing to keep the skin open until the abscess cavity heals. Following adequate drainage, antibiotics are rarely needed. Patients should be discharged with fiber supplements (stool softeners), pain medications, and instructions for sitz baths two to three times daily.

FISTULA IN ANO

An anal fistula is a communication from the anal canal to the perianal skin. Fistulas are identified in 40 to 80% of anorectal abscesses. The fistula usually begins in a crypt at the dentate line and follows a course between the internal and external sphincters (the most common location), resulting in a perianal abscess; across the external sphincter, resulting in an ischiorectal abscess; or above the sphincters, leading to a supralevator abscess.

Following acute drainage of an abscess, one of three things may occur if a fistula is present: (1) the fistula may heal spontaneously, and the patient experiences no further symptoms; (2) the abscess may heal only to recur in the future; or (3) the abscess may heal, leaving a chronic draining anal fistula or fistula in ano. Only the third scenario is discussed here. Following the drainage of one or more abscesses, a fistula is usually associated with chronic serosanguineous to seropurulent drainage. As long as the fistula remains open and draining, patients report little pain. But should the fistula close externally, an anorectal abscess may develop. Physical

examination reveals a 2- to 3-mm opening in the perianal skin, with surrounding induration. Often, a fistula tract can be palpated as a firm cord running between the external opening and the anal canal.

Essentially, all chronic fistulas require surgical treatment, which consists of unroofing the entire fistula track (fistulotomy) and leaving the wound open to heal secondarily. Rarely, fistulas that course through significant amounts of sphincter muscle cannot be opened entirely because incontinence will result. These fistulas are partially opened, and the anal musculature is left intact and is encircled with a seton. Another option involves closing the internal fistula opening with a rectal advancement flap.

GASTRITIS

method of
BRIAN J. SWANSIGER, M.D., and
MICHAEL C. DUFFY, M.D.
William Beaumont Hospital
Royal Oak, Michigan

"Gastritis" is a poorly defined term, as there are no generally accepted definitions that apply to the endoscopic, histologic, and clinical diagnosis. Infection of the gastric antrum with *Helicobacter pylori*, a spiral, urease-producing bacterium, is perhaps the most common chronic bacterial infection in humans and accounts for most cases of histologic gastritis, but the degree to which this histologic inflammation causes clinical symptoms is the subject of much debate. Although the conventional wisdom of patients and their physicians is that an irritated, inflamed stomach lining should produce dyspeptic symptoms, the majority of studies in this area have shown poor correlation between endoscopic appearance and the presence or absence of dyspeptic symptoms. An erythematous or friable gastric mucosa of whatever cause, often termed "gastritis" by the endoscopist, is generally asymptomatic, and there is great interobserver variability in the endoscopic diagnosis. Furthermore, up to 30% of all individuals undergoing upper endoscopy are labeled as having gastritis by gross examination, although there is poor correlation between the gross endoscopic appearance of the mucosa and histologic evidence of inflammation. Finally, to add to the confusion, dyspepsia is extraordinarily common in the general population, with only a minority of symptomatic individuals seeking medical attention. This chapter focuses on the management of dyspepsia, followed by a discussion of specific types of gastritis.

DYSPEPSIA

Dyspepsia, defined as the presence of recurrent or chronic upper abdominal discomfort or nausea without typical features of biliary colic or gastroesophageal reflux, is an extraordinarily common symptom, affecting up to 30% of the population. When dyspeptic patients are investigated by endoscopy, approximately 20% prove to have peptic ulcer disease, 25% have gastroesophageal reflux, and 50% have no precise etiology determined (nonulcer dyspepsia). Only

TABLE 1. **Empirical Treatments for Dyspepsia**

Antacids
H₂-receptor antagonists—low-dose over-the-counter
H₂-receptor antagonists—prescription-strength (cimetidine,
   ranitidine, famotidine, nizatidine)
Sucralfate
Prokinetic drugs (cisapride, metoclopramide)

1 or 2% have gastric neoplasia. Various algorithms and clinical strategies are currently being developed to allow cost-effective evaluation of this problem, but as yet there is no consensus on the best way to manage a dyspeptic patient. The goal is to identify individuals with serious medical conditions (i.e., neoplasia, peptic ulcer disease) early and provide effective treatment, while limiting the evaluation and providing effective empirical treatment for patients with less serious diseases such as gastroesophageal reflux, irritable bowel syndrome, and nonulcer dyspepsia.

Prior to embarking on empirical treatment for a dyspeptic patient, a careful history and physical examination should be performed and baseline laboratory studies (complete blood count, biochemistry panel) should be obtained. Symptoms such as weight loss, blood in the stool, fever, or onset of symptoms after age 50 should prompt immediate evaluation, which generally involves either upper endoscopic examination or upper gastrointestinal x-rays. Failure to respond to empirical therapy within a few weeks or recurrent symptoms after 8 weeks of therapy should also prompt additional diagnostic studies.

Standard treatments for dyspepsia are listed in Table 1. For most patients, a trial of an H₂ blocker is the preferred empirical therapy. There is no evidence that the combination of an H₂ receptor antagonist and sucralfate is more effective than either agent alone. The use of combination therapies that increase the cost of treatment without therapeutic benefit should be avoided. The role of proton pump inhibitors (omeprazole [Prilosec], lansoprazole [Prevacid]) in the management of dyspeptic patients has not been well studied, but because of the higher cost of these drugs, this approach is not currently recommended. Similarly, the role of prokinetic drugs as primary empirical therapy for dyspeptic patients has not been studied, but they may be appropriate in selected patients with symptoms suggesting delayed gastric emptying. Moderation or elimination of smoking and alcohol use may also be beneficial.

HELICOBACTER PYLORI

Helicobacter pylori infection of the gastric antrum is generally a lifelong infection unless treated. The prevalence of infection increases with age, with up to 70% of individuals over age 60 being infected. The diagnosis can be established by serology, urea breath test, endoscopic biopsy with staining, or rapid urease testing or culture. The currently preferred methods are serology and endoscopic biopsy. *H. pylori* is the cause of most of the superficial antral gastritis seen on endoscopic examination and is usually present in ulcer patients not taking nonsteroidal anti-inflammatory drugs (NSAIDs). Eradication of the infection in such patients prevents recurrent ulcer disease. Chronic infection leads to atrophic gastritis, which is of particular concern, since there is an association between *H. pylori* infection and gastric carcinoma and lymphoma. The World Health Organization recently classified *H. pylori* as a Class I carcinogen.

Although anti-*Helicobacter* treatment is now standard therapy for patients with ulcer disease and is effective in preventing recurrence of ulcer disease if the organism is eradicated, there are few data to support the treatment of gastritis alone in the absence of ulcer disease. Clinical trials in patients with nonulcer dyspepsia infected with *H. pylori* have generally shown no benefit from anti-*Helicobacter* treatment. Successful eradication of the infection results in healing of the histologic gastritis but little improvement in dyspeptic symptoms. However, in selected dyspeptic patients who have failed other empirical therapy, anti-*Helicobacter* treatment may be warranted if no other cause for symptoms has been found and the patient has a documented *H. pylori* infection.

Many regimens for *Helicobacter* treatment exist, none of which is ideal. Cost, side effects, and poor compliance are major obstacles to effective treatment. Treatment with a single antimicrobial agent is generally unsuccessful and should be avoided due to the rapid development of resistant organisms. Most effective regimens require the use of one or two antibiotics in combination with either bismuth or a proton pump inhibitor to achieve eradication. Table 2 lists some of the currently available treatment regimens. The Food and Drug Administration has re-

TABLE 2. *Helicobacter pylori* **Treatment Regimens**

Drug	Dose	Frequency/ Duration	Total Cost*
Standard Triple Therapy			
Bismuth subsalicylate	2 tablets (262 mg/tablet)	qid × 14 days	
Metronidazole (Flagyl)	250 mg	qid × 14 days	$25
Tetracycline†	500 mg	qid × 14 days	
Dual Therapy			
Omeprazole (Prilosec)‡	20 mg	bid × 14 days	$240
Clarithromycin (Biaxin)§	500 mg	tid × 14 days	
"MOC" Therapy			
Metronidazole	500 mg	bid × 7 days	
Omeprazole	20 mg	bid × 7 days	$100
Clarithromycin	250 mg	bid × 7 days	

*Costs are estimates based on a survey of retail prices in suburban Detroit pharmacies, Oct. 1995.
†Amoxicillin 500 mg tid may be substituted for tetracycline.
‡Preliminary data suggest that lansoprazole (Prevacid) is as effective as omeprazole.
§Less effective if not started concomitantly.

cently approved a combination of clarithromycin (Biaxin) and a proton pump inhibitor for the treatment of *Helicobacter* infection.

NSAID GASTRITIS

Aspirin and NSAIDs are known to cause gastric mucosal injury by inhibition of cyclooxygenase, which is responsible for prostaglandin synthesis. In the gastric mucosa, prostaglandins have a number of potentially beneficial effects, including maintenance of mucosal blood flow, mucus production, and bicarbonate secretion. Patients on chronic NSAID therapy may present with a variety of gastric endoscopic lesions ranging from petechiae and diffuse erythema to frank ulceration. Small, contact-induced erosions are typically seen after immediate ingestion but bear no relationship to the ultimate development of gastritis or ulcer disease. Although NSAIDs are taken by almost 8% of the U.S. population, most injury is seen in people who consume large amounts of alcohol or are more than 60 years of age. The risk of injury is also higher with acute ingestion than with chronic therapy (greater than 6 months), presumably because of adaptive cytoprotection by the gastric mucosa. Unfortunately, dyspeptic symptoms do not correlate with the presence of ulcer disease in patients taking NSAIDs. Serious complications such as bleeding or perforation frequently occur in asymptomatic patients. Patients who develop dyspeptic symptoms on NSAIDs should be advised to discontinue the NSAID if feasible. Transient dyspepsia can be treated with antacids or H_2 blockers. Endoscopy is generally reserved for patients with persistent symptoms or bleeding. Ulcers associated with NSAIDs can be treated with H_2 antagonists or proton pump inhibitors (omeprazole, lansoprazole) for 8 weeks if the NSAID is discontinued or longer if the NSAID therapy is required.

Misoprostol, the oral prostaglandin congener that is FDA approved for the prevention of NSAID-induced gastric ulcer, can prevent gastric ulcer formation in patients who must continue NSAIDs and reduces the incidence of complications such as bleeding or perforation by 40%. Misoprostol (Cytotec), is usually administered in a dosage of 100 to 200 μg orally four times daily, although recent studies suggest that a dosage of 200 μg twice or three times a day may provide the same benefit with fewer side effects such as diarrhea. The abortifacient property of this drug prevents its use in pregnancy; women of childbearing age should be cautioned to use effective birth control methods while taking misoprostol. Because of the cost associated with long-term use and potential side effects, misoprostol should be reserved for patients requiring NSAIDs who are at high risk for the development of ulcer disease. Risk factors for NSAID-induced ulcer disease include advanced age, female sex, prior history of ulcer disease or gastrointestinal bleeding, and history of cardiac disease. Misoprostol therapy should be considered for patients with one or more of these risk factors, realizing that the pro-tection against serious complications is only partial, and only after the patient's need for continued NSAIDs is carefully assessed.

With recent advances in drug therapy, newer NSAIDs have appeared on the market with the promise of reduced rates of gastric injury. Prodrugs, for example, decrease topical injury by breaking down to an active moiety only after absorption. In time, however, the risk of ulceration approaches that associated with older NSAIDs, reflecting the systemic nature of NSAID-induced damage. Since the discovery of two isoforms of cyclooxygenase (COX-1 and COX-2), NSAIDs specific for the latter have been developed and may be safer than nonselective anti-inflammatory agents. NSAIDs have also been linked to nitric oxide by an ester bond and are termed NO-NSAIDs. The nitric oxide moiety exerts cytoprotective effects similar to prostaglandins, thereby improving the safety profile of the parent compound. These agents are currently investigational but may eventually fulfill the requirement for a "safe" NSAID.

STRESS GASTRITIS

Upper gastrointestinal hemorrhage occurring in patients in the intensive care unit (ICU) is often due to multiple erosions of the proximal stomach, sometimes referred to as stress gastritis or stress ulcers. The incidence of this condition has been steadily decreasing, primarily due to advancements in intensive care treatment of these critically ill patients. Trials of prophylactic treatment have shown that acid suppression with H_2 antagonists, acid neutralization with antacids, and topical therapy with sucralfate are equally effective in reducing the incidence of overt hemorrhage but do not affect the overall mortality. Concerns about an increased incidence of nosocomial pneumonia in patients treated with acid suppression have not been substantiated. Stress gastritis prophylaxis should be used only in patients who are at high risk of bleeding, including medical patients requiring prolonged mechanical ventilation who have coagulopathy and surgical patients with head injury, extensive burns, or multiple trauma. The majority of ICU patients do not appear to benefit from empirical therapy. Effective treatment regimens are listed in Table 3. At present, either continuous intravenous infusion of H_2 antagonists or oral sucralfate is the preferred prophylactic regimen. There is no rationale for combining therapy with an H_2 antagonist and sucralfate. Gastric pH should be measured periodically and kept above 4.0 if H_2 antagonists or

TABLE 3. **Prophylaxis for Stress Gastritis**

Histamine H_2 antagonist
Cimetidine (Tagamet) 50 mg/h IV
Ranitidine (Zantac) 6.25 mg/h IV
or
Sucralfate (Carafate) 1 g PO q 6 h
or
Antacids 20 mL/h

antacids are utilized. Proton pump inhibitors may prove to be effective, especially when an intravenous formulation is available.

ATROPHIC GASTRITIS

Any persistently active gastritis may eventually lead to gastric atrophy. Atrophic gastritis is characterized by inflammation into the deepest portions of the mucosa and loss of glandular activity, resulting in hypo- or achlorhydria. Atrophy is classified according to the site of involvement, which is determined in part by etiology. Type A gastritis, involving the fundus and gastric body, is an autoimmune disease that is frequently associated with other autoimmune diseases and pernicious anemia. Type B gastritis involves the gastric antrum and is usually caused by *H. pylori*. Although treatment is not required for atrophic gastritis, therapy aimed at the sequelae of chronic achlorhydria may be necessary. Iron and calcium supplementation may be useful to prevent iron-deficiency anemia and osteoporosis. Patients with pernicious anemia should receive 100 µg of vitamin B_{12} intramuscularly each month.

ALKALINE REFLUX GASTRITIS

Alkaline or bile reflux gastritis refers to the gastric mucosal damage caused by contact with bile salts, generally due to duodenal-gastric reflux. This occurs most commonly in a patient who has undergone gastric surgery with gastrojejunostomy but can be seen in normal subjects and in patients with disruption of the pyloric sphincter due to prior ulcer disease. The endoscopic appearance is characterized by an erythematous, friable mucosa. Histologically, there is minimal inflammatory infiltrate, leading to the suggestion that this injury should be termed "gastropathy" rather than gastritis. As with other types of gastritis, there is a poor correlation between symptoms and the presence or absence of endoscopic and histologic changes. However, patients may complain of bilious vomiting, nausea, and a bitter taste in the mouth.

For patients with dyspeptic symptoms associated with alkaline gastritis, therapy is largely empirical and not entirely satisfactory. Cholestyramine (Questran)* should be of theoretical benefit, but few patients respond well and the medication is poorly tolerated. Sucralfate (Carafate) 1 gram orally four times daily or ursodeoxycholic acid (Actigall)* 300 mg orally twice daily may provide symptomatic relief. Prokinetic agents such as metoclopramide (Reglan) 10 mg orally before meals and at bedtime or cisapride (Propulsid) 10 to 20 mg orally before meals and at bedtime may be helpful, particularly in patients with nausea as a predominant symptom. There is little role for H_2-receptor antagonists or proton pump inhibitors in the therapy of these conditions, since the majority of patients are achlorhydric due to the pre-

---

*Not FDA-approved for this indication.

vious surgery. Refractory symptoms may require a surgical biliary diversion.

ACUTE AND CHRONIC VIRAL HEPATITIS

method of
JEROME B. ZELDIS, M.D., PH.D.
Janssen Research Foundation
Titusville, New Jersey

and

LAWRENCE S. FRIEDMAN, M.D.
Massachusetts General Hospital and
Harvard Medical School
Boston, Massachusetts

The clinical manifestations of acute infections with the hepatitis viruses are indistinguishable despite the biologic diversity of the causative agents (Table 1). Often, particularly in children, the episode of acute hepatitis is clinically silent. Jaundice does not develop in most patients, and the illness is often interpreted as a nonspecific viral syndrome unless liver biochemical tests and serologic assays for viral hepatitis are obtained. Prodromal immune-complex phenomena, including arthritis, a serum sickness–like illness, vasculitis, and glomerulonephritis, may occur with acute hepatitis A, B, or C. In the elderly and in those with immunologic disorders, however, acute illness can be severe or protracted beyond the typical 6 months that usually demarcates acute, self-limited hepatitis from chronic hepatitis.

After an incubation period characteristic of each virus, symptoms of the acute viral hepatitis may develop, including malaise, anorexia, nausea, vomiting, low-grade fever, alteration in taste and smell, and right upper quadrant or epigastric discomfort. These symptoms typically last 1 to 2 weeks and coincide with peak elevations in serum aminotransferase levels. Jaundice may appear as the prodromal symptoms abate and probably reflects the degree of liver injury or a cholestatic phase in patients with acute hepatitis A. After approximately 6 to 8 weeks of symptomatic illness, most patients recover fully without residual hepatic impairment.

Six viruses—labeled A, B, C, D, E, and G—have been designated as hepatitis viruses, and many others are known to infect the liver and cause acute hepatitis as part of a systemic illness. What distinguishes the six hepatitis viruses from the others is their predilection to infect the liver and evitably cause clinical or subclinical biochemical hepatitis. Over 95% of all cases of viral hepatitis in the United States are caused by one of these six agents.

The major issues that clinicians must address during the acute phase of viral hepatitis are whether the hepatitis will lead to liver failure (fulminant hepatic failure, subfulminant hepatic failure) and whether the infection will be self-limited or will become chronic. Once the infection becomes chronic (chronicity usually being defined as an infection that persists for over 6 to 12 months in individuals with normal immune function), the major issues confronting the clinician are related to the natural history of the infection, the patient's infectivity to others, and the potential responsiveness to antiviral therapy.

TABLE 1. **The Hepatitis Viruses**

Characteristic	Hepatitis A	Hepatitis B	Hepatitis C	Hepatitis D	Hepatitis E	Hepatitis G
Nucleic acid	RNA	DNA	RNA	RNA	RNA	RNA
Incubation period (days)	15–45	30–180	15–160	21–140	14–63	15–160
Fecal-oral transmission	+ + +	−	−	?	+ + +	−
Percutaneous transmission	+ (rarely)	+ + +	+ + +	+ + +	?	+ + +
Chronic hepatitis (frequency)	No	Yes (1–90%)*	Yes (>90%)	Yes	No	Yes
Fulminant hepatitis	~0.1%	<1%	<0.1%†	Up to 17%	10–20% in pregnant women	<1%
Risk of hepatocellular carcinoma	No	Yes	Yes	Yes	No	Possibly

*Depends on age and immunocompetence of patient.
†No case of fulminant hepatitis C has yet been documented.

Overall, mortality from acute viral hepatitis is well below 1%, but in patients with acute hepatitis D, the mortality rate may be as high as 5%; in pregnant women with hepatitis E, the mortality rate is 10 to 20%. In the majority of cases, acute viral hepatitis is a self-limited illness; approximately 85% of hospitalized patients and over 95% of outpatients recover completely and uneventfully within 3 months. Rarely, acute hepatitis can lead to rapid hepatic deterioration associated with coagulopathy and encephalopathy, a condition known as fulminant hepatic failure. All the hepatitis viruses can cause fulminant hepatic failure, although fulminant hepatitis C appears to be rare. Fulminant hepatic failure is an indication for liver transplantation, since the survival after liver transplantation is better than the natural history of this rare complication.

Of the six hepatitis viruses, four (hepatitis B virus [HBV], hepatitis C virus [HCV], hepatitis D virus [HDV or delta agent], and hepatitis G virus [HGV]) can cause chronic infection. The probability that the infection will become chronic varies with the virus (see Table 1). Chronic viral hepatitis presents a spectrum of clinical and biochemical manifestations. Patients may be entirely asymptomatic, mildly or moderately symptomatic, or have symptoms and signs of severe liver disease, and the course may be uncomplicated, relapsing, unrelenting, or progressive. Serum aminotransferase levels may be normal, mildly elevated, or markedly elevated. In some patients, chronic infection can be detected only by the presence of viral nucleic acid or antigens in serum and liver.

Chronic hepatitis has traditionally been classified as either chronic persistent hepatitis, in which mononuclear cell inflammation is limited to portal tracts, or chronic active hepatitis, in which the mononuclear cell portal infiltrate extends beyond the portal tracts into the adjacent periportal space and results in erosion of the limiting plate of periportal hepatocytes—so-called piecemeal necrosis. The distinction between chronic persistent and chronic active hepatitis is not absolute, in part because percutaneous needle biopsy of the liver is associated with some degree of sampling error and in part because the course of chronic hepatitis, whether persistent or active, is unpredictable and variable. Because of this, a newer classification of chronic hepatitis based on etiology, grade of portal inflammation (none, mild, moderate, or severe), and stage of fibrosis (none, mild, moderate, severe, or cirrhosis) has been introduced. The implication is that the milder the inflammation, the better the prognosis.

ETIOLOGIC AGENTS AND DIAGNOSIS

Hepatitis A Virus

Hepatitis A virus (HAV) is a picornavirus distantly related to poliovirus that causes acute but not chronic hepatitis. Like other enteroviruses, HAV is almost always transmitted by the fecal-oral route. HAV is associated with both sporadic cases of acute hepatitis and larger outbreaks traced to contaminated food, water, milk, and shellfish. Acute hepatitis A is most likely to occur in the late fall and early winter. Symptoms usually appear after an incubation period of approximately 1 month. Because fecal virus shedding is maximal during the late incubation period, patients are most infectious just before or shortly after the onset of symptoms of liver disease. The patient's age affects both the clinical presentation and the severity of illness. In young children, especially those under age 2, acute hepatitis A is frequently asymptomatic and often passes unnoticed. Most adults develop a symptomatic illness that may be associated with jaundice.

Diagnosis of acute hepatitis A is based on detection of serum IgM antibody to HAV (anti-HAV) at the time symptoms appear. IgM anti-HAV is typically short-lived, persisting for approximately 3 to 6 months after the onset of acute illness. Occasionally, IgM anti-HAV remains detectable for longer periods. False-positive IgM anti-HAV results due to rhematoid factor are rare. During convalescence, anti-HAV persists indefinitely as an IgG antibody and the IgM antibody is no longer detectable. The presence of IgG anti-HAV signifies recovery and immunity to reinfection.

The prognosis of acute hepatitis A is excellent. With resolution of the acute infection, liver function invariably returns to normal. Only about 0.1% of patients with jaundice develop fulminant hepatic failure. In a small proportion of cases, biochemical and serologic relapse can occur weeks or occasionally months after apparent recovery, but ultimate recovery is the rule. Occasional cases of acute hepatitis A are associated with profound cholestasis, mimicking biliary obstruction. In all these persistent forms of infection, IgM anti-HAV remains positive.

Management of acute hepatitis A involves supportive care and protection of contacts who are not immune to the virus. Corticosteroid therapy for the cholestatic form of acute HAV infection is of no proven benefit.

Hepatitis B Virus

HBV is a DNA virus (hepadnavirus) associated with a wide spectrum of clinical outcomes. HBV is spread percutaneously from contaminated needles, sexually, or perinatally from an infected mother to her infant.

As many as 90% of acute hepatitis B cases are clinically silent, particularly when infection is acquired early in life. The risk of fulminant hepatic failure is less than 1% in patients with acute hepatitis B, and jaundice is more common in those with HDV co-infection (see below) or with chronic hepatitis C.

The probability that acute hepatitis B will become chronic depends, in part, on the patient's age, sex, and immunocompetence. Chronic hepatitis B occurs in less than 2% of immunocompetent adult males over age 18 but in over 90% of neonates infected at birth. The rate of chronic infection in infants and children decreases as the age at acquisition of the initial infection increases. In immunocompromised individuals, the duration of acute hepatitis B is prolonged, and the likelihood of developing chronic hepatitis is increased (5 to 10%). Women are one-quarter as likely as men to develop chronic hepatitis B.

In patients with chronic hepatitis B, the lifetime risk of cirrhosis may be as high as 40%. The rate of progression to cirrhosis depends, in part, on the severity of chronic hepatitis, the immune status of the infected individual, the presence of specific viral mutations, co-infections with other hepatitis viruses (especially hepatitis D and C), and concomitant exposure to hepatotoxins (e.g., alcohol). End-stage liver disease and, in some cases, hepatocellular carcinoma generally occur many decades after initial infection, although rarely they may occur within 10 years or less.

Many serologic markers for HBV infection are available. Judicious use of these tests permits rapid and inexpensive diagnosis and determination of the stage (acute, chronic, resolved) of the disease (Table 2). Hepatitis B surface antigen (HBsAg) becomes detectable in serum before the onset of acute illness and persists through early convalescence. In typical cases of acute hepatitis B, HBsAg becomes undetectable as acute hepatitis resolves, and the antibody to HBsAg (anti-HBs) appears in the serum. Anti-HBs is a neutralizing antibody that confers lifelong immunity and is the sole antibody produced in response to hepatitis B vaccination. Most patients in whom liver enzymes normalize after acute hepatitis B become negative for HBsAg and positive for anti-HBs and can be considered to have recovered and no longer be infectious for HBV. HBsAg may be detected in serum for weeks after viral protein synthesis abates, due to its long half-life (7 to 14 days; longer in men than in women), its high concentrations in serum (up to 3 mg per mL), and the extreme sensitivity of most commercial assays (as low as 10 pg per mL). Following the return of serum aminotransferases to normal, HBsAg testing need not be repeated more often than every 3 months to confirm resolution of acute hepatitis B. Persistence of circulating HBsAg is suggestive of progression to chronic hepatitis B.

Hepatitis B core antigen (HBcAg) is a nucleocapsid protein contained in the inner core of the hepatitis B virus and usually does not circulate freely in serum. However, antibody to HBcAg (anti-HBc) appears in serum early in the course of infection, just after HBsAg, and persists indefinitely. During acute hepatitis B, anti-HBc of the IgM class predominates; as the infection resolves, levels gradually decline and are often undetectable within 6 months. Thereafter, anti-HBc of the IgG class predominates and remains detectable indefinitely. Unlike anti-HBs, anti-HBc is not neutralizing. In a patient with acute hepatitis, the detection of IgM anti-HBc in serum suggests acute hepatitis B, whereas the detection of only IgG anti-HBc is more consistent with acute hepatitis due to another agent superimposed on chronic hepatitis B. In approximately 10% of cases, patients with acute hepatitis B are negative for HBsAg and positive for anti-HBs at the time of clinical presentation. Diagnosis of acute hepatitis B may be made by detecting IgM anti-HBc.

Hepatitis B e antigen (HBeAg) is usually detected in serum when the liver is making large quantities of HBcAg during viral replication. Typically, HBeAg is detectable early in acute infection and disappears after several weeks, as the acute hepatitis resolves. When HBeAg persists for more than 3 to 4 months, progression to chronic hepatitis B is likely. In chronic hepatitis B, HBeAg may remain detectable for months or even years, signifying continued active replication of the virus. Testing for HBeAg is of little value during acute infection but is useful for managing patients with chronic hepatitis B, in whom HBeAg is an important marker of viral replication and ongoing liver injury. Antibody to HBeAg (anti-HBe) appears as HBeAg becomes undetectable in serum. The detection of anti-HBe is associated with a high likelihood of spontaneous resolution of acute infection. In patients with chronic hepatitis B, seroconversion from HBeAg to anti-HBe positivity is often associated with a flare mimicking acute hepatitis and may be associated with transiently positive IgM anti-HBc and, in some cases, liver failure or decompensation. Often this chronic lobular hepatitis is associated with a significant decline in serum viral concentration.

Regardless of their HBeAg and anti-HBe status, all HBsAg-positive patients should be considered potentially infectious for HBV. In general, patients with HBV infection who are positive for HBeAg have a higher serum level of HBV DNA than anti-HBe–positive patients. However, variant forms of HBV have been identified that contain mutations in the pre-core region of the viral genome and are incapable of making HBeAg. Patients infected with these pre-core mutants may have high serum levels of HBV DNA, despite the absence of HBeAg and the presence of anti-HBe in serum. These viral variants may arise during the course of chronic infection by wild-type HBV and appear to be more common in Mediterranean countries than elsewhere. Although patients infected with pre-core mutants have been reported to have rapidly progressive and severe chronic hepatitis B, often fulminant hepatic failure, and a limited response to antiviral therapy, the precise significance of these mutants with respect to the natural history of HBV infection remains to be determined. Currently, no commercial assay is available to identify HBV pre-core mutants.

Sensitive tests to detect serum HBV DNA allow a quanti-

TABLE 2. **Common Serologic Patterns of Hepatitis**

Type of Hepatitis	Anti-HAV	HBsAg	Anti-HBs	Anti-HBc	HBeAg	Anti-HBe	Anti-HCV	Anti-HDV
Acute hepatitis A	IgM	−	−	−	−	−	−	−
Acute hepatitis B	−	+	−	IgM	+	−	−	−
Resolved hepatitis B	−	−	+	IgG	−	±	−	−
HBV vaccine response	−	−	+	−	−	−	−	−
Chronic hepatitis B	−	+	−	IgG	+/−	−/+	−	−
Acute or chronic hepatitis C	−	−	−	−	−	−	+	−
Acute hepatitis D and B	−	+	−	IgM	+	−	−	+
Chronic hepatitis D and B	−	+	−	IgG	−	±	−	+

tative estimate of the level of HBV replication and may identify low levels of viremia even in the absence of positive test results using commercial serologic assays. Determination of serum HBV DNA concentrations may also be used to identify patients who are likely to respond to antiviral treatment and to monitor response to therapy (see later discussion).

Hepatitis C Virus

HCV is similar to flaviviruses and accounts for a substantial proportion of cases previously designated as parenterally transmitted non-A, non-B hepatitis. This RNA virus has at least six subtypes based on nucleotide sequence and serologic testing. The prevalence of each genotype varies among geographic locations, and in certain localities, responsiveness to antiviral therapy correlates with genotype (see the later discussion). Acute hepatitis C is clinically silent in approximately 95% of cases. The role of HCV in causing fulminant hepatic failure appears to be limited. Acute hepatitis C leads to chronic HCV infection in as many as 90% of cases, although not all cases are associated with persistent serum aminotransferase elevations. A characteristic waxing and waning pattern of serum aminotransferase elevations is seen in many patients with chronic hepatitis C. Chronic hepatitis C may slowly progress to cirrhosis and, in some cases, hepatocellular carcinoma. In some localities, the rate of progression correlates with viral genotype and serum viral titer; however, there are no universally accepted markers for determining disease progression. Cofactors for the development of cirrhosis in patients with chronic hepatitis C include a history of heavy sustained alcohol consumption and exposure to other hepatotoxins. Overall, approximately 20% of patients with chronic hepatitis C develop cirrhosis after 10 to 20 years. Extrahepatic complications of HCV infection include mixed cryoglobulinemia, membranoproliferative glomerulonephritis, lymphocytic sialoadenitis, and autoimmune thyroiditis. In addition, HCV appears to be a contributory factor to the liver disease associated with porphyria cutanea tarda.

Transmission of HCV is primarily by the percutaneous route. Hepatitis C accounts for most cases of transfusion-associated hepatitis, but transfusion-associated cases make up only about 4% of all cases of hepatitis C. Presumably, most cases of hepatitis C are the result of intravenous drug use. Perinatal and sexual transmission of HCV is not common but has occurred when circulating levels of HCV RNA are high, especially in immunocompromised individuals. Transmission via homosexual activity is also rare. The risk of sexual transmission may correlate with the duration of marriage: in one study, less than 10% of spouses of infected persons were infected after 10 years of cohabitation, but more than 50% were infected after 50 years. It is not clear whether the mode of transmission in these cases was sexual or exposure to contaminated razors and toothbrushes.

Diagnosis of HCV infection is based on immunoassays to specific HCV antigens (see Table 2). In addition to a recombinant polypeptide called C100-3 used in the first-generation enzyme immunoassays (EIAs), currently available second-generation EIAs utilize HCV-related antigens designated C200 (a composite of C100-3 and C-33c, an adjacent segment of the nonstructural protein) and C-22-3 (a segment of the nucleocapsid core protein). Typically during acute hepatitis C, antibodies against the C-22-3 and C-33c viral antigens are detected 30 to 90 days before antibody to C100-3. Therefore, the overall sensitivity of the second-generation assay is 10 to 20% higher than that of the first-generation assay. Newer third-generation EIAs incorporate an additional peptide from the RNA polymerase gene of HCV and are likely to be even more sensitive and specific for HCV infection.

Confidence in the specificity of the second-generation anti-HCV EIA can be improved with the use of a supplemental recombinant immunoblot assay (RIBA-II), which uses a nitrocellulose strip impregnated with separate bands of the same recombinant viral polypeptides (C100-3, C-33c, and C-22-3) utilized in the EIA. The primary use of RIBA-II testing is to confirm positive anti-HCV results on EIA testing when there is a high likelihood of a false-positive result. For example, RIBA-II testing is useful in confirming positive anti-HCV EIA results in low-risk populations such as asymptomatic blood donors with normal serum aminotransferase levels who have no risk factors for HCV.

In the past year, a number of diagnostic tests for HCV RNA have become available commercially. The most sensitive method of detecting HCV RNA is by polymerase chain reaction (PCR), which may detect between 100 and 1000 viruses per milliliter. Most patients with acute hepatitis C become positive for HCV RNA by PCR within 10 days of virus exposure. A branched chain DNA test is useful for quantifying the amount of virus in serum or plasma, but it is less sensitive than PCR. The HCV RNA assays may ultimately have a role in diagnosing patients with suspected HCV infection who are negative for anti-HCV by EIA and in monitoring the efficacy of antiviral therapy (see the later discussion).

Hepatitis D Virus

HDV is an RNA virus that requires HBV for its infection and propagation. Therefore, HDV infection is encountered only in the setting of acute (co-infection) and chronic (superinfection) hepatitis B. HDV superinfection tends to cause a more severe, rapidly progressive hepatitis than chronic hepatitis B alone. HDV co-infection may be associated with an increased risk of fulminant hepatic failure compared with hepatitis B alone.

HDV is endemic in the Mediterranean countries and other regions, where transmission usually occurs by nonpercutaneous routes, presumably by intimate contact. In nonendemic areas such as North America and Western Europe, HDV transmission is primarily through percutaneous routes and is generally confined to specific high-risk groups such as intravenous drug users and multiply transfused hemophiliacs.

The diagnosis of HDV infection is based on the detection of a serum antibody to HDV (anti-HDV) (see Table 2). In acute HDV and HBV co-infection, anti-HDV may be present in serum only transiently or in low titers. In HDV superinfection of a patient with chronic hepatitis B, however, anti-HDV titers are high and sustained. Prevention of HDV infection occurs by preventing HBV infection (see the later discussion).

Hepatitis E Virus

Hepatitis E virus (HEV) is a calicivirus that causes acute, self-limited hepatitis but not chronic hepatitis. Like HAV, this RNA virus is spread primarily by the fecal-oral route. HEV is an important cause of epidemic and sporadic hepatitis in Asia, Africa, and Central America. For unknown reasons, the mortality rate is particularly high (10 to 20%) in pregnant women. Although 1 to 2% of U.S.

volunteer blood donors react positively to immunoassays for HEV, the role of this virus in sporadic hepatitis in North America remains to be determined. Specific serologic tests for HEV infection should become commercially available in the near future.

Hepatitis G Virus

HGV is a flavivirus unrelated to HCV and causes acute, self-limited hepatitis and chronic infections. Because HGV infection may be detected in persons infected with HCV, it is assumed that HGV is spread parenterally in a manner similar to HCV. However, chronic hepatitis develops in a lower percentage of HGV-infected patients than HCV-infected patients. Chronic HGV carriers often have normal serum aminotransferase levels. Currently, the only reliable diagnostic test for HGV infection is a PCR assay that is not yet commercially available. The clinical importance of HGV infection, including its contribution to the development of cirrhosis, is as yet unknown.

PRINCIPLES OF MANAGEMENT

Clinically apparent acute viral hepatitis is usually benign and self-limited. In most cases it can be managed on an outpatient basis. Hospitalization should generally be reserved for patients with severe illness or for high-risk patients such as the elderly, immunocompromised persons, and patients with underlying illnesses that may be difficult to manage in the setting of acute hepatitis. Severe illness is suggested by marked prolongation of the prothrombin time (>5 seconds prolonged), encephalopathy, ascites, edema, inability to maintain adequate hydration or oral intake, and hypoglycemia. No specific therapy for acute viral hepatitis exists that shortens the symptomatic phase or prevents complications from occurring. Therefore, management centers on maintenance of adequate nutrition, amelioration of symptoms, avoidance of further hepatic injury, and prevention of the spread of infection to others. Any patient hospitalized for severe acute viral hepatitis should be considered a possible candidate for liver transplantation if the clinical course progresses toward fulminant hepatic failure.

There is no evidence that dietary manipulations or strict bed rest affects the course of acute viral hepatitis. Many clinicians recommend a high-calorie diet that is low in protein, and because many patients experience nausea late in the day, larger meals are usually tolerated best in the morning. Exercise does not interfere with convalescence, although many patients feel better with restricted physical activity. Corticosteroid therapy has no value in acute viral hepatitis and in some cases may be hazardous. The value of corticosteroids in treating cholestatic hepatitis A, as suggested by some authorities, has not been proved. Alcohol intake should be avoided, and the use of drugs associated with liver injury should be avoided or closely monitored; in general, however, oral contraceptives need not be discontinued.

The symptoms associated with acute viral hepatitis can be quite debilitating and may require pharmacologic intervention. Nausea and vomiting can be controlled by judicious use of antiemetics. Because phenothiazines can cause cholestatic hepatitis in up to 1% of patients, other agents such as trimethobenzamide (Tigan) or metoclopramide (Reglan) should be used. In patients with cholestasis and pruritus, cholestyramine (Questran) or colestipol (Colestid),* up to 1 packet in a glass of water four times a day, may give relief.

Patients with acute viral hepatitis usually do not need to be isolated, except perhaps in the case of a fecally incontinent patient with hepatitis A or a bleeding patient with hepatitis B or C. Although fecal shedding of virus is minimal or absent during the symptomatic phase of HAV infection, it is still prudent to recommend simple hygienic precautions to the patient, including thorough handwashing, particularly after a bowel movement. For patients with acute hepatitis B or C, caregivers should follow universal precautions to avoid direct contact with blood or other body fluids. Sexual activity should be avoided until the illness resolves; chronic HBV carriers, regardless of their HBeAg and anti-HBe status, should practice "safe sex."

After the initial presentation of acute hepatitis, an office visit in 2 to 3 weeks is generally advisable in ambulatory patients with mild to moderate symptoms. Thereafter, the frequency of follow-up visits depends on how well the patient is managing. More frequent visits and telephone contact may be necessary for very symptomatic patients to assess their ability to manage the chores of daily living and to detect any evidence that they are failing to thrive. Serum aminotransferase and bilirubin levels and the prothrombin time may need to be assessed several times a week in severely ill patients or every few weeks in stable patients. Serum aminotransferase levels are particularly helpful in detecting ongoing liver inflammation, but the absolute values do not correlate with the severity of disease in the acute phase of illness. In the setting of acute hepatitis, the prothrombin time and serum glucose levels are good determinants of hepatocellular function. If symptoms or laboratory values of disease activity persist beyond 3 months after presentation, repeated assessments at monthly intervals are warranted. In cases of hepatitis B, HBsAg should be repeated after clinical and biochemical resolution of acute illness and then every 3 months until seroconversion. Liver biopsy as a prelude for antiviral therapy may be considered in patients with evidence of hepatitis B or C persisting for longer than 6 months but is not usually necessary in patients with acute hepatitis (see the later discussion).

IMMUNOPROPHYLAXIS

To prevent the spread of infection, immunoprophylaxis should be considered for contacts of patients with viral hepatitis. For hepatitis A, passive immunization of all household and institutional contacts

---

*Not FDA-approved for this indication.

with serum immune globulin (sIG) (Gamastan, Gammar) in a dose of 0.02 mL per kg intramuscularly is indicated. Because sIG is safe and inexpensive, potential recipients need not be tested for anti-HAV before immunoprophylaxis. Passive immunization may be effective even when administered as late as 2 weeks after exposure. Generally, prophylaxis with sIG is not necessary for casual contacts, such as coworkers. In some areas of the world, elderly individuals are almost invariably immune to HAV and may not need to receive immune globulin.

Several vaccines derived from inactivated HAV have been shown to be highly effective in providing protection from clinically apparent disease in both adults and children. One vaccine (Havrix) is commercially available in the United States. The dose for children ages 2 to 18 is two 360 ELISA unit (EL.U.) (0.5 mL) intramuscular doses given a month apart, which results in a seroconversion rate of over 99% after the second dose. In adults, a single 1440 EL.U. (1 mL) intramuscular dose confers immunity in 80 to 98% of vaccinees within 15 days of immunization and in greater than 96% within a month. A booster immunization at 6 to 12 months is recommended to attain a higher antibody titer. One month after the booster immunization, 100% of subjects are anti-HAV positive. Vaccination should be completed at least 2 weeks prior to expected exposure to HAV. Persons in whom vaccination should be considered include travelers to areas of high HAV endemicity, persons at increased risk due to their employment (institutional workers, employees of day care centers, veterinary assistants who handle primates, laboratory personnel who work with HAV), and persons engaged in high-risk behaviors such as homosexually active males, intravenous drug users, residents of a community experiencing an outbreak of hepatitis A, and military personnel.

HBV infection may be prevented by both passive immunoprophylaxis with high-titered anti-HBs immune globulin (HBIG) and active immunization with an HBV vaccine (Recombivax HB, Engerix-B) (Table 3). Pre-exposure prophylaxis to prevent infection in persons at high risk due to frequent or occupational exposure consists of three intramuscular injections (deltoid, not gluteal) of the HBV vaccine at 0, 1, and 6 months. One month after the third injection, greater than 95% of immunized subjects have neutralizing titers of anti-HBs. If protection is needed in a shorter time span, the vaccine may be given at 0, 1, and 2 months; to achieve high antibody titers, a fourth intramuscular injection should be administered at 12 months. Persons at high risk of HBV infection include health care workers exposed to blood products, dialysis patients, intravenous drug users, hemophiliacs, persons with a history of sexual promiscuity, and household and sexual contacts of chronic HBV carriers. Because many persons who contract HBV infection do not fall into a defined high-risk group, it is now recommended in the United States that HBV vaccination be incorporated into the standard immunization program for all children, preferably before adolescence, when risk-taking behavior often begins.

The currently available HBV vaccine is a genetically engineered recombinant vaccine, and the recommended dose for each injection is 10 to 20 µg for adults (the precise dose depending on the formulation) and 40 µg for immune suppressed persons. Because there is a small but significant failure rate (about 5%) in achieving protective antibody titers after a three-dose course of the vaccine, particularly in older recipients and hemodialysis patients, serum anti-HBs titers should be determined approximately 1 month after the third injection if confirmation of seroconversion is considered desirable. Adverse effects from the vaccine are uncommon and are usually limited to soreness at the injection site, malaise, and occasionally low-grade fever.

For unvaccinated persons who are exposed to HBV, postexposure prophylaxis with both HBIG and the HBV vaccine is recommended (see Table 3). The dose of HBIG in adults is 0.06 mL per kg intramuscularly. For persons experiencing a direct exposure of HBV, such as from a needle stick with HBsAg-positive blood or body fluids, a single dose of HBIG administered as soon after exposure as possible followed by a complete course of HBV vaccine beginning in the first week is recommended. The first dose of vaccine and HBIG can be administered simultaneously at different sites. Another dose of HBIG can be repeated a month later. Similar guidelines are recommended for persons exposed by sexual contact to a patient who is a chronic HBV carrier or to an infant born to an HBsAg-positive mother. In the event that an unvaccinated person is exposed to serum for which the HBV status is unknown, administration of the complete course of hepatitis B vaccine is indicated. If the exposed individual has been previously vaccinated against HBV, serum anti-HBs levels should be

TABLE 3. **Guidelines for Immunoprophylaxis Following Percutaneous Exposure to Hepatitis B**

Status of Exposed Individual	Source of Exposure			
	HBsAg +	HBsAg −	Unknown Serologic Status	Anti-HCV +
Unvaccinated	Hepatitis B immune globulin + HBV vaccine	HBV vaccine	HBV vaccine	Immune globulin
Previously vaccinated	Test for anti-HBs; if titer less than 10 mIU/mL, treat as unvaccinated	No treatment	No treatment	—

HBsAg = hepatitis B surface antigen; HBV = hepatitis B virus; HCV = hepatitis C virus.

obtained prior to vaccination to determine whether protective antibody levels are still present. An individual with an antibody level of less than 10 mIU per mL should be treated as an unvaccinated person.

Administration of sIG probably has no role in preventing HCV infection after an exposure, but sIG is often advised (without proof of efficacy) in persons who sustain percutaneous, sexual, or perinatal exposure to the virus. One regimen consists of two intramuscular injections of 0.06 mL per kg within the first 2 weeks of exposure.

A vaccine for preventing HEV infection is currently under development.

MEDICAL THERAPY OF CHRONIC VIRAL HEPATITIS

The only drug approved for the treatment of chronic viral hepatitis in the United States is interferon-alfa-2b (IFN-α) (Intron A). Because of their immunomodulatory and antiviral properties, interferons have been administered in pharmacologic doses for the treatment of chronic hepatitis B and C (Table 4). A 4-month course of subcutaneous IFN-α in a dose of 5 million units daily or 10 million units three times a week induces remission in 25 to 40% of patients with chronic hepatitis B infection, compared with a spontaneous remission rate of 5 to 15% in untreated controls. Remission is defined as the loss of HBV DNA and HBeAg from serum, events that are almost invariably associated with resolution of symptoms, normalization of serum aminotransferase levels, and decrease in liver inflammation. Typically, response to interferon is heralded by an elevation, or "flare," in serum aminotransferase levels, most commonly after approximately 8 to 10 weeks of treatment. This characteristic response is thought to represent immune clearance of HBV-infected hepatocytes and generally predicts long-term remission. Responders to IFN-α may ultimately clear HBsAg from serum and develop anti-HBs, indicating resolution of infection. In one study, the apparent "cure" rate in responders was 65% at 5 years. Unfortunately, not all patients who develop a hepatitis flare

TABLE 4. Suggested Regimens of Interferon-alfa-2b (Intron A) for Chronic Hepatitis B and C

Hepatitis B

5 million units daily or 10 million units three times a week
Treat for 4 months
Monitor serum aminotransferase, HBeAg, HBV DNA levels

Hepatitis C

3–5 million units three times a week
Treat for 6–12 months if serum aminotransferase levels improve by 3 months and if HCV RNA is decreasing or absent
If serum aminotransferase levels do not improve by 3 months and HCV RNA is not decreasing, consider either discontinuing therapy or increasing interferon dose to 5 million units three times a week for another 3 months

Abbreviations: HBeAg = hepatitis B e antigen; HBV = hepatitis B virus; HCV = hepatitis C virus.

TABLE 5. Side Effects of Interferon-alfa

Constitutional	Immunologic
Flulike symptoms	Autoantibodies
Fever	Thyroid disease
Myalgias	**Neuropsychiatric**
Arthralgias	
Headache	Decreased concentration
Fatigue	Depression
Hematologic	Irritability
Granulocytopenia	
Leukopenia	
Thrombocytopenia	

with IFN-α therapy clear HBeAg and enter into remission.

Factors that correlate with the greatest likelihood of responding to IFN-α include female sex, serum alanine aminotransferase level greater than 100 units per liter, serum HBV DNA level less than 200 pg per mL, liver histology consistent with chronic active hepatitis, onset of disease in adulthood, absence of antibody to human immunodeficiency virus, and absence of anti-HDV antibody. However, the presence of one or more of these variables need not preclude a therapeutic trial in any patient. Because IFN-α induces a hepatitis flare, therapy should not be administered to patients with marginal liver function, in whom such a flare might lead to hepatic failure.

In an effort to increase the likelihood of response to IFN-α therapy, patients with serum aminotransferase levels of less than 100 units per liter have been treated with a tapering course of prednisone for 6 weeks prior to IFN-α treatment. The rationale is that a brief dose of prednisone is often followed by a biochemical and clinical flare of hepatitis, resulting in greater responsiveness to IFN-α. However, this strategy is not recommended outside controlled trials, since it may precipitate a fatal deterioration in liver function, especially in patients with marginal liver function. Higher than recommended doses of IFN-α are associated with increased toxicity without a substantially increased response rate.

Common initial side effects to IFN-α therapy are dose dependent and include chills, malaise, myalgia, headache, and fever (Table 5). These flulike symptoms usually last for 24 hours after each injection, can be ameliorated by the administration of acetaminophen before each dose, and usually do not persist beyond the first few weeks of treatment. Additional side effects of IFN-α include diarrhea, alopecia, lethargy, anorexia, nausea, and vomiting. Adverse neuropsychiatric effects, including irritability, insomnia, difficulty in concentrating, depression, and, rarely, delirium and suicidal ideation, occur in approximately 5% of treated patients. IFN-α can induce autoimmune disease, including autoimmune thyroiditis, although this may be less common in patients with chronic hepatitis B than in those with chronic hepatitis C.

Blood counts need to be monitored during IFN-α

treatment, weekly for 2 to 4 weeks and monthly thereafter. Typically, the granulocyte and platelet counts drop by 25 to 40% in a dose-dependent manner. The dose of IFN-α should be decreased by 50% when the granulocyte count drops below 1000 per mm^3 or the platelet count drops below 60,000 per mm^3; the drug should be discontinued when these counts fall below 500 and 50,000 per mm^3, respectively. Usually, the granulocyte and platelet counts return to pretreatment values within 3 days of discontinuing therapy.

The decision to treat a patient with chronic hepatitis B with interferon must be individualized. The patient should be fully informed about the potential merits and shortcomings of therapy. Interferon is a carefully tested therapy that can eradicate the virus in a minority of individuals, presumably lessening the potential for progression to cirrhosis or primary liver cancer. Remission can also result in recovery from the often incapacitating symptoms of chronic viral hepatitis. However, interferon fails to produce a sustained response in most patients and can have potentially serious side effects in patients who were previously asymptomatic. Additionally, IFN-α is expensive, with a 4-month course of therapy costing over $1500.

IFN-α therapy is also used to treat chronic hepatitis C (see Table 4). Three million units three times a week administered for 6 months results in normalization of serum aminotransferase levels and improvement in liver histology in approximately 50% of patients with chronic hepatitis C. However, approximately 50% of responders relapse within 6 months of stopping therapy. The percentage of subjects who have a sustained remission may be increased by prolonging therapy for 12 months instead of 6 months, and by gradually tapering the subject off the drug instead of abruptly stopping therapy. Subjects who are positive for serum HCV RNA at the end of therapy are more likely to relapse than those who are negative. Many clinicians discontinue therapy if serum aminotransferase levels do not return to normal by 3 months. Variables that may correlate with responsiveness to IFN-α include the absence of cirrhosis, shorter duration of infection, low pretreatment serum HCV RNA levels, and HCV genotype; however, excellent responses may be observed in patients who do not meet this profile.

IFN-α therapy is effective only transiently for treating chronic hepatitis D. Because of the usually excellent prognosis, no antiviral therapy is recommended for acute hepatitis A or E. Because the percentage of acute HBV infections that become chronic is usually small (less than 2%), IFN-α treatment is not indicated for acute hepatitis B. Although rarely observed, acute hepatitis C is as responsive to therapy with IFN-α as chronic hepatitis C is.

Other antiviral agents are actively being investigated for use in chronic hepatitis B and C. These include interferon-beta and nucleoside analogues such as ribavirin and lamivudine. None of these is yet approved for routine use. Ribavirin may have limited efficacy in the treatment of chronic hepatitis C, and lamivudine has shown promise in chronic hepatitis B.

MALABSORPTION

method of
CHARLES E. KING, M.D.
Digestive Disorders Associates
Annapolis and Glen Burnie, Maryland

Malabsorption of nutrients is a clinically important condition that is more common than is appreciated. It can lead to difficulties as a result of symptoms related to the passage of unabsorbed food through the gastrointestinal tract and to problems of malnutrition and vitamin deficiency. If one thinks of the body as a group of organs requiring energy to function, failure to absorb digested energy-rich nutrients is an important phenomenon affecting the health of the whole individual. In addition, if malnutrition occurs from malabsorption (or from any other cause such as fasting or during severe illness), protein deficiency can lead to additional malabsorption due to enzyme deficiency, cell loss, or both. Thus, one may have to treat the secondary malnutrition first before the patient can benefit from simplified, specific therapy of the underlying cause of the malabsorption. In fact, treatment of the malnutrition may be required before testing for specific causes of the malabsorption.

This article is organized in the same way as one would think through the clinical evaluation of malabsorption: Is it present? How can I confirm its presence? How can I diagnose the specific cause? How can I treat the specific cause? In practical terms, these questions can be answered in a different order; for example, if a therapeutic trial is chosen and successful, this supports the need for that specific therapy.

GENERAL CATEGORIES OF MALABSORPTION

Because most ingested nutrients require processing (digestion) prior to absorption, impaired absorption may occur as a result of maldigestion, impaired absorption by the mucosa, impaired exit from the cell, or a combination thereof. It is helpful to think of maldigestion and postdigestive malabsorption as two broad categories when undertaking the clinical evaluation. Another broad splitting of malabsorption is based on whether only isolated nutrients are malabsorbed (due to either digestive or absorptive defects) or generalized malabsorption (e.g., involving carbohydrate, protein, and fat) is occurring (again, due to either digestive or absorptive defects). Tests performed to evaluate the absorption of various substances enable one to categorize the absorptive problem as either maldigestive or malabsorptive and as either specific or generalized malabsorption. Making these distinctions is discussed in the sections on tests of malabsorption.

CLINICAL FEATURES

Because ingested nutrients that are not absorbed pass through the colon in larger than normal quantities, increased volume and/or watery stool is a frequent presenting feature of malabsorption. This may be manifest as increased frequency of stooling, diarrhea (loose stools), and/or crampy abdominal pain. The failure to absorb energy-rich nutrients can lead to weight loss. Poor absorption of protein by-products can lead to malnutrition, with a secondary deficiency of both visceral and serum proteins. Postprandial pain can lead to decreased nutrient intake, further magnifying weight loss and malnutrition. Vitamin malabsorption can be manifest by deficiencies of both water-soluble and fat-soluble vitamins (A, D, E, and K). Diarrhea coupled with malabsorption can lead to high-grade electrolyte disturbances and intravascular volume depletion (with associated renal and vascular dysfunction), as well as deficiencies of micronutrients such as zinc and magnesium. Anemia may be multifactorial, including deficiencies of iron, folate, and/or cobalamin (vitamin B_{12}).

PHYSIOLOGY

Fat Absorption. Triglyceride, the major dietary form of fat, is an important energy source, supplying 9 kcal per gram. The assimilation of triglyceride is the most demanding of all nutrients; generalized malabsorption, even when minor, is thus most manifest by the effects of malabsorption of fat. Triglyceride requires digestion by intraluminal lipase, which originates primarily from the pancreas but is also derived from oral secretions. Conjugated bile salts, derived from the liver and stored by the gallbladder, are required for micelle formation to solubilize triglyceride and the products of its digestion (glycerol, free fatty acids, and mono- and diglycerides). Mucosal cells have to not only absorb the fatty acids and glycerol but also repackage the absorbed products back into triglyceride form. Finally, the re-esterified triglyceride is passed into the lymphatics (in contrast to the portal venous passage of products of carbohydrate and protein absorption).

Failure to absorb triglyceride leads not only to loss of 9 kcal per gram of energy but also to impaired absorption of fat-soluble vitamin A (affecting vision and skin), D (affecting serum calcium and calcification of bone), E (antioxidant deficiency), and K (coagulation factor deficiency). Passage of malabsorbed triglyceride and/or fatty acid to the normal bacterial flora of the colon leads to production of hydroxy–fatty acids (with a castor-oil effect and secretory diarrhea).

Carbohydrate Absorption. Carbohydrates are ingested primarily as complex polysaccharides and disaccharides. Intraluminal carbohydrases break apart the complex carbohydrates sequentially to disaccharides, which are then digested to monosaccharides by mucosal disaccharidases such as lactase, sucrase, isomaltase, and maltase. Once absorbed, the monosaccharides are passed without repackaging directly to the portal venous system.

Failure to absorb carbohydrate most commonly occurs as a result of deficient mucosal disaccharidases, with lactase being the most easily disturbed and clinically apparent disaccharidase deficiency. Carbohydrate that is passed to the bacteria of the colon undergoes breakdown from 6-carbon monosaccharides to twice as many 3-carbon organic acids (which doubles the osmotic effect), ethanol (which leads to electrolyte and water secretion), and gases such as hydrogen and methane (with secondary abdominal cramping and flatulence).

Protein Absorption. Ingested protein undergoes digestion by proteases and peptidases derived from the stomach and (most importantly) the pancreas. The end products of protein digestion are small peptides containing two to four amino acids (di-, tri-, and tetrapeptides) and free amino acids; the ability to absorb incompletely digested products (e.g., dipeptides) makes the absorption of protein less demanding than that of either carbohydrate or fat. Amino acids absorbed from the lumen or produced by the intracellular breakdown of small peptides are passed into the portal venous system, just as occurs with carbohydrates (and in contrast to fat absorption via lymphatic channels).

Failure to absorb protein most commonly occurs as a result of intraluminal protease-peptidase deficiency or marked loss of absorptive cell number. Consequences of protein malabsorption lead not only to protein deficiency affecting all parts of the body but also to worsening mucosal absorption due to development of both intraluminal and intracellular enzyme deficiency.

Diarrhea Due to Malabsorption. As noted above, malabsorbed nutrients are passed to the colon, which has a luxuriant bacterial flora (10^{10} to 10^{11} organisms per mL, as contrasted to 10^6 to 10^7 [millions] less present in the proximal intestinal tract). These bacteria can produce diarrhea by creating an osmotic effect (e.g., breaking down 6-carbon sugars to twice as many 3-carbon by-products); this is exemplified by the osmotic diarrhea one sees when a lactase-deficient subject ingests too much lactose. The second mechanism by which the colonic bacteria can produce diarrhea is through the production of chemicals that cause secretion of water and electrolytes. The production of castor-oil–like hydroxy–fatty acids was noted earlier in the section on fat absorption. Production of ethanol from malabsorbed carbohydrate can also lead to increased secretion of water and electrolytes by the colonic mucosa. Similarly, deconjugation of malabsorbed bile acids can lead to a secretory diarrhea from a "Carter's Little Liver Pills" secretory effect on the colon.

CAUSES OF MALABSORPTION

Maldigestive Malabsorption

The most common cause of maldigestion leading to malabsorption is pancreatic insufficiency. The most common cause of pancreatic insufficiency in the United States is chronic pancreatitis due to alcohol-induced injury. Pancreatic duct obstruction due to malignancy can lead to a similar inadequate flow of pancreatic enzymes to the duodenal lumen. Other less common causes include pancreatic insufficiency due to surgical resection and/or massive necrosis following acute gallstone or instrumental or traumatic pancreatitis. A subtle pancreatic insufficiency can occur in the setting of duodenal-jejunal mucosal atrophy, where inadequate release of cholecystokinin-pancreozymin (CCK–PZ) from enterocytes leads to secondary inadequate release of pancreatic enzymes. As mentioned earlier, protein malnutrition can lead to deficiency of both pancreatic and mucosal enzymes.

Biliary obstruction, occurring as a result of neoplastic or inflammatory extrahepatic obstruction or intrahepatic cholestatic disease, can lead to decreased triglyceride digestion due to impaired micelle formation. Abnormal enterohepatic circulation, such as is seen in ileal inflammatory disease or following small bowel surgical bypass or resection, can also lead to maldigestion from inadequate levels of conjugated bile salts in the small intestinal lumen. Deconjugation of bile salts by excessive bacteria in the small intestine is one of the mechanisms leading to fat maldigestion and malabsorption in the bacterial overgrowth syndrome. A less common cause of inadequate luminal levels of conjugated bile salts is seen in the setting of massive acid hypersecretion (e.g., Zollinger-Ellison syndrome), where the acid pH precipitates bile salts out of the luminal solution.

Malabsorptive Malabsorption

The prototype of malabsorption occurring as a result of mucosal dysfunction is that seen in gluten enteropathy (celiac sprue, nontropical sprue). In this syndrome, injury to cells leads to severe flattening of the mucosa and tremendous loss in villus surface area. In addition to the loss of absorptive columnar epithelial cells, there is a relative increase in secretory crypt cells, with a secondary secretory flux of water and electrolytes to the lumen. The injury is more severe in the proximal small intestine (where highest concentrations of ingested gluten are found after ingestion); thus, nutrients absorbed primarily in the proximal small intestine, such as iron and folic acid, may be severely deranged in this setting. Likewise, since release of the mucosal hormone CCK–PZ occurs primarily in the duodenum and proximal jejunum, secondary luminal bile acid and pancreatic enzyme deficiency is seen in celiac sprue.

Partial villous atrophy is seen in tropical sprue, where maturation of villi is disrupted probably by a combination of intraluminal toxins (derived in part from ingested bacteria) and vitamin deficiency (particularly folate). A similar picture of partial villous atrophy is occasionally seen in the syndrome of bacterial overgrowth of the small intestine, which may occur as a result of decreased killing of ingested bacteria by acid, slowed small intestinal or gastric motility, and/or altered anatomy (e.g., strictures, small intestinal diverticula, and/or surgical creation of blind intestinal loops). Altered maturation of small intestinal cells with secondary partial villous atrophy may occur as a result of any cause of folic acid (dietary, sulfa drugs) or vitamin B_{12} (pernicious anemia, dietary, pancreatic insufficiency, bacterial overgrowth) deficiency. Partial villous atrophy may also be seen during chemotherapy or radiation therapy, during protein malnutrition, or with the use of colchicine. Cell damage can also occur as a result of ethanol intake and from certain drugs, such as neomycin and certain laxatives. Loss of total surface area is also seen with surgical resection of the bowel—the short bowel syndrome.

The final step of assimilating fat is the passage of triglyceride from the enterocyte into the lymphatics. Marked fat malabsorption may be seen in congenital or acquired dilatation of the lymphatics, or intestinal lymphangiectasia. Acquired causes include obstruction due to neoplastic (lymphoma) or infectious (tuberculosis) disease or in the setting of Crohn's disease. In addition, lymphatic obstruction and decreased surface area are seen in Whipple's disease, where bacilli-laden macrophages swell the enterocyte and obstruct the lymphatics intracellularly.

CLINICAL TESTS TO DETERMINE THE PRESENCE OF MALABSORPTION

Blood Tests. Screening for malabsorption can be done with commonly used blood tests. Serum iron and folate or red blood cell folate can be used to screen for proximal small intestinal malabsorption. Serum vitamin B_{12} can screen generally for malabsorption; if it is depressed, this points to long-standing malabsorption leading to depletion of body vitamin B_{12} stores. Vitamin B_{12} malabsorption may be related to gastric hyposecretion of acid and/or intrinsic factor (pernicious anemia or abnormal release of protein-bound B_{12} from foods), pancreatic insufficiency, bacterial overgrowth of the small intestine, ileal disease (e.g., Crohn's disease), or resection. Serum screening for fat malabsorption can be done by determining serum carotene (vitamin A), serum calcium (vitamin D), and prothrombin time and partial thromboplastin time (vitamin K).

Fecal Fat. Because the absorption of fat is more compli-

cated than that of carbohydrate or protein, screening for fat malabsorption is commonly helpful in detecting generalized malabsorption. Staining a microscopic fecal smear with Sudan stain is a useful qualitative screening test for fat malabsorption. It involves the microscopic evaluation of a slide for fat globules when Sudan stain is mixed with stool (staining malabsorbed fatty acids); if negative, a second slide should be examined after the addition of stool, Sudan stain, and ethanol to the slide and following warming of the slide with a flame to look for malabsorption of undigested triglyceride. When this test is coupled with Wright's stain to look for excessive leukocytes and testing of the stool for reducing substance, one can quickly screen for common causes of chronic diarrhea (fat malabsorption with Sudan stain, invasive bacteria or inflammatory bowel disease with Wright's stain, and carbohydrate malabsorption with reducing substance). Although quantitative 72-hour stool collection for fat analysis is more accurate and reliable than the qualitative Sudan stain, it is not practical for the nonresearch evaluation of malabsorption because of the unpleasantness of handling 3 days of stool collection. When it is performed, however, 24-hour quantitative fat above 6 grams (indicating less than 95% fat absorption when 100 grams of dietary fat per day is administered for the test) and stool weight greater than 200 grams are considered abnormal.

D-xylose Absorption Test. Measurement of 5-hour urine excretion and 2-hour plasma levels of D-xylose after drinking 25 grams of xylose solution is an excellent screen for simple sugar malabsorption. D-xylose is a 5-carbon simple sugar absorbed in the proximal small intestine. Abnormal values point to mucosal disease and/or bacterial overgrowth. Values can be easily followed to assess response to therapy. The plasma value is particularly helpful as a backup to the 5-hour urine determination when there is unreliable urine collection and/or renal dysfunction.

Vitamin B_{12} Absorption Test (Schilling Test Stage I). Determination of excretion of ^{57}Co-labeled vitamin B_{12} in a 24-hour urine sample is a simple and sensitive test of vitamin B_{12} absorption. It involves ingestion of a tracer amount of ^{57}Co-labeled vitamin B_{12}, administration of a parenteral dose of vitamin B_{12} (to "flush" absorbed ^{57}Co-labeled B_{12} into the urine), 24-hour urine collection (with a backup serum value for possible incomplete urine collection or inadequate renal function), and simple gamma counting of an aliquot of urine for ^{57}Co content. Because test results can be available soon after completion of the 24-hour urine collection, and because vitamin B_{12} absorption reflects a number of different intestinal functions, this test is an excellent one to screen for malabsorptive disorders. An abnormal Stage I B_{12} absorption test can be followed up with other tests, including administration of gastric intrinsic factor (Stage II) or pancreatic enzymes (Stage III), and/or following antibiotic therapy (Stage IV), to isolate the specific cause of the malabsorptive disorder.

Hydrogen Breath Tests. Ingested carbohydrate that is not absorbed by the small intestine (because of maldigestion and/or altered mucosal absorption) can be metabolized by bacteria in the colon to hydrogen gas. Since approximately 17% of hydrogen produced in the colon is absorbed and excreted in the breath, a rise in breath hydrogen content can be used to detect malabsorption of carbohydrate. Although originally developed to test for malabsorption of the disaccharide lactose, this technique can be used to test for the malabsorption of simple monosaccharides (e.g., glucose) as well as complex carbohydrate-containing mixtures (e.g., liquid nutritional supplements) to see if they are causing diarrhea or flatulence. A false-negative rise in hydrogen content can occur following recent antibiotic therapy or electrolyte purging of the colon, and false elevation of breath hydrogen can occur with cigarette smoking prior to collection of the breath specimen.

TESTS TO DETERMINE THE CAUSE OF MALABSORPTION

Vitamin B$_{12}$ Absorption Test (Schilling Test Stages II–IV). As mentioned earlier, an abnormal vitamin B$_{12}$ absorption test can be followed up with other tests, including co-administration of gastric intrinsic factor and/or pancreatic enzymes, or following antibiotic therapy of suspected bacterial overgrowth. Normalization of the ^{57}Co–vitamin B$_{12}$ absorption test specifies which gastrointestinal dysfunction or deficiency was causing the vitamin B$_{12}$ malabsorption.

Mucosal Biopsy. Suction biopsy and, more recently, endoscopically obtained mucosal biopsies from the proximal small intestine allow microscopic evaluation for partial or complete villous atrophy; protozoal infestations such as *Giardia, Cryptosporidium,* or *Strongyloides* on the surface of the mucosa; infection of enterocytes with *Isospora, Eimeria,* or *Microsporidia*; presence of macrophages laden with periodic acid Schiff (PAS)–positive granules (Whipple's disease) or acid-fast staining particles (*Mycobacterium avium-intracellulare,* particularly in the immunodeficient setting); lymphangiectasia; and other infiltrative diseases such as Crohn's disease, lymphoma, eosinophilic gastroenteritis, and amyloidosis. Use of this test should be considered whenever the xylose absorption (or glucose-hydrogen breath) test is abnormal, since mucosal malabsorption is suggested (especially if bacterial overgrowth has been ruled out). Limitations of the test include the expensive nature of biopsy collecting, the spotty character of many of the lesions, and the many different causes of villous atrophy, particularly partial villous atrophy. The recent clinical availability of antigliadin, antireticulin, and antiendomysial serum antibody testing has decreased the requirement for small intestinal biopsies when gluten enteropathy (celiac sprue) is suspected.

Pancreatic Function Testing. The "gold standard" of pancreatic function testing—small intestinal intubation to collect secretions for bicarbonate analysis (secretin test) or to analyze enzyme output (CCK–PZ test)—is a very sensitive test but is available only at specialized centers. More practical but less sensitive is a determination of urinary excretion of para-aminobenzoic acid (PABA) following administration of PABA conjugated with peptide (bentiromide test). A similar lack of sensitivity is seen with the serum testing of trypsinogen for pancreatic insufficiency. Perhaps the most practical pancreatic function test is assessing clinical improvement (weight gain, improvement in diarrhea) during a therapeutic trial of antecibal pancreatic enzyme supplementation. Although pancreatin tablets are inexpensive, adequate dosing requires six to eight tablets prior to each meal. Newer pancreatic enzyme preparations (e.g., Creon 20) protect against acid denaturation in the stomach, are micronized to optimize release in the proximal small intestine, and more predictably improve malabsorption due to pancreatic insufficiency. It should be noted that intensive acid blockade (e.g., proton-pump blockers such as omeprazole and lansoprazole) may actually decrease the effectiveness of enteric-coated pancreatic enzyme preparations; if they are required, moderation to nocturnal H$_2$ blockade therapy may be desirable.

TESTS TO EVALUATE FOR BACTERIAL OVERGROWTH

Small intestinal intubation with anaerobic collection of jejunal juice for anaerobic and aerobic culturing is the "gold standard" for detecting bacterial overgrowth of the small intestine. Normal jejunal content of bacteria is 10^4 organisms per mL or less and includes no coliforms or anaerobic bacteria. When bacterial overgrowth occurs as a result of lessened acid production by the stomach, slowed transit through the stomach and small intestine, or altered anatomy, growth up to 10^7 to 10^8 organisms per mL (including both anaerobic and aerobic bacteria) can be seen. Because specimen collection is time-consuming and good anaerobic-aerobic quantitative culturing is cumbersome, small bowel culturing is infrequently accomplished in clinical practice.

Because excessive bacteria in the small intestine can lead to gas production from the interaction of bacteria and carbohydrate, breath analysis testing has been developed to detect bacterial overgrowth. Breath hydrogen analysis after the ingestion of 50 to 80 grams of glucose (which requires no digestion and is avidly absorbed by the small intestine, making colonic bacterial contact with the test sugar less of a problem) is probably the best readily available breath test for bacterial overgrowth. An early rise in hydrogen after the ingestion of lactulose (a disaccharide not digested by mammals) is an alternative breath hydrogen test for bacterial overgrowth of the small intestine. Tests that detect the production of labeled carbon dioxide (labeled with either radioactive ^{14}C or stable isotopic ^{13}C) as a marker for bacterial overgrowth are more sensitive than the breath hydrogen tests (e.g., 1-gram labeled xylose test, labeled bile acid breath test). However, equipment to measure the labeled carbon dioxide is not available in most hospitals, and waiting for test results from a specialized center is less desirable than using the more readily available breath hydrogen results.

TRIAL OF DIET

If lactase insufficiency is suspected (either as an isolated defect or as part of a generalized malabsorption), lactose restriction in the diet, use of lactase-treated milk, and use of lactase tablets with meals containing cheese or other dietary lactose should be encouraged. Ingestion of any nonabsorbed substance in the diet increases the rapidity of passage through the small intestine. This intestinal "hurry" magnifies any defect in digestion or absorption that is already present, increasing overall malabsorption. Obviously, improvement in symptoms (diarrhea, flatulence, cramps) with a trial of lactose restriction or lactase supplementation solidifies the diagnosis of lactase insufficiency.

Trial of a gluten-free diet can be made in patients suspected of having celiac sprue by either antigliadin antibodies or mucosal biopsy. A longer period of observation is required with this diet than with the lactose-restricted diet. In addition, compliance needs to be as close to 100% as possible, since small amounts of dietary gluten can have deleterious effects on the mucosa for weeks.

TREATMENT OF MALABSORPTION

Since the primary clinical problems related to malabsorption are caused by side effects from the passage of malabsorbed nutrients to the colon and by deficiencies related to the malabsorption, treatment revolves around three treatment principles: (1) dietary restriction of nutrients that have limited absorption, (2) compensation for malabsorbed nutrients by alternative (e.g., parenteral) means, and (3) specific therapy directed at the cause of the malabsorption.

Restrictive

The diet should include quantities of nutrients that can be absorbed by the small intestine to minimize colonic bacterial degradation of malabsorbed substances and secondary diarrhea and electrolyte losses due to osmotic factors, production of castor-oil–like hydroxy–fatty acids, and ethanol. The extreme example of this principle is the use of slow-rate, around-the-clock enteral feeding by tube of predigested nutrients, which is often required in patients with severe malabsorption, short bowel syndrome, and/or complicating malnutrition. An intermediate example would be the use of multiple small oral feedings with limited triglyceride and disaccharides (particularly lactose), possibly supplemented with more easily absorbed medium chain triglyceride oil and liquid nutritional supplements containing no lactose. A less severe example of this principle is the use of a lactose-restricted diet for a patient with low-grade, nongeneralized lactose malabsorption.

Compensatory

Malabsorption of long chain triglycerides, with secondary calorie deficiency, can be compensated by supplementing the diet with more readily absorbed medium chain triglyceride. This fat requires no digestion prior to absorption and no re-esterification once absorbed, and it is assimilated via the portal venous system rather than via lymphatics. It can thus be helpful in the setting of bile acid deficiency, villous atrophy, and lymphatic obstruction.

Digestive abnormalities of protein and carbohydrate can be compensated with liquid nutritional supplements utilizing lactose-free carbohydrate and protein hydrolysate mixtures of amino acids and small peptides.

Compensation for vitamin deficiency accompanying malabsorption may require parenteral administration (e.g., vitamin B_{12} for noncorrectable vitamin B_{12} malabsorption) or the use of water-miscible vitamin formulations of fat-soluble vitamins.

Specific

Maldigestion due to pancreatic insufficiency can usually be adequately treated with antecibal administration of pancreatic enzymes (e.g., pancreatin, Creon, Pancrease). Malabsorption due to gluten enteropathy responds, albeit slowly, to strict adherence to a diet devoid of gluten. At times, severe involvement requires the administration of corticosteroids during initiation of therapy. Malabsorption due to bacterial overgrowth can usually be managed with a combination of periodic oral broad-spectrum antibiotic therapy (e.g., tetracycline, amoxicillin, chloramphenicol), along with the above-noted restrictive and compensatory therapy.

ACUTE PANCREATITIS AND ITS COMPLICATIONS

method of
GENE D. BRANUM, M.D.
*Emory University School of Medicine
Atlanta, Georgia*

The diagnosis and management of acute pancreatitis have steadily improved over the past 2 decades. Appropriate clinical suspicion can lead to an early diagnosis, and aggressive monitoring can lead to improved physiologic support and the prompt recognition of complications. Complications such as abscesses and infected necrosis are the leading cause of mortality in acute pancreatitis, and their early identification and treatment may lead to a reduction in morbidity and mortality in this devastating disease. Current methods of diagnosis and management of pancreatitis, including serologic studies, radiologic imaging techniques, medical support, endoscopic interventions, and surgical management are discussed. In addition, the current international classification system for acute pancreatitis is emphasized and integrated throughout the article.

PATHOGENESIS

Approximately 45% of all cases of acute pancreatitis are caused by gallstones and 35% by alcohol use. These percentages vary by 30 to 40% among series. Approximately 10% of cases have miscellaneous etiologies, and another 10% are idiopathic.

The events that incite acute pancreatitis remain unclear. Although it is known that necrosis and intraglandular vascular damage are caused by autodigestion of the pancreas by various proteolytic enzymes within the organ, the specific role of various factors such as ductal obstruction or overdistention, exposure to alcohol, hypertriglyceridemia, hypercalcemia, and hyperstimulation of the gland is unclear. Intra-acinar activation of trypsin is an important common feature of the several etiologies of acute pancreatitis. Several investigators have shown that small amounts of intracellular trypsin can be inactivated by pancreatic trypsin inhibitor. However, this defense mechanism may be overwhelmed when larger amounts of the enzyme are released. Moreover, there are no inhibitors of phospholipase A. Other enzymes such as lactases, when activated, lead to digestion of intrapancreatic vascular components, causing further instability, vascular permeability, and liberation of enzymes into peripancreatic tissues. Once trypsin inhibitors become depleted, vascular insufficiency and local vascular damage prevent repletion by circulating inhibitors, further aggravating the process.

Numerous theories have been advanced as to the initiating event of pancreatitis. The classic hypothesis of common channel obstruction with reflux of bile into the pancreatic duct and subsequent activation of pancreatic enzymes is one such theory. Bile injected into the pancreatic ducts of some animals may cause pancreatitis, but bile does not by itself activate pancreatic zymogens. Bile acids, however, do activate lipases, and recent studies have shown obesity to be a major risk factor for severe pancreatitis. Decades of experimentation have failed to prove the bile reflux theory of acute pancreatitis.

Obstruction of the pancreatic duct leading to ductal hypertension, ductal disruption, and activation of pancreatic enzymes is an attractive theory. However, ligation of the pancreatic duct in most species results only in pancreatic edema. Partial obstruction of the pancreatic duct in some animal models may induce pancreatic hypertension, intraacinar activation of enzymes, and ultimately inflammation.

A third classic hypothesis of pancreatitis is the reflux of duodenal contents into the pancreatic duct. This theory is unproved, and the fact that patients who have endoscopic retrograde cholangiopancreatography (ERCP) and sphincterotomy, allowing free reflux of duodenal contents into the pancreatic duct, do not suffer recurrent acute pancreatitis counters this theory.

Recent investigations have shown that trypsin and other proteolytic enzymes may be activated intracellularly in acinar cells. In several animal models, including diet induced, secretagogue induced, and duct obstruction induced, pancreatic digestive enzyme zymogens and cathepsin B become co-localized within the acinar cell. An attractive theory, then, is that an initiating stimulus (e.g., duct obstruction or reflux of bile or duodenal contents) leads to ductal hypertension, which, by an as yet unknown mechanism, leads to acinar cell dysfunction with co-localization of digestive enzymes and hydrolysis within the acinar cell, causing digestive enzyme activation, destruction of the acinar cell from within, and subsequent acute pancreatitis. EtOH may play a significant role in this process, as it has been shown to prevent fusion of secretory components to the cell membrane. Intracellular zymogens are then released, leading to the above-mentioned co-localization. Numerous questions remain unanswered about the pathogenesis of acute pancreatitis, and intense investigation is ongoing.

CLASSIFICATION

The literature is rife with terms describing the radiologic appearance of acute pancreatitis. The variations in terminology make comparisons of studies essentially impossible. A recent international symposium was held at which a classification system of acute pancreatic inflammation was established. The terminology agreed upon at this symposium is based on computed tomography (CT) and clinical findings and includes (1) acute pancreatitis, (2) severe acute pancreatitis, (3) mild acute pancreatitis, (4) acute fluid collections, (5) pancreatic necrosis, (6) pseudocysts, and (7) pancreatic abscess. This terminology is useful not only during the critical 1 to 3 days after the onset of the process but also throughout the course of the disease. Various components of this system are discussed throughout this article. Several advantages of the classification system are noteworthy. Severe acute pancreatitis is defined based on the presence or absence of organ failure. This is important, since a CT scan may not be obtained immediately after an episode begins, and criteria such as Ranson's or the second version of the Acute Physiology and Chronic Health Enquiry (APACHE II) may be misleading as to the severity of the disease. Moreover, some patients defined by CT scan to have pancreatic necrosis may not develop clinically severe pancreatitis despite their CT findings.

Since the classification system requires CT scanning with rapid bolus injection of CT contrast, interstitial pancreatitis and pancreatic necrosis can be differentiated. It is clear that patients with pancreatic necrosis have a much higher risk of severe disease, septic complications, and organ failure than patients with interstitial pancreatitis. Recognizing such patients should lead to more appropriate aggressive monitoring and therapy.

The simplification and standardization of terminology offered by the classification system are of great advantage. For example, the fact that acute fluid collections occur early in the course of the disease, lack a defined wall, and usually regress spontaneously, whereas pseudocysts take at least 4 weeks to form and have defined walls, is an important distinction. The practical result of this clarification is the assurance that acute fluid collections require no intervention and become pseudocysts in less than half of cases.

Pancreatic abscess has been more clearly defined as a collection of pus near the pancreas resulting from acute pancreatitis or pancreatic trauma. Such an abscess may be an infected pseudocyst but is not pancreatic necrosis. Pancreatic phlegmon has been removed from the terminology of acute pancreatitis because it is so vague and may be applied to either edematous or necrotizing pancreatitis. Phlegmon has been replaced by more specific terms such as interstitial pancreatitis, sterile necrosis, or infected necrosis. Other confusing terms such as hemorrhagic pancreatitis and persistent acute pancreatitis have been deleted as well.

DIAGNOSIS

The clinical presentation of patients with acute pancreatitis is highly variable. Patients may have minimal upper abdominal pain or may present in circulatory shock. A history and physical examination are critical to the diagnosis. Upper abdominal pain is the most common complaint, is usually acute in onset, is of a burning, boring quality, and may radiate to the back. Nausea is very common, and vomiting may occur as well. A history of alcohol use, known biliary tract disease or gallstones, use of medications, and a prior history of pancreatitis may be obtained. Physical findings may range from mild upper abdominal tenderness to an acute-appearing abdomen with rigidity and exquisite tenderness. Physical findings are attributable to pain and the hypovolemia caused by retroperitoneal inflammation. Rare physical findings such as flank hematoma (Grey Turner's sign) or periumbilical discoloration (Cullen's sign) are indicative of severe pancreatitis with retroperitoneal hemorrhage.

Pancreatic amylase and lipase are usually released systemically by the inflammatory process. The serum half-life of amylase is shorter than that of lipase and returns to normal more rapidly. Although serum levels of pancreatic alpha-amylase, phospholipase A, and C-reactive protein are touted as highly sensitive and specific, applications of these tests are not widespread.

Serum lipase levels are more sensitive and specific than serum amylase. This is especially true in diagnosing acute alcoholic pancreatitis, in which serum amylase is often normal or only mildly elevated. Serum lipase levels in alcoholic pancreatitis typically are dramatically high, with a sensitivity approaching 100%, versus only 50 to 60% for serum amylase (Table 1). A serum lipase/amylase ratio may be helpful in determining an etiology, with alcoholic pancreatitis usually having a ratio of greater than 2.

Leukocytosis, hyperglycemia, hypocalcemia, elevated lactate dehydrogenase, and metabolic acidosis are not specific to pancreatitis and may or may not be present. Ele-

TABLE 1. **Comparison of Diagnostic Tests for Acute Pancreatitis**

	Total Amylase	Lipase	P-Isoamylase	Ultrasonography	Contrast-Enhanced
Sensitivity	Very good, 95–100%	Very good, 90–100%	Good, 84–100%	Low, 62–95%	Good, 85%
Specificity	Low, 70%; influenced by "cutoff value"	Very good, 99% at upper limit of normal	Good, 40–97%; influenced by "cutoff value"	Good, 98%	Very good, 100%
Predictive value (positive test)	Very low, 15–72%	Very good, 90%	50–96%	Good	Good
Predictive value (negative test)	97–100%	95–100%	70–100%	Poor	Indicates mild disease if present
Reliability	Methodologic differences	Good	Methodologic differences	Operator dependent	Excellent
Feasibility	Good	Good	Poor	Good	Poor
Cost per test	Low ($10)	Low ($9)	Moderate ($40)	Expensive ($300)	Very expensive ($800)
Clinical significance	No relationship to severity of disease	No relationship to severity of disease	No relationship to severity of disease	Not accurate for necrosis; no relationship to severity; main value in assessment of biliary tree	Accurate in demonstrating necrosis and extent of disease; very accurate when combined with clinical criteria

Reprinted from The Gastroenterologist V2, 2:119–130, 1994. By permission of Little, Brown and Company Inc.

vated alkaline phosphatase and bilirubin may be present in biliary pancreatitis.

Radiographic findings in acute pancreatitis are quite variable. Plain radiographs may be normal or show displacement of the stomach or small bowel by the mass effect of pancreatic inflammation. A chest radiograph may show a pleural effusion, and an abdominal radiograph may show a sentinel loop with local intestinal ileus.

The usefulness of ultrasonography in acute pancreatitis is limited by the presence of bowel gas, and the test is relatively nonspecific. Ultrasonography may be useful for the detection of choledocholithiasis or biliary ductal dilatation.

CT is the imaging modality of choice for assessing acute pancreatitis (see Table 1). The CT scan is important for both diagnosing the severity of the disease and guiding therapy. In mild cases of pancreatitis, findings may range from a normal gland to glandular edema. More severe signs include blurring of the pancreatic borders and stranding or edema along the retroperitoneal tissue planes within the right and left retrocolic gutters and perirenal and peripsoas spaces. In severe circumstances, acute hemorrhage into and around the gland as well as acute fluid collections in and around the pancreas may be noted. Perhaps most critically, rapid bolus contrast-enhanced CT scans may reveal various degrees of nonperfused necrotic pancreas. Patients with necrosis or hemorrhage clearly have a higher risk of morbidity and a greater potential need for surgical intervention.

Diagnostic peritoneal lavage (DPL) may be helpful when CT scanning is not available. DPL may also help diagnose acute abdomen in conditions other than pancreatitis, such as gastrointestinal perforation. If prune juice–colored fluid is found, severe disease and an increased likelihood of complications are suggested. Trypsinogen activation peptide (TAP) in peritoneal fluid is suggestive of pancreatic necrosis. Free air, bile, and vegetable matter do not rule out pancreatitis but indicate gastrointestinal perforation and mandate exploration.

ASSESSMENT OF SEVERITY

The early prediction of the severity of an episode of acute pancreatitis is challenging. Multiple systems have been developed in an attempt to increase the accuracy of this prediction. The prediction of severity is important, since the likelihood of complications increases with the severity of the illness.

Ranson's criteria were developed in the mid-1970s and had predictive value both retrospectively and prospectively (Table 2). Eleven criteria were evaluated either at admission or 48 hours after admission. Patients with acute pancreatitis and one to two Ranson risk factors had a mortality of 1%; those with three to four risk factors, a 15% mortality; and those with six or more risk factors, a mortality approaching 100%. These criteria were developed before the era of CT scanning but are still quite valuable today in assessing severity. The mortality associated with the number of positive Ranson's criteria has decreased as critical care techniques have improved.

The modified Glasgow, or Imrie, criteria were distilled from the Ranson risk factors. These are assessed within the first 48 hours of hospitalization and are slightly more specific but less sensitive than Ranson's criteria. The positive and negative predictive values of the Imrie and Ranson criteria are nearly identical.

APACHE II is based on an index of 12 physiologic variables as well as a patient's age and history of major organ system diseases. This index is used in a wide range of critical care settings to assess disease severity. The APACHE II score has been applied in multiple studies to acute pancreatitis and has been shown to be more sensitive and specific than either the Ranson or Glasgow scales in predicting the severity of pancreatitis. Another advantage of the APACHE scoring system is that it is useful on a daily basis from the initial assessment to well beyond the 48 hours that define the limit of the Ranson and Imrie systems. The APACHE II score in acute pancreatitis may be particularly useful in assessing the severity of an attack soon after admission; if calculated daily, the peak

APACHE II score accurately assesses mild versus complicated versus fatal pancreatitis in many cases.

The most common cause of death in patients with acute pancreatitis who survive the initial resuscitation is multiple organ system failure (MOSF) secondary to local or systemic complications of the disease. The mortality of patients who develop MOSF is greater than 50%. A scoring system based on the objective assessment of multiple organ system function has been shown to be accurate in predicting the severity of and the development of complications in acute pancreatitis. The developers of the MOSF system applied these criteria to a large group of patients and concluded that it is more sensitive than either the Ranson or the Imrie system or the APACHE II score for predicting severity (Table 3). Like the APACHE II score, the MOSF score is available soon after the patient is admitted and allows repetitive assessment throughout the hospitalization. Moreover, the MOSF score is organ specific and may thus be better than the APACHE II score in reflecting specific sites of disease activity.

The early identification of patients with acute pancreatitis at risk for developing complicated or fatal disease is of great importance, since intensive monitoring in such cases and early surgical or endoscopic intervention may prevent complications and improve outcome. Moreover, it is im-

TABLE 2. Adverse Prognostic Factors in Severe Acute Pancreatitis

Ranson's Criteria

Pancreatitis not due to gallstones
　On admission
　　Age >55 years
　　White-cell count >16,000/mm³
　　Glucose >200 mg/dL
　　Lactic dehydrogenase >350 U/L
　Within 48 hours of hospitalization
　　Decrease in hematocrit >10 points
　　Increase in blood urea nitrogen >5 mg/dL
　　Calcium <8 mg/dL
　　Partial pressure of oxygen <60 mmHg
　　Base deficit >4 mmol/L
　　Fluid deficit >6 L
Gallstone-induced pancreatitis
　On admission
　　Age >70 years
　　White-cell count >18,000/mm³
　　Glucose >220 mg/dL
　　Lactic dehydrogenase >400 U/L
　　Aspartate aminotransferase >250 U/L
　Within 48 hours of hospitalization
　　Decrease in hematocrit >10 points
　　Increase in blood urea nitrogen >2 mg/dL
　　Serum calcium <8 mg/dL
　　Base deficit >5 mmol/L
　　Fluid deficit >4 L

Modified Glasgow Criteria

　Within 48 hours of hospitalization
　　Age > 55 years
　　White-cell count >15,000/mm³
　　Glucose >180 mg/dL
　　Blood urea nitrogen >45 mg/dL
　　Lactic dehydrogenase >600 U/L
　　Albumin <3.3 gm/dL
　　Calcium <8 mg/dL
　　Partial pressure of oxygen <60 mmHg

Reprinted by permission of The New England Journal of Medicine. Steinberg W, Tenner S: Acute pancreatitis. N Engl J Med 330:1198–1210, 1994. Copyright 1994, Massachusetts Medical Society.

TABLE 3. Criteria for Organ System Failure

Organ System	Criteria
Cardiovascular	Mean arterial pressure ≤ 50 mmHg; need for volume loading and/or vasoactive drugs to maintain systolic blood pressure above 100 mmHg; heart rate ≤50 beats/min; ventricular tachycardia/fibrillation; cardiac arrest; acute myocardial infarction
Pulmonary	Respiratory rate ≤5/min or ≥50/min; mechanical ventilation for 3 or more days or fraction of inspired oxygen (F_1O_2) >0.4 and/or positive end expiratory pressure >5 mmHg
Renal	Serum creatinine ≥280 μmol/L (3.5 mg/dL); dialysis/ultrafiltration
Neurologic	Glasgow Coma Scale ≤6 (in the absence of sedation)
Hematologic	Hematocrit ≤20%; leukocyte count ≤0.3 × 10⁹/L; thrombocyte count ≤50 × 10⁹/L; disseminated intravascular coagulation
Hepatic	Total bilirubin level ≥51 μmol/L (3 mg/dL) in the absence of hemolysis; serum glutamic-pyruvic transaminase >100 U/L
Gastrointestinal	Stress ulcer necessitating transfusion of more than 2 units of blood per 24 h; acalculous cholecystitis; necrotizing enterocolitis; bowel perforation

From Tran DD, Cuesta MA: Evaluation of severity of patients with acute pancreatitis. Am J Gastroenterol 87:604–608, 1992.

portant to avoid intensive monitoring and/or invasive interventions in patients with mild or moderate disease. A scoring system should be used that allows ongoing accurate assessment of the patient's disease severity.

Disease severity may also be assessed by CT scan. The combination of a CT scoring system and a clinical scoring system can be highly predictive of severe complications. Ranson and Balthazar developed a grading system based on CT scans: Grade A, normal pancreas; Grade B, pancreatic enlargement; Grade C, inflammation confined to the pancreas and peripancreatic fat; Grade D, one peripancreatic fluid collection; and Grade E, two or more pancreatic fluid collections. Patients with Grade A or B scans rarely develop infectious complications, whereas 12% of Grade C, 17% of Grade D, and 61% of Grade E patients develop infectious complications. Combining this index with Ranson's criteria can accurately predict which patients are at high risk for complications and mortality.

MANAGEMENT

Acute pancreatitis is often considered the equivalent of retroperitoneal burn. Massive amounts of fluid may be sequestered in the retroperitoneum, where capillary permeability has been lost, inflammatory cells recruited, and vasoactive substances (tumor necrosis factor, interleukins-6 and -8, and polymorphonuclear elastase) released into the circulation. The goal in the management of pancreatitis is adequate intravascular fluid repletion to ensure effective oxygenation of organs most at risk for injury (i.e., kidney, lung, gut, and liver). Evaluation of this support may be as simple as monitoring urine output and capillary refill, or it may require Swan-Ganz catheterization and intra-arterial pressure monitoring, since the volumes of intravenous fluid may be very large and physical findings may not accurately reflect intravascular volume.

Controversies related to the medical management of pancreatitis still exist, including the effectiveness of nasogastric suction, gastric acid neutralization, or peritoneal lavage, as well as the necessity of enteral or parenteral nutrition. Mild disease (as defined by <3 Ranson criteria, APACHE II score <7, and/or MOSF score <1) accounts for 85% of cases and can usually be managed outside of the intensive care unit setting. Most such cases resolve within 3 to 4 days. Patients should initially be given nothing by mouth, although no studies have shown a definite advantage to nasogastric suction. The discomfort associated with the nasogastric tube is best avoided unless significant nausea and vomiting are present. Patients should typically take nothing by mouth until they are pain free and preferably until the serum amylase, if elevated, returns to normal. The patient's urine output should be monitored and maintained with sufficient intravenous fluid to produce a urine output of 0.5 to 1 mL per kg per hour.

Moderate or severe disease (i.e., >3 Ranson criteria, APACHE II score >7, or MOSF score ≥1) should be managed in the intensive care unit. A urinary catheter is mandatory, and either central venous pressure monitoring or Swan-Ganz catheterization should be employed, depending on the severity of disease and co-morbid conditions, to objectively assess the adequacy of fluid resuscitation. Depending on organ function and systemic vascular resistance, vasoactive or inotropic agents may be necessary to support end-organ perfusion. Oxygen delivery and consumption should be measured in selected situations to ensure adequate tissue perfusion. Daily assessment of the APACHE II or MOSF score is useful in the assessment of improvement or progression of systemic manifestations of the disease.

Intestinal ileus often accompanies the onset of acute pancreatitis. Enteral nutrition therefore may not be appropriate during the first several days of an episode of pancreatitis. If clinical pancreatitis continues beyond 5 days, enteral or parenteral nutrition should be employed, especially if a prolonged course is anticipated. Parenteral formulas need not be specialized but should be formulated to deliver approximately 35 kcal per kg per day and 1.5 to 2 grams of protein per kg per day. Standard lipid formulas may be used, but they should be avoided in patients with hypertriglyceridemia. Standard parenteral lipid solutions have not been shown to stimulate exocrine pancreatic secretion.

Once ileus has resolved, enteral feeding should begin in patients with moderate to severe disease. Standard low-fat formulas infused distal to the ligament of Treitz cause minimal exocrine pancreatic secretion and can be safely used. Such formulas may be infused via nasojejunal feeding tube or, in patients who require exploration for complications of the disease, via an operatively placed jejunostomy feeding tube.

Numerous substances have been used to attempt to decrease the severity of acute pancreatitis. Somatostatin* is one such agent that is attractive because of its potential to shut down pancreatic exocrine secretion. Trials to date have not proved its efficacy, although meta-analyses suggest that somatostatin may be of value if started sufficiently early in the disease. Larger randomized trials are needed to clarify this issue. Enzyme inhibitors such as aprotinin (Trasylol)† have not yet proved beneficial. Calcitonin, H_2 blockers, and atropine have all been studied and proved ineffective.

The use of antibiotics to prevent septic complications in acute pancreatitis is controversial. The risk of infective complications in patients with mild to moderate acute pancreatitis is very low, and the use of prophylactic antibiotics may increase the prevalence of resistant strains and should be avoided. Patients with severe interstitial pancreatitis are at intermediate risk for the development of infective complications, and the use of antibiotics such as ciprofloxacin (Cipro), ceftazidime (Fortaz), and clindamycin (Cleocin) may be appropriate. There is evidence from some investigators that the use of imipenem/cilastatin (Primaxin) in patients with necrotizing pancreatitis can reduce the rate of infective complications. No survival benefit has been shown to date in these studies. The use of such broad-spectrum antibiotics may lead to superinfection with *Candida*, and it is prudent to cover such patients with an antifungal agent such as fluconazole (Diflucan). Prospective randomized, placebo-controlled, double-blinded multicenter studies are still needed to determine the role of antibiotics in the prevention of infective complications of severe pancreatitis.

Peritoneal lavage is a controversial treatment for severe acute pancreatitis. Studies in the 1970s and early 1980s of short-term peritoneal lavage ranging from 2 to 4 days showed no benefit in severe acute pancreatitis. Recent studies using lavage for 5 to 7 days, however, suggest that this therapy may lead to a decrease in mortality due to sepsis. Prospective randomized trials are clearly needed to re-evaluate the role of long-term lavage in severe acute pancreatitis. Moreover, the role of protease inhibitors such as aprotinin and gabexate nesylate must be studied to determine whether their addition to peritoneal irrigant leads to greater efficacy.

ENDOSCOPIC INTERVENTION

Acute pancreatitis is caused in many cases by the passage or impaction of gallstones at the ampulla of Vater. Patients without a history of alcohol ingestion and no other cause for their pancreatitis should be investigated for gallstones. Patients who present with hyperbilirubinemia and/or an elevated alkaline phosphatase should be investigated for choledocholithiasis or choledochal dilatation. Neither ultrasonog-

---

*Investigational drug in the United States.
†Not FDA-approved for this indication.

raphy nor CT is very sensitive for the detection of choledocholithiasis. ERCP is clearly superior at detecting common bile duct stones and other anatomic variants (e.g., pancreas divisum or pancreatolithiasis) that predispose to pancreatitis. The safety of ERCP in the setting of pancreatitis (if performed by experienced operators) has been shown by several investigators.

In cases of severe acute biliary pancreatitis, ERCP with endoscopic sphincterotomy is the treatment of choice. Sphincterotomy allows extraction of an impacted gallstone and prevents the subsequent episodes of pancreatitis that might be induced by the passage of other gallstones. ERCP and endoscopic sphincterotomy are recommended in patients with clearly diagnosed biliary pancreatitis, whereas ERCP alone should be used in patients with a suspected biliary etiology. In general, ERCP should not be used in patients in whom a biliary etiology is not suspected.

COMPLICATIONS OF ACUTE PANCREATITIS

Numerous scoring systems (described previously) are used to predict the likelihood of complications of acute pancreatitis. Variable periods of observation and testing are needed to identify patients at risk. The early recognition and treatment of complications are critical to a patient's survival. Locoregional complications of pancreatitis are discussed using the terminology agreed on at the international symposium. Such complications are based on specific anatomic derangements, including necrosis, fluid collections (acute, pseudocysts, and abscess), and gastrointestinal and vascular complications.

Routine surgical intervention in acute pancreatitis is unwarranted. There are subsets of patients, however, who do benefit from surgical intervention. At present, surgery is reserved for the management of complications of pancreatitis and for the prevention of future episodes. In biliary pancreatitis, cholecystectomy serves such a preventive role, although endoscopic sphincterotomy may serve the same purpose with a lower morbidity and mortality.

Pancreatic Necrosis

Pancreatic necrosis occurs as a result of ductal and cellular disruption and autodigestion of the gland. Once the process has begun and the vascular supply and drainage of the gland are destroyed by the digestive process, the stage is set not only for glandular necrosis but also for leakage of pancreatic enzymes into surrounding retroperitoneal fatty tissues, with peripancreatic necrosis and digestion. Necrotic pancreatic and peripancreatic tissues are at high risk for infection. Thus, operative débridement of devitalized or necrotic tissue has been shown to be beneficial for the prevention of septic complications. Moreover, a disrupted ductal system that continues to secrete

predisposes to further periglandular secretion and necrosis.

Current CT scanning techniques can clearly define pancreatic necrosis. After a rapid bolus injection of contrast material, selected views through the pancreas may demonstrate failure of the gland to enhance with contrast material, suggesting the presence of nonperfused pancreas. An estimate of the site and amount of pancreatic necrosis can be made, and these findings generally correlate well with subsequent anatomic and histologic findings at surgery.

Pancreatic necrosis can be either sterile or infected. Infected necrosis is suggested by air within the necrotic tissue and can be reliably diagnosed by fine-needle aspiration under CT guidance. There is an approximate 10% false-negative rate associated with this procedure.

The resolution of small to moderate amounts of pancreatic necrosis without surgical intervention has been documented. It is therefore safe to closely observe such patients in the intensive care unit using support of organ systems, as discussed previously. Such patients may exhibit the sepsis syndrome (hyperdynamic hemodynamics, low systemic vascular resistance, shock) despite the absence of invasive infection. This results from the release and absorption of various cytokines and leukotrienes and may require aggressive hemodynamic support. If improvement does not ensue or if there is evidence of clinical deterioration (such as organ failure or the sepsis syndrome), patients should undergo surgical débridement. Any patient with documented infection of pancreatic necrosis should be treated surgically. Patients with moderate to large amounts of pancreatic necrosis should undergo surgical treatment early in the course whether or not the material appears to be infected if clinical deterioration occurs.

Numerous methods for the surgical treatment of pancreatic necrosis have been suggested and investigated. Each has its proponents, but all fall into three major categories: (1) débridement with placement of drains and selective reoperation; (2) multiple, staged débridements with open packing; and (3) multiple débridements with subsequent placement of drains and continuous lavage.

Some clinicians advocate radical one-time débridement followed by placement of large-bore multilumen catheters. These catheters are then irrigated with various solutions in large volumes to continuously débride residual necrotic material. Once the irrigant is free of particulate matter, the irrigation can cease and the drains are gradually withdrawn. Although attractive and useful in patients with relatively small amounts of necrosis, this method is difficult to apply in patients with massive pancreatic and peripancreatic necrosis.

Patients with large amounts of pancreatic and peripancreatic necrosis who are explored for necrosectomy often have more nonviable tissue than can be removed at the first exploration. Such patients are débrided and packed with laparotomy pads or gauze rolls and returned to the operating room for staged removal of all dead tissue. Once the dead tissue is removed and granulation begins, some authors have proposed daily packing in the intensive care unit, with gradual contraction of the wound. Of the three treatments, this carries a higher rate of gastrointestinal complications from colonic or duodenal perforation, as well as bleeding complications such as erosion by the packing process into the splenic or mesenteric veins. This can be prevented in some cases by lining the base of the wound with a nonadhesive gauze bandage.

The treatment currently advocated by most authors is a combination of these two methods. The patient is explored, with débridement of necrotic pancreas and peripancreatic tissues. Staged re-explorations are undertaken every 24 to 48 hours until all nonviable tissue is removed surgically. At the last exploration, a cholecystectomy is performed, if needed, for the prevention of future attacks of biliary pancreatitis. Because of the possibility of ongoing necrosis and infection, large-bore multilumen sump drains are placed into the lesser sac and any retroperitoneal cavities, and the abdomen is closed over these drains. Irrigation is then begun and continues until there is minimal particulate matter in the effluent.

Each of these three methods has a place in the management of particular patients with necrosis. The most important principle is to remove all necrotic material to prevent septic complications. Modern intensive care practices and attention to nutritional therapy should limit the mortality rate to 15 to 20% after the development of severe pancreatic necrosis.

Fluid Collections

Fluid collections occur in 50 to 60% of episodes of acute pancreatitis. Acute fluid collections are very common, and most of these resolve spontaneously, do not coalesce, and become circumscribed by a well-formed capsule. These acute fluid collections should not be aspirated or treated in any way unless the patient appears septic; then percutaneous aspiration can be used to rule out infection. The fluid in acute collections may be amylase-rich, indicating that its source is pancreatic exocrine secretion, or it may be low in amylase, indicating peripancreatic or interstitial edema fluid. Asymptomatic fluid collections should be followed at 1- to 2-week intervals until the pancreatitis resolves. If clinical improvement occurs, a CT scan should be performed 1 to 3 months after the acute episode to confirm resolution of fluid collections.

Pancreatic ascites occurs when there is erosion of an acute fluid collection or a portion of the pancreatic ductal system into the peritoneal cavity. The abdominal examination is usually benign, and the ascites fluid is rich in amylase. Pancreatic ascites should be treated with intermittent large-volume paracentesis and the administration of octreotide to decrease pancreatic exocrine secretion. The condition usually resolves with these measures, but if ascites persists, ERCP is indicated to define the pancreatic ductal anatomy. Persistent ascites is usually due to a pancreatic ductal stricture distal to the leak. An endoscopically placed stent may facilitate pancreatic ductal drainage and allow resolution of the ascites. Rarely, the rupture of an acute fluid collection with pancreatic ascites causes the clinical picture of an acute abdomen. Prompt exploration is necessary to rule out visceral perforation in the setting of high-amylase ascitic fluid. The pancreas should be examined, and if a ruptured duct is identified, it should be drained externally. Fluid collections may also rupture into the pleural cavity. This usually presents as an acute pleural effusion with mild to moderate respiratory distress. Pleurocentesis and octreotide usually allow resolution of the leak.

The operative therapy of choice for nonresolved pancreatic ascites or pancreaticopleural fistula entails identification of the site of the leak by ERCP, with subsequent distal pancreatectomy, since most leaks occur from this portion of the pancreas. Alternatively, Roux-en-Y pancreaticojejunostomy may be used for well-identified ductal leaks amenable to this therapy.

Pancreatic pseudocysts develop from acute fluid collections that persist longer than 1 month after the episode of acute pancreatitis and develop a wall of fibrous or granulation tissue. Pseudocyst fluid is typically rich in amylase due to either ongoing or prior connection with a pancreatic ductal system. Previously, it was thought that pseudocysts present for longer than 6 to 8 weeks should be drained to prevent the development of complications. Numerous studies have now shown that asymptomatic pseudocysts that are observed for 1 year resolve in over half of cases. Moreover, most pseudocysts remain asymptomatic and can be safely observed. Pseudocysts greater than 6 cm in size are less likely to spontaneously resolve and are more likely to be symptomatic.

Complications of pseudocysts include bleeding, infection, pain, or compressive symptoms. Bleeding into a pseudocyst is typically manifest by acute pain with varying hemodynamic instability. The pseudocyst most commonly erodes into the splenic artery. If the patient remains stable, angiography is the test of choice for confirmation of the diagnosis, with therapeutic embolization of the offending artery. If the patient is unstable, exploration with direct ligation of the artery and drainage of the pseudocyst is necessary.

Infection of a pseudocyst may occur at any time in its existence. Bacterial contamination of a pseudocyst that is discovered at the time of its enteric or percutaneous drainage is not considered a pancreatic abscess. Under the new terminology of the international symposium, however, a pseudocyst containing pus is a pancreatic abscess. Internal drainage of a colonized pancreatic pseudocyst is appropriate. However, a pseudocyst containing pus should be drained externally either by CT-guided catheter placement or by external operative drainage. CT-guided drainage is appropriate if the fluid contained in the abscess can be completely removed and if there is no residual necrotic material within the abscess. Operative drainage is often necessary to provide adequate removal of debris from the abscess cavity and removal of tenacious contents from within the abscess. Antibiotic treatment should be directed toward the offending organisms cultured at the time of aspiration or exploration.

Pseudocysts may cause abdominal pain or obstructive symptoms and must be evaluated thoroughly prior to treatment. Multiple options are available for pseudocyst drainage, including internal or external surgical drainage, radiographically placed catheter drainage, and endoscopic or radiographic internal drainage. If possible, drainage of a pseudocyst should be delayed 6 to 8 weeks to allow adequate maturity of the pseudocyst wall to develop. ERCP should be performed prior to drainage of any pseudocyst to assess its anatomy and any communication with the main pancreatic duct. Pseudocysts that are in continuity with the main pancreatic duct should not be drained externally because of the probability that a pancreaticocutaneous fistula will develop.

Surgical enteric drainage of pancreatic pseudocysts (cystogastrostomy, cystoenterostomy) is successful in more than 90% of cases in achieving definitive drainage and carries a mortality of less than 5%. Radiographic and endoscopic methods for internal drainage of pseudocysts are successful in 40 to 100% of cases but are extremely operator dependent. Procedural morbidity is reported to be low, but long-term follow-up is needed to evaluate the effectiveness of these methods. Small series of laparoscopic cystogastrostomies have been reported with good success rates, but advanced laparoscopic expertise is required, and long-term follow-up is lacking.

Multiple pseudocysts occur simultaneously in a minority of cases. Such pseudocysts that are not in continuity with the main pancreatic duct can be treated with external catheter drainage. Surgical options for the treatment of such complicated cases include Roux-en-Y limbs with multiple cystoenterostomies or cystoenterostomy in combination with cystoduodenostomy or cystogastrostomy. If all the pseudocysts are located in the tail of the pancreas, distal pancreatectomy is the procedure of choice with or without a pancreaticojejunostomy, depending on the presence and location of any pancreatic ductal stricture.

Gastrointestinal

Gastrointestinal complications secondary to pancreatitis usually involve obstruction or perforation. Gastrointestinal obstruction may occur at the gastric outlet or in the duodenum secondary to compression by a pseudocyst. Such obstruction is usually resolved by drainage of the pseudocyst. Transverse colonic obstruction occurs either from an inflammatory stricture or from middle colic arterial thrombosis secondary to inflammation. Although resolution of inflammation and pericolonic edema may lead to resolution of the stricture, segmental colectomy is often needed to relieve the obstruction. Patients with such colonic complications from acute pancreatitis are at very high risk for ongoing necrosis, sepsis, and abscess formation. If pseudocyst drainage fails to relieve the gastric or duodenal obstruction, gastrojejunostomy or duodenojejunostomy is the treatment of choice for relief of the obstruction.

Perforation associated with acute pancreatitis occurs most often in the transverse colon, secondary to occlusion of the middle colic artery. Proximal diversion with ileostomy and mucous fistula is the treatment of choice to deviate the fecal stream well away from the inflamed pancreatic bed. Gastric or duodenal perforation due to inflammation or injury from repeated débridements is treated with primary repair or controlled drainage. Occasionally, duodenal exclusion with gastrojejunostomy or gastrostomy is required for long-term diversion.

Vascular

Vascular complications of acute pancreatitis may affect either the arterial or the venous system. As mentioned earlier, thrombosis of the middle colic vessels may lead to ischemic strictures or perforation of the transverse colon. The splenic and gastroduodenal arteries may have their structural components weakened by pancreatic enzymes, leading to aneurysmal dilatation and rupture. If this is discovered prior to rupture, angiographic embolization may be performed and used as definitive therapy, although operative exclusion of the aneurysm is often necessary. Splenic vein thrombosis is relatively common and may lead to left-sided portal hypertension, with the development of transgastric varices. Splenectomy is curative in such cases. Portal and superior mesenteric venous occlusion is unusual even in the most severe cases of pancreatitis.

CHRONIC PANCREATITIS

method of
RICARDO L. ROSSI, M.D.
Pontificia Catholic University of Chile
Santiago, Chile

RODRIGO L. VALDERRAMA, M.D.
University of Chile
Santiago, Chile

and

GUILLERMO S. WATKINS, M.D.
Pontificia Catholic University of Chile
Santiago, Chile

Chronic pancreatitis (CP) implies irreversible and usually progressive changes in the pancreas, whereas the acute forms imply reversible changes. The Marseille-Rome classification of 1988 defined acute pancreatitis as a spectrum of inflammatory lesions in the pancreas and in the peripancreatic tissues (edema, necrosis, hemorrhagic necrosis, fat necrosis). Chronic pancreatitis was defined as the presence of chronic inflammatory lesions characterized by the destruction of exocrine parenchyma and fibrosis and, at least in the later stages, the destruction of endocrine parenchyma. This classification is not always easy to apply clinically because of the overlap that frequently occurs on clinical presentation, especially in the early stages of chronic pancreatitis, in which acute attacks of pain may be the only clinical symptom. Because biopsy specimens are not readily available, attempts have been made to classify pancreatitis according to clinical or radiologic criteria. For example, the Cambridge classification uses changes in the pancreatic ducts as seen on endoscopic pancreatography. The incidence and prevalence of chronic pancreatitis are not well known. The prevalence is estimated to be 4 in 100,000 inhabitants older than 20 years, according to studies in Sweden and the United States. In autopsy reports, the ranges are from 0.04% to 5%.

The natural history of CP is not well known. Recently, a French study of 240 patients with CP of any etiology, with a 9-year follow-up, observed that this disease is more frequent in men, and that alcohol is the main cause. Around 50% of the cases developed diabetes, 40% presented some kind of associated liver disease, most of them showed pancreatic calcifications, and 40% required surgical treatment. The mortality rate reached 24%, and the probability of staying alive after 20 years was 70%, this probability being significantly lower than the reference population.

ETIOLOGY

Many causative factors have been identified in pancreatitis (Table 1). Alcohol consumption is the main factor, associated with up to 70% of the cases of CP in developed countries. It has been suggested that the use of alcohol to produce CP should be of more than 100 gr. a day for over 6 years, associated with a diet rich in fats. The obstruction of the pancreatic drainage (trauma, tumors, pancreas divisum) can be associated with CP. Other causes include cystic fibrosis, autoimmune diseases (Sjögren's syndrome), and hyperparathyroidism. Gallstone disease has not been proved as a definitive cause of CP. Up to 40% of cases fall into the group of idiopathic CP.

The basic pathogenic mechanism remains obscure, and in most instances, management continues to be empirical and directed to the treatment of symptoms, sequelae, and complications. Our limited knowledge of the mechanisms of pain and of the natural history of the disease hampers successful treatment. Longitudinal studies suggest that pain is completely relieved in more than 60% of the patients when the follow-up period is long enough, irrespective of cause. It has been shown that at least half the patients became diabetic and that one third of the patients with alcohol-induced pancreatitis had nonprogressive disease with preservation of endocrine function. However, the concept that the disease may "burn itself out" may be flawed by a methodologic bias, because the higher earlier

TABLE 1. Causative Factors of Chronic Pancreatitis

Alcohol	Congenital abnormalities
Obstruction	Autoimmune
Trauma	Idiopathic

TABLE 2. Presenting Features of Chronic Pancreatitis

Pain
Exocrine or endocrine insufficiency or both
Complications
Pseudocyst
Infection
Biliary or duodenal obstruction or both
Fistula (ascites, pleural effusion)
Obstructed splenic (left-sided) portal hypertension

mortality in patients with severe disease may reduce the incidence of pain in the late follow-up groups. Other studies have not clearly shown this "burnout" phenomenon. Unifactorial and multifactorial analyses of death associated with CP in a series of 240 French patients showed that the mortality rate after 20 years of illness was 35.8% higher than the mortality rate of the matched population. The main causes of death were alcoholic liver disease, carcinoma, and postoperative complications. That CP was less frequently the direct cause of death contrasted with the multivisceral consequences of alcoholism and smoking. It was suggested, but not well documented, that abstinence from alcohol improved long-term survival.

DIAGNOSIS

Pain is the most common symptom (Table 2). The diagnosis of CP relies on a clinical history of characteristic pain and some objective evidence of disease, which includes elevation in the level of serum amylase, the presence of calcifications, abnormalities of the pancreas seen on computed tomography (CT), ductal changes consistent with pancreatitis seen on retrograde pancreatography, or the presence of a firm, fibrotic white pancreas found at previous abdominal exploration with or without biopsy of the pancreas. The presence of endocrine or exocrine insufficiency strengthens the diagnosis. A small number of patients with the characteristic pain of pancreatitis fail to have objective signs of disease, although these patients have an abnormal pancreas at the time of exploration and biopsy.

Clinical Findings

Abdominal pain is the main and commonly the first symptom. It is characterized by recurrent pain attacks in the upper abdomen, occasionally radiated to the back, often exacerbated with meals, at intervals of months or years. These attacks tend to become more frequent until pain becomes persistent. The incidence of pain ranges between 70% and 90% of the diagnosed cases, being severe in half of them. This disease starts clinically with an episode of acute pancreatitis in approximately 50% of patients, whereas in 40% of cases the onset of pain is quite insidious. Painless CP accounts for 10% to 20% of patients and is more likely to present in older patients. In advanced stages of the disease, when exocrine function is reduced by 90%, diarrhea and weight loss may appear. Diabetes may also occur in these stages as a manifestation of endocrine insufficiency, with a prevalence ranging between 28% and 70%. Other manifestations of CP are cholestasis caused by common bile duct stenosis, occurring in 27% of cases; duodenal stenosis; ascites, described in 3% (commonly from a ruptured pseudocyst or pancreatic duct); and associated liver disease, described in about 40% of cases.

For assessment of pancreatic disease there are two main groups of studies: imaging techniques and functional tests.

Imaging Techniques

The development of imaging techniques, such as ultrasonography, CT scanning, and endoscopic retrograde cholangiopancreatography (ERCP), has allowed for a better morphologic evaluation of the pancreatic gland.

Plain abdominal radiography shows pancreatic calcifications in 30% to 50% of patients. Abdominal ultrasonography is often the first study to be carried out for suspected CP, because of its efficacy and low cost. We are interested in the size of the pancreas, its characteristics, peripancreatic changes, calcifications, cysts, fluid collections, biliary tree, pancreatic duct, and portal system. For these changes, ultrasound has a sensitivity ranging between 60% and 70%, and a specificity between 75% and 90%. The role of endoscopic ultrasound is being evaluated.

Abdominal CT scanning is today the favored imaging technique for pancreatic pathology. Although more expensive and requiring radiation, it provides the most reliable overall assessment of the pancreas and peripancreatic area in CP with a sensitivity of between 75% and 90% and a specificity between 94% and 100%. It should be considered in all patients in whom surgery is contemplated. Additional data are necessary to define the role of MRI in the evaluation of CP and pancreatic masses.

Finally, ERCP allows for visualization of the papilla of Vater, and the opacification of the common bile duct and pancreatic ducts. ERCP is useful to evaluate the state of the CP, to outline the ductal morphology when considering surgery, and in some cases to help in differentiating CP from a neoplasm. The sensitivity of ERCP in the diagnosis of CP goes from 71% to 93%, and its specificity from 81% to 100%. It is abnormal in most of the cases with calcifications, and an inverse correlation between the degree of ductal alterations and the exocrine pancreatic function has been observed. However, there is a poor correlation between the degree of ductal changes and pain.

Functional Tests

It is rare that one requires functional studies of the pancreas for the diagnosis of CP. One possible case is that of the patient with chronic pain suggestive of pancreatic origin but with negative imaging studies.

Pancreatic Exocrine Function Tests

TESTS REQUIRING DUODENAL INTUBATION. These tests involve stimulating exocrine pancreatic secretion through the intravenous administration of secretin, cholecystoquinine, or cerulein. The concentration of the pancreatic enzymes amylase, lipase, trypsin, and chymotrypsin, and of bicarbonates is quantified from the drainage collected from the duodenum. These concentrations are significantly reduced in advanced stages of CP. However, in early disease, a decrease in only one or two enzymes may be detected, with lipase being the first one to drop. The sensitivity and specificity are over 90%. Nevertheless, these studies are invasive, expensive, and performed only in highly specialized centers.

ORAL TESTS. These are based upon use of a test meal to stimulate pancreatic secretion, as well as administration of a synthetic pharmaceutical preparation that requires the action of certain pancreatic enzymes to be hydrolyzed. Part of the hydrolyzed product is absorbed by the intestine and excreted through the kidney. The proportion of the synthetic preparation in the urine reflects the intraluminal pancreatic enzyme activity.

The most widely used techniques are those measuring urinary excretion of para-aminobenzoic acid (N-benzoyl-L-tyrosyl-p-amino benzoic acid [NBT-PABA] test) and fluorescein (pancreolauril test). These substances are released from substrates within the intestinal lumen through the action of chymotrypsin and esterase, respectively. Both tests have a high accuracy in detecting pancreatic exocrine insufficiency, but their value decreases in mild pancreatic disease. Malabsorption and renal failure may interfere with the results. The sensitivity and specificity of the described oral tests in severe pancreatic insufficiency range from 70% to 90% and from 72% to 80%, respectively, both being very similar to those done by direct stimulation.

SERUM PANCREATIC ENZYMES QUANTIFICATION. Serum quantification of some pancreatic enzymes (P-isoamylase and trypsin) is highly specific but has a low sensitivity for CP. Abnormally low values appear when there is an important functional deterioration of the gland. High values reflect a reduction in the pancreatic secretion flow to the duodenum. Serum levels of trypsin associated with the BT-PABA test have allowed distinction of three different secretor patterns in CP: normal BT-PABA and serum trypsin, low BT-PABA and serum trypsin, and low BT-PABA and normal or high serum trypsin. Serum levels of trypsin are directly correlated with the functional pancreatic reserve. An abnormal BT-PABA test associated with a low serum trypsin has been suggested as a predictive factor of the nonreversibility of pancreatic exocrine function, whereas low values of BT-PABA together with normal or high trypsin levels suggest a possible improvement of the pancreatic function, especially in relation to alcohol abstinence and surgical treatment.

FECAL FAT QUANTIFICATION. The fecal fat content is useful only in the final stages of pancreatic exocrine insufficiency, since it appears when 90% of the exocrine function is lost. Typical values in steatorrhea are those over 7 grams per 24 hr. This test may be useful in control of the therapeutic effect of oral administration of substitutive pancreatic enzymes in pancreatic exocrine insufficiency. A breath test with ^{14}C-triolein has been introduced recently. This test consists of measuring the proportion of ^{14}C exhaled after the ingestion of ^{14}C-marked triolein. It is a sensitive, simple, and noninvasive technique, but, like fecal fat determination, it does not distinguish between different etiologies of steatorrhea. The main disadvantage of this test is that it is qualitative, so it does not determine the amount of fat loss.

Pancreatic Endocrine Function Tests.

Endocrine pancreatic function abnormalities are frequently observed in advanced CP stages. Plasma levels of glucagon after arginine infusion are useful to distinguish primary from secondary diabetes in CP, as they are decreased in secondary diabetes. On the other hand, the integrated response of plasma pancreatic polypeptide to a meal, secretin, or cerulein seems to be a reliable test in the diagnosis of CP and also in distinguishing mild and severe stages of the disease. However, the sensitivity of this test is very low in early disease.

THERAPY

Medical therapy, for the most part, is limited to control of the pain, removal of a causative factor when identified (e.g., alcohol), and management of diabetes or exocrine insufficiency when present (pancreatic enzymes). Behavioral modifications and personal and family support are crucial in the management of related alcoholism and drug addiction and in facilitating control of pain and rehabilitation.

Etiologic Factors

Alcohol represents the main etiologic factor in CP. Therefore, it is important that the patients be managed by a multidisciplinary group that includes a comprehensive program for alcoholism. In areas of the world (South India, Indonesia) where nutritional deficiencies appear to play a role in the pathogenesis, adequate nutrition should be a goal. The role of antioxidant agents (selenium, β-carotene, vitamins C and E, methionine) and the use of zinc supplements remain controversial and under evaluation.

Pancreatic Endocrine Insufficiency

Vascular complications of diabetes are infrequent; however, neuropathy can be seen more often, probably because of the associated effects of alcohol and malnutrition. Treatment of diabetes in CP does not differ substantially from that of diabetes mellitus. Oral hypoglycemic agents are usually not very effective. Patients may require low doses of exogenous insulin and are more susceptible to develop hypoglycemia because of inappropriate insulin release, glucagon deficiency, and a low hepatic glycogen reserve.

Pancreatic Exocrine Insufficiency

A major loss of exocrine function is required for malabsorption of pancreatic origin to occur. Steatorrhea appears when pancreatic function has been reduced to less than 10% to 15% of its capacity. The end points of treatment are fitting the diet to the digestive capacity and metabolic requirements; supplementing fat-soluble vitamins (e.g., B_{12}), trace elements such as zinc, selenium, and folic acid if required; and finally, treating protein, carbohydrate, and fat malabsorption with administration of exogenous pancreatic enzymes. It is advisable to restrict fats and vegetable fiber; in severe cases, use medium-chain triglycerides. The end point of the substitutive therapy with exogenous pancreatic enzymes is to restore the physiologic intraluminal digestion.

The result of pancreatic enzyme administration depends on several intraluminal factors: (1) gastric pH, (2) appropriate mixture of the alimentary bolus (granules rather than tablets give better results), (3) duodenal pH, and (4) appropriate enzymatic concentration in the intestinal lumen, the concentration of lipase being especially important. It is well known that pancreatic enzymes given orally, and especially lipase, are inactivated at a pH lower than 4. To avoid this effect, a histamine H_2 receptor antagonist can be added to increase gastric as well as duodenal pH. It is important to use preparations high in lipase concentration. A minimum of 11,000 to 30,000 lipase units per meal is recommended, adjusting the dose to the clinical improvement of the steatorrhea. Pancreatic enzymes are supplied as conventional tablets, as enteric-coated pills, or as microspheres. Microspheres are the most suitable presentation, since they mix better with the alimentary bolus and have a greater gastric pH resistance.

Finally, in some selected patients, such as those with severe malnutrition or with complications, total parenteral nutrition may be required.

Pain Management

Increased ductal and interstitial pressure, perineural fibrosis, an increase in the number and diameter of pancreatic nerves, the role of various neuropeptides in processing the information concerning pain, and the possibility of a neuroimmunologic disorder have all been suggested as mechanisms for pain. The first step in pain management is to exclude any complication as responsible for this symptom, such as an acute exacerbation of the pancreatitis, a pseudocyst, biliary obstruction, and so on. Often a computed tomogram will give this information. It is important to insist on alcohol abstinence, since it has been proved that such abstinence can relieve pain. A retrograde pancreatogram can suggest a possible pathogenic mechanism (pancreas divisum, ampullary stenosis, ductal dilatation with pancreatic stones, and so on). A negative feedback mechanism between the duodenal trypsin content and the pancreatic exocrine secretion has been suggested. This phenomenon justifies a trial of exogenous pancreatic enzyme preparations high in trypsin. They would decrease intraductal pressure in these patients through an inhibition of the exocrine pancreatic secretion. Significant relief of pain after exogenous pancreatic enzyme administration in comparison with placebo has been proved.

When pain does not respond to analgesics and/or enzyme administration, a celiac plexus block by percutaneous alcohol injection may be tried. However, the benefits may last only a few months, and repeated injections tend to be less effective.

Early results of endoscopic removal of pancreatic stones and the use of stents in main pancreatic ducts in selected cases appear good. Nevertheless, longer follow-ups are required and a critical analysis of the cases needed.

Surgery

The indications for surgery are summarized in Table 3. Severe intractable pain, complications of the disease that require surgical management, and the inability to rule out a neoplasm are some of these reasons.

The factors that should be considered in the assessment of a patient as a possible candidate for operation are listed in Table 4. The first category, clinical information, deals with the severity of the pain, previous treatments, the presence of drug or substance abuse, the presence or absence of diabetes, and an estimation of the patient's willingness and ability

TABLE 3. **Indications for Surgery in Chronic Pancreatitis**

Disabling pain
Multiple relapses during year
Considerable lost time from work during year
Prevention of drug addiction
Complications
  Pseudocyst
  Gastrointestinal tract or biliary tract obstruction or both
  Fistula
  Infection
  Left-sided portal hypertension
Inability to rule out neoplasm

to manage the condition postoperatively, which may include the apancreatic state. In the second category, studies are outlined that will define the morphologic characteristics of the pancreas and the surgical options available. Retrograde pancreatography and imaging techniques, such as CT and ultrasonography, are helpful in obtaining information.

In general, for patients with severe disabling disease and dilated pancreatic duct, side-to-side pancreaticojejunostomy is the procedure of choice; for patients with a pseudocyst, internal drainage is recommended; and for the rare instance of ampullary stenosis, sphincterotomy is recommended. For patients with a nondilated pancreatic duct in whom previous decompressive operations have failed, when a mass effect is present, or when the disease appears to be lateralized, therapy usually entails some form of pancreatic resection.

No standard protocol for assessing and reporting results of the various surgical treatments exists. Comparison of the results reported in the literature is difficult because frequently the patient population, type of disease, length of follow-up study, and criteria for improvement vary. However, relief of pain cannot be the only criterion for success, especially when the results of pancreatic resection are reviewed. The metabolic consequences of the therapy, i.e., endocrine and exocrine insufficiency, the related late morbidity and mortality, and the possibility for rehabilitation with return to a productive life, should be considered. To optimize results, a multidisciplinary team approach that includes gastroenterologists, consultants in behavioral medicine, nutritionists, and surgeons is preferable.

TABLE 4. **Basic Considerations for Surgical Therapy in Chronic Pancreatitis**

Clinical information
  Symptoms
  Personality
  Addiction to drug, or substance abuse
  Diabetes
  Associated diseases
  Previous operations
Structural changes found on
  Pancreatography
  Computed tomography or ultrasonography or both
  Operative finding

The surgical procedures available in the management of patients with CP are listed in Table 5.

Pancreaticojejunostomy

This procedure is indicated in patients with a dilated pancreatic duct and usually requires a duct of 8 mm or more in diameter. The technique requires extensive opening of the pancreatic duct from the tail to the head of the pancreas. When present, calculi should be removed.

The operative risk associated with the procedure is low, and the remaining glandular tissue is preserved. At 5 years after operation, about two thirds of all patients experience relief of pain. Some reported results are included in Table 6. The proportion of patients who achieved relief of pain is inversely related to the length of the postoperative period. In our experience, only 54% of patients had improvement of pain at 5 years. Good results after pancreaticojejunostomy have been reported in the management of patients with chronic relapsing pancreatitis and in children with an associated dilated pancreatic duct. In this latter group, CP has increasingly been recognized as a cause of abdominal pain, and unlike the case in adults, alcoholism is rarely the cause of the disease.

If pain recurs, endoscopic retrograde pancreatography is indicated to assess the patency of the anastomosis. When the anastomosis is obstructed, a repeat pancreaticojejunostomy can result in improvement of pain in about half the patients.

Sphincterotomy and Spincteroplasty

In the past, patients who had disabling pain and laboratory findings suggestive of pancreatitis, often with minimal evidence of pancreatic parenchymal or ductal disease, frequently underwent ampullary procedures because of the belief that impaired outflow of pancreatic secretions was responsible for the disease. This procedure is used rarely now for the management of patients with CP because the true incidence of ampullary stenosis is thought to be extremely small.

A series from the Lahey Clinic reported that by 6

TABLE 5. **Surgical Procedures**

Direct to pancreas
  Anastomosis to intestinal tract (jejunum, stomach, duodenum)
  Drainage of cysts and abscesses
  Resection
    Distal
    Subtotal
    Pancreatoduodenectomy
    Duodenum preserving
    Total
  Resection and autotransplantation (islet cells, segmental)
  Occlusion of pancreatic duct (surgical, endoscopic)
Indirect to pancreas
  Sphincterotomy, sphincteroplasty
  Biliary enteric anastomosis
  Gastroenterostomy
  Nerve interruption

TABLE 6. **Results of Pancreaticojejunostomy for Relief of Pain**

	Pain		Operative	
	No. of Patients	Improvement (%)	Follow-up (Year)	Mortality (%)
Prinz, 1981	86	71	24.0	4
Taylor, 1981	20	54	5.0	0
Hart, 1983	75	63	4.0	0
Morrow, 1984	46	80	6.6	0
Holmberg, 1985	51	72	8.2	0
Crombleholme, 1990*	10	80	4.0	0

*In children.

months after operation, more than 60% of patients had improvement of pain, but by 5 years after operation, only 40% of the patients noted some degree of relief of pain. The more complex sphincteroplasty appeared to offer no advantage over the simpler sphincterotomy and, in patients who were alcoholic, avoidance of alcohol appeared to be the major determinant of a better outcome after operation.

Sphincteroplasty of the minor papilla in patients with CP and pancreas divisum offers no benefit. Successful results are seen with recurrent acute pancreatitis and a normal gland. Some endoscopists use endoscopic papillotomy and stenting in patients with CP. This procedure is likely to reproduce the limited results associated with open sphincteroplasty.

Cystogastrostomy, Cystoduodenostomy, and Cystojejunostomy

Pancreatic cysts associated with chronic pancreatitis are unlikely to resolve spontaneously and in most instances have mature walls that permit internal drainage. Therefore, it is usually not necessary to delay resolution for pseudocysts in patients with chronic pancreatitis. Operation is delayed for 4 to 6 weeks only in selected patients—specifically, in patients with a recent identifiable acute relapse. Although internal drainage of a pseudocyst usually results in resolution of the cyst, persistent or recurrent pain is common in patients with chronic pancreatitis because of persistence of the underlying disease. In our experience, only one third of patients with cysts in the head of the pancreas achieved long-term pain improvement. Therefore, retrograde pancreatography is performed preoperatively to assess the pancreatic ductal system. This procedure identifies patients who are candidates for more definitive treatment, such as concomitant drainage of a dilated main pancreatic duct or pancreatic resection.

When the cyst is in the retrogastric position, cystogastrostomy is the treatment of choice. With cysts in the head of the gland, Roux-en-Y cystojejunostomy or transduodenal drainage is preferred. Endoscopic transgastric and transduodenal drainage have been performed; however, perforation and bleeding have been described. The long-term results after these procedures require further assessment. In our experience, external drainage performed for selected cysts in the head of the pancreas and in difficult locations has been associated with resolution of the cysts in most patients and with minimal morbidity and mortality. The high morbidity and mortality associated with external drainage reported by surgeons may be in part the result of treating patients with acute pseudocysts.

Not all cysts need to be treated. When a patient is asymptomatic or has minimal symptoms and the cyst is small (5 cm or less), treatment is probably unnecessary. Follow-up study with serial ultrasonography is advisable. When cystic neoplasms are suspected, resection is required.

Pancreatic Resection

Resection is indicated in patients with disabling disease and a small pancreatic duct, in patients in whom previous decompression operations have failed, in patients with disease that is lateralized or dominant to the head or the tail of the gland, in some patients with pseudocysts or pancreatic fistulas, and in patients in whom a neoplasm cannot be ruled out.

Pancreatic resections consist of standard distal resection that divides the pancreas at the level of the superior mesenteric vessels and removes approximately 60% of the gland; near-total or 80% to 95% resection, in which the pancreas is divided to the right of the superior mesenteric vessels, leaving a rim of tissue of variable size attached to the duodenum to preserve the pancreaticoduodenal vessels and common bile duct; and pancreatoduodenectomy, in which the head of the gland and the duodenum are removed, leaving the pancreas in place distal to the superior mesenteric vessels. We prefer the pylorus-preserving technique. Total pancreatectomy removes the entire gland.

In the assessment of the results of resective operations, one has to consider that removal of pancreatic tissue can precipitate or accelerate the development of endocrine or exocrine insufficiency and therefore increase the morbidity and mortality associated with the procedure. The surgical treatment of patients with pancreatitis is based on the preservation of as much pancreatic function as possible while attempting to improve the patient's symptoms. It must be kept in mind, however, that diabetes mellitus eventually occurs in about 40% of patients with chronic pancreatitis even without surgery. Therefore, the incidence of diabetes after resection should be compared with the incidence in medically treated patients and patients who have undergone decompression procedures and not with members of the population at large. On occasion, in patients whose personality may preclude the management of an apancreatic state, it is better to accept some degree of pain and disability rather than the metabolic complications.

Distal Resection

Usually, lesser forms of distal resection are associated with a lower incidence of endocrine (30%) and exocrine insufficiency but tend to achieve less pain relief (50%). With maximal distal resection (90% to 95% of the gland), the pain is relieved more often (90%), but the incidence of metabolic complications increases substantially (70%). Limited distal resection achieved relief of pain by 5 years in only 20% of our patients. Other surgeons have reported better results, perhaps because of a different or better selection of patients. When we extended resection to near-total pancreatectomy, long-term improvement of pain occurred in approximately two thirds of patients but with an appreciable rise in metabolic complications. Distal resection appears to be best suited for patients with disease lateralized to the tail of the gland, for some patients with cysts in the body and tail, for patients with severe disease in the body and tail with ductal obstruction at the neck of the gland, and for patients with previous ductal injury from blunt abdominal trauma with fracture of the pancreas and stenosis of the duct at the midbody level. When the pancreatic duct is patent toward the head of the gland, the transected surface of the pancreatic duct is managed by suture ligation. When the pancreatic duct is obstructed proximally, pancreaticojejunostomy to the transected pancreas is favored. The patency of the duct can be assessed by retrograde pancreatography before operation or at the time of operation either by operative pancreatography or by probing the duct, preferably with a Fogarty catheter. Of patients who underwent 80% to 95% resection, those with simultaneous segmental pancreatic autotransplantation had the lowest incidence of insulin-dependent diabetes in the late postoperative period.

Total Pancreatectomy

Complete removal of the pancreas is associated with pain relief in 60% to 100% of patients. However, exocrine and endocrine insufficiency will occur in all these patients. Most total pancreatectomies are staged and are done in patients who previously underwent partial resection. Although the operative mortality is low, the late mortality in the Lahey Clinic experience was 46% at the median follow-up time of 5 years, and 40% in the Mayo Clinic series with a median follow-up time of 9 years. The short- and long-term morbidity was significant. In the Lahey Clinic experience, 24 of 26 patients required multiple readmissions, uncontrolled diabetes being the most common reason. Related late operations were common. Causes of death included cardiovascular problems, carcinoma at other sites (esophagus, larynx), hypoglycemia, suicide, complications of narcotic addiction, and alcohol-related death and disease. Because of the appreciable morbidity and mortality that results from an apancreatic state, especially in a patient with substance addiction or alcoholism, total pancreatectomy should be performed only as a last resort in patients whose previous operations have failed and who appear capable of managing their apancreatic state. In patients who already have insulin-dependent diabetes, indications for extensive pancreatectomy can be less rigid. When total pancreatectomy is performed, the pylorus-preserving technique is used. In postoperative management, we avoid the strict regulation of glucose levels and favor levels between 150 and 200 mg per dL to decrease the number of hypoglycemic episodes. All patients require exocrine pancreatic replacement therapy.

Proximal Pancreatic Resection

Increasing evidence in the literature suggests that resection of the head of the pancreas and uncinate process results in a higher degree of relief of pain than does distal resection. The better results obtained with proximal resection, together with the gradual decrease in the operative mortality associated with pancreatoduodenectomy and the realization of the limited results of distal resection, explain the increase in the frequency of proximal pancreatic resection in the management of patients with CP. This procedure is advocated for patients with severe disabling pain and a pancreatic duct of small diameter, for patients with a mass in the head of the pancreas with or without biliary and duodenal obstruction, and when the possibility of a neoplasm cannot be ruled out. The procedure is also used in patients in whom previous decompression operations and ampullary procedures have failed. In the Lahey Clinic experience, approximately 80% to 90% of patients continued to have relief of pain 5 years after the procedure. Of the insulin-independent patients before operation, 40% required insulin within 5 years after operation. However, the diabetes was stable and easy to control in most instances. Although the late mortality was 26%, only in 5.4% of patients was it related to the underlying pancreatic disease. By 5 years after operation, half the patients were maintaining a normal lifestyle, and an additional 30% claimed to do so intermittently. The use of narcotics had decreased from 85% before operation to 28% by 5 years after operation.

Pylorus-preserving pancreatoduodenectomy has been used extensively because it facilitates the procedure, avoids gastric resection, preserves gastric capacity, minimizes postgastrectomy syndromes, and may be associated with better absorption of fat than if gastric resection had been performed. Beger and coworkers have reported extensively on the technique of duodenum-preserving resection of the head of the pancreas with pain relief in 89% of the patients with a median follow-up time of 3.6 years: confirmatory data from other centers are required to determine the value of this procedure.

Techniques of Preservation of Endocrine Function

Implantation of islet cells into the portal system after extensive pancreatic resection has been reported. However, the low yield of isolation of islet cells in a fibrotic and calcified pancreas and the decreased mass of islet cells in these patients are in part responsible for the fact that in most of these patients, insulin is required within a few months after operation. Our experience with extensive distal pancreatic resection and segmental autotransplantation suggests that this technique is effective in preventing or delaying the onset of diabetes in these patients. However, because of the limited relief of pain provided by distal resection, in most of these patients we favor initial pancreatoduodenectomy, and we defer distal resection and autotransplantation for the patients whose proximal resection would fail.

Nerve Interruption Techniques

Relief of pain is the main goal of therapy for most patients with CP. Mallet-Guy reported extensive experience with splanchnicectomy and celiac ganglionectomy in 127 patients, with a minimum follow-up time of 5 years. Mallet-Guy's preferred method is a lumbar approach with resection of the twelfth rib, followed by removal of the great splanchnic nerve and celiac ganglion. Poor results were reported in only 10% of his patients. These results, however, have not been duplicated. Leger and associates reported relief of pain in only about one third of patients over a 2-year period of observation. White and associates achieved long-term reduction of pain in only 4 of 27 patients. The good initial results reported by Stone and associates for bilateral vagotomy with left splanchnicectomy through a thoracic approach needs confirmation by other groups. Anesthetic agents, alcohol, or phenols have achieved relief of pain in up to half of patients with CP; however, this relief lasts for only a couple of months after performance of this technique. For the most part, nerve ablation procedures have a minimal role in the management of patients with CP.

ASSOCIATED PROBLEMS

Pancreatic Ascites and Pancreatic Pleural Effusion

Pancreatic ascites and pancreatic pleural effusion result from disruption of the pancreatic duct either into the peritoneal cavity or through the retroperitoneum to the chest. Patients with pancreatic ascites present with a distended abdomen. A history of alcoholism or previous abdominal pain from pancreatitis may occasionally be absent. Patients with pleural effusion of pancreatic origin present with the nonspecific symptoms common to a patient with pleural effusion, the severity of which depends on the accumulation of fluid in the chest. Analysis of fluid in these patients discloses whether the ascitic or pleural fluid has a high concentration of amylase and protein (2.5 grams per dL). Medical therapy for patients with this condition includes the usual measures for ascites plus somatostatin, total parenteral nutrition, paracentesis, and no oral intake. Although a trial of this therapy is probably justifiable, failure is common in more than half of patients. Because medical therapy is accompanied by serious morbidity and mortality, perseverance is not justified when the patient's condition is failing and no progress is noted.

Retrograde pancreatography is essential in the work-up of these patients before operation because it permits determination of the site of leakage in the pancreatic ductal system and thus facilitates surgical exploration and selection of therapy. Depending on the location of the leakage and the characteristics of the ductal system, Roux-en-Y anastomosis to the site of the fistula or pancreatic resection, with or without pancreaticojejunostomy, may be selected for treatment. The placement of an endoscopic stent has been reported useful in selected cases.

Biliary Obstruction in Patients with Chronic Pancreatitis

Obstruction of the distal biliary tree may be the result of progressive fibrosis, formation of a pseudocyst, acute inflammatory changes, common bile duct calculi, or underlying carcinoma. An elevated level of alkaline phosphatase, which precedes jaundice, appears to be the most sensitive assay in detecting such obstruction. The incidence of stenosis of the distal bile duct in alcoholic pancreatitis has been reported to be at least 8%.

Obstruction of the biliary tree can be transient, recurrent, or persistent, depending on the basic mechanism causing the obstruction. The characteristics of the clinical course, results of cholangiography, and characteristics of the head of the pancreas, such as the presence of a pseudocyst, are factors that determine the need for therapy. Because fibrosis is the most common cause of distal biliary stricture in these patients, it should not be assumed that drainage of a cyst in the head of the gland will necessarily relieve the obstruction. Patients with a severely dilated common duct, recurrent or persistent obstruction as determined by continued elevation in the level of serum alkaline phosphatase, persistent jaundice, or recurrent episodes of cholangitis benefit from biliary enteric anastomosis. A patient with transient obstruction during an episode of acute relapse may be observed. Operative cholangiography after drainage of a cyst in the head of the pancreas can help assess the role of the cyst in the obstruction of the distal common duct. In well-selected patients with disabling pain and with disease lateralized to the head, pseudocyst in the head, and biliary obstruction, pancreatoduodenectomy may be the procedure of choice. Chronic stenosis of the common bile duct can cause cholangitis and biliary cirrhosis.

TRENDS

The management of patients with CP continues to achieve limited success. The diagnosis is usually based on a history of classic pain and some objective finding of pancreatic disease. Morphologic information provided by endoscopic retrograde pancreatography and ultrasonography or CT is essential in selecting the procedure that may achieve the result with the lowest morbidity and mortality. Other than morphologic data, clinical information regarding characteristics of personality, drug or substance abuse, presence of exocrine and endocrine insufficiency, and the patient's ability to manage the disease is essential in determining who is a surgical candidate and what procedure to perform. The basic surgical principles are to be conservative and to try to preserve as much pancreatic tissue as possible. The operation should be tailored to each patient according to the clinical and morphologic characteristics. Although management of pain is the primary goal of treatment in most patients, the morbidity and late mortality that can result from different procedures must be a major consideration in the selection of therapy. Pancreaticojejunostomy is the procedure of choice at this time for patients with a dilated pancreatic duct and internal drainage for a pseudocyst. Different forms of pancreatic resection are indicated for patients with severe disease and small pancreatic ducts, in patients in whom decompression operations have failed, in patients with lateralized disease to the tail of the gland, in some patients with pseudocysts or pancreatic fistulas, and, for some patients, when carcinoma cannot be ruled out. Procedures on the ampulla (sphincterotomy, sphincteroplasty) are now rarely performed. Of the resective procedures, operations that remove the head of the pancreas and uncinate process appear to achieve the best long-term results. This result, plus the decreased operative morbidity and mortality associated with operations on the head of the pancreas, explains the increase in use of these procedures. Endoscopic procedures are being used more often, and their results will need further evaluation.

GASTROESOPHAGEAL REFLUX DISEASE

method of
ADRIAN P. IRELAND, M.D., and
TOM R. DeMEESTER, M.D.
University of Southern California School of Medicine
Los Angeles, California

Gastroesophageal reflux disease is the spectrum of diseases due to excess reflux of gastric content into the esophagus. Diagnostic testing is required to confirm the diagnosis and plan the optimal mode of therapy. In up to 25% of patients with esophagitis the disease follows a recurrent, progressive course necessitating lifelong therapy. The reasons for this are that acid suppression therapy may fail to suppress acid production owing to inadequate dosage or poor compliance and does not address the nonacid components of the disease. The most effective treatment in these patients is a technically adequately performed antireflux operation that eliminates esophageal exposure to all refluxed material.

The role of the physician is to identify those patients at highest risk of recurrent or progressive disease and to halt the disease process prior to the point of end-stage disease when medical therapy is considered a failure and surgical therapy gives less satisfactory results. This approach should reduce the prevalence of complications, in particular specialized intestinal metaplasia, a premalignant condition that may progress to esophageal adenocarcinoma.

MAGNITUDE OF THE PROBLEM

Gastroesophageal reflux disease is the most common disease of the foregut in the western hemisphere. There is a wide spectrum of disease from patients with occasional symptoms without mucosal damage to patients with complications. More than 30% of the population experience heartburn on a frequent basis, and 10% experience heartburn daily. Results from a long-term follow-up of a group of 701 adult patients with esophagitis in Lausanne, Switzerland, were reported in 1993 and give the best available information on the natural history of reflux esophagitis. This "natural history" is in patients treated with a variety of medical agents such as antacids, H_2-receptor antagonists, omeprazole, and prokinetic agents and as such represents the course of the patients undergoing medical therapy. Seventy-seven percent of patients have an isolated episode of esophagitis or have recurrent, nonprogressive disease. These patients may be viewed as having a "benign" form of reflux disease in that they have only one episode of esophagitis, or when they do relapse they do so to the same or a less severe grade of esophagitis. The remaining 23% of patients have recurrent, progressive disease. These have a more severe form of reflux disease, because the degree of esophagitis worsens despite medical therapy.

Specialized intestinal epithelium (Barrett's esophagus) develops in 10% to 18% of patients with chronic gastroesophageal reflux disease. A postmortem study has shown that the age- and sex-adjusted prevalence of Barrett's esophagus is 376 per 100,000 population, compared with the clinically diagnosed prevalence of 22.6 per 100,000. This represents a 20-fold increase and indicates that the majority of patients with reflux never seek medical attention. Concomitantly and for unknown reasons, the incidence of esophageal adenocarcinoma is increasing at a faster rate than any other cancer, and in many centers esophageal adenocarcinoma outnumbers squamous cancer.

Several investigators have reported an increase in the incidence of reflux esophagitis. It was thought that this reflected an increase in the availability of endoscopy, but deaths from nonmalignant esophageal disease are also on the increase. These data indicate that reflux disease is becoming more common. This is reflected in drug sales, with a large share due to the sales of antacids and acid suppressants. Most who suffer with symptoms of gastroesophageal reflux disease treat themselves prior to seeking the advice of a physician. This self-treatment has been confined to the use of antacids in the past, but H_2-receptor antagonists have recently become available as over-the-counter medications. It is anticipated that fewer patients will seek medical attention for reflux symptoms because of this.

MANIFESTATIONS

The physician suspects that gastroesophageal reflux disease may be present when the patient presents with reflux symptoms, or investigation reveals complications of the disease. Typical symptoms of reflux include heartburn (sensation of retrosternal discomfort due to the reflux of gastric content into the esophagus), regurgitation (reflux of gastric content into the mouth), and dysphagia (sensation of swallowed material sticking in the esophagus). Regurgitation of gastric content into the mouth must be differentiated from regurgitation of bland material that has never reached the stomach. This may be seen in patients with esophageal motility disorders or a pharyngeal (Zenker's) diverticulum. The typical patient with gastroesophageal reflux disease complains of heartburn and regurgitation that are aggravated by a large meal (especially fatty) and by lying down. The patient has usually noted that antacids partially relieve heartburn but have less effect on regurgitation. Some patients experience excess salivation (waterbrash). The atypical presentations of reflux include dental erosions, chronic cough, hoarseness, asthma, and noncardiac chest pain. Eighty percent of patients with asthma or chronic hoarseness have reflux. Reflux is present in 50% of patients with noncardiac chest pain. It has been noted that gastroesophageal reflux disease is frequently present in patients who present with Zenker's diverticulum and cricopharyngeal dysphagia. In some patients, reflux is precipitated by exercise, which may lead to diagnostic confusion. The sensation of postprandial abdominal bloating, often described as a complication of antireflux surgery, is as common in patients treated with medication as in those who have undergone surgery. Complications of reflux disease include ulceration, stricture, short esophagus, Barrett's epithelium, high-grade dysplasia, and esophageal adenocarcinoma.

INVESTIGATION

Patients who have just one episode of heartburn and respond to lifestyle modification and a course of acid suppressant therapy require no further investigation or treatment. Indications for investigation are summarized in Table 1. Investigation should be tailored to the patient and available resources along the following guidelines.

Barium Esophagogram

If dysphagia is a primary symptom, then a barium esophagogram should precede endoscopy. Barium esophago-

TABLE 1. Indications for Investigation of the Patient with Suspected Gastroesophageal Reflux Disease

Prior to surgery
Incomplete response to treatment, recurrent disease, or
  prolonged acid suppressant therapy
Atypical symptoms; laryngeal, pulmonary, or noncardiac chest
  pain
Idiopathic pulmonary fibrosis or recurrent aspiration pneumonia
Presence of complications prior to or while on therapy

TABLE 2. Endoscopic Grading of Esophagitis

Grade	Endoscopic Findings
I	Erythema and friability
II	Linear erosions
III	Deeper and wider erosions with islands of edematous mucosa between erosive furrows
IV	Fibrous stricture or large ulcer

gram provides complementary information to stationary esophageal motility and endoscopy. The anatomy of the pharynx and esophagus are outlined so that there is less chance of iatrogenic injury upon instrumentation. It permits assessment of esophageal motility and demonstrates the presence and reducibility of a hiatal hernia. Provocative testing for the presence of reflux on barium esophagogram is often positive in normal subjects and should not be used. Video recording of the study increases usefulness to the clinician and provides a basis for the radiologist to compare studies.

Endoscopy and Biopsy

Endoscopy will reveal the presence of esophagitis and permit acquisition of tissue for histologic examination. All patients with dysphagia should have endoscopy with biopsy of mucosal abnormalities to rule out cancer. The degree of esophagitis should be classified using one of the published systems. Our preferred grading system is given in Table 2. Biopsy is essential to diagnose specialized intestinal epithelium that may be invisible on endoscopy or interpreted as esophagitis. In cases of macroscopic Barrett's esophagus, four-quadrant biopsies every 2 cm and biopsy of any mucosal abnormality should be made to confirm the diagnosis and sample for the presence of high-grade dysplasia or cancer. In view of the rising incidence of adenocarcinoma of the cardia and the recent reports of specialized intestinal epithelium on biopsy specimens taken from this location, we advocate routine biopsy of the cardia in all patients undergoing endoscopy for the investigation of foregut symptoms. The detection of specialized intestinal metaplasia at this location may be associated with an increased risk of malignant degeneration as it is in the esophagus. Patients with this finding should be enrolled in a surveillance program so that dysplasia or early cancer in the cardia may be detected and cured by surgical resection.

Histologic examination of squamous epithelium may show signs associated with reflux disease, such as basal cell hyperplasia ($>15\%$ of the thickness of the epithelium comprising the basal zone where cells are separated by <1 nuclear diameter), increase in the number of papillae, and papillary elongation (papillae extending $>65\%$ of the thickness of the epithelium). These changes indicate irritation of the squamous epithelium and are not specific for reflux disease. The presence of microscopic ulceration or an intraepithelial accumulation of neutrophils or eosinophils is more specific for reflux but may be due to other causes of esophageal inflammation. Further, these changes are not found in equal intensity in adjacent biopsies, which may range from normal to inflamed.

Manometry and pH Testing

All patients should undergo stationary esophageal motility prior to ambulatory pH testing to ensure accurate placement of the pH probe. The motility test also provides information on the characteristics of the lower esophageal sphincter and function of the esophageal body, which are important to rule out achalasia and plan the optimal mode of surgical repair.

Ambulatory pH monitoring will detect pathologic reflux in the majority of patients with reflux disease. False-negative results are rare. Technical failures may cause a false-negative test. The pH probe should be calibrated in suitable buffers both prior to and after the test to ensure that there has been no electrode drift. The physician should check the pH tracing for evidence of technical failure. Misplacement of the pH probe at too high a position may cause a false-negative result. Rarely the probe is displaced after initial satisfactory placement by an episode of coughing or vomiting. Low acid content in the stomach, from medication or chronic gastric atrophy, in pernicious anemia, and following surgery, may result in a negative pH test in a patient with reflux. Antacids and H_2-receptor antagonists should be discontinued at least 48 hours and proton pump inhibitors at least 2 weeks prior to the test. In some patients a marked degree of duodenogastric reflux may be increasing gastric pH. This would require a large amount of duodenogastric reflux such that 40% to 70% of gastric content would have to consist of duodenal juice to maintain gastric pH greater than 4. It is possible that a patient may eat a smaller amount and therefore reflux less, or the tubing may cause an increase in salivation so that the esophageal pH profile is shifted to the alkaline range. Strictures may cause false-negative tests and should be dilated prior to the test. The stricture may prevent reflux of gastric content into the esophagus, and with associated poor contractility pooling of saliva shifts the pH profile in the alkaline direction.

If the patient's symptoms are typical for reflux disease and the pH test is negative, then the physician should search for causes of false-negative results. If the investigator suspects that there is hypochlorhydria, this can be assessed with gastric secretion studies. If there is hypochlorhydria, then an alternative to pH monitoring, such as ambulatory monitoring for the presence of duodenal juice using the Bilitec device, should be considered. The pH test should be repeated if there has been an avoidable failure or when there are no reasons for a false-negative test in a patient with esophagitis or typical symptoms. If the second test is negative, then a nonreflux cause for the patient's symptoms or esophagitis should be sought.

Bilitec Device

The recently introduced Bilitec device combines a data logger with a spectrophotometer that is carried on the patient's belt. The probe consists of a white Teflon reflector, a sampling area, and a bundle of optical fibers that carry alternating light signals (blue reference and green sampling) to the device. The light signal travels down the probe through the sampling area (and any material in it) and is reflected by the Teflon back up the probe, where the intensity of the reflected signal is measured. Absorbance at a wavelength of 453 nm is compared with the absorbance of the reference light to ensure that a reduction in absorbance is not due to blockage of the sampling area or loss of light from another cause. The maximal absorbance of bilirubin is close to 453 nm, which is used as a marker for the presence of duodenal juice in the same way as pH is used as a marker for the presence of gastric content. The Bilitec device is a useful method to detect increased esophageal exposure to duodenal juice and may help predict those patients at greatest risk of progression to Barrett's esophagus. The role of this device in clinical decision making is under evaluation.

Other Investigations

In certain circumstances other tests may be added to these basic investigations to provide additional information. Ambulatory pH monitoring with dual pH probes placed in the proximal and distal esophagus can provide objective evidence of reflux into the upper esophagus in patients with laryngeal and pulmonary symptoms. Some investigators have shown drops in tracheal pH in association with pulmonary symptoms. Assessment of esophageal motility over the circadian cycle permits correlation of motility abnormalities with symptoms in patients with noncardiac chest pain. It also shows the response of the esophagus to a meal, which is a more physiologic situation than the conventional assessment using swallows of water in the supine position.

The acid perfusion test lacks the sensitivity and specificity of ambulatory pH monitoring and for this reason has fallen out of favor. A worrying aspect of this test is that it may be negative in patients with Barrett's esophagus who have a reduced sensitivity to acid. As part of the ambulatory pH test the examiner may look for correlation between symptoms noted in the patient's diary and reflux episodes on the pH record; this is the essence of the Bernstein test. A standard or modified acid reflux test similarly lacks the sensitivity and specificity of ambulatory pH monitoring. This test may be useful in cases of decreased acid content of the stomach when pH testing is likely to give a false negative result and ambulatory monitoring for duodenal juice using the Bilitec device is not available.

MEDICAL THERAPY

The nonsurgical therapies for gastroesophageal reflux disease are lifestyle modifications and drugs to neutralize acid, suppress acid secretion, or enhance motility in the foregut. It is conventional to start with lifestyle modifications and add the minimal drug therapy that will keep the patient free from symptoms and complications.

Lifestyle modifications form part of conservative management of the patient. Advice may be given to lose weight, stop smoking, elevate the head of the bed, avoid recumbency for 3 hours after eating, and avoid fat, chocolate, peppermint, and onions. Treatment with medication should be accompanied by advice on lifestyle modifications.

Histamine-receptor antagonists were the first drugs to have a marked impact on gastroesophageal reflux disease. Results in trials are variable, with about 60% amelioration of symptoms and 50% initial healing in esophagitis. However, relapse is common upon cessation of therapy. Lifelong maintenance therapy is required in a group of patients. The efficacy of maintenance therapy with ranitidine (Zantac), 150 to 300 mg daily, in maintaining the patient free from esophagitis varies between 10% and 83%.

Proton pump inhibitors are more effective than H_2-receptor antagonists and give symptom relief and initial healing of esophagitis in 80% of patients. Discontinuation of omeprazole (Prilosec) is frequently followed by return of the patient's symptoms. In patients who have been free from heartburn, the return of symptoms is less tolerable. In these patients and in those whose esophagitis relapses upon cessation of therapy, lifelong maintenance therapy is required. Maintenance therapy with omeprazole, 20 mg daily, is associated with a relapse rate in esophagitis of 11% to 33% within 1 year. A higher dose of 40 mg a day gives better results, with a relapse rate of 0% to 14%.

The main prokinetic agent in clinical use for the treatment of gastroesophageal reflux disease is cisapride (Propulsid), 10 mg 15 to 30 min before meals and at bedtime. Cisapride is superior to placebo for the relief of symptoms and healing of esophagitis. The effect of cisapride is comparable to that of cimetidine or ranitidine. When used in conjunction with cimetidine, there is a 46% to 70% improvement in the rate of healing of esophagitis. It is unknown whether the addition of cisapride to omeprazole increases symptom relief and healing of esophagitis.

Acid suppressant medications have their beneficial effects in gastroesophageal reflux disease by reducing the volume of gastric secretion and increasing gastric pH so that pepsin's activity is minimized. This reduces the injurious effects of the acid/peptic component of the refluxate and the volume of gastric content refluxed. Heartburn appears to be largely due to the effects of acid in the esophagus. Long-term acid suppressant therapy effectively relieves heartburn in the majority of patients. This lulls the patient and physician into a false sense of security while the reflux of gastric juice with a higher pH continues. Duodenal components of gastric juice have most of their deleterious effects in a nonacid pH range and as a consequence may be potentiated by acid suppressant therapy. In addition, acid may protect the esophagus against the effects of bile salts by causing their irreversible precipitation. Consequently some patients progress to Barrett's esophagus while taking acid suppressant medication. Other patients remain symptomatic, and esophagitis persists despite increasing doses of acid suppressant medications.

SURGICAL THERAPY

The prerequisites for surgical therapy in a patient with suspected gastroesophageal reflux disease are objectively proven reflux, a mechanically defective lower esophageal sphincter, and proof that the patient's symptoms are caused by increased esophageal exposure to gastric content. The patient should have had a course of medical therapy, consisting of lifestyle modifications and acid suppressant therapy, for at least 8 to 12 weeks.

In patients with these prerequisites whose symptoms and esophagitis are controlled by medication, there is a choice between continued maintenance medical treatment and surgery. If the patient shows an incomplete response to medication with continued symptoms or persistent esophagitis, then surgery should be considered. When complications develop in a patient under medical therapy, there is clearly a treatment failure and surgery is indicated.

It is unfortunate that the patient is referred to surgery at this late stage, because the results are less satisfactory than for disease without complications. How can one tell which patients will go on to develop complications? Indications for surgery that are too liberal will result in unnecessary operations with a small but significant morbidity and perhaps mortality. Too restrictive a policy will result in many missed opportunities to prevent the complications of chronic gastroesophageal reflux disease. This is a difficult balance and more research is needed. From the data available at present, the following risk factors appear to be important.

Male Sex. There is a marked male preponderance in esophageal adenocarcinoma, with a slightly less marked male preponderance in Barrett's esophagus. Men are also more likely to have erosive esophagitis than women.

Family History. There are several reports in the literature of Barrett's esophagus or esophageal adenocarcinoma in many members of the same family. This may be due to a hereditary factor or to similar lifestyles or both. It is prudent to investigate and treat patients aggressively with such a family history.

Mechanical Defect in the Lower Esophageal Sphincter. The presence of a mechanically defective sphincter is a well-recognized poor prognostic indicator. These patients respond less well to medical therapy and commonly relapse.

Presence of Severe Esophagitis. Patients with Savary-Miller grade 3 or 4 esophagitis respond less well to medical therapy than patients with lesser grades of esophagitis. If the esophagitis does not heal after 4 weeks of medical therapy, then consideration should be given to surgery.

Pattern of Reflux. A combined upright and supine reflux pattern on ambulatory pH monitoring is associated with more advanced disease. Some investigators have reported that an isolated upright reflux pattern is associated with early disease. Caution should be observed in offering surgery to patients with a competent sphincter. If the patient has an incompetent sphincter, then the pattern of reflux is unimportant when there is increased esophageal exposure to acid.

Composition of the Refluxate. Increased esophageal exposure to duodenal juice is associated with advanced disease. Experimental evidence and clinical observation link esophageal exposure to duodenal juice to Barrett's esophagus and esophageal adenocarcinoma. It is possible that patients without complications who have increased esophageal exposure to duodenal juice are more likely to develop progressive disease.

In patients with these risk factors, the choice between continued medical therapy and surgery should be swayed in the direction of surgery. It is wise to ask specifically about symptoms of gastric dysfunction in a patient being considered for antireflux surgery; if the patient complains of nausea, early satiety, or postprandial abdominal bloating, then preoperative assessment should include gastric emptying studies and an assessment for the presence of duodenogastric reflux.

Patients with extraesophageal manifestations of reflux disease, particularly pulmonary ones, are best managed by surgery.

THE TAILORED APPROACH TO SURGERY

With the wide spectrum of pathology in gastroesophageal reflux disease, no single operation is suitable for all cases (Figure 1). Factors to consider in the selection for the best operation in the patient with gastroesophageal reflux disease are the presence of complications, force of esophageal contraction, acid hypersecretion or history of peptic ulcer disease, duodenogastric reflux, delay in gastric emptying, and the presence of hiatal hernia. Patients who have had previous gastric or antireflux surgery are especially complex and should be treated in a center with the facilities for complete assessment of foregut physiology and the expertise to apply the optimal surgical procedure tailored to the patient's pathophysiology. The chance of a satisfactory result in this group of patients is indirectly related to the number of previous attempts at repair. A thoracic approach should be considered when there has been previous gastric or antireflux surgery, severe stricture, short esophagus, obesity, or when thoracic access is required to deal with concomitant pulmonary pathology.

The transabdominal Nissen fundoplication is the procedure of choice for the straightforward patient with gastroesophageal reflux disease. The long-term results for this procedure in appropriately selected patients show that the actuarial success rate is greater than 90% at up to 10 years. These results are for the open procedure with an upper midline incision. Provided the operative indications are the same and that the operation is performed in the same manner, the recently introduced laparoscopic Nissen fundoplication should have the same long-term results. Early reports are encouraging, but long-term results are not yet available.

The main contraindication to abdominal Nissen fundoplication is poor motility in the esophageal body. In our laboratory, this is assessed from 10 wet swallows performed with the patient supine. Sensors are placed 1, 6, 11, 16, and 21 cm below the lower border of the upper esophageal sphincter. A median contraction amplitude less than the 2.5 percentile of normals (20 mm Hg) in any of the sensors placed at 11, 16, or 21 cm is used to define poor contractility. If there is greater than 20% simultaneous waves (peak to peak velocity greater than 20 cm per second) between these levels or poor contractility in all three sensors, then the patient has poor motility. Patients with poor motility have an inadequate force of esophageal contraction to overcome the resistance of a full fundoplication. If a full fundoplication is applied in this situation, there is a risk of dysphagia. A transthoracic Belsey partial fundoplication, along with full mobilization of the esophageal body to reduce tension on the repair, will give a good result in most of these patients, but the procedure is not as effective in eliminating reflux as a complete fundoplication.

Esophageal shortening is defined as the presence of greater than 5 cm between the crura and the gastroesophageal junction on endoscopy or an irreducible hiatal hernia on barium esophagogram. In this situation, an attempt to perform an abdominal Nissen fundoplication will result in a plication placed

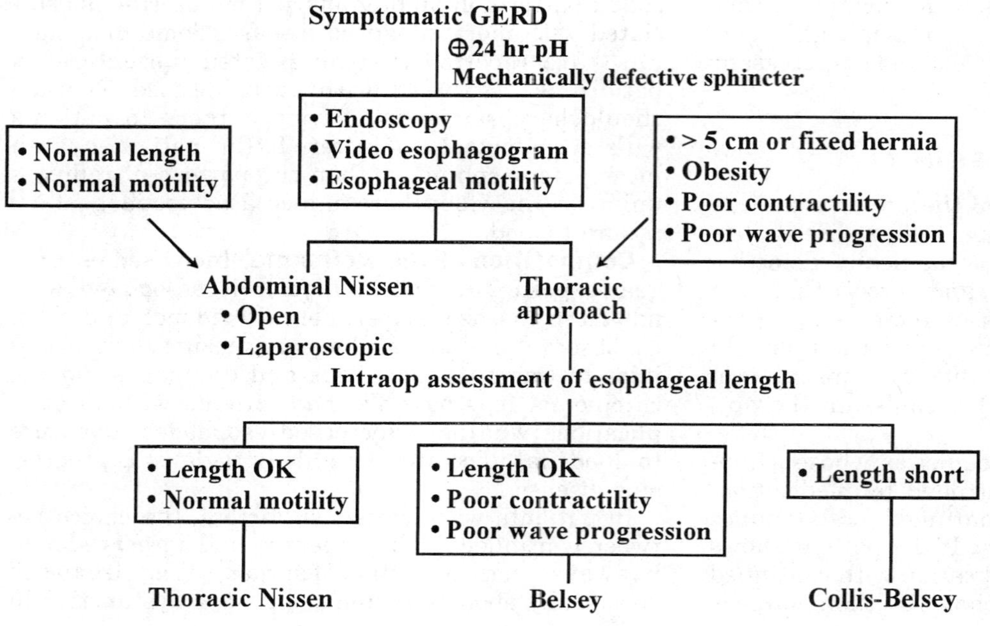

Figure 1. Clinical algorithm for the tailored approach to surgery for gastroesophageal reflux disease (GERD).

around the proximal stomach ("slipped Nissen") or around the esophagus under undue tension; the result is a failed antireflux procedure. A thoracic approach is necessary first to mobilize the esophagus. If the repair can be easily placed within the abdomen, then a transthoracic Nissen is the best option, provided esophageal contractility is adequate. If the repair cannot be easily placed in the abdomen, then a lengthening procedure in the form of a Collis gastroplasty is needed. After the new distal esophagus is constructed from the proximal stomach, a partial fundoplication is used to halt further reflux.

COMPARISON OF MEDICAL AND SURGICAL THERAPY

Many reports of long-term follow-up of patients undergoing antireflux surgery are a testament to its effectiveness. Such reports on the long-term follow-up of medically treated patients are lacking. There have been two trials of medical therapy compared with surgical therapy for chronic reflux disease. In the first, which compared the then optimal medical therapy of lifestyle modifications and antacids with Nissen fundoplication, surgery was clearly superior. When H_2 blockers were introduced, the trial was repeated and surgery was again superior. A cost benefit analysis showed that surgery was cheaper than medical therapy for patients less than 49 years of age. No comparison of surgical therapy with long-term omeprazole therapy has been carried out to date.

Despite the available data, many physicians are reluctant to consider surgery for chronic reflux disease and look upon it as the last resort. This attitude is unfair to both the physician and the patient. A referral to surgery by the physician does not represent a failure but a recognition of the need for a mechanical improvement of the patient's failing antireflux mechanism and is the best treatment option for the patient with severe disease.

COMPLICATIONS

Stricture

Reflux-induced stricture of the esophagus represents one of the end-stages of gastroesophageal reflux disease, and treatment is less satisfactory than for patients with erosive esophagitis. Prevention is better than cure. Recent improvements in treatment options are the availability of proton pump inhibitors and better dilatation systems. Schatzki's ring consists of mucosal hyperplasia and is not a true stricture. It is associated with reflux disease and may progress to stricture, particularly in patients who have esophagitis. Stricturing occurs when healing is accompanied by fibrosis. In most patients fibrosis is confined to the submucosa, but in others it extends into the muscularis propria. Besides the depth of fibrosis, other important characteristics of reflux-induced strictures are their location in the esophagus,

luminal diameter, and length. The lower border of the stricture is located just above the squamocolumnar junction so that when the junction is displaced orally, as in Barrett's esophagus, the stricture is found at a more proximal location. The internal luminal diameter of the stricture may be measured endoscopically and classed as mild (12 mm), moderate (10 to 12 mm) and severe (<10 mm). An open-biopsy forceps (7.5 mm diameter for the 2.5 mm forceps) or the size of the endoscope may be used to measure the diameter of the stricture. Most reflux-induced strictures are short, under 1 cm in length, but may be longer particularly when associated with a superimposed drug injury.

In some patients there is no history of gastroesophageal reflux disease; instead, the history may be that after taking some medication for a headache the patient lay down to sleep and the next day had some chest pain that resolved but was followed by dysphagia. The pill usually lodges at one of the narrow areas in the esophagus such as the aortic arch, the level of the left main bronchus, or the gastroesophageal junction. The history and location of the stricture may suggest the possibility of pill injury to the clinician. Esophageal function testing may reveal an esophageal motor disorder and show no evidence of increased esophageal exposure to acid on ambulatory pH testing.

Associated pathologies include Zollinger-Ellison syndrome (10% have strictures), scleroderma, previously treated achalasia, and Barrett's esophagus. Some patients develop a stricture after a period of nasogastric intubation. Patients with stricture tend to be older with a long history of gastroesophageal reflux disease. Diagnostic testing reveals markedly impaired competence of the lower esophageal sphincter and subnormal contractility in the distal esophagus. Ambulatory pH testing following dilatation shows markedly increased esophageal exposure to acid.

It is of paramount importance to rule out a malignant cause of any stricture regardless of how benign it may appear. Most patients presenting with a stricture have a neoplasm.

Investigation of Stricture

Barium esophagogram should be obtained prior to endoscopy when possible. A possible exception to this is a bolus obstruction when a contrast examination may cause aspiration, show little mucosal detail in the presence of retained food particles, and make extraction of the bolus more difficult. Careful endoscopy prior to the contrast study is needed and should be therapeutic and diagnostic. In cases of mild stricture it is necessary to distend the esophagus to identify the stricture. This may be accomplished by asking the patient to swallow solid contrast agents ("barium burgers and marshmallows") or by positioning the patient prone and asking him or her to swallow liquid barium while fluoroscoping the esophagus. The barium study may overestimate the length of tight strictures due to streaming of the barium below the stricture.

All patients with a stricture should have urgent endoscopy to ensure that there is not an underlying malignancy. This may require several attempts at dilatation and biopsy. More biopsy specimens should be taken if there is a suspicion that this is a malignant stricture. Brush cytology is a useful adjuvant to forceps biopsy. Clues to a malignant stricture are abnormal location, long length, asymmetry on endoscopy, or heaped-up margins on the contrast study.

Management of Reflux-Induced Stricture

In the elderly frail patient, the best course of action is dilatation accompanied by maximal medical therapy. Dilatation needs to be repeated on a regular basis in most of these patients. Placement of an endoprosthesis across the stricture is contraindicated; reflux continues and the patient will develop esophagitis and a further stricture proximal to the prosthesis, which becomes stuck and cannot be removed.

The optimal operative intervention needs to be tailored to the patient, depending on the underlying pathophysiology. The best predictor of the patient's response to surgery is dilatation. When possible the esophagus should be preserved, as the function of the natural esophagus is better than that of a substitute. Esophagectomy is required when there is transmural esophageal fibrosis, indicated by an undilatable stricture or persistent dysphagia following dilatation. If there is associated Barrett's epithelium, then all the esophagus containing Barrett's epithelium should be resected to eliminate the possibility of subsequent adenocarcinoma. A short distal esophagectomy with gastric pull-up into the left chest will provide only temporary relief of dysphagia, as reflux is aggravated with early restricturing at the esophagogastrostomy. In this situation we prefer a colon interposition.

For the dilatable stricture, progressive preoperative dilatation to a No. 60 French bougie is recommended. Coexisting pathophysiology includes esophageal foreshortening and poor motility in the esophageal body. In these circumstances, an abdominal Nissen fundoplication is contraindicated. The mission of the surgeon is to safely restore swallowing and prevent restricturing by eliminating further reflux. There are two surgical strategies in this situation. The first, favored by many European surgeons, is to dilate the stricture and leave the esophagus alone but eliminate injurious agents by suppressing acid and diverting duodenal content. Acid suppression is accomplished by vagotomy and antrectomy, duodenal juice diversion by a Roux-en-Y reconstruction. The second approach, preferred by us, is to operate upon the esophagus and tailor the repair to the underlying pathophysiology, as previously discussed.

The results of surgery for stricture are more effective and durable than continued medical therapy. With continued medical therapy, there is usually a need for repeated dilatations. With each dilation there is a risk of perforation and other complications.

Antireflux surgery is followed by excellent results in 65% to 92% of patients, with a rate of repeat dilatations (usually only once) of 1% to 30%. When esophageal resection is required for advanced disease results are not as good, indicating the need for earlier effective treatment.

BARRETT'S ESOPHAGUS

Barrett's esophagus is an acquired condition that represents a peculiar form of healing that occurs at any stage in reflux disease. The squamous epithelium of the terminal esophagus is replaced by a columnar epithelium containing goblet cells. This specialized intestinal epithelium warrants special attention because it is the initiating step in a metaplasia to dysplasia to carcinoma sequence. Barrett's metaplasia is accepted to be a complication of gastroesophageal reflux disease and links this common malady to one of the most lethal cancers.

The relative risk of a patient with benign Barrett's esophagus progressing to esophageal adenocarcinoma is 30 to 125 times the risk in the general population. The actual risk is about 500 adenocarcinomas per 100,000 patients with Barrett's esophagus per year.

Dysplasia and Barrett's Esophagus

Histologically, Barrett's epithelium may be classified as without dysplasia, indefinite for dysplasia, low-grade dysplasia, and high-grade dysplasia. An experienced pathologist is required to make the diagnosis. There is good pathologic agreement for the presence of high-grade dysplasia (86%), but for the lower grades of dysplasia agreement is less, with 75% for low-grade dysplasia and 58% for indefinite dysplasia. The main diagnostic difficulty for the pathologist regarding the presence of dysplasia is differentiation of the findings from those due to inflammation and regeneration. High-grade dysplasia looks like cancer but there is no evidence of invasion beyond the basement membrane of the epithelium. Some investigators refer to high-grade dysplasia as intraepithelial cancer.

Dysplasia is the best marker for the risk of progression to adenocarcinoma. Recent innovations like cell flow cytometry to search for aneuploidy and immunohistochemistry to look for overexpression of the tumor suppressor gene p53 have not been shown to have greater predictive benefit than high-grade dysplasia. In patients who undergo esophagectomy for high-grade dysplasia, adenocarcinoma is present in the resected specimen in 50% of cases.

Role of Surgery in Patients Free of Dysplasia

Many patients with Barrett's esophagus seen in our surgical clinic have developed Barrett's epithelium while under medical therapy. Experimental evidence supports a pathogenetic role for duodenal juice in the genesis of Barrett's esophagus and esophageal adenocarcinoma. Reflux of duodenal content into the esophagus continues despite medical therapy aimed at acid suppression. There are no prospective trials that compare the prognosis of patients with Barrett's esophagus randomized to either medical or surgical therapy, but one report has shown a lower rate of progression to cancer in patients with Barrett's epithelium following surgery than in those who continue with medical therapy. For these reasons we recommend that patients with Barrett's esophagus should be considered for antireflux surgery rather than being managed by continued medical therapy. Surgery restores lower esophageal sphincter function and abolishes reflux of both gastric and duodenal juice into the esophagus. This eliminates further damage to the Barrett's epithelium and normal esophageal mucosa. It is still recommended that after surgical therapy the patient should continue with annual endoscopic surveillance.

Management of the Patient with Low-Grade Dysplasia

Low- or indefinite-grade epithelial dysplasia means that the pathologist cannot be sure whether the changes in the specimen represent a neoplastic process or are due to regeneration and inflammation. If not previously done, the patient should receive an intensive course of medical therapy, and the endoscopy should be repeated, with biopsy of the four quadrants of the esophagus every two cm of macroscopic Barrett's and areas of mucosal abnormality. If there is no evidence of high-grade dysplasia, then the patient should be treated with an antireflux procedure followed by surveillance every 6 months until the low-grade dysplasia regresses.

Management of the Patient with High-Grade Dysplasia

Management decisions about a patient with high-grade dysplasia should not be made until two experienced pathologists have reviewed the slides and agreed upon the diagnosis. Some investigators feel that the patient with high-grade dysplasia can be safely followed up with repeated biopsy and referred for esophagectomy when adenocarcinoma develops. The idea behind this approach is that some patients will not progress to adenocarcinoma or will die from another cause before adenocarcinoma develops.

Another approach is to treat all patients with high-grade dysplasia and who are fit for surgery with an esophagectomy. We reviewed our own experience with 17 patients referred from surveillance programs. Seven of 11 patients referred with the diagnosis of high-grade dysplasia had adenocarcinoma in the resected specimen. The tumor was intramucosal in five, submucosal in one, and in one patient who had ulceration the tumor reached the muscularis propria. None of these patients had lymph node metastases. The patients were all alive and well at

follow-up, a median of 12 (range, 4 to 66) months. Aggressive rebiopsy of these patients prior to surgery revealed only two of the seven adenocarcinomas found in the surgical specimen. For this reason we feel that it is not possible to be sure that there is no adenocarcinoma when the patient has high-grade dysplasia.

Because of the difficulty in ensuring that a patient with high-grade dysplasia does not have adenocarcinoma, the future risk of the patient developing adenocarcinoma if it is not present, and the relative safety with which elective esophagectomy can be performed in expert hands, we advocate esophagectomy for the patient with high-grade dysplasia. A careful continued surveillance policy should be adopted only for the patient who is judged unfit for surgery. The aim of surveillance in patients with Barrett's esophagus is to detect adenocarcinoma at an early curable stage. Once high-grade dysplasia is found, surveillance has performed its aim and has detected the patient who will benefit from esophagectomy.

PEPTIC ULCER

method of
DOUGLAS K. REX, M.D.
Indiana University School of Medicine
Indianapolis, Indiana

INCIDENCE

Over the past 3 decades, the incidence of duodenal ulcer has declined in the United States, presumably the result of declining rates of *Helicobacter pylori* infection and changing cigarette smoking patterns. The incidence of gastric ulcer has remained stable as a result of increasing use of nonsteroidal anti-inflammatory drugs (NSAIDs). The point prevalence of peptic ulcer in the United States is between 1 and 2%, with about 4 million affected individuals and 350,000 incident cases per year. Rates of hospitalization for bleeding and perforated peptic ulcer have remained largely unchanged over the past 3 decades, again due to continued high-volume NSAID use.

PATHOPHYSIOLOGY

Three types of peptic ulcer are encountered in clinical practice: *Helicobacter*-related ulcer, NSAID–related ulcers, and Zollinger-Ellison ulcers. Since Zollinger-Ellison ulcers account for less than 0.1% of all ulcers, *Helicobacter*- and NSAID–related ulcers constitute the overwhelming majority of peptic ulcers. Idiopathic ulcers are now considered rare. The classification of ulcers into one of these three categories is clinically useful, since it leads directly to appropriate therapy.

Under normal circumstances, the integrity of the gastric and duodenal mucosa is maintained by a balance between "aggressive" factors, such as acid and pepsin, and the normal defense mechanisms of the gastric and duodenal epithelium, including secretion of mucus and bicarbonate, normal mucosal blood flow, and regeneration of new epithelial cells. These defense mechanisms are dependent on mucosal synthesis of prostaglandins.

H. pylori establishes a chronic infection during which the bacterium attaches itself to gastric epithelial cells, releasing a variety of extracellular enzymes, including urease, which break down the mucous layer and facilitate diffusion of bacterial antigens into the mucosa. An inflammatory response, including IgG and IgA antibodies and cellular infiltrate, is present in virtually all infected persons. Basal and postprandial hypergastrinemia develops, probably related to suppression of somatostatin-producing D cells by cytokines released in the inflammatory response.

Although chronic active gastritis is present in all infected persons, only a minority develop actual duodenal ulcers. Critical events in the development of duodenal ulcer include development of gastric metaplasia in the duodenal bulb (which may result from hyperacidity induced by hypergastrinemia), colonization of duodenal bulb metaplasia by *H. pylori*, and secretion of cytotoxic proteins by certain strains. Strains producing cytotoxins have been associated with an increased severity of gastritis and a higher risk of developing peptic ulcer disease. Eradication of *H. pylori* infection restores basal and postprandial gastrin levels to the normal range and essentially eliminates the risk of recurrent ulcer disease.

NSAID–related ulcers are caused primarily by systemic prostaglandin synthesis inhibition by the NSAID. Thus peptic ulcer disease (PUD) may follow intrarectal or parenteral administration of NSAIDs. Some NSAIDs also have a direct topical toxic effect, which has been best characterized for aspirin. Aspirin facilitates the back-diffusion of acid through the gastric mucosa.

Zollinger-Ellison ulcers are caused by hypersecretion of acid, which results directly from high circulating levels of gastrin produced by endocrine tumors arising in the pancreas or wall of the small intestine.

In general, *Helicobacter* infection, NSAIDs, and Zollinger-Ellison syndrome appear to be independent risk factors for PUD. Thus, the prevalence of *Helicobacter* infection in Zollinger-Ellison patients with ulcer is no different from the prevalence in those without ulcer. Likewise, patients infected with *Helicobacter* are not more likely to develop ulcers when administered NSAIDs. However, patients with *Helicobacter*-related ulcers are more likely to suffer bleeding after ingestion of NSAIDs, because of their antiplatelet effect.

Other factors traditionally thought to be important in the causation of PUD can now be said to modify the risk of ulcer disease, but in themselves are insufficient to result in ulcers. Of these, the most important is cigarette smoking. The risk of development of duodenal ulcer, the risk of failure to heal on antisecretory therapy, and the risk of recurrence are directly proportional to the number of cigarettes smoked. However, eradication of *H. pylori* infection eliminates the risk of recurrent ulcer disease in both smokers and nonsmokers. There remains no definable increased risk of PUD related to chronic alcohol ingestion, diet, or psychological stress.

DIAGNOSIS

History and physical examination cannot be relied on as an accurate diagnostic method for PUD. Thus, only one-third of patients with "classic" ulcer symptoms have PUD at endoscopy. Nevertheless, the presence of an ulcer is usually suggested initially by symptoms compatible with an ulcer. The classic symptoms of duodenal ulcer include burning epigastric pain that awakens the patient at night and is relieved by meals and antacids. Gastric ulcer patients are more likely to experience early satiety, nausea and vomiting, exacerbation of pain by eating, and atypical pain location, such as left upper quadrant. However, no symptom complex can be considered either sensitive or specific for the diagnosis of PUD.

In clinical practice, patients with PUD most commonly present with a subset of symptoms known collectively as dyspepsia. Dyspeptic symptoms include burning epigastric pain, upper abdominal gas, bloating, and nausea. Most patients with dyspepsia have the poorly understood syndrome of nonulcer dyspepsia, the etiology of which is likely multifactorial. Some dyspeptic patients have an atypical epigastric presentation of gastroesophageal reflux disease. The most cost-effective and appropriate diagnostic approach to dyspepsia remains unsettled. Endoscopy should be performed promptly in patients over age 50 with new-onset dyspepsia or in those who have associated dysphagia, odynophagia, weight loss, anemia, or severe pain. For young patients with uncomplicated dyspepsia, several approaches are under evaluation. One is empirical therapy with H_2 antagonists followed by review of symptoms in 2 to 3 weeks, with endoscopy performed in those who fail to improve or who develop recurrent symptoms after one or two 8-week courses of H_2 antagonists. A second approach under evaluation is prompt endoscopic evaluation of all dyspeptic patients, with specific therapy reserved for those with endoscopic diagnoses. This approach leads to a higher number of endoscopies but fewer medication courses. A third approach under evaluation is to perform *H. pylori* serologic testing on uncomplicated dyspeptic patients. Serologic-negative patients are treated symptomatically, since they have little chance of having PUD; those who are positive undergo endoscopy to determine whether they have ulcers. Patients with ulcers are then treated for *Helicobacter*; ulcer-negative patients with *Helicobacter* gastritis are treated symptomatically. A fourth approach is to perform *H. pylori* serologic testing on all uncomplicated dyspeptic patients, with treatment of *Helicobacter* in all serologic-positive patients. Using this approach, ulcer patients would be expected to improve, but some nonulcer dyspepsia patients would return later with persistent symptoms despite eradication of *Helicobacter*. In this approach, endoscopy is reserved for patients returning with persistent symptoms after eradication of *Helicobacter*. The relative costs, benefits, and weaknesses of these approaches differ, but all of them are currently acceptable in clinical practice.

Double-contrast barium radiography is an acceptable alternative to endoscopy for the diagnosis of ulcer disease. However, endoscopy is preferred because it is more accurate in the detection of ulcers, allows the differentiation of active and inactive ulcer disease, allows biopsy of gastric ulcers to rule out malignancy, and allows documentation of histologic gastritis and *Helicobacter* infection.

MANAGEMENT

Helicobacter-Related Ulcers

Management of PUD is based on etiology. *Helicobacter*-related ulcers are managed primarily by eradication of *Helicobacter* infection. For optimal symptomatic response, an antisecretory agent is generally given in combination with anti-*Helicobacter* therapy. Proton pump inhibitors (PPIs) are the preferred antisecretory agents, since they also have anti-*Helicobacter* activity; when given in conjunction with triple therapy, they increase bacterial eradication rates. However, it is not essential to give antisecretory therapy, since ulcers heal with eradication of *Helicobacter* alone.

The current "gold standard" for eradication of *Helicobacter* is triple therapy with Pepto-Bismol 2 tablets or 30 mL four times daily, metronidazole (Flagyl) 250 mg four times daily, and tetracycline hydrochloride 500 mg four times daily, all given for 2 weeks. The eradication rate of this regimen when analyzed by meta-analysis is approximately 93%. For children, amoxicillin 500 mg four times daily can be substituted for tetracycline, but the eradication rate is lower—approximately 73%. Adults who have previously received metronidazole or have been refractory to previous courses of anti-*Helicobacter* therapy should be presumed to have *Helicobacter* strains that are metronidazole resistant, and clarithromycin (Biaxin) 500 mg three times daily should be substituted for metronidazole. The single most effective therapy is standard triple therapy plus concurrent administration of double-dose PPI given as a split dose (omeprazole [Prilosec]) 20 mg twice daily or lansoprazole [Prevacid] 30 mg twice daily). This "quadruple therapy" is associated with eradication rates of approximately 98%.

The principal alternative to bismuth-based triple or quadruple therapy is PPI-based triple therapy. PPI-based triple therapy involves administration of double-dose PPI given in split doses for 1 week (omeprazole 20 mg twice daily or lansoprazole 30 mg twice daily, plus clarithromycin 250 to 500 mg twice daily, plus either metronidazole 500 mg twice daily or amoxicillin 500 to 1000 mg twice daily). Eradication rates with PPI-based triple therapy are approximately 90% and have the advantage of twice-daily dosing of all medications, which could lead to superior compliance. However, this has not been proved in clinical trials. With any therapy for *Helicobacter*, it is necessary to emphasize the importance of patient compliance.

Regimens consisting of a PPI and one antibiotic are not appropriate for clinical use. Eradication rates with a PPI plus amoxicillin alone have been as low as 50%. Likewise, a PPI plus clarithromycin is associated with eradication rates of only 75%. Thus, at the present time, all forms of *Helicobacter* therapy require the use of three or four medications.

The healing of *Helicobacter*-related ulcers by antisecretory therapy or the administration of sucralfate (Carafate) alone is possible but is generally inadvisable, since failure to eradicate *Helicobacter* is associated with recurrence of PUD. However, administration of one of these therapies along with *Helicobacter* eradication therapy is likely to improve symptom relief. If these therapies are utilized as the sole treatment for *Helicobacter*-related ulcers, the following guidelines are appropriate. First, the PPIs (omeprazole 20 mg per day or lansoprazole 15 to 30 mg per day) produce faster healing of PUD than H_2-receptor antagonists. However, the clinical importance of this may be minimal. More than 90% of ulcers are healed by a single daily dose of PPI administered in the morning for 4 weeks.

Four H_2-receptor antagonists are available in the United States. For duodenal ulcer, the effective doses are cimetidine (Tagamet) 800 mg at bedtime, 400 mg twice daily, or 300 mg four times daily; ranitidine (Zantac) or nizatidine (Axid) 300 mg at bedtime or 150 mg twice daily; and famotidine (Pepcid) 40 mg at bedtime or 20 mg twice daily. For gastric ulcer, only the split-dose regimens should be used.

The dose of sucralfate for healing duodenal ulcers is 1 gram four times daily. Sucralfate has comparable effectiveness to H_2-receptor antagonists and should not be considered superior to H_2-receptor antagonists for healing duodenal ulcers in smokers or in the elderly. The effectiveness of sucralfate for healing gastric ulcers is less well established.

NSAID–Related Ulcers

Ingestion of NSAIDs has been associated with ulceration and stricture formation in the esophagus, ulceration of the stomach and duodenum, and ulceration and stricture formation in the small bowel and colon. The most common sites of NSAID–related gastrointestinal tract injury are the stomach and duodenum. Unlike *Helicobacter*-related ulcers, which are most common in the duodenal bulb, NSAID–related ulcers are most common in the stomach. Although only approximately 20% of NSAID–related ulcers are located in the duodenal bulb, bleeding and perforation associated with NSAID ingestion occur as commonly from duodenal ulcers as from gastric ulcers. Thus, a given NSAID–related duodenal ulcer is more likely to bleed than an NSAID–related gastric ulcer. This may relate in part to the rich vascular supply of the duodenal bulb.

NSAID–related ulcers are common, occurring in 10 to 15% of patients chronically ingesting NSAIDs. About 1 to 3% of persons chronically ingesting NSAIDs suffer a complication of bleeding or perforation. It has been estimated that approximately 2600 persons with rheumatoid arthritis die each year in the United States because of NSAID–related gastrointestinal tract complications. Approximately one-third of the cost of arthritis management in the United States is consumed by the diagnosis and treatment of NSAID–related gastrointestinal tract complications.

NSAIDs vary in their ulcerogenic potential. As mentioned earlier, the principal mechanisms by which NSAIDs cause ulcers are systemic inhibition of prostaglandin synthesis and their direct topical toxic effect. In general, the ulcerogenicity of NSAIDs is related to their potency and, to a lesser extent, their duration of action. Thus, the relative risk of ulcer from piroxicam is about three times higher than from ibuprofen. NSAIDs diminish prostaglandin synthesis by inhibition of cyclooxygenase. Two cyclooxygenase isoenzymes, designated COX-1 and COX-2, have been described. Recently, NSAIDs have been developed that specifically inhibit COX-2 and have considerably decreased ulcerogenic potential. However, these agents should still be considered to have ulcerogenic potential, particularly in high-risk individuals.

The development of NSAID–related ulcers in patients on chronic therapy is unpredictable, but certain clinical features are associated with increased risk. The clearest risk factor is a history of previous PUD. Concomitant use of corticosteroids is also a major risk factor, and it is likely that some increased risk is associated with cigarette smoking and advanced age. Patients in these categories may be considered candidates for prophylactic therapy to prevent PUD when started on chronic NSAID therapy. H_2-receptor antagonists are well-tolerated prophylactic agents and have been proved to prevent NSAID–related duodenal ulcers but are not effective in the prevention of NSAID–related gastric ulcers. H_2-receptor antagonists should be used in full split doses when given for prophylaxis of NSAID–induced duodenal ulcers. The prostaglandin analogue misoprostol (Cytotec) has been shown to prevent NSAID–related duodenal and gastric ulcers and also to prevent NSAID–related complications, particularly perforation. However, the agent is often poorly tolerated because of abdominal cramping and diarrhea.

NSAID–related ulcers are notorious for their tendency to remain asymptomatic until the development of a complication. There is a remarkable association between the presence of symptoms and endoscopic findings in patients taking NSAIDs. Thus, most patients who develop dyspepsia while taking NSAIDs have either normal endoscopic findings or the presence of only superficial erosions. Conversely, most patients with NSAID–related PUD are asymptomatic. Diagnostic endoscopy in dyspeptic patients on NSAIDs can be reserved for those with evidence of bleeding, dysphagia, odynophagia, weight loss, vomiting, or severe pain.

Management of apparent NSAID–related ulcers should include testing for the presence of *Helicobacter* and eradication of the infection if it is present. The rationale for *Helicobacter* eradication in patients with PUD on NSAIDs is that in clinical practice it is impossible to determine whether *Helicobacter* was a factor in the pathogenesis of the patient's PUD. Patients with apparent NSAID–related duodenal ulcers should be treated with a full 8-week course of H_2-receptor antagonists or full-dose sucralfate or with a 4-week course of a PPI. NSAID–related duodenal ulcers are relatively easy to heal, and healing can often be achieved even while the patient continues NSAID ingestion. Proper treatment of NSAID–related gastric ulcers depends on whether the patient continues the NSAID. In most clinical cases, the NSAID is discontinued. In this instance, gastric ulcers can be treated with either full-dose H_2-receptor antagonists or a PPI. If the ulcer is larger than 5 mm, the PPI provides superior healing rates and is preferred. Patients with NSAID–related gastric ulcers who must continue taking NSAIDs pose a difficult treatment problem. These patients require pro-

found suppression of acid secretion to heal their ulcers, and H_2-receptor antagonists are frequently unsuccessful. PPIs are preferred, and if the ulcer is large (>5 mm), the PPI should be given in a double dosage. NSAID–related gastric ulcers may be quite large at the time of diagnosis and require several months or longer to heal, even with double-dose PPI.

GASTRIC TUMORS

method of
GERARD V. ARANHA, M.D.
Loyola Stritch School of Medicine
Maywood, Illinois

and

G. ROBERT MASON, M.D.
Hines Veterans Administration Hospital
Hines, Illinois

BENIGN GASTRIC TUMORS

Benign tumors of the stomach can originate from any tissue in the stomach. These tumors are rare, constituting less than 5% of gastric tumors. Those most commonly seen arising from mesenchymal origin are the leiomyomas and neurofibromas. From the endoderm, various forms of polyps can be found. These can be of various histologic types, including hyperplastic, adenomatous, hamartomatous, and juvenile polyps, as well as villous adenomas.

Leiomyoma

Leiomyoma of the stomach, though rare, is the most common benign mesenchymal tumor of the stomach, constituting almost half of benign gastric tumors. These tumors are usually asymptomatic, with a majority being found either at autopsy or incidentally at laparotomy for other disease. However, virtually all leiomyomas greater than 3 cm are symptomatic, causing either gastrointestinal hemorrhage or abdominal pain. Rarely, if they develop a pedunculated stalk, these large leiomyomas will present with gastric outlet obstruction. Almost 50% of leiomyomas are located in the body of the stomach, anteriorly. Leiomyomas may be submucosal, intramucosal, or subserosal. As the tumor grows toward the mucosa, it can outgrow its blood supply thus resulting in avascular necrosis of the overlying mucosa with subsequent bleeding.

The most useful test in making a diagnosis of leiomyoma is an upper gastrointestinal series. Since these lesions can be submucosal, endoscopy with biopsy can frequently miss the lesion. Enucleation has been suggested as adequate treatment; however, the gross features of leiomyosarcoma can resemble benign leiomyoma, and frozen-section diagnosis of malignancy in these tumors can be difficult. The only proper way to treat them is complete surgical excision with a normal margin. Recently attention has been directed to leiomyoblastoma of the stomach. These lesions may be benign or malignant. The treatment of benign leiomyoblastoma is the same as that for leiomyoma—that is, complete surgical resection.

Polyps

Hyperplastic polyps are the most common type of benign gastric polyp (Japanese types I and II) and appear to have no malignant potential specific to the polyp but are associated with atrophic gastritis, which does have a premalignant potential. Adenomatous polyp (Japanese types III and IV) appear to have malignant potential, since foci of carcinoma can be found in approximately 40% of the villous polyps, 24% in adenomatous polyps greater than 2 cm in diameter, and 4% in those less than 2 cm. Patients with gastric polyps will usually present with an iron deficiency anemia. Endoscopic polypectomy is indicated in all gastric polyps. If the polyps are found to be hyperplastic or tubular adenomas, no further treatment is necessary. However, if the polyp is found to be a villous adenoma, a complete resection is mandatory. If invasive carcinoma is found in the polyp, then gastric resection according to anatomic guidelines is indicated. Surgical excision is also indicated for those polyps that are greater than 2 cm and for multiple polyps, either sporadically or as part of a polyposis syndrome. Most forms of sporadic adenomatous polyps in the stomach are limited to the antrum and will be treated effectively by distal gastrectomy. Rarely, polyps with invasive adenocarcinoma are found in the proximal stomach and total gastrectomy will be necessary.

MALIGNANT GASTRIC TUMORS

Gastric Leiomyosarcoma

Leiomyosarcomas account for 1 to 3% of all malignant gastric tumors. Their most common presentation is gastrointestinal bleeding and abdominal pain. Bleeding with either melena or hematemesis occurs in greater than 50% of patients. Weight loss is frequent. Occasionally these tumors will reach a large size, and physical examination will reveal a palpable mass. The primary diagnostic modality for these patients is an upper gastrointestinal series. Because these lesions can be submucosal, endoscopy with biopsy can often be negative. In one series, computed tomography (CT) scan was found to be useful in 25% of patients.

The choice of operation for gastric leiomyosarcomas depends on the size of the tumor and its invasiveness. In most series, subtotal or partial gastrectomy was used in over 70% of individuals. The difficulty in recommending a particular surgical approach is that the requirements for margin of resection are not known for gastric leiomyosarcoma. Anywhere from a 2- to a 10-cm margin has been proposed to be adequate. Several studies have shown that the extent of resection was not statistically associated with survival after adjusting for tumor size and grade. Thus routine total or subtotal gastrectomy is not warranted for gastric leiomyosarcoma. Partial gastrectomy or wedge resection is a reasonable alternative as long as a 2- to 4-cm margin can be obtained. In some cases, the entire stomach will be replaced by tumor. In this situation, a total gastrectomy can be undertaken. Sometimes adjacent organs are also involved and may require removal, e.g., spleen and tail of pancreas. En bloc resection of adjacent organs when carried out has not decreased the local recurrence rate and does not lead to long-term survival. Lymph node dissection is not routinely performed in these patients since there is a low rate of lymph node metastasis. There have been no randomized perspective studies using adjunctive radiation and chemotherapy in these patients. For the moment it is safe to assume that the addition of chemotherapy and radiation therapy does not result in significant prolongation of survival in the face of advanced disease.

The same treatment guidelines are recommended for the malignant variety of leiomyoblastoma. The median survival of patients undergoing curative resection for gastric leiomyosarcoma is 14 months, compared with 8 months for those having palliative procedures. The estimated 5-year survival rates are 34% and 10%, respectively.

Gastric Lymphoma

Gastric lymphoma is an uncommon tumor comprising less than 5% of all primary gastric malignancies. It is the most frequent type of extranodal, non-Hodgkin's lymphoma. It is thought that the incidence of gastric lymphoma is rising whereas the incidence of gastric adenocarcinoma has not been completely established as yet. Gastric lymphoma can occur in any age group, but most patients are over 50 years of age at the time of presentation. This tumor predominates in men by a ratio of 2:1. The usual presenting symptoms are upper abdominal pain, nausea and vomiting, and weight loss. Other symptoms include weakness, gastrointestinal bleeding, and loss of appetite. Sometimes gastric lymphoma will present as a gastric perforation. Because symptoms are vague, many patients will not be seen until they have developed large, bulky tumors. Because of the upper gastrointestinal symptoms, these patients frequently undergo endoscopy and biopsy, which will often establish the diagnosis.

Once primary gastric lymphoma has been diagnosed, every effort should be made to rule out the presence of systemic lymphoma. The staging tests include routine blood examination, with complete blood count (CBC) and sequential multiple analyses, chest radiograph, abdominal computed tomography (CT), and bone marrow biopsy. The Ann Arbor Staging System is most commonly used. Gastric lymphoma will spread to the regional lymph nodes and contiguous organs, followed by distant metastasis. Historically, surgery has been the treatment of choice for gastric lymphomas. During abdominal exploration the extent of disease is assessed. Every effort is made to obtain a curative resection. Traditionally, a radical total gastrectomy with splenectomy and en bloc lymph node dissection has been performed to assure adequate margins. However, more recent reports indicate that lesser gastric resections are sufficient. The goal of a curative resection should be the removal of all gross disease, along with regional lymph nodes. Resectability rates range from 66% to 88%. The mortality is higher in those undergoing palliative procedures. The 5-year survival rate after curative resections ranges from 50% to 90%. This compares to 25% when palliative procedures are performed. This obviously reflects a selection: those patients having earlier stage disease undergo curative resections whereas those with advanced disease have palliative resections.

Although the goal of surgical therapy is complete resection, one needs to proceed with caution if the lymphoma extends into the duodenum distally or the esophagus proximally. In these situations an extensive procedure in an attempt to achieve clear margins is not indicated. Further biopsy is indicated for abnormalities seen in the liver at the time of surgery or for direct extension. Likewise, splenectomy is also indicated only with the direct extension of the lymphoma into the spleen. Radiation therapy has been proposed as primary therapy for eradication of local disease and as adjunctive to complete or palliative surgical resection. In one study from Memorial Sloan-Kettering Hospital in New York, patients undergoing surgery alone had a 5-year survival of 33%, whereas those with adjunctive radiation had a 5-year survival of 65%. However, all other studies of adjunctive radiotherapy have not shown any benefit over complete curative gastric resection.

A significant proportion of patients with gastric

lymphoma develop systemic disease. To address this problem, several centers have used chemotherapy after local therapy or as primary treatment. The most commonly used chemotherapy regimen has been cyclophosphamide (Cytoxan), doxorubicin (Adriamycin), vincristine (Oncovin), prednisone and bleomycin (Blenoxane) (CHOP-BLEO), and radiotherapy. In one recent report, patients with stage IE and stage IIE gastric lymphoma were treated by endoscopic or open biopsy followed by alternating chemotherapy and radiation therapy. They received four cycles of CHOP-BLEO followed by 3000 to 5000 cGy and subsequent eight additional cycles of chemotherapy. The 5-year survival in this group was 73%, and the disease-free survival was 62%. There were two treatment-related deaths for a mortality rate of 6%.

It is difficult to determine the ideal treatment of gastric lymphoma from a review of the literature. Our approach is that patients who have stage IE and stage IIE gastric lymphoma undergo complete resection. If complete resection is possible, no further therapy is necessary. However, if this is not possible, then radiation therapy would assist local control. Chemotherapy is given for those who have diffuse disease and for those who have curative resections but poor prognostic factors, i.e. large tumor size, increased tumor penetration, lymph node involvement, and a poorly differentiated histology.

Gastric Adenocarcinoma

The incidence of gastric adenocarcinoma has been steadily decreasing in the United States: in 1995, there were estimated to be 22,800 new cases and 14,700 deaths from the tumor. Gastric adenocarcinoma accounts for over 95% of gastric malignancies. Gastric carcinoma is more common in men than in women, with a 2:1 ratio. A high incidence of carcinoma of the stomach is reported from Japan, Iceland, Chile, Costa Rica, Poland, Hungary, Portugal, Czechoslovakia, Bulgaria, Austria, Italy, and Rumania. Several entities are thought to be precursors of gastric carcinoma: (1) chronic gastritis, (2) intestinal metaplasia, (3) adenomatous polyps, (4) gastric remnants (postgastrectomy state), (5) Ménétrier's disease, and (6) gastric epithelial dysplasia. The difference in incidence of gastric carcinoma from country to country supports an environmental etiology. Studies of Japanese migrants to the United States show that the migrant population carries the same risk as the indigenous population. Diets high in salt and smoked fish and meat that contains nitrates have been associated with an increase in gastric carcinoma in countries such as Japan and Iceland. Recently studies have shown that 60% to 70% of patients with gastric carcinoma reveal *Helicobacter pylori* in biopsy specimens of the gastric mucosa. At present, it is felt that blood Group A and pernicious anemia have a minor relationship to the development of gastric adenocarcinoma.

PATHOLOGY

Pathologically, gastric adenocarcinoma falls under two separate classifications. One is that of Lauren, a histologic system in which two carcinoma types are seen—intestinal (well-differentiated) and diffuse (infiltrating or poorly differentiated). The intestinal type of tumor is more common in populations at high risk and has a strong environmental component. It arises in areas of gastric mucosa altered by chronic gastritis or intestinal metaplasia, carries a better prognosis, and is the type that has shown decreased incidence in Western industrialized countries. The diffuse type or endemic form is predominant in populations at low risk. The second type of pathologic classification of gastric adenocarcinoma is based on the Borrmann classification, a macroscopic system containing five types. Type 1 includes polypoidal or fungating cancers; 2, ulcerating lesions surrounded by elevated borders; 3, ulcerating lesions infiltrating the gastric wall; 4, tumors with diffuse infiltrating carcinoma; and 5, unclassifiable cancers. In addition, a separate type of gastric carcinoma is seen, early gastric cancer. This is a unique form of gastric neoplasm that is histologically confined to the mucosa but is highly curable following adequate resection. The TNM staging system defined by the International Union Against Cancer and the American Joint Committee on Cancer has been widely adopted by Western nations for staging of gastric adenocarcinoma.

DIAGNOSIS

The presence of gastric adenocarcinoma can be variable and vague. Early gastric carcinoma may have no symptoms, and most patients who have symptoms already have advanced disease. This leads to a poor 5-year survival rate. The most common symptoms at presentation, in decreasing frequency, are weight loss, abdominal and epigastric pain, vomiting, and bowel symptoms such as anorexia, dysphagia, nausea, weakness, hematemesis, regurgitation, and early satiety. Therefore, unexplained symptoms of fatigue and dyspepsia associated with weight loss or anemia in patients older than 40 years of age should be viewed with suspicion and require investigation.

Clinical findings may be minimal or may denote advanced disease. These will include an abdominal mass, loss of weight, liver enlargement, the presence of a supraclavicular node, ascites, pelvic mass, and Blumer's (rectal) shelf. The two oldest methods for confirming the presence of gastric adenocarcinoma are the upper gastrointestinal series and fiberoptic gastroscopy. We favor upper GI endoscopy as a cost-saving measure. Endoscopy, in addition to obtaining a diagnosis, also allows the differential of a malignant ulcer from a benign ulcer of peptic origin.

Once diagnosis is made, further staging is conducted, and we support the use of an abdominal CT and endoscopic ultrasound. Both tests, we feel, could be used in conjunction, the CT to assess distant metastasis and the endoscopic ultrasound to asses the depth of invasion of the primary tumor and the lymph node status. At present there are no useful biochemical markers for gastric carcinoma.

TREATMENT

Gastric cancer can be treated by three different therapeutic modalities: surgery, radiation therapy, and chemotherapy. The choice of whether to use these singly or in combination depends upon the stage of the disease. Patients with localized gastric cancer are candidates for surgery with curative intent with or without adjunctive chemotherapy or irradiation. Patients with unresectable or partially resectable or disseminated cancer require treatments that include chemotherapy with or without radiation therapy or palliative surgery. Resection provides the most effective relief of symptoms and constitutes the only modality for potential cure of adenocarcinoma of the stomach. Operations for gastric carcinoma include resection of all or part of the stomach (total or subtotal gastrectomy, respectively), removal of the regional lymph nodes adjacent to the stomach and along the arterial branches of the celiac axis, and omentectomy.

The radical nature of the operation for gastric cancer refers primarily to the extent of lymph node dissections. An R_1 resection refers to removing nodes along the stomach wall. An R_2 resection refers to nodes removed along the branches of the celiac artery—that is, the hepatic, splenic, and left gastric arteries. An R_3 resection refers to lymph nodes removed along the portal vein. Because extensive lymphadenectomy is thought to be associated with high complication rates, many surgeons have adopted a conservative approach, that is, gastrectomy without extensive lymphadenectomy. However, recent data from Memorial Sloan-Kettering Cancer Center suggest that the resection of one lymph level beyond that involved by metastatic tumor was associated with significantly improved survival, accomplished with only a minimal increase in postoperative complications.

We support the recommendation of radical gastrectomy based on the "R-N" formula. Using this formula, most patients with N1 disease would be treated with R_2 gastrectomy, and patients with no demonstrable lymph node metastases would not undergo a radical lymphadenectomy. Patients with lymph node metastases beyond the N1 echelon would not be candidates for curative resection. Our recommendation for gastric resection of tumors of the stomach are as follows:

1. Tumors of the distal third of the stomach. These patients undergo radical subtotal gastrectomy. Resection usually involves between 75% to 90% of the distal stomach and 2 to 3 cm of the first portion of the duodenum, the hepatogastric omentum, and all of the greater omentum. In addition an R_1 and R_2 lymphadenectomy is performed.

2. Tumors of the middle third of the stomach. Frequently, tumors of the upper part or middle third may require total gastrectomy. Those in the true middle part of the stomach or the lower part of the middle of the body of the stomach will be treated adequately by a radical subtotal gastrectomy as just outlined. Preserving a small cuff of stomach in these patients makes for a safer anastomosis.

3. Tumors of the upper third and cardia. These patients undergo a total gastrectomy plus omentectomy, the removal of the hepatogastric mesentery, 2 to 3 cm of duodenum, and reconstruction by Roux-en-Y esophagogastrectomy. An R_1 and R_2 lymph node resection is also included. We feel that extended radical gastrectomy has substantial postoperative morbidity and mortality and is unlikely to improve survival; therefore, removal of the spleen and distal pancreas is not routinely recommended unless these are involved by the gastric tumor.

The 5-year survival following gastrectomy according to the American Joint Committee on Cancer is stage I—50%, stage II—29%, stage III—13%, and stage IV—3%. Palliative surgery is sometimes required for bleeding and obstruction. This may be undertaken as a simple distal gastrectomy even in the presence of liver metastasis. Patients with ascites, carcinomatosis, and extensive liver metastasis and those who have high operative risk due to heart disease or other co-morbid conditions are generally not considered for palliative operations because of their high risk of postoperative complications and expected short survival.

Because gastric adenocarcinoma shows a propensity for local, regional, and distant failure, several studies have investigated the role of adjunctive radiation therapy and chemotherapy. Results with 5-fluorouracil used alone have been disappointing. Currently, 5-FU is usually administered in combination with radiotherapy as a sensitizing agent. Chemotherapy has been used in various combinations for gastric adenocarcinoma. These drugs have included 5-fluorouracil, mitomycin (Mutamycin), doxorubicin (Adriamycin), cytarabine (Cytosar-U), and cisplatin (Platinol). Increased survival has not been demonstrated with adjunctive therapy. One study from Seoul has suggested that a long survival can be obtained with the adjunctive use of systemic immuno-chemo-surgery, that is, a resection, a radical gastrectomy followed by 5FU, mitomycin, and cytarabine for chemotherapy, and OK 432* *(Streptococcus pyogenes)* for immunotherapy. The efficacy of this regimen has to be confirmed by other centers.

Radiation therapy as a primary curative therapy is not helpful in patients suitable for resection. It is generally considered as an adjunct to surgical treatment or chemotherapy or in the palliation of obstructing or bleeding, unresectable tumors. Intraoperative radiotherapy has been demonstrated to have definite effects on locally advanced gastric carcinoma in combination with external beam radiotherapy. However, the modality of adjunctive therapy requires further evaluation. More recently, in the hope of improving survival for patients with gastric adenocarcinoma, neoadjuvant therapy has been used. In one Phase II study, etoposide, doxorubicin, and cisplatin were used prior to surgery. The overall response rate was 73%. Twenty-one percent of those patients with locally advanced gastric carcinoma had complete responses. Because of the small number of patients treated, no definite statements can be made about the role of neoadjuvant therapy in the treatment of gastric adenocarcinoma. This approach, however, deserves further investigation and should possibly be part of a large cooperative group trial.

---

*Investigational drug in the United States.

TUMORS OF THE COLON AND RECTUM

method of
DONALD G. KIM, M.D.,
ROBERT D. MADOFF, M.D., and
STANLEY M. GOLDBERG, M.D.

University of Minnesota
Minneapolis, Minnesota

Colon and rectal carcinoma is the fourth most common cancer (excluding skin cancer) in the United States and is the second most common cause of cancer-related deaths in men and women. Lifetime risk of developing colon or rectal carcinoma is 1 in 16 for males and 1 in 17 for females. Approximately 133,500 new cases are diagnosed annually in the United States: 94,500 are colon cancer and 39,000 are rectal cancer. An estimated 54,900 people will die of colon and rectal cancer this year. In men, colorectal carcinoma constitutes approximately 9% of the estimated cancer deaths, surpassed only by lung and prostate carcinomas. Among women, colorectal carcinoma accounts for approximately 10% of cancer-related deaths, following lung and breast carcinomas in frequency. The overall 5-year survival rate for colorectal carcinoma is 61 and 58%, respectively, for men and women. Although there has been a decrease in incidence and mortality rates nationwide, with an overall increase in survival, there has been no change in survivorship by stage.

Colorectal carcinoma affects predominantly the elderly. The incidence begins to rise in the sixth decade and peaks in the seventh and eighth decades, with an average age of 67 years. Approximately 6 to 8% of colorectal carcinomas are diagnosed in persons under 40 years of age.

EPIDEMIOLOGY AND PATHOGENESIS

Environmental and genetic factors appear to play a role in the etiology of colorectal cancer. The incidence and mortality rates for colorectal cancer vary throughout the world. The United States was ranked twentieth for males and nineteenth for females among 62 industrialized nations reporting colorectal cancer mortality. Reported age-adjusted death rates per 100,000 population for colorectal carcinoma were lowest in Mexico and Ecuador, whereas the highest rates were noted in Czechoslovakia and Hungary. Of the environmental factors, diet appears to be the most important. Studies have suggested a relationship between a low-fiber diet, bile salts, and dietary fat and a higher incidence of colorectal carcinoma. Increased intake of dietary fiber has been associated with a lower risk of colorectal carcinoma. Other dietary factors—including calcium; selenium; vitamins A, D, C, and E; and sulfur-containing compounds derived from garlic and onion—may play a role in the chemoprevention of colorectal carcinoma.

It is generally believed that colorectal carcinomas arise from benign neoplastic polyps. The notion of an adenoma-carcinoma sequence has become a well-accepted concept. Polyps recognized as precursor lesions are defined pathologically as tubular, tubulovillous, or villous adenomas (Table 1). The most common type is the tubular adenoma, which constitutes 75% of neoplastic colon polyps. Tubulovillous adenomas account for 15%, and pure villous adenomas for 10% of neoplastic colon polyps. The malignant potential of an adenomatous polyp is based on the histology and size of the lesion. The risk of malignancy increases with increasing villous component. Five percent of tubular adenomas harbor a malignancy, versus 22% of tubulovil-

TABLE 1. Neoplastic Colorectal Polyps

Type of Polyp	Incidence (%)	Malignancy (%)
Tubular adenoma	75	5
Tubulovillous adenoma	15	22
Villous adenoma	10	40

lous and 40% of villous adenomas. Invasive malignancy is uncommon in polyps under 1 cm in diameter, but there is a substantial increase in risk in polyps greater than 2 cm. Over 50% of villous adenomas larger than 2 cm are malignant.

Once diagnosed, polyps should be removed. The method of removal depends on polyp size, morphology, and location. The vast majority can be removed via the colonoscope. Those lesions that reveal a focus of carcinoma must be assessed as to the level of invasion, polyp morphology, and adequacy of the polypectomy margin. Further surgical management is based on these factors.

Several recent studies have stressed the existence of small flat adenomas, distinct from the typical adenomatous polyps, that have a strong propensity for malignant degeneration and invasiveness. These flat colorectal neoplastic lesions, even when invasive, are difficult to detect with conventional colonoscopy. This difficulty may be compounded by a lack of awareness of the existence and significance of these lesions. These lesions may be more common than anticipated due to the difficulty in detecting them; however, because the majority of reports have come from Japan, their existence in Western countries has been debated. Lynch and coworkers recently described a rare variant of familial adenomatous polyposis (FAP) in which affected individuals develop multiple flat adenomas and are at high risk for colorectal cancer. Further investigation of small, flat colorectal neoplasms is warranted to elucidate the clinical importance of these lesions in Western countries.

Although most colorectal cancer is considered to be sporadic (70 to 80%), 5 to 10% of colorectal carcinomas are considered to be inheritable. The role of genetics is most striking in the adenomatous polyposis syndromes, accounting for 1% of colorectal carcinomas, and in hereditary nonpolyposis colon cancer (HNPCC), accounting for an additional 6%. These syndromes are conferred in an autosomal dominant inheritance pattern.

The adenomatous polyposis syndromes include FAP, Gardner's syndrome (related osteomas, sebaceous cysts, and desmoid tumors), and Turcot's syndrome (related central nervous system tumors). The syndromes are characterized by hundreds to thousands of colorectal polyps that develop after puberty. Colorectal carcinoma develops by 40 years of age in virtually 100% of untreated patients.

HNPCC syndromes are manifested by a family history of colon cancer that typically occurs at an early age. The diagnosis of HNPCC has relied on pedigree analysis. Consensus criteria popularly known as the Amsterdam criteria have been established (Table 2). Modification has resulted in the Copenhagen criteria, which permit substitution of uterine or small bowel cancer for colon cancer. These cancers are frequently located in the proximal colon and are related to replication errors and microsatellite instability. HNPCC has been divided further into Lynch Type I syndrome, in which cancers are confined to the colon, and Lynch Type II (cancer family syndrome), in which cancers occur in the colon and related organs (uterus, ovary, breast, stomach, and pancreas, among others).

TABLE 2. Hereditary Nonpolyposis Colon Cancer (HNPCC): Amsterdam Criteria*

1. Greater than three histologically verified cases of colorectal cancer† in which two of the cases are first-degree relatives of the third
2. Colon cancer† occurring in more than one generation
3. Colon cancer† diagnosis under the age of 50 years in one case
4. Familial adenomatous polyposis is ruled out

*Diagnosis of HNPCC requires all four criteria.
†Copenhagen criteria permit the substitution of uterine or small bowel cancer for colon cancer.

The adenoma-carcinoma sequence has been well established for the development of colorectal carcinoma, and the molecular biology of colorectal neoplasia is among the best understood of human malignancies. Both oncogenes and tumor-suppressor genes are altered somatically in colorectal neoplasia. Oncogenes include *ras, src,* and *myc*; suppressor genes include the adenomatous polyposis coli (APC) gene, deleted in colorectal carcinoma (DCC) gene, mutated in colorectal cancer (MCC) gene, and p53. Two major genetic pathways have been identified leading to colorectal cancer. The "loss of heterozygosity" (LOH) pathway, implicated in adenomatous polyposis syndromes and sporadic colorectal cancers, describes the somatic gene mutations that accompany the adenoma-carcinoma sequence. These mutations tend to occur in a characteristic order, with APC mutation (long arm of chromosome 5, 5q) occurring early in the sequence, followed by K-*ras* gene mutation (short arm of chromosome 12, 12p), DCC deletion (long arm of chromosome 18, 18q), and p53 mutation or deletion (short arm of chromosome 17, 17p) as later events. However, it is the accumulation of mutations rather than their specific order that appears to be critical in carcinogenesis. The LOH pathway accounts for greater than 70% of sporadic colorectal carcinoma and all adenomatous polyposis syndromes. The second pathway, "replication error" (RER), occurs sporadically and is a characteristic of HNPCC. Mismatch repair genes involved in this pathway include DNA repair genes, four of which have been identified to date (MSH2, MLH1, PMS1, and PMS2). These genes are required by cells to repair DNA replication errors and spontaneous base-pair loss. Tumors developing along the RER pathway are characterized by a marked increase in replication errors within short segments of the genome containing repeating base pairs, termed microsatellites. Microsatellite instability is caused by inactivation of the mismatch repair pathway. Approximately 20% of colorectal carcinomas develop along the RER pathway.

Clinical application of the molecular genetics of colorectal carcinoma is in its infancy. Recent clinical applications include the determination of APC gene mutations in familial polyposis kindreds and studies demonstrating a poorer prognosis associated with allelic loss of 18q and 17p. Four areas of potential applications are beginning to emerge: (1) prognostication and selection of patients for adjuvant therapy, (2) genetic diagnosis of inherited syndromes and presymptomatic testing, (3) fecal screening tests, and (4) gene and molecular therapy of colorectal neoplasia. As clinical applications are beginning to emerge, further research is necessary to clearly define how the various molecular genetic abnormalities can be useful.

SCREENING

The ultimate goal of a screening program is to identify an individual in an asymptomatic population in the early stages of a neoplastic process, thus increasing the likelihood of a successful therapeutic outcome. Colorectal cancer is ideal for screening: it is sufficiently common, with significant morbidity and mortality, to warrant the health care expenditure; it has a prolonged curable preclinical phase (adenoma-carcinoma sequence); safe and accurate diagnostic tests are available; and detection of early lesions increases survival. To be a successful screening tool, the test not only must be simple and effective, with benefits outweighing detriments, but also should have a favorable cost/benefit ratio. Potential screening tests include digital examination, fecal occult blood testing (FOBT), flexible sigmoidoscopy, colonoscopy, and barium enema. Of these, FOBT and flexible sigmoidoscopy may meet the criteria for an effective mass screening test. Despite the popularity of these screening methods, there continues to be a degree of uncertainty regarding the effect of mass screening programs on colorectal cancer mortality and morbidity.

Screening for colorectal cancer has been recommended by the American Cancer Society, the National Cancer Institute, the World Health Organization, and the American College of Physicians. The United States Preventive Services Task Force has neither recommended nor discouraged screening. Screening recommendations for colorectal cancer have been outlined by the American Cancer Society (Table 3). Screening programs include digital examination, FOBT, and flexible sigmoidoscopy, with colonoscopy and barium enema reserved for selected patients.

Digital Examination

Digital examination is an integral part of a routine physical examination but it cannot be relied on as an accurate screening tool for colorectal carcinoma. Realistically, only a few rectal cancers are within reach of the examining finger.

FOBT

FOBT utilizes the peroxidase test (Hemoccult) to detect occult bleeding. Major problems with the test include suboptimal sensitivity (nonbleeding or intermittently bleeding cancers) and poor specificity (altered by ingestion of red meats, broccoli, turnips, red radishes, cauliflower, cantaloupe, and other foods). The only randomized study with definitive mortality results from the use of FOBT is the

TABLE 3. American Cancer Society Recommendations for Colorectal Cancer Screening

Population	Age	Procedure	Frequency
Asymptomatic, no risk factors	40	Digital rectal examination	Yearly
	50	Fecal occult blood test	Yearly
	50	Sigmoidocopy, preferably flexible	Every 3–5 years
First-degree relative of patient with colorectal cancer diagnosed at age ≤55	35–40	Colonoscopy or double-contrast barium enema	Every 5 years

University of Minnesota trial. A 33% reduction in mortality from colorectal cancer was reported when annual FOBT of rehydrated slides was combined with colonoscopy of those patients testing positive. Other studies failed to find such a decrease in mortality.

Flexible Sigmoidoscopy

Flexible sigmoidoscopy performed by an experienced, well-trained examiner allows visualization of up to 60 cm of the distal colon, reaching as far as the splenic flexure, and detection of 50 to 70% of all colorectal neoplasia. Case-controlled studies have documented that sigmoidoscopy can result in a 60% mortality reduction in rectosigmoid cancer, but randomized controlled trials have yet to be performed. For screening of asymptomatic individuals, current recommendations are for a flexible sigmoidoscopy at age 50 and repeated at 3- to 5-year intervals (see Table 3). With a presentation of Hemoccult-positive stools or a high-risk patient based on past medical history, proctosigmoidoscopy alone is insufficient. In these cases, full colonoscopy is the preferred examination.

Colonoscopy

Colonoscopy is currently the most accurate and complete examination of the large bowel. In addition to its diagnostic role, it has therapeutic potential in the management of many benign-appearing colonic neoplasms. Colonoscopy should not be used for screening low-risk patients but is useful as a definitive evaluation of selected high-risk patients. Colonoscopy is advised for those patients with a previous history of neoplastic polyps or colorectal cancer, a family history of adenomatous polyposis syndromes or colorectal cancer, or chronic ulcerative colitis or long-standing Crohn's colitis. Colonoscopy is recommended for patients in whom a polyp or cancer was recently diagnosed on proctosigmoidoscopy to rule out synchronous lesions.

Barium Enema

In general, a double-contrast barium enema is preferred over a single-column barium enema for diagnostic accuracy. A double-contrast barium enema is a less invasive and less expensive alternative to colonoscopy. A good-quality study can detect lesions as small as 0.5 cm. Although the diagnostic yield is less than for colonoscopy, each modality has its place, and the two tests should be considered complementary rather than competitive. When a complete examination of the colon is mandated, the double-contrast barium enema remains essential in patients with incomplete colonoscopic examinations. Also, a water-soluble contrast enema may be used in the evaluation of an obstructing lesion, where an endoscopic examination may be impossible. Because the diagnostic accuracy of the barium enema drops significantly in the rectum, a rigid or flexible proctosigmoidoscopy should be performed to complete the examination.

High-Risk Screening

Screening guidelines for the management of colorectal polyps have been recommended as a result of the National Polyp Study. After initial resection of an adenomatous polyp, the first follow-up examination does not usually have to be performed until 3 years later. The guidelines also advise that if the first follow-up is negative at 3 years, the second follow-up should be done in 5 years.

Screening in FAP should commence at puberty. Because colonic polyps rarely develop in the absence of rectal polyps, initial screening can be accomplished with annual flexible sigmoidoscopy. If polyps are identified, they should be biopsied to confirm their histologic type. Initial medical management of FAP patients may include sulindac, a nonsteroidal anti-inflammatory drug demonstrated to produce polyp regression. All patients with FAP should ultimately undergo prophylactic surgery, because the risk of developing colorectal carcinoma is 100%. The timing of the procedure and the type of procedure should be approached individually, based on factors such as age, extent of polyposis, extracolonic manifestations, associated morbidities, and social factors. Because of the complexity of surgical management, FAP patients are best served by referral to a specialized center interested in the care of these patients. Surgical options include colectomy with ileorectal anastomosis, restorative proctocolectomy, mucosectomy and pouch-anal anastomosis, or total proctocolectomy with ileostomy.

Chronic ulcerative colitis also carries a risk of cancer that increases with the duration of disease. The risk of cancer becomes significant after 10 years, with long-term risk estimates varying considerably. Current estimates of cancer risk vary from 1.3% at 18 years' duration to 24.2% at 20 years' duration. Screening methods consist of colonoscopic surveillance and random biopsies assessing for mucosal dysplasia. Although mucosal dysplasia has been used as a marker of colorectal carcinoma in ulcerative colitis screening, its accuracy is questionable. Dysplasia does not always precede cancer development and is not evenly distributed throughout the colon. Despite these drawbacks, no other effective screening method exists currently, and colonoscopy with random biopsies continues to be the screening method of choice in chronic ulcerative colitis.

Patients with Crohn's disease have an increased risk of gastrointestinal malignancies, but to a lesser degree than do chronic ulcerative colitis patients. The calculated risk is between 4 and 20 times that of the general population. Unlike in ulcerative colitis, in Crohn's disease the risk factors for the development of colorectal carcinoma are not well defined. In general, colorectal carcinoma developing in Crohn's colitis seems to occur in bypassed loops and fistulas, in sites of active macroscopic disease, in extensive colitis, and in patients with long-standing disease. The value of a rigorous surveillance program with random biopsies of the colon is unknown for Crohn's colitis patients, and such surveillance is generally not pursued. Because the cancers tend to develop in segments with active disease, biopsies assessing for cancer or dysplasia could be limited to these areas.

CLINICAL MANIFESTATIONS

Although detection of early asymptomatic colorectal carcinoma is the ideal scenario, the majority of patients present with cancers large enough to cause symptoms. The signs and symptoms of colorectal cancer are nonspecific and vary depending on the location and size of the lesion and the stage of disease. The typical symptoms of change in bowel habits and rectal bleeding first noted by the patient do not necessarily indicate an early lesion. Occult bleeding may present as mild iron-deficiency anemia or significant hypochromic, microcytic anemia, often associated with symptoms of progressive fatigue or new cardiac symptoms such as angina or congestive heart failure. A change in bowel habits may take the form of diarrhea, constipation, or alternating diarrhea and constipation and is usually noted in the later stages of tumor progression. Abdominal pain, another significant symptom of colon cancer, is also a late symptom. Rectal carcinoma may cause a feeling of incomplete evacuation or tenesmus. Bleeding is probably the most common symptom of colorectal cancer. The blood can be bright red or dark maroon. Most of the visible bleeding comes from left-sided lesions, whereas bleeding from the right side or transverse colon is usually occult. Clinical manifestations associated with right-sided or transverse colon lesions include anemia and weakness from occult bleeding. In left-sided lesions, pain and bleeding are accompanied by thin, narrow stools and a change in bowel habits. Obstruction is more common in left-sided lesions, usually in the region of the sigmoid or rectosigmoid. Weight loss, anorexia, and fatigue are often late symptoms of colorectal carcinoma.

PREOPERATIVE EVALUATION

Once the diagnosis of colorectal carcinoma has been made, preoperative evaluation should be initiated. The purpose of a preoperative work-up is to rule out synchronous carcinomas and polyps, stage the tumor, and assess the patient's perioperative risk factors. It is important to stress the management differences between colonic tumors and rectal tumors. Surgical resections for colonic tumors are standard for the tumor's location, regardless of the depth of invasion or the presence of nodal metastasis. Palliative resection is usually indicated in patients with distant metastasis. In rectal tumors, management options vary and include local therapy for selected lesions as well as preoperative adjuvant therapy in certain cases. Clinical staging in rectal tumors has become an important factor in determining the overall management. Therefore, preoperative staging of colonic tumors is not as important as it is for rectal tumors.

Colonoscopy

Total colonoscopy should be performed to fully evaluate the colon, ruling out synchronous lesions. Synchronous colorectal cancer has been reported in 2 to 8% of patients, and synchronous adenoma has been reported in 12 to 62% of patients. If total colonoscopy is unsuccessful or impractical, air-contrast barium enema can be used to complete the colon evaluation. In certain cases of obstructive colorectal carcinomas, a full colonic evaluation is impossible preoperatively by colonoscopy or Gastrografin enema. These patients should undergo an on-the-table colonoscopy at the time of operation or a colonoscopy postoperatively to rule out synchronous lesions. Colonoscopy at the time of operation has the advantage of identifying those synchronous lesions that require further resection.

Carcinoembryonic Antigen

Carcinoembryonic antigen (CEA) remains the most widely used diagnostic marker for colorectal cancer. Initial enthusiasm for CEA as a prognostic marker and a herald to undetectable recurrent disease has waned, however. Although CEA levels are often obtained preoperatively and may indicate an adverse prognosis if elevated, their utility is controversial. Many surgeons and oncologists do not routinely obtain CEA levels preoperatively or in routine follow-up of colorectal cancer patients.

Computed Tomography

Preoperative computed tomography (CT) scans are not routinely obtained. They may be helpful in documenting liver metastasis in the presence of abnormal liver function tests, but they usually do not alter the management of the primary lesion. They also may be helpful in advanced rectal lesions by documenting the extent of the lesion and adjacent organ invasion.

Magnetic Resonance Imaging

The role of magnetic resonance imaging (MRI) in the preoperative evaluation of colorectal carcinoma is undefined. MRI may become useful in the staging of rectal carcinoma with the development of rectal coils that enhance pelvic imaging. It may also be helpful in detecting recurrent disease within the pelvis, distinguishing tumor from fibrosis or postsurgical changes. It provides no advantage over CT in the evaluation of liver metastasis.

Endorectal Ultrasonography

Endorectal ultrasonography (ERUS) has proved invaluable in the evaluation of rectal cancer. ERUS can determine the depth of tumor penetration through the rectal wall and the presence of metastatic lymph nodes in the perirectal tissues. In experienced hands, ERUS has an accuracy rate of 80 to 90% for depth of wall invasion and a 70 to 80% accuracy rate for predicting lymph node status. With the trend toward more conservative local therapy of rectal cancer (local excision, endocavitary radiation, fulguration) and the availability of preoperative adjuvant therapy, preoperative staging of rectal carcinoma is becoming increasingly important in selecting the optimum therapy.

STAGING

In 1932, Cuthbert Dukes, a pathologist at St. Mark's Hospital in London, developed his classic classification of rectal cancer. Many modifications have followed, and the modified Astler-Coller classification is commonly used today. The TNM system has also been introduced into the classification of colorectal cancers (Table 4). The TNM system more accurately defines bowel wall penetration and nodal metastasis in order to stage colorectal carcinoma. This system has been widely adopted and has the advantage of including clinical observations rather than just pathologic findings. Rectal cancers staged clinically by ERUS are denoted by a uT, uN designation.

TABLE 4. **Staging Systems for Colorectal Cancer**

Primary Tumor (T)

Stage	Description	Stage	Dukes
Tis	Carcinoma in situ	0	A
T1	Tumor invades submucosa	I*	A
T2	Tumor invades muscularis propria	I*	B1/C1
T3	Tumor invades through muscularis propria into subserosa, or into nonperitonealized pericolic or perirectal tissues	II*	B2/C2
T4	Tumor directly invades other organs or structures and/or perforates visceral peritoneum	II*	B3/C3

Lymph Nodes (N)

Stage	Description	Stage	Dukes
N0	No regional lymph node metastasis		
N1	Metastasis in 1 to 3 pericolic or perirectal lymph nodes	III†	C1, 2, 3
N2	Metastasis in 4 or more pericolic or perirectal lymph nodes	III†	C1, 2, 3
N3	Metastasis in any lymph node along course of a named vessel, and/or metastasis to apical node(s) (when marked by the surgeon)	III†	C1, 2, 3

Distant Metastasis (M)

Stage	Description	Stage	Dukes
M0	No distant metastasis		
M1	Distant metastasis	IV‡	D

*N0, M0.
†Any T, M0.
‡Any T, any N.

SURGICAL THERAPY

The surgical treatment of colorectal cancer is based on the predictable behavior of the primary lesion and its spread to regional lymph nodes. The only effective curative therapy for carcinoma of the colon is complete operative removal. Rectal carcinoma is managed predominantly by operative resection, but endocavitary radiation can be used in selected early lesions. As discussed above, the differences in the management of colon and rectal tumors and neoplastic polyps warrant a separate discussion of the options available.

With widespread use of the laparoscope in abdominal surgery, laparoscopic techniques have been developed for the management of colorectal carcinoma. But with the alarming reports of port-site recurrences noted in the literature and the lack of survival data, it is premature to recommend "routine" laparoscopic resection for colorectal carcinoma. Final recommendations should await the results of ongoing prospective, randomized trials, and use of laparoscopic techniques should be limited to enrollment in these trials.

Polyps

Colonoscopic snare polypectomy is the procedure of choice in the management of colorectal polyps. Most polyps within the colon and rectum are accessible with a colonoscope and can be resected with minimal morbidity. Most pedunculated and small sessile polyps are easily removed with the snare. Large sessile polyps can be excised in a piecemeal fashion using the snare.

Management of polyps with invasive cancer is based on polyp morphology and the extent of invasion. Haggitt and coworkers have developed a polyp classification scheme (Table 5). For a pedunculated polyp with invasion into the head or upper part of the stalk (Levels 1 through 3), the risk of lymph node invasion is low, and no further surgery is indicated. If invasion extends to the base of the stalk (Level 4), there is a significant risk of lymph node metastasis, and bowel resection should be considered. Other adverse factors that mandate further resection include incomplete excision, a poorly differentiated tumor, lymphatic or vascular invasion, or invasion at the cautery margin. It must be stressed that the polyp must be totally removed to achieve a cure.

Colon Cancer

Surgical resection is the modality of choice for the management of colon carcinoma. This includes the

TABLE 5. **Haggitt Classification of Colorectal Polyps**

Level	Description
0	Carcinoma in situ, mucosal lesion without invasion into the muscularis mucosae
1	Carcinoma invading through the muscularis mucosae into the submucosa but limited to the head of the polyp
2	Carcinoma invading to the level of the junction between the adenoma and the stalk
3	Carcinoma invading any part of the stalk
4	Carcinoma invading into the submucosa of the bowel wall but above the muscularis propria

primary tumor and the associated mesentery that bears the regional lymphatics. For tumors involving the cecum and ascending colon, a right hemicolectomy encompassing the ileocolic, right colic, and right branch of the middle colic vessels is recommended. For lesions involving the hepatic flexure, an extended right hemicolectomy, including the distribution of the middle colic vessel, is indicated. Tumors involving the transverse colon and splenic flexure require complete excision of the distribution of the middle colic vessel and may include the right colon or descending colon to encompass an adequate drainage basin and/or achieve a tension-free anastomosis. Sigmoid lesions are appropriately treated by sigmoid colectomy. Primary anastomosis is almost always possible with colonic lesions. No benefit has been demonstrated from the no-touch isolation technique.

Tumors that invade neighboring structures such as the small bowel, bladder, ovaries, or uterus should be removed en bloc. In patients with multiple synchronous colon cancers or a colon cancer and multiple adenomatous polyps in different colonic segments, a subtotal colectomy is recommended.

Rectal Cancer

A variety of management options are available for rectal cancer patients and are based on the size, stage, mobility, location, and distance from the dentate line of the rectal tumor. Of all these variables, tumor distance from the dentate line has the greatest impact on the ability to achieve a primary anastomosis and avoid a permanent stoma.

Transanal local excision is ideally suited for lesions with low risk of nodal metastasis—T1 and selected T2 lesions. These lesions must be located within 10 cm of the anal verge, be less than 3 cm in size, be well to moderately differentiated, and involve less than 50% of the wall circumference. Above the 8- to 10-cm level, local excision is possible using transanal endoscopic microsurgery (TEM), which is available at centers specializing in this technique. Endocavitary radiation using a special proctoscope can be used in selected T1 and T2 lesions within 10 cm from the anal verge. This therapy is effective and well tolerated, but it is available only in centers specializing in this technique. Local therapy is ideally suited for early lesions, but it may be used in more advanced lesions in high-risk patients. ERUS is crucial in the selection of patients for these local techniques.

Standard resections of rectal carcinoma include anterior resection, sphincter-preserving coloanal resection, and abdominoperineal resection. Circular stapling devices have simplified the creation of low-lying distal colorectal and coloanal anastomoses, enabling the preservation of sphincter function. Controversial issues regarding resection of rectal carcinoma include level of mesenteric ligation, distal margin of resection, mesorectal excision, lateral margin of resection, radical pelvic lymphadenectomy, and role of covering stoma.

High ligation of the inferior mesenteric artery was initially advocated, but no controlled studies demonstrate a survival benefit. The traditional 5-cm distal margin rule has come under scrutiny, with several investigators demonstrating that cure is not compromised with a distal margin of 2 cm. Total mesorectal excision has been advocated, based on the belief that local recurrence in rectal carcinoma is due to microscopic spread of tumor into the distal mesorectum. This technique, without radiation therapy, has resulted in a local recurrence rate as low as 5%, with an average follow-up of 10 years. Clearance of the lateral margin has also been demonstrated to be critical in the prevention of local recurrence. Radical pelvic lymphadenectomy has been advocated by Japanese surgeons, but there is no clear evidence that this technique confers any survival benefit. The technique, requiring a substantial increase in operative time and accompanied by high morbidity, has not gained wide acceptance in the United States.

The level of the anastomosis after resection determines the need for covering stoma. Data from the University of Minnesota demonstrated increased leak rates in patients receiving double-stapled anastomoses less than 4 cm from the anal verge. As a result, patients with anastomoses less than 4 cm from the anal verge usually receive temporary proximal diversion. Patients with higher anastomoses who have received preoperative radiation therapy should also be considered for temporary diversion.

ADJUVANT THERAPY

Colon Cancer

For the past 40 years, 5-fluorouracil (5-FU) has been used with some success in the management of colon cancer. In 1989, the North Central Cancer Treatment Group reported that 5-FU in combination with levamisole increased disease-free survival in patients with Stage III (node-positive) colon cancer. Although this regimen has become standard therapy for patients with node-positive disease, the validity of the approach continues to be debated. There is no evidence to suggest that preoperative radiation or chemotherapy offers any survival benefit for colon cancer, and their use is limited to clinical trials.

Rectal Cancer

Adjuvant therapy of rectal carcinoma includes radiation therapy and chemotherapy as a means of decreasing local recurrence rates and improving survival. Controversy exists as to the timing of radiation therapy (preoperative, intraoperative, or postoperative), the radiation dosage schedule, and the effectiveness of chemotherapy. Although survival studies have documented reduced rates of local recurrence, no improvement in survival has been definitively demonstrated. Whereas postoperative radiation therapy has been the standard in the adjuvant setting, preoperative radiation is better tolerated and associated with fewer complications. Traditional radiation schedules deliver a dose of 40 to 50 Gy in a 5-week period, followed by surgery after a 5- to 6-week hiatus. In Sweden, short-term (5 to 7 days) high-dose radiation therapy delivering the bioequivalent dose of radiation is used, followed by surgery without a waiting period. Ongoing Swedish trials, refining the technique of short-term, high-dose preoperative radiation therapy, are beginning to show a survival benefit.

Preoperative radiation therapy combined with chemotherapy is also useful for improving the resectability of locally advanced rectal cancers. Combinations of adjuvant chemotherapy and radiation therapy have demonstrated advantages in survival when compared with surgery alone or postoperative radiation therapy alone. Important trials using 5-FU and leucovorin with either preoperative or postoperative radiation therapy are ongoing and may provide the answer to some of the existing controversies. Use of ERUS improves patient selection for preoperative adjuvant therapy through accurate staging, thereby diminishing the problem of overtreating patients with early lesions who would not require adjuvant therapy.

FOLLOW–UP

Patients who have had a colorectal cancer resected may or may not be cured. Local recurrences, metachronous lesions, and isolated pulmonary and liver metastases are potentially curable. The great majority of all recurrences occur within 3 years of the initial operation.

The most appropriate follow-up for resected patients has not been determined and remains controversial, because several studies have failed to demonstrate significant patient salvage despite intensive follow-up surveillance regimens. Rectal carcinomas have a much higher propensity for local recurrence and may warrant closer surveillance. The role of ERUS has yet to be established. Close ERUS follow-up of postoperative rectal cancer patients may detect local recurrences early, allowing timely intervention, but the benefits of the approach remain to be proved. Current rectal cancer follow-up regimens may include ERUS at 3- to 4-month intervals for the first 2 years postoperatively.

CEA determinations are commonly obtained at varying intervals postoperatively, but routine CEA monitoring has not been definitively shown to be of benefit, much less cost effective. Colonoscopy should be performed at 1 year and then at 3- to 5-year intervals thereafter to identify metachronous neoplasms. Routine CT scan is not recommended unless recurrence or metastasis is suspected based on the physical examination or abnormal laboratory tests.

INTESTINAL PARASITES

method of
ELIZABETH PHILLIPS, M.D., and
JAY S. KEYSTONE, M.D.
The Toronto Hospital
Toronto, Ontario, Canada

INTESTINAL PROTOZOA

Giardia intestinalis is an important cause of acute and chronic diarrhea in North Americans. Large water-borne outbreaks have been reported from communities in the Rocky Mountains and the Appalachian Mountains. Infection is occasionally acquired by hikers who drink unboiled ground water. *G. intestinalis* is a relatively common pathogen among children in day care centers; approximately 10% of children attending day care centers are asymptomatic carriers. Giardiasis can be acquired during international travel. Historically, giardiasis has been a problem for North Americans who visit St. Petersburg and other cities in the former Soviet Union. Although *G. intestinalis* is prevalent among children living in the developing world, it does not appear to be a significant cause of disease among them except in the first 2 years of life.

Metronidazole (Flagyl), administered at 250 mg three times a day for 5 days, is the drug of choice for the treatment of adults with giardiasis (it has not been approved for this specific indication by the FDA). Single-dose therapy appears to be equally well tolerated as multiple daily doses. In adults, 2 grams in a single dose is given daily with food for 3 days. Children less than 25 kg in weight receive 35 mg per kg per dose; those who weigh between 25 and 40 kg receive 50 mg per kg per dose for 3 days. Patients must be warned against the use of alcohol while taking metronidazole because of its disulfiram-like effect. Gastrointestinal disturbances, headache, dry mouth, and a metallic taste are frequent side effects. Metronidazole rarely has been associated with seizures, encephalopathy, peripheral neuropathy, ataxia, and pancreatitis. Clinical resistance to metronidazole has been described. Tinidazole (Fasigyn),* a nitroimidazole derivative similar to metronidazole, is effective when given as a single dose of 2 grams. It is well tolerated but occasionally can cause nausea, vomiting, rash, or a metallic taste. Furazolidone (Furoxone) is available in liquid form and therefore is often used to treat children. It is frequently associated with nausea and vomiting. Allergic reactions, hypoglycemia, and headache occur occasionally. Rarely, hemolytic anemia may be induced in those with glucose-6-phosphate dehydrogenase deficiency. Paromomycin (Humatin), an oral aminoglycoside that is poorly absorbed, can be used in dosages of 25 to 30 mg per kg per day in three divided doses for 7 days. It is not highly effective against *G. intestinalis* (approximately 50% efficacy) but has been used by

---

*Not available in the United States.

some to treat giardiasis during pregnancy. Albendazole,* a benzimidazole that has not been licensed for use in the United States, has been shown to be as effective as metronidazole in two randomized trials. It is administered as 400 mg daily for 5 days, has few adverse effects, and may be useful to treat patients with suspected clinical resistance to metronidazole. More recently, bacitracin zinc,† 120,000 U twice daily for 10 days, has been shown to have cure rates similar to those of metronidazole for the treatment of giardiasis. The major side effects are unpleasant taste and, less commonly, nausea, abdominal pain, and diarrhea. Quinacrine is no longer available for the treatment of giardiasis.

Entamoeba histolytica is an important cause of colitis and liver abscesses in areas of crowding, low socioeconomic status, and poor sanitation. Stools are almost always positive for gross or occult blood in persons with amebic colitis, but fecal leukocytes are frequently absent because they are lysed by trophozoites. It has recently been discovered that two distinct species of *Entamoeba* exist that are morphologically identical. *E. dispar* is the most prevalent species in North America and is associated with an asymptomatic carrier state. Serology may be useful to differentiate *E. histolytica* from *E. dispar*, since antibodies develop only during *E. histolytica* infection. No treatment is currently recommended for asymptomatic *E. dispar* infection. Asymptomatic infection with *E. histolytica* is treated with a luminally active agent such as iodoquinol (Yodoxin) or paromomycin. Iodoquinol uncommonly causes rash, thyroid enlargement, or gastrointestinal side effects and, very rarely, optic neuritis, optic atrophy, and loss of vision after prolonged use at high doses. It is contraindicated in patients with known iodine sensitivity. The usual dose should not exceed 650 mg three times per day for 20 days. Paromomycin is generally well tolerated but has been associated with eighth nerve and renal damage in patients with renal insufficiency. Diloxanide furoate (Furamide)* is not licensed for use in the United States but is a well-tolerated alternative. Flatulence is relatively frequent, and, on rare occasions, the drug is associated with diplopia, dizziness, urticaria, or pruritus. Invasive colitis or liver abscess should be treated with high-dose metronidazole, 750 mg three times per day for 10 days, followed by treatment with a luminally active agent described previously. Metronidazole, 2.5 grams in a single dose, has been shown to be very effective in the treatment of uncomplicated amebic liver abscesses. Outside the United States, tinidazole* is often used to treat *E. histolytica*; the dose and duration depend on the severity of infection as shown in Table 1. Tinidazole appears to be at least as effective as metronidazole and better tolerated.

Other intestinal protozoa are occasionally identified in the stools of asymptomatic persons and those with diarrhea. The significance of *Blastocystis hom-*

inis is controversial, but clinical responses have been anecdotally reported with metronidazole, 750 mg three times a day for 10 days; iodoquinol, 650 mg three times a day for 20 days; or paromomycin, 30 mg per kg per day for 7 days. Symptomatic infections with *Dientamoeba fragilis* may respond to iodoquinol, paromomycin, or tetracycline. *Dientamoeba fragilis* is thought to be transmitted within the eggs of *Enterobius vermicularis* (pinworm), and infections may not remit until the pinworm infection is treated.

Over the past decade, *Cryptosporidium parvum* has been increasingly recognized as a cause of enteric disease. It is endemic throughout the world and was recently responsible for a large water-borne epidemic in Wisconsin. *Cryptosporidium* has emerged as a major pathogen in patients with human immunodeficiency virus (HIV) infection. The organism typically causes self-limited diarrhea in immunocompetent persons, but it can cause severe, large-volume, chronic diarrhea in persons with concurrent HIV infection. Despite extensive studies of a large number of drugs, none has emerged as the treatment of choice for cryptosporidiosis. Paromomycin, 500 mg four times a day, may have some initial efficacy in the treatment of HIV-infected individuals with intestinal disease. Other agents such as octreotide (Sandostatin), to decrease the volume of diarrhea, or azithromycin (Zithromax),* 1250 mg per day for 2 weeks followed by 500 mg daily, have been used with variable success.

The HIV epidemic has brought attention to several other enteric protozoa. *Isospora belli*, which is common in some tropical areas but encountered infrequently in the United States, can produce self-limited disease in immunocompetent patients and severe, chronic diarrhea in patients with concurrent HIV infection. *I. belli* is susceptible to trimethoprim-sulfamethoxazole. Relapses are common in patients with HIV infection, and long-term suppressive therapy may be necessary. In sulfonamide-sensitive individuals, pyrimethamine, 50 to 75 mg daily, has been effective. Microsporidiosis due to *Enterocytozoon bieneusi* or *Septata intestinalis* has been identified in HIV-infected persons with diarrhea. Although the precise pathogenic role of microsporidia in persons with HIV and diarrhea has been questioned, albendazole,† 400 mg per day for 28 days, has brought symptomatic relief with decreased fecal excretion of *Septata intestinalis*. However, cessation of treatment has commonly resulted in symptomatic recurrences, raising the issue of the need for long-term suppressive therapy.

Cyclospora cayatenensis is a recently described coccidian parasite that microscopically appears as a larger version of *Cryptosporidium parvum*. It has been implicated in prolonged, severe diarrhea in normal and immunocompromised hosts locally and abroad. A recent placebo-controlled trial of immunocompetent *Cyclospora*-infected expatriates in Nepal

---

*Not available in the United States.
†Not FDA-approved for this indication.

*Not FDA-approved for this indication.
†Not available in the United States.

TABLE 1. **Drugs for the Treatment of Protozoal Infections**

Infection	Drug	Adult Dosage	Pediatric Dosage
Amebiasis (*Entamoeba histolytica*)			
Asymptomatic			
Drug of choice	Iodoquinol	650 mg tid × 20 d	30–40 mg/kg/d in 3 doses × 20 d
	or		
	Paromomycin	25–30 mg/kg/d in 3 doses × 7 d	25–30 mg/kg/d in 3 doses × 7 d
Alternative	Diloxanide furoate*	500 mg tid × 10 d	20 mg/kg/d in 3 doses × 10 d
Mild to moderate intestinal disease			
Drug of choice	Metronidazole	750 mg tid × 10 d	35–50 mg/kg/d in 3 doses × 10 d
	or		
	Tinidazole*	2 gm/d × 3 d	50 mg/kg (max 2 gm) once daily × 3 d
Followed by iodoquinol, paromomycin, or diloxanide furoate as above			
Severe intestinal disease			
Drugs of choice	Metronidazole	750 mg tid × 10 d	35–50 mg/kg/d in 3 doses × 10 d
	or		
	Tinidazole*	500 mg bid × 5 d	50 mg/kg (max 2 gm) once daily × 3 d
Followed by iodoquinol, paromomycin, or diloxanide furoate as above			
Blastocystis hominis Infection			
Drug of choice	See text		
Cryptosporidiosis (*Cryptosporidium parvum*)			
Drug of choice	See text		
Cyclospora species			
Drug of choice	Trimethoprim-sulfamethoxazole	TMP 160 mg, SMX 800 mg bid × 7 d	TMP 5 mg/kg, SMX 25 mg/kg bid × 7 d
Dientamoeba fragilis			
Drug of choice	Iodoquinol	650 mg tid × 20 d	40 mg/kg/d in 3 doses × 20 d
	or		
	Paromomycin	25–30 mg/kg/d in 3 doses × 7 d	25–30 mg/kg/d in 3 doses × 7 d
	or		
	Tetracycline	500 mg qid × 10 d	40 mg/kg/d (max 2 gm/d) in 4 doses × 10 d (not recommended for children less than 8 yr)
Entamoeba polecki Infection			
Drug of choice	Metronidazole	750 mg tid × 10 d	35–50 mg/kg/d in 3 doses × 10 d
Giardiasis (*Giardia lamblia*)			
Drug of choice	Metronidazole	250 mg tid × 5 d or 2 gm daily × 3 d	15 mg/kg/d in 3 doses × 5 d
Alternatives			or <25 kg—35 mg/kg once d × 3 d
			25–40 kg—50 mg/kg once d × 3 d
	Tinidazole*	2 gm once	>40 kg—adult dose
	or		
	Furazolidone	100 mg qid × 7–10 d	6 mg/kg/d in 4 doses × 7–10 d
	or		
	Paromomycin	25–30 mg/kg/d in 3 doses × 7 d	
Isosporiasis (*Isospora belli*)			
Drug of choice	Trimethoprim-sulfamethoxazole	160 mg TMP, 800 mg SMX qid × 10 d, then bid × 3 wk	
Microsporidiosis			
Intestinal (*Enterocytozoon bieneusi, Septata intestinalis*)			
Drug of choice	See text		

*Not available in the United States.

Modified from Drugs for parasitic infections. Med Lett Drugs Ther 37:99–108, 1995; Pearson RD: Intestinal parasites. *In* Rakel RE (ed): Conn's Current Therapy, 1995. Philadelphia, WB Saunders Co, 1995, pp 479–486.

suggests that trimethoprim (160 mg)/sulfamethoxazole (800 mg) (Bactrim, Septra), given twice a day for 7 days, is the treatment of choice. In HIV-infected patients, long-term suppressive therapy may be needed.

INTESTINAL NEMATODES

The intestinal helminths can be classified as nematodes (roundworms) or platyhelminths (flat worms); the latter are further subdivided into trematodes (flukes) and cestodes (tapeworms). This classification is helpful not only in organizing these parasites but also in planning chemotherapy, since members of these groups are frequently susceptible to the same drugs or family of drugs.

Ascaris lumbricoides, hookworms, *Trichuris trichiura,* and *Strongyloides stercoralis* are prevalent throughout the world in areas where sanitation is poor. In North America, they are most frequently encountered among immigrants and returning travelers, but on occasion they are found in North Americans who have not traveled abroad. Ova of *A. lumbricoides,* hookworms, and/or *T. trichiura* are often found in the stool of the same person. The benzimidazoles, which are generally well tolerated but are contraindicated in pregnancy, are widely used for the treatment of these nematodes. Mebendazole (Vermox), 100 mg twice a day for 3 days, is effective against all three parasites. Although it is usually well tolerated, on occasion it is associated with diarrhea, abdominal pain, or migration of *Ascaris* through the mouth or nose. Rarely, mebendazole has been associated with leukopenia, agranulocytosis, or hypospermia.

Albendazole* is also active against these nematodes and has the advantage that it can be given as a single dose (400 mg). Albendazole has been used successfully as a single dose in mass treatment programs, resulting in an increased rate of weight gain and physical performance by children with *A. lumbricoides, T. trichiura,* and/or hookworms. However, in the case of a heavy *T. trichiura* infection, it may be necessary to give albendazole, 400 mg daily for 3 days. Albendazole is usually well tolerated but sometimes causes diarrhea, abdominal pain, or migration of *Ascaris* through the mouth or nose. Rarely, leukopenia, reversible alopecia, or elevated serum transaminase levels have been reported. Pyrantel pamoate (11 mg per kg body weight to a maximum daily dose of 1.0 gram), a depolarizing neuromuscular blocker, is effective against *A. lumbricoides* and hookworms, but it is not active against *T. trichiura.* It is generally well tolerated, although gastrointestinal disturbances, headache, dizziness, rash, or fever occur on occasion.

Enterobius vermicularis, the pinworm, is a common finding in North America and other industrialized countries among children of all socioeconomic classes. The diagnosis is usually made by finding ova or adult worms in the perianal region. Ova are occasionally identified in the stool or in ectopic sites in the urogenital tract of females. Pinworms can be treated with a dose of either pyrantel pamoate (11 mg per kg body weight to a maximum daily dose of 1.0 gram), mebendazole (100 mg), or albendazole* (400 mg) followed by a second dose 2 weeks later. If pinworm infections recur and there is more than one young child in the household, empirical therapy for all children should be considered. At the beginning of therapy, undergarments and bedding must be washed and the house thoroughly cleaned to prevent reinfection. In addition, between treatments infected individuals should wear pajamas and underwear to bed and bathe in the morning to remove eggs that have been deposited on the perianal surface during the night.

Strongyloides stercoralis is found in the southern part of the United States and in many developing areas of the world. Periodically, it is diagnosed in immigrants, returning travelers, military personnel including former prisoners of war, and residents of endemic areas in North America. *S. stercoralis* is important because it produces autoinfection, can persist for decades after a person leaves an endemic area, and, in immunocompromised patients, can produce life-threatening disseminated hyperinfection. The hyperinfection syndrome has been associated with steroid use, immunosuppression following organ transplantation, and malnutrition. Hyperinfection with *S. stercoralis* has not been as prevalent in HIV-infected persons, as might have been predicted on the basis of their T cell defects.

Thiabendazole (Mintezol) has been the treatment of choice for strongyloidiasis. The dose is 50 mg per kg body weight (maximum 3 grams per day) administered in two divided doses for 2 days for intestinal disease and at least 5 days for hyperinfection syndrome. Thiabendazole is well absorbed, but significant side effects such as nausea, vomiting, and vertigo are frequent. Rash, erythema multiforme, leukopenia, hallucinations, and olfactory disturbances are occasionally seen. Less common side effects include shock, tinnitus, intrahepatic cholestasis, convulsions, angioneurotic edema, and the Stevens-Johnson syndrome.

Recent studies suggest that ivermectin,* a macrocyclic lactone, at a dose of 200 μg/kg for 1 or 2 days, is highly effective for chronic intestinal strongyloidiasis and is much better tolerated than thiabendazole. Albendazole* is also well tolerated but appears to be less effective than ivermectin when given at a dose of 400 mg daily for 3 days. Longer courses with higher doses (e.g., 400 mg twice daily for 7 days) may be more effective. However, data are lacking on the efficacy of albendazole for hyperinfection syndrome.

Trichinella spiralis is acquired through ingestion of inadequately cooked or raw pork, bear, walrus, or other contaminated meat. Abdominal pain and diarrhea can occur during the early phases of infection. Invading larvae are responsible for the classic picture of myalgia, periorbital edema, and eosinophilia. Chronic diarrhea due to *Trichinella nativa* has been reported among Inuit populations in Canada who have evidence of prior *Trichinella* infection. Mebendazole, 200 to 400 mg three times a day for 3 days, then 400 to 500 mg three times a day for 10 days, is recommended. It eradicates adult *Trichinella* in the intestinal tract, and animal studies suggest that mebendazole has activity against invading larvae in the muscle. Albendazole* may also be effective. Steroids are frequently used to reduce the severe symptoms that accompany heavy degrees of larval invasion.

A number of less common intestinal nematodes may be encountered among returning travelers, immigrants, or residents of endemic areas. *Capillaria philippinensis* is acquired by ingesting improperly cooked, contaminated fish in the Philippines or other endemic areas. Infection is associated with malabsorption, diarrhea, and severe wasting. High-dose, prolonged treatment with mebendazole (Vermox), 200 mg twice a day for 20 days, is the treatment of choice based on studies in animals; albendazole,* 200 mg twice a day for 10 days, or thiabendazole

---

*Not available in the United States.

TABLE 2. **Drugs for the Treatment of Helminth Infections**

Infection	Drug	Adult Dosage	Pediatric Dosage
Angiostrongyliasis (*Angiostrongylus costaricensis*)			
Drug of choice	Thiabendazole	75 mg/kg/d in 3 doses × 3 d (max 3 gm/d); toxicity may require dosage reduction	75 mg/kg/d in 3 doses × 3 d (max 3 gm/d); toxicity may require dosage reduction
Anisakiasis (*Anisakis* and other genera)			
Treatment of choice	Surgical or endoscpic removal		
Ascariasis (*Ascaris lumbricoides*)			
Drug of choice	Mebendazole	100 mg bid × 3 d	100 mg bid × 3 d
	or		
	Pyrantel pamoate	11 mg/kg once (max 1 gm)	11 mg/kg once (max 1 gm)
	or		
	Albendazole*	400 mg once	400 mg once
Capillariasis (*Capillaria philippinensis*)			
Drug of choice	Mebendazole	200 mg bid × 20 d	200 mg bid × 20 d
Alternative	Albendazole*	200 mg bid × 10 d	200 mg bid × 10 d
	or		
	Thiabendazole	25 mg/kg/d in 2 doses × 30 d	25 mg/kg/d in 2 doses × 30 d
Cysticercosis; see Tapeworm Infection			
Enterobius vermicularis (Pinworm) Infection			
Drug of choice	Pyrantel pamoate	11 mg/kg once (max 1 gm); repeat after 2 wk	11 mg/kg once (max 1 gm); repeat after 2 wk
	or		
	Mebendazole	A single dose of 100 mg; repeat after 2 wk	A single dose of 100 mg; repeat after 2 wk
	or		
	Albendazole*	400 mg once; repeat in 2 wk	400 mg once, repeat in 2 wk
Flukes (Intestinal Infection)			
Fasciolopsis buski			
Drug of choice	Praziquantel	75 mg/kg/d in 3 doses × 1 d	75 mg/kg/d in 3 doses × 1 d
	or		
	Niclosamide	A single dose of 4 tablets (2 gm) chewed thoroughly	11–34 kg: 2 tablets (1 gm); >34 kg: 3 tablets (1.5 gm)
Heterophyes heterophyes			
Drug of choice	Praziquantel	75 mg/kg/d in 3 doses × 1 d	75 mg/kg/d in 3 doses × 1 d
Metagonimus yokogawai			
Drug of choice	Praziquantel	75 mg/kg/d in 3 doses × 1 d	75 mg/kg/d in 3 doses × 1 d
Nanophyetus salmincola			
Drug of choice	Praziquantel	60 mg/kg/d in 3 doses × 1 d	60 mg/kg/d in 3 doses × 1 d
Hookworm Infection (*Ancylostoma duodenale, Necator americanus*)			
Drug of choice	Mebendazole	100 mg bid × 3 d	100 mg bid × 3 d
	or		
	Pyrantel pamoate	11 mg/kg (max 1 gm) × 3 d	11 mg/kg (max 1 gm) × 3 d
	or		
	Albendazole*	400 mg once	400 mg once
Pinworm; see *Enterobius vermicularis*			
Schistosomiasis (Bilharziasis)			
Schistosoma haematobium			
Drug of choice	Praziquantel	40 mg/kg/d in 2 doses × 1 d	40 mg/kg/d in 2 doses × 1 d
S. japonicum			
Drug of choice	Praziquantel	60 mg/kg/d in 3 doses × 1 d	60 mg/kg/d in 3 doses × 1 d
S. mansoni			
Drug of choice	Praziquantel	40 mg/kg/d in 2 doses × 1 d	40 mg/kg/d in 2 doses × 1 d
Alternative	Oxamniquine	15 mg/kg once	20 mg/kg/d in 2 doses × 1 d
S. mekongi			
Drug of choice	Praziquantel	60 mg/kg/d in 3 doses × 1 d	60 mg/kg/d in 3 doses × 1 d
Strongyloidiasis (*Strongyloides stercoralis*)			
Drug of choice	Thiabendazole	50 mg/kg/d in 2 doses (max 3 gm/d) × 2 d; ≥5 d for hyperinfection	50 mg/kg/d in 2 doses (max 3 gm/d) × 2 d; ≥5 d for hyperinfection
	or		
	Ivermectin†	200 µg/kg/d × 1–2 d	
Tapeworm Infection—Adult (Intestinal Stage)			
Diphyllobothrium latum (fish), *Taenia saginata* (beef), *Taenia solium* (pork), *Dipylidium caninum* (dog)			
Drug of choice	Praziquantel	5–10 mg/kg once	5–10 mg/kg once
	or		
	Niclosamide	A single dose of 4 tablets (2 gm), chewed thoroughly	11–34 kg: a single dose of 2 tablets (1 gm); >34 kg: a single dose of 3 tablets (1.5 gm)

TABLE 2. **Drugs for the Treatment of Helminth Infections** *Continued*

Infection	Drug	Adult Dosage	Pediatric Dosage
Hymenolepis nana (Dwarf Tapeworm)			
Drug of choice	Praziquantel	25 mg/kg once	25 mg/kg once
Alternative	Niclosamide	A single daily dose of 4 tablets (2 gm), chewed thoroughly, then 2 tablets daily × 6 d	11–34 kg: a single dose of 2 tablets (1 gm) × 1 d, then 1 tablet (0.5 gm)/d × 6 d; >34 kg: a single dose of 3 tablets (1.5 gm) × 1 d, then 2 tablets (1 gm) × 6 d
Cysticercus cellulosae (Cysticercosis)			
Treatment of choice	Albendazole* or	15 mg/kg/d in 3 doses × 28 d, repeated as necessary	15 mg/kg/d in 3 doses × 28 d, repeated as necessary
	Praziquantel	50 mg/kg/d in 3 doses × 15 d	50 mg/kg/d in 3 doses × 15 d
Alternative	Surgery		
Trichinosis *(Trichinella spiralis)*			
Drug of choice	Steroids for severe symptoms plus mebendazole	200–400 mg tid × 3 d, then 400–500 mg tid × 10 d	
Trichostrongylus Infection			
Drug of choice	Pyrantel pamoate	11 mg/kg once (max 1 gm)	11 mg/kg once (max 1 gm)
Alternative	Mebendazole or	100 mg bid × 3 d	100 mg bid × 3 d
	Albendazole*	400 mg once	400 mg once
Trichuriasis *(Trichuris trichiura,* Whipworm)			
Drug of choice	Mebendazole or	100 mg bid × 3 d	100 mg bid × 3 d
	Albendazole*	400 mg once; may require 3 d for heavy infection	400 mg once; may require 3 d for heavy infection

*Available in the U.S. only from the manufacturer.

†Available from the CDC Drug Service, Centers for Disease Control and Prevention, Atlanta, GA 30333; 404-639-3670 (evenings, weekends and holidays, 404-639-2888).

Modified from Drugs for parasitic infections. Med Lett Drugs Ther 37:99–108, 1995; Pearson RD: Intestinal parasites. *In* Rakel RE (ed): Conn's Current Therapy 1995. Philadelphia, WB Saunders Co, 1995, pp 479–486.

(Mintezol), 25 mg per kg body weight daily in two divided doses for 30 days, is an alternative.

Trichostrongylus species are important pathogens of cattle, which are periodically acquired through fecal-oral contamination by people living in cattle-raising areas. Human infection is usually mild or asymptomatic. The drug of choice is pyrantel pamoate (Antiminth), 11 mg per kg body weight to a maximum daily dose of 1 gram. Mebendazole, 100 mg twice a day for 3 days, or albendazole,* 400 mg, is an alternative.

Anisakiasis follows ingestion of raw or inadequately treated fish that are infected with *Anisakis* species or related genera. The larvae elicit painful, inflammatory responses when they attempt to invade the wall of the stomach, small intestine, or colon. On many occasions larvae can be visualized and removed endoscopically, but some cases require surgery.

CESTODES (TAPEWORMS)

Humans are the definitive host for a number of tapeworms that reside in the human gastrointestinal tract. *Diphyllobothrium latum,* the fish tapeworm, which is acquired by eating raw or inadequately cooked freshwater fish, competes with humans for vitamin B_{12}. *Taenia saginata,* which is acquired from contaminated beef, grows to incredible lengths in the human intestine but usually does so without

producing significant symptoms. On occasion, the dog tapeworm, *Dipylidium caninum,* is acquired by children. Praziquantel (Biltricide), 5 to 10 mg per kg body weight as a single dose, or niclosamide (Niclocide), 2 grams chewed thoroughly, is effective for the treatment of these cestodes. Praziquantel is reasonably well tolerated and without serious long-term sequelae. Short-term side effects, including malaise, headache, and dizziness, are common; sedation, abdominal pain, sweating, fever, nausea, and fatigue occur occasionally. Since very little niclosamide is absorbed, it is usually well tolerated; occasionally patients experience nausea and abdominal pain.

Hymenolepis nana, the dwarf tapeworm, is among the most prevalent of the human cestodes. Although a single dose of praziquantel, 25 mg per kg body weight, is effective, niclosamide can also be used. However, a 7-day course is required (2 grams chewed thoroughly the first day followed by 1 gram daily for 6 days) because the worm is capable of autoinfection, during which time the larval stage develops in the submucosa for several days. Thus, to be effective, niclosamide, a lumen-active agent, must be given until the larval stage re-enters the lumen.

Humans can be both the definitive and the intermediate host for *Taenia solium,* the pork tapeworm. When adult worms are present in the human intestine, a single dose of praziquantel, 5 to 10 mg per kg body weight, or niclosamide, 2 grams, is effective. When humans ingest *T. solium* ova in fecally contaminated food or water, they excyst in the intestine,

*Not available in the United States.

releasing larvae that invade the brain, resulting in neurocysticercosis, or other organs. Indications for treatment of neurocysticercosis depend on the stage of the disease, and adjunctive treatment with steroids and anticonvulscents is often necessary. Albendazole (15 mg per kg body weight per day in three doses for 28 days) is the treatment of choice. Alternatively, praziquantel (50 mg per kg body weight per day for 15 days) can be used. Albendazole*, 10 mg/kg daily for 3 to 6 months, is the treatment of choice for inoperable echinococcal liver cysts. Absorption of albendazole is enhanced with fatty meals, and concurrent cimetidine administration increases the levels of an active metabolite, albendazole sulfoxide, in echinococcal cyst fluid. Cure rates of *Echinococcus granulosus* infection, approach 40%, while clinical improvement may reach 75%. Surgery remains the treatment of choice; however, recent studies show percutaneous cyst aspiration with scolicidal instillation and re-aspiration to be a reasonable alternative in selected cases.

INTESTINAL TREMATODES AND SCHISTOSOMIASIS

Trematodes have complex life cycles involving snails and additional intermediate hosts. Several trematode species reside in the lumen of the human gastrointestinal tract. They include *Fasciolopsis buski,* which is acquired by eating contaminated water plants such as the water chestnut; *Heterophyes*

---

*Not available in the United States.

heterophyes and *Metagonimus yokogawai,* which are acquired through ingestion of contaminated freshwater fish; and *Nanophyetus salmincola,* which is acquired by eating raw or uncooked salmon or other fish. All of these trematodes are thought to be susceptible to praziquantel, although treatment data are anecdotal in some instances. The recommended dosage and duration of therapy are summarized in Table 2. As noted, praziquantel is associated with a number of transient side effects but has no known major long-term toxicity. The abdominal discomfort, fever, eosinophilia, and rash that are occasionally associated with praziquantel are probably due at least in part to the release of worm antigens during worm death.

Adult *Schistosoma* species live in the vesical plexus or mesenteric venules of humans, where they produce ova that pass through the mucosa into the lumen of the bowel. Egg trapping in tissues results in mucosal inflammation, hypertrophy, and ulceration. The most important intestinal pathogens are *Schistosoma mansoni,* which is endemic in many areas of Africa, Latin America, and the Middle East; and *Schistosoma japonicum* and *Schistosoma mekongi,* which are endemic in Southeast Asia. *Schistosoma hematobium,* endemic in Africa and the Middle East, typically resides in the vesical plexus producing urinary tract pathology. All of the *Schistosoma* species are susceptible to praziquantel. Oxamniquine (Vansil), an alternative drug for the treatment of *S. mansoni,* is occasionally associated with headache, dizziness, nausea, diarrhea, rash, and orange-red discoloration of the urine. Seizures and neuropsychiatric disturbances are rare side effects (see Table 2).

Metabolic Disorders

DIABETES MELLITUS IN ADULTS

method of
PAULOS BERHANU, M.D.
University of Colorado Health Sciences Center
Denver, Colorado

Diabetes mellitus is a complex syndrome characterized by abnormalities of carbohydrate, lipid, and protein metabolism resulting from either a deficiency of insulin or its cellular metabolic effects. The syndrome is manifested by sustained hyperglycemia and the development of chronic microvascular complications (retinopathy, nephropathy, and neuropathy) and macrovascular complications (accelerated atherosclerosis of the coronary and peripheral vasculature). This general metabolic and clinical manifestation is common to the diabetic state regardless of the underlying etiology, although differences can occur in the rate and extent of the metabolic and clinical derangements, depending on the type of diabetes.

Diabetes is the most common endocrine-metabolic disorder. In the United States, it affects approximately 14 million people, and the incidence of new cases is rapidly increasing in association with the aging of the population and the increasing prevalence of overnutrition and obesity in the country. In addition, demographic factors are important, since diabetes is known to affect various ethnic groups differently. For example, African Americans, Hispanics, and Native Americans are two to four times more likely than whites to get diabetes. Diabetes is also becoming a growing health problem worldwide, where it is estimated to affect 5 to 7% of the adult population. The global estimate in 1994 was that 110 million people had diabetes, and this is projected to increase to 280 million people by the year 2010. This rapid rise is thought to be due to a combination of factors, including increasing urbanization around the world, adoption of Western diet and lifestyle, and increasing life expectancy.

Diabetes and its complications constitute the third leading cause of death in the United States, and the associated economic costs are substantial. In 1992, the total cost (including direct and indirect costs) was estimated to be $92 to $105 billion. This translates into one out of seven health care dollars being spent on individuals with diabetes. Thus, it is anticipated that the effective management of diabetes and the prevention of its many complications will decrease morbidity and mortality and result in significant savings.

CLASSIFICATION AND DIAGNOSIS

The current classification of disorders of glucose metabolism consists of three specific diagnoses: diabetes mellitus (includes Type I and II diabetes), impaired glucose tolerance (IGT), and gestational diabetes mellitus (GDM). The three major types of diabetes are summarized in Table 1.

IGT is a special category characterized by blood glucose values that are higher than normal but lower than those considered diagnostic for clinical diabetes mellitus. This condition is associated with increased risk for cardiovascular disease, and many subjects with IGT, particularly those who are obese, eventually progress to overt diabetes. This indicates that IGT is most likely an early subclinical stage of non–insulin dependent diabetes. Accordingly, studies are under way to determine whether progression of IGT to diabetes can be prevented through dietary and other lifestyle modifications. GDM refers to the condition in which glucose intolerance first develops during pregnancy. It occurs in about 2% of pregnant women and is associated with increased risk of fetal morbidity and mortality if appropriate glycemic control is not maintained during pregnancy. Glucose tolerance usually returns to normal after delivery, but a significant percentage of women with GDM eventually develop non–insulin dependent diabetes mellitus. Again, this suggests that subjects with GDM have an underlying disorder of glucose metabolism and a susceptibility for diabetes that is unmasked by pregnancy.

Insulin-dependent diabetes mellitus (IDDM), or Type I diabetes, accounts for 5 to 10% of diagnosed cases of diabetes mellitus in the United States (see Table 1). IDDM is characterized by absolute insulin deficiency that results from chronic autoimmune destruction of the pancreatic beta cells in genetically susceptible individuals. Such individuals are prone to the development of ketoacidosis and are absolutely dependent on the administration of exogenous insulin to sustain life. The development of IDDM has a variable course, ranging from aggressive autoimmune destruction of the beta cells early in life to a more indolent course in which beta cell loss may occur over years to decades. However, in general, IDDM most often manifests itself within the first 2 decades of life, with a peak incidence at around 12 years of age.

Non–insulin dependent diabetes mellitus (NIDDM), or Type II diabetes, is by far the most common form of diabetes mellitus and accounts for 90 to 95% of the 14 million people with diabetes in the United States. NIDDM is characterized by insulin resistance rather than absolute insulin deficiency, and plasma insulin levels are generally either normal or high. Accordingly, patients with NIDDM are not prone to ketosis and are not absolutely dependent on exogenous insulin to sustain life. It is a slowly evolving condition that is diagnosed in adulthood, usually after 40 years of age.

The diagnosis of IDDM is relatively straightforward, since most patients generally present with abrupt onset of the classic symptoms of polyuria, polydipsia, weight loss, and/or ketoacidosis in association with unequivocal hyperglycemia. In contrast, the manifestations of NIDDM can be subtle, and the disease may exist for several years without producing overt symptoms. In part, this factor accounts for the current estimation that approximately 50% of NIDDM cases remain undiagnosed. The standard criteria for the diagnosis of diabetes mellitus are based on

TABLE 1. **Classification and Characteristics of Diabetes Mellitus (DM)**

Type	% of All DM	Age at Diagnosis	Defect	Insulin Level	Ketosis Proneness
I (IDDM)	5–10	<30 years (mean, 12 years)	Insulin deficiency (absolute)	Absent	+
II (NIDDM)	90–95	>30 years	Insulin resistance, relative insulin deficiency	Normal or high	−
Gestational DM	2% of pregnancies	Second to third trimester of pregnancy	Insulin resistance	Normal or high	−

Abbreviations: IDDM = insulin-dependent diabetes mellitus; NIDDM = non–insulin dependent diabetes mellitus.

the levels of plasma glucose attained either in the fasting state and randomly in the postprandial state, or following a standard 75-gram glucose load during performance of the oral glucose tolerance test (OGTT). The diagnostic criteria are summarized in Table 2. OGTT is rarely utilized now, since the majority of patients present with unequivocal hyperglycemia in the fasting and/or postprandial state. Since almost all cases of new-onset diabetes in adults are NIDDM, the remainder of this article is limited to discussions of the pathophysiology and management of this major metabolic disorder.

PATHOPHYSIOLOGY OF NIDDM

NIDDM represents a group of disorders with different underlying causes but generally similar clinical presentations. Furthermore, NIDDM in a given patient can pass through various stages of hormonal, biochemical, and clinical profiles throughout the patient's life. Accordingly, an understanding and appreciation of the major pathophysiologic features of NIDDM is important for the proper individualization of therapeutic choices and for long-term management. Genetic factors play a prominent role in the pathogenesis of NIDDM, as shown by the high degree of familial aggregation of the disease, the high concordance rate in identical twins, and the markedly increased prevalence in certain population groups. However, for the most part, neither the nature of the genetic defects nor the mode of inheritance is known, and it is likely that NIDDM is a polygenic disease, the expression of which in genetically susceptible individuals is strongly influenced by environmental factors. Such factors include intake of high-calorie/high-fat diets, obesity, physical inactivity, and aging. These are all features that typically accompany economic development and affluence, thus potentially explaining the dramatic increase in the prevalence of NIDDM around the world, especially in developing and developed countries.

Insulin resistance is a cardinal feature and the earliest identifiable abnormality in NIDDM. In nondiabetic individuals who have inherited the "diabetic genotype" (e.g., offspring of diabetic parents), the presence of insulin resistance can be demonstrated using sophisticated techniques (e.g., the euglycemic insulin clamp technique) well before any changes occur in plasma glucose levels. The insulin resistance occurs at the level of the liver and peripheral tissues, primarily muscle. In whole-body measurements, this resistance has been attributed to defects in insulin-mediated nonoxidative glucose disposal. With increasing duration, the insulin resistance gets progressively worse due to a combination of factors. These include the increasing hyperglycemia and the diabetic milieu, obesity, physical inactivity, and the aging process, all of which are known to be associated with or contribute to insulin resistance. The hepatic insulin resistance is manifested by fasting hyperglycemia and is due to impairment of insulin-mediated suppression of hepatic glucose output (i.e., impairment of insulin-mediated suppression of gluconeogenesis and glycogenolysis). Peripheral tissue insulin resistance is manifested by postprandial hyperglycemia, principally resulting from impairment in insulin-stimulated glucose uptake by muscle.

Various candidate genes of the insulin action pathway have been evaluated for possible mutations causing the NIDDM syndrome. Although certain mutations of the insulin receptor gene have been identified, these are relatively few and occur in special syndromes of extreme insulin resistance that are usually associated with specific phenotypes, such as acanthosis nigricans and hirsutism. However, in ordinary cases of NIDDM, including those of the Pima Indians, who have the highest prevalence of diabetes in the world, the coding sequence for the insulin receptor is normal. Similarly, the gene coding for the insulin-sensitive glucose transporter (GLUT4) is also normal. Therefore, at present, the nature of the genetic defects leading to the insulin resistance of ordinary NIDDM is not known.

In addition to insulin resistance, NIDDM is accompanied by varying alterations of insulin secretory function. Subjects with IGT, or those with early and mild NIDDM, generally have augmented insulin production by pancreatic beta cells and are hyperinsulinemic in the basal state. This is thought to be a compensatory mechanism to overcome resistance to insulin-mediated glucose metabolism by target tissues. With progressive insulin resistance and sustained hyperglycemia over many years, beta cell function eventually declines and leads to relative hypoinsulinemia. This process has been termed "beta cell exhaustion," although the specific mechanism is not known. However, in one special form of NIDDM, maturity-onset diabetes of the young (MODY), the insulin secretory defect is linked to mutation of the gene for the glucokinase enzyme. This enzyme is expressed both in the liver and in the pancreatic beta cell, and in the latter tissue it serves

TABLE 2. **Diagnostic Criteria for Diabetes Mellitus**

Random plasma glucose >200 mg/dL *plus* classic signs and symptoms of diabetes

or

Fasting plasma glucose >140 mg/dL on at least two occasions

or

Fasting plasma glucose <140 mg/dL *plus* sustained elevated plasma glucose levels during at least two oral glucose tolerance tests: plasma glucose ≥200 mg/dL both at 2 h after ingestion of a 75-gm oral glucose dose and at some time between 0 and 2 h as part of the glucose-sensing mechanism for glucose-stimulated insulin release. However, in most cases of ordinary NIDDM, the insulin secretory defect is most likely acquired, since it can be corrected, at least temporarily, with normalization of hyperglycemia by appropriate therapeutic means.

In consideration of the factors discussed earlier, the final common pathogenetic pathway leading to NIDDM can be viewed as a composite of insulin resistance (primary defect) and variable defects in insulin secretion (secondary defect). The insulin resistance is the underlying defect that gets progressively worse with the superimposition of chronic hyperglycemia and the diabetic milieu, as well as environmental factors such as obesity, physical inactivity, and the aging process. The changes in beta cell function in NIDDM go through a bimodal phase throughout the life of a diabetic subject. In the early phases of the disease, beta cell function may be normal, and there is sufficient capacity to augment insulin production and compensate for the insulin resistance. However, in the advanced stages of the disease, progressive loss of beta cell function occurs presumably as a consequence of the chronic and sustained hyperglycemia. Thus, recognition and appreciation of the changing interplay between insulin resistance and insulin secretion throughout the life of a patient with NIDDM have important implications for the choice of appropriate management strategies for each stage of the disease.

MANAGEMENT OF NIDDM

Goals of Therapy

There are three major objectives for the treatment of diabetes mellitus: (1) to resolve the symptoms attributable to the disease, including polyuria, polydipsia, fatigue, and weight loss, and restore the patient's sense of well-being; (2) to prevent the acute metabolic complications of the disease, including diabetic ketoacidosis, hyperglycemic hyperosmolar nonketotic coma, and hypoglycemia; and (3) to prevent the chronic microvascular, macrovascular, and neuropathic complications in an effort to reduce or eliminate the associated morbidity and mortality and to achieve increased life expectancy for the patient. The first two objectives are straightforward and relatively easy to achieve, but there has been a long-standing uncertainty regarding the feasibility of obtaining and maintaining normal or near-normal metabolic control and whether such efforts reduce or prevent the long-term complications of diabetes. This issue is especially pertinent in NIDDM, because other factors such as dyslipidemia, hypertension, and smoking also contribute to cardiovascular disease, which is the predominant cause of morbidity and mortality. Nevertheless, with respect to glycemic control per se, there is now growing evidence that improved metabolic control translates into reduced risk of chronic complications.

Relationship of Glycemic Control to Chronic Diabetic Complications

The Diabetes Control and Complications Trial (DCCT), which was reported in 1993, has settled a long-standing question on the relationship between glucose control and diabetic complications. In this landmark study, 1441 patients with IDDM were randomized to receive intensive or conventional insulin treatment regimens and were then followed for up to 9 years, with the average follow-up being 6.5 years. The results conclusively demonstrated that in the areas of retinopathy, nephropathy, and neuropathy, the risk of developing new complications can be significantly reduced (primary prevention), and the progression of pre-existing complications can be slowed (secondary prevention). When compared with the conventional treatment group, the intensive glucose control group attained a combined risk reduction of 63, 54, and 60% for the development of retinopathy, nephropathy, and neuropathy, respectively. The major risk associated with intensive insulin therapy was a threefold increase in the development of severe hypoglycemia. Of note, the DCCT results also demonstrated that the relationship between microvascular complications (as assessed by retinopathy) and the levels of glycemia (measured by hemoglobin A_{1C} levels) was continuous over the entire spectrum of measurements. Thus, there was no "glycemic threshold" above which complications occurred and below which patients were protected. This has important implications for diabetes management, since it indicates that any diabetic patient with suboptimal glycemic control can reduce the risk of complications by attaining a better glycemic level.

Since the DCCT was limited to IDDM patients, questions have been raised whether the results can be extrapolated to NIDDM. However, since it is believed that the same or similar underlying pathogenetic mechanisms mediate the retinopathic, nephropathic, and neuropathic complications of both IDDM and NIDDM, there is no reason to believe that the beneficial effects of better glycemic control do not also apply to NIDDM. Furthermore, other studies published subsequent to completion of the DCCT have indicated that the degree of glycemic control in NIDDM is an important predictor for the incidence and progression of retinopathy and for the risk of developing coronary heart disease. It is also hoped that completion of the ongoing U.K. Prospective Diabetes Study will shed further light in this area.

On the basis of the proven benefits of optimization of glycemic control, the current standards of diabetes care require that appropriate patient-specific therapeutic modalities be utilized, with the goal of achieving near-normal or normal blood glucose levels. The recommended targets for glycemic control are the same in IDDM and NIDDM and are summarized in Table 3. These targets serve as idealized guidelines and should be modified in accordance with the patient's needs and his or her ability to carry out tight glycemic control. A major determinant of the glycemic target is the frequency and/or severity of hypoglycemia. Although insulin is the mainstay of therapy for achieving glycemic targets in IDDM, the therapeutic choices in NIDDM are diverse and include nonpharmacologic as well as pharmacologic

TABLE 3. **Targets for Glycemic Control in Diabetes**

Biochemical Index	Nondiabetic	Diabetic	
		Goal	*Action Suggested*
Pre-meal glucose (mg/dL)	<115	80–120	<80 >140
Bedtime glucose (mg/dL)	<120	100–140	<100 >160
HbA$_{1c}$ (%)	<6	<7	>8

These values are for nonpregnant individuals. HbA$_{1c}$ is referenced to a nondiabetic range of 4.0 to 6.0%.
Adapted from ADA—Standards of medical care for patients with diabetes mellitus. Diabetes Care *19*(Suppl 1):S8–S15, 1996.

therapy, including oral agents and insulin or various combinations of these modalities.

Nonpharmacologic Therapy of NIDDM

Nonpharmacologic therapy, consisting of diet, exercise, and weight control, is the cornerstone of NIDDM management and should be instituted early in the disease process. The main rationale for this is that each of these nonpharmacologic maneuvers favorably influences insulin resistance, which plays a major role in the pathophysiology of NIDDM. It is known that a high-calorie/high-fat diet, physical inactivity, and the development of obesity are major risk factors for the progression from simple glucose intolerance to clinical NIDDM.

In view of the heterogeneity of the NIDDM population and their nutritional needs, the institution of dietary therapy and weight-loss programs must be individualized and requires the participation of a registered dietician. An effort should be made to avoid the rapid loss-regain cycles that frequently occur. Modest restriction in calories with modest weight loss that is sustainable and can be incorporated into the patient's lifestyle is preferred and has been shown to improve glucose control in NIDDM. The dietitian is invaluable for individualizing the levels of caloric intake; distributing calories among carbohydrates, fat, and protein; and monitoring individualized weight-loss programs.

Exercise is an important adjunct to diet therapy in the management of NIDDM. In addition to its overall benefit in enhancing the diet plan and promoting and maintaining weight loss, a program of regular exercise also improves insulin sensitivity and glycemic control. Exercise can also improve physical fitness and hypertension and reduce cardiovascular risk factors. Although a modest exercise program can be undertaken by most patients with NIDDM, many subjects are elderly and may have pre-existing conditions that are aggravated by unregulated exercise. Therefore, a pre-exercise evaluation is advised to check for hypertension, neuropathy, retinopathy, nephropathy, and peripheral vascular disease. Stress exercise tolerance testing to look for silent ischemia is also advised in middle-aged and older individuals. In general, the exercise program should be individualized; when indicated, it should be instituted and monitored by a trained exercise physiologist, preferably in a setting that specializes in cardiovascular fitness programs under medical supervision.

Oral Antidiabetic Agents

Three classes of oral antidiabetic agents are currently available in the United States for the management of NIDDM: sulfonylureas, a biguanide, and an alpha-glucosidase inhibitor. The agents in each class work by different and independent mechanisms to lower fasting and/or postprandial hyperglycemia. The sulfonylurea drugs have the longest documented safety and efficacy. The agents in the other two classes were approved for use in the United States in 1995.

Sulfonylureas. Sulfonylurea drugs have been the mainstay of oral antidiabetic therapy for the past 4 decades. The drugs in this class are listed in Table 4, along with some of their properties. The first-generation compounds are now used less frequently, primarily because of their low intrinsic potency, which necessitates large doses and multiple daily dosing regimens. The second-generation compounds, glyburide and glipizide, are more potent and more bioavailable, so smaller doses are required. All sulfonylurea compounds lower blood glucose by the same mechanism: stimulation of endogenous insulin secretion. It is thought that this process is mediated by binding of the drugs to a specific protein (sulfonylurea receptor) on the surface of pancreatic beta cells. Glyburide and glipizide show subtle differences in their effects on the insulin secretory profile. Although much overlap exists, glyburide has greater effect on fasting insulin levels, and glipizide has greater effect on postprandial insulin levels. Such subtle differences can be taken into account when choosing a drug for individual patients, based on their fasting and postprandial glycemic profiles. Finally, although much has been written about the possible extrapancreatic effect of sulfonylureas, such effects are probably secondary to the improved glycemic control resulting from the augmented insulin secretion rather than from the drug's direct effect on peripheral tissues. Therefore, therapeutic response to sulfonylurea therapy in NIDDM is dependent on the presence of endogenous insulin secretory capacity.

Certain general principles should be followed in using sulfonylurea drugs in the management of NIDDM. Maximum effect is obtained with these

TABLE 4. **Characteristics of Sulfonylurea Drugs**

Drug	Dose Range (mg/Day)	Duration of Action (Hours)	Doses/Day
First Generation			
Tolbutamide (Orinase)	500–3000	6–12	2–3
Tolazamide (Tolinase)	100–1000	12–24	1–2
Acetohexamide (Dymelor)	250–1500	12–24	1–2
Chlorpropamide (Diabinese)	100–500	60	1
Second Generation			
Glipizide (Glucotrol)	2.5–40	12–24	1–2
Glipizide-GITS (Glucotrol XL)	5–20	24	1
Glyburide (Micronase, DiaBeta)	1.25–20	12–24	1–2
Glyburide, micronized (Glynase)	0.75–12	12–24	1–2

drugs when their use is combined with adherence to appropriate diet, exercise, and weight-control programs. Therefore, in most cases, the drugs should be started only after a reasonable trial (6 to 8 weeks) of appropriate diet therapy fails to achieve the desired level of glycemic control. Therapy should be started with a low dose and titrated upward every 1 to 2 weeks. The objective should be to use the lowest dose that is optimally effective. Rapid escalation of doses and the use of inappropriately high doses of sulfonylureas can lead to desensitization or to hypoglycemia, the latter being the main side effect of these drugs. Appropriate selection of NIDDM patients for sulfonylurea therapy is important, since the best response occurs early in the disease process, when endogenous insulin secretory reserve is present. The patients who fall into this category tend to be normal weight or obese subjects with a relatively recent onset of disease and mild hyperglycemia. Thin NIDDM subjects with moderate to marked hyperglycemia are unlikely to respond to sulfonylurea therapy and are best treated with insulin. Thus, most of the reported 20% primary failure rate of sulfonylurea therapy is likely due to inappropriate patient selection. Patients who initially respond to sulfonylurea therapy may manifest secondary failure at the rate of 5 to 10% per year after 5 or more years of therapy. Some of these represent true failures due to the natural course of progressive beta cell deficiency that occurs in NIDDM. However, before deciding that sulfonylurea therapy is no longer effective, it is important to rule out treatable causes such as noncompliance, dietary indiscretion, infection, other systemic illnesses, or concurrent use of other medications (e.g., glucocorticoids) that interfere with carbohydrate metabolism.

Metformin. Metformin (Glucophage) and phenformin* are biguanide compounds that were introduced in the late 1950s for the treatment of NIDDM. Phenformin (the only biguanide previously available in the United States) was removed from the market in the late 1970s because of its association with the development of lactic acidosis. The use of metformin was continued in other countries but not in the United States, where it was only recently introduced.

Metformin lowers blood glucose concentrations to a similar extent as the sulfonylureas but does so by a different mechanism. Unlike sulfonylureas, metformin does not stimulate insulin secretion. Instead, its antihyperglycemic effect is mediated via potentiation of insulin effect by decreasing hepatic glucose production and enhancing glucose utilization by muscle. Thus, metformin appears to decrease the insulin resistance of NIDDM, and the presence of adequate circulating levels of insulin is necessary for the manifestation of its antihyperglycemic effects.

Because of metformin's effect in reducing insulin resistance, certain secondary advantages may be gained from its use in the treatment of NIDDM. These include modest weight loss, decrease in plasma insulin levels, and variable degrees of improvement in the plasma lipid profile (decrease in triglycerides and LDL-cholesterol, and increase in HDL-cholesterol). Monotherapy with metformin is not associated with hypoglycemia. The side effects of metformin therapy are primarily gastrointestinal and include diarrhea, nausea, abdominal discomfort, and anorexia. These symptoms can be reduced by administering the drug with food and by dose reduction. Although subnormal vitamin B_{12} levels have been reported in some patients, these have not been associated with anemia or other clinical manifestations. In clinical trials in the United States, metformin therapy was not associated with significant effect on plasma lactate levels, and no cases of lactic acidosis were reported. However, since certain conditions can predispose to lactic acidosis, specific exclusion criteria for the use of metformin have been established. These are listed in Table 5 and should be followed.

In NIDDM patients, metformin can be used as monotherapy or in combination with sulfonylureas. Although either agent can be used as initial monotherapy in patients who have failed an adequate trial of diet therapy, metformin may be preferred in obese patients because of its effects of reducing insulin resistance and the secondary benefit of potential weight reduction. However, in patients who are already on maximal doses of sulfonylureas without adequate glycemic control, metformin can be added. In either case, metformin therapy should be started at a low dose (500 mg with morning and evening meals),

---

*Not available in the United States.

TABLE 5. **Exclusion Criteria for the Use of Metformin**

Renal impairment: plasma creatinine values ≥ 1.5 mg/dL
  for men and ≥ 1.4 mg/dL for women
Cardiac or respiratory insufficiency that is likely to cause
  central hypoxia or reduced peripheral perfusion
History of lactic acidosis
Severe infection that could lead to decreased tissue
  perfusion
Liver disease, including alcoholic liver disease, as
  demonstrated by abnormal liver function tests
Alcohol abuse with binge drinking sufficient to cause acute
  hepatic toxicity*
Use of intravenous radiographic contrast agents

*Moderate alcohol intake is not a contraindication if liver function is normal.

Adapted from Bailey CJ, Turner RC: Metformin. N Engl J Med *334*:574–579, 1996. Copyright 1996, Massachusetts Medical Society. All rights reserved.

with further adjustments made at 1- to 2-week intervals to the maximal dose of 2550 mg per day. As with sulfonylurea therapy, treatment with metformin should be coupled with strict adherence to appropriate diet, exercise, and weight-control measures, since these nonpharmacologic measures enhance the efficacy of antidiabetic drug therapy.

Acarbose. Acarbose (Precose) is an alpha-glucosidase inhibitor that was recently introduced in the United States for the management of NIDDM. Its main effect is to reduce the postprandial rise in blood glucose levels, and its mechanism of action is different from that of the other oral antidiabetic agents. Acarbose competitively inhibits the alpha-glucosidase enzymes located in the brush border cells of the small intestine. These enzymes cleave oligosaccharides and complex carbohydrates into monosaccharides, including glucose, which are subsequently absorbed. By competitively inhibiting these enzymes, acarbose delays the breakdown and absorption of carbohydrates and thereby decreases postprandial glycemic excursion. Carbohydrate that escapes digestion in the small intestine in the presence of acarbose spills into the lower gastrointestinal tract, where it is metabolized by bacteria. Accordingly, the major side effects of acarbose therapy are gastrointestinal in nature and include abdominal fullness, discomfort, flatulence, and occasional diarrhea. Because of the local effect of acarbose in the small intestine, therapy with this drug is not accompanied by the development of hypoglycemia or significant change in body weight.

Acarbose can be used in NIDDM as monotherapy or in combination with sulfonylureas, metformin, or insulin to control postprandial glycemia. Monotherapy is likely to be limited to patients with mild fasting hyperglycemia and moderate postprandial hyperglycemia. Since most patients with NIDDM have significant elevations in both fasting and postprandial blood glucose levels, it is more likely that acarbose will be used in combination with other agents. Because of the nature of its mechanism of action, the drug is administered three times daily, with each dose being taken with the first mouthful of each major meal. Since gastrointestinal side effects of acarbose are dose related, therapy is initiated with low doses (25 mg three times daily). The doses are then gradually increased to the maximum recommended dose of 50 mg three times daily for patients weighing 60 kg or less and 100 mg three times daily for patients weighing more than 60 kg. Doses higher than these may be associated with an increased risk of elevation in serum transaminase levels.

Oral Antidiabetic Agents on the Horizon. Two new oral antidiabetic agents have recently been undergoing clinical trials. One of these, glimepiride (Amaryl),* is a third-generation sulfonylurea. As such, its primary mechanism of action is stimulation of insulin release from functioning pancreatic islet cells. The other drug that is under development is troglitazone, which is a member of the thiazolidinedione class of compounds; these drugs do not stimulate insulin release but act by improving insulin resistance.

Insulin Therapy

When appropriate diet therapy in combination with oral antidiabetic agents eventually proves to be insufficient for adequate glycemic control in NIDDM, it is most likely that progressive beta cell failure has occurred and that the level of endogenous insulin secretion is no longer sufficient to maintain proper glycemic control. At this stage, therapy with exogenous insulin is indicated.

Certain special features of insulin therapy in NIDDM should be discussed with patients. First, it should be emphasized that insulin is an adjunct to and not a substitute for proper diet, exercise, and weight-control measures. Indeed, the patient should be forewarned that poor adherence to diet during insulin therapy will most likely lead to weight gain, worsening of insulin resistance, and escalation of insulin requirements to inordinately high dosage levels. Frank discussion of these issues with patients results in improved compliance with dietary recommendations. Second, patients should be advised that chronic hyperglycemia can aggravate the impairment in insulin secretion and insulin action in NIDDM, and that many of these acquired defects can be reversed following optimization of glycemic control with insulin therapy. Thus, it is possible for some insulin-treated NIDDM patients to return to therapy with diet and oral agents or diet alone. This possibility is a strong incentive for patient compliance with diet, exercise, and weight-control regimens.

The specific insulin regimen should be individualized for each patient by taking into account the patient's glycemic profile throughout the day (derived from finger stick blood glucose measurements performed in the fasting state, before each meal, and at bedtime), the amount and distribution of meals, and the level of physical activity. Most patients require

---

*Glimepiride (Amaryl) was approved for use in the U.S. in April 1996.

insulin dosing twice a day, given before breakfast and before the evening meal. Initially, intermediate-acting insulin (NPH or Lente) can be used, although the addition of short-acting (regular) insulin to each of the two doses is often necessary to control postprandial glycemia. In many cases, premixed insulin such as the 70/30 preparation (i.e., 70% intermediate-acting and 30% short-acting insulin) is used because of convenience in administration. Other insulin regimens, including dosing more than two times per day, can be instituted for more intensive therapy, depending on the daily glycemic profile and the specific needs of the patient.

In estimating the starting dose of insulin for NIDDM patients, it is helpful to first calculate the expected range of total eventual dose and then use about 50% of this level as the starting dose. Further adjustments can be made based on the patient's monitored glycemic profile. The total expected eventual dose for nonobese NIDDM patients is 0.5 to 0.7 U per kg per day; for obese patients (those weighing >20% above normal weight), the total eventual dose is estimated to be 1.0 to 1.2 U per kg per day. For most patients, two-thirds of the total daily dose is given before breakfast, and one-third is given before supper. About two-thirds of each dose should be intermediate-acting insulin and one-third should be short-acting insulin, although this can vary based on individual patient requirements. The main side effect of insulin therapy is hypoglycemia, and this can be minimized or eliminated by appropriate glycemic monitoring of the patient.

Combination Therapy

Since the sites and mechanisms of action of the three classes of oral antidiabetic agents are different (Table 6), it should be possible to use combination therapy to maximize glycemic control. In patients with suboptimal glycemic control while on maximal doses of sulfonylureas, the addition of metformin significantly improves control. Presumably, this occurs because of the combined effects of augmented insulin secretion (sulfonylurea effect) and increased peripheral glucose uptake and decreased hepatic glucose production (metformin effects). It is important to note that combination therapy should be considered only after first maximizing therapy with one agent. Acarbose can also be added to sulfonylurea therapy, especially in patients who experience significant

postprandial hyperglycemia. In this setting, the acarbose dose is titrated by following the 1-hour-postprandial plasma glucose levels. There is presently insufficient information regarding the efficacy of acarbose-metformin combination therapy.

The use of sulfonylureas in combination with insulin therapy has produced variable results. In NIDDM patients requiring very large doses of insulin, sulfonylureas have been added in an effort to decrease the insulin requirement. However, for the most part, the benefits obtained have been limited. A sequential sulfonylurea-insulin therapy regimen has also been utilized. In this setting, intermediate-acting insulin is administered at bedtime to decrease nocturnal hepatic glucose production and improve fasting blood glucose levels. The sulfonylureas are then administered in the morning to control the daytime glycemia. This regimen, termed BIDS (bedtime insulin daytime sulfonylurea), can be used as an intermediate therapeutic step in patients who are secondary sulfonylurea failures before such patients are switched to insulin therapy alone. If this regimen proves to be unsuccessful after a trial of 1 to 2 months, the sulfonylureas are stopped and the patients are switched to twice-daily administration of insulin. Anecdotal reports indicate that the addition of metformin to insulin therapy in NIDDM helps reduce the large insulin dose requirements in some patients. Although the rationale for this is evident, controlled studies are needed to conclusively establish the general usefulness of metformin-insulin combination therapy.

Monitoring of Therapy

The availability of practical methods for monitoring the glycemic status of patients with diabetes mellitus has greatly facilitated effective patient management. Self-monitoring of blood glucose (SMBG) should be a component of all diabetes management, since it is essential not only for therapeutic decision making but also for monitoring patient safety. With this method, blood glucose readings can be obtained using either a color chart or a glucose meter. The latter is the preferred method because of its reliability and accuracy. The frequency of performance of SMBG can be quite variable and should be individualized, taking into account the profile and stability of the glycemic control, the nature of the therapeutic regimen, and the presence or absence of intercurrent

TABLE 6. **Comparison of Oral Antidiabetic Agents**

Drug	Site of Action	Mechanism of Action	Side Effects
Sulfonylureas (see Table 4)	Pancreas (beta cell)	↑ insulin secretion	Hypoglycemia, weight gain
Metformin (Glucophage)	Liver, peripheral tissues	↓ glucose production ↑ glucose uptake	Gastrointestinal symptoms, lactic acidosis (rare)*
Acarbose (Precose)	Small intestine	↓ carbohydrate digestion and absorption	Gastrointestinal symptoms

*In susceptible subjects (see exclusion criteria in Table 5).

illnesses or other stressful situations. For a patient who is well managed on diet therapy alone, SMBG once or twice a week can be sufficient; for an insulin-treated patient, the frequency can be two to four times daily or more. Overall, the most important consideration is that the patient has the ability and the means to perform SMBG and can appropriately respond to the glucose data obtained (with appropriate input from his or her diabetes care team).

For estimation of the average level of blood glucose over the preceding 2- to 3-month period, measurements of glycated hemoglobin fractions should be used. The levels of these fractions in diabetic patients increase in proportion to the duration and degree of hyperglycemia. Different assay methods are used to measure different fractions (HbA$_{1C}$, HbA$_1$, or fast hemoglobin), and the appropriate reference ranges for each of these should be used in patient monitoring and decision making. The optimal frequency for obtaining these assays in NIDDM patients is variable and ranges from two to four determinations per year, based on the stability of the glycemic control and the treatment modalities being used.

INTEGRATION OF THE MANAGEMENT PLAN

Providing effective care for a patient with diabetes requires a multidisciplinary approach that is based on the participation of a management team. The core team consists of the patient and his or her family, the physician, a diabetes educator, and a nutritionist. To the extent feasible, input and participation by an exercise physiologist, clinical psychologist, and other related health care providers should also be sought. Based on the stage of the disease and the patient's specific needs, one should also enlist the help of specialists in podiatry, ophthalmology, nephrology, urology, neurology, and cardiology. The success of this multidisciplinary management effort is highly dependent on the extent to which the patient has been educated about the disease process and encouraged and empowered to be an active participant in his or her own care. Accordingly, patient education is extremely important, and this should be provided not only at the beginning of therapy but also as an ongoing process. Patient education is an effective means of enhancing compliance with the treatment plan and facilitating active participation in SMBG and institution of follow-up recommendations. The level of patient education and the formulation of treatment and monitoring plans should be individualized, taking into account the age of the patient, stage of the disease, and educational, socioeconomic, and psychosocial factors. The frequency of follow-up visits should also be individualized, based on patient needs. The details of clinical practice recommendations for diabetics have been addressed elsewhere.*

Finally, it is important to emphasize that in addi-

---

*See American Diabetes Association—clinical practice recommendations. Diabetes Care 19 (Suppl 1):S1–S118, 1996.

tion to glycemic control, the management of NIDDM also involves the identification and treatment of cardiovascular risk factors. Cardiovascular disease is the major cause of morbidity and mortality in NIDDM; its major modifiable risk factors, in addition to diabetes mellitus, include dyslipidemia, hypertension, and smoking. Appropriate management of these risk factors in conjunction with optimization of glycemic control should go a long way toward minimizing or even eliminating the macrovascular and microvascular complications of NIDDM.

DIABETES MELLITUS IN CHILDREN AND ADOLESCENTS

method of
JOSEPH I. WOLFSDORF, M.B., B.Ch., and
CHRISTINA LUEDKE, M.D., Ph.D.
Children's Hospital
Boston, Massachusetts

Type I diabetes mellitus or insulin-dependent diabetes mellitus (IDDM) results from insulin deficiency caused by chronic progressive autoimmune destruction of the insulin-producing beta cells of the islets of Langerhans. In the United States, the prevalence of IDDM in people younger than 20 years is about 1.7 cases per 1000; it is estimated that there are about 125,000 children and teenagers with IDDM.

Hyperglycemia occurs when at least 90% of the beta-cell mass has been destroyed. The most common symptoms are polyuria, polydipsia, and weight loss. Dehydration results from the osmotic diuresis induced by hyperglycemia. More severe insulin deficiency causes unrestrained lipolysis and ketoacid production that leads to an anion gap acidosis characterized by nausea, vomiting, abdominal pain, and hyperpnea (Kussmaul's respiration).

At diagnosis, most children have residual beta cells whose function is impaired by hyperglycemia. Reversal of the metabolic derangements restores function of the remaining beta cells for months to years until they are destroyed by progression of the autoimmune process. Similarly, correction of hyperglycemia restores tissue sensitivity to insulin. These two factors account for the period of partial remission, often called the "honeymoon," during which normal or nearly normal glycemic control is easily maintained with a relatively low dose of insulin, on the order of less than 0.3 to 0.5 U per kg per day. After destruction of the remaining beta cells, the insulin dose gradually increases until the full replacement dose is reached.

At our center, most children are briefly hospitalized to initiate therapy. Even when the child is not gravely ill, the emotional impact of the diagnosis on the child and family often causes great distress. Therefore, we prefer to begin the program of diabetes education and self-care training in a safe and supportive environment. This enables grieving and overwhelmed parents to acquire survival skills while they are coping with the emotional upheaval caused by the crisis resulting from the discovery of this incurable disease in their child.

The initial goals of therapy are to stabilize the metabolic state with insulin, fluid, and electrolyte replacement and to provide basic diabetes education and self-care training to the patient, in an age-appropriate fashion, and to parents and other important caregivers.

DIABETIC KETOACIDOSIS

Approximately one-third of newly diagnosed children referred to Children's Hospital, Boston, arrive in diabetic ketoacidosis (DKA). The principles of the treatment protocol used at this center are presented here.

Initial Evaluation

1. Perform a clinical evaluation to establish the diagnosis and determine its cause (especially any evidence of infection) and to assess the patient's degree of dehydration. Weigh the patient and measure height or length.

2. With a glucose meter, determine the blood glucose concentration at the bedside.

3. Obtain a blood sample for measurement of plasma glucose, electrolytes, total CO_2, BUN, serum osmolality, arterial or venous pH, P_{CO_2}, P_{O_2}, hemoglobin, hematocrit, white blood cell count and differential, calcium, magnesium, and phosphorus. Calculate the anion gap.

4. Perform a urinalysis and obtain appropriate specimens for culture (blood, urine, throat) even if the patient is afebrile.

5. Perform an electrocardiogram for baseline evaluation of potassium status.

6. Determine baseline neurologic status.

Supportive Measures

1. In semiconscious or unconscious patients, secure the airway and empty the stomach by nasogastric suction to prevent aspiration.

2. Give supplementary oxygen to patients who are cyanosed or in shock or when the PaO_2 is less than 80 mm Hg.

3. Measure urine output accurately; use bladder or condom catheterization if necessary.

4. Record in a flow chart the patient's clinical and laboratory data, details of fluid and electrolyte therapy, administered insulin, and urine output. Successful management of diabetic ketoacidosis requires meticulous monitoring of the patient's clinical and biochemical response to treatment so that timely adjustments in the treatment regimen can be made when necessary.

5. Measure plasma glucose, serum electrolytes (and corrected sodium), pH, P_{CO_2}, T_{CO_2}, anion gap, calcium, and phosphorus every 2 hours for the first 8 hours and then every 4 hours until they are normal.

6. Admit to an intensive care unit infants, toddlers, and severely ill older children with DKA, especially those with central nervous system obtundation or cardiovascular instability.

7. Administer broad-spectrum antibiotics to febrile patients after appropriate cultures of body fluids have been obtained.

Fluid and Electrolyte Treatment

All patients with DKA are dehydrated and suffer total body depletion of sodium, potassium, chloride, phosphate, and magnesium. Patients with mild-to-moderate DKA are usually about 5% (50 mL per kg) dehydrated, and those with severe DKA are up to 10% (100 mL per kg) dehydrated.

1. Start an intravenous infusion using a large-bore cannula and infuse 10 mL per kg of isotonic saline solution (0.9%) within 60 minutes. In the severely dehydrated patient or the patient in shock, initially give 20 mL per kg followed by an additional 10 mL per kg over 60 minutes if hypotension or shock persists.

2. Once the circulation has been stabilized, change to half-normal saline solution and aim to replace the calculated fluid deficit at an even rate over 24 to 36 hours. Aim to achieve slow correction of the serum hyperosmolality and to avoid a rapid shift of water from the extracellular to the intracellular compartment. The sodium concentration of the solution should be increased to 100 to 130 mEq per liter if the corrected serum sodium concentration fails to rise as the plasma glucose concentration decreases. The corrected sodium is calculated:

$$Na^+ + (1.6 \times [\text{plasma glucose mg per dL} - 100]/100)$$

3. Maintenance fluid is given as half isotonic saline solution at a rate of 1500 mL per m^2 per day.

4. Add 5% dextrose to the infusion fluid when the plasma glucose concentration reaches 300 mg per dL and attempt to maintain the plasma glucose concentration at approximately 200 mg per dL for the first 36 to 48 hours. To avert hypoglycemia, 10% dextrose may be needed.

5. Continue intravenous fluid administration until acidosis is corrected and the patient can eat and drink without vomiting.

Insulin

After an intravenous priming dose of 0.1 U per kg, insulin is diluted in saline solution (50 U regular insulin in 50 mL saline solution) and is given intravenously at a rate of 0.1 U per kg per hour, controlled by an infusion pump. Insulin has a serum half-life of approximately 5 to 7 minutes; therefore, insulin deficiency develops rapidly if the insulin infusion is interrupted. Intravenous insulin therapy should not be used unless it can be closely supervised.

When DKA has resolved (venous pH greater than 7.32, total CO_2 greater than 18 mEq per liter) and the change to subcutaneous insulin is planned, the first injection should be given 60 to 120 minutes before stopping the infusion, to allow sufficient time for the injected insulin to be absorbed.

Potassium Replacement

All patients with DKA are potassium depleted (4 to 6 mEq per kg) despite an initial serum potassium concentration that may be normal or increased. With the administration of fluid and insulin, serum potassium may decrease abruptly, predisposing the patient to cardiac arrhythmias. Patients whose serum potassium level is initially low are the most severely depleted. They should receive potassium after urinating, and the serum potassium concentration should be measured hourly. The serum potassium level should be maintained in the normal range. Half the potassium is given as potassium acetate and the other half as potassium phosphate; this reduces the total amount of chloride administered and partially replaces the phosphate deficit.

Acidosis

Routine administration of bicarbonate neither hastens resolution of acidosis nor improves survival and may impair tissue oxygenation and cause hypokalemia. Its routine use is not recommended; however, when acidosis is severe (arterial pH less than 7.0) or there is hypotension, shock, or an arrhythmia, sodium bicarbonate, 1 to 2 mEq per kg or 40 to 80 mEq per m^2, is infused over 2 hours.

Cerebral Edema

This is an uncommon complication of DKA that can cause acute brain herniation and death. It typically develops abruptly within 2 to 12 hours of starting treatment and manifests as headache, vomiting, altered level of consciousness, delirium or restlessness, incontinence, bradycardia, increased blood pressure, unequal pupils, papilledema, respiratory arrest, and sudden onset of polyuria from acute diabetes insipidus. Computed tomography scan of the brain confirms brain swelling. When cerebral edema is suspected, the following steps should be taken immediately: administer mannitol, 1 gram per kg intravenously, and repeat as necessary; reduce the rate of fluid administration; insert an endotracheal tube; and hyperventilate the patient.

INSULIN THERAPY

The three major categories of insulin preparations differ in their absorption kinetics (Table 1). Several insulin regimens can be used: each has the same goal, namely, to provide basal insulin throughout the

TABLE 2. **Insulin Regimens**

Doses	Breakfast	Lunch	Dinner	Bedtime
Two	R + NPH/L		R + NPH/L	
	R + NPH/L		R + UL	
	R + UL		R + UL	
Three	R + NPH/L		R	NPH/L
	R + UL	R	R + UL	
Four	R	R	R	NPH/L
	R + NPH/L	R	R	NPH/L

Abbreviations: R = regular insulin; L = lente insulin; UL = ultralente insulin; NPH/L = either intermediate-acting insulin may be selected for use with this regimen.

day and more with meals (Table 2). The most commonly used regimen consists of a combination of short- and intermediate-acting (NPH or Lente) insulin given twice daily, before breakfast and before the evening meal. A modification of this regimen that involves three doses per day, with intermediate-acting insulin given at bedtime instead of before supper, is especially recommended for adolescents. The child's age, weight, and pubertal status guide the initial choice of dose.

Subcutaneous insulin is started in a newly diagnosed child who is not significantly dehydrated, is not vomiting, and either does not have ketoacidosis or has mild ketoacidosis (arterial pH greater than 7.25, venous pH greater than 7.20). In a child diagnosed early with moderate hyperglycemia and no ketonuria, the recommended starting dose of insulin is 0.3 to 0.5 U per kg per day. When metabolic decompensation is more severe (ketonuria but without acidosis or dehydration), the initial dose is 0.5 to 0.75 U per kg, supplemented, if necessary, with 0.1 U per kg of regular insulin subcutaneously at 4- to 6-hour intervals. The upper end of each suggested range is used for pubertal patients and for those who are physically inactive and overweight. The total daily dose (TDD) is divided so that two-thirds is given before breakfast and one-third in the evening. The ratio of short- to intermediate-acting insulin at both times is 1:2. Target blood glucose levels for different ages are shown in Table 3. The insulin dose is adjusted until satisfactory blood glucose control is achieved.

For toddlers and young children, we use U10 (U100 insulin diluted 1:10) regular insulin; children of this age typically require a smaller fraction of regular

TABLE 1. **Insulin Preparations***

Type	Action	Onset of Action (h)	Peak Action (h)	Duration of Action (h)
Regular	Short-acting	0.5	2–4	6–8
NPH (isophane)	Intermediate-acting	1–2	6–12	18–24
Lente	Intermediate-acting	1–3	6–12	18–24
Ultralente	Long-acting	4–6	8–20	24–28

*These figures are for human insulins and are approximations from laboratory studies in test subjects. The times of onset, peak, and duration of action vary greatly within and between patients and are affected by many factors, including size of dose, site of injection, exercise of the injected area, temperature, and insulin antibodies.

TABLE 3. **Target Blood Glucose Levels for Children and Adolescents***

	Fasting (mg/dL)	Premeal (mg/dL)	2–4 A.M. (mg/dL)
Infant/toddler	80–180	100–200	80–180
School-age	80–150	80–180	80–150
Adolescent	70–120	70–180	70–150

*Target blood glucose levels for patients with normal counterregulatory mechanisms who practice intensive insulin therapy are 70–120 mg/dL fasting and before meals, <180 mg/dL 90–120 minutes after meals, and 70–100 mg/dL at 2–4 A.M.

insulin (10 to 20%) with proportionately more inter-mediate-acting insulin.

The optimal ratio of rapid- to intermediate-acting insulin for each patient is determined empirically, guided by the results of frequent blood glucose measurements. Five measurements daily: before each meal, before the bedtime snack, and at 2 to 4 A.M., are initially required to determine the effects of each prescribed dose. Adjustments are made to each dose at 3- to 5-day intervals, usually in 10% increments or decrements, in response to patterns of consistently elevated or low blood glucose levels, respectively. The daily insulin requirements of patients with complete insulin deficiency ("total" diabetes) is 0.5 to 1.0 U per kg before puberty and 0.8 to 1.5 U per kg during puberty.

Good glycemic control is impossible to achieve without strict attention to the other important factors that influence blood glucose levels: namely, diet and physical activity.

NUTRITION

Attention must be paid to the timing and content of meals in order to match food intake with the availability of injected insulin. The registered dietitian is an important member of the diabetes treatment team. Starting with the initial hospitalization and continuing with intermittent visits in the outpatient setting, the dietitian is responsible for instructing patients on the principles of nutritional management of diabetes and formulating an individualized meal plan that attempts to minimize postprandial hyperglycemia and avoid hypoglycemia between meals.

General Principles

The nutritional needs of children with diabetes do not differ from those of healthy children. Newly diagnosed children, however, typically have lost weight, and the initial diet prescription aims to restore a desirable weight for height. Once this has been achieved, the total intake of calories and nutrients must be sufficient to balance the daily expenditure of energy and satisfy the requirements for normal growth and development. A method commonly used to estimate energy requirements is based on age and is useful as a crude approximation for children up to 12 years of age: to 1000 kcal, add 100 × the patient's age in years.

The American Diabetes Association currently recommends that carbohydrate provide 50 to 60% of the total calories, with protein and fat making up 15 and 30%, respectively. The diet prescription has to be periodically adjusted to achieve an ideal or desirable body weight and to maintain a normal rate of physical growth and maturation. The main objective of dietary therapy in obese patients is to lose weight.

People with diabetes are predisposed to atherosclerosis and should follow a prudent fat diet; the amount of fat should not exceed 30% of the total daily calories. Dietary cholesterol is reduced to 300 mg per day or less and saturated fat to less than 10% of calories by consumption of less beef and pork and leaner cuts of meat, chicken, turkey, fish, low-fat milk, and vegetable proteins.

Dietary fiber may benefit the diabetic patient by blunting the rise in blood glucose after meals. Unrefined or minimally processed foods, such as grains, legumes, and vegetables, should replace highly refined carbohydrates. To avoid abrupt increases in blood glucose, children should eat fruit whole and avoid fruit juices, which should be reserved for treating episodes of hypoglycemia.

Because insulin is released continuously from the injection site, hypoglycemia, exacerbated by exercise, may occur if snacks are not eaten between the main meals. Hence, most children who receive twice-daily injections of insulin (split-mixed insulin regimen) have a snack between each meal and at bedtime; adolescents usually prefer to omit the midmorning snack. Meals and snacks should be eaten at approximately the same time each day, and the total consumption of calories and the proportions of carbohydrate, protein, and fat in each meal and snack should be consistent from day to day.

Exchange System

The meal plan is formulated using the system of food exchanges and is individualized to meet the ethnic, religious, and economic circumstances of each family and the food preferences of the individual child. The diet prescription must take into account the child's school schedule, gym classes, and after-school physical activity. The exchange system is based on six food groups—milk, fruit, vegetable, bread/starch, meat/protein, and fat—and the meal plan contains the number of exchanges from each food group to be included in each meal and snack. Parents should learn to calculate exchanges from the information on food labels.

EXERCISE

Exercise acutely lowers the blood glucose concentration by increasing utilization of glucose to a variable degree, depending on the intensity and duration of physical activity and the concurrent level of insulinemia. Children and teenagers with diabetes are encouraged to participate in sports and to exercise throughout the year. In addition to normalizing the child's life and promoting a positive self-image, exercise promotes good health practices, facilitates weight control, and may improve glycemic control.

Young children's activities tend to be spontaneous; bursts of activity are covered with a snack before and, if the exercise is prolonged, during the activity. A useful guide is to provide 15 grams of carbohydrate (one bread or fruit exchange) per 30 to 60 minutes of vigorous physical activity. Strenuous exercise in the afternoon or evening should be followed by a 10 to 20% reduction in the presupper or bedtime dose of intermediate-acting insulin and a larger bedtime snack, to reduce the risk of nocturnal or early-morning hypoglycemia from the lag effect of exercise.

Acute vigorous exercise in the face of poorly controlled diabetes can aggravate hyperglycemia and ketoacid production. Therefore, a child with ketonuria should not exercise. Exercising the limb into which insulin has been injected accelerates the rate of insulin absorption. If exercise is planned, it is recommended that the preceding insulin injection be given in a site that is least likely to be affected by exercise. Youngsters who participate in organized sports are advised to reduce the dose of insulin predominantly active during the period of sustained physical activity. The size of such reductions is determined by measuring blood glucose levels before and after exercise and are generally in the range of 10 to 30% of the usual insulin dose.

DIABETES CARE IN THE OUTPATIENT SETTING

The child is discharged from the hospital as soon as she or he is medically stable and the parents (or other care providers) have learned the essentials of diabetes management: insulin administration, self-monitoring of blood glucose (SMBG), urine ketone measurement, basic meal planning, and recognition and treatment of hypoglycemia. Frequent telephone contact, often daily, is initially needed to help parents interpret SMBG data and adjust insulin dose(s) necessitated by the home schedule of activity and meals. Within the first few weeks of diagnosis, two-thirds of children enter partial remission, and the dose of insulin usually has to be reduced considerably.

The patient is seen frequently in the first month, primarily by the nurse specialist/educator and dietitian, to review and consolidate the skills and principles taught in the hospital. Thereafter, follow-up visits with members of the diabetes team occur every 3 months. The purpose of regular clinic visits is to ensure that the child's diabetes is being appropriately managed at home and that the goals of therapy are met. A focused history should obtain information about self-care behaviors, the child's daily routines, the frequency, severity, and circumstances surrounding hypoglycemic events, and evidence of hyperglycemia (polyuria, polydipsia, nocturia, weight loss, blurry vision, perineal candidiasis).

At every visit, height and weight are measured and plotted on a growth chart. The weight curve is especially helpful in assessing adequacy of therapy, since a significant weight loss usually indicates that the prescribed dose is insufficient or the patient is omitting injections. A physical examination should be performed at least twice per year and includes measurement of blood pressure, pubertal staging, signs of thyroid disease, skin examination, and an evaluation of the organs most affected by long-standing diabetes. The injection sites are inspected for evidence of lipohypertrophy from overuse of the site.

Insulin therapy must be viewed as a dynamic process that takes into account growth and development, changes in lifestyle and activity, intercurrent illness, and other factors that influence insulin requirements. Doses are adjusted with the goal of maintaining blood glucose levels within the target range as much as possible. The target range varies with the age of the patient (see Table 3). For infants and toddlers, who cannot understand or easily express symptoms of hypoglycemia, the target range is higher to minimize the risk of severe hypoglycemia.

Regular clinic visits are opportunities to reinforce and expand on the diabetes self-care training that began in the hospital. Optimal care of diabetes depends on the patient's intimate understanding of the interplay of medication and lifestyle. At each visit, the goal is to increase the patient's and family's understanding of diabetes management, so that as the child becomes more independent, he or she can assume increasing responsibility for daily self-care. Mature and motivated teenagers are encouraged to use intensified insulin management techniques that involve multiple daily insulin injections, use of algorithms for insulin dose selection, and target blood glucose levels in or near the normal range (see Table 3).

Self-Monitoring of Blood Glucose

This is routinely taught to all patients with IDDM, and the ability of patients to obtain accurate results is confirmed at clinic visits, when patients are asked to compare results obtained with their meters with simultaneous blood glucose determinations in the clinical chemistry laboratory. SMBG is the cornerstone of any intensive diabetes management program, and frequent SMBG in conjunction with urine tests for ketones is essential to manage intercurrent illnesses and prevent ketoacidosis. A variety of meters with a digital display are available that enable the user to obtain measurements of blood glucose concentration within 10% of the value obtained in a clinical chemistry laboratory.

Patients ideally should test before each meal and at bedtime. If this is impractical or intolerable, patients should be encouraged to test before each dose of insulin and perform additional tests before lunch and at bedtime at least twice each week. Alternatively, for patients who cannot tolerate such frequent monitoring or who cannot afford the cost of the reagent strips, a period of intensive monitoring before each meal, at bedtime, and between 2 and 4 A.M. for several consecutive days before an office visit often provides sufficient information to confirm satisfactory control or serve as a basis for modifying the insulin regimen.

Urine should be tested for the presence of *ketones* whenever the child is sick, when the blood glucose level exceeds 250 mg per dL, and when blood glucose levels are high before breakfast and the possibility of unrecognized nocturnal hypoglycemia is suspected.

Glycosylated Hemoglobin (Hemoglobin A$_1$ or A$_{1c}$). The level of glycosylated hemoglobin, formed when glucose is bound nonenzymatically to the hemoglobin molecule, is directly proportional to the time-integrated mean blood glucose concentration over the preceding 2 to 3 months. Quarterly determinations of glycosylated hemoglobin should be used to provide an objective measure of average glycemia in the intervals between office visits.

PSYCHOSOCIAL ISSUES

A social worker performs a psychosocial assessment on all newly diagnosed patients and their families. Thereafter, patients are referred to the mental health specialist on the diabetes team when emotional, social, or financial concerns are identified that may be obstacles to achieving and maintaining acceptable glycemic control. Common problems encountered in a diabetes clinic are financial hardship affecting the ability to purchase costly supplies, parental guilt, the child's rebellion against treatment, noncompliance with medication, family adjustment problems, and frequently missed appointments. Recurrent ketoacidosis is the most extreme indicator of psychosocial stress.

HYPOGLYCEMIA

Occasional episodes of hypoglycemia are an unavoidable consequence of insulin therapy aimed at maintaining blood glucose levels near normal. The goal is to minimize the frequency and severity of hypoglycemia while maintaining blood glucose levels as close to normal as possible.

Patients and family members must be taught to recognize the early symptoms of hypoglycemia and to treat it promptly with a suitable form of concentrated carbohydrate. Because infants and toddlers may be unable to recognize the symptoms of hypoglycemia and cannot verbalize their symptoms, parents are advised to measure the blood glucose concentration whenever the child's behavior is unusual. Most episodes of hypoglycemia are satisfactorily treated with 10 to 20 grams of glucose; 5 grams is sufficient for an infant or toddler. Suitable forms of rapidly absorbed carbohydrate for treatment of hypoglycemia are glucose tablets (each contains 5 grams of glucose), Lifesavers candy (3 grams each), granulated table sugar (4 grams per teaspoon), orange or apple juice (10 to 12 grams per 120 mL). Family members are taught to use glucagon (which should be available at home) to treat an episode of severe hypoglycemia in which the child is unconscious or unable to swallow or retain ingested carbohydrate. Glucagon (0.02 to 0.03 mg per kg, maximum dose 1.0 mg) is injected intramuscularly or subcutaneously and raises the blood glucose level within 5 to 15 minutes. Nausea and vomiting may follow the administration of glucagon. After consciousness has been regained, oral carbohydrate should be given to prevent further hypoglycemia. If the patient cannot take it orally or retain sugar-containing fluids, glucose, 0.5 gram per kg, is injected intravenously followed by a continuous infusion at a rate that maintains a normal blood glucose concentration.

A Medic Alert bracelet or necklace should always be worn to identify the patient as having diabetes mellitus.

SCREENING FOR COMPLICATIONS

The organs most affected by diabetes are the eyes, kidneys, circulatory system, and peripheral nervous system. Diabetic complications develop insidiously but can be detected years before they become symptomatic. Systematic screening is performed to detect abnormalities early, when intervention to arrest, reverse, or retard complications is most beneficial. Both diabetic retinopathy and nephropathy are rare before puberty and in patients who have had IDDM for less than 5 years. Therefore, beginning 5 years after diagnosis, patients annually should have a dilated retinal examination and measurement of albumin and creatinine concentrations in a timed overnight or first-morning urine specimen to detect microalbuminuria. Circulatory and neurologic complications of diabetes are seldom clinically significant in the pediatric and adolescent population.

CONCLUSION

Advances in the treatment of diabetes in children in the past 2 decades now make it possible to ensure normal growth and development and safely achieve a level of blood glucose control that previously was unattainable. It is reasonable to expect that the benefits of sustained improvement in glycemic control will prevent, or at least delay, the appearance of the chronic complications of diabetes. It is important, however, to remember that the arduous task of controlling blood glucose in a child is difficult and frustrating. The members of the diabetes team must set realistic and attainable goals for each patient and constantly provide encouragement and support. The resources of a multidisciplinary health care team—physician, nurse educator, dietitian, mental health specialist, and ophthalmologist—are essential for the successful management of IDDM by the child or adolescent and family.

DIABETIC KETOACIDOSIS

method of
MONICA E. DOERR, M.D., and
JOHN B. BUSE, M.D., Ph.D.
University of North Carolina at Chapel Hill
School of Medicine
Chapel Hill, North Carolina

PATHOPHYSIOLOGY OF DIABETIC EMERGENCIES

Currently, the majority of patients with diabetes can be classified as having type I (juvenile-onset or insulin-dependent) diabetes or type II (adult-onset or non–insulin-dependent) diabetes. Type I diabetes results from the auto-immune destruction of the insulin-secreting beta cells in the pancreas leading to insulin deficiency. Most patients with type I diabetes present in childhood or early adult-hood though well-documented cases have been described in the geriatric population. In times of stress (either physiologic or emotional), insulin requirements increase and often precipitate metabolic decompensation because of inadequate insulin secretory reserve. The half-life of insulin in the circulation is only 7 minutes; therefore, treatment of insulin deficiency requires continuous delivery to the circulation by infusion or by diffusion of insulin from depot injections.

Diabetic ketoacidosis (DKA) is the life-threatening metabolic consequence of insulin deficiency. Insulin deficiency in concert with excess secretion of primarily glucagon as well as catecholamines, glucocorticoids, and growth hormone produces hyperglycemia by stimulating glycogenolysis and gluconeogenesis and impairing glucose disposal. This hormonal milieu also results in lipolysis and unrestrained fatty acid oxidation, producing acetone, β-hydroxybutyrate, and acetoacetate, and thereby ketoacidosis.

DKA AND ITS DIFFERENTIAL DIAGNOSIS

The cases of DKA that are not recognized quickly usually occur in patients with new-onset diabetes. All patients with nonspecific complaints such as fatigue, dizziness, and malaise should be asked about more specific symptoms of diabetes. Polyuria or nocturia and weight loss are commonly present, though often not reported by the patient. Measurement of glucose and electrolytes is indicated in any patient with a severe illness and new-onset neurologic changes.

History and Physical Examination

In DKA, the metabolic decompensation usually develops over a period of hours to a few days. The classic presentation of DKA includes lethargy and a characteristic hyperventilation pattern known as Kussmaul's respirations with deep slow breaths associated with the fruity odor of acetone. Complaints of nausea and vomiting are very common, with abdominal pain somewhat less frequently reported. The abdominal pain can be severe and may be associated with distention, ileus, and tenderness without rebound. Unless there is underlying abdominal pathology, the abdominal pain should resolve fairly quickly with therapy. Most patients are normotensive and tachycardic with signs of mild-to-moderate volume depletion. Patients in DKA with underlying infection may not manifest fever; in fact, hypothermia has been described. Cerebral edema may develop during therapy.

Laboratory Studies and Differential Diagnosis

Once DKA is considered, the diagnosis can be quickly made with routine laboratory studies. It is important to differentiate DKA from other causes of ketosis and metabolic acidosis. This can be quite difficult since these disorders often coexist.

The sine qua non of DKA is ketoacidosis. Two ketoacids are produced in DKA—β-hydroxybutyrate and acetoacetate—as well as the neutral ketone acetone. Patients with DKA will almost always have large amounts of ketones in their urine. The nitroprusside reaction commonly used to detect ketone bodies does not react with β-hydroxybutyrate. In severe DKA, the predominant ketone is often β-hydroxybutyrate; therefore, it is possible though unusual to have a minimal serum nitroprusside reaction despite the presence of severe ketosis. Fortunately, the "anion gap" (normal <14 mEq per L) provides a readily available index for unmeasured anions in the blood:

$$anion\ gap = sodium - (chloride + bicarbonate).$$

Most patients with DKA will have an anion gap greater than 20 mEq per L and some as high as greater than 40 mEq per L at presentation.

The serum glucose in DKA is usually in the 500 mg per dL range. Euglycemic DKA has been described in the presence of decreased oral intake or pregnancy. In these cases, the serum glucose is near normal, but the patient requires insulin therapy for the clearance of acidosis.

The arterial pH is commonly less than 7.3 and can be as low as 6.5. Tachypnea with hypocapnia causing partial respiratory compensation is to be expected. Hyperosmolality is typically mild; osmolalities greater than 330 mOsm per kg are unusual without mental status changes.

The combination of hyperglycemia, metabolic acidosis, and an increased anion gap is not always due to DKA. Lactic acidosis usually occurs with decreased tissue oxygen delivery and often arises as a consequence of dehydration or shock and complicates other primary metabolic acidoses. The presentation is identical to DKA; however, in pure lactic acidosis, the serum glucose and ketones should be normal unless diabetes coexists.

Starvation ketosis occurs as a result of physiologically appropriate lipolysis and ketone production to provide fuel for muscle metabolism. Starvation ketosis is essentially never associated with ketoacidosis as ketone bodies are not produced in sufficient quantities to accumulate in the plasma. Alcoholic ketoacidosis is a more severe form of starvation ketosis. In these patients, who are typically long-standing alcoholics for whom ethanol has been the main caloric source for days to weeks, the ketogenic response to poor carbohydrate intake is increased. The ketoacidosis presents when alcohol and caloric intake decrease for any reason but generally as a result of abdominal pain. In alcoholic ketoacidosis, the patient will usually be normoglycemic or hypoglycemic though occasionally mild hyperglycemia is present.

It should be kept in mind that patients will often present with more than one of these processes. DKA can present with hyperosmolarity and coma. Hyperglycemic hyperosmolar nonketotic coma (HHNC) can have mild-to-moderate ketonemia and acidosis. Alcoholic ketoacidosis can complicate either DKA or HHNC; furthermore, lactic acidosis is common in severe DKA and HHNC. *We recommend that any patient with a serum glucose over 250 mg per dL and an anion gap metabolic acidosis should be treated by the general principle outlined below. Consideration should be given to the possible contributions of other metabolic acidoses.*

THERAPY

In the past 50 years, numerous controversies have arisen regarding the optimum management of DKA. The guidelines we propose are based in large part on prospective studies of DKA by Kitabchi and coworkers and are readily applicable to HHNC. The general approach (Table 1) is to (1) follow the patient carefully, (2) restore the circulation by providing neces-

TABLE 1. **Treatment of Diabetic Ketoacidosis**

Fluids (Usual Deficit 5–10 L)

If hypotensive: 1 L 0.90% NaCl in first h
If normotensive: 1 L 0.45% NaCl in first h
In subsequent hours:
    Match urine output with 0.45% NaCl
    If hypotensive, 200–1000 mL/h 0.9% NaCl (consider Swan-
      Ganz catheter and colloid solutions)
    Otherwise, calculate free water deficit and replace 50% over
      12 h
    After glucose reaches 250–300 mg/dL, add glucose to IV fluids

Insulin (Regular)

10-U IV bolus
0.1 U/kg/h IV continuously or 0.2 U/kg IM hourly
Check glucose hourly and adjust drip to decrease glucose 10%
    per h to a level of 250 mg/dL

Potassium (Usual Deficit 200–1000 mEq)/Phosphate

Establish that the patient is not oliguric
ECG monitoring for hyperkalemia, hypokalemia, and arrhythmia
If hyperkalemic, follow hourly
If normokalemic, 10–20 mEq/h
If hypokalemic, 40 mEq/h and avoid rapid reversal of acidosis
$^1/_2$ to $^2/_3$ as chloride salts and the balance as phosphate salts

Bicarbonate

None if pH > 7.1
NaHCO$_3$ 1 mEq/kg IV for pH < 6.9
For pH 6.9–7.1, consider for hyperkalemia or shock
In general, avoid > 50 mEq/h

Search for Underlying Cause

Monitor for Complications of Therapy

Judicious use of laboratory studies
Flow sheet
Frequent mental status checks
Patient education

Modified from Buse JB, Polonsky KS: Diabetic ketoacidosis, hyperglyce-
mic hyperosmolar non-ketotic coma and hypoglycemia. *In* Hall JB, Schmidt
GA, Wood LDH (eds): Principles of Critical Care. With the permission of
The McGraw-Hill Companies, 1992.

sary fluids, (3) use continuous insulin to treat insulin deficiency, (4) correct electrolyte abnormalities, and (5) evaluate possible underlying causes of metabolic decompensation.

Fluids

Volume contraction is one of the hallmarks of DKA. Fluid deficits in the range of 5 to 10 L are common in DKA, and the urine produced during the osmotic diuresis caused by hyperglycemia is roughly equivalent to half-normal saline. Therefore, free water deficits are relatively greater than sodium deficits. In the past, large volumes of isotonic intravenous fluids have often been rapidly administered to patients in DKA. We advise a more cautious approach.

When there is clear evidence of dehydration such as hypotension, decreased skin turgor, or dry mucous membranes, we generally infuse 1 L of normal saline over the first hour. In subsequent hours, we continue normal saline at a rate of 200 to 500 mL per hour until significant hypotension resolves and an adequate circulation is restored. If hypotension is severe, with clinical evidence of hypoperfusion, and does not respond quickly to crystalloid, therapy with colloid is considered, often in combination with invasive hemodynamic monitoring. If there is no hypotension and no concern of renal failure, we administer 1 L of half-normal saline over the first hour.

By the end of the first hour, laboratory data usually return and are often helpful in directing further therapy. Despite the fact that water losses exceed those of sodium, the measured sodium is usually low due to osmotic effects of glucose. This simple formula allows for correction of this osmotic effect:

Corrected sodium concentration =
    measured sodium + 0.016 (glucose − 100)
when glucose is reported in mg/dl.

Severe hypertriglyceridemia, which is common in poorly controlled diabetes, can falsely lower the serum sodium concentration by approximately 1 mEq per L at a serum lipid concentration of 460 mg per dL. Using the corrected sodium, the patient's free water deficit can be estimated:

Water deficit in liters =
    0.6 (weight in kg) [(sodium/140) − 1].

Using these formulas, a 70-kg patient with a measured sodium of 140 mEq per L and a glucose of 800 mg per dL would have a calculated water deficit of 3.4 L.

If the patient is normotensive after the first liter of fluids, our goal is to replace urinary losses with one-half normal saline. In addition, we provide approximately one-half the water deficit as 5% dextrose over the first 12 to 24 hours (using the example above, 1.7 L) and the remainder during the following 24 hours. Fluid replacement strategy should be frequently re-evaluated depending on the patient's clinical and laboratory responses. When the serum glucose approaches the range of 250 to 300 mg per dL, all fluids should contain 5% dextrose. At this point, the goal of treatment should be maintaining the serum glucose in the range of 200 to 300 mg per dL for 24 hours to permit gradual equilibration of osmotically active substances across cell membranes. Early feeding once ileus and nausea resolve should be considered, as increased caloric intake in concert with increased insulin therapy will result in quicker clearance of ketones. When the patient is drinking in an unrestricted fashion, intravenous fluids can be discontinued.

Insulin

Because DKA is essentially an insulin-deficient state, insulin therapy is an absolute requirement. Recent studies have shown that low-dose insulin therapy (0.1 U per kg per hour) is equally effective at decreasing serum glucose and promoting the clearance of ketones as the previously employed higher-dose regimens. Furthermore, low-dose insulin therapy reduces the incidence of hypoglycemia and hypokalemia, which are responsible for most of the morbidity associated with higher doses of insulin.

It is well established that intravenous insulin is significantly more effective than intramuscular or subcutaneous insulin in lowering serum ketone concentrations during the first 2 hours of therapy. The subcutaneous route is contraindicated in the critically ill patient due to its slower absorption kinetics and the possibility of tissue hypoperfusion. However, when there is insufficient nursing monitoring or venous access to allow for safe intravenous administration, intramuscular therapy (beginning at 0.2 U per kg per hour) is a reasonable alternative.

It has been shown that a 10-U priming dose of insulin given intravenously when starting a patient on intravenous insulin therapy significantly enhances the glycemic response to the first hour of treatment by fully saturating insulin receptors prior to beginning continuous therapy. When mixing insulin in normal saline, the intravenous tubing should be flushed with the insulin infusate prior to use to prevent insulin absorption onto the infusion set.

In an unusual case, when the glucose does not decline by at least 10% or 50 mg per dL in an hour, the insulin infusion rate should be increased by 50% to 100% and a second bolus of intravenous insulin given. As the glucose level decreases, it is often necessary to decrease the rate of infusion. After the glucose reaches approximately 250 mg per dL, the insulin infusion rate sometimes needs to be lowered despite the addition of dextrose to intravenous fluids. An additional 12 to 24 hours is normally required to clear ketones from the circulation after hyperglycemia is corrected. This process can be accelerated by providing more carbohydrate and insulin as tolerated (e.g., early feeding).

When the patient is ready to resume eating, insulin administration should be switched to subcutaneous therapy. The first dose of subcutaneous insulin should be given before a meal, and the insulin drip then stopped about 30 minutes later. The glucose should be checked in 2 hours and at least every 4 hours afterward until a maintenance insulin regimen can be determined.

Potassium

Potassium losses arising in the development of DKA are typically quite high (3 to 10 mEq per kg). These losses are mediated by shifts from the intracellular to the extracellular space caused by acidosis, osmotic diuresis, protein catabolism, and hyperaldosteronism. Most patients with DKA have deceptively normal or even high serum potassium levels at presentation due to these electrolyte shifts. It is vitally important to be aware that initial therapy with fluids and insulin will invariably cause serum potassium levels to drop. Our approach is to administer potassium with the intravenous fluids provided there are no electrocardiographic signs of hyperkalemia, such as peaked T waves or QRS widening initially, and the patient is capable of brisk diuresis. If the patient is oliguric, we do not administer potassium unless the serum concentration is less than 4 mEq per L or if there are ECG signs of hypokalemia (U wave) and even then only with extreme caution. With treatment of DKA, the potassium level usually reaches a nadir after several hours. We usually replace potassium at 10 to 20 mEq per hour, one-half to two-thirds as potassium chloride and one-third to one-half as potassium phosphate. Initially, we monitor serum levels at least every 2 hours and follow ECG morphology. A certain small but significant percentage of patients with DKA and protracted courses with vomiting will present with hypokalemia and acidosis; they may require 40 mEq per hour by central line to avoid precipitating potentially life-threatening hypokalemia. Some practitioners will postpone insulin therapy until the degree of hypokalemia is known and therapy has been initiated to reverse this problem, as insulin therapy and the resolution of acidosis would be associated with a further lowering of serum potassium and has precipitated rhythm disturbances in rare cases.

Phosphate

Like potassium, phosphate is depleted in patients with DKA; in addition, its serum level also declines with therapy. As potential complications of hypophosphatemia include cardiac dysfunction, skeletal muscle weakness, and respiratory depression, it seems advisable to administer phosphate replacement in the treatment of DKA. Though no clinical benefit of phosphate use has been demonstrated in prospective studies, most authorities recommend phosphate therapy as discussed earlier and monitoring for its possible complications—hypocalcemia and hypomagnesemia.

Bicarbonate

Serum bicarbonate is always low in DKA but does not represent a true deficit because the ketoacid and lactate anions are metabolized to bicarbonate during therapy. The use of bicarbonate in the therapy of DKA is highly controversial. No benefit of bicarbonate therapy has been shown in clinical trials; in fact, two trials reported that hypokalemia was more common in bicarbonate-treated patients. We reserve bicarbonate therapy for use (1) in patients with severe acidosis (pH <6.9) and (2) in the presence of hemodynamic instability if the pH is less than 7.1 or (3) in cases of hyperkalemia with ECG findings. If bicarbonate is used, it should be used sparingly and considered a temporizing measure only. Approximately 1 mEq per kg of bicarbonate can be given as a rapid infusion over 10 to 15 minutes, with further therapy based on repeat arterial blood gases (ABG) every 30 to 120 minutes. Unless the bicarbonate is being used for severe hyperkalemia, potassium should be given prior to the bicarbonate, since transient hypokalemia is a common complication of bicarbonate treatment and can precipitate fatal dysrhythmias.

Monitoring

Many cases of mild DKA can be managed without intensive care unit (ICU) admission, depending on nursing staff availability. We routinely admit patients with DKA to the ICU if they have a pH of less than 7.3 unless they respond quickly to initial therapy in the clinic or emergency ward. If mental status is compromised, prophylactic intubation is considered. In lethargic patients, nasogastric suctioning is always performed because of frequent ileus and danger of aspiration. Bladder catheterization is often necessary to follow urine output adequately. ECG monitoring should be continuous in severe DKA or DKA complicated by significant electrolyte abnormalities. Initially, we measure serum glucose, electrolytes, BUN, creatinine, calcium, magnesium, phosphate, ketones, lactate, creatine phosphokinase, and liver function tests, and obtain a urinalysis, ECG, upright chest radiograph, CBC, and ABG. If there is any possibility of a toxic ingestion, we add a toxicology screen to the initial studies. Glucose and electrolytes are then generally measured hourly, with calcium, magnesium, and phosphate repeated every 2 hours. The BUN, creatinine, and ketones are rechecked every 6 to 24 hours. Serum bicarbonate and anion gap are relatively good indices of the response to therapy. Urine ketones are more sensitive indicators of inadequate insulin therapy and carbohydrate metabolism than serum ketones. Frequent arterial pH and serum ketone determinations are not needed. In the severely ill patient with obvious underlying disease, the course is often more protracted. Flow sheets to keep track of laboratory data, mental status, vital signs, insulin dose, fluid and electrolytes administered, and urine output allow for easy analysis of response to therapy. Laboratory use should be curtailed once the acidosis begins to resolve and electrolyte abnormalities are consistently improving. If cardiovascular status becomes a concern in terms of fluid therapy, invasive hemodynamic monitoring should be used. The goal should be to quickly restore hemodynamic stability and to correct DKA completely in 12 to 36 hours.

Search for Underlying Causes

Once the patient has been initially stabilized, a thorough history and physical examination should be directed at determining any precipitating factors. The two most common causes of DKA are noncompliance with insulin therapy and infection. The most frequent infections consist of viral syndromes, urinary tract infection, pelvic inflammatory disease, and pneumonia. Determining whether the patient is infected initially can be challenging due to the absence of fever in a significant proportion of these patients. The white blood cell count can be in the range of 20,000 or higher even in the absence of infection. We therefore perform cultures on most patients with DKA. If reasonable concern about infection exists, we cover the patients empirically with broad-spectrum antibiotics pending microbiologic results. Meningitis should be strongly considered in any patient with altered mental status. Lumbar punctures should be performed in all patients with meningismus; in cases with a lower index of suspicion, we will cover bacterial meningitis with antibiotic therapy and perform a lumbar puncture only if the mental status does not improve in parallel with the DKA. Cerebrospinal fluid (CSF) glucose determinations are of little value in this setting, and the protein levels are usually high. Pancreatitis and pregnancy are well-known precipitating causes and need to be considered when evaluating abdominal pain, which is common at presentation. The serum amylase is often nonspecifically elevated. An elevated lipase should lead to strong consideration of pancreatitis. Moderate elevations of creatine kinase and transaminases are also common. The more insulin resistant the patient seems to be, the more likely one is to find a precipitating cause. If a precipitating cause is found, treatment is essential if adequate metabolic control is to be achieved.

Complications and Prognosis

At the close of the twentieth century, it should be possible to treat successfully almost all cases of DKA. The most troublesome complication is cerebral edema. It is unusual except in children and can be fatal. In most series, specific causes could not be found; however, aggressive hydration (particularly with hypotonic fluids) may contribute. In 50% of patients with DKA and cerebral edema who later had a respiratory arrest, premonitory symptoms were present; in spite of early intervention, only half of them survived without severe or fatal brain damage. Hypokalemic cardiac arrest is a rare problem that warrants very careful consideration of how therapy (insulin, bicarbonate, and fluids) affects serum potassium levels. Arterial and venous thromboembolic events are quite common. Standard prophylactic low-dose heparin is certainly reasonable in patients with DKA, but no indication currently exists for full anticoagulation. Unfortunately, almost 50% of cases of DKA will occur in patients with recurrent episodes. All patients should have access or be referred to teams of health care providers who can provide adequate individualized education and follow-up. This can prevent future admissions and allow the patient to become a confident self-manager of his or her diabetes.

HYPERURICEMIA AND GOUT

method of
N. WILSON HOLLAND, M.D., and
CARLOS A. AGUDELO, M.D.
Emory University School of Medicine
Atlanta, Georgia

Podagra, pain in the foot, was first described clinically in the fourth century B.C. Although there are other causes for podagra, gouty arthropathy is the most commonly recognized. Its prevalence ranges between 0.3% and 1% in the United States, depending on the population studied. It is much more common in men than in women and increases in women in the postmenopausal period. The peak age for acute gout is in the fifth decade. Approximately 12% of patients have a family history of gout.

Hyperuricemia and gout must be differentiated. Hyperuricemia alone is a biochemical abnormality and not a disease. Saturation of the serum with uric acid occurs at around 7 mg%. Approximately 25% of patients with persistent levels of uric acid above this will develop gouty arthritis after a period of years, and the prevalence of the disease increases with increasing uric acid levels. Uric acid levels in the body are regulated by diet, purine metabolism, and renal clearance.

What causes crystallization of monosodium urate in the synovial fluid after years of hyperuricemia is not totally clear. Microtophaceous deposits may be present for years along the synovial surfaces. Trauma or other factors, such as changes in the pH of synovial fluid, set the stage for the release of or de novo crystallization of monosodium urate into the joints. These crystals then set up a cascade of events: coating of crystals with immunoglobulin and ingestion by polymorphonuclear cells that subsequently release their contents, including lysosomal enzymes, which further lower the pH of synovial fluid and are involved in the production of various mediators like interleukin-1, leukotrienes, prostaglandins, and kinins.

Gout is usually classified into primary and secondary forms. Underexcretion of uric acid occurs in approximately 75% of patients with primary gout and is caused by increased tubular resorption, decreased tubular secretion, or a combination. Approximately 25% of patients with primary gout are overproducers of uric acid. Important enzyme abnormalities have been described in a small percentage of these latter patients. Complete and partial deficiencies of hypoxanthine-guanine phosphoribosyltransferase (HGPRT) occur in young men. The former, also known as Lesch-Nyhan syndrome, is an X-linked disorder associated with hyperuricemia, self-mutilation, arthritis, and spasticity. 5-Phosphoribosyl-1-pyrophosphate (PRPP) synthetase overactivity is another disorder associated with hyperuricemia and arthritis.

Most cases of primary gout tend to fall into an idiopathic category without a definitive genetic defect. These patients tend to have hypertension and obesity.

Secondary gout accounts for most cases seen in a hospital setting. It can also result from either overproduction of uric acid secondary to increased purine catabolism or impaired excretion of uric acid (Table 1).

The first attack of gout occurs in the great toe in over 50% of cases. Gouty arthritis is generally monarthric in presentation but can have a polyarthric, usually asymmetrical presentation, especially in those with renal insufficiency, advanced age, or diuretic therapy. In chronic stages the presentation can be confused with rheumatoid arthritis with symmetrical hand involvement and nodules (tophaceous changes). In older women on diuretics with underlying renal insufficiency, gout can be confused with erosive osteoarthritis and other inflammatory arthropathies.

Chronic gouty arthritis with tophaceous changes usually develops after many years in patients with persistently elevated uric acid levels above 8 mg%. Tophaceous deposits usually occur on the toes, elbows, hands, and ears but have been described in more unusual locations, such as the finger pads, spinal cord, vocal cords, and cardiac valves.

The diagnosis of gout is based on the clinical history,

TABLE 1. **Classification of Secondary Hyperuricemia**

Overproduction (24-hour urinary uric acid level > 600 mg on purine restriction or > 800 mg on regular diet)
  Myeloproliferative disorders
    Polycythemia vera
  Lymphoproliferative disorders
    Chronic lymphocytic leukemia
    Multiple myeloma
    Chronic myelocytic leukemia
  Psoriasis
  Hemolytic anemias, including sickle cell, pernicious anemia
  Paget's disease
  Disseminated carcinoma
  Cytotoxic drugs (acute tumor lysis syndrome)

Underexcretion
  Chronic renal insufficiency
  Lead intoxication (saturnine gout)
  Acidosis
    Lactic acidosis—ethanol
    Ketoacidosis—diabetes mellitus, starvation
  Drug ingestion
    Low-dose salicylates
    Diuretics
    Cyclosporine
    Ethambutol
    Pyrazinamide
    Nicotinic acid
    Levodopa
  Down syndrome
  Bartter's syndrome

Uncertain etiology
  Hyperparathyroidism
  Hypoparathyroidism
  Hypothyroidism
  Adrenal insufficiency
  Type I glycogen storage disease (Von Gierke's)

physical examination, and laboratory documentation, including serum uric acid and synovial fluid analysis. It is important to remember that not all monarthric arthritis in the great toes or even other areas is caused by gout, and therefore synovial fluid analysis is extremely important not only to identify and confirm monosodium urate crystals (needle-shaped, negatively birefringent, blue at right angles, yellow in parallel to the polarizing plane) but also to exclude other etiologies, including infection, hemarthrosis, or other crystals. Although rare, gout may coexist in the same joint with infections, especially in the more debilitated patient. Uric acid levels alone should not be used as a sine qua non, since in 20% to 30% of patients they can be normal in the face of an acute gouty flare. Additionally, hyperuricemia in a young man, premenopausal woman, or teenager should prompt a more extensive search for underlying secondary causes, as listed. In these latter patients, quantification of 24-hour urine uric acid measurements is important. We rarely feel that quantification is useful in the otherwise typical adult man with gout.

THERAPY FOR AN ACUTE ATTACK

The treatment mainstays for an acute gouty flare include nonsteroidal anti-inflammatory agents (NSAIDs), intra-articular microcrystalline corticosteroid injections, intramuscular microcrystalline corticosteroids, intramuscular or subcutaneous adrenocorticotropic hormone (ACTH), oral corticosteroids, or colchicine.

In those patients who are otherwise healthy with

normal renal function, NSAIDs can be used. Indomethacin (Indocin) in doses of 50 mg every 6 to 8 hours for the first several days is highly effective in relieving the acute symptoms. The dosage can then be tapered to 100 mg daily for the next 10 to 14 days. NSAIDs must be used with extreme caution if at all in elderly patients (more than 70 years of age); in the setting of underlying renal insufficiency, congestive heart failure, cirrhosis, gastrointestinal bleeding, or peptic ulcer disease; and in those with concomitant anticoagulant therapy. Additionally, indomethacin can occasionally be associated with headache and other central nervous system manifestations, including alteration in mental status and dizziness. Other NSAIDs can be used in place of indomethacin with similar precautions (Table 2). Intra-articular microcrystalline corticosteroids such as methylprednisolone (Depo-Medrol) can be used in the setting of a monarthric gouty flare. Typically, in large joints, such as the knee, 40 to 80 mg of Depo-Medrol can be used; in intermediate joints (ankles, wrists), 20 mg; and in small joints (metatarsophalangeal), 5 to 10 mg. Patients should be warned about the possibility of infection and a possible postinjection flare within the first 24 hours. Success has been found with ACTH, especially in those with risk factors such as underlying renal insufficiency in whom NSAIDs should be avoided. ACTH is given as a gel, either 40 or 80 units intramuscularly or subcutaneously, and can be repeated if necessary within 24 hours. Alternatively, intramuscular microcrystalline corticosteroids such as Depo-Medrol, 40 to 60 mg, can be used. Oral corticosteroids like prednisone, starting at 30 to 40 mg daily with a rapid taper over 7 to 10 days, are also acceptable. The usual associated side effects of corticosteroids may be seen. Some patients may be best managed with the use of analgesics alone, such as acetaminophen (Tylenol), acetaminophen with codeine, or propoxyphene (Darvocet), when the corticosteroid regimens are felt to be clinically contraindicated.

Lastly, although colchicine has long been a favored initial treatment of an acute gouty flare, it is now being used less frequently. It is usually given as 1

tablet (0.6 mg) every hour until relief occurs, gastrointestinal toxicity develops (nausea, vomiting, diarrhea), or a maximum of 6 mg has been reached. Intravenous colchicine can also be used although the potential for toxicity, especially marrow suppression and local tissue damage if extravasation occurs, is greater. Once given, further colchicine should not be used for the next 7 days. Because of the frequent side effects, narrow therapeutic:toxic ratios, and availability of other agents, we avoid either of the preceding regimens in the acute setting. The older patient with renal or hepatic insufficiency is especially prone to colchicine toxicity.

INTERVAL GOUT AND ASYMPTOMATIC HYPERURICEMIA

Therapy after the acute episode resolves might include weight loss, dietary counseling (avoidance of organ meats of sweetbreads and liver), minimizing alcohol consumption, and substituting or discontinuing, if possible, precipitating medications. Many patients with this management will never have another attack or will have very infrequent attacks.

The natural history of asymptomatic hyperuricemia is not totally clear, but it does not appear that renal function is adversely affected by hyperuricemia alone, and studies have shown that correction of hyperuricemia does not have an apparent effect on renal function.

Prophylaxis

In those patients who continue to experience acute gouty flares despite the foregoing measures, prophylactic therapy is indicated. Colchicine can be used in doses of 0.6 mg orally twice daily if renal function is normal. Side effects to monitor and make the patient aware of include nausea, diarrhea, or worsening weakness. The latter may indicate the development of a neuromyopathy that has been described in patients on maintenance colchicine therapy, especially with underlying renal insufficiency. Alternatively, a small dose of an NSAID can be used prophylactically (e.g., naproxen [Naprosyn], 250 mg orally twice daily). Prophylactic therapy should be started before adding a uricosuric agent or allopurinol (Zyloprim) to prevent flares.

CHRONIC GOUT

Uric acid–lowering therapy is indicated in those patients who have recurrent episodes of gout despite prophylactic therapy. Other indications include severe joint deformities clinically or radiographically, tophaceous changes, renal stones, or enzyme deficiencies.

Uricosuric agents such as probenecid (Benemid) or sulfinpyrazone (Anturane) decrease the tubular reabsorption of uric acid and can be used in patients with normal renal function. Uricosuric agents should not be used in patients who have a history of renal

TABLE 2. **Nonsteroidal Anti-Inflammatory Agents**

	Frequency (Times/Day)	Maximum Dose (mg)
indomethacin (Indocin)	3–4	200
fenoprofen (Nalfon)	3–4	3200
flurbiprofen (Ansaid)	3–4	300
ibuprofen (Motrin)	3–4	2400
ketoprofen (Orudis)	3–4	300
meclofenamate (Meclomen)	3–4	400
etodolac (Lodine)	3–4	1200
tolmetin (Tolectin)	3	1800
naproxen (Naprosyn)	2	1000
diclofenac (Voltaren)	2	200
sulindac (Clinoril)	2	400
nabumetone (Relafen)	1	1500
oxaprozin (Daypro)	1	1200
piroxicam (Feldene)	1	20

stones or in overexcretors. Salicylates block the uricosuric effects of these agents. Probenecid is the drug of choice. Initial dosage is 250 mg orally twice daily for 1 week, with the dose then increased to 500 mg orally twice daily up to 2 grams daily, depending on the serum uric acid levels. Adequate hydration should be maintained. Sulfinpyrazone is an alternative agent. Initial dosage is 50 mg orally twice daily for 1 week, increased to a maximum of 800 mg daily in three to four divided doses. Allopurinol (Zyloprim) is a xanthine-oxidase inhibitor used to lower serum uric acid levels. It is indicated in the following situations: (1) underlying renal insufficiency, (2) in the setting of nephrolithiasis, (3) in the setting of tophaceous gout, (4) in those who have enzymatic defects (HGPRT deficiency or PRPP overactivity), (5) in those who are "overproducers" (24-hour urinary uric acid level more than 800 mg on a regular diet), (6) in those allergic to uricosuric agents or who have failed this treatment, and (7) to prevent the tumor lysis syndrome prior to starting cytotoxic therapy. In those patients with normal renal function, allopurinol can be started at 300 mg daily.

Adjustments need to be made with starting dosages in the setting of renal insufficiency. In those with a creatinine clearance rate of less than 50 mL per minute, start with 50 mg orally daily. The dose can then be gradually increased over months depending on the clinical assessment and serum uric acid level. Preferably, the serum uric acid level should be lowered to less than 6 mg per dL. Allopurinol is not without potential toxicity, and patients should be carefully informed of this. Hypersensitivity reactions, including fever, rash, eosinophilia, nephrotoxicity, bone marrow suppression, and hepatic abnormalities, have been reported. These can occasionally be associated with significant morbidity and mortality. The latter reactions have been reported especially in patients taking diuretics who have underlying renal insufficiency and are given full doses (300 mg daily) initially. Allopurinol must be used with caution and at decreased dosages in those patients on azathioprine (Imuran) and 6-mercaptopurine (Purinethol). For these patients, these drug dosages should be reduced by two-thirds. The maximum dose of allopurinol varies widely with individual patients; some patients ultimately require more than 300 mg daily.

GOUT IN TRANSPLANTATION

Acute gouty flares are increasingly seen in patients postheart and renal transplantation. These patients typically are receiving cyclosporine (Sandimmune) and prednisone at the time of an acute flare. NSAIDs in this setting are generally contraindicated. Once an infection is excluded, the treatment of choice is either a local intra-articular microcrystalline corticosteroid injection for monarthric flares or, anecdotally, parenteral ACTH for polyarthric flares. Another option is a temporary increase in the maintenance prednisone dosage, although this may not be as effective.

HYPERLIPOPROTEINEMIAS

method of
DONALD B. HUNNINGHAKE, M.D.
University of Minnesota
Minneapolis, Minnesota

Cholesterol and triglycerides are insoluble in water and circulate in the blood in lipoprotein complexes. The two lipoproteins of greatest clinical interest are low-density lipoprotein (LDL) and high-density lipoprotein (HDL). Increased LDL levels are associated with increased risk for coronary heart disease (CHD), and reduced levels of HDL are associated with increased CHD risk. Very-low-density lipoprotein (VLDL) is the major triglyceride-carrying lipoprotein, and elevated levels also predict increased risk for CHD. Chylomicrons contain triglycerides derived from dietary sources, and elevated levels may be associated with the development of pancreatitis.

METABOLISM AND SIGNIFICANCE OF LIPOPROTEINS

All lipoproteins contain cholesterol, triglycerides, phospholipids, and proteins. However, the amount of each of these in the individual lipoproteins varies considerably, and this results in specific physicochemical and functional differences for each lipoprotein. The lipoproteins are spherical particles, and the more hydrophobic or water-insoluble components, triglycerides and cholesterol esters, are contained in the core. The more hydrophilic components, including free cholesterol, phospholipids, and the apoproteins (many different proteins), are located on the surface. The apoproteins promote the solubilization of lipoproteins in plasma and serve as ligands for receptors and as cofactors for many of the enzymes in lipid metabolism.

Low-Density Lipoprotein. LDL is the major cholesterol-carrying lipoprotein and accounts for about 70% of the total plasma cholesterol in population studies. It is removed from the plasma primarily by LDL receptors, which are heavily concentrated in the liver. LDL receptor numbers can be decreased in genetic disorders such as familial hypercholesterolemia, and their activity can be reduced by high-fat, high-cholesterol diets and genetic factors. Circulating LDL levels are definitely correlated with risk for CHD, and reducing LDL levels is associated with reductions in CHD risk. LDL may be modified to form oxidized forms of LDL. These oxidized derivatives are avidly taken up by scavenger receptors and probably account for most of the atherogenicity of LDL.

High-Density Lipoprotein. HDL is the other major cholesterol-containing lipoprotein, but it also contains large amounts of protein. It is derived from the liver and intestine. The exact mechanism for its protective effect is poorly understood. It may promote transport of cholesterol from cells to the liver and increase the endothelial synthesis of prostacyclin, and it is very important in the exchange of various lipids between different lipoproteins.

Very-Low-Density Lipoprotein. VLDL is the major carrier for endogenously synthesized triglycerides. It is synthesized by the liver. The enzyme lipoprotein lipase catalyzes the hydrolysis of the triglycerides in the core of this lipoprotein with the release of fatty acids. The resultant smaller remnant particles are then either removed by receptor mechanisms or converted to LDL. Elevated triglycerides or VLDL is a definite risk factor for CHD. However, they may not be an independent risk factor but simply a marker for other metabolic abnormalities associated with increased risk.

Chylomicrons. Chylomicrons are generally not found in the plasma in the fasting state but may appear in the postprandial state. They can also occur with genetic abnormalities or in disease states such as uncontrolled diabetes mellitus. They are the major carrier for triglycerides exogenously derived from the diet. They are also broken down to the smaller remnant particles by lipoprotein lipase. These remnants are then removed by receptor mechanisms, and they may be atherogenic.

DIAGNOSIS OF THE HYPERLIPOPROTEINEMIAS

Although total cholesterol has been used for screening, the overall assessment of risk for CHD in a physician's office should include an assessment of other risk factors and a lipoprotein profile. The latter includes measurement in the fasting state of total and HDL-cholesterol (HDL-C) and triglycerides (Tg) and an estimate of LDL-cholesterol (LDL-C). The cholesterol in blood in the fasting state is found in LDL, HDL, and VLDL. LDL is calculated from the formula LDL-C = Total-C − (HDL-C + Tg/5). The usual composition of VLDL is such that triglycerides divided by five provides the VLDL-C level. The estimated LDL-C value is adequate, provided the specimen is fasting and the triglycerides are 400 mg per dL or less. If the triglycerides are 400 mg per dL or more, the initial approach to therapy is to reduce the triglyceride level and then to re-evaluate the LDL-C level.

Although lipoprotein phenotyping according to the Frederickson and Lees classification was popular, current practice is to simply quantitate the absolute levels of LDL-C, HDL-C, and triglycerides. These levels, in association with other risk factors, provide the basis for therapeutic decisions. Patients with high LDL-C or triglyceride levels or low HDL-C levels may have a genetic basis for the hyperlipoproteinemia. This should increase the intensity of screening of family members for evidence of hyperlipoproteinemia.

Before initiating intense dietary or pharmacologic therapy, one should consider secondary causes of hyperlipoproteinemia. Diet, obesity, hypothyroidism, nephrotic syndrome, and a variety of drugs are some of the common secondary causes of elevated LDL-C levels. Hypothyroidism can also develop during chronic hypolipidemic therapy, and increasing LDL-C levels or nonresponsiveness to drug therapy should increase the index of suspicion. In patients with hypertriglyceridemia, diet, obesity, excessive ethanol intake, diabetes mellitus, estrogen, hypothyroidism, uremia, and a variety of drugs should be considered as contributing causes. If the triglycerides are greater than 1000 mg per dL, the patient has chylomicronemia, which is a risk factor for developing pancreatitis. The initial treatment is to control the hypertriglyceridemia and chylomicronemia to reduce the risk of pancreatitis, and later to reassess whether there is an increased risk of CHD.

LIFESTYLE MODIFICATIONS

The recommendations for initiating intense dietary therapy are included in Table 1. Increased dietary intake of saturated fat and cholesterol increases blood LDL-C levels because they decrease LDL receptor activity and removal of LDL from the blood. Obesity (excess calories or physical inactivity) increases the hepatic secretion of VLDL, which is a major precursor of LDL. The current recommendations are to restrict saturated fat to less than 10% of total calories, with additional restriction to less than 7% (Step II diet) if the target LDL-C is not obtained. Similarly, dietary cholesterol intake is limited to less than 300 mg per day and progresses to less than 200 mg per day (Step II) if required. Restricting total fat calories to less than 30% of total calories is recommended for both Step I and Step II diets. The cholesterol intake goal is most readily achieved by patients, followed by the saturated fat goal; it is most difficult to achieve the total fat intake goal. Attempts should also be made to increase physical activity and to achieve a desirable body weight. Increased consumption of fruits, vegetables, cereals, and grains should be encouraged. The reduced risk of CHD associated with a healthier diet is not exclusively due to the reduction in LDL-C. Thus, dietary modifications should be encouraged and maintained irrespective of changes in LDL-C levels.

In patients with hypertriglyceridemia, weight loss, increased physical activity, and ethanol restriction may be especially helpful. In patients with chylomicronemia, restricting total fat intake to 20% or even 10% may be helpful and even necessary. Increased physical activity and weight loss may also be helpful in controlling hypertension, diabetes mellitus, and low HDL-C levels. Discontinuance of smoking may also result in modest increases in HDL-C levels.

TABLE 1. Treatment of High LDL-C in Adults

CHD Risk Status	LDL-C Level to Initiate		LDL-C Goal
	Diet Therapy	*Drug Therapy*	
CHD or other atherosclerotic disease	>100 mg/dL	≥130 mg/dL*	≤100 mg/dL
No CHD and ≥2 other risk factors	≥130 mg/dL	≥160 mg/dL	≤130 mg/dL
No CHD and <2 other risk factors	≥160 mg/dL	≥190 mg/dL†	≤160 mg/dL

*Clinical judgment is indicated to initiate therapy if LDL-C is 100–129 mg/dL.
†In men under 35 years old or in premenopausal women, consideration should be given to delaying drug therapy if the LDL-C is < 220 mg/dL and there are no other risk factors.
Abbreviations: LDL-C = low-density lipoprotein cholesterol; CHD = coronary heart disease.

TREATMENT OF ELEVATED LDL-C LEVELS

Adults. The primary goal of lipid-lowering therapy is to control LDL levels. A large number of clinical trials have demonstrated that lowering LDL-C levels with either diet or drug therapy reduces the risk of CHD. Generally, a 1% reduction in total cholesterol is associated with a 2% reduction in risk in trials lasting up to 5 years, and more prolonged therapy may result in a 3% reduction in risk. The HMG CoA reductase inhibitors (HMGRIs) have been used in recent trials, and clinically significant reductions in total mortality, fatal and nonfatal myocardial infarction (MI), and the need for revascularization procedures have been demonstrated in patients either with or without prior MI. Additionally, aggressive cholesterol lowering in angiographic trials reduces the rate of progression of the atherosclerotic lesions and may result in regression in some cases.

The Adult Treatment Panel of the National Cholesterol Education Program (NCEP) has consistently recommended that LDL-C be the primary target for therapy. Its recommendations for both the initiation of and the target goals for dietary and drug therapy are illustrated in Table 1. Patients with CHD or other clinically evident atherosclerotic disease are the highest priority for treatment and should have the most aggressive therapy. The suggested target LDL-C goal is less than 100 mg per dL. Patients with a prior stroke or transient ischemic attacks, abdominal aneurysm, or evidence of lower extremity atherosclerosis are treated with similar intensity. Their risk of dying of CHD is nearly as high as that of someone with a previous MI. Cholesterol-lowering therapy is also a very cost-effective treatment when clinical evidence of atherosclerosis is present.

The second priority for treatment is patients who do not have CHD but have two or more risk factors for CHD as defined in Table 2. If the HDL-C level is 60 mg per dL or more, one risk factor is subtracted. Also, physical inactivity and obesity should be corrected, if possible, in all patients, because they increase risk by multiple mechanisms. Thus, they are not included as specific risk factors to determine the aggressiveness of LDL-C reduction. Patients without CHD and fewer than two risk factors have the lowest priority for treatment. This is especially true for men 35 years of age and younger and for premenopausal women. In the absence of other risk factors, it is suggested that an LDL-C of 220 or greater should be present to initiate drug therapy. The risk of a clinical CHD event is very low in the next 10 years, but more aggressive therapy is indicated with increasing age.

Children. Children have lower levels of total and LDL cholesterol than adults. The official pediatric guidelines indicate that acceptable levels of LDL-C are less than 110 mg per dL; 110 to 129 mg per dL is borderline, and 130 mg per dL or more is high. Approximately 5% of individuals less than 20 years of age have an LDL-C level greater than 130 mg per dL. Lipid screening in children is recommended if a first-degree relative has premature CHD, a parent has a cholesterol level greater than 240 mg per dL, or two or more CHD risk factors are present.

No cholesterol measurements or dietary restrictions are recommended for children less than 2 years of age. In older children, reasonably healthy eating patterns are recommended, and very restrictive diets, which could influence growth and development, should be avoided. After age 2, the Step I diet has no adverse effects if there are no serious caloric restrictions and is an appropriate diet whether or not the child has an elevated cholesterol level. Drug therapy is rather controversial. The pediatric guidelines suggest that drug therapy can be considered after age 10 if the LDL-C is 190 mg per dL or more or if it is 160 mg per dL with two or more risk factors. If drug therapy is considered, only the bile acid sequestrants can be considered safe for routine use. However, patient compliance with these drugs is very difficult in children.

The pediatric guidelines for drug therapy are more aggressive than the adult guidelines. The major consideration is whether drug therapy should be initiated based on lifetime risk or short-term risk of a clinical event, perhaps in the next 10 years. The pediatric guidelines are based on lifetime risk. The significant reduction in clinical events in adults and the evidence that drug therapy can slow the rate of progression of atherosclerotic disease suggest that drug therapy should be very limited in children. There are only a few children with very high LDL-C levels, multiple other risk factors, or a history of very early clinical CHD events in a nonsmoking, nondiabetic parent who should receive drug therapy. These children should probably be referred to a lipid specialist for consideration of the use of an HMGRI. The long-term safety of this class of drugs has not been carefully studied in large numbers of children. Also, these drugs must be used cautiously in women with childbearing potential, because the marked cholesterol-lowering effect could have an adverse effect on the fetus.

TABLE 2. **Risk Factors for Coronary Heart Disease**

Positive Risk Factors

Low HDL-C (<35 mg/dL)
Current cigarette smoking
Hypertension (BP ≥140/90 mmHg or drug treatment for
   hypertension)
Family history of premature CHD (myocardial infarction or
   sudden death in male first-degree relative <55 years of age or
   female <65 years of age)
Diabetes mellitus
Age (male ≥45 years of age, female ≥55 years of age or
   menopausal without estrogen replacement)

Negative Risk Factor

High HDL-C (≥60 mg/dL)

Abbreviations: HDL-C = high-density lipoprotein cholesterol; BP = blood pressure; CHD = coronary heart disease.

AVAILABLE DRUGS

The major drugs for lowering LDL-C levels are the bile acid sequestrants and the HMG CoA reductase inhibitors. Nicotinic acid must generally be given in large doses to achieve reductions in LDL-C of 25% or more. Estrogen reduces LDL-C levels by 10 to 15% in postmenopausal women and also increases HDL-C levels. Nicotinic acid reduces both LDL-C and triglyceride levels and also increases HDL-C levels. The fibric acids are used primarily to decrease triglyceride levels.

HMG CoA Reductase Inhibitors. These drugs are currently the most widely used class of lipid-lowering drugs. They are most effective for lowering LDL-C levels, are easy to use, and have few side effects or drug interactions; their long-term safety has been demonstrated in clinical trials. There are four drugs currently available: lovastatin (Mevacor), simvastatin (Zocor), pravastatin (Pravachol), and fluvastatin (Lescol). The relative potency for LDL-C lowering per milligram of drug administered is simvastatin, lovastatin, pravastatin, and fluvastatin. Reductions in LDL-C of 20 to 40% with currently recommended dosages can be achieved. Modest increases in HDL-C and reductions in triglycerides are noted. Their primary mechanism of action is to stimulate LDL receptor activity. The most important side effects are the rare occurrence of clinically significant transaminase elevations, which are frequently transient, and very rare cases of myositis and rhabdomyolysis.

Bile Acid Sequestrants. The two drugs that are currently available are cholestyramine (Questran) and colestipol (Colestid). Both drugs are available in several forms containing different flavor additives, and colestipol is also available in tablet form. The effects on LDL-C are dose dependent, with reductions ranging from 10 to 30%. The drugs increase LDL-C receptor activity by decreasing the enterohepatic circulation of bile acids, which lowers the hepatic cholesterol content. They are not absorbed systemically and thus are considered very safe. However, they can alter the absorption of many other drugs. The most common side effects are gastrointestinal, especially constipation, and patients frequently dislike the granular consistency. They are occasionally used as monotherapy to achieve modest reductions in LDL-C but are used most frequently in combination with an HMGRI. They can be used in combination with all lipid-lowering drugs. They can increase triglyceride levels, however, and are usually used in patients with triglyceride levels of less than 250 mg per dL.

Nicotinic Acid. Nicotinic acid (niacin) is a B vitamin that is used in pharmacologic doses to achieve its lipid effects. Nicotinamide has no lipid-altering effect. Nicotinic acid lowers VLDL or triglycerides and LDL and increases HDL levels. Crystalline niacin at levels of 1.5 grams per day or less may increase HDL-C by 25% or more and modestly decreases triglycerides and LDL-C. Higher doses of 3.0 to 4.5 grams are rarely tolerated but may decrease LDL-C by 25 to 30% and decrease triglycerides by 50%. Cutaneous flushing and gastrointestinal symptoms frequently limit its use. Nicotinic acid should be administered during or after meals to minimize the flushing, and aspirin pretreatment may also be of benefit. There are many other adverse effects, including hepatitis, hyperglycemia, and hyperuricemia. Sustained-release niacins are occasionally used because of less flushing, but the risk of hepatotoxicity is greater. They are less effective in increasing HDL-C levels but do lower LDL-C levels.

Estrogen. Estrogen administration in postmenopausal women is usually associated with 10 to 15% decreases in LDL-C and 10 to 15% increases in HDL-C. Estrogen may be considered as the initial drug in postmenopausal women if there are no contraindications. Concomitant administration of progestin, which is essential in a woman with a uterus to prevent endometrial cancer, negates the increase in HDL-C produced by estrogen. Epidemiologic studies suggest that CHD risk is reduced by 50% with estrogen, and the reduction in risk is even greater in women with clinically evident CHD. However, these findings have not been proved in controlled clinical trials. There is little information on the estrogen-progestin combination's effect on CHD risk, but combination therapy also appears to reduce CHD risk.

Fibric Acid Derivatives. Gemfibrozil (Lopid) is used primarily in the United States. The use of clofibrate (Atromid-S) was essentially discontinued because of concerns about potential toxicity in earlier clinical trials. Many other fibric acids are available in other countries. The fibric acids are used primarily to lower triglyceride levels. Although multiple mechanisms may be involved, a major effect is to increase lipoprotein lipase activity. In patients without hypertriglyceridemia, decreases in LDL-C of 10 to 15% and increases in HDL-C of 10 to 15% are observed. With higher pretreatment triglyceride levels, the decrease in LDL-C progressively decreases, and there may actually be an increase in LDL-C levels. The side effects are primarily gastrointestinal in nature. These drugs also increase the lithogenicity of bile and may increase the risk of cholelithiasis. When administered concomitantly with the HMGRIs, there is an increased risk of myopathy.

Probucol. The marketing of probucol (Lorelco) was recently discontinued. It modestly lowered LDL-C levels but reduced HDL-C levels by 20 to 25%. The major interest was in the antioxidant properties of this drug. A single, small, short-term clinical trial in patients with ileofemoral atherosclerosis did not reveal significant benefit.

SELECTION OF DRUGS

When drug therapy is initiated according to the NCEP guidelines, significant clinical benefit can be expected. Many patients who should be receiving drug therapy are not treated. This is still true even in patients with CHD. If patients are treated, the treatment is frequently inadequate, because there is no attempt to achieve target LDL-C levels. Patients who are treated with drugs frequently discontinue the drugs within the first 12 months for a variety of reasons, including lack of follow-up. Compliance with drug therapy should be encouraged, and this is more frequently achieved when nonphysician health professionals monitor the therapy.

Recent clinical trials have shown a reduction in clinical events beginning within months of initiating therapy. Many patients have also made lifestyle modifications prior to seeking a health professional's assistance for lipid management. Thus, there should not be an arbitrary period of diet therapy before initiating drug therapy. In patients with CHD or multiple risk factors, drug therapy should be initiated at the time of diagnosis. Lifestyle modification can then be encouraged at all follow-up visits. If the target LDL-C level is surpassed, the dose of drug can be reduced. Most lipid and lipoprotein abnormalities can be categorized into four groups.

Elevated LDL-C and Triglycerides 200 mg per dL or Less. Elevated LDL-C levels are defined as those requiring drug therapy according to the NCEP guidelines. The primary focus is on lowering the LDL-C levels, but some patients also have low HDL-C levels. The HMGRIs are the first consideration for patients with CHD or multiple risk factors. Estrogen may be considered in postmenopausal women. The bile acid sequestrants are usually then combined with an HMGRI, if needed. Many patients tolerate 2 scoops or packets, which results in an additional 10 to 15% reduction in LDL-C. The sequestrants are given with the evening meal and the HMGRI at bedtime. If HDL-C is low, niacin can be combined with the HMGRI.

Elevated LDL-C and Triglycerides 200 to 400 mg per dL. When triglycerides are elevated, the risk associated with the same LDL-C level is much higher. These patients frequently have low HDL-C levels and underlying genetic or secondary causes for their hyperlipidemia. These patients almost always need combination therapy, and some require triple therapy or referral for management. The initial drug is an HMGRI, and then niacin is added. If adequate doses of niacin are not tolerated, gemfibrozil may be considered. The risk of myopathy is increased, and patients should be instructed to report symptoms immediately and have a creatine kinase measurement. Many patients who are not on drug therapy have modest elevations of creatine kinase, and drug therapy need not be discontinued for minor, asymptomatic increases. Some patients may require the addition of a bile acid sequestrant, if the triglyceride level has been controlled, to reach target LDL-C goals.

Estrogen therapy can also be considered in postmenopausal women. Higher estrogen doses are more likely to cause additional hypertriglyceridemia. Modest increases in triglycerides are not considered atherogenic. If severe hypertriglyceridemia occurs, estrogen can be administered transdermally. The transdermal preparations have minimal effects on lipids and lipoproteins, but it is not known whether they reduce CHD risk.

Triglycerides 400 mg per dL or More. Lifestyle modification is very important, but high-risk patients with CHD or multiple risk factors also require drug therapy. Gemfibrozil is usually the first-line drug, because these patients frequently have hyperglycemia and hyperuricemia in addition to low HDL-C levels. Niacin can be used as the first drug in selected patients or combined with gemfibrozil. Adequate control of diabetes in diabetic patients with hypertriglyceridemia is essential. Elevated LDL-C levels are frequently discovered when the triglyceride levels are controlled, and they should be treated appropriately.

Low HDL-C Levels. Some patients have low HDL-C levels without LDL-C levels requiring drug therapy according to the NCEP guidelines. If the patient has CHD or a strong family history of CHD, drug therapy is justified. Greater increases in HDL-C will be achieved if elevated triglycerides are present and treated or if an obese patient loses weight. Crystalline niacin is the most effect drug for increasing HDL-C. If niacin is not tolerated in hypertriglyceridemic patients, gemfibrozil should be used. If niacin is not tolerated and the patient does not have hypertriglyceridemia, an HMGRI should be used. If target HDL-C levels cannot be achieved, more aggressive lowering of LDL-C is indicated.

OBESITY

method of
FRANK L. GREENWAY, M.D.
Pennington Biomedical Research Center
Baton Rouge, Louisiana

The incidence of obesity is on the rise. The National Health and Nutrition Examination Survey III showed that the incidence of obesity increased from 28% of the U.S. population in 1980 to more than one-third in 1995. This increase is in spite of the obsession that Americans have about being thin and the estimated $30 to $50 billion per year that they spend on the diet industry. This increase is taking place in teenagers as well as adults, and African Americans, Hispanics, women, and the economically disadvantaged are most afflicted. This increase in the incidence of obesity despite national priorities to reduce its incidence suggests that weight is physiologically controlled and that obesity is a regulatory disorder caused by more than bad habits or a lack of willpower.

DEFINITION

Obesity is an increase in body fat. Although it would seem logical to measure body fat directly, the methods of doing so are too expensive, too complex, or too inaccurate to substitute in clinical practice for indirect measures derived from height and weight, which are easy, noninvasive, and inexpensive. The relationship between body fat and other indirect measures of obesity is illustrated in Table 1. The Metropolitan Life Insurance tables, a commonly used standard, define desirable weight as the weight at which mortality is the least. Tables such as the one derived from the National Research Council, 1989, do not include differences based on frame size (Table 2). The percentage of

TABLE 1. **Desirable Levels of Weight and Fat**

Weight	Body Mass Index	Fat
<120% of desirable*	<25 (<37 years of age) <27 (>37 years of age)	15–25% (men) 20–30% (women)

*Calculated from standard weight tables (see Table 2).

desirable or ideal body weight is a person's weight divided by the desirable weight from the weight table. The body mass index (BMI) is the person's weight in kilograms divided by their height in meters squared. The BMI is the expression of height and weight that best reflects body fat and allows people of different heights and sexes to be compared in terms of obesity risk. By plotting the BMI against mortality for people between 19 and 34 years of age, one can see that there is a flat area between 19 and 25 that is considered the desirable weight range (Figure 1). Desirable BMI for women over 34 years of age is between 20 and 27. Overweight can be defined as a BMI between 25 or 27 and 30. Mortality risk at a BMI of 30 is increased, is almost always associated with an increase in body fat, and can therefore be considered obesity. Above a BMI of 30, the mortality risk rises sharply and increases to over two times normal with a BMI of 40 (Figure 1).

Not only the amount of body fat is important in defining the risks of obesity, but the distribution of that fat is important as well. Intra-abdominal fat is correlated with insulin resistance, which is associated with the major metabolic risks of obesity. In fact, intra-abdominal fat is a stronger predictor of mortality than either BMI or body weight. Although intra-abdominal fat can best be measured by computed tomography (CT) scan or magnetic resonance imaging (MRI), the waist to hip ratio or the waist circumference is most often used in clinical practice because of the relatively low cost and ease of measurement. A fat distribution that predominates about the abdomen, typical of men, is associated with higher medical risks, whereas a female fat distribution that predominates around the hips and thighs is much less dangerous. A waist to hip ratio of more than .95 in males or more than .8 in females is associated with an increased health risk.

OBESITY RISKS

The increased risks of obesity are in large measure due to the diseases associated with it. Obesity is associated with insulin resistance, Type II diabetes mellitus, hypertension, gallstones, cardiovascular disease, skin problems, abnormal menses, and some types of cancer. Obesity can aggravate arthritis, gout, reflux esophagitis, back pain, and sleep apnea. Although more difficult to quantitate, the great psychological burden of being obese should not be overlooked. The obese are discriminated against socially as well as in competition for jobs and mates, because they are viewed as lazy and weak-willed and are frequently despised. These medical and psychological liabilities can all improve with weight loss.

The risks of obesity are low with a BMI of 25 to 30 (Class 1), moderate with a BMI of 30 to 35 (Class 2), high with a BMI of 35 to 40 (Class 3), and very high with a BMI above 40 (Class 4). The presence of medical problems associated with obesity that would be expected to improve with weight loss, a waist to hip ratio greater than .95 in men or .8 in women, and an age less than 40 are all factors that would increase the risk by one class above the actual BMI (Table 3).

MECHANISMS

Rarely, there are identifiable underlying causes for obesity. Obesity can result from hypothalamic injury, Cushing's syndrome, hypothyroidism, gonadal failure, and unusual genetic syndromes such as Prader-Willi or Bardet-Biedl. These causes of obesity are rare and are important only because some of them have specific treatments. A more common and potentially reversible cause of obesity is taking medications that either increase appetite or decrease metabolic rate. Psychotrophic drugs, insulin, corticosteroids, cyproheptadine, beta blockers, and the cessation of smoking can all be associated with weight gain.

Dietary or exogenous obesity, a situation in which the caloric intake exceeds the caloric expenditure for unexplained reasons, is clearly the most important cause of obesity. There is much recent work that sheds light on obesity as a chronic medical disorder. Research studies have demonstrated that the body defends its usual weight, whether fat or thin. With overfeeding, the body gets rid of

TABLE 2. **Good Body Weights for Adults***

Height	19–34 Years		Over 35 Years	
	Average (lb)	Range (lb)	Average (lb)	Range (lb)
In feet and inches				
5'0"	112	97–128	123	108–138
5'1"	116	101–132	127	111–143
5'2"	120	104–137	131	115–148
5'3"	124	107–141	135	119–152
5'4"	128	111–146	140	122–157
5'5"	132	114–150	144	126–162
5'6"	136	118–155	148	130–167
5'7"	140	121–160	153	134–172
5'8"	144	125–164	158	138–178
5'9"	149	129–169	162	142–183
5'10"	153	132–174	167	146–188
5'11"	157	136–179	172	151–194
6'0"	162	140–184	177	155–199
6'1"	166	144–189	182	159–205
6'2"	171	148–195	187	164–210
6'3"	176	152–200	192	168–216
6'4"	180	156–205	197	173–222
6'5"	185	160–211	202	177–228
6'6"	190	164–216	208	182–234
In centimeters	Average (kg)	Range (kg)	Average (kg)	Range (kg)
152	51	44–58	55	49–62
155	53	46–60	58	50–65
157	54	47–62	59	52–67
160	56	49–64	61	54–69
163	58	51–66	64	56–72
165	60	52–68	65	57–74
168	62	54–71	68	59–76
170	64	55–72	69	61–78
173	66	57–75	72	63–81
175	67	58–77	74	64–83
178	70	60–79	76	67–86
180	71	62–81	78	68–88
183	74	64–84	80	70–90
185	75	65–86	82	72–92
188	78	67–88	85	74–95
191	80	69–91	88	77–99
193	82	71–93	89	78–101
196	85	73–96	92	81–104
198	86	75–98	94	82–106
BMI (kg/m²)	22	19–25	24	21–27

*Without clothes. Derived from National Research Council, 1989.

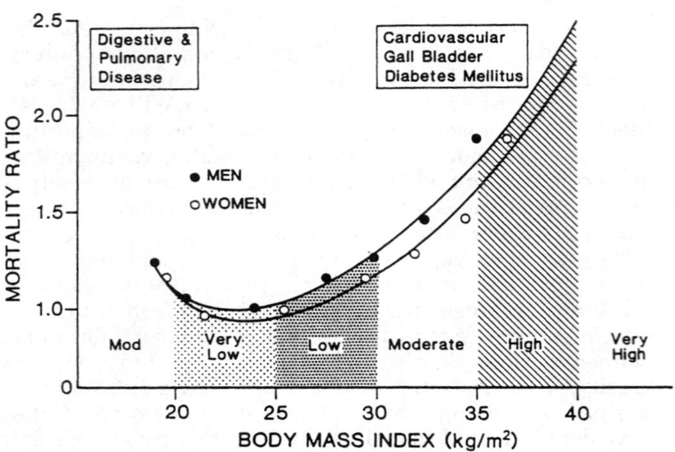

Figure 1. Relationship of BMI to risk. The curvilinear plot is based on data adapted from the American Cancer Society study. As BMI increases, the excess risk rises. A healthy or good body weight range is between 19 and 27 kg/m². (From Bray GA: Pathophysiology of obesity. Am J Clin Nutr 55:488S–494A, 1992. © American Society for Clinical Nutrition.)

extra heat energy; with underfeeding, it conserves calories. Mutations in the beta$_3$ receptor are associated with an earlier onset of Type II diabetes and possibly obesity as well. The *ob* gene in genetically obese mice has led to the discovery of a protein, leptin, that comes from fat and feeds back on the brain in both mice and humans. Genetics clearly plays a role in the regulation of body weight. Pima Indians are more likely to become fat if their family's metabolic rate is in the low-normal range. Genetics and environment are interactive, as can be seen in Japan, where the incidence of obesity is on the rise with Westernization of the diet. These insights into the mechanisms responsible for obesity should help us view the problem as a chronic malregulation of body fat rather than a moral weakness or lack of willpower.

ASSESSMENT

The medical history should include the onset of obesity, its pattern of progression, and the history of previous attempts to lose weight—the different weight loss programs tried, as well as the amount of weight lost and the time that the weight loss was maintained. Aspects of the dietary history that are important include the pattern of dietary intake and any evidence of compulsive overeating or bulimia. Lifestyle factors such as occupation, food habits, and beliefs about food also affect obesity. A physical activity history to find out the current and past levels of physical activity as well as any barriers to exercise or physical limitations is important. A history should also explore psychological factors such as depression, anxiety, or stress. A family history of premature coronary heart disease or diabetes mellitus should be sought as well.

The physical examination should include a measurement of weight, height, blood pressure, waist to hip ratio, and BMI (kg/m²). Medical testing that is appropriate in the evaluation of obese patients includes blood tests such as a thyroid panel, fasting glucose, lipid panel, uric acid, liver enzymes, electrolytes, and complete blood count. A urinalysis and often an electrocardiogram are indicated as well.

TREATMENT

As with any medical problem, the appropriate treatment reflects the relative risk/benefit ratio of the treatment in relation to the disease. The risk of obesity increases with severity and associated conditions, as reflected in Table 3. Treatments can also be categorized by risk, with balanced deficit dieting of more than 800 kcal per day, exercise, and behavior modification being low risk. Very low calorie dieting of less than 800 kcal per day and drug treatment are moderate-risk treatments, and surgery is a high-risk therapy (see Table 3). With the exception of surgery, treatments for obesity have been disappointing in terms of weight maintenance, but recent experience with drugs has been encouraging, and the other treatment modalities have been improving. A sug-

TABLE 3. **Obesity Risk Categories and Treatments**

Class	Risk	Body Mass Index	Low-Calorie Diet (>800 cal/day)	Exercise	Behavior Modification	Very-Low-Calorie Diet	Drugs	Surgery
0	Very low	20–27	√	√	√			
1	Low	25–30	√	√	√			
2	Moderate	30–35	√	√	√	√	√	
3	High	35–40	√	√	√	√	√	
4	Very high	>40	√	√	√	√	√	√

The following risk factors increase class by one: serious medical problems requiring weight loss, age less than 40 years, and waist to hip ratio >.80 in women and >.95 in men.

gested treatment scheme that is based on risks and benefits is illustrated in Table 3.

Fads

Fad treatments have been associated with obesity for decades. Since our society discriminates against the obese, it is not surprising that they are tempted to turn to fad treatments that offer magical solutions. Unfortunately, these magical solutions are usually ineffective and may be harmful. Chronic diseases such as obesity need chronic treatment. It is important that these magical solutions, which are often based on scientifically questionable claims, be discouraged.

Conventional Diets

The standard dietary approach to weight loss has been a balanced, calorically restricted diet based on the food exchange lists developed by the American Diabetes Association and individualized to the patient's dietary preferences. Recommendations have been that 20 to 30% of calories be derived from fat, 55 to 60% be derived from carbohydrate, and 15 to 20% come from protein. Since the typical American diet contains 37% fat, this represents a change for most people. A diet that is high in complex carbohydrate and fiber has more bulk in relation to calories and is therefore more satiating than a diet with more fat but an equal amount of calories. The dietary pyramid that was developed by the U.S. Department of Agriculture is a visual way of emphasizing the goals of increasing complex carbohydrates while reducing fat calories.

The calorie level of a conventional weight-loss diet can be calculated in a number of ways, but most are predicated on supplying approximately the number of calories needed to support basal metabolic needs so that the calories used above basal metabolic requirements will come from stored fat. Conventional weight-loss diets should cause 1 to 2 pounds of weight loss per week, not exceeding 1% of body weight per week after the first 2 weeks. Although calorie levels of 1200 to 1500 per day in women and 1500 to 1800 per day in men usually result in a weight loss in the desired range in sedentary or moderately active people, one can also use standard formulas to predict metabolic requirements, and a deficit of 500 kcal per day is equivalent to 1 pound of weight loss per week (Table 4).

Weight loss is predicated on a calorie deficit based on the total calories derived from food and those expended in basal metabolism and energy expenditure as activity. Although the calorie exchange system theoretically allows one to keep this type of calorie balance sheet, in practice, due to the multiple food items that must be memorized and the many foods that are mixtures of other foods, this accounting is difficult to the point of being impossible for most people. Steve Silva, who was once very obese, uses a calorie balancing system that has allowed him to maintain a 200-pound weight loss for over 17 years. This system, which uses anchor points that are memorized for both food and activity calories, may be easier to put into practice (Figure 2). In this system, maintenance calories without physical activity are estimated to be 11 calories per pound in women and 12 calories per pound in men. There are seven sheets that must be committed to memory: baked goods; meat, poultry, and fish; fresh fruits; vegetables; condiments; beverages; and prepared food (see Figure 2). Once these sheets are memorized, one can intelligently estimate virtually all foods by noting their similarities to the anchor-point foods. For example, the baked goods list goes from a low of 75 calories per ounce for bread to a high of 200 calories per ounce for butter. To estimate the caloric value of a bagel, which is not on the list, one would note that bread is 75 calories per ounce and muffins are 100 calories per ounce. Since a bagel would be in between these two foods if it had been included on the list, one can estimate that bagels would be 85 calories per ounce, which is an acceptable approximation. The system also requires users to learn the amount represented by an ounce or a cup. There are two food goals in addition to keeping a running total of the calories consumed each day: to eat a minimum of 5 cups of fruits or vegetables per day, and to eat less than a 25% fat diet 80% of the time.

Physical Activity

Physical activity must be distinguished from exercise. Physical activity is based on the principle of moving the mass of one's body through space and thus burning calories (mass $\times$ distance = work). Exercise is an activity designed to increase fitness in terms of either strength or maximal oxygen consumption. Although exercise in individuals whose cardiovascular systems are able to withstand the strain is a healthy pursuit, increasing the calories burned

TABLE 4. **Metabolic Requirements**

Basal Metabolic Rate (BMR): 18 to 30 years (men) = [(.063 $\times$ wt. in kg) + 2.8957] $\times$ 240 = kcal/day
31 to 60 years (men) = [(.0484 $\times$ wt. in kg) + 3.6534] $\times$ 240 = kcal/day
over 60 years (men) = [(.0491 $\times$ wt. in kg) + 2.4587] $\times$ 240 = kcal/day
18 to 30 years (women) = [(.0621 $\times$ wt. in kg) + 2.0357] $\times$ 240 = kcal/day
31 to 60 years (women) = [(.0342 $\times$ wt. in kg) + 3.5377] $\times$ 240 = kcal/day
over 60 years (women) = [(.0377 $\times$ wt. in kg) + 2.7545] $\times$ 240 = kcal/day
Total daily energy expenditure: mild to moderate activity = BMR $\times$ 1.3 = kcal/day
strenuous activity = BMR $\times$ 1.5 = kcal/day

Each category of food has a floor (least) and ceiling (most) number of calories per unit of measure.

Each number represents an anchor point or reference point for like foods. By using anchor points, you can problem-solve foods that are not on these sheets.

Cal/cup	Vegetables
135	Corn
100	Winter squash
65	Carrots
40	Mixed veg. Broccoli Cauliflower
20	Mushroom
10	Lettuce

Cal/oz	Veg/fruit
45	Avocado
25	Banana
20	Potato
15	Apples
10	Melons
5	Tomato

Cal/oz	Protein
125	Prime rib
100	Steak/cheese
75	Hamburger/ham
50	Poultry/dark fish
25	Egg white protein

Cal/oz	Baked Foods
200	Butter
175	Nuts
150	Chocolate
125	Crackers, cookies cake, pastry
110	Dry carbs, sugar Pretzels
100	Muffins, pancakes
80	Bagels, English muff.
70	Whole wheat bread

Important Note: Remember to check the unit of measure. Also note that some of the foods are lower in calories per cup than others are per ounce.

SPECIAL NOTE: CALORIES PER OUNCE AND CUP ARE NOT THE SAME AS PORTION SIZE OR PACKAGE.

Cal/Tbl	Condiments
125	Oil
100	Butter, mayo Margarine
75	Salad dressing
50	Sugar, gravy Cream cheese
30	Sour cream Soy sauce
15	Catsup, mustard
5	Salsa
2	Vinegar

Cal/oz	Beverages
100/oz	Heavy cream/liquor (800/cup)
65/oz	Lt cream 80% proof (520/cup) Gin, rum, whisky
40/oz	Egg nog, sherry (320/cup)
20/oz	Whole milk, wine (160/cup)
12/oz	Soft drinks, OJ (96/cup)
5/oz	Tomato juice (40/cup)

Figure 2. Calorie sheets. (Copyright Silva's Life Steps 1995.)

through physical activity is most important for the treatment of obesity. A study of high-density lipoprotein (HDL) cholesterol levels showed similar improvements in both slow walkers and joggers, as long as they traversed the same distance. Increasing physical activity can improve glucose intolerance and physical fitness as well as increase HDL levels, but it obviously takes longer to walk a mile than to jog it. In spite of the time pressures of our society, increasing the duration rather than the intensity of the activity minimizes the dropout rate in physical activity programs. Clearly, physical activity pro-

grams to treat chronic diseases must be maintained for a lifetime. Therefore, encouraging increased physical activity is the primary goal, with exercise being reserved for those who wish to participate in a fitness program after being medically cleared to do so. One of the most effective physical activities for weight loss is walking, because it is a cost-free activity that almost everyone can do, and walking distance can easily be converted into calories.

The increasing incidence of obesity may be related to a decreasing energy expenditure in this country and other industrial societies. The percentage of fat

Cal/cup	Soups	Cal/cup	Vegetables/Fruits	Cal/cup	Starch with Protein
				800	Cheese sauce/gravy
					Nuts and seeds 600-800 cal/cup
				600	Starch protein, high fat
					Meat, 400-600/cup Pasta with cheese sauce
					Fried rice, 400/cup
350		350	Mixed veg., high fat	350	Starch protein, medium fat
	Heavy cream butter Cheese N.E. clam chowder		Sauteed onions Veg. with cheese sauce		Potato salad
250	French onion	250		250	Beans, 250/cup
	Milk solids/corn starch Cream of mushroom Split pea, tomato Manhattan clam		Mixed veg., medium fat Mixed veg., with oil Cole slaw Mixed veg. with protein		Chicken, 250/cup Tunafish, 210/cup Rice, 200/cup Pasta, 150-200/cup Whitefish,150/cup
100		100		100	
	Water based soups Chicken noodle Wonton		Mixed veg., low fat Mixed fruits Mixed steamed veg.		
50		50			

Figure 2 *Continued*

in the diet has been decreasing, but the incidence of obesity has been rising. Studies in children relate the incidence of obesity to the amount of time spent watching television. As animals are confined in progressively smaller cages that restrict their physical activity, their food intake decreases up to a point, but at low levels of activity, the food intake actually increases as activity declines. Calorie intake has risen in this country in spite of the reduction of fat in the diet.

Aerobic activity to promote physical fitness has been stressed. But resistance exercises such as weight lifting, which are anaerobic activities, are much more efficient in increasing muscle mass. Muscle is a metabolically active tissue that decreases with age unless measures are taken to counteract this natural trend. Therefore, a physical activity that combines both aerobic activities such as walking and resistance activities such as weight lifting is ideal. The health benefits of activity or exercise are realized with an energy output of 2000 to 2500 calories per week, and a gradual, stepwise approach should be taken to increasing the amount of activity. Increasing the time spent walking by minutes a day and stressing the duration rather than the intensity of the activity are most likely to be successful in maintaining active habits over the long haul. Activity calories, like food calories, can be estimated by the anchor point system (Figure 3). The calories burned in walking can be estimated as two-thirds of a person's body weight in pounds per mile. Since a normal walking pace is 3 miles per hour, a 150-pound man burns approximately 300 calories per hour walking at a comfortable pace; if done daily, this would be 2100 calories per week. Regular physical activity appears to be one of the most important factors in weight maintenance.

Behavior Modification

The principles of behavior modification draw from research in the field of psychology. Behavior modification attempts to analyze the behaviors surrounding eating and to modify those behaviors while monitoring whether the changes result in a decrease in calorie balance. Behaviors that appear to decrease calorie balance are incorporated into daily habit patterns and are reinforced; those behaviors that do not favorably modify calorie balance are discarded. Examples of this approach are chewing each bite 10 times to slow the rate of eating, removing high-calorie foods from the house to reduce the stimulus to eat, and implementing a self-reward system for achieving behavior goals. The interface between eating and emotions is explored, and coping strategies are designed. Examples include relaxation training for anxiety-associated eating, development of a support system of people that can help in achieving behavior goals, and reinforcing the knowledge that imperfect adherence to behavior goals should not cause abandonment of attempts to lose weight. Over the years, behavior modification programs have become progressively longer, and weight losses of approximately 10 pounds have been maintained for longer periods (Table 5).

Commercial Programs

Commercial programs are, for the most part, based on variations of a low-calorie diet, increased physical

Calories per minute	Calories per hour		Intensity
20 cal/min.	1200 cal	Run 12 miles Climb 400 flights of stairs (1 cal/5 steps—15 steps/flight)	Very high
13 cal/min.	800 cal	Run 8 miles Cross-country skiing	
10 cal/min.	600 cal	Run 6 miles	
8 cal/min.	500 cal	Swimming Walk 5 miles	High
6.5 cal/min.	400 cal	Tennis, competitive Walk 4 miles	
5 cal/min.	300 cal	Walk 3 miles Bike 12 miles (10-speed) Aerobics	Medium
3.5 cal/min.	200 cal	Gardening	Low
1.5 cal/min.	100 cal	Weight-lifting, shopping Housework	

All of these numbers are estimates. They are for the purpose of tracking physical activity calories.
This sheet is based on a 150-pound person's weight. If you weigh more or less, just divide weight by 150 to get your multiplying factor for the page.

Figure 3. Physical activity sheet. (Copyright Silva's Life Steps 1995.)

activity, and behavior modification principles. One strategy is meal replacements, which usually consist of a drink or a food bar that substitutes for one or two meals a day. This approach is designed to provide the full supplement of nutrients, vitamins, and minerals to maintain health. The advantage of this approach is that it isolates a person from the usual food choices and encourages a regimen of 1000 to 1200 calories per day. Prepackaged food is a similar approach and also has the advantage of eliminating food choices while ensuring adequate nutrition. The disadvantage over time is the monotony and the inability to learn the food choices that are necessary for long-term weight maintenance. Therefore, this approach is designed to be temporary; regular food is gradually reintroduced as the educational process proceeds. Because behavior modification principles and nutrition education are best delivered by another person, commercial programs that offer these services along with the food products have an advantage over purchasing the products in isolation.

Very-Low-Calorie Dieting

Very-low-calorie diets contain between 400 and 800 calories per day and are an attempt to maximize weight loss while minimizing the loss of lean tissue. There is little evidence that diets of less than 800 calories result in better weight loss. These diets are indicated in individuals who have a medical need to

TABLE 5. **Summary Analysis of Selected Studies Providing Treatment by Behavior Therapy and Conventional Reducing Diet**

	1974	1978	1984	1985–1987	1988–1990
Number of studies included	15	17	15	13	5
Sample size	53.1	54.0	71.3	71.6	21.2
Initial weight (kg)	73.4	87.3	88.7	88.7	91.9
Initial % overweight	49.4	48.6	48.1	56.2	59.8
Length of treatment (wk)	8.4	10.5	13.2	15.6	21.3
Weight loss (kg)	3.8	4.2	6.9	8.4	8.5
Loss per week (kg)	0.5	0.4	0.5	0.5	0.4
Attrition (%)	11.4	12.9	10.6	13.8	21.8
Length of follow-up (wk)	15.5	30.3	58.4	48.3	53
Loss at follow-up	4.0	4.1	4.4	5.3	5.6

The data, adapted and updated, are from Wadden TA: Evidence for success of caloric restriction in weight loss and control: Summary data from clinical research studies. *In* Methods for Voluntary Weight Loss and Control. NIH Technology Assessment Conference, March 30 to April 1, 1992, Bethesda, Maryland.

lose fat rapidly and have a BMI greater than 30 kg/m². Individuals with a BMI less than 30 kg/m² do not conserve protein as well and may lose more lean tissue, which can lead to cardiac disturbance, among other side effects.

Very-low-calorie diets should contain at least 1 gram of high biologic value protein per kilogram of desirable body weight, and 10 grams of fat in one meal is sufficient to cause the gallbladder to contract. Gallstones are one of the risks of very-low-calorie diets, and this risk is probably due in part to gallbladder stasis. These diets should be administered under medical supervision after a thorough medical examination, including vital signs and blood tests such as electrolytes and uric acid. Patients are encouraged to drink at least 2 quarts of noncaloric fluid per day to prevent uric acid precipitation or dehydration. Contraindications to very-low-calorie dieting include myocardial infarction in the previous 6 months, prolonged QT interval, serious arrhythmias, protein wasting states, serious renal or hepatic disease, cerebrovascular disease, Type I diabetes, or significant psychiatric disorders. Complications associated with these diets include dizziness, fatigue, muscle cramping, headache, gastrointestinal disturbances, cold intolerance, dehydration, orthostatic hypotension, electrolyte imbalance, elevated uric acid levels, and cholesterol gallstones.

These very-low-calorie diets are usually dispensed in powder form and reconstituted with water. The length of treatment is usually from 12 to 16 weeks. Average weight losses are around 20 kg and amount to 1.5 to 2.5 kg per week, which is three to five times that seen with low-calorie dieting. Combining behavior modification increases the weight loss and slows the subsequent weight gain. At 1 year, the weight loss with very-low-calorie diet alone is about 5 kg; with the addition of behavior modification, it increases to about 10 kg. At 5 years, however, the weight in both groups had returned to baseline or above.

Psychiatric Counseling

Obesity is not a psychiatric disorder, but binge eating is seen in a subset of obese patients and is an indication for a psychological evaluation. Depression is not uncommon in the obese population, and evaluation and specific treatment may be indicated. Psychological counseling can be helpful in improving an individual's mental health but has been disappointing in terms of reducing the obese state. Obesity is not classified as a psychological disorder or an eating disorder.

Pharmacologic Therapy

The medications presently approved for obesity are all appetite suppressants. Most were developed and approved at a time when obesity was thought to be a habit problem. The medications were used like training wheels on a bicycle that were removed after 2 or 3 months. Obesity is now understood to be a regulatory problem of body fat, in the same way that hypertension is a regulatory problem of blood pressure. If medications are to be effective for a chronic medical problem, they need to be given chronically, but since most of the medications presently available are approved for a period of only a few weeks (usually interpreted to be 12 or less), chronic use of these drugs is investigational. There is still much controversy about this class of medication both within and outside the medical community, making it prudent for practitioners who wish to use these medications for more than 12 weeks to go through the physician-sponsored investigational new drug process with the Food and Drug Administration (FDA).

There are two drugs approved for use on a nonprescription basis. Although there is little support for the use of benzocaine in the scientific literature, support for the safety and efficacy of phenylpropanolamine (Acutrim, others) is substantial. Over the first 4 weeks of treatment with phenylpropanolamine, weight loss is similar to that achieved with prescription medications and approximately .5 pound per week more than placebo, but it may be less effective than prescription drugs after that point. The prescription medications have two mechanisms of action. Racemic fenfluramine (Pondimin) works through serotonin, and the other medications work through noradrenergic pathways. Fenfluramine, mazindol (Mazanor, Sanorex), phentermine (Ionamin), and diethylpropion (Tenuate) have a low potential for abuse and are in a lower category of regulatory restriction. Long-term studies of these medications are few but seem to indicate that the use of one medication results in an average weight loss of 8% over 6 months and maintains it thereafter if the medication is continued. A study published in 1992 that combined diet, activity, and behavior modification with fenfluramine 60 mg per day and phentermine 15 mg per day demonstrated that a 16% weight loss could be achieved over 6 months and was maintained on the drug treatment. Another study combining diet, activity, and behavior modification with ephedrine 20 mg and caffeine 200 mg given three times a day also resulted in a 16% weight loss over 6 months that was maintained over the next 6 months of treatment. These encouraging results suggest that in the future, obesity will be successfully treated with chronic medication in much the same way that hypertension is treated when diet, exercise, and behavior modification alone are insufficient. Several drugs are presently in the development process for the long-term treatment of obesity. One of these, dexfenfluramine (Redux), has recently been marketed and is the only medication approved by the FDA for the long-term treatment of obesity.

Surgery

Surgery is reserved for patients who have been unsuccessful with other forms of treatment and have a BMI of 40 kg/m² or a BMI of 35 kg/m² and serious medical problems that require weight loss for adequate treatment. There are two surgical procedures for obesity that were recommended by the National Institutes of Health consensus conference. The vertically banded gastroplasty is technically easier to perform, makes the stomach smaller (60 cc stomach capacity), makes the outlet from the stomach smaller (1 cm diameter) and works as a mechanical barrier to eating rapidly or in large amounts. The Roux-en-Y gastric bypass, in which the food bypasses the majority of the stomach and approximately 50 cm of the upper intestinal tract, is more difficult to perform and can be complicated by malabsorption of iron and vitamin B_{12}. The Roux-en-Y gastric bypass results in more weight loss than the vertically banded gastroplasty, and weight loss seems to be maintained better in studies lasting up to 10 years. These surgical procedures should be performed only when an experienced team of medical, surgical, psychiatric, and nutritional professionals is working closely together. These patients require lifelong follow-up to manage the reinstitution of liquid and solid foods, as well as monitoring for medical complications such as anemia, vomiting, and vitamin deficiencies and for psychological problems in adjusting to the changes induced by surgery. Patients should be well informed about the surgery and its risks, and the surgery should be done by a surgeon who is experienced in the procedures and in a clinical setting that is prepared to handle all aspects of the unique clinical problems of these patients.

VITAMIN NUTRITION

method of
LARRY E. JOHNSON, M.D., PH.D.
University of Cincinnati Medical Center
Cincinnati, Ohio

GENERAL PRINCIPLES

Diagnosis of vitamin disorders can be difficult because deficiency and toxicity often present subtly. More obvious classic deficiency states, like pellagra, beriberi, and scurvy, are not recognized because they are relatively rare in developed countries. This contributes to a frequent lack of recognition by health care workers. A high degree of suspicion is needed, therefore, to make a diagnosis of deficiency or toxicity before permanent damage or even death occurs. Vitamin and other nutritional deficiencies play a role in many persons who become ill or who respond poorly to medical or surgical treatment. A nutritional history and risk assessment, including vitamin intake, should be part of a complete evaluation of every patient.

Two major risk categories are associated with vitamin deficiency. Social and psychological risk factors include social isolation, depression, alcohol abuse, elder abuse and neglect, institutionalization, poverty, inadequate assistance with eating or marketing, eating disorders (such as anorexia and bulimia), and loss of a spouse or other caregiver. Physical risk factors include poor dental hygiene, poorly fitting or missing dentures, decreased calorie intake with advanced age, impaired mobility, memory and attention disorders, neurologic impairments of chewing and swallowing, chronic disease (particularly vascular disease, pulmonary disease, and cancer), and medications causing anorexia or drug-nutrient interactions.

In contrast, persons likely to have high, and potentially toxic, vitamin use are those with chronic diseases, particularly those associated with pain and disability (such as arthritis, diabetes mellitus, and Parkinson's disease), incurable or potentially fatal disease (such as cancer, AIDS, and progressive neurologic diseases), those who distrust the medical establishment, and those who prefer homeopathic or naturopathic therapy.

Approximately one third of the adult population in the United States regularly consumes vitamin supplements. Vitamin supplementation should not be a substitute for a well-rounded diet, which includes a *minimum* of five to six servings of fruits and vegetables daily. Only 10% of adults and 15% of high school students meet this requirement on any given day. Studies suggest that simple daily multiple vitamin supplementation in healthy older adults may positively influence health and immune status. In addition, one should not automatically presume that persons receiving "complete" artificial diets are receiving adequate nutrition. Up to 6 cans or more of protein nutritional supplements may be needed just to achieve the Recommended Dietary Allowance (RDA) for vitamins.

A barrier to proper vitamin nutriture is understanding how to use the RDA (or the US RDA, the simplified dietary intake recommendations by the Food and Drug Administration used for labeling food and dietary supplements). The RDAs were developed as scientific estimates of the amount of specific nutrients most healthy persons need to prevent known classic deficiency states. However, some vitamins may have important disease-preventing and health-promoting effects at intakes higher than the RDAs. That is, the amount of certain vitamins required for optimum health may be greater than that needed to prevent deficiency states. The RDAs were designed for population groups; there are many conditions that require adjustments for specific individuals. In addition, the current RDAs continue to include all elderly persons within the category of all persons above 51 years of age, which may not be appropriate.

VITAMIN A AND CAROTENE

Vitamin A represents a variety of synthetic and natural compounds, termed retinoids, necessary for vision, growth, cellular differentiation and proliferation, maintaining the integrity of epithelial tissues (skin, cornea, gastrointestinal tract, lungs, urinary tract, and so on), reproduction, and immune system function. A protective role for vitamin A and provitamin A carotenoids against various cancers remains controversial. The body's vitamin A requirements can be obtained by consuming preformed retinoids in liver, fish, eggs, and fortified whole milk products or by consumption of carotenoid precursors (termed provitamins) of vitamin A, such as alpha and beta carotene and cryptoxanthin in vegetables (carrots, spinach, sweet potatoes, broccoli, tomatoes, and squash) and fruits (pink or red grapefruits, apricots, cantaloupes, mangoes, papayas, and dried prunes). Of the more than 600 naturally occurring carotenoids, only one tenth can be converted into vitamin A; beta carotene is the most prevalent provitamin A carotenoid. Many of the carotenoids not converted into vitamin A have significant biologic activity, including antioxidant properties. High intakes of foods rich in carotenoids may decrease the risk of age-related macular degeneration.

Vitamin A deficiency is common in the developing world, particularly in young children. It can also result from chronic fat malabsorption or cystic fibrosis. Nonspecific signs of deficiency include anorexia; apathy; dry, rough skin; and increased susceptibility to infection. Anemia, with or without hepatosplenomegaly, is often present. Eye disease (termed xerophthalmia) is common, and includes night blindness and conjunctival and corneal xerosis; corneal ulceration and keratomalacia may become irreversible, leading to partial or total blindness. Small, gray, foamy lesions on the conjunctiva (Bitot's spots) are a common clinical sign. Vitamin A intake decreases with age but hepatic levels generally do not change and hypovitaminosis is uncommon in adults, even in the very old.

Vitamin A activity in foods is expressed as retinol equivalents (RE); 1 RE is defined as 1 μg of all-*trans* retinol. Beta carotene has one sixth the vitamin A activity of retinol, and the other provitamin carotenoids have one twelfth the activity. International units (IU) are often used for both vitamin A and the carotenoids and are frequently confusing and inaccurate. One RE equals 3.33 IU of retinol and 10 IU of provitamin A carotenoids, but food composition tables often assume that retinol IU and carotenoid IU are the same. It is important to emphasize that vitamin A is not an antioxidant and that REs do not express the antioxidant and other healthful properties of the various carotenoids in fruits and vegetables.

The current RDA for vitamin A for infants under 1 year of age is 375 μg RE, gradually increasing to 1000 μg RE in men and 800 μg RE in women, including pregnancy. Vitamin A is a powerful teratogen and should not be consumed in doses above the RDA during pregnancy. Related compounds, such as isotretinoin for acne, should not be taken by women who may become pregnant. Lactation increases women's requirements to 1300 μg RE. Serum retinol levels correlate with vitamin A status only at the extreme ranges. There are no RDAs for the carotenoids.

Vitamin A can be highly toxic, both acutely and after long-term ingestion. Acute toxic effects present as headaches, drowsiness, irritability, dizziness, nausea, vomiting, and diarrhea. Toxicity has been seen with intakes as little as 15,000 RE per day, although when monitored carefully many persons can tolerate 50,000 to 300,000 RE per day as treatment for various skin diseases. Chronic toxic effects nonspecifically present as desquamation and redness of the skin and mucous membranes, disturbed hair growth, anorexia, fatigue, irritability, thyroid suppression, pseudotumor cerebri, and elevations of liver enzyme levels. Infants may have increased irritability, poor

weight gain, and tender bone swelling; x-ray films can show hyperostosis of long bones. Toxicity increases in patients with renal failure or pre-existing hepatic dysfunction. Hypercalcemia and a negative calcium balance similar to that seen with vitamin D toxicity may occur.

Fruits and vegetables do not contain preformed vitamin A. The provitamin A carotenoids they contain are not efficiently absorbed at high intakes and are converted slowly into vitamin A, which is why carotenoid ingestion does not cause vitamin A toxicity. However, high intakes (30 mg of beta carotene daily) may cause a yellow-orange discoloration of the skin (particularly nasolabial folds, palms, and soles), which is distinguished from jaundice because the sclera remain normal. High-dose beta carotene supplementation should be discouraged because of an association with an increased incidence of cancer.

VITAMIN D

The most important vitamin in bone metabolism is vitamin D, which also acts as a hormone. It enables bone mineralization, facilitates intestinal calcium and phosphorus absorption, regulates renal reabsorption and homeostasis of amino acids and phosphorus, and influences the activity of parathyroid hormone (PTH) on bone and in the kidney. Vitamin D can stimulate both osteoblastic and osteoclastic activity in the bone. It has many other roles, and receptors for vitamin D are found in many tissues. Vitamin D may directly influence beta-cell function in the pancreas and thyroid hormone function, affect cellular proliferation and differentiation of skin (e.g., some forms may have a role in the treatment of psoriasis), participate in a paracrine system affecting macrophage, cytokine and immunoglobin synthesis by lymphocytes, and modulate muscle function.

Vitamin D deficiency classically causes osteomalacia in adults and rickets in children (most commonly at 1 to 2 years of age). Bone is soft and easily deformed, resulting in bone pain, difficulty rising from a chair or climbing stairs, a waddling gait, and decreased mobility. Adults show muscle tenderness and weakness, as well as anorexia and weight loss. Signs of rickets in children are beaded swellings along the costochondral junction (rachitic rosary), misshapen head with widened sutures, pot belly (muscle hypotonia), bowed limbs, and joint swelling. Highly characteristic radiologic features are pseudofractures in both children and adults, or widened epiphyseal plates and frayed bone, particularly at the wrist. A deficiency of calcium or phosphorus can cause deficient mineralization identical to that seen in osteomalacia.

Vitamin D is not plentiful in food; major sources are *fortified* dairy products (milk, 100 IU per 8 ounces; margarine, 21 IU per teaspoon), fatty fish (like salmon, mackerel, sardines), liver, fish liver oils, and egg yolks. Dietary intake of these is often low in adolescents, young women, and the older adult; lactose intolerance in some ethnic groups may also be a factor. Vitamin D is stable in foods; storage, processing, and cooking do not appear to affect its activity. The RDA for vitamin D is 400 IU (10 μg) for persons from age 6 months to 24 years and for pregnant or lactating women of all ages, and 200 IU for all others above 24 years of age. Breast-fed infants who are not exposed to sunlight should receive a daily supplement of 300 to 400 IU. The RDAs for vitamin D are particularly controversial for elderly people who commonly have osteopenia; many experts now recommend that older adults above 65 years of age receive 400 to 800 IU of vitamin D daily to permit adequate calcium absorption.

Vitamin D may be ingested as ergocalciferol (D_2) or cholecalciferol (D_3), both found in foods or nutritional supplements, or synthesized from 7-dehydrocholesterol in the skin after sun exposure. To become physiologically active, vitamin D must undergo 25-hydroxylation in the liver [to calcidiol; 25(OH)D], followed by 1-hydroxylation in the kidneys [to calcitriol; 1,25(OH)$_2$D]. As oral intake decreases, endogenous skin production becomes more important. Sunlight exposure commonly decreases in older adults, particularly during winter months at higher latitudes, and 7-dehydrocholesterol concentrations decrease in the aging epidermis. Darkly pigmented skin (black children are particularly susceptible) and the use of sunscreens further reduce skin capacity to synthesize vitamin D. Thirty minutes of daily morning or late afternoon sun exposure (not through window glass) to heads, forearms, and legs can significantly increase calcidiol levels in elderly persons. Direct sunshine is not absolutely essential as UV-B radiation can penetrate light cloud cover fairly well. There is a marked decrease in 1-hydroxylation by the aging kidney and in kidney failure; calcitriol supplementation in the latter may be the only effective form of replacement. Conditions that cause chronic small intestinal malabsorption or fat malabsorption increase the risk for vitamin D deficiency. Phenytoin, phenobarbital, and glucocorticoids interfere with vitamin D metabolism or calcium transport or absorption.

Osteoporosis and osteomalacia are common in older adults and frequently coexist. A common feature of type I (postmenopausal) and type II (senile or old age) osteoporosis is calcium malabsorption, attributable both to decreased vitamin D levels and intestinal unresponsiveness to calcitriol. Estrogen may improve calcium absorption by affecting vitamin D receptors in the intestine. Vitamin D facilitates the action of parathyroid hormone to maintain ionized calcium concentration in its proper and narrow range; vitamin D deficiency is therefore associated with secondary hyperparathyroidism, which can accelerate bone loss.

Although calcitriol is the active form of vitamin D, serum calcitriol levels correlate poorly with body stores and most clinical diseases. The most reliable indicator of vitamin D status is the calcidiol [25(OH)D] serum level. Levels of serum calcium and phosphorus (which may decline) and alkaline phosphatase (which may elevate) are not sensitive measures for vitamin D deficiency. In the future, new serum parathyroid hormone (PTH) assays may serve as better markers of vitamin D deficiency.

Vitamin D has different effects depending upon whether it is given in vitamin D-depleted (promoting bone mineralization) or replete states (where it can stimulate demineralization). Persons with osteomalacia require 2000 to 4000 IU of vitamin D daily for several months, accompanied by adequate calcium (1.5 grams daily). The use of vitamin D in osteoporosis requires doses that do not increase bone resorption (by its calcemic action) but rather reduce it. Persons at risk for osteoporosis should receive 1.0 to 1.5 grams of calcium in their diet or as supplements daily, plus not more than 400 to 800 IU of vitamin D. Coffee-associated osteoporosis may be minimized by drinking at least one cup of milk a day.

Vitamin D deficiency can be prevented in high-risk persons (institutionalized, homebound on marginal diets, and those with malabsorption, hepatic, or renal disease) by giving 50,000 IU once or twice monthly.

Chronic vitamin D ingestion of 25,000 to 50,000 IU a day may be extremely toxic, increasing calcium absorption from the intestines and calcium mobilization from bone. The resulting hypercalcemia can cause calcification of the heart (aortic stenosis), blood vessels, lungs, joints and kidney (leading to renal insufficiency). Children may present with hypotonia, irritability, and pallor. Persons with hypercalcemia, parathyroid disorders, and chronic renal insufficiency are at greatest risk. All supplemented persons should have periodic renal and serum calcium assessments.

VITAMIN E

Vitamin E (alpha tocopherol is the most abundant and active isomer) generally functions as a lipid-soluble antioxidant, helping protect the body from the damaging effects of free radicals and other unstable molecules generated during normal oxygen metabolism or from environmental exposure to cigarette smoke, ozone, and radiation. More subtle deficiency states may place persons at risk for coronary artery disease. Population studies suggest that vitamin E serum levels correlate more strongly with ischemic heart disease than either cholesterol levels or diastolic blood pressure.

Commonly recognized vitamin E deficiency states occur primarily in premature, very-low-birthweight infants and in conditions associated with fat malabsorption. In children, these are normally congenital disorders, including cystic fibrosis, biliary atresia, and lipid transport abnormalities (e.g., abetalipoproteinemia). Vitamin E deficiency in children may be associated with anemia. The role for vitamin E in the prophylaxis or treatment of retrolental fibroplasia remains controversial. Adults at higher risk for deficiency include those with stomach resection, gluten enteropathy, regional enteritis, and chronic pancreatitis. Neuropathy may occur in adults with vitamin

E deficiency but generally requires many years of severe malabsorption. Drugs that may interfere with vitamin E absorption include mineral oil, cholestyramine, and colestipol.

The RDA for vitamin E is 3 to 4 mg for infants under 1 year of age, increasing to 10 mg of natural alpha-tocopherol equivalents for men and 8 mg for women (10 mg for pregnant women; 12 mg for lactating women)(natural vitamin E, 1 mg = 1.5 IU; synthetic vitamin E, 1 mg = 1 IU). Vitamin E decreases platelet adhesion, which may also be protective in thromboembolic disease, enhances cell-mediated immunity in healthy older persons, and improves abnormal movement ratings in persons with recent-onset tardive dyskinesia. Studies examining the role of vitamin E and cardiovascular disease, in which vitamin E appears to decrease low-density lipoprotein (LDL) oxidation and subsequent atherogenesis, generally show a protective effect for populations who consume 60 to 800 IU daily as supplements. Larger intakes have *not* been more protective.

Dosage in cystic fibrosis is 25 to 50 IU for infants, increasing to 200 IU for those over 18 years of age. Vitamin E therapy does *not* appear to affect either the physical or cognitive changes associated with Parkinson's disease, treat fibrocystic disease of the breast, or reduce nocturnal leg cramps. Studies are ongoing to examine any role for vitamin E in insulin resistance and cancer prevention.

The richest sources of vitamin E are common vegetable oils, products made from them (e.g., margarine and shortening), and wheat germ. Large losses of vitamin E occur during storage, processing, and preparation of food. Red meats, fish, animal fats, fruits, and vegetables have little vitamin E. It is difficult to consume high doses of vitamin E from natural foods without also consuming large amounts of fat. Although the synthetic form of vitamin E is less active than naturally occurring vitamin E, both forms provide equal antioxidant protection to LDL. Vitamin E status can be assessed by measuring the ratio of serum vitamin E to total serum lipids.

Toxic effects of vitamin E may present as diarrhea or fatigue, but even huge intakes are usually well tolerated. However, vitamin E can potentiate warfarin and increase the risk for bleeding in persons receiving this anticoagulant. A vitamin history is necessary for all persons taking anticoagulants.

VITAMIN B₁ (THIAMINE)

Thiamine plays a role in carbohydrate metabolism as a coenzyme in the decarboxylation of pyruvate and alpha-ketoglutarate and in the pentose phosphate cycle. It also affects nerve conduction. Food sources for thiamine include whole grains, legumes, pork, liver, and enriched flour products; it is absent from fats, oils, and refined sugars. Dairy products, fruits, and vegetables are poor sources. The covering (bran) on cereal grains contains most of the vitamin; polished grains, therefore, have reduced availability. The vitamin is degraded by heat and lost in discarded cooking water. Freezing does not affect thiamine content.

Thiamine requirements are increased with increasing carbohydrate intake, pregnancy, lactation, in the presence of folate or protein deficiency, and in hypermetabolic states such as strenuous physical exertion, fever, and thyrotoxicosis. Hemodialysis and peritoneal dialysis, diuretic therapy, and diarrhea increase thiamine loss while chronic malnutrition and intestinal disease decrease absorption. Alcohol impairs both absorption and metabolism. Some foods, such as raw fish, shellfish, coffee (regular and decaffeinated), and tea, contain thiaminases that can destroy thiamine.

In the United States, thiamine deficiency occurs primarily in alcoholics or in special clinical situations, such as in chronic dialysis, or when refeeding after starvation or after providing glucose to alcoholics with subclinical deficiency (as carbohydrate intakes rapidly increase). Early signs and symptoms of deficiency include tachycardia, weakness, irritability, anorexia, headache, malaise, nausea, and muscle aching. Hoarseness due to laryngeal nerve involvement may occur. If deficiency continues, more classic manifestations of beriberi can appear, related to a combination of cardiovascular (wet beriberi) and neurologic (dry beriberi and Wernicke-Korsakoff syndrome) symptoms. Beriberi heart disease includes peripheral vasodilatation with high-output (biventricular) congestive failure and edema. Dry beriberi manifests as a peripheral polyneuropathy (impairing sensory, motor, and tendon reflex functions), with a noninflammatory nerve degeneration.

Wernicke's syndrome is often associated with alcoholism and consists of a progression of symptoms: vomiting, nystagmus (usually horizontal), unilateral or bilateral sixth nerve ophthalmoplegia, fever, ataxia (weakness and a staggering drunken gait), and progressive global confusion. Not all patients with Wernicke's syndrome have a demonstrable vitamin B₁ deficiency, and most thiamine-deficient patients do not develop the syndrome. The disease may be dependent upon individual genetic variations in thiamine-dependent enzyme systems. The encephalopathy may develop into Korsakoff's syndrome: retrograde amnesia, decreased learning ability, and confabulation.

The most reliable biochemical test to detect thiamine deficiency is measurement of red blood cell (RBC) transketolase activity, although this may be less accurate in older adults. Assessment of clinical response to thiamine administration is most important. Beriberi is treated with 50 to 100 mg of thiamine intramuscularly for 1 to 2 weeks, followed by 2.5 to 10 mg per day orally until recovery. Improvement should occur rapidly in cardiovascular beriberi with an increase in blood pressure, a decrease in heart rate, and improved pulmonary congestion within 12 hours of beginning therapy. Eye signs generally improve quickly; other neurologic findings improve more slowly. The RDAs for thiamine begin at 0.3 to 0.4 mg for infants under 1 year of age, increasing to 1.2 mg for men and 1.0 mg for women (pregnant women need 1.5 mg; lactating women 1.6 mg).

Thiamine has minimal toxicity, but large parenteral intakes (>400 mg) may be accompanied by mental status changes (acute vigilance or lethargy), mild ataxia, and nausea.

VITAMIN B₂ (RIBOFLAVIN)

Riboflavin is necessary for the formation of two coenzymes (flavin adenine dinucleotide and flavin mononucleotide) involved in hydrogen transport and oxidation. Riboflavin deficiency almost invariably occurs in combination with deficiencies in other B vitamins. Deficiency can interfere with vitamin B_6 metabolism and conversion of tryptophan to niacin. Persons receiving probenecid, phenothiazines, excess thyroid hormone, or oral contraceptives may be more susceptible to deficiency. Neonatal phototherapy increases riboflavin destruction. Signs and symptoms of vitamin B_2 deficiency include cheilosis, sore throat, glossitis, angular stomatitis, seborrheic dermatitis (especially around the nasolabial folds), and a normocytic, normochromic anemia. Eye signs include lacrimation and superficial, interstitial keratitis, often associated with conjunctivitis and photophobia.

The RDA for vitamin B_2 is 0.4 to 0.5 mg for infants under 1 year of age, increasing to 1.4 mg for men and 1.2 mg for women (pregnant women need 1.6 mg per day; lactating women, 1.8 mg per day). Persons suspected of riboflavin deficiency (physical findings, poor intakes, small intestine disease) require 3 to 10 mg per day; other B vitamins should also be supplemented. Measurement of RBC riboflavin or glutathione reductase may help assess riboflavin status. Riboflavin is plentiful in dairy products, meats, poultry, fish, green vegetables, and enriched flour products. It is lost in cooking water. High intakes of riboflavin have no known toxicity.

VITAMIN B₆ (PYRIDOXINE)

Vitamin B_6 (pyridoxine and related compounds) is involved in the formation of brain metabolites such as epinephrine and norepinephrine, tyramine, dopamine, 5-hydroxytryptamine, serotonin, and gamma-aminobutyric acid (GABA). Vitamin B_6-dependent coenzymes play a role in the Krebs' cycle, protein and lipid metabolism, and melanin, cysteine, glycine, glutamate, serine, niacin, and porphyrin synthesis. It is involved in heme and arachidonic acid synthesis, stabilizes muscle phosphorylase, and participates in amino acid transport across membranes. Pyridoxine content is affected by food processing, cooking, and freezing. Good food sources are chicken, fish, kidney, liver, pork, and eggs.

The RDAs for vitamin B_6 in infants under 1 year of age are 0.3 to 0.6 mg, increasing to 2.0 mg for men and 1.6 mg for women, or 0.016 mg per gram of protein. Pregnant women need 2.2 mg; lactating women need 2.1 mg. Pyridoxine deficiency is associated with general malnutrition, chronic alcoholism, and a deficiency in other B-complex vitamins. However, pyridoxine metabolism or bioavailability may be specifically affected by over 40 drugs, including isoniazid, hydralazine, cycloserine, and penicillamine. Pyridoxine status may be estimated by measuring xanthurenic acid (a tryptophan metabolite) in the urine following tryptophan loading; measurement of RBC amino transaminases may prove a better indicator.

As with many B-vitamin deficiencies, pyridoxine deficiency is associated with seborrheic dermatitis, cheilosis, glossitis, and angular stomatitis. Some of the drug-associated deficiencies present as a peripheral neuropathy or a pyridoxine-responsive, microcytic, hypochromic anemia. Infants with deficiency exhibit gastrointestinal distress and irritability. Infants with a seizure disorder should be assessed for pyridoxine deficiency or dependency if more common causes have been ruled out. Supplementation with 30 mg per day of pyridoxine is recommended in persons taking isoniazid and estrogens. Up to 100 mg per day may be required in persons taking penicillamine. Any role for pyridoxine in treating nausea and vomiting associated with irradiation, anesthesia, and travel sickness remains unproved. Low doses (10 mg three times a day) may help the nausea and vomiting in early pregnancy. Vitamin B_6 can reduce elevated serum homocysteine levels, though not as effectively as folate.

Vitamin B_6 intakes up to 2000 mg have been tolerated without adverse side effects, although a sensory neuropathy (perioral numbness, hand and foot clumsiness, ataxia, and loss of position and vibratory sense) can occur at prolonged doses of 100 mg per day. Pyridoxine increases the peripheral decarboxylation of levodopa, reducing its effectiveness as a treatment for Parkinson's disease, and may antagonize the anticonvulsant effect of phenytoin and barbiturates.

NIACIN

Niacin is the generic name for nicotinic acid and its derivatives. It is an essential component of two coenzymes (NAD and NADP) necessary for many oxidation-reduction reactions. It can be formed from the essential amino acid tryptophan (about 60 mg of tryptophan is needed to form 1 mg of niacin), so dietary estimates of niacin must consider the tryptophan content as well. Vitamins B_2 (riboflavin) and B_6 (pyridoxine) are also required for the conversion of tryptophan to niacin. Good sources of niacin are meats, liver, fish, legumes, and enriched flour products. Niacin is poorly bioavailable from many cereal grains.

Pellagra (*pellis*, skin; *agra*, rough) is the classic form of niacin deficiency. Although commonly associated with a high dietary intake of maize and millet, it is more likely caused by food-processing and preparation techniques that decrease niacin bioavailability. Today, pellagra is associated with two rare disorders of tryptophan metabolism: carcinoid syndrome and Hartnup's disease. The 4 Ds of pellagra are dermatitis, dementia, diarrhea, and, finally, death. Early signs and symptoms are vague: anorexia, weakness, and paresthesias. The dermatitis tends to be bilaterally symmetrical and on areas of the body (neck, forehead, backs of hands) exposed to sunlight, with chronic inflammation, hyperkeratosis, red or dark pigmentation, and desquamation. The neurologic manifestations are nonspecific, with headache, depression, fatigue, and malaise preceding an encephalopathy with confusion and memory loss, hallucinations, and psychosis. Widespread inflammation of the mucosa leads to diarrhea, stomatitis, glossitis, and vaginitis.

There is no convenient biochemical measure to assess niacin status accurately; diagnosis is based upon clinical suspicion and response to replacement therapy. In the presence of adequate dietary tryptophan, 10 mg per day of niacin should adequately treat pellagra. In cases of suspected deficiency, other B vitamins should also be supplemented. Higher amounts (40 to 300 mg per day) are usually needed in Hartnup's disease and carcinoid syndrome, or with more severe symptoms. The RDAs for niacin are 5 to 6 NE (1 NE equals 1 mg of niacin) for infants below 1 year of age, gradually increasing to 15 NE for men and 13 NE for women, or 6.6 NE per 1000 kcal with no less than 13 NE per day. Pregnant women need 17 NE per day; lactating women need 20 NE per day.

High doses of nicotinic acid (1 to 8 grams per day) are necessary to see an effect on cholesterol levels. This anticholesterol effect is not seen with nicotinamide or nicotinic acid metabolites. Doses of nicotinic acid above 200 mg per day are frequently associated with flushing and pruritus due to histamine release and may increase pain in peptic ulcer disease, elevate serum uric acid and glucose, and cause liver toxicity. The side effect of flushing may often be reduced by starting at low doses, increasing slowly, taking an aspirin before the niacin, or taking it with foods.

VITAMIN B$_{12}$ (COBALAMIN)

Vitamin B$_{12}$ is bound to animal proteins such as meat (particularly organ meats), fish, and egg yolks; it is associated with some plants contaminated by microorganisms that contain vitamin B$_{12}$. Acid and digestive enzymes extract vitamin B$_{12}$ from food, and it attaches to R-binding proteins found in gastric juices, saliva, and bile. Pancreatic enzymes in the duodenum and jejunum degrade the R-proteins and allow intrinsic factor (IF), made by the stomach's parietal cells, to bind to vitamin B$_{12}$. The vitamin B$_{12}$-IF complex continues down the small bowel and attaches to receptors in the ileum. Vitamin B$_{12}$ is transported through the bowel mucosa and then throughout the body attached to the transport protein, transcobalamin II. The liver is the major storage site for vitamin B$_{12}$. Vitamin B$_{12}$ lost in the bile is efficiently recovered via the enterohepatic cycle. This recycling ability is so good that, in the presence of a normal gastrointestinal tract and large liver

reserves, the half-life of vitamin B$_{12}$ is approximately 4 years. Vitamin B$_{12}$ deficiency secondary to inadequate intake, therefore, takes 10 years or more to develop. Strict vegetarians should be monitored periodically for deficiency and counseled appropriately.

Vitamin B$_{12}$ malabsorption can be caused by prolonged use of histamine (H$_2$)-receptor antagonists and other antacids (particularly in marginally nourished persons), pancreatic insufficiency, intestinal bacterial overgrowth syndromes and parasitic infections including fish tapeworm and *Giardia lamblia*, and any disease or surgery affecting the stomach or distal small bowel. Cobalamin deficiency appears to be most common in older adults (prevalence ranges from 3% to 44%), in persons with AIDS, and in pernicious anemia. Most cases of vitamin B$_{12}$ deficiency in older adults are probably due to atrophic gastritis rather than pernicious anemia.

The development of vitamin B$_{12}$ deficiency passes through several stages following negative nutrient balance. The earliest serum marker is low holotranscobalamin II (the combined B$_{12}$-transport molecule), then low holohaptocorrin (a storage carrier), followed (as RNA and DNA synthesis are disrupted) by abnormalities in the deoxyuridine (dU) suppression test and an increase in hypersegmentation in the nuclei of polymorphonuclear leukocytes. Finally, serum and urine homocysteine and methylmalonic acid (MMA) levels rise and serum vitamin B$_{12}$ levels fall.

It is well established that macrocytosis (elevated mean corpuscular volume) and megaloblastic anemia are insensitive and late markers of vitamin B$_{12}$ deficiency that may be absent even in pernicious anemia. Depletion of vitamin B$_{12}$ may occur more rapidly in one tissue than another, and neurologic damage may not be synchronized with the hematologic changes. Neurologic and neuropsychiatric damage may occur before or after hematologic changes. The Schilling test may be used to detect malabsorption of vitamin B$_{12}$ (but not to diagnose deficiency). It is recommended only for younger persons or for those in whom the diagnosis of pernicious anemia is critical; this is not necessary for most older adults. Many errors are possible in performing or interpreting the Schilling test. Free vitamin B$_{12}$, as given in the classic Schilling test, may be easily absorbed, but vitamin B$_{12}$ bound to protein, as it is normally consumed in the diet, may not be available due to inadequate stomach acidity. Atrophic gastritis and hypochlorhydria are common in older adults, occurring in up to 50% of people over age 65 years. In such persons, the Schilling test may be falsely normal if the patient is unable to absorb cobalamin in foods despite being able to absorb free vitamin B$_{12}$ during the test. A "food Schilling test," using protein-bound cobalamin, should be used to mimic normal vitamin B$_{12}$ ingestion.

The most common peripheral symptoms of cobalamin deficiency are paresthesias (tingling, numbness, pins and needles sensation), usually bilaterally in the feet or hands. Some patients also have a gait ataxia and extremity weakness. Other findings include diminished or absent vibration and/or proprioceptive sense in the lower extremities; touch and pain sensation may also be reduced. Severity of neurologic findings may be worse when there is minimal anemia, and vice versa.

Serum cobalamin levels remain the most practical and widely available screening tool for vitamin B_{12} deficiency. Screening is recommended in persons with characteristic hematologic abnormalities and in persons with unexplained peripheral neuropathy, psychopathology, or difficulty ambulating.

Advanced age alone probably should not be the sole reason to screen. It is reasonable to consider persons with a serum vitamin B_{12} of less than 200 pg per mL to be deficient. One should measure MMA in persons whose cobalamin levels are 200 to 350 pg per mL, as well as in any patient with compatible neurologic or neuropsychiatric signs or symptoms, regardless of their cobalamin levels. A trial of therapy (parenterally in symptomatic patients) in enigmatic cases, while monitoring MMA or homocysteine levels, can be done; elevated levels should fall in true deficiency states.

Mental impairment as the sole manifestation of cobalamin deficiency is rare. However, confusion, memory loss, disorientation, and slowed thinking (symptoms hard to distinguish from dementia) have been shown to improve in persons known to be vitamin B_{12} deficient. Overall, however, dementia in elderly people is rarely caused by cobalamin deficiency. Evaluating a person with a dementia for vitamin B_{12} deficiency should be based on risk factors (including AIDS), the presence of suspicious neurologic or hematologic findings, or the likelihood that the dementia is due to reversible causes. Persons with low cobalamin levels and cognitive changes suggestive of dementia may show cognitive improvement with cobalamin replacement, especially if treatment is begun early. Overall, however, most demented persons who have evidence of vitamin B_{12} deficiency show no intellectual or behavioral improvement with cobalamin replacement.

Dosing schedules for vitamin B_{12} replacement are anecdotal. The adult RDA for vitamin B_{12} is 2 μg (2.2 μg in pregnancy; 2.6 μg during lactation). A dietary history should be done on all vitamin B_{12}-deficient persons. Once inadequate intake is ruled out, patients with uncomplicated inadequate absorption should achieve complete remission following a single injection of 100 μg of vitamin B_{12}.

Patients with continuing absorption problems will need monthly injections of 100 μg for life. Patients with multiple or severe coexisting medical problems, evidence of more severe deficiency such as neurologic findings, or symptoms that do not completely resolve should have higher initial and/or monthly injections (1000 μg). Reticulocytosis, a decrease in hypersegmentation, or a fall in MMA or homocysteine should occur by 10 days. Oral vitamin B_{12}, given in large doses (1000 to 2000 μg per day), is also usually effective even with intrinsic factor deficiency. There is insufficient experience at this time to determine the role of sublingual or intranasal vitamin B_{12} replacement. Vitamin B_{12} is generally nontoxic even in large doses. This low toxicity, however, does not justify its use as a placebo.

The more severe the neurologic symptoms or the longer their duration, and the less anemic the patient, the less complete the neurologic response to treatment. Advanced age may also decrease the likelihood of complete recovery. Neurologic evidence of response to treatment should be seen within the first 3 months. Nonresponders should be re-evaluated for evidence of continued vitamin B_{12} tissue deficiency (re-evaluating MMA or homocysteine levels), or for other causes of neuropathy. Axonal recovery can take years with peripheral injury or may never occur with CNS disease.

FOLIC ACID

Folic acid (or folate) is required for many methylation and nucleotide biosynthetic reactions. Folate is present in many foods and is especially concentrated in spinach, liver, and kidney. It is easily degraded by heat and storage, and leached and lost into cooking water.

Folate, like vitamin B_{12}, is excreted into the bile and reabsorbed from the gut in an enterohepatic cycle. Decreased small bowel mucosal transport, caused by general sepsis, uremia, and the mucosal edema that accompanies heart failure, can reduce folate absorption. Increased metabolic rate (such as hyperthyroidism) increases requirements. Alcohol decreases absorption, blocks utilization, and interferes with the enterohepatic cycle. Phenytoin both decreases absorption and increases excretion. Folate losses also increase in renal dialysis. Folate deficiency alone may be associated with irritability, hostility, or forgetfulness, but it probably does not cause a neuropathy or myelopathy; low folate is more commonly a coexisting problem in dementia, and folate assessment should not be a standard test in the work-up of dementia.

Low serum folate represents negative folate balance but does not diagnose tissue folate deficiency. An early sign of tissue depletion is a decreasing erythrocyte (RBC) folate, followed by an abnormal dU suppression test (indicating a slowing of DNA synthesis) and hypersegmentation of neutrophil nuclei. Macrocytosis and anemia, as in vitamin B_{12} deficiency, appear late. Serum folate decreases rapidly when folate intake or absorption decreases and quickly increases as intake resumes. RBC folate changes more slowly, reflecting folate nutriture at the time the red cell is developing; it may take 2 to 3 months before RBC folate becomes deficient (because of liver folate stores and RBC life span). Serum folate increases and RBC folate decreases in the presence of coexisting vitamin B_{12} deficiency. RBC folate also increases in the presence of other types of anemia. However, as a screening tool, when diet has not dramatically changed, serum folate measurement is generally sufficient.

Vitamins B_{12}, B_6, and folate each play a role as either coenzymes or substrates in the metabolism of homocysteine. Epidemiologic studies suggest that elevated homocysteine is an independent risk factor for accelerated arteriosclerotic disease. The relative risk for cardiovascular disease associated with hyperhomocysteinemia may be greater than that caused by smoking or elevated low-density lipoprotein (LDL) cholesterol. Elevated levels of homocysteine can also be caused by renal disease, psoriasis, some malignancies, and several drugs (e.g., antifolates and nitrous oxide). Folate supplementation may reduce elevated homocysteine regardless of etiology. The role of folate supplementation in cardiovascular disease prophylaxis remains intriguing, but unclear. Folic acid supplements (5 mg per week) may reduce methotrexate toxicity but not its efficacy in patients with rheumatoid arthritis.

The RDA for folate is 25 to 35 μg in infants below 1 year of age, gradually increasing to 200 μg for men and 180 μg for women (280 μg for lactating women). The U.S. Public Health Service recommends that all women who are or might become pregnant consume 400 μg daily to lower the incidence of neural tube defects. Folate can be replaced orally from a good diet with lots of dark green leafy vegetables, legumes, or liver. Infant requirements can generally be met from human milk or cow milk, but not from boiled or evaporated milk or from goat milk.

Large doses of folate are generally safe, although they potentially mask the hematologic signs of coexisting vitamin B_{12} deficiency (a major argument against widespread food fortification). They can also antagonize anticonvulsant therapy and may interfere with zinc metabolism. Vitamin B_{12} and folate supplementation have generally not been proved useful in preventing zidovudine-induced bone marrow suppression.

VITAMIN C (ASCORBIC ACID)

Vitamin C is a water-soluble vitamin with diverse biochemical properties, including acting as an antioxidant (e.g., stabilizing folic acid and vitamin E) and participating in the synthesis of collagen, carnitine, and neuropeptides such as norepinephrine and serotonin. It inhibits nitrosamine formation (associated with gastrointestinal cancers), activates intracellular drug-metabolizing systems, and increases nonheme iron absorption. It promotes wound healing and affects the function of leukocytes, macrophages, and other immune system modulators.

Vegetables and fruits contain relatively high amounts of vitamin C, particularly oranges (80 to 100 mg for a medium orange or 8 ounces of juice) and other citrus fruits (medium guava, 165 mg; one cup of cantaloupe, 68 mg; medium papaya, 188 mg), red sweet peppers (0.5 cup, 95 mg), tomato (24 mg), broccoli (0.5 cup, 58 mg), potatoes (medium baked, 26 mg), and strawberries (one cup, 85 mg). Red meat, fish, poultry, eggs, and dairy products contain much less, and grains contain none. Large amounts are lost in cooking water or when foods are heated or exposed to oxygen. Groups at special risk for vitamin C deficiency include smokers, diabetics, and frail or isolated older adults. Infants fed with nonfortified formula need vitamin C supplementation.

The classic vitamin C deficiency is scurvy, characterized by swollen or bleeding gums (in persons with teeth), perifollicular papules and petechial hemorrhages, and joint pains. Anemia is common. Vague weakness and malaise may precede classic signs and symptoms, and poor wound healing may also be a subtle marker for deficiency.

Most cases of scurvy in children occur between 6 and 24 months of age. Symptoms include irritability, anorexia, and bone tenderness; legs may assume a "frog" position with the hips and knees semiflexed and feet rotated outward. Long bone x-ray films, especially of the knees, reveal very thin cortex and a "ground glass" appearance of the bone. A linear rarefaction or break in the bone just proximal to the metaphysis may also be seen. Vitamin C intakes of approximately 10 mg per day will prevent scurvy, and the RDAs begin at 30 to 35 mg for infants up to 1 year of age, increasing to 60 mg in adults (70 mg during pregnancy, 90 to 95 mg during lactation, and 100 mg for smokers). The RDA for vitamin C is *not* based on its antioxidant properties. Treatment for diagnosed or clinically suspected scurvy is 500 to 1000 mg of vitamin C daily. Spontaneous bleeding and muscle and bone pain should resolve quickly; gums should begin to heal in 2 to 3 days. Vitamin C status can be measured in plasma or leukocytes.

Epidemiologic dietary studies strongly suggest a protective effect of fruits and vegetables against cancer. Because these foods contain carotenoids, folic acid, soluble and insoluble fiber, and various phytochemicals in addition to vitamin C, it is not yet known which dietary factor is most responsible or how synergic the interactions are. In addition, persons who consume this type of diet may have other lifestyle behaviors that also lower their risk. Vitamin C intakes of 300 to 500 mg per day appear protective against senile cataract formation. Vitamin C may also be protective against urinary tract infections. Its use as a treatment or prophylaxis for viral colds remains controversial; there is no scientific evidence for its use as cancer therapy.

Vitamin C can increase the absorption of nonheme iron. This can prove quite useful as an adjuvant for iron absorption in persons on a vegetarian diet or who are consuming iron supplements for iron deficiency. However, iron can act as a pro-oxidant, increasing free radical formation; high serum ferritin levels reflect the body's iron load and correlate with an increased relative risk for coronary artery disease. Vitamin C supplementation should be specifically discussed with persons at risk for iron overload (e.g., persons with thalassemia and hemochromatosis) and those with a history of renal oxalate stones. Vitamin C may also interfere with tests for fecal occult blood and glycosuria. Abruptly discontinuing high vitamin

C intake may make some persons deficient (rebound scurvy), but this is rare.

In general, vitamin C supplementation of less than 1000 mg per day currently appears to be associated with few adverse consequences. Because vitamin C is rapidly excreted in the urine, it is recommended that any supplementation be spread throughout the day.

VITAMIN K DEFICIENCY

method of
MAMMO AMARE, M.D., and
JOHN V. COX, D.O.
Texas Oncology, P.A.
Dallas, Texas

Vitamin K exists in two natural forms differing from one another in the structure of their side chains. Phylloquinone (vitamin K_1) is mainly found in green plants, and the menaquinones (vitamin K_2), which include a spectrum of molecular forms, are produced by intestinal flora. Menadione (vitamin K_3) is a synthetic vitamin that is converted in the liver to vitamin K_2.

Vitamin K is a cofactor in the gamma carboxylation of a diverse group of proteins present in various tissues. The most widely known vitamin K–dependent proteins are the four clotting factors—Factors II, IX, X, and VII—and the natural inhibitors of coagulation proteins C and S. After being assembled in the liver as inert precursor molecules, these coagulation factors undergo post-translational modifications in hepatocytes including a unique vitamin K–dependent gamma carboxylation of specific glutamic acid residues. Gamma-carboxyglutamic acid confers metal-binding properties to the proteins, which, in the presence of calcium, attach to cell membranes, especially platelet surfaces, where they form complexes with other clotting factors to carry out their biologic activity.

The carboxylase that catalyzes the gamma carboxylation of vitamin K-dependent proteins requires a steady supply of reduced vitamin K, derived from two sources. First, vitamin K obtained from the diet and intestinal bacteria is reduced in the liver by hydroquinone reductase to functionally active vitamin K hydroquinone. Second, during the process of carboxylation, reduced vitamin K is oxidized to vitamin K epoxide. A liver microsomal epoxide reductase then converts vitamin K epoxide to vitamin K quinone, which is reduced and recycled in the carboxylation process. Oral anticoagulants produce their effect by inhibiting vitamin K reductases, particularly epoxide reductase. Inhibition of the reductases depletes reduced vitamin K and curtails gamma carboxylation of the vitamin K-dependent clotting factors, which accumulate as nonfunctional uncarboxylated forms, collectively known as "protein induced by vitamin K antagonists" (PIVKAs).

Vitamin K is also necessary for the functional integrity of noncollagenous proteins, particularly osteocalcin, important for bone formation. Hence the distinct chondrodysplasia seen in infants born to women exposed to warfarin during early pregnancy is believed to be due to the drug-induced vitamin K deficiency leading to the formation of defective hypocarboxylated osteocalcin. A similar embryopathy has been described in an infant with a congenital absence of vitamin K epoxide reductase, the enzyme selectively inhibited by warfarin, in the liver.

The daily requirement of vitamin K is unknown, but it is generally recommended that adults consume 70 to 200 μg per day. Green leafy vegetables such as spinach, broccoli, brussels sprouts, and lettuce are important sources of phylloquinone, which accounts for the major portion of the vitamin normally found in the liver. Menaquinones (vitamin K_2) synthesized by intestinal bacteria may be additional sources of the vitamin.

The precise mechanisms of absorption of vitamin K are not fully understood. Dietary vitamin K_1, phylloquinone, is mainly absorbed from the proximal small bowel in the presence of bile salts. Animal studies have shown that menaquinones may be absorbed by simple diffusion in the distal ileum and the colon. Recent observations, however, suggest that a bile-mediated absorption from the terminal ileum may be more important. Once absorbed, vitamin K is mostly transported by chylomicrons via lymphatics to its primary storage site in the liver. The storage pool is small and may be depleted within days to weeks.

CAUSES OF VITAMIN K DEFICIENCY

The major categories of vitamin K deficiency are listed in Table 1. Sensitive assays indicate that poor dietary intake leads to a progressive depletion of vitamin K, despite the lack of clinically overt vitamin deficiency. When poor intake coexists with a reduced endogenous bacterial source, clinical deficiency occurs more rapidly. The contribution of menaquinones to the overall body store of vitamin K remains controversial, and it is uncertain if selective depletion of menaquinones results in clinically significant vitamin K deficiency. The hypoprothrombinemic coagulopathy seen with certain antibiotics that contain the methyltetrazole thiol (e.g., aztreonam, cefoperazone) results from direct inhibition of vitamin K rather than from alternation in the intestinal flora.

Diseases associated with disruption of bile flow to the intestinal lumen (e.g., obstructive biliary disease) and malabsorptive disorders due to intrinsic small intestinal disease or short-bowel syndrome lead to vitamin K deficiency of variable severity within days or weeks.

Vitamin K antagonists block the conversion of vitamin K to its biologically active reduced form (see earlier), in effect producing a vitamin K–deficiency state.

HEMORRHAGIC DISEASE OF NEWBORN

Hemorrhagic disease of the newborn (HDN) is a self-limited but at times fatal bleeding disorder caused by deficiency of vitamin K-dependent factors. Three clinical forms are known: early, classic, and late. Early HDN occurs within the first 24 hours of birth and is frequently associated with exposure of the mother to vitamin K antagonists

TABLE 1. **Causes of Vitamin K Deficiency**

Decreased ingestion
Poor dietary intake
Decreased endogenous (intestinal) production
Impaired absorption
Obstructive biliary disease
Intrinsic intestinal disease; short bowel syndrome
Impaired utilization
Oral anticoagulant
Anticonvulsant

such as warfarin or anticonvulsants. Classic HDN has its onset in the first 7 to 14 days after birth. Bleeding commonly occurs from the skin, gastrointestinal tract, and circumcision site. Inadequate intake, poor transplacental transfer of vitamin K, a lack of intestinal bacteria, and immaturity of the liver may contribute to the negative vitamin K balance. Late HDN becomes manifest between 2 and 12 weeks after birth and is associated with a higher incidence of intracranial bleeding.

LABORATORY TESTS

The prothrombin time (PT) and activated partial thromboplastin time (aPTT) are standard screening tests for coagulopathy of vitamin K deficiency. Prolongation of the PT occurs early, and abnormality of the aPTT indicates a more severe deficiency. Correction of the PT and aPTT when the patient's plasma is mixed with an equal volume of normal plasma confirms the deficiency of factor(s) and excludes the presence of inhibitor. Direct measurement of individual vitamin K-dependent clotting factors shows a variable decrease in the functional activities of Factors II, VII, IX, and X, and proteins C and S.

Routine laboratory tests do not discriminate between early hepatocellular disease and vitamin K deficiency. The distinction can be made by measuring both factor activity and antigen level. Vitamin K deficiency shows a decreased factor activity and a normal antigen level, whereas liver disease is manifested by a proportional decrease in the antigen and functional activity level. "Ecarin test" provides similar information. Ecarin, a snake venom, converts normal and uncarboxylated prothrombin molecules to thrombin. The test is normal in vitamin K deficiency and prolonged in liver disease. Diagnosis of the coagulopathy induced by the accidental ingestion or surreptitious use of warfarin may require measurement of the plasma drug level.

PREVENTION

The routine administration of vitamin K_1, 0.5 to 1 mg parenterally or 2 to 5 mg orally, to newborn babies has significantly reduced the incidence of HDN. Repeated doses may be necessary with oral prophylaxis.

Patients with poor oral intake or on long-term parenteral nutrition benefit from vitamin K supplementation, especially if they are concurrently receiving a broad-spectrum antibiotic. In patients with malabsorption syndrome, the periodic (every 1 to 4 weeks) administration of vitamin K_1, 5 to 10 mg intramuscularly or subcutaneously, is appropriate. When clinically applicable, oral vitamin K, 5 to 10 mg daily, may be used.

TREATMENT

The treatment of the coagulopathy caused by vitamin K deficiency is dependent on the site and severity of the bleeding. For a patient who has active bleeding or needs an immediate correction of the coagulopathy, the therapeutic options include fresh-frozen plasma (FFP) and/or vitamin K replacement. FFP is usually reserved for life-threatening bleeding and is infrequently used for surgical emergencies when prompt control of the coagulopathy is critical. It is administered at a dose of 15 to 20 mL per kg of body weight together with parenteral vitamin K. If the PT remains prolonged at 6 to 8 hours, a second dose may be necessary. FFP carries the risk of viral transmission and should be used with caution.

Vitamin K_1 (AquaMEPHYTON), 5 to 10 mg intramuscularly, is sufficient to correct the PT within 6 to 24 hours. An identical dose of intravenous vitamin K_1 is used if there is a contraindication to intramuscular injection or if a more rapid correction of the coagulopathy is desired. Intravenous vitamin K has been associated with anaphylactic reaction and should be given with care after the necessary precautions are taken. Oral vitamin K (Mephyton), 10 to 20 mg, may be used for less severe bleeding.

In a patient on oral anticoagulant therapy, withholding the drug corrects the prolonged PT and PTT within hours to days. In contrast, treatment of the coagulopathy caused by ingestion of long-acting "superwarfarins" (e.g., brodifacoum) may require the administration of high daily doses of vitamin K_1 over weeks to months for normalization of the PT.

OSTEOPOROSIS

method of
MICHAEL R. McCLUNG, M.D., and
BETSY LOVE McCLUNG, R.N., M.N.
Oregon Osteoporosis Center
Portland, Oregon

Osteoporosis has been thought of as a disorder characterized by fractures in older women. Based on recent studies of the natural history of postmenopausal and age-related bone loss, we now view osteoporosis as a disorder of skeletal fragility due principally to low bone mass that renders a patient susceptible to fracture after only minor injury. In this context, fractures are the complications of osteoporosis, much as strokes are the complications of hypertension. Both osteoporosis and increased blood pressure are usually asymptomatic conditions until or unless complications (fractures or strokes) occur. The asymptomatic phase of osteoporosis can now be recognized. A World Health Organization panel recently defined osteoporosis in women as a bone mass value more than 2.5 standard deviations (SD) below the average values measured in young women. In recognition of the fact that one osteoporotic fracture increases the likelihood of experiencing subsequent fractures, patients with bone density values in the osteoporotic range and who have already had one fracture are said to have severe osteoporosis. Individuals with bone mass values between 1 and 2.5 SD below peak young adult values are described as having osteopenia or low bone mass. Although these patients are not at significantly increased risk of experiencing a fracture at the time of testing, they may be at increased risk for the development of osteoporosis in the future.

With the availability of sensitive and precise measurements of bone mass, patients who have osteoporosis can be readily identified even before fractures occur. Therapeutic intervention can prevent or decrease further bone loss and will minimize the likelihood of fractures occurring over the remainder of the patient's lifetime. The decision to begin pharmacologic therapy for the prevention or treatment of osteoporosis is based upon several factors, including the patient's bone density value, age, lifestyle, risk factors for bone loss, and other medical problems. Although this review focuses on the treatment of patients with established osteoporosis, many of the points regarding the use of calcium and antiresorptive drugs will pertain to their use for prevention as well.

Bone turnover in patients with osteoporosis is unbalanced such that bone resorption exceeds bone formation. Bone loss can be attributed to an excessive rate of bone resorption, a decreased rate of bone formation, or a combination of these two problems. Until recently it was thought that bone loss in early menopause was related primarily to high rates of bone resorption whereas osteoporosis in elderly men and women was primarily due to impaired osteoblastic function and decreased bone formation. States of "high turnover" and "low turnover" osteoporosis were described, with the implication that different treatments might be more effective in one type of patient over another. With the use of new biochemical markers of bone turnover and from studies monitoring interval changes in bone density in older adults, we now recognize that high rates of bone turnover and progressive bone loss persist into old age. In recent clinical trials evaluating new treatments for postmenopausal osteoporosis, baseline assessment with biochemical markers does not demonstrate a bimodal distribution of bone turnover rates. Bone resorption and formation markers are normal or high but are very rarely below normal premenopausal values. Furthermore, estimates of baseline bone turnover rate do not predict response to treatment. Thus, the concept of high versus low turnover osteoporosis is not so helpful in choosing therapeutic strategies for osteoporosis in postmenopausal women. Furthermore, these data support the use of antiresorptive therapy in all patients with osteoporosis rather than attempting to segregate patients into those who benefit more from antiresorptive versus bone-forming therapy on the basis of bone turnover. This is fortuitous, for we now have several effective antiresorptive drugs from which to choose whereas we have not had a safe and effective drug that stimulates bone formation.

The primary objective of treating patients with osteoporosis is to decrease the occurrence of new fractures (Table 1). Bone density and the presence of previous fractures are the major influences on fracture risk. In the absence of osteoporosis, fragility fractures are uncommon, even when injuries such as falls occur. As patients with osteoporosis grow older, however, extraskeletal factors play an increasingly important role in fracture risk. Principal among these nonskeletal factors are the occurrence of and the response to injury. Thus, a therapeutic strategy to decrease fracture frequency must address both the skeletal and the injury components of fracture risk.

PRESERVING AND IMPROVING BONE MASS

Correction of Secondary Factors That Contribute to Bone Loss

Factors other than decreased calcium intake, estrogen deficiency, and aging frequently contribute to or amplify rates of bone loss. The initial step in an effective program of treatment is to identify and correct, when possible, these secondary factors, listed in

TABLE 1. **Osteoporosis: Management Objectives**

Decrease risk of fracture
Prevent further bone loss
Correct secondary factors
Adequate calcium and vitamin D intake
Antiresorptive therapy
Estrogen
Calcitonin
Bisphosphonates
Prevent injury
Minimize symptoms
Improve functional status

Table 2. This requires careful clinical and laboratory evaluation and the recognition of clinically silent problems such as intestinal malabsorption, renal calcium leak, and hyperparathyroidism or subclinical hyperthyroidism.

Adequate Calcium and Vitamin D

Although calcium alone cannot prevent bone loss in early menopause, calcium is effective in decreasing bone turnover, rates of bone loss, and fracture incidence in patients with osteoporosis. The importance of adequate calcium intake increases in older patients because of the gradual impairment in vitamin D metabolism and calcium absorption that occurs with aging. For patients with osteoporosis, a total daily intake (diet plus supplement) of 1500 mg is recommended. For patients who are unable to consume two to three servings of dairy products daily, supplements are required. Most clinical studies have used calcium in the form of calcium carbonate (calcium carbonate tablets, Tums, or oyster shell cal-

TABLE 2. **Correctable Causes of Bone Loss**

Lifestyle Factors
Smoking
Excessive alcohol intake
Inadequate physical activity
Defects in Calcium Balance
Decreased intake
Vitamin D deficiency
Malabsorption of calcium and/or vitamin D
Renal calcium leak
Drugs
Glucocorticoids
Anticonvulsants
Thyroid hormone
Endocrinopathies
Hyperparathyroidism
Hyperthyroidism
Hypogonadism
Acromegaly
Cushing's syndrome
Hyperprolactinemia
Other Medical Problems
Multiple myeloma
Renal insufficiency
Hepatic disease

cium). Preparations are available containing 100 to 600 mg of elemental calcium per tablet in forms that can be swallowed or chewed. Although calcium carbonate is poorly absorbed when given on an empty stomach in achlorhydric patients, the absorption of calcium from this salt is excellent and predictable when administered with food. No single dose should exceed 600 mg. Some patients experience mild gastrointestinal symptoms with calcium carbonate. Switching to tricalcium phosphate (Posture) or calcium citrate (Citracal) may alleviate these symptoms. Other sources of calcium such as lactate or gluconate are not practical because so many tablets must be taken to achieve an appropriate calcium intake.

Vitamin D is necessary for adequate calcium absorption, bone formation, and muscle strength. Vitamin D deficiency without clinical manifestations of osteomalacia is common in elderly patients, especially those who live in northern latitudes and have restricted exposure to sunlight. For patients with vitamin D deficiency (assessed by serum 25-hydroxyvitamin D levels), treatment with 50,000 units of vitamin D each week for 6 months is usually sufficient to replenish vitamin D stores. If the level of 25-hydroxyvitamin D does not at least normalize, further evaluation of small bowel function is indicated. When vitamin D deficiency does not or no longer exists, the provision of 400 to 800 units of vitamin D daily is usually sufficient to prevent the development of deficiency. The combination of 1200 mg calcium plus 800 units of vitamin D daily substantially decreased hip fracture incidence in very elderly women in a French nursing home after 18 months of therapy. Adequate calcium and vitamin D is the keystone of any therapeutic plan for osteoporosis.

Antiresorptive Therapy

Estrogen. The importance of estrogen therapy in the prevention of bone loss in early menopause is well understood. It is not so well recognized that estrogen is also effective as a treatment for older women with established osteoporosis. In several studies, estrogen administration to women in their sixties and seventies was found to suppress bone resorption, preserve bone mass, and decrease the incidence of vertebral and hip fractures. There seems to be no significant difference in skeletal effectiveness among oral and transdermal estrogens, and several preparations are approved for the treatment of osteoporosis (Table 3). Although full discussion of hormonal replacement therapy is beyond the scope of this article, estrogen should not be given to women with unexplained uterine bleeding or breast masses of unknown significance. The use of estrogen in women with a history of previous breast or endometrial cancer involves medicolegal as well as clinical and scientific concerns. With the availability of new antiresorptive agents, the use of estrogen in these patients for the treatment of osteoporosis is not necessary, although estrogen therapy may be indicated

TABLE 3. Therapeutic Agents for Osteoporosis

Drug	Dose(s)
Estrogens	
conjugated estrogens (Premarin)	0.625 mg daily
estropipate (Ogen)	0.625 mg daily
estradiol (Estrace)	0.5, 1.0 mg daily
estradiol (Estraderm)	0.05, 0.1 mg TDS twice weekly
Salmon calcitonin	
Calcimar	100 U SC daily
Miacalcin	100 U SC daily
Miacalcin Nasal Spray	200 U daily
Bisphosphonates	
alendronate (Fosamax)	10 mg daily
etidronate (Didronel)*	400 mg daily for first 14 days q 3rd month

*Not FDA-approved for this indication.

for the control of menopausal symptoms or reduction in risk of heart disease.

Attention to endometrial safety is necessary in women with an intact uterus. Progestational agents administered cyclically or continuously are indicated with estrogen therapy. Annual endometrial biopsy may be used for women who choose not to take progestins. For older women who have not taken estrogen for many years, breast swelling and tenderness is a frequent early symptom when hormone therapy is begun. Beginning treatment with small doses (0.3 mg of conjugated estrogen (Premarin) or its equivalent every other day) and gradually increasing the dose will minimize the frequency of these symptoms and will enhance long-term compliance. Education about the medication is necessary and will enhance compliance with the therapeutic regimen.

The target dose of estrogen preparations is listed in Table 3. Smaller doses (e.g., 0.3 mg of conjugated estrogen) are often sufficient to prevent bone loss in women whose calcium intake is adequate and may be ideal to minimize side effects of estrogen therapy in older women.

Bone loss resumes quickly when estrogen therapy is discontinued. Because hip fracture frequency continues to increase exponentially with age, continuous long-term therapy with estrogen or one of its alternatives to be discussed is indicated in women with osteoporosis.

Calcitonin. Calcitonin directly inhibits osteoclast activity and has been shown to reduce bone loss in both early postmenopausal women and in patients with established osteoporosis. In some studies, the effect of calcitonin seems to wane after 18 to 24 months of therapy, and the long-term usefulness of this treatment is not known. The effectiveness of calcitonin for fracture prevention has not been adequately explored.

The preparations available for use are salmon calcitonin, which is more potent and more effective than human calcitonin. Subcutaneous administration has been the only method available until recently. One hundred units (0.5 mL) of salmon calcitonin (Calcimar, Miacalcin) administered daily is the approved dose. A reduced dosing schedule has been suggested, in part to minimize the expense of injectable calcitonin. However, it is not known whether reducing the dose to 50 units daily or to 100 units three times each week provides adequate protection from bone loss.

The nasal spray form of calcitonin (Miacalcin Nasal Spray) has recently received FDA approval for the treatment of women with established postmenopausal osteoporosis. The appropriate dose is 200 units administered once each day. Systemic side effects such as nausea and flushing occur much less often than with the injected calcitonin. Nasal symptoms such as stuffiness and rhinitis are infrequent side effects of this approach to therapy.

Bisphosphonates. Bisphosphonates are derivatives of pyrophosphate in which the oxygen ether linkage between two phosphate groups is substituted with a carbon atom. All members of this drug class are poorly absorbed from the intestinal tract and are not metabolized. Approximately half of the absorbed doses is deposited in the skeleton, and the other half is excreted in the urine. These agents bind to the surface of bone and inhibit osteoclastic bone resorption by mechanisms that are not well understood.

Etidronate (Didronel)* is the parent member of this drug class and is approved for the treatment of Paget's disease of bone and hypercalcemia of malignancy. At doses of etidronate that suppress osteoclast activity, mineralization of bone is also impaired. Continuous therapy is associated with the accumulation of unmineralized bone and the development of osteomalacia. Cyclic administration of etidronate has been evaluated for the treatment of osteoporosis. A usual schedule is 400 mg daily for the first 2 weeks of every third month. Several studies show that etidronate therapy prevents bone loss in women with postmenopausal osteoporosis. Therapy also decreases the incidence of vertebral fractures in patients at highest risk in these studies. These results, however, have not satisfied the new FDA guidelines for new osteoporosis treatments, and etidronate has not received FDA approval for this indication. Nonetheless, etidronate has frequently been used off-label for the treatment of osteoporosis in women who cannot or choose not to take estrogen.

Alendronate (Fosamax) is a new, potent aminobisphosphonate that does not impair bone mineralization at doses that suppress bone resorption. In a very large set of clinical trials in women with postmenopausal osteoporosis, alendronate therapy decreased indices of bone turnover to levels seen in premenopausal women. Bone density values in the spine and hip, sites rich in trabecular bone, increased progressively over 3 years of therapy. Cortical bone mass was also preserved by alendronate therapy. The increase of spinal bone density of 9% compared with the calcium-treatment control group was associated with a 48% reduction in the number of patients who experienced fractures over the interval study and a significant reduction of height loss. The risk of nonvertebral fractures was also decreased, by 29%. On the basis of these data, alendronate received FDA approval for the treatment of postmenopausal women with osteoporosis. The approved dose of alendronate (10 mg) is administered once daily upon arising each morning, on an empty stomach after an overnight fast. To ensure adequate absorption, the drug should be taken with a full glass of water at least 30 minutes before breakfast, other beverages, or medications, including vitamins and mineral supplements. To minimize upper gastrointestinal side effects, patients should not lie down for at least 30 minutes after taking the drug. Like estrogen, continuous therapy seems to be required for maximum benefits.

Patients in the alendronate clinical trials all received calcium supplements, and none had vitamin D deficiency at the beginning of the study. Providing adequate calcium and vitamin D is very important with the use of potent antiresorptive drugs such as alendronate.

There are theoretical concerns about the very long-term use of a drug like alendronate, which accumulates in the skeleton in an active form. These concerns are being addressed in longer studies of alendronate's effect.

Combination Therapy. A recent study demonstrated that the combination of estrogen and etidronate produced a greater increase in bone mineral density (BMD) than did either therapy alone. Studies combining estrogen and alendronate are underway. The concurrent use of estrogen, for control of menopausal symptoms and protection from heart disease, and bisphosphonate therapy for added skeletal protection, will undoubtedly occur frequently.

Bone-Forming Agents

The ultimate therapeutic goal in patients who have already developed osteoporosis would be to stimulate new bone formation and to repair the qualitative and quantitative changes in bone. No drug is available that accomplishes this objective safely. Sodium fluoride (NaF)* stimulates osteoblast activity in trabecular bone. No form of sodium fluoride is approved for the treatment of osteoporosis. A dose of 20 to 75 mg daily increases bone mass in the spine but not in the hip or in cortical bone. However, vertebral fracture incidence is only minimally changed, and there is concern that long-term therapy with sodium fluoride might actually increase the risk of hip fracture. With these doses of NaF, GI symptoms are frequent, and some patients experience pain in the lower extremities due to stress fractures and possible osteomalacia. Recent studies with a slow-release form of sodium fluoride are encouraging. At this writing, the routine

---

*Not FDA-approved for this indication.

*Not FDA-approved for this indication.

use of sodium fluoride therapy in clinical practice is not recommended until more data about its use are available.

Future Therapies

Several new therapeutic agents are currently being evaluated for the treatment of osteoporosis, including other new bisphosphonate drugs and different combinations of estrogen and progestins. Parathyroid hormone and growth hormone both promote bone growth and are being studied as potential treatments for established osteoporosis. Several agents in the antiestrogen class of drugs are also being evaluated. These drugs inhibit estrogen activity in the breast and uterus while acting as estrogen agonists in the skeleton and on serum lipid levels. If preliminary findings are confirmed in longer studies, these drugs may soon be available for the management of menopause and as therapy for osteoporosis.

Monitoring Therapy

Routine clinical evaluation (symptoms, examination, height measurement, spinal radiographs) is adequate to assess whether new fractures occur in patients with osteoporosis but is not sufficient to assess the skeletal response to pharmacologic therapy. Repeat BMD measurements at intervals of 1 to 2 years are the only way to monitor therapy currently. Because of variations among types of bone density measuring devices, serial BMD measurements must be made with the same machine. Meticulous attention to quality control of the BMD device and of technician performance is necessary for bone density measurements to be clinically useful.

Monitoring the levels of the new biochemical markers of bone turnover may prove useful in evaluating the skeletal response to therapy. Changes in biochemical markers have been associated with subsequent changes in BMD in clinical research studies. Whether clinicians can use the markers to evaluate or predict an individual patient's response to treatment awaits further study.

INJURY AND FALL PREVENTION

Although osteoporosis is associated with increased fracture risk, not all patients with osteoporosis experience a fracture. Usually osteoporotic fractures follow an injury, albeit minor. Patients with vertebral osteoporosis must avoid spinal loading in the flexed position. Education regarding body mechanics, proper lifting techniques, and safe strategies for household chores is important.

Falls are the major injury associated with fractures of the radius or the hip and sometimes contribute to vertebral or pelvic fractures as well. Weakness, impaired balance, and unsteady gait are important risk factors for falls. These problems may be improved with an appropriate program of exercise and physical activity. Visual and other neuromuscular impairments need to be minimized as much as possible, and hazards in the patient's living environment also should be corrected to avoid falls and injury. Drugs that impair balance or cause postural changes in blood pressure, like alcohol, sedatives, tranquilizers, and some antihypertensive medications, also contribute to falls and fractures and should be reduced or avoided when possible. Despite these efforts, all falls cannot be prevented in frail elderly patients with osteoporosis. Padded hip protection has been shown to reduce substantially the frequency of hip fractures in such patients. New, less bulky designs will soon be available and may be the most useful and important short-term approach toward the prevention of hip fractures in patients with severe osteoporosis.

SYMPTOM RELIEF

Osteoporosis usually develops without symptoms until or unless fractures occur. Patients with generalized or prolonged bone pain should be evaluated for other skeletal problems, such as osteomalacia, multiple myeloma, or focal bone diseases such as Paget's disease. Chronic back discomfort, however, occurs commonly in patients who have previously experienced vertebral fractures. These chronic symptoms are rarely due to spinal root compression but may be related to facet joint arthritis, which occurs as a consequence of vertebral deformity. More often, patients complain of muscle aches or tiredness due to a combination of decreased extensor muscle strength and increased demand for muscle function to maintain posture in the face of height loss. Symptoms often occur in the low back, especially in patients with fractures of the lumbar vertebrae or those with significant thoracic kyphosis that requires an accentuation of lumbar lordosis for postural stability. Other patients experience muscle symptoms in the interscapular region, especially while performing activities that require forward bending. Pharmacologic agents that alter bone turnover are generally not effective in alleviating these symptoms. Mild analgesics and nonsteroidal anti-inflammatory drugs are occasionally helpful, but the most important approach to symptom relief is a program of exercises targeting the muscles of the back. Appropriate exercises to stretch and then to strengthen the extensor musculature of the back often result in a salutary effect. Instruction by an experienced physical therapist is a very important component of the treatment of such patients. Examples of appropriate exercises are described in "Boning Up on Osteoporosis," a booklet distributed by the National Osteoporosis Foundation.

PSYCHOSOCIAL ISSUES

Patients with osteoporosis must frequently deal with a variety of emotional and psychosocial issues. For many patients, osteoporosis is the first objective evidence of age-related deterioration. Patients who have experienced fractures, the complications of osteoporosis, often visualize themselves as "crumbling" or in a state of extreme fragility. Pain and fear of future limitations in functional ability limit their activities and often cause increased dependence on others for transportation or help in the home. Progressive withdrawal from interactions with family and friends is often the consequence. Anger and frustration regarding inability to perform routine daily activities, anxiety and fear of future fractures, and depression and dismay over height loss, spinal curvature, and abdominal protrusion may occur.

Recognizing, validating, and even anticipating these problems in patients with symptomatic osteoporosis is an important component of comprehensive patient management. Just learning about what osteoporosis is and its consequences and that therapeutic strategies are available to reduce the risk of subsequent fractures, to improve symptoms, and to regain and maintain functional and social activities is often very helpful and reassuring to patients. Educating the patient's family about osteoporosis, the patient's limitations, and, more importantly, what the patient can do is also important. Finally, engaging a patient with osteoporosis with a member of a local support group can be helpful, reassuring, and therapeutic for those who are frightened, anxious, or depressed.

ACUTE VERTEBRAL FRACTURES

Acute fractures of the thoracolumbar spine usually occur as a result of minor trauma such as a fall in the seated position or lifting while the back is in flexion. The pain associated with a fracture is usually localized to the region of the fracture and may be very intense, requiring bed rest for a few days. Prolonged bed rest is to be avoided because of the progressive muscle weakness and bone loss that accompany immobility. Spasm of adjacent musculature, sometimes with radiation in a dermatomal distribution, may occur. These patients often benefit from either ice or heat treatments to the affected part of the back. Other physical therapy modalities such as ultrasound and massage may be helpful in this phase. Analgesics, including narcotics, may be necessary in the first several days following the fracture. Constipation, a common consequence of bed rest and analgesics, is perhaps avoided by increasing fluid and fiber intake and by early ambulation.

Fortunately, the acute pain following a fracture gradually improves and almost invariably abates in 4 to 12 weeks as the fracture heals. Maintaining as much mobility and physical activity as possible during the period of fracture healing is essential, for it may minimize the intensity and duration of chronic back symptoms following a spinal fracture. Lumbar support corsets are frequently helpful during the phase of acute back pain for patients with lower thoracic or lumbar fractures. Back braces should be reserved only for patients who are very weak and frail and whose symptoms are not controlled by other means. The use of braces should be envisioned as a short-term solution during which appropriate rehabilitation efforts are made. Clearly the best back brace is a set of strong back muscles.

Calcitonin* may provide analgesic effect in some patients with acute vertebral fractures. Although not FDA-approved for its analgesic effect, a therapeutic trial of 100 units subcutaneously or 200 units intranasally daily for 7 to 10 days is often used in patients whose activities are markedly limited by their bone pain. If significant improvement in symptoms is noted, therapy is continued for a total of 6 to 8 weeks. If no acute response occurs, calcitonin therapy is stopped unless it is to be used long-term for its antiresorptive effect.

Patients who have had one or more vertebral fractures are at very high risk of experiencing subsequent fractures. The occurrence of one vertebral fracture in a patient with osteoporosis is a strong indication for careful evaluation and correction of secondary causes and for beginning treatment with antiresorptive agents.

HIP FRACTURES

The treatment of a hip fracture is almost always an orthopedic procedure. Following the surgical repair of the fracture, appropriate rehabilitation is usually accomplished. Virtually all patients who experience nontraumatic hip fractures have osteoporosis, and these patients are at substantial risk for having another hip fracture or other complications of skeletal fragility. Beyond their postoperative rehabilitation program, however, drug therapy to preserve or increase bone mass and nonpharmacologic strategies to avoid recurrent injury are indicated.

OSTEOPOROSIS IN MEN

Men experience age-related bone loss at a rate almost as great as do women. Because men develop greater bone mass during their growth years than do women, and because men do not have an accelerated phase of bone loss corresponding to the early menopausal years, osteoporosis and the occurrence of fractures are less frequent in men. Men over age 75 years often have osteoporosis due to their age, possible abnormalities of calcium balance, and perhaps androgen deficiency. With the exception of estrogen therapy, the approach to a man with osteoporosis is similar to that of women. Correction of secondary causes of bone loss, the use of antiresorptive therapy, and both education and exercise to avoid injury and to improve symptoms are appropriate for men, although studies evaluating the use of antiresorptive therapy in men are just being performed. Younger men who have osteoporosis frequently have secondary causes such as hypogonadism, glucocorticoid use, previous gastrointestinal surgery, or excessive alcohol use. Other young men with osteoporosis seem to

---

*Not FDA-approved for this indication.

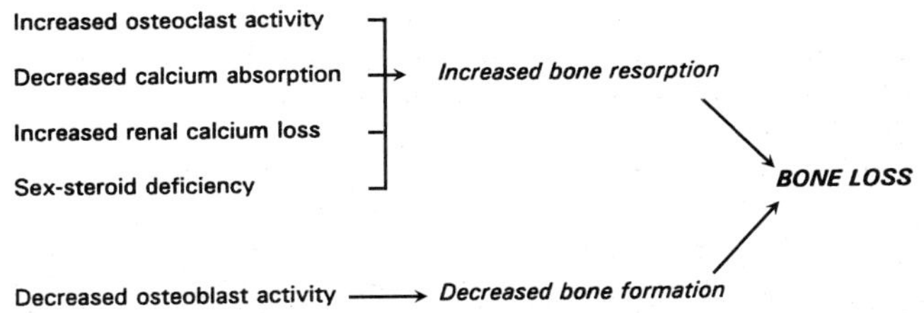

Figure 1. Pathophysiology of glucocorticoid-induced osteoporosis.

have low bone mass because of poor bone formation and may have a mild form of osteogenesis imperfecta. Bone density values in these men usually remain stable. Other than avoiding secondary causes of bone loss, the proper approach to therapy of these men has not been determined.

STEROID-INDUCED BONE DISEASE

Glucocorticoids adversely affect skeletal health through several mechanisms (Figure 1). The combination of suppressed bone formation and increased bone resorption may lead to very rapid bone loss, but the skeletal response to steroid therapy is quite variable. The steps in the management of patients on long-term steroid therapy are outlined in Table 4. The target for calcium intake is 1200 to 1500 mg daily, and for vitamin D, 400 to 800 units daily. Estrogen replacement is appropriate for postmenopausal women or younger women with amenorrhea or menstrual irregularity. Androgen deficiency is common in men receiving 10 mg or more of prednisone daily. Androgen replacement (testosterone cypionate [Depo-Testosterone] or transdermal testosterone [Testoderm]) is indicated in men with clinical or laboratory evidence of hypogonadism. Neither estrogen nor testosterone should be used if strong contraindications exist. Bone density testing is very helpful in determining whether additional therapy is indicated. For patients with osteoporosis (BMD more than 2.5 standard deviations below young normal values) or who exhibit progressive bone loss, therapy with calcitonin or bisphosphonates is frequently used. Although none of these therapies are FDA-approved for the treatment of steroid-related osteoporosis, several clinical studies have documented the effectiveness of antiresorptive therapy to minimize bone loss in these patients.

For patients beginning extended therapy (3 months or more) with glucocorticoids, bone density testing is also useful. Patients with low BMD values

are at increased risk of experiencing fractures in the first few months of steroid therapy. Treatment with estrogen in postmenopausal women or with calcitonin or bisphosphonates in men and premenopausal women seems very reasonable, although prospective studies do not yet exist documenting the ability of such therapy to prevent bone loss when steroid therapy has been recently begun. Patients with organ transplants (especially heart and liver) who are begun on steroids and other immunosuppressive drugs have a very high incidence of osteoporosis and fractures. Because this constellation of events can be a major disabling problem for transplant patients, antiresorptive therapy with calcitonin or bisphosphonates at the time of transplantation seems reasonable, especially if bone density is low. However, prospective studies evaluating these treatments have yet to be completed. In patients on chronic steroid therapy and those recently begun on steroids, serial bone density measurement every 6 to 12 months is of value in monitoring skeletal response and guiding therapeutic decisions.

PAGET'S DISEASE OF BONE

method of
BART L. CLARKE, M.D.
University of Chicago Medical Center
Chicago, Illinois

Paget's disease is a localized disorder of bone remodeling caused by an initial increase in osteoclast-mediated bone resorption, coupled to an increase in osteoblast-mediated bone formation. Accelerated bone resorption and formation result in a disorganized mosaic of abnormal woven and normal lamellar bone with increased vascularity at affected skeletal sites. After osteoporosis, Paget's disease is the second most common disorder affecting bone in the United States.

Epidemiologic surveys have demonstrated Paget's disease to be relatively common in northern Europe, North America, Australia, and New Zealand but uncommon elsewhere. The highest prevalence rates are reported from Lancashire, England, where as many as 6% to 8% of the adult population over age 55 years have radiographic evidence of the disease. Paget's disease probably affects about 3% of the United States population over age 55 years, with most affected individuals having European ancestry.

Paget's disease affects slightly more men than women. The average age of diagnosis is in the fifth to sixth decade, but it may be diagnosed as early as the second decade. The great majority of patients are asymptomatic and are diagnosed incidentally on radiographic studies obtained for other purposes, but a small percentage have symptomatic disease.

The pathogenesis of Paget's disease remains unknown. Genetic predisposition to the disease, as reflected by positive family history, is a factor in as many as 15% to 30% of patients. Analysis of multiple affected families suggests an autosomal dominant pattern of inheritance. Individuals with an affected first-degree relative have a sevenfold increased risk of developing the disease. Paget's disease has been linked with HLA-DQW 1, even in patients without

TABLE 4. **Management of Glucocorticoid-
Induced Osteoporosis**

Lowest possible steroid dose
Adequate calcium and vitamin D intake
Maintain physical activity as much as possible
Correct sex-steroid deficiency
Antiresorptive therapy if bone mass is low or decreases

family history of the disease. Current evidence suggests that genetically predisposed individuals develop Paget's disease after slow viral infection of their osteoclasts. Viruses identified within pagetic osteoclasts have included respiratory syncytial virus, measles virus, and canine distemper virus. Virally infected osteoclasts form multinucleated giant cells rapidly, accelerating bone resorption in affected bones, and virally infected osteoclast progenitor cells differentiate into mature osteoclasts more rapidly as well. Presumably slow viral infection occurs early in life, but the factors responsible for osteoclast susceptibility to slow viral infection remain unclear.

CLINICAL FEATURES AND DIAGNOSIS

Paget's disease is most often diagnosed incidentally when radiographic studies are performed for other reasons. Only a minority of patients present with clinical symptoms and signs of active Paget's disease. Bone involvement may be monostotic or asymmetrically polyostotic. Paget's disease rarely spreads to bones other than those initially involved at diagnosis, although it may progress within bones over time. The most common sites of involvement are the pelvis, femur, spine, skull, and tibia. Bones of the upper extremities, clavicles, scapulae, ribs, and facial bones are less commonly involved.

The most common symptom of Paget's disease is bone pain, which may result from pagetic bone involvement or from degenerative arthritis in joints adjacent to pagetic bone. Pain may be due to microfractures or swelling of the cortices of bones due to advancing lytic lesions and is usually dull, aching, and fairly localized. Pain may occur at rest but is typically made worse with ambulation or activity. Pagetic bone is often swollen or warm due to hypervascularity; some patients perceive the increased warmth as uncomfortable. Weight-bearing bones, especially the femur or tibia or both, may become deformed, resulting in gait abnormality. Degenerative arthritic changes may occur at joints adjacent to deformity or in joints in the contralateral normal limb.

Back pain may be due to pagetic involvement of vertebrae, vertebral collapse fractures due to coexisting osteoporosis, or spinal stenosis or neural compression. Skull pain may be associated with warmth, tenderness, bandlike headache, or increasing head size with or without frontal bossing or deformity. Hearing impairment may be due to isolated or combined conductive (due to otosclerosis) or neurosensory abnormalities. Nerve palsies may affect cranial nerves II, VI, VII, or others. Platybasia (flattening of the base of the skull) may occur with subsequent basilar invagination, resulting in brain stem compression or obstructive hydrocephalus. Facial bone involvement may result in deformity, dental problems, or, rarely, narrowing of the airway.

Pagetic bone fractures more easily than normal bone. Fractures may be traumatic or pathologic, causing considerable blood loss when they occur. Long bones with advancing lytic lesions are most susceptible to fracture. Small, stable, asymptomatic partial cortical fractures along the convex surfaces of bowed lower extremity bones may occasionally extend through the cortex and cause complete fractures. Pagetic fractures typically heal normally.

Late malignant transformation occurs rarely. Patients present with increased pain and swelling of pagetic bone. Sites most commonly affected are the pelvis, femur, and humerus, with lytic lesions superimposed on pagetic bone. Treatment is difficult, with the preferred course being wide local excision of tumor, followed by either chemotherapy or radiation therapy. Survival is usually limited to 1 to 3 years. Patients may also develop benign giant cell tumors in pagetic bone that usually respond well to glucocorticoid therapy.

Patients with newly diagnosed Paget's disease should have a total body bone scan, with roentgenograms of affected bones, to document the extent of disease. This will eliminate confusion later regarding new pagetic activity if other bones become symptomatic. Follow-up bone scans or other roentgenograms are generally not necessary unless the patient develops new or worsening symptoms.

Patients with active Paget's disease typically have increased serum alkaline phosphatase activity, which is a marker of osteoblast function. Since alkaline phosphatase activity may come from sources other than bone, it should always be fractionated during initial evaluation to ensure that it is the bone fraction that is increased. Specific assays are now available to measure the bone isozyme. Evaluation of other biochemical markers of bone turnover, such as urinary pyridinium cross-links, is generally not useful unless these markers will be followed during treatment. Serum alkaline phosphatase correlates reasonably well with activity and extent of the disease. Patients having the highest levels of serum alkaline phosphatase often have polyostotic involvement, including the skull. Patients with mildly to moderately increased alkaline phosphatase levels may have monostotic involvement or relatively inactive ("burned-out") Paget's disease. In some cases, patients with long-standing inactive disease may have completely normal serum alkaline phosphatase levels. During effective treatment, markers of bone turnover typically decline by 50% within the first few weeks to months and may normalize within 3 to 6 months of therapy. Urinary markers such as pyridinium cross-links decrease within days to weeks of beginning therapy, whereas serum alkaline phosphatase responds more slowly.

Serum calcium is typically normal in Paget's disease except when patients with relatively widespread disease are immobilized, or when Paget's disease and primary hyperparathyroidism coexist. Secondary hyperparathyroidism may develop in 15% to 20% of Paget's disease patients with normal serum calcium and significantly increased serum total alkaline phosphatase levels. Such individuals are advised to maintain an oral calcium intake of at least 1000 mg each day.

TREATMENT

All agents currently used to specifically treat Paget's disease suppress osteoclast activity. Drugs approved for this indication by the U.S. Food and Drug Administration include the bisphosphonates alendronate sodium (Fosamax) and etidronate disodium (Didronel), and calcitonin-salmon (Calcimar, Miacalcin) and calcitonin-human (Cibacalcin). Parenteral pamidronate (Aredia) and plicamycin (mithramycin [Mithracin]) have not been approved for treatment of Paget's disease. Other bisphosphonates, such as risedronate* and Tiludronate,* may eventually be useful.

Major indications for treatment of Paget's disease are relief of bone pain and prevention of fracture or deformity. Asymptomatic individuals generally do not require treatment. Calcitonins or bisphospho-

---

*Investigational drug in the United States.

nates are effective in decreasing bone pain and warmth, headache, and low back or hip pain due to pagetic activity. These agents may also improve compression radiculopathies, slowly progressive brain stem or spinal cord compression, joint pain, and lytic lesions in long bones (preventing pathologic fractures). Bone deformity or hearing loss will generally not improve with treatment, although hearing loss may be slowed. Other indications for treatment remain controversial.

The bisphosphonates are orally available, tend to be less expensive than the calcitonins, and are associated with tolerable side effects, whereas the calcitonins may improve bone pain more rapidly, decrease risk of impending pathologic fracture more effectively, and decrease bone vascularity prior to surgery more rapidly. Initial selection of either type of agent does not preclude use of the other type of agent if the initial agent does not provide effective relief within a reasonable period of time, and either type of agent may be substituted for the other even after years of effective therapy by the other agent.

Bisphosphonates

Alendronate sodium (Fosamax) is available in 40-mg tablets and is usually taken as 1 tablet each day for 6 months. Recent United States and multinational double-blind, placebo-controlled, randomized trials in patients with moderate-to-severe Paget's disease (baseline serum alkaline phosphatase at least twice the upper limit of normal) showed alendronate, 40 mg each day, to suppress serum alkaline phosphatase more effectively than etidronate, 400 mg each day, at 6 months. About 85% of patients improved with alendronate, and the drug was effective regardless of age, gender, ethnicity, prior use of other bisphosphonates, or baseline serum alkaline phophatase level. No osteomalacia was seen in 33 patients treated with alendronate for 6 months, and new bone formed had normal lamellar structure, suggesting that patients form new bone of normal quality and strength when treated with alendronate.

Etidronate (Didronel) is available in 200- and 400-mg tablets. Five mg per kg per day will usually reduce serum alkaline phosphatase by 50% and improve symptoms in as many as 70% of patients within 6 months. The major risk with etidronate is osteomalacia, which may develop if used in higher doses or for longer than 6 months. Osteomalacia presents with increased bone pain or fractures at sites of weakened bone.

In general, most investigators recommend 6-month cycles of treatment with bisphosphonates. Several years of cyclical therapy controls symptoms and signs of Paget's disease effectively in many patients. Side effects, other than osteomalacia seen with etidronate, include occasional upper gastrointestinal or esophageal distress or diarrhea, which usually resolves upon withholding the drug for several days, and short-lived bone pain when first starting therapy, which usually resolves over several days of continued

therapy. Patients who develop a sudden or marked increase in pain while on therapy should temporarily stop the drug and be evaluated for progression of lytic lesions or impending fracture.

Pamidronate (Aredia) is currently being investigated in the United States for use in Paget's disease. One regimen infuses 60 mg in 1 liter of fluid over 8 hours. Mild-to-moderate Paget's disease may respond to a single infusion, whereas moderate-to-severe Paget's disease may require several weekly or biweekly infusions over the course of weeks to months. Side effects include low-grade fever or flulike symptoms the day after infusion; hypocalcemia, hypophosphatemia, or lymphopenia several days after infusion; and venous irritation if low fluid volumes are infused.

Calcitonins

Calcitonin is currently available as parenteral synthetic salmon calcitonin and parenteral human calcitonin. Intranasal calcitonin (Miacalcin Nasal Spray) has recently been approved for treatment of osteoporosis, but is not yet approved for the treatment of Paget's disease.

Parenteral salmon calcitonin is available in 2-mL vials containing 200 units per mL. The initial dose is 100 units (0.5 mL) injected subcutaneously each day, with reduction to 50 units (0.25 mL) each day if necessary. Parenteral human calcitonin is available in prefilled syringes containing 0.5 mg, which is equivalent to 150 to 200 units of salmon calcitonin. Symptoms typically improve within a few weeks of beginning therapy, with biochemical parameters improving by 3 to 6 months of treatment. Once improvement has occurred, the maintenance dose may be reduced to 50 to 100 units every other day or three times each week. The initial course of therapy is usually 6 months, although patients with severe involvement may benefit from more prolonged treatment. Despite salmon calcitonin being about 20 times more potent than human calcitonin, salmon calcitonin may lose effectiveness due to down-regulation of calcitonin receptors or development of neutralizing antibodies. Human calcitonin is often effective in this situation.

Side effects of parenteral calcitonin include nausea and/or flushing about the face and ears lasting minutes to hours after injections, and transient hypocalcemia during the first few months of therapy. Patients may minimize nausea or flushing by taking calcitonin at bedtime or with meals, decreasing the dose, or taking an aspirin 30 minutes before doses. The nausea or flushing is not harmful, and patients may develop tolerance to either.

Other Treatments

Parenteral plicamycin (mithramycin [Mithracin])* has previously been used to treat patients with se-

---

*Not FDA-approved for this indication.

vere or refractory Paget's disease or individuals with neurologic syndromes requiring immediate relief, usually at 15 to 25 μg per kg over 6 to 8 hours. Doses are repeated every 2 to 3 days as required. Patients with spinal cord compression may have relief with a regimen combining plicamycin and dexamethasone but should undergo surgical decompression if symptoms persist. Side effects include nausea, vomiting, hepatotoxicity, nephrotoxicity, thrombocytopenia, and mild transient hypocalcemia and hypophosphatemia.

Nonspecific treatments used to decrease pain due to Paget's disease include analgesics and nonsteroidal anti-inflammatory drugs (NSAIDs). These may be used alone or in combination with specific antipagetic agents, especially to decrease arthritic symptoms. Shoe lifts, canes, or walkers may stabilize or improve gait abnormalities. Patients should be advised against prolonged immobilization due to the risk of hypercalcemia.

Orthopedic surgery may stabilize or prevent impending fracture in long bones, and hips and knees affected by pagetic arthritis may be electively replaced. Deformed bone may be straightened with osteotomies. Neurosurgical decompression may relieve spinal cord compression, spinal stenosis, or basilar skull invagination with neural compromise. All cases of serious neurologic compromise should receive immediate neurologic and neurosurgical consultation.

The patient is often best served by a multidisciplinary approach to treatment. This includes the primary care practitioner and physical therapist, as well as the orthopedic surgeon and neurosurgeon when appropriate. Patients may also benefit from association with other patients with Paget's disease. The Paget's Disease Foundation (200 Varick Street, Suite 1004, New York, NY 10014) is an excellent resource of information about diagnosis and treatment of Paget's disease.

PARENTERAL NUTRITION IN ADULTS

method of
ALFONS POMP, M.D.
Hôtel-Dieu de Montréal
Montréal, Québec

and

JORGE E. ALBINA, M.D.
Rhode Island Hospital
Providence, Rhode Island

It is well established that protein-calorie malnutrition is common in hospitalized patients. Although the severity of illness and of intercurrent complications correlate best with the nature and extent of the primary disease and, in surgery, with the type of operation performed, the coexistence of protein-calorie malnutrition leads to increased morbidity and mortality. The malnutrition-dependent component of excess morbidity should be reduced by the provision of adequate nutritional support. This corollary is the basis for the provision of specialized nonvolitional nutritional support to hospitalized patients.

The development of total parenteral nutrition (TPN) almost 30 years ago promised to revolutionize the care of medical and surgical patients by expediently correcting existing nutritional abnormalities, preventing the deterioration of body composition associated with acute and chronic illness, and improving nutritional status. While it has been well shown by daily experience that many patients can be maintained indefinitely on intravenous nutrition, the expectation has been unrealized that nutritional support would dramatically improve outcome in critically ill subjects and alter the course of patients with cancer, AIDS, and other processes frequently accompanied by significant weight loss and alterations of body composition. Current opinion justifiably champions the use of enteral nutrition in a large number of patients who would, in the recent past, be fed preferentially intravenously.

Some relative advantages of enteral nutrition over parenteral nutrition are obvious. Beyond the use of a more "physiologic" route of nutrient delivery, enteral nutrition is less expensive than TPN, can probably be delivered with a lower rate of complications, and avoids the need for surgically inserted central venous catheters. Other putative advantages of enteral feedings are more controversial and ill defined. It has been proposed, in this connection, that enteral nutrition protects and enhances the role of the gut as an immunologic barrier and prevents the translocation of bacteria or their products into the portal circulation. Additionally, it has been suggested that the delivery of nutrients through the gastrointestinal tract, compared with the parenteral route, decreases the overall incidence of systemic infections unrelated to the presence of a venous catheter in parenterally fed patients. Thus the belief in TPN as a magic bullet has been, in some environments, replaced by the perception of enteral feedings as the ultimate power lunch. This has led to practices not totally supported by solid data, like the provision of homeopathic doses of enteral feedings to critically ill patients to "feed the gut" and the perseverance on enteral nutrition in patients with severe diarrhea, in whom little if any information is available about the quality of nutrient digestion and absorption.

It remains true, however, that a significant number of hospitalized patients will better meet their nutritional needs when fed intravenously. When properly instituted and managed, TPN can be delivered safely and economically and allows a unique route to guarantee nutrient delivery and provide fluid and electrolyte therapy, mainly in patients who require central venous access for reasons independent of their need for nutritional support.

Clinical judgment must play a major role in deciding when to offer parenteral nutritional support. In patients with pre-existing malnutrition, nutritional therapy must be instituted early if a prolonged period of limited intake is foreseen. This same conduct applies to all patients who have postoperative complications that compromise oral or enteral food intake. The use of TPN in the critically ill patient should complement instead of compete with the use of enteral feeding. The dictum, "If the gut works, use it," is valid, but the prescription of a diet or a tube-feeding regimen does not guarantee its delivery or the patient's tolerance. Perseverance in feeding through the GI tract in the presence of recurrent vomiting, diarrhea, or other forms of digestive intolerance is not warranted if TPN can be delivered safely. However, TPN should be used only in institutions in which the incidence of mechanical, metabolic, and septic complications is acceptably low. This precondition usually requires the existence of a nutritional support service and of firmly enforced patient care protocols to provide IV nutrition at minimal cost both in terms of complications and of dollars.

INDICATIONS AND CONTRAINDICATIONS FOR PARENTERAL NUTRITION

Parenteral nutritional support encompasses the assessment of nutritional status, the determination of nutrient requirements, and the provision of intravenous nutritional therapy when these needs cannot be met voluntarily through food intake or involuntarily through enteral feedings. The indications for the use of parenteral nutritional support are summarized in Table 1. Major considerations for selecting the type of nutritional support include gastrointestinal function, the expected duration of nutritional therapy, the presence of pre-existing protein caloric

TABLE 1. **Guidelines for the Use of Parenteral Nutrition**

Clinical settings in which TPN should be a part of routine care

  Massive small-intestinal resection or disease
  Radiation enteritis
  Intractable vomiting or diarrhea
  Severe peritonitis
  Severe acute pancreatitis
  Severe malnutrition in the face of a nonfunctional GI tract
  Severe catabolic state in which GI tract is not usable
    within 5–7 d

Clinical settings in which TPN should be considered

  Major surgical procedure in a severely malnourished patient
  Enterocutaneous fistulas
  Inflammatory bowel disease
  Situations in which adequate enteral nutrition cannot be
    established within 7–10 d of hospitalization

Clinical settings in which TPN is of limited value

  Patients in whom the GI tract is usable within a 10-d period
    following moderate stress or trauma

Clinical settings in which TPN should not be used

  A functional and usable gastrointestinal tract that is capable
    of absorbing adequate nutrients
  Duration on TPN anticipated to be less than 5 d

malnutrition, the possibility of increased metabolic demands due to sepsis or major trauma, and the potential for or the actual development of organ dysfunction. Certain patient groups, including alcoholics and patients taking medication with nutrient or catabolic side effects (immunosuppressants or chemotherapy), are associated with an increased nutritional risk. Malnutrition is easier to prevent than to cure. Poor prognosis makes the burden of intravenous nutritional support outweigh its potential benefits. It is unwise to initiate TPN against the informed patient's or family's wishes. Hemodynamic instability; poor peripheral tissue oxygen consumption, which will limit substrate synthesis; and severe metabolic imbalances (hyperglycemia, hyperkalemia) may preclude the installation of TPN.

NUTRITIONAL ASSESSMENT

The nutritional assessment is based on clinical history, physical examination, and biochemical determinations that provide an objective evaluation of nutritional status. Current methods used for nutritional assessment are summarized in Table 2. Severe protein-calorie malnutrition is evident even on cursory physical examination. At present, however, there is no single reliable marker for moderate malnutrition or for monitoring the course of nutritional repletion.

Our approach to nutritional assessment combines elements of history (changes in body weight, dietary intake, and gastrointestinal function), physical examination (muscle mass and tone, subcutaneous fat, and external signs of specific nutrient deficiencies), and the determination of plasma protein concentrations (serum albumin, transferrin, thyroxine-binding prealbumin, and retinol-binding protein). The response to nutritional therapy is monitored by the magnitude and direction of change of these measurements and serial determinations of nitrogen balance.

NUTRIENT REQUIREMENTS

The purpose of nutritional support is to maintain or improve body composition and to prevent or correct nutritional deficiencies. Nutrient intake, therefore, must meet or reasonably exceed requirements. However, the delivery of excess nutrients can be harmful. Excessive glucose or protein intakes can result in hypertonic dehydration. Liver function abnormalities and carbon dioxide retention were reported after the administration of high-carbohydrate loads. Thus, more is not necessarily better. Nutrient requirements must be estimated when planning nutritional support, and therapy must be tailored to meet these needs.

ENERGY REQUIREMENTS

Daily energy expenditure in health can be divided conceptually into two major components. The resting metabolic expenditure (RME), the amount of energy used in maintaining the metabolic processes of the

TABLE 2. **Nutritional Assessment Before Total Parenteral Nutrition**

Test	Advantages	Disadvantages
Clinical history and physical examination (subjective global assessment)	Rapid, inexpensive, noninvasive; good correlation with morbidity and mortality; identifies patients at risk	Requires some nutritional training and index of suspicion; body weight may be altered by dehydration or third-space fluid accumulation
Anthropometrics	Rapid, inexpensive, noninvasive; serial measurements provide good evaluation	Insensitive to short-term changes; poor reproducibility; subject to measurement error
Biochemical measurements		
Serum albumin	Low concentrations correlate with inadequate protein intake	Large body pool with intercompartmental shifts according to fluid status; long half-life
Serum transferrin	Small body pool; short half-life	Concentration affected in iron deficiency, sepsis, liver disease, neoplasia, nephrotic syndrome
Serum thyroxine-binding prealbumin, serum retinol-binding protein	Short half-life; small body pool; respond quickly to refeeding	Better as indicators of dietary intake than of nutritional status; affected by stress, sepsis, renal failure, hyperthyroidism, vitamin A deficiency, and zinc
Balance studies		
Nitrogen balance	Clinically useful; norm for protein accretion	Incomplete urine collection or underestimation of nonurinary nitrogen losses tends to overestimate nitrogen retention
Immunocompetence studies		
Serum immunoglobulin	Rapid synthesis in response to nutritional therapy	Maintained even in the presence of undernutrition
Cellular immunity, delayed cutaneous hypersensitivity, total lymphocyte count	—	Low specificity

body in the absence of external work, accounts for 65% to 75% of daily energy expenditure. The RME is approximately 20 to 25 kcal per kg per day and can be measured directly or estimated using published regression equations. The most widely used predictive equations were generated by Harris and Benedict in 1909:

$$\text{Women: RME (kcal/day)} = 655 + (9.6 \times W) + (1.8 \times H) - (4.7 \times A)$$

$$\text{Men: RME (kcal/day)} = 65 + (13.7 \times W) + (5 \times H) - (6.8 \times A)$$

where W = weight in kg, H = height in cm, and A = age in years.

The second component of daily energy expenditure is the thermic effect of exercise (TEE), that is, the energy used in physical activity. The TEE in a sedentary person accounts for 15% to 20% of daily energy expenditure. Admission to a hospital generally results in a marked decrease in physical activity. Hospital activity in a patient not confined to bed increases the RME by only 20% to 30%.

Illness adds an additional component to the daily energy expenditure. The magnitude of this hypermetabolism of stress has been debated. Although it has been reported that major fractures and sepsis were followed by a 15% to 30% increase in RME for a period of 2 to 3 weeks, we have found that energy expenditure measured by indirect calorimetry closely agrees with the predictions of the Harris and Benedict equation in nontrauma patients with a variety of disease processes. In patients in whom it is possible that RME may be significantly different from the predicted values, energy expenditure is better measured either by indirect calorimetry or by using a Swan-Ganz catheter. This group includes potentially hypermetabolic, severely traumatized patients and elderly malnourished patients, who are frequently hypometabolic. When energy expenditure is calculated rather than measured, we routinely increase the calculated values by about 20% to account for individual variability when estimating the daily energy requirements of patients.

Body weight is the most significant determinant of the results obtained using the Harris and Benedict equation. Most patients referred to the nutritional support service have lost weight. In these situations we use the higher of either the patient's usual body weight or the ideal body weight to calculate energy expenditure. For persons in whom weight gain is desirable, we empirically add 500 to 1000 kcal per day to this estimate. Even with these additions, few patients require more than 3000 calories per day. For persons with important obesity we calculate resting energy expenditure on the basis of ideal body weight plus 50% of excess weight (excess weight = current weight − ideal weight).

Energy can be provided through carbohydrates and fats. The minimum amount of carbohydrate in the diet sufficient to prevent the ketosis of fasting is 100 to 150 grams per day. Net protein catabolism is inversely proportional to energy intake, and carbohydrates have a larger protein-sparing capacity than fats. Maximal nitrogen economy is obtained with a carbohydrate intake of 5 to 7 mg per kg per minute. Fats are a high-caloric-density energy source and should be used in both enteral and parenteral nutrition. The minimal dietary fat intake is that which provides the daily requirements of essential fatty acids. This requirement can be met by delivering 2% to 4% of daily caloric intake as linoleic acid.

In parenteral nutrition we approximate the composition of a normal diet by providing 20% to 30% of nonprotein calories in the form of fat emulsions. This practice guarantees the delivery of essential fatty acid requirements and allows a decrease in the amount of dextrose contained in TPN solutions. Although there has been much controversy regarding the relative efficacies of glucose and fat as energy sources in TPN, it appears that the delivery of 20% to 30% of nonprotein calories in the form of fat emulsions has no adverse effects on nitrogen balance. The currently available soybean or safflower oil emulsions have a remarkable safety record.

Although circulating triglyceride levels do not necessarily reflect the ability to clear exogenous fats, we determine serum triglyceride concentrations before we administer fat emulsions. In patients with serum triglyceride concentrations of less than 250 mg per dL, fats are delivered at a maximal dose of 2 grams of fat per kg per day and infused at a rate that does not exceed 0.2 grams of fat per kg per hour. In our institutions, fat emulsions are always infused at 40 mL per hour over 12 hours. In patients with triglyceride concentrations between 250 and 350 mg per dL in whom the use of intravenously administered fat is desirable because of the projected duration of TPN or the presence of glucose intolerance, we infuse 500 mL of 10% fat emulsion over 12 hours and determine peak (end of infusion) and 6-hour postinfusion triglyceride concentrations. In most instances, we find no elevation of triglyceride concentration above preinfusion levels, indicating adequate clearance of the emulsion. Essential fatty acid requirements in patients with impaired exogenous fat clearance or severe hypertriglyceridemia are met by small amounts of intravenous fat emulsion (2% to 4% of total calories as linoleic acid).

PROTEIN REQUIREMENTS

The recommended daily allowance (RDA) for protein is 0.8 gram per kg per day. This figure includes allowances for variability in protein quality, digestibility, and absorbability. Few data are available on protein requirements in hospitalized patients. Amino acid solutions used in TPN have a high biologic value; in addition, TPN solutions do not require digestion or absorption. Therefore, protein intakes of 0.8 to 1.0 gram per kg per day will probably provide an adequate protein intake for most patients.

Commercially available parenteral solutions enriched with branched chain amino acids (leucine, isoleucine, and valine) that can be metabolized by skeletal muscle, and largely omitting aromatic and sulfur-containing amino acids, have not been shown to improve the clinical outcome nor reverse the encephalopathy of patients with severe liver dysfunction or trauma. Encephalopathy, however, is not worsened by branched-chain, amino acid–enriched products even when moderately high protein intakes are provided. Because the alternative treatment is to restrict protein intake severely, with consequent negative nitrogen balance, we prescribe the modified amino acid formulas for patients with severe liver dysfunction or encephalopathy with abnormal plasma amino acid profiles.

Glutamine is a nonessential amino acid that is not present in commercially available amino acid solutions. In animal studies, glutamine-enriched formulas stimulate lymphocyte reproduction, hepatic regeneration, and impact on skeletal muscle synthesis. Parenteral glutamine is currently available in Europe as synthetic dipeptides (alanine glutamine and glycine glutamine), which are relatively stable in solution and are rapidly hydrolyzed after intravenous infusion but are expensive. Glutamine-enriched TPN formulas are still not available for clinical use other than in a few research centers.

ELECTROLYTES, VITAMINS, AND TRACE ELEMENTS

A complete nutrient mixture is necessary for positive nitrogen balance during TPN. The requirements for electrolytes, vitamins, and trace elements in disease and injury have not been fully established. This lack of complete information is compounded by the clinical unavailability of simple laboratory techniques to establish micronutrient status and the low specificity of the clinical signs associated with deficiency states. Furthermore, the circulating concentrations of minerals and vitamins may not reflect body stores, because these nutrients can be redistributed within body compartments during acute illness. For example, plasma levels of zinc and iron are reduced during sepsis whereas those of copper and B_{12} are elevated. Table 3 shows the clinical circumstances in which mineral requirements may be altered by disease.

The AMA has published guidelines for the delivery of vitamins and trace elements during parenteral nutrition (Table 4). These doses probably meet the vitamin and trace element requirements of most persons receiving TPN when provided daily. We maintain a high degree of awareness of the potential for specific deficiencies. Whenever there is clinical suspicion of a specific deficiency, such as macrocytosis, oral mucosal alterations, or a history of prolonged malabsorption, we perform the specific functional diagnostic tests for the nutrient in question.

Deficiencies of trace elements and vitamins during TPN have been described. These deficiencies gener-

TABLE 3. Disease-Related Alterations in Mineral Requirements

	May Increase Requirements	May Decrease Requirements
Sodium	Diarrhea, GI fistulas, diuretics	Congestive heart failure, renal failure, edematous syndromes
Potassium	Malnutrition, diarrhea, diuretics, nasogastric suction, alcoholism	Renal failure, potassium-sparing diuretics, glucocorticoid therapy
Calcium	Osteoporosis	Hypercalcemia from multiple metastases, hyperparathyroidism, or sarcoidosis
Magnesium	Alcoholism, malabsorption, inflammatory bowel disease, diuretics, aminoglycosides, cisplatin, amphotericin B	Renal failure
Phosphorus	Refeeding, alcoholism, antacids	Renal failure

ally occurred when the nutrient in question was totally absent from the solution and, in most instances, when the duration of therapy was prolonged (home TPN). Zinc deficiency is characterized by acrodermatitis enteropathica, anergy, and slow wound healing. Zinc is the micronutrient abnormality most frequently found in the acute care setting and has been described as early as in the third week of zinc-free TPN in patients with inflammatory bowel disease. We empirically provide additional zinc (10 to 15 mg per day) to patients with alcoholic liver disease, in-

TABLE 4. Daily Vitamin and Trace Element Dose Recommendations in Total Parenteral Nutrition

Vitamin/Trace Element	Recommended Daily Allowance	AMA Recommendations
A	4000–5000 IU	3300.0 IU
D	400 IU	200.0 IU
E	12–15 IU	10.0 IU
Ascorbic acid (C)	45 mg	100.0 mg
Folacin	400 µg	400.0 µg
Niacin	12–20 mg	40.0 mg
Riboflavin (B_2)	1.1–1.8 mg	3.6 mg
Thiamine (B_1)	1.0–1.5 mg	3.0 mg
Pyridoxine (B_6)	1.6–2.0 mg	4.0 mg
Cyanocobalamin (B_{12})	3 µg	5.0 µg
Pantothenic acid	5–10 mg	15.0 mg
Biotin	150–300 µg	60.0 µg
Zinc	15 mg	2.5–4 mg
Copper	2–3 mg	0.5–1.5 mg
Chromium	0.05–0.2 mg	10–15 µg
Manganese	2.25–5 mg	0.15–1.8 mg
Selenium	0.05–0.2 mg	
Iron	10–15 mg	
Iodine	150 µg	
Fluoride	1.5–4 mg	
Molybdenum	0.15–4 mg	
Cobalt	As part of B_{12} requirements	

flammatory bowel disease, and malabsorption. These patients are predisposed to suffer zinc deficiency because of poor dietary intake and increased zinc losses, since diarrheal stools contain about 15 mg of zinc per kg, and urinary zinc excretion is increased in hypoalbuminemia and in stress. Vitamin K is not included in IV vitamin preparations and must be provided by parenteral injection (1 to 10 mg per week).

PERIPHERAL PARENTERAL NUTRITION

We rarely use peripheral veins for parenteral nutrition. Formulations presumably capable of delivering adequate nutritional intake through peripheral veins have been developed. In most of our patients, nutrient requirements can be met only through peripheral veins by delivering unacceptably large volumes of dilute nutrient solutions. Even then, thrombophlebitis develops rapidly in most patients fed through peripheral veins. We use the peripheral venous route almost exclusively to supplement enteral nutrition with intravenous fat emulsions in patients with limited GI tolerance. Intravenous fats cannot be used as the only source of nutritional intake because fat has no protein-sparing capacity. Therefore, adequate protein intake and enough carbohydrates to prevent ketosis must be provided simultaneously through the GI tract.

ACCESS FOR DELIVERY OF TPN

Percutaneously inserted subclavian vein catheters advanced into the superior vena cava are the route of choice for delivery of TPN. Other forms of central venous access are less satisfactory. In our experience, internal jugular vein catheters are associated with a higher rate of infection, probably because of difficulty in maintaining a sterile dressing in the neck. A high incidence of venous thrombosis is associated with long catheters inserted through the antecubital fossa. The insertion of central venous catheters is a surgical procedure and should be performed under ideal conditions. We do not allow the placement of central venous catheters for TPN at the bedside in our institutions. All catheters are placed in either the operating room or in a separate special procedures room by a modification of the Seldinger technique. We have found that many of the initial J wire insertions were malpositioned, more frequently when the right subclavian vein was cannulated. In all instances, the J wires were repositioned under fluoroscopy, prompting us to promote, if available, the use of fluoroscopy during catheter placement. We continue to obtain a chest roentgenogram immediately after catheter placement because pneumothoraces are not easily detected by fluoroscopy. Multilumen catheters may be associated with a high risk of septic complication per catheter; however, patient and nursing acceptance of these catheters is optimal. We currently exchange triple-lumen catheters over a guidewire every 14 days with an acceptable incidence (<5%) of line sepsis.

DELIVERY OF TPN

Total parenteral nutrition is delivered in our institutions in a single, variable volume bag per day (1000 to 3000 mL), containing dextrose, amino acids, minerals, vitamins, and trace elements. Intravenous fat emulsions are infused through a Y connector into the TPN delivery system. We do not use in-line filters. Alternatively, all components of TPN can be mixed in one container (three-in-one system).

We found that a standard solution of 30% dextrose with 5% amino acids can be used to meet nutrient requirements in most patients. The infusion of 1.5 L of this solution with 500 mL of 10% intravenous fat emulsion provides 75 grams of protein and 2080 nonprotein kcal per day. Our average patient weighs 60 kg and with this regimen receives approximately 35 kcal per kg per day, 1.25 grams of protein per kg per day, and 25% of nonprotein calories as intravenous fat.

COMPLICATIONS OF TPN

The complications of TPN can be mechanical, septic, or metabolic and are summarized in Table 5. The incidence and severity of these potential complications can be reduced effectively by careful patient monitoring, strict adherence to protocols, and the presence of a nutritional support service.

Catheter-related sepsis occurs in 1% to 27% of patients receiving TPN and is defined by positive cultures of the catheter tip, concurrent positive blood cultures, and defervescence of the clinical signs of sepsis following catheter removal. Several patient-related factors have been suggested to increase the rate of central line infection: age greater than 60 years, neutropenia, a loss of skin integrity (burns), and acquired immunodeficiency syndrome (AIDS). Only 20% to 40% of catheters removed for suspicion of sepsis will prove to be the cause of infection. The availability of the technique of catheter replacement over a guidewire has modified our approach to the diagnosis and treatment of this complication. There is no indication to remove the central line in initial studies of a febrile episode in a patient receiving TPN who is in an otherwise stable condition. We reserve immediate catheter removal for patients presenting signs of systemic sepsis with hemodynamic instability and for patients with clear signs of local inflammation or infection at the catheter entry site. Otherwise, we exchange the existing catheter over a guidewire for a new catheter, culture the distal 2 inches of the catheter by a semiquantitative technique, and complete the work-up for fever. If the catheter cultures are positive, the new catheter is removed, antibiotic therapy is started, and a new catheter is inserted in the contralateral subclavian vein 24 hours later. When catheter cultures are negative and blood cultures are positive, we empirically exchange the new catheter over a guidewire every 3 to 4 days until sepsis resolves.

Common metabolic complications of TPN include disorders of glucose metabolism, liver dysfunction, and respiratory complications. Hyperglycemia is encountered during nutritional support in diabetic patients and in patients with stress-related glucose intolerance. Both groups may require insulin therapy. Maintaining blood glucose concentrations between 150 and 200 mg per dL generally prevents glycosuria while providing an adequate margin of safety to prevent acute hypoglycemia. Higher glucose concentrations result in glycosuria, accelerated fluid losses, and progressive hyperosmolar dehydration.

Patients with moderate hyperglycemia taking 5% dextrose solutions who are to start parenteral nutrition receive 1 unit of regular insulin for each 20 grams of glucose contained in the initial TPN solution. After TPN is started, additional regular insulin can be used to achieve a stable glucose concentration and prevent glycosuria. We use regular insulin therapy only during TPN and discontinue both long-acting insulin preparations and oral hypoglycemic agents. The intravenous route is used preferentially for insulin treatment, mainly in subjects with edema or dehydration in whom the absorption of subcutaneous insulin is unpredictable. Once the daily insulin requirements for a given TPN dextrose content are known, approximately 75% of the total dose is added to the solution. In patients with severe glucose intolerance requiring more than 50 units of insulin per day for intakes below 0.5 gram of glucose per kg per day, an insulin drip is probably the most expedient way safely to maintain euglycemia.

TABLE 5. **Potential Complications of Total Parenteral Nutrition**

Mechanical Complications

Pneumothorax
Subclavian artery injury
Air embolism
Venous thrombosis
Catheter tip misplacement

Septic Complications

Catheter-related sepsis

Metabolic Complications

Glucose metabolism
  Hyperglycemia
  Hyperosmolar nonketotic dehydration
  Hypoglycemia
  Carbon dioxide retention
Protein metabolism
  Prerenal azotemia
  Encephalopathy
Fat metabolism
  Essential fatty acid deficiency
  Hypertriglyceridemia
Mineral metabolism
  Hypo- or hyperkalemia
  Hypophosphatemia
  Trace element deficiencies
Vitamin deficiencies

Liver Function Abnormalities

In adults, a broad spectrum of liver function derangements occurring during TPN has been reported in 20% to 30% of patients, especially in those with inflammatory bowel disease and short bowel syndrome. The biochemical abnormalities are predominately elevated levels of serum glutamic oxaloacetic transaminase (SGOT) and serum glutamic pyruvic transaminase (SGPT); only later and less commonly encountered are elevated alkaline phosphatase and bilirubin levels. TPN-associated liver dysfunction is probably a process of multifactorial etiology. It has been suggested that continuous translocation of endotoxin originating from gram-negative bacterial overgrowth during bowel rest and TPN activate Kupffer's cells to produce and release tumor necrosis factor alone or in combination with interleukin-6 with resultant liver damage. Deficiencies of glutamine, essential fatty acids, taurine, cysteine, and carnitine have all been implicated in TPN-associated liver function derangement. There is, however, little conclusive evidence to prove that one or more of these uncommon deficiency states play a causative role in hepatocyte dysfunction. There seems to be ample evidence to suggest that a macronutrient combination that avoids the infusion of excess calories, uses a low glucose-fat distribution (30% of nonprotein calories as fat), and provides an adequate calorie-to-nitrogen ratio (100:1) will reduce liver dysfunction during TPN.

The delivery of high-glucose intakes results in excess CO_2 production, which may precipitate respiratory failure or prevent weaning from mechanical ventilation in patients with severe pre-existing pulmonary disease. It is also recognized, however, that adequate nutritional intake is essential for optimal respiratory function. In our experience, the syndrome of CO_2 retention and respiratory failure induced by nutritional therapy occur infrequently. This may be related to our practice of adjusting caloric intake to a patient's requirements and providing 20% to 30% of daily energy intake as fat. If, however, a patient's weaning from a respirator is compromised by CO_2 retention and no other mechanism for ventilatory insufficiency is evident, we stop TPN overnight to decrease CO_2 production maximally and attempt weaning in the morning. Although theoretically CO_2 production and respiratory quotient can be modulated by alterations in the carbohydrate-to-fat ratio of TPN, significant changes in these factors are obtained practically only through total fasting. If weaning is successful, TPN is restarted and advanced cautiously while CO_2 production is monitored.

Severe acute hypophosphatemia and hypokalemia can be precipitated by TPN infusion, especially in patients being refed after severe weight loss. This is primarily because during malnutrition intracellular stores have become depleted to maintain circulating serum levels, and with TPN-induced anabolism these cations migrate intracellularly. Electrolyte homeostasis must be maintained during TPN infusion. Hyponatremia is most often dilutional and secondary to fluid overload. Factitial hyponatremia due to high blood glucose levels must be ruled out. Disorders in magnesium and calcium metabolism have been reported, including metabolic bone disease associated with long-term TPN. Although the etiology and management of this clinical syndrome need further study, there is some evidence that increased sensitivity to vitamin D_2 and aluminum toxicity may play an etiologic role. Present TPN formulations do not necessarily cause worsening of bone health and in some cases may be beneficial to bone. Copper, chromium, and selenium deficiencies are rarely, if ever, encountered during short-term parenteral feeding but may develop insidiously in home TPN patients if adequate trace elements are not supplied.

HOME TOTAL PARENTERAL NUTRITION

A select group of patients who are unable to maintain nutritional homeostasis may benefit from home TPN. These patients include those with radiation enteritis, chronic bowel obstruction or pseudo-obstruction, short bowel syndrome, or severe inflammatory bowel disease. Although TPN corrects malnutrition and allows or prevents deferred surgery in some of these patients, these diseases remain poorly predictable and progressive, with numerous relapses and rehospitalizations.

The clinical considerations requiring home TPN are the same as those for in-hospital treatment, except that the patient no longer requires acute hospital care. Patients are rigorously evaluated and are trained to administer TPN themselves. Consideration is given to the patient's ability to adjust to the change in lifestyle and demands of the therapy. Access to the central venous circulation is necessary and is accomplished using a surgically implanted infusion device, such as a silicone-tunneled catheter or a subcutaneously implanted port. The patient must be monitored closely following discharge and re-evaluated periodically to determine whether continued TPN therapy is needed. Nutritional components may need readjustment if oral or enteral intake is begun. The goals of home TPN are to provide adequate and appropriate nutritional support in the home and to minimize the complications associated with the therapy. TPN technology is highly valued as life-sustaining and therapeutic by these patients and their families.

PARENTERAL FLUID THERAPY FOR INFANTS AND CHILDREN

method of
JONATHAN D. HEILICZER, M.D.
University of Illinois College of Medicine
Chicago, Illinois

When considering intravenous fluid therapy in any patient, we can divide the body into two parts: solids and body water. The water component is further divided by membranes into a series of compartments. Intravenous (IV) fluids allow access to the plasma compartment only. Therefore substances in relatively high concentration in plasma can change and be changed rapidly (minutes to hours). Intracellular substances must be manipulated more slowly (hours to days).

Na^+, the major plasma cation, can change and be changed rapidly. Conversely, the extracellular concentration of K^+ (the major intracellular cation) can only be changed slowly, as K^+ must pass through several membranes before reaching its area of highest concentration.

Keeping everything in place, maintaining compartment concentrations, are osmotic gradients. These are regulated by osmolality, the first line of cellular defense. Osmolality, defined as the number of particles dissolved per unit of fluid, can be measured in the laboratory by freezing point depression. Simply, a substance freezes at a higher temperature if it has more particles dissolved in its fluid state. One can calculate osmolality in clinical medicine by the following formula:

$$Osm = 2 \times Na + \frac{glucose}{20} + \frac{BUN}{3}$$

$$= (2 \times 140) + \frac{100}{20} + \frac{9}{3}$$

$$= 280 \text{ mOsm/L}$$

Two times Na equaling 280 mOsm per liter can estimate osmolality when blood urea nitrogen (BUN) and glucose contribute very little to the overall osmolality. Therefore, under normal conditions, Na is the body's "osmometer," or put another way, the body's "hydrometer." The major etiology of hyponatremia is *dilutional*, caused by an excess of free water, whereas hypernatremia is due to *contraction*, losses of free water. However, in three situations hyponatremia occurs without an excess of free water. The first situation occurs during hyperlipidemia. The laboratory directly measures the Na^+ found in plasma water and then indirectly determines the Na^+ in the solid (cells) phase of blood, to arrive at a total serum Na. In hyperlipidemia, there are three phases of blood (solids, water, and lipid), and only the Na^+ in the water can be measured directly. The Na^+ "trapped" in the lipid phase cannot be measured, yet the laboratory still uses the smaller measurement over the entire volume. This is "factitious" hyponatremia and does not signify actual loss of Na^+. The other two conditions causing hyponatremia are chronic hyperglycemia and uremia; they occur because of Na^+ shifts to maintain osmolar integrity. Again, this may not signify actual loss of Na^+.

Beyond the cellular level, a number of organ groups account for control of normal fluid and electrolyte homeostasis (Table 1).

With this very basic understanding of normal homeostasis, we can now contemplate IV maintenance fluids. The goal in maintenance is to maintain euvolemia. Recognizing that all the formula calculations for maintenance are estimates of the fluid needs of the average-sized patient, it is very important that the following three statements be documented as correct for each individual patient:

Child is neither wet nor dry, but in *zero* water balance.

Child has a normal *cardiovascular system,* able to pump and retain within the system the fluid you are going to deliver.

Child has a normal *renal-endocrine system,* able to "fine-tune" the fluid you deliver.

If these statements describe your patient, then whichever method is used will get the patient "into the ball park" and the patient's organ-hormonal system will balance things appropriately. Two methods are in popular use: milliliters per kilogram of body weight and milliliters per square meter of body area. Either is correct (as long as the preceding three statements are also correct).

Pediatrics is a growth and development specialty, and fluid-electrolyte balance in children is therefore similar. Both methods of fluid calculation take the fluid changes during growth into account, varying with age (growth) and development.

We first review maintenance fluid (i.e., water) requirements and then add electrolytes to the fluid.

MAINTENANCE FLUID CALCULATIONS

The milliliters per kilogram of body weight method and the milliliters per square meter method are outlined in Table 2. Surface area can be calculated by a

TABLE 1. Normal Homeostasis

Kidney	Renin
Liver	Angiotensin I
Lung	Angiotensin II
Adrenal	Aldosterone
Hypothalamus/pituitary	Antidiuretic hormone
Heart	Atrial natriuretic peptide

TABLE 2. Methods of Calculating Maintenance Fluids

Milliliters per Kilogram of Body Weight	
100 mL/kg for each of the first 10 kg	
50 mL/kg for each kg from 10.1–20 kg	
20 mL/kg for each kg over 20 kg	
Milliliters per Square Meter	
Metabolic loss	1000 mL/m²/day
Insensible loss	400 mL/m²/day
Fecal loss	100 mL/m²/day
Minimal urine loss	400 mL/m²/day
TOTAL	1900 mL/m²/day (~2000)

TABLE 3. Fluid Maintenance Calculations

7-kg child = 0.36 m²	
mL/kg	mL/m²
7 × 100 = 700 mL/day	0.36 × 1900 = 684 mL/day

nomogram found in many pediatric reference texts, or it can be estimated using the following formula:

$$m^2 = \frac{4 \times (\text{wt in kg}) + 7}{90 + (\text{wt in kg})}$$

If our three statements are true, then either is correct. The difference in a 7-kg child who is 0.36 m² is less than 1 mL per hour (Table 3) and can easily be retained in the cardiovascular system and fine-tuned by the kidney and endocrine system.

If the three statements cannot be affirmed, then an alternative method for maintenance fluids must be used. One can examine the patient and determine that the child is neither wet nor dry. Then maintaining that zero balance state can be accomplished by estimating any ongoing losses and replacing those losses (Table 4). The appropriate output replacement fluid can be scientifically determined by sending an aliquot to the laboratory for electrolyte determinations. A reasonable starting estimate for urine and gastrointestinal fluid is 0.45 normal saline (NS), which contains 77 mEq of NaCl (see next section). Replacement of cerebrospinal fluid (e.g., lost through ventricular drains) is best accomplished with NS.

ELECTROLYTE REQUIREMENTS

To this point, we have dealt mainly with water. Now something needs to be mixed into the maintenance water, namely Na and K as cations, in addition to Cl as the major anion. Following are the maintenance requirements for Na and K (each usually balanced with Cl):

Na: 3 to 4 mEq/kg/day
K: 1 to 2 mEq/kg/day

However, a maximum of only 40 mEq per liter of K is used clinically, K being an intracellular ion, and therefore its extracellular concentration can be changed only slowly (over hours to days). Additionally, K is very caustic to peripheral veins in concentrations greater than 40 mEq per liter.

Therefore, a 7-kg child would require the following to be mixed into the daily maintenance water of 700 mL per day (using mL per kg for water):

7 kg × 3 mEq Na/day = 21 mEq NaCl
kg × 2 mEq K/day = 14 mEq KCl

Although one could ask the pharmacist to place the sodium chloride concentration into a liter bag of a D5W solution, economic necessity requires that we use some commercial solutions. The most common shelf solutions are

0.9% NaCl = 154 mEq Na per liter
0.45% NaCl = 77 mEq Na per liter
0.3% NaCl = 51 mEq Na per liter
0.2% NaCl = 34 mEq Na per liter

In our example, the closest fluid would be D5.2NS. As long as the *three statements are true*, then the small amount of extra Na per day is not a problem. Bear in mind that D5.2NS is the most commonly used pediatric solution because it fits the majority of children requiring intravenous fluids. However, in older (larger) children, the correct fluid might be 0.45 NS (containing 77 mEq per liter). In the example, our final order would be D5.2NS adding 20 mEq KCl per liter (after the child voids) to run at 29 mL per hour (Table 5).

Adding the potassium chloride after the child voids assures us that there is continued good renal function. Again, with the three statements being true and K being an intracellular ion (changing over hours to days), adding maintenance K later poses no risks.

Remember, maintenance fluid calculations are estimates, all based on the average-sized child under "ideal" conditions. Therefore, one cannot just "set it and forget it" but must reassess the patient to see that the fluid estimates remain reasonable in what might be a changing situation. The following conditions might alter fluid requirements and should be considered at the initial assessment and the frequent reassessments:

Fever will increase fluid requirements (12% for each 1° over 37.8° C, or 8% for each 1° over 100° F); hypothermia will similarly decrease needs.

Seizures due to constant and repetitive muscle activity will increase fluid requirements.

Changes in insensible losses will increase with tachypnea, low humidity, or burns and will decrease with mechanical ventilation, high humidity, or extensive casting.

Unusual sweating, such as with cystic fibrosis pa-

TABLE 4. The Safest Maintenance for Fluids

Insensible H₂O loss = 400 mL/m²/day
plus
All output—urine, nasogastric, diarrhea, etc.

Insensible loss contains no electrolytes; therefore use D5W solution and then
Replace output with "appropriate" fluid

TABLE 5. Calculations for Electrolytes

$$\frac{21\ \text{mEq/NaCl}}{700\ \text{mL H}_2\text{O}} = \frac{X\ \text{mEq/NaCl}}{1000\ \text{mL H}_2\text{O}} = X = 30\ \text{mEq NaCl/L}$$

$$\frac{14\ \text{mEq/KCl}}{700\ \text{mL H}_2\text{O}} = \frac{X\ \text{mEq/KCl}}{1000\ \text{mL H}_2\text{O}} = X = 20\ \text{mEq KCl/L}$$

Abbreviation: X = total amount of Na per liter.

tients, will need increased water (10 to 25 mL per kg per day) and Na (1 to 2 mEq per kg per day). However, alterations in urine volume (increased in glycosuria, diabetes insipidus, and sickle cell disease and decreased in the syndrome of inappropriate antidiuretic hormone [SIADH]) require previously noted "safest maintenance."

Again, anyone without a normal renal-endocrine axis should not be placed on maintenance fluids.

DEFICITS

Fluid deficits are the most common reason that children require hospitalization. Gastrointestinal disorders (mostly viral) can cause rapid fluid losses. These losses are magnified in the pediatric patient, who is proportionately "wetter" and has larger fluid requirements relative to adults. Being able to determine deficit fluid requirements added to maintenance fluids is an important pediatric skill.

To determine a fluid deficit accurately, subtract the patient's dry weight from the preloss weight. Thus a child who weighed 10 kg yesterday and is 9.5 kg today has a fluid deficit of 500 mL (i.e., 0.5 kg equals 0.5 liter). However, this ideal situation is rarely encountered clinically. In most cases, the fluid (and electrolyte) deficit will need to be estimated.

Any clinical problem requires a good history and physical examination. The child's hydration status is emphasized, as outlined in Table 6. In laboratory evaluation of children with fluid and electrolyte deficits, the laboratory value of water or the effect of water loss is the major issue. In evaluating hemoglobin (Hgb) and hematocrit (Hct), we look at the ratio of solids (Hgb) to fluid (Hct). The normal ratio is 1:3 (i.e., 12 grams to 36%). In dehydration, the Hct will theoretically rise because of concentration (less fluid). The reverse would be true in fluid overload situations. Serum osmolality and Na (and Cl) are the body's hydrometers. BUN will vary more with water content than will creatinine. Creatinine should in theory rise only when the glomerular filtration rate (GFR) falls. In simple dehydration, the GFR should remain relatively constant until fluid loss is severe enough to drop blood pressure (and thus renal blood flow). BUN, however, is a function not only of production (liver) and excretion (kidney) but also of volume concentration (hydration).

During fluid depletion, peripheral perfusion decreases in an effort to preserve the central circulation. Peripherally, O_2 delivery decreases and an increase in anaerobic metabolism occurs. The byproduct of anaerobic metabolism is lactic acid. Thus, the possibility of a metabolic acidosis during dehydration requires evaluation of acid-base status. Checking a blood pH by venous blood gas (VBG) and either a bicarbonate (HCO_3) (from the VBG) or a $_tCO_2$ (from a sequential multiple analyzer) allows us to further assess the severity of dehydration. Clinically, there is no need to use an arterial blood gas determination unless the child is suspected to have a concurrent pulmonary or cardiac problem.

Usually no accurate weight change is available to calculate deficits, so a *subjective* estimate must be made. Table 7 is a general guideline for this estimate, which will vary from observer to observer. The goal is to estimate a deficit so as to calculate a replacement plus maintenance fluid requirement. We assume (from the history) that prior to the acute illness the child had normal water balance, a normal cardiovascular system, and a normal renal-endocrine axis. We want to get the child back to the starting point. Again, this estimate must be re-evaluated periodically to ensure that the child is responding appropriately.

The majority of deficits are isotonic (e.g., normal serum sodium). However, this can be determined only by laboratory evaluation.

For our purpose, the estimate of "% dry" can be used to obtain the milliliters of fluid deficit by multiplying the percent by the child's weight in kilograms. Example: a child weighing 7 kg and estimated at 10% dry has a fluid deficit of 700 mL (i.e., 7 kg $\times$ 10% = 0.7 kg; or, since a kilogram equals a liter, then 0.7 liter, or 700 mL). This is a subjective estimate, but if the assessment is 15% or more, the patient is in shock! A patient in hypovolemic shock has a deficit of at least 15%. Hypovolemic shock must be treated (as in Table 8) immediately via a largebore IV line (*not a 25-gauge butterfly*).

TABLE 6. Evaluation of Fluid Deficits

Deficit History

Fluid loss from vomiting, diarrhea
Frequency
Amount
Most recent weight
Replacement fluids/diet

Physical Examination

Tears and saliva	Skin color
Skin turgor	Peripheral perfusion
Mucous membranes	Anterior fontanelle
Blood pressure	Heart rate
Respiratory rate	Urine

Laboratory Evaluation

Hgb, Hct	HCO_3
K	BUN/creatinine
Serum osmolality	VBG
Na (plus Cl)	

Abbreviations: Hgb = hemoglobin; Hct = hematocrit; HCO_3 = bicarbonate; BUN = blood urea nitrogen; VBG = venous blood gas.

TABLE 7. Estimating Isotonic Deficits

	5%	10%	15%
Urine specific gravity	>1.030	>1.035	anuric
Membranes	moist	dry	parched
Skin color	pale	mottled	cyanotic
Heart rate	+ +	+ + +	+ + + +, thready
Peripheral perfusion	±	−	almost none
Fontanelle	within normal limits	±	sunken
Blood pressure	within normal limits	Low	*SHOCK*

TABLE 8. **Shock (Deficit 15% or Over)**

Rx: *Immediately treat with isotonic solution*
        and
Blood
Lactated Ringer's solution
Albumin
Normal saline

At a rate of at least 20 mL/kg/h until blood pressure is adequate

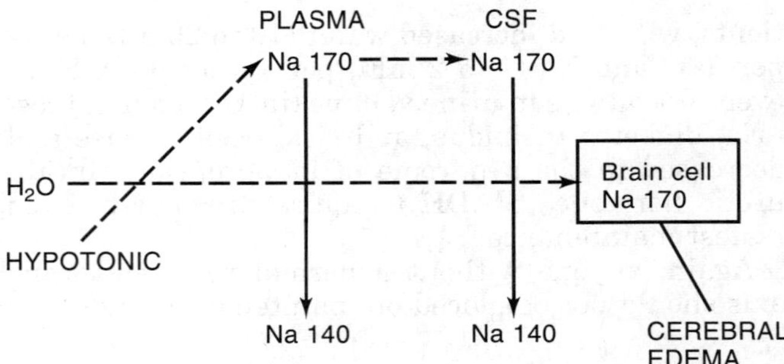

Figure 1. The problem in hypertonic dehydration. *Abbreviation:* CSF = cerebrospinal fluid.

ISOTONIC DEHYDRATION

When calculating fluid requirements in any deficit condition, the patient requires a deficit replacement plus usual maintenance and may also require concurrent replacement of ongoing losses. In the previous example, 7 kg × 10% dry, the child will need a maintenance of 700 mL per day (mL per kg method) and need to make up a deficit of 700 mL (10% of 7 kg) (Table 9). The total fluid for 24 hours is 1400 mL. The child will also require maintenance Na (21 mEq per liter) and deficit Na.

Deficit losses (most commonly gastrointestinal) can be estimated as requiring 0.45 NS (77 mEq per liter). In our example, 700 mL of 0.45 NS contains 54 mEq of sodium chloride. This, added to maintenance Na, totals 75 mEq of sodium chloride added to 1400 mL for the day. The initial order would be D5.3NS per liter and add 10 mEq of potassium chloride per liter after the child voids twice. Start at 88 mL per hour for 8 hours, then 44 mL per hour for the balance of the 24 hours. Once again, this is an estimate, and you should reassess the patient's response.

HYPERTONIC DEHYDRATION

The problem in hypertonic (hypernatremic) dehydration is essentially a greater amount of solvent (water) loss than solute (Na) loss. The major issue is, what fluid replacement would be best to utilize? Historically, this clinical entity accounted for approximately one-third of dehydrated children. However, with better oral replacement regimens that avoid the use of hypertonic solutions such as boiled milk, hypertonic dehydration has become less common. Physical examination in these children discovers extreme irritability and a lesser degree of circulatory collapse than one might expect because of the hypertonicity. The clinical problem is as follows:

$$\text{Osmolality} = (2 \times \text{Na}) + \frac{\text{Glucose}}{20} + \frac{\text{BUN}}{3}$$

$$\text{that is,} = (2 \times 170) + \frac{100}{20} + \frac{30}{3} = 355 \text{ mOsm}$$

As noted in Figure 1, the serum Na concentration can easily be decreased using a hypotonic solution (D5W or D5.2NS). However, the resulting rapid fluid shifts to other compartments will potentially cause cerebral edema, seizures, and death! Therefore, one must decrease the Na slowly at a rate no faster than 10 mEq per liter per day, using a solution allowing for a much more gradual gradient. Of the most common commercially available fluids, NS (154 mEq per liter) and 0.45 NS (77 mEq per liter) have the least steep gradients. Figure 2 illustrates this gradient differential.

D5.2NS, the most commonly used "pediatric" fluid, has an extremely steep and dangerous gradient if used in hypertonic dehydration. Thus a good rule to follow is: if you do not yet have the electrolyte results from the laboratory, use *normal saline* as the initial fluid. No one will ever be harmed by NS—the rate the fluid is given might be harmful (too fast or too slow), but not the content. The same cannot be said for any other fluid.

TABLE 9. **Isotonic Deficit Calculations for a 7-kg Child Estimated 10% Dry**

	Water	Na	K
Maintenance	7 × 100 = 700	7 × 3 = 21	2 × 7 = 14
Deficit	7000 × 10% = 700	$\frac{77}{1000} = \frac{X}{700} = {\sim}54$	*None*
TOTAL	700 + 700 = 1400 *mL*	54 + 21 = 75 $\frac{75}{1400} = \frac{X}{1000} = 54/L$ *or D5.3NS*	$\frac{14}{1400} = \frac{X}{1000} = 10$ *Add 10 mEq of KCl after 2 voids*

Replace half in the first 8 h
Replace the second half in the next 16 h

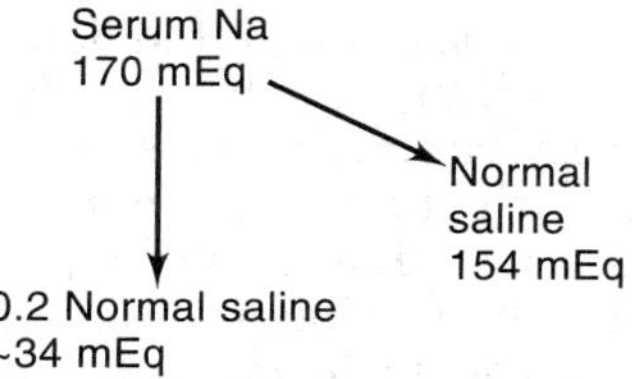

Figure 2. Fluid gradient differentials in hypernatremia.

The goal is to lower serum Na slowly to less than 150 mEq per liter at a rate of approximately 10 mEq per liter per day. In a child with a serum Na of 170 mEq per liter, fluid calculation is based on the percent deficit plus two times the maintenance (water, sodium chloride, and maintenance K) to be replaced over 48 hours (half given in the first 16 hours, the rest over the following 32 hours). The initial fluid should be either NS (if the Na is greater than 170) or 0.45 NS (if the Na is less than 170). When the Na has decreased to less than 150, then the Na content should be adjusted for the amount that would be given in an isotonic patient. It is important to follow electrolytes and make frequent clinical reassessments so as not to allow the Na to drop too fast (Figure 3).

Hypotonic Dehydration

The problem in these patients is the theoretical loss of more solute (Na) than solvent (water). In actuality this rarely causes hypotonic dehydration in pediatric patients. Rather, children develop fluid loss, and the fluid is abnormally replaced. This is the mother who takes the advice to place her child on a "clear fluid" diet to the extreme, using water exclusively (or forms of water such as tea or Kool-Aid). Clinically, such a child may be profoundly hypotensive due to the low serum osmolality.

Treatment depends on symptoms and the serum Na level. Without central nervous system (CNS) symptoms and a serum Na level of more than 120 mEq per liter, replacement with NS over a period of 24 hours will suffice. However, if the child manifests CNS symptoms (particularly seizures) or the serum Na is less than 120 mEq per liter, then hypertonic 3% sodium chloride should be infused rapidly to raise the serum Na to approximately 125 mEq per liter. This is accomplished as in Table 10. Since fluid is not as significant an issue as osmolar content, rapid

TABLE 10. **Hypotonic Dehydration**

Amount of Na required: weight in kilograms × Na space (0.6) × deficit = mEq Na

10-kg child with Na level of 115 mEq/L: deficit here is 10 mEq/dL (the Δ of 125 − 115)

$$10 \times 0.6 \times 10 = 60 \text{ mEq Na}$$
or
$$\frac{X}{60} = \frac{1}{0.518} = \text{approximately 116 mL of 3\% NaCl}$$

Given over 60–90 minutes

repletion of the initial Na deficit is possible. Full correction for fluid is then made over 48 hours.

ACID–BASE THERAPY

Our emphasis here is to address *acute* acid-base disturbances. Chronic pH, H^+ ion, or P_{CO_2} changes and their work-up are involved subjects beyond the scope of the present review. This includes chronic metabolic acidosis (e.g., inborn errors of metabolism, renal tubular acidosis, renal failure).

The first step in evaluating any acid-base problem is differentiating respiratory etiology from metabolic causes. We essentially evaluate lung function (P_{CO_2}) and kidney function (HCO_3).

$$(7.4) \text{ Serum pH} = \frac{HCO_3}{P_{CO_2}} = \frac{\text{Kidney}}{\text{Lung}}$$

$$7.3 - 7.49 = \frac{18 - 24}{35 - 45}$$

Clinical acid-base concerns differ from academic theory. Not every pH abnormality needs to be immediately corrected. For example, the most common type of metabolic acidosis encountered in pediatrics occurs during routine fluid-losing illnesses such as gastroenteritis. As previously discussed, in "clamping down" on the peripheral circulation to maintain central perfusion, lactic acid is produced. In most cases, just stopping the fluid loss by stopping any oral intake and beginning to replenish the deficit will be sufficient to shut off the lactic acid production and resolve the acidosis. Therefore, in most clinical pediatric situations, treatment with alkali is not undertaken unless the serum pH is less than 7.20.

Clinical Acid-Base Determinations

Respiratory Acidosis

$$\text{pH} < 7.30 = \frac{HCO_3}{P_{CO_2}} = \frac{\text{nl or} > 24}{> 45}$$

Respiratory Alkalosis

$$\text{pH} > 7.45 = \frac{HCO_3}{P_{CO_2}} = \frac{\text{nl or} < 24}{< 35}$$

Metabolic Acidosis

$$\text{pH} < 7.30 = \frac{HCO_3}{P_{CO_2}} = \frac{< 18}{\text{nl or} < 45}$$

Metabolic Alkalosis

$$\text{pH} > 7.45 = \frac{HCO_3}{P_{CO_2}} = \frac{> 24}{\text{nl or} > 35}$$

In respiratory acidosis, a ventilator may be needed

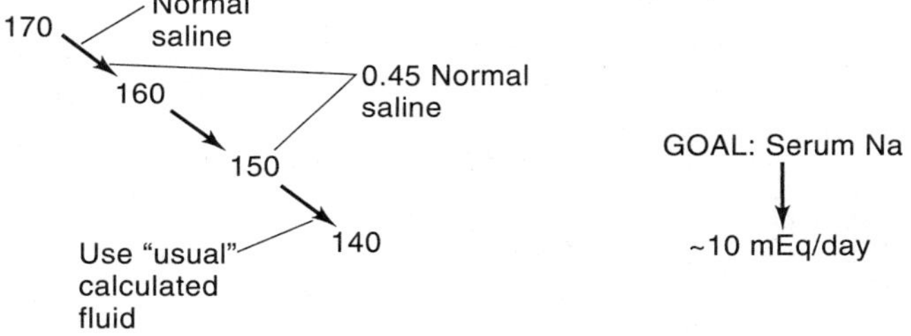

Figure 3. Treatment plan in hypernatremia.

but *not* HCO_3. Unless one suspects a pulmonary or cardiac problem (when an accurate PO_2 is necessary), VBGs are sufficient for our purpose, namely serum pH. Alkalosis is just as harmful to body homeostasis as is acidosis; therefore a pH of over 7.49 should be addressed with the same degree of urgency as a pH of less than 7.20 (more on alkalosis later).

TREATMENT OF UNCOMPENSATED METABOLIC ACIDOSIS

pH <7.2   kg × 0.6 × deficit

deficit to >18 mEq/dL

Give only partial correction

When you have decided to help the patient compensate for an acute metabolic acidosis, the deficit is the difference between the child's present HCO_3 and the lower normal for HCO_3 of 18 mEq per dL. Only a third or a fourth of the calculated deficit is given over the first hour. Sodium bicarbonate ($NaHCO_3$) should not be given very rapidly as it is very hyperosmolar. In any event, with the most common form of metabolic acidosis—that due to poor peripheral perfusion—reversing the perfusion problem with rehydration will resolve the acidosis.

Metabolic alkalosis is most commonly seen in the following pediatric conditions: chronic vomiting (e.g., pyloric stenosis, anorexia or bulimia), nasogastric suction, and chronic diuretic therapy. Each of these conditions has as major components loss of Cl^- and K^+, in addition to H^+. Thus the usual treatment is Cl^- and K^+. These children will need higher concentrations of Cl^- as supplied by NS and probably a higher amount of KCl.

The preceding pages have been meant as an overview of parenteral fluid therapy in children. The clinician is cautioned to use this as a guideline. Specific clinical problems may require more complex solutions.

The Endocrine System

ACROMEGALY

method of
IVOR M. D. JACKSON, M.D.
Brown University School of Medicine
Rhode Island Hospital
Providence, Rhode Island

Acromegaly (Gr. 'ακρος, extremity; μεγαλη, large) results from chronic hypersecretion of growth hormone (GH), most often due to an adenoma of the somatotroph cells in the anterior pituitary. This condition leads to a kaleidoscopic array of clinical and metabolic manifestations that include large hands and feet, prognathism, coarsening of the facial features, hyperhidrosis, oiliness of the skin, macroglossia, arthralgias, carpal tunnel syndrome, sleep apnea, hypertension, cardiomyopathy, diabetes mellitus, headache, and an increased propensity for the development of neoplastic change, especially in the colon. If the disorder occurs before the epiphyses have closed, gigantism occurs. Acromegaly is not a common disorder, having an incidence of around four new cases per million population and a prevalence of about 80 per million. It is possibly slightly more common in females than males, but almost all cases of gigantism occur in males.

GH induces secretion of somatomedin C (IGF-1), a protein with a molecular weight of approximately 7650 produced in the liver, and it is through IGF-1 that many of the effects of GH are mediated. Measurement of IGF-1, which has a long half-life in the circulation, in essence reflects integrated serum GH levels over the previous 24 hours. GH release is regulated by the hypothalamic releasing factors growth hormone–releasing hormone (GHRH) (which is stimulatory) and somatostatin (which is inhibitory), both of which bind to specific receptors on the surface of the somatotroph. The activation of the somatotroph is normally transduced by a guanosine triphosphate (GTP)-binding or G protein, which leads to activation of adenyl cyclase and cyclic AMP as a second messenger. In the stimulatory or Gs protein that normally mediates the effect of GHRH, a somatic mutation has been identified in about 30 to 40% of acromegalic tumors, designated as a *gsp* (for Gs protein) ongene. The *gsp* oncogene in adenomas is constitutively activated, leading to a high level of GH secretion not subject to the normal physiologic restraints. In the McCune-Albright syndrome, a hypersecretory endocrinopathy with polyostotic fibrous dysplasia and café au lait pigmented lesions, the genetic abnormality appears to be an activating mutation within the Gs gene in the germ line, giving rise to an oncogene identical to *gsp*. The acromegaly that occasionally occurs as part of this syndrome is associated with either hyperplasia or tumor of the somatotrophs. Although a eutopic hypophysial adenoma is by far the most common cause of acromegaly, ectopic pituitary adenomas can occur in the sphenoid or parapharyngeal sinus.

Rarely, acromegaly can be caused by excess GHRH secretion either from the hypothalamus (e.g., a gangliocytoma) or elsewhere in the body (ectopic GHRH syndrome) from neuroendocrine tissue such as an islet cell tumor of the pancreas or bronchial carcinoid. In these cases, the acromegaly results from GH secretion by hyperplastic pituitary somatotrophs stimulated by the high circulating levels of GHRH. Ectopic GH secretion from other than a pituitary gland giving rise to acromegaly is extraordinarily rare. Acromegaly may rarely occur as part of the multiple endocrine neoplasia Type I (MEN I) syndrome, an autosomal dominant disorder resulting from a mutation on the long arm of chromosome 11 (11q;13). Other associated disorders that are part of the MEN I syndrome include hyperparathyroidism and islet cell tumors of the pancreas. The pathogenesis of acromegaly is summarized in Table 1.

DIAGNOSIS

The diagnosis of acromegaly depends on a high index of clinical suspicion. Patients with acromegaly may present with carpal tunnel syndrome, diabetes mellitus, or sleep apnea, features that may mask the underlying disorder. Confirmation of the diagnosis requires an elevated serum GH level that fails to fall below 2 μg per liter within 2 hours following ingestion of a 100-gram oral load of glucose. In about 10 to 20% of cases, a paradoxical rise in the serum GH occurs in response to the glucose. A random serum GH above 10 μg per liter accompanied by an elevated serum IGF-1 and/or insulin-like growth factor binding protein 3 (IGF-BP3) is virtually diagnostic of the disorder. It must be emphasized that an elevated serum GH can occur in a number of disorders other than acromegaly, including renal failure, hepatic failure, and anorexia nervosa, but these conditions do not usually resemble acromegaly clinically; also, in these disorders, IGF-1 is generally low. During the rapid growth phase of puberty, the normal range for IGF-1 is increased, and in some boys, it may be difficult to unequivocally distinguish a normal subject from one with acromegalic gigantism. In pregnancy, IGF-1 may be elevated as a result of stimulation by placental GH, which is not detected by the usual pituitary GH radioimmunoassay (RIA). The raised IGF-1, in turn, suppresses GH release from the pituitary somatotroph so that the circulating GH may be low in the RIA.

TABLE 1. **Pathogenesis of Acromegaly**

Pituitary adenoma
  Eutopic
  Ectopic
Somatotroph hyperplasia
  Hypothalamic GHRH
  Ectopic GHRH
McCune-Albright syndrome
Ectopic GH secretion

A paradoxical GH response to thyrotropin-releasing hormone (TRH; protirelin) stimulation (200 to 500 μg intravenously) occurs in 25 to 50% of acromegalics. Persistence of this TRH responsivity can be useful in determining whether acromegaly is still present following trans-sphenoidal surgery, especially when the basal GH level is under 5 μg per liter. Hyperprolactinemia is found in 30 to 40% of acromegalic subjects and may result in the patient being mistakenly diagnosed as having a prolactinoma. Although ectopic GHRH production is a cause of acromegaly in 1% or less of patients, the diagnosis can be made by measurement of plasma GHRH (normal <50 ng per liter), which is markedly elevated in such cases (usually above 1 μg per liter).

As part of the clinical evaluation, other components of pituitary function need to be investigated, including thyroid status, pituitary-adrenal axis, and gonadal function. Appropriate replacement therapy should be provided as required. Impairment of gonadal function can result from damage to normal gonadotrophs by a pituitary tumor or by inhibition from the associated hyperprolactinemia. The patient should be screened for MEN I syndrome by measurement of serum calcium to rule out hyperparathyroidism, as well as have various gastrointestinal peptides such as insulin and gastrin levels (measured in the fasting state) tested if there is clinical suspicion of hypoglycemia from an insulinoma or peptic ulcer disease from Zollinger-Ellison syndrome, respectively.

TUMOR LOCALIZATION

Once acromegaly has been confirmed biochemically, the pituitary should be imaged, preferably by magnetic resonance imaging (MRI) with gadolinium enhancement. If MRI is not available, high-resolution computed tomography (CT) scanning may be used. In over 85% of cases, at the time of initial presentation the tumor is greater than 10 mm in size (macroadenoma), with suprasellar extension that may encroach upon the optic chiasm or extend laterally into the cavernous sinus. Sometimes a magnetic resonance angiogram is helpful to the neurosurgeon in delineating anatomic relationships when pituitary surgery is planned for a large macroadenoma. In less than 15% of cases is a microadenoma (<10 mm) found. This may reflect the slow, insidious onset of acromegaly, which may be present for an average of 5 to 10 years before being recognized. If an ectopic GHRH syndrome is considered, a CT scan of the chest and abdomen should be performed to identify the presumptive bronchial carcinoid or islet cell tumor of the pancreas. A radioisotope scan with [111]indium-octreotide (OctreoScan) is sometimes helpful in the localization of neuroendocrine tumors.

TREATMENT

Surgery

Trans-sphenoidal surgery with selective adenomectomy is the treatment of choice for GH-secreting adenomas that are intrasellar and subdiaphragmatic. In such cases, an immediate cure of the acromegaly with normalization of GH and IGF-1 secretion can be obtained by a skilled surgeon in over 70% of cases. Suprasellar extension and cavernous sinus invasion markedly limit the probability of cure with preservation of intact anterior pituitary function. Nevertheless, surgical decompression may still be worthwhile,

especially if there is tumor encroachment on the optic chiasm. In such cases, as well as in those with extension of tumor into the brain, a transcranial-subfrontal approach may allow the surgeon better access to the tumor and achieve significant debulking. The mortality rate is very low with the trans-sphenoidal procedure (under 1%) but may rise to 3 to 4% with the transcranial approach. With trans-sphenoidal surgery, complications include transient diabetes insipidus, which may occur in up to 25% of patients and responds to fluid adjustment and/or desmopressin (DDA VP) 1 to 4 μg (0.25 to 1 mL) given subcutaneously usually once or twice daily. Other complications include cerebrospinal fluid (CSF) rhinorrhea, meningitis, and wound infection, which are observed in less than 4% of cases. Hypopituitarism as a complication of trans-sphenoidal surgery is influenced by the adequacy of pituitary function preoperatively as well as by the extent of the surgical resection. In most instances, surgery does not lead to recovery of pituitary function unless there is concomitant hyperprolactinemia that is inhibiting the pituitary-gonadal axis.

It is recommended that glucocorticoids be administered over the surgical period even if the pituitary-adrenal axis appears adequate. On the day of surgery, hydrocortisone 300 mg or dexamethasone (Decadron) 10 mg may be given parenterally. Glucocorticoids are reduced to maintenance doses by 5 days postoperatively. Efficacy of the surgery should be determined 2 to 4 weeks later by measuring a fasting GH and an IGF-1. The necessity of continuing glucocorticoid replacement may be determined by measuring a morning serum cortisol after stopping glucocorticoids for 24 to 48 hours. Simultaneously, other components of pituitary function may be monitored. If there is persistence of the acromegaly, a second trans-sphenoidal procedure may be considered, but a total hypophysectomy is probably necessary to obtain remission of the acromegaly. Even then, the cure rate is only about 20%.

If an ectopic GHRH syndrome has been identified, cure of the acromegaly can be achieved by surgical removal of the neuroendocrine tumor.

Radiation Therapy

Acromegaly can be treated with conventional supervoltage radiotherapy delivered to the pituitary by a linear accelerator in which 4000 to 5000 cGy are given as fractional doses of 180 cGy per day, 5 days per week, over a 5- to 6-week period. Such treatment is generally considered for patients who have persistent acromegaly following surgery. Radiotherapy is most effective when the GH level is under 30 ng per mL. The disadvantage of this treatment is the slow onset of therapeutic effect—50% reduction in GH levels after 2 years, and 75% after 5 years—and the high incidence of anterior pituitary failure. Complications of radiotherapy include cranial nerve damage, cerebral radionecrosis, and cognitive defects. Other forms of radiotherapy include Bragg peak proton beam therapy utilizing a cyclotron, which is currently available in only one center in the United States. In this modality, the radiation is delivered in a single dose rather than in fractions. The efficacy of this form of therapy over conventional radiation is controversial, and it may be associated with a higher prevalence of cranial nerve damage.

Most recently, stereotactic radiosurgery (gamma knife therapy) has been introduced for the treatment of pituitary tumors. This involves the delivery in a single session of a high dose of ionizing radiation (cobalt 60) as precise, narrow, collimated beams through multiple ports. Since the dose gradient is very steep, surrounding tissues receive minimal irradiation. The resulting lesion is sharply circumscribed, and the rest of the pituitary may receive little irradiation. The limiting factor with respect to the dose of radiation administered is the proximity of the tumor to the optic chiasm. The role of gamma knife therapy as a primary or secondary treatment of pituitary tumors is currently under investigation; this treatment modality has a number of advantages over conventional radiotherapy, including absence of significant irradiation of surrounding brain tissue. It is our current practice to utilize gamma knife therapy rather than conventional radiotherapy when radiation treatment is being considered for acromegaly.

Medical Therapy

Dopaminergic Agonists

Bromocriptine (Parlodel), the only dopaminergic agonist approved for use in acromegaly, is administered orally in divided doses. It is less effective than in hyperprolactinemia, and its efficacy is not usually enhanced by increasing the dose beyond 20 mg per day. The side effects of nausea, constipation, nasal stuffiness, dizziness, and digital vasospasm are intolerable in some patients. It should be initiated in a dose of 1.25 mg (1/2 tablet) with the evening meal. Taking the medication with food and gradually increasing the dose by no more than 1.25 mg every 3 to 4 days improves tolerance of the medication. When the daily dose reaches 5 mg, it should be taken in four divided doses for maximum efficacy. As an alternative, pergolide (Permax)* may be used, and it is sometimes better tolerated than bromocriptine. Pergolide is not, however, approved by the Food and Drug Administration (FDA) for the treatment of acromegaly. Dopaminergic agonists provide benefit in approximately 10 to 15% of cases of acromegaly, usually the milder forms, but rarely produce significant reduction in tumor size.

Somatostatin Analogues

Because of its short half-life of around 2 minutes, native somatostatin has not been useful as a therapeutic agent for acromegaly. It needs to be administered by continuous intravenous infusion, and when

the infusion is stopped, there is rebound hypersecretion. The development of an octapeptide analogue of somatostatin (octreotide [Sandostatin]; SMS 201–995) with a D-phenylalanine at the N-terminus and an amino alcohol (threonol acetate) at the C-terminus has given rise to a substance that is much more resistant to enzymatic degradation, with a half-life of around 2 hours. Octreotide has been utilized extensively in a large number of centers as a therapeutic agent for the treatment of acromegaly. In a double-blind trial involving 104 acromegalic subjects from 14 university-affiliated medical centers, GH and IGF-1 levels were normalized in 50 to 70% of patients utilizing doses of 100 or 250 μg three times per day by subcutaneous injection. Although most patients do not benefit from further increases in the octreotide dose, some require 1500 μg or more per day for maximum benefit. Pituitary tumor size was reduced by 20 to 30% on MRI with the 750-μg-per-day dose. The medication was well tolerated in most cases, although transient diarrhea occurred in 10 to 15% of patients. Tolerance or tachyphylaxis does not generally occur. The major side effect of concern is the development of gallstones, which occurred in about 20% of cases. Ultrasound of the gallbladder is recommended prior to starting therapy and every 6 months thereafter. Octreotide is often effective in relieving headache and arthralgias, even if the GH and IGF-1 cannot be normalized. Some patients, because of persistent headaches, need to take octreotide every 6 hours. Despite the necessity of administration by injection (two to four times per day), octreotide therapy is readily accepted by most acromegalic patients. Some patients have been treated by continuous subcutaneous infusion, which allows the total dose administered over a 24-hour period to be reduced. The mechanism allowing octreotide to inhibit GH secretion and reduce pituitary tumor size is the binding to specific somatostatin receptors (Type 2) on the surface of the tumor cell. In some cases, an additive effect from bromocriptine can be obtained. However, ineffectiveness of octreotide occurs in about 10% of acromegalics and likely reflects reduced affinity or density of the somatostatin receptor on the tumor surface for octreotide.

Octreotide has been utilized in patients for 3 to 6 months prior to pituitary surgery, since there is some evidence that this approach makes the subsequent surgical procedure easier either by reducing the size of the macroadenoma or by making it softer and easier to resect. Octreotide may be used following radiation therapy, in view of the delay before the full effect of this procedure is attained. It is also therapeutically effective in the treatment of ectopic GHRH syndrome and is given long term when the primary tumor is unresectable. Octreotide acts at the tumor site to inhibit GHRH secretion, as well as directly on the pituitary somatotroph. It is probably the treatment of choice in the McCune-Albright syndrome, where the alternative may be total hypophysectomy or radiotherapy.

Most recently, a depot long-acting somatostatin an-

---

*Not FDA-approved for this indication.

TABLE 2. **Treatment of Acromegaly**

Surgery

Trans-sphenoidal adenomectomy
Subfrontal craniotomy
Other (for ectopic syndromes)

Radiation

Conventional supervoltage radiotherapy
Stereotactic radiosurgery (gamma knife)

Pharmacologic Agents

Dopaminergic agonists
  Bromocriptine (Parlodel)
  Pergolide (Permax)*
Somatostatin analogues
  Octreotide (Sandostatin)
  Octreotide LAR†

*Not FDA-approved for this indication.
†Investigational drug in the United States.

alogue (Sandostatin LAR)* was prepared. It is a formulation that incorporates octreotide in microspheres of a biodegradable polymer and is administered by injection once a month in a dose of 10 to 30 mg. It has been shown to be effective in maintaining suppressed GH levels in acromegalic subjects. It is likely to be several years before it is available and approved for the treatment of acromegaly.

The various treatment options indicated for the management of acromegaly are given in Table 2.

SUMMARY

Acromegaly is usually caused by a pituitary adenoma that, if not invasive, may be resectable by the trans-sphenoidal route, with cure of the disorder. However, if it is large and there is suprasellar or parasellar extension, surgery may only be palliative, and other forms of treatment are required. Radiotherapy, including gamma knife surgery, has a therapeutic role, but because the onset of benefit is generally delayed, pharmacologic therapy is indicated in the interim. Dopaminergic agonists may be tried initially because they are taken orally and are less expensive than octreotide, but their efficacy is limited. Somatostatin analogue is generally effective in doses of 300 to 750 µg per day, but occasional patients require higher doses in order to normalize GH secretion. Octreotide is also effective in the treatment of acromegaly due to somatotroph hyperplasia caused by GHRH stimulation or the McCune-Albright syndrome.

*Investigational drug in the United States.

ADRENOCORTICAL INSUFFICIENCY

method of
ROBERT J. ANDERSON, M.D.
*Creighton University School of Medicine and
  VAMC
Omaha, Nebraska*

Adrenal insufficiency encompasses endocrine disorders of high morbidity that are fatal if the patient is left undiag-

nosed and untreated. Patients' dramatic response to treatment underscores the necessity for accurate and timely diagnosis and treatment. Adrenal insufficiency is divided into two categories based on the anatomic location of the deficit in the hypothalamic-pituitary-adrenal axis. Primary adrenal insufficiency refers to the loss of cortisol and mineralocorticoid due to destruction or drug-induced dysfunction of the adrenal gland. Secondary adrenal insufficiency refers to lack of adrenocorticotropic hormone (ACTH) due to pituitary damage or destruction. Hypothalamic etiologies that lead to corticotropin-releasing hormone (CRH) loss (tertiary insufficiency) are included in the secondary group for convenience, because the differentiation is often difficult and the treatment is the same.

PRIMARY ADRENOCORTICAL INSUFFICIENCY

Etiology

Primary adrenocortical insufficiency (Addison's disease) is an uncommon but urgent clinical problem that has multiple causes (Table 1). The most common cause (approximately 80% of cases) is autoimmune destruction of the adrenal glands. The autoimmune disease can occur as an isolated disorder, or it can be associated with other autoimmune deficiencies in polyglandular failure syndrome Type I (primary adrenal insufficiency, hypoparathyroidism, chronic mucocutaneous candidiasis, and pernicious anemia) and polyglandular failure syndrome Type II (primary adrenal insufficiency, primary hypothyroidism, Type I diabetes mellitus, and vitiligo). The second most common etiology is infection (approximately 20% of cases). Within this group, tuberculosis and histoplasmosis are the most frequent. Fungal infections with blastomycosis, cryptococcosis, and coccidioidomycosis have also been reported as causes. With the resurgence of tuberculosis today, the classic presentation of primary adrenal insufficiency described by Addison in 1855 may be more frequent. The adrenal necrosis commonly seen in acquired immune deficiency syndrome (AIDS) patients is usually caused by associated opportunistic infections, especially cytomegalovirus (CMV) and tuberculosis. Numerous other causes of primary adrenal insufficiency exist, and each is potentially fatal if un-

TABLE 1. **Causes of Primary Adrenal Insufficiency**

Autoimmune adrenalitis—up to 80% of cases

Infectious—up to 20% of cases
  Tuberculosis
  Histoplasmosis
  Blastomycosis
  Cryptococcosis
  Coccidioidomycosis
  Bacterial
  AIDS-associated opportunistic infections

All other causes
  Bilateral adrenal hemorrhage—postoperatively,
    trauma, heparin
  Surgical—bilateral adrenalectomy
  Metastatic disease—lung, breast, gastric
  Congenital adrenal hyperplasia
  Adrenoleukodystrophy (X-linked)
  Drugs—*decreased cortisol biosynthesis:* mitotane
    (Lysodren), ketoconazole (Nizoral), aminoglutethimide
    (Cytadren), metyrapone (Metopirone)*; *accelerated
    cortisol metabolic clearance:* rifampin (Rifadin),
    phenytoin (Dilantin), phenobarbital

*Not available in the United States.

recognized (see Table 1). Increased awareness and better imaging techniques have led to more frequent reports of bilateral adrenal hemorrhage in patients after abdominal surgery or trauma. Table 1 includes drugs that may lead to partial or complete cortical dysfunction and adrenal insufficiency either by decreasing cortisol biosynthesis (metyrapone,* mitotane [Lysodren], aminoglutethimide [Cytadren], ketoconazole [Nizoral]) or by enhancing cortisol catabolism via induction of hepatic microsomal enzymes (rifampin [Rifadin], phenytoin [Dilantin], phenobarbital). Patients on corticosteroid replacement have increased corticosteroid requirements when treated with rifampin or similar agents.

Clinical Presentation

Acute and chronic courses are the major modes of presentation of adrenal insufficiency. The presentation may be confusing if it is acute primary (e.g., disseminated histoplasmosis or postoperative bilateral adrenal hemorrhage), before the typical features of chronic primary adrenal insufficiency have had time to develop. A patient with a rapid onset of primary adrenal insufficiency is usually ill enough with the underlying disease to present in adrenal crisis. Major manifestations are dehydration, fever, and hypotension, with cardiovascular collapse associated with hyponatremia, hyperkalemia, and hypoglycemia. The patient responds to fluid resuscitation, glucose, and blood pressure maintenance initially but often expires if the cortisol lack is unrecognized. If acute primary adrenal insufficiency is suspected, it should be treated first, and the diagnostic testing completed when the patient is stable.

Chronic primary adrenal insufficiency, the second major mode of presentation, may include more clues to the diagnosis. Such patients decline in health over months, with gradual weakness, fatigue, anorexia, weight loss, and postural hypotension. They develop hyperpigmentation of the skin (described by Addison as "a dingy or smokey appearance of various tints or shades of deep amber or chestnut brown"), especially at the palmar creases, extensor surfaces (particularly the knuckles, elbows, and knees), buccal mucosa, recent scars, and sun-exposed areas. Vitiligo that is either stippled or expansive in confluent areas may be present. These findings, together with hyperkalemia, hyponatremia, fasting hypoglycemia, possible hypothyroidism, pernicious anemia, and other deficiencies, assist in the diagnosis. Patients may have difficulty with minor illnesses. They are always at risk for the third major mode of presentation—catastrophic acute adrenal crisis concomitant with the underlying chronic insufficiency—if the stress is severe enough. Vigilance, early diagnosis, and timely treatment are lifesaving for these patients.

SECONDARY ADRENOCORTICAL INSUFFICIENCY

Etiology

Causes of secondary adrenal insufficiency commonly involve hypothalamic-pituitary tumors and accompanying anatomic and therapeutic sequelae (Table 2). Other causes include trauma, infarction, infiltrative and infectious diseases, and autoimmune disease. The most common cause of secondary adrenal insufficiency is iatrogenic—the use and withdrawal of exogenous glucocorticoid preparations. Patients who have received a course of high-dose glucocor-

---

*Not commercially available in the United States.

TABLE 2. Causes of Secondary Adrenal Insufficiency

Iatrogenic
  Discontinuation of exogenous glucocorticoid treatment or inadequate coverage during stress in patients on long-term or intermittent glucocorticoids by any route
Tumor
  Pituitary adenoma—functioning plus nonfunctioning
  Craniopharyngioma
Isolated ACTH deficiency
Trauma
Infarction/vascular
  Ischemic necrosis
  Sheehan's syndrome (postpartum pituitary necrosis), diabetes mellitus, sickle cell disease
  Pituitary apoplexy—necrosis of tumor
Radiation of pituitary
  Usually gradual and progressive decline in function
Infiltrative and infectious disease
  Sarcoidosis
  Hemochromatosis
  Meningitis
  Tuberculosis
Autoimmune
  Lymphocytic hypophysitis
Idiopathic

---

ticoids for a month or more within the previous year can have variable degrees of suppression and recovery of the hypothalamic-pituitary-adrenal axis. The possibility of secondary adrenal insufficiency must be considered in these individuals.

Clinical Presentation

General malaise, fatigue, weakness, hypotension, and lack of skin hyperpigmentation are suggestive findings. Hyponatremia can occur, and some patients may present with symptomatic hypoglycemia as the main finding. Female patients may have loss of pubic and axillary hair because of the lack of adrenal androgens. Patients may also present with other manifestations of pituitary disease, such as mass effect of the lesion with headache and cranial nerve paralysis. The loss of growth hormone (GH), thyroid-stimulating hormone (TSH), follicle-stimulating hormone (FSH), luteinizing hormone (LH), and antidiuretic hormone (ADH) leads to the accompanying lack of GH effects, hypothyroidism, hypogonadism, and diabetes insipidus, respectively. Hyperfunctioning tumors may produce excess GH, prolactin, TSH, gonadotropins, or their subunits. The combined effects of one or more overproduced hormones may occur with variable pituitary hormone losses due to tumor compression or destruction of normal pituitary cells. Patients on exogenous glucocorticoids may be cushingoid but may present in the interesting situation of having secondary adrenal insufficiency with clinical Cushing's syndrome if the corticosteroid is withheld or withdrawn. Careful review of the patient's history and drug records should help avoid secondary adrenal insufficiency due to patient noncompliance or inadvertent omission of corticosteroids in the perioperative period or in the intensive care unit.

DIAGNOSIS

Clinical

Typical skin hyperpigmentation and vitiligo help establish the diagnosis of chronic primary adrenocortical insufficiency or acute adrenal crisis if they occur in a patient with underlying chronic primary insufficiency. Because isolated ACTH deficiency is rare, the diagnosis of chronic secondary adrenal insufficiency can be assisted by the finding of accompanying pituitary hormone hypofunction and/or hyperfunction. Skin hyperpigmentation is not present. Diagnosis of acute adrenal crisis, whether due to the rapid onset of primary disease or to decompensated secondary adrenal insufficiency, depends on laboratory results. A careful history is useful to detect exogenous glucocorticoid administration and subsequent interruption of treatment. Exogenous glucocorticoid suppression of the hypothalamic-pituitary-adrenal axis is the most common cause of secondary adrenal insufficiency.

Laboratory

In primary adrenal insufficiency, the simultaneous serum cortisol and ACTH levels are diagnostic. The serum cortisol is low (usually <10 μg per dL), and the ACTH is high (>200 pg per mL). If it is possible to draw these values in the acute situation or before treatment is initiated in chronic disease, the diagnosis can be documented. Treatment should not be withheld if the diagnosis is suspected, however. Frequently, further testing with ACTH stimulation is required (see the later discussion). The presence of hyponatremia, hyperkalemia, and hypoglycemia adds to the diagnostic information. The usual findings in secondary hypoadrenalism are a low or "normal" ACTH level (0 to 50 pg per mL) in association with a serum cortisol level of less than 10 μg per dL in the morning or during severe stress. The patient may present in an acute crisis with cardiovascular collapse. A serum cortisol level of less than 20 μg per dL in this situation is highly suggestive of adrenal dysfunction.

To evaluate any patient suspected of adrenal insufficiency when the ACTH value is not immediately available, a rapid adrenocortical screen with the synthetic α^{1-24}-ACTH (cosyntropin [Cortrosyn]) should be done. A baseline cortisol is drawn, 250 μg of ACTH is given intravenously, and cortisol levels are obtained at 30 and 60 minutes. A normal response is a cortisol level of at least 18 μg per dL at 30 minutes. Cortisol levels show little or no response in primary adrenal insufficiency. Simultaneous aldosterone levels do not rise to 16 ng per dL at 30 minutes. In secondary adrenal insufficiency, the response of cortisol is usually less than 18 μg per dL at 30 and 60 minutes. A normal response excludes primary but does not exclude secondary adrenal insufficiency. If the patient has already been treated with glucocorticoids and the clinical picture is not clear, the use of a 1- to 3-day intravenous ACTH infusion documents a rise in cortisol and the presence of adrenal cortical function in secondary adrenal insufficiency. There is no cortisol response or only a minimal response in primary adrenal insufficiency. The metyrapone test or insulin-induced hypoglycemia test may be needed to confirm secondary adrenal insufficiency by demonstrating a lack of cortisol response associated with low ACTH. Both tests entail risks and can precipitate an adrenal crisis. They should be used with appropriate precautions. CRH can be obtained on an investigational basis for stimulation testing to differentiate primary from secondary adrenal insufficiency. The delays currently involved in procuring the CRH make it less practical. The reader is referred to standard endocrinology texts for detailed protocols of these tests.

Computed tomography (CT) or magnetic resonance imaging (MRI) scans of the adrenals can be helpful in the differential diagnosis of primary adrenal insufficiency. In autoimmune adrenalitis, the glands are small, atrophied, and difficult to visualize, whereas chronic granulomatous adrenal disease or hemorrhage is associated with high-density areas or calcifications. Bilateral enlarged adrenals are present in hemorrhage, metastases, and subacute granulomatous diseases. MRI scanning is equally informative in hemorrhage and may be superior in differentiating inflammatory from metastatic disease.

TREATMENT

Acute Adrenal Crisis

The treatment for acute adrenal insufficiency is the same whether it is primary or secondary (Table 3). Hydrocortisone sodium succinate (Solu-Cortef) 100 mg intravenously every 6 hours should be given for the first 24 hours, with full fluid resuscitation with dextrose and normal saline. Mineralocorticoid replacement is not needed because of the adequate mineralocorticoid effect with a glucocorticoid dose of 100 mg per day or greater. The dose of Solu-Cortef can be reduced by half each day as the patient improves. Oral treatment can be resumed rapidly once the patient has recovered. An aggressive review is required to define and treat the precipitating event and associated illnesses.

Chronic Primary and Secondary Adrenal Insufficiency

Corticosteroid replacement in both chronic disorders is the same. The major goal in treatment is to restore normalcy by attempting to reproduce the diurnal rhythm of cortisol production with a glucocorticoid preparation. ACTH is not used in secondary insufficiency because it is parenteral and immunogenic, and it is more difficult to mimic the diurnal pattern. I prefer to use cortisone acetate (Cortone) 25 mg in the morning and 12.5 mg in the late afternoon or prednisone (Deltasone) 5 mg in the morning and 2.5 mg in the late afternoon. Hydrocortisone (Hydrocortone tablets) at a dose of 20 mg in the morning and 10 mg in the late afternoon can also be used. The standard hydrocortisone replacement dose is 12 to 15 mg per m² per day. I avoid longer-acting preparations, such as dexamethasone (Decadron, Hexadrol), because of the higher occurrence of exogenous Cushing's syndrome. In primary adrenal insufficiency, the mineralocorticoid preparation fludrocortisone (Florinef) is used at a dose of 0.05 to 0.2 mg per day (usual dose, 0.1 mg per day). Too little fludrocortisone leads to hyperkalemia, hyponatremia, and dehydration. Too much causes upright and supine hypertension and hypokalemia. Rarely, a patient does not require the mineralocorticoid due to an adequate effect from the glucocorticoid or residual adrenal mineralocorticoid production. In most cases of secondary adrenal insufficiency, a mineralocorticoid preparation is not required, because the renin-angiotensin system is intact.

How do we know how much glucocorticoid replacement is enough? Urine free cortisol or serum cortisol

TABLE 3. **Treatment of Adrenal Insufficiency**

	Treatment	Items to Monitor
Acute		
Primary and secondary	Solu-Cortef 100 mg IV q 6 h Dextrose 5%/normal saline Treat underlying illness, precipitating event	Blood pressure, electrolytes, glucose
Chronic		
Primary	Cortisone acetate 25 mg PO, A.M., 12.5 mg PO, P.M. *or* Prednisone 5.0 mg PO, A.M., 2.5 mg PO, P.M. *or* Hydrocortisone 20 mg PO, A.M., 10 mg PO, P.M. *and* Fludrocortisone 0.05–0.2 mg/day (usual dose 0.1 mg/day)	Sense of well-being, strength, blood pressure, electrolytes Avoid cushingoid changes Skin pigmentation Blood pressure, electrolytes
Secondary	Same as primary except no fludrocortisone	Same as primary except skin changes do not occur and potassium is usually normal

measurements are not reliable indicators of adequate cortisol replacement. In primary adrenal insufficiency, progressive increases in the skin hyperpigmentation may serve as an indication of inadequate replacement. The ACTH level is not a good measure of adequate replacement because it may not be suppressed into the normal range in some patients with primary adrenal insufficiency. Likewise, in secondary insufficiency, there are no special laboratory tests for defining the adequacy of replacement. In both primary and secondary adrenal insufficiency, the best approach is to follow the clinical examination and history for a sense of well-being and good appetite and to monitor blood pressure and serum electrolytes. The peripheral tissue response is helpful. Occasionally, patients become cushingoid on the estimated doses and require a smaller twice-per-day dose or a once-per-day dose. In some situations, the afternoon dose has to be given earlier or later in the day to allow the patient to function as normally as possible. In secondary adrenal insufficiency, the corticosteroids may unmask underlying mild diabetes insipidus in some patients.

The patient must understand the need to increase the glucocorticoid dose during sick days. Each patient receives a detailed sheet that lists how to adjust the medicine. The patient should double the dose during the 1 to 3 days of a moderate illness such as the "flu" with a low-grade fever ($\leq$100° F) and triple the dose if fever (>100° F) is present. Patients are given prefilled syringes with injectable dexamethasone (Decadron Phosphate 4 mg per mL in 2.5-mL disposable syringes) to use if they are vomiting and cannot get to medical care quickly. Patients administer half the dose intramuscularly (5 mg) and repeat if necessary every 8 to 12 hours before arriving at the hospital. They frequently keep one syringe at work and one in the car, taking care to renew them as needed. Patients must get medical information bracelets or necklaces that detail their need for cortisol (Medic

Alert Foundation International, 2323 Colorado Ave., Turlock, California 95382; telephone 1-800-432-5378).

Glucocorticoid Coverage

Glucocorticoid coverage for surgery and stressful procedures is the same for primary and secondary adrenal insufficiency. I give a depot of 100 mg hydrocortisone sodium succinate (Solu-Cortef) intramuscularly on call to surgery and then 50 to 100 mg hydrocortisone intravenously every 6 hours (starting in surgery) the first 24 hours. The intramuscular dose is given to ensure a depot in case the intravenous access is interrupted. The dose is decreased by 50% each postoperative day as indicated by patient progress until the oral glucocorticoid (and mineralocorticoid for primary adrenal insufficiency) can be resumed. An intravenous preparation of prednisolone sodium phosphate (Hydeltrasol) can be used if less mineralocorticoid effect is desired. Prednisolone 40 mg intramuscularly is given on call, then 20 to 40 mg intravenously every 8 hours for the first 24 hours. The dose is tapered to 50% of the previous day's dose as tolerated and is given every 8 to 12 hours until oral glucocorticoids can be used.

CUSHING'S SYNDROME

method of
LYNNETTE K. NIEMAN, M.D.
National Institutes of Health
Bethesda, Maryland

Optimal treatment of Cushing's syndrome in 1996 involves targeted surgical resection of the specific tissue causing excessive adrenocorticotropic hormone (ACTH) secretion or autonomous cortisol production, to reverse the

All material in this article is in the public domain, with the exception of any borrowed figures or tables.

chemical and biochemical abnormalities of the syndrome. Three obstacles limit the realization of this goal: (1) inappropriate diagnosis of Cushing's syndrome, (2) incorrect assignment of the cause of Cushing's syndrome, hence inappropriate surgical procedures, and (3) inoperability or incomplete resection. Hence, this article discusses these clinical therapeutic challenges: the initial diagnosis of Cushing's syndrome, the differential diagnosis, surgical management, and the choice of second-line therapy.

DIAGNOSIS OF CUSHING'S SYNDROME

Cushing's syndrome reflects excessive tissue exposure to exogenous or endogenous glucocorticoids. Iatrogenic Cushing's syndrome, an adverse side effect of administration of exogenous glucocorticoids or ACTH, is largely reversible by discontinuation of the medications.

The diagnosis of endogenous Cushing's syndrome requires demonstration of both physical and biochemical features of glucocorticoid excess. Many of the signs of hypercortisolism, such as obesity, hypertension, mood changes, menstrual irregularities, and hirsutism, are common in the general population; screening for Cushing's syndrome is not cost effective in these patients unless there are additional features of the syndrome. Conversely, mild glucocorticoid excess (urine cortisol threefold normal) is seen in patients without cushingoid features who have affective disorders, strenuous exercise, chronic alcoholism and withdrawal from alcohol, renal failure, and hypoglycemia, the so-called pseudo-Cushing's states.

The biochemical diagnosis of Cushing's syndrome rests on documentation of excessive glucocorticoid levels in blood or urine. Although morning plasma cortisol values may be normal, an increased nighttime nadir blunts or obliterates the normal diurnal rhythm. This increase in mean 24-hour plasma values is reflected in increased levels of free, or unbound, cortisol in urine and saliva.

Measurement of a complete 24-hour free cortisol excretion by immunoassay or by high-pressure liquid chromatography (HPLC) is probably the best urine screening test for Cushing's syndrome. Unlike 17-hydroxysteroids, these assays are not affected by medications, obesity, or other medical conditions. Urine free cortisol (UFC) excretion greater than fourfold normal is rare except in Cushing's syndrome; lesser values are compatible with pseudo-Cushing's states, which must be excluded. If conditions associated with pseudo-Cushing's states are found, treatment or avoidance should result in eucortisolism. Up to 15% of patients with pseudo-Cushing's states, obesity, or chronic illness are misdiagnosed as having Cushing's syndrome by the 1- or 2-mg dexamethasone suppression tests. A combined dexamethasone-CRH (corticotropin-releasing hormone) test has better diagnostic accuracy (98%). When UFCs are normal in the setting of clinical features that suggest the diagnosis, repeated measurement of urine cortisol may demonstrate cyclicity or progression.

ETIOLOGY OF CUSHING'S SYNDROME

The differential diagnosis of endogenous Cushing's syndrome can be divided into ACTH-dependent and ACTH-independent causes. ACTH-dependent etiologies, characterized by excessive ACTH production, account for 70% to 75% of patients and include pituitary adenoma (Cushing's disease, 80%) or nonpituitary (ectopic, 20%) ACTH-producing tumors; very rarely, CRH production from a tumor stimulates normal corticotrophs to cause ACTH-dependent

Cushing's syndrome. ACTH-independent causes of Cushing's syndrome, characterized by autonomous cortisol production from adrenal tissue, account for about 25% of patients and include unilateral disease (adenoma and carcinoma), and, rarely, bilateral disease (primary pigmented nodular adrenal disease, PPNAD; McCune-Albright syndrome; massive macronodular adrenal disease; and food/GIP[gastric inhibitory polypeptide]-induced hyperplasia), and hyperfunction of adrenal rest tissue. In this setting, the excessive amount of cortisol inhibits the CRH neuron and the corticotroph so that basal ACTH secretion is subnormal ($\leq$10 pg per mL) when assessed by sensitive radioimmunoassay or immunoradiometric assay. Because nonautonomous adrenal tissue atrophies when ACTH support is subnormal, CT scans of adrenal adenoma and carcinoma show a unilateral adrenal mass, with atrophy of the adjacent and contralateral tissue. The rare ACTH-independent forms show normal or slightly lumpy glands (PPNAD) or huge (>5-cm) nodular or hyperplastic glands (massive macronodular adrenal disease). Iodocholesterol scanning may discriminate whether or not the contralateral gland is metabolically inactive (due to lack of ACTH support) in patients with unilateral masses. Thus, measurement of plasma ACTH concentration, followed by adrenal CT scan when the ACTH value is low, is the usual initial approach to classification of the cause of Cushing's syndrome.

Basal ACTH values greater than 10 pg per mL indicate that Cushing's syndrome is caused by ACTH. In contrast to ACTH-independent Cushing's syndrome, where imaging is the next step, biochemical tests must be used to identify the source of ACTH, because imaging of the pituitary gland is normal in up to 60% of patients with corticotropinomas and may be abnormal in up to 10% of patients with ectopic ACTH secretion. I recommend using conservative criteria for interpretation of the biochemical tests that result in 100% specificity, to minimize the chance of misdiagnosing a patient who has ectopic ACTH secretion. Patients with positive responses to two tests (ovine CRH, 6 day or overnight 8 mg dexamethasone, or metyrapone) would be classified as having Cushing's disease. These patients then undergo gadolinium-enhanced MR imaging of the pituitary gland to identify the tumor. If the pituitary MR scan is normal, and the surgeon would do a "blind" hemihypophysectomy based on localization data from inferior petrosal sinus sampling (IPSS), then this test may be performed. If the biochemical data are not congruent, the patient most likely has Cushing's disease, which can be confirmed by IPSS.

If the endocrine test results are consistent with ectopic ACTH secretion, imaging of possible tumor sites follows. CT and MR scans of the chest may identify the most common ACTH-producing tumors, small cell carcinoma, and bronchial or thymic carcinoid. Measurement of serum calcitonin and gastrin, and urinary catecholamines, as well as imaging of the neck, pancreas, and adrenals, may detect medullary carcinoma of the thyroid, gastrinoma, or pheochromocytoma. Octreotide scintigraphy is a promising new option for identification of tumors having somatostatin receptors, including pancreatic tumors, carcinoids, glomus tumors, and small cell cancer of the lung. Imaging studies may be repeated every 6 to 12 months until tumor is found.

DIAGNOSIS-SPECIFIC TREATMENT OPTIONS FOR CUSHING'S DISEASE

Transsphenoidal adenomectomy is the preferred treatment of microadenomas, with up to a 90%

chance of postoperative cure in experienced hands. When no tumor is found, hemihypophysectomy of the side of the gland with an ACTH gradient on petrosal sinus sampling may induce remission in up to 80% of patients. The likelihood of a successful outcome decreases in less experienced hands or when the diagnosis of Cushing's disease is incorrect. Because of this, I recommend that this procedure be performed only by surgeons with significant experience in the treatment of patients with Cushing's disease, preferably in consultation with endocrinologists familiar with the vagaries of these diagnostic tests.

The success of resection of macroadenomas, recurrent tumor, or tumor invading the cavernous sinus decreases dramatically so that surgical therapy is not clearly superior to treatment with radiation therapy and adrenolytic agents or adrenalectomy.

Alternative treatments of Cushing's disease include radiation therapy and adrenalectomy. Radiation therapy to the pituitary gland with adjunctive medical therapy to normalize cortisol levels is a good option for patients who cannot undergo surgery, and for those in whom the risk of Nelson's syndrome is deemed great. Adrenalectomy may be chosen over radiation therapy by young patients desiring fertility who have concerns about radiation-induced hypopituitarism and loss of reproductive function. Adrenalectomy is preferred also if rapid normalization of hypercortisolism is needed. Medical therapy alone is rarely appropriate, as it requires close monitoring and adjustment of dose and has low long-term efficacy. When this approach is chosen, mitotane may be the best agent if an adrenolytic dose can be tolerated.

Conventional radiation therapy (45 Gy) alone achieves a remission in a minority of adults (20%) but the majority of children (80%). The reason(s) for this difference is not known. The response of adults increases to 90% with the adjuvant use of steroidogenesis inhibitors, usually mitotane (Lysodren) or ketoconazole (Nizoral).* Medical therapy is initiated with radiation therapy and increased as needed to normalize cortisol values; when the urine free cortisol value is around 50 μg per day, the dose of adrenal blockade should be reduced and biochemical parameters monitored frequently to avoid hypocortisolism. Some patients require mitotane (250 mg to 4 grams/ daily, or on alternate days) up to 15 years after radiation therapy. Since remission has not been reported upon discontinuation of medical therapy beyond 11 years after radiation, it is reasonable to consider adrenalectomy at that time.

Stereotactic radiosurgery of the pituitary gland (60 to 150 Gy in four doses) with heavily-charged particles from proton or helium beams is available only at a few centers. It appears to give an improved response compared with conventional radiation therapy but has not been studied as extensively. Adverse effects include injury to the optic nerves (<5%) and hypopituitarism (33%).

In contrast to radiation therapy, bilateral adrenal-ectomy provides rapid resolution of hypercortisolism without risk of hypopituitarism. The major disadvantage is a lifelong requirement for glucocorticoid and mineralocorticoid therapy. The reported mortality (3%) and morbidity (1% to 20%) reflect the severity of Cushing's syndrome, the presence of associated conditions such as cardiovascular disease, and the choice of incision. The adrenal glands in Cushing's disease are usually amenable to open resection via bilateral flank incisions or to the promising newer laparoscopic approach, which avoids the technical problems associated with massive intra-abdominal obesity.

Ectopic ACTH/CRH Secretion

Patients with ACTH and/or CRH secretion from an ectopic source can be cured if the tumor is not metastatic, and if it can be found and removed. If the source of ACTH cannot be localized, or if metastatic disease precludes surgery, alternative treatment of hypercortisolism must be chosen. Intermittent surveillance for occult tumors must continue because of their malignant potential.

Medical therapy (discussed later) for the patient with occult disease allows for interval tumor surveillance with the goal of eventual tumor resection. As some tumors remain occult for up to 20 years, this may not prove practical for all patients. Long-term medical therapy is indicated for the patient with widely disseminated disease who is not a good surgical candidate for adrenalectomy. Short-term medical therapy may be used to prepare a patient for adrenalectomy. I recommend adrenalectomy when maximal daily doses of ketoconazole, aminoglutethimide, and metyrapone given in combination do not render the patient eucortisolemic, when previously effective medical therapy must be discontinued because of significant medical side effect or intolerance, and when a severely hypercortisolemic patient is unable to take oral medications.

Although some of the neuroendocrine islet cell tumors decrease ACTH secretion during somatostatin or interferon treatment, experience with these agents is limited.

Primary Adrenal Disease

Nonmalignant causes of Cushing's syndrome deriving from the adrenal gland(s) are cured by resection of the abnormal tissue, whether unilateral or bilateral. An anterior incision, allowing for en bloc tumor resection and abdominal exploration, is indicated for resection of adrenal carcinoma and tumors larger than 6 cm, whereas a posterior open or laparoscopic approach avoids the technical problems associated with intra-abdominal obesity and is recommended for smaller glands.

Surgery is the mainstay in the treatment of adrenal cancer; more aggressive surgical approaches directed to local recurrences and metastases probably account for the increase in lifespan reported in this

---

*Not FDA-approved for this indication.

disease. Adjuvant treatment with suramin,* keto-conazole,* gossypol,† and combination chemotherapy has not been uniformly successful. Mitotane is the treatment of choice for patients requiring control of hypercortisolism after surgery, as it may provide chemotherapeutic benefit.

Perioperative and Postoperative Considerations

Preoperative Evaluation and Treatment. Preoperative adrenal blockade is necessary only if wound healing would be compromised by severe hypercortisolism and is given empirically to achieve a minimum of one month of eucortisolism before surgery. The associated medical conditions of hypercortisolism, especially diabetes, hypertension, and cardiovascular disease, should be assessed and treated to decrease perioperative morbidity and mortality. Spironolactone blockade of mineralocorticoid action, a good theoretical choice for blood pressure reduction, is often insufficient. However, spironolactone may reverse hypokalemia at doses up to 400 mg per day.

Postoperative Evaluation and Treatment. Patients typically receive supraphysiologic doses of glucocorticoids after all surgical procedures, at initial daily doses of up to 300 mg of hydrocortisone (4 mg of dexamethasone), tapering off within two days (after transsphenoidal surgery) or when the patient can take oral medication (after abdominal or thoracic procedures). Morning serum cortisol and daily urine free cortisol measurements are then obtained for three days without glucocorticoid administration, while watching for signs of adrenal insufficiency.

Plasma cortisol values that remain unchanged from preoperative values reflect surgical failure. Eucortisolemic patients with morning cortisol values of 6 to 9 μg per dL have a greater risk of recurrence compared with hypocortisolemic patients.

Postoperative hypocortisolism reflects adequate removal of the cause of hypercortisolism, which then unmasks the underlying suppression of the hypothalamic-pituitary-adrenal axis. Morning cortisol values of less than 3.6 μg per dL and daily urine free cortisol excretion of less than 20 μg suggest cure. If cortisol values are consistently below 5 μg per dL, dexamethasone replacement, 0.5 mg per day in the morning, is begun to allow continued assessment of cortisol secretion. Prior to discharge, hydrocortisone, at a physiologic replacement dose of 12 to 15 mg per m², is substituted for dexamethasone. This agent, in contrast to prednisone, hydrocortisone acetate, or dexamethasone, is consistently absorbed and has biologic effects identical to those of cortisol. Additionally, the available tablet formulations provide great flexibility in dose adjustment and scheduling. Most patients do well with a single morning dose of steroids taken before getting out of bed; a split-dose strategy in which one third of the total daily dose is taken be-tween 3 and 6 P.M. may be effective for those complaining of extreme evening fatigue.

Patients with preoperative adrenal steroidogenesis blockade or episodic hypercortisolism may have had partial recovery of the adrenal axis so that postoperative cortisol cannot be used to assess surgical efficacy. The diurnal cortisol rhythm can be used, however, as it will be normal after successful surgery.

After bilateral adrenalectomy, hydrocortisone (at about twice replacement) and saline 0.9% are given intravenously, to provide sodium and sufficient mineralocorticoid activity until fludrocortisone (Florinef) (100 μg per day) can be given by mouth. Cortisol secretion to confirm adequacy of resection is then assessed while the patient receives dexamethasone and fludrocortisone. Discharge orders should substitute hydrocortisone and retain fludrocortisone. The dose of fludrocortisone is adjusted according to the patient's blood pressure, exposure to heat, and salt intake; the usual dose is 100 μg daily but ranges from 50 to 400 μg. A normal plasma renin activity measurement provides evidence for adequate mineralocorticoid replacement and can be used to gauge therapy. Adjustments in hydrocortisone dosage above 15 mg per m² are rarely necessary if mineralocorticoid replacement is adequate.

The patient should wear an identification bracelet noting the requirement for glucocorticoids. Education should stress the effects of glucocorticoid withdrawal, the need for compliance with the daily dose of glucocorticoid, the need to double the oral dose for nausea, diarrhea, and fever, and the need for parenteral administration and medical evaluation during emesis, trauma, or severe medical stress. I instruct patients to self-inject hydrocortisone before seeking medical attention if advanced signs of adrenal insufficiency are present.

The components of the hypothalamic-pituitary-adrenal axis gradually recover within 3 to 24 months of surgical cure of Cushing's syndrome, if at least one adrenal gland remains. The time until recovery may be shorter in patients with mild hypercortisolism and those who ultimately recur, and longer after resection of an adrenal adenoma. Recovery of the axis can be monitored by the cortisol response to synthetic ACTH (cosyntropin [Cortrosyn], 250 μg intravenously) administered at intervals, beginning at 6 to 9 months. Glucocorticoid replacement can be discontinued abruptly when the cortisol response at 30 to 60 minutes exceeds 18 μg/dL.

Glucocorticoid replacement during recovery of the axis may be managed in a variety of ways, as long as adrenal insufficiency and iatrogenic Cushing's syndrome are avoided. The Cortrosyn test and clinical assessment of the patient's sense of well-being, blood pressure, weight, and regression of cushingoid features provide useful measures of recovery. The hydrocortisone dose should be recalculated and adjusted as the patient loses weight. Hydrocortisone may also be weaned, beginning at around 6 months if the cortisol response to cosyntropin exceeds 9 μg per dL, by reducing the total daily dose by 5 mg

---

*Investigational drug in the United States.
†Not FDA-approved for this indication.

every 4 to 8 weeks. One disadvantage of weaning is that patients may complain of intolerable symptoms of glucocorticoid withdrawal. If this occurs, the daily dose of hydrocortisone may be increased by 2.5 or 5 mg, and the steroid taper may be reinitiated two months later.

The question of recurrence arises in a minority of patients after successful surgery. Patients who say that the Cushing's syndrome has returned are often correct. Measurement of urine free cortisol is warranted in these patients and those with recurrent physical signs characteristic of their hypercortisolemic phase. This should be done initially on dexamethasone, 0.5 mg per day, if the patient is not yet weaned from glucocorticoids. If the UFC excretion is increased, evaluation of hypercortisolism should proceed. If the result is subnormal or low, the patient should be questioned about the actual dose of glucocorticoid that has been taken. Often patients take additional hydrocortisone and have a suppressed axis and very slow regression of cushingoid features because of exogenous hypercortisolism. They require education and support along with reduction in the daily dose of hydrocortisone to recommended levels.

MEDICAL THERAPY

Medical therapy is indicated if the patient cannot safely undergo surgery or if the tumor is occult or metastatic. A major disadvantage is the need for lifelong therapy; in general, recurrence follows discontinuation of treatment. These agents have two broad mechanisms of action. One class of compounds modulates ACTH release from a pituitary tumor and is restricted to the treatment of Cushing's disease. The second class of agents reduces cortisol levels or action through adrenolytic activity, inhibition of steroidogenesis, or antagonism of cortisol action at the level of the receptor. These compounds are used in the treatment of all forms of Cushing's syndrome.

Agents That Modulate Pituitary ACTH Release

Compounds that affect CRH or ACTH synthesis or release, including cyproheptadine, bromocriptine, somatostatin, and valproic acid, have been examined as single therapeutic agents for Cushing's disease. Response rates are poor, but no large-scale, placebo-controlled trials have been reported. Daily doses and side effects are shown in Table 1.

Agents That Inhibit Steroidogenesis

Mitotane, trilostane, ketoconazole, aminoglutethimide, and metyrapone decrease cortisol by inhibition of steroidogenesis at one or more enzymatic steps (Table 2). There is little clinical experience with other agents, such as etomidate and other imidazole derivatives with a similar mechanism of action. Unfortunately, apart from etomidate, no available agent can be given parenterally.

TABLE 1. **Agents That Modulate ACTH Release**

Agent	Daily Dose*	Major Side Effects
Bromocriptine (Parlodel)	3–30 mg	Postural hypotension, nausea
Cyproheptadine (Periactin)	4–24 mg	Sedation, weight gain
Valproic acid (Depakene)	250–2000 mg	Sedation, nausea, hepatic toxicity
Octreotide acetate	600–3000 mg, SC	Diarrhea, gallstones

*Medications are given PO and in divided doses, except as indicated.

Steroidogenesis blockade can be titrated to complete or partial inhibition of cortisol production, as judged by urine cortisol excretion. Full adrenal blockade requires glucocorticoid replacement to avoid symptoms of adrenal insufficiency in patients with variable cortisol production. Often complete inhibition of cortisol production is not achieved, and the additive effects of exogenous and endogenous cortisol render the patient hypercortisolemic. This approach also requires higher doses of medications, with concomitant greater costs and adverse effects. For these reasons I recommend partial inhibition of cortisol production, which aims to render the patient eucortisolemic without additional exogenous hydrocortisone. Patients and their physicians must be alert for the signs and symptoms of adrenal insufficiency, which are treated by reduction or brief discontinuation of the agent(s), and with hydrocortisone if necessary.

Ketoconazole, the most recent addition to this class of compounds, is the best tolerated. It inhibits cytochrome P450 enzymes, including side-chain cleavage, 17,20 lyase, 11 β-hydroxylase, and 17α-hydroxylase. Therapy is initiated at a daily dose of 600 mg and increased to 1600 mg in four divided doses. Side effects of gastrointestinal distress and gynecomastia occur in less than 15% of patients. Menstruant women may experience irregular menses. Reversible hepatic dysfunction, manifest by increased hepatocellular enzymes, is common and need not provoke discontinuation of the agent if levels remain below two- to threefold normal. Although reports of idiosyncratic hepatic dyscrasia, occurring in about 1 in 15,000

TABLE 2. **Agents That Inhibit Steroidogenesis**

Agent	Daily Dose*	Major Side Effects
Ketoconazole (Nizoral)	600–1600 mg	Hepatic toxicity, GI disturbance, gynecomastia
Aminoglutethimide (Cytadren)	0.5–2 gm	Neurologic complaints, rash, sedation
Metyrapone (Metopirone)†	1–4.5 gm	Hypertension, acne, hirsutism, nausea
Trilostane (Modrastane)†	120–960 mg	GI disturbance, paresthesias
Mitotane (Lysodren)	0.5–8 gm	GI disturbance, neurologic complaints

*Medications are given PO and in divided doses, except for mitotane, which may be given once daily.
†Investigational drug in the United States.

cases, have diminished enthusiasm for its use, a relatively benign spectrum of side effects and the potential for single-agent therapy make ketoconazole a first choice for many patients. Ketoconazole is not an option in patients treated with H_2 antagonists because gastric acidity is necessary to metabolize it into the active compound.

Metyrapone* or aminoglutethimide may be useful as sole treatment for ectopic ACTH secretion or adrenal adenoma, in combination with radiation therapy of the pituitary for Cushing's disease, or in combination with other agents for the treatment of ectopic ACTH secretion. Metyrapone is begun at a daily dose of 1 gram (in four divided doses) and increased every few days to a maximal daily dose of 4.5 grams, although often no further gain is obtained beyond a daily dose of 2 grams. Its inhibition of 11β-hydroxylase increases androgenic and mineralocorticoid precursors, resulting in dose-dependent hypertension, acne, and hirsutism during long-term treatment at daily doses of 2 to 3 grams per day. Nausea and dizziness may also limit its use.

Aminoglutethimide is begun at a dose of 500 mg daily, in four divided doses, and may be increased by 250 to 500 mg every 3 to 4 days to a total dose of 2 grams. Neurologic complaints, including somnolence, dizziness, depression, and blurred vision, are common (30%), especially at daily doses greater than 1 gram. A transient morbilliform rash and fever are seen in about 20% of patients within the first 2 weeks of therapy; therapy need not be discontinued.

Mitotane, or o,p'-DDD, inhibits steroidogenesis at the steps of side-chain cleavage, 11- and 18-hydroxylase and 3β-hydroxysteroid dehydrogenase. Its additional adrenolytic action has led to its chemotherapeutic use in the treatment of adrenal cancer, but the contribution of the agent to improved survival remains unclear. Therapy begins at 0.5 to 1 gram per day, given with food, and is increased gradually, by 0.5 to 1 gram every one to four weeks. The utility of mitotane is limited by its gastrointestinal and neurologic toxicity, which may persist because of the long half-life (18 to 159 days). Nausea and diarrhea are common at doses greater than 2 grams per day. At the higher doses, neurologic findings, including gait disturbances, dizziness or vertigo, confusion, and problems with expressive language, are common. Fatigue, gynecomastia, skin rash, hyperlipidemia, hypouricemia, and elevated liver enzymes also occur. Mitotane is relatively contraindicated in women desiring fertility within 2 to 5 years, as it is an abortifacient and a teratogen. If adrenal crisis or gastrointestinal symptoms occur, the drug should be stopped. Usually symptoms improve within a week, and mitotane can be restarted at a previously tolerated lower dose.

Trilostane* is a relatively weak inhibitor of steroidogenesis that rarely induces remission, even at maximal daily doses. It may prove useful in combination treatment strategies.

*Investigational drug in the United States.

The anesthetic etomidate (Amidate),* is an imidazole derivative that inhibits cholesterol side-chain cleavage and 11β-hydroxylase. Its use is limited by its sedating properties and the necessity for intravenous administration.

RU 486 is a steroid that binds competitively to the glucocorticoid and progestin receptors and inhibits the action of the endogenous ligands. Its use in Cushing's syndrome has been limited to a few investigational studies of patients with ectopic ACTH secretion, and it is not available presently in the U.S.

---

*Not FDA-approved for this indication.

DIABETES INSIPIDUS

method of
DAVID R. BROOKER, M.D., and
LAWRENCE S. WEISBERG, M.D.
*UMDNJ/Robert Wood Johnson Medical School
at Camden, Cooper Hospital/University
Medical Center*
Camden, New Jersey

Approximately 60% of the weight of the human body derives from water. Total body water (TBW) is divided into an extracellular fluid (ECF) compartment, constituting one-third of TBW, and an intracellular fluid (ICF) compartment, constituting the remaining two-thirds. For example, the TBW of a 70-kg adult is calculated as 0.60×70, or 42 liters, of which 14 liters are extracellular and 28 liters are intracellular. The intravascular space makes up only one-fourth of the ECF and, therefore, only one-twelfth ($\frac{1}{4} \times \frac{1}{3}$) of TBW. Because solute-free water readily equilibrates across all fluid compartments, the loss of 1 liter of solute-free water from the body is experienced as an intravascular loss of only 83 mL; the gain of 1 liter of solute-free water results in expansion of the intravascular space by only 83 mL. Thus, the loss or gain of large volumes of solute-free water tends to have a relatively small effect on an individual's volume status. In contrast, such changes in water balance result in proportionate changes in body fluid osmolality, seen as alterations in the concentration of ECF (plasma) sodium, the predominant extracellular solute.

The osmolality of body fluids is maintained within a very narrow range around a set point, normally about 280 mOsm per kg. Such tight regulation is achieved by two cooperative homeostatic mechanisms: the action of vasopressin or antidiuretic hormone (ADH), and thirst. Slight increases (1 to 2%) in plasma osmolality (e.g., as a result of water deprivation) are sensed by osmoreceptors in the anterior hypothalamus, which stimulates synthesis of ADH and its release into the circulation by the posterior pituitary. Circulating ADH binds to receptors on the collecting duct, leading to an increase in water permeability of that segment of the nephron. Filtered water may then be reabsorbed down its concentration gradient from the duct lumen into the concentrated medullary interstitium and is returned to the circulation via the vasa recta, thus mitigating the rise in plasma osmolality. By the time plasma osmolality reaches 290 mOsm per kg, the circulating ADH concentration will have risen to 4 to 5 pg per mL, a level that induces maximal urinary concentration (about 1200 mOsm per kg). Further increases in plasma osmolality stimulate thirst and water ingestion, which returns plasma osmolality to normal.

PATHOPHYSIOLOGY OF DIABETES INSIPIDUS

Diabetes insipidus (DI) is a state of inadequate urinary concentration. This results in excessive urinary loss of solute-free water and a tendency toward total-body hyperosmolality and hypernatremia. Owing to an intact thirst mechanism, most individuals with DI are able to replace their urinary water losses and thus maintain a near-normal serum sodium concentration.

There are three general types of DI. Nephrogenic DI (NDI) is caused by renal unresponsiveness to appropriate circulating levels of ADH. Alternatively, DI may result from inadequate levels of circulating ADH, either from deficient pituitary release of ADH (termed central DI, or CDI) or from accelerated degradation of circulating ADH. The latter syndrome occurs in pregnancy and is caused by increased vasopressinase activity, leading to so-called vasopressin-resistant DI.

The specific causes of CDI and NDI are summarized in Table 1.

CLINICAL PRESENTATION

Patients with DI present most commonly with polyuria, defined as a urine volume of greater than 30 mL per kg per 24 hours. Hypernatremic hyperosmolality develops when water intake does not match urinary water losses (e.g., in patients with severe DI or in comatose, bed-bound, or demented patients). Hyperosmolality of the ECF results in transcellular water movement, leading initially to cellular dehydration. The accompanying cerebral dehydration may lead to fatigue, lethargy, confusion, seizures, and even coma. The brain adapts to cell volume contraction by generating new intracellular osmotically active solutes (idiogenic osmoles), causing shift of water back into the cells and restoration of normal brain volume after several days. This sequence of adaptive events has important therapeutic implications (see "Treatment").

Volume contraction, manifested by tachycardia and hypotension, becomes manifest only when intravascular fluid losses exceed 10 to 15%. Because of the uniform distribu-

TABLE 1. **Causes of Diabetes Insipidus**

Central

Idiopathic
Postsurgical
Head trauma
Neoplastic—craniopharyngioma, lymphoma, metastatic disease
Hypoxic/ischemic—cardiopulmonary arrest, shock, Sheehan's
  syndrome
Granulomatous—hysticytosis X, sarcoidosis
Infection—encephalitis, meningitis
Autoimmune
Familial

Nephrogenic

Familial
Chronic renal disease
Hypokalemia
Hypercalcemia
Postobstruction
Drugs—lithium, demeclocycline, methoxyflurane anesthesia
Sickle cell anemia
Sjögren's syndrome

tion of body water, this occurs in an adult after TBW losses of 4 to 6 liters, at which point the serum sodium concentration will have reached 155 to 160 mEq per liter.

Most cases of CDI, especially those following trauma or surgery, are self-limited, lasting 3 to 5 days. A classic triphasic syndrome may be seen following severe head trauma. Initially, there is abrupt cessation of ADH release from the posterior pituitary, accompanied by polyuria. After about a week, an antidiuretic phase ensues, characterized by urinary concentration and water retention with a tendency toward hyponatremia, lasting 5 to 6 days. This appears to result from the release of stored ADH from degenerating hypothalamic neurons. CDI recurs when the ADH stores are depleted.

Both CDI and NDI may be complete or partial, the degree of polyuria being dependent on the extent of the defect.

DIAGNOSIS

Care must be taken in making a diagnosis of DI, since irrationally based treatment may be futile or catastrophic. For example, erroneous administration of vasopressin to a polyuric patient with primary polydipsia can lead to rapid water retention, profound hyponatremia, and attendant neurologic sequelae.

A diagnostic strategy for evaluating a polyuric patient is outlined in Figure 1. Patients undergoing water deprivation must be supervised carefully, since those with complete DI may become dehydrated quickly. A water deprivation test is unnecessary and may be dangerous in a patient who is already hypertonic. Reliably distinguishing partial NDI from primary polydipsia often requires a detailed medical history and close clinical observation; at the end of the water deprivation test, the plasma ADH concentration may be similarly elevated in both disorders.

TREATMENT

The goals of treatment in DI are to correct volume depletion, correct the water deficit, replace ongoing urinary water losses, and limit the degree of polyuria. Volume depletion is diagnosed at the bedside by the presence of tachycardia, hypotension, or orthostatic changes in the vital signs. Volume resuscitation is performed with 0.9% NaCl solution (normal saline), even in patients who are hypernatremic.

The following formula is used to estimate a hypernatremic patient's water deficit:

$$\text{water deficit} = 0.6 \times BW \times (1 - [140/\text{current } S_{Na}])$$

where BW is the estimated premorbid body weight in kg, and S_{Na} is the current serum sodium concentration in mEq per liter. This formula is based on the questionable assumptions that TBW is 60% of body weight and that there is no net loss of solute during the development of the hypertonic state. As such, it provides only a rough estimate of the TBW deficit.

When the water deficit is greater than 10% (i.e., the serum sodium concentration is greater than 155 mEq per liter) and the disorder has been present for days, care should be taken to avoid overly rapid water replacement. Once the brain has adapted to hyperosmolality, the shift of rapidly administered water

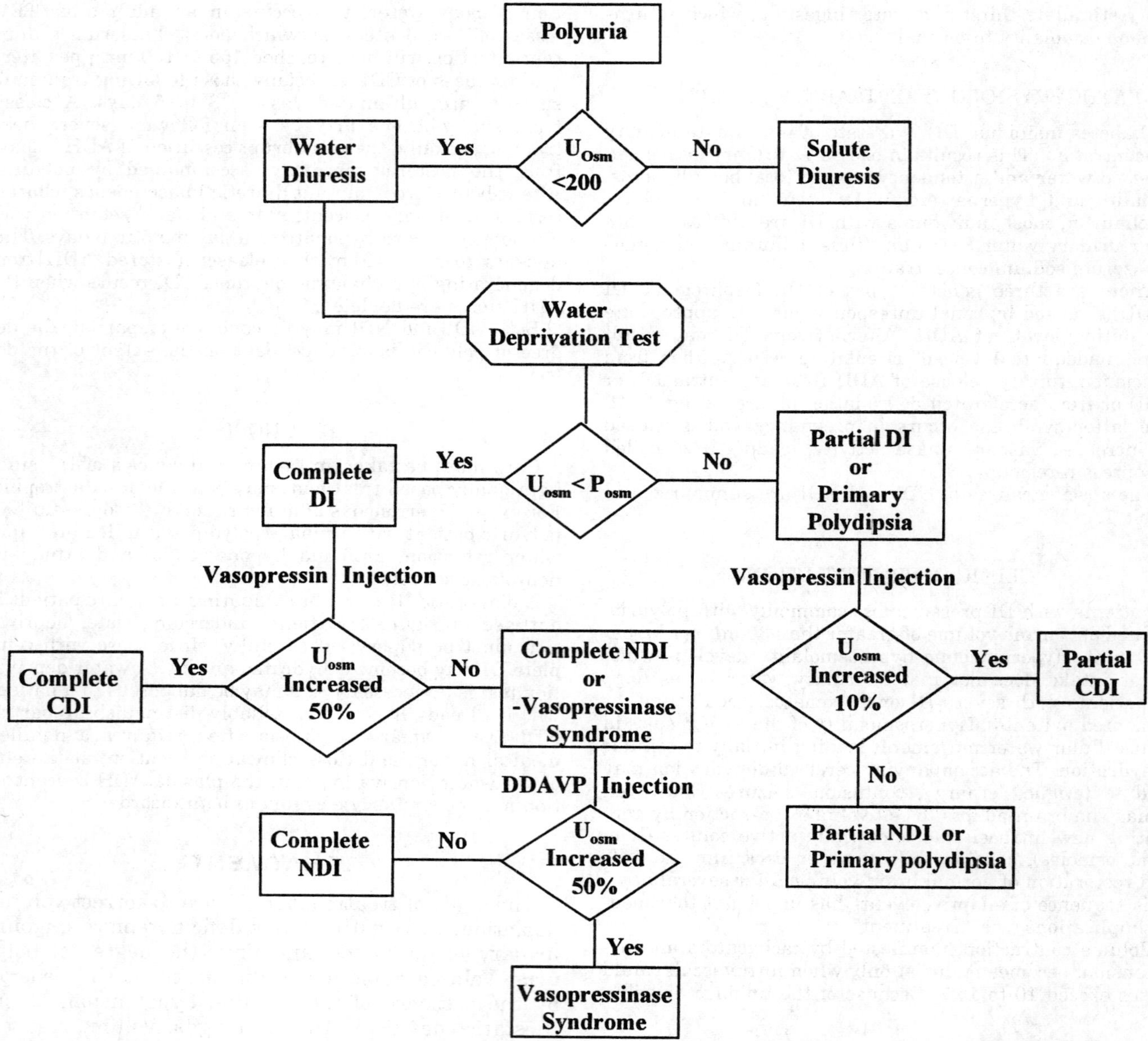

Figure 1. Diagnostic strategy for the evaluation of a polyuric patient. U_{osm}, P_{osm}, DI, CDI, and NDI are defined in the text. Vasopressin injection: subcutaneous injection of 5 U aqueous vasopressin. DDAVP injection: intravenous injection of 1 µg desmopressin.

into cells can lead to cerebral edema, accompanied by seizures, permanent neurologic damage, or death. The recommended rate of reduction of the serum sodium concentration is no more than 0.5 mEq per liter per hour, or 12 mEq per liter in the first 24 hours. Ignoring ongoing water losses, the amount of water needed over the first 24 hours to achieve that reduction may be estimated by:

$$[12 \div (\text{current } S_{Na} - 140)] \times \text{water deficit}$$

Because this formula provides only a rough estimate of the water deficit, serum electrolytes should be monitored frequently during therapy.

Several fluids are clinically available for water replacement therapy. Tap water administered enterally

is the preferred modality. For patients who cannot tolerate enteral water administration, the intravenous route is available. Usually a 5% dextrose solution (D5W) is given by peripheral vein. With the large quantities of fluid required in many hypernatremic patients, the glucose load may be substantial and may cause hyperglycemia in patients with diabetes mellitus. Volume overload rarely complicates D5W administration, since only 83 mL of every liter remains in the intravascular space (compared with normal saline solution, of which 250 mL of every liter remains in the intravascular space). A 0.45% NaCl solution (half-normal saline) may be ineffective in lowering the serum sodium concentration if the urinary sodium concentration is lower than that in the intravenous solution. Furthermore, the sodium load can be substantial and could result in volume overload and pulmonary edema, especially in patients with ventricular dysfunction.

Urine is composed of water and solute. The daily urinary solute-free water losses may be estimated by the following formula:

$$C_{H20} = V (1 - [U_{osm}/P_{osm}])$$

where C_{H20} is urinary solute-free water excretion, V is the urinary volume in 24 hours, U_{osm} is the urine osmolality, and P_{osm} is the plasma osmolality. Thus, if the urine volume is 4000 mL in 24 hours, the plasma osmolality is 310 mOsm per kg, and the urine osmolality is 100 mOsm per kg, the urinary solute-free water excretion is calculated as:

$$4000 \text{ mL} (1 - [100/310]) = 2709 \text{ mL}$$

This amount must be added to the quantity calculated to correct the existing water deficit in order to prevent further dehydration.

At this point, attention should be turned to reducing the degree of polyuria by addressing the specific disorder.

Treatment of CDI (Table 2). Hormone replacement is the mainstay of therapy in patients with CDI. In the acute (postsurgical or post-traumatic) setting, L-arginine vasopressin (Pitressin) may be used either subcutaneously or intravenously. The advantage of vasopressin in this setting is its short half-life, which allows the physician to repeatedly assess the need for continued hormone replacement in a disorder that is often self-limited. Because vasopressin targets both the V1 (vascular) and V2 (collecting duct) receptors, its use may be complicated by hypertension and myocardial ischemia; it should therefore be administered with caution to elderly patients or patients with known heart disease. Desmopressin (DDAVP) is a synthetic analogue of L-arginine vasopressin whose altered structure confers the advantages of a longer half-life and attenuated vasoconstrictive properties. The injectable form may be given subcutaneously or intravenously and is supplied in 2-mL vials at 4 μg per mL. It is the agent of choice in patients with chronic CDI and is most often self-administered intranasally by means of a calibrated rhinal tube. This requires a degree of dexterity not possessed by all patients. A more convenient metered-dose nasal spray is available but does not allow for dose adjustment. An oral form of desmopressin is available in Europe but is not yet approved for use in the United States. Regardless of the modality of hormone replacement, therapy should be reduced or withdrawn intermittently to check for polyuria. This is especially important in patients with acute post-traumatic CDI, who may undergo a transient antidiuretic phase.

A variety of adjuvant agents may allow for a reduced hormone dose in patients with complete CDI or may obviate the need for hormonal therapy in patients with partial CDI. Chlorpropamide (Diabinese), a sulfonylurea oral hypoglycemic agent, potentiates the effect of ADH on the collecting duct and thus decreases urinary dilution. It is ineffective in complete CDI or in NDI. The antidiuretic effect requires at least 4 days of treatment to become fully manifest. Hypoglycemia is the most important side effect and is most common in children and patients with concurrent hypopituitarism. The other sulfonyl-

TABLE 2. **Pharmacologic Treatment of Diabetes Insipidus**

Drug	Usual Total Daily Dose	Usual Frequency	Duration (Hours)
CDI—Hormonal			
Desmopressin (DDAVP)			
4 μg per mL for injection	2–4 μg IV or SC	qd or bid	8–12
10 μg per mL nasal spray	10–40 μg intranasally	qd or bid	8–12
100 μg per mL with calibrated rhinal tube	10–40 μg intranasally	qd or bid	8–12
Vasopressin (Pitressin)			
20 U per mL	5–10 U SC	q 2–4 h	2–6
Lypressin (Diapid)			
185 μg per mL nasal spray	7–14 μg intranasally	q 4–8 h	3–8
CDI—Nonhormonal			
Chlorpropamide (Diabinese)*			
100- and 250-mg tablets	100–500 mg PO	qd or bid	24–48
Clofibrate (Atromid-S)*			
500-mg tablets	1000–4000 mg PO	bid to qid	12–24
Carbamazepine (Tegretol)*			
100- and 200-mg tablets	400–1200 PO	bid	12–24
NDI			
Hydrochlorothiazide (HydroDIURIL)			
25-, 50-, and 100-mg tablets	25–100 mg PO	qd or bid	24–48
Amiloride (Midamor)			
5-mg tablets	5–20 mg PO	qd or bid	24
Indomethacin (Indocin)*			
25- and 50-mg tablets	50–200 mg PO	bid or tid	6–8

*Not FDA-approved for this indication.

urea hypoglycemic agents have less antidiuretic potency, and the later-generation oral hypoglycemic agents have no antidiuretic effect. Hydrochlorothiazide (HydroDIURIL), a thiazide diuretic, acts in two ways to decrease urinary solute-free water excretion. First, by causing volume depletion, it enhances reabsorption of glomerular filtrate in the proximal tubule, thus reducing delivery of filtrate to the diluting sites of the nephron. Second, it impairs urinary dilution by blocking sodium reabsorption in the distal tubule. All thiazide diuretics are similarly efficacious in this regard. The major side effects are volume depletion and hypokalemia. Carbamazepine (Tegretol)* is an anticonvulsant that has been shown to enhance ADH release in patients with partial CDI. Serious bone marrow toxicity (aplastic anemia and agranulocytosis) limits the use of this medication in the treatment of CDI. Similarly, clofibrate (Atromid-S),* an antihyperlipidemic agent, may stimulate ADH release, but its long-term side effects contraindicate its use in CDI.

Treatment of NDI (Table 2). Thiazide diuretics (HydroDIURIL) are the first line of treatment for NDI, for reasons discussed previously. Patients taking lithium must have drug levels monitored closely when starting a thiazide diuretic, since the diuretic-induced volume depletion will reduce renal lithium elimination and may result in toxicity. The diuretic amiloride (Midamor) may block lithium uptake by the distal nephron and may therefore ameliorate lithium-induced NDI. Renal prostaglandins increase urinary water excretion by antagonizing the effect of ADH and increasing medullary blood flow. The prostaglandin synthesis inhibitor indomethacin (Indocin)* may thus reduce urinary dilution in NDI.

Treatment of Vasopressinase Excess. Because desmopressin is resistant to degradation by vasopressinase, it is the agent of choice in this setting. The dosing guidelines for CDI are applicable to patients with this disorder. Because this is a complication of pregnancy, it is self-limited.

---

*Not FDA-approved for this indication.

GOITER

method of
CHARLES H. EMERSON, M.D.
University of Massachusetts Medical Center
Worcester, Massachusetts

A goiter is an enlarged thyroid gland. In lay usage, the term refers to visible enlargement of the thyroid gland. For clinical purposes, a goiter is present regardless of whether thyroid enlargement is ascertained by inspection, palpation, or imaging procedures. Enlargement of the thyroid may be focal or generalized. If focal, it usually has the characteristics of a thyroid nodule. If generalized, the enlargement may be symmetrical or asymmetrical and either diffuse or nodular. It is useful to describe these features, since they have diagnostic implications. The nature of thyroid enlargement is not completely specific for any disorder, however. Most importantly, although thyroid cancer usually presents as a thyroid nodule, it can occur in any type of goiter, be it focal or generalized, symmetrical or asymmetrical, diffuse or nodular.

PATHOGENESIS AND CLASSIFICATION

Table 1 presents a pathophysiologic classification of goiter. Thyroid enlargement is caused by processes that are intrinsic to the thyroid (primary goiter) or by those originating outside the thyroid (secondary goiter).

Primary Goiter

In the United States, the most common forms of primary goiter are colloid goiter (simple goiter) and multinodular goiter; both are probably variants of the same disorder. An early concept was that colloid and multinodular goiters were related to the induction of subclinical hypothyroidism by unidentified goitrogens. With the development of methods for measuring serum thyroid-stimulating hormone (TSH) concentrations, this view has not received support, at least from studies of goitrous patients in the United States. The theory that nodular thyroid disease is caused by somatic mutations and that these, in turn, induce neoplastic transformation is being actively pursued.

Thyroid cancer is the most important, though not the most common, cause of primary goiter. Although most thyroid cancers present as a solitary nodule, this is not always the case; one reason is that thyroid cancer sometimes coex-

TABLE 1. **Pathophysiologic Classification of Goiter**

Primary

Neoplastic
  Malignant tumors
    Epithelial cell thyroid carcinoma (papillary and
      follicular)
    Anaplastic thyroid carcinoma
    Medullary thyroid carcinoma
  Benign tumors
    Epithelial cell thyroid adenoma (papillary and
      follicular)
    Multinodular goiter (sporadic nontoxic goiter)
Other
  Colloid goiter

Secondary

Thyroinvasive
  Metastatic solid tumors
  Lymphoma
  Granulomatous diseases
  Hashimoto's thyroiditis
  Riedel's thyroiditis
  Subacute thyroiditis
  Painless thyroiditis
  Amyloid goiter
Thyrostimulatory
  Thyrotropin (TSH) mediated
    Hashimoto's thyroiditis
    Endemic, iodine-deficiency goiter
    Hereditary goiter
    Colloid goiter
  Thyroid-stimulating immune globulin (TSI) mediated
    Graves' disease
  Human chorionic gonadotropin (hCG) mediated
    Goiter of pregnancy
  Growth hormone (GH) mediated
    Goiter of acromegaly

ists with other conditions that cause goiter. It is not rare, for example, for papillary thyroid cancer to occur in Hashimoto's thyroiditis. Occasionally, thyroid cancer develops within a long-standing multinodular goiter. Another reason that goiters other than solitary nodules may harbor a cancer is that some types of thyroid cancer, such as papillary and medullary carcinoma, are sometimes multicentric.

Secondary Goiter

Thyroinvasive Goiter. One mechanism for the development of secondary goiters is invasion of the thyroid by "foreign" cells—referred to here as "thyroinvasive goiter." Hashimoto's thyroiditis is the most important form of thyroinvasive goiter. In this condition, the thyroid is infiltrated with lymphoid cells, giving rise to focal areas of inflammation and a "bumpy" texture on palpation. This feature is sometimes so pronounced that a discrete nodule is noted. Other causes of thyroinvasive goiter are metastatic cancer, infection, and systemic diseases such as sarcoidosis. Fibrosclerosis is a disease of unknown etiology. When it involves the thyroid it is known as Riedel's struma. In some unusual disorders, such as the goiter of systemic amyloidosis, the invading cells produce enough material to enlarge the thyroid.

Thyrostimulated Goiter. The other fundamental mechanism for the development of secondary goiter is stimulation of the thyroid by circulating hormones—referred to here as "thyrostimulated goiter." Many drugs and chemicals cause goiters by this mechanism and, as such, are called goitrogens. Their primary action is to inhibit thyroid hormone secretion. The ensuing hypothyroidism, even if mild, causes serum TSH concentrations to increase. This, in turn, promotes generalized thyroid growth. The antithyroid drugs propylthiouracil and methimazole are strong goitrogens. Other drugs with weaker goitrogenic properties include *p*-aminosalicylic acid, tolbutamide, and resorcinol. Because of its widespread use and inherent antithyroid properties, lithium is an important goitrogenic drug. The pathogenesis of lithium-induced goiter may be complex, however, because lithium is also concentrated by the thyroid, perhaps causing a reaction in surrounding thyroid tissue. Hashimoto's thyroiditis, a form of thyroinvasive goiter, is also a form of thyrostimulated goiter because of the eventual development of hypothyroidism in many patients. In the United States, the incidence of Hashimoto's thyroiditis is high, making it the most prevalent cause of TSH-mediated thyrostimulated goiter. In global regions where there is iodine deficiency, endemic goiter is the most important cause of TSH-mediated thyrostimulated goiter. Serum TSH concentrations need not be elevated to cause endemic goiter, because iodine deficiency sensitizes the thyroid to the growth-promoting effects of TSH. In some endemic goiter regions, the population is exposed to goitrogens in the water or diet. This potentiates the effects of iodine deficiency. In a few localities, environmental goitrogens may be the major cause of goiter. Other causes of TSH-mediated thyrostimulated goiter are TSH-producing pituitary tumors, congenital goiter due to inborn errors of thyroid hormone synthesis, and the thyroid hormone resistance syndromes.

Not all forms of thyrostimulated goiter are caused by TSH. The goiter of Graves' disease is produced by thyroid-stimulating autoantibodies that recognize and activate the TSH receptor. Human chorionic gonadotropin (hCG) is another thyroid-stimulating substance. Its thyroid-stimulating effects are much weaker than TSH, but in some disorders such as hydatidiform mole and choriocarcinoma, it is produced in large enough quantities to cause goiter and even hyperthyroidism. Human chorionic gonadotropin also causes thyroid enlargement in pregnancy. This is usually so mild that it is not apparent on physical examination but can be documented by ultrasound. Mild thyroid enlargement, along with similar changes in other visceral organs, occurs in acromegaly due to the growth-stimulating effects of somatotropin.

EVALUATION OF GOITER

There are two fundamental issues that must be addressed in a patient who presents with goiter. One concerns the thyroid function, the other the pathology of the goiter.

Thyroid Function

A free thyroxine index (FTI) and a third-generation serum TSH assay are sufficient in most patients with goiter to uncover subclinical thyroid dysfunction or, when signs and symptoms are present, to confirm the clinical impression of thyrotoxicosis or hypothyroidism. Obviously, the major reason for thyroid function testing is to determine whether treatment for hypothyroidism or thyrotoxicosis is indicated. However, thyroid function tests can also provide a sense of the pathologic nature of the goiter (but not definitive information). If the patient is thyrotoxic, a thyroid malignancy is unlikely to be the cause of the goiter. Hyperthyroidism may be caused by primary thyroid cancer or by a cancer that has metastasized to the thyroid, but this is rare. More likely, a thyrotoxic patient has Graves' disease if the goiter is diffuse and antithyroid antibodies are positive, or a toxic multinodular goiter if the thyroid examination is consistent with this and the antithyroid antibodies are negative. Silent thyroiditis, subacute thyroiditis, and toxic solitary adenoma are other common causes of thyrotoxicosis and thyroid enlargement. The first two conditions, in contrast to Graves' disease, are associated with a low thyroid radioactive iodine uptake (see elsewhere). If thyroid function testing shows that the patient is hypothyroid and the serum test for antithyroid antibodies is positive, the presumptive diagnosis is Hashimoto's thyroiditis. If there is a distinct thyroid nodule, however, the possibility of associated thyroid cancer must be considered. Rapid enlargement of the thyroid in a patient with Hashimoto's thyroiditis may be due to thyroid lymphoma.

Thyroid Morphology

The most important reason for ascertaining the pathology of goitrous tissue is to detect and treat thyroid cancer. In an afebrile patient with painless thyroid enlargement, there is rarely the need to determine whether a specific infection is present unless the patient has human immunodeficiency virus (HIV) or another cause of severe immune deficiency. Whereas serum tests are generally used to evaluate thyroid function, information relevant to thyroid morphology is obtained by examining the thyroid itself. There are several exceptions. Determination of antithyroid antibodies is extremely useful if a sensitive test is ordered. A test for antibodies against thyroid peroxidase should be ordered in almost all patients with goiter. Another useful serum test is the determination of serum calcitonin concentrations after pentagastrin and/or calcium infusion. A rise in serum calcitonin is highly suggestive of medullary thyroid carcinoma (MTC). This test is generally limited to selected patients, including patients with a family history of MTC or those with physical features of multiple endocrine adenomatosis Type IIb, or when the needle biopsy suggests MTC (see the later discussion).

Thyroid Imaging. The thyroid can be imaged by radionuclide scanning, ultrasound, computed tomography (CT) scan, and magnetic resonance imaging (MRI). The most useful of these is the thyroid scan with [123]I. This scan should be performed in almost all nonpregnant patients who present for the first time with nodular thyroid disease. A thyroid scan should also be done in patients with diffuse goiter if there is a history of rapid thyroid enlargement or if the thyroid is so large that a sizable nodule would be difficult to palpate. The most crucial issue that the scan is concerned with is whether a palpable nodule is actively concentrating iodine or if there are focal regions of decreased iodine uptake. Thyroid cancers, along with many other lesions, are typically "cool" or "cold" on scan. Their decreased radioactive iodine uptake may be masked, however, if they are small or surrounded by normal tissue. If there are regions within the thyroid that are concentrating iodine, it is important to determine whether they are dependent on TSH secretion. Therefore, a scan after thyroid hormone suppression can be performed unless the patient's TSH secretion is already suppressed in the basal state. Suppression scans should usually be avoided, however, if the patient is elderly or has cardiac disease. Nodules that actively concentrate iodine in the presence of low serum TSH concentrations are referred to as "hot nodules." They are almost always benign follicular adenomas.

Ultrasound is a sensitive method for detecting and localizing thyroid nodules. It can distinguish thyroid cysts from solid lesions, but it does not provide information concerning their iodide-concentrating ability. Although ultrasound has been part of some algorithms for the evaluation of goiter, I limit its use to carefully selected patients.

Needle Biopsy. Needle biopsy is the best method for evaluating the malignant potential of goiters. In most patients, fine-needle aspiration biopsy (FNAB) is performed, a technique that yields cells and clusters of cells for cytologic examination. If the lesion is cystic, fluid can be obtained for cell block and, in selected instances, analysis of the fluid proteins. Not all apparent thyroid nodules are composed of thyroid tissue. For example, some parathyroid cysts accumulate large amounts of fluid and are clearly palpable in the neck. They can be diagnosed by showing that the aspirated fluid contains high levels of parathyroid hormone.

FNAB may yield a large variety of readings. Of those that provide useful information, the three most common are colloid nodule, follicular neoplasm, and epithelial cell thyroid cancer. Hashimoto's thyroiditis can also be strongly suspected on the basis of the FNAB sample. Metastatic tumors from other organs are rare but usually distinctive. MTC is highly likely if stains for calcitonin are positive. Unfortunately, sometimes the aspirate is nondiagnostic, suggesting that normal tissue around the nodule was sampled or that the amount of cellular material in the aspirate was inadequate.

TREATMENT OF GOITER

Patients who present with goiter should have their thyroid function evaluated. If thyrotoxicosis is present, its etiology should be determined and appropriate treatment instituted (see elsewhere). If hypo-

thyroidism is detected and the test for antithyroid antibodies is positive, the etiology is probably Hashimoto's thyroiditis. In goitrous patients with hypothyroidism, thyroid hormone treatment should reduce the tendency for further thyroid enlargement and may even cause regression of the goiter. With the exception of a pregnant woman, a thyroid scan should be performed in most patients with nodular thyroid disease. This test is also indicated if thyroid enlargement has been rapid, in goitrous patients who received external head and neck radiation during their childhood, or in those with goiter and a family history of thyroid cancer. FNAB is also indicated in these patients unless the nodule is "hot." FNAB is useful even in patients who are certain to have thyroid surgery, because the results influence the nature of the operation. In some cases, ultrasound can be helpful in guiding the biopsy. FNAB is well tolerated in most patients. Care must be taken, and supplementation of coagulation factors may be necessary, if the patient has a coagulation disorder.

Thyroid surgery and examination of the resected tissue is the only procedure that provides definitive information on the pathology of goiter. Nonetheless, the usual practice is to select only a fraction of patients with goiter for surgery. There are many reasons for this. In patients with diffuse goiters, the incidence of cancer is low unless there is a history of very rapid thyroid enlargement. Even in this case, the diagnosis is likely either subacute or silent thyroiditis if the enlargement is accompanied by thyrotoxicosis. Nodular thyroid disease is very common. Although it is more likely to be associated with thyroid cancer than diffuse goiter, the incidence of thyroid cancer within these goiters is still relatively low. More importantly, perhaps, the biologic behavior of the common thyroid cancers is less aggressive than that of most other malignancies.

Clinical judgment and the FNAB are probably the best tools for deciding who should have thyroid surgery to rule out biologically meaningful thyroid cancer. Regardless of the results of the FNAB, surgery is usually recommended for patients with rapidly enlarging noncystic solitary nodules, for patients with thyroid nodules and biochemical evidence of MTC, and for patients with thyroid nodules who received external head and neck radiation during infancy or childhood. Thyroid surgery is indicated in all but the poorest operative candidates if the FNAB is consistent with thyroid cancer. It must be emphasized that thyroid surgery in this setting is a therapeutic as well as a diagnostic procedure. The initial surgery must be more extensive than merely resecting the thyroid nodule itself and usually involves removing at least the involved lobe and isthmus.

Thyroid surgery is also indicated in most patients in whom the FNAB is consistent with a follicular neoplasm, provided the scan does not show that the nodule is "hot." If the FNAB is consistent with a colloid nodule, it is reasonable not to operate, but individual judgment must be exercised. The patient should also be apprised of the pros and cons of surgery and the reliability of diagnostic procedures so that he or she can participate in the decision. A decision not to operate is not a permanent decision, even in the case of "hot" nodules. Patients must understand that they should have long-term follow-up so that the need for surgery can be reconsidered and thyroid dysfunction treated if it develops. In some cases, repeating the FNAB may be worthwhile. If a nodule continues to grow, surgery is usually recommended unless it is a pure cyst that is reaccumulating fluid.

If the nodule is not "hot," thyroid hormone treatment can be considered. I treat selected patients with apparent benign nodular thyroid disease with L-thyroxine but do not give enough hormone to suppress serum TSH concentrations below about 0.6 µU per mL. I favor thyroid hormone treatment if serum antithyroid antibodies are positive, if the TSH is in the high-normal range, and if the nodules do not appear to be long-standing. I avoid thyroid hormone in elderly patients and those with cardiac disease.

HYPERPARATHYROIDISM AND HYPOPARATHYROIDISM

method of
LORRAINE A. FITZPATRICK, M.D.
Mayo Medical School
Mayo Clinic and Mayo Foundation
Rochester, Minnesota

HYPERPARATHYROIDISM

Enlargement and hyperfunction of one or more of the parathyroid glands result in hyperparathyroidism. Primary hyperparathyroidism may be produced by an adenoma, hyperplasia of multiple glands, or, rarely, parathyroid carcinoma. Ectopic production of parathyroid hormone (PTH) by a nonparathyroid malignancy is rare but can mimic primary hyperparathyroidism. The major actions of PTH—mobilization of calcium from bone and conservation of the reabsorption of calcium in the kidney—lead to the major hallmark of the disorder, hypercalcemia. PTH also increases serum calcium by enhancing production of 1,25-dihydroxyvitamin D, which, in turn, increases gastrointestinal absorption of calcium. The incidence of primary hyperparathyroidism increased dramatically in the late 1960s and early 1970s due to the introduction of the multichannel autoanalyzer for the measurement of serum calcium. The incidence of primary hyperparathyroidism in residents of Rochester, Minnesota, increased fivefold in the first year after the routine availability of serum calcium measurements. It is difficult to estimate the true incidence of primary hyperparathyroidism, but estimates of 27.7 per 100,000 person-years are identical in the United States and Europe. The incidence of hyperparathyroidism peaks in the middle years, and women predominate by a 2:1 to 3:1 margin compared with men.

A well-established predisposing factor for primary hyperparathyroidism is a history of neck irradiation.

Eighty to 85% of patients with primary hyperparathyroidism have a single adenoma, and 15 to 20% of patients have hyperplasia of all four parathyroid glands. Parathyroid hyperplasia is seen in conjunction with multiple endocrine neoplasia (MEN) Types I and II. Parathyroid carcinoma is a rare disorder and is present in less than 1% of cases.

The signs and symptoms of primary hyperparathyroidism are related to the degree of hypercalcemia. Physical signs are usually unremarkable. The common occurrence of hypertension has not been established to be directly related to primary hyperparathyroidism. Band keratopathy, calcium phosphate deposition in the medial and lateral limbic margins of the cornea, is rarely noted. Parathyroid gland enlargement in the neck is notable in cases of parathyroid carcinoma.

Initially, hyperparathyroidism was manifest by specific abnormalities in target organs. With the advent of widespread screening of serum calcium levels, most patients are asymptomatic. The classic bone disease of primary hyperparathyroidism is osteitis fibrosis cystica. Excessive PTH is associated with subperiosteal bone resorption of distal phalanges, and pathologic fractures may occur in association with parathyroid bone disease. A mothy or salt-and-pepper pattern of the skull has been described, and the distal one-third of the clavicles may appear to be tapered. Bone cysts and brown tumors are local lesions consisting of osteoclasts mixed with poorly mineralized woven bone. Generalized skeletal demineralization is evident in some cases. The number of patients who present with frank bone disease has diminished.

The incidence of nephrolithiasis in primary hyperparathyroidism has also diminished with increased general screening of serum calcium levels. Kidney stones occur in 15 to 20% of patients with primary hyperparathyroidism, and approximately 2 to 5% of stone formers will be shown to have primary hyperparathyroidism. Nephrolithiasis may occur due to deposition of calcium phosphate crystals throughout the parenchyma. Hypercalcuria occurs in 35 to 40% of patients with primary hyperparathyroidism. Hypercalcuria is caused by the large load of filtered calcium, which exceeds the kidneys' reabsorption capacity, despite the conservative action of PTH on renal calcium handling.

Other organ systems may also be effected. Neuromuscular spasm, characterized by atrophy of Type II muscle fibers, results in weakness and easy fatigability. Proximal muscle weakness can sometimes be detected on physical examination. Peptic ulcer disease was reported as a frequent complication in patients with MEN Type I and coexisting primary hyperparathyroidism. A pathophysiologic link between these two relatively common disorders is debated. Gout or pseudogout may affect the joints, and asymptomatic chondrocalcinosis of the knees and bones of the wrist can occur. Normochromic, normocytic anemia may occur and is associated with marrow replacement by fibrosis.

Recent studies indicated that the incidence of specific radiographic manifestations of primary hyperparathyroidism has dropped from 23 to 2%. In a similar manner, the incidence of nephrolithiasis has dropped from approximately 57% in 1965 to 19% in recent years.

Biochemical Assessment of Primary Hyperparathyroidism

Hypercalcemia and elevated levels of PTH are hallmarks of primary hyperparathyroidism. Because of improvements in immunoradiometric and immunochemilluminetric assays, the diagnosis can be established with great certainty. Occasionally, repeat testing is necessary to prove definite hypercalcemia or elevated PTH levels. In 90% of patients with primary hyperparathyroidism, PTH levels are elevated. In the remaining 10% of patients, concentrations of PTH are inappropriately elevated and are usually at the upper limit of normal. Serum phosphorous levels are usually in the lower range of normal and are usually less than 3.5 mg per dL in patients with normal renal function. The serum alkaline phosphatase level may be modestly elevated due to an increase in bone turnover that is associated with the disorder. The 25-hydroxyvitamin D level tends to be in the lower range of normal, and the 1,25-dihydroxyvitamin D concentration is generally in the upper range of normal. In 30 to 35% of patients, 1,25-dihydroxyvitamin D levels are elevated, illustrating the ability of PTH to stimulate its production. Total urinary calcium excretion is elevated in approximately 35 to 40% of patients, and the concentration of urinary pyridinoline cross-links of collagen is at the upper limit of normal. Measurements of bone densitometry indicate that bone density is reduced more markedly at the radius than at the lumbar spine. Reductions in cortical bone density reflect the preferential effect of PTH on cortical bone.

In the outpatient setting, primary hyperparathyroidism is the most common cause of hypercalcemia. Another common cause of hypercalcemia is hypercalcemia of malignancy. PTH levels are suppressed due to inhibition by the hypercalcemia associated with the malignancy. When hypercalcemia of malignancy is caused by PTH-related protein (PTHrP), PTH levels remain suppressed, as PTHrP is not detected in the currently available assays. Uncommon causes of hypercalcemia, including granulomatous disease, vitamin D or A toxicity, immobilization, and thyrotoxicosis, are all associated with reduced levels of PTH. Elevated PTH levels may be found with hypercalcemia associated with diazide or lithium use and in familial hypocalcuric hypercalcemia. Additional testing and appropriate historic information can rule out these disorders.

Management of Primary Hyperparathyroidism

Surgery is currently the treatment of choice for patients with symptomatic primary hyperparathyroidism. A National Institutes of Health consensus conference presented guidelines for surgical indications, which are listed in Table 1. Hyperparathyroid-induced bone disease such as bone cysts, brown tumors, or subperiosteal resorption warrants neck exploration and parathyroidectomy. Documented demineralization of the skeleton is a guideline for surgical intervention. Surgical extirpation of the parathyroid gland is recommended in patients with nephrolithiasis, nephrocalcinosis, and impaired renal function with or without hypercalcuria. Vague neuromuscular symptoms such as weakness are prevalent in patients with primary hyperparathyroidism, but the ability of surgery to guarantee amelioration of these symptoms is problematic.

The treatment of a patient with asymptomatic hyperparathyroidism is also problematic. Medical treatment of symptomatic hypercalcemia and primary hyperparathyroidism is the same as the treatment of any symptomatic hypercalcemia, regardless of etiology. Rehydration and treatment of nausea and vomiting are important for volume repletion. Saline diuresis (after volume repletion) usually results in a rapid decrease in serum calcium levels. Treatment of this kind in the outpatient setting can be difficult because of prerenal azotemia and worsening of hypercalcemia with diuretics and electrolyte abnormalities. Thiazide diuretics should be discontinued, as they can decrease calcium excretion. Immobilization also results in hypercalcuria and hypercalcemia, and sustained bed rest should be avoided. Specific therapies include the use of oral phosphate, which has the potential side effect of precipitation of calcium phosphate deposits in the kidney and other organs. Its long-term effects on renal function and bone metabolism are not well established, and the possibility of ectopic calcification limits its usefulness.

Oral conjugated estrogen (Premarin) has been used in the treatment of postmenopausal women with osteoporosis, with a notable decrease in serum calcium

TABLE 1. **Guidelines for Surgical Intervention in Primary Hyperparathyroidism**

Serum calcium >1 mg/dL above the upper limit of normal
Hyperparathyroid-induced bone disease (osteitis fibrosa cystica)
Nephrolithiasis or nephrocalcinosis
History of life-threatening hypercalcemia
Creatinine clearance reduced by 30% compared with age-matched normals
Calcium excretion >400 mg/24 h
Bone mineral density <2.5 D compared with age-, gender-, and race-matched controls

Additional considerations:
Patient is unlikely or unwilling to return for follow-up
Management complicated by coexistent illness
Patients <50 years of age

levels. No changes were noted in serum PTH or 1,25-dihydroxyvitamin D levels, consistent with the antagonistic effects of estrogen on the PTH-mediated skeletal resorption. Estrogen replacement therapy has many benefits in postmenopausal women and may lower serum calcium levels and urinary calcium excretion in primary hyperparathyroidism. However, hormone therapy should be individualized, based on risk and benefit assessments.

The bisphosphonates, pyrophosphate analogues that bind to hydroxyapatite, have been used to inhibit osteoclast-mediated bone resorption. Their usefulness has been restricted by their poor absorption, however. Overall, administration of the bisphosphonates results in lowered serum calcium in patients with primary hyperparathyroidism, with minimal side effects. The long-term benefits of second-generation bisphosphonates in the medical management of primary hyperparathyroidism are promising but not yet proved. Calcitonin is a peptide hormone that inhibits osteoclastic bone resorption and increases renal calcium excretion. Chronic use of calcitonin for treatment of primary hyperparathyroidism is limited by its low potency, short-term efficacy, and intermittent response to administration.

Secondary Hyperparathyroidism

In response to hypocalcemia, parathyroid glands are stimulated, resulting in an increased release of PTH, which, through actions noted above, works to increase serum calcium to its normal levels. This disorder of secondary hyperparathyroidism is associated with syndromes of vitamin D deficiency, vitamin D resistance, gastrointestinal disorders associated with malabsorption of calcium or vitamin D, renal insufficiency, and PTH resistance. In these cases, serum calcium levels are low or normal, with an elevated PTH level.

Parathyroid Crisis

In patients with untreated primary hyperparathyroidism, the risk of developing hypercalcemic crisis is low. One patient among a group of 47 patients followed over a 5-year interval developed acute primary hyperparathyroidism. In a prospective series of patients in Rochester, Minnesota, followed for 10 years, 1 of 142 (0.7%) developed hyperparathyroid crisis. In this disorder, serum calcium levels average 17.5 mg per dL, and PTH levels are strikingly elevated, averaging 20 times normal levels. Treatment of severe, life-threatening hypercalcemia must be instituted. Definitive treatment of acute hyperparathyroidism is surgical extirpation of the abnormal parathyroid gland or glands. This is a reversible, curable, and life-threatening disorder that can be confused with humeral hypercalcemia of malignancy. An antecedent history of primary hyperparathyroidism or an incapacitating illness has been confirmed in several cases. Recognition, rapid diagnosis, aggressive medical management, and successful surgery can result in a favorable outcome.

Parathyroid Carcinoma

Parathyroid carcinoma is an uncommon cause of PTH-dependent hypercalcemia and accounts for less than 1% of patients with primary hyperparathyroidism. There are several distinguishing clinical features, including serum calcium generally greater than 14 mg per dL. This marked elevation of serum calcium is invariably associated with signs and symptoms, including fatigue, weakness, weight loss, nausea, emesis, polyuria, and polydipsia. Bone pain, fractures, and renal colic are also frequently reported. A palpable neck mass has been reported in 30 to 76% of patients, and this finding is unusual in primary hyperparathyroidism. The most effective therapy is complete resection of the primary lesion in this indolent tumor. Parathyroid carcinoma is not radiosensitive, and experience with chemotherapy is limited due to the rarity of the condition.

HYPOPARATHYROIDISM

In hypoparathyroidism, the relative or absolute lack of PTH causes hypocalcemia from the reduced release of calcium from bone and the reduced renal tubular resorption of calcium. Calcium absorption from the gastrointestinal tract is impaired due to decreased 1α-hydroxylation of 25-hydroxyvitamin D in the kidney. Several categories of hypoparathyroidism exist: postoperative, sporadic, and familial.

Hypocalcemic symptoms include perioral numbness, paresthesia of the extremities, and muscle cramps. Other common symptoms include fatigue, hyperirritability, and anxiety. Symptoms can vary in relation to absolute levels of ionized calcium. Severe signs include carpopedal spasm, laryngeal stridor, laryngeal spasm, and focal or generalized seizures. A clinical sign of neuromuscular irritability is Chvostek's sign, produced by tapping the skin over the facial nerve anterior to the external auditory meatus, resulting in ipsilateral contraction of the facial muscles. Normal adults may have a positive reaction, however. Trousseau's sign—thumb adduction, metacarpophalangeal joint flexion, and interphalangeal joint extension—is elicited in response to ischemia of nerves in the upper arm, usually created by inflating a sphygmomanometer to 20 mmHg above the systolic blood pressure for 3 to 5 minutes. The neuronal irritability caused by hypocalcemia can be present as nonspecific electroencephalographic changes, increased intercranial pressure, and papilledema. Seizure activity has also been described and can include subclinical epilepsy and cerebral tetany.

On the electrocardiogram, the QT interval may be prolonged, and hypocalcemia-induced congestive heart failure has been reported. Calcium replacement in patients with hypocalcemia results in improved cardiac output and exercise duration. Smooth muscle involvement is due to irritability of the autonomic ganglia and can include dysphasia from esophageal involvement, abdominal pain and biliary colic from small intestine and sphincter of Oddi involvement, and wheezing and dyspnea from involvement of pulmonary tree.

With the presence of chronic hypocalcemia, ectodermal changes include dry skin, coarse hair, and brittle nails. In children, delayed dentition and enamel hypoplasia may be manifestations of hypocalcemia. Alopecia has been noted in surgically induced hypoparathyroidism and is associated with autoimmune hypoparathyroidism. Other skin lesions include ectopic eczema, exfoliative dermatitis, psoriasis, and impetigo herpetiformis. Subcapsular cataracts are a common sequela of hypocalcemia and are distinct from senile cataracts. Paravertebral ligamentous ossification has been noted in up to 50% of patients with hypoparathyroidism, and antalgic gate may be present. Calcification of the basal ganglia, cerebral cortex, and cerebellum is found on computed tomography (CT) scans, and the relationship to preexisting epilepsy or convulsive disorders is not well understood. Organic brain syndrome, psychosis, and psychoneurosis have been associated with chronic hypoparathyroidism, and subnormal intelligence has been noted in some children. Treatment may improve intelligence and personality, but amelioration of symptoms is not guaranteed. Some patients remain asymptomatic despite a lack of therapy for chronic hypoparathyroidism.

By definition, PTH levels are low, resulting in abnormally low levels of serum calcium. PTH concentration is often undetectable. Most patients have a serum phosphorus level that is at the upper limit of normal or elevated.

Surgically Induced Hypoparathyroidism

Surgically induced hypoparathyroidism can result from various types of neck surgery, including thyroid, parathyroid, and radical neck operations for esophageal or laryngeal carcinoma. Damage to the vascular supply or direct injury of the parathyroid glands may result in decreased release of PTH. In a series of 500 patients operated on at the Mayo Clinic, permanent hypoparathyroidism was noted in 2%. In other studies, symptomatic postoperative hypoparathyroidism requiring treatment was noted in 10%, but permanent hypoparathyroidism occurred in only 1%. Risk factors include repeated neck surgery for persistent or recurrent hyperparathyroidism or partial bilateral parathyroidectomy for parathyroid hyperplasia. Permanent hypoparathyroidism after parathyroid surgery is rare and occurs in up to 3% of patients. The risk of hypoparathyroidism is greater after total thyroidectomy than after partial thyroidectomy and is greater after surgery for thyrotoxic goiter compared with surgery for euthyroid goiter. After total thyroidectomy for thyroid cancer, up to 33% of patients experience transient postoperative hypoparathyroidism. The incidence of postoperative tetany is higher in women than in men and diminishes with

age. Transient hypoparathyroidism can occur due to edema of neck tissues or exposure to anesthesia or may be a nonspecific response to surgery.

Transient, reversible hypocalcemia may occur after removal of a hyperfunctioning parathyroid gland due to suppression of the remaining normal parathyroid tissue. This hypocalcemia may be exaggerated in patients with pre-existing hyperparathyroid bone disease ("hungry bones"). The sudden reduction in PTH release after removal of the abnormal parathyroid gland results in increased movement of calcium and phosphorous into the remineralizing skeleton. Symptoms are easily relieved with oral administration of calcium and vitamin D.

Hypomagnesemia and Hypermagnesemia

Impaired release of PTH with severe magnesium deficiency occurs and is reversed by rapid magnesium repletion. In the presence of severe magnesium deficiency, resistance to PTH at its target organs occurs and exacerbates the effect. Impaired intestinal absorption and increased intestinal or urinary loss of magnesium may result in hypomagnesemia. In children, selective gastrointestinal malabsorption of magnesium may occur, leading to hypocalcemia and seizures. PTH levels are low or near the detection limit of the assay and return to normal with magnesium repletion. In adults, magnesium depletion may result from intestinal malabsorption or reduced renal tubular reabsorption (drug-induced or idiopathic). In vitro and in vivo studies indicate that supraphysiologic increased concentrations of magnesium suppress PTH secretion. In obstetric patients receiving magnesium therapy for toxemia of pregnancy and suppression of premature labor, supraphysiologic levels of magnesium were associated with hypocalcemia and acute suppression of PTH. This group of patients did not have overt signs or symptoms of hypocalcemia, despite marked elevations in serum magnesium.

Hypoparathyroidism Associated with Radiation, Drugs, or Sepsis

Chronic hypoparathyroidism has occasionally been associated with the administration of radioiodine for the treatment of hyperthyroidism. Onset is usually within 4 to 18 months of radioiodine administration, and the incidence is unrelated to dose. Chemotherapeutic agents are rarely associated with hypoparathyroidism. Some compounds are associated with alterations in parathyroid gland function. Administration of asparaginase has been associated with hypocalcemia, but it is uncertain if this is due to a direct effect on parathyroid glands. Commonly used medications such as calcitonin, bisphosphonates, oral phosphate, gallium nitrate (Ganite), and plicamycin (Mithracin) lower serum calcium levels but are associated with the inhibition of osteoclastic bone resorption and not with direct effects on the parathyroid glands. The aminoglycoside class of antibiotics causes hypocalcemia as a result of drug-induced hypomagnesemia. Chronic alcoholism is frequently associated with hypocalcemia and hypomagnesemia. Acute administration of intoxicating levels of alcohol to normal volunteers results in decreased PTH levels. Acquired parathyroid gland insufficiency has been associated with sepsis, and the basis for hypocalcemia in these patients is multifactorial.

Infiltrative processes such as hemochromatosis, Wilson's disease, metastatic neoplasia, granulomatous disease, amyloidosis, and syphilis have been described as infiltrative disease of the parathyroid glands. Chronic hypoparathyroidism can occur with iron overload. Progressive systemic sclerosis may cause fibrosis of the parathyroid glands, manifest by clinical hypoparathyroidism.

Neonatal Hypoparathyroidism

Although hyperparathyroidism during pregnancy is rare, children with hypocalcemia have been described, probably due to compensatory intrauterine atrophy of parathyroid glands due to maternal hypercalcemia.

Developmental Disorders of the Parathyroid Gland

The DiGeorge syndrome, also known as the third and fourth pharyngeal pouch syndrome, is characterized in its full form by aplasia or hypoplasia of the thymus, aplasia or hypoplasia of the parathyroids, and conotruncal cardiac malformations. Partial forms of the syndrome can occur, and use of an ethylenediaminetetraacetic acid (EDTA) challenge test to unmask clinically silent hypoparathyroidism and familial partial DiGeorge syndrome has been reported. Due to the associated immunodeficiency, T cell function is compromised, and many children succumb to infection. Most cases are sporadic, but heritable forms occur, and it is unknown whether the DiGeorge syndrome is caused by mutation or deletion of a single gene or is a contiguous gene syndrome responsible for the different phenotypic manifestations.

Idiopathic Hypoparathyroidism

Idiopathic hypoparathyroidism refers to forms of hypoparathyroidism not due to surgery or acquired causes. This is a heterogeneous group of rare and often sporadic disorders. In cases of isolated hypoparathyroidism, association with Kearns-Sayre syndrome or Kenny-Caffey syndrome has occasionally been described. Coexistence of several autoimmune endocrinopathies is unusual. The association of hypoparathyroidism with other autoimmune disorders, including adrenal disease and moniliasis, is termed polyglandular autoimmune syndrome Type I. Inheritance is autosomal recessive and not associated with a particular human leukocyte antigen (HLA) locus. Clinical presentation is initiated by candidal infection of nails and mucous membranes. Hypoparathy-

roidism develops several years after the onset of candidiasis, with a mean age ranging from 7 to 10 years. Addison's disease and other associated autoimmune abnormalities may follow years later. Intestinal malabsorption occurs in 25% of these patients and complicates pharmacologic intervention.

Molecular Genetic Aspects of Hypoparathyroidism

Familial isolated hypoparathyroidism is defined as a subcategory of idiopathic hypoparathyroidism with a clearly inherited basis. Autosomal dominant, autosomal recessive, and X-linked recessive forms have been described. Possible molecular explanations for PTH deficiency in these families include mutations of the coding region of the prepro-PTH gene or its regulatory regions. Because the prepro-PTH gene is located on chromosome 11, only X-linked forms of isolated hypoparathyroidism can be automatically judged to have a gene defect outside the prepro-PTH locus as their primary cause. In one kindred, an abnormal prepro-PTH allele that contained one identified mutation, a substitution of C for T in codon 18 at the prepeptide encoding region, has been described. The mutation provided a plausible explanation for the inactivity of the product of the mutant allele due to inability of the sequence to provide translocation of the nascently formed peptide through the endoplasmic reticulum. In another family, a prepro-PTH gene splice site mutation was described in autosomal recessive hypoparathyroidism. Two kindreds have been reported with isolated hypoparathyroidism inherited in an X-linked recessive manner. The responsible X-linked gene or genes have not been identified, although DNA polymorphisms indicate that the disease-causing gene in these families is probably in the XQ26–XQ27 region.

Pseudohypoparathyroidism

Pseudohypoparathyroidism is due to resistance to the action of PTH. A varying number of clinical and genetic abnormalities are present in this category of disorders. Biochemical diagnosis has been confirmed by hypocalcemia, hyperphosphatemia, and elevated levels of PTH.

Type IA pseudohypoparathyroidism is associated with a phenotype known as Albright's hereditary osteodystrophy, which is represented by short stature, rounded facies, and foreshortened metacarpal and metatarsal bones. These patients have a deficiency in the guanine nucleotide–binding protein G_s. This protein couples the signal from the PTH receptor to adenylate cyclase. Absence of the G_s results in resistance to the action of PTH at the cellular level. Pseudohypoparathyroidism Type IB is not associated with Albright's hereditary osteodystrophy, and guanine nucleotide regulatory hormone binding is not deficient. In both Types IA and IB, administration of intravenous PTH (the Ellsworth-Howard test) does not result in expected phosphaturia and increased urinary cyclic AMP excretion.

In pseudohypoparathyroidism Type II, response to PTH is normal in terms of an increase in cyclic AMP, but phosphaturia does not occur following infusion of PTH. Pseudopseudohypoparathyroidism presents with normal serum biochemical parameters, but it has the phenotype of Albright's hereditary osteodystrophy, as described above.

Differential Diagnosis of Hypocalcemia

Characterization of the severity of symptoms of underlying medical conditions directs important laboratory investigations. Pseudohypocalcemia can be diagnosed by calculation of the true serum calcium value in relation to the serum protein concentration. Hypoalbuminemia is one of the most common causes of apparent hypocalcemia, especially in acutely ill patients. Measurement of PTH is useful in the differential diagnosis. Levels of PTH are usually normal or high in pseudohypoparathyroidism and in vitamin D–deficient states. Diagnosis of pseudohypoparathyroidism can be readily confirmed by the lack of a brisk increase in urinary excretion of cyclic AMP and phosphate in response to infusion of PTH (Ellsworth-Howard test). In hypoparathyroidism due to other causes, serum levels of PTH are usually low or undetectable. If hypomagnesemia is the cause of hypocalcemia, magnesium levels are usually less than 0.5 mmol per liter. Urine calcium excretion is low in patients with hypoparathyroidism due to the low filtered load of calcium. Measurement of vitamin D metabolites can be helpful in documenting abnormalities of vitamin D action or metabolism as a cause of hypocalcemia.

Treatment of Hypocalcemia

The ideal treatment of hormone-deficient endocrinopathies is replacement of the absent hormone with natural analogue. The clinical experience with synthetic human PTH is limited because parenteral administration prevents widespread patient acceptance and efficacy of long-term use has not been widely explored. Currently, administration of supplemental

TABLE 2. **Commonly Prescribed Calcium Salts**

Oral Calcium Preparation	% Elemental Calcium
Calcium carbonate	40
Calcium citrate	21
Calcium bionate 1.8 g/5mL	6.5
Calcium gluconate	9
Calcium lactate	13
Calcium phosphate dibasic	23
Tricalcin phosphate	39

TABLE 3. **Dosages of Common Treatments for Hypoparathyroidism**

Preparation	Dose
Cholecalciferol (Delta-D, vitamin D_3)	400–1000 U
Ergocalciferol (Calciferol, Drisdol)	25,000–100,000 U tiw to qd
Calcifediol (Calderol)	20–50 μg tiw to qd
Calcitriol (Rocaltrol, Calcijex)	0.25–1.0 μg qd to bid
Dihydrotachysterol (DHT, Hytakerol)	0.2–1.0 mg qd

calcium and vitamin D is the mainstay of therapy for hypoparathyroidism. In acute hypocalcemia, the decision to treat may depend on the degree of hypocalcemia. Serum calcium levels less than 7.5 mg per dL (after correction for hypoalbuminemia and resolution of hypomagnesemia) in symptomatic patients warrant treatment. Calcium gluconate (10%) is available for intravenous administration; 10 mL of calcium gluconate contains 90 mg of elemental calcium and can be infused over 5 to 10 minutes. The half-life is short and depends on glomerular filtration rate and tubular reabsorption.

In chronic hypocalcemia, any underlying cause of malabsorption and malnutrition should be corrected. Maintenance therapy with calcium involves a delicate balance, because the lack of PTH results in hypercalcuria with long-term consequences of nephrocalcinosis and nephrolithiasis. Insufficient replacement is associated with subcapsular cataract formation. Dietary and supplemental calcium should approximate 1000 to 2000 mg per day. Oral calcium supplements are better absorbed in smaller doses in an acidic environment (with meals). Table 2 lists the commonly prescribed calcium salts. In patients with decreased parathyroid reserve, oral calcium supplementation may suffice to alleviate symptoms. In most patients, however, the addition of vitamin D or one of its metabolites is required. In hypoparathyroidism, regulation of conversion of the precursors of 1,25-dihydroxyvitamin D_3 does not occur because PTH is absent. The advantages of 1,25 dihydroxyvitamin D administration include rapid onset of action and short half-life in case of toxicity. The cost of this agent and the relative ease of management of patients with other preparations of vitamin D have limited its use. Dihydrotachysterol, vitamin D_2 (ergocalciferol [Calciferol, Drisdol]), and 25-hydroxyvitamin D (calcifediol [Calderol]) are less expensive preparations that are effective in the treatment of hypoparathyroidism. The usual doses are listed in Table 3, but doses must be individualized. Serum concentrations of vitamin D metabolites may be monitored to assess absorption and compliance. In the event of toxicity, a prolonged period is required for the resolution of drug effects.

PRIMARY ALDOSTERONISM

method of
MYRON H. WEINBERGER, M.D.
Indiana University School of Medicine
Indianapolis, Indiana

Primary aldosteronism is an unusual cause of hypertension, occurring in less than 5% of an unselected hypertensive population, but it is often overlooked as a potentially curable form of elevated blood pressure. The frequency of hypertension makes it likely that most physicians will encounter such patients in their practices, and the subtle abnormalities found in this syndrome require a high index of suspicion and an understanding of how to establish the diagnosis, differentiate among the different causes, and pursue the most appropriate treatment.

MECHANISM

Primary aldosteronism results from any of several abnormalities of the adrenal cortex leading to the excessive production of aldosterone or other mineralocorticoids independent of the traditional stimuli for steroid production. This state of increased mineralocorticoidism then induces excessive sodium and water reabsorption by the distal portion of the renal tubules and collecting ducts, resulting in expansion of extracellular fluid volume and elevated blood pressure. The sodium reabsorption occurs by steroid-induced exchange for potassium and/or hydrogen ions, leading to potassium loss, hypokalemia, and metabolic alkalosis. The volume expansion typically results in profound suppression of the renin-angiotensin system, which is normally the primary stimulus of aldosterone production by the adrenal glomerular zone. Although excessive aldosterone production can often be identified as an elevation in the plasma level or urinary excretion of aldosterone or its major metabolites, this is not invariably the case, since "normal" levels are occasionally observed. However, such values are inappropriate given the marked suppression of the renin-angiotensin system and the expanded fluid volume status seen in primary aldosteronism.

SIGNS AND SYMPTOMS

The symptoms associated with primary aldosteronism are nonspecific. Headaches are commonly reported, as is fatigue, muscle weakness, and, occasionally, muscle cramps. Rarely, severe muscle weakness and tetany are observed. Hypokalemia is often, but not always, found. Serum sodium levels are usually greater than 139 mEq per liter, but rarely are values above the normal range. Alkalosis, reflected by elevated serum bicarbonate values, is also common, as well as decreased serum ionized calcium levels, usually attributed to alkalosis. This appears to be responsible for the tetanic muscle contractions occasionally observed. Although it is not often measured, the serum magnesium level may also be reduced and can contribute to muscle cramps. The blood pressure elevation can range from mild to severe, and even malignant hypertension has been reported. Despite significant blood pressure elevation and, frequently, a long duration of hypertension, retinopathy is usually conspicuously absent. Although renal function is typically normal when measured by blood urea nitrogen and serum creatinine levels, creatinine clearance is often above normal, presumably reflecting glomerular hyperfiltration resulting from the expansion of extracellular fluid volume, the increased renal perfusion pressure, and the relative lack of angiotensin II–mediated efferent arteriolar tone. Polyuria and nocturia are also common, probably related to hypokalemia; proteinuria is not unusual.

SCREENING AND DIAGNOSIS

Traditionally, hypokalemia has been used as the initial screening test for primary aldosteronism, but this has proved to be of inadequate sensitivity and specificity. The majority of hypertensive patients with hypokalemia have secondary hyperaldosteronism resulting from diuretic administration or excessive renin production (renal vascular hypertension, "high-renin" essential hypertension, renal parenchymal disease, or, rarely, renin-producing tumors). As many as 25% of patients with primary aldosteronism have "normal" serum potassium levels for a variety of reasons. Thus, the most accurate screening test for primary aldosteronism is the measurement of plasma renin activity, being careful that the patient has *not* been receiving medications known to suppress renin secretion, such as beta blockers or antisympathetic agents, when the peripheral blood sample is obtained. However, the finding of renin suppression alone does not ensure the diagnosis of primary aldosteronism, since reduced renin levels are also observed in "low-renin" essential hypertensives. It is also necessary to demonstrate evidence of normal or elevated aldosterone production in the face of suppressed renin levels. This can be done most easily by measurement of plasma aldosterone concentration. In the past, it was necessary to apply maneuvers that normally reduce aldosterone production, such as a high-salt diet, intravenous saline administration, or exogenous steroids, to demonstrate inappropriate aldosterone levels. The most sensitive approach currently is the simultaneous measurement of plasma renin activity and plasma aldosterone and the calculation of the ratio between aldosterone and its primary stimulus (renin) under conditions free of the suppressive effect of medication. When this ratio exceeds 20 (disregarding the units of measurement), the diagnosis can be made. In addition, this ratio has been helpful in discriminating between the two most commonly encountered forms of primary aldosteronism (discussed later).

FORMS OF PRIMARY ALDOSTERONISM AND OTHER MINERALOCORTICOID EXCESS SYNDROMES

Approximately two-thirds of patients with primary aldosteronism have a solitary adrenal adenoma, usually from 0.3 to 2.0 cm in diameter. Removal of such adenomas is usually associated with correction of both the metabolic and the blood pressure abnormalities. About 30% of patients have bilateral adrenal macro- and/or micronodular hyperplasia; in these individuals, even complete bilateral adrenalectomy, which corrects the hyperaldosteronism and the metabolic abnormalities, is typically not associated with a sustained reduction in blood pressure. Thus, differentiation of these most common forms of primary aldosteronism is important, since the treatment is obviously different. Rarely, primary aldosteronism results from bilateral solitary adrenal adenomas or from adrenal carcinoma.

In addition, there are other less common forms of hyperaldosteronism or mineralocorticoid excess syndromes. Several families have now been identified in which a genetic mutation has resulted in a hybrid gene, combining the

11-beta-hydroxylase and aldosterone synthase genes, that produces aldosterone under the control of corticotropin (ACTH) rather than angiotensin II, which is the normal stimulus. In this syndrome, called dexamethasone-remediable (or suppressible) aldosteronism, the excessive aldosterone production can be treated by administration of a glucocorticoid to reduce the ACTH-dependent hyperaldosteronism. Other genetic abnormalities can also produce mineralocorticoid excess. For example, 17-alpha-hydroxylase or 11-beta-hydroxylase deficiency leads to excessive production of desoxycorticosterone at levels that produce the mineralocorticoid excess syndrome, mimicking primary aldosteronism but without excessive production of aldosterone, due to the enzymatic block.

Another genetic abnormality producing clinical manifestations that mimic primary aldosteronism has recently been elucidated. Liddle's syndrome, a form of salt-sensitive hypertension with marked renin suppression and hypokalemia but very low aldosterone levels, has been found to result from a mutation in the beta subunit of the epithelial sodium channel. This syndrome is responsive to triamterene administration. In addition, despite the fact that cortisol circulates in plasma at levels at least a thousand times greater than that of aldosterone, the renal mineralocorticoid receptor recognizes only aldosterone, because cortisol is converted to cortisone by the action of 11-beta-hydroxysteroid dehydrogenase, and cortisone has only weak affinity for the receptor. The candy licorice, which is metabolized to glycyrrhizic acid, and carbenoxolone have both been shown to competitively inhibit 11-beta-hydroxysteroid dehydrogenase and thus permit cortisol to occupy the mineralocorticoid receptor and produce the effects of mineralocorticoid excess.

DIFFERENTIATION AND TREATMENT OF PRIMARY ALDOSTERONISM

For the majority of patients with primary aldosteronism, the differentiation is between a solitary adrenal adenoma and bilateral adrenal hyperplasia. The differentiation of these forms has involved a variety of anatomic and physiologic procedures, none of which provides sufficient sensitivity and specificity to be relied on.

Adrenal isotope scanning with a radio-labeled precursor of steroid synthesis (^{131}I-iodocholesterol) has been used by some groups with variable results. Because adrenal adenomas are often small, most centers have found this approach to have inadequate sensitivity or specificity, and we have not used it for 20 years. Computed tomography (CT) scanning is often more useful but may miss small adenomas or misidentify large hyperplastic nodules as representing solitary adenomas. Thus, CT cannot be used as the sole differentiating test. Adrenal venography can be useful in identifying relatively large adenomas (>2 cm in diameter) but can be associated with hemorrhage or infarction of the adrenal.

The technique that provides the greatest accuracy in differentiating unilateral from bilateral disease is adrenal venous sampling for the measurement of both aldosterone *and* cortisol, which permits correction for dilution of adrenal venous blood by nonadrenal sources, and sampling from the inferior vena cava. Both tests are conducted during intravenous

ACTH infusion (cosyntropin [Cortrosyn] 25 U in 500 mL dextrose/5% saline at a rate of 100 mL per hour) begun 30 minutes prior to blood sampling. However, since no single test is sufficiently accurate, we rely on at least two procedures that provide consistent results.

Additional helpful tests include examining the postural response of plasma aldosterone in peripheral blood samples obtained at 8 A.M., following overnight recumbency, and then at noon after 4 hours of upright posture. The normal response is an increase in plasma aldosterone at noon, reflecting the two- to fourfold increase in plasma renin activity that typically occurs following assumption of the upright posture. In many patients with a solitary adrenal adenoma, an anomalous postural decline in plasma aldosterone levels is seen; in those with bilateral adrenal disease, no change or an increase in plasma aldosterone levels is observed at noon. Many investigators have found that patients with a solitary adrenal adenoma have plasma concentrations of an aldosterone precursor steroid, 18-hydroxycorticosterone, that exceed 100 ng per dL, whereas lower values are found in those with bilateral adrenal disease. Patients with adrenal carcinoma often have other manifestations of malignancy and evidence of excessive production of a variety of steroids and steroid metabolites in addition to aldosterone. An additional benefit of localization of a solitary adrenal adenoma is that it permits a simpler surgical approach, since a flank incision or laparoscopic technique can be used rather than the abdominal approach, with its attendant increase in morbidity and prolonged recovery time.

Medical treatment is available for primary aldosteronism when it is caused by bilateral adrenal disease or when the patient is not a surgical candidate. The most effective treatment is administration of the mineralocorticoid receptor antagonist spironolactone (Aldactone). The doses required for blood pressure reduction in primary aldosteronism range from 100 to 800 mg per day, and a period of 7 to 10 days is required for optimal effects on potassium and blood pressure. Unfortunately, side effects are frequent at the doses required. Painful gynecomastia and impotence are frequent in men, and breast tenderness and menstrual abnormalities occur in women. If spironolactone cannot be tolerated, potassium-sparing diuretic combinations (Dyazide, Maxzide, Moduretic) can be used but will likely be associated with persistent hypokalemia. This can be treated with supplemental triamterene (Dyrenium) or amiloride (Midamor) or potassium supplementation, but the latter may require as much as 150 to 200 mEq per day. In addition to drug therapy, salt restriction can enhance the antihypertensive effects and limit the magnitude of potassium loss by reducing steroid-induced sodium-for-potassium exchange in the kidney. Calcium channel entry blockers have also been shown to be effective in the treatment of primary aldosteronism. In some patients with bilateral adrenal hyperplasia, the syndrome appears to be related to exquisite sensitivity of the adrenal to angiotensin II. Thus angiotensin-converting enzyme (ACE) inhibitors may be effective in a small number of patients.

Inquiry regarding the ingestion of licorice or carbenoxolone usually identifies this form of aldosteronism and permits elimination of the contributing factor. When the syndrome is present without evidence of excessive aldosterone production, one of the rare genetic abnormalities should be considered. The finding of elevated desoxycorticosterone levels should prompt a trial of dexamethasone (Decadron 0.25 to 0.5 mg every 8 hours) alone or in combination with a potassium-sparing diuretic agent. For long-term treatment, diuretics are preferred. In subjects with Liddle's syndrome, both renin and aldosterone levels are markedly suppressed, and no evidence of other mineralocorticoid excess is observed. Triamterene (Dyrenium) 25 to 100 mg per day is the most effective treatment. When a family history of hypertension is obtained and the onset is early in life, dexamethasone-remediable aldosteronism should be considered and a trial of dexamethasone (Decadron 0.25 to 0.5 mg every 8 hours) initiated. If the blood pressure, steroid, and metabolic abnormalities are responsive to glucocorticoid administration, which may take up to 6 weeks to ascertain, chronic treatment with a potassium-sparing diuretic combination such as triamterene-hydrochlorothiazide (Dyazide, Maxzide 1 to 2 tablets per day) or amiloride-hydrochlorothiazide (Moduretic 1 tablet per day) is preferable to long-term steroid therapy. If the potassium-sparing diuretic combination is not adequate for control of blood pressure, the addition of a calcium channel entry blocker or other antihypertensive agents may be required.

HYPOPITUITARISM

method of
BAHA M. ARAFAH, M.D.
*Case Western Reserve University School of
    Medicine and University Hospitals of
    Cleveland
Cleveland, Ohio*

Hypopituitarism is a clinical disorder characterized by diminished secretion of some (partial hypopituitarism) or all (panhypopituitarism) of the hormones secreted by the anterior pituitary gland. Although less frequent, selected deficiency of a single pituitary hormone (monotropic hypopituitarism) can also occur. In most instances, loss of pituitary hormone secretion is a slow and progressive process, occurring over months or years and involving more than one hormonal axis. Often, patients present with several years' history of nonspecific complaints and remain compensated until they experience a major illness, infection, accident, or trauma. Any stressful experience can result in clinical decompensation and the need for urgent medical attention. Occasionally, hypopituitarism develops acutely, leading to a rapid onset of symptoms, as is often seen in patients with pituitary tumor apoplexy.

Hypopituitarism has been considered a permanent and irreversible process that requires lifelong hormone replacement therapy. Although this may be the case in some instances, recent studies have documented that recovery of pituitary function can be demonstrated in a significant number of patients with hypopituitarism. Furthermore, reversibility of various functional forms of hypopituitarism has been demonstrated repeatedly. For example, recovery of gonadal function after medical or surgical treatment of hyperprolactinemia has been demonstrated.

DIAGNOSIS OF HYPOPITUITARISM

Dynamic pituitary hormone testing has been a valuable tool in defining the pathophysiologic mechanisms involved in the development of hypopituitarism. Although dynamic studies are useful in documenting hypopituitarism and demonstrating pituitary hormone reserve, they should be interpreted along with other clinical and/or neuroimaging studies. In some instances, dynamic studies may provide an approximation of the functional reserve of the pituitary gland rather than the site of injury causing impaired hormone secretion. A thorough understanding of the physiology of pituitary hormone secretion and appropriate correlation with additional anatomic and clinical data are essential in the interpretation of dynamic studies.

Although the diagnosis of hypopituitarism can often be made by measurements of basal hormone levels, dynamic studies are sometimes needed for confirmation. Both the target gland hormone product and the pituitary hormone in question should be measured simultaneously to assess the appropriateness of serum values. Each axis should be assessed in patients suspected of having partial or complete loss of pituitary function. The following is a summary of the approach in establishing the diagnosis of hypopituitarism. Evaluation of the function of each axis is presented separately.

Thyroid-Stimulating Hormone (TSH) Secretion. This can be evaluated by measurements of serum thyroxine (total or free) and TSH levels. Deficiency of TSH results in a low serum thyroxine, associated with a normal or low serum TSH level as well as clinical hypothyroidism.

Corticotropin (ACTH) Function. Measurements of ACTH plasma levels are not helpful in establishing the diagnosis of hypopituitarism or secondary adrenal insufficiency. The levels are, however, useful in differentiating primary from secondary adrenal insufficiency in a patient whose adrenal function is already shown to be impaired. The diagnosis of adrenal insufficiency can be suspected in patients with clinical symptoms who also have low serum cortisol levels (<3 to 4 μg per dL) in the absence of exogenous glucocorticoid intake. In evaluating a single serum cortisol value, one needs to take into consideration many of the known limitations influencing the level, such as the time of the day, degree of stress at the time of measurement, and any other associated illnesses. Patients with borderline serum cortisol levels may need further testing using insulin-induced hypoglycemia. In some instances, the cosyntropin (Cortrosyn) stimulation test is recommended as a screening test. It evaluates adrenal responsiveness to exogenous, synthetic ACTH. Although the test is an excellent screening tool, it is often unreliable in excluding the diagnosis of secondary or tertiary forms of adrenal insufficiency that one would expect to see in patients with hypopituitarism. Many patients with documented ACTH deficiency have "normal" cortisol responses to exogenous ACTH. This is particularly true if the ACTH deficiency is recent in onset or if it is partial rather than complete.

The most reliable test for establishing the diagnosis of ACTH deficiency in patients with borderline serum cortisol levels is the assessment of cortisol or ACTH response to insulin-induced hypoglycemia (0.05 to 0.2 U per kg insulin intravenously). This test represents the "gold standard" for establishing the diagnosis of adrenal insufficiency. The test should be performed in the presence of an experienced physician to minimize potential side effects. Prolonged hypoglycemia can be avoided if lower doses of insulin are given to patients strongly suspected of having deficiency of growth hormone or ACTH. In centers with experienced staffs and where patients are carefully screened and monitored, the test is rarely associated with complications. The test is generally contraindicated in elderly patients and those with coronary artery disease.

Gonadotropin Secretion. Clinical assessment of gonadal function, particularly in women, is valuable in the proper interpretation of biochemical tests. In a premenopausal, amenorrheic woman, measurements of serum gonadotropins (follicle-stimulating hormone [FSH] and luteinizing hormone [LH]) and estradiol levels can be helpful in establishing the diagnosis of hypogonadotropism. A clinical history of normal, regular menses almost always indicates normal gonadotropin function. In postmenopausal women, in whom serum gonadotropin levels are expected to be high, measurements of the serum FSH and LH levels, in the absence of exogenous estrogen intake, help confirm the diagnosis of impaired gonadotropin function. In men, the simultaneous determination of testosterone and gonadotropin serum levels can establish the diagnosis.

Growth Hormone (GH) Secretion. A single determination of serum GH level is of no clinical significance. Measurements of serum GH levels during insulin-induced hypoglycemia or after an infusion of arginine are the most reliable tests to assess GH secretion. With few exceptions, measurement of plasma levels of insulin-like growth factor-1 (previously known as somatomedin C) is a reasonably reliable method for the rapid assessment of GH secretion.

Prolactin Secretion. Measurements of basal prolactin levels, on more than one occasion, are often adequate to assess secretion of this lactogenic hormone.

Antidiuretic Hormone (ADH) Secretion. ADH deficiency occurs when the neurosecretory cells of the hypothalamus (supraoptic and paraventricular nuclei) are damaged. Patients with hypopituitarism rarely have ADH deficiency, unless they have hypothalamic disease. Loss of ADH secretion can lead to excessive free water excretion by the kidneys and the clinical diagnosis of diabetes insipidus (DI). Patients with DI have increased free water loss by the kidneys, resulting in dilute urine despite an associated increase in serum sodium and osmolality. Patients with total DI can lose several liters of water a day in the urine and, in the absence of adequate water intake, may become dehydrated. Diagnosis of DI is established by the presence of dilute urine (low osmolality) despite hypernatremia and/or increased serum osmolality. The diagnosis can be confirmed by measurement of serum ADH levels, although this is not necessary. Instead, one can determine the response to the administration of exogenous ADH or one of its analogues (e.g., DDAVP). The latter test differentiates patients with central DI, in whom a drop in urinary volume is promptly noted, from those with nephrogenic DI, in whom no such response is expected.

Considering the physiology of normal pituitary hormone secretion and its dependence on hypothalamic regulation, at least three different mechanisms can lead to the development of hypopituitarism. Although there are specific examples that apply to each of the three mechanisms, it is important to point out that in most patients, more than one mechanism contributes to the development of hypopituitarism. In each instance, there is often a predominant mechanism that dictates not only the degree of impairment but also whether the process is potentially reversible. Postulated mechanisms include:

1. Diminished release and/or secretion of hypothalamic hormone(s). This can be congenital (e.g., gonadotropin-releasing hormone [GnRH] deficiency in Kallmann's syndrome) or acquired as a result of primary or metastatic tumors, inflammation, infection, mass lesions, or ischemia.

2. Interruption of the delivery of hypothalamic hormones to the anterior pituitary. This is commonly seen as a result of parasellar mass lesions such as craniopharyngioma, meningioma, pituitary tumor, and aneurysm. Hypopituitarism in these instances can occur as a result of mechanical compression of the pituitary stalk and portal vessels. In addition, inadvertent damage, injury, or transection of the pituitary stalk can occur intraoperatively and lead to hypopituitarism.

3. Loss or destruction of hormone-producing cells of the pituitary gland. This can occur as a result of an ischemic event (e.g., Sheehan's syndrome), inflammation (lymphocytic hypophysitis), or infiltrative diseases (amyloidosis, hemochromatosis, metastatic cancer) and in response to an expanding pituitary mass lesion such as an adenoma.

The clinical manifestations of hypopituitarism are diverse and variable, depending to a large degree on the extent and duration of pituitary hormone deficits. In addition to the signs and symptoms of specific hormone deficits, patients often present with symptoms and signs related to the cause of hypopituitarism. The clinical manifestations in patients presenting with hypopituitarism can therefore be divided into two categories: signs and symptoms of hormone deficits (Table 1) and signs and symptoms related to the etiology of hypopituitarism. Such latter symptoms include headaches and visual disturbances in patients with perisellar mass lesions, as would be expected in patients with pituitary macroadenomas, meningiomas, or craniopharyngiomas. Patients with functioning pituitary adenomas also have clinical manifestations related to and caused by excessive hormone secretion (e.g., a patient with a GH-secreting adenoma presenting with hypopituitarism). Such a patient has signs of hormone excess from the functioning tumor (acromegaly) and signs and symptoms of loss of normal pituitary function, in addition to possible mechanical symptoms such as headache and visual disturbances.

Occasionally, hemorrhage and/or necrosis (i.e., pituitary tumor apoplexy) are the first reported clinical manifestations of a previously undiagnosed pituitary mass. In this instance, hypopituitarism develops acutely after hemorrhagic infarction of the tumor and often contributes to the associated morbidity of this syndrome.

PRACTICAL MANAGEMENT

Understanding the pathophysiology of hypopituitarism and recognizing the probability for recovery of function are important issues to be emphasized in the management of patients with this disease. Patients' education is an essential aspect of the management that is often overlooked. Patients need to

TABLE 1. **Symptoms and Signs of Hypopituitarism**

Axis Deficit	Symptoms	Signs
ACTH	Tiredness; fatigue; low energy, especially in P.M.; nausea; weight loss	Pale skin, loss of pubic and axillary hair (women)
FSH/LH	In men, loss of libido and potency, infertility, and hot flashes; in women, amenorrhea, hot flashes, dyspareunia, and infertility	In men, loss of facial or body hair, gynecomastia, increased body fat, soft or small testes; in women, vaginal atrophy or dryness
Growth hormone	Short stature in children; unknown symptoms in adults	Short stature, increased body fat in children; unknown signs in adults
Prolactin	Absence of lactation in women; no symptoms in men	None
TSH	Cold intolerance, tiredness, slow mentation, constipation, weight gain	Pale, waxy, dry skin; delayed relaxation of tendon reflexes

understand the impact of pituitary hormone deficiency on their daily lives and activities and must be fully aware that treatment may need to be modified in the event of intercurrent illnesses, accidents, or surgical procedures. Patients should wear Medic Alert bracelets or necklaces identifying them as being hypopituitary or receiving replacement glucocorticoid therapy. Each patient should, in addition, carry a card providing the diagnosis, list of medications, and name and telephone number of the treating physician. Management of patients with hypopituitarism starts with suspecting the diagnosis and determining the extent of pituitary hormone deficit. The managing physician should appreciate the variable clinical manifestations of the disease and the possible occurrence of other associated neuroendocrine, neurologic, and neuro-ophthalmic signs and symptoms.

HORMONE REPLACEMENT

Hormone replacement should be initiated as soon as the diagnosis of hypopituitarism is made. This is especially true for glucocorticoid replacement, where a delay in treatment can be life-threatening. Treatment should not be rigid but should always be individualized, taking into consideration the patient's age, sex, education, original disease process, and clinical history. Theoretically, one can provide the deficient hypothalamic or pituitary hormone, which in turn can stimulate other hormones in the periphery and result in clinical benefit. Although this approach may be applicable in certain instances, it is impractical in others. For instance, a patient with central hypothyroidism responds to the administration of thyrotropin-releasing hormone (TRH) if the cause of hypothyroidism is hypothalamic deficiency and to TSH injections if his or her disease involves the pituitary. Neither approach is as practical as the oral administration of levothyroxine. The same argument can be made for ACTH deficiency, for which oral glucocorticoid therapy is the appropriate choice. The use of hypothalamic hormones in the management of patients with various forms of hypopituitarism has been limited primarily to those with GnRH deficiency. Some patients with GH deficiency secondary to growth hormone–releasing hormone (GHRH) deficiency were similarly treated with the hypothalamic hormone, with reasonable success.

ACTH DEFICIENCY

Either hydrocortisone (cortisol) or cortisone in two or preferably three divided doses, totaling 15 to 30 mg of the former steroid, is the usual glucocorticoid replacement therapy. The dose is titrated individually, using primarily clinical symptoms as a guideline. Measurement of serum or urinary hormone levels is of no clinical value in determining the proper dose unless poor gastrointestinal absorption or poor compliance with drug intake is suspected. In the author's experience, the vast majority of patients require 20 mg of hydrocortisone or less per day to control symptoms. Although hyponatremia is sometimes seen in patients with ACTH deficiency, mineralocorticoid replacement is rarely, if ever, necessary in patients with hypopituitarism, since the function of the adrenal glomerular zone is maintained. Serum sodium levels return to normal a few days after hydrocortisone therapy is initiated.

TSH DEFICIENCY

L-thyroxine (Synthroid) therapy is the preferred replacement therapy in patients with TSH deficiency. Although measurement of total thyroxine and free thyroxine index serum levels is sometimes helpful in determining the optimal dose of L-thyroxine in these patients, physicians should rely primarily on clinical signs and symptoms before adjustments are made. In contrast to patients with primary hypothyroidism, in whom serum TSH measurements are used to titrate the dose of thyroid hormone replacement, similar determinations in patients with TSH deficiency are of no value and need not be performed. The optimal dose of thyroxine is variable (0.05 to 0.20 mg per day) and depends on the patients' age, other illnesses, and concurrent medications. It is important to point out that thyroxine replacement therapy in hypopituitary patients can unmask signs of ACTH deficiency that may have been unrecognized previously. Symptomatic patients should be tested and treated appropriately.

FSH/LH DEFICIENCY

Effective treatment of hypogonadism in postpubertal adults can be achieved by giving gonadal steroid replacement. Delay in the treatment of men and women with documented hypogonadism increases the risk for osteoporosis and heart disease. Treatment of such patients is usually oral estrogen/progestin for women and long-acting testosterone for men. Oral equine estrogen preparations are the most widely used form of gonadal steroid replacement in women. The average dose of equine estrogen (Premarin), is 0.625 mg every day. Younger women and those taking antiseizure medications require higher doses of estrogen to provide clinical benefit. Women with intact uteri also need a progestational agent to minimize the development of estrogen-induced endometrial hyperplasia. The latter can be given orally as medroxyprogesterone acetate (Provera) every day (2.5 to 5 mg) or for 12 days of each month. Intermittent spotting often occurs initially in patients using combined daily therapy with estrogen and Provera. This is often followed by the development of amenorrhea, with minimal risk for endometrial cancer. In contrast, women given Provera for 12 days of the month are likely to have a monthly menstrual bleed. Women receiving estrogen replacement therapy should have annual mammograms and Pap smears and should also be educated about routine breast self-examination.

Testosterone therapy in men is often superphysiologic when given in the currently prescribed doses of 200 to 300 mg every 2 to 3 weeks. Such doses provide superphysiologic concentrations of gonadal steroids and are likely to be associated with side effects. A common yet frequently overlooked complication of testosterone therapy is hyperlipidemia, which can increase the risk for cardiovascular disease. Symptoms of prostatism and progression of previously unrecognized prostate cancer can occur with testosterone therapy. For these reasons, particular attention should be paid to any potential abnormalities in the prostate before and during androgen therapy. Similarly, attention should be directed at potential alterations in plasma lipids in treated patients. Excessive snoring and even obstructive sleep apnea can occur after androgen replacement, especially in obese men. Every effort should therefore be made to give the lowest possible dose to minimize these and other potential side effects. In the author's experience, most men can be adequately replaced with 120 to 150 mg of testosterone enanthate (Delatestryl) or cypionate (Depotest) intramuscularly every 2 weeks. Testosterone skin patches (Testoderm), that can be applied directly on the scrotum were introduced for clinical use a few years ago. These preparations have been reported to provide a stable and physiologic serum testosterone concentration throughout the day. However, with the increased activity of the enzyme 5-alpha-reductase in the scrotum, higher circulating serum levels of dihydrotestosterone were noted in such patients. These changes have caused some concern among physicians. A more recently introduced preparation of transdermal testosterone, Androderm, appears to be more practical to use, as it can be applied on other areas of the body, such as the thighs and back. When used at the recommended doses of 5 mg per day, these preparations provide stable serum testosterone and dihydrotestosterone levels throughout a 24-hour period. Although these preparations appear to provide testosterone replacement in physiologic doses, there are currently no long-term studies addressing their use, particularly in comparison with other approaches.

Loss of libido is a common symptom in women with hypopituitarism, as a result of diminished adrenal androgen production. Small doses of androgens in the form of parenteral testosterone (15 to 25 mg intramuscularly every 2 weeks) can be used to restore libido in such patients, under strict and careful follow-up.

Male patients desiring the restoration of fertility require a different approach that aims at stimulating intratesticular, endogenous testosterone production using human chorionic gonadotropin (hCG) (A.P.L.). The latter hormone is similar in structure to LH and, at the recommended doses (600 to 1000 U intramuscularly three times per week), can stimulate testosterone secretion by the testes and support spermatogenesis. Often, however, human menopausal gonadotropin (hMG) (menotropins [Pergonal]) also must be used in these patients to restore spermatogenesis. This preparation contains equal amounts of human FSH and LH isolated from menopausal women. In many patients in whom the hypogonadism is of recent onset, hCG alone is sufficient to restore fertility. Patients with more prolonged hypogonadism require both hCG and hMG injections to restore fertility.

In both male and female patients in whom the cause of hypopituitarism is a hypothalamic disease process (e.g., Kallmann's syndrome or a hypothalamic disease), the administration of the hypothalamic releasing hormone GnRH can be more effective in restoring fertility and gonadal function. The hypothalamic hormone has to be injected in a pulsatile manner through a portable implantable pump designed to mimic the natural rhythm of GnRH secretion.

GH DEFICIENCY

Treatment of GH deficiency is essential in children with documented deficiencies. The availability of synthetic GH has significantly increased its clinical use in children as well as in adults. Although there is an extensive experience in the treatment of GH deficiency in children, only limited data are available in adults. Recent studies demonstrated the beneficial effects of GH treatment in elderly patients with deficiency.* An increase in lean body mass and a decrease in body fat were shown during short-term therapy with exogenous GH. The available studies are primarily short term and should therefore be viewed with caution. An additional issue of concern is the cost of prolonged treatment with GH in adults. It is not clear whether persistent, untreated states of GH deficiency in adults have any impact on the long-term morbidity of patients with hypopituitarism, as was recently suggested. If this is confirmed, and if treatment can be given without significant side effects, GH can be offered to all patients with deficits, regardless of age. Additional studies are necessary before a firm recommendation can be given. Treatment of GH deficiency in adults is considered experimental at the present time.

The potential for recovery of pituitary function should always be considered, since it can prevent the unnecessary use of lifelong hormone replacement therapy. This is becoming particularly important in view of recent data suggesting increased morbidity in treated as well as untreated patients with hypopituitarism. The cause or causes of increased morbidity and mortality in treated patients are not known. It is reasonable to speculate that overtreatment with gonadal steroids, glucocorticoids and/or thyroid hormone contributes to the increased morbidity. Some reports, however, have implicated persistence of GH deficiency in these patients as a potential cause. Until more firm data are available, treatment with GH should be considered experimental and should be given under specific research protocols. Furthermore, patients with permanent hypopituitarism should be followed regularly, and their hormone replacement doses should be adjusted, as necessary, to avoid overtreatment.

---

*Not FDA-approved for this indication.

HYPERPROLACTINEMIA

method of
ROMA GIANCHANDANI, M.D., and
ARIEL BARKAN, M.D.
University of Michigan Medical Center
Ann Arbor, Michigan

In healthy men and women, serum prolactin is usually below 20 ng per mL. Hyperprolactinemia is the most common disorder of the anterior pituitary gland. Prolactin is necessary for the initiation and maintenance of lactation and serves as a natural contraceptive, inhibiting secretion of gonadotropin-releasing hormone (GnRH). The resultant suppression of pituitary luteinizing hormone (LH) and follicle-stimulating hormone (FSH) secretion leads to hypogonadism. Thus, amenorrhea (in women) or impotence (in men) and often galactorrhea are the cardinal manifestations of hyperprolactinemia of any etiology. The pituitary secretion of prolactin is controlled predominantly by inhibitory influences exerted by the hypothalamus via numerous prolactin-inhibiting factors (PIFs), the most important physiologically being dopamine. Dopamine is produced by the ventromedial and arcuate nuclei of the hypothalamus and is transported to the pituitary via the hypothalamic-pituitary portal vessels. There it binds to D_2 receptors on lactotroph cell membranes to tonically inhibit prolactin production. Therefore, interference with hypothalamic dopamine synthesis, hypothalamic-pituitary portal blood flow, or dopamine action on the lactotrophs leads to an elevated level of prolactin.

Numerous mechanisms may lead to excessive prolactin production. These include:

1. Prolactin hyperproduction by pituitary tumors (prolactinomas, growth hormone [GH]- and rarely corticotropin [ACTH]-producing pituitary tumors).
2. Disorders of dopamine, including deficient dopamine synthesis (e.g., hypothalamic disease, dopamine synthesis blockers such as methyldopa and reserpine), deficient delivery of dopamine to the pituitary (e.g., pituitary stalk section or compression by pituitary and parapituitary masses), deficient action of dopamine on the pituitary (e.g., dopamine receptor antagonists such as metoclopramide), and desensitization of pituitary lactotrophs to dopamine by estrogens.
3. Excessive stimulation of prolactin secretion by hypothalamic thyrotropin-releasing hormone (TRH) (e.g., primary hypothyroidism).
4. Neurogenic hyperprolactinemia from any chest irritation (e.g., broken ribs, thoracotomy, mastectomy, herpes zoster, burns).
5. Diminished prolactin clearance, as in chronic renal failure.

CAUSES OF HYPERPROLACTINEMIA

The numerous causes of hyperprolactinemia can be grouped into the following broad categories: physiologic, pharmacologic, and pathologic. A detailed list of causes is outlined in Table 1.

Physiologic

Prolactin increases with sleep, stress, meals, and postictally, probably from input of higher centers to the hypothalamus. In pregnancy, prolactin levels rise due to stimulation of pituitary lactotrophs by estrogen, and the pituitary gland may enlarge, sometimes to double its size. Prolactin starts to decline post partum, with a peak during each suckling episode. Although lactation may continue, 4 to 6 months post partum, both basal and suckling-associated prolactin levels usually normalize.

Pharmacologic

Obtaining an accurate drug history is important for patients with hyperprolactinemia. Psychotropic agents usually raise prolactin, especially dopamine-blocking agents (e.g., phenothiazines and butyrophenones). All tricyclic antidepressants may raise serum prolactin, but newer antidepressants working on the serotoninergic system (fluoxetine [Prozac], sertraline [Zoloft]) do not normally elevate prolactin. Additionally, dopamine depletors such as reserpine can raise prolactin. The calcium channel blocker verapamil (Isoptin) may produce mild hyperprolactinemia through a poorly understood mechanism. Opioids and estrogens have similar effects on prolactin levels.

Pathologic

Prolactinomas are the most common pituitary tumors. Prolactin may be co-secreted in acromegaly and Cushing's

TABLE 1. Causes of Hyperprolactinemia

Physiologic States

Pregnancy
Lactation
Suckling
Sleep
Stress
Postprandial state

Pharmacologic

Neuroleptics: phenothiazines—chlorpromazine (Thorazine), prochlorperazine (Compazine), thioridazine (Mellaril), trifluoperazine (Stelazine), thiothixene (Navane); butyrophenones—haloperidol (Haldol), loxapine (Loxitane)
Tricyclic antidepressants—amitriptyline (Elavil), nortriptyline (Pamelor), desipramine (Norpramin), imipramine (Tofranil)
Dibenzepin antidepressants—amoxapine (Asendin)
Antihypertensives—methyldopa (Aldomet), reserpine (Serpasil), verapamil (Calan, Isoptin, Verelan)
Monoamine oxidase inhibitors—phenelzine (Nardil), tranylcypromine (Parnate)
Opioids—morphine, meperidine (Demerol)
Estrogen (including birth control pills)
H_2-receptor blockers—cimetidine (Tagamet), ranitidine (Zantac), famotidine (Pepcid)
Antimotility agents—metoclopramide (Reglan), cisapride (Propulsid), domperidone

Pathologic

Pituitary
Prolactinoma
Nonsecretory pituitary adenoma
Cushing's disease
Empty sella
Acromegaly
Lymphocytic hypophysitis
Pituitary stalk section
Hypothalamic
Craniopharyngioma
Dysgerminoma
Sarcoidosis
Eosinophilic granuloma
Neuroaxis radiation

Other

Chest wall injury
Chronic renal failure
Cirrhosis
Hypothyroidism
Primary adrenal insufficiency
Pseudocyesis
Spinal cord lesions

Idiopathic

May have a microadenoma too small to be identified by current radiologic techniques

---

disease. Nonsecretory pituitary or parapituitary tumors increase prolactin by associated stalk compression. Hypothalamic tumors or granulomas (e.g., sarcoid) can also raise prolactin.

Other

Primary hypothyroidism raises prolactin by increasing TRH levels or decreasing dopaminergic tone. There may be associated sellar enlargement, which normalizes with thyroid replacement. In renal failure, there may be decreased clearance or breakdown of prolactin or impaired hypothalamic regulation. Correction of renal failure or renal transplant may normalize prolactin levels. Cirrhotics may have high prolactin due to disordered hypothalamic regulation and a relatively increased estrogen level. Breast stimulation, chest wall trauma, and cervical cord lesions stimulate prolactin via signals transmitted through afferent neural pathways.

When no specific cause for hyperprolactinemia can be identified, the elevation is considered idiopathic. Idiopathic hyperprolactinemia may be secondary to a tumor too small to be detected by current radiographic techniques or due to minor stalk abnormalities. On long-term follow-up of these patients, 30% normalize their prolactin, 15% have a rise in prolactin and may develop microadenomas, and the remaining continue to have an elevated but stable level of prolactin.

CLINICAL PRESENTATION

Hyperprolactinemia functionally interferes with the hypothalamic-gonadal axis and suppresses pulsatile gonadotropin secretion. Its clinical presentation varies, depending on the degree of hypogonadism present. Adolescent girls may have primary amenorrhea or delayed puberty. Women usually present with menstrual disturbances that range from mild menstrual irregularities to oligomenorrhea, an-

ovulation, and amenorrhea. Galactorrhea is present in 30 to 80% of these women, but in a population of women with amenorrhea and galactorrhea, the incidence of prolactinoma is up to 75%. Other problems of estrogen insufficiency such as decreased libido, vaginal dryness, and dyspareunia may occur. Men usually come to clinical attention due to headaches, visual disturbances, and field defects, namely, temporal hemianopsia. When sexual disturbance is the presenting complaint in a male, it is usually partial or complete impotence, lack of libido, or, rarely, oligospermia and gynecomastia. It is of note that men with prolactinoma come to medical attention much later than women and have larger tumors at diagnosis.

The physical examination of a patient with prolactin excess should include a fundus examination; visual field testing by confrontation; assessment of cranial nerve III, IV, and VI function; and assessment of breast milk discharge in women by manual expression, gynecomastia and testicular atrophy in men, body hair distribution, chest wall lesions, signs of hypothyroidism (including goiter), acromegaly, or Cushing's disease.

LABORATORY EVALUATION

Before interpreting an elevated prolactin level, it is necessary to confirm normal liver and kidney functions, thyroid indices (thyroid-stimulating hormone [TSH] and free thyroxine [T_4]), and a negative pregnancy test in premenopausal women. A history of interfering drugs needs to be obtained. Prolactinomas are the most common secretory pituitary tumors, although prolactin may be co-secreted by GH- and ACTH-producing tumors.

Because of both the episodic secretion of prolactin and its sensitivity to meals and physical exercise, it is often useful to measure two separately drawn prolactin levels (especially if the level is borderline). Since prolactin secretion is physiologically augmented in the early morning hours, blood samples for prolactin should optimally be drawn after 10 A.M. In the absence of pregnancy, a prolactin level over 200 ng per mL is virtually always associated with a prolactinoma. Since serum prolactin is usually proportional to tumor size, smaller lesions may be associated with levels less than 100 ng per mL. In hyperprolactinemia secondary to drugs or physiologic excess states, the prolactin level is often less than 50 ng per mL and usually below 150 ng per mL. If no cause for hyperprolactinemia is identified on routine testing, a pituitary imaging study—either a contrast-enhanced computed tomography (CT) scan or, preferably, a magnetic resonance imaging (MRI) scan with gadolinium—is warranted to detect a pituitary or hypothalamic lesion. An MRI, although more expensive, is preferred to a CT scan because it provides better anatomic detail of the pituitary, especially of the surrounding structures.

Formal dynamic pituitary function testing is usually not necessary for microadenomas, which, due to their small size, do not compromise pituitary reserve. For macroadenomas, preoperative pituitary function testing is not necessary either, because steroid coverage needs to be provided perioperatively. In macroadenomas that are medically managed or if any suspicion of hypopituitarism is present, formal pituitary function tests need to be obtained. Formal visual field testing is performed in patients with symptoms of field defects or if a macroadenoma is in proximity to or is invading the optic chiasm. In pregnancy, formal visual field testing is performed in each trimester for women with macroadenomas, especially those on no medical treatment. Additionally, other baseline hormones that may need assessment in appropriate clinical situations include GH/somatomedin C (insulin-like growth factor 1) to exclude acromegaly.

CLASSIFICATION AND NATURAL HISTORY

Radiologically, pituitary tumors are divided into microadenomas (<10 mm), macroadenomas (>10 mm), and macroadenomas with extrasellar extension. This distinction is important for predicting the natural history of the tumor and for outlining the management plan. Microadenomas are slow-growing tumors, and more than 90% do not enlarge over a 4- to 6-year follow-up. Some microadenomas appear to vanish spontaneously. Macroadenomas demonstrate a propensity to grow from the start and need to be managed aggressively.

MANAGEMENT OF HYPERPROLACTINEMIA

In addition to lowering the prolactin level, management goals include release of mass effect and normalization of pituitary function. Absolute indications for the treatment of hyperprolactinemia include the request for improved sexual function or fertility and the presence of a macroadenoma with or without mass effect. Other indications for treatment include troublesome galactorrhea, irregular menses, and the risk of osteoporosis. The effects of hyperprolactinemic hypogonadism on the skeleton of both men and women have been recognized recently. In hyperprolactinemia, bone mineral density (of cancellous more than cortical bone) is reduced and may be restored with treatment. The associated hypogonadism is the major cause of bone demineralization, although the

contribution of a high prolactin level is presently unclear.

In pharmacologic hyperprolactinemia, the drugs that elevate prolactin should be stopped (if possible), and prolactin should be remeasured and confirmed to be normal. If it is imperative to continue the offending agent, dopamine agonists (as described later) can be added to the medical regimen. Bromocriptine use has recently been shown to be safe and effective in hyperprolactinemic patients in combination with antipsychotic medications. In primary hypothyroidism, replacement with levothyroxine lowers TSH and reduces prolactin levels and pituitary size, if it was initially increased.

Drugs

Since drugs are extremely efficacious in the treatment of prolactinomas, they are the primary mode of therapy for both macro- and microadenomas. Bromocriptine (Parlodel), an ergot-derived dopamine agonist, is the only agent licensed for the treatment of hyperprolactinemia in the United States. It normalizes ovulatory menses in 80 to 90% of premenopausal women by binding to lactotroph D_2 receptors and reducing prolactin levels. In prolactinomas, it reduces lactotroph DNA synthesis, cell multiplication, and tumor size. This relieves mass effect and often improves visual field abnormalities dramatically. The drug is initially started in very small doses of 1.25 mg taken at bedtime with a snack. The dose is increased slowly (by about 1.25 mg every 3 to 4 days) and may be as high as 25 mg per day, although most patients do not require more than 7.5 mg per day (2.5 mg three times a day). Side effects of the drug include nausea, vomiting, abdominal pain, dizziness, lightheadedness, nasal stuffiness, and orthostatic hypotension. In up to 5% of patients, these symptoms are severe enough to warrant discontinuation of the drug. Although not licensed for intravaginal use, bromocriptine* has been prescribed by this route for patients with severe gastrointestinal symptoms on oral therapy. Long-acting preparations of bromocriptine (Parlodel LAR)† are not yet available for use in the United States.

Pergolide (Permax),* another ergot-derived dopamine agonist commonly used in parkinsonism, may be useful in some patients who cannot tolerate bromocriptine and is administered in the dose range of 0.05 to 1 mg. This drug is not approved by the U.S. Food and Drug Administration (FDA) for the treatment of hyperprolactinemia but is widely used for this purpose in other countries. Pergolide is 10 to 1000 times more potent than bromocriptine, has fewer side effects, has a longer duration of action (12 to 24 hours), and is about five times cheaper on a dose basis. Newer non–ergot-derived dopamine agonists that are well tolerated by most patients include

---

*Not FDA-approved for this indication.
†Not available in the United States.

quinagolide* (CV 205-502) and cabergoline.* These drugs need to be administered daily and weekly, respectively, but at present can be obtained only on a compassionate-need basis.

In women with microadenomas who tolerate drugs, normal menses resume within 2 months and rarely may be delayed for up to a year. Although the drug effects are not permanent, in a few patients with microadenomas, prolactin levels normalize and remain low after stopping all medications. In both micro- and macroadenomas, bromocriptine decreases tumor size. Prolactin usually declines before tumor shrinkage is detected, and the maximal effect is usually seen within the first 3 to 6 months of treatment. Usually 50% of macroadenomas shrink by more than 50%, 20% by less than 50%, and the rest by 25% of their original size. Tumor shrinkage is maximal in the first 6 weeks of treatment but can often take up to 6 months, after which an additional gradual decline in size may be noted. Visual fields improve after 1 to 3 months of therapy. After discontinuing bromocriptine, macroadenomas rapidly enlarge and prolactin levels rise, necessitating continued medical treatment.

Surgery

Surgery is sometimes necessary in patients unable or unwilling to use medical therapy. Additionally, it may be required in patients with persistent field defects or large tumors with a cystic or hemorrhagic component to relieve local symptoms. The usual surgical approach to the pituitary is via the trans-sphenoidal route, but a craniotomy may rarely be necessary. Trans-sphenoidal surgery has low mortality and morbidity rates, with prolactin levels normalizing within 24 hours in 70% of patients. Its few side effects include transient diabetes insipidus, cerebrospinal fluid rhinorrhea, and central nervous system infections. The major drawback of surgery is its poor cure rate: 70% for microadenomas, and 30% for macroadenomas. Recurrence of hyperprolactinemia usually occurs within the first 6 months, and even when not documented radiologically, it necessitates medical therapy.

Radiation

Radiotherapy is used in rare patients with unusually aggressive residual tumors who are unable to tolerate or respond to drugs after surgery. Normal prolactin levels are achieved 5 to 10 years after therapy. The major side effect of radiation is hypopituitarism and the need for replacement hormones. Patients must therefore be monitored for extended periods of time.

Treatment of Prolactinomas During Pregnancy

Pregnancy induces lactotroph hyperplasia in normal pituitaries, although its effect on prolactinomas is variable. The incidence of tumor enlargement during pregnancy is 2% for microadenomas and 16% for macroadenomas. Prolactin levels rise during pregnancy, making them a poor indicator of concomitant tumor regrowth, unless the levels are higher than 400 to 500 ng per mL. The usual recommendation is to discontinue bromocriptine at the first missed period in patients with either macro- or microadenomas. If tumor-related symptoms recur, the drug can be restarted. Additionally, formal visual field testing is performed every trimester in women with macroadenomas, and an MRI needs to be obtained if marked regrowth is suspected. An alternative approach is to continue the use of bromocriptine during pregnancy. Although experience with bromocriptine in pregnancy is limited, no increases in congenital malformations, spontaneous abortions, ectopic pregnancies, or ill effects on children have been noted on long-term follow-up.

Bromocriptine and Lactation

Bromocriptine's indication for aborting lactation in normal women has recently been withdrawn due to numerous reports of vascular sequelae. The postpartum treatment of prolactinomas is a different problem. Therapy with bromocriptine should be resumed after childbirth in women with prolactinomas. Although some of these women wish to lactate post partum, the practice should be discouraged, and bromocriptine administration should be reinstituted as soon as possible.

SUMMARY

Hyperprolactinemia is the most common disorder of the anterior pituitary gland. The cardinal symptoms include amenorrhea in women and impotence in men. Galactorrhea and, less often, other symptoms of hypogonadism are often present. After obtaining a detailed drug history, physicians need to assess patients for renal and liver disease, hypothyroidism, and pregnancy. A negative work-up mandates assessment for a pituitary or hypothalamic lesion. Treatment goals include lowering prolactin levels, reducing tumor size, and restoring fertility. These are usually achieved with bromocriptine therapy. Surgery is reserved for patients who are unable to respond to or tolerate drugs. Women with hyperprolactinemia, especially those with macroadenomas, need close follow-up during pregnancy.

HYPOTHYROIDISM

method of
RONALD J. KOENIG, M.D., PH.D.
University of Michigan Medical Center
Ann Arbor, Michigan

Hypothyroidism is a common condition, especially in women, affecting up to 5% of females in the United

---

*Investigational drug in the United States.

States. Clinical severity can range from an asymptomatic state to coma. Common symptoms include lethargy, mild weight gain, cold intolerance, constipation, and menstrual irregularities. Primary thyroid gland failure accounts for the overwhelming majority of cases and is most commonly due to autoimmune destruction (Hashimoto's thyroiditis) or ablative treatment of hyperthyroidism (radioiodine or surgical thyroidectomy). The most sensitive assay for primary hypothyroidism is the measurement of serum thyroid-stimulating hormone (TSH), which is elevated even in asymptomatic cases. Thyroxine (T_4) levels fall below normal after the TSH rises. (In this article, measurement of the serum T_4 level is presumed to take the strength of serum T_4 binding proteins into account either by a test such as the triiodothyronine (T_3) resin uptake or by measurement of free T_4.) T_3 levels are not useful to diagnose hypothyroidism due to poor sensitivity and specificity.

A minor fraction of cases of hypothyroidism are due to pituitary or hypothalamic disease (secondary or tertiary hypothyroidism, respectively). These cases are usually associated with other anterior pituitary hormone deficiencies (especially growth hormone and gonadotropins) and generally occur in the setting of already known or clinically suspected pituitary or hypothalamic disease. Since TSH is either low or inappropriately normal in secondary and tertiary hypothyroidism, diagnosis requires measurement of T_4.

Treatment of hypothyroidism is with L-thyroxine (Levothroid, Levoxyl, Synthroid). Patients may take L-thyroxine any time of day, but establishing a standard routine helps maximize compliance. If a patient forgets to take a dose one day, he or she can take two pills the following day. The average full replacement dose is about 0.8 µg per pound of body weight, although the range is considerable. It is prudent to start with a lower dose (50 µg per day or less) in the elderly or in individuals with cardiac disease (see the later discussion). The intestinal absorption of L-thyroxine is impaired by cholestyramine (Questran), colestipol (Colestid), iron sulfate, and sucralfate (Carafate). The goals of treatment in primary hypothyroidism are to alleviate symptoms and normalize the serum TSH. It is generally not necessary to follow the serum T_4 level during therapy. However, it should be recognized that there are occasional conditions that confound interpretation of the serum TSH. For example, severe nonthyroidal illness and high-dose glucocorticoid therapy can themselves suppress the serum TSH.

Since the circulating half-life of T_4 is approximately 1 week, it takes 4 to 6 weeks of a given L-thyroxine dose to achieve a new steady state. Therefore, the TSH is generally not measured until a given dose of L-thyroxine has been maintained for at least that length of time. The normal range for TSH spans an order of magnitude (approximately 0.5 to 5 µU per mL in most assays). Most patients are asymptomatic if the TSH falls anywhere within the normal range, although there are exceptions. Once the correct dose of L-thyroxine has been determined, TSH need be measured only once per year, unless the patient develops symptoms compatible with thyroid hormone deficiency or excess. Patients who have been maintained on a steady dose of L-thyroxine with a mid-normal TSH are sometimes found to have a borderline abnormal TSH (such as 0.3 or 6 µU per mL) on routine follow-up. These individuals are generally asymptomatic, and it is not clear if this modest abnormality represents an indication for a change in dosage. A reasonable approach is to repeat the TSH in 2 to 3 months and make a dosage adjustment if the abnormality persists. Phenytoin (Dilantin), carbamazepine (Tegretol), and rifampin (Rifadin) increase the metabolism of T_4, and patients taking these drugs may need an increase in L-thyroxine dosage.

In secondary and tertiary hypothyroidism, one must follow the serum T_4 rather than the TSH. Normal individuals derive about 80% of their circulating T_3 from peripheral deiodination of T_4 and about 20% from direct thyroidal secretion. Since individuals on L-thyroxine therapy generally lack direct thyroidal secretion, slightly more circulating T_4 is needed to produce a given serum T_3 level. Thus, when using the serum T_4 level as a guide to replacement therapy in secondary and tertiary hypothyroidism, it is generally reasonable to maintain the T_4 in the upper half of the normal range.

Hypothyroid women who are infertile may have their fertility restored by L-thyroxine treatment, and they should be advised of this in advance. L-Thyroxine therapy in hypothyroid diabetics may necessitate an increase in insulin dose. Patients on anticoagulants may need to lower the dose following L-thyroxine replacement therapy. Since T_4 stimulates the metabolism of cortisol, L-thyroxine replacement therapy may exacerbate cortisol deficiency in patients with Schmidt's syndrome (combined thyroid and adrenal insufficiency). Patients with suspected adrenal insufficiency should be evaluated and treated prior to or concomitant with initiation of L-thyroxine therapy.

SPECIAL CIRCUMSTANCES

Replacement Therapy During Pregnancy. In many women, the L-thyroxine dose requirement rises by 25 to 50% during pregnancy. The reason for this is not entirely clear, but the increased need becomes manifest during the first trimester and continues until shortly after delivery. In primary hypothyroidism, this is best judged by following the TSH, which should be checked at around 8 weeks gestation and, if no changes are made, again at around 20 to 24 weeks. The L-thyroxine dose should be decreased to prepregnancy levels immediately after delivery. Therapy with L-thyroxine is not a contraindication to nursing.

Replacement Therapy in Individuals with Cardiac Disease. A subset of hypothyroid individuals with cardiac disease has an exacerbation of angina or arrhythmias if L-thyroxine replacement is instituted too vigorously. In such individuals, it is generally wise to begin therapy with low doses of L-thyroxine, such as 12.5 to 25 μg per day, and increase by about 25 μg per day every 4 to 6 weeks. Such individuals also may best be managed by maintaining the serum TSH in the upper portion of the normal range.

Individuals with Subclinical Hypothyroidism. Many individuals have serum TSH levels just slightly above normal (about 6 to 10 μU per mL) and few, if any, symptoms of hypothyroidism. These patients might have transient subacute thyroiditis or early Hashimoto's thyroiditis. It is generally reasonable to repeat the TSH in a couple of months to assess whether the abnormality persists. If it does, institution of L-thyroxine therapy should be considered. The approach should be individualized. Presuming the patient had nonspecific symptoms such as fatigue that prompted the initial TSH measurement, it is reasonable to give L-thyroxine therapy to normalize TSH for several months. If the symptoms resolve, therapy can be maintained indefinitely. If the symptoms do not resolve, they were not caused by hypothyroidism. In such cases, continuation of L-thyroxine therapy is optional, but in any case, the TSH needs to be followed periodically, since the rate of progression of Hashimoto's thyroiditis is unpredictable. Mild hypothyroidism occasionally contributes to hypercholesterolemia; this is an additional reason to treat selected patients with mildly elevated TSH and no overt symptoms.

Surgery in Hypothyroid Patients. Although it is logical to postpone elective surgery in hypothyroid individuals, it is occasionally necessary to perform emergency surgery in such patients. Retrospective analyses indicate that general anesthesia and surgery are usually well tolerated by hypothyroid individuals. However, there may be an increased risk of perioperative complications, so these patients require careful observation. Hypothyroid individuals are less likely to mount a fever in response to infections. They may require lower doses of anesthetic and may be prone to postoperative fluid and electrolyte abnormalities and ileus.

Treatment of Myxedema Coma. The rarity of myxedema coma virtually precludes prospective trials comparing different forms of therapy. In most anecdotal reports of successful treatment, intravenous L-thyroxine was used, although there are also reports of using T_3. A common treatment schedule would be 500 μg L-thyroxine intravenously as initial treatment, followed by 100 μg L-thyroxine intravenously per day. The exact form and dose of thyroid hormone replacement may not be the key determinant of patient outcome. It is critical to search for and treat associated illnesses such as infections. It is equally important to monitor the patient's respiratory status carefully, since these patients have diminished respiratory drive and may succumb to apnea. Patients with myxedema coma due to Hashimoto's thyroiditis may have other autoimmune diseases, most prominently Addison's disease. Therefore, it is wise to treat these patients empirically with glucocorticoids until their adrenal status has

been determined. Patients with myxedema coma are generally hypothermic; warming should be passive, since active warming could result in peripheral vasodilatation and cardiovascular collapse.

Treatment of Subacute Thyroiditis. Subacute thyroiditis is a self-limited condition that can cause transient hyperthyroidism followed by transient hypothyroidism. Each of these phases may be asymptomatic or may be symptomatic for up to 2 to 3 months. Subacute thyroiditis can be painful or painless. Since the hypothyroid phase is usually mild and short-lived, treatment with L-thyroxine is usually not necessary. In patients who are bothered significantly by symptoms of hypothyroidism, L-thyroxine may be given to normalize the serum TSH. After 3 to 6 months, the dose should be decreased by 50% and the TSH rechecked in approximately 4 weeks. If the TSH remains normal, the L-thyroxine dose can be decreased by another 50% for 4 weeks and then discontinued entirely, again using TSH as a guide.

Continuation of Thyroxine Therapy in Patients with Questionable Hypothyroidism. Physicians occasionally encounter patients who have been on thyroid hormone replacement for many years but for whom the initial diagnosis of hypothyroidism is not well documented. In such patients, the physician can determine whether such therapy is still warranted by decreasing the dose by 50% and checking the TSH in 4 to 6 weeks. If the TSH remains normal, the L-thyroxine dose can be decreased by another 50% for 4 to 6 weeks and then discontinued entirely, again using TSH as a guide to the patient's thyroid status.

HYPERTHYROIDISM

method of
DOUGLAS S. ROSS, M.D.
Massachusetts General Hospital
Boston, Massachusetts

The classic symptoms of overt hyperthyroidism include weight loss, increased appetite, palpitations, tremulousness, heat intolerance, fatigue, dyspnea on exertion, frequent bowel movements, oligomenorrhea, muscle weakness, insomnia, and irritability. Mild hyperthyroidism may paradoxically be associated with weight gain due to appetite stimulation. Elderly patients may present with weight loss and cachexia without tachycardia or tremulousness. Exacerbation of angina or congestive heart failure is common. Occasional patients have minimal symptoms despite marked chemical hyperthyroidism. Physical examination classically reveals tachycardia, a widened pulse pressure, tremor, stare, hyper-reflexia, and onycholysis. Goiter may be absent, especially in elderly patients. Exophthalmos, orbital inflammation, and pretibial myxedema are specific for Graves' disease.

LABORATORY DIAGNOSIS

Serum thyroid-stimulating hormone (TSH) concentrations are now utilized as the primary screening test for thyroid disease. Hyperthyroid patients have subnormal serum TSH concentrations. A low serum TSH cannot distinguish degrees of hyperthyroidism, which requires determination of both a serum free thyroxine (T_4) level (free T_4 index, "direct" free T_4 measurement, or free T_4 by dialysis) and a serum triiodothyronine (T_3) level. *Subclinical hyperthyroidism* is defined as a subnormal serum TSH associated with a normal serum free T_4 and T_3 concentration and is the least severe form of hyperthyroidism. Patients with subclinical hyperthyroidism have a threefold increased prevalence of atrial fibrillation, and postmenopausal women with subclinical hyperthyroidism have reduced bone density. Therefore, older men and postmenopausal women with subclinical hyperthyroidism may benefit from treatment. All patients with *overt hyperthyroidism* (elevated serum free T_4 or T_3 with subnormal serum TSH) require treatment.

A low serum TSH level does not always indicate hyperthyroidism. Low serum TSH, when associated with low or low-normal serum free T_4 concentrations, may indicate secondary or central hypothyroidism, severe nonthyroidal illness, corticosteroid excess, depression, or concurrent dopamine therapy. Rarely, hyperthyroidism is caused by a TSH-producing adenoma or partial pituitary resistance to thyroid hormone; these patients have normal or elevated serum TSH levels.

ETIOLOGY OF HYPERTHYROIDISM

Conceptually, there are two groups of thyroid disorders (Table 1). Hyperthyroidism associated with a high radioiodine uptake is consistent with de novo intrathyroidal synthesis of hormone, and primary treatment modalities are antithyroid drugs and radioiodine. Hyperthyroidism associated with a low radioiodine uptake occurs either when there is inflammation and destruction of thyroid tissue with release of preformed hormone into the circulation or when the source of thyroid hormone is extrathyroidal. These entities are generally not treated with antithyroid drugs or radioiodine (see the later discussion).

THERAPY FOR HYPERTHYROIDISM WITH A HIGH RADIOIODINE UPTAKE

Graves' disease is the most common form of hyperthyroidism, an autoimmune disorder characterized by immune globulin–mediated stimulation of the TSH receptor. Treatment options include a course of antithyroid drugs with the hope of attaining a

remission, ablation of the gland with radioiodine, and surgical removal of the gland. *Toxic adenoma* and *toxic multinodular goiter* result from autonomous function of thyroid tissue and are treated similarly to Graves' disease, except that remissions are not anticipated following a course of antithyroid drugs. Therapy of trophoblastic disease and TSH-producing adenomas is directed primarily against the neoplastic process, but antithyroid drugs may provide useful adjunctive therapy. Pituitary resistance is difficult to treat; some patients have improved with liothyronine (Cytomel) or 3,5,3′-triiodothyroacetic acid (TRIAC). The following discussion addresses treatment for Graves' disease and toxic nodular goiter.

Beta-Adrenergic Blocking Agents

Because hyperthyroidism increases beta-adrenergic receptors in many tissues, beta-adrenergic blocking agents ameliorate the tachycardia, palpitations, tremulousness, heat intolerance, and anxiety associated with hyperthyroidism and are therefore useful adjunctive therapy for all patients without specific contraindications. Propranolol (Inderal) in high concentrations also decreases serum T_3 concentrations by inhibiting serum T_4 to T_3 conversion. However, propranolol must be given every 6 hours to be effective. I therefore prefer the use of long-acting beta$_1$-selective drugs such as atenolol (Tenormin), 25 to 50 mg or more daily, usually as a single daily dose.

Thionamides (Antithyroid Drugs)

Methimazole (Tapazole) and propylthiouracil (PTU) are the two thionamides available in the United States; carbimazole,* which is metabolized to methimazole, is available in Europe. Thionamides inhibit organification of iodine and therefore prevent de novo hormone synthesis. Thionamides may be given in both Graves' disease and toxic nodular goiter to control the hyperthyroidism in advance of definitive therapy with surgery or radioiodine, or they may be used in Graves' disease for a prolonged time with the hope of achieving a permanent remission. Controversy exists as to whether thionamides have immunomodulatory effects that make remission more likely or whether they simply control the hyperthyroidism until spontaneous remission occurs. Remission rates in the United States are approximately 20 to 35% after 1 to 2 years of thionamide therapy. In Japan, remission rates of 75 to 80% have been reported after 10 years.

There are significant differences in the pharmacology of methimazole and PTU. The serum half-life of PTU is 75 minutes, versus 4 to 6 hours for methimazole. More importantly, intrathyroidal methimazole concentrations remain high for over 20 hours after a single dose, resulting in a more prolonged organification blockade compared with PTU. As a result, methimazole is initially effective as a single daily

TABLE 1. **Types of Hyperthyroidism**

Hyperthyroidism with a High Radioiodine Uptake

Graves' disease
Toxic adenoma or toxic multinodular goiter
Trophoblastic disease
TSH-mediated hyperthyroidism

Hyperthyroidism with a Low Radioiodine Uptake

Subacute thyroiditis
    Subacute granulomatous (de Quervain's) thyroiditis
    Subacute lymphocytic (painless) thyroiditis
    Postpartum thyroiditis
Ectopic hyperthyroidism
    Factitious
    Struma ovarii
    Metastatic follicular thyroid cancer

Abbreviation: TSH = thyroid-stimulating hormone.

---

*Not available in the United States.

dose; PTU requires divided doses to be equally effective. PTU, but not methimazole, inhibits conversion of T_4 to T_3. This theoretical advantage is not realized unless serum PTU concentrations are maintained at therapeutic levels by frequent dosing. Consequently, patients given methimazole normalize their serum T_3 concentrations weeks earlier than those given PTU. I therefore prefer methimazole for initial therapy.

Initial Therapy

Thionamides only prevent new hormone synthesis. It takes weeks for patients given thionamides to become euthyroid, because existing hormone stores must first be exhausted. Traditionally, high doses of thionamides are given initially: 30 to 40 mg of methimazole in single or divided doses, or 300 mg of PTU in divided doses. Once euthyroidism is restored, lower maintenance doses are substituted, e.g., 5 to 15 mg of methimazole daily. Recent studies have demonstrated that lower "maintenance" doses of methimazole, when given as initial therapy, result in attainment of chemical euthyroidism equally rapidly as the traditional higher doses, although occasional patients with severe hyperthyroidism, especially those with large glands, require higher doses. Accordingly, I treat patients with mild hyperthyroidism and small glands (up to twice normal size) with 10 to 15 mg of methimazole, patients with moderate hyperthyroidism and moderately enlarged glands (two or three times normal) with 15 to 20 mg of methimazole, and patients with more severe hyperthyroidism and large glands with 30 mg of methimazole. Single daily dosing with methimazole and a long-acting beta blocker markedly improves compliance. For patients who have minor side effects from methimazole, PTU may be substituted at an initial dose of 100 mg three times daily. Once euthyroidism is achieved (usually after 3 to 12 weeks), patients may go on to radioiodine or surgery, or patients with Graves' disease may opt for long-term maintenance therapy.

Maintenance Therapy

With the control of chemical hyperthyroidism, the thionamide dose may need to be tapered to lower levels, especially if the initial dose of methimazole was greater than 10 to 15 mg. TSH measurements may be misleading during the acute therapy of hyperthyroidism, since subnormal serum TSH concentrations may persist for weeks to occasionally months after euthyroidism has been attained. It is essential to monitor both serum free T_4 and T_3 concentrations during titration of the thionamide dose. Patients are initially seen at 4- to 6-week intervals but may be seen at 3- to 6-month intervals once stability has been achieved. Patients with Graves' disease in the United States who opt for long-term therapy are traditionally treated for 1 to 2 years, but there is no compelling reason not to treat longer. After the desired interval, the thionamide dose is cautiously tapered to assess whether a remission has been attained. Relapses may occur 1 to 26 weeks or longer after stopping thionamide therapy. A recent Japa-

nese study suggested that the co-administration of levothyroxine (Synthroid, Levothroid, Levoxyl) and methimazole increased the chance of remission after 4 to 5 years of treatment, but preliminary reports have been unable to confirm these findings. Patients who do achieve a prolonged remission (greater than 6 months) still have a 5 to 10% chance of late relapse, which may occur years later.

Side Effects and Toxicity

Both thionamides have significant side effects. Approximately 5 to 13% of patients cannot tolerate thionamide therapy because of rashes, hives, fever, joint pain, or nausea. Patients allergic to one thionamide may tolerate the other, but cross-reactivity may occur in up to 50%. Agranulocytosis occurs in 0.2 to 0.5% of patients; it may be slightly less common with doses of methimazole under 30 mg and occurs most commonly during the first 3 months of therapy. Controversy exists as to whether monitoring the white blood cell count is useful. One study detected agranulocytosis early when white counts were obtained every 2 weeks, but most endocrinologists in the United States check white blood cell counts only at follow-up visits. If patients develop fever or sore throat, they are instructed to obtain a white blood cell count immediately before taking any additional thionamide. Leukopenia (3000 to 4000 cells per mm^3) in Graves' disease due to antineutrophil antibodies is common and should not be confused with agranulocytosis. When agranulocytosis occurs, recovery usually takes 2 to 10 days and might be shortened with granulocyte colony-stimulating factor (filgrastim [Neupogen]). Prolonged bone marrow suppression and fatal sepsis are infrequent complications. Agranulocytosis precludes further thionamide therapy. Cholestatic jaundice (methimazole) and hepatocellular necrosis (PTU) are less common toxicities of thionamides.

Use During Pregnancy and Lactation

Because PTU is less soluble than methimazole and bound to serum proteins, it crosses the placenta only one-fourth as well as methimazole and is concentrated in breast milk only one-tenth as well. Methimazole has also been associated with a rare fetal scalp defect, aplasia cutis. PTU is therefore the thionamide of choice during pregnancy. Fetal goiter and hypothyroidism can be minimized by using the smallest dose necessary to control maternal hyperthyroidism. When monitoring thyroid function during pregnancy, it is important to note the effects of estrogen-induced thyroxine-binding globulin (TBG) excess on total serum T_4 and T_3 concentrations and rely on free hormone levels to titrate the dose. Nursing during maternal thionamide therapy has traditionally been discouraged but remains controversial; no side effects in neonates have yet been reported.

Iodinated Radiocontrast Agents and Iodine

Ipodate (Oragrafin)* and iopanoic acid (Telepaque),* two drugs marketed as oral cholecysto-

---

*Not FDA-approved for this indication.

graphic agents, are increasingly used by endocrinologists for patients with severe hyperthyroidism or when rapid amelioration of hyperthyroid symptoms is essential. These agents are the most potent inhibitors of T_4 to T_3 conversion and normalize serum T_3 concentrations within 5 days. Additionally, they provide a source of iodine. Iodine blocks the release of thyroid hormone, and in Graves' disease it blocks its own organification. However, iodine may provide a substrate for hormone synthesis in patients with toxic nodular goiter. Therefore, iodine-containing drugs should not be administered to patients with toxic nodular goiter unless thionamide therapy is initiated at least 2 hours earlier. They should also not be used routinely, since the iodine content precludes the use of radioiodine for up to 6 weeks and may therefore limit therapeutic options if the patient is allergic to thionamides. Indications for the use of these agents include thyroid storm, severe hyperthyroidism, preoperative preparation of hyperthyroid patients who are allergic to thionamides, and symptomatic hyperthyroidism from subacute thyroiditis. Most studies have used doses of 500 mg or 1 gram daily.

Iodine may also be given alone for adjunctive therapy of severe hyperthyroidism as potassium iodide (SSKI), 5 drops two to four times daily, or intravenously as sodium iodide, 1 to 2 grams every 24 hours. Iodine (SSKI 10 drops daily) has been used as adjunctive therapy 1 week following radioiodine treatment of Graves' disease to normalize thyroid hormone concentrations more rapidly and is routinely used preoperatively in Graves' disease to reduce gland vascularity.

Radioiodine

Radioiodine is widely used in the United States as definitive therapy for hyperthyroidism and recommended as the therapy of choice by two-thirds of thyroid specialists. It is administered as an oral solution or capsule and has no immediate aftereffects. Patients are advised to avoid close contact with young children and pregnant women for several days after treatment. The biologic half-life of radioiodine is 2 to 3 days. Radioiodine slowly destroys thyroid tissue over a period of 6 to 24 weeks or longer. One percent of patients develop transient painful radiation thyroiditis. Ten percent require a second treatment. There is no increased risk of leukemia, cancer, or birth defects. There may be worsening ophthalmopathy following radioiodine, and I generally defer radioiodine treatment in patients with severe inflammatory eye findings until the eyes have been stable for 6 months to 1 year.

There are two reasons to pretreat patients with thionamides prior to giving radioiodine. First, thionamides result in euthyroidism in 3 to 8 weeks, whereas radioiodine works much more slowly. Patients who are poorly tolerating their hyperthyroid symptoms should be rendered euthyroid before proceeding with ablation. Second, thyroid hormone levels may increase during the first few weeks after radioiodine administration due to release of hormone from radioiodine-induced inflammation. Thionamide pretreatment depletes thyroid hormone stores and prevents exacerbation of hyperthyroid symptoms. Thionamide pretreatment is indicated in elderly patients or in those with serious heart disease. Otherwise, patients with mild or moderate hyperthyroidism whose symptoms are controlled with beta-adrenergic blocking agents can be given radioiodine as initial therapy. If hyperthyroid symptoms worsen after radioiodine, patients may be treated with either iodine or thionamides.

Hypothyroidism is a common outcome following radioiodine. The prevalence of postradioiodine hypothyroidism can be reduced by utilizing smaller doses, but the trade-off is an increased need for two or more radioiodine treatments, a more prolonged duration of hyperthyroidism, and a higher risk of late recurrent hyperthyroidism. I prefer to use doses of radioiodine that result in rapid control of the hyperthyroidism and are associated with a 60% rate of hypothyroidism within a few months after therapy. Patients who are euthyroid after radioiodine administration develop late hypothyroidism at a rate of 2 to 3% annually.

Surgery

Surgery is rarely chosen as therapy for hyperthyroidism. It is appropriate therapy in patients with large obstructive goiters, patients with very large glands who might require multiple radioiodine doses for adequate ablation, patients with coexistent suspicious cold nodules, pregnant hyperthyroid women who are allergic to thionamides, and patients who fear radioiodine.

It is critical that the surgeon be skilled at near-total thyroidectomy. Complications include permanent hypoparathyroidism and recurrent laryngeal nerve injury. If an excessively large surgical remnant remains, persistent or recurrent hyperthyroidism may occur. Many surgeons prefer the risk of postoperative hypothyroidism to failure to control the hyperthyroidism. Therefore, postoperative hypothyroidism occurs in 10 to 90% of patients.

Ideally, patients are rendered euthyroid with thionamides preoperatively. In patients with Graves' disease, iodine is given for 10 days preoperatively to reduce gland vascularity. In patients allergic to thionamides, ipodate or iopanoic acid and beta-adrenergic blocking agents are used preoperatively in those with Graves' disease, and beta blockers alone are used in those with toxic nodular goiter. Ideally, beta blockers are given in sufficient doses to reduce the heart rate to less than 80 beats per minute after moderate exercise. Long-acting agents such as atenolol persist in the immediate postoperative period when the patient is unable to take medication orally. If necessary, intravenous propranolol can be used intraoperatively.

Thyroid Storm

True thyroid storm with severe hyperthyroidism, fever, and altered mental status is rare, but severe hyperthyroidism is not uncommon and is treated similarly. Beta-adrenergic blocking agents are administered when tolerated. In patients who are hemodynamically unstable, shorter-acting agents should be used initially. Propranolol is most commonly given orally or intravenously, but ultra-short-acting agents such as esmolol (Brevibloc) can be used when there is concern about the hemodynamic or pulmonary effects of beta blockade. Many endocrinologists prefer to use PTU 200 mg every 4 hours because of its ability to reduce T_4 to T_3 conversion. Because ipodate and iopanoic acid are considerably more potent than PTU at blocking T_4 to T_3 conversion, and because methimazole has a longer duration of action than PTU, both allowing for persistent blockade if doses are missed and providing for simplified dosing and compliance once the patient is discharged, I prefer to treat severe hyperthyroidism with methimazole 10 to 15 mg every 6 hours and an iodinated radiocontrast agent 500 mg twice daily. Methimazole is absorbed equally well through the rectal mucosa and can be prepared by the hospital pharmacy for administration as a rectal suppository if the oral route is unavailable. Iodine can be given intravenously as sodium iodide 1 to 2 grams per day. Corticosteroids have traditionally been used for thyroid storm, although there is little evidence for their efficacy. Cholestyramine (Questran)* reduces the enterohepatic circulation of thyroid hormones. Plasmapheresis and peritoneal dialysis have also been used in this setting.

TREATMENT OF HYPERTHYROIDISM WITH A LOW RADIOIODINE UPTAKE

Hyperthyroidism is associated with a low radioiodine uptake in patients with subacute thyroiditis (see Table 1) or when the source of thyroid hormone is not the thyroid gland (factitious hyperthyroidism, struma ovarii, or functional metastatic thyroid cancer). Thionamides may be useful adjunctive therapy in struma ovarii or functional thyroid cancer, but therapy is directed primarily against the neoplasm. It is critical to appreciate that neither thionamides nor radioiodine has a role in the treatment of subacute thyroiditis, since there is no ongoing hormone synthesis. In subacute thyroiditis, hormone is leaking into the circulation from an inflamed gland. Since the hyperthyroidism is usually mild, beta-adrenergic blocking agents are the primary therapy. When hyperthyroidism is severe, the use of iodinated radiocontrast agents may be of considerable benefit. The treatment of thyroiditis is discussed in a separate chapter.

---

*Not FDA-approved for this indication.

THYROID CANCER

method of
CHARLES G. WATSON, M.D.
University of Pittsburgh School of Medicine
Pittsburgh, Pennsylvania

Thyroid cancers are relatively uncommon and, with a few notable exceptions, carry a favorable prognosis. They constitute 1% of all newly diagnosed malignancies in the United States. It is anticipated that in 1997, 12,000 to 13,000 clinically significant thyroid cancers will be diagnosed, with an incidence of 40 thyroid cancers per 1 million population per year. Slightly more than 10% of patients with clinically overt thyroid cancers will succumb to their disease, the majority after a prolonged and asymptomatic interval.

The following classification of thyroid cancer is widely accepted. Thyroid malignancies are either differentiated or undifferentiated; the two differentiated forms are papillary thyroid cancer (PTC) and follicular thyroid cancer (FTC), and the undifferentiated forms are medullary thyroid cancer (MTC) and anaplastic thyroid cancer (ATC). Hürthle cell carcinomas are considered a variant of FTC, and other thyroid malignancies in descending order of frequency include primary thyroid lymphoma, metastatic cancer to the thyroid, and, rarely, squamous carcinoma of the thyroid. PTCs are subclassified on the basis of characteristics of the primary tumor: the *occult* form, measuring less than 1 cm in diameter and without evidence of capsular invasion; the *intrathyroidal* form, being greater than 1 cm in diameter and once again failing to breach the thyroid capsule; and the *extrathyroidal* form, which, regardless of size, breaches the thyroid capsule to involve adjacent structures. In autopsy series, the incidence of occult PTC varies from 13% (United States) to 38% (Scandinavia). All three variants of PTC may be associated with or present with regional nodal metastases, and the extrathyroidal variant is most likely to be associated with hematogenous spread to lung, liver, brain, and bone. By and large, the presence of nodal metastases in PTC does not adversely influence a patient's prognosis, a fact unique to this cancer. Patients with the occult and intrathyroidal forms of PTC generally enjoy a normal life expectancy.

Head and neck irradiation (6.5 to 2000 cGy) is associated with a 10% risk of developing thyroid cancer. The risk is greatest for those exposed when less than 20 years of age, but such exposure up to the age of 50 is associated with an increased risk. The vast majority (90% +) of radiation-induced thyroid cancers are papillary. The incidence of thyroid cancer in Ukrainian children exposed to the 1986 Chernobyl nuclear fallout increased 100-fold over baseline.

Although most hereditary thyroid carcinomas are MTC, occasional patients with PTC have a positive family history for this disease. Two uncommon hereditary disorders, familial polyposis and Cowden's (multiple hamartoma) syndrome, are associated with an increased incidence of PTC.

Most thyroid carcinomas present as a dominant hypofunctioning (by radioiodine scan) nodule, and the diagnosis can at least be suspected on the basis of a thorough history, physical examination, and fine-needle aspiration biopsy (FNAB) for cytology. Patients with a history of head and neck irradiation presenting with a dominant thyroid nodule have a 30% likelihood of harboring a differentiated thyroid cancer. In any patient with a prior or family history suggesting the possibility of multiple endocrine neoplasia (MEN) Type IIa or IIb or with a family history of MTC, the dominant nodule is an MTC until proved otherwise. The likelihood of a dominant nodule being malignant varies significantly with age and gender. Solitary "cold" nodules in patients under the age of 30 should be strongly suspected of being carcinoma, with a likelihood of greater than 30%. Most dominant cold thyroid nodules occur in middle-aged females, however, with the likelihood of a malignancy being less than 5%. Beyond the age of 60 in both males and females, a solitary cold thyroid nodule is increasingly likely to be malignant. In general, a solitary nodule in a male is more likely to be malignant than one in a female, regardless of age.

EMBRYOLOGY AND PHYSIOLOGY

In understanding the clinical presentation and optimal management of a thyroid malignancy, a brief review of the embryologic descent and physiology of the thyroid gland is in order. The human thyroid is a conglomerate of three embryologic sources. The lateral anlagen arise bilaterally from the fourth branchial clefts (along with the superior parathyroids), consist of parafollicular or C cells, and descend and ultimately fuse with the median anlage. The median anlage arises from the base of the tongue, consists wholly of follicular cells, and descends in the midline to the low anterior neck. C cells (and therefore C cell malignancies) are concentrated primarily in the upper two-thirds of both thyroid lobes.

Normal follicular cells are stimulated by thyroid-stimulating hormone (TSH) to trap and concentrate iodine and to facilitate the iodinization of tyrosine molecules in the thyroglobulin matrix within the thyroid follicle. TSH also stimulates follicular cell mobilization of triiodothyronine (T_3) and thyroxine (T_4) from thyroglobulin and secretion of T_3 and T_4 into the circulation. Differentiated thyroid cancer cells (both papillary and follicular) are capable of trapping and organifying iodine and synthesizing thyroglobulin, but they do so far less efficiently than normal thyroid follicular cells. Therefore, considerably greater concentrations of TSH are required to drive these processes (i.e., iodine uptake) in malignant thyroid cells. Differentiated thyroid cancers can therefore be staged and patients periodically screened for recurrent disease with serial whole-body radionuclide iodine scans and serum thyroglobulin levels, but only in the setting of maximal TSH stimulation.

The parafollicular or C cell normally produces calcitonin and has the potential to produce other polypeptides such as carcinoembryonic antigen (CEA), corticotropin (ACTH), somatostatin, histaminase, neuron-specific enolase, calcitonin gene-related peptide, thyroglobulin, thyrotropin-stimulating hormone, serotonin, chromogranin, and substance P. Individuals at risk for developing MTC can be screened with either a pentagastrin or a pentagastrin-calcium stimulated calcitonin assay, and those patients operated on for MTC should be followed periodically with basal or stimulated calcitonin and/or CEA assays. The less well differentiated MTCs are more likely to produce more CEA and less calcitonin.

PAPILLARY THYROID CANCER

PTCs constitute at least 70% of thyroid malignancies and have far and away the best outlook. Although usually presenting as a solitary thyroid nodule, they are frequently microscopically multicentric and often (especially in children) metastasize to regional nodes, which is thought to be of little clinical consequence. The biologic behavior and therefore the prognosis of PTC relate to the nature of the primary tumor. The occult and intrathyroidal forms are generally curable. Having the potential to metastasize hematogenously, the extrathyroidal form entails a worse prognosis. Mixed papillary-follicular carcinomas represent a variant of PTC, are more likely to take up radioactive iodine, and generally have an excellent overall prognosis. In patients over the age of 60, PTC may become locally more aggressive, with an increased likelihood of direct infiltration of the trachea, larynx, and other contiguous structures.

The management of PTC remains somewhat controversial, as it relates to the scope of surgery for the primary tumor, how to approach regional nodal metastases, and the role of postoperative treatment with radioactive iodine 131. There is universal agreement that postoperatively all patients with PTC should be fully TSH-suppressed for life with adequate doses of L-thyroxine (Synthroid). To minimize the likelihood of L-thyroxine–induced osteoporosis, the daily dose should not exceed 1.6 µg per kg of body weight. In the vast majority of patients, this dose adequately suppresses TSH (i.e., less than 0.1 µIU per mL). Under "ideal" circumstances, a total thyroidectomy should be performed. When all normal as well as abnormal thyroid tissue is removed, endogenous TSH levels rise significantly postoperatively, facilitating disease staging by the uptake of radioiodine by metastatic PTC cells. The risks of total thyroidectomy relate to recurrent and superior laryngeal nerve injury, resulting in laryngeal dysfunction, and hypoparathyroidism, necessitating the lifelong administration of calcium and vitamin D to prevent tetany. In experienced hands, both these complications are minimized. Theoretically, the postoperative administration of radioactive iodine 131 for scanning and treatment purposes in patients with primary lesions greater than 1.5 cm in diameter is desirable, once they are fully TSH stimulated. Most if not all malignant PTC cells capable of taking up iodine concentrate radioactive iodine and self-destruct. Controversy surrounding the optimal management of differentiated thyroid cancer can be resolved only by carefully constructed prospective clinical trials comparing one option with another. Such clinical trials have yet to be performed. Regarding lymph node dissection, there is no demonstrated treatment advantage for central compartment, modified radical, or radical neck dissection. There is general agreement that palpably involved nodes should be excised at the time of a thyroidectomy.

There are two particularly aggressive histologic variants of PTC: tall cell carcinoma of the thyroid and insular thyroid carcinoma. Both lesions are uncommon, have characteristic histologic appearances, are biologically more aggressive, tend not to take up iodine, and generally have an unfavorable prognosis.

For PTC, prognostic indices have been devised based on multivariant analyses, the most reliable being based on age (less or greater than 40 years), histologic grade, extent of the primary tumor with or without metastases, and size of the primary lesion. In general, patients under the age of 40 without thyroid capsular involvement have a better prognosis the smaller the primary lesion.

FOLLICULAR THYROID CANCER

FTC is usually unifocal and uncommonly involves lymph nodes (5 to 10%). The prognosis of FTC primarily depends on age (worse over the age of 50), degree of angioinvasiveness of the primary tumor, and presence or absence of metastatic disease at the time of diagnosis. In and of themselves, the existence of adjacent tissue involvement and DNA ploidy appear not to impact survival. Patients with FTC are at low risk for recurrent disease if none or only one of the three variables mentioned above is present (20-year tumor-related mortality of 15%). With two or more of the variables present, the likelihood of recurrence is much higher (20-year mortality of 92%). Again, the ideal therapeutic approach is a total thyroidectomy to facilitate whole-body radioiodine scanning for staging purposes and radioiodine therapy while fully TSH stimulated, and then TSH suppression with L-thyroxine for life.

A Hürthle cell carcinoma is difficult to differentiate from an adenoma histologically and is thought to represent a variant of FTC. It differs from FTC, however, by more frequently involving regional nodes, more readily involving both thyroid lobes, and rarely taking up radioactive iodine. Hürthle cell carcinomas can produce thyroglobulin as a biologic marker for recurrence (following a total thyroidectomy). They appear to be less influenced than PTC and FTC by circulating TSH. The primary determinants of the prognosis of a Hürthle cell carcinoma are the clinical stage at the time of initial presentation and its DNA ploidy. In the absence of aneuploidy, the prognosis is excellent for 20-year survival; in the presence of aneuploidy, 20-year mortality is 32%. Hürthle cell carcinoma does not respond to adjuvant chemotherapy or irradiation.

MEDULLARY THYROID CARCINOMA

MTCs are of neural crest origin as part of the amine precursor uptake decarboxylation (APUD) system of neuroendocrine cells. There are four variants of MTC, each with its own biologic behavior and prognosis: sporadic, familial MTC, MTC as a component of MEN Type IIa, and MTC as a component of MEN Type IIb. As mentioned above, MTCs arise from the parafollicular or C cell and therefore are more likely to be found in the upper two-thirds of a thyroid lobe. The sporadic variant is unifocal; the hereditary forms are generally multifocal and associated with C cell hyperplasia. MTCs generally spread both via the regional lymphatics and hematogenously. Being of C cell origin, they are unresponsive to TSH stimulation and do not trap or concentrate radioiodine. Calcitonin and CEA are the most commonly employed biologic markers in screening for the

disease and testing for recurrent disease. Generally, patients with the very uncommon hereditary pure MTC have an excellent prognosis. Patients with MTC as a component of MEN Type IIa syndrome do reasonably well. Those with sporadic MTC do less well, and those with MTC in the context of MEN Type IIb have a generally poor prognosis unless the disease is detected very early in life (i.e., at 5 years or younger). For any patient with MTC, the prognosis is worse if preoperative basal calcitonin levels are high (greater than 10,000 pg per mL), if the percentage of tumor cells staining for calcitonin is low, if CEA levels are high, or if there is evidence of metastatic disease to regional nodes or beyond. With recurrent disease, rising calcitonin levels may ultimately be associated with cutaneous flushing and diarrhea. These symptoms may respond to the administration of somatostatin analogue and/or interferon-alfa* and to debulking of disease capable of being imaged.

As surgery is the only cure for MTC, the currently recommended approach is a total thyroidectomy and a central compartment node dissection on the involved side or sides. If there is palpable lymphadenopathy, a more generous (ipsilateral functional) node dissection with the excision of both parathyroids is recommended. Any patient undergoing surgery for MTC should be followed up with calcitonin and CEA levels for life. If they are elevated and there is no palpable residual disease, neck ultrasound or neck and mediastinal computed tomography scanning is indicated.

Specific genetic defects for MEN Type IIa and isolated familial MTC have been identified at the RET proto-oncogene locus on chromosome 10. Potentially afflicted family members can therefore be screened directly for these disorders by analysis of lymphocyte DNA. It is hoped that those without the genetic defect need not be tested clinically, but the possibility of genetic heterogenicity does exist.

ANAPLASTIC THYROID CANCER

ATC usually presents as a rapidly growing mass lesion rather than a discretely palpable nodule. At the time of diagnosis, contiguous structures are invariably involved. By and large, this is an untreatable and incurable disorder. Anaplastic carcinoma must be differentiated from small cell lymphoma, as the latter can and frequently does respond to chemotherapy with or without irradiation. Tissue for histology and flow cytometry (rather than cells for cytology) is required for the diagnosis. If a pathologist is incapable of differentiating ATC from primary thyroid lymphoma, a trial of external beam irradiation is indicated. Attempts at debulking may be undertaken, but with few exceptions, patients with ATC succumb to the locally invasive effects of the disease within 6 months of diagnosis. The role of surgery is primarily to control the airway and provide tissue for diagnosis.

---

*Not FDA-approved for this indication.

PRIMARY THYROID LYMPHOMA

Primary non-Hodgkin's thyroid lymphoma constitutes less than 5% of thyroid neoplasms and less than 2% of all extranodal lymphomas. It generally presents as a thyroid-related mass rather than a discrete nodule, and in general, a core needle or open tissue biopsy is indicated rather than an FNAB for cytology. Cure rates vary with the type of lymphoma. Generally, the best results are obtained with combined modality therapy (i.e., chemotherapy and x-ray therapy).

SUMMARY

Thyroid cancer is an uncommon disorder with a generally good prognosis. The management of most thyroid cancers is based on the experience of individual physicians or institutions and, regrettably, not on controlled clinical trials. There is therefore lingering controversy over the "ideal" scope of surgery and the indications for radioiodine therapy in the management of the differentiated forms of thyroid cancer (PTC and FTC). The diagnostic and therapeutic approaches to PTC, FTC, and MTC are generally logical, usually successful, and have withstood the test of time. In general, the following statements are true: (1) The earlier the diagnosis, the better the prognosis. (2) The scope of surgery and the role of radioiodine therapy have yet to be scientifically defined, although thoughtfully constructed guidelines for each exist. (3) For the hereditary thyroid cancers, direct gene testing simplifies screening and facilitates early diagnosis. (4) Thyroid cancers deserve the multimodality input of an endocrinologist, surgeon, pathologist, and nuclear radiologist. To fine-tune the management of differentiated thyroid cancers, multi-institutional clinical trials are essential.

PHEOCHROMOCYTOMA

method of
JEROME M. FELDMAN, M.D.
Duke University Medical Center
Durham, North Carolina

Pheochromocytomas are tumors composed of chromaffin cells that originate from neuroectodermal tissue. The hallmark of pheochromocytomas is the production of catecholamines such as dopamine, norepinephrine, and epinephrine. The symptoms of pheochromocytomas are caused by the particular combination of catecholamines they excrete. Sustained secretion of norepinephrine can result in sustained hypertension, intermittent secretion of norepinephrine or epinephrine can result in episodic hypertension, sustained secretion of epinephrine can result in anxiety and tachycardia, and secretion of dopamine alone may not produce any vascular symptoms.

Pheochromocytomas occur in fewer than 1% of patients with hypertension. Although this percentage is small, there are estimated to be 36,000 patients in the United States with pheochromocytomas. The diagnosis of these tumors frequently eludes physicians. In one series, only 13 of 54 patients (24%) found to have pheochromocytomas at autopsy had been correctly diagnosed during life. This is unfortunate, because pheochromocytoma represents a potentially "curable" form of hypertension; if patients with undiagnosed pheochromocytoma have surgery or an accident, they may die of a hypertensive crisis, and certain medications used in the treatment of hypertension or depression such as reserpine, guanethidine, propranolol, and imipramine may produce severe paroxysms of hypertension.

Approximately 90% of pheochromocytomas are located in the adrenal glands. The rule of 10% is a handy way to recall information about pheochromocytomas: 10% are in both adrenal glands (bilateral), 10% are extra-adrenal, and 10% are malignant. This rule of 10% can vary from population to population. Patients with multiple endocrine neoplasia (MEN) have a higher percentage of bilateral pheochromocytomas. In one recent series of 100 patients with pheochromocytomas, 26 patients had malignant tumors.

MEDICAL MANAGEMENT

Once the diagnosis of pheochromocytoma is made, the physician should establish adrenergic blockade, carry out appropriate studies to localize the pheochromocytoma, and then, if possible, have it resected by an experienced surgeon. Occasionally one encounters a patient who is a poor operative risk because of advanced age, other serious illnesses, or the anatomic location of the pheochromocytoma. Although such patients can be managed by chronic medical therapy, there is always the risk that one is following a malignant pheochromocytoma.

The cornerstone of both preoperative and, if necessary, long-term medical management of pheochromocytomas is establishment of adequate adrenergic blockade with phenoxybenzamine (Dibenzyline). Phenoxybenzamine covalently binds to the alpha-adrenergic receptors and blocks the hypertensive effects of catecholamines. This drug is given to all patients with norepinephrine- and epinephrine-secreting pheochromocytomas, even if they do not have sustained hypertension or any hypertension under basal conditions. These nonhypertensive patients may develop dangerous elevations of blood pressure with induction of anesthesia and manipulation of the pheochromocytoma. The initial dose of phenoxybenzamine is 10 mg orally twice a day. The dose is increased by 10 mg per day at 3-day intervals until the patient's blood pressure has been reduced to normal levels. The usual dose for effective alpha-adrenergic blockade is 30 to 60 mg per day in divided doses three times a day. Some patients with pheochromocytoma require as much as 150 mg per day,* a dose that is higher than that listed in the manufacturer's official directive. The critical factor is not to increase the dose of phenoxybenzamine until the patient has been on a given dose for 3 days, as it may take this long for it to exert its full effect. If the patient has only intermittent and infrequent bouts of hypertension and sustained hypertension cannot

---

*Exceeds dosage recommended by the manufacturer.

be used as an end point to judge the adequacy of therapy, one usually gives the patient 30 to 60 mg of phenoxybenzamine per day.

Phenoxybenzamine does not interfere with measurement of vanillylmandelic acid (VMA) and catecholamines when good methodology is employed. The most frequent side effects of phenoxybenzamine are nasal congestion, sedation, dry mouth, and orthostatic hypotension. The latter is due to relaxation of the patient's chronically constricted blood vessels, with a resulting decreased blood volume. If the patient is maintained on a generous salt diet, the contracted blood volume will expand and the orthostatic hypotension will decrease. The patient should be maintained on adequate alpha-adrenergic blockade for at least 2 weeks prior to surgery.

There are now a number of other medications with alpha-adrenergic blocking effects, such as phentolamine (Regitine), prazosin (Minipress),* terazosin (Hytrin),* and doxazosin (Cardura),* that have been used in patients with pheochromocytomas. The combination alpha- and beta-blocking agent labetalol (Normodyne, Trandate)* has also been used in treating patients with pheochromocytomas. However, there are a number of reports in the literature that these medications do not provide consistent effects in patients with pheochromocytomas. Thus, I prefer to use the reliable agent phenoxybenzamine for this important role.

In most patients with pheochromocytomas, beta-adrenergic blockade is not as important as the absolutely essential alpha-adrenergic blockade. Beta-adrenergic blockade is indicated in any patient with a pheochromocytoma who has a heart rate greater than 110 beats per minute, a history of arrhythmias, persistent ventricular extrasystoles, or a pheochromocytoma that is secreting predominantly epinephrine. In a substantial number of other patients without these initial findings, the pulse rate increases to 110 beats per minute after initiation of phenoxybenzamine, and these patients should also be treated with a beta-adrenergic blocker. It cannot be emphasized too strongly that one should not initiate therapy with a beta-adrenergic blocker until establishing at least a partial alpha-adrenergic blockade with phenoxybenzamine. If one blocks the vasodilating beta-adrenergic effects of catecholamines, one may unmask the vasoconstricting alpha-adrenergic effects, resulting in a dangerous increase in blood pressure.

Although there are a number of beta-adrenergic blocking agents available, I have had the most experience with the noncardioselective agent propranolol (Inderal). Patients with pheochromocytomas are usually fairly sensitive to propranolol, and the starting dose should not exceed 10 mg three times daily. Usually, 30 to 60 mg of propranolol per day controls the patient's tachycardia and arrhythmia. Side effects of propranolol include bradycardia, lightheadedness, epigastric distress, and bronchospasm. Patients with

a history of bronchospastic disease should not receive propranolol. If a patient with a pheochromocytoma and a history of bronchospastic disease needs a beta-adrenergic blocker, one could cautiously try the cardioselective beta-blocker metoprolol (Lopressor) or atenolol (Tenormin). It is probably prudent to start therapy with these drugs at a lower than usual dose, as the cardioselective beta-blocking property is relative and may still have some beta-blocking effects on bronchial dilatation.

A new medication that is now available for clinical use in patients with pheochromocytomas is metyrosine (Demser). This drug blocks the conversion of tyrosine to L-dopa, the rate-limiting step in the synthesis of catecholamines. The usual initial dose is a 250 mg capsule orally four times a day. The dose is increased by 250 to 500 mg daily until the patient's blood pressure is reduced to the normal range. The usual dose of 1 to 4 grams per day is given in four divided doses. Although metyrosine produces an artifactual elevation in urinary catecholamine excretion as measured by fluorometry, most clinical catecholamine measurements are now made by more specific methods that minimize such interference. Metyrosine usually does not interfere with the urinary measurement of VMA or metanephrines. Metyrosine can cause as much as an 80% reduction in the urinary excretion of catecholamines in patients with pheochromocytomas. Side effects include sedation in almost all patients and extrapyramidal symptoms in 10% of patients. The latter is probably caused by depletion of dopamine in the patient's basal ganglia. In addition, occasional patients develop anxiety and psychiatric disturbances and sometimes crystalluria. The latter can probably be avoided by maintaining a large fluid intake. Metyrosine seems particularly valuable in patients who are in such poor condition that they cannot undergo resection of their pheochromocytomas. In some cases, this is due to catecholamine-induced myocardiopathy that is improved after chronic metyrosine therapy. The drug is also useful in patients with unresectable malignant pheochromocytomas (described later). For the time being, it seems prudent in the management of most patients with pheochromocytomas to reserve metyrosine for those who cannot tolerate phenoxybenzamine's side effects or when phenoxybenzamine does not adequately control the patient's hypertension in the preoperative period.

OPERATIVE MANAGEMENT

The successful removal of a pheochromocytoma remains one of the most demanding surgical procedures. It requires skillful preoperative, intraoperative, and postoperative management with pharmacologic agents as well as the technical skills of an experienced surgeon and anesthesiologist. When the patient has MEN with medullary carcinoma of the thyroid and a pheochromocytoma, it is important to remove the pheochromocytoma and schedule a second operation to remove the thyroid tumor.

---

*Not FDA-approved for this indication.

The usual approach for the removal of a pheochromocytoma is either the abdominal approach or a flank incision through the bed of the twelfth rib. In recent years, there have been a series of reports of laparoscopic removal of pheochromocytomas. Although the operative time is longer than in traditional approaches, the postoperative hospitalization is usually shorter. The traditional approach is preferable for suspected malignant pheochromocytomas, multiple pheochromocytomas, or large pheochromocytomas. As is always the case in pheochromocytoma resection, an experienced laparoscopic surgeon who is familiar with retroperitoneal surgery is essential.

In general, either abdominal computed tomography (CT) or magnetic resonance imaging (MRI) is a good technique for the preoperative localization of pheochromocytomas. Abdominal CT is less expensive and is more acceptable to patients with claustrophobia than is MRI. However, MRI is particularly useful in distinguishing right-sided pheochromocytomas that are in contact with the liver from hepatic masses. Because of the possibility of multiple or malignant pheochromocytomas, I prefer to do a more specific preoperative imaging procedure as well, with agents that are more specific for neuroendocrine tumors. I prefer ^{131}I-metaiodobenzylguanidine or iobenguane sulfate I-131 injection (I-131 MIBG) to indium In 111 pentetreotide (OctreoScan), as it is more specific. However, there are occasional pheochromocytomas that concentrate one and not the other of these two agents.

If there is any likelihood that bilateral pheochromocytomas will be found, the patient is given intramuscular injections of cortisone acetate 48 and 24 hours prior to surgery as well as on the morning of surgery. This should be done in all cases of pheochromocytoma in patients with MEN Type II, as there is a high frequency of bilateral pheochromocytomas. Patients should receive their phenoxybenzamine and, if warranted, propranolol on the morning of surgery.

In past years, one of the major operative problems was hypotension after removal of the pheochromocytoma. This can now be avoided if one allows the patient 2 weeks of therapy with phenoxybenzamine prior to surgery and carefully replaces blood loss with appropriate fluids during surgery. In addition, it is the practice of some anesthesiologists to place the patient in a slight reversed Trendelenburg's position, so that the lower extremities can be used as volume capacitors during surgery. After ligation of the renal veins or removal of the pheochromocytoma, the table can be tilted to the horizontal position to increase the circulating blood volume if this proves necessary.

When it is important to examine both adrenals as well as other areas of the abdomen, most surgeons prefer an anterior transabdominal approach for pheochromocytomas. This is usually done with bilateral subcostal incisions. The adrenal gland with the known pheochromocytoma is resected first. Each pheochromocytoma should be handled as a potentially malignant lesion and removed with the capsule intact. It is usually impossible to remove the tumor and spare the adrenal in extra-adrenal pheochromocytomas. After the known pheochromocytoma is removed, the surgeon examines the contralateral adrenal, the paraspinal area, the organ of Zuckerkandl, and the bladder for additional tumors.

Palpation and resection of the pheochromocytoma result in dramatic increases in the plasma catecholamine concentration, with increases in blood pressure and heart rate, even in patients with seemingly adequate adrenergic blockade. The hypertensive episodes can be treated by intermittent intravenous injections of the alpha-adrenergic blocking agent phentolamine. However, phentolamine's hypotensive action can persist for 30 to 60 minutes after the plasma catecholamines have fallen toward the premanipulation level, and phentolamine has some actions other than alpha-adrenergic blockade. Thus, one can get into repeated cycles of hyper- and hypotension. I prefer to control the surges of blood pressure with a sodium nitroprusside (Nipride) drip. The nitroprusside powder is reconstituted with 5% dextrose in water to give a concentration such as 50 mg in 1000 mL of 5% dextrose in water (50 μg per mL). The reconstituted solution is protected from light. In response to manipulation of the pheochromocytoma with resulting hypertension, the patient receives 0.5 to 10 μg per kg body weight per minute with an average infusion rate being 3 μg per kg body weight per minute using an infusion pump or a microdrip regulator. The potential side effects of nitroprusside include hypotension and cyanide poisoning. The great advantage of this agent is that its effect is rapidly dissipated when its administration is discontinued.

Tachycardia and arrhythmia during surgery can be treated with intravenous injections of small amounts of propranolol. The usual dose of intravenous propranolol in patients with pheochromocytomas is 0.5 to 2.0 mg, with the rate of administration not to exceed 1 mg per minute. This reduces the possibility of lowering the blood pressure and causing cardiac standstill. If a vasopressor should be needed in a patient undergoing surgery for a pheochromocytoma, one should avoid the indirect-acting agents, as they can release an unpredictable amount of norepinephrine from the nerve endings. Direct-acting vasopressors such as norepinephrine and phenylephrine are the drugs of choice. If the patient has had an adequate preoperative period of alpha-adrenergic blockade and if fluids and blood are administered appropriately during surgery, it is usually not necessary to administer vasopressor amines.

Patients who have undergone resections of pheochromocytomas require careful monitoring in the immediate postoperative period. If they have had bilateral adrenalectomy or unilateral adrenalectomy with significant manipulation of the second adrenal gland, they should be continued on glucocorticoid replacement. In the immediate postoperative period, hypertension may recur; however, this usually reflects fluid shifts and autonomic instability and does not necessarily indicate a persistent pheochromocytoma. Some patients develop transitory hypoglycemia. Urinary VMA excretion and sometimes plasma norepinephrine may remain elevated for 3 days after complete removal of all pheochromocytoma tissue. This probably represents elimination of the large stores of extra pheochromocytoma norepinephrine in the tissues of the body. One week or more after surgery, the preoperative biochemical tests should be repeated to ascertain whether the patient remains hypertensive because of either irreversible renal damage or essential hypertension.

MALIGNANT PHEOCHROMOCYTOMA

About half of patients who ultimately prove to have malignant pheochromocytomas appear to have benign tumors at the time of initial diagnosis; the other half have obviously malignant tumors. Patients with malignant pheochromocytomas experience a slow but usually downhill course. Eventually, metastases can appear in lung, liver, brain, or bone. Ultimately, the majority of patients with malignant pheochromocytomas die from their tumors.

Bone metastasis can usually be ameliorated by external radiation therapy; the metabolic effects of excessive catecholamine production can be reduced by chronic therapy with phenoxybenzamine, propranolol, or metyrosine. Although not helpful in all patients, the two most useful methods of treating the generalized tumor have been therapy with the radiopharmaceutical agent iobenguane sulfate I-131 (I-131 MIBG) and combined chemotherapy. The chemotherapy combination that has been used most successfully is cyclophosphamide (Cytoxan, Neosar), vincristine (Oncovin, Vincasar), and dacarbazine (DTIC-Dome). Both I-131 MIBG and combination chemotherapy should be given in a specialized center.

THYROIDITIS

method of
STEVEN A. SMITH, M.D.
Mayo Clinic
Rochester, Minnesota

Histologic and immunologic changes have typified the morphologic classifications of thyroiditis, whereas the rapidity of onset, severity, and duration of illness have been used in clinical diagnosis. Acute, subacute (granulomatous and lymphocytic), and chronic (lymphocytic and sclerosing) thyroiditis are the traditional clinical classification schemes.

ACUTE THYROIDITIS

The sudden onset of unilateral anterior neck pain, dysphagia (particularly with pharyngitis), fever, and signs of systemic toxicity associated with an extremely tender neck on examination and skin erythema should suggest acute thyroiditis. Leukocyto-

sis, thyroid function testing (which is usually normal), and radioactive iodine uptake (which can be normal or low) overlap with other conditions that cause a painful thyroid. The diagnosis can be confirmed and initial cultures can be obtained by fine-needle aspiration (FNA) of the thyroid.

Bacteria (most frequently *Streptococcus pyogenes*), viruses (in particular, cytomegalovirus), fungi, mycobacteria, *Pneumocystis carinii*, and other parasites can cause acute thyroiditis. Treatment should include parenteral antimicrobials and the possibility of surgical resection or drainage of complicating abscesses. Although permanent sequelae are rare if the condition is recognized early, hypothyroidism can result from diffuse destruction of the gland. Recurrences can occur when thyroglossal duct or other fistulas exist.

SUBACUTE GRANULOMATOUS THYROIDITIS

Subacute granulomatous thyroiditis (SGT) can mimic acute thyroiditis and other causes of acute painful thyroid. The acute presentation of unilateral (often progressing to bilateral) neck pain with signs and symptoms of hyperthyroidism, associated with an elevated sedimentation rate, elevated thyroid function, and low radioactive iodine uptake (RAIU), clinically defines the disorder. Only FNA can confirm the distinct histologic findings of disrupted follicular structure, acute inflammatory cells with histiocytes, and particles of colloid-producing structures that resemble giant cells.

Because of its seasonality and often preceding self-limited upper respiratory illness, SGT is thought to be viral in origin, and treatment is supportive. Salicylates and nonsteroidal anti-inflammatory drugs maybe useful for pain in mild cases. The response to steroids (starting dose, 1 mg per kg per day equivalent prednisone) is so dramatic that if the patient is not all but cured of the neck discomfort within 24 hours, the diagnosis should be questioned. Unless there is a contraindication to the use of steroids—and especially if the diagnosis is supported by FNA—they are the treatment of choice, with a taper over 4 weeks. Recurrent pain may result during the steroid taper (in <20% of patients), necessitating dose adjustment to the smallest dose providing relief and a slower taper. The course of thyroid dysfunction in SGT is believed to correlate with the acute destruction of the gland (and release of stored thyroxine), hormone depletion, and then recovery (hyperthyroidism, hypothyroidism, followed by the euthyroid state). Each patient varies with respect to the severity, duration, and time of each stage (with recovery usually taking less than 6 months and rarely over 1 year). Treatment should depend on the patient's symptoms. When symptoms of hyperthyroidism are significant, beta-adrenergic blocking drugs are useful. Treatment with antithyroid drugs is generally not helpful because of the release of preformed hormone, but in severe cases, propylthiouracil has been used to block thyroxine (T_4) to triiodothyronine (T_3) conversion. Rarely, thyroidectomy is required. T_3 has been suggested by some for SGT because it is believed that thyroid-stimulating hormone (TSH) suppression benefits the acute inflammatory phase, but because hyperthyroidism is often seen at this initial phase, this is not recommended. Thyroid hormone is useful in the treatment of symptomatic patients with hypothyroidism during the later phases of this illness. Because less than 5% of patients develop permanent hypothyroidism, if thyroid hormone is required, its use should be reassessed after 1 year. Recurrence of SGT after recovery is rare.

SUBACUTE LYMPHOCYTIC THYROIDITIS

The clinical presentation of subacute lymphocytic thyroiditis (SLT) is similar to that of SGT, except that it is more often "subacute" because of the protean nature of the symptoms of thyroid dysfunction and the lack of a painful thyroid. It can present sporadically or post partum. Antithyroid antibodies, increased T_4 to T_3 ratio, and low RAIU help support the diagnosis. There is a small nontender goiter (in 50%), and histologic or cytologic features (from FNA) show follicular disruption and lymphocytic infiltration similar to chronic autoimmune thyroiditis (often resolving following recovery). Patients taking the antiarrhythmic amiodarone and the chemotherapeutic drug interleukin-2 and lymphokine-activated killer cell treatments can have thyroiditis that mimics SLT.

Because of the lack of neck pain, treatment is directed primarily toward symptomatic hyper- or hypothyroidism. Hyperthyroidism is best managed with beta blockers; as with SGT, antithyroid drugs are generally not helpful. Glucocorticoids do not shorten the duration of thyroid dysfunction and should not be used. T_4 replacement is useful in symptomatic hypothyroidism and can often be discontinued, as in SGT. Although the clinical course of hyperthyroidism, hypothyroidism, followed by euthyroidism in SLT is similar to that of SGT, sequelae such as goiter (50%), hypothyroidism (6%), and recurrence (11%) are more common. Following recovery from *severe* recurrent episodes of hyperthyroidism, ablative ^{131}I followed by T_4 replacement has been recommended by some to prevent further recurrences.

CHRONIC LYMPHOCYTIC THYROIDITIS

This autoimmune disease, often called Hashimoto's thyroiditis, is associated with the presence of antibodies (thyroglobulin, microsomal thyroid peroxidase, thyroid hormone, and the TSH receptor), but they are not specific. Histologic and cytologic changes confirm the diagnosis and consist of lymphocytic infiltration, fibrosis, epithelial cell atrophy, and Hürthle cells. Hashimoto's thyroiditis most commonly presents with an irregular "bosselated" goiter, which can be large enough to give local symptoms of discomfort or dysphagia. Hypothyroidism (20%) can be transient (secondary to TSH receptor blocking antibodies) or permanent (secondary to persistent blocking antibodies or fibrosis and thyroid follicular cell loss). Hyperthyroidism (5%) can occur with a clinical presentation that is indistinguishable from Graves' disease (hashitoxicosis).

Treatment of chronic lymphocytic thyroiditis (CLT) has been to correct associated abnormalities in thyroid hormone levels and to reduce the size of enlarged thyroid glands. Symptomatic thyroid hormone deficiency should be treated with T_4 replacement at a dose that normalizes the serum TSH. Average replacement therapy with levothyroxine is 1.5 to 1.7 µg per kg per day. The elderly and those at risk for coronary heart disease should start at 12.5 to 25 µg per day and slowly increase to replacement, monitoring for the onset of angina or other cardiac signs or symptoms. This should be considered lifelong replacement therapy until further studies clarify the incidence of TSH receptor blocking antibodies and the patient population that might benefit from a reassessment of the long-term need for this replacement therapy. It is less certain whether mild elevations of TSH (<15 mIU per mL) should be treated. Many asymptomatic individuals with CLT have TSH levels that are modestly elevated and remarkably stable over time. The incidence of symptomatic hypothyroidism in this group has been reported from 5 to 15% per year. Although some use this as justification for treatment of all patients with mildly elevated TSH levels, a more conservative approach is to recognize the predictive nature of the laboratory tests and counsel the patient regarding the signs and symptoms of hypothyroidism and the appropriate follow-up. The treatment of hyperthyroidism associated with CLT is similar to that of Graves' disease. The choice of antithyroid drugs, radioactive iodine, surgery, or combinations is complicated and dependent on the age and clinical stability of the patient, the RAIU, and the preferences of the physician and the patient. A full discussion of each treatment option is not possible in this section but is addressed elsewhere in this text. T_4 therapy has been used in euthyroid patients with CLT and significant thyroid enlargement. It is reported that T_4 decreases the size of enlarged glands by 35% (and more in those patients with associated hypothyroidism). When the physician chooses to prescribe T_4 because of a patient's enlarged gland, it is best to consider the value of this limited response. Clinical judgment is required before prescribing lifelong therapy for small goiters. In patients with very large glands, particularly those with symptoms of compression, surgery is more appropriate. Periodic neck examination is important in the long-term follow-up of an individual with CLT. Changes in the size of the gland should always raise the suspicion of an incorrect diagnosis or concurrent carcinoma or lymphoma.

CHRONIC SCLEROSING THYROIDITIS

Although rare, another form of chronic thyroiditis is characterized histologically by replacement of the thyroid by dense fibrous tissue. This condition can be a primary event (Riedel's thyroiditis or struma), a fibrosing variant of CLT, or associated with more generalized sclerosing syndromes. It presents with a subacute (weeks to years) painless enlargement of the thyroid, often with local (esophageal and tracheal) compression symptoms. The thyroid is "woody" and can be a localized or diffuse process, with invasion and fixation into adjacent tissue. Thyroid function, antibody profiles, visualization studies, and FNA are often inadequate to make the diagnosis. Surgery is usually required to confirm a histologic diagnosis.

Although surgery is often necessary to secure a diagnosis, limited resection to relieve compressive symptoms is preferred if there is infiltration of surrounding tissue. Extensive surgery is not recommended because of the high incidence of inadvertent laryngeal nerve injury and bleeding. Recurrences after resection are believed to be rare, and the process often stabilizes with a favorable prognosis. Extensive destruction of the gland can compromise thyroid hormone production. Thyroid hormone therapy is recommended if there is hypothyroidism.

The Urogenital Tract

BACTERIAL INFECTIONS OF THE URINARY TRACT IN MEN

method of
BENJAMIN A. LIPSKY, M.D.
University of Washington
*Veterans Administration Puget Sound Health
    Care System*
Seattle, Washington

EPIDEMIOLOGY

Urinary tract infections (UTIs) most often occur in female patients, but at certain ages and in specific circumstances the male sex is also affected. UTIs are actually more common in infant boys than girls, but in elderly or institutionalized men the rate is similar to that in women. UTIs also occur with similar frequency in men and women after urethral catheterization or other genitourinary instrumentation. Factors that appear to increase the risk of UTIs in men include being uncircumcised; having the acquired immunodeficiency syndrome (AIDS); engaging in insertive anal intercourse or in vaginal intercourse with a woman colonized with uropathogens. Bladder outlet obstruction caused by prostatic hypertrophy is associated with an increased risk of bacteriuria, although the mechanism for this is unclear. In fact, unlike the well-defined pathophysiologic sequence of events leading to UTIs in women, little is known about the causes of bacteriuria in men. Nevertheless, UTIs in men are classified by most authorities as almost always being "complicated," i.e., associated with obstruction, a foreign body, or other genitourinary abnormalities.

DIAGNOSTIC EVALUATION

UTIs in men cause similar symptoms to those in women, i.e., dysuria and urinary frequency or urgency. In addition to these irritative symptoms, some men present with new or worsened obstructive symptoms, e.g., hesitancy, nocturia, and slowed or diminished stream, or with pyuria or hematuria. Physical examination is of limited value but may disclose a urethral discharge or tender epididymis or prostate gland.

A specimen of urine should be obtained for culture from most men in whom a UTI is suspected. The etiologic agents causing infection, and therefore the appropriate antibiotic therapy, are much less predictable in men than in women. Although *Escherichia coli* is the commonest uropathogen, it causes less than half of all infections. *Providencia* species, and gram-negative cocci, especially enterococci, as well as streptococci, are often isolated. *Staphylococcus saprophyticus,* although the second most common uropathogen

in women, rarely causes UTIs in men. Fastidious organisms, which require special media for growth, e.g., *Haemophilus influenzae* or *Gardnerella vaginalis*, occasionally cause UTIs. These, and other rare pathogens like *Mycobacterium tuberculosis* or *Trichomonas vaginalis*, should be sought in men with urinary symptoms and/or pyuria but sterile routine cultures.

Because urine specimens from men are less likely to be contaminated with periurethral flora than those from women, the clean-catch midstream void procedure for obtaining a specimen is less important. Studies have shown that growth from a single voided specimen of 10^3 or more colony-forming units per mL of a single or predominant pathogen is indicative of true bacteriuria. Urine colony counts do not reliably correlate with the anatomic site or severity of infection. Pyuria ($\geq$1000 leukocytes per mL) has both an approximate 75% sensitivity and specificity in predicting bacteriuria.

LOCALIZATION STUDIES

Procedures are available to help distinguish cystitis from pyelonephritis (ureteral catheterization, bladder wash-out, radionuclide scans) or prostatitis (four-cup test), but these are rarely clinically indicated. Structural or functional abnormalities of the urinary tract are frequent in men with UTIs. Diagnostic studies, e.g., renal ultrasound, excretory urography, and sometimes cystoscopy and retrograde uroradiography, are indicated in all young boys and many elderly men. Older men will often have abnormalities, but the clinical importance of these may be unclear. Most older men should be evaluated for bladder outlet obstruction with urinary flow studies and a measurement of postvoid residual urine.

TREATMENT

The choice of antimicrobial therapy of UTIs in male patients should take into consideration the age of the patient, severity of the infection, possibility of underlying systemic or genitourinary disorders, and the likely pathogen. Initial therapy is often empiric, and a change in agents may be indicated based on culture and sensitivity results, as well as the clinical response to therapy.

Cystitis. The treatment of cystitis has been less well studied in men than in women. Available data suggest that 7 to 10 days of therapy with any of several antibiotics (Table 1) is usually effective. When a Gram-stained smear of the urine is available, it can guide the choice of agents: if gram-positive cocci are the likely pathogen, amoxicillin should be prescribed; if gram-negative rods, cotrimoxazole or a fluoroquinolone may be indicated. Because the prostate may be involved in urinary infections in men, agents that penetrate this gland, e.g., trimethoprim or fluoroquinolones, are often recommended.

All material in this article is in the public domain, with the exception of any borrowed figures or tables.

TABLE 1. **Antibiotic Therapy for Male Urinary Tract Infections**

Antibiotic	Recommended Dose*	
	Adult	*Child*
Oral Therapy		
Amoxicillin	250 mg PO q 8 h	10 mg/kg PO q 8 h
Trimethoprim-sulfamethoxazole (Bactrim, Septra)	1 DS tablet PO q 12 h	4 mg/kg of trimethoprim and 20 mg/kg sulfamethoxazole bid
Fluoroquinolone (e.g., ofloxacin [Floxin])	200–500 mg PO q 12 h	Not recommended for children
Parenteral Therapy		
Gentamicin sulfate† (Garamycin)	1–1.5 mg/kg IV q 8 h	2 mg/kg IV q 8 h
Ampicillin	1–2 gm IV q 6 h	25–50 mg/kg IV q 6 h
Fluoroquinolone	200–500 mg q 12 h	Not recommended for children
***Candida* Infections**		
Amphotericin B bladder irrigation (Fungizone)	250 mL of 5–10 mg/L concentration for 1–1.5 h q 8 h	Not recommended for children
Fluconazole (Diflucan)	200 mg PO on first day, then 100 mg q d for 3–5 d	Not recommended for children

*See text for duration of therapy.
†Dose must be adjusted with renal failure.

If a recurrent infection appears to be a relapse, i.e., caused by the same microorganism, treatment for 6 to 12 weeks (for possible bacterial prostatitis) is indicated (see the article "Prostatitis"). Epididymitis may complicate cystitis and in older men is usually caused by uropathogens (see the article "Epididymitis"). Pyelonephritis presumably most often results from ascending infection, as it does in women, and treatment guidelines (see the article "Pyelonephritis") are similar.

Asymptomatic Bacteriuria. In elderly men, as in women, bacteriuria in the absence of genitourinary or systemic symptoms does not require antimicrobial therapy. The risks of adverse drug reactions and the tendency to induce antibiotic resistance are not outweighed by any potential advantages of therapy. Exceptions to this include patients who are undergoing genitourinary instrumentation or who have urinary tract abnormalities, immunocompromising conditions, or organisms with special morbidity (e.g., urea-splitters).

Urethritis. Urethritis is defined as the presence of a urethral discharge or 5 or more leukocytes per oil immersion field on a Gram-stained urethral smear. Urethral infections are usually caused by sexually transmitted pathogens, especially in younger men. These include *Neisseria gonorrhoeae, Chlamydia trachomatis, Ureaplasma urealyticum,* and occasionally *Trichomonas vaginalis.* Uropathogens, especially *E. coli,* may also cause urethritis, most often in patients using urinary catheters or who have undergone other urogenital instrumentation. Uncommon causes of urethritis include intraurethral herpes simplex or papilloma virus infections, and urethral strictures or other anatomic abnormalities.

Treatment depends on identifying the cause and administering appropriate antimicrobial therapy. For nongonococcal urethritis, the most common sexually transmitted disease among men in the United States, an oral tetracycline (e.g., doxycycline [Vibramycin], 100 mg twice a day, for 1 week, or azithromycin [Zithromax], 1.0 gram as a single dose), is the best regimen.

Patients with Urinary Catheters. After several days, nearly all men with an indwelling urethral catheter will develop bacteriuria, and some of these men will ultimately have UTIs. Condom catheters, intermittent urethral catheterization, and wearing diapers can reduce this risk. Neither prophylactic antibiotics nor treatment of asymptomatic bacteriuria is indicated for catheterized patients, but the catheter should be replaced at regular intervals.

BACTERIAL INFECTIONS OF THE URINARY TRACT IN WOMEN

method of
JAMES R. JOHNSON, M.D.
University of Minnesota
Minneapolis, Minnesota

Urinary tract infection (UTI) is one of the commonest bacterial infections of adult women. This article describes an approach to the diagnosis, treatment, and prevention of UTI that is designed to maximize efficacy while minimizing costs and adverse effects.

UTI is not a unitary entity but is rather a group of diverse clinical syndromes, each with its own requirements for optimal management. In adult women, in order to select the appropriate diagnostic evaluation and treatment regimen, the clinician must determine whether a patient's UTI is complicated or uncomplicated and must differentiate between the syndromes of acute cystitis, acute pyelonephritis, and asymptomatic bacteriuria.

TYPES OF UTI AND THEIR TREATMENT

"Complicated" Versus "Uncomplicated" UTI.

A UTI is considered complicated when the patient has underlying conditions associated with resistant pathogens or an increased likelihood of therapeutic failure. These conditions include diabetes mellitus, anatomic or functional abnormalities of the urinary tract, urinary catheterization (indwelling or intermittent), urinary calculi, renal transplantation, immunosuppression, nonambulatory status, and advanced age. Complicated UTI generally requires more aggressive and prolonged antimicrobial therapy than does uncomplicated UTI and often is associated with relapse or reinfection even after seemingly successful initial therapy.

Acute Cystitis. The commonest form of symptomatic UTI, acute cystitis is characterized by symptoms suggesting inflammation within the lower urinary tract, such as frequency, dysuria, urgency, hematuria, and alterations in the odor or appearance of the urine. Onset of symptoms is typically abrupt, and dysuria is perceived as internal, i.e., arising from the urethra or bladder. In the differential diagnosis, consideration should be given to the possibility of a vaginitis syndrome if dysuria is the only voiding symptom and is accompanied by a vaginal discharge, or if the patient perceives the dysuria as external (vulvar origin) rather than internal. Similarly, a sexually transmitted urethritis due to herpes simplex virus, *Chlamydia trachomatis*, or *Neisseria gonorrhoeae* should be suspected if the dysuria is internal but is of gradual onset and is accompanied by a vaginal discharge, and when the patient has a new or multiple sexual partners. It is important to remember that patients who in addition to the irritative symptoms of cystitis also have constitutional symptoms such as malaise, fever, and nausea or symptoms localizing to anatomic sites other than the lower urinary tract (e.g., abdominal pain or flank pain) should be suspected of having an alternative diagnosis, such as acute pyelonephritis, and should be evaluated accordingly.

The traditional approach to the diagnosis of acute cystitis has included routine pretherapy urine cultures. However, in uncomplicated cases of cystitis in young adult women, it is more cost effective to test the urine for the presence of excess numbers of white cells (pyuria), either with a dipstick test or with urine microscopy, and to treat presumptively for cystitis based on the clinical impression if pyuria is present. Nonetheless, culture remains an important component of the evaluation for possible cystitis when the diagnosis is unclear from the history; when, despite a history suggesting cystitis, pyuria is absent; when there are complicating factors (as listed earlier); and when the patient has recently received antimicrobial therapy (which might select for a resistant pathogen). If quantitative urine culture is used to confirm the diagnosis of cystitis, the colony count must be interpreted in light of the fact that approximately one-third of young women with true bacterial cystitis have "low-count" bacteriuria, i.e., between 10^2 and 10^5 colony-forming units (cfu) per mL of a uropathogen in the urine, rather than exceeding the conventional cutoff of more than 10^5 cfu per mL.

The optimal therapy for uncomplicated acute cystitis in women currently appears to be 3 days of a highly active oral agent such as trimethoprim-sulfamethoxazole (Bactrim, Septra) or a fluoroquinolone (Noroxin, Cipro, Floxin, Maxaquin, Penetrex) (Table 1). On the whole, 3-day regimens give slightly better cure rates than the single-dose regimens that were popular a decade ago, but still avoid the excess costs and side effects associated with longer, traditional courses of therapy. Historical features such as prolonged pretherapy symptoms, recent UTI, and diaphragm use are predictive of failure with short-course therapy, however, and may warrant consideration of a 7-day treatment course (Table 1).

Although the net costs of a 3-day trimethoprim-sulfamethoxazole regimen and 3-day fluoroquinolone regimens are similar when drug cost, efficacy, and adverse effects are considered, trimethoprim-sulfamethoxazole may be preferable because of the desirability of minimizing the use of fluoroquinolones so as to forestall the emergence of resistant organisms. Amoxicillin (Amoxil) and narrow-spectrum cephalosporins (cephalexin [Keflex], cephradine [Velosef]) have long but comparatively poor track records in the treatment of UTI and generally should be avoided except when patients are intolerant of alternative agents and during pregnancy.

For acute cystitis in patients with complicating factors, an oral fluoroquinolone usually can be used empirically to initiate therapy (Table 1), with subsequent modification based on the results of susceptibility tests. Treatment should be given for at least 10 days in most cases.

Post-therapy urine cultures can be omitted in most cases of uncomplicated acute cystitis, since with the suggested regimens failure is highly unlikely, asymptomatic recurrences do not necessarily need to be treated, and symptomatic recurrences will bring the patient back for re-evaluation and retreatment. However, post-therapy cultures probably are advisable in patients with complicating factors.

Acute Pyelonephritis. Clinicians must be alert for symptoms or signs suggesting upper urinary tract involvement (such as fever, malaise, and flank pain) in women presenting with symptoms of lower UTI, since such patients require more intensive diagnostic evaluation and treatment than do women with simple cystitis alone. Pretherapy urine culture is recommended in all cases of suspected pyelonephritis because of the importance of matching the treatment regimen to the patient's urine organism. The culture can be expected to yield 10^5 or more cfu per mL of a recognized uropathogenic organism in nearly all cases. Urinalysis, which usually serves as the basis for a presumptive diagnosis (pending culture results), almost invariably shows pyuria. Additional laboratory tests or imaging studies may be war-

TABLE 1. **Treatment Regimens for UTI in Women**

Condition	Characteristic Pathogens	Mitigating Circumstances	Recommended Empirical Treatment*
Acute uncomplicated cystitis	*Escherichia coli, Staphylococcus saprophyticus, Proteus mirabilis, Klebsiella pneumoniae*	None	3-d regimens: oral trimethoprim-sulfamethoxazole (Bactrim, Septra), trimethoprim (Proloprim, Trimpex), norfloxacin (Noroxin), ciprofloxacin (Cipro), ofloxacin (Floxin), lomefloxacin (Maxaquin), or enoxacin (Penetrex)†
		Symptoms for >7 d, recent UTI, use of diaphragm, age > 65 yr	Consider 7-d regimen with drugs listed above
		Pregnancy	Consider 7-d regimen: oral amoxicillin (Amoxil), macrocrystalline nitrofurantoin (Macrodantin, Macrobid), cefpodoxime proxetil (Vantin), cefixime (Suprax), or trimethoprim-sulfamethoxazole (Bactrim, Septra)†
Acute uncomplicated pyelonephritis	*E. coli, P. mirabilis, K. pneumoniae, S. saprophyticus*	Mild-to-moderate illness, no nausea or vomiting: outpatient therapy acceptable	Oral‡ trimethoprim-sulfamethoxazole (Bactrim, Septra), norfloxacin (Noroxin), ciprofloxacin (Cipro), ofloxacin (Floxin), lomefloxacin (Maxaquin), or enoxacin (Penetrex)† for 10–14 d
		Severe illness or possible urosepsis: hospitalization required	Parenteral§ trimethoprim-sulfamethoxazole (Bactrim, Septra), ceftriaxone (Rocephin), ciprofloxacin (Cipro), gentamicin (Garamycin) with or without ampicillin (Omnipen, Polycillin), or ampicillin-sulbactam (Unasyn) until patient is better; then oral‡ trimethoprim-sulfamethoxazole (Bactrim, Septra), norfloxacin (Noroxin), ciprofloxacin (Cipro), ofloxacin (Floxin), lomefloxacin (Maxaquin), or enoxacin (Penetrex) to complete 14 d of therapy
		Pregnancy: hospitalization recommended	Parenteral§ ceftriaxone (Rocephin), gentamicin (Garamycin) with or without ampicillin (Omnipen, Polycillin), or ampicillin-sulbactam (Unasyn), or trimethoprim-sulfamethoxazole (Bactrim, Septra) until patient is better; then oral‡ amoxicillin (Amoxil), amoxicillin-clavulanate (Augmentin), a cephalosporin, or trimethoprim-sulfamethoxazole (Bactrim, Septra) for 14 d

Table continued on opposite page

ranted depending on the severity of illness and the presence of specific underlying illnesses. Blood cultures, although positive in a significant proportion of women with acute pyelonephritis, generally do not provide useful prognostic information or influence management decisions and need not be collected routinely.

Although patients with pyelonephritis traditionally have been admitted to the hospital for several days for initial intravenous antibiotic therapy, abundant recent experience has demonstrated the safety and efficacy of outpatient management and oral therapy. Some patients with very mild pyelonephritis can be sent home to take oral therapy from the outset (see Table 1). Others who are more than mildly ill or who appear somewhat dehydrated but who are not so ill as to require immediate hospitalization can be given intravenous fluids and an initial parenteral dose or two of antibiotic in an Emergency Department or clinic, then discharged to home with a supply of oral antibiotic if they appear stable and are able

TABLE 1. **Treatment Regimens for UTI in Women** *Continued*

Condition	Characteristic Pathogens	Mitigating Circumstances	Recommended Empirical Treatment*
Complicated UTI	*E. coli; Proteus, Klebsiella, Pseudomonas,* and *Serratia* spp; enterococci; staphylococci	Mild-to-moderate illness, no nausea or vomiting: outpatient therapy acceptable	Oral‡ norfloxacin (Noroxin), ciprofloxacin (Cipro), ofloxacin (Floxin), lomefloxacin (Maxaquin), or enoxacin (Penetrex) for 10–14 d
		Severe illness or possible urosepsis: hospitalization required	Parenteral§ ampicillin (Omnipen, Polycillin) and gentamicin (Garamycin), ciprofloxacin (Cipro), ofloxacin (Floxin), ceftriaxone (Rocephin), aztreonam (Azactam), ticarcillin-clavulanate (Timentin), piperacillin-tazobactam (Zosyn), or imipenem-cilastatin (Primaxin) until patient is better; then oral‡ trimethoprim-sulfamethoxazole (Bactrim, Septra), norfloxacin (Noroxin), ciprofloxacin (Cipro), ofloxacin (Floxin), lomefloxacin (Maxaquin), or enoxacin (Penetrex) for 14–21 d

*Treatments listed are those to be prescribed before the etiologic agent is known (Gram's staining can be helpful); they can be modified once the agent has been identified. The recommendations are mine and are limited to drugs currently approved by the Food and Drug Administration, although not all the regimens listed are approved for these indications. Fluoroquinolones (Noroxin, Cipro, Floxin, Maxaquin, Penetrex) should not be used in pregnancy. Trimethoprim-sulfamethoxazole (Bactrim, Septra), although not approved for use in pregnancy, has been widely used. Gentamicin (Garamycin) should be used with caution in pregnancy because of its possible toxicity to eighth-nerve development in the fetus.

†Multiday oral regimens for cystitis are as follows: trimethoprim-sulfamethoxazole (Bactrim, Septra), 160–800 mg q 12 h; trimethoprim (Proloprim, Trimpex), 100 mg q 12 h; norfloxacin (Noroxin), 400 mg q 12 h; ciprofloxacin (Cipro), 250 mg q 12 h; ofloxacin (Floxin), 200 mg q 12 h; lomefloxacin (Maxaquin), 400 mg q d; enoxacin (Penetrex), 400 mg q 12 h; macrocrystalline nitrofurantoin (Macrodantin, Macrobid), 100 mg 4 times/d; amoxicillin (Amoxil), 250 mg q 8 h; cefpodoxime proxetil (Vantin), 100 mg q 12 h; and cefixime (Suprax), 400 mg q d.

‡Oral regimens for pyelonephritis and complicated UTI are as follows: trimethoprim-sulfamethoxazole (Bactrim, Septra), 160–800 mg q 12 h; norfloxacin (Noroxin), 400 mg q 12 h; ciprofloxacin (Cipro), 500 mg q 12 h; ofloxacin (Floxin), 200–300 mg q 12 h; lomefloxacin (Maxaquin), 400 mg q d; enoxacin (Penetrex), 400 mg q 12 h; amoxicillin (Amoxil), 500 mg q 8 h; cefpodoxime proxetil (Vantin), 200 mg q 12 h; and cefixime (Suprax), 400 mg q d.

§Parenteral regimens are as follows: trimethoprim-sulfamethoxazole (Bactrim, Septra), 160–800 mg q 12 h; ciprofloxacin (Cipro), 200–400 mg q 12 h; ofloxacin (Floxin), 200–400 mg q 12 h; gentamicin (Garamycin), 1 mg/kg q 8 h, 1.5 mg/kg q 12 h, or 3 mg/kg q 24 h; ceftriaxone (Rocephin), 1–2 gm q d; ampicillin (Omnipen, Polycillin), 1 gm q 6 h; imipenem-cilastatin (Primaxin), 250–500 mg q 6–8 h; ampicillin-sulbactam (Unasyn),1.5 gm q 6 h; ticarcillin-clavulanate (Timentin), 3.2 gm q 6–8 h, 1.5 mg/kg q 12 h, or 3 mg/kg q 24 h; piperacillin-tazobactam (Zosyn), 3.375 gm q 6–8 h; aztreonam (Azactam), 1 gm q 8–12 h.

Adapted from Stamm WE, Hooten TM: Management of urinary tract infections in adults. N Engl J Med *329*:1328–1334, 1993. Copyright 1993, Massachusetts Medical Society; all rights reserved. Johnson JR: Treatment and prevention of urinary tract infections. *In* Mobley HLT, Warren JW (eds): Urinary Tract Infections. Washington, DC, A.S.M. Press, 1996, pp 95–118.

to take medication and fluids by mouth. Hospitalization is still appropriate for unstable patients, patients with complicating factors, and pregnant women.

Initial therapy for acute pyelonephritis is almost always selected empirically, taking into consideration the patient's underlying host status and local antimicrobial susceptibility patterns. Suggested initial regimens for different situations are shown in Table 1. Once susceptibility results are known, the regimen can be modified accordingly.

Patients given intravenous therapy initially in the hospital can be switched to oral therapy when they are able to take medications well by mouth, and they can be discharged home when they are clearly responding to therapy, even if fever and symptoms have not completely resolved. Failure to improve by 48 hours suggests a resistant organism, a mistaken diagnosis, or an unsuspected complication such as obstruction, stone, or abscess.

The optimal duration of therapy for acute pyelonephritis in women is undefined; duration of therapy must be individualized. Fourteen days total is suffi-

cient for women without complicating factors, and even shorter courses are successful in some cases. Longer courses may be needed in patients with complicating factors, a slow response to therapy, or relapse after a shorter initial course. Post-therapy urine cultures remain part of the standard management of acute pyelonephritis.

Asymptomatic Bacteriuria. The presence of bacteria in the urine in the absence of symptoms, irrespective of the degree of inflammatory response, is termed "asymptomatic bacteriuria" (ABU). Circumstances in which treatment of ABU in adults is clearly warranted include during pregnancy (in which without treatment there is a substantial risk of severe pyelonephritis and possibly of prematurity or low-birthweight infants) and prior to invasive procedures involving the urinary tract (which may precipitate bacteremia if the urine is infected). In most other settings the risk/benefit ratio for treating ABU is less favorable, and it generally is preferable not to obtain the urine culture in the first place, so as to avoid discovering the presence of a UTI that may not need to be treated.

Recurrent UTI. Following an initial episode of UTI, some women go on to have multiple subsequent episodes, sometimes for years. Only rarely are such recurrent infections due to anatomic or functional abnormalities of the urinary tract that warrant urologic investigation, so a routine search for such predisposing factors in all women with recurrent UTI is not warranted. Instead, recurrent UTI in women is more often attributable to behavioral factors such as sexual intercourse (particularly with the use of spermicide-diaphragm contraception) or biologic factors such as a predisposition to vaginal colonization with uropathogenic bacteria. Management options include the use of postcoital antibiotics (for women with intercourse-associated UTI), use of an alternative method of contraception (for spermicide users), chronic low-dose antibiotic prophylaxis (Table 2), and self-administered home antibiotic therapy (as for acute cystitis: see Table 1) for early treatment of self-diagnosed UTI. In postmenopausal women, restoration of the normal premenopausal vaginal microflora and acidic pH by topical application of estrogen cream reduces vaginal colonization with *Escherichia coli* and decreases the frequency of UTI. The optimal approach for an individual woman will depend on the relevant risk factors in the particular case and the patient's preferences.

Catheter-Associated UTI. In women with a chronic indwelling bladder catheter, bacteriuria is almost universally present, usually without causing symptoms. When such infections become symptomatic, therapy is indicated (as for complicated UTI: see Table 1). In the absence of symptoms, it is best to ignore catheter-associated bacteriuria in chronically catheterized patients, since treatment will not make the patient feel better at the time, will render the urine sterile only temporarily (if at all), and will select for more resistant organisms, which may complicate the therapy of a subsequent symptomatic UTI episode.

In women who undergo short-term urinary catheterization (such as during an acute hospital admission), careful attention to maintenance of a closed drainage system reduces the likelihood of developing bacteriuria. Drainage bag additives contribute little, and routine meatal cleansing and application of antibacterial ointments to the meatus are without proven benefit and may promote UTI. Prophylactic antibiotic therapy for patients with short-term bladder catheter use is effective in preventing UTI, but whether this benefit is worth the associated expense, adverse effects, and potential for selection of resistant organisms is unclear.

BACTERIAL INFECTIONS OF THE URINARY TRACT IN GIRLS

method of
JONATHAN H. ROSS, M.D.
Cleveland Clinic Foundation
Cleveland, Ohio

Approximately 5% of girls will develop a urinary tract infection prior to the age of 18 years. The incidence in infants is approximately 1%, and the peaks of incidence are at the time of toilet training and in late adolescence. Urinary tract infections can result in significant morbidity, particularly in the presence of associated urologic anomalies. Vesicoureteral reflux is the most commonly associated anomaly, and reflux nephropathy is an important cause of end-stage renal disease in children and adolescents.

DIAGNOSIS

Urinary tract infections in girls do not always present with the classic symptoms of irritative voiding or flank pain. Infants often present with fever and irritability. Even older girls may have nonspecific symptoms, such as abdominal pain or an unexplained fever. Any child with symptoms suggestive of a urinary tract infection or unexplained fever should undergo a urinalysis and urine culture. Because a documented infection warrants thorough radiographic evaluation, empiric treatment on the basis of symptoms or urinalysis alone should be avoided. The most accurate means of obtaining a urine culture is by suprapubic aspiration. A 21- or 22-gauge needle is introduced 1 or 2 cm above the pubic symphysis into a full bladder while aspirating with a sterile syringe. Although this technique is generally safe and effective, there have been anecdotal reports of significant complications, and it can be an anxiety-provoking procedure for the child, parent, and physician. Urine cultures are therefore most often obtained from urine collected by placing a plastic bag over the perineum of infants, and from urine from a voided specimen in older children. Catheter specimens are another alternative, but these may introduce infection. If a catheter is used, a single dose of oral antibiotic should be given to prevent iatrogenic infection. Because "bag" and voided specimens may be contaminated, they must be interpreted in conjunction with the urinalysis and clinical setting. Pyuria and/or classic symptoms support the diagnosis of a urinary tract infection, whereas a positive culture in the face of a normal urinalysis and/or atypical symptoms may represent contamination.

Although the presence or absence of a true urinary tract infection is occasionally difficult to determine, the distinction between cystitis and pyelonephritis is even more problematic. The presence of neither fever nor flank pain is sensitive or specific. Acute phase reactants such as erythro-

TABLE 2. **Oral Regimens for Daily Prophylaxis of UTI in Women**

Agent	Daily Dose (mg)
Trimethoprim (Proloprim, Trimpex)*	100
Trimethoprim-sulfamethoxazole (Bactrim, Septra)*	40 + 200†
Nitrofurantoin (generic)*	50
Nitrofurantoin macrocrystals (Macrodantin, Macrobid)*	100
Cephalexin (Keflex), cephradine (Anspor, Velosef), or cefaclor (Ceclor)	250
Norfloxacin (Noroxin)	200

*Preferred agent.
†Also effective as 40 + 200 mg 3 times/wk.

cyte sedimentation rate (ESR) are also inaccurate. A [99m]technetium dimercaptosuccinic acid (DMSA) renal flow scan is the best study for confirming pyelonephritis and the risk of subsequent renal scar formation. Patients with a normal scan during an acute infection will not develop scarring, whereas an area of photopenia on a DMSA scan identifies a region of the affected kidney at risk for eventual scar formation. Because this test is invasive, expensive, and exposes the child to radiation, it is not routinely used.

TREATMENT

Because urinary tract infections are usually caused by gram-negative rods, particularly *Escherichia coli*, any oral antibiotic with good gram-negative coverage is a reasonable choice for treatment. Trimethoprim/sulfamethoxazole (Bactrim, Septra) offers good coverage and is inexpensive. It is given in suspension form at 4 mg of trimethoprim per kg twice daily. Other commonly used antibiotics include amoxicillin (Amoxil), 10 mg per kg three times a day, and nitrofurantoin (Furadantin, Macrodantin), 2.5 mg per kg three times a day. Cephalosporins may be indicated if infection with a more resistant organism is suspected. Ciprofloxacin (Cipro) is the only oral agent effective against *Pseudomonas*, but it is not approved for use in children.

Children requiring hospitalization should be placed on broad-spectrum intravenous antibiotics pending the results of the urine culture. The usual regimen is gentamicin (Garamycin), 2 mg per kg every 8 hours for gram-negative coverage, and ampicillin 20 mg per kg every 6 hours for coverage of enterococci.

EVALUATION

A renal ultrasonogram is obtained to rule out obstructive uropathy in girls presenting with a urinary tract infection. An ultrasonogram can also detect gross renal scarring or marked asymmetry of renal size in patients with vesicoureteral reflux. When accurate detection of renal scarring is important, a DMSA renal flow scan is the best study.

A cystogram is also obtained in girls with a urinary tract infection to rule out vesicoureteral reflux, which is present in 30% to 50%. Because an ultrasonogram is normal in 50% to 75% of patients with significant reflux, it is a poor study for excluding it. A cystogram performed by an experienced pediatric radiologist is well tolerated by most children. A few doses of antibiotics should be given around the time of the cystogram to prevent an iatrogenic infection.

Two types of cystogram are currently available. A standard voiding cystourethrogram (VCUG) is accomplished by instilling radiopaque contrast into the bladder and imaging the bladder and renal fossae with x-ray during filling and voiding. The severity of vesicoureteral reflux is graded on a scale of 1 to 5 depending on the degree of distention of the collecting system.

Alternatively, a nuclear cystogram can be obtained by instilling a radionuclide into the bladder and imaging with a gamma camera. Nuclear cystography is at least as sensitive for the detection of reflux as a standard VCUG and exposes the child to less radiation. However, grading of reflux is less precise, and associated bladder abnormalities cannot be detected with nuclear cystography. Therefore, a VCUG is preferred as the initial study in the evaluation of a girl with a urinary tract infection. Nuclear cystography is used in follow-up of patients with vesicoureteral reflux who are on an observation protocol and for screening siblings and children of refluxers.

MANAGEMENT OF VESICOURETERAL REFLUX

Reflux will resolve spontaneously in some patients. It is more likely to resolve if it is low grade, unilateral, and not associated with other anomalies. The grade of reflux is the most important factor. Over several years of observation, reflux will resolve in approximately 80% of patients with grade 1 or 2 reflux, 50% of patients with grade 3 reflux, and 25% of patients with grade 4 reflux. Because of this tendency to resolve, most patients with reflux are initially treated on an observation protocol. Renal scarring usually occurs only with the reflux of infected urine. Therefore, prevention of urinary tract infections in children with reflux is essential, and the mainstay of medical management is antibiotic prophylaxis. The most frequently used agents are nitrofurantoin (Furadantin, Macrodantin), 1 to 2 mg per kg once daily, and trimethoprim/sulfamethoxazole (Bactrim, Septra), 2 to 4 mg of trimethoprim per kg once daily. Patients on observation should have periodic urine cultures (e.g., every 3 months) to detect asymptomatic bacteriuria. Cystograms are obtained annually, and chemoprophylaxis is discontinued when reflux resolves. Upper tract studies are obtained periodically as dictated by the patient's clinical course. Bladder instability and constipation should be treated when present (see next section).

Any patient on observation who develops a breakthrough urinary tract infection or new renal scarring should undergo surgical correction of her reflux. Surgery is also appropriate in patients who cannot comply with close follow-up and long-term antibiotic prophylaxis. This includes patients who wish to avoid repeated cystograms and office visits. Patients with high-grade reflux may be considered for immediate surgical intervention.

RECURRENT URINARY TRACT INFECTIONS

Some children without a discernible anatomic anomaly develop recurrent urinary tract infections. Many of these children present after toilet training, when normal reflex voiding is interfered with by social constraints. The risk of renal scarring in these patients is low, though not absent. Some of these children will have symptoms of bladder instability, such as urge incontinence or squatting behavior in the absence of an infection. These voiding symptoms often respond to anticholinergic agents such as oxybutynin chloride (Ditropan), 0.15 mg per kg three times a day. Even when the symptoms are subtle and not in themselves troublesome, the recurrent infections can be prevented, or reduced in frequency, by anticholinergic therapy in conjunction with antibiotic prophylaxis. Constipation can predispose to bladder instability and recurrent urinary tract infections. It should therefore be aggressively managed.

Even an anatomically and functionally normal urinary tract may be predisposed to recurrent infections. Certain host factors may play a role, such as antigen expression on the bladder epithelium. However, there is no specific therapy for these host factors, and so girls with frequent infections are managed with antibiotic prophylaxis administered in the same fashion as for patients with vesicoureteral reflux. However, in the absence of reflux, upper tract monitoring and routine urine cultures are rarely indicated, as treatment of asymptomatic bacteriuria in this setting is unnecessary.

CHILDHOOD ENURESIS

method of
R. DUANE CESPEDES, M.D., and
MICHAEL L. RITCHEY, M.D.
University of Texas–Houston Medical School
Houston, Texas

Enuresis is the involuntary voiding of urine after the expected age when urinary control is ordinarily achieved. Although prevalence varies among different racial and ethnic groups, enuresis is clearly the most common voiding disorder in children, with 15% to 20% of 5-year-olds affected to a variable degree. It is helpful to divide enuresis into its various types, since evaluation, treatment, and prognosis are frequently different. The most prevalent form of enuresis is *nocturnal enuresis*, defined as bedwetting that occurs more than twice a month after the age of 5 years. *Diurnal enuresis* is wetting that occurs during the day. If the child is 5 years or older and has never been dry for any significant period of time, the enuresis is primary. *Primary enuresis* is much more common than *secondary enuresis*, which is the onset (or recurrence) of enuresis after a 6-month dry interval. Approximately 15% to 20% of patients with nocturnal enuresis have concurrent daytime wetting. Nocturnal enuresis is more common in boys by a 1.5:1 ratio and diurnal enuresis is slightly more common in girls. The great majority of primary enuretics are wet usually only at night, with rare daytime enuresis, and have no definable urologic or neurologic etiology. Since the etiologic theories, evaluation, and treatment considerations are somewhat different between nocturnal and diurnal enuresis, it is helpful to discuss each type separately.

NOCTURNAL ENURESIS
Etiology

Many factors have been reported as causing or contributing to nocturnal enuresis. Possible etiologies include inherited factors, psychological maladjustment, sleep disorders, delayed central nervous system maturation, abnormal bladder storage and function, food allergies, and inadequate nocturnal secretion of antidiuretic hormone (ADH). The prevalence of enuresis is increased if a parental history of nocturnal enuresis exists. The prevalence may be as high as 77% if both parents and 44% if one parent had nocturnal enuresis. Psychological problems were once believed to be the major cause of nocturnal enuresis; however, no correlation has been found in prospective studies.

Many parents and early investigators believed that children with nocturnal enuresis were "heavy sleepers" and were not awakened by the need to void. Subsequent sleep studies revealed that enuretics are essentially normal sleepers with the enuretic episodes occurring throughout the night. Additionally, recent evidence shows that children with nocturnal enuresis have essentially normal bladder capacity and no increased incidence of detrusor instability. A large percentage of enuretics have been shown to produce excessive amounts of urine at night secondary to abnormally low nocturnal ADH secretion; however, this does not explain why enuretics do not wake up once their bladder is full. It is possible that nocturnal enuresis is due to several factors, with some playing a more predominant role in one group of children versus another.

Evaluation

The initial interview of the patient with nocturnal enuresis (and parents) should include a familial history of enuresis, duration and degree of enuresis, and a complete profile of any associated daytime voiding dysfunction, previous urinary tract infections, or urologic procedures. The physical examination should be directed toward identifying genitourinary abnormalities and neurologic lesions. The abdomen is examined for a distended bladder or enlarged kidneys. A complete examination of the genitalia, including a rectal examination, is essential. Cutaneous abnormalities of the sacral region, including hair patches, lipomas, or pigmented or vascular lesions, may suggest occult abnormalities of the spinal cord. Finally, a urinalysis should be performed to rule out diabetes insipidus/mellitus or a urinary tract infection. If the results of a directed evaluation are normal (as they typically are in nocturnal enuresis), additional diagnostic tests are not indicated.

Treatment

The age at which treatment begins needs to be individualized for each family. For the younger child, patience and understanding are the best things to offer. However, by 7 years of age the social cost of bedwetting begins to rise, and the enuresis will start to interfere with the child's participation in activities such as sleepovers. In the older child, these latter factors serve as motivation for behavioral modification therapy, which requires active participation and cooperation to succeed. Our initial management for all children with nocturnal enuresis is fluid restriction. We recognize that the majority of children will not be dry with this alone, but it may be sufficient for some children. However, even if not successful, fluid restriction is continued when other treatment programs are started.

Several types of behavioral modification have been advocated for the treatment of nocturnal enuresis, including positive reinforcement therapy, bladder retention training, and conditioning therapy. We believe the most important factor is to avoid negative reinforcement and not punish the child for wetting. A reward system for dry nights is helpful. We have not found an appropriate role for bladder retention training. Some parents find that waking the child at night may solve the problem. This is generally done randomly in relation to bladder filling, usually when the parent goes to bed later than the child. We have not found tremendous success with this approach, but that is because most children referred to us have usually failed this method.

One of the most successful forms of treatment consists of an alarm system that awakens the child when contact with urine occurs. Current systems are self-contained units with sensor and alarm sewn into the bed clothes. These are battery-operated devices that produce either a buzzing noise or a vibration of the device to awaken the child. This therapy presumably is based upon repetitively awakening the child when urinary leakage occurs, which ultimately conditions the child to recognize that voiding is about to occur. However, we see success in some children who do not wake up at night but still remain dry. The main advantage of the alarm systems is that they have a very good success rate (70%), comparable to that reported for pharmacologic therapy. The alarm must be used for a period of at least 3 to 4 months before it can be considered to be a failure. Reasons for failure include lack of motivation by the child and parent, and subsequently noncompliance. It is important that the parent awaken the child when the alarm goes off initially, if the child seems to sleep through it. Once the child achieves dryness, the alarm is continued for another 4 to 6 weeks to reinforce the success. Relapse does occur in about 20% to 30% of patients, but they can be treated again with another alarm trial. This rate of relapse is much lower than that seen after pharmacologic treatment.

Drug Therapy

The pharmacologic agents that have been used for treatment of nocturnal enuresis include anticholinergics, tricyclic antidepressants, and drugs that decrease urine output. Despite the proven effectiveness of behavioral modification and alarms, many children are initially started on drug therapy. Although this may offer some children quick short-term success, there are several disadvantages. After the medications are stopped, relapse is frequent, requiring that the medications be restarted. Many children are maintained long-term on medication. Other disadvantages include side effects of the medications and cost.

The most frequently used tricyclic antidepressant is imipramine (Tofranil). The exact mechanism of action of the tricyclics is unknown; however, four theories have been proposed: (1) antidepressant action, (2) alteration of sleeping patterns, (3) decreasing detrusor instability and increasing bladder capacity, and (4) increase in the amount of ADH secreted. The usual dose of imipramine is 25 mg taken 1 hour before bedtime for 6- to 8-year-olds (50 to 75 mg in older children). Imipramine should not be used in children less than 6 years old. Results are usually seen within 1 week, with the highest success rates in older children. Treatment should continue for 3 to 6 months before the dosage is gradually decreased. If relapse occurs, another 3- to 6-month treatment course should be initiated. Initial success rates are approximately 50%, with long-term results closer to 25% once the medication is stopped. One advantage of this medication is that it is relatively inexpensive. Side effects from treatment are common and include gastrointestinal disturbances, anxiety, insomnia, dry mouth, and emotional instability. Most importantly, an overdose can lead to fatal cardiac arrhythmias, hypotension, and convulsions. Parents must be warned about the potential danger so they can take action to prevent accidental overdoses in the enuretic patient and other children in the family.

Desmopressin acetate (DDAVP) nasal spray is an ADH analogue with a long-acting and highly specific antidiuresis action. The use of this drug is based upon the premise that some children have decreased nocturnal ADH secretion with excess urine output that exceeds the functional capacity of the bladder, with resultant enuresis. Several different regimens have been employed in initiating therapy with DDAVP. The drug is administered intranasally. It is very important that the child be instructed not to sniff the medication. The drug is absorbed in the nasal mucosa; if it goes farther back into the upper pharynx or GI tract, absorption is markedly decreased. Our initial starting dose is 10 μg, or 1 spray from the metered container. We instruct the child to use the medication about an hour before bedtime. The child has also been instructed to restrict fluids for 2 hours before bedtime. We reinforce the need to empty the bladder at the time the child does go to bed. After the child has been maintained on this dose for several weeks, we monitor the response. If there has been no success rate, then we double the dose every few weeks until a maximum of 40 μg (2 sprays in each nostril) is reached. The medication needs to be kept in a refrigerator. It can be left out for several days if the child is going on a short trip, but it is not stable at room temperature for long periods of time.

Side effects of DDAVP are fortunately uncommon. We see occasional nasal irritation and nose bleeds. Nasal congestion is common in children and will decrease the effectiveness of the medicine, but it is not generally caused by the treatment. One serious complication reported after the use of intranasal DDAVP is hyponatremia. The number of reported cases is few and in some cases it can be attributable to the drinking of fluids after the DDAVP is administered. It is recommended that after treatment of DDAVP is instituted, serum electrolyte levels of the child be measured during the first week of usage to be sure that there is no occult drop in the serum sodium. However, in our years of use of this medication we have not found any abnormal serum chemistries. The severe manifestations of hyponatremia are seizures, which can be life-threatening. This might be more of a concern in children with cystic fibrosis, in whom DDAVP may be contraindicated, and in children who are treated with combinations of medications, such as imipramine and DDAVP. Evidence shows that imipramine can potentiate nocturnal secretion of ADH. This must be taken into consideration when using combination therapy.

Once the child has achieved success with DDAVP, we usually continue therapy for several more weeks before tapering the medication. The children who relapse after stopping the medication can be restarted and treated for several months before again tapering the medication to determine whether the enuresis has resolved. DDAVP is also used by many physicians on an "as needed" basis. The medication is used at times when bedwetting will be especially embarrassing and inconvenient, such as on sleepovers or visits with relatives. Because of its prompt action it seems to be effective in these circumstances. A major disadvantage of DDAVP is that it is considerably more expensive than the other aforementioned modalities. However, we do find it to be effective and therefore recommend it to many of our patients who have failed conditioning therapies such as the alarm.

Despite the effectiveness of imipramine, other bladder antispasmodics and anticholinergics such as oxybutynin (Ditropan) have not been successful in treating monosymptomatic nocturnal enuresis. Sedatives and stimulants are also ineffective.

DIURNAL ENURESIS

Like nocturnal enuresis, the incidence of diurnal enuresis is also age dependent. Diurnal enuresis occurs in 5% to 10% of children aged 5 to 8 years. There is a higher prevalence of daytime accidents in girls than boys. The etiology for diurnal enuresis is varied. For most children, this represents a general delay in the achievement of daytime control. The children often have a decreased perception of bladder filling. They are very focused on their play activities and do not tune in to the early signals of bladder fullness until it is too late (for the Nintendo players, we call it Super Mario enuresis). Many of the children also appear to lack the ability to inhibit the bladder centrally from contracting. Many of these children will learn at an early age that contraction of the external sphincter will inhibit the detrusor contraction. This is the only mechanism they have at

their disposal to stay dry. Unusual posturing such as squatting to compress the urethra with the heel (Vincent's curtsy) or crossing the legs may be seen. Urodynamic studies of enuretic patients have shown that these symptoms are associated with sudden detrusor contractility that is provoked by filling. However, very few children with diurnal enuresis have underlying physical abnormalities of the urinary tract or nervous system. Therefore, the initial evaluation before beginning treatment consists of careful history, physical examination, and urinalysis.

We reserve further work-up for those children who have more "complicated" enuresis, which includes those with a history of urinary tract infection, an abnormal urologic or neurologic evaluation, associated encopresis, or diurnal enuresis that fails to respond to initial treatment measures as outlined subsequently. Although the majority of these children will not demonstrate anatomic or neurologic abnormalities upon further evaluation, additional diagnostic studies are necessary. In children with daytime enuresis and urinary tract infections, a renal and bladder ultrasonogram and voiding cystourethrogram are recommended. The ultrasonogram will rule out hydronephrosis, bladder thickening, duplication anomalies, or increased postvoid residual. Even if the ultrasonogram is normal, further evaluation with a voiding cystourethrogram is indicated to rule out vesicoureteral reflux. Some have advocated more extensive evaluation of the spine to exclude occult abnormalities. However, the incidence of tethered cord or lipoma is low. For children with obvious abnormalities on physical examination, lipoma or hairy patches over the sacral area, or abnormal neurologic findings, we proceed with spine imaging with magnetic resonance imaging (MRI). However, for all other children we proceed with treatment. Those who fail to respond to standard therapy undergo urodynamic evaluation of bladder function. If abnormalities are noted on this examination, further evaluation of the spine is then obtained.

Nonpharmacologic management is the preferred initial therapy in the child. When these children are asked to document their voiding activities, we find that many of them are infrequent voiders. The children are instructed to void by the clock every 1 to 2 hours. We try to have them void before they get an urge to void since they have such a short time interval between the first desire to void and the actual enuretic episode. Another advantage of the frequent voiding schedule is that the children are voiding when they are relaxed and not trying to contract the external sphincter to inhibit voiding or enuretic episodes. By retraining them to void while they are relaxed, the amount of postvoid residual urine in the bladder is decreased.

A timed voiding program is sometimes difficult to initiate in young children. They frequently lose track of the time and do not keep to the agreed-upon schedule. A watch with an alarm is often very helpful. We also ask the children to keep a diary so they can objectively document the frequency of voiding. This reinforces the fact that they need to void every 2 hours. It is another way for us to evaluate whether persistent enuresis is a failure of the timed voiding or just poor compliance with the program. For those children who have difficulty relaxing the external sphincter to initiate voiding by the clock, biofeedback programs can be used. These are more time consuming and expensive, but worthwhile in a child who is unresponsive to simple measures.

If the child continues to have wetting episodes once the timed voiding schedule has been implemented, we then institute anticholinergic therapy. The most common drug used is oxybutynin (Ditropan) at a maximum daily dose of 0.5 mg per kg. The medication is started in a low dose twice daily then gradually titrated to the maximum dosage over 6 to 8 weeks. Side effects are common with anticholinergics. These include facial flushing, constipation, and dry mouth. Less common complaints are headache and palpitations. The minor side effects will often abate with prolonged usage, but the dosage of the medication has to be altered or stopped in 20% of our patients.

Children with a history of urinary tract infection are maintained on antibiotic prophylaxis. Also, if there is a history of constipation or encopresis, this should be treated with lactulose to restore regular bowel habits. For those children who fail to respond to pharmacologic treatment, we recommend more extensive diagnostic studies, including urodynamic evaluation of bladder function.

URINARY INCONTINENCE

method of
TABINDA NAZIR, M.D.
Elmhurst Hospital Center
Elmhurst, New York,

ZAFAR KHAN, M.D.
Beth Israel Medical Center
New York, New York,
                    and

HUGH BARBER, M.D.
Lenox Hill Hospital
New York, New York

Urinary incontinence is a costly and prevalent problem. Up to 7% of children over the age of 5 years suffer from incontinence. The incidence ranges from 1.4% in the 15- to 24-year age group to 2.9% in the 55 to 64 year age group. Studies of elderly subjects living at home demonstrate a prevalence of 14% to 18%. The average prevalence in institutionalized elderly subjects is estimated to be 45% and as much as 50% to 55% by some investigators. The oldest subjects (over the age of 80 years) have a higher prevalence of incontinence both at home and in institutions. Dementia, restricted mobility, and depression are some of the factors frequently associated with urinary incontinence in elderly people. The overall prevalence of urinary incontinence in a given population is very important for estimating the cost of this disorder, which has been calculated to be over $10 billion.

In Western countries, 4% to 8% of the population can be considered to suffer from significant urinary incontinence —that is, to require treatment or protection or even admission to a long-stay unit for elderly patients. A precise medical diagnosis is established in only 5% of cases.

DIAGNOSTIC EVALUATION

The history is the most important step in the evaluation of urinary incontinence. A detailed description should be obtained, focusing on the type (urge, reflex, stress, overflow, or mixed), onset, frequency, severity, duration, pattern (diurnal, nocturnal, or both), precipitants (medications, including nonprescription drugs), palliating features, associated symptoms (straining to void, incomplete emptying, dysuria), and conditions (cancer, diabetes, acute illness, neurologic disease, alteration in bowel/sexual function, pelvic or lower urinary tract surgery). Physical examination is essential to rule out transient causes and to evaluate co-morbid disease and functional ability. The examination should check for signs of neurologic diseases, spinal column deformities, stress leakage, and general medical illnesses. On rectal examination, look for skin irritation, resting tone, voluntary control of anal sphincter, prostate, and fecal impaction. Pelvic examination should focus on atrophic vaginitis, masses, and muscle laxity.

Investigations include a voiding diary prepared by the patient, metabolic survey (measurement of electrolytes, calcium, glucose, and urea nitrogen), urinalysis and culture, renal ultrasound measurement of postvoiding residual volume, and urine cytology. Bladder and urethral function can be assessed via urodynamic evaluation.

Urodynamic Study. Urodynamic study of the lower urinary tract can provide useful clinical information about the function of the urinary bladder, the sphincteric mechanism, and the voiding pattern. Cystometry is used in the studies. The activity of the smooth muscle sphincter and the voluntary sphincter can be recorded urodynamically by pressure measurements; the activity of the voluntary sphincter can be recorded by electromyography.

Urinary Flow Rate. The normal flow rate from a full bladder is about 20 to 25 mL per sec in men and 25 to 30 mL per sec in women. Obstruction should be suspected in any adult voiding with a full bladder at a rate of less than 15 mL per sec. A flow rate of less than 10 mL per sec is considered definite evidence of obstruction. A normal flow pattern is represented by a bell-shaped curve. The flow rate is more often recorded electronically: The patient voids into a container on top of a measuring device that is connected to a transducer, the weight being converted to volume and recorded on a chart in milliliters per second. The overall appearance of the flow curve may disclose unsuspected abnormalities.

Flow rates in mechanical obstruction are totally different, classically in the range of 5 to 6 mL per sec; flow time is greatly prolonged, and there is sustained low flow with minimal variation. Reduced flow rate in the absence of mechanical obstruction is due to some impairment of sphincteric or detrusor activity.

Bladder Function. The basic factors of normal bladder function are bladder capacity, accommodation, sensation, contractility, voluntary control, and response to drugs. All can be evaluated by cystometry. If all are within the normal range, bladder physiology is assumed to be normal.

Cystometry can be done by either of two basic methods: filling the bladder with water and recording the intravesical pressure against the volume of water introduced into the bladder, or gas cystometry, which is being used in some laboratories as a substitute for water cystometry. A cystometrogram is obtained during the phase of bladder filling; the volume of fluid in the bladder is plotted against the intravesical pressure to show bladder wall compliance to filling. Normally, the sensation of fullness is first perceived when the bladder contains 100 to 200 mL of fluid and is strongly felt as the bladder nears capacity; the desire to void occurs when the bladder is full (normal capacity being 400 to 500 mL). The bladder normally shows no evidence of contractility or activity during the filling phase. However, once it is filled to capacity and the subject perceives the desire to urinate and consciously allows urination to proceed, strong bladder contractions will occur and will be sustained until the bladder is empty. Whether the patient can inhibit urination with a full bladder and initiate urination when asked—aspects of voluntary detrusor control—must be assessed during cystometric study to rule out uninhibited bladder activity. Low pressure with a very large capacity might imply sensory loss or flaccid lower motor neuron lesion, a chronically distended bladder, or a large bladder due to myogenic damage. High pressure (usually associated with reduced capacity) that rises rapidly with bladder filling is most commonly due to inflammation, enuresis, or reduced bladder capacity. However, uninhibited bladder activity during this high-pressure filling phase might indicate neuropathic bladder or an upper motor neuron lesion.

The most valuable part of the cystometric study is the determination of voiding activity or voiding contraction. Normal voiding contractions are about 20 to 40 cm of water, and a higher voiding pressure indicates possible increase in outlet resistance. The quality of bladder pressure can also be informative, even without simultaneous recording of flow rate. Cystometric study may disclose complete absence of detrusor contractility due to motor or sensory deficits or conscious inhibition of detrusor activity. Detrusor hyperactivity is shown as uninhibited activity, usually due to interruption of the neural connection between spinal cord centers and the higher midbrain and cortical centers.

Evaluation of Sphincteric Function

Urinary sphincteric function can be evaluated by the following methods.

Profilometry. The urethral pressure profile is determined by recording the pressure in the urethra at every level of the sphincteric unit from the internal meatus to the end of the sphincteric segment. Profilometry has been performed by gas or water perfusion techniques.

Electromyographic Study of Sphincteric Function. Electromyography gives useful information about sphincteric function when done in conjunction with cystometry. Direct needle electromyography of the urethral sphincter provides the most accurate information. Recording via needle electrodes can be obtained from the anal sphincter, from the bulk of the musculature of the pelvic floor, or from the external sphincter itself, though in the latter case the placement is difficult and the accuracy of the results is questionable.

Electromyography study makes use of the electrical activity that is constantly present within the pelvic floor and external urinary sphincter at rest, which increases progressively with bladder filling. If the bladder contracts for voiding, electrical activity ceases completely. Urethral closure pressure is the difference between intravesical pressure and urethral pressure, that is, the net closure pressure.

ENURESIS

Enuresis is described as bedwetting after age 3 years. Most children have achieved normal bladder control by that time, girls earlier than boys. At age 6 years, 7% of children have enuresis. Even at age 14 years, 5% still wet the bed. The cause is thought to be delayed maturation of the nervous system or an intrinsic myoneurogenic bladder dysfunction. Few cases are of psychic origin, and 20% are secondary to organic disease. Most children with functional enuresis spontaneously gain nocturnal control by age 10 years.

A child may wet the bed occasionally or regularly. Many void frequently and are found to have a diminished vesical capacity. General physical and urologic examinations are normal. Excretory urograms show no abnormality. Urethrocystoscopy is normal. Cytometric studies are usually abnormal, and a curve typical of the *uninhibited* (hyperirritable) neuropathic bladder is often obtained.

Treatment

Treatment should be considered if enuresis persists after age 3 years. Fluids should be limited after supper. The bladder should be completely emptied at bedtime. Drug therapy includes (1) Imipramine (Tofranil); (2) parasympatholytic drugs, e.g., oxybutynin (Ditropan); and (3) desmopressin (DDAVP, Stimate), which is an antidiuretic that increases renal reabsorption of water. Use of mechanical devices such as metal-covered pads that when wet cause an alarm to ring may be of benefit in cases of delayed maturation by setting up a conditioned reflex. Analytic evaluation and treatment may be indicated for some enuretic children and their parents.

STRESS URINARY INCONTINENCE

Stress incontinence is the inability to hold urine when intra-abdominal pressure is increased. Activities that commonly precipitate episodes of stress urinary incontinence include coughing, laughing, straining, dancing, sneezing, lifting, bending, and jogging. Stress urinary incontinence (SUI) must be distinguished from *giggle* incontinence, a cerebrospinal reflex phenomenon seen in some adolescent girls who experience leakage of urine when they giggle but not during other activities related to stress urinary incontinence.

Stress urinary incontinence is most often associated with a history of vaginal delivery, aging (e.g., in women it may be associated with estrogen deficiency), obesity, chronic cough (asthma, smoking), sneezing, running, or chronic constipation. Hypertensive patients treated with alpha-adrenergic blocking agents (e.g., prazosin) may also develop stress urinary incontinence.

Laboratory studies include the following:

Dynamic cystourethroscopy. If the bladder neck and proximal urethra are observed to be open, the presence of sphincter incompetence is confirmed.

Uroflowmetry. In stress urinary incontinence, enhanced flow is expected because of the reduced urethral resistance.

Cystometrography study is normal in stress urinary incontinence.

Urethral pressure profile shows poor transmission of abdominal pressure to the proximal urethra.

Electromyography of the external urethral sphincter. Abnormal motor potentials (e.g., fibrillations, positive waves) indicate neurologic damage to the sacral nerves. Nerve potentials are not affected by stress urinary incontinence.

Videofluoroscopy of micturition demonstrates stress urinary incontinence radiographically.

Treatment

Pelvic Floor Rehabilitation. Also called Kegel exercises, this is designed to improve the strength of the pelvic floor musculature, which in turn will suspend the proximal urethra. Kegel exercises consist of frequent voluntary contractions of the pubococcygeus muscle. Alternatively, the patient may be taught to interrupt the urinary stream for a few seconds during each voiding before continuing to empty the bladder. The exercises should be repeated five times every waking hour, every day. They can be done anywhere without interfering with normal activity and without others being aware. Improvement in stress urinary incontinence (SUI) requires 8 to 12 weeks of exercises. Maximum benefit is realized at 3 to 6 months. The patient may also report that the improved muscle tone heightens sexual enjoyment.

Pharmacologic Therapy

1. Estrogen therapy. A vaginal estrogen creme such as conjugated equine estrogens,*† 2.5 grams three times a week for 12 weeks, may be prescribed for postmenopausal women in stress urinary incontinence.

2. Alpha-adrenergic agonists. Phenylpropanolamine (Entex LA),* 75 to 100 mg daily in slow-release form, may improve the symptoms of mild stress urinary incontinence.

3. Discontinuation of alpha-adrenergic blockers.

Surgery. A wide variety of operations continue to be used for stress urinary incontinence. Most surgical corrections are aimed at elevating the bladder neck and bringing the proximal urethra back into the abdominal cavity. If a proper diagnosis is made, the success rate is approximately 85% to 90%. Surgical procedures used are anterior colporrhaphy, retropubic urethropexy, cystoscopically controlled bladder neck suspension, and the pubovaginal sling procedure.

---

*Not FDA-approved for this indication.
†Not available in the United States.

URGE (REFLEX) INCONTINENCE

Urge incontinence is sudden voiding caused by involuntary bladder contraction. Besides sudden loss of urine, which is perceived by the patient, symptoms include frequency and urgency. In contrast to SUI, in which loss of urine is associated only with activities that increase intra-abdominal pressure, urine loss can occur at any time.

Involuntary bladder contractions occur without a known neurologic lesion. Such idiopathic urge incontinence is termed *detrusor instability.* Involuntary bladder contraction may result from a known underlying neurologic condition (e.g., cerebrovascular accident, Parkinson's disease, prolapsed intervertebral disc, spinal cord injury, or multiple sclerosis). This is termed *hyperreflexic bladder.* Urge incontinence can also accompany outflow obstruction. No specific physical findings are associated with this clinical entity. The history provides important clues, which may be further confirmed by urodynamic studies. Cystoscopy provides useful information regarding the state of the bladder. Differential diagnosis includes interstitial cystitis, urinary tract infection, stress incontinence, and urinary fistula.

Treatment

Drugs used to control detrusor instability or hyperreflexia are primarily anticholinergic agents such as oxybutynin (Ditropan), 2.5 to 10 mg orally three or four times daily, or propantheline bromide (Probanthine), 7.5 to 30 mg orally three or four times daily. The dosage needed to control bladder contractions may lead to side effects such as dryness of the mouth or constipation. Stool softeners may be necessary to manage the constipation. Intraocular pressure should be followed carefully by an ophthalmologist when anticholinergic drugs are used in patients with glaucoma. These drugs must be used with great care in patients suffering from cardiac conditions.

OVERFLOW INCONTINENCE

The most common cause of overflow incontinence is diabetes mellitus, which greatly reduces detrusor activity. Other neurologic deficits that may cause detrusor atony (neurogenic bladder) include lumbosacral nerve disease (e.g., compression from prolapsed intervertebral disc, spinal tumors, myelomeningocele, multiple sclerosis) and high spinal cord injury. The causes of outflow obstruction include enlarged prostate, urethral stricture, urethral scarring resulting from surgery, urethral angulation caused by prolapse, and meatal stenosis. Severe outflow obstruction can lead to urinary retention that can result in overflow incontinence if chronic. It is usually associated with hydronephrosis and azotemia. Sometimes an elderly patient may present with azotemia and urinary incontinence, and work-up reveals an enlarged prostate.

The history should be carefully noted. On physical

examination, bladder distention is often seen to mimic pelvic or abdominal tumors. Catheterization of the bladder with subsequent disappearance of the mass establishes the diagnosis.

Laboratory studies include the following:

Catheterization. Postvoiding residual urine volume is over 500 mL. This finding distinguishes overflow incontinence from stress incontinence.

Ultrasonography can detect a large, urine-filled bladder without catheterization.

Cystourethroscopy is helpful in defining urethral scarring, strictures, or meatal stenosis, all of which can cause outflow obstruction.

Cystoscopy is done for an enlarged prostate.

Urodynamics. These studies include *uroflowmetry.* The pattern of voiding is interrupted, and a high postvoiding residuum is found. *Cystometrography.* The bladder capacity is usually in excess of 600 mL. The sense of proprioception associated with bladder distention is greatly reduced. Bladder is either absent or considerably weaker than normal. *Electromyography* of the external sphincter will diagnose external sphincter dysynergia caused by spinal cord injury. *Videofluoroscopy.* Of all these techniques, observation of micturition under fluoroscopy provides the most useful information regarding configuration of the bladder and the urethra. Urethral abnormalities can be clearly visualized. The site of obstruction or angulation can be determined precisely.

Treatment

Outflow Obstruction. Urethral stricture may need dilation if the patient has an enlarged prostate. A prostatectomy can be performed provided bladder contraction is reasonable. Otherwise, intermittent catheterization, an indwelling catheter, or a suprapubic tube to drain the bladder may be necessary. When the bladder contraction recovers, prostatectomy can then be performed.

Neurogenic Bladder. Clean, intermittent self-catheterization four times daily is the only feasible treatment for patients with neurogenic bladder.

CONTINUOUS (TOTAL) INCONTINENCE

In sharp contrast to the preceding types of incontinence, in which the patient can always tell when urine loss occurs, leakage of urine is imperceptible to the patient with continuous or total incontinence. The patient is generally unaware of the incontinence as it occurs, and finds the undergarments wet.

Etiology

Multiple operations on the urethra may cause severe periurethral fibrosis, precluding proper closure of the urethra and resulting in urethral incompetence. *Pelvic irradiation* may induce bladder fibrosis, which severely limits bladder capacity and renders the bladder noncompliant. *Lower motor neuron disease* (e.g., low lumbosacral meningomyelocele) can result in paralysis of the urethral sphincter and loss of sensation. Ureterovaginal, vesicovaginal, and urethrovaginal *fistulas* result in urinary incontinence. In *ectopic ureteral orifice*, one or both ureters open into the vaginal vestibule. The patient is a child who should have outgrown nocturnal enuresis but continues to wet the bed and be incontinent during the day, without perceiving the loss of urine.

Postprostatectomy incontinence. (1) Post-transurethral resection of prostate (TURP). Approximately 2% of patients suffer from continuous incontinence after the procedure due to urethral sphincter damage. (2) Postradical prostatectomy. Approximately 30% of patients suffer from continuous incontinence of urine after radical prostatectomy for carcinoma of the prostate. It is due to the sacrifice of the urethral sphincter that sometimes is necessary for complete removal of carcinoma.

Diagnosis

Findings on the physical examination depend upon etiologic factors. Urine may be seen dripping continuously from the urethra while the patient is relaxed. When vesico-vaginal fistula is suspected in a female patient, a *dye test* may be carried out. In the simple form the patient is given phenazopyridine (Pyridium) tablets, and she may be asked to use tampons. If bright orange staining is seen at the proximal end of the tampon (in the region of the vaginal vault), a fistula is present. Cystourethroscopy is useful in both sexes to evaluate the condition of the bladder, the presence of a fistula, and intactness of the urethral sphincter. Urodynamic studies may be needed to evaluate the bladder compliance. Videofluoroscopy is an extremely valuable test in these patients. It will reveal the configuration of the bladder, location of a fistula, and functioning of the urethral sphincter, as well as the condition of the entire urethra during voiding.

Treatment

This is determined by the specific cause. Continuous incontinence resulting from urethral fibrosis may be managed by the pubovaginal sling procedure, periurethral injection, or an artificial urinary sphincter. Continuous incontinence caused by a noncompliant bladder can be treated with augmentation cystoplasty to increase bladder capacity, unless the bladder has been irradiated heavily. Urinary fistulas are generally treated by surgical correction.

MIXED INCONTINENCE (STRESS AND URGE)

In many patients, a history of severe urgency and loss of urine may be concomitant with a history of loss of urine during coughing, sneezing, or walking. Such a combination of symptoms may result from an overactive detrusor in combination with an incompetent urethra. Therefore, the investigations previously described for each of these entities are necessary.

FUNCTIONAL INCONTINENCE

Some patients with incontinence may have normal bladder and urethral function with no detectable abnormality on urodynamic testing or cystourethroscopy. Patients with Alzheimer's disease, Parkinson's disease, or severe arthritis may find it difficult to reach the bathroom and undress themselves in time to urinate in the appropriate place. Easy accessibility and availability of toilet facilities as well as possible clothing modifications are important factors in maintaining continence, and thereby dignity, in this group.

EPIDIDYMITIS

method of
JOHN N. KRIEGER, M.D.
University of Washington School of Medicine
Seattle, Washington

EPIDEMIOLOGY AND CLINICAL PRESENTATION

Epididymitis is an inflammatory reaction of the epididymis to infection or to local trauma. Epididymitis is common, accounting for over 600,000 visits to physicians per year in the United States. Acute epididymitis is responsible for more days lost from military service than any other disease and is responsible for 20% of urologic admissions in the military.

Men with epididymitis usually complain of painful swelling of the scrotum. In most cases the pain and swelling are unilateral. The onset may be acute over 1 or 2 days or more gradual. Pain may radiate along the spermatic cord and into the lower abdomen. Dysuria or irritative lower urinary tract symptoms are characteristic. Many patients have a urethral discharge. Particular attention should be directed to eliciting a history of genitourinary tract disease or sexual exposure. Some men may have only a nonspecific finding of fever or other signs of infection. This is especially common in hospitalized men who have had urinary tract manipulation and may be obtunded by medication.

Tender swelling, generally unilateral and often accompanied by erythema, may occur in the posterior aspect of the scrotum. Early in the course, the swelling may be localized to one portion of the epididymis. Later, there is involvement of the ipsilateral testis, producing an epididymoorchitis. At this point it is difficult to distinguish the testicle from the epididymis within the inflammatory mass. Scrotal examination reveals the characteristic hydrocele caused by secretion of inflammatory fluid between the layers of the tunica vaginalis. Urethral discharge may be apparent on inspection or stripping of the urethra.

PATHOGENESIS AND HOST DEFENSES

Acute epididymitis occurs when genitourinary tract pathogens overcome the host defenses of the male lower genitourinary tract to establish infection of the epididymis. Most cases result from retrograde ascent of organisms through the urethra, prostate, ejaculatory duct, and vas deferens. Therefore, infections of the urethra, bladder, or prostate are important risk factors for development of epididymitis. Mechanical factors, such as the flushing action of micturition and ejaculation, should provide some protection against infection, although the relative significance of such defenses is unclear. However, extensive clinical experience indicates that structural or functional abnormalities of the lower urinary tract increase the risk of epididymitis.

Prostatic antibacterial factor is an important defense of the male lower genitourinary tract against ascending infections. This zinc-containing polypeptide is secreted by the prostate. Men with chronic bacterial prostatitis have significantly lower levels of zinc in their prostatic fluid than healthy men, but their serum zinc levels are normal. It is unclear whether reduced zinc concentrations precede the development of prostatic infection or represent a secretory dysfunction resulting from such infections. Prostatic secretions of men with well-documented genitourinary infections contain high concentrations of immunoglobulins. Several studies demonstrated antigen-specific antibody coating of bacteria isolated from men with genitourinary tract infections. The antigen-specific antibody response in prostatic secretions is predominantly secretory IgA and is significantly greater than is the serologic response. Increased concentrations of leukocytes occur in many conditions of the male lower urinary tract, including prostatitis and epididymitis. These humoral and cellular immune responses are important for resolution of tissue-invasive genitourinary infections.

CLASSIFICATION AND CLINICAL MANAGEMENT OF ACUTE EPIDIDYMITIS

There are two common types of epididymitis, nonspecific bacterial epididymitis and sexually transmitted epididymitis. In addition, epididymitis may occur after genital trauma or with disseminated infections.

Clinical evaluation begins with a thorough history, specifically eliciting recognized risk factors, and a physical examination. Initial laboratory tests include urinalysis, culture, and sensitivity testing for men with presumed nonspecific bacterial epididymitis. Men at risk for sexually transmitted epididymitis should also have a Gram-stained urethral smear, culture for *Neisseria gonorrhoeae*, and testing for *Chlamydia trachomatis*. In the latter group, serologic testing is also recommended for syphilis and for human immunodeficiency virus infection.

Nonspecific Bacterial Epididymitis

Genitourinary infection with coliform or *Pseudomonas* species is the most common cause of epididymitis in men over 35 years old. In most series, gram-negative rods caused over two thirds of the cases of bacterial epididymitis. However, gram-positive cocci are also important pathogens and were the most common organisms in other reports.

Many men with bacterial epididymitis have underlying urologic pathology or have a history of genitourinary tract manipulation. Epididymitis after surgery or urethral catheterization may occur weeks or rarely months after the manipulation. Epididymitis is particularly likely in men who undergo urinary tract surgery or instrumentation while they are bacteriuric. Both acute and chronic bacterial prostatitis are other important predisposing conditions for development of bacterial epididymitis.

Medical management is appropriate for most men with bacterial epididymitis. Most men with uncomplicated epididymitis are managed as outpatients. Indications for hospitalization include systemic symptoms, such as leukocytosis and fever, complications, or associated medical conditions. In such severe cases, parenteral antimicrobial therapy, using the combination of an aminoglycoside plus a beta-lactam agent, or a third-generation cephalosporin, is continued until the patient defervesces, followed by a longer course of oral therapy.

Initial empirical treatment is started with agents appropriate for both gram-negative rods and gram-positive cocci pending urine culture and sensitivity results. Our first choice for empirical management of nonspecific epididymitis in outpatients is the combination of trimethoprim and sulfamethoxazole (Bactrim, Septra), one double-strength tablet twice daily for 10 to 14 days. The fluoroquinolones, such as ciprofloxacin (Cipro), ofloxacin (Floxin), and norfloxacin (Noroxin), are alternative medications. If there is evidence of bacterial prostatitis, antimicrobial therapy is continued for 6 to 12 weeks. This initial empirical therapy may be changed, if necessary, after culture results are available.

Nonspecific measures are worthwhile, including bed rest, scrotal elevation, analgesics, and local ice packs. A spermatic cord block with bupivacaine (Marcaine) may be helpful for management of severe pain. We recommend urologic evaluation because structural or functional abnormalities are common among men with nonspecific bacterial epididymitis.

Sexually Transmitted Epididymitis

Sexually transmitted epididymitis is most common in young men. *C. trachomatis* and *N. gonorrhoeae* are the major pathogens. In most series, chlamydiae were identified as the most common cause of epididymitis in younger, sexually active populations. For example, in our institution, chlamydiae were documented in 17 of 34 cases of epididymitis in men less than 35 years of age but in only 1 of 16 cases of epididymitis in men older than 35 years. In the past, these patients were considered to have "idiopathic" nonspecific epididymitis. Sexually transmitted *Escherichia coli* infection also occurs among men who are the insertive partners during anal intercourse.

Frequently patients with chlamydial epididymitis do not complain of urethral discharge. However, 11 of 17 patients with epididymitis caused by chlamydiae had demonstrable discharge, usually the scant, watery discharge characteristic of nongonococcal urethritis. The median interval from the last sexual exposure was 10 days and ranged from 1 to 45 days. Thus, urethral *C. trachomatis* may be carried for

long periods before development of overt epididymitis.

In the preantibiotic era, epididymitis occurred in 10% to 30% of men with gonococcal urethritis. However, in contemporary series, *N. gonorrhoeae* was identified in 16% of men with epididymitis in military populations and in 21% of men with epididymitis in civilians less than 35 years old. Many men with epididymitis do not have a history of urethral discharge, and a discharge may be demonstrable in only 50% of such patients. Diagnosis depends on a high index of clinical suspicion, evaluation for the presence of urethritis (that may be asymptomatic), and appropriate cultures.

Empirical therapy is indicated before culture results are available. Appropriate coverage is necessary for both gonorrhea and *C. trachomatis* infection. Our first choice is the combination of ceftriaxone (Rocephin), 250 mg intramuscularly in a single dose, plus doxycycline (Vibramycin), 100 mg orally two times a day for 10 days. Alternatives for coverage of *N. gonorrhoeae* include spectinomycin (Trobicin), 2 grams intramuscularly in a single dose; ciprofloxacin (Cipro), 500 mg orally in a single dose; or norfloxacin (Noroxin), 800 mg orally in a single dose. Alternatives for coverage of *C. trachomatis* include azithromycin (Zithromax), 1 gram orally as a single dose, or tetracycline HCl, 500 mg orally four times a day for 10 days. Nonspecific measures are helpful, including bed rest, scrotal elevation, analgesics, and local ice packs. A spermatic cord block with bipuvacaine (Marcaine) may reduce the need for analgesics in men with severe pain.

Patients should be evaluated for other sexually transmitted pathogens, and treatment of sexual partners is important. Underlying genitourinary tract abnormalities are uncommon in this population. Thus, a complete urologic work-up rarely is indicated for patients with uncomplicated, sexually transmitted epididymitis.

Uncommon Causes

Tuberculous epididymitis is the most common manifestation of male genital tuberculosis, with orchitis and prostatitis less common. The usual symptom is heaviness or swelling. There is a characteristic scrotal swelling with "beadlike" enlargement of the vas deferens. Chronic draining scrotal sinuses may be present. The systemic mycoses rarely cause epididymitis; blastomycosis is the most common pathogen and may also cause a draining sinus through the scrotal wall. Men with HIV infection and uncomplicated epididymitis should receive the same treatment as those without HIV. However, fungal and mycobacterial causes of epididymitis are more common among patients who are immunocompromised.

In the pediatric population, epididymitis may occur with congenital anatomic abnormalities, such as ectopic ureter or posterior urethral valves. Epididymitis occasionally occurs after testicular trauma. Many of these men have evidence of genitourinary tract infections with the aforementioned organisms, but occasional men develop traumatic epididymitis that is not associated with positive cultures or inflammation. We also described an unusual syndrome of noninfectious epididymitis associated with amiodarone (Cordarone) therapy for refractory ventricular arrhythmias.

DIFFERENTIAL DIAGNOSIS

Severe inflammation can lead to an enlarged, indurated epididymis that is indistinguishable from the testicle. This can present difficulties in the differential diagnosis of epididymitis from testicular torsion or testicular cancer. The epididymis lies posterior to the testis, and this demarcation is often preserved in cases of epididymitis. "Reactive" hydrocele formation may render the palpation of intrascrotal structures difficult. Although transillumination frequently identifies hydroceles, color-flow Doppler ultrasonography is our preferred imaging study when the diagnosis is in doubt. Acute epididymitis must be distinguished from testicular torsion at the initial evaluation because uncorrected torsion results in testicular death within 24 hours. Men with swelling and tenderness that persist after completing therapy should be reevaluated for testicular cancer, tuberculosis, or fungal epididymitis.

COMPLICATIONS

Most patients experience relief of their symptoms within 48 hours, but swelling and discomfort may persist for weeks or months following eradication of the infecting organism. In some cases the epididymis remains enlarged and/or indurated indefinitely. Such men may develop chronic epididymitis, characterized by pain and occasionally by recurrent swelling.

Bacterial epididymitis may be an important focus of organisms causing both local morbidity and bacteremia in men with indwelling transurethral catheters. Genitourinary tract complications of acute epididymitis include testicular infarction, scrotal abscess, pyocele of the scrotum, a chronic draining scrotal sinus, chronic epididymitis, and infertility. Ultrasonography, particularly color-flow Doppler ultrasonography, is useful for the differential diagnosis of complicated cases. Surgery may be necessary for complications of acute epididymal infections but has no role in treatment of tuberculous or fungal epididymitis.

PRIMARY GLOMERULAR DISEASES

method of
STEPHEN M. KORBET, M.D.
Rush Medical College
Chicago, Illinois

Glomerular diseases are defined by their histologic, clinical, and laboratory features. Patients with these diseases initially present as a result of clinical symptoms or signs of edema, hematuria, hypertension, and/or nausea and vomiting, or as a result of abnormal renal function studies and proteinuria in asymptomatic patients. With an initial laboratory evaluation, which should consist of a biochemistry profile, urinalysis, and 24-hour urine specimen for protein and creatinine clearance tests, the physician is able to localize the problem as being primarily renal. However, the renal biopsy ultimately allows the physician to define the problem as being glomerular in origin, since no laboratory feature, with the possible exception of red blood cell casts or proteinuria in excess of 3.5 grams per 24 hr, is pathognomonic for glomerular diseases, and even these are not universally found in all patients with glomerular diseases.

Patients with glomerular diseases have been categorized into essentially four major groups: nephrotic syndrome, asymptomatic proteinuria with or without hematuria, acute nephritic syndrome, and chronic glomerulonephritis. Ultimately, a renal biopsy is required to secure a diagnosis, which becomes critical for the patient as the prognosis and therapy associated with many of these diseases are quite different.

The distinction of "primary" and "secondary" glomerular disease is important because the histology of the glomerular lesions is descriptive in nature and gives no insight into pathogenesis. Primary (or idiopathic) glomerular disease implies that the disease process affects only the kidney without extrarenal or systemic involvement. Since glomerular disease may be a manifestation of a number of secondary causes, these must be evaluated prior to classifying a patient as having a primary glomerular disease since the course, treatment, and prognosis may differ substantially. These secondary glomerulopathies are usually the result of systemic diseases, medications, acute or chronic infections, or malignancy.

I will review the major clinical categories of primary glomerular disease and the presentation, course, treatment, and some secondary causes associated with the specific glomerular lesions within these groups.

NEPHROTIC SYNDROME

The nephrotic syndrome is defined by proteinuria of 3.5 or more grams per 24 hr, hypoalbuminemia, edema, hypercholesterolemia, and lipiduria. As a result of the loss of glomerular integrity and thus its charge and size selectivity, proteinuria in patients with glomerulopathies resulting in the nephrotic syndrome is predominantly composed of albumin but also includes other large-molecular-weight proteins, such as immunoglobulins, lipoproteins, and proteins involved with anticoagulation. The significant loss of these proteins leads to the complications associated with the nephrotic syndrome.

Proteinuria of 3.5 or more grams per 24 hr may occasionally be observed in the absence of glomerular disease. This results from the loss of low-molecular-weight proteins, which are being produced in excess and freely filtered by the normal glomerulus, thus leading to what is termed "overflow" proteinuria. This type of proteinuria is classically observed in patients with multiple myeloma and can be confirmed by finding free light chains in the urine by immunofixation. In this setting, larger-molecular-weight proteins are not lost, and hypoalbuminemia is therefore not observed.

The goal in treating patients with the nephrotic syndrome is to achieve a remission in the underlying glomerular disease. Achieving such a remission involves disease-specific therapy that will be discussed with each glomerular lesion. However, general supportive measures should be applied to all patients with the nephrotic syndrome.

Hypoalbuminemia can be quite severe (<2.0 grams per dL) in nephrotic patients. This is the result not only of albumin loss in the urine, which can be quantified, but also from increased catabolism by the proximal tubules, which is not measurable. Thus, even though the hepatic production of albumin increases by as much as 300%, protein loss that should be within the range of hepatic synthesis of albumin (i.e., 5 grams per 24 hr) can still be associated with significant hypoalbuminemia. Previously, a high-protein diet had been recommended in order to compensate for protein losses in the urine, maintain positive nitrogen balance, and increase albumin synthesis. However, it has been shown that this actually results in augmentation of proteinuria and ultimately an overall decrease in serum albumin concentration. Thus, it is presently recommended that a moderate protein intake of 0.8 to 1.0 gram per kg per day (based on edema-free weight) be prescribed.

A major complication resulting from the retention of sodium and water is the formation of *edema*. This is often dependent, involving the lower extremities, but can be quite extensive, extending up to the sacrum. This can lead to problems in mobility, breakdown of skin, and cellulitis. Facial swelling may be present in some patients; in others, the volume expansion results in ascites or pleural effusions. Classically, edema has been attributed to the decrease in oncotic pressure resulting from the low serum albumin levels. This leads to transudation of fluid into the interstitial space, thereby decreasing intravascular volume (or effective arterial blood volume), resulting in an increase in salt and water retention by the kidneys. It is now recognized, however, that only 30% to 40% of all patients with the nephrotic syndrome are hypovolemic. Another mechanism to explain the formation of edema in nephrotic patients is one of a primary salt- and water-retaining state that leads to an expansion of intravascular volume and an increase in hydrostatic pressure and edema formation. Most likely both processes are acting in concert.

The mainstay of therapy in treating edema is a combination of salt and water restriction as well as diuretics. Patients should be restricted to 1000 mL of fluids and dietary sodium intake decreased to 2 grams (86 mEq) per day (1 gram of sodium equals 43 mEq and 1 gram of sodium chloride has 17 mEq of sodium). Dietary adjustments alone are not usually sufficient to treat edema successfully, and most patients require diuretics. The loop diuretics like furosemide (Lasix) work best and are usually started at 20 mg per day orally and titrated up in dose by doubling, as well as increasing from a once-a-day to twice-a-day regimen (up to 240 mg per day). Due to the avid sodium-retaining state, the addition of a distal tubule diuretic (metolazone [Zaroxolyn], 2.5 to 5 mg per day orally) is sometimes required to complement the effect of the loop diuretic. In extremely compromised patients, hospitalization and intravenous administration of diuretics may be required. The goal is to achieve a diuresis resulting in the loss of 1 to 2 kg of water weight per day until the desired end point is reached. Ideally, an edema-free state is sought; however, this may not be tolerated in some patients because the resultant decrease in intravascular volume in combination with a low oncotic pressure may lead to intolerably low blood pressure or orthostatic hypotension. Hypokalemia may result from aggressive diuresis: it should be sought and treated by either diet or pharmacologic potassium supplementation. Persistent hypokalemia may require the addition of a potassium-sparing diuretic. In patients with severe diuretic-refractory edema, salt-poor albumin infusions have been used as a temporary measure. This should be done only in combination with diuretics, in a hospital setting with close supervision, as these infusions can precipitate pulmonary edema (remember, 60% to 70% of nephrotic patients may be intravascularly euvolemic or volume expanded even though they are hypoalbuminemic).

In response to hypoalbuminemia, cholesterol synthesis increases, leading to *hypercholesterolemia*. This is associated with an increase in hydroxymethylglutaryl CoA (HMG CoA) reductase activity, the rate-limiting step for hepatic cholesterol synthesis. Defects in lipid catabolism have also been identified. As a result, low-density lipoprotein (LDL) levels are increased. This, in association with a decrease in high-density lipoprotein (HDL) levels due to urinary loss, contributes to the increased risk of atherosclerotic cardiovascular disease (2.5-fold increase in coronary artery disease and fivefold increase in myocardial infarction) observed in nephrotic patients. Although difficult to treat, hypercholesterolemia is managed with a combination of a low-fat (high in polyunsaturated fats) diet and HMG CoA reductase inhibitors (lovastatin [Mevacor] or pravastatin [Pravachol]). These produce significant decreases in serum cholesterol and LDL levels. This therapy is generally well tolerated, but an increase in liver transaminases and myalgias/myositis, although rare, may occur and should be monitored.

Hypercoagulability in nephrotic patients results from the urinary loss of naturally occurring anticoagulants such as antithrombin III, protein-S, and protein-C. This leads to an increased risk for thromboembolic complications, such as renal vein or deep venous thrombosis and pulmonary embolism. Renal vein thrombosis can be acute or chronic in nature and is said to complicate the nephrotic syndrome in 35% of cases. This is most frequently described in patients with membranous glomerulonephritis. Renal vein thrombosis should be suspected and a venogram performed (diagnostic procedure of choice) in nephrotic patients with unexplained rapid deterioration in renal function, acute flank pain, macroscopic hematuria, pleuritic chest pain, or any symptom suggestive of a thromboembolic event. The treatment is that of standard acute (heparin) and chronic (warfarin) anticoagulation therapy. For patients felt to be at high risk of thromboembolic complications, such as those with membranous glomerulonephritis and severe hypoalbuminemia (<2 grams per dL), prophylactic anticoagulation with warfarin has been suggested.

A predisposition to *infection* exists for nephrotic patients owing to the loss of immunoglobulins and complement. Patients are particularly prone to infections with encapsulated organisms such as *Streptococcus pneumoniae*. It is therefore recommended that persistently nephrotic adults receive the pneumococcal vaccine. The efficacy of immunoglobulin infusions is unknown, and no definite recommendations currently exist for nephrotic patients.

Hypertension is commonly associated with many of the primary glomerular diseases resulting in the nephrotic (as well as nephritic) syndrome. The mechanism for this is most likely multifactorial but often is attributed to intravascular volume expansion. In general, blood pressure control starts with dietary restriction of sodium and diuretics as outlined earlier. If these measures fail to normalize blood pressure to 130/80 mm Hg or less, an antihypertensive agent will be required. An angiotensin-converting enzyme (ACE) inhibitor is usually effective and well tolerated (captopril [Capoten], 25 to 50 mg orally three times daily or enalapril [Vasotec], 5 to 10 mg orally twice daily). An ACE inhibitor has the additional potential benefits of not only lowering proteinuria but also being renoprotective, as observed in diabetic nephropathy. Since a significant reduction in the decline in glomerular filtration rate has been observed in nephrotic patients attaining a blood pressure of 125/75 mm Hg, this has become the recommended target.

The ultimate goal in treating patients with the nephrotic syndrome is in achieving a remission in the underlying disease. This results not only in the reversal of the aforementioned complications associated with the nephrotic state but also improves the renal prognosis, as the majority of the glomerular diseases associated with the nephrotic syndrome progress to end-stage renal disease without a remission.

Remissions are usually referred to as "complete" or "partial," generally based on the degree to which the proteinuria has decreased in association with stable or improved renal function. A complete remission occurs when proteinuria falls below 300 mg per 24 hr, and a partial remission when proteinuria is greater than 300 mg per 24 hr but less than 2.5 grams per 24 hr. A complete remission is associated with significant improvement in renal prognosis. Less is known about the overall benefit of a partial remission as this has been inconsistently defined and therefore less well evaluated, but even this type of

TABLE 1. Glomerular Lesions in Adults with Idiopathic Nephrotic Syndrome

Histology	Black (%)	White (%)
Minimal change disease (MCD)	15	15
Focal segmental glomerular sclerosis (FSGS)	60	20
Membranous glomerulonephropathy (MGN)	20	45
Membranoproliferative glomerulonephritis (MPGN)	2	5
Other (IgA, immunotactoid glomerulopathy (ITG), and so on)	3	15

remission appears to confer a more favorable prognosis compared with patients who remain nephrotic. Although the glomerular lesions resulting in the nephrotic syndrome all seem to be immunologically mediated, their pathogenesis, while unknown, appears to differ for each. As a result, the response to various immunotherapies is quite different for each even though the drugs used are similar. We will now look at the individual glomerular lesions associated with the nephrotic syndrome in adults (Table 1).

Until recently, membranous glomerulonephritis was considered the most common primary glomerular lesion associated with the nephrotic syndrome in adults (40%). As can be seen in Table 1, however, there are definite differences in the racial distribution of the glomerular lesions in adults. Membranous glomerulonephropathy is the most common lesion seen in white patients. In nephrotic black patients, however, focal segmental glomerular sclerosis (FSGS) is the predominant lesion, accounting for 60% of cases. The renal biopsy is critical in the evaluation of patients with the nephrotic syndrome as there is nothing unique about the clinical presentations of these glomerular diseases (Table 2). Identifying the lesion allows the physician to make knowledgeable decisions regarding prognosis and treatment.

Minimal Change Disease

Minimal change disease (MCD) is the most frequent lesion associated with the nephrotic syndrome in children, accounting for over 75% of cases. The experience in the pediatric population accounts for much of the understanding of the clinical and morphologic implications of this lesion. As more informa-

TABLE 2. Presenting Features in Adults with Idiopathic Nephrotic Syndrome

	MCD (%)	FSGS (%)	MGN (%)	MPGN (%)	ITG (%)
Male	50	60	60	50	60
Hypertension (blood pressure > 140/90)	25	40	30	40	65
Renal insufficiency (creatinine > 1.3 mg/dL)	25	50	20	70	50
Microscopic hematuria	25	40	30	90	75
Hypocomplementemia	0	0	0	50	0

Abbreviations: Refer to Table 1.

tion on adult MCD is reported, we see that there are differences, particularly in the response to treatment, between these two patient populations. In adults with MCD, hypertension and microscopic hematuria may each be a presenting feature in 25% of cases (Table 2). Furthermore, renal insufficiency, usually acute in nature and attributed to hemodynamic factors, is a common presenting feature in up to 25% of patients. Thus, in adult MCD, the clinical presentation may be indistinguishable from that of focal segmental glomerular sclerosis (FSGS).

Pathology

Minimal change disease is a T cell–mediated disorder in which circulating lymphokines result in altered glomerular epithelial cell function. The histology of the glomeruli is normal when evaluated by light microscopy, and no immunoglobulins are found in the glomeruli by immunofluorescence microscopy. The characteristic feature is fusion of the epithelial cell foot processes seen by electron microscopy.

Therapy

Spontaneous remissions occur in up to 50% of patients, but this may take months to years. Since idiopathic MCD is exquisitely sensitive to steroid therapy, it does not make sense to allow patients to be exposed to the deleterious effects of the nephrotic state for prolonged periods of time. Thus, nephrotic patients with idiopathic MCD should be treated.

Treatment of MCD in children is outlined in Table 3. With this regimen over 95% of children will respond by 8 weeks. By contrast, only 50% to 60% of adults respond by 8 weeks. At 16 weeks, approximately 78% of adult patients will have gone into remission, but not until 28 weeks will over 80% of adults have attained a remission. Ultimately, over 90% of adults will achieve a remission if treated long enough. Thus, adults appear to need a more prolonged course of therapy to achieve the optimal outcome observed in children.

As in children, relapses will occur in 65% to 85% of adults. The majority of patients relapse within the first 12 months after withdrawal of steroid therapy. After an initial relapse, a remission can usually be reestablished with a second course of steroid treatment.

Treatment of Frequent Relapsers or Steroid-Dependent Patients. Some patients may become frequent relapsers (>two relapses within 6 months or >four within 12 months) or ultimately steroid-dependent (two relapses occurring with steroid taper or a relapse within 1 month of ending treatment). Of adult patients that relapse, 16% are frequent relapsers and 14% are steroid-dependent. A course of cytotoxic therapy (oral cyclophosphamide [Cytoxan], 2 mg per kg per day for 8 weeks) can be beneficial in inducing a more sustained remission than that observed with steroids alone. Adverse events from the use of cytotoxic agents over this short period are unlikely. We have the patient take the medication in the morning to prevent the possibility of hemorrhagic cystitis that is associated with a metabolite of cyclophosphamide (acrolein) and is related to the contact time of this metabolite to the bladder wall (this would be greatest if taken at night as urine accumulates and sits in the bladder). Infertility and the potential for malignancy are also concerns with the use of cytotoxic agents. In a 70-kg patient, the cumulative dose of cyclophosphamide given over 2 months is 120 mg per kg, or 8.4 grams. This is well below the cumulative dose of cyclophosphamide that has been associated with infertility ($\geq$300 mg per kg) or the development of acute leukemia/lymphoma (>10 grams). Nonetheless, these agents should be used with caution, especially in children or young adults, for whom it is recommended that they receive no more than a cumulative dose (<250 mg per kg) to prevent gonadal toxicity. A second remission with cytotoxic treatment seems to be achieved more rapidly when steroids are used concomitantly. In this setting prednisone is given orally at 1 mg per kg per day up to 80 mg per day until a remission is attained or for up to 4 weeks and then rapidly tapered off over an additional 4 weeks.

Patients who continue to relapse after a trial of cytotoxic therapy may respond to cyclosporin* (Sandimmune). Cyclosporin A in dosages of 5 to 6 mg per kg per day has led to sustained remissions in 60% to 80% of MCD patients who were otherwise frequent relapsers or steroid-dependent. In most patients, if a response to CSA is not observed by 4 to 6 months, it is unlikely to occur. A concern with the use of CSA is that patients usually become CSA-dependent, relapsing within 2 months of taper or discontinuation. Thus, steroid dependency is replaced by CSA dependency with its potential long-term renal complications. This is of particular concern as it has recently been shown that histologic evidence of nephrotoxicity may occur in patients with MCD on prolonged CSA therapy even though, clinically, renal function is unchanged. This may, in part, be dose related as the degree of nephrotoxicity was significantly associated with a CSA dose of more than 5.5 mg per kg per day. It is now recommended that repeat renal biopsies be performed in patients with MCD in remission, on CSA for 12 months or more, irrespective of the stability of the renal function. Based on the histologic findings, it can then be determined whether it is

TABLE 3. **Treatment in Minimal Change Disease**

Children	Prednisone, 60 mg/m²/d (up to 80 mg/d) in divided doses for 4 wk
	Prednisone, 40 mg/m²/d (up to 60 mg/d), alternate d, for 4 wk
	Taper off over 4 wk
Adults	Prednisone, 1 mg/kg/d (up to 80 mg/d) for 8–12 wk
	Prednisone, 0.5 mg/kg/d (or 60 mg qod) for 6–8 wk
	Taper off over 8 wk

From Korbet SM: Management of idiopathic nephrosis in adults, including steroid-resistant nephrosis. Curr Opin Nephrol Hypertens 4:169–176, 1995.

---

*Not FDA-approved for this indication.

advisable to continue on CSA. Of note is that sustained remissions of 1 year or more after discontinuation of CSA have been reported. Patients who are refractory to steroid therapy or have become steroid-resistant should have the first biopsy re-evaluated or undergo a second biopsy evaluating the possibility of FSGS.

Secondary Causes of Minimal Change Disease

The minimal change lesion in adults may be secondary (e.g., lymphoma, carcinoma, nonsteroidal anti-inflammatory drugs [NSAIDs], lithium) in as many as 13% of adult cases. Consequently, these conditions must be thoroughly evaluated since remission of the nephrotic syndrome depends on treatment of the underlying malignancy or discontinuation of the causative drug. The combination of acute renal failure (due to interstitial nephritis) and nephrotic syndrome secondary to MCD is associated with NSAIDs. This can occur after only 4 to 8 weeks of NSAID use, and discontinuation of the medication results in spontaneous remission of the nephrotic syndrome and acute renal failure by 2 to 4 weeks in most cases.

Focal Segmental Glomerulosclerosis

Primary FSGS has been reported in only 7% to 20% of children and adults with the idiopathic nephrotic syndrome. Even though the majority of adults with primary FSGS present with the nephrotic syndrome, one third have a non-nephrotic presentation (proteinuria of <3.0 grams per 24 hr without hypoalbuminemia). Hypertension and microscopic hematuria are common presenting feature in FSGS, and renal insufficiency is present in 40% of patients (see Table 2). These clinical features have prognostic significance. Patients with nephrotic-range proteinuria reach end-stage renal disease (ESRD) over 6 to 8 years. Patients with massive proteinuria (>14 grams per 24 hr) have an even more malignant course, with end-stage renal disease occurring within 2 to 3 years. Non-nephrotic patients, however, have a 10-year renal survival of over 80%. Finally, patients presenting with evidence of chronic renal insufficiency (serum creatinine >1.3 mg per dL) have significantly poorer renal survival than those without.

Pathology

Focal segmental glomerulosclerosis is also considered a T cell–mediated disorder in which a circulating "permeability factor" results in altered glomerular epithelial cell function. This leads to irreversible damage and glomerular scarring. Upon light microscopy some glomeruli appear normal; however, other glomeruli have segmental areas of scarring with hyalinosis. The segmental scars may first only be apparent in glomeruli at the cortical-medullary junction, but ultimately glomeruli in the outer cortex will also be involved. Immunofluorescence is generally nega-

tive, but granular deposits of IgM and complement may be seen in areas of segmental scars; they are considered to be trapped there rather than of pathogenic importance. Epithelial foot process fusion and segmental scarring are seen on electron microscopy.

A number of histologic features have been considered important in predicting outcome: the location of the segmental scar, mesangial proliferation, the presence of IgM, "collapsing glomerulopathy," and interstitial fibrosis. However, only the extent of interstitial fibrosis consistently predicts a poor prognosis.

Therapy

Spontaneous remissions are rare in FSGS, seen in less than 5% of nephrotic patients, with the majority of patients progressing to ESRD. Since the clinical course for patients with non-nephrotic proteinuria is quite good in contrast to nephrotic patients, non-nephrotic patients do not usually receive specific therapy with steroids or cytotoxic agents. It is the nephrotic patients in whom a therapeutic trial of these drugs has been focused in an attempt to achieve a remission. This is based on the finding that nephrotic patients who achieve a remission have a significantly improved clinical course. This improvement in outcome depends on a sustained remission, as recurrence of the nephrotic syndrome portends a prognosis similar to that of primary nonresponders. Even the outlook for patients with partial remissions is optimistic when compared with nonresponders. Thus, the best clinical indicator of outcome in a nephrotic patient with FSGS is the response to therapy. Unfortunately, no reliable clinical or histologic features at presentation predict which patients will respond to therapy.

As a consequence of its steroid nonresponsiveness relative to MCD, nephrologists have been reluctant to treat patients with primary FSGS aggressively. This is understandable when one finds that complete remission rates of less than 20% were observed in virtually every study in adult FSGS prior to 1980. In half of these studies no patient attained a complete remission. Since 1980, most studies demonstrate complete remission rates in excess of 30%, with the majority being more than 40%. Since the initial dose of prednisone was similar among these studies, ranging from 0.5 to 2 mg per kg per day, the most obvious difference in those reporting higher complete remission rates was the duration of therapy: remissions over 30%, 5 to 8 months; less than 20%, under 2 months.

Less than one third of adults who ultimately achieve a complete remission do so by 8 weeks of therapy. Complete remission takes 3 to 4 months on average, with the majority of patients reaching a complete remission by 6 months. Based on experience in adults with FSGS and MCD, it has now been proposed that steroid resistance in adults be defined as the persistence of the nephrotic syndrome after a 4-month trial of therapy with prednisone at a dose of 1 mg per kg per day. An initial course of treatment with prednisone for nephrotic adults with FSGS is

TABLE 4. Treatment of Focal Segmental Glomerular Sclerosis in Nephrotic Adults

Prednisone, 1 mg/kg/d (up to 80 mg/d) for 12–16 wk
Prednisone, 0.5 mg/kg/d (or 60 mg qod) for 6–8 wk
Taper off over 8 wk

outlined in Table 4. Significant side effects from this prolonged course of steroid therapy have not been routinely encountered.

The use of cytotoxic drugs along with steroids as initial therapy appears to confer no added benefit in attaining a complete remission when compared with steroids alone. However, fewer relapses occur in those patients receiving immunosuppressive agents as part of the initial therapy (20% versus 60% for steroids alone), thus inducing a more stable remission. For patients who sustain a prolonged remission (longer than 10 years), the likelihood of subsequent relapse is extremely remote.

Steroid-Resistant and Relapsing or Steroid-Dependent Patients. Relapses are frequent in adults with FSGS. The majority of relapsers are able to re-achieve a remission with retreatment using steroids alone or in combination with a cytotoxic agent (cyclophosphamide, 2 mg per kg per day for 8 to 12 weeks). As with MCD, the greatest benefit of cytotoxic therapy is in the ability to attain a more sustained remission in patients initially responsive to steroids. For patients who are steroid resistant, the added advantage of treatment with cytotoxic agents such as cyclophosphamide is minimal, with less than 15% achieving a remission.

Cyclosporin A* has also been used for steroid-resistant or steroid-dependent FSGS patients, with results similar to those of cytotoxic agents. The steroid-responsive patients demonstrate the best response to CSA. Complete or partial remissions are generally seen in 20% or less of steroid-resistant patients. For those patients responsive to CSA, the remission is maintained only with continuous therapy, and the concerns of prolonged therapy are as described for patients with MCD. An additional consideration is the recent observation that CSA may actually accelerate the course of FSGS to ESRD. The risk of CSA nephrotoxicity is greatest in patients with a higher percentage of glomeruli with segmental scars on the initial biopsy, renal insufficiency at the time of biopsy, and receiving CSA doses of greater than 5.5 mg per kg per day. Thus, CSA could be detrimental for patients with FSGS, particularly those with pre-existing renal insufficiency and tubulointerstitial disease, and it should be avoided or used with caution in this setting.

Other Treatment Considerations. NSAIDs and angiotensin-converting enzyme (ACE) inhibitors have each been shown to reduce proteinuria in patients with nephrotic syndrome. The use of these drugs in FSGS, however, has not been promising.

The combined use of NSAIDs and ACE inhibitors requires caution. Even though the effects of these two drugs on the reduction in proteinuria can be additive, a marked decline in glomerular filtration rate (as much as 27%) may result, as well as significant hyperkalemia.

Plasmapheresis or a protein adsorption device has been proposed based on the premise that the circulating "factor(s)" responsible for FSGS will be removed. Recent trials in transplant patients with recurrent FSGS (known to occur in up to 33% of patients) have promising results. Whether these results can be recreated in patients with primary FSGS is yet to be seen.

Secondary Causes of FSGS

It is now well recognized that HIV-associated nephropathy may occur not only in patients with acquired immune deficiency syndrome (AIDS) but also in HIV carriers. It is more frequently seen in men, blacks, and intravenous drug abusers. Clinically, the patients present with the nephrotic syndrome and varying degrees of renal insufficiency, and the course is one of rapid deterioration in renal function, resulting in ESRD. The renal lesion most commonly identified in these patients is FSGS. Compared with primary FSGS, a significantly greater (>50%) proportion of glomeruli demonstrate global collapse. Preliminary and limited experience with treating HIV-associated nephropathy using zidovudine (AZT), Retrovir or steroids suggests that progression of the renal insufficiency may be retarded with these agents.

Recently, a similar glomerular lesion (glomerular capillary collapse, visceral epithelial cell swelling, and hyperplasia) was observed in a group of patients who were HIV-negative with no evidence of immune deficiency. As in HIV-associated nephropathy, the patients were characterized by a black racial predominance and massive proteinuria with rapidly progressing renal insufficiency. Of the few patients treated, essentially all have been steroid resistant. These patients were thought to represent a distinct clinicopathologic entity termed "collapsing glomerulopathy." Whether this is truly a variant of FSGS with a different pathogenetic significance is yet to be determined.

Membranous Glomerulonephritis

Membranous glomerulonephritis (MGN) has classically been considered the most common lesion associated with the nephrotic syndrome in adults, but recent data demonstrate this is not necessarily the case (see Table 1). As with the other primary glomerulopathies, patients can present with hypertension, renal insufficiency, and microscopic hematuria (see Table 2). In up to one third of patients, the proteinuria at presentation may be non-nephrotic in nature, and these patients have a more favorable prognosis. A poor prognosis in patients with MGN is associated with male sex, older age at presentation, proteinuria

---

*Not FDA-approved for this indication.

greater than 10 grams per day, hypertension, renal insufficiency at presentation, and the degree of interstitial fibrosis.

Pathology

Membranous glomerulonephritis is an immune complex–mediated disease. The deposits develop in situ in the subepithelial space and are felt to be the result of an antibody response to an altered preexisting antigen in this location or an antigen that has been "planted" or trapped (such as viral, DNA, or tumor antigens) in this location. This explains why circulating immune complexes are rarely found in patients with primary MGN. By light microscopy, diffuse thickening of the capillary walls is the most prominent feature. Characteristic "spikes" in the capillary walls are seen on the silver stain (this specifically stains the mesangium and glomerular basement membrane) and represent the reaction of the glomerular basement membrane to the immune deposits in the subepithelial space. The immunofluorescence is positive for IgG, and complement is seen in a characteristic granular pattern around the capillary walls. In idiopathic membranous glomerulonephropathy the mesangium is negative for immunoglobulin deposits. If the mesangium is positive by immunofluorescence for immunoglobulins, a secondary cause of MGN should be considered, such as systemic lupus erythematosus (SLE). Early on in this disease electron microscopy demonstrates electrondense deposits in a subepithelial location and encircling the glomerular capillary. In time, the underlying basement membrane incorporates the deposits, at which point they are referred to as being intramembranous.

Therapy

Left untreated, the prognosis for most patients with MGN is quite good, with 5- and 10-year renal survivals of 90% and 70% respectively. The likelihood of a spontaneous remission is excellent at 60% over 5 years (20% complete remission, 40% partial remissions). The potential for a spontaneous remission is greatest among women and young adults. As a result of the favorable prognosis for a majority of patients with idiopathic MGN, the value of treating all patients with potentially toxic therapies has come into question.

A subset of patients, however, are at significant

TABLE 6. Treatment Approach in Adults with Idiopathic Membranous Glomerulopathy

Approach	Patient Characteristics
1. Treat early	Proteinuria >10 gm/d Severe symptomatic nephrotic syndrome Progressive renal insufficiency
2. Delay treatment	Proteinuria 3.5 to 10 gm/d with normal renal function
3. Observe	Normal renal function and non-nephrotic Female with <5 gm/d proteinuria
4. No treatment	Creatinine >4 mg/dL

From Glassock RJ: Therapy of idiopathic nephrotic syndrome in adults. Am J Nephrol 13:422–428, 1993. With permission from S. Karger AG, Basel.

risk of progressive renal failure with MGN. The "high-risk" patients are those with heavy proteinuria (>10 grams per 24 hr), men, age greater than 50 years at onset, renal insufficiency at presentation, and hypertension. The 5-year probability for renal survival in patients with proteinuria of more than 10 grams per day decreases to 50%. Even patients with lesser degrees of proteinuria may be at risk if it persists. Patients with persistent proteinuria (>6 grams per day for >6 months) have over a 60% probability of developing ESRD within 5 to 10 years and should also be considered as high risk. The use of immunosuppressive therapy with or without steroids is now being recommended in these high-risk patients and those with progressive loss of renal function.

A number of therapeutic regimens have been tried in patients with MGN: high-dose oral prednisone taken daily or on alternate days, oral cytotoxics plus steroids, and cyclosporin* (Table 5). It is now accepted that oral prednisone alone is of little value in the treatment of MGN. Recent experience from controlled studies favors the use of cytotoxic therapies, showing a complete or partial remission in 60% of patients treated compared with only 30% of controls. Furthermore, the 10-year renal survival improves to over 90% for treated patients compared with 50% for controls. Even though the response has been promising, there is a significant risk of complications resulting from the prolonged courses of the cytotoxic drugs utilized, which must be taken into account and discussed with the patient. Cyclosporin* has also been used in MGN patients with evidence of progressive loss of renal function and has been associated with a significant reduction in the rate of decline in creatinine clearance and improved proteinuria in 75% of patients treated.

A reasonable approach to the treatment of patients with MGN is outlined in Table 6. For those patients at highest risk of progressing to ESRD treatment should begin immediately. In those patients most likely to remit spontaneously, a period of observation and symptomatic treatment are all that is required. In one group of patients the risk is intermediate, and treatment may be delayed but ultimately will be

TABLE 5. Treatment Protocols for Membranous Glomerulopathy

1. Cyclophosphamide (Cytoxan),* 1–2 mg/kg/d PO, plus steroids, 30 mg qod for 6–12 mon
2. Month 1: Methylprednisolone, 1 gm intravenously for 3 d, then prednisone, 0.5 mg/kg/d for 27 d
   Month 2: Chlorambucil (Leukeran), 0.2 mg/kg/d for 30 d
   Cycle 3 times (6 mon of total therapy)
3. Cyclosporin (Sandimmune)* 3–4 mg/kg/d PO, in 2 divided doses for 12 mon

*Not FDA-approved for this indication.

*Not FDA-approved for this indication.

instituted if a spontaneous remission does not occur or renal insufficiency develops. Finally, in those patients with advanced renal failure (creatinine >4 mg per dL), aggressive immunosuppressive treatment is best withheld as the benefit of therapy is marginal and does not outweigh the risks.

Secondary Causes

Common secondary causes of MGN are shown in Table 7. Malignancy can be found in up to 10% of patients with presumed idiopathic MGN. In 45% of cases the nephrotic syndrome precedes the recognition of the tumor by more than 4 months. In another 40% of cases, the nephrotic syndrome and tumor have been identified simultaneously. In only 15% of patients has the recognition of the tumor preceded the discovery of proteinuria. Thus, it is prudent to evaluate all patients with idiopathic MGN for the possibility of malignancy at presentation and at follow-up over 6 to 12 months. In some cases, the successful removal of the tumor results in a remission of the nephrotic syndrome.

Membranous glomerulonephritis from chronic infection with hepatitis B has been successfully treated with alfa-interferon, resulting in a complete remission of the nephrotic syndrome. This therapy has also lead to seroconversion of HBeAg- and HbsAg-positive patients.

Membranoproliferative Glomerulonephritis

Of all the primary glomerular diseases resulting in the nephrotic syndrome, MPGN is one of the more uncommon. Of these patients, 50% are nephrotic at presentation, 30% non-nephrotic, and up to 20% having a presentation consistent with an acute glomerulonephritis. Membranoproliferative glomerulonephritis is divided into three types based on subtle histologic differences, with types I and II accounting for the majority of the lesions seen. Since the presentation and course of patients with the various types of MPGN are similar, they are usually discussed as a group. The presenting features are comparable to the other primary glomerulopathies (see Table 2), with renal insufficiency and microscopic hematuria being somewhat more common. Unlike the other diseases, however, macroscopic hematuria is observed

TABLE 7. **Secondary Causes of Membranous Glomerulopathy**

Systemic diseases	Systemic lupus erythematosus Rheumatoid arthritis
Drugs	Penicillamine Gold Captopril
Infections	Hepatitis B or C Syphilis Malaria Schistosomiasis
Malignancy	Solid tumors

in 10% of cases. Additionally, a serologic finding unique to MPGN is hypocomplementemia. In 50% of cases, a low 3rd component of complement (C3) is observed, a finding more common in type II MPGN. The extremely depressed C3 levels observed in MPGN have been associated with the presence of C3 nephritic factor (an IgG autoantibody that stabilizes C3 convertase, protecting it from inhibitor proteins, allowing ongoing degradation of C3), and this too is more frequently seen in type II patients. Low levels of C4 are observed much less frequently (<15%) in all forms of MPGN. It is also well recognized that type II MPGN may be associated with partial lipodystrophy.

Pathology

Membranoproliferative glomerulonephritis is an immune complex–mediated disease whose pathogenesis is unknown. By light microscopy there is marked thickening of the glomerular capillary wall with mesangial proliferation and expansion, which gives the glomerulus a "lobular" appearance. On silver stain the characteristic "tram tracking" or "double contour" of the glomerular capillary wall is seen and represents interposition of the mesangial cell cytoplasm between the glomerular basement membrane and endothelial cell which lays down new basement membrane resulting in the split appearance. The three forms of MPGN are distinguished by their ultrastructural features. In type I MPGN, subendothelial electron-dense deposits are observed and correspond to granular deposits of immunoglobulin (IgG and IgM) and complement (C3). In type II MPGN, electron-dense deposits are seen within the glomerular basement membrane, hence the name "dense deposit disease." Immunoglobulins may be entirely absent in type II MPGN; however, C3 is invariably present in the mesangium and capillary walls. In type III MPGN, both subendothelial and subepithelial deposits are found.

Therapy

Patients with a non-nephrotic picture have a significantly more favorable course, with a 5-year renal survival of 90% compared with 55% for nephrotic patients. Spontaneous remissions are uncommon among nephrotic patients, and so a number of therapies have been evaluated. Since platelet activation is felt to be a factor in many forms of glomerulonephritis, platelet-inhibition therapy has been tried in MPGN. Aspirin, (325 mg, three tablets daily), along with dipyridamole (Persantine),* 75 mg, three tablets daily, has been used for up to 1 year. An initial decrease in the rate of loss of renal function resulted from this therapy, but at 10 years the renal survival (50%) was ultimately no different for patients with or without treatment. A number of other treatments have been tried: high-dose alternate-day prednisone;

---

*Not FDA-approved for this indication.

cyclophosphamide,* warfarin,* and dipyridamole;* and warfarin and dipyridamole, but the results have not been encouraging. At present, symptomatic therapy, including good control of hypertension, is considered the mainstay of treatment. Renal transplantation is associated with a high recurrence rate, particularly for patients with type II disease, but this rarely leads to graft loss.

Secondary Causes

Secondary conditions associated with an MPGN-like lesion include autoimmune diseases (SLE, Sjögren's syndrome, rheumatoid arthritis), chronic bacterial or viral infections (bacterial endocarditis, infection of ventriculoatrial shunt, hepatitis B or C), and sickle cell disease. Membranoproliferative glomerulonephritis can develop in patients with mixed essential cryoglobulinemia (MEC). The cause of MEC was previously unknown but is now attributed to infection with hepatitis C, since serologic evaluation demonstrates antibodies to hepatitis C in more than 85% of patients and the presence of hepatitis C RNA in more than 80% of patients. Over the past 20 years, the therapy for patients with MEC and renal disease has consisted of a combination of prednisone, cytotoxic agents (cyclophosphamide* or chlorambucil*), and plasmapheresis. This has led to an improvement in renal symptoms in 70% to 100% of patients, with fewer than 10% of patients progressing to ESRD within 5 to 10 years. In light of recent observations, interferon-alfa, an agent with antiproliferative, immune regulatory, and antiviral effects, has now become the therapy of choice for patients with hepatitis C virus–associated MEC. Its use has been associated with significant improvement in symptoms, with resolution of purpura, improvement in renal function, reduction in cryoglobulin levels, and normalization in liver function studies. Treatment consists of 2 to 3 million units of recombinant interferon-alfa-2b subcutaneously three times weekly for 6 months, monitoring patient symptoms, liver function studies, white blood counts and platelet counts, and adjusting the dose accordingly. Unfortunately, in the majority of studies with interferon-alfa, patients relapse shortly after therapy has been discontinued. Side effects include a flulike syndrome, fatigue, and headache. A suggested approach to therapy for MEC patients is to treat patients who have acute nephritis or signs of vasculitis with a combination of immunosuppression and plasmapheresis, saving antiviral therapy for the treatment of chronic stages of renal disease.

Immunotactoid Glomerulopathy

Immunotactoid glomerulopathy (ITG) is a relatively new clinicopathologic entity defined by its glomerular pathology of immunoglobulin-associated microfibrils. It has no specific clinical or serologic features, and it is diagnosed only after the exclusion

of diseases known to be associated with organized glomerular immune deposits, such as amyloidosis, cryoglobulinemia, systemic lupus erythematosus, and light chain deposition disease. There is no doubt that some patients with ITG have been misdiagnosed as having amyloidosis, based on the similar ultrastructural features of the renal biopsy, even though the Congo red stain (the diagnostic test for amyloid) was negative. This distinction is an important one, as the prognosis of ITG is significantly better than that for amyloidosis (5-year patient survival for ITG is over 80%, compared with 15% for primary amyloidosis).

On clinical grounds, patients with immunotactoid glomerulopathy do not appear to have a systemic disease; furthermore, extrarenal involvement has been described only in two reports out of the more than 150 cases identified to date. Thus, ITG is best classified as a primary glomerular process distinct from the other diseases known to be associated with organized glomerular immune deposits. On clinical grounds there is nothing unique about the presentation or course of immunotactoid glomerulopathy that would allow one to distinguish this disorder from other primary glomerulopathies (see Table 2). Progression to ESRD is a common finding, occurring in almost 50% of patients over 4 to 5 years.

Pathology

By light microscopy, the mesangium is prominent with only mildly increased cellularity, and the capillary walls may be thickened. Immunoglobulins and complement (predominantly IgG and C3) are demonstrated within the mesangium and along the glomerular capillary walls in a granular pattern and correspond to electron-dense deposits seen in the mesangium as well as along the glomerular capillary wall in subepithelial, intramembranous, and sometimes subendothelial locations. Ultrastructurally, the morphology of the deposits varies among patients with ITG. Some biopsies have highly organized deposits composed of microtubules arranged in parallel bundles, whereas in other patients the deposits have a microfibrillar appearance and are randomly arranged. There is variability in the size or diameter of the fibrils among patients, but in a patient with ITG the size is fairly constant. The majority of cases have fibrils that measure 18 to 22 nm.

The microfibrils in ITG contain immunoglobulins and complement, but their precise composition is not known. Using immunoelectron microscopy, it has been shown that the fibrils in patients with ITG do, in fact, contain immunoglobulins (both heavy and light chains) as well as amyloid P component but do not contain other basement membrane–associated (type IV collagen and heparan-sulfate proteoglycans) or microfibril-associated (fibronectin and fibrillin) proteins. In essentially all cases, microfibrils contain IgG and complement, and in those cases in which light chains were evaluated, 75% contained both kappa and lambda light chains. Although the pathogenesis of ITG is not known, the presence of comple-

---

*Not FDA-approved for this indication.

ment and polyclonal IgG raises the possibility that deposits in some cases of ITG are immune complexes. In other cases, however, monoclonal immunoglobulin deposition may be involved, as only kappa light chains are identified in association with a heavy chain (usually IgG) in 25% of cases.

Therapy

Very little information exists regarding the response to therapy in patients with immunotactoid glomerulopathy. In the few patients that have been treated, steroids alone, steroids with plasma exchange, and steroids with cyclophosphamide* generally have not altered the clinical course. Renal transplantation has been successful. However, the disease recurred with the development of the nephrotic syndrome after 2 to 5 years in several cases.

ASYMPTOMATIC PROTEINURIA WITH OR WITHOUT HEMATURIA

Patients in this category present with persistent (found on more than one occasion) proteinuria of less than 2 grams per 24 hr and are by definition clinically asymptomatic with otherwise normal renal function and normal blood pressure. The urine sediment may be normal but typically will demonstrate microscopic hematuria.

This presentation, as discussed earlier, can be seen in patients with focal segmental glomerulosclerosis, membranous glomerulonephritis, membranoproliferative glomerulonephritis, and immunotactoid glomerulopathy and carries a more favorable prognosis than that associated with patients having similar histology and the nephrotic syndrome. Probably the most common glomerular disease in this category is IgA nephropathy.

Orthostatic or postural proteinuria should be sought in patients with asymptomatic proteinuria. This is diagnosed by demonstrating that protein excretion is normal (<50 mg over 8 hours) in the recumbent position, even though the daily (upright) protein excretion may be as high as 1.5 grams. To do this, two separate urine collections must be obtained. The first is collected from 7 A.M. (after discarding the first morning void) to 11 P.M., during which time the patient is upright and carrying out normal activities. The patient should remain recumbent after 9 P.M. and begin the second collection at 11 P.M., completing it at 7 A.M. with the first morning void. Patients with orthostatic proteinuria are not felt to have a primary glomerular disease as they have essentially normal glomeruli on biopsy. The prognosis is excellent, with the degree of proteinuria decreasing over time in many patients. Due to its benign nature, no therapy is required.

Patients with persistent, asymptomatic proteinuria of 1 to 2 grams per 24 hr do not routinely require a renal biopsy as this is often associated with a benign course. However, patients should be followed

every 6 months checking biochemistry, urinalysis, and 24-hour urine protein quantification; a biopsy should be performed if there is evidence of progressive renal disease as demonstrated by reduced renal function, proteinuria of over 2 grams per 24 hr, concurrent hematuria, hypoalbuminemia, or hypertension.

IgA Nephropathy

IgA nephropathy is common in young adults, with 80% of patients between the ages of 16 and 35 years. It is uncommon in blacks. Asymptomatic proteinuria of less than 1 gram per 24 hr with microscopic hematuria is the most common presentation. This is usually associated with a normal serum creatinine level and normal blood pressure. The classic presentation is recurrent macroscopic hematuria, with or without flank pain, preceded by 24 to 48 hours by an upper respiratory tract infection. This usually resolves within 1 day but may last as long as a week. Up to 10% of patients will present with the nephrotic syndrome, and 10% will present with rapidly progressive glomerulonephritis associated with crescentic glomerulonephritis. Serum IgA levels are elevated in 50% of cases, but this has neither diagnostic nor prognostic significance. With the exception of finding IgA deposited in dermal vessels on skin biopsy, patients classified as having IgA nephropathy have a primary glomerular disease since they have no other systemic manifestations.

Pathology

The pathogenesis of IgA nephropathy is thought to be the result of an increased production of polymeric IgA by mucosal surfaces, such as the respiratory tract, in response to infection, along with a decrease in the removal of IgA complexes by the reticuloendothelial system. The circulating IgA immune complexes are then deposited in the glomerular mesangium. The lesion is defined by demonstrating IgA in the mesangium as the sole or primary immunoglobulin (IgG and IgM may be seen but are less prominent). This corresponds to electron-dense deposits in the same location. By light microscopy, expansion of the mesangial matrix and increase in mesangial cellularity are commonly observed. However, focal or diffuse proliferative forms of glomerular lesion can be seen and, rarely, crescentic glomerulonephritis has been described.

Therapy

IgA nephropathy generally follows a benign course. However, progressive renal insufficiency may develop in 20% to 30% of patients over the course of 20 years. Risk factors for progressive disease are male sex, older age at presentation, hypertension, renal insufficiency, proteinuria of more than 1.5 grams per day, and glomerulosclerosis, interstitial fibrosis or crescentic glomerulonephritis.

The use of fish oil (MaxEPA,* Sundown Vitamins,

---

*Not FDA-approved for this indication.

*Not FDA-approved for this indication.

Del Ray Beach, FL) has been shown to be beneficial in high-risk patients (proteinuria greater than 1 gram per 24 hr and/or renal insufficiency). This is given in 1-gram gelatin capsules in a dose of 6 grams twice daily and has resulted in a significant decrease in the rate of decline in renal function, with progression to ESRD one fourth that of patients on placebo. Control of hypertension is important in slowing the rate of progressive renal disease and may be achieved with diuretics and ACE inhibitors, as described earlier. The use of phenytoin (Dilantin)* (lowers IgA levels), antibiotics, or prednisone and cytotoxic agents has not proved to be of any significant benefit in most IgA patients. A short course of steroids (prednisone, 60 mg per day for 2 to 4 days) may reduce the severity of symptoms (flank pain) and the duration of macroscopic hematuria. These episodes are otherwise self-limited and rarely result in the need for transfusion of blood products or the use of antifibrinolytic agents. In rapidly progressive/crescentic glomerulonephritis, aggressive treatment with prednisone, cytotoxic drugs and plasmapheresis, as described later, has been utilized with variable results. In patients presenting with the nephrotic syndrome, treatment with prednisone similar to that described for adults with MCD has been beneficial. Recurrence of IgA nephropathy in transplanted patients may be as high as 50%, but this rarely leads to loss of the allograft.

Secondary Causes

Henoch-Schönlein purpura is associated with a renal biopsy picture identical to that of IgA nephropathy and in the clinical spectrum is considered to be a systemic form of the disease associated with abdominal pain, palpable purpura, and arthralgias. Mesangial deposits of IgA may also be seen in patients with hepatic cirrhosis or gluten enteropathy. The pathogenetic significance of this finding may not be the same as in patients with idiopathic IgA nephropathy.

ACUTE NEPHRITIC SYNDROME

The acute nephritic syndrome is defined by the presence of an "active" urinary sediment containing red blood cells and classically, red blood cell casts (which are pathognomonic for this entity), proteinuria of 2 to 3 grams per 24 hr, and renal insufficiency with a rising serum creatinine level. As a result of the decreased glomerular filtration rate and sodium and water retention, patients develop edema, hypertension, anemia, and hypoalbuminemia. Oliguria may ensue as the renal function worsens. In its most severe form, the presentation can be one of rapidly progressive glomerulonephritis (RPGN). Patients progress to end-stage renal disease (ESRD) over a very short course, weeks to months, if not identified early and treated aggressively. The classic example of acute glomerulonephritis is that associated with streptococcal infections (poststreptococcal glomerulo-

nephritis), but it can be seen after other bacterial, viral, or parasitic infections (postinfectious acute glomerulonephritis). In addition, a number of systemic diseases may first manifest as acute glomerulonephritis (SLE, cryoglobulinemia).

Diffuse Proliferative Glomerulonephritis (Poststreptococcal Glomerulonephritis)

A result of infection from group A β-hemolytic streptococci, poststreptococcal glomerulonephritis may follow either a pharyngeal or skin infection with a nephrogenic strain. The glomerulonephritis presents after a latent period of 1 to 2 weeks (in contrast to IgA nephropathy), allowing the production of soluble immune complexes similar to serum sickness. It is considered primarily a disease of children but occurs in adults as well. In addition to the features just described, patients may present with oliguria, gross hematuria (smoky-appearing urine), and congestive heart failure due to severe intravascular volume expansion. In 25% of patients proteinuria will be greater than 3 grams per day. At presentation, antibody titers to streptococcal enzymes (antistreptolysin O-[ASO], antideoxyribonuclease B-[ADNase B], and antihyaluronidase-[AHT]) are elevated, and the level of the 3rd component of complement (C3) is decreased to less than 50% of normal, with C4 levels being normal (suggesting alternate complement pathway activation). In 90% of patients with pharyngeal infections ASO titers will be elevated, whereas elevations of AHT and ADNase B are more common (>90%) in glomerulonephritis secondary to skin infections.

Pathology

This is an immune complex–mediated disease resulting from an antibody response to streptococcal antigen(s) such as M-protein or other cell membrane proteins. Autologous immunoglobulin that has been altered by a streptococcal enzyme has also been suggested as the antigen in the immune complexes in some patients. Light microscopy demonstrates a diffuse proliferative and exudative glomerulonephritis with endocapillary proliferation and infiltration of the glomeruli with polymorphonuclear leukocytes. A characteristic finding on electron microscopy is the presence of distinct, subepithelial, electron-dense deposits referred to as "humps." Deposits may also be found within the mesangium. By immunofluorescence, granular deposits of IgG and C3 are noted in a similar distribution as the electron-dense deposits.

Therapy

Over 90% of patients with poststreptococcal glomerulonephritis have a spontaneous and complete remission over the course of several weeks, with no long-term sequelae. Complement levels and antibody titers return to normal within 8 to 16 weeks. Renal function and volume-related problems (hypertension, edema) normalize over this same period of time, but urinary abnormalities (microscopic hematuria and

---

*Not FDA-approved for this indication.

mild proteinuria) may persist for 6 to 12 months in some patients. Antibiotic therapy (penicillin or erythromycin) for the patient and immediate family should be provided to treat and limit the spread of infection. This does not prevent the development of glomerulonephritis but may diminish its severity. Treatment is primarily supportive, with the use of loop diuretics and dietary restriction of salt and water to control hypertension, edema, and vascular congestion. Approximately 5% of patients, adults more commonly than children, have a rapidly progressive glomerulonephritis/crescentic glomerulonephritis. Treatment in these patients is more aggressive, as discussed under crescentic glomerulonephritis next.

Idiopathic Crescentic Glomerulonephritis

Crescentic glomerulonephritis is a pathologic term defined by having 30% to 50% or more of glomeruli involved with cellular crescents. Clinically, patients present with an acute deterioration in renal function over 2 to 6 weeks and are referred to as having a rapidly progressive glomerular nephritis (RPGN). Since crescentic glomerulonephritis is generally seen with the clinical picture of RPGN, the terms are often used synonymously. Crescentic glomerulonephritis is subdivided into three types based on immunopathologic features (Table 8). As Table 8 shows, each category of crescentic glomerulonephritis has secondary causes that must be considered before the diagnosis of idiopathic crescentic glomerulonephritis is applied. This classification has significant diagnostic, prognostic, and therapeutic implications. As a result, the timely performance of a renal biopsy is critical in patients with RPGN. An elevated erythrocyte sedimentation rate is found in all patients, and serologic evidence of disease can be demonstrated by elevated titers of antiglomerular basement membrane (GBM) antibodies (anti-GBM nephritis), cryoglobulins (idiopathic, immune complex–mediated RPGN), or antineutrophil cytoplasmic antibodies (ANCA) (idiopathic, pauci-immune RPGN), depending on the underlying disease.

Pathology

Crescentic glomerulonephritis can be the result of glomerular inflammation due to anti-GBM antibodies, immune complexes, or cellular immune mechanisms. Crescents are defined by the accumulation of parietal epithelial cells and macrophages in Bowman's space, occupying at least one third the circumference of the Bowman's capsule, and being at least three cell layers deep. The crescents may be associated with an underlying segmental necrotizing or proliferative glomerular lesion. In addition to the defining immunofluorescence findings outlined in Table 8, fibrin can be demonstrated within the crescents.

Therapy

Untreated, over 90% of patients will progress to ESRD within 3 to 6 months, but with aggressive immunosuppressive therapy renal survival can be significantly improved to over 70% of patients at 1 year. Factors at presentation portending a poor prognosis include oliguria/anuria, a serum creatinine level greater than 6.5 mg per dL, and more than 75% crescents. Although the level of anti-GBM antibodies, cryoglobulins, or ANCAs does not correlate with the severity of disease, the titer declines with improvement in disease activity. Following these serologic markers, along with the serum creatinine level, urinalysis, and erythrocyte sedimentation rate, is useful in monitoring response to therapy. In addition to supportive measures, such as control of blood pressure and fluid and electrolyte balance, treatment of idiopathic (immune complex and pauci-immune) crescentic glomerulonephritis consists of "pulse" methylprednisolone, 0.5 to 1.0 gram per day given intravenously every other day for a total of three doses, followed by oral prednisone, 1 mg per kg per day up to 80 mg per day for 1 to 2 months, and then tapered over 4 months. Oral cyclophosphamide (Cytoxan),* 2 mg per kg per day is used in combination with this therapy, particularly in patients with underlying necrotizing glomerular lesions, and is continued for 6 months. Leukocyte counts should be checked weekly until stable and then every other week throughout the course of therapy and the cyclophosphamide dose adjusted to maintain the leukocyte count between 3000 and 5000 per mm³.

In patients with anti-GBM nephritis, plasmapheresis (daily for 2 to 3 treatments and then every other day for a total of 12 treatments) has been beneficial in rapidly decreasing the anti-GBM titer and achieving an improvement in renal function. This is combined with oral prednisone (1 mg per kg per day up to 80 mg per day) for 1 to 2 months, then tapered off over 4 months, and cyclophosphamide (2 mg per kg per day) for 3 to 6 months. As discussed earlier, these prolonged courses of cytotoxic therapy

---

TABLE 8. **Immunopathologic Classification of Crescentic Glomerulonephritis**

I. Antiglomerular basement membrane antibodies (linear immune deposits): 20%
   Goodpasture's syndrome (with pulmonary hemorrhage)
   Nephritis without pulmonary hemorrhage
II. Immune complex–mediated nephritis (granular immune deposits): 40%
   Idiopathic
   Associated with systemic diseases (SLE, Henoch-Schönlein purpura, mixed essential cryoglobulinemia)
   Postinfectious (poststreptococcal glomerulonephritis)
   Complicating primary glomerular diseases (MPGN, IgA, MGN)
III. Pauci-immune nephritis (no or few immune deposits): 40%
   Idiopathic
   Systemic vasculitis (Wegener's granulomatosis, microscopic polyarteritis nodosa)

From Couser WG: Rapidly progressive glomerulonephritis: Classification, pathogenic mechanisms, and therapy. Am J Kidney Dis 11:449–464, 1988.

---

*Not FDA-approved for this indication.

place the patient at increased risk of infertility and malignancy as well as infection, resulting in the need for close follow-up. In addition, the high dose and prolonged course of steroids place the patients at risk of hyperglycemia, exacerbating or developing hypertension, peptic ulcer, weight gain, cushingoid facies, and striae. For patients in whom transplantation is being considered it is recommended that clinical or serologic evidence of disease activity (anti-GBM antibody or ANCA titer) be absent for 6 to 12 months prior to proceeding with transplantation, as the recurrence rate may be as high as 50% in some patients (primarily those with anti-GBM nephritis).

CHRONIC GLOMERULONEPHRITIS

Patients with chronic glomerulonephritis present with advanced renal failure. They are often asymptomatic but can have symptoms and signs related to advanced renal disease, including hypertension, edema, easy fatigability, nausea, pruritus, and decreased mental acuity. In addition to an elevated serum creatinine level (often over 4 mg per dL), microscopic hematuria and mild proteinuria (1 to 3 grams per 24 hr) may be present. In addition, anemia, hyperphosphatemia, and mild acidosis may be evident. Ultrasound of the kidney will demonstrate small kidneys with increased echogenicity consistent with the advanced irreversible nature of the underlying disease. It is often not possible to determine the cause of the glomerular process, but it may be the result of any of the primary glomerular diseases.

Pathology

The histologic picture is one of advanced glomerular scarring, often referred to as chronic sclerosing glomerulonephritis associated with tubular dilatation and severe interstitial fibrosis. The findings are nonspecific, making the diagnosis of the underlying primary glomerular process impossible. A renal biopsy is usually not performed in these patients owing to the probability that a specific diagnosis will be unlikely, and that intervention with immunosuppressive therapy would offer greater risks than benefit at this stage of renal failure.

Therapy

Therapy is primarily supportive. Patients often require dietary restriction to control fluid and electrolyte abnormalities and azotemia. When the serum creatinine level is greater than 6 mg per dL, this restriction may consist of 2 grams of sodium, 2 grams of potassium, and 1 gram per kg per day of protein. Fluid may need to be restricted to 1.0 to 1.5 liters per day in patients with urine volumes of less than 750 mL per day. Blood pressure control is also important and may reduce the rate of decline in renal function. Whether or not ACE inhibition is renoprotective in advanced stages of renal insufficiency is less clear, but hyperkalemia may be a significant side effect if used in this setting and should be monitored closely. Drugs that may further precipitate loss of renal function, such as NSAIDs, should be avoided. Ultimately, when the serum creatinine level reaches 8 mg per dL or more or creatinine clearance is 10 mL per min or less, renal replacement therapy (dialysis or transplantation) will be required.

PYELONEPHRITIS

method of
PHILLIP M. PINELL, M.D.
*Baylor College of Medicine and Houston
  Perinatal Associates
Houston, Texas*

Pyelonephritis is a urinary tract infection involving the renal parenchyma that is clinically characterized by pyuria, fever, and flank pain. Urinalysis, urine culture, and microscopic examination of the urine usually yield the offending organism. Pyelonephritis can be classified as ascending, intrinsic, or hematogenous.

ASCENDING INFECTION

Ascending infection is the most common cause of pyelonephritis. The ascending infection may occur because of vesicoureteral reflux through an incompetent vesicoureteral orifice.

Men

Pyelonephritis in the young adult man is rare. In the absence of prior surgery, intrinsic and hematogenous sources should be investigated by culture and radiographic techniques. Pyelonephritis in a previous healthy young man may be a sign of the presence of another serious underlying disease. When renal calculi are found, their elimination may be necessary if positive cultures persist or obstructive changes are noted in order to eradicate the source of infection.

Obstructive or neurologic conditions should be investigated in young men with ascending infection as the etiology of pyelonephritis. In men under the age of 45 years, prostatic cancer is uncommon; however, prostatic or epididymal infections are not uncommon and need to be ruled out. Other tumors that may cause obstruction in this age group that must be ruled out include bowel and renal cancer.

In older men, the most common etiology of obstruction is prostatic enlargement; other causes include neurologic causes, cancer (particularly prostatic cancer), and renal calculi. Medical conditions that may lead to a neurologic cause should also be considered, including diabetes mellitus.

Diagnosis and treatment of the underlying cause are essential in the management of pyelonephritis in men. Antimicrobial therapy should be directed against the specific etiologic organism. Chronic catheterization is a common cause of recurrent pyelonephritis. If obstruction is an essential cause of infection and the patient's medical condition does not permit surgical correction, then chronic catheterization may be needed. Continuous antibiotic prophylaxis is usually not successful in the long term to treat this condition and may lead to colonization and infection by multiple resistant organisms. Frequent and meticulous changes of the catheter, accompanied by antibacterial irrigation along with hygienic handling, decrease this problem.

When uncomplicated pyelonephritis has been diagnosed and the organism and sensitivity studies have been obtained, outpatient treatment may be instituted. In the past, treatment of acute pyelonephritis required hospitalization and intravenous antibiotic therapy. In uncomplicated cases, oral antibiotics may be instituted for a 14-day period. If the patient is stable but considered to need intravenous antibiotics, home intravenous therapy may be an option.

A variety of antibiotic regimens may be used successfully to treat pyelonephritis. Empiric choices may be initiated and altered on the basis of culture and sensitivity results. If an aminoglycoside is to used, it is important to check the patient's aminoglycoside levels and renal status routinely to ensure the integrity of renal function. Decreasing renal function may result in elevated or toxic levels of the aminoglycosides. Alternative antibiotics to the aminoglycosides include the quinolones, aztreonam (Azactam), and third-generation cephalosporins.

Women

Young women frequently have urinary tract infections. Acute episodes of pyelonephritis are not uncommon in women. Approximately 1% to 2% of all young women have asymptomatic bacteriuria; a condition in which the individual chronically harbors bacteria in the urine without symptoms. Incidence appears to increase with increasing age in women. Asymptomatic bacteriuria and urinary tract infections possibly are much more common in women secondary to a shorter urethra and hormonal changes affecting mucosal adherence of bacteria.

Asymptomatic bacteriuria appears to be a source of ascending infection predisposing to pyelonephritis in young women. Several strategies may used to prevent or decrease colonization of bacteria in the bladder and ascending infection to the kidneys. Antibiotic prophylaxis with single oral doses of trimethoprim-sulfamethoxazole (Bactrim, Septra), 80/400 mg, or nitrofurantoin (Macrodantin), 100 mg, following intercourse; immediate urination following intercourse; increased hydration; and acidification of the urine through oral intake have been used to decrease asymptomatic bacteriuria.

The most common risk factor for developing pyelonephritis in young women is pregnancy. Acute pyelonephritis has been reported to occur in 1% to 2.5% of pregnancies. The incidence increases with gestational age, with approximately 90% of cases occurring in the second and third trimesters. Pregnant women with asymptomatic bacteriuria have an approximate 25% chance of developing acute pyelone-

phritis. This risk increases even before the uterus grows out of the pelvis and is thought to be secondary to the effect of pregnancy hormones on ureteral function and genital urinary tissue receptors for bacterial adherence. Compression of the ureters and bladder by an enlarging uterus is also thought to play a role. Right-sided pyelonephritis is more common than left-sided pyelonephritis in pregnancy.

The bacteria responsible for pyelonephritis in pregnancy are predominantly the Enterobacteriaceae, especially *Escherichia coli*. Gram-positive bacteria, including group B streptococcus and enterococcus, comprise approximately 5% of etiologic organisms contributing to pyelonephritis in pregnancy.

Pyelonephritis is a common infectious cause of hospitalization during pregnancy. There is an association of pyelonephritis in pregnancy with preterm labor and sepsis, and a small risk of adult respiratory distress syndrome. Pregnant patients with fever should have a urinalysis and culture to rule out urinary tract infection as a source. A urinalysis with positive pyuria in the presence of fever and flank pain or costovertebral angle tenderness is diagnostic for pyelonephritis. White blood cell casts found with microscopic evaluation of urine are pathognomonic for pyelonephritis. A Gram stain may be used to determine whether the etiologic organism is gram-positive or gram-negative. Parenteral ampicillin demonstrates excellent activity against enterococcus and group B streptococcus infections, and cephalosporins display a good gram-negative coverage. Aminoglycosides have been used to treat pyelonephritis in pregnancy, but careful monitoring of the levels and renal function is important.

All pregnant patients with the diagnosis of pyelonephritis should be hospitalized for evaluation and treatment. Antibiotic therapies that are considered safe and effective in pregnant patients with pyelonephritis include cefazolin (Ancef), the third-generation cephalosporins including cefotaxime (Claforan), ceftriaxone (Rocephin), antipseudomonal penicillins including piperacillin (Pipracil), beta-lactamase inhibitor containing pencillins including ampicillin-sulbactam (Unasyn), ticarcillin-clavulinate (Timentin), and piperacillin-tazobactam (Zosyn). Ampicillin and gentamicin (Garamycin) in combination have also been used effectively to treat pyelonephritis in pregnancy. The quinolones are contraindicated in pregnancy. Sulfa-containing compounds are generally not recommended late in pregnancy because of safety considerations.

There is an increased incidence of urogenital anatomic abnormalities in patients with pyelonephritis in pregnancy. In light of this fact, it is suggested by some to consider radiographic or ultrasound evaluation of the urinary tract in pregnant patients. If a pregnant patient fails to respond to therapy or if she develops recurrent infections, this evaluation is useful in detecting urogenital anatomic abnormalities.

Catheterization in older women, particularly those in nursing homes, is not uncommon secondary to descensus bladder that has occurred after childbearing. Anyone who requires long-term or frequent catheterizations, including women who have undergone surgical procedures that may denervate the bladder, may acquire an ascending infection, just as in men, from bacteria colonizing the urinary tract.

To treat catheter-related infections effectively, it is important to note the culture and sensitivity reports at the time of infection and the history of previous organisms and their sensitivity pattern. Empiric treatment may be based on previous organisms and sensitivity patterns. Culturing urine samples with each new infection is important because of the potential of resistance to antibiotic therapy that occurs frequently.

INTRINSIC INFECTION

Surgical interventions, including transplantation, often cause intrinsic infection. The etiologic organisms and clinical syndromes vary widely, depending on the manipulations that have been done and the host immune system. For the immunocompromised patient, including patients who have received immunosuppressive agents, organisms that are considered even mildly pathogenic may be a cause of infection and should be taken seriously when cultured out. Yeast on urinalysis in an immunosuppressed patient may be a formidable pathogen. As with ascending infections, treatment of intrinsic infections should be based on culture and sensitivity reports. Drugs effective for fungal infections include amphotericin and fluconazole.

HEMATOGENOUS INFECTION

Pyelonephritis from hematogenous spread occurs most often in the setting of septicemia or infective endocarditis, which is frequently due to staphylococcus or *E. coli* and is worsened by urinary obstruction. Bacteria that have been introduced to the kidney secondary to these insults may help form an abscess or progress to a chronic infection and inflammatory response representing chronic pyelonephritis. Chronic pyelonephritis is a major cause of renal failure in the elderly. It may be difficult to make the diagnosis with noninvasive techniques.

It is important to obtain blood and urine cultures to determine the etiologic organism causing hematogenous infection. Although initial treatment may be empiric, continued treatment should be based on the results of culture and sensitivity testing of the blood and urine specimens. Repeat cultures are recommended even after clinical improvement is noted because if a follow-up culture is positive, persistent infection requires longer treatment. In the case of a positive urine culture with a positive blood culture and a clinically improving patient, formation of a renal abscess or intermittent bacterial seeding of the blood secondary to endocarditis may be considered. This can be confirmed by ultrasound and selected radiography, including computed tomography and magnetic resonance imaging. Treatment of persistent infection may require long-term therapy for up to 6 weeks with a parenteral regimen. If abscess formation is found, drainage along with parenteral antibiotic therapy may be necessary.

TREATMENT OPTIONS (Table 1)

The most important aspect of treating pyelonephritis is to diagnose the cause, which is usually treatable. Although antibiotic therapy is often initiated

TABLE 1. **Treatment Options for Pyelonephritis**

Fluoroquinolones			
Ciprofloxacin (Cipro)	500 mg	PO	q 12 h for 14 d
Ofloxacin (Floxin)	400 mg	PO	q 12 h for 14 d
Norfloxacin (Noroxin)	400 mg	PO	q 12 h for 14 d
Lomefloxacin (Maxaquin)	400 mg	PO	once daily for 14 d
Enoxacin (Penetrex)	400 mg	PO	q 12 h for 14 d
Ciprofloxacin	400 mg	IV	q 12 h
Ofloxacin	400 mg	IV	q 12 h
Cephalosporins			
Cefazolin (Ancef)	1–2 gm	IV	q 6–8 h
Ceftriaxone (Rocephin)	1–2 gm	IV	q 12–24 h
Cefotaxime (Claforan)	1–2 gm	IV	q 6–12 h
Ceftizoxime (Cefizox)	1–2 gm	IV	q 8–12 h
Ceftazidime (Fortaz)	1–2 gm	IV	q 8–12 h
Pencillins			
Piperacillin (Pipracil)	3 gm	IV	q 6 h
Ampicillin-sulbactam (Unasyn)	3 gm	IV	q 6 h
Ticarcillin-clavulinate (Timentin)	3.1 gm	IV	q 6 h
Piperacillin-tazobactam (Zosyn)	3.375	IV	q 6 h
Sulfa Drugs			
Trimethoprim-sulfamethoxazole (Bactrim, Septra)	160/800 mg	PO	q 12 h for 14 d
Trimethoprim-sulfamethoxazole	2 mg/kg trimethoprim	IV	q 6 h
Monobactams			
Aztreonam (Azactam)	1–2 gm	IV	q 6–8 h
Combination therapy: ampicillin and gentamicin			

empirically, Gram stain results, culture results, and resistant patterns in previous infections should help determine proper antimicrobial therapy.

Although some clinicians advocate oral antimicrobial therapy for uncomplicated pyelonephritis, it may be more beneficial to treat true pyelonephritis with initial parenteral therapy followed by oral therapy to complete a 2-week course. It may take up to 6 weeks of therapy to treat chronic or recurring pyelonephritis adequately.

In select cases of uncomplicated pyelonephritis in relatively healthy nonpregnant patients, outpatient oral therapy may be advantageous. Oral agents that are deemed effective include the quinolones, the penicillins, cephalosporins, and sulfa agents.

Pyelonephritis may be a serious bacterial infection, but with early diagnosis and appropriate and expeditious antimicrobial therapy, the prognosis is excellent. Follow-up examination and cultures are an important factor in preventing chronic pyelonephritis and other serious sequelae.

TRAUMA TO THE GENITOURINARY TRACT

method of
MICHAEL COBURN, M.D.

Baylor College of Medicine and Ben Taub
General Hospital
Houston, Texas

Urologic trauma may occur as an isolated injury to a genitourinary organ or as part of multisystem trauma. Injuries may be readily apparent, as in injuries to the external genitalia, or may be less obvious on initial patient assessment, as in renal injuries from blunt trauma. While urinary tract injury is an uncommon direct cause of mortality in the trauma patient, significant morbidity can result from delayed diagnosis or injudicious management. Urologic injury may be categorized as blunt versus penetrating, upper tract versus lower tract, isolated injury versus multiple injuries. This discussion will center on the mechanism, diagnosis, appropriate imaging studies, and management of the most commonly encountered and important varieties of urologic injury.

RENAL INJURY

Mechanism and Pattern of Injury

Renal injury most commonly results from blunt trauma, from mechanisms such as motor vehicle or industrial accidents, direct blows to the flank or abdomen, or falls. Renal parenchymal injuries may range from minimal cortical contusions to major lacerations and crush injuries with destruction of the organ. Parenchymal disruption and laceration may result from sudden compression of the kidney against the posterior ribs or spine at the time of abdominal impact. Deceleration injuries, as seen in high-speed motor vehicle accidents or falls from a height, may

classically result in renal pedicle injuries with intimal arterial disruption, thrombosis, and resultant infarction of the kidney. Patterns of injury from blunt trauma often include concomitant injury to other solid abdominal viscera, such as liver injury on the right or splenic injury on the left. The kidney with an underlying abnormality, such as congenital ureteropelvic junction obstruction or other hydronephrotic process, or tumor, is more vulnerable to injury because of the disordered anatomy and is more prone to injury from seemingly minor trauma.

Clinical Presentation

The presentation of a patient with renal injury may be subtle, with no obvious sign of trauma, or may be dramatic, with hemodynamic instability from major renal bleeding. Prevalent symptoms may include flank or abdominal pain, a sense of fullness of flank mass, symptoms of hemodynamic instability such as lightheadedness or syncope, and hematuria. Possible signs of renal injury include flank ecchymosis, tenderness, and flank or abdominal mass effect. Rare injuries such as bilateral renal pedicle trauma with arterial occlusion may result in anuria. In a patient with concomitant head injury or other process affecting mental status, diagnosis may be more challenging because of the absence of the ability to report pain or other symptoms.

Diagnosis

When renal injury is suspected based on history, physical findings, or mechanism of injury, additional studies should be performed to identify and carefully stage the injury and select a management approach for the patient. Relevant laboratory studies include urinalysis, complete blood count, electrolytes, blood urea nitrogen and creatinine levels, and urinary tract imaging studies. Hematuria is a cardinal sign of urinary tract injury, although it is important to appreciate that the presence of hematuria is variable, and the magnitude of the hematuria does not consistently correlate with the seriousness of the injury. In general, patients with blunt abdominal trauma who have had no hypotension at any time after injury and have had only microscopic hematuria have a low risk of major renal injury, and recent data suggest that routine imaging of such patients has a low yield of significant injury. This rule needs to be tempered by individual case assessment, however. Pediatric patients, or patients with other signs of major associated trauma (deceleration mechanism, closed head injury, long bone fracture), are best routinely imaged to avoid missing significant injuries.

Renal imaging studies useful in assessment of patients with possible urinary tract trauma include intravenous pyelography, abdominal computed tomography (CT) scanning, and possibly renal and abdominal ultrasound in experienced hands. Intravenous pyelography (IVP) for assessment of trauma is performed by bolus infusion, with films obtained at intervals to demonstrate the nephrographic and excretory phases of contrast excretion. Loss of the cortical outline, significant contrast extravasation, and nonfunction of a kidney may be noted on IVP, prompting further assessment and staging of the injury. Although this study is readily available in the emergency center and is excellent for demonstrating the presence of two functional renal units prior to surgery, and for demonstration of renal perfusion and rapid imaging of the parenchyma and collecting system, often IVP is lacking in anatomic detail adequate for detailed staging of the injury. CT scanning has become the study of choice for such precise imaging of renal trauma. It provides the advantages of clearly demonstrating the renal parenchyma, including any subcapsular or perirenal hematoma or laceration, absent perfusion as seen with arterial injury, and any contrast extravasation, while also providing useful information regarding other abdominal viscera such as the liver, spleen, or pancreas.

Arteriography has been utilized in renal trauma primarily to study the renal arteries when pedicle injury is suspected, as when nonvisualization of a kidney is noted on IVP. It has largely been supplanted by CT scanning but is still occasionally useful when other less invasive studies fail to provide adequate anatomic detail for clinical decision making.

In addition to these designated urinary tract imaging studies, signs such as spinal transverse process fracture, loss of the psoas margin, and fracture of lower ribs may raise the suspicion of renal injury in certain patients, and such findings may be noted on simple chest and abdominal radiographs obtained in the emergency center.

Renal imaging studies should allow precise staging of renal injuries to allow one to select a management strategy intelligently. Most injuries may be described as contusions, minor parenchymal injuries, major parenchymal injuries, pedicle injuries, or severe crush or parenchymal destruction injuries. Less common injuries that may be encountered include complete forniceal avulsion or ureteropelvic disruption, more commonly seen in the pediatric age group. The patient's clinical condition, stage of renal injury, and presence and nature of other injuries will largely determine the management approach.

Management

The approach to blunt renal trauma has evolved such that nonoperative management is considered appropriate for the majority of injuries; renal contusion, subcapsular or small perinephric hematomas, and minor parenchymal lacerations, comprising over 80% of renal trauma, may be managed nonoperatively with a low rate of complications. Major, life-threatening hemorrhage from renal injury is generally obvious clinically and is managed with urgent operative exploration and reconstruction, partial nephrectomy, or nephrectomy. The major challenge in selecting nonoperative versus operative management

arises in cases of major parenchymal laceration with moderate blood loss. Current literature on the topic focuses on the issue of hemodynamic stability as the primary factor in selecting nonoperative therapy for such cases. Radiographic findings, such as minimal-to-moderate contrast extravasation, small areas of devitalized parenchyma, or moderate-sized perinephric hematomas, are not absolute operative indications, although such injuries require close observation for the possibility of sudden or progressive clinical deterioration requiring operative or other forms of intervention. Patients with significant renal injuries who are initially managed nonoperatively should be closely observed in an inpatient hospital setting, often in an intensive care unit setting, with frequent clinical assessment including vital signs, abdominal examination, and hematocrit determination, along with initial bed rest. The occurrence of clinical deterioration, significant blood replacement requirements, and worsening physical examination findings may require urgent intervention, possibly including surgery, repeat imaging, or selective angiographic embolization, depending on the specific aspects of the case.

Renal pedicle injuries resulting in arterial thrombosis may be successfully revascularized surgically if encountered and operated in the early hours after injury, though other aspects of the patient's condition and the prioritization of other injuries have an impact on the appropriateness of selecting aggressive surgical reconstructive attempts in these patients.

Complications

Complications of renal trauma may occur early, or possibly weeks to months after injury. Progressive or delayed bleeding, urinary extravasation with urinoma formation, and renal or perinephric infection may develop. Late complications may include hypertension due to parenchymal ischemia, or loss of renal function.

Penetrating Injury—Special Considerations

Urinary tract injury may be found in approximately 10% to 15% of penetrating abdominal trauma, and a high index of suspicion is required to avoid missed injuries. Any degree of hematuria should prompt appropriate urinary tract imaging after penetrating trauma, and although controversial, some investigators suggest routine intravenous pyelography after all penetrating abdominal injury. If laparotomy is required for general surgical management, injured kidneys are typically assessed intraoperatively and repaired if indicated. Some penetrating injuries, particularly some of those resulting from posterior or flank stab wounds, can be managed nonoperatively if the patient is hemodynamically stable, has a peripheral or superficial parenchymal injury, and has no other indication for laparotomy after assessment by the trauma surgeon. As with blunt trauma, nonoperative management of penetrating renal injury requires close patient observation and frequent reassessment, with a low threshold for intervention if deterioration occurs.

URETERAL INJURY

Mechanism and Pattern of Injury

Ureteral injury from blunt trauma is rare, as the ureter is generally protected from the forces of major blunt trauma. Occasionally, ureteropelvic disruption or avulsion may be seen after blunt trauma, more commonly in pediatric patients or in the presence of underlying anatomic abnormalities. More commonly seen forms of ureteral injury include iatrogenic trauma and penetrating trauma. Iatrogenic ureteral injury may complicate open or endoscopic surgery; nearly every abdominal or retroperitoneal operation may result in ureteral injury. Some of the most common procedures during which ureteral injuries occur include hysterectomy, cesarean section, and lower colonic or rectal surgery, particularly when neoplastic or inflammatory disease results in abnormal anatomy. Retroperitoneal surgical procedures such as sympathectomy, spinal or pelvic orthopedic reconstructions, and surgery for aortoiliac reconstruction may also place the ureter at risk. In the penetrating trauma setting, the ureter may be injured at any level and requires a high degree of suspicion to avoid missing such injuries.

Clinical Presentation

Iatrogenic ureteral injury may be recognized at the time of surgery, or noted later either when complications of urinary obstruction or extravasation develop, or when the ureter is unexpectedly recognized in a pathologic specimen. When presenting in a delayed fashion, the patient may develop flank pain, abdominal distention, pain, ileus, fever, or signs of intraabdominal sepsis. Some ureteral injuries result not from direct injury but from ischemia induced by the surgical dissection or abnormal anatomy or both; late presentations, sometimes weeks after surgery, may be noted in such cases. Alternatively, hematuria may be observed postoperatively, or fistulas from a surgical wound or vaginal cuff may be noted.

Diagnosis

Regardless of the mechanism of injury, when ureteral injury is suspected, laboratory studies and radiographic imaging studies are indicated for diagnosis. If ureteral obstruction or extravasation is occurring, progressive acidosis, hyperkalemia, and worsening renal function may be noted on serum chemistry studies. Hematuria or pyuria may be present on urinalysis. Useful imaging studies may include renal ultrasonography or IVP. If ureteral ligation has occurred, hydronephrosis or nonfunction of the involved kidney may be noted; after ureteral laceration or transection, contrast extravasation may be seen on IVP, or an abdominal mass from urinoma formation may be apparent. Abdominal CT scanning may be useful for general assessment of the abdomen when abdominal findings suggest the possibility of a postoperative complication reflecting an operative injury. Percutaneous aspiration of an abdominal fluid collection under ultrasound or CT guidance may be diagnostic—fluid should be analyzed for creatinine concentration and sent for culture, Gram stain, and other relevant studies. After such initial assessment, further urologic imaging may be necessary. Cystoscopy and retrograde pyelography are generally viewed as the "gold standard" for diagnosis of ureteral trauma and can demonstrate whether complete ligation or transection has occurred. When the level of injury, length of ureteral loss if any, complete versus partial nature of injury, and condition of surrounding tissues are determined diagnostically, a sensible treatment approach may be selected.

Management

When recognized intraoperatively, immediate repair is generally indicated. When diagnosed in the hours or days after iatrogenic injury, the decision to re-explore the patient immediately or on a delayed basis must be addressed. In general, ureteral injuries diagnosed in the early days after injury may be repaired at the time of recognition if the patient is believed to be in acceptable condition to tolerate the additional surgery. When recognized greater than 5 to 7 days after injury, the degree of inflammation present may make further surgery at that time difficult, and delayed reconstruction may be preferable. If the patient is ill, with impending sepsis, azotemia, or significant postoperative debilitation, delayed reconstruction is generally favored.

If initial endoscopic assessment reveals ureteral continuity, retrograde ureteral stent placement may provide temporary or even definitive therapy. Alternatively, percutaneous nephrostomy tube placement may be performed to halt continued urinary extravasation, providing temporary urinary diversion while also allowing access for an attempt at antegrade stent placement across the injured area. Percutaneous drainage of urinomas may also be performed radiographically.

When definitive reconstruction for ureteral injuries is performed, several options exist. Lower ureteral injuries are often managed by ureteroneocystostomy or ureteral reimplantation into the bladder, to avoid the problems of possible ischemia of the distal ureteral stump. This may be combined with a psoas hitch, in which the bladder is mobilized and sewn to the ipsilateral psoas muscle fascia, when limited proximal ureteral length is problematic. Mid and upper ureteral injuries are typically managed with primary anastomosis when possible. In cases of extensive ureteral loss or other complicating factors such as pelvic inflammation or neoplasm, more elaborate ureteral reconstruction techniques may be indicated, including transureteroureterostomy (anastomosis of the proximal injured ureter to the opposite normal ureter), ileal ureteral replacement, or renal auto-transplantation into the pelvis. Nephrectomy may also need to be considered when the function of the involved kidney and the risk/benefit ratio of a complex reconstruction suggest that removal may be the least morbid course of action.

Complications

Complications, as alluded to earlier, relate to the effects of continued urinary extravasation or obstruction. Late stenosis may result in pain, loss of renal function, chronic infection, or stone formation.

Penetrating Injuries—Special Considerations

Penetrating ureteral injuries are best repaired surgically, most often at the time of abdominal exploration for management of associated intra-abdominal injuries, present in over 80% of cases. Conservative débridement and primary anastomosis are usually possible; for distal injuries, ureteral reimplantation is often preferable.

BLADDER INJURY

Mechanisms and Pattern of Injury

Bladder injury may occur due to blunt or penetrating forces. Bladder rupture is generally classified as intraperitoneal or extraperitoneal. Intraperitoneal bladder rupture generally occurs when a full bladder sustains a sudden pressure increase, as from a direct blow to the lower abdomen or motor vehicle accident. A large laceration through the dome results, with free communication of urine to the peritoneal cavity. Extraperitoneal bladder ruptures most commonly accompany pelvic fractures; due to shear forces and its fascial attachment in the pelvis, the bladder tears in the lower segment, most often anterolaterally. Urine may extravasate into the pelvis or within the deeper layers of the abdominal wall but does not directly communicate with the peritoneal cavity. Concomitant injury to adjacent structures, including the vagina, rectum, or perineum, may complicate such pelvic fractures and bladder ruptures, with an impact on the management approach. Iatrogenic bladder injury may be either intra- or extraperitoneal, depending on the mechanism and location of the injury.

Clinical Presentation

Common presenting signs and symptoms of bladder injury include hematuria, pain with voiding or inability to void, abdominal distention, and pelvic pain. Delayed diagnosis of bladder rupture may result in a presentation characterized by local or intra-abdominal infection or azotemia.

Diagnosis

When bladder injury is suspected, either based on history, physical findings, or the presence of hematuria, the study of choice for documentation is a stress cystogram. This is performed by inserting a Foley catheter into the bladder and filling the bladder by gravity until the patient reports a sense of fullness, or until a reasonable full bladder capacity is reached, at which point plain radiographs or fluoroscopic images are obtained. After the contrast is drained from the bladder via the catheter, the bladder is lavaged with saline and a "washout" film is obtained. Extravasation of contrast on the cystogram is diagnostic of bladder injury; the washout film is needed to be sure extravasation anterior or posterior to the plane of radiographic projection was not missed when the bladder was distended with contrast. Intraperitoneal extravasation can be recognized as contrast outlining loops of bowel, filling the paracolonic gutters or cul-de-sac, or outlining the liver. Extraperitoneal contrast appears as flame-shaped patterns, usually in the perivesical region.

Cystoscopic examination may occasionally be useful diagnostically in suspected bladder rupture, although the cystogram is generally more easily accessible in the emergency setting. In the setting of suspected iatrogenic injury, performing cystoscopy and obtaining retrograde pyelograms may be an expeditious means of assessing all the anatomy at risk.

With a complex injury, indicated by the presence of blood per rectum or vagina, or an open perineal laceration, careful physical examination using a vaginal speculum and possibly proctoscopic examination may be required to assess the injury fully. Performing such assessment in an operating room setting with appropriate sedation or anesthesia, and the capability to progress to surgical management, may be necessary.

Management

Intraperitoneal bladder ruptures are most often managed with open surgical repair, to prevent continued extravasation of urine into the peritoneal cavity with resultant peritonitis. Extraperitoneal bladder ruptures most often can be managed by Foley catheter drainage, commonly healing within 10 days. Typically, a repeat cystogram is performed at that point to document healing prior to catheter removal. More complex injuries, such as those mentioned earlier involving concomitant vaginal or rectal trauma, or injuries that fail catheter drainage (due to continued bleeding, catheter occlusion, or some extensive disruptions involving the bladder neck) may require operative repair. One should exercise great caution in approaching the injured bladder surgically in the setting of a pelvic fracture, in which inadvertently entering the retropubic hematoma may result in severe bleeding from a previously contained site.

Complications

Persistent extravasation, gross hematuria with inadequate catheter drainage from clot formation, urinary or local pelvic infection, and pseudodiverticulum or fistula formation represent some of the potential complications of bladder trauma, which may require delayed operative management or prolonged catheter drainage for full resolution.

Penetrating Injuries—Special Considerations

Penetrating bladder injuries are most often repaired surgically at the time of abdominal exploration, typically performed due to the high likelihood of associated nonurologic visceral or vascular injury requiring operative management.

URETHRAL INJURIES

Mechanisms and Pattern of Injury

Urethral injuries may result from blunt or penetrating trauma and are generally described as involving the anterior or posterior urethra. Posterior urethral disruption is a classic complication of certain types of pelvic fractures, in which the prostatomembranous urethra separates from the anterior urethra, near the level of the pelvic floor or urogenital diaphragm. Such injuries can be complete, involving complete separation, or partial, involving stretching or incomplete laceration of the membranous urethra. Blunt injuries to the anterior urethra (the portion below the urogenital diaphragm, including the bulbous and pendulous urethra) commonly result from straddle injuries, with direct impact to the perineum from falls or kicks, when there is a contusion or crush injury to the urethra between the perineum and pubis. Similarly, such injuries may be partial-thickness or full-thickness lacerations. Injuries to any portion of the urethra may also result from penetrating trauma.

Injuries to the female urethra are less common than in the male but may occasionally complicate pelvic fracture, gynecologic surgery, or penetrating trauma to the pelvis or perineum.

Clinical Presentation

Typical findings after urethral injury include hematuria, inability to void, pain with voiding, blood at the urethral meatus, perineal hematoma, or pelvic or perineal extravasation of urine.

Diagnosis

Retrograde urethrography should be performed whenever urethral injury is suspected, prior to any attempt to pass a urethral catheter into the bladder. Blood at the urethral meatus or urethral bleeding represents a cardinal sign of urethral injury which should prompt urethrography, but any setting in which such an injury is suspected should be evaluated even in the absence of overt urethral bleeding. The urethrogram is most often performed by placing the tip of a Foley catheter into the distal penile urethra (fossa navicularis) and gently instilling 1 to 2 mL of fluid into the balloon to maintain its position and extend the penis, then injecting contrast through the catheter to fill the urethra. Plain radiographs are obtained upon adequate instillation to determine whether extravasation is present and to identify the level and completeness of any injury. In the setting of suspected urethral or bladder injury, if the urethrogram is normal, the catheter balloon is deflated and passage into the bladder is performed, followed by appropriate cystography as mentioned above.

Management

Posterior urethral disruptions are most commonly managed with placement of a suprapubic cystostomy tube, either percutaneously or by open cystotomy, followed after several months with a delayed urethral reconstruction if an obliterated stricture forms. For partial injuries and for selected complete disruptions, some urologists will attempt endoscopically guided realignment of the disruption over a catheter, in the hope that the injury may heal, obviating the need for subsequent reconstructive surgery. This management decision represents an area of some controversy currently.

Anterior urethral injuries may be managed with suprapubic tube diversion, urethral catheter placement, or immediate surgical repair, depending on the details of the injury and the patient's general condition.

Complications

Stricture formation is a common event after urethral injury, often requiring subsequent endoscopic or surgical intervention. Infection, stone formation, diverticulum formation, and problems related to catheter malfunction may also occur, requiring further urologic intervention.

Penetrating Injuries—Special Considerations

Penetrating urethral injuries may require complex reconstructive techniques, if involving the prostate and rectum, for example, or may be simply managed with primary repair if involving the anterior urethra. Often coexisting with injury to other genital structures, such injuries typically require operative management.

EXTERNAL GENITAL INJURIES

Mechanisms and Pattern of Injury

External genital trauma may result from blunt or penetrating forces and may range from simple contusions or lacerations to extensive avulsion or amputation injuries requiring specialized microsurgical or plastic surgical expertise for successful management. Blunt injuries to the genitalia include penile fracture and testicular rupture. Penile fracture involves laceration of the tunica albuginea, the tough, fibrous sheath that encloses the erectile tissues, during erection—either due to sexual activity or other bending or torquing of the erect penis. Testicular rupture involves laceration of the surrounding tunica albuginea with resultant extrusion of testicular parenchyma.

Clinical Presentation

Patients who present with penile rupture during erection typically report a snapping sound or sensation upon penile bending, resulting in immediate loss of erection and penile swelling due to extravasation of blood in the tissues, often accompanied by a mass effect in the penile shaft and angulation. Blunt testicular trauma resulting in testicular rupture causes scrotal swelling, pain and tenderness, along with a mass effect. Significant scrotal swelling may also result from scrotal wall bleeding from blunt or penetrating trauma in the absence of testicular rupture, sometimes making specific diagnosis difficult.

Diagnosis

Diagnosis of genital injury is generally based on history and physical examination findings, though scrotal ultrasound may be useful in distinguishing true testicular rupture from simply scrotal wall edema or hematoma. Retrograde urethrography, as mentioned, may also be needed to rule out concomitant urethral injury in the setting of genital trauma.

Management

Penile fracture is best managed by early operative repair, with closure of the tunica albuginea defect and evacuation of the hematoma. Similarly, testicular rupture is best approached surgically, with débridement of devitalized parenchyma and repair of the tunica albuginea. Orchiectomy may be necessary if the testicle is not salvageable by reconstructive techniques. Avulsion or amputation injuries of the genitalia usually are managed by attempted replantation using microsurgical techniques.

Complications

Bleeding and local infection are the potential early problems, and loss of erectile function or of endocrine or reproductive function are the potential delayed consequences of genital injury. In most cases, functional results after repair of penile or testicular injuries, from the sexual or reproductive function viewpoint, are very good.

Penetrating Injuries—Special Considerations

Penetrating and blunt genital injuries are handled similarly, usually with surgical exploration and repair when testicular or penile penetration is suspected. The possiblity of concomitant vascular (femoral, iliac) or abdominal injury should not be overlooked.

PROSTATITIS

method of
JEFFREY D. REICH, M.D., and
PHILIP M. HANNO, M.D.
Temple University
Philadelphia, Pennsylvania

Prostatitis describes a complex array of symptoms in adult men that is caused by prostatic inflammation or infection. These complaints can include back or genitourinary pain, irritative or obstructive voiding symptoms, or a number of nonspecific symptoms. About 25% of men seen by physicians for genitourinary complaints will have prostatitis, and 95% of men will experience some symptoms of prostatitis during their lifetime.

Prostatitis has been divided into four forms: acute bacterial prostatitis, chronic bacterial prostatitis, nonbacterial prostatitis, and prostatodynia (Table 1). These types can be differentiated through a thorough work-up, including a careful history, physical examination, appropriate cultures, and microscopic examination of expressed prostatic secretion (EPS). Symptoms of prostatitis can also mask other disease entities, such as carcinoma in situ of the bladder and interstitial cystitis, making a complete evaluation necessary. Once the type of prostatitis is determined, appropriate treatment can be implemented.

A number of symptoms should initiate a prostatitis evaluation: perineal, genital, low back, or ejaculatory pain; dysuria; urethral discharge; recurrent urinary tract infections; obstructive voiding complaints; and occasionally sexual dysfunction. A review of prior genitourinary complaints and abnormalities and a sexual history should be obtained. A generalized physical examination should be performed with special attention to the urogenital organs, including the prostate.

Since all prostate infections are associated with infected urine, it is usually necessary to do localization cultures to pinpoint the source of the infection and help differentiate the types of prostatitis. A simple method is to obtain a midstream urine sample and a sample of prostatic secretions after a prostatic massage, sending both to a laboratory for culture. If the colony counts of the prostatic secretions are ten times greater than the midstream urine counts, then bacterial prostatitis should be suspected. If the counts are greater in the midstream urine than in the EPS, cystitis should be suspected. If neither sample grows any colonies and the EPS shows significant inflammation (>10 to 15 white blood cells per high-power field), then nonbacterial prostatitis is likely. For a more definitive diagnosis, additional formal localization cultures should be done.

TABLE 1. **Prostatitis: Types, Causes, and Treatment**

Type	Definition	Organism/Cause	Treatment
Acute and chronic bacterial prostatitis	Urine and expressed prostatic secretion (EPS) culture positive for bacteria (avoid EPS in acute cases)	*Escherichia coli* *Klebsiella* spp *Pseudomonas aeruginosa* *Proteus* spp *Staphylococcus epidermidis* *Staphylococcus aureus* *Streptococcus faecalis* Non–group D streptococci Diphtheroids	If very ill: intravenous ampicillin/aminoglycoside or intravenous ciprofloxacin If stable: oral trimethoprim/sulfamethoxazole (Bactrim DS, Septra DS), 160 mg/800 mg twice daily), or oral fluoroquinolone (ofloxacin [Floxin], 300 mg twice daily), or ciprofloxacin (Cipro), 500 mg twice daily for 30 days
Nonbacterial prostatitis	EPS shows inflammation, but culture is negative for bacteria	Unknown etiology *Chlamydia trachomatis* *Ureaplasma urealyticum* *Mycoplasma hominis* *Trichomonas vaginalis* *Mycobacterium tuberculosis* (rare) Various fungi (rare)	2–4 wk doxycycline (100 mg twice daily) or erythromycin (500 mg four times daily); sitz baths; NSAIDs; normal sexual activity; avoid spicy foods, caffeine, alcohol
Prostatodynia	Symptoms, but urine and EPS show no infection or inflammation	Unknown etiology (most likely) Urinary sphincter dyssynergia Pelvic tension myalgia Stress Emotional distress	Sitz baths; NSAIDs; avoid spicy foods, caffeine, alcohol; alphablockers; muscle relaxants; benzodiazepines; psychological counseling

Abbreviation: NSAIDs = nonsteroidal anti-inflammatory drugs.

TYPES OF PROSTATITIS AND THEIR TREATMENT

Acute bacterial prostatitis is the least common form of prostatitis and the easiest to diagnose. It is characterized by the abrupt onset of fever, low back pain, perineal pain, malaise, arthralgia, or myalgia. It can also be associated with irritative voiding or obstructive voiding complaints and usually occurs in younger men. Physical examination will reveal an ill-appearing man in moderate distress. A rectal examination can be performed and it usually reveals a large, warm, tender, and boggy prostate. Prostatic massage should not be done to avoid seeding the bloodstream and causing a more global sepsis. A urinalysis and urine culture should be obtained, along with blood cultures, if indicated. Blood studies may reveal a leukocytosis with a left shift. If the patient is in urinary retention, it is best to place a suprapubic tube rather than a urethral catheter.

Empirical antibiotics should be started immediately. Eighty percent of identified pathogens will be *Escherichia coli*, although *Klebsiella* species, *Pseudomonas aeruginosa*, *Proteus* species, and various gram-positive organisms can also be involved. During an acute prostate infection, most antibiotics will have good penetration into the prostate owing to the inflammation. If the patient is not acutely ill, a course of oral antibiotics, such as trimethoprim-sulfamethoxazole (Bactrim, Septra), 160 mg/800 mg twice daily, or a fluoroquinolone (ofloxacin [Floxin]), 300 mg twice daily, or ciprofloxacin (Cipro), 500 mg twice daily, can be prescribed, and the patient can be sent home. The patient should be instructed to rest, hydrate himself, and use analgesics as necessary. A 30-day course of antibiotics will complete therapy.

If the patient is very ill or septic, he should be admitted to the hospital and placed on intravenous antibiotics, such as an ampicillin/aminoglycoside combination or an intravenous fluoroquinolone. Again, the patient should be placed at bed rest and given intravenous hydration and round-the-clock analgesics. Once the acute phase of the illness is over, the patient can be sent home on oral antibiotics to complete a 30-day course. If symptoms do not resolve or leukocytosis persists, a prostatic abscess should be suspected. This can be diagnosed by transrectal ultrasound or computed tomography scan and drained appropriately.

Once the patient is over the acute event, an intravenous urogram should be obtained to rule out any anatomic or other abnormality. Also, prostatic localization cultures should be obtained after completion of antibiotic therapy to rule out conversion to chronic bacterial prostatitis.

Chronic bacterial prostatitis should be suspected when older men present with recurrent urinary tract infections or asymptomatic bacteriuria. It is extremely unlikely in the absence of a history of recurrent episodes of bacterial cystitis. Other presentations can include perineal or low back pain, suprapubic fullness or pain, and irritative voiding symptoms and/or pain during or after ejaculation. Any or all of these symptoms may be present, and they may wax and wane. Fever does not usually occur, and the prostate examination is normal, although a boggy, indurated gland may be found. Prostatic crepitus may also be a sign of chronic bacterial infection.

Diagnosis is made by performing a prostatic massage and finding inflammation (>10 to 15 white blood cells per high-power field) and a culture-positive prostatic fluid. A urinalysis and urine culture specimen should also be obtained. Gram-negative organisms, as in acute bacterial prostatitis, are most common. Several gram-positive organisms that commonly colonize the anterior urethra have recently been implicated by some investigators. These include *Staphylococcus epidermidis, Staphylococcus aureus, Streptococcus faecalis*, non–group D streptococci, and diphtheroids. The mechanism by which bacteria infect the prostate has not been conclusively proved. Some theories include direct infection from the urethra, reflux of infected urine into the prostate via the prostatic ducts, hematogenous or lymphatic spread, and extension of rectal bacteria.

Treatment involves a 12- to 16-week course of oral trimethoprim-sulfamethoxazole (Bactrim, Septra), fluoroquinolones (ofloxacin, ciprofloxacin), or tetracyclines. Relapse occurs most commonly with *P. aeruginosa* infection. Prostatic stones found on transrectal ultrasound examination of the prostate can occasionally harbor infection. If the infection persists after antibiotic treatment and prostatic calculi exist, unroofing and removal of the stones may be indicated. Some patients who have recurrent symptoms or experience relief only while on antibiotics may benefit from chronic suppressive therapy with low-dose antibiotics. Trimethoprim-sulfamethoxazole or doxycycline can be used.

Nonbacterial prostatitis is the most common form of prostatitis, occurring eight times more often than bacterial prostatitis. Like other forms of prostatitis, it can be characterized by perineal, suprapubic, or low back pain and irritative or obstructive voiding symptoms. Unlike bacterial prostatitis, patients do not have urinary tract infections or positive cultures from urine or prostatic secretions after prostatic massage. However, these prostatic secretions do show inflammation (>10 to 15 white blood cells per high-power field).

The etiology of this symptomatology and inflammation has not been conclusively identified. Various organisms, such as *Chlamydia trachomatis, Ureaplasma urealyticum, Mycoplasma hominis,* and *Trichomonas vaginalis*, have been implicated, but many of these organisms can be found in the normal male urethra. Rare organisms such as *Mycobacterium tuberculosis* or fungi such as *Coccidioides, Histoplasma,* and *Candida* must also be ruled out. Therapy is still directed at these organisms.

A 2- to 4-week course of doxycycline (100 mg twice daily) or erythromycin (500 mg four times daily) may give some relief. Nonsteroidal anti-inflammatory drugs (NSAIDs) and sitz baths should be prescribed and normal sexual activity encouraged. The patient should be counseled to avoid spicy foods, caffeine, and alcohol, as they can aggravate symptoms. Furthermore, the patient should be reassured that nonbacterial prostatitis is not life-threatening and is usually self-limiting. If symptoms do persist, then the patient should be referred to a urologist to rule out more serious entities, such as carcinoma in situ of the bladder, interstitial cystitis, or stricture disease.

Prostatodynia is a symptom complex of unknown etiology that occurs in young to middle-aged men that may be the result of multiple pelvic disorders. These patients have back, perineal, and pelvic pain, as in prostatitis, but do not have urinary tract infections or inflammation in EPS. They also have a normal physical examination. These patients should have a full urodynamic evaluation and cystoscopy to identify specific entities and rule out other bladder, prostatic, or urethral pathology. A careful rectal examination and sigmoidoscopy may be necessary to rule out rectal pathology such as fistulas.

The differential diagnosis of this entity includes urinary sphincter dyssynergia, tension myalgia of the pelvic musculature, stress, and emotional disorders. Sphincter dyssynergia is a lack of coordination between the urinary sphincter and the bladder that can cause significant voiding dysfunction. This can be treated with alphablockers or incision of the bladder neck. Pelvic tension myalgia is increased tension of the musculature of the pelvic floor and is treated with muscle relaxants and benzodiazepines. Usually, however, a concrete diagnosis cannot be identified, and treatment is targeted to the symptoms. Again, as in most forms of prostatitis, NSAIDs and sitz baths should be prescribed. Also, the avoidance of spicy foods, caffeine, and alcohol along with engagement in normal sexual activity should be encouraged. Stool softeners may also help. The patient should be reassured that prostatodynia is usually self-limiting and not life-threatening. Psychological evaluation and counseling may enhance treatment in certain patients.

BENIGN PROSTATIC HYPERPLASIA

method of
ROBERT R. ISACKSEN, M.D., and
JOHN S. WHEELER, JR., M.D.
Loyola University Medical Center
Maywood, Illinois

Benign prostatic hyperplasia (BPH) is a common histologic finding in men and a common cause of voiding symptoms leading men to seek treatment. Histologic evidence of BPH is found in more than 50% of 60-year-old men and in 90% of men by age 85 years. Although many men are not afflicted with urinary symptoms related to BPH, it is estimated that one in four men will have received surgical treatment for BPH by age 80 years. In 1990, more than 300,000 operations were performed for BPH at a cost of over two billion dollars. Subsequent scrutiny has revealed wide variation in practice patterns across the United States. These factors, coupled with the emergence of new medical and surgical therapies, necessitate that all providers of care to this patient population reassess critically their approach to the diagnosis and management of BPH.

ETIOLOGY AND PATHOPHYSIOLOGY

The exact etiology and pathogenesis of BPH are not completely understood. The two most clearly defined risk factors are advancing age and the presence of androgens. Autopsy studies have shown that the incidence of BPH increases steadily as men grow older. Deprivation studies have proved a role for androgens in both the establishment and maintenance of BPH.

Three factors are believed to contribute to clinically significant BPH, the constellation of symptoms known as prostatism: mechanical urethral outlet obstruction, dynamic urethral outlet obstruction, and detrusor dysfunction.

Hyperplastic nodules consisting primarily of glandular elements develop in the transition or periurethral zone of the prostate gland. As these nodules enlarge they compress both the surrounding prostatic tissue and the urethra, leading to bladder outlet (urethral) obstruction. In addition to this static, mechanical component of obstruction, the prostatic capsule and proximal urethra are rich in smooth muscle, and in alpha-adrenergic and cholinergic innervation. This creates a dynamic component of obstruction that fluctuates with autonomic stimulation.

Changes in detrusor function account for some of the symptoms associated with BPH. It is believed that the high voiding pressures required to overcome outlet obstruction lead to decreased bladder compliance, detrusor instability, and hypertrophy and trabeculation of the bladder. Eventually, detrusor failure may lead to upper urinary tract pathology.

SYMPTOMS

Symptoms of prostatism are commonly classified as either obstructive or irritative in nature. Irritative symptoms are attributed to alterations in detrusor function and include frequency, urgency, urge incontinence, dysuria, and nocturia. Obstructive symptoms include decreased force and caliber of the urinary stream, hesitancy in initiating micturition, straining to void, postvoid dribbling, and the sensation of incomplete bladder emptying. Occasionally, an asymptomatic patient with "silent prostatism" will be discovered by finding a palpable bladder on physical examination, bilateral hydronephrosis as an incidental radiologic finding, or previously unsuspected azotemia.

Treatment for clinical BPH is guided largely by the patient's symptoms and the degree to which they impair quality of life. The development of scoring systems allows for the accurate assessment of the severity of symptoms attributed to BPH. The American Urological Association (AUA) symptom-scoring system accurately and reproducibly assesses seven common symptoms of prostatism (Table 1). This provides a reliable method of quantification of voiding symptoms for the initial evaluation and for subsequent assessment, whether to monitor results of therapy or to follow the course of watchful waiting.

Although BPH is the most common cause of the voiding symptoms measured by the AUA score, these symptoms are nonspecific, and 15 to 20% of symptomatic men will have a diagnosis other than BPH. An elevated AUA symptom score is not necessarily diagnostic of bladder outlet obstruction due to BPH. A thorough history and physical examination are essential in directing the diagnosis and to rule out other causes of voiding dysfunction (Figure 1).

DIAGNOSIS

The history should begin with the onset, duration, and severity of the chief complaint. Completion of the AUA symptom index questionnaire will be valuable in patients with symptoms of prostatism. Detailed urologic history should include inquiry regarding urinary tract infection, hematuria, urethritis, strictures, stones, dysuria, incontinence, and prior urologic surgery or instrumentation. Comorbid illness such as diabetes and neurologic disease and a history of spine surgery or trauma are important considerations in directing a more in-depth work-up. The physical examination should specifically include a careful digital rectal examination and a focused neurologic examination. In the absence of specific indications, initial laboratory work-up should be limited to urinalysis and serum blood urea nitrogen and creatinine. This will rule out hematuria, infection, glucosuria, and occult renal insufficiency. The AUA recommends annual serum prostate-specific antigen (PSA) testing in men over 50 years of age to screen for prostate cancer.

Two simple diagnostic measurements that may easily be performed in the urologist's office are postvoid residual urine volume and urinary flow rate. Measuring the urinary flow rate is helpful in confirming a decreased force of stream. Men with significant symptoms but a normal urinary flow rate may have a diagnosis other than bladder outlet obstruction. The postvoid residual urine volume is easily measured by urethral catheterization or by office ultrasonography, a less invasive technique. This information may be useful for serial examinations or to guide initial treatment.

Critical evaluation of the benefits of further diagnostic studies has called into question the need for tests that in the past have been routine. Radiologic studies such as renal ultrasound, intravenous pyelography, and transrectal ultrasound (TRUS) of the prostate are not routinely indicated. Similarly, cystometric studies add little to the diagnosis and are rarely indicated in patients with simple BPH.

Complete urodynamic evaluation with bladder pressure–urinary flow studies is indicated in patients with significant symptoms but a normal flow rate. These studies are also helpful in patients with low flow rates who are suspected of having significant detrusor failure due to diabetes or other neurologic disease, thereby differentiating those with outlet obstruction from those with bladder dysfunction. Pressure-flow studies, combined with fluoroscopy, are the "gold standard" for evaluating and differentiating urethral obstruction and should be utilized in complex cases.

Cystourethroscopy is not routinely indicated. However, a history of transurethral surgery or urethral strictures, or the presence of infection or hematuria is an indication for cystoscopy. Cystoscopy may also be used to rule out bladder carcinoma in situ in patients with predominantly irritative voiding symptoms. In the absence of specific indications, cystourethroscopy is most appropriately used to guide the surgeon in choosing a surgical approach based on the cystoscopic appearance of the prostate in patients for whom surgical therapy has been selected. In such cases, cystoscopy should be performed immediately prior to the planned surgical procedure.

TREATMENT OPTIONS

Watchful Waiting

The natural history of untreated prostatism is variable. A substantial proportion of patients will have symptomatic improvement over time, whereas others will experience stable or worsening symptoms. Watchful waiting consists of reassurance, counseling,

TABLE 1. **American Urological Association Symptom Index**

Questions to Be Answered	Not at All	Less Than 1 Time in 5	Less Than Half the Time	About Half the Time	More Than Half the Time	Almost Always
Considering the past month:						
1. How often have you had a sensation of not emptying your bladder completely after you finished urinating?	0	1	2	3	4	5
2. How often have you had to urinate again less than 2 hours after you finished urinating?	0	1	2	3	4	5
3. How often have you found you stopped and started again several times when you urinated?	0	1	2	3	4	5
4. How often have you found it difficult to postpone urination?	0	1	2	3	4	5
5. How often have you had a weak urinary stream?	0	1	2	3	4	5
6. How often have you had to push or strain to begin urination?	0	1	2	3	4	5
7. How many times did you most typically get up to urinate from the time you went to bed at night until the time you got up in the morning?	0 (none)	1 (1 time)	2 (2 times)	3 (3 times)	4 (4 times)	5 ($\geq$5 times)

The sum of 1 through 7 responses is the AUA symptom score (0–35).

Adapted from McConnell JD, Barry MJ, Bruskewitz RC, et al: Benign prostatic hyperplasia: Diagnosis and treatment. Clinical Practice Guideline, No. 8. AHCPR Publication No. 94-0582. Rockville, MD, Agency for Health Care Policy and Research, Public Health Service, U.S. Department of Health and Human Services, 1994.

annual re-evaluation with the AUA symptom score, digital rectal examination, and appropriate laboratory studies. The risk of an adverse event such as a urinary tract infection or acute urinary retention is low, and many patients with mild-to-moderate symptoms will appropriately choose watchful waiting.

Medical Management

Alpha Antagonists. Doxazosin (Cardura) and terazosin (Hytrin) are selective alpha$_1$-adrenergic antagonists approved by the Food and Drug Administration for the treatment of BPH. Selective alpha antagonists have more favorable side effect profiles than nonselective alpha blockers. Most patients will experience modest improvement in urinary flow rate and a decrease in symptom scores. These changes are durable at 4 years' follow-up, but a significant number of patients may discontinue therapy because of side effects, inadequate response to therapy, or for other reasons. Side effects occur in 10% to 15% of patients and include dizziness, asthenia, and somnolence.

Finasteride. Finasteride (Proscar) is a 5-alpha-reductase inhibitor that blocks the conversion of testosterone to dihydrotestosterone, the active form of testosterone in the prostate. Serum testosterone levels are not affected. It is effective in decreasing prostate size by approximately 20% to 25% after 3 to 6 months of therapy, thereby reducing the mechanical component of outlet obstruction. Improvement in maximum urinary flow rate and symptom scores has

been demonstrated, and in patients electing to continue therapy these findings appear durable at 3 years' follow-up. Finasteride decreases serum prostate-specific antigen (PSA) by about 50%, and it is not known how this will alter PSA effectiveness as a screening tool for cancer. Serum PSA should be determined prior to initiating finasteride therapy and again after 6 months of treatment. Side effects are minimal but include diminished ejaculate volume or decreased libido in approximately 5% to 10% of patients.

Other Hormonal Therapies. Several other forms of androgen deprivation therapy have been evaluated for the treatment of BPH, including gonadotropic hormone–releasing hormone (GnRH) agonists, true antiandrogens such as flutamide (Eulexin),* and progestational agents. Significant side effects and insufficient treatment efficacy prevent the use of this class of drugs for BPH.

Combination Medical Therapy. Given the mechanical and dynamic element of symptomatic BPH, it has been theorized that some patients might benefit from combined alpha blockade and hormonal treatment. A large multi-institutional study is currently underway to evaluate the efficacy of terazosin combined with finasteride for the treatment of BPH. Outcome data are not yet available.

Surgical Therapy

Transurethral Resection of the Prostate. TURP is the standard by which other surgical and medical

---

*Not FDA-approved for this indication.

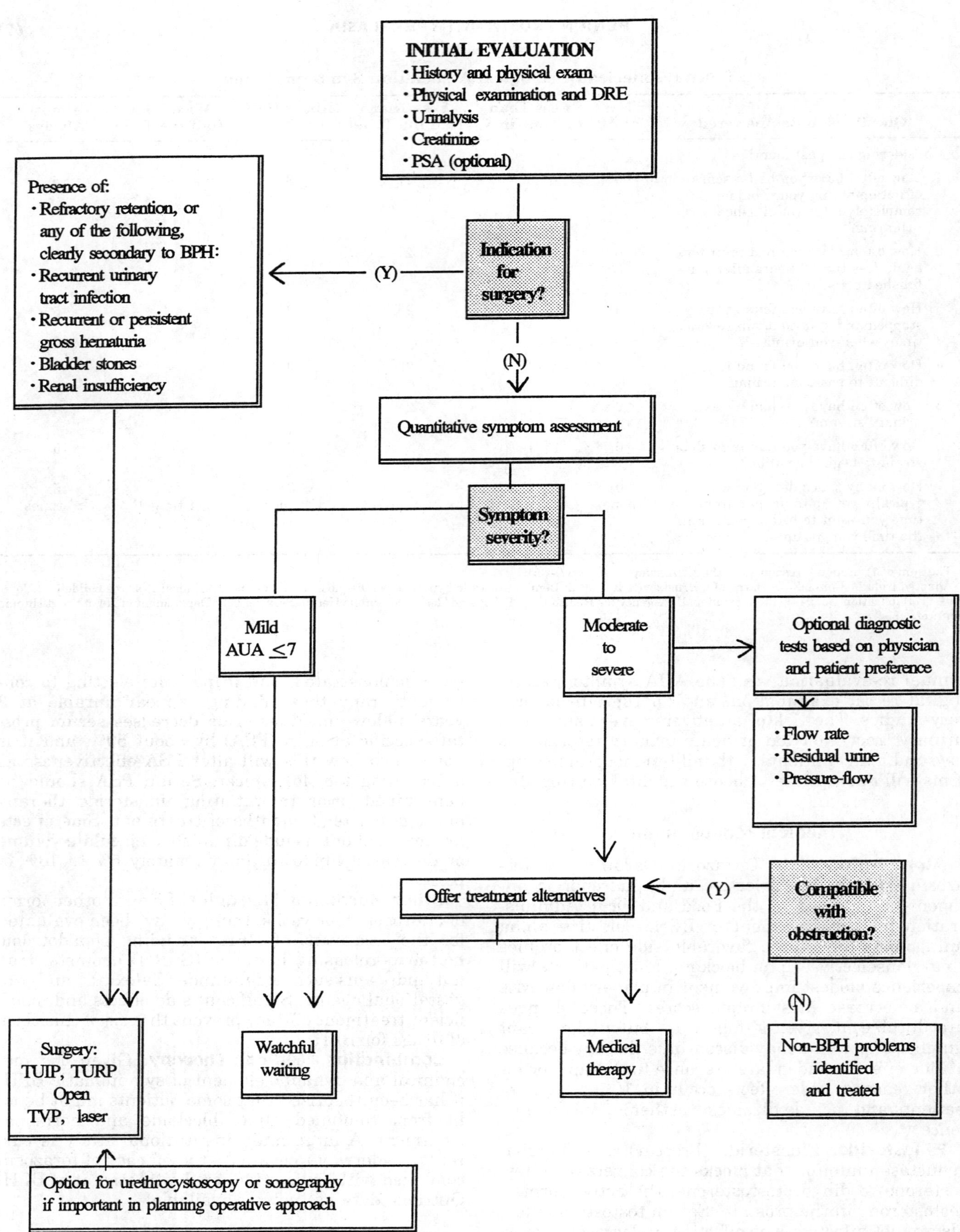

Figure 1. Benign prostatic hyperplasia; treatment options for patients with moderate to severe symptoms. (Adapted from McConnell JD, Barry MJ, Bruskewitz RC, et al: Benign prostatic hyperplasia: Diagnosis and treatment. Clinical Practice Guideline, No. 8. ACHCPR Publication No. 94-0582. Rockville, MD, Agency for Health Care Policy and Research, Public Health Service, U.S. Department of Health and Human Services, 1994.)

therapies are measured. Under spinal or general anesthesia, a resectoscope is used to remove the adenomatous hyperplastic tissue obstructing the urethra. Urethral catheterization and hospitalization are typically required for 3 days. Of all therapies, TURP is most likely to produce substantial symptomatic improvement, with approximately 90% of patients reporting significant reduction in symptom scores. Complications include retrograde ejaculation in 70%, incontinence in 1% to 2%, strictures or bladder neck contracture in 3%, and retreatment rates (for recurrent BPH or other complications) of 10% at 5 years postoperatively. Additional risks include the need for blood transfusion in up to 10%, transurethral resection syndrome (excess absorption of irrigant) in 2%, and impotence in 10% to 15% of patients.

Transurethral Incision of the Prostate. TUIP is an ideal procedure for men with outlet obstruction but a small prostate gland that is estimated to be less than 30 grams of resectable tissue. The prostate is endoscopically incised, rather than resected, extending from the bladder neck to the verumontanum. In appropriately selected patients, TUIP is nearly as effective as TURP in relieving symptoms. It can be performed as outpatient surgery and has significantly lower risks of retrograde ejaculation (25%), incontinence (0.1% to 1%), and blood transfusion (1%). Retreatment rates are similar to those of TURP.

Transurethral Electrovaporization of the Prostate. TVP is a modification of TURP that utilizes standard resectoscope equipment and a specially designed grooved roller element to vaporize prostatic tissue. High-power cutting current allows vaporization of tissue with little or no bleeding and no significant fluid absorption. Potential advantages over TURP include shorter hospitalization, early catheter removal, and less risk of bleeding. Short-term improvements in symptom scores and urinary flow rate are similar to those of TURP. Long-term controlled studies are underway for this promising new modality.

Open Prostatectomy. This is performed via a lower abdominal midline incision, and either a transvesical (suprapubic) or extravesical (retropubic) approach may be used. This procedure relieves symptoms in nearly all patients, but it is associated with the morbidity and longer recovery time inherent to an open surgical procedure. It is usually reserved for patients with very large prostates or with another indication for open bladder surgery, such as a large bladder stone or diverticulum.

Laser Ablation. Laser energy has been used with increasing frequency to treat symptomatic BPH. The fiber can be directed either by transrectal ultrasound guidance or cystoscopically under direct vision. Depending on the type of fiber used, tissue may be either directly vaporized or allowed to slough postoperatively from laser-induced coagulation necrosis. Laser prostatectomy has been shown to reduce symptoms, although not as effectively as TURP. Long-term success rates and retreatment rates are un-

known. Laser prostatectomy can be performed as outpatient surgery and is not associated with significant risk of bleeding or TUR syndrome. Long-term controlled studies are needed to further evaluate this modality.

Balloon Dilatation. Balloon dilatation of the prostate was met with initial enthusiasm as a minimally invasive, low-morbidity treatment for BPH. Long-term outcomes have been disappointing, however, and some data suggest it has no more efficacy than simple cystoscopy. It is not a widely used therapy for BPH.

Stents. Prostatic stents have been utilized for the treatment of BPH, particularly in individuals who are poor candidates for more invasive surgery. These expandable prostheses are placed transurethrally using a cystoscope and delivery device. Problems have included irritative voiding symptoms, stent encrustation, and stent migration. The majority of patients experience symptomatic improvement, but long-term data are not yet available. Prostatic stents remain an experimental modality at present.

Experimental Therapies. Numerous other techniques are being studied for the treatment of BPH: microwave thermotherapy, transurethral needle ablation using radiofrequency energy, ultrasonic ablation, and cryosurgery. These experimental techniques are not available for general clinical use.

SELECTING APPROPRIATE THERAPY

A significant number of patients will have an absolute indication for surgery at the time of their initial presentation. These indications include persistent or recurrent gross hematuria, urinary tract infection, bladder stones, uremia due to obstruction, and refractory urinary retention. Those patients with minimal symptoms—that is, an AUA score less than or equal to 7—should be followed with watchful waiting. The disadvantages of any medical or surgical intervention outweigh the possibility of improving such minimal symptoms.

Many more treatment options exist for those patients with an AUA score greater than or equal to 8 who have moderate-to-severe symptoms (see Figure 1). The selection of therapy for these patients will largely be determined by their expectations, preferences, and the degree to which they are bothered by their symptoms. It is the physician's responsibility to elicit this information from an informed patient. The risks and benefits of each form of medical and surgical treatment must be presented. Specifically, each therapy must be considered in terms of the likelihood and degree of symptom improvement, the durability of treatment, retreatment and failure rates, and the risk of morbidity or side effects.

ERECTILE DYSFUNCTION

method of
SANSERN BORIRAKCHANYAVAT, M.D., and
TOM F. LUE, M.D.
University of California, San Francisco
San Francisco, California

Erectile dysfunction (impotence) is defined as the inability to achieve and maintain adequate penile erection for satisfactory sexual intercourse. It has been estimated that approximately 10 to 18 million men in the United States suffer from erectile dysfunction. Recent advances in the understanding of erectile physiology have led to improvements in both the diagnostic and therapeutic approaches to the treatment of erectile dysfunction. Historically, it had been thought that the development of erectile dysfunction was normal to the aging process or due to poorly defined psychological causes. We now understand that in most cases, an organic etiology can be found. This discussion outlines the current diagnostic and therapeutic approaches to the treatment of the patient with erectile dysfunction.

ERECTILE PHYSIOLOGY

The erectile bodies of the penis can best be thought of as specialized vascular structures. Histologically, the erectile tissue is composed of vascular spaces within a smooth muscle and connective tissue stroma. The erectile tissue is encased within a relatively nondistensible connective tissue sheath called the tunica albuginea. Arterial blood flows into the corpora cavernosa by way of the paired penile arteries that are derived from the internal pudendal arteries. Venous outflow occurs by way of a complex intercommunicating venous system. During appropriate stimulation, neurotransmitters (among them, nitric oxide is believed to be the most important) are released, which produce arterial dilatation and smooth muscle relaxation and thus engorgement of the erectile bodies. Concurrently, venous outflow from the penis is severely restricted by compression of the subtunical venules. The sequential combination of neurotransmitter release, increased arterial inflow, and restriction of venous outflow is necessary to produce a normal penile erection.

CLASSIFICATION OF ERECTILE DYSFUNCTION

As previously noted, erectile dysfunction can be roughly classified into those cases due to *organic* etiologies and those arising from *psychogenic* causes (Table 1). Owing to a better understanding of erectile physiology, it is not surprising that organic erectile dysfunction can be further divided into many subcategories. *Hormonal deficiencies* may occasionally present with erectile dysfunction. Patients with Klinefelter's syndrome or prolactin-secreting pituitary tumors can initially present with erectile dysfunction. *Neurogenic erectile dysfunction* most commonly occurs as a result of trauma to the cavernous nerves following pelvic surgery, pelvic fracture, or spinal cord injury. *Vasculogenic erectile dysfunction* is likely the most common form of organic impotence and can be further classified into arteriogenic and venogenic. *Arteriogenic erectile dysfunction* occurs as a result of insufficient arterial inflow into the penis. Arteriogenic insufficiency can result from many causes, including atherosclerotic disease, diabetes mellitus, and traumatic disruption of the penile arteries. *Venogenic erectile dysfunction* is defined as the inability to trap blood within the corpora cavernosa in order to achieve and maintain an adequate erection. Venogenic erectile dysfunction may be congenital due to abnormal communicating veins or acquired secondary to sinusoidal fibrosis, smooth muscle atrophy, or priapism. Although these categories are helpful in the assessment of each patient, in many cases more than one contributing etiology can be found.

Although its prevalence has been undoubtedly overestimated in the past, *psychogenic factors* have long been known to contribute to the pathogenesis of erectile dysfunction. To aid in the treatment of these patients, the authors have further classified psychogenic factors into the following categories: (1) marital/partner conflict; (2) ignorance/misinformation regarding normal sexual function; (3) sexual deviancy, anhedonia; and (4) fear, performance anxiety. Early recognition of the presence of psychogenically based impotence can help avoid the costly evaluation of an extended organic erectile dysfunction work-up.

HISTORY AND PHYSICAL EXAMINATION

The evaluation of patients with erectile dysfunction begins with a thorough history and physical examination. A general medical history should be obtained, including all medical illnesses and past surgeries. A detailed sexual history is crucial to the evaluation of erectile dysfunction. Sexual history should include the onset and duration of erectile dysfunction, changes in libido, and an inventory of all sexual partners. Common medical illnesses such as hypertension, coronary artery disease, diabetes mellitus, and renal insufficiency can lend important clues to the organic etiology of erectile dysfunction. Medications such as antihypertensives and histamine receptor (H_2) blockers may occasionally produce erectile dysfunction as a side effect. On the other hand, a healthy young patient with an extensive psychiatric history is much more likely to have a psychogenic component contributing to erectile dysfunction. Surgical history of radical pelvic surgery (e.g., abdominoperineal resection, radical prostatectomy) or severe pelvic trauma can often result in neurogenic and/or vasculogenic erectile dysfunction. A recent history of erectile dysfunction associated with decreased libido suggests an underlying endocrinopathy.

Although physical examination is often normal, it may nevertheless yield important information regarding the etiology of erectile dysfunction. Physical examination may reveal an obvious impediment to intercourse such as a micropenis or penile curvature. Gynecomastia, decreased libido, and erectile dysfunction are often the first presenting sign of a prolactin-secreting tumor. The presence of small atrophic testes is an indication of hypogonadism. Congenital syndromes such as Klinefelter's syndrome and Kallman's syndrome may also present with obvious physical characteristics and body habitus.

LABORATORY EVALUATION

The laboratory evaluation is directed at finding treatable medical conditions that may be contributing to the develop-

TABLE 1. **Classification of Erectile Dysfunction**

Organic Etiology	Psychogenic Etiology
Vasculogenic	Marital conflict
Arteriogenic	Ignorance/misinformation of normal
Venogenic	sexual function
Neurogenic	Sexual deviancy/psychiatric disturbances
Hormonal deficiency	Performance anxiety

ment of erectile dysfunction. Screening laboratory tests include urinalysis, serum electrolytes, glucose, lipid profile, and renal panel. Conditions such as renal insufficiency and undiagnosed diabetes may contribute to the development of erectile dysfunction. A screening hormonal evaluation with serum testosterone and prolactin is helpful in ruling out an underlying endocrinopathy. Due to the low incidence of endocrine dysfunction in the impotent patient population, some investigators suggest that a hormonal evaluation need only be performed in patients with physical signs of hypogonadism. However, erectile dysfunction can occasionally be the first presenting symptom of a serious life-threatening illness such as a prolactin-secreting tumor. For this reason, the authors believe that most patients with erectile dysfunction should undergo a baseline screening hormonal evaluation.

Although the range of normal testosterone levels is quite large, an abnormally low testosterone level may indicate an underlying endocrinopathy. Due to the cyclical nature of testosterone secretion, abnormal levels (<200 ng/dL) should be repeated and confirmed. Persistently elevated serum prolactin (>22 ng/ml) levels should prompt a search for a prolactin-secreting pituitary tumor.

DIAGNOSTIC EVALUATION OF ERECTILE DYSFUNCTION

Owing to recent advances in the understanding of erectile physiology and imaging technology, the authors perform much of the evaluation of erectile dysfunction in the privacy of an office setting. Following the completion of a detailed history, physical examination and screening laboratory evaluation, the etiology of erectile dysfunction may still be unclear. Since the penile erectile bodies can be thought of as a specialized vascular organ, it is often helpful to obtain information regarding the vascular status of the penis. As previously mentioned, penile erection requires the sequential increase in penile arterial blood flow followed by a decrease in the penile venous return. Intracavernous injection of vasodilators such as papaverine or alprostadil (prostaglandin E_1) mimic the natural neurotransmitter release required for erection. Therefore, a simple screening evaluation for vasculogenic erectile dysfunction consists of an intracavernous injection of a vasodilating agent. The patient is then instructed to perform self-stimulation to achieve an erection. This particular method is known as the *combined injection and stimulation (CIS) test*. A full erection following intracavernous injection indicates the presence of an intact veno-occlusive mechanism. A small percentage of patients with marginal penile arterial flow can also produce a full erection, although the response may be somewhat delayed. However, a prompt and full response to intracavernous injection makes further evaluation for vasculogenic erectile dysfunction unnecessary.

An abnormal CIS test should prompt an evaluation directed at identifying a vascular or psychogenic cause of erectile dysfunction. Currently, *color-coded duplex ultrasonography* is the most useful examination in making the diagnosis of arteriogenic erectile dysfunction. The duplex ultrasound probe allows simultaneous high-resolution imaging of the three branches of the penile artery (dorsal, cavernosal, and spongiosal) as well as accurate measurement of arterial flow velocity. The ultrasound examination is performed before and after the injection of a vasodilating agent and self–genital stimulation. Normal peak systolic blood flow velocity in the cavernosal arteries during early erection should exceed 30 cm per second. In young patients who are candidates for surgical reconstruction of traumatic penile arterial injury, additional anatomic information can be gained by performing a *selective pudendal arteriography*. However, due to its invasive nature and high cost, arteriography should be restricted to only those patients who would clearly benefit from vascular reconstruction.

Venogenic erectile dysfunction is a difficult diagnosis to confirm. Often, venogenic erectile dysfunction is suspected only after a complete vascular evaluation has ruled out the possibility of arteriogenic erectile dysfunction. Currently, the most commonly used study to make the diagnosis of venogenic erectile dysfunction is *pharmacologic cavernosometry and cavernosography*. Similar to other functional studies of the penis, cavernosometry is performed following the intracavernous injection of a vasodilating agent. *Cavernosometry* consists of infusion of saline into the corpora cavernosa to generate an artificial erection and simultaneous monitoring of intracorporeal pressure. Venogenic erectile dysfunction is characterized by an inability to produce or maintain an erection even at high rates of saline infusion. *Cavernosography* consists of the infusion of dilute contrast material into the penis to radiographically detect the various sites of venous leakage.

Some investigators have recommended the use of *nocturnal penile tumescence (NPT)* studies in the routine evaluation of erectile dysfunction. In the authors' practice, NPT is used to help identify those patients with erectile dysfunction due to psychogenic causes. A normal nocturnal penile tumescence study indicates a probable psychogenic cause. Sophisticated nocturnal erection monitoring devices have been developed that measure the number of erection episodes, the rigidity of the penis, and the change in diameter of the penis. However, despite its long history and substantial cost, nocturnal penile tumescence studies have not proven to be adequately specific or sensitive in making the diagnosis of psychogenic erectile dysfunction. Therefore, the authors do not routinely use nocturnal penile tumescence studies in the evaluation of patients with erectile dysfunction.

TREATMENT OF ERECTILE DYSFUNCTION

Understanding the various pathophysiologic mechanisms of erectile dysfunction has allowed the clinician to offer a greater range of therapeutic modalities. In general, the treatment of erectile dysfunction can be subdivided into the nonsurgical and surgical modalities.

Nonsurgical Modalities

Many patients will opt for nonsurgical treatment of erectile dysfunction. It is the authors' practice to offer nonsurgical treatment to the patient initially. If these treatments prove to be unsatisfactory, surgical approaches can be offered. Elimination of offending medications and treatment of reversible causes are the first steps in the management of erectile dysfunction. Change of lifestyle such as instituting a regimen of regular exercise, appropriate diet, and cessation of smoking and excessive alcohol use may also be of benefit.

Vacuum constriction devices (VCD) are a popular and effective treatment for many patients. These devices employ a vacuum chamber to generate negative

TABLE 2. **Treatment Options for Erectile Dysfunction**

Nonsurgical Modalities
Vacuum Constriction Device (VCD)
Oral Pharmacologic Therapy

	Dose Range
Yohimbine (Yocon)	5.4 mg PO tid
Trazodone (Desyrel)*	150 mg PO qhs
Pentoxifylline (Trental)*	400 mg PO tid
Bupropion (Wellbutrin)*	100 mg PO bid

Intracavernous Injection (ICI)

	Dose Range
Prostaglandin E_1 (Caverject)	1–60 µg IC PRN
Papaverine*/phentolamine*	0.1–1.0 mL IC
PGE_1/papaverine*	
Phentolamine*	0.1–1.0 mL IC

Hormonal Replacement

	Dose Range
Testosterone	200 mg IM q 2–3 wk
Transdermal testosterone (Testoderm)	5 mg qd

Psychosexual Therapy

Surgical Modalities
Penile Prosthesis
Arterial Revascularization
Penile Venous Surgery

*Not FDA-approved for this indication.

pressure and draw blood into the erectile bodies. The artificial erection is then maintained by a constriction ring placed around the base of the penis and can be safely maintained for up to 30 minutes at a time. The success of the device is dependent on the presence of adequate arterial flow to the corporeal bodies. Therefore, patients with severe penile arterial insufficiency may not be able to employ the device successfully. Some patients and their partners may find the necessity of the constriction ring unacceptable.

Pharmacologic treatments such as oral yohimbine, trazodone, Trental, and Wellbutrin have been used with marginal positive effect. Others such as oral phosphodiesterase inhibitors, sublingual apomorphine, and intraurethral alprostadil (PGE_1) are currently in clinical trials and may provide more effective treatment.

Pharmacologic *intracavernous injection (ICI)* of a vasodilating agent has revolutionized the nonsurgical treatment of impotence. Currently, the regimens most commonly prescribed are alprostadil (prostaglandin E_1), (Caverject), papaverine* with phentolamine* (Regitine),* or a combination of all three agents (Table 2). Intracavernous injection bypasses the natural neurotransmitter release of the intracavernous nerves and produces penile erection. A solution of the vasodilating agents is injected into a corporeal body using a 28- or 29-gauge needle. The area of injection is then massaged to prevent hematoma formation. An erection is usually produced within 15 minutes of the injection and is maintained for 30 to 40 minutes. Intracavernous injection is well tolerated and effective in up to 80% of patients. Adverse effects of ICI include priapism, hematoma formation, pain, and scarring at the injection site. Successful treatment using intracavernous injection also requires adequate penile arterial inflow and a competent veno-

*Not FDA-approved for this indication.

occlusive mechanism. Therefore, patients with severe arteriogenic or venous leak impotence may respond poorly to intracavernous injection.

For those patients with impotence secondary to hypogonadism, *hormonal replacement* with testosterone injection or transdermal (Testoderm) patches may improve libido and quality of erections. It is generally believed that testosterone influences the quality of erections mainly through central effects on libido rather than direct effects on the penile tissue itself. As previously mentioned, due to the cyclical secretion of the hormone, the diagnosis of hypogonadism should be confirmed by several serum testosterone measurements. Repeat measurements of serum testosterone levels should be obtained during the treatment period to confirm a therapeutic level. Only patients with the diagnosis of hypogonadism should be treated with hormonal replacement.

Erectile dysfunction owing to fear, anxiety, partner conflict, and sexual misinformation can be successfully treated with *psychosexual therapy*. Erectile dysfunction owing to severe depression or psychological disturbances is more resistant to treatment and often requires pharmacologic treatment of the underlying psychiatric disorder. In these more resistant cases, psychosexual therapy can be used in combination with nonsurgical modalities such as vacuum constriction devices or intracavernous injection.

Surgical Modalities

Surgical treatment of erectile dysfunction is safe and successful in the appropriately selected patient. Surgical treatment of impotence is generally reserved for those patients who fail to respond to nonsurgical therapy. The most commonly used surgical modality is the placement of a *penile prosthesis*. Although there are many different types of prostheses available, the choice of the particular device is dependent primarily on patient needs and preferences. The placement of a penile prosthesis offers a long-term solution to impotence for many patients. Complications of penile prostheses are relatively rare but include device failure, erosion through the penis or urethra, and infection.

For carefully selected patients with arteriogenic erectile dysfunction, *arterial revascularization* can be used to restore blood flow to the penis. A selective pudendal arteriogram is required to delineate the vascular anatomy and plan the operative approach. Surgical revascularization is primarily reserved for younger patients with discrete traumatic disruption of the penile arteries. In contrast, the older patient with diffuse atherosclerotic disease is unlikely to benefit from arterial revascularization. Arterial revascularization most commonly employs the inferior epigastric artery as the donor vessel, which is then anastomosed to the recipient vessel. For some patients with venous leak erectile dysfunction, *penile venous surgery* procedures have been employed with some success. However, the long-term results of penile venous ligation procedures to correct venogenic erectile dysfunction have been disappointing due to the development of venous collaterals.

ACUTE RENAL FAILURE

method of
JIM REICHMAN, M.D., and
MAYER BREZIS, M.D.
Hadassah University Hospital
Jerusalem, Israel

Acute renal failure (ARF) is a clinical entity characterized by an abrupt (hours to days) decline in renal function resulting in the retention of nitrogenous waste products and a perturbation of water, electrolyte, and acid-base balance. It is typically associated with daily increments in serum urea and creatinine levels greater than 10 and 0.5 mg per dL, respectively. ARF is frequently encountered, occurring in approximately 5% of all hospitalized patients and in up to 30% of intensive care unit admissions. Oliguria (urine output <400 mL per day) is observed in 50% of cases of ARF, with an associated mortality of 50 to 80%. Nonoliguric ARF portends a better prognosis, with mortality rates of 15 to 40%. Many cases of ARF are iatrogenic, induced by unnecessary procedures or medications. If primary care and hospital physicians are cognizant of the indications and potential nephrotoxicities of each medication and invasive procedure prescribed, the incidence of ARF may be curbed.

The etiologies of ARF are divided into three categories: prerenal, intrinsic, and postrenal (Table 1). This classification facilitates the diagnostic process and the application of therapeutic modalities. Prerenal ARF is consequent to renal hypoperfusion and denotes a functional impairment without renal parenchymal damage. It is responsible for 55 to 70% of cases of ARF. Renal hypoperfusion is often due to an absolute decrease in blood volume (hemorrhage, diarrhea, vomiting, diuretics) or a relative decrease in effective blood volume (cardiac failure, hypoalbuminemia, cirrhosis). Careful balance of the volume status in these patients may obviate progression to the prerenal state. Renal arterial occlusion (thromboemboli) and systemic vasodilatation (sepsis, anaphylaxis) also impair kidney perfusion. Drug-induced renal vasoconstriction (cyclosporine, norepinephrine) and hypoperfusion (nonsteroidal anti-inflammatory drugs [NSAIDs]) constitutes a widespread iatrogenic cause of prerenal ARF. These medications, particulary angiotensin-converting enzyme (ACE) inhibitors, are extremely hazardous in the presence of hypoperfusion or high renin output and should be supplanted by alternative drugs in these settings.

Between 25 and 40% of cases of ARF may be ascribed to intrinsic renal damage. Primary glomerular disease and secondary glomerulonephritis (systemic lupus erythematosus [SLE], postinfectious) reduce renal blood flow, and ARF may ensue. Vascular etiologies of intrinsic ARF (malignant hypertension, vasopressors, contrast, thromboemboli) are more prevalent in patients with hypertension, coronary artery atherosclerosis, or peripheral vascular disease. Prolonged renal ischemia (as for prerenal ARF), endogenous toxins (myoglobin, hemoglobin, uric acid), and exogenous toxins (aminoglycosides, amphotericin B, contrast) can all produce acute tubular necrosis, accounting for about 90% of cases of intrinsic ARF. Acute tubulointerstitial nephritis following various infections, malignancies, or drug use may

precipitate intrinsic ARF. Patients with chronic renal failure, volume depletion, or oliguria have a predilection for the development of intrinsic ARF, which typically evolves in the setting of combined risk factors and additional insults (contrast). Recognition of these predisposing conditions prior to ordering diagnostic tests and administering drugs will discourage indiscriminate imaging with radiocontrast and encourage scrupulous risk/benefit analysis.

Postrenal ARF, constituting 5% of cases of ARF, indicates obstruction of the urethra or bladder neck, bilateral ureteric obstruction, or unilateral ureteric obstruction in patients with one functioning kidney or chronic renal failure. Common etiologies include ureteral calculi, blood clots, neoplasms, prostatic hypertrophy or malignancy, retroperitoneal fibrosis, or neurogenic bladder. Analgesic-induced papillary necrosis is a cause of postrenal ARF seen in patients with rheumatoid arthritis or chronic lower back pain.

DIAGNOSIS

History

A thorough history is crucial to the diagnosis and stratification of ARF. Weight gain, edema, or a reduction in urine output are early indices of renal insufficiency. Excessive diarrhea, vomiting, bleeding, sweating, or diuretic use accompanied by dizziness implies a prerenal state. Osmotic diuresis should be suspected in brittle or noncompliant diabetics. A diagnosis of adrenal insufficiency should be considered in a chronic steroid user whose steroids were abruptly stopped. A careful drug history is essential. Complaints of chest pain and/or shortness of breath may indicate pulmonary emboli, myocardial ischemia, atrial fibrillation, and/or congestive heart failure with subsequent renal hypoperfusion. Alcoholism may implicate cardiomyopathy, cirrhosis, or rhabdomyolysis as the cause of ARF. Weight loss or fever suggests underlying infection or malignancy. Recent procedures such as angioplasty or surgery support a thromboembolic etiology. Complaints of hematuria, purpura, hemoptysis, or a malar rash imply a systemic vasculitis. Finally, symptoms of prostatism or nephrolithiasis implicate postrenal failure as the culprit.

A fundamental part of the history is the inquiry into past medical diseases, focusing on hypertension, diabetes, congestive heart failure, atrial fibrillation, cirrhosis, vasculitides, malignancy, prostatism, nephrolithiasis, and chronic renal disorders. Previous measures of renal function help determine the acuteness of the renal insufficiency.

Physical Examination

A detailed physical examination is a vital part of the diagnostic evaluation. Orthostatic hypotension, tachycardia, dry mucous membranes, or poor skin turgor suggests a decrement in effective blood volume. Elevated jugular venous pressure, moist rales, a displaced point of maximal intensity, a third heart sound, a positive hepatojugular reflex, pitting edema, shifting dullness, fluid waves, and Cullen's (bluish discoloration of the umbilicus) or Grey Turner's (blue or green ecchymoses of the flank) sign all reflect a state of ineffective vascular blood volume. Hypotension in tandem with hyper- or hypothermia implies sepsis or adrenal insufficiency. Abdominal bruits indicate renal artery atherosclerosis, whereas flank tenderness denotes nephrolithiasis, renal vein thrombosis, or pyelonephritis. Roth's spots, fever, and a new or changing cardiac murmur support a diagnosis of endocarditis. A malar rash

TABLE 1. Causes of Acute Renal Failure

Prerenal Failure

Absolute Decrease in Blood Volume

Hemorrhage
Skin losses (burns, sweating)
Gastrointestinal losses (diarrhea, vomiting, surgical gastric drainage)
Renal losses (diuretics, diabetes insipidus, salt-losing nephropathy, osmotic diuresis, adrenal insufficiency)
Burns

Decrease in Effective Blood Volume

Cardiac dysfunction and/or low cardiac output (myocardial infarction, tamponade, valvular disease, arrhythmias, pulmonary
 embolism, cor pulmonale, positive pressure mechanical ventilation)
Liver disease with ascites
Hypoalbuminemia
Fluid pooling (pancreatitis, peritonitis)

Peripheral Vasodilatation

Sepsis
Anaphylaxis
Antihypertensive drugs
Anesthesia

Renal Vasoconstriction

Hypercalcemia
Norepinephrine, epinephrine
Cyclosporine
Amphotericin B
Cirrhosis with ascites

Renal Hypoperfusion with Impairment of Renal Autoregulatory Responses

Cyclooxygenase inhibitors, angiotensin-converting enzyme inhibitors

Hyperviscosity Syndrome

Multiple myeloma, macroglobulinemia, polycythemia

Renal Arterial Occlusion

Bilateral thromboembolism, renal artery stenosis, surgery, trauma, angioplasty, dissecting aneurysm, vasculitis

Intrinsic Renal Failure

Glomerular

Primary glomerulonephritis (membranoproliferative)
Secondary glomerulonephritis (hemolytic uremic syndrome, thrombotic thrombocytopenic purpura, disseminated intravascular
 coagulation, toxemia of pregnancy, postinfectious, accelerated hypertension, radiation nephritis, scleroderma, systemic lupus
 erythematosus, Goodpasture's syndrome, Wegener's granulomatosis)

Vascular

Vasculitis, malignant hypertension, renal vein thrombosis, vasopressors, eclampsia, hyperviscosity syndrome, iodinated
 contrast agent, NSAIDs

Acute Tubular Necrosis

Ischemia (as for prerenal failure)
Toxins (contrast, aminoglycosides, heavy metals, cyclosporine, amphotericin B, cisplatin, ethylene glycol, acetaminophen
 intoxication)
Pigments (hemoglobin, myoglobin)
Proteins (in multiple myeloma)
Crystals (uric acid, oxalate, sulfonamides)

Tubulointerstitial Nephritis

Allergic (beta-lactams, sulfonamides, trimethoprim, rifampin, cyclooxygenase inhibitors, diuretics, captopril)
Infectious (pyelonephritis, cytomegalovirus, human immunodeficiency virus, candidiasis, tuberculosis)
Infiltration (lymphoma, leukemia, sarcoidosis)
Radiation

Renal Allograft Rejection

Postrenal Failure

Ureteric

Calculi, blood clot, papillary necrosis, neoplasm, retroperitoneal fibrosis or hemorrhage, fungus balls, ligation, inflammatory
 aortic aneurysm

Bladder Outflow Obstruction

Prostatic hypertrophy, calculi, blood clot, neurogenic bladder, neoplasm, prostatitis

Urethra

Phimosis, meatal stenosis, stricture, neoplasm, congenital valve suggests SLE, whereas concomitant fever, neurologic signs, and purpura implicate thrombotic thrombocytopenic purpura. A systemic blanching rash warrants an investigation of all past and recent medication use, focusing on a potential agent inducing allergic interstitial nephritis. An enlarged prostate associated with dullness on complete bladder percussion reflects postrenal ARF. Uveitis suggests the diagnosis of sarcoidosis.

Laboratory Analysis

Urinalysis. Examination of the sediment and supernatant of an early-morning fresh urine specimen may further elucidate the etiology of ARF. Several agents affect supernatant urine color. Bilirubin and melanin induce a dark brown or yellow color. Red urine may result from porphyria, hemoglobinuria, hematuria, or myoglobinuria; using rifampin, phenazopyridine, or phenolphthalein; or eating beets. A blue-green color suggests *Pseudomonas* infection, the use of methylene blue or amitriptyline, or biliverdin. Turbid white implies pyuria, crystalluria, or chyluria. Hematuria may reflect trauma, nephrolithiasis, neoplasm, cystitis, vasculitis, coagulation defects, or menstruation.

Specific gravity (SG—determined by both the mass and the number of solute particles) provides a rough estimation of urine osmolality (determined by the number of osmotically active particles) except in the setting of excess high-density substances (contrast, protein, or glucose) or low-density substances (urea). Urine that is iso-osmotic with plasma has an osmolality of 285 mOsm per kg and an SG of 1.010. A high SG (>1.020) reflects the kidney's ability to concentrate urine and implies a prerenal state. An SG of 1.010 is seen in concert with intrinsic ARF and evidence of tubular and concentrating dysfunction.

Urine pH is normally below 7, but this varies with diet, respiration, infection, and systemic acid-base balance. A urine pH greater than 7 suggests a bicarbonate diuresis or the presence of urease-producing bacteria. Acidic urine is associated with uric acid or cystine stones, whereas alkaline urine accompanies struvite stones. Glucose detected by urine dipstick implies hyperglycemia or proximal tubular dysfunction. Bacteria may reduce nitrates to nitrites, yielding a positive nitrite test in approximately 50% of bacteriuric specimens. Urinary ketones may be seen with diabetic ketoacidosis, starvation, volume depletion, and chronic or acute alcohol intoxication.

Normal adults excrete between 40 and 80 mg of protein per day, with the upper limit of normal being 150 mg per day. The urine dipstick detects predominantly albumin. Detection of immune globulins in suspected cases of multiple myeloma, amyloidosis, lymphoma, or macroglobulinemia can be assessed by mixing 2.5 mL of urine with 7.5 mL of 3% sulfosalicylic acid, which precipitates all proteins. Interpretation must also take into account the concentration of urine; a 1+ protein result in a concentrated specimen with an SG of 1.030 may have no significance, whereas the same result combined with an SG of 1.010 may warrant further investigation.

A more accurate assessment of proteinuria is obtained by the spot urine protein-to-creatine ratio, which readily yields an accurate estimate of a 24-hour urine collection. Factors causing false-positive dipstick results include gross hematuria, urine pH greater than 8, phenazopyridine, and contamination with an antiseptic. False-positive tests with sulfosalicylic acid may be due to gross hematuria, radiographic contrast agents, beta-lactam antibiotics, and sulfonamides. Mildly increased protein excretion, typically less than 1 gram per day, is common in acute tubular necrosis, whereas 1 to 3 grams per day is observed in tubulointerstitial nephritis. Nephrotic-range proteinuria, greater than 3.5 grams per day, is compatible with glomerulonephritis and atheroembolic disease.

Urinary sediment is obtained via centrifugation of 10 to 15 mL of urine at 2000 to 3000 rpm for 3 to 5 minutes and then decanting the supernatant. Microscopic examination must not be delayed, since erythrocytes and casts degenerate rapidly, especially in alkaline or dilute urine. Moreover, urine pH may change and bacteria may proliferate with time. The normal range of erythrocytes is 0 to 2 per high-power field. Dysmorphic erythrocytes are often associated with glomerular disease, whereas normal erythrocyte morphology suggests an extraglomerular source. The normal range of leukocytes is 0 to 2 per high-power field. Leukocyturia usually implies cystitis, pyelonephritis, glomerulonephritis, or interstitial nephritis. Pyuria with negative urine cultures (sterile pyuria) denotes partially treated urinary tract infection, tuberculosis, urethritis, prostatitis, interstitial nephritis, calculi, or papillary necrosis. Eosinophiluria (between 1 and 50% of urine leukocytes) is detected in 90% of cases of drug-induced allergic interstitial nephritis when using Hansel's stain. Wright's stain is less sensitive, detecting approximately 20% of cases. Eosinophiluria is 85% specific for allergic interstitial nephritis, occurring less commonly in atheroembolization, glomerulonephritis, pyelonephritis, cystitis, prostatitis, and ischemic and toxin-induced ARF.

Red blood cell casts suggest glomerulonephritis but may also be seen with pyelonephritis, tubulointerstitial nephritis, trauma, thromboemboli, and malignant hypertension. White blood cell casts imply pyelonephritis, glomerulonephritis, or tubulointerstitial nephritis. Hyaline casts, devoid of cellular elements, do not reflect renal disease and are visualized in concentrated urine following exercise, fever, or diuretic use. Renal tubular epithelial cells indicate tubular damage and are seen in acute tubular necrosis, tubulointerstitial nephritis, and glomerulonephritis. These cells are 1.5 to 3 times the size of a leukocyte and contain a large round nucleus. In nephrotic-range proteinuria, degenerating tubular epithelial cells may be manifested as oval fat bodies with a Maltese cross appearance under polarized light. Coarsely granular or waxy casts represent progressive degeneration of cellular elements or aggregated proteins within a cast, denoting tubular injury. Broad casts indicate chronic renal failure, reflecting stasis in the collecting tubules draining diseased nephrons. They may contain cellular elements. Finally, the presence of squamous epithelial cells reflects vaginal contamination, and a new midstream clean-catch specimen should be obtained. The presence of urinary crystals in ARF may facilitate the diagnostic process. Calcium oxalate crystals may indicate excessive exposure to ethylene glycol, methoxyflurane, or high-dose vitamin C. Uric acid crystals may follow tumor lysis, rhabdomyolysis, or the prerenal state.

Blood Tests. Hepatic catabolism of amino acids generates ammonia, which is subsequently converted to urea. Several factors influence blood urea nitrogen (BUN), so it is not a reliable index of the glomerular filtration rate. Conditions that increase BUN include gastrointestinal bleeding, a high-protein diet, tissue trauma, glucocorticoids, tetracycline, and reduction of effective circulating blood volume. Factors that decrease BUN include malnutrition and liver disease. The serum creatinine is a more specific measurement of renal function. ARF secondary to atheroemboli, ischemia, or contrast results in rapid elevation of the serum creatinine (24 to 48 hours), with peak levels in contrast nephropathy appearing earlier (3 to 5 days) than in ischemic or atheroembolic disease (7 to 10 days). Aminoglycosides typically induce a rise in the creatinine during the second week of therapy. Spurious elevations in serum creatinine due to the production of noncreatinine chromogens may be seen in ketoacidosis, cephalosporin administration, and methanol or isopropyl alcohol intoxication. Ingesting large amounts of cooked meat containing creatinine may generate a rise in serum creatinine. Various drugs (aspirin, cimetidine, trimethoprim, triamterene, spironolactone, amiloride) inhibit tubular creatinine secretion and may increase serum creatinine, especially in the presence of renal insufficiency. Decrements in serum creatinine levels appear with cachexia and increasing age due to pathologic and physiologic decreases in muscle mass, respectively. Although the BUN creatine ratio is often cited as a useful measure for distinguishing prerenal from intrinsic ARF, urinary indices are more reliable measurements.

A complete blood count and smear may provide evidence of infection (leukocytosis, leukopenia), hematologic malignancy (blasts, plasma cells, anemia), allergic response (eosinophilia), vasculitis (eosinophilia, anemia, schistocytes, thrombocytopenia), or malignant hypertension (anemia, schistocytes). Abnormal liver function tests may reflect hepatic disease or congestive heart failure, whereas a low albumin may indicate chronic liver or cardiac disease, nephrotic-range proteinuria, or malnutrition. Electrolyte disturbances such as hypokalemia may be secondary to diarrhea, vomiting, hyperosmotic diuresis, or drug-induced diuresis, whereas hyponatremia may be consistent with diuresis, adrenal insufficiency, cirrhosis, nephrosis, or congestive heart failure. Hyperkalemia associated with hyperphosphatemia, hyperuricemia, and hypocalcemia following chemotherapy suggests a tumor lysis syndrome. Severe hypercalcemia can induce ARF. Elevated creatinine kinase (MM isoenzyme) levels are observed with tumor lysis or rhabdomyolysis. The presence of antinuclear antibody, antineutrophil cytoplasmic antibody, or antiglomerular basement membrane antibody supports a diagnosis of SLE, Wegener's granulomatosis, or Goodpasture's syndrome, respectively. A low complement level suggests SLE, postinfectious glomerulonephritis, cryoglobulinemia, or membranoproliferative glomerulonephritis. Finally, monitoring blood levels of aminoglycosides and cyclosporine should be routine when these drugs are administered.

Urine Diagnostic Indices. The most sensitive urinary index applied for distinguishing prerenal from intrinsic ARF is the fractional excretion of sodium (FENa), the percentage of filtered sodium that is excreted (Table 2). A FENa of less than 1% is seen with avid proximal tubular reabsorption of sodium and is consistent with the prerenal state. Intrinsic renal damage disrupts tubular function, diminishing sodium reabsorption and producing an FENa of greater than 1%. The FENa in early and late postrenal ARF resembles prerenal and intrinsic ARF, respectively. Conditions of partial tubular preservation (nonoliguric ischemia, aminoglycoside or contrast nephrotoxicity, rhabdomyolysis, hemolysis, sepsis, burns, hepatorenal syndrome, acute interstitial or glomerulonephritis) may result in a low FENa. Furthermore, the FENa may occasionally be greater than 1% in the prerenal state (diuretics, adrenal insufficiency, chronic renal failure with salt wasting, bicarbonaturia associated with natriuresis). The FENa is a useful diagnostic tool that may reveal the classification of the ARF. It does not pinpoint the etiology but serves to complement the history and physical examination. The renal failure index (RFI) is a measurement similar to the FENa, excluding the serum sodium. Indices of urinary concentrating ability such as urine osmolality, urine specific gravity, and urine to plasma creatinine or urea ratios are less useful measures for differentiating the prerenal, intrinsic, and postrenal ARF states (see Table 2).

Radiology

Ultrasound imaging of the kidney in ARF is warranted to rule out obstruction. Information regarding kidney size, cyst formation, anatomic abnormalies, stones, neoplasms, retroperitoneal masses, and asymmetry is also provided. Reduction in kidney size is typically seen in chronic renal failure, although several chronic diseases may exhibit normal-size or enlarged kidneys (multiple myeloma, amyloidosis, diabetes, polycystic kidneys, renal vein thrombosis, infiltrative lesions). Ultrasound imaging provides a noninvasive and rapid anatomic assessment of the kidney, and it can be performed at the bedside in an unstable patient. Doppler ultrasonography may be utilized to assess the patency of the renal vasculature, although angiography is the "gold standard." Angiography carries the added risks of contrast nephropathy, dislodgment of atherosclerotic plaques, and thromboembolic events. Preliminary observa-

TABLE 2. **Urine Diagnostic Indices**

Diagnostic Index	Prerenal	Intrinsic*	Postrenal†
Fractional excretion of sodium‡ FENa (%) $$\left[\left(\frac{\text{Urine Na} \times \text{plasma creatinine}}{\text{Plasma Na} \times \text{urine creatinine}}\right) \times 100\right]$$	<1	>1	>1
Renal failure index‡ $$\left[\frac{\text{Urine Na}}{(\text{Urine creatinine/plasma creatinine})}\right]$$	<1	>1	>1
Urine sodium (mmol/L)	<10	>20	>20
Urine creatinine/plasma creatinine	<40	<20	<20
Urine urea/plasma urea	>8	<3	—
Urine specific gravity	>1.020	<1.010	—
Urine osmolality (mmol/kg H_2O)	>500	<350	<350

*Many conditions causing intrinsic ARF are associated with renal hypoperfusion, resulting in urine diagnostic indices similar to those observed in prerenal ARF.

†Diagnostic indices in early obstruction can mimic prerenal indices.

‡More sensitive indices.

tions using magnetic resonance imaging (MRI) suggest that it may become the procedure of choice for evaluating renal vasculature, hence avoiding the hazards of angiography. Computed tomography (CT) affords similar visualization as ultrasonography but often requires radiocontrast.

Biopsy

Indications for renal biopsy in the setting of ARF are controversial. Prerenal and postrenal causes of ARF do not require biopsy, and most etiologies of intrinsic ARF (acute tubulointerstitial nephritis, contrast, endogenous and exogenous toxins, ischemia) can be diagnosed without a biopsy. In cases of intrinsic ARF in which the diagnosis has not been ascertained and the suspected disease is amenable to therapy (Goodpasture's syndrome, Wegener's granulomatosis, thrombotic thrombocytopenic purpura), renal biopsy is indicated. Contraindications to kidney biopsy include a solitary or ectopic kidney, horseshoe kidney, uncorrected bleeding disorder, severe uncontrolled hypertension, renal infection, renal neoplasm, or uncooperative patient.

MANAGEMENT AND COMPLICATIONS

Prevention

Despite significant advances in supportive care, mortality rates in the setting of ARF have not changed over the past 3 decades. Therein lies the importance of preventive therapy. Foremost, physicians are obliged to know the indications, interactions, and adverse side effects of all medications and procedures prescribed. The need to adjust the drug dosage and/or dose interval in patients with reduced creatinine clearance should be routinely assessed (Table 3). There are myriad alternative medications (cephalosporins instead of aminoglycosides) and procedures (ultrasound instead of contrast CT) for the treating physician to utilize. Recognizing the risk factors for ARF (volume depletion, chronic renal failure) and the synergistic effect of combined insults should discourage the use of potential nephrotoxic agents (NSAIDs, ACE inhibitors) in high-risk patients.

Hydration and salt loading are the mainstay of prophylactic treatment against ischemic and nephrotoxic injury. This protective effect has been demonstrated in recipients of cisplatin, amphotericin, and radiocontrast, as well as in postoperative patients. There is no convincing evidence that dopamine, loop diuretics, mannitol, or calcium channel blockers prevent ARF in high-risk patients. Moreover, increased risk of ARF has been shown with furosemide and mannitol treatment. Forced diuresis and alkalinization of urine can limit renal injury due to uric acid, methotrexate, and myoglobin toxicity. The early administration of acetylcysteine sodium (Mucomyst) in acetaminophen overdose and the use of dimercaprol in heavy metal intoxication may obviate renal injury.

Supportive Care

ARF is complicated by intravascular volume overload consequent to reduced water and sodium excre-

TABLE 3. Dosage and Interval Adjustment for Commonly Prescribed Drugs

Drugs Not Requiring Adjustment

Alprazolam	Furosemide	Miconazole
Amiodarone	Gemfibrozil	Minoxidil
Amitriptyline	Glipizide	Nifedipine
Bromocriptine	Griseofulvin	Nitroglycerin
Carbidopa	Haloperidol	Pentobarbital
Cefoperazone	Heparin	Pentoxifylline
Ceftriaxone	Ibuprofen	Phenytoin
Chloramphenicol	Indomethacin	Piroxicam
Clindamycin	Imipramine	Prazosin
Clonazepam	Isosorbide	Propafenone
Clonidine	Isradipine	Propranolol
Diazepam	Itraconazole	Rifampin
Diazoxide	Ketoconazole	Secobarbital
Dicloxacillin	Labetolol	Semisodium valproate
Diltiazem	Levodopa	Steroids
Diphenhydramine	Lidocaine	Streptokinase
Dipyridamole	Lorazepam	Sulindac
Dobutamine	Lovastatin	Theophylline
Esmolol	Metolazone	Verapamil
Flurazepam	Metoprolol	

Dose Interval Adjustment for Commonly Prescribed Drugs

	Dose Interval (Hours)	
Drug	GFR 10–50 mL/min	GFR <10 mL/min
Acetazolamide*	12	—
Acyclovir	12	24
Amantadine	48	96
Amikacin	12	24–48
Amphotericin	24	24–36
Cefazolin	12	24–48
Cefotaxime	12	24–48
Cefoxitin	12	24–48
Ceftazidime	12	24–48
Cefuroxime	12	24–48
Cephalexin	6	8–12
Chlorpropamide*	24	—
Ethacrynic acid*	8–12	—
Ethambutol	24–36	48
Digoxin	36	48
Fluconazole	24–48	48–72
Gentamicin	12	24–48
Methyldopa	12	24
Pentamidine	24–36	48
Procainamide	6–12	8–24
Spironolactone*	12–24	—
Sulfamethoxazole	18	24
Tobramycin	12	24–48

*Avoid if glomerular filtration rate (GFR) is <10 mL/min.

From Bennett WM, Aronoff GR, Golper TA, et al: Drug prescribing in renal failure, dosing guidelines for adults, 2d ed. 1991.

tion. Careful assessment of volume status should be obtained by the physical examination and by monitoring fluid input and output and weighing the patient daily. Prerenal ARF due to hemorrhage should be corrected with packed red blood cells or whole blood, and isotonic saline should be administered for replacement of plasma losses (peritonitis, burns). Hypotonic solutions (0.45% saline) are satisfactory repletion for hemodynamically stable patients with urinary or gastrointestinal losses. Cardiac failure complicated by ARF often requires salt and water restriction. Salt and water limitation is also warranted for ARF due to intrinsic renal disease, and careful matching of input and output (urinary, gastrointestinal, insensible, and drainage site losses) is required. Postrenal causes of ARF should be dealt with promptly, conferring with a urologist, nephrologist, and radiologist for the optimal means of relieving the obstruction. Most patients experience diuresis following relief of obstruction, with potential severe volume and electrolyte depletion. Refractory volume overload complicated by intractable hypertension or congestive heart failure or pulmonary edema mandates dialysis treatment.

Oliguric ARF portends a worse prognosis than non-oliguric ARF, perhaps reflecting more severe disease. Pharmacologic methods, particularly diuretics, dopamine, and mannitol, are commonly precribed to augment urinary output. Nonetheless, their efficacy in enhancing patient survival or attenuating renal injury has not been demonstrated. Atrial natriuretic peptide is potentially beneficial in the treatment of oliguric ARF.

Metabolic Acidosis

ARF is frequently complicated by an elevated anion gap metabolic acidosis. The metabolism of dietary protein produces approximately 1 mmol per kg (patient's weight) per day of nonvolatile acids, which is excreted by the kidney. Acidosis may be compounded by other causes of increased endogenous acid production (diabetes, starvation, or alcholic ketoacidosis). Bicarbonate repletion is required when serum bicarbonate levels fall below 15 mmol per liter. Bicarbonate should be administered cautiously, since it may precipitate metabolic alkalosis, hypokalemia, hypocalcemia, and volume overload. Refractory acidosis is an indication for dialysis.

Hypo- and Hypernatremia

Hyponatremia often accompanies ARF due to the excess retention of water in comparison to sodium. Overzealous ingestion or administration of water (hypotonic fluids) may be contributing factors. Water restriction is recommended. Hypernatremia, reflecting absolute volume depletion, may complicate the prerenal state. Treatment options include water or hypotonic or isotonic solutions, depending on the severity of volume loss.

Hypo- and Hyperkalemia

Hyperkalemia due to impaired potassium excretion and concomitant acidosis is common in ARF, characterized by daily increments of 0.5 mmol per liter in oliguric and anuric patients. Hyperkalemia may be exacerbated in patients with ARF associated with rhabdomyolysis, hemolysis, or tumor lysis syndrome. Management of hyperkalemia requires limitation of dietary potassium and elimination of dietary supplements, potassium-sparing diuretics, and ACE inhibitors. Early electrocardiographic abnormalities, typically developing with levels greater than 6 mmol per liter, include peaked T waves, P wave flattening, first- and second-degree heart block, QRS widening, and ST elevation. Potential lethal cardiac arrhythmias include asystole, bradycardia, complete heart block, and ventricular tachycardia or fibrillation. Neurologic manifestations of hyperkalemia include paresthesias, hyporeflexia, weakness, ascending flaccid paralysis, and respiratory failure. Emergency measures, as illustrated in Table 4, should be employed for potassium levels greater than 6.5 to 7.0 mmol per liter or with evidence of cardiac or neurologic abnormalities.

Initial therapy consists of calcium gluconate (10 to 20 mL of a 10% solution infused over 5 to 10 minutes), which rapidly antagonizes the cardiac and neurologic effects of hyperkalemia; the onset of action is 1 to 2 minutes, and transient effects last approximately 15 to 20 minutes. Calcium administered in solutions containing bicarbonate precipitates, so this combination should be avoided. Sodium bicarbonate (1 to 2 ampules or 44.6 to 89.2 mmol intravenously over 5 to 10 minutes) promotes an extracellular to intracellular potassium shift, with a rapid onset of action (10 to 20 minutes) and effects lasting from 1 to 2 hours. Furthermore, bicarbonate combats the metabolic acidosis of ARF. Additional doses can be given at 15-minute intervals if symptoms or signs persist. Circulatory overload, hypernatremia, and symptomatic hypocalcemia may complicate bicarbonate treatment. Intravenous glucose (50 mL of 50% dextrose) and insulin (5 to 10 U regular insulin) induce intracellular potassium uptake within 30 to 60 minutes, with effects persisting for several hours. Hypoglycemia may ensue, so periodic glucose measurements should be obtained. Glucose therapy should be omitted in patients with hyperglycemia.

Albuterol (Ventolin)* 10 to 20 mg nebulized or 0.5 mg intravenously, a beta$_2$-adrenergic agonist, effectively redistributes potassium to the intracellular space 30 minutes after administration. The cation exchange resin sodium polystyrene sulfonate (Kayexalate) binds potassium in exchange for sodium (1 mEq of potassium for 1 to 2 mEq of sodium) in the intestinal tract, thereby effectively reducing total body potassium. Onset of action is 1 to 2 hours, and the duration is 4 to 6 hours. Recommended oral doses are 15 to 30 grams, which may be repeated every 2 to 4 hours. Each gram of resin binds 1 mEq of potassium, and 50 grams decreases the serum potassium by approximately 0.5 to 1 mEq per liter. Since resin is constipating, the osmotic agent sorbitol (50 to 100 mL of a 20% solution) is administered concurrently to hasten gastrointestinal transit time. Adverse side effects include nausea, vomiting, hypernatremia, volume overload, calcium and magnesium depletion, and, rarely, intestinal necrosis. If oral administration is not feasible, retention enemas may be given (50 grams in 200 mL of a 20% dextrose solution). A rectal catheter is inflated to ensure retention of the enema

---

*Not FDA-approved for this indication.

TABLE 4. **Treatment of Hyperkalemia**

Therapy	Mechanism	Onset	Duration	Side Effects
Calcium gluconate 10%, IV, 1–2 ampules or 10–20 mL over 5–10 min	Antagonism	1–2 min	15–20 min	Calcium load
Sodium bicarbonate IV, 1–2 ampules or 44.6–89.2 mEq over 5–10 min	Redistribution	10–20 min	1–2 h	Sodium and volume load, alkalosis, symptomatic hypocalcemia
Glucose 50% 50 mL and regular insulin 5–10 U IV	Redistribution	30–60 min	Hours	Hyperglycemia, hypoglycemia, volume expansion
Albuterol, beta$_2$ agonist, 10–20 mg nebulized or 0.5 mg IV, or salbutamol	Redistribution	30 min	Hours	Arrhythmias
Sodium polystyrene sulfonate (potassium exchange resin) 15–30 gm PO 2–4 h plus sorbitol 50–100 mL of a 20% solution, or 50 gm rectally plus 200 mL of a 20% dextrose solution	Elimination	1–2 h	4–6 h	Nausea, vomiting, sodium and volume load, calcium and magnesium depletion, intestinal necrosis
Dialysis	Elimination	Hours	Hours	See Table 6

for 30 to 60 minutes. Onset of action is 1 to 2 hours, and enemas can be repeated every 4 to 6 hours. Colonic necrosis and perforation have been rarely reported with the use of resin exchange enemas in humans (animal studies suggest that sorbitol may be the responsible agent; thus sorbitol solutions are not recommended for use in enema preparations).

Intractable hyperkalemia is an indication for dialysis treatment, preferably hemodialysis, which extracts potassium more rapidly than peritoneal dialysis. Cation exchange resins combined with dietary restriction of potassium provide adequate therapy for asymptomatic moderate hyperkalemia (less than 6.5 mmol per liter). Hypokalemia is a rare occurrence in ARF, complicating nonoliguric cisplatin or amphotericin nephrotoxicity.

Hyperphosphatemia and Hypocalcemia

Hyperphosphatemia consequent to impaired phosphate excretion is frequently observed in ARF. ARF due to rhabdomyolysis, tumor lysis, or acute leukemia may result in severe hyperphosphatemia. Clinical manifestations include ectopic calcifications of soft tissues such as blood vessels, cornea, skin, kidney, and periarticular tissue, particularly when the calcium phosphorus by-product exceeds 70 mg per dL. Moreover, the excess phosphate binding of calcium precipitates hypocalcemia. Phosphate lowering involves dietary phosphate restriction (800 to 1000 mg per day) and administering oral phosphate binders such as aluminum-containing antacids (15 to 30 mL or 1 to 3 capsules orally with meals), calcium carbonate (500 to 1000 mg every 8 hours with meals), or calcium acetate. Side effects of short-term use of aluminum-containing antacids are limited to nausea and constipation, whereas prolonged use may result in osteomalacia, encephalopathy, and anemia. Because calcium carbonate and acetate can elevate se-

rum calcium levels, they should be employed only when the calcium phosphorus by-product is less than 70 mg per dL.

Hypocalcemia is a typical finding in ARF, induced by phosphate binding, skeletal resistance to parathyroid hormone, and reduced levels of 1,25-dihydroxyvitamin D. It is often asymptomatic and is alleviated by the concomitant acidosis of ARF, which reduces calcium protein binding and augments ionized serum calcium levels. Hypocalcemia may be more pronounced in ARF associated with rhabdomyolysis, pancreatitis, or excessive bicarbonate infusions. Clinical sequelae of hypocalcemia include paresthesias, tetany, Trousseau's and Chvostek's signs, lethargy, confusion, laryngospasm, seizures, prolonged QT interval, cardiac failure, and hypotension. Symptomatic hypocalcemia necessitates immediate treatment with 2 ampules (20 mL) of 10% calcium gluconate over 10 minutes, followed by a continuous infusion of 60 mL of calcium gluconate in 500 mL of 5% dextrose at 0.5 to 2 mg per kg per hour if symptoms persist. Subsequently, oral calcium supplements may be utilized. Dialysis should be instituted for refractory hyperphosphatemia.

Hyperuricemia and Hypermagnesemia

Elevated uric acid and magnesium levels are common in ARF, rarely warranting treatment. ARF combined with rhabdomyolysis or tumor lysis may dramatically increase uric acid levels. Acute gouty attacks infrequently complicate hyperuricemia in ARF, and colchicine or steroids are sufficient therapy; NSAIDs are prohibited. Clinical manifestations of hypermagnesemia include areflexia, lethargy, weakness, paralysis, respiratory failure, hypotension, bradycardia, prolonged PR, QRS, and QT intervals, complete heart block, and asystole. Magnesium-containing antacids and laxatives should be avoided in patients with ARF. Emergency treatment of symptomatic hypermagnesemia entails infusion of 10 to 20 mL of a 10% calcium gluconate solution over 10 minutes. Intractable hypermagnesemia requires immediate dialysis.

Uremia

Manifestations of uremia include pericardial effusions, pericarditis, anorexia, nausea, vomiting, ileus, lethargy, confusion, stupor, agitation, psychosis, asterixis, myoclonus, hyper-reflexia, restless legs syndrome, focal neurologic deficits, seizures, coma, and bleeding. Symptomatic uremia is an indication for dialysis.

Hematologic Abnormalities

Uremia causes platelet dysfunction and a reduction in platelet survival time, constituting the predominant bleeding diathesis observed in ARF. Severe anemia may result, compounded by stress-induced bleeding ulcers in this patient population. Temporizing measures include intravenous 1-deamino-8-D-arginine vasopressin (DDAVP, 0.3 µg per kg), conjugated estrogens (0.6 mg per kg per day for 5 days), or cryoprecipitate (1 to 2 U per 10 kg per day). The hemostatic effect of DDAVP occurs after 1 hour and persists for 6 hours. Histamine$_2$-receptor antagonists or sucralfate are advocated prophylactically to curtail episodes of gastrointestinal hemorrhage, although reductions in overall mortality have not been demonstrated. Uncontrollable bleeding mandates dialysis treatment. Since hemodialysis reduces platelet counts, involves puncturing a major venous blood vessel, and requires heparin administration, peritoneal dialysis may be preferred in this setting.

Cardiovascular Complications

Cardiac failure, pulmonary edema, and hypertension may evolve in ARF due to volume overload. Electrolyte abnormalities may cause refractory arrhythmias in the setting of persistent acidosis. Initial treatment of cardiac failure, pulmonary edema, and hypertension entails fluid and sodium restriction. Antihypertensive medications should be instituted judiciously; ACE inhibitors are generally prohibited. Intractable cardiac failure, pulmonary edema, and hypertension are indications for dialysis. Uremic-induced pericarditis warrants emergent dialysis treatment. Pulmonary embolism is an infrequent complication, despite prolonged immobilization.

Infection

Infection complicates 50 to 90% of cases of ARF, accounting for up to 75% of deaths. The high prevalence of infection is attributed to the combination of impaired host immunity due to uremia and the excessive number of indwelling instruments (urinary, arterial, and venous catheters; endotracheal and di-

alysis tubes) breaching mucocutaneous barriers. Furthermore, manifestations of infection in ARF are limited, as urea displays antipyretic properties and may impede the body's ability to elevate white blood cell counts. Abdominal signs may be absent in cases of peritonitis. Hence, daily physical evaluations and the removal of all unnecessary indwelling instruments are critical to the early identification and to the forestallment of infectious complications, respectively. The need for dose and/or interval adjustments of antibiotics and antifungal drugs should be routinely assessed.

Nutrition

Malnutrition in ARF is characteristically multifactorial in origin, consequent to diminished intake and enhanced catabolism induced by uremia and the underlying disease state. Nutrient depletion in drainage fluids or dialysate may further aggravate the state of malnutrition. The role of hyperalimentation in ARF is controversial. A consistent benefit has not been demonstrated, and parenteral nutrition may cause serious complications, including infections, electrolyte abnormalities, acid-base disturbances, and increased urea and fluid load. Consequently, adequate oral or nasogastric tube feeding should be implemented if use of the gastrointestinal tract is feasible. Sufficient calories should be provided (minimum of 30 kcal per kg per day), increasing the caloric input according to the increment in catabolism. To minimize the production of nitrogenous waste, ARF patients should be restricted to 0.6 to 0.8 grams per kg per day of protein of high biologic value. Protein ingestion should be increased to 1 to 1.4 grams per kg per day when dialysis is instituted, since dialysis enhances protein catabolism. In addition, significant quantities of protein are lost across peritoneal dialysis membranes.

Dialysis

The optimal timing, frequency, and intensity of dialysis are unclear. Since dialysis does not expedite recovery or alter the prognosis in ARF, its use should probably be limited to absolute indications, as illustrated in Table 5. The primary modes of dialysis are hemo- and peritoneal dialysis, with neither method proved to be superior in the management of ARF. Variations of hemodialysis include ultrafiltration, continuous arteriovenous hemofiltration dialysis (CAVHD), and continous venovenous hemofiltration

TABLE 5. **Indications for Dialysis**

Refractory
Fluid overload
Acidosis
Hyperkalemia, hyperphosphatemia, hypermagnesemia
Symptomatic uremia
Some overdoses and intoxications (e.g., methanol)

TABLE 6. **Methods of Dialysis**

Hemodialysis
  Advantages: efficiency, intermittent use, easy access for blood sampling and medication administration
  Complications and disadvantages: bleeding, infection, pneumothorax, hypotension, hypertension, nausea, vomiting, cramps, headache, hypoxia, arrhythmias, disequilibrium syndrome, venous stenosis, venous thrombosis, heparin administration

CAVHD or CVVHD
  Advantages: more physiologic (continuous), better titration of volume and electrolyte status, minimizes cardiovascular instability
  Complications and disadvantages: continuous anticoagulation, supervision in intensive care setting, repeated manipulation of a potential infectious access site, slow removal of filtrate, bleeding, infection

Peritoneal Dialysis
  Advantages: no complex machinery, minimal anticoagulation, limited cardiovascular and neurologic disturbances
  Complications and disadvantages: peritonitis, protein depletion, hyperglycemia, pulmonary compromise, low efficiency

---

dialysis (CVVHD). The advantages and disadvantages of each technique are listed in Table 6.

Hemodialysis

Hemodialysis for ARF is performed via percutaneous cannulation of the subclavian, internal jugular, or femoral vein. Subclavian and internal jugular cannulation provides a cleaner milieu than the femoral approach, so femoral insertion should be limited to short-term dialysis (<48 hours). Moreover, femoral catheters are more uncomfortable for the patient. Major advantages, disadvantages, and complications are depicted in Table 6. Hemodynamically unstable patients are not candidates for hemodialysis. A disadvantage of hemodialysis is the need for heparin administration, adding another risk for bleeding in patients who are already harboring bleeding diatheses.

Ultrafiltration

Ultrafiltration, except for the lack of dialysate, is similar to hemodialysis. It is employed exclusively to extract volume, resulting in fewer hemodynamic changes.

CAVHD and CVVHD

CAVHD and CVVHD entail a more physiologic mode of renal replacement, relying on continuous ultrafiltration. This affords better titration of volume and electrolyte status and reduces the incidence of cardiovascular instability. CAVHD involves cannulation of the femoral artery and vein or insertion of an arteriovenous shunt. The patient's arterial pressure suffices to promote blood flow through the extracorporeal circuit. CVVHD requires insertion of a double-lumen venous catheter and is contingent on a pump for blood flow. Disadvantages of hemofiltration include continuous anticoagulation, constant supervision in an intensive care setting, repeated manipulation of a potential infectious access site, and the relative slow removal of filtrate.

Peritoneal Dialysis

Access for peritoneal dialysis is achieved by a cannula inserted percutaneously at the bedside or via a minilaparotomy for more permanent usage. Advantages, disadvantages, and complications are delineated in Table 6. Absolute contraindications to peritoneal dialysis include significant peritoneal fibrosis or a pleuroperitoneal leak; relative contraindications include colostomy or nephrostomy, severe catabolism, peritonitis, recent abdominal surgery, extensive abdominal adhesions, or inguinal or abdominal hernia.

OUTCOME

Of those patients recovering from ARF, less than 5% require long-term dialysis or renal transplantation. Approximately 50% of survivors of ARF exhibit subclinical renal functional or anatomic abnormalities. Furthermore, 5% of survivors display progressive deterioration in renal function subsequent to an initial recovery period. It is important to recognize that ARF is often a marker of severe subclinical disease (cardiovascular) and reflects overall patient prognosis. Despite profound advances in supportive care, mortality rates in ARF have not changed over the past 30 years. The best treatment is preventive care. Patient education and physician awareness of the factors contributing to ARF formulate the optimal means of combating ARF.

CHRONIC RENAL FAILURE

method of
GLENN M. CHERTOW, M.D., and
J. MICHAEL LAZARUS, M.D.
Harvard Medical School
Boston, Massachusetts

MEASUREMENT OF RENAL FUNCTION AND DIAGNOSIS OF CHRONIC RENAL FAILURE

The most common measure used to estimate kidney function is the serum creatinine. The serum creatinine is a useful, albeit imperfect measure, because of its physical characteristics and handling by the human nephron. Within intact nephrons, creatinine is freely filtered, not reabsorbed, and only minimally secreted. Unlike creatinine, the blood urea nitrogen (BUN) is a relatively poor surrogate for renal function. Many factors may increase the BUN independent of intrinsic renal function, including gastrointestinal bleeding, drugs that promote catabolism (e.g., glucocorticoids, tetracyclines), and impaired renal perfusion (e.g., volume depletion, hepatic cirrhosis).

The creatinine clearance (CrCl) can be determined using the following formula:

$$\text{CrCl (mL per minute)} = \frac{\text{Urine concentration of creatinine (mg per dL)} \times \text{urine volume (mL per minute)}}{\text{Plasma concentration of creatinine (mg per dL)}}$$

The creatinine clearance closely approximates the glomerular filtration rate (GFR) when the GFR exceeds 50 to 60 mL per minute. However, as renal function deteriorates, the CrCl tends to overestimate GFR because of the relative contribution of secreted creatinine and nonrenal routes of creatinine excretion. In contrast, the urea nitrogen clearance (calculated as in the preceding equation but using urine and serum urea) tends to underestimate GFR because of tubular urea reabsorption. The average of the creatinine and urea clearances is reasonably accurate when the GFR falls below 20 mL per minute.

An approximation of CrCl can be obtained using the Cockcroft-Gault formula:

$$\text{CrCl (mL per minute)} = \frac{(140 - \text{age} \times \text{ideal body weight} \, [\times \, 0.85 \text{ if female}])}{\text{Serum creatinine} \times 72}$$

Additional methods of assessing renal function are outlined in Table 1.

The urinalysis is an important diagnostic tool that is rapid, inexpensive, and relatively easy to perform. Urine dipsticks can detect modest degrees of hematuria, pyuria, and proteinuria and are often the first clue to the presence of acute or chronic renal disease. A microscopic analysis may provide insight into the severity and/or duration of renal disease. Radiographic studies are also helpful. The abdominal plain film and intravenous urogram are useful in the work-up of nephrolithiasis but are rarely sufficient in a patient with renal insufficiency. Rather, renal ultrasound is the preferred diagnostic screening study. Ultrasound can be used to assess kidney structure (e.g., the presence of cysts, hydronephrosis), size (e.g., reduced size with long-standing disease), and integrity (i.e., echogenicity). Occasionally, computed tomography, magnetic resonance imaging, and nuclear medicine studies are used in the diagnosis of chronic renal failure (CRF), particularly when associated with hypertension and vascular disease.

CAUSES OF CHRONIC RENAL FAILURE

The most common causes of CRF are outlined in Table 2. Although many patients progress to end-stage renal disease (ESRD) without a definitive diagnosis, it is important to investigate the cause(s) of CRF, as associated complications may develop in future years.

TABLE 1. **Methods Used to Estimate Renal Function**

Serum creatinine
Blood urea nitrogen
Cockcroft-Gault equation
24-hour urine collection for creatinine and/or urea nitrogen
DTPA renal scan
Radiolabeled iothalamate clearance

Abbreviation: DTPA = diethylenetriaminepenta-acetic acid.

TABLE 2. **Most Common Causes of Chronic Renal Failure and End-Stage Renal Disease**

Glomerulonephritis, glomerulosclerosis, glomerulopathy
  Diabetic nephropathy
  Hypertensive nephrosclerosis
  Primary renal
    Focal segmental glomerular sclerosis
    Membranous nephropathy
    IgA nephropathy
  Systemic disease
    Systemic lupus erythematosus
    Human immunodeficiency virus–associated
      nephropathy
    Vasculitis
Tubulointerstitial disease
  Chronic pyelonephritis
  Papillary necrosis, analgesic nephropathy
  Interstitial nephritis
  Multiple myeloma
Hereditary renal disease
  Polycystic kidney disease
  Hereditary nephritis (Alport's disease)
  Vesicoureteral reflux
Decreased renal perfusion, vascular disease
  Renovascular disease
  Atheroembolic disease
  Renal infarction
  Cyclosporine nephrotoxicity
Urinary tract obstruction
  Prostate, bladder pathology
  Retroperitoneal fibrosis, lymphadenopathy
  Irreversible ureteral obstruction
Nephrectomy or partial nephrectomy for malignancy
Renal transplant failure

Conditions associated with prerenal failure, owing to frank volume depletion (e.g., blood loss, gastrointestinal fluid loss, overzealous use of diuretic agents) or to reduced renal perfusion (e.g., congestive heart failure, hepatic cirrhosis, renovascular disease), are the most common causes of acute renal failure in hospitalized adults. However, with the possible exception of renovascular disease, these pathophysiologic states are relatively uncommon causes of CRF and ESRD (i.e., they are reversible). Likewise, postrenal failure, i.e., urinary tract obstruction, infrequently causes CRF or ESRD unless it remains undiagnosed and is bilateral, severe, and prolonged. Rather, the great majority of cases of CRF or ESRD are due to intrinsic renal diseases, which can be broadly categorized as predominantly glomerular or tubulointerstitial in origin.

Glomerular diseases, including diabetic nephropathy and hypertensive nephrosclerosis, account for the majority of cases of CRF that progress to ESRD. Glomerular diseases can be broadly categorized as nephrotic or nephritic. The term "nephrotic" refers to the loss of large (greater than 3 to 5 grams per day) quantities of protein (usually albumin) in the urine. When full-blown, the nephrotic syndrome includes edema owing to salt and water retention, hypoalbuminemia, hypercholesterolemia, and occasionally a predisposition to venous thrombosis. In contrast, the term "nephritic" refers to the presence of hematuria, hypertension, and mild to moderate proteinuria, usually with associated loss of renal function. Several of the glomerular diseases are associated with systemic disease, such as bacterial endocarditis, systemic lupus erythematosus, and vasculitis; others are primary, often idiopathic, and somewhat less aggressive, such as membranous or IgA nephropathy. Among the glomerular diseases, systemic lupus erythematosus, focal segmental glomerulosclerosis (FGS), and human immunodeficiency virus (HIV)–associated nephropathy are associated with frequent progression to ESRD. Although diabetic nephropathy and hypertensive nephrosclerosis are common causes of ESRD, it is important to recognize that some patients with diabetes and/or hypertension with renal failure suffer from other conditions, such as atherosclerotic vascular disease, that may be the actual cause of renal failure, and that among all persons with diabetes and/or hypertension, advanced renal failure develops in the minority.

Tubulointerstitial diseases are somewhat less common but important causes of CRF, particularly among women. Chronic pyelonephritis, mostly when associated with reflux nephropathy or other congenital abnormalities, can result in a substantial loss of renal function. In this case, CRF results from the effects of repeated infections, leading to scarring and loss of functional renal mass. Papillary necrosis may occur in the setting of diabetes mellitus or sickle cell anemia or as a result of prolonged exposure to nonsteroidal anti-inflammatory drugs (NSAIDs), so-called analgesic nephropathy. Acute interstitial nephritis is usually due to drug exposure. Antibiotics (e.g., penicillins, cephalosporins, sulfonamides) are the most common culprits. Although anecdotal reports have suggested a benefit of glucocorticoids, empirical therapy is usually ill-advised, especially in the setting of an underlying infection. Renal function usually improves after withdrawal of the offending agent, although some degree of CRF develops in 20 to 40% of patients.

COMPLICATIONS OF CHRONIC RENAL FAILURE

Fluid, Electrolytes, and Hypertension

Several characteristic fluid and electrolyte abnormalities manifest during the course of CRF, although they vary widely, depending on the primary disease. Owing in part to reduced functional renal mass, hypertension and edema often occur as a consequence of sodium retention. Diabetic renal disease and many forms of glomerulonephritis are associated with this phenomenon. Ironically, arterial vasodilators prescribed for hypertension (e.g., nifedipine [Procardia], prazosin [Minipress], hydralazine [Apresoline], minoxidil [Loniten]) often contribute to further salt and water retention. The addition of a diuretic agent to an antihypertensive regimen consisting of sympatholytics or vasodilators is often required to achieve adequate blood pressure control in individuals with CRF. It is important to manage hypertension aggressively in the presence of renal insufficiency, as uncontrolled hypertension can accelerate the loss of renal function, particularly among hypertensive African Americans.

Hyponatremia may accompany fluid retention, especially with nephrotic syndrome and hypoalbuminemia, or with concurrent cardiac or hepatic failure. In contrast, patients with interstitial renal disease less frequently develop fluid retention or hyponatremia because of an associated disruption in tubular reabsorptive function, owing to tubular inflammation or fibrosis.

Mild hyperkalemia (5 to 6 mEq per liter) is ex-

tremely common among patients with advanced renal failure. However, life-threatening hyperkalemia (more than 7 mEq per liter) rarely occurs until the GFR drops below 5 to 10 mL per minute. Hyperkalemia is diet dependent (potassium is abundant in many fruits and vegetables) and is more common among diabetics and patients taking certain drugs (Table 3). Hyperkalemia can almost always be controlled with withdrawal of offending agents and other conservative measures, including the administration of a cation exchange resin (sodium polystyrene sulfonate [Kayexalate]), insulin and glucose, sodium bicarbonate, and/or beta$_2$-adrenergic receptor agonists. Frequently coincident with hyperkalemia, metabolic acidosis usually results from insufficient ammoniagenesis and an accumulation of organic and inorganic acids.

CRF associated with hypokalemia is rare but can be seen in association with certain nephrotoxic agents, including amphotericin B (Fungizone), cisplatin (Platinol), and aminoglycosides; excessive doses of loop or thiazide diuretics; or, rarely, hypouricemia, glycosuria, and aminoaciduria (the Fanconi syndrome). Similarly, CRF associated with metabolic alkalosis is uncommon; if it is observed, one should carefully rule out excessive vomiting, overzealous diuretic use, or excessive base ingestion, as in the milk-alkali syndrome.

Disorders of calcium, phosphorus, and parathyroid hormone (PTH) are almost universally present as the GFR drops below 25 mL per minute. Phosphorus tends to accumulate with worsening renal function. Hyperphosphatemia itself drops the serum calcium, as does the reduced intestinal absorption of calcium owing to vitamin D deficiency. PTH secretion is regulated by calcium (increased with decreased serum calcium), phosphate (increased with increased serum phosphate), and 1,25-OH vitamin D (increased with decreased serum 1,25-OH vitamin D). Although hyperparathyroidism tends to increase the serum calcium toward the normal range, it does so at the expense of bone integrity. This vicious circle of calcium dysmetabolism and secondary hyperparathyroidism results in osteitis fibrosa cystica, the most common form of bone disease in patients with renal failure. Aluminum overload may also be present in ESRD patients, owing to increased aluminum intake (in the form of phosphate binders) and reduced excre-

TABLE 3. **Drugs Associated with Hyperkalemia**

Salt substitutes
Potassium-sparing diuretic agents
  Spironolactone (Aldactone)
  Amiloride (Midamor)
  Triamterene (Dyrenium)
Angiotensin-converting enzyme inhibitors
Nonsteroidal anti-inflammatory drugs
Beta-adrenergic antagonists
Cyclosporine (Sandimmune)
Heparin
Digoxin

tion, and may result in a unique form of bone disease (aluminum osteomalacia).

Stepwise management of calcium metabolism includes modest dietary phosphate restriction (e.g., dairy products, especially cheeses, beans, animal proteins) and calcium supplementation with or just after meals. Calcium carbonate (Tums E-X and others) and calcium acetate (PhosLo) are beneficial in that they bind dietary phosphate and provide calcium for systemic absorption. Additionally, these agents provide a small quantity of base equivalents without the additional administration of sodium, such as with sodium bicarbonate. Calcium citrate (Citracal) should be avoided, as citrate markedly enhances the intestinal absorption of aluminum. Likewise, aluminum-based products (e.g., aluminum hydroxide [Amphogel], sucralfate [Carafate]) should be avoided if at all possible. After hyperphosphatemia has been controlled, a vitamin D analogue may be added to improve intestinal absorption of calcium and to directly inhibit PTH secretion.

Hematologic Effects

Anemia and platelet dysfunction are the most common hematologic effects of reduced renal function. The anemia associated with advanced renal failure is usually normocytic and normochromic in type and is caused by a reduction in the production of erythropoietin, a growth factor produced within the kidney. However, the usual causes of anemia should not be ignored in patients with renal failure. Gastrointestinal blood loss owing to peptic ulcer disease, gastritis, esophagitis, malignancy, hemolysis (autoimmune vs. other), and/or nutrient deficiencies (e.g., iron, folate, vitamin B_{12}) is more common among persons with CRF than in the general population and is usually responsive to appropriate therapeutic measures. Aluminum toxicity may result in a microcytic, hypochromic anemia; fortunately, this complication is now rare with diminished administration of aluminum-based phosphate binders.

The anemia associated with reduced erythropoietin production rarely occurs until the GFR drops below 10 to 15 mL per minute. However, this reduction in erythropoietin production is highly variable among individuals and renal diagnoses. For instance, individuals with polycystic kidney disease are less likely to develop severe anemia, presumably owing to the effects of cyst compression on renal tissue, resulting in local ischemia and a relative excess of erythropoietin production. Furthermore, it is important to recognize that, like the reticulocyte count, a level of circulating erythropoietin within the normal range indicates a suboptimal and distinctly abnormal response in a patient with anemia.

Hemostasis can be impaired with severe reductions in GFR (5 to 10 mL per minute). CRF does not appear to affect the clotting cascade, and the prothrombin time and partial thromboplastin time are usually normal except with severe malnutrition or coexistent liver disease. Rather, the hemostatic defect involves platelet dysfunction, which can be diagnosed by an abnormal bleeding time, often exceeding 10 minutes (normal 5 to 7 minutes). Prior to performing any invasive procedure on a patient with renal failure, including renal biopsy, a bleeding time should be assessed. The patient should be off all aspirin products for 1 week and off NSAIDs for several days. If the bleeding time is abnormal, administration of desmopressin acetate (DDAVP), cryoprecipitate, erythropoietin (Epogen) and/or transfusion, or conjugated estrogens (Premarin) or the initiation of dialysis may be needed to improve hemostasis.

Erythropoietin therapy has resulted in the maintenance of adequate hematocrits in most dialysis patients without the need for blood transfusions and has been shown to improve quality of life. Iron stores must be sufficient to support erythropoiesis. Administration of subcutaneous erythropoeitin (Epogen, 2000 to 4000 U once or twice weekly) to individuals with CRF has also been effective.

Gastrointestinal Effects

The most common gastrointestinal manifestations of uremia are nausea and vomiting. These symptoms are attributable to uremia, but other causes of nausea and vomiting, such as myocardial ischemia, diabetic gastropathy, peptic ulcer disease, and other primary gastrointestinal diseases, should be investigated if dialysis does not lead to resolution. Inflammation and edema of the gastrointestinal tract are also relatively common. These changes cause blood loss, altered drug and nutrient availability, and excess absorption of the intracellular constituents of blood, such as nitrogen (derived from hemoglobin), potassium, and phosphorus.

Dialysis markedly improves the nausea and vomiting of uremia. H_2-receptor antagonists, such as ranitidine (Zantac), can be used to reduce dyspepsia. Alternatively, calcium carbonate (Tums E-X and others) can be used, as long as hypercalcemia is not present. Over-the-counter antacids containing magnesium and aluminum (Mylanta) should be avoided.

Serositis

Serositis, or inflammation of the epithelial surfaces of internal organs with altered serosal porosity, can occur with severe reductions in renal function (GFR 5 to 10 mL per minute). The most frequent manifestations are pericarditis, pleuritis, and enteritis (serositis involving the heart, lung, and gastrointestinal tract, respectively). Uremic pericarditis can be life-threatening. If combined with a bleeding diathesis, hemorrhagic pericarditis can develop; at the extreme, this could result in pericardial tamponade. All patients with advanced azotemia should be carefully examined for the presence of a pericardial friction rub. Typically, a three-component rub can be heard best with the patient leaning forward. Intestinal serositis can contribute to nausea and vomiting as well as to hemorrhagic gastritis, esophagitis, and ascites.

A pleural rub or pleural effusion should be carefully evaluated. An infectious (e.g., bacterial, especially *Staphylococcus* spp, or mycobacterial, e.g., tuberculous), malignant (e.g., lung or breast carcinoma), or autoimmune (e.g., systemic lupus erythematosus, rheumatoid arthritis) cause should be excluded in all patients.

Central Nervous System Effects

The internist or nephrologist is often asked to evaluate a hospitalized patient with CRF or ESRD and altered mental status. However, unless the GFR is markedly reduced (below 5 mL per minute), an altered mental state is much more commonly due to other causes, such as medication (e.g., benzodiazepines, ethanol, narcotic analgesics, anticholinergic [including antihistaminic] drugs), infection, cerebrovascular disease, hypoxemia, and/or underlying mental illness. Uremia rarely causes seizures, except when accompanied by profound hypocalcemia (less than 5 to 6 mg per dL). The characteristic encephalopathy of uremia is a gradual reduction in mental alertness and attention capacity, extending from lethargy to stupor and finally, at end-stage, to coma. The central nervous system manifestations of uremia typically respond quite rapidly to the institution of dialysis.

Dementia in patients with CRF is most often due to strokes secondary to cerebrovascular disease or severe systemic hypertension and/or Alzheimer's disease. "Dialysis dementia" refers to a specific condition associated with severe aluminum poisoning. The recognition of this syndrome, improved water quality control, and the decreased use of aluminum-based phosphate binders have markedly reduced the incidence. "Dialysis disequilibrium" refers to a distinct syndrome associated with the rapid removal of urea and other extracellular solutes with dialysis initiation after the chronic progression of renal failure. Clinically, the syndrome is characterized by headache, confusion, and occasionally seizures and is presumably caused by acute cerebral edema (owing to the removal of extracellular osmolar equivalents). Gradual solute removal with diminished blood and dialysate flow rates can usually prevent the occurrence of dialysis disequilibrium. If more aggressive dialysis is otherwise indicated, an osmotically active substance, such as mannitol and/or phenytoin (Dilantin), for anticonvulsant prophylaxis can be administered.

Peripheral neuropathy associated with CRF can affect any or all of the sensory, motor, or autonomic nervous systems. Neuropathy can be particularly disabling in individuals with concurrent diabetic or alcohol-associated neuropathy and may or may not improve with dialysis therapy. Common complications of neuropathy in CRF patients include pain typically involving the lower extremities, altered sensation leading to unrecognized trauma, and orthostatic hypotension. Although tricyclic antidepressant agents such as amitriptyline (Elavil) may be successful in

TABLE 4. **General Effects of Uremia**

Pruritus
Fatigue
Weight loss
Malnutrition
Sleep disturbance (altered day-night cycle, central sleep apnea)
Depression
Musculoskeletal complaints
Nitrogenous fetor
Hair loss

reducing pain and disability, these drugs may exacerbate autonomic nervous dysfunction and/or contribute to fatigue and are often poorly tolerated.

General Effects

Additional associated signs and symptoms of uremia are outlined in Table 4.

METHODS OF RENAL REPLACEMENT THERAPY

It is advisable to refer a patient with chronic renal insufficiency (GFR of approximately 50) to a nephrologist well before renal replacement therapy is required. Adequate blood pressure control and attention to various hormonal and metabolic disturbances may ameliorate some of the long-term complications of chronic renal disease and attenuate the progression of renal failure. Several clinical criteria mandate the prompt institution of renal replacement therapy in persons with advanced CRF (Table 5). However, the provision of dialysis under urgent circumstances places the patient at undue and unnecessary risk; it is best to prepare an individual carefully and deliberately for what will become a major change in lifestyle, employing either dialysis or transplantation. Sufficient time should be allowed for patient reflection and discussion with family and friends regarding treatment options. Likewise, the creation of a native arteriovenous fistula or placement of an artificial arteriovenous graft requires several weeks to months to heal and mature. Although no strict laboratory criteria define uremia, a BUN greater than 150 mg per dL and a serum creatinine greater than 12 to 15 mg per dL are often associated with the development

TABLE 5. **Absolute Indications for Initiation of Chronic Renal Replacement Therapy**

Volume overload refractory to sodium restriction and diuretic therapy
Hyperkalemia refractory to dietary restriction and intestinal binders
Uremia
Pericarditis, serositis
Encephalopathy, neuropathy
Bleeding diathesis
Severe nausea and vomiting
Malnutrition associated with foregoing

of advanced uremic symptoms. Diabetic patients and elderly persons may become symptomatic with less dramatic elevations of serum chemistries.

No one modality can be considered superior in all respects; each method of renal replacement carries its own advantages and disadvantages. It is imperative that the nephrologist assist the patient and family in medical decision making and allow for individualization of care, considering additional issues such as quality of life and emotional and social role function.

Hemodialysis

Hemodialysis is the most common form of renal replacement therapy. Most persons undergo treatment at outpatient centers; fewer are dialyzed at hospital-affiliated units; and a small number dialyze at home with the assistance of a nurse or family member. The procedure is performed as follows. A vascular access (usually a native arteriovenous fistula or polytetrafluoroethylene graft) is needed to provide the obligate blood flows (approximately 350 to 400 mL per minute) required to cleanse the blood efficiently. The clearance of solutes associated with uremia, such as urea nitrogen, creatinine, and other unmeasured or unknown solutes, is achieved primarily by diffusion across a semipermeable membrane, as well as by convection, i.e., solute transfer with ultrafiltration or fluid removal. Whereas low-molecular-weight solutes are very efficiently cleared by diffusion, larger solutes—the so-called middle molecules—are cleared more efficiently by convection. Depending on the size, permeability, and other characteristics of the dialyzer (artificial kidney), increases in blood flow and dialysate flow increase solute clearance.

A typical hemodialysis prescription includes 3 to 5 hours of therapy three times weekly, with blood flows of 300 to 400 mL per minute and dialysate flows of 500 to 800 mL per minute. The dialysate, or fluid against which the blood is bathed, can be individualized to fit the needs of the particular patient. Typically, it is composed of the following electrolytes (concentrations): sodium (138 to 145 mEq per liter), potassium (0 to 4 mEq per liter), chloride (100 to 110 mEq per liter), bicarbonate (35 to 45 mEq per liter), calcium (1.5 to 3.5 mEq per liter), magnesium (1.5 mEq per liter), and glucose (2 grams per liter). An anticoagulant, usually heparin, is required to prevent clotting of blood within the hollow fibers of the dialyzer. The dialysis machine, or delivery system, is not in contact with the blood or dialysate. Rather, its pumps, controls, and safety devices provide precision to the hemodialysis procedure by ensuring proper dialysate composition and temperature and by monitoring the transmembrane pressure required to perform ultrafiltration, or net fluid removal. Complications commonly observed in hemodialysis are listed in Table 6.

TABLE 6. **Common Complications of Dialysis**

Hemodialysis
  Hypotension
  Arrhythmia
  Catheter-related or endovascular infection
  Hemorrhage
  Pyrogen reaction
  Hypoxemia
  Leukopenia
  Catabolism
  Dialysis disequilibrium

Peritoneal dialysis
  Peritonitis
  Ultrafiltration failure
  Hyperglycemia
  Hypertriglyceridemia
  Weight gain
  Elevated intra-abdominal pressure
  Constipation

Peritoneal Dialysis

Like hemodialysis, peritoneal dialysis is achieved by diffusion, using a semipermeable membrane—in this case, the peritoneum rather than the dialyzer. Peritoneal dialysis is less commonly employed than hemodialysis in the United States (approximately 15% of patients), although the fraction of patients who choose peritoneal dialysis varies widely from center to center and among physicians. In addition, a substantial fraction of patients initiated on peritoneal dialysis switch to hemodialysis as residual renal function deteriorates or if recurrent peritonitis renders the peritoneum ineffective as a dialysis membrane. The technique failure rate due to all causes is approximately 50% at 3 years.

Peritoneal dialysis is delivered in one of three major ways. Continuous ambulatory peritoneal dialysis (CAPD) is provided by four to six fluid exchanges throughout the day. Generally, these exchanges (2 to 3 liters) are instilled into the peritoneal cavity through a surgically placed Silastic catheter and drained every 3 to 4 hours during waking hours; a 2-liter bag is instilled overnight to provide additional solute clearance. Continuous cyclical peritoneal dialysis (CCPD) utilizes a machine that automatically performs fluid exchanges during the night. Patients on CCPD may retain a dry abdomen during waking hours but receive better dialysis with 1 to 2 liters to dwell during the daytime. Both continuous techniques must be performed daily and require responsible patients with a strong desire for self-care. Intermittent peritoneal dialysis (IPD), or frequent exchanges on alternate days or thrice weekly, may be employed short term, for instance, during hospitalization. However, IPD rarely provides adequate time-averaged clearance unless substantial residual renal function remains.

Among the peritoneal dialysis regimens, CCPD may be more convenient for some patients, particularly those with children or whose work precludes the ability to perform sterile exchanges. However, the absence of around-the-clock clearance limits dialysis efficiency, particularly for middle molecules. Likewise, because the fluid is instilled while the patient is supine, large volume exchanges (over 2.5 liters) are often poorly tolerated. For all peritoneal dialysis regimens, an increase in the frequency and/or volume of peritoneal exchanges usually results in increased solute clearance. The percentage of dextrose in the peritoneal dialysate in large part determines the ultrafiltration rate—the higher the concentration of dextrose (1.5, 2.5, or 4.25%), the greater the quantity and rate of ultrafiltration.

Peritoneal dialysis exerts important effects on the nutritional status of a patient with ESRD. The instillation and absorption of glucose result in the delivery of 400 to 500 kcal per day, which may augment nutrition in patients with poor appetite but may worsen pre-existent hypertriglyceridemia, particularly among diabetic patients. In contrast, the loss of protein through the peritoneum can contribute to protein malnutrition (discussed later).

Unlike hemodialysis, a reliable measure of delivered dialysis dose in peritoneal dialysis has not been validated. A peritoneal equilibrium test can be used to assess the transport properties of the membrane and does correlate somewhat with dialysis adequacy.

Peritonitis is the most important complication of peritoneal dialysis. It is most often caused by a break in sterile technique and is usually (80 to 90% of the time) associated with the introduction of bacteria colonizing the pericatheter skin (e.g., *Staphylococcus epidermidis, S. aureus, Streptococcus* spp). Peritonitis may also be caused by enteric gram-negative rods, hydrophilic gram-negative rods (e.g., *Pseudomonas* spp), mycobacteria, or fungi. Antimicrobial agents can be administered systemically or directly into the peritoneal cavity. Most cases of peritonitis can be resolved without interruption of dialysis or impairment of peritoneal function. However, repeated gram-negative infections or fungal peritonitis usually require removal of the indwelling catheter. Additional complications of peritoneal dialysis are listed in Table 6.

Transplantation

Kidney transplantation, a third option in renal replacement, is considered by most patients and nephrologists to be the treatment of choice for ESRD. Its major advantages are freedom from long-term dialysis, more complete reversal of uremia and nephroendocrine functions, and an overall reduction in health care costs. However, transplantation is better considered a trade-off rather than a panacea for ESRD, as the agents used to combat rejection have many important short- and long-term adverse effects (Table 7).

Most allografts are derived from cadaver donors. The waiting time ranges from 3 months to years, depending largely on blood type, human leukocyte antigen (HLA) matching, and donor organ availability. In contrast, related-donor transplantation can be performed with a healthy, immunologically compati-

TABLE 7. Immune Suppressive Drugs Used in Renal Transplantation

Drug	Major Side Effects	Cost
Cyclosporine (Sandimmune)	Infection Hypertension Hyperkalemia Hyperuricemia and gout Renal dysfunction Lymphoid malignancy Hirsutism Gingival hypertrophy	Very high
Azathioprine (Imuran)	Infection Squamous cell carcinoma of skin Leukopenia	High
Prednisone or methylprednisolone	Infection Hypertension Fluid retention Hyperglycemia and diabetes Osteoporosis Cataracts Hirsutism Depression	Low
Muromonab-CD3 (Orthoclone OKT3)*	Infection Lymphoid malignancy Aseptic meningitis Capillary leak syndrome	Extremely high
Lymphocyte immune globulin (antithymocyte globulin [ATG]) (Atgam)*	Infection Lymphoid malignancy Hypersensitivity	Extremely high

*Used for acute rejection or induction therapy.

ble, willing family member at almost any time, even before the initiation of dialysis. The short-term outcome of renal transplantation has gradually improved: 80 to 85% of all cadaveric kidneys and more than 90% of living-related kidneys transplanted are functional at the end of a year. Unfortunately, the long-term "survival" of allografts has remained modest (7 years for cadaveric allografts, 14 years for living related allografts), presumably due to recurrence of underlying disease, poor adherence to immune suppressive therapy, cyclosporine nephrotoxicity, hyperfiltration-induced injury (i.e., nonimmunologic damage to remnant nephrons), and financial and other psychosocial constraints. In addition, the supply of donor organs has remained stable over several years, whereas the number of eligible potential recipients rises with the treated incidence of ESRD.

NUTRITION AND CHRONIC RENAL FAILURE

The roles of dietary protein and other nutrients in CRF have been investigated intensely in the past decade. Long ago it was recognized that dietary protein intake was associated with uremic symptoms in persons in advanced kidney failure. Before the advent of renal replacement therapy (pre-1950s), uremia was often managed with diets consisting of minimal protein, such as rice, certain vegetables, and fruit juice. Indeed, the reduction in dietary protein intake reduced nausea, vomiting, and some other uremic symptoms. Although life was prolonged for some patients who followed these dietary modifications, many others developed severe protein malnutrition. Later, similar diets supplemented with small quantities of proteins of high biologic value were shown to result in far less protein catabolism. Meanwhile, several investigators suggested that the restriction of dietary protein (and phosphorus) might attenuate the progression of various types of renal disease. Soon after, the administration of low-protein diets became commonplace among patients with CRF and ESRD.

Only recently, however, has the importance of malnutrition been highlighted in several well-designed studies in dialysis patients. A striking association has been demonstrated between mortality and diminished levels of serum albumin (a proxy for visceral protein mass) and creatinine (after adjustment for dialysis intensity, a proxy for somatic protein mass). In addition, results of a prospective trial of protein restriction in patients with chronic renal insufficiency (the Modification of Diet in Renal Disease Study) showed only modest overall benefit in terms of rate of progression of renal failure among patients on a low-protein (or very-low-protein) diet. Although some benefit of protein restriction cannot be excluded, it is advisable to exercise caution with this therapeutic modality. Indeed, attention to blood pressure control may be equally if not more effective and has fewer potential hazards. If protein restriction is prescribed, nutritional status should be carefully monitored. Several methods of nutritional assessment are serial measurements of body weight, anthropometry, serum chemistries (e.g., albumin, transferrin, total lymphocyte count), and functional assessment (e.g., exercise tolerance).

MALIGNANT TUMORS OF THE UROGENITAL TRACT

method of
JOHN D. SEIGNE, M.B., and
H. BARTON GROSSMAN, M.D.
The University of Texas M.D. Anderson
Cancer Center
Houston, Texas

Genitourinary neoplasms encompass a broad spectrum of human cancers ranging from the most common tumor, adenocarcinoma of the prostate, to some of the rarest. These cancers are generally accessible to a variety of diagnostic modalities and can be detected and staged by physical examination, blood tests, and/or diagnostic imaging. The range of therapeutic options is broad, depending on the type and extent of the neoplasm, and can include observation, surgery, radiation, chemotherapy, and immunotherapy. Goals of therapy include eradication of the neoplasm and preservation of quality of life by maintaining organ function whenever possible.

ADRENAL TUMORS

Adrenocortical Carcinoma

Adrenal cancers are rare tumors that occur with an incidence of 1 per 1.7 million population. Approximately 80% of tumors are functional, producing biologically active adrenal hormones that result in a variety of disorders including, in order of decreasing frequency, Cushing's syndrome, virilization, feminization, and hyperaldosteronism. Adrenocortical carcinoma has a slight female preponderance and occurs in all age groups, with a slightly higher incidence after the age of 40 years. Endocrinologic symptoms are the most common presentation. However, many patients present with nonspecific symptoms such as weight loss, anorexia, or an abdominal mass. Increasingly, these tumors are discovered as incidental adrenal masses on computed tomography (CT) or ultrasonography images.

All patients should undergo endocrinologic evaluation, including 24-hour urine collections for 17-ketosteroids (screens for excess cortisol, androgens, and estrogens), vanillylmandelic acid (VMA), metanephrins, and catecholamines (screens for pheochromocytoma) and have the serum potassium level measured. Routine radiologic staging studies include chest radiograph and abdominopelvic CT scan. The staging of adrenal tumors is shown in Table 1.

Management

The primary therapy of adrenocortical tumors is complete surgical resection. Surgical excision should be performed even if resection of adjacent organs, such as the kidney, pancreas, or spleen, is necessary. Median disease-free survival after complete surgical resection is 12 months, with 22% of patients surviving 5 years. Patients should be followed every 3 months with an abdominal CT scan, chest radiograph, and liver function tests. Fifty to eighty percent of patients present with metastatic disease. Patients with metastatic adrenocortical carcinoma have a poor prognosis. Chemotherapy with mitotane (o,p'-DDD [Lysodren]) can induce partial tumor regression and control endocrinologic symptoms. Unfortunately, few responses are durable, and mitotane can have significant gastrointestinal side effects. Radiation therapy is indicated only for palliation.

TABLE 1. **Staging of Adrenal Cancer**

T1	Confined to adrenal, tumor diameter < 5 cm
T2	Confined to adrenal, tumor diameter > 5 cm
T3	Tumor outside adrenal into fat
T4	Tumor invading adjacent organs
N0	No regional node metastasis
N1	Regional node metastasis
M0	No distant metastasis
M1	Distant metastasis

Pheochromocytoma

Pheochromocytomas are rare tumors of paraganglionic chromaffin cells. Patients with multiple endocrine neoplasia syndrome type II and von Hippel–Lindau disease have a higher incidence of pheochromocytoma. Pheochromocytomas occur primarily in the adrenal gland but can be found anywhere paraganglionic cells are located, from the mediastinum to the bladder wall. Most pheochromocytomas are benign functional tumors, and less than 10% are malignant. Excessive production of catecholamines by these tumors is responsible for the classic symptoms of paroxysmal or sustained hypertension associated with headaches, flushing, and palpitations. Pheochromocytoma is a causative factor in less than 0.2% of hypertensive patients.

Metabolic evaluation consists of a 24-hour urine collection for VMA, metanephrins, and catecholamines and a serum sample for catecholamines (drawn at rest). Abdominal magnetic resonance imaging (MRI) usually shows a bright tumor on T2-weighted images. ^{131}I-meta-iodobenzylguanidine (MIBG) nuclear scanning can be used to localize tumors that are not evident on radiologic images.

Management

The primary treatment is surgical excision following appropriate control of blood pressure. Alpha-adrenergic blockade with phenoxybenzamine (Dibenzyline), initial dose 10 mg twice daily, and volume expansion are achieved before surgery. Surgical excision is performed through a midline incision, which provides access to the retroperitoneum and opposite adrenal gland (up to 10% of pheochromocytomas are bilateral). The alpha blocker metyrosine (Demser), initial dose 250 mg four times daily, can be used to control symptoms in the rare patient with metastatic pheochromocytoma.

Neuroblastoma

Neuroblastoma is the most common extracranial solid tumor of infants and children, with an incidence of 9 per 1 million children. The tumor arises from the sympathetic nervous system and can occur anywhere along the sympathetic chain. The most common site is the adrenal gland. Most children present with an abdominal mass or symptoms of metastatic disease. Hypertension is uncommon despite the fact that 95% of patients have elevated urinary levels of VMA and homovanillic acid. Initial evaluation consists of 24-hour urine collection for VMA, MRI of the abdomen, chest radiograph, skeletal survey, and bone marrow aspiration (abnormal in up to 70% of cases). Staging is illustrated in Table 2.

Management

Children with stage I or stage II neuroblastomas undergo primary surgical excision. Postoperative chemotherapy is administered for pathologic stage II disease. Survival is approximately 80%. Children

TABLE 2. Staging of Neuroblastoma (Evans' System)

Stage I	Confined to organ of origin
Stage II	Extends beyond organ of origin but not across the midline
Stage III	Extends across the midline
Stage IV	Metastatic disease
Stage IV-S	Local stage I or II with metastases confined to the bone marrow, skin, and liver

with stage III or stage IV neuroblastomas are treated with radiation and combination chemotherapy. Survival rates of 37% and 5% have been reported for stage III and stage IV diseases, respectively (children younger than 1 year of age have a better prognosis). In patients with stage IV-S disease the tumor usually undergoes spontaneous regression, and treatment is used only to alleviate symptoms before this occurs.

Evaluation and Management of an Incidental Adrenal Mass

Incidental adrenal masses are discovered on up to 2% of abdominal CT scans performed for an unrelated reason. The differential diagnosis of a solid adrenal mass includes, in order of decreasing frequency, benign nonfunctional adenoma, metastatic carcinoma, functional adenoma, pheochromocytoma, and adrenocortical carcinoma. Adrenal cyst, hemorrhage, and myelolipomas can usually be distinguished by radiologic criteria alone and do not require further evaluation. In the absence of findings on history and physical examination suggestive of excessive hormonal production, we recommend a 24-hour urine collection for VMA, metanephrins, and catecholamines to exclude a pheochromocytoma. The level of serum potassium should be measured in hypertensive patients to exclude excessive mineralocorticoid production. Masses that are hormonally active or larger than 5 cm should be excised. Smaller, hormonally inactive masses can be followed with repeat CT scanning at 3, 9, and 21 months. If the mass grows, it should be excised; otherwise, radiographic follow-up can be discontinued.

KIDNEY TUMORS

Renal Cell Carcinoma

Renal cell carcinoma is an uncommon malignancy, representing approximately 2% of all new cancer cases. The tumor has a 2:1 male to female predominance and occurs primarily in the fifth through seventh decades of life but can occur in any age group. Patients with von Hippel–Lindau disease (an autosomal dominant condition that manifests by retinal angiomas, cerebellar hemangioblastomas, and renal cell carcinomas) have a high incidence of renal cell carcinoma. Recent molecular studies have indicated that loss of function of a tumor suppressor gene on the short arm of chromosome 3 contributes to the development of renal cell carcinoma. Most renal cell carcinomas arise from the cells of the proximal tubule. However, evidence from immunohistochemical studies suggests that some renal cell carcinomas arise from more distal portions of the nephron.

Presentation and Diagnosis

Renal cell carcinoma presents in a variety of ways. The classic triad of flank pain, abdominal mass, and gross hematuria occurs in fewer than 20% of patients. A more common presentation includes nonspecific symptoms such as anorexia, weight loss, and night sweats. These tumors are being increasingly discovered as incidental renal masses on ultrasonogram or abdominal CT scan performed for an unrelated reason. Renal cell carcinoma may produce a variety of hormones or hormone-like substances (e.g., erythropoietin, renin, and parathyroid hormone), and patients with renal tumors may present with an assortment of paraneoplastic syndromes. Evaluation of the patient with renal cell carcinoma includes a complete blood count and alkaline phosphatase, creatinine, calcium, and liver function tests. Radiologic evaluation includes a chest film and abdominal CT scan. MRI can provide additional information in cases of suspected renal vein and inferior vena cava involvement by tumor thrombus. Needle biopsy of a renal mass is rarely indicated. The American Joint Committee on Cancer (AJCC) staging system for renal carcinoma is shown in Table 3.

Management

Localized Disease. The treatment of localized (T1–T3) renal cell carcinoma is surgical excision. Radical nephrectomy involves removal of the kidney, the surrounding fat, and the adrenal gland. The surgical approach depends on the preference of the surgeon and can be through the flank or abdomen. For particularly large tumors or tumors involving the inferior vena cava, a thoracoabdominal approach can be utilized. Tumor thrombus extending into the vena cava and right atrium can be safely removed by an experienced surgical team with the help of cardiopulmonary bypass and total circulatory arrest. The value of routine regional lymphadenectomy at the

time of radical surgery is unclear. We feel that regional lymphadenectomy should be performed because it provides prognostic information and may be therapeutic. Partial nephrectomy is as effective as radical nephrectomy in selected patients. Partial nephrectomy is indicated in patients with a solitary kidney, bilateral tumors, or compromised renal function. The use of partial nephrectomy in patients with small tumors and a normal contralateral kidney remains controversial.

The 5-year survival rate for patients (after radical nephrectomy) with T1–T2 disease is approximately 80% and decreases to approximately 50% in patients with T3a disease. Tumor thrombus extension into the vena cava has little impact on survival. Patients with nodal disease (N1) have a poor prognosis, with a 5-year survival rate of between 10% and 20%.

Following surgery, patients should have a chest radiograph and creatinine determination every 3 to 4 months for the first year and twice annually thereafter. Evaluation of the tumor bed and contralateral kidney with CT scan should be performed on patients with high-stage tumors every 6 months for the first 2 years, with a renal ultrasonogram done annually thereafter.

Metastatic Disease. Patients with metastatic renal cell carcinoma have an extremely poor prognosis, with a median survival of 6 to 8 months. In general, radical nephrectomy does not prolong the survival of patients with metastatic renal cell carcinoma. However, in patients with a solitary metastasis, surgical resection of the primary tumor and the metastasis can lead to prolonged survival. Nephrectomy is occasionally necessary for control of pain or hemorrhage from the kidney. However, angioinfarction and radiation therapy are effective palliative methods and are less invasive alternatives to surgery.

In general, radiation therapy and cytotoxic chemotherapy are relatively ineffective in the treatment of renal cell carcinoma. The single most effective agent is vinblastine (Velban), with an objective response rate of 10% to 12%. Initial favorable reports using hormonal therapy with medroxyprogesterone acetate have not withstood more rigorous testing. Biologic response modifiers have shown the greatest potential for effective treatment of metastatic renal cell carcinoma. Interferons are glycoproteins produced by mammalian cells in response to viral infection. Of the three classes of interferons, alfa-interferon has shown the most potential, with response rates of up to 17%; major side effects are flulike symptoms. Interleukin-2* (IL-2) is a potent T cell growth factor that causes T cell proliferation and enhances natural killer cell function. IL-2 alone or in combination with activated lymphocytes (LAK cells) has shown response rates of up to 30% in patients with renal cell carcinoma. High-dose IL-2 can have significant cardiopulmonary toxic effects that require admission into an intensive care unit. Newer approaches using tumor-infiltrating lymphocytes, gene-modified lym-

TABLE 3. **American Joint Committee on Cancer Staging of Renal Cell Carcinoma**

T1	Confined to kidney, <2.5 cm in diameter
T2	Confined to kidney, >2.5 cm in diameter
T3	Extends into veins or outside kidney, but not beyond Gerota's fascia
T3a	Tumor in perinephric fat or adrenal gland, but confined by Gerota's fascia
T3b	Tumor in renal vein or vena cava below the diaphragm
T3c	Tumor extends into supradiaphragmatic vena cava
T4	Tumor extends beyond Gerota's fascia
N0	No regional node metastasis
N1–3	Regional node metastasis
M0	No distant metastasis
M1	Distant metastasis

*Investigational drug in the United States.

phocytes (gene therapy), and gene-modified tumor vaccines are currently being investigated. Our practice is to treat patients with 5-fluorouracil and alfa-interferon,* or IL-2 based regimens.

Renal Oncocytoma

Renal oncocytoma accounts for 5% to 7% of all solid renal masses. These tumors have a typical gross and histologic appearance and usually behave in a benign fashion. Grossly, the tumors are well encapsulated, tan in color, and classically have a central scar. Histologically, they consist of large cells with intensely eosinophilic granular cytoplasm. Although a central scar on a CT scan and a spoke-wheel pattern on an arteriogram have been associated with oncocytomas, the radiologic differentiation of oncocytoma and renal cell carcinoma is extremely difficult. In rare cases, when an oncocytoma is strongly suspected, partial nephrectomy can be utilized. However, radical nephrectomy is the usual diagnostic and therapeutic method.

Angiomyolipoma

Angiomyolipomas account for about 3% of solid renal lesions and are frequently bilateral. They are hamartomas that consist of smooth muscle, blood vessels, and mature adipose tissue. Angiomyolipomas occur in 40% to 80% of patients with tuberous sclerosis. However, fewer than 20% of patients with angiomyolipoma have tuberous sclerosis. There is an 8:1 female to male ratio, and presentation usually occurs in the fifth through seventh decades of life. The most common presentation is flank pain, with 50% of patients having a palpable mass on abdominal examination. Between 10% and 25% of patients will present with acute retroperitoneal hemorrhage and shock. Abdominal CT scanning is usually diagnostic. Angiomyolipomas are solid tumors that contain areas of fat with a density of between -10 and -80 Hounsfield units. MRI can also be used. The major complication associated with angiomyolipoma is retroperitoneal hemorrhage, a complication that occurs more frequently in pregnant women. Lesions that are smaller than 4 cm in diameter are unlikely to bleed and can be followed with biannual renal ultrasonograms. Lesions that are larger than 4 cm in size or that occur in women of childbearing age are at increased risk of hemorrhage and should be treated by partial nephrectomy or angioinfarction. We favor renal-sparing surgery for this benign tumor. Acute hemorrhage and very large tumors can often be controlled with selective angioinfarction.

Wilms' Tumor

Wilms' tumor is the most common malignant urinary tract neoplasm of childhood, with an incidence of 1 per 100,000 children younger than 5 years of age. Five to ten percent of Wilms' tumors are bilateral. Two forms of the disease are recognizable, heritable and nonheritable forms. The heritable form accounts for 15% to 20% of cases and is associated with specific congenital abnormalities, including aniridia and hemihypertrophy. Loss of function of the WT1 and WT2 tumor suppressor genes on the short arm of chromosome 11 are factors in the development of Wilms' tumor.

Presentation and Diagnosis

Most patients are younger than 5 years of age and present with a palpable abdominal mass. Intravenous urography and abdominal ultrasonography are the tests of choice used to differentiate Wilms' tumor from the other benign and malignant causes of abdominal masses in children. Chest x-ray film and abdominal MRI are the staging investigation methods of choice. Tumors are staged using the National Wilms' Tumor Staging System (Table 4). Wilms' tumors are also subdivided according to whether they have favorable or unfavorable histology. Tumors of unfavorable histology are present in 5% of patients and are manifested by the presence of anaplasia. Patients with anaplastic histology have a death rate nine times greater than those who have a favorable histology.

Management

Treatment has been determined by the National Wilms' Tumor Studies, which are currently in their fourth generation. Patients with a stage 1 or stage 2 tumor that has a favorable histology undergo surgical resection followed by 26 weeks of chemotherapy with actinomycin D (dactinomycin [Cosmegen]) and vincristine (Oncovin). The 2-year disease-free survival rate is 90%. Patients with stage 3 tumors that have a favorable histology undergo surgical resection followed by 1000 cGy of flank irradiation and 26 weeks of chemotherapy with actinomycin D, doxorubicin (Rubex), and vincristine. The 2-year disease-free survival rate is 78%. Patients with stage 4 disease and those whose tumors have an unfavorable histology undergo surgical resection followed by 1200 cGy of pulmonary irradiation and 65 weeks of chemotherapy with actinomycin D, doxorubicin, and vincristine. The 2-year disease-free survival rate is 20%. Patients with bilateral Wilms' tumor should have both tumors biopsied followed by primary chemother-

TABLE 4. **Staging of Wilms' Tumor (National Wilms' Tumor Study 3)**

Stage I	Tumor confined to kidney and completely resected
Stage II	Tumor extension beyond the kidney but tumor completely resected
Stage III	Residual nonhematogenous tumor confined to the abdomen (nodes, peritoneal implants)
Stage IV	Hematogenous metastatic disease
Stage V	Bilateral Wilms' tumor at diagnosis

*Not FDA-approved for this indication.

apy. Nephron-sparing surgical resection of residual disease should be performed following chemotherapy. Survival depends on initial tumor stage and histology.

UROTHELIAL TUMORS

Bladder Cancer

Bladder cancer is the fourth most common cause of cancer in men, with an incidence of 29 per 100,000. Bladder cancer has a 2.5 times greater incidence in men than in women and is a disease that occurs primarily in the sixth and seventh decades of life. Transitional cell carcinoma is the most common histologic type (95%), with squamous cell carcinomas and adenocarcinomas occurring infrequently. A variety of chemical carcinogens have been shown to cause bladder cancer in both animals and man. Occupational exposure to aromatic amines, especially beta-naphthylamine, has been documented to produce an increased incidence of bladder cancer. Workers in the textile, dye, rubber, and printing industries are at increased risk. However, the most important etiologic agent is cigarette smoke.

Presentation and Diagnosis

The hallmark of bladder cancer is gross, painless hematuria. However, hematuria does not have to be persistent or visually obvious to be of clinical significance. A minority of patients present with irritable voiding symptoms (e.g., frequency and dysuria), symptoms that occur frequently in patients with carcinoma in situ. A high degree of suspicion is required to detect carcinoma in situ in patients when it presents in this manner. It is not cost effective to go through a complete diagnostic evaluation in everyone with irritative voiding symptoms, because the incidence of cancer in this patient population is low. However, urine cytology combined with flow cytometry or image analysis is an effective, noninvasive way to screen this group of patients.

All patients who present with hematuria should be evaluated with intravenous urography (IVU) and cystoscopy. IVU and tomography will effectively evaluate the kidneys and ureters for most surgically treatable conditions likely to cause hematuria. Renal ultrasonography is an alternative imaging modality that has greater sensitivity in detecting small renal cell carcinomas but is less able to detect transitional cell carcinomas. The bladder is poorly evaluated by radiologic studies, so cystoscopy is the diagnostic study of choice. Urine cytology occasionally detects tumors before they are grossly visible and may provide useful additional information.

Patients with bladder tumors should have cystoscopy, and all visible tumor should be resected whenever possible. Deep biopsies that include bladder muscle will facilitate tumor staging. Bimanual examination while the patient is under anesthesia will increase the accuracy of staging muscle-invasive tumors. Patients with muscle-invasive tumors should

also be evaluated for metastatic disease with liver function tests, alkaline phosphatase, abdominopelvic CT scan, and chest radiograph. Bladder tumors are staged using the AJCC system (Table 5).

Management

Bladder cancers can be functionally divided into two groups: (1) superficial bladder cancer (Ta, T1, Tis), which makes up approximately 70% of bladder tumors, usually requires local therapy, and has a good prognosis; and (2) invasive bladder cancer (T2 to T4), which accounts for 30% of bladder tumors, usually requires aggressive surgical treatment, and has a poorer prognosis.

Superficial Disease. The treatment of superficial bladder cancer is transurethral resection. The recurrence rate for patients with superficial bladder cancers exceeds 50%. Therefore, regular follow-up with cystoscopy and cytology studies every 3 months for 2 years, 6 months for 2 years, and annually thereafter is necessary. Patients with multiple recurrences of low-grade Ta lesions are candidates for intravesical chemotherapy. We recommend thiotepa (Thioplex), 6 weekly instillations of 60 mg of thiotepa in 60 mL of water retained intravesically for 60 minutes, because it is an effective agent that is well tolerated and relatively inexpensive. A white blood cell count should be performed before each administration because thiotepa can cause leukopenia. Patients who present with high-grade (grade 3), T1, or Tis tumors are at high risk for tumor recurrence and progression to muscle invasion. These patients should be treated with intravesical therapy commencing 1 to 2 weeks after initial transurethral resection. We recommend using bacillus Calmette-Guérin (BCG) (6 weekly courses of lyophilized BCG solubilized in 50 mL of saline retained intravesically for 120 minutes) as initial therapy in this high-risk group. Additional "maintenance" therapy may be efficacious. Intravesical BCG can decrease the rate of local recurrence to less than 25% at 2 years. A second course of BCG can be effective in 50% of patients in whom disease recurs after an initial course. BCG administration can cause significant irritative voiding symptoms.

TABLE 5. **American Joint Committee on Cancer Staging of Bladder Cancer**

Ta	Noninvasive papillary tumor
Tis	Carcinoma in situ, noninvasive flat carcinoma
T1	Tumor invades lamina propria
T2	Tumor invades superficial muscle (inner half of muscularis propria)
T3	Tumor invades deep muscle or perivesical fat
T3a	Tumor invades deep muscle (outer half of muscularis propria)
T3b	Tumor invades perivesical fat
T4	Tumor invades adjacent structure (prostate, vagina, pelvic side wall)
N0	No regional node metastasis
N1–3	Regional node metastasis
M0	No distant metastasis
M1	Distant metastasis

BCG is a live, attenuated tuberculosis bacterium (*Mycobacterium bovis*), and systemic infections and deaths have been reported after BCG administration following traumatic catheterization. **BCG should not be administered if there is difficulty in catheterization**. Patients with persistent fevers unresponsive to antipyretics 48 hours after BCG administration should be treated with isoniazid at 300 mg per day. Patients who become critically ill should also be treated with steroids, rifampin at 600 mg daily, ethambutol at 1200 mg daily, and cycloserine at 500 mg twice daily.

Invasive Disease. Patients with invasive bladder cancer have a high likelihood of developing significant local complications and metastatic disease. Therefore, aggressive surgical treatment with removal of the lymph nodes, bladder, and prostate in men and the uterus, urethra and anterior vaginal wall in women with urinary diversion is the treatment of choice for patients with clinically localized disease (T2, T3, and T4a). Five-year survival rates after radical cystectomy are 75%, 44%, 36%, and 5% for pathologic stage T2, T3, T4, and node-positive tumors, respectively. The operative mortality rate is less than 2%. Postoperative chemotherapy appears to improve survival in patients with stage T3b disease. Primary radiation therapy is often associated with local failure. Bladder-sparing with transurethral resection, chemotherapy, and radiation therapy is an alternative treatment being investigated in patients with T2 disease.

Following cystectomy, the urinary tract is traditionally reconstructed by anastomosing the ureters to an isolated segment of ileum brought to the abdominal surface as a stoma that drains into an external collection device. Recently, reconstructive techniques have been developed that reconfigure a segment of isolated bowel into a pouch. The pouch can be attached to the urethral stump to create a neobladder (which allows most patients to void per urethra) or brought to the abdominal wall as a continent, catheterizable stoma. Nocturnal incontinence is a problem in 20% to 30% of patients following neobladder construction. Continent diversions are associated with a higher incidence of complications and a reoperation rate of approximately 15%.

Follow-up after cystectomy consists of a chest film, liver function tests, and determination of creatinine level every 6 months for 2 years and annually thereafter. Patients with continent diversions should also have vitamin B_{12} and electrolytes monitored. Intravenous urography (IVU) is usually performed 6 weeks after surgery. Upper urinary tract imaging studies should be performed annually.

Metastatic Disease. Currently, the most effective chemotherapeutic regimen is methotrexate, vinblastine (Velban), doxorubicin (Adriamycin), and cisplatin (MVAC protocol). The complete response rate is 30%, with an additional 20% achieving a partial response. Approximately 15% of patients will enjoy a long duration of unmaintained complete responses. MVAC chemotherapy has significant toxicity.

TABLE 6. **American Joint Committee on Cancer Staging of Renal Pelvis and Ureteral Cancers**

Ta	Noninvasive papillary tumor
Tis	Carcinoma in situ, noninvasive flat carcinoma
T1	Tumor invades subepithelial connective tissue
T2	Tumor invades muscle
T3 (renal pelvis)	Tumor beyond muscularis into peripelvic fat or renal parenchyma
T3 (ureter)	Tumor beyond muscularis into periureteral fat
T4	Tumor invades adjacent organs
N0	No regional node metastasis
N1–3	Regional node metastasis
M0	No distant metastasis
M1	Distant metastasis

Carcinoma of the Ureter and Renal Pelvis

Transitional cell carcinoma of the upper urinary tract accounts for 5% of all transitional cell carcinomas. Tumors occur most frequently in the renal pelvis and appear with decreasing frequency as one progresses toward the bladder. Synchronous or metachronous bladder tumors occur in 40% to 80% of patients. Contralateral ureteral tumor will be present or subsequently develop in 2% to 4% of patients. The most common presentation of upper tract tumors is gross hematuria, often with the passage of stringlike clots (ureteral casts) in the urine. Other presentations include flank pain, palpable mass, systemic symptoms of malignancy, and an incidental filling defect on IVU (differential diagnosis includes tumor, radiolucent stone, blood clot, and fungus ball). Initial evaluation should include IVU, retrograde pyelography, and ureteral washings. Further studies, including flexible or rigid ureteroscopy and abdominal CT scanning, are often necessary. Tumors are staged by the AJCC system (Table 6).

Treatment depends on tumor stage, grade, and location, as well as contralateral renal function. High-grade and high-stage (T2 or greater) tumors have a greater propensity for local recurrence and multicentricity. Therefore, in the presence of a normal contralateral kidney, treatment consists of nephroureterectomy (excision of the kidney and ureter with a cuff of bladder) and a regional node dissection. Surgical removal of the distal ureter is critical because tumors recur in up to 65% of retained ureteral stumps. Low-grade and low-stage tumors in the mid and distal ureter can be treated by segmental resection or distal ureterectomy. Low-grade and low-stage renal pelvic and upper ureteral tumors usually require nephroureterectomy. When upper tract tumors occur in a solitary kidney or in association with a compromised contralateral kidney, endoscopic resection or laser tumor ablation are additional treatment options. Topical therapy with mitomycin (Mutamycin),* and BCG (TICE BCG)* can be used in a fashion similar to intravesical therapy

---

*Not FDA-approved for this indication.

for bladder cancer, albeit with a higher complication rate. Prognosis is related to tumor grade and stage. T0-T1 Grade 1, T2 grade 2, and T3–T4 grade 3 tumors have 5-year survival rates of 80% to 90%, 60% to 70%, and 10% to 15%, respectively. Patients with nodal or metastatic disease are treated with MVAC chemotherapy and rarely survive 5 years.

Female Urethral Cancer

The female urethra is 3 to 5 cm in length and lies anterior to the vagina. The lymphatic drainage of the distal one third of the urethra is to the inguinal nodes. The more proximal two thirds of the urethra drains to both the inguinal and deep pelvic lymph nodes. Urethral tumors are rare and occur more frequently in women than in men. The most common histologic type is squamous cell carcinoma (75%), followed by adenocarcinoma (15%) and transitional cell carcinoma (10%). The most common presenting features are urethral bleeding, irritative or obstructive voiding symptoms, and a palpable mass. Diagnosis requires cystoscopy and biopsy. Evaluation of patients with urethral cancer should include a careful inguinal node examination, abdominopelvic CT scan, and chest radiograph. Tumors are staged by the AJCC system (Table 7). Treatment depends on location, stage, and grade of the tumor. Tumors of the distal urethra are usually superficial and can be managed by local excision. Prognosis is excellent, with 70% to 100% of patients surviving 5 years. Tumors of the proximal two thirds of the urethra are usually of higher stage and grade and frequently require cystourethrectomy. Inguinal lymphadenectomy should be performed only in patients with palpably enlarged nodes. The prognosis for women with proximal urethral tumors is poor because most patients present with advanced disease.

Male Urethral Tumors

The male urethra is divided into the prostatic, membranous, bulbar, and penile portions. Lymphatic drainage of the penile urethra is to the inguinal nodes. The more proximal portions of the urethra drain to both the inguinal and deep pelvic lymph nodes. The majority of tumors occur in the bulbar urethra and are squamous cell carcinomas (80%).

TABLE 7. **American Joint Committee on Cancer Staging of Urethral Cancer (Male and Female)**

Tis	Carcinoma in situ, noninvasive flat carcinoma
T1	Tumor invades subepithelial connective tissue
T2	Tumor invades corpora spongiosum, prostate, or periurethral muscle
T3	Tumor invades corpus cavernosum, bladder neck, or anterior vaginal wall
T4	Tumor invades other adjacent organs
N0	No regional node metastasis
N1–3	Regional node metastasis
M0	No distant metastasis
M1	Distant metastasis

Transitional cell carcinoma occurs in the prostatic urethra and accounts for approximately 15% of urethral cancers. The remaining 5% of tumors are adenocarcinomas and other tumors of rare histologic types. Urethral tumors are usually locally invasive and present with symptoms of bladder outlet obstruction, urethral bleeding, and a palpable mass. Diagnosis requires cystoscopy and biopsy. Evaluation of patients with urethral cancer should include a careful inguinal node examination, abdominopelvic CT scan, and chest radiograph. Tumors are staged according to the depth of local invasion by the AJCC system (see Table 7). Treatment depends on location, stage, and grade of the tumor. Most distal urethral tumors (pendulous urethra) are of low stage and grade and can be managed by partial penectomy. Prognosis is generally good, with a mean survival of more than 6 years. Proximal urethral tumors (bulbomembranous) tend to present late and are of higher stage and grade. We recommend wide resection, which frequently consists of total penectomy and cystoprostatectomy. Inguinal lymphadenectomy should be performed only in patients with palpably enlarged nodes. Prognosis is poor despite aggressive treatment. Transitional cell carcinoma of the prostatic urethra is usually a manifestation of a concurrent bladder cancer. Treatment is that of the underlying bladder cancer but also includes total urethrectomy at the time of cystectomy. Patients who have stromal involvement of the prostate by transitional cell carcinoma have a poor prognosis.

PROSTATE CANCER

Prostate cancer is the most common tumor and second most common cause of cancer deaths in men in the United States, with an estimated 244,000 new cases diagnosed in 1995. Prostatic tumors spread to the regional pelvic lymph nodes and via the bloodstream to the bones, where they classically cause osteoblastic metastases in the axillary skeleton. Thirty per-cent of men older than the age of 50 years have histologic evidence of prostate cancer. However, only one fourth of these cancers are estimated to be clinically significant. At presentation 60% of patients have incurable prostate cancer (stage T3 or higher). A further 25% have clinically insignificant disease. Therefore only 15% of patients have the potential to be cured of their tumor. The high incidence of incidental tumors combined with the fatal nature of advanced prostate cancer dictates that there be a selective approach to treatment. Determining which cancers require treatment depends on the patient's physiologic age and the grade and stage of the tumor.

Prostate-Specific Antigen

The diagnosis and treatment of prostate cancer have been revolutionized by the discovery of prostate-specific antigen (PSA). PSA is a serine protease that is produced by prostatic epithelial cells, the function of which is to liquefy semen. The serum PSA level represents the summation of PSA produced by normal prostate, benign prostatic hyperplasia, prostatitis, prostatic trauma, and cancer. Gram for gram, prostatic carcinoma produces approximately 10 times as much serum PSA as benign prostatic hyperplasia. Therefore, as the PSA level increases, the likelihood that the PSA elevation is caused by prostate cancer increases. In the presence of a normal digital rectal examination, approximately 1.4%, 25%, and 60% of patients with a PSA level of less than 4, between 4 and 10, and greater than 10 ng/mL respectively, will have prostate carcinoma. To compensate for the increased prevalence of benign prostatic hyperplasia as men become older, an age-specific reference range for serum PSA can be utilized (Table 8). Before therapy, PSA is a useful prognostic marker. After treatment, progressive elevation of the PSA level indicates recurrent disease.

Presentation and Diagnosis

Prostate cancer does not usually cause symptoms unless the tumor is relatively advanced. The most frequent symptoms are those of hematuria, bladder outlet obstruction, and vesical irritation caused by local tumor growth. Many patients present with symptoms of metastatic disease, especially bony metastases. Increasingly, patients are presenting because of an incidentally discovered elevated serum PSA level or a palpable abnormality on digital rectal examination. Thirty percent of patients with a nodule on digital rectal examination will have prostate cancer. Prostatic biopsy is indicated for patients in whom a diagnosis of prostate cancer is suspected by elevated serum PSA level and/or abnormal digital examination. Transrectal ultrasound (TRUS)–guided biopsy can be performed as an office procedure with minimal patient discomfort and risk. The major complications of prostate biopsy are infection and bleeding, which occur less than 1% of the time. The prostate is visualized with a TRUS probe and any hypoechoic areas are biopsied. A total of six systematic prostate biopsies are then performed at the apex, midgland, and base of both right and left lobes of the prostate. If the initial biopsy specimens are negative and there is a high suspicion of cancer, the patient should undergo another biopsy, because 15% of these patients will be found to have cancer.

If at presentation the PSA level is less than 10 ng/mL and the patient has no symptoms suggestive of metastatic disease, no other radiologic staging studies are necessary. If the PSA level is greater than 10

TABLE 8. **Age-Specific Prostate-Specific Antigen Reference Range**

Age (years)	PSA Range (ng/mL)
40–49	0.0–2.5
50–59	0.0–3.5
60–69	0.0–4.5
70–79	0.0–6.5

TABLE 9. **American Joint Committee on Cancer Staging of Prostate Cancer**

T0	No evidence of primary tumor
T1	Impalpable tumor, not visualized on TRUS
T1a	Incidental tumor, <5% of tissue resected at prostatectomy
T1b	Incidental tumor, >5% of tissue resected at prostatectomy
T1c	Tumor identified by needle biopsy alone (because of elevated PSA)
T2	Tumor confined within prostate
T2a	Tumor involves less than half of one lobe
T2b	Tumor involves more than half of one lobe
T2c	Tumor involves both lobes
T3	Tumor extends through prostatic capsule
T3a	Unilateral extracapsular tumor
T3b	Bilateral extracapsular tumor
T3c	Tumor involves seminal vesicles
T4	Tumor fixed to adjacent structures, e.g., bladder neck or pelvic wall
N0	No regional node metastasis
N1–3	Regional node metastasis
M0	No distant metastasis
M1	Distant metastasis

ng/mL, a radionuclide bone scan should be performed. Pelvic CT scanning is rarely indicated because of its low sensitivity and specificity in the detection of nodal metastases. Prostate cancer is staged by the AJCC system (Table 9). Prostate cancers are graded 1 to 5, depending on the architecture of the tumor, using the Gleason grading system. Grading is commonly reported as a Gleason score (2–10) which is the sum of the Gleason grade of the major and minor patterns within the tumor. A Gleason score of 2 is the best-differentiated, and 10 is the most poorly differentiated tumor.

Management

Organ-Confined Tumors (T1–T2)

The management options for patients with clinically organ-confined disease (T1–T2) include observation, radiation therapy, and radical prostatectomy. The choice of therapy depends on the tumor volume, Gleason score, patient's physiologic age, and patient preference. Patients presenting with low-grade (Gleason score <5) and low-stage tumors (T1a) are unlikely to experience tumor-related complications for 10 years or more. These patients are particularly suitable for observation unless they have a very long life expectancy. Patients with higher stage (T1b and higher) and grade tumors (Gleason 7 or greater) are likely to have symptoms of local progression and/or metastasis in a shorter time frame and are suitable candidates for definitive therapy.

Observation and Delayed Hormone Therapy. Several retrospective studies have reported excellent 10-year survival rates (85% to 90%) with observation and delayed hormonal therapy for clinically localized prostate cancer. However, a significant proportion of men treated in this fashion will experience local progression (75%), and some will develop metastatic disease (20%). Therefore, it appears that given sufficient time most prostate cancers will become symptomatic. Observation is recommended for patients who are likely to die of other causes before their prostate cancer progresses.

Radical Prostatectomy. This should be reserved for healthy men with clinically localized prostate cancer and a projected survival of greater than 10 years. The operation consists of removal of the prostate, ampulla of the vas deferentia, and seminal vesicles, with reanastomosis of the bladder neck to the membranous urethra. The operation can be performed equally effectively via the retropubic (abdominal) or perineal approach. Several series indicate that 15-year survival rates of 86% to 93% can be achieved in patients with clinically localized disease (T2 or less). Operative morbidity is low, with a mortality rate of less than 1% in most centers. Intraoperative complications include blood loss, necessitating a transfusion in 5% to 10% of patients, and rectal injuries, occurring in less than 1% of cases. The major long-term complications are urinary incontinence, impotence, and bladder neck contracture. Bladder neck contracture requiring dilatation or internal urethrotomy occurs in 3% to 12% of patients. Eighty to ninety percent of patients are dry 1 year after radical prostatectomy. In the remaining 10% to 20%, most experience stress urinary incontinence that requires the use of a protective pad. Approximately 4% of patients have total incontinence that may require the placement of an artificial sphincter. The cavernosal nerves, which control erectile function, travel in neurovascular bundles alongside the prostate. The neurovascular bundles can be preserved by performing a nerve-sparing prostatectomy. Unilateral nerve-sparing prostatectomy can result in potency preservation in 30% to 60% of patients. Removal of the cavernosal nerves does not affect penile sensation or the ability to achieve orgasm. Therapeutic options for the impotent patient include the vacuum erection device, intracorporal injection therapy, and penile prosthesis placement.

Radiation Therapy. This has been used extensively in the treatment of clinically localized prostate cancer. The best results have been achieved by delivering approximately 70 cGy of external-beam irradiation to the prostate bed in 2-cGy daily increments over 7 weeks. Fifteen-year disease-specific survival rates of up to 85% have been reported for clinically localized disease (T1–T2). Complications are minor, with 30% to 40% of patients experiencing transient gastrointestinal symptoms. Approximately 10% of patients will have prolonged gastrointestinal (chronic diarrhea and rectal bleeding) and genitourinary (urinary frequency, urgency, and hematuria) symptoms. Impotence occurs in approximately 50% of patients and urinary incontinence in 3% to 5% of patients.

Interstitial radiation therapy with implantation of gold-198 and iodine-125 seeds has fallen into disfavor because variable seed placement resulted in uneven radiation delivery, causing an unacceptably high rate of local recurrence. Recent technologic advances, including new isotopes, seed stabilization, and TRUS-guided seed placement, have led to a resurgence of interest in this treatment. No long-term results are available.

Cryotherapy. Transperineal prostatic freezing has recently gained some popularity as a treatment of clinically localized prostate cancer. Early results suggest that cryotherapy results in effective local tumor control with moderate side effects. No long-term results are available.

Follow-Up of Organ-Confined Tumors. Follow-up of patients with clinically localized prostate cancer should consist of a digital rectal examination and measurement of PSA level every 3 months for 1 year and every 6 months thereafter. The PSA level should be undetectable 6 weeks after radical prostatectomy. Any subsequent rise in the PSA level indicates recurrent tumor. The PSA level should drop to less than 1 ng/mL 1 year after radiation therapy. If the PSA level fails to drop below 1 ng/mL or starts to rise, there is a high probability of residual or recurrent tumor.

Locally Advanced Tumors (T3)

Many patients with locally advanced tumors have occult metastatic disease at diagnosis. There is little evidence to suggest that most patients whose tumors have spread beyond the prostate can be cured by more aggressive surgery or radiation therapy alone. Although the optimum treatment of T3 prostate cancer has not been defined, we treat these patients with a combination of local radiation therapy and androgen ablation.

Node-Positive Disease (T1–T3)N1–3

Patients who are discovered to have positive pelvic lymph nodes at exploration before radical prostatectomy are unlikely to be cured by performing an extended lymph node dissection combined with surgical removal of the prostate. Several treatment options are advocated, including hormonal therapy alone, radical prostatectomy combined with hormonal therapy, and radiation therapy combined with hormonal therapy. Although there are no definitive data supporting combination therapy, our early experience with local irradiation to control the primary tumor combined with androgen ablation to treat the metastatic disease has been promising.

Metastatic Disease (M1)

The observation by Huggins that most prostate cancers are androgen dependent and regress on androgen withdrawal led to the development of hormonal therapy. Androgen ablation is the primary treatment for patients with metastatic prostatic carcinoma. Eighty-five percent of patients will have a response to androgen ablative treatment. There is debate as to whether hormone therapy should be administered at the time of diagnosis of metastatic disease or withheld until the patient becomes symptomatic. There is some evidence suggesting that early hormone therapy prolongs survival, and we favor this approach. Although most androgens come from the testes, a small but significant amount is derived from the adrenal secretion of androstenedione and peripheral conversion to testosterone. Standard hormonal therapy has been targeted at the elimination of testicular androgens by surgical or medical means. Several studies have suggested that combined androgen blockade directed at both testicular and adrenal sources of androgens results in a modest prolongation of survival. Limited data suggest that patients with low-volume metastatic disease may derive the most benefit from combination therapy. Nevertheless, the use of combined androgen blockade remains controversial.

Testicular androgens can be eliminated by surgical castration (an outpatient procedure) or medical castration with estrogens or luteinizing hormone–releasing hormone (LHRH) agonists. There is little benefit to combining surgical castration with estrogens or LHRH agonists. Diethylstilbestrol is a cheap, effective method of medical castration but has fallen out of favor because of the potential for cardiovascular toxicity. Breast enlargement is common with estrogen therapy but can be prevented by pretreatment breast irradiation. LHRH agonists initially result in an increase in testosterone production followed by a decrease to castrate levels. An antiandrogen, flutamide (Eulexin) at 250 mg three times daily, or bicalutamide (Casodex) at 50 mg once daily for 2 weeks, should be administered with LHRH agonists when initiating androgen ablation to prevent a "flare" of the prostate tumor associated with the initial stimulation of androgen production. LHRH agonists can be administered as depot injections once per month (leuprolide [Lupron] at 7.5 mg or goserelin [Zoladex] at 3.6 mg) and are expensive. Side effects include hot flushes, which can be treated with megestrol acetate (Megace) at 20 mg twice daily, and diminished muscle mass, libido, and sexual potency. The median survival of patients with metastatic prostate cancer treated with androgen ablation is 28 months.

Combined androgen ablation involves using orchiectomy or medical castration to decrease testicular androgens and an antiandrogen (flutamide [Eulexin] at 250 mg three times daily or bicalutamide [Casodex] at 50 mg once daily) to block adrenal androgens. Flutamide can cause diarrhea in a minority of patients. An extremely rare but potentially fatal complication associated with antiandrogens is hepatitis. These rare events most commonly occur early in the course of treatment and usually respond to withdrawal of the antiandrogen. Patients starting on a course of antiandrogen therapy should have blood drawn at the initiation of therapy and during the first few months of treatment to monitor the serum glutamic pyruvic transaminase (alanine aminotransferase) level.

Median survival of patients with metastatic prostate cancer treated with combined androgen ablation is 36 months. A decline in the PSA level indicates a response to therapy. Patients who do not respond to initial hormonal therapy should have the level of serum testosterone measured to ensure that it is indeed at the castration level (<50 ng/dL). A subsequent increase in the PSA level is an indicator of tumor progression. If a patient on combined hormonal therapy has a rising PSA, the antiandrogen should be withdrawn because up to 75% of patients will show another, usually short, response.

Adenocarcinoma of the prostate is resistant to most chemotherapeutic regimens, but trials of single and multiple-agent chemotherapy for hormone-refractory prostate cancer are ongoing. Current trials are focusing on ketoconazole, estramustine phosphate, vinblastine, and suramin. The combination of etoposide and estramustine phosphate is an active but toxic regimen. Symptomatic treatment of bone metastasis can be achieved with palliative local radiation or intravenous strontium-89. Bladder outlet obstruction can be treated with transurethral resection but may result in urinary incontinence.

Screening for Prostate Cancer

No curative treatment is available for advanced prostate cancer. However, radical prostatectomy is a curative treatment for organ-confined cancer. Early detection of prostate cancer has the potential to affect the mortality rate of this tumor by identifying organ-confined tumors before the development of extracapsular and metastatic disease. A combination of annual PSA and digital rectal examination appears to be the most effective method for the early detection of prostate cancer and is recommended by the American Cancer Society and American Urological Association for all men over the age of 50 years. African Americans and men with a family history of prostate cancer are at increased risk and should be screened from the age of 40 years. Men who have a life expectancy of less than 10 years are unlikely to benefit from early detection and therefore should not be screened. Screening for prostate cancer remains controversial because no study has demonstrated a decrease in the prostate cancer mortality rate as a result of screening. Such studies are underway, but the results will not be available for many years. We think that the preliminary evidence suggests a benefit and that prostate cancer screening should be offered to men over the age of 50 years.

PENILE CANCER

Penile cancer is an uncommon tumor with an incidence of 1 to 2 per 100,000 population. The majority are squamous cell carcinomas. The peak incidence is in the sixth decade, but tumors can occur in men as young as 30 years of age. Phimosis and poor hygiene play a role in the development of penile cancers.

Presentation and Diagnosis

Penile cancer presents as a lesion on the glans or prepuce. Frequently, patients present late with fungating masses. However, early cases may present as a red irritative area that resembles local inflam-

TABLE 10. **American Joint Committee on Cancer Staging of Penile Cancer**

Tis	Carcinoma in situ
Ta	Noninvasive verrucous carcinoma
T1	Tumor invades subepithelial connective tissue
T2	Tumor invades corpora spongiosum or corpus cavernosum
T3	Tumor invades urethra or prostate
T4	Tumor invades other adjacent structures
N0	No regional node metastasis
N1–3	Regional node metastasis
M0	No distant metastasis
M1	Distant metastasis

mation. Diagnosis is established by performing a biopsy. Careful attention should be paid to evaluating the regional lymph nodes (inguinal nodes) for metastatic disease. Tumors are staged by the AJCC system (Table 10).

Management

T1 lesions of the foreskin can be treated by circumcision. T1 and small T2 lesions of the glans penis can be treated by local excision using Mohs' microsurgery or CO_2 laser ablation. Larger T2 and T3 lesions require excision of the tumor with a 2-cm margin. Tumor excision can be performed by partial penectomy if sufficient penis will remain for the patient to stand to void. Otherwise, total penectomy with perineal urethrostomy is performed.

In addition to treatment of the primary tumor, all patients require continued assessment of the inguinal nodes. Enlarged inguinal nodes may result from infection or neoplasm. We prefer to evaluate enlarged nodes immediately with aspiration cytology. Alternatively, patients can be treated with 6 weeks of antibiotics followed by re-evaluation. Patients with persistent nodal enlargement should have bilateral inguinal node dissections. Patients whose primary tumor is poorly differentiated or invades the corpora spongiosum or cavernosa should undergo prophylactic node dissection because 78% will have nodal metastasis. Prognosis is excellent for patients with T1–T2 tumors and negative inguinal nodes. Patients who undergo immediate node dissection and have less than two positive nodes have an 80% 5-year survival rate. Patients with more than two positive nodes have a 5-year survival rate of 10% to 30%. Close follow-up is essential and consists of clinical examination every 3 months for 2 years and every 6 months thereafter. Patients with metastatic disease are treated with combination chemotherapy (bleomycin, methotrexate, and cisplatin).

Unusual Tumors

Sarcomas, melanomas, lymphomas, and Kaposi's sarcomas all occasionally occur on the penis. Treatment depends on tumor type and the stage of disease. Up to 20% of AIDS patients with Kaposi's sarcoma will have genital involvement. Kaposi's sarcoma responds well to low-dose irradiation.

TESTICULAR CANCER

Testicular cancer is the most common tumor of young adult males, with an incidence of 3.7 per 100,000 population. The tumor is uncommon in African Americans. A history of cryptorchidism increases the risk of testis cancer between 3 and 48 times. The increased risk of testis cancer is not eliminated by orchidopexy. However, orchidopexy is valuable in preserving testicular function and permits easy examination of the testicle. Germ cell tumors are the most common malignant tumors of the testis and for therapeutic purposes can be divided into seminomas and nonseminomatous germ cell tumors (NSGCT).

Presentation and Diagnosis

The most common presenting feature is a testicular mass that may be first recognized after minor trauma. Physical examination usually reveals a firm testicular mass. Occasionally the tumor may be obscured by a reactive hydrocele. A testicular ultrasonogram is useful if the diagnosis is unclear. All patients with suspected testicular tumors should have blood drawn for measurement of beta-human chorionic gonadotropin (βhCG), alpha-fetoprotein (AFP), and lactate dehydrogenase. Ten percent of patients with seminoma will have an elevated βhCG level. Fifty to ninety percent of patients with NSGCT will have an elevated level of either or both βhCG and AFP. Patients with a primary tumor that is histologically a pure seminoma but who have an elevated level of AFP are classified for treatment purposes as having NSGCT. Testicular tumors spread through both the lymphatic and vascular systems. The lymphatics of the left testicle primarily drain to the left para-aortic nodes and the right testicle to the interaortocaval group. The most common site of hematogenous metastasis is the lung. Surgical exploration of a possible testicular tumor should be performed through an inguinal incision to permit early control of the spermatic cord and to prevent contamination of the inguinal lymphatics. After the testicle has been removed, metastatic work-up should be performed consisting of an abdominal CT scan to evaluate the para-aortic nodes and a chest x-ray film to rule out pulmonary metastases. The staging system for testis cancer is shown in Table 11. Treatment depends on histologic tumor type and stage of disease.

Management

Seminomas. The treatment of stage I and stage IIa seminomas is radical orchiectomy combined with

TABLE 11. **Staging of Testicular Cancer**

Stage I	Tumor confined to the testis
Stage II	Nodal metastases
IIA	Limited nodal metastases
IIB	Bulky nodal metastases
Stage III	Tumor involving lymphatics above the diaphragm
Stage IV	Hematogenous metastases

30 cGy of radiation therapy to the retroperitoneum. Prognosis is excellent, with a greater than 95% 5-year survival rate. Historically, stage IIb and stage III tumors were treated with abdominal and mediastinal irradiation. Currently, cisplatin-based chemotherapy is curative for most patients and is the treatment of choice. Prognosis is excellent, with more than 90% of patients achieving long-term survival. Adjuvant radiation therapy is indicated only for bulky lesions that do not respond adequately to chemotherapy. Follow-up consists of a physical examination and chest radiograph every 6 months. Patients should be taught testicular self-examination because 2% to 3% of testicular tumors are bilateral.

Nonseminomatous Germ Cell Tumors. The treatment of patients with stage I NSGCT is controversial. Twenty to twenty-five percent of patients with stage I disease will have occult retroperitoneal nodal metastasis. These patients can be identified and potentially cured by retroperitoneal lymph node dissection (RPLND). However, to identify the 20% to 25% of patients who have occult metastasis, 75% of the patients have to be subjected to an unnecessary operation. The major long-term complication of RPLND is failure of antegrade ejaculation (resulting in infertility) from injury to the lumbar sympathetics. The use of template dissection and nerve-sparing surgery has decreased the frequency of this complication. An alternative approach to RPLND for patients with stage I disease is observation with tumor markers and chest radiograph monthly for 1 year, every 3 months for 1 year, and then every 6 months thereafter. Abdominal CT scanning is performed every 3 months for the first year and then every 6 months for two additional years. The potential for rapid undetected tumor growth on surveillance protocols underscores the need for close follow-up. Early treatment in the case of recurrence is important because prognosis is related to tumor volume. The presence of vascular invasion and involvement of the epididymis or cord structures are associated with a higher risk of metastasis, and patients bearing tumors with these features are not suitable for observation protocols and should undergo RPLND. Patients who are discovered to have lymph node metastasis at the time of RPLND and who receive two cycles of postoperative chemotherapy have a tumor recurrence rate approaching zero. The long-term survival rate associated with both methods (observation and initial RPLND) is greater than 95% at 5 years.

Patients with higher stages of disease (stages II, III, and IV) should undergo primary chemotherapy (bleomycin, etoposide, and cisplatin), with resection of residual tumor masses after chemotherapy. We continue chemotherapy until maximum tumor shrinkage has been achieved and then resect any residual masses. The most common site for residual disease is in the retroperitoneum. However, patients should undergo resection of residual masses in other organs, e.g., lung and liver, if tumor stabilization and normalization of tumor markers is achieved by chemotherapy. Residual masses are fibrous scar in 40% of patients, benign teratoma in 40%, and viable tumor in 20%. RPLND after chemotherapy is more difficult than a primary dissection because residual masses are often adherent to the surrounding structures, including the aorta and vena cava. Occasionally aortic replacement and vena caval resection are necessary to achieve clear margins. Full bilateral node dissections are performed for residual masses after chemotherapy. Therefore, postchemotherapy RPLND is associated with a greater likelihood of complications, including intraoperative blood loss, chylous ascites, pancreatitis, and failure of ejaculation. Prognosis depends on tumor volume, with 95% of patients with low-volume disease achieving long-term survival. Using modern multidisciplinary approaches, long-term survival is possible in 40% to 60% of patients who have massive metastatic disease.

SCROTAL TUMORS

Squamous cell carcinoma of the scrotum became the first cancer known to be caused by an industrial carcinogen when it was identified as a disease of chimney sweeps by Pott in 1775. Scrotal cancer exhibiting other than squamous histology is rare. Scrotal cancers metastasize via the lymphatics to the inguinal nodes. Treatment is similar to that for penile carcinoma, with local excision and management of the regional nodes. Prognosis is good, with a 60% to 70% 5-year survival rate in the absence of positive nodes.

Malignant intrascrotal tumors (excluding testicular cancer) are rare, and most are sarcomas.

GENITOURINARY SARCOMAS

Sarcomas are rare tumors of diverse histologic types that can arise from any mesenchymal tissue in the body. The percentage of patients presenting with local disease depends on the histologic type and organ of origin. Sarcomas are staged by careful physical examination, MRI of the affected organ (MRI defines tumor margins more accurately than CT), and CT of the chest. Careful pathologic review by an experienced pathologist is important to determine the histologic type and tumor grade. The mainstay of therapy for clinically localized tumors is wide local excision. The roles of pre- or postoperative irradiation and chemotherapy are unknown. Patients with clinically localized tumors less than 5 cm in size and of low histologic grade have a 3-year relapse-free survival rate of 89%. Locally advanced and metastatic tumors are treated with combination chemotherapy (doxorubicin, dacarbazine, and cyclophosphamide), followed by surgical excision and postoperative irradiation. The 3-year relapse-free survival rate in this group of patients is less than 25%.

Retroperitoneal Sarcomas

Retroperitoneal sarcomas account for 10% to 15% of all sarcomas. Liposarcoma is the most common histologic type. Most tumors present late with a large retroperitoneal mass that should be differentiated from retroperitoneal lymphoma. Surgical excision is the primary therapy. The 5-year survival rate is 50% after complete local excision. However, more than 90% of patients will develop local recurrence if followed for 10 years.

Renal Sarcomas

Sarcomas constitute 1% to 2% of all renal tumors. Leiomyosarcomas are the most common type. Three-year survival is dismal even after complete resection. Chemotherapy and radiation therapy are ineffective.

Bladder and Prostatic Sarcomas

Sarcomas account for 0.5% of all bladder and prostate tumors. Sarcomas should be differentiated from benign spindle cell nodules that can occur after transurethral surgery. Rhabdomyosarcomas are the most common histologic type and occur primarily in children. Modern approaches using combination chemotherapy and irradiation permit an organ-sparing approach in 35% of these patients. Long-term survival is achieved in 75%. Leiomyosarcomas are the most common histologic type in adults. The survival rate is worse for adults than it is for children.

Paratesticular Sarcomas

Rhabdomyosarcomas of the paratesticular tissues are the most common paratesticular tumor of children and are treated by orchiectomy, retroperitoneal node dissection, and combination chemotherapy. Radiation therapy is administered to patients who have residual disease after surgery. Prognosis is good, with 60% of patients achieving long-term survival. Leiomyosarcomas are the most common tumor type in adults.

URETHRAL STRICTURES

method of
RONALD T. KODAMA, M.D.
University of Toronto
Sunnybrook Health Science Center
Toronto, Ontario, Canada

A urethral stricture is a narrowing of the urethral lumen. It results from fibrosis and scarring of normal urethral tissue. Patients present with symptoms when the urethral lumen becomes significantly stenosed. Although these strictures occasionally occur in females, they are much more common in the male patient.

The male urethra is divided into anterior and posterior segments. The posterior portion includes the prostatic and membranous urethras. The prostatic urethra traverses the substance of the prostate gland. Located at its entrance is the smooth muscle internal sphincter mechanism. The two ejaculatory ducts enter dorsally on an elevated ridge of tissue, the verumontanum. On either side of the verumontanum, the multiple ducts of the prostate open. The prostatic urethra is commonly obstructed by benign and malignant diseases of the prostate. Distal to the prostatic

urethra, traversing the urogenital diaphragm, is the membranous urethra. This urethral segment contains the distal or external sphincter mechanism. It is surrounded by both smooth and striated muscle. The striated portion is under voluntary control through the pudendal nerve.

The anterior urethra is composed of the bulbous and penile urethra. This portion of the urethra is essentially a conduit for urinary passage. The penis is composed of three erectile bodies: the paired corpora cavernosa and the corpus spongiosum. The ventrally located corpus spongiosum contains the urethra and terminates as the glans penis. Buck's fascia surrounds these three erectile bodies. Within this fascia lies the neurovascular bundle: the deep dorsal vein, the paired dorsal arteries, and the branches of the dorsal nerve of the penis. Superficial to Buck's fascia is the dartos fascia. This is a loose areolar layer that allows the penile skin to slide easily on the penile shaft. This fascia is continuous with the dartos muscle layer of the scrotum, Colles' fascia of the perineum, and Scarpa's fascia of the anterior abdominal wall.

The arterial blood supply to the penis is from the paired internal and external pudendal arteries. The internal pudendal artery is a terminal branch of the anterior division of the internal iliac artery. It sends branches to the perineum and the erectile bodies before it terminates as the dorsal artery of the penis. The corpus spongiosum is supplied by the bulbar urethral arteries and the dorsal arteries of the penis. The urethra is also supplied by perforating vessels between the corpus spongiosum and the corpus cavernosa. The external pudendal artery, a branch of the common femoral artery, supplies the skin to the penis. This supply occurs ventrally and dorsally in a coaxial pattern. The venous drainage of the penis is through three intercommunicating systems. The deep system is through the corpora cavernosal and spongiosal veins. This system communicates with the deep dorsal vein of the penis through emissary veins. The deep dorsal vein and the erectile bodies drain into the prostatic venous complex. The superficial venous complex drains the penile skin, and the majority of this system drains into the left saphenous vein.

Histologically, the prostatic and membranous urethra is lined with transitional epithelium. The anterior urethra is lined with pseudostratified columnar epithelium. The glandular urethra, including the fossa navicularis, is lined by nonkeratinizing squamous epithelium. The glands of the anterior urethra are the paired Cowper's glands, whose ducts enter the proximal bulbar urethra, and the multiple glands of Littre, which are located along the entire urethra.

ETIOLOGY

Strictures of the anterior urethra can be caused by blunt or penetrating trauma. Blunt injuries are usually caused by straddle injuries to the bulbar urethra. This occurs when there is a direct blow onto the perineum such a fall onto a workhorse with outstretched legs. Although gonococcal infections were a major infective cause of urethral strictures, this entity is decreasing in incidence because of the use of modern antibiotics. It is unknown whether chlamydial infections will lead to urethral strictures. Iatrogenic causes for strictures are common. These include previous catheterization and endoscopic manipulation. However, often there is no definite cause and the patient presents only with obstructive voiding symptoms.

Posterior urethral strictures are usually secondary to blunt pelvic trauma. Approximately 2 to 5% of patients suffering a pelvic fracture will have a concomitant urethral injury. Although there is controversy to the initial management of the urethral injury, the author believes that a trial of primary realignment should be attempted in order to possibly decrease the stricture rate. In a review of the literature, Herschorn and colleagues (J Urol *148*:1428, 1992) found that when patients were treated with a suprapubic tube alone, a very high percentage of the patients required a delayed reconstruction for the resulting stricture. In those patients who had successful early realignment, the stricture rate and subsequent need for repair were significantly reduced. A urethral stricture after a pelvic fracture usually occurs at the bulbomembranous junction. The resulting urethral fibrosis is secondary to the violent shearing forces that the soft tissue structures of the pelvis and the urogenital diaphragm suffer when a pelvic fracture occurs. Strictures of the membranous urethra from infective or iatrogenic causes are very uncommon.

SIGNS AND SYMPTOMS

The evaluation of patients with urethral stricture disease begins with a thorough history. Patients' symptoms may vary greatly and may not at times be correlated with the degree of occlusion. Patients usually describe varying degrees of obstructive and irritative voiding symptoms, including frequency, urgency, and nocturia. They often describe a decrease in the force and caliber of their urinary stream. With detrusor hypertrophy, some men can have a forceful urinary stream and complain only of a prolonged voiding time. A recurrent history of lower urinary tract infections or epididymitis in a young male patient should also prompt further investigations. Occasionally a patient may present with anterior urethral bleeding. Because the anterior urethra is a conduit with no sphincter function, any lesion that bleeds will cause bleeding that is not associated with micturition. A previous history of urethritis, instrumentation, or perineal trauma should be elicited. One should always be aware of the possibility of silent urinary retention with secondary bilateral hydroureteronephrosis and obstructive renal failure. Often the first time a stricture is discovered is when a catheter cannot be inserted for fluid monitoring.

Examination of the abdomen may reveal a distended bladder with urinary retention. Penile inspection will reveal evidence of chronic infection or sexually transmitted diseases. The glans penis should be exposed in uncircumcised patients to rule out meatal stenosis, balanitis xerotica obliterans, and premalignant and cancerous lesions of the penis. Palpation of the entire length of the corpus spongiosum, including the bulbar portion within the scrotum, is essential. One may sometimes feel a cord of fibrotic spongy tissue indicative of a scarred urethra. Palpable hard masses may indicate a urethral stone or cancer. A urethral diverticulum may present as a soft midline mass that can be decompressed with manual pressure. Palpation of both testicles and epididymi is necessary to rule out evidence of chronic inflammation. Finally, a rectal examination should be performed to rule out concomitant prostatic hypertrophy or carcinoma.

In more acute situations, patients may present to the emergency department with urinary retention and sepsis. Physical examination may reveal a distended bladder and an inflamed scrotum with a tender scrotal mass draining pus and/or urine. This represents a urethral abscess with the development of a urethrocutaneous fistula. Although uncommon, these occur in the debilitated elderly patient or spinal cord–injured patients. Most of these patients have a chronic urethral stricture and inflammation, and their abscess develops when there is acute exacerbation of their infected urethra. In patients with blunt pelvic trauma, a urethral injury should always be suspected. The classic signs of urethral trauma include the presence of blood at the urethral meatus, the inability to void, the presence of scrotal and perineal ecchymoses, a suprapubic mass, and a "high riding" or nonpalpable prostate. From the experience of the author and colleagues, blood at the meatus appears to be the most reliable sign. The treatment of these injuries is not within the scope of this discussion, but the importance of the possibility of urethral injury must be stressed. The early diagnosis and the correct acute management of these injuries may decrease the incidence of stricture formation and may facilitate the subsequent repair.

DIAGNOSIS

In any patient with irritative and obstructive voiding symptoms, certain laboratory investigations should be carried out. These include a urinalysis, urine culture, and a serum creatinine. A quantitative measurement of urine flow tells the physician the amount of urine voided, the maximum and mean urinary flow rate, and the time required to void. These figures can be compared with normative values. Uroflowmetry in itself does not establish obstruction because a weak detrusor muscle may give the same pattern and flow rates as a urethral stricture. Cystourethroscopy is performed to examine the urethra for strictures. This procedure allows direct observation of the affected area. If cancer of the urethra is suspected, a transurethral biopsy of the stricture should be performed. Once a urethral stricture is diagnosed and its extent cannot be delineated, a retrograde urethrogram and voiding cystourethrogram should be performed to delineate the extent of the disease. This examination is performed by inserting a urethral catheter into the meatus and injecting radiopaque dye retrogradely into the bladder. This portion of the examination delineates the distal extent of the stricture. After the bladder has been filled, the patient voids under fluoroscopy and spot radiographs are taken. These x-rays may show the degree of bladder hypertrophy, diverticular formation, the presence of vesicoureteral reflux, and the presence of intravesical lesions including bladder stones or neoplasms. In the voiding phase of the examination, there is dilatation of the urethra proximal to the stricture.

TREATMENT

The treatment of urethral strictures depends on several factors, including the etiology of the stricture, its location, the length and depth of the stricture, and previous treatments. Finally, one must take into account the patient's age and general medical condition. Devine and coworkers (see Campbell's Urology, 6th ed., 1992, pp 2957–3032, WB Saunders) have suggested that those strictures of the anterior urethra that are limited to the mucosa or the superficial spongy tissue may be amenable to relatively easy methods of treatment with good results. Those with deep fibrosis of the corpus spongiosum usually require reconstructive techniques.

The simplest technique is urethral dilatation. This should be performed only by trained personnel who are familiar with urethral anatomy, the instruments, and the potential complications of the procedure. Graduated metal sounds may be used to gently dilate the narrowed area. Alternatively, filiforms and urethral followers may be used. These are a set of instruments that include a filiform catheter and a set of graduated stiff catheters that can be screwed onto the end of the filiform catheter. Initially, the filiform catheter is placed into the urethra. Because of its small caliber, it is able to negotiate its way through the strictured area into the bladder. Once in, the smallest "following" catheter is secured to the filiform catheter and dilatation of the urethra is performed by advancing the stiffer catheter into the bladder. The filiform acts as the guiding catheter. Gradual dilatation of the urethra using larger catheters can then be performed under relatively careful conditions. One of the potential complications of this technique is the failure to recognize the improper placement of the initial filiform catheter. Thus, subsequent dilatation with the stiff catheters can lead to creation of false urethral passages.

There are essentially three endoscopic techniques that are at present available for the treatment of urethral strictures. These procedures are usually performed under general anesthesia. The principle of two of the techniques is to cut the stricture in a controlled fashion. The oldest method is called a visual internal urethrotomy. A cold knife or urethrotome is placed into the urethra, and under direct vision the stricture can be identified and incised with the sharp blade. This is usually performed at the 12 o'clock position of the urethra, and the depth of the incision is carried into normal spongy tissue. A catheter is placed after the procedure and is kept in for several days to a week while the urethra is healing. The principle is to allow the epithelium to cover the spongy tissue at the new larger circumference. More recently, with use of contact laser technology, direct visual vaporization of the scar tissue is possible. The purported advantage of this method is the relatively bloodless surgical field because the delivered laser energy coagulates and vaporizes the tissue simultaneously. Because of the relatively superficial depth of penetration, injury to adjacent structures is minimized. The scar tissue is actually removed in this technique in order to increase the circumference. However, long-term data regarding the efficacy of this new laser technique are limited. The third endoscopic technique is to place an expandable meshed metal stent into the urethra to keep the stricture open. Using this technique, the stricture is initially dilated and then the stent is deployed under direct vision along the entire length of the stricture. The expanded meshed stent gradually becomes epithelialized over 6 to 12 months. To date, there has been fairly good success with this method. There are, however, several disadvantages of this stent, including malplacement of the stent, persistent pain, urethral leakage, and ingrowth of fibrous tissue through the stent requiring periodic endoscopic resection of the tissue. If the stent has to be removed, the resulting stricture is usually longer than the one that was initially treated. At present, these stents can be used only in the bulbous urethra because they do not expand with erections.

The preceding techniques, with the possible exception of stent implantation, should be considered management tools only. Because of their nature, the scar tissue usually recurs with recurrence of the patients' symptoms. Persistent use of these techniques depends on the patients' medical conditions, their symptoms, and the time interval between required interventions. Another simple alternative is self–intermittent dilatation. In those patients who are poor medical risks or in whom conservative or even reconstructive measures have failed, self–intermittent catheterization is a viable option. Patients must be motivated to perform this daily because, if stopped for a short period of time, the stricture recurs.

With the advent of tissue transfer techniques, operative reconstructive techniques may be offered to these patients with good long-term success rates. Reconstruction of the urethra should be performed by surgeons who are familiar with all of the possible reconstructive surgical options. Previously, staged procedures were performed, usually in two operations. In the first stage, the urethral stricture was opened and marsupialized to the penile or scrotal skin depending on the length of the stricture. The patient would then urinate from a proximal ostium at the base of the penis or in the perineum. The second stage or closure of the urethra was performed approximately 6 months later. This involves incorporating some of the genital skin into the urethra to make a larger lumen.

However, with the development of newer tissue transfer techniques and the use of surgical magnification, finer instruments, and suture material, the majority of reconstructive procedures can be carried out in a one-stage procedure. Techniques that may be employed include removing the diseased portion of urethra and reanastomosing the healthy ends together again. In longer strictures, patching of the urethra to make a larger lumen is necessary. Local hairless penile and scrotal skin flaps may be reliably elevated on a vascular pedicle and sutured to the diseased urethra. In patients who do not have enough available or appropriate local skin for flap reconstruction, it may be necessary to use grafts. The more commonly used grafts include extragenital full-thickness skin, bladder mucosa, and buccal mucosa. Grafts, by their inherent nature, tend not to be as reliable, because they must revascularize in order to survive. All these methods have allowed the reconstructive surgeon to rebuild the urethra reliably and in a one-stage procedure. Occasionally, patients require a staged procedure because of inadequate available tissue. Using a split-thickness skin graft harvested from the thigh, this skin is grafted onto the penis or scrotum at the time of their first stage. At the time of their closure in 6 months, the previously grafted skin can be elevated as a local flap for closure and incorporation into the urethra.

In patients with bulbomembranous strictures from a pelvic injury, an end-to-end anastomosis of the bulbar urethra to the apex of the prostate is usually performed. This usually involves a partial pubectomy and separation of the corporeal cavernosal bodies, to gain sufficient length and mobilization so that a tension-free anastomosis may be performed. Other methods of bridging the gap include rerouting the urethra around the corporeal body and reconstructing a portion of the urethra with a tubularized skin flap. The long-term success rate with an end-to-end anastomosis is in the order of 95%. Another surgical alternative that should be considered is the creation of a urethral ostium proximal to the urethral stricture. This scrotal or perineal urethrostomy is a viable alternative in those patients who are elderly or debilitated, or in whom previous reconstructive procedures have failed.

Urethral strictures may cause a great deal of patient suffering. With the advent of newer reconstructive techniques, it is possible to reliably decrease patient morbidity and increase quality of life.

RENAL CALCULI

method of
MICHAEL A. GLASS, M.D., and
PARAMJIT S. CHANDHOKE, M.D., PH.D.
University of Colorado Health Sciences Center
Denver, Colorado

Renal calculi are a major source of morbidity and account for a significant number of emergency department visits. The majority of stones contain calcium. The peak incidence of stone disease occurs in the third to fifth decades of life; men are affected three times more often than women. Geographically, stones are more prevalent in the mountainous northwest, tropical southeast, and the arid southwest of the United States. Symptomatic kidney stones present more frequently in the months of July, August, and September, presumably due to increased dehydration.

SIGNS AND SYMPTOMS

Kidney and ureteral stones commonly cause renal colic: severe, intermittent, unilateral flank pain that may radiate around the anterior abdominal wall down to the ipsilateral testicle, scrotum, or labia. This pain is due to distention of the renal collecting system and renal capsule. Patients may also have nausea, vomiting, abdominal distention, and even an ileus due to common autonomic innervation of the kidneys and the gastrointestinal tract via the celiac ganglia. As the stone approaches the bladder, irritative symptoms of urinary frequency and urgency and dysuria may develop. In contrast to patients with peritonitis who lie still, renal colic patients generally are unable to find a comfortable position; costovertebral angle tenderness is common. Abdominal examination may show mild tenderness to deep palpation over the lower abdominal quadrants without peritoneal signs.

LABORATORY FINDINGS

Urinalysis reveals microscopic hematuria in more than 90% of patients with urolithiasis. Significant pyuria (greater than 5 white blood cells per high-power field) should alert the clinician to the possibility of infection. Urinary pH is always documented, and the urine is cultured if significant WBCs or bacteria are present. A low urinary pH (<6.0), and a radiolucent filling defect on an intravenous pyelogram (IVP) suggest uric acid urolithiasis. Patients should have a complete blood count and renal panel. These tests may corroborate clinical suspicion of a significant upper tract urinary infection. A serum creatinine level is obtained to evaluate renal function as well as to prepare for subsequent intravenous contrast administration as necessary for an IVP or computed tomography.

RADIOGRAPHIC EXAMINATION

Approximately 80% of renal calculi are radiopaque and easily visualized on plain films of the kidneys, ureters, and bladder (KUB). The radiopacity of renal calculi varies with stone type. Stones composed of calcium phosphate are the most radiopaque, followed by calcium oxalate, struvite, and cystine. Uric acid stones are radiolucent and therefore not seen on a KUB film. Patients who have a history consistent with an acute stone episode should undergo a radiographic examination to document the stone size, type, and location.

Intravenous pyelography is the study of choice for evaluating patients with probable kidney stones. This study will not only document the size and location of the stone but also the degree of obstruction. The most consistent finding on IVP is delayed contrast excretion on the affected side. The length of delay in contrast excretion correlates with the degree of obstruction; delayed KUBs may be necessary to document the anatomic site of obstruction. Ureteral stones will often create filling defects with columnization of contrast behind the stone on an upright film. Radiolucent stones may be suspected as a negative shadow or a filling defect. A postvoid film will help visualize the distal ureter, which is often obscured by contrast in the bladder.

An ultrasound examination of the kidneys, ureter, and bladder should be reserved for patients who cannot have an IVP for reasons of renal failure, severe contrast allergy, or the need to reduce radiation exposure, such as in pregnancy. Ultrasound is useful for documenting hydronephrosis and visualizing large kidney or upper ureteral stones. However, ultrasound is poor for the visualization of mid and lower ureteral stones. If the stone is within the intramural ureter, it may be seen during bladder ultrasonography.

MANAGEMENT

Once the diagnosis of urolithiasis has been established, management of the acute stone episode will depend on several factors. The characteristics of the stone and the seriousness of the patient's illness will determine the timing and type of subsequent treatment. Initial therapy should be directed toward relieving the patient's pain, which usually responds well to parenteral morphine (5 to 15 mg) or intramuscular meperidine (50 to 100 mg). Patients should also receive intravenous fluid resuscitation as necessary. Most patients can be managed as outpatients; however, there are some indications for hospitalization and close observation (Table 1). Diabetic, elderly, and

TABLE 1. **Indications for Hospitalization**

Intractable pain requiring parenteral medication
Inability to tolerate oral fluids
High grade fever (>101°F)
Solitary renal unit with obstruction
Obstruction with infection

immunocompromised patients are a unique population who must be monitored very closely due to their increased risk of developing complications.

The size and location of the stone greatly influence the timing and the type of intervention. Almost all stones that are 2 mm or less will pass spontaneously. Stones of 4 mm or less have an 80% chance of spontaneous passage. Stones measuring 4 to 6 mm have a 50% chance, and stones over 6 mm have a 10% chance of spontaneous passage. Stone location also influences the probability of spontaneous passage. For a particular stone size, the likelihood of spontaneous stone passage is increased when the stone is located in the distal ureter. All patients should be given a strainer to catch the stone for chemical analysis. Knowledge of the stone composition is critical in the subsequent metabolic evaluation and medical management of recurrent urolithiasis.

Kidney stone patients who are afebrile and tolerating oral fluids, and whose pain can be controlled with oral analgesics, need not be hospitalized at the time of the acute stone episode. They are treated as outpatients with analgesics and hydration and told to strain their urine for stones. Febrile kidney stone patients whose urine appears to be infected should be hospitalized. Their urine should be cultured and intravenous antibiotics administered. If there is significant renal obstruction, either a percutaneous nephrostomy (preferably) or a ureteral stent should be placed (Figure 1). Insertion of a ureteral stent may also be necessary when patients have continued pain that is not relieved by parenteral analgesics.

Stones that are radiolucent and suspected to be uric acid calculi are initially treated with dissolution therapy. Radiopaque stones cannot be treated with dissolution and need surgical management. Generally, kidney and upper ureteral stones 3 cm or less in size are most suitable for treatment by extracorporeal shock wave lithotripsy (SWL). In this noninvasive treatment, shock waves are used to fragment the stones into small pieces that pass spontaneously. Stones located in the mid and lower ureter that have not passed spontaneously after a period of 6 weeks are best treated by ureteroscopic manipulation. Small-caliber ureteroscopes are passed retrograde from the bladder up into the ureter until the stone can be visualized. Under direct visualization, a laser or an electrohydraulic probe can then be used to fragment the stone into small pieces. If the stone is small enough, it may be engaged within a basket and removed from the ureter with great care.

Large stones (>3 cm) that are located in the kidney should be removed by percutaneous nephrolithotomy as the treatment of choice. During this procedure, a percutaneous tract is developed from the patient's flank to the kidney, large enough to allow the placement of a No. 24 French nephroscope. The stone is fragmented using ultrasonic lithotripsy and removed through the same tract. Open surgical stone removal is rarely necessary in this era of SWL and endoscopic lithotripsy. However, large ureteral stones (>2 cm) and some complex staghorn calculi may be best treated with open surgery.

Uric Acid Stones

Uric acid stones account for 5% to 10% of urinary stones. Patients at risk for uric acid stones are those with gout, chronic diarrhea, an ileostomy, and those who have had cytotoxic therapy for malignant conditions. However, most patients have a normal 24-hour urinary uric acid excretion. The predisposing condition to the formation of uric acid stones is a persistently acidic urine (pH <5.5). Approximately 25% of patients with symptomatic gout will form uric acid stones, and 25% of patients with uric acid stones will have gout.

Uric acid exists in two forms: as uric acid, which

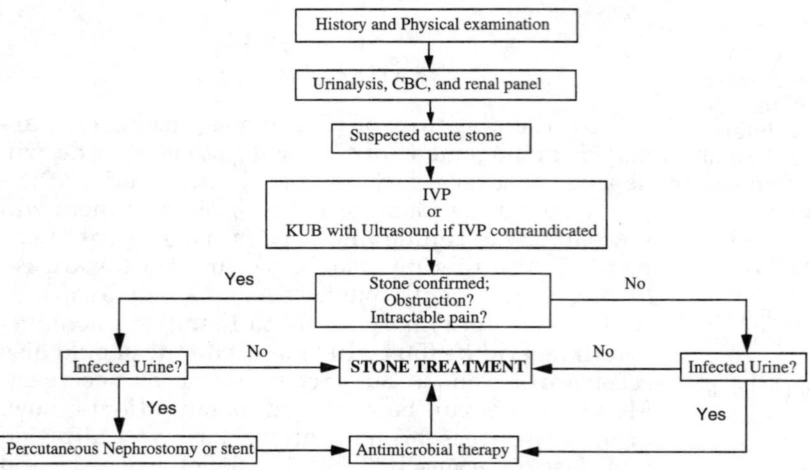

Figure 1. Flow diagram for the management of acute stone episode.

is insoluble, and as urate salt, which is 20 times more soluble in water. Thus, the solubility of uric acid is dependent upon the pH of the urine. The dissociation constant, pKa, of uric acid is 5.75. At a pH of 5.75, half of the urinary uric acid is in the insoluble non-ionized form and half is in the soluble ionized form. Therefore, treatment of uric acid stones is aimed at increasing the pH above the pKa, thereby increasing its solubility.

Patients should maintain a urine volume greater than 2 liters per day, decrease purine-rich foods (meat, poultry, fish), and use urine alkalinization to dissolve the stone. The amount of alkali used should be titrated to raise the urinary pH to between 6.5 and 7.0; this will result in a tenfold increase in the solubility of uric acid. Urinary alkalinization greater than 7.0 may precipitate a calcium phosphate shell on a uric acid stone. Commonly used alkali agents are sodium bicarbonate and potassium citrate. Potassium citrate should be avoided in patients with renal insufficiency. Sodium bicarbonate may be contraindicated in patients with heart disease due to the increased sodium load. If dissolution therapy fails, uric acid stones can be treated with SWL, ureteroscopy, or percutaneous techniques.

Finally, the prevention of uric acid stones should include a metabolic evaluation. Serum and 24-hour urine samples should be sent to the laboratory for uric acid determination. If serum or urinary uric acid is elevated, the patient can be treated with allopurinol, 300 mg per day. Patients with a normal serum or urinary uric acid determination are best managed by alkali therapy alone.

Struvite Stones

Struvite stones form in an alkaline urine caused by urea-splitting bacteria that hydrolyze urea into ammonia, increasing the urinary pH. This sets up a unique environment in the urine to precipitate magnesium, ammonium, and phosphate to form struvite stones (10%). Urea-splitting bacteria are *Proteus, Klebsiella, Pseudomonas*, staphylococci, and *Mycoplasma*. Struvite stones are more common in women and in patients with urinary diversion (ileal conduit), chronic catheter drainage, or a neurogenic bladder. These stones frequently enlarge rapidly and can fill the entire collecting system (staghorn calculus). Primary treatment is complete removal of the stone and concurrent eradication of the urinary tract infection. Failure to do both will result in higher stone recurrence rates. Surgical options include SWL and percutaneous nephrolithotomy. Stones less than 3 cm are initially treated with SWL. Percutaneous stone removal is preferable for larger stones. After stone removal, patients should be followed closely for recurrent infections. Underlying anatomic abnormalities that predispose patients to recurrent kidney infections should be corrected. Metabolic evaluation should be undertaken in most patients, especially if a calcium stone coexists with the struvite stone.

Cystine Stones

Cystine stones (2%) are formed because of an autosomal recessive disorder affecting the transport across epithelium of cystine, ornithine, lysine, and arginine (COLA). Cystine stones are faintly opaque and have a ground-glass, smooth-edged appearance on KUB. Heterozygous patients excrete 200 mg per day of cystine (normal: 100 mg per day), whereas homozygous patients excrete more than 500 mg per day of cystine. The diagnosis is made with a 24-hour urinary cystine excretion measurement.

Cystine solubility, as uric acid, is dependent upon urinary pH. As the pKa of cystine is 8.1, the goal of alkali therapy is to achieve a urinary pH close to its pKa. Cystine stones are very hard and not easily fragmented with SWL. Percutaneous procedures obtain the best results, especially if the stone size exceeds 2 cm.

The metabolic evaluation of cystine stones includes a 24-hour urine sample for cystine determination. Prevention of cystine stones is aimed at reducing urinary cystine concentration by hydration, increasing the solubility of cystine by alkalinization, and decreasing urinary excretion. Urinary volume should exceed 2 liters per day. D-Penicillamine (Cuprimine) has been shown to complex with the cysteine component of cystine, thereby decreasing cystine excretion. However, due to the side effects of agranulocytosis and nephrotic syndrome, it is not often used. Alpha-mercaptopropionylglycine (Thiola) acts in a similar fashion to D-penicillamine but has fewer side effects. The dosage of Thiola is 0.5 to 1.0 gram per day in divided doses. The dose should be titrated to obtain the urinary concentration of cystine below 300 mg per liter.

Calcium-Containing Stones

Calcium stones (75% to 80%) are the most common renal calculi and present either as calcium oxalate or calcium phosphate stones. Calcium oxalate is the sole or major component of approximately 70% of all stones. Approximately 50% of patients after the first calcium stone will have a recurrence within the next 5 years. Most of the recurrent stone-forming patients have an underlying metabolic abnormality or an anatomic abnormality predisposing them to the formation of stones. First-time stone-formers with a single stone and no family history do not need extensive metabolic evaluation and may be encouraged solely to increase fluids. Patients who need metabolic evaluation are those with bilateral stones, recurrent stones, or a family history of stones. Children, African Americans, and patients with a solitary kidney who have urolithiasis should also have a metabolic evaluation. Calcium oxalate stones can occur from a multitude of metabolic abnormalities: increased urinary calcium excretion (hypercalciuria), increased urinary oxalate excretion (hyperoxaluria), increased urinary uric acid excretion (hyperuricosuria), and de-

TABLE 2. **Limited and Comprehensive Metabolic Evaluation of Calcium Stones**

Limited Metabolic Evaluation

1. Serum calcium, ionized calcium, sodium, potassium, BUN, creatinine, carbon dioxide, chloride
2. Two random 24-hour urine analyses for volume, creatinine, calcium, oxalate, uric acid, citrate, sodium

Comprehensive Metabolic Evaluation

1. Two 24-hour urine analyses for volume, creatinine, calcium, oxalate, uric acid, citrate, sodium, potassium, BUN, phosphate, magnesium
2. One week of low-calcium and low-oxalate diet, followed by another 24-hour urine on a restricted diet. Serum calcium, ionized calcium, sodium, potassium, BUN, creatinine, carbon dioxide, chloride
3. Calcium load test:
   6 A.M.–8 A.M. (2 h)—Fasting urinary Ca/Cr ratio
   8 A.M.–1 gm oral Ca load (45mL neo-calcium gluconate)
   8 A.M.–10 A.M.—urinary Ca/Cr ratio
   10 A.M.–noon—urinary Ca/Cr ratio

Abbreviations: BUN = blood urea nitrogen; Ca = calcium; Cr = creatinine.

creased urinary citrate excretion (hypocitraturia). Treatment includes increasing fluid intake to achieve a urine volume in excess of 2 liters per day and correction of the underlying metabolic abnormality.

There are two types of metabolic evaluation for calcium stones: a limited evaluation and a comprehensive evaluation (Table 2). A limited evaluation is best suited for most private practices, whereas the comprehensive evaluation is used within the framework of Metabolic Stone Clinics. The major difference in the two types is the further differentiation of the hypercalciurias in the comprehensive evaluation.

Upon completion of the metabolic evaluation, patients can be divided into those with hypercalciuria and those with normocalciuria (Figure 2). Patients with normal calcium excretion can be further subdivided into three groups: those with hyperoxaluria, hyperuricosuria, or hypocitraturia. Hypercalciuria is further divided into those with absorptive (three types), resorptive, or renal leak.

Hyperoxaluria (Figure 3). Inherited primary hyperoxaluria is a rare metabolic disorder that causes renal oxalosis in childhood that is usually fatal. In adults, hyperoxaluria is considered secondary to increased oxalate absorption from the gastrointestinal tract. Hyperoxaluria is defined as urinary oxalate exceeding 40 mg per day. This condition is frequently found in patients with inflammatory bowel disease and in patients following small bowel bypass surgery for the treatment of morbid obesity. Foods with a high oxalate content are spinach, rhubarb, tea, carbonated beverages, and nuts. In the gastrointestinal tract, oxalate binds normally with calcium, limiting its absorption. However, in malabsorption syndromes, excess fatty acids bind calcium in the intestines and leave more free oxalate for absorption. Treatment for this condition is dietary restriction of oxalate. If this fails to lower the urinary oxalate, then calcium supplementation may be given to bind oxalate in the intestine.

Hyperuricosuria (Figure 3). Hyperuricosuria, defined as excretion of greater than 700 mg per day of uric acid in the urine, is associated with calcium oxalate stones in 20% of patients. Uric acid may bind stone inhibitors or promote calcium oxalate stone formation on a uric acid nidus. The treatment is low purine diet and allopurinol (Zyloprim), 300 mg per day.

Hypocitraturia (Figure 3). Citrate is an important inhibitor of calcium oxalate stone formation. Hypocitraturia is defined as excretion of less than 300 mg per day of urinary citrate. Citrate complexes with calcium and thus decreases the amount of ionic calcium available for stone formation. In addition, it has a direct inhibitor activity on calcium oxalate nucleation. Treatment is best accomplished with po-

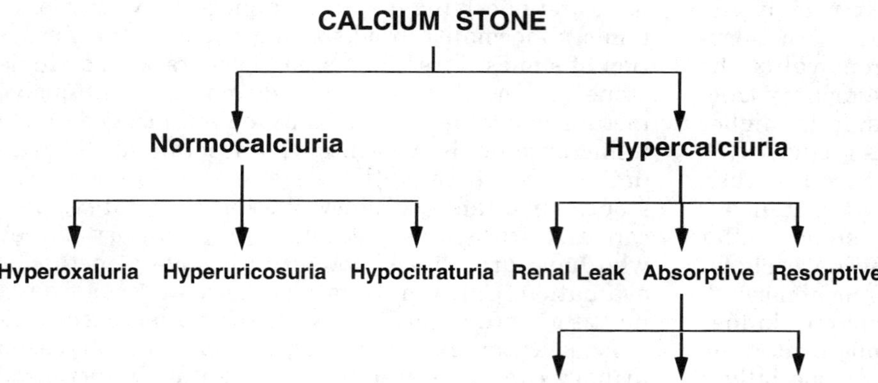

Figure 2. Comprehensive evaluation to determine patients with hypercalciuria or normocalciuria.

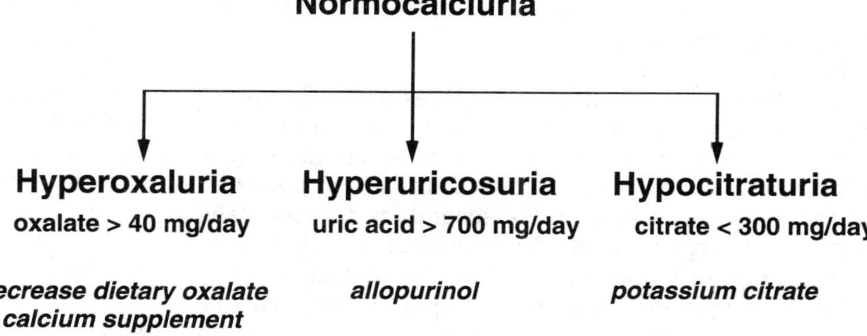

Figure 3. Limited and comprehensive evaluation of hyperoxaluria, hyperuricosuria, and hypocitraturia.

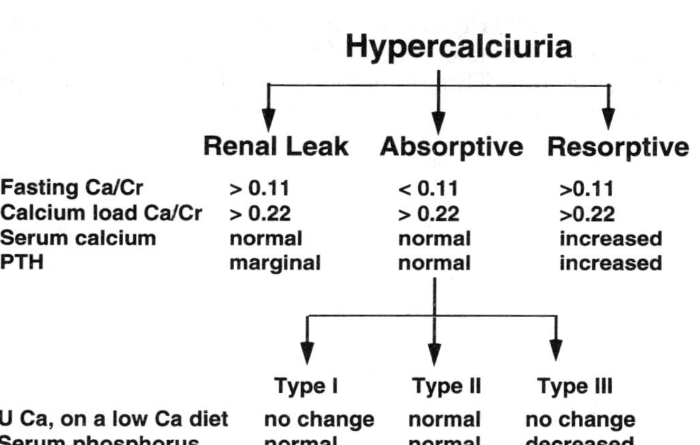

Figure 4. Comprehensive evaluation of types I, II, and III absorptive hypercalciuria.

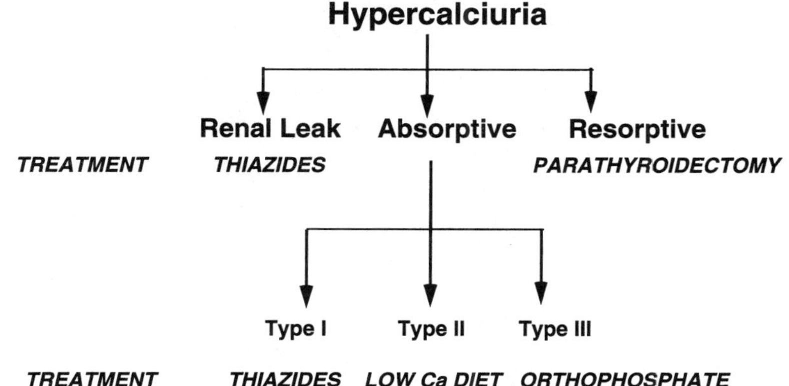

Figure 5. Treatment of the various hypercalciurias.

tassium citrate supplementation, 60 to 120 mEq daily in divided doses.

Hypercalciuria

ABSORPTIVE (TYPES 1, 2, 3) (Figures 4, 5). Hypercalciuria is defined as urinary calcium excretion greater than 300 mg per day. This is the most common type of metabolic abnormality found in stone patients. Absorptive hypercalciuria is secondary to increased calcium absorption from the intestine, which results in a higher excretion of calcium. With the comprehensive evaluation, absorptive hypercalciuria can be differentiated from other forms of hypercalciuria using the calcium load test (Figure 4). In absorptive hypercalciuria, the fasting urinary calcium excretion is normal.

In Type I absorptive hypercalciuria, patients have an increased urinary calcium excretion even on a calcium-restricted diet. Treatment is hydrochlorothiazide* 25 to 50 mg per day, or cellulose phosphate, 5 grams orally three times daily. Hydrochlorothiazide increases the renal reabsorption of calcium from both the proximal and distal tubules, causing decreased

---

*Not FDA-approved for this indication.

excretion of calcium. Cellulose phosphate prevents calcium absorption from the intestine.

Type II absorptive hypercalciuria is the most common type and is dependent on dietary calcium. Patients should therefore limit their calcium intake to 400 to 600 mg per day. If diet fails to lower the urinary excretion of calcium, then thiazides may be used.

Type III absorptive hypercalciuria is secondary to a renal phosphate leak. Low phosphate increases 1,25-vitamin D, increasing the absorption of phosphate as well as calcium from the intestine. Treatment is dietary phosphate supplementation with orthophosphate, 250 to 2000 mg three times daily.

RESORPTIVE (Figure 5). Resorptive hypercalciuria accounts for less than 5% of calcium stones. These patients have hypercalciuria due to increased calcium bone loss, as in hyperparathyroidism. The parathyroid hormone level is elevated, along with urinary phosphate. Treatment is removal of the parathyroid adenoma.

RENAL LEAK (Figure 5). Hypercalciuria due to renal leak is an intrinsic defect of the renal tubule to reabsorb calcium. This condition is effectively treated with a thiazide.

The Sexually Transmitted Diseases

CHANCROID

method of
STEPHEN J. KRAUS, M.D.
Georgia Clinical Research
Atlanta, Georgia

Effective chancroid therapy depends on an accurate diagnosis. Although there are distinguishing clinical features for chancroid, genital herpes, syphilis, lymphogranuloma venereum (LGV), and granuloma inguinale (GI), it is not unusual for one sexually transmitted genital ulcer to mimic another. In addition, two different causes of genital ulcers can coexist in up to 10% of genital ulcer cases. Laboratory tests are crucial to an accurate diagnosis: darkfield examination or direct immunofluorescence for *Treponema pallidum,* culture for *Haemophilus ducreyi,* culture or antigen detection for herpes simplex virus (HSV), serology or culture for LGV, and histology for GI.

TREATMENT

First-line therapeutic regimens for chancroid are ceftriaxone (Rocephin), 250 mg intramuscularly in a single dose, azithromycin (Zithromax), 1 gram orally in a single dose, and erythromycin base, 500 mg orally four times a day for 7 days (Table 1). Single-dose therapy with ceftriaxone or azithromycin is advantageous in the poorly compliant population frequently seen with chancroid. Erythromycin is the least expensive regimen, and its more prolonged therapy is advantageous in treating human immuno-

deficiency virus (HIV)-positive patients with chancroid. Alternative regimens for chancroid therapy are amoxicillin, 500 mg, plus clavulanic acid, 125 mg (Augmentin), orally three times a day for 7 days, and ciprofloxacin (Cipro), 500 mg orally two times a day for 3 days. Pregnant women with chancroid can be treated with ceftriaxone, erythromycin, or amoxicillin/clavulanic acid. Ciprofloxacin is contraindicated for pregnant or lactating women and in children less than 18 years of age.

The healing time for chancroid ulcers is related to ulcer size: large ulcers may require several weeks to heal. Fluctuant inguinal lymphadenopathy responds more slowly than the genital ulcers and may require large-bore needle aspiration through adjacent normal skin. The nodes should not be treated by incision and drainage.

Patients treated for chancroid should be re-examined 3 to 7 days after the start of therapy and then weekly until the ulcers have healed. With effective therapy, the lesions are less painful within 3 days and smaller in size within 7 days. When no clinical improvement is evident or the ulcers fail to heal, the clinician should consider compliance with medication, the correctness of the diagnosis, co-infection with another genital ulcer sexually transmitted disease, HIV infection, or a resistant *H. ducreyi* organism. Sexual contacts for a period of up to 10 days before the onset of the chancroid ulcer should be treated regardless of symptoms. Patients with chancroid are at increased risk of contracting HIV; therefore, HIV testing should be done at the time of chancroid therapy. If negative, the test should be repeated at 3 and 6 months.

TABLE 1. **Antibiotic Therapy for Chancroid**

Recommended Regimens

Azithromycin (Zithromax), 1 gm PO in a single dose,
or
Ceftriaxone (Rocephin), 250 mg IM in a single dose,
or
Erythromycin base, 500 mg PO qid for 7 d

Alternative Regimens

Amoxicillin, 500 mg, plus clavulanic acid, 125 mg (Augmentin), PO bid for 7 d,
or
Ciprofloxacin (Cipro),* 500 mg PO bid for 3 d.

*Ciprofloxacin is contraindicated for pregnant and lactating women, children, and adolescents under 18 years of age.
From Centers for Disease Control: 1993 Sexually Transmitted Diseases Treatment Guidelines. MMWR 42, 1993.

GONORRHEA

method of
JONATHAN M. ZENILMAN, M.D.
Johns Hopkins University School of Medicine
Baltimore, Maryland

Gonorrhea is the most commonly reported infectious disease in the United States, with 500,000 cases reported annually. Over the past 2 decades, the disease has increasingly assumed a "core group distribution"; areas where disease rates are extraordinarily high are typically impoverished inner-city or rural areas.

Recent studies from the United States as well as developing countries have established that heterosexual transmission of human immunodeficiency virus (HIV) is facilitated by the exudative sexually transmitted diseases (STDs) gonorrhea and chlamydia. Since these infections are common, especially in individuals at high risk for HIV, a large proportion of heterosexually transmitted HIV may be attributable to facilitation by STDs. This finding has made treatment of STDs an imperative in HIV prevention strategies.

CLINICAL MANIFESTATIONS

Neisseria gonorrhoeae causes a primary mucosal infection that is almost exclusively acquired through sexual exposure. In men, the most common syndrome is urethritis. The patient typically experiences dysuria and urethral discharge within 24 to 48 hours of exposure. Symptoms eventually develop in 95% of patients; however, 5% of patients remain asymptomatic. The major differential diagnosis is nongonococcal urethritis due to chlamydia and other organisms.

In women, endocervical disease is the most common syndrome. Symptoms such as vaginal discharge, lower abdominal discomfort, and dyspareunia occur in only approximately 50% of patients; these symptoms are often nonspecific, and onset is often associated with menses. On physical examination, findings may include cervical edema, discharge, friability, and erythema. Untreated, approximately one-third of patients develop pelvic inflammatory disease (PID), which often results in tubal scarring and consequent increased risk for ectopic pregnancy and infertility. PID is characterized by lower abdominal pain, cervical motion tenderness, and fever. However, PID is clinically difficult to diagnose, and because of the severity of complications, the practice is to treat aggressively for PID if lower abdominal pain or any suggestion of cervical motion tenderness is present.

Gonococcal proctitis is seen in two different populations. In homosexual men who have had receptive rectal intercourse, the disease presents symptomatically in half of cases. Symptoms include mucopurulent discharge, tenesmus, and constipation. In about 5 to 10% of women with gonococcal cervicitis, asymptomatic rectal infection is present and is not usually associated with rectal sexual exposure. It is assumed to be caused by tracking of secretions across the perineum.

Gonococcal pharyngitis is seen in patients who have had oral sexual exposure. Signs and symptoms are not distinguishable from any other cause of bacterial or viral pharyngitis. In a small proportion of patients (estimated to be <0.5%), disseminated gonococcal infection (DGI) occurs. DGI is a sign-symptom complex resulting from gonococcal sepsis that presents with fever, arthralgia, tenosynovitis, oligoarticular septic arthritis, and a skin rash characterized by sparse pustular lesions on the extensor surfaces. DGI should be suspected in any sexually active individual presenting with fever and joint symptoms. These patients should receive three site cultures for *N. gonorrhoeae* (rectum, throat, and genitalia), even in the absence of local symptoms.

DIAGNOSIS

Diagnosis of gonococcal infection is made most often by culture. However, with the advent of newer non–culture-based diagnostic tests using genetic probes and newer DNA amplification technology, culture may be supplanted by these other methods. Often, the clinician has to make a presumptive diagnosis and formulate treatment on the basis of a clinical syndrome. In men, the differential diagnosis of urethritis is gonococcal or nongonococcal urethritis (NGU); in women, cervicitis may be gonococcal or nongonococcal mucopurulent cervicitis (MPC). When previous culture results or exposure histories are not available, Gram's stains may be a useful adjunct. When available, Gram's stains are 90 to 95% sensitive and specific in men; in women, sensitivity drops to 30 to 50%, but specificity remains high. Because Gram's stains are often not available in the typical clinical practice setting, presumptive treatment is often given, based on the prevalence of gonococcal diseases in the local community.

ANTIMICROBIAL RESISTANCE

Since 1986, the Centers for Disease Control and Prevention (CDC) has maintained a gonococcal isolate surveillance system that periodically assays systematic samples of clinical isolates for susceptibility to currently used antimicrobials. Current treatment strategies are based on the susceptibility data obtained through this system. For example, in the late 1980s, the program noted an increased proportion of organisms with high-level plasmid-mediated resistance to penicillin and tetracycline; therefore, these have been eliminated as single-drug treatment options. Since 1992, isolates with decreased susceptibility to ciprofloxacin and ceftriaxone have been detected. These trends are being observed very closely.

PUBLIC HEALTH ISSUES IN THE TREATMENT OF GONORRHEA

Treatment strategies are based on a number of practical and logistical issues, including:

1. *Single-dose oral treatment regimens.* Single-dose regimens ensure compliance; oral regimens ensure ease of administration.

2. *Co-treatment for chlamydia.* In the mid-1980s, a number of studies demonstrated that coexistent chlamydia infection was present in 30 to 50% of patients with gonorrhea. Although these levels have dropped in many areas, most authorities believe that it is still cost effective to co-treat for chlamydia in all patients treated for gonorrhea.

3. *Efficacy against antimicrobial-resistant strains.* It is more cost effective to treat with antimicrobials that are effective against resistant strains than to test all isolates for susceptibility.

4. *Presumptive treatment of partners.* Current public health practice is to presumptively treat all sexual partners of patients with diagnosed gonorrhea, even if the individual does not have clinical evidence of disease. The rationale of this approach is to prevent incubating disease from developing and to reduce transmission to the next generation of sexual partners.

In the late 1980s, in the wake of large syphilis epidemics in the United States, some authorities believed that all patients with gonorrhea should be treated with regimens that were also effective against incubating syphilis, such as beta-lactam–based drugs. For example, the quinolones and spectinomycin have no activity against *Treponema pallidum.* Large-scale studies in major urban centers where syphilis outbreaks occurred demonstrated that incubating syphilis in gonorrhea patients is not an important consideration. Furthermore, regimens used to co-treat for chlamydia infection (tetracyclines and macrolides) have antitreponemal activity. Therefore, efficacy against syphilis does not have to be a consideration in formulating antigonococcal therapy.

TREATMENT

Uncomplicated Urogenital, Rectal, or Pharyngeal Infections (Table 1)

As noted above, the principles of treatment include single-dose, preferably oral administration, and efficacy against all known types of antimicrobial-resistant gonococci. The quinolones and oral third-generation cephalosporins are used for most gonococcal treatment.

In Baltimore, our group has been using quinolones since 1989 for the treatment of routine gonococcal infection. CDC recommendations currently include ciprofloxacin (Cipro) 500 mg and ofloxacin (Floxin) 400 mg as therapy options. Clinical trial data suggest very high efficacy rates for uncomplicated genital infection (urethritis, cervicitis). For rectal and pharyngeal infection, the data are more limited; however, most authorities believe that the efficacy of these drugs is greater than 90%. Oral single-dose cephalosporins are also highly efficacious. The largest clinical experience to date has been with cefixime (Suprax) 400 mg, which has been extensively evaluated for genital infections. Ceftriaxone (Rocephin) has been used at both 125- and 250-mg doses for over 10 years. Current recommendations are 125 mg for all uncomplicated syndromes. Because this drug can be given only parenterally, ceftriaxone has been largely supplanted by the oral single-dose regimens cited above.

Pelvic Inflammatory Disease

Women with suspected PID who do not require hospitalization should be treated with ceftriaxone 250 mg intramuscularly, followed by co-treatment for chlamydia. Repeat clinical evaluation, including a bimanual examination, should be performed within 48 to 72 hours, and if no improvement is noted, the patient should be referred to a gynecologist.

TABLE 1. **Treatment of Uncomplicated Gonorrhea in Adults**

Oral Single-Dose Regimens
Ciprofloxacin (Cipro) 500 mg
Ofloxacin (Floxin) 400 mg
Cefixime (Suprax) 400 mg
Parenteral
Ceftriaxone (Rocephin) 125–250 mg IM

TABLE 2. **Treatment of Disseminated Gonococcal Infection**

Inpatient Phase (IV)
Ceftriaxone (Rocephin) 1 gm q 24 h
Cefotaxime (Claforan) 1 gm q 8 h
Ceftizoxime (Cefizox) 1 gm q 8 h
Ciprofloxacin (Cipro) 400 mg q 12 h
Outpatient Phase (PO)
Cefixime (Suprax) 400 mg bid
Ciprofloxacin (Cipro) 500 mg bid

Disseminated Gonococcal Infection

No large-scale clinical trial of DGI has been performed since the mid-1970s. Therapy recommendations are therefore based on expert opinion rather than clinical trial data. Our group has used the approach to DGI treatment outlined in Table 2. Briefly, patients with documented or suspected gonococcal septicemia should be treated with parenteral third-generation cephalosporins or quinolones until defervescence, followed by oral outpatient antibiotics to complete a full 1-week course of therapy.

Chlamydia Co-Treatment

All patients with gonococcal disease should be co-treated for chlamydia, except if a chlamydia diagnostic test is being performed routinely. The two major treatment options for chlamydia are doxycycline and azithromycin (Table 3). Azithromycin (Zithromax) is a new macrolide with an extremely long half-life; therefore, patients can be given 1 gram as single-dose observed therapy. In patients who are unable to take doxycycline or azithromycin, erythromycin (either erythromycin-based ethylsuccinate formulation) is an acceptable alternative but is often accompanied by gastrointestinal side effects.

SPECIAL SITUATIONS

Test of Cure (Post-Therapy Evaluation). Under current recommendations and using approved regimens, routine post-therapy evaluation is not necessary unless patients continue to be symptomatic or suspected high-level resistant strains are present within the community.

Gonorrhea in HIV-Infected Patients. It appears that standard treatment regimens are efficacious in HIV-infected patients and that no change in management is required. However, incident STD represents objective evidence of unprotected sexual activity, highlighting a need for intensive counseling.

Gonorrhea in Pregnancy. Gonorrhea in preg-

TABLE 3. **Treatment of Chlamydia Infections**

Doxycycline 100 mg bid for 7 days
Azithromycin 1 gm (single-dose)
Erythromycin base 500 mg qid for 7 days

nancy should be treated aggressively. Quinolones are contraindicated in pregnancy; therefore, patients should be treated with either oral or injectable cephalosporin regimens. Chlamydia co-treatment can be with either erythromycin or azithromycin (which is currently classified as Class B). Patients who are pregnant and who have a severe allergy to penicillin should be treated with spectinomycin 2 grams intramuscularly as a single dose.

Gonorrhea in the Perinatal and Neonatal Period. Infants born to women with known gonococcal infection should be treated presumptively with ceftriaxone 25 to 50 mg per kg intravenously or intramuscularly in a single dose. All infants should routinely receive recommended ophthalmic prophylaxis immediately after parturition.

Gonorrhea in Preadolescent Children. Gonococcal infections in this population are almost always a result of child abuse. Treatment is relatively straightforward in these cases (ceftriaxone 125 mg), but it is critical that specimens be obtained to ensure that forensic procedures are appropriately followed and specimens are archived. Confirmed gonococcal infection in preadolescent children is prima facie evidence of sexual exposure.

PUBLIC HEALTH MANAGEMENT ISSUES

Referral of Sexual Partners. Sexual partners exposed within the previous 30 days (prior to evaluation and treatment) should be referred for clinical evaluation and treated presumptively. Local health departments can often facilitate partner notification. Patients should not be prescribed antimicrobials to be given to their sexual partners.

Reporting. Gonorrhea is a reportable disease in all 50 states. Local health authorities should be notified with the appropriate information.

Other STDs. All patients with gonococcal infection should be assessed for other STDs. All patients with an STD should receive HIV counseling and be offered HIV testing.

Counseling. Prevention counseling is an integral part of primary care and includes promoting condom use, reducing high-risk sexual behaviors, and reducing the numbers of sexual partners. Contraceptive counseling should be offered (or referred) as part of any reproductive health care evaluation.

NONGONOCOCCAL URETHRITIS

method of
MANOJ MONGA, M.D., and
WAYNE J. G. HELLSTROM, M.D.
Tulane University School of Medicine
New Orleans, Louisiana

Urethritis is a clinical diagnosis, based on signs and symptoms that include dysuria, urethral pruritus, penile discharge, meatal erythema, and hematuria on initiation of the urinary stream. A presumptive diagnosis of nongonococcal urethritis requires a Gram's stain of a urethral swab specimen to document the absence of intracellular gram-negative diplococci. Recent advances in the ability to culture *Chlamydia* and *Ureaplasma* have facilitated identification of the cause of nongonococcal urethritis; however, therapy is often empirical, especially in large urban centers, because of the expense and specialization of these diagnostic techniques.

Chlamydia trachomatis is the causative organism in 25 to 50% of cases, and *Ureaplasma urealyticum* (15 to 40%), *Trichomonas vaginalis* (2 to 20%), and herpes simplex virus are implicated in a smaller proportion of cases. *Mycoplasma genitalium* may be detected in 15 to 25%, but further studies are needed to establish a causal relationship. An organism cannot be identified in over 25% of cases.

A recent change in sexual partners (within 3 months) and multiple sexual partners are risk factors for nongonococcal urethritis. Foreign bodies, urethral instrumentation, and chemical detergents (soaps, shampoos, vaginal douches, spermicidal formulations) may be implicated in certain cases. Urethritis may be a manifestation of systemic diseases such as Reiter's syndrome, Stevens-Johnson syndrome, and Wegener's granulomatosis. Smoking has been suggested as an independent risk factor for urethritis. Of interest, circumcised men are 1.6 times more likely than uncircumcised men to contract nongonococcal urethritis.

LABORATORY EVALUATION

The leukocyte esterase dipstick test may be utilized as a sensitive screening test for urethral inflammation. In general, the first 10 mL of a voided urine specimen (VB_1) should be centrifuged and examined for pyuria (>15 polymorphonuclear leukocytes per 400× field). Localization of inflammation to only the urethra and confirmation of a diagnosis of urethritis can be achieved by demonstrating a significantly higher ratio of white blood cells per high-power field in the first voided urine (VB_1) compared with the midstream urine (VB_2) or the voided urine following prostatic massage (VB_3).

In practice, a specimen obtained by urethral swab should be examined by Gram's stain for evidence of urethritis (>5 polymorphonuclear leukocytes per 1000× field) and the presence of intracellular gram-negative diplococci (indicative of *Neisseria gonorrhoeae*) and cultured for *Chlamydia, Ureaplasma,* and gonococcus. Obtaining the urethral swab in the morning, prior to the first urine void, may increase the diagnostic yield. Cultures for *Chlamydia,* an obligate intracellular parasite, require a sampling of the endourethral columnar epithelium instead of the urethral exudate. *Trichomonas* can be detected by wet mount examination in less than 50% of culture-positive cases.

More sophisticated tests may be utilized if financial resources permit or in cases of recurrent or refractory urethritis. These techniques include indirect hemagglutination titers for *Trichomonas,* direct immunofluorescence methods for *Chlamydia* detection utilizing monoclonal antibodies, an enzyme-amplified immunoassay for *Chlamydia* detection, and polymerase chain reaction methods utilizing DNA probes for *Chlamydia, Trichomonas,* and *Mycoplasma.*

TREATMENT

Treatment of urethritis should include therapy of both the patient and the cohort. The patient should

TABLE 1. **Treatment Options for Nongonococcal Urethritis**

Drug	Dose	Duration	Estimated Cost*
Doxycycline	100 mg bid	7 days	$ 6.00
Erythromycin	500 mg q 6 h	7 days	$ 9.00
	250 mg q 6 h†	14 days	$10.00
Ofloxacin (Floxin)‡	300 mg bid	7 days	$51.00
Azithromycin (Zithromax)	1000 mg single dose	—	$27.00
Minocycline	100 mg qd	7 days	$12.00
Tetracycline	500 mg q 6 h	7 days	$ 6.00
	250 mg q 6 h†	14 days	$ 6.00

*Retail price based on a survey of New Orleans outpatient pharmacies.
†If higher dose not tolerated.
‡Contraindicated in pregnancy and children less than 16 years of age.

be instructed to avoid unprotected intercourse during the treatment period. Counseling on safe sexual practices and the option of testing for syphilis and human immunodeficiency virus should be incorporated in the patient discussion. The incidence of other concomitant sexually transmitted diseases in patients with nongonococcal urethritis is 10 to 15%.

Empirical treatment options that are effective against *C. trachomatis, U. urealyticum,* and *M. genitalium* are summarized in Table 1. A 7-day course of doxycycline 100 mg twice daily is the most common initial therapy.

If the causative organism is known to be *Chlamydia,* amoxicillin (500 mg every 8 hours for 10 days), clindamycin (Cleocin, 450 mg every 8 hours for 10 days), and sulfisoxazole (500 mg every 6 hours for 10 days) are alternative therapeutic regimens. These agents may be used in pregnancy, *with the exception of sulfisoxazole,* which should be avoided in late pregnancy because of the risk of kernicterus. Erythromycin is the agent of choice in the treatment of nongonococcal urethritis during pregnancy and lactation.

Fluoroquinolones are highly effective therapy for gonococcal urethritis, but in this class of antimicrobials, only ofloxacin (Floxin, 300 mg twice daily for 7 days) has a 90 to 95% cure rate for nongonococcal urethritis.

Azithromycin (Zithromax) is a novel azalide antibiotic that achieves sustained high tissue levels and is transported by migratory leukocytes to areas of inflammation. Azithromycin administered in a single dose (1000 mg) provides a 90 to 98% cure rate for nongonoccal urethritis and a 95% cure rate for gonococcal urethritis. A 3-day regimen (500 mg on day 1, followed by 250 mg on days 2 and 3) has been suggested to improve efficacy. Empirical therapy with this agent may prove cost effective by decreasing the need for extensive laboratory studies and the need for retreatment because of poor patient compliance.

T. vaginalis should be treated with a single 2-gram dose of metronidazole or a 7-day course of 250 mg three times daily. Treatment failures should undergo a course of metronidazole 2 grams daily for 5 days. The patient should be counseled to avoid alcohol during the treatment period. Instead of metronidazole, vaginal suppositories of clotrimazole 100 mg daily for 2 weeks should be used during pregnancy.

Adverse reaction profiles for these antimicrobial agents are similar: gastrointestinal side effects occur in approximately 15%, and central nervous system side effects (headache, dizziness) occur in 2 to 5%.

Persistent or recurrent urethritis may be caused by poor patient compliance, reinfection, relapse, or antibiotic resistance. The incidence of tetracycline-resistant *Ureaplasma* is 6 to 10%. *Ureaplasma* may be detected in 30 to 40% of initial treatment failures. Doxycycline treatment failures should undergo a course of erythromycin or a single dose of azithromycin. Relapse may indicate the presence of pathogens in "protected" sites, such as the prostate, and longer courses of antibiotic therapy (4 to 6 weeks) may be indicated in this instance. Examination of the sexual cohort may assist in identifying the pathogen responsible for persistent or recurrent urethritis.

The presence of condylomata acuminata or urethral obstruction should be evaluated by urethroscopy in cases of urethritis refractory to therapy. Significant structural abnormalities, such as urethral diverticula, meatal stenosis, or urethral strictures, may be present in 10% of patients with nongonococcal urethritis and in up to 25% of those with persistent urethritis following antibiotic therapy. Uroflow studies may assist in identifying these patients. Additional diagnostic considerations in patients with persistent irritative voiding symptoms include urinary cytology and the use of acid-fast bacilli cultures.

ACKNOWLEDGMENTS

The authors would like to thank Mrs. June Banks Evans and Mrs. Michon Breisacher Shinn for their help with the preparation of this manuscript.

GRANULOMA INGUINALE
(Donovanosis)

method of
THOMAS A. CHAPEL, M.D.
Wayne State University
Detroit, Michigan

and

JOHANNA CHAPEL, M.D.
Oakwood Hospital
Dearborn, Michigan

Granuloma inguinale (GI) is a slowly progressive, ulcerative anogenital infection caused by a gram-negative, obligate intracellular bacillus *Calymmatobacterium granulomatis*. The disease is rare in the United States but common in certain tropical and subtropical regions. It begins as a subcutaneous nodule that erodes through the skin, producing erythematous, painless ulcers. Inguinal or genital masses may appear as a result of subcutaneous granulomatous inflammation. The disease may be confused with syphilis, chancroid, cancer, cutaneous amebiasis, and fungal or mycobacterial infections.

Diagnosis is made by microscopic examination of crush or touch preparations of tissue obtained by punch biopsy from the margins of active lesions. Specimens are air-dried and methanol fixed and stained with Giemsa or Wright's stain. GI is confirmed by demonstrating *C. granulomatis*, the Donovan body, in mononuclear cells.

TREATMENT

The treatment of choice is tetracycline 500 mg four times daily for at least 3 weeks or until lesions have completely healed. In cases of tetracycline resistance, effective alternative therapies include streptomycin 1 gram intramuscularly every 12 hours for 10 to 15 days, chloramphenicol (Chloromycetin) 500 mg every 8 hours orally for 2 weeks, or gentamicin (Garamycin) 1 mg per kg intramuscularly twice daily for 14 to 21 days. The combination of trimethoprim 160 mg and sulfamethoxazole 800 mg (Bactrim) twice daily for 10 to 14 days is effective. In pregnant women, erythromycin 500 mg every 6 hours for 14 to 21 days may be effective.

LYMPHOGRANULOMA VENEREUM

method of
THOMAS A. CHAPEL, M.D.
Wayne State University
Detroit, Michigan

and

JOHANNA CHAPEL, M.D.
Oakwood Hospital
Dearborn, Michigan

Lymphogranuloma venereum (LGV) is a systemic sexually transmitted disease caused by serovar L1, L2, or L3 of *Chlamydia trachomatis*. The disease, rare in the United States, is common to areas of Africa, Asia, India, and the Caribbean.

LGV has an incubation period that ranges from days to several weeks. The initial lesion, an evanescent vesicle, papule, or ulcer of the genitalia or perineum, is followed in 2 to 6 weeks by multiocular suppurative regional lymphadenopathy. Acute LGV is usually associated with systemic symptoms such as fever and leukocytosis. Late complications include genital elephantiasis due to lymphatic involvement and strictures and fistulas of the penis, urethra, and rectum.

The diagnosis of LGV is confirmed by either serologic tests or culture. Detection of antibody in serum by fixation titer at a dilution of 1:64 or greater is considered diagnostic. A microimmunofluorescence test with *C. trachomatis* antigens is more sensitive but not yet widely available. This test is considered positive in a titer of 1:512 or greater. Also, isolation of appropriate strains of *Chlamydia* from lymph nodes, rectum, urethra, or cervix is confirmative.

TREATMENT

In general, chlamydial infections should be treated with antibiotics for 2 to 3 weeks or until all signs and symptoms have resolved. Standard regimens include tetracycline hydrochloride 500 mg four times a day for at least 14 days or minocycline (Minocin) or doxycycline (Vibramycin) 100 mg twice a day for 14 days. Sulfisoxazole 1 gram four times a day for 3 weeks is usually effective, and erythromycin base 500 mg four times a day for 14 to 21 days is the therapy of choice for pregnant women.

Buboes requiring surgical treatment should be aspirated rather than excised and drained, to avoid formation of fistulous tracts.

SYPHILIS

method of
STEVEN C. JOHNSON, M.D.
University of Colorado Health Sciences Center
Denver, Colorado

Syphilis is a common systemic disease caused by the spirochete *Treponema pallidum*. It is most often transmitted sexually and is characterized by a wide variety of clinical manifestations that have traditionally been divided into disease stages. The number of cases of primary and secondary syphilis reported to the Centers for Disease Control and Prevention (CDC) has varied from a high of over 50,000 cases in 1990 to approximately 20,000 cases in 1994, the last year for which data are available. Including all stages of syphilis, over 80,000 cases were reported in 1994. In recent years, this illness has been especially common in urban areas associated with intravenous drug use and the commercial sex industry. However, syphilis may be seen in many other patient populations where sexual activity is present. Consequently, the index of suspicion for this illness, with its protean clinical presentations, should remain high.

CLINICAL MANIFESTATIONS

Proper recognition of the various stages of syphilis is important, as treatment recommendations are based on these stages. The term "early syphilis" includes primary, secondary, and early latent syphilis and implies relatively recent acquisition of infection. Primary syphilis is characterized by an indurated skin ulcer (chancre) frequently located on the genitals, although it may occur at other sites. The ulcer is generally nontender and may be associated with regional lymphadenopathy. Occasionally, multiple chancres are seen. Secondary syphilis is an extremely varied illness that is most frequently identified by a generalized skin rash that may include the palms and soles. Other manifestations include fever, mucous patches, condylomata lata, generalized lymphadenopathy, and aseptic meningitis. Many other findings are seen less commonly, including alopecia, anterior uveitis, nephrotic syndrome, arthritis, and hepatitis. Individuals with early latent syphilis have positive serologic tests for syphilis in the absence of any clinically apparent disease, and there is evidence to support acquisition of infection within the last year.

The term "late syphilis" includes late latent syphilis, latent syphilis of unknown duration, and the various forms of tertiary syphilis, including neurosyphilis, cardiovascular syphilis, and gummatous syphilis. Neurosyphilis can be symptomatic or asymptomatic. Symptomatic forms of neurosyphilis include meningitis, meningovascular syphilis, parenchymal brain disease (including general paresis), and spinal cord disease (tabes dorsalis). Cardiovascular syphilis is typically associated with an ascending aortic aneurysm. The other form of tertiary syphilis is rarely seen today but involves granulomatous-like (gummatous) inflammation involving skin, bones, mucous membranes, or potentially any other tissue.

DIAGNOSIS

T. pallidum cannot be cultivated in vitro. Consequently, the diagnosis of syphilis is suggested by epidemiologic clues, clinical symptoms, and physical examination findings and confirmed either by directly visualizing the bacteria with dark-field microscopy or biopsy or by serologic testing for syphilis. Serologic tests for syphilis include nontreponemal tests and treponemal tests. The most common nontreponemal tests are the Venereal Disease Research Laboratory (VDRL) test and the rapid plasma reagin (RPR) test. These tests detect the presence of antibodies directed against a cardiolipin-cholesterol-lecithin antigen and are not specific for syphilis. Both tests are useful screening tests but may be falsely positive in 1 to 2% of individuals. The most common treponemal tests are the fluorescent treponemal antibody absorption (FTA–ABS) test and the microhemagglutination assay for antibody to *T. pallidum* (MHA–TP) test. These tests detect antibodies directed against *T. pallidum* and are useful in confirming a serologic diagnosis of syphilis in individuals with reactive nontreponemal tests.

Primary and secondary syphilis are generally recognized based on symptoms and physical findings. Dark-field microscopy is useful for chancres and moist lesions of secondary syphilis. Skin biopsy with silver staining or immunofluorescent staining may be useful in other skin lesions of secondary syphilis. Serologic tests of syphilis are nearly always positive in these forms of syphilis, with the exception that these tests may be negative very early in the course of primary syphilis. The prozone phenomenon may occasionally produce false-negative nontreponemal tests, most commonly in secondary syphilis.

Latent syphilis implies an absence of symptoms or physical findings in the setting of positive serologic tests for syphilis. If serologic tests for syphilis have been negative within the last 12 months or if the individual has had an illness compatible with primary or secondary syphilis within the last 12 months, early latent syphilis can be diagnosed. Otherwise, the diagnosis of latent syphilis in asymptomatic individuals requires lumbar puncture with cerebrospinal fluid (CSF) examination to exclude asymptomatic neurosyphilis.

The various forms of tertiary syphilis are uncommon but important to recognize, given their associated morbidity and mortality. As mentioned above, cardiovascular syphilis most commonly presents as an ascending aortic aneurysm, with associated aortic insufficiency and positive serologic tests for syphilis. The diagnosis of symptomatic and asymptomatic forms of neurosyphilis depends greatly on lumbar puncture results. CSF examination should include the VDRL test, protein, and cell count. The CSF VDRL is a specific but insensitive test for neurosyphilis. In certain cases of neurosyphilis, nonspecific evidence of inflammation (i.e., elevated CSF protein or white blood cells) is the only finding and must be interpreted with other clinical findings and serologic test results.

The diagnosis of syphilis (except congenital disease) implies sexual activity that may lead to the acquisition of another sexually transmitted disease (STD). Individuals with syphilis should be counseled and tested for HIV infection.

TREATMENT

Early syphilis may resolve without treatment. However, treatment is indicated in all individuals to resolve clinical disease, prevent transmission, and prevent late complications. *T. pallidum* is susceptible to many classes of antibiotics, including penicillins, cephalosporins, macrolides, and tetracyclines. Penicillin is the treatment of choice for all stages of syphilis. Table 1 outlines the latest recommendations for treatment from the 1993 CDC STD treatment guidelines, including treatment of choice and alternative treatments. In the setting of penicillin allergy, alternative therapies such as doxycycline are effective in early syphilis and benign forms of late syphilis. However, penicillin desensitization is recommended in neurosyphilis, congenital syphilis, and syphilis in pregnancy.

SPECIAL CONSIDERATIONS FOR TREATMENT

Syphilis in Pregnancy. Given the risk of congenital syphilis from untreated syphilis, all pregnant women with syphilis should be treated at the time the illness is recognized. Penicillin is the treatment of choice, and the standard regimens for the particular stage of syphilis are used. In the setting of penicillin allergy, the tetracyclines are clearly contraindicated. Most authorities recommend desensitization to penicillin in this setting. Close follow-up of the mother and infant is important.

Congenital Syphilis. With the recent resurgence in syphilis among adults, an increase in congenital syphilis has been an unfortunate consequence. This

TABLE 1. **Recommended Treatment Regimens for Syphilis**

Type of Syphilis	Treatment of Choice	Alternative Treatment*
Primary, secondary, and early latent syphilis	Benzathine penicillin 2.4 million U IM as one dose	Doxycycline 100 mg PO bid for 14 days
Late latent, cardiovascular, or gummatous syphilis†	Benzathine penicillin 2.4 million U IM weekly for 3 doses	Doxycycline 100 mg PO bid for 28 days
Neurosyphilis	Aqueous penicillin G 2–4 million U IV every 4 h for 10–14 days	Procaine penicillin G 2.4 million U IM daily for 10–14 days, plus probenecid 500 mg PO qid for 10–14 days
Syphilis in pregnancy	As listed above for the appropriate stage	Desensitization to penicillin
Congenital syphilis	Aqueous penicillin G 50,000 U/kg IV every 8–12 h for 10–14 days‡	Procaine penicillin G 50,000 U/kg IM daily as a single dose for 10–14 days

*Alternative treatments are often used in patients with penicillin allergy. However, penicillin desensitization is recommended for the treatment of neurosyphilis, congenital syphilis, and all stages of syphilis in pregnancy.

†In most individuals with late syphilis, a cerebrospinal fluid examination is necessary to exclude neurosyphilis (see text).

‡Aqueous penicillin G 50,000 U/kg IV is administered every 12 hours during the first 7 days of life and every 8 hours thereafter. Expert consultation is advised.

Adapted from the 1993 CDC STD treatment guidelines.

form of syphilis presents special diagnostic challenges, and consultation with experts in this area is recommended. Penicillin is the treatment of choice (see Table 1).

Syphilis in HIV Infection. The epidemiology of syphilis and HIV infection overlaps significantly. Over the last 10 years, a series of case reports and case series have raised concerns that individuals with HIV infection may be more likely to fail standard syphilis treatment. Some of these failures have been dramatic, including the rapid development of neurosyphilis, relapses of secondary syphilis, and the development of uncommon complications such as ocular syphilis. For this reason, the proper approach to a co-infected patient is unclear. Although standard regimens appropriate to the stage of syphilis are currently recommended in the CDC treatment guide-lines, many experts favor more aggressive therapy such as that used for neurosyphilis. Regardless of the treatment used, close follow-up with serial serologic testing to assess the clinical and serologic response to therapy is strongly recommended.

Lumbar Puncture in an Asymptomatic Patient with Serologic Evidence of Syphilis. An asymptomatic patient with positive nontreponemal and treponemal tests for syphilis is a common clinical problem. As mentioned above, patients with a documented negative test within the last 12 months or with an illness compatible with primary or secondary syphilis within the last 12 months can be treated as having early latent syphilis, as outlined in Table 1. All other patients have a finite risk of having asymptomatic neurosyphilis. Standard treatment with benzathine penicillin may not be adequate for individuals with asymptomatic neurosyphilis. The risks and benefits of performing a lumbar puncture should be discussed with the patient in this setting. Individual physicians and patients may be willing to accept the small risk of undertreating asymptomatic neurosyphilis in selected situations. The CDC guidelines identify circumstances in which a lumbar puncture is likely to be of higher yield and should always be performed: documented treatment failure, a serum VDRL or RPR greater than or equal to 1:32, individuals with HIV infection, individuals with unexplained neurologic or ophthalmic signs or symptoms, or individuals in whom a nonpenicillin treatment regimen is planned.

ASSESSING THE RESPONSE TO TREATMENT

In all treated patients, follow-up to document clinical and serologic resolution of infection is important. The nontreponemal tests (RPR, VDRL) should be titered and should fall with treatment. In most individuals with early syphilis, titers fall to low levels or negativity with time (typically 1 year for primary syphilis, 2 years for secondary and early latent syphilis). A rise in titer or a failure to fall suggests primary treatment failure or reinfection. The serologic response to therapy is less predictable in later forms of syphilis. However, most treated individuals exhibit a gradual fall in titer over time before reaching a "serofast" state (usually 1:8 or less). Individuals with neurosyphilis should have a subsequent CSF examination in 6 months to monitor the response to therapy.

Diseases of Allergy

ANAPHYLAXIS AND SERUM SICKNESS

method of
STEPHEN L. WINBERY, Ph.D., M.D.
University of Tennessee Medical Group
Memphis, Tennessee

and

PHILIP L. LIEBERMAN, M.D.
University of Tennessee
Cordova, Tennessee

ANAPHYLAXIS

Anaphylaxis is a systemic, allergic reaction. In the strictest sense, anaphylaxis refers to an antigen-stimulated, IgE-mediated degranulation of mast cells and/or basophils. Degranulation of these cells releases a host of inflammatory mediators and chemotactic cytokines. An anaphylactoid reaction is a clinically similar syndrome in which release of inflammatory mediators is independent of IgE. Inflammatory mediators exert effects on smooth muscle and vasculature, resulting in increased capillary permeability, vasodilatation, and bronchoconstriction.

Incidence

The incidence of anaphylaxis is increasing in the general population, perhaps because of increased environmental and medical exposure to drugs, latex, food additives, and other biologic agents. The exact incidence is unknown and is probably under-reported. On average, anaphylactic reactions occur once for every 2000 to 3000 hospitalized patients and with 1 of 100 doses of penicillin and 8 of 1000 Hymenoptera stings. There are about 500 deaths due to anaphylaxis in the United States each year. Of concern in the medical arena is the increasing incidence of latex hypersensitivity among health care workers and patients with chronic illnesses, most likely a result of increased exposure to latex-containing products. Also, elevated serum levels of the inflammatory mediator, histamine, have been shown to be associated with many perioperative medications, plasma expanders, and some procedures such as cardiac bypass and dialysis.

Pathophysiology

Classic anaphylaxis involves a complex formed between a foreign antigen and IgE antibody. The antigen cross-links IgE receptors on the surface of mast cells and basophils, causing a calcium-dependent degranulation and release of preformed mediators as well as active synthesis of other mediators. These events require prior exposure to the antigen, but clinically, many anaphylactic reactions occur without history of prior exposure.

Many drugs and hyperosmolar solutions can cause release of mast cell contents independent of IgE. Other biologically active substances can activate complement and indirectly stimulate mast cells and basophils. These reactions appear clinically identical to anaphylaxis because the same mediators of inflammation are involved. Common causes of anaphylaxis and anaphylactoid reactions are listed in Table 1.

Mediators of Anaphylaxis

Many of the symptoms of anaphylaxis can be mimicked by histamine infusion in both experimental animals and humans. However, anaphylaxis is quite complex. The host of mediators that are directly released or indirectly generated includes heparin, prostaglandins, leukotrienes, platelet-activating factor, interleukins, tumor necrosis factor, other lymphokines, neuropeptides, and even nitric oxide. Chemotactic factors (mainly the leukotrienes) can cause migration of cells into areas of inflammation, releasing even more mediators. Mast cell and basophil contents are capable of activating a number of inflammatory pathways, including the complement system, the kinin system, the clotting system, and the clot lysis system. The clinical implication of all these substances is that the anaphylactic reaction can perpetuate itself. Therapeutically, it is important to plan for the biphasic nature of anaphylactic reactions. In the late phase, there is a recurrence of symptoms 3 to 12 hours after the initial symptom complex, often after initial improvement or apparent resolution. The transition between early and late phase may be less dramatic, so that the late phase appears as a prolongation of symptoms rather than a recurrence after improvement.

Anesthesia-Related Release of Histamine

Histamine can be released from mast cells perioperatively. The clinical signs of histamine release may be different from the classic reaction because of the effects of anesthesia and other drugs. For instance, urticaria and angioedema may not be present, and

TABLE 1. **Pathophysiologic Classification of Anaphylaxis and Anaphylactoid Reactions**

Anaphylaxis (IgE-Mediated Reaction)
A. Food
  1. Peanuts
  2. Seafood (shellfish)
  3. Eggs
  4. Milk
  5. Grains
B. Drugs
  1. Penicillins
  2. Cephalosporins
  3. Sulfonamides
C. Venoms
  1. Hymenoptera
  2. Fire ants
  3. Snakes
D. Human proteins
  1. Insulin
  2. Corticotropin
  3. Vasopressin
  4. Serum and seminal proteins
E. Exercise anaphylaxis (food-allergen dependent)

Anaphylactoid (Non–IgE-Mediated Reaction)
A. Direct release of mediators from mast cells or basophils
  1. Drugs
    a. Opiates
    b. Paralytic agents
    c. Vancomycin
    d. Fluorescein
    e. Dextran
  2. Hyperosmolar solutions
  3. Idiopathic
  4. Exercise
  5. Physical factors such as cold and sunlight
B. Disturbances in arachidonic acid metabolism
  1. Aspirin
  2. Other nonsteroidal anti-inflammatory drugs
C. Immune aggregates
  1. Gamma globulin
  2. IgG-anti-IgA
D. Cytotoxic: transfusion reactions to cellular elements
E. Miscellaneous and multimediator activity
  1. Nonantigen-antibody-mediated complement activation
    a. Radiocontrast material
    b. Some protamine reactions
    c. Dialysis membranes
  2. Activation of contact (kinin) system
    a. Dialysis membranes
    b. Radiocontrast material

From Winbery S, Lieberman P: Anaphylaxis. Immunol Allergy Clin North Am 15:447–475, 1995.

hypotension, bronchospasm, or cardiac arrhythmias may appear as isolated manifestations. Elevated plasma histamine concentrations are associated with arrhythmias, increased thrombosis, stress ulceration, increased intrapulmonary shunt, hypotension, bronchospasm, and even adult respiratory distress syndrome. Plasma histamine concentrations from 0.2 to 1.0 ng per mL must be considered elevated, and their significance cannot be dismissed because of the absence of cutaneous or classic signs. Perioperative prophylaxis with H_1- and H_2-receptor antagonist has been proposed and used for patients with previous perioperative anaphylactoid reactions and atopic individuals undergoing anesthesia. The doses are similar to those for radiocontrast media (RCM) reaction prophylaxis.

Route of Administration

Anaphylaxis is possible with all routes of administration. General reactions following parenteral administration are more frequent, more rapid, and more severe than those following oral administration. The most severe reactions generally follow intravenous administration of the causative agent. To minimize the severity of anaphylatic reactions, drugs should be administered orally whenever feasible.

Atopy and Anaphylaxis

Atopic patients appear to be predisposed to anaphylaxis in general, although the relative risk varies with the antigen. Atopic individuals do not seem to be at increased risk for reactions to Hymenoptera stings, insulin, and penicillin. They do have an increased risk of idiopathic reactions and reactions to latex, RCM, and food, however. Predisposition to anaphylactic reaction in atopy may be due to a state of hyper-releasability of mast cells and basophils in the atopic individual.

Symptoms of Anaphylaxis

Signs and symptoms of anaphylaxis range from mild urticaria to fatal cardiac collapse. The onset of symptoms is usually within 5 to 30 minutes after exposure but can be hours later, especially after antigen ingestion. Generally, the likelihood and severity of an anaphylactic response decrease with increasing time between the exposure and the start of the reaction. The severity of an individual's response is dependent on rate, amount, and site of mediator release, as well as individual risk factors such as underlying cardiac disease, atopy, asthma, or therapy with angiotensin-converting enzyme (ACE) inhibitors or beta blockers. Initial signs and symptoms may include a feeling of warmth, itching with or without rash, erythematous rashes, lightheadedness or weakness, shortness of breath, upper airway congestion or swelling sensation in the throat, and palpitations. Anaphylaxis most commonly affects the skin, the respiratory system, the gastrointestinal system, and the heart (see Table 2). Urticaria and angioedema are by far the most frequent manifestations of anaphylaxis and anaphylactoid reactions. The other common signs include orthostatic changes with or without hypotension, gastrointestinal symptoms, and lower respiratory tract symptoms. The most dramatic and severe symptom of an anaphylactic reaction is shock due to rapid loss of intravascular volume. Up to 50% of intravascular volume can shift to extravascular spaces during the first few minutes of anaphylaxis. The frequencies of symptoms of anaphylaxis are listed in Table 3.

TABLE 2. **Organ System–Related Symptoms of Anaphylaxis**

Organ System	Symptoms
Skin	Urticaria, angioedema, pruritus, erythema, increased warmth
Eye	Pruritus, conjunctival injection, lacrimation
Nose	Pruritus, rhinorrhea, congestion
Respiratory	Upper airway congestion and swelling, lower tract bronchospasm (wheezing)
Cardiac	Palpitations, arrhythmias, hypotension, cardiac ischemia
Gastrointestinal	Cramping, nausea, vomiting, diarrhea
Central nervous	Confusion, dizziness, lethargy, seizures (rarely)

Death from Anaphylaxis

Death from anaphylaxis is usually due to cardiovascular collapse or respiratory obstruction leading to respiratory failure. Autopsy may reveal no characteristic findings of death due to anaphylaxis, but in the majority of cases, myocardial damage and dilatation of the right ventricle can be detected. In 50% of anaphylactic deaths, upper airway edema, bronchial obstruction, and hyperinflation of the lungs can be found. Determination of specific IgE (radioallergosorbent test [RAST]) for suspected antigens and/or high levels of serum tryptase may aid in postmortem diagnosis of anaphylaxis. The mast cell tryptase level peaks 60 to 90 minutes after the onset of anaphylaxis and has about a 3-hour half-life.

Differential Diagnosis

The differential diagnosis of anaphylaxis includes flush syndromes, restaurant syndromes, types of acute shock, panic attacks, and syndromes in which excess endogenous histamine is produced (see Table 4). Once the diagnosis of anaphylaxis has been made, a specific agent may not be identifiable in many cases. The search should begin with a detailed, temporal-oriented history and include foods, environ-

TABLE 3. **Frequency of Symptoms in Anaphylaxis**

Symptoms	Frequency Out of 100%
Urticaria and/or angioedema	88
Upper airway edema	56
Dyspnea or wheeze	47
Flush	46
Dizziness, hypotension, orthostasis, or syncope	33
Gastrointestinal symptoms (nausea, vomiting, diarrhea, abdominal pain or cramping)	30
Rhinitis	16
Headache	15
Itch without rash	4.5
Seizure	1.5

From Winbery S, Lieberman P: Anaphylaxis. Immunol Allergy Clin North Am 15:447–475, 1995.

TABLE 4. **Differential Diagnosis of Anaphylaxis**

   I. Anaphylaxis and anaphylactoid reactions
     A. Exogenous agents—foods, drugs, stings, biologicals
     B. Physical factors—exercise, cold, heat, sunlight
     C. Idiopathic
  II. Vasodepressor reactions
 III. Flush syndromes
     A. Carcinoid
     B. Oral hypoglycemic agents with alcohol
     C. Postmenopausal symptoms
     D. Medullary carcinoma of the thyroid
     E. Autonomic epilepsy
  IV. "Restaurant syndromes"
     A. Sulfites
     B. Monosodium glutamate (MSG)
     C. Scombroidosis
   V. Other types of shock
     A. Hemorrhagic
     B. Cardiogenic
     C. Endotoxin
  VI. Excess endogenous production of histamine
     A. Systemic mastocytosis
     B. Urticaria pigmentosa
     C. Basophilic leukemia
     D. Acute promyelocytic leukemia (tretinoin treatment)
 VII. Nonorganic disease
     A. Panic attacks
     B. Münchausen's stridor
     C. Vocal cord dysfunction syndrome
     D. Globus hysterica
VIII. Miscellaneous
     A. Hereditary angioedema
     B. "Progesterone" anaphylaxis
     C. Pheochromocytoma
     D. Pseudoanaphylaxis
     E. Urticarial vasculitis
     F. Hyperimmune globulin E, urticaria syndrome
     G. "Red man syndrome" (vancomycin)

From Winbery S, Lieberman P: Anaphylaxis. Immunol Allergy Clin North Am 15:447–475, 1995.

mental exposure, preservatives, dyes, vegetable gum products, and drugs, where appropriate.

Treatment of Anaphylaxis

Anaphylaxis is a potentially fatal but treatable event. Rapid diagnosis or at least suspicion leading to prompt treatment is essential. Treatment of the acute event begins with rapid assessment of airway, breathing, and circulation. Oxygen may help prevent cardiac ischemia secondary to hypoperfusion, bronchospasm, cardiac arrhythmias, or coronary vasospasm.

Epinephrine is the drug of choice for the acute anaphylactic event. It should be administered coincidental with the initial assessment as soon as anaphylaxis is suspected. With the availability of prescription self-injection devices, patients at risk can initiate their own treatment. The dose of epinephrine (1:1000) is 0.3 to 0.5 mL (0.3 to 0.5 mg) in adults and 0.01 mg per kg for children. Epinephrine can be administered subcutaneously or intramuscularly. If the antigen responsible for anaphylaxis was injected, the injection of epinephrine into the site may slow absorption of the antigen. For severe hypotension, epinephrine can be administered intravenously. The intravenous dose of epinephrine should start at 100 μg, and the patient should be monitored for cardiac arrhythmias. In the most severe cases, intravenous constant infusion of epinephrine may be used to counteract hypotension.

Hypotension is the most threatening manifestation of anaphylaxis and can be protracted and resistant to therapy. The mainstay of acute treatment is rapid administration of large volumes of intravenous fluids. Initial infusion rates may necessarily be as high as 5 to 10 mL per kg in the first 10 minutes of therapy.

Vasopressors are indicated for refractory hypotension and shock. Their effectiveness may be diminished because hypotension frequently occurs in patients who also have increased peripheral resistance from compensatory mechanisms. For hypotension, dopamine is the vasopressor of choice, administered at a rate of 2 to 20 μg per kg per minute. This rate is titrated against blood pressure.

If the offending antigen was injected at a distal site, a tourniquet proximal to the portal of entry may slow the systemic propagation of anaphylaxis. Caution should be taken not to produce cyanosis and hypoperfusion distal to the tourniquet.

Not uncommonly, bronchospasm can be part of an anaphylactic reaction, especially in asthmatic patients. If bronchospasm is present, aerosolized beta-adrenergic agonists may be a useful adjunct. The doses are the same as those used to treat acute bronchospasm in asthmatic patients.

A patient experiencing anaphylaxis after administration of a beta-adrenergic antagonist presents a special therapeutic challenge, because symptoms are often resistant to epinephrine. Atropine is useful for bradycardia and bronchospasm but often does not reverse hypotension. The catabolic hormone glucagon is the drug of choice for hypotension in these situations. The dose of glucagon is 1 to 5 mg by intravenous bolus, followed by an intravenous infusion of 5 to 15 μg per minute titrated to blood pressure. Nausea and vomiting may limit glucagon therapy.

Antihistamines (H_1-receptor antagonists) should be administered early and repeated every 4 to 6 hours as dictated by the clinical course. Diphenhydramine (Benadryl) 25 to 75 mg intramuscularly or intravenously is an example of appropriate H_1 antagonist therapy. H_2 antagonists may have added benefit in the treatment of anaphylaxis. Cimetidine (Tagamet)* (200 to 300 mg or ranitidine (Zantac)* 50 mg can be given intramuscularly or intravenously.

The action of glucocorticoids may be delayed for several hours. However, the anti-inflammatory steroids may lessen or even abort the late phase of anaphylaxis. In severe reactions, corticosteroids, such as hydrocortisone 5 to 10 mg per kg intravenously up to 500 mg every 4 to 6 hours, may prevent a protracted course of anaphylaxis and decrease sequelae. Other glucocorticoids include methylprednis-

---

*Not FDA approved for this indication.

TABLE 5. Acute Treatment of Anaphylaxis

Remove offending agent if present
Activate emergency medical service or transport system if in the field
Rapid assessment
  Secure airway and breathing (oxygen)
  Assess level of consciousness
  Monitor cardiac function
  Monitor vital signs and blood pressure
  Assess perfusion and cutaneous signs
Treatment
  Epinephrine (SC, IM, IV, endotracheal)
  Rapid volume resuscitation for hypotension
  If the antigen was injected, place a proximal tourniquet
  Positioning (supine, Trendelenburg)
  H_1 and/or H_2 antagonists
Conditional actions
  Vasopressors for hypotension (dopamine)
  Glucagon and/or atropine (patient on beta antagonists)
  Corticosteroids (prevent late response)
  Aerosolized beta agonists for bronchospasm

From Winbery S, Lieberman P: Anaphylaxis. Immunol Allergy Clin North Am 15:447–475, 1995.

olone 60 to 125 mg intramuscularly or intravenously every 4 to 6 hours and prednisone 40 to 60 mg orally every 12 to 24 hours. A patient with significant symptoms should be observed in the emergency room or in the hospital for 4 to 8 hours, since the secondary phase of the allergic response can mimic the original symptoms. Treatment of anaphylaxis is summarized in Table 5. A consensus list of equipment and drugs for office management of anaphylaxis is presented in Table 6.

Treatment of Mild to Moderate Reactions

It is common for an anaphylactic or anaphylactoid reaction to include mild urticaria and/or angioedema without hypotension, upper airway compromise, or bronchospasm. These patients require observation until the symptoms are no longer progressing. Many of these reactions can be self-limited. However, most symptoms respond to epinephrine plus parenteral or oral H_1 antagonists with or without glucocorticoids and H_2-receptor antagonists.

Addition of H_2-Receptor Antagonists

Experimentally, the combination of an H_1 and H_2 antagonist is needed to maximally reduce histamine-induced peripheral vasodilatation, hypotension, and mucous secretion. Combinations of antagonist are more effective in preventing the decrease in diastolic blood pressure and the widening pulse pressure caused by histamine. In several instances, the addition of an H_2 antagonist reversed anaphylactoid symptoms that did not respond to an H_1 antagonist alone. Combination antagonist therapy is more effective than either antagonist alone for the prevention of reactions to chymopapain, perioperative agents, morphine, and plasma expanders. H_2 antagonists should be added to the acute therapy of anaphylaxis,

TABLE 6. **Recommended Drugs and Equipment for the Management of Anaphylaxis in an Office Setting**

Drugs

Epinephrine solution (aqueous) 1:1000
Diphenhydramine (injectable)
Cimetidine (Tagamet)* or ranitidine (Zantac)* (injectable)
Corticosteroids (hydrocortisone or methylprednisolone, injectable)
Beta$_2$-adrenergic bronchodilator and compressor nebulizer
 (albuterol [Proventil, Ventolin] or terbutaline [Brethine])
Glucagon (injectable)
Dopamine for intravenous infusion
Sodium bicarbonate (injectable)
Atropine (injectable)
Calcium gluconate (injectable)
Lidocaine for intravenous infusion
Sedative hypnotics (lorazepam [Ativan] or diazepam [Valium] for
 seizure)

Intravenous Fluids and Equipment

Crystalloid (normal saline)
Hydroxyethyl starch
Intravenous set-up with large-bore (18-gauge) catheters

Other Equipment

Oxygen delivery apparatus and masks/nasal prongs
Tourniquet
Syringes
Bag mask apparatus
Laryngoscope and endotracheal tubes
Electrocardiogram with or without defibrillator
Suction apparatus

especially when the patient is hypotensive, and H$_2$ antagonists probably add to the therapeutic efficacy of most prophylactic regimens.

Prevention of Anaphylaxis with Antihistamines

In experimental models, pretreatment with antihistamines can prevent or attenuate anaphylactic symptoms and prevent anaphylactic death. In patients, pretreatment with H$_1$ antagonists prevents bronchoconstriction due to histamine challenge, nonisotonic aerosols, exercise, and microvascular leak in the skin wheal response to histamine and allergen provocation tests. Theoretically, H$_2$ antagonists alone may be deleterious in the event of histamine release, because of increased and unopposed H$_1$ receptor stimulation. The regimen listed in Table 7 has been successfully applied to prevent anaphylaxis in patients with previous reaction to RCM who must be

TABLE 7. **Prophylactic Regimen for Patients with History of Reaction to Radiocontrast Media (RCM)**

Prednisone 50 mg PO 13, 7, and 1 h before
Diphenhydramine 50 mg IM 1 h before
Ephedrine 25 mg PO 1 h before*
Ranitidine† 150 mg or cimetidine† 300 mg PO 3 h before‡
Use low-osmolar RCM agents

*Omit if patient has contraindication to sympathomimetics.
†Not FDA-approved for this indication.
‡Optional.

given RCM again. Although not as well studied, antihistamine therapy with or without glucocorticoids has been successfully applied to prevent anaphylaxis associated with volume expanders, plasma exchange, fluorescein, latex, exercise, anesthesia, perioperative medications, and chymopapain.

Preventing and Minimizing Anaphylactic Events

Every patient should have a complete history of allergic-type reactions to drugs, chemicals, latex, food, creams, ointments, drops, and so forth. Any positive information should be displayed prominently in the patient's records. This information should be updated frequently.

Anaphylactic reactions to parenterally administered antigens are more severe and rapid than reactions to orally administered agents. The clinician should consider oral rather than parenteral route of administration whenever possible. A patient should wait in the office at least 20 to 30 minutes after parenteral administration of a drug. Once a medication or other substance is suspected as the cause of anaphylaxis, the patient should discard the potentially harmful substance.

One should also know about cross-reactions. For example, there is a 7 to 15% incidence of reaction to cephalosporins in penicillin-allergic individuals. There are also cross-reactions among other drug classes, such as the nonsteroidal anti-inflammatory agents and sulfa-containing agents.

Once the causative agent is identified, the primary method of prophylaxis is to avoid exposure, especially in food, drug, and latex allergies. Any patient with a history of systemic anaphylaxis should receive and be trained in the use of an epinephrine autoinjection system (EpiPen, Ana-Kit, Ana-Guard) and provided with a Medic Alert bracelet or tag. Patients with systemic reactions to Hymenoptera should be referred to an allergist for possible desensitization.

Patients at risk who must undergo procedures should receive pretreatment with antihistamines and steroids. Low-osmolar RCM should be used for patients with a history of reaction to RCM.

Several drugs should be avoided in patients at risk for anaphylactic reactions. Beta-adrenergic antagonists blunt the effect of epinephrine on the heart and vasculature and may induce bronchospasm, even when given as ocular medications. Angiotensin is counter-regulatory to shock. ACE inhibitors prevent the mobilization of angiotensin II, which is an endogenous compensatory mechanism to counteract hypotension. Monoamine oxidase inhibitors and certain tricyclic antidepressants (such as amitriptyline) make the use of epinephrine hazardous because they interfere with its degradation.

Desensitization can be undertaken for appropriate antigens when there is proven benefit and administration cannot be avoided.

TABLE 8. **Some Causes of Serum Sickness**

Antibiotics
  Penicillins
  Cephalosporins
  Sulfonamides
  Metronidazole
Antihypertensives
  Thiazide diuretics
  Propranolol
Nonsteroidal anti-inflammatory drugs
  Naproxen
  Phenylbutazone
Other
  Phenytoin (other hydantoins)
  Blood products
  Heterologous serum

SERUM SICKNESS

The name "serum sickness" was derived from the observation that a large percentage of patients receiving heterologous serum developed the syndrome. Today, however, the majority of serum sickness is due to medications (see Table 8). Serum sickness is very different from anaphylaxis. It is a form of immune complex disease in which soluble, circulating antibody-antigen complexes activate complement and subsequently release inflammatory mediators. Antigen binds with circulating IgG and IgM. The soluble immune complexes can migrate into vasculature walls, where they can fix and activate complement. Inflammatory cells are called into the site by chemotactic autocoids, causing inflammation, tissue damage, and vasculitis. The characteristic symptoms include fever, rash, lymphadenopathy, hepatosplenomegaly, arthralgias, arthritis, and myalgias. Cutaneous eruptions, including urticaria, maculopapular and purpuric lesions, and erythema multiforme, occur in 90% of patients with serum sickness. A band or erythema at the palmar and plantar junctions on the hands and feet has been described with serum sickness. Other symptoms are listed in Table 9. Rarely, glomerulonephritis, mononeuritis multiplex, or Guillain-Barré syndrome may occur with serum sickness.

Diagnosis and Treatment of Serum Sickness

The diagnosis of serum sickness is largely based on history and clinical presentation. There are no

TABLE 9. **Symptoms of Serum Sickness**

Symptom	Frequency (%)
Fever	100
Erythematous rash	90
Arthralgia	75
Myalgia	50
Arthritis	25
Lymphadenopathy	20
Glomerulonephritis	<1
Guillain-Barré syndrome	<1
Mononeuritis multiplex	<1

TABLE 10. **Laboratory Changes with Serum Sickness**

Complete blood count
  Peripheral eosinophilia
  Peripheral leukocytosis
  Peripheral leukopenia
  Elevated sedimentation rate (mild to moderate)
Urinalysis
  Proteinuria
  Hematuria
Complement
  Decreased CH_{50}
  Decreased C3
  Decreased C4

specific laboratory tests to confirm the diagnosis of serum sickness. Nonspecific laboratory abnormalities are listed in Table 10. Symptoms occur in 1 to 2 weeks after exposure to the offending agent and may occur within 24 hours with re-exposure.

The syndrome is usually a self-limited illness and subsides in 1 to 3 weeks. If the patient is still receiving potential offending agents, they should be stopped immediately. Treatment is largely directed toward symptomatic relief. Antihistamines (diphenhydramine or hydroxyzine [Atarax]) are given for pruritus and hives. Nonsteroidal anti-inflammatory agents (naproxen, ibuprofen, aspirin) are given for fever and pain. If symptoms persist, glucocorticoids may provide additional relief. Prednisone can be given orally starting at 1 to 2 mg per kg per day (maximum dose, 60 mg) and tapering over 5 to 10 days.

ASTHMA IN ADOLESCENTS AND ADULTS

method of
D. W. COCKCROFT, M.D.
Royal University Hospital
Saskatoon, Saskatchewan, Canada

Asthma is a common disease affecting 5 to 10% of the population. It may be defined as a syndrome characterized by symptoms, variable airflow obstruction, airway hyper-responsiveness, and airway inflammation, particularly with eosinophils, metachromatic cells, and lymphocytes. Current views in the pathogenesis of asthma regard airway inflammation as the primary event and airway hyper-responsiveness and variable airflow obstruction as secondary and symptomatic events. Consequently, therapy in asthma at all ages and in all situations (ambulatory, emergency, and so forth) is directed toward both prevention and treatment of the airway inflammation. Patient education and environmental control are probably more important in the long-term management of asthma than is the use of pharmacologic agents.

PATIENT EDUCATION

Patient education is crucial to establishing control of asthma. Patients initially must understand the nature of the disease. Concepts such as airway inflammation and bronchoconstriction should be taught to them. They, like we, must recognize the importance of airway inflammation in the pathogenesis of asthma. The nature of the medications is also important. Asthmatics must understand that some medications such as bronchodilators are *symptom relievers* and should be used only as needed, whereas other medications (inhaled corticosteroids, nedocromil, cromolyn) are anti-inflammatory *preventers* and should be used regularly or, in the case of cromolyn or nedocromil, as needed *before* certain exposures.

The goals of treatment must be understood by both patient and physician. If not, it is unlikely that the goals will be achieved. For the vast majority of patients, the goals of therapy should be nil to minimal symptoms, nil to minimal use of *reliever* medications, normalization of lifestyle (except those exposures contraindicated by environmental control, as noted later), and normalization of expiratory flow rates.

Recognizing exacerbations is critical to the prevention of morbidity (hospitalizations, emergency visits, time lost from work and school, and even death) in asthma. Asthma generally exacerbates gradually over a period of days. The most important causes of gradual asthma exacerbations are inflammatory and include exposure to allergens or low-molecular-weight chemical sensitizers, viral or *Mycoplasma* respiratory tract infection, and tapering (either by design or by noncompliance) of anti-inflammatory therapies. Asthmatics can be taught to recognize exacerbations early chiefly by recognizing that they are no longer meeting the goals of treatment outlined above. Symptoms, inhaled beta$_2$ agonist requirements, and, where relevant, self-measured peak expiratory flow (PEF) rates can all be used to identify an exacerbation early.

Self-treatment of exacerbations is the corollary of early recognition. Asthmatics should have the knowledge and the wherewithal to treat exacerbations on their own. This is done by adding or stepping up anti-inflammatory medications. For treatment of exacerbations, this usually involves corticosteroids in adults. Inhaled corticosteroids can be added or increased by a factor of two to four (doubled or quadrupled) very early in the course of an exacerbation. In this setting, we occasionally allow an inhaled beta$_2$ agonist to be used prior to an inhaled corticosteroid, but only for a few days. Otherwise, we no longer recommend this practice routinely. More severe exacerbations, or those not responding within a few days to inhaled corticosteroids, can be treated by self-administration of ingested prednisone 25 to 60 mg per day until symptoms have *completely* resolved to baseline, followed by rapid tapering or, in fact, abrupt discontinuation.

The action plan is recognized as a useful tool. Action plans may be written or verbal and contain recommendations for what steps to take based on the occurrence and frequency of symptoms, beta$_2$ agonist requirements, and PEF measurements. The actions, which must be individualized, could include the addition or increase in inhaled corticosteroids, recommendations regarding the timing and dose of ingested corticosteroids, and recommendations on when to go to the nearest emergency room.

PEF rate measurements can be a useful educational tool, allowing asthmatics to correlate symptoms with the degree of airflow obstruction. A small number of asthmatics, generally those with chronic and suboptimally controlled disease, may fail to perceive airflow obstruction and thus superficially appear to develop sudden but otherwise unexplained exacerbations. These patients may benefit from home-measured PEF as a guide to therapy. Since failure to perceive airflow obstruction is usually an acquired adaptation to the chronic obstruction, once the asthma is controlled, the ability to perceive lesser degrees of airflow obstruction frequently returns.

ENVIRONMENTAL CONTROL

Environmental control is also important to the control of asthma. Stimuli involved in the pathogenesis of asthma and its symptoms can be divided into *inducers* and *triggers*. Inducers are those stimuli that cause airway inflammation and thereby cause or heighten airway hyper-responsiveness. Examples of inflammatory inducers include allergens, low-molecular-weight chemical sensitizers, and viral or *Mycoplasma* respiratory tract infections. Triggers are those stimuli that cause bronchoconstriction in asthmatics without truly worsening the condition. In this regard, the response to triggers is symptomatic of the underlying asthma severity. Examples of common triggers include exercise, cold air, hyperventilation, laughter, inhaled irritants, and anxiety.

Clearly, the inflammatory inducers are much more important than the bronchospastic triggers in the pathogenesis of asthma. However, paradoxically, the relationship between triggers and symptoms is frequently much more obvious to the patient and the physician. The relationship between inducers (for example, allergens) and symptoms may be much more subtle. Although allergens may cause acute bronchoconstriction, it is more common, especially with chronic low-grade exposure, that they cause airway inflammation and gradual worsening of asthma. It is probably fairly common for exercise-induced bronchoconstriction during sports events to actually be caused by airway inflammation, which is caused by exposure to an allergen in the home. This requires a great deal of understanding by both the physician and the patient in order to put forth a convincing argument.

Physicians must be concerned with not only the home but also the workplace, school, and recreational activities with regard to identifying inhaled allergens and other sensitizers. Allergy prick skin testing can be a useful adjunct to the history to clarify the possible role of allergens to which patients are exposed. Relevant animals should be removed from the home. If subjects are proved to have sensitization to an allergen or a chemical at work, a job change is in order, and worker's compensation should look after the financial burden. In subjects allergic to house dust mites, there are many measures that have been shown to reduce house dust mite exposure. Review of environmental control and reassessment for possible new exposures should be a regular part of follow-up. This is particularly important for subjects whose asthma has worsened.

PHARMACOTHERAPY

The approach to drug treatment in asthma has been outlined in numerous consensus guidelines, generally in a *stepwise* approach. It now appears that this well-intentioned stepwise design is too restrictive, in that it tends to peg individuals at a given treatment level. Asthma is inherently variable, and there is a continuum of severity. Therefore, our current approach to asthma treatment is to regard the treatment program as a *continuum* rather than a number of *steps* or *levels*.

Ambulatory asthma therapy is started with the symptomatic use of inhaled beta$_2$ agonists in the lowest dose possible. These drugs are referred to as symptom relievers and are prescribed exclusively as needed, not as regularly scheduled doses. The beta$_2$ agonist requirement is one of the keys to determining control, identifying exacerbations, and determining the need for additional treatment. As soon as the beta$_2$ agonist is required in excess of twice a week, inhaled anti-inflammatory agents are added for regular use. Inhaled corticosteroids are most often used in adults and adolescents. The two preparations with the best benefit–systemic effect ratio appear to be fluticasone (Flovent)* and budesonide (Pulmicort),* followed closely by beclomethasone dipropionate (BDP; Beclovent, Vanceril). Flunisolide (AeroBid) and triamcinolone (Azmacort) are infrequently used outside of the United States. The high-dose preparations include BDP 250* μg per puff, fluticasone* 125 and 250 μg per puff, and budesonide* 200 and 400 μg per puff. Unfortunately, fluticasone, budesonide, and high-dose BDP are not yet available in the United States. High-dose inhaled corticosteroid preparations are used to administer *low doses* by administering 1 or 2 puffs per day. Approximate equivalence in efficacy is seen for fluticasone* at 125 μg per puff, budesonide* at 200 μg per puff, and BDP at 250 μg per puff.* These drugs are frequently added in medium to high doses and tapered to find the lowest dose that will maintain control. Exacerbations can be treated by increasing the inhaled corticosteroid by a factor of two to four (doubling to quadrupling). Treating exacerbations with the same medication that is used for chronic control is an easily

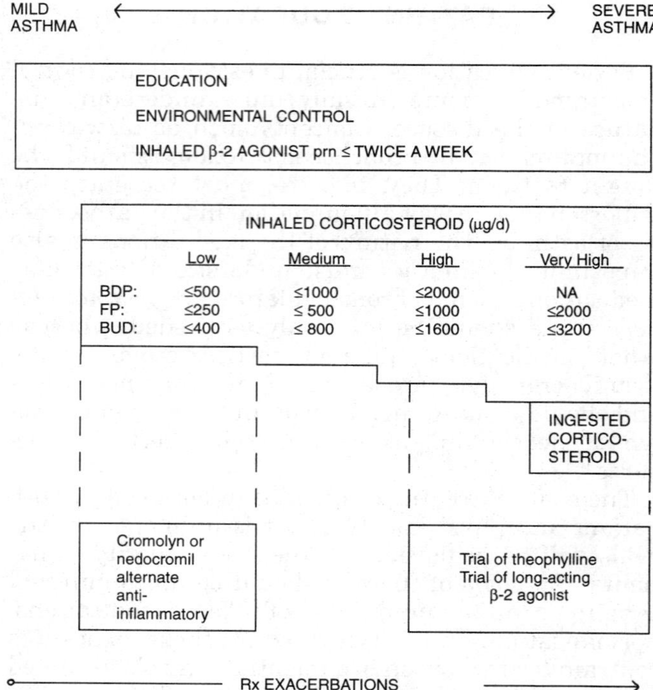

Figure 1. Chronic asthma therapy: a continuum. Abbreviations: BDP = beclomethasone dipropionate (Beclovent, Vanceril); FP = fluticasone (Flovent); BUD = budesonide (Pulmicort). (FP and BUD are not available in the United States.)

understandable approach to asthma management for the layperson. The fact that patients do not have to speak to a physician or add another inhaler or a pill improves compliance.

The continuum of asthma treatment by this approach (Figure 1) has mild to moderate asthmatics receiving low-dose inhaled corticosteroids (<2 puffs per day—e.g., fluticasone* ≤250 μg per day, budesonide* ≤400 μg per day, BDP ≤500 μg per day) to very high-dose inhaled corticosteroids (fluticasone* 2000 μg per day, budesonide* 3200 μg per day).

For subjects at the milder end of the continuum, cromolyn or nedocromil may be substituted as the anti-inflammatory agent. At this level, inhaled corticosteroids are virtually free of systemic side effects, but a number of physicians still prefer to try these other agents first. This is particularly relevant for younger patients. Cromolyn (Intal) is more effective as an anti-inflammatory in young, allergic asthmatics than it is in nonallergic asthmatics. Nedocromil (Tilade) may have a somewhat broader spectrum. These agents are also useful as prophylaxis against exercise- or cold air–induced bronchoconstriction when used immediately prior to exposure. Addition of either of these agents prior to a known allergen exposure (and regularly, as long as exposure continues) can also prevent allergen-induced bronchoconstriction and allergen-induced inflammation.

---

*Not available in the United States.

TABLE 1. Causes of Poor Asthma Control and Poor Response to Asthma Treatment

Beta agonist overuse
Untreated sinus disease
Untreated gastroesophageal reflux
Psychogenic issues, including paradoxical vocal cord dysfunction

In subjects at the more severe end of the spectrum, additional therapy is sometimes required. Before embarking upon any other therapy, it is important to exclude causes of poor control that will not respond well to more intensive asthma therapy. This includes asthma worsening due to overuse of inhaled beta$_2$ agonists, gastroesophageal reflux, untreated sinus disease, and psychological factors (Table 1). Once these have been excluded and, if relevant, dealt with, asthmatics whose symptoms are not well controlled on medium- to high-dose inhaled corticosteroids may be considered for additional therapy. Long-acting theophylline preparations may help prevent nighttime bronchoconstriction. Likewise, the long-acting inhaled beta$_2$ agonist salmeterol (Serevent) may be added at this stage. Neither of these agents should be used in asthma without concomitant anti-inflammatory therapy.

At the very severe end of the asthma continuum, patients may require recurrent or chronic ingested corticosteroid to maintain control. In this setting, remittive agents such as gold, methotrexate,* azathioprine,* cyclophosphamide,* cyclosporin,* hydroxychloroquine,* and dapsone,* have been tried. The use of any or all of these agents requires referral to an expert and inclusion in an investigational treatment program.

The goals of treatment of asthma are the same at all levels and are only modified or liberalized in the case of more severe asthmatics. Therefore, it is not appropriate to use symptoms, flow rates, and morbidity to assign asthma severity. Asthma severity should be determined by the minimum amount of medication required to achieve ideal control. At the very severe end of the spectrum, there are a small number of asthmatics in whom ideal control cannot be achieved despite intensive therapy; under these circumstances, the goals of therapy are modified for these patients alone.

EMERGENT MANAGEMENT OF ASTHMA

Acute, severe episodes of asthma occur from time to time despite compliance with the best asthma therapy. Such exacerbations are much more common in poorly controlled and poorly treated asthmatics, whether from inadequate access to treatment or from noncompliance. The key points in the management of acute, severe asthma are outlined in Table 2.

Assessment of a patient having an acute, severe

*Not FDA-approved for this indication.

asthmatic episode must be done rapidly and in an ongoing fashion, generally concurrently with the commencement of treatment. A rapid assessment of the severity of the *exacerbation* (note that this is not synonymous with severity of *asthma*) includes vital signs (respiratory rate, pulse, blood pressure, pulsus paradoxus), assessment for cyanosis, ability to speak in complete sentences, and level of consciousness. Factors in the clinical examination suggesting a severe attack are rapid respiratory rate ($\geq$32), rapid pulse ($\geq$120), low blood pressure, pulsus paradox greater than 15 to 18 mm Hg, inability to speak more than a few words without pausing for breath, and altered level of consciousness. Oxygenation should be rapidly assessed with a pulse oximeter. Note that this simple noninvasive device does *not* allow assessment of arterial carbon dioxide and when it is important to know this; in subjects who are critically ill or not responding, it is necessary to perform an arterial blood gas measurement. If possible, assessment of expiratory flow rates prior to administration of medication can be helpful in assessing the response. PEF can be measured by a bedside portable peak flowmeter. A spirometer should be available in the emergency room so that the forced expiratory volume in 1 second (FEV$_1$) can be assessed.

Asthma treatment should be started promptly—almost concurrently with the initial assessment, and while the assessment is continuing. The principles of asthma therapy are the same in acute, severe asthma as they are in chronic asthma. The cornerstone of acute asthma therapy is the administration of corticosteroids to reverse the inflammation while bronchodilators are administered to achieve symptomatic relief. Inhaled beta$_2$ agonists are given either by nebulizer or by repeated doses from a metered dose inhaler and a spacer. At the same time, oral or intravenous corticosteroids are given promptly. These two classes of drugs suffice for most cases. If the inhaled beta$_2$ agonist affords adequate symptomatic relief and the patient is objectively in no danger, the inhaled beta$_2$ agonist is repeated as often as necessary—even continuously, if required. If symptomatic relief is not achieved or if the patient is objectively not responding, then a combination of an inhaled beta$_2$ agonist and an anticholinergic (e.g., albuterol [Proventil, Ventolin] and ipratropium [Atrovent]) is administered. The usual dose of corticosteroids is 60 to 120 mg of oral prednisone or 40 to 125 mg of intravenous methylprednisolone sodium succinate (Solu-Medrol) initially. Subsequent corticosteroid treatment, both the nature of the drug and the route of administration, is determined based on the patient's response and disposition.

Supportive treatment is important and includes

TABLE 2. Emergency Management of Asthma

Assessment	Complications
Asthma treatment	Precipitating cause
Supportive treatment	Disposition—follow-up

attention to oxygenation, hydration, electrolytes, anxiety, and occasionally assisted ventilation. Oxygen can be given with high-flow nasal cannulas, as there is no concern about suppression of ventilation in an acute asthmatic. Attention to hydration and electrolytes (particularly potassium) is important. Nonmedicinal relief of anxiety by a confident and caring staff is important. When the patient is in severe respiratory failure or deteriorates despite adequate treatment, endotracheal intubation and mechanical ventilation are occasionally necessary. The key to successful assisted ventilation is intubation by the best available person in the facility, followed by assisted ventilation with the lowest pressure and lowest volume possible to achieve adequate oxygenation. Hypercapnia is not a problem, and permissive hypercapnia has become the standard for ventilation of acutely ill individuals, particularly those with bronchospasm. The low pressures and low volumes reduce the risk of barotrauma (pneumothorax, pneumomediastinum, air embolus, and hypotension), which is so common in acute ventilated asthmatics.

Complications should be looked for and treated promptly. They include respiratory failure (noted earlier), barotrauma (noted earlier), atelectasis, and pneumonia. Performance of a chest radiograph is not routinely indicated for exacerbations of asthma, but when atelectasis, pneumonia, or pneumothorax is suspected, a chest radiograph can be invaluable. Immediate rapid insertion of a chest tube in an acute asthmatic with a pneumothorax can be life-saving.

The precipitating cause of an asthma exacerbation should be ascertained as a guide to the prevention of future episodes (i.e., the beginnings of patient education). On some occasions, the nature of the cause of the acute exacerbation dictates primary therapy. For example, when a severe asthma exacerbation is part of a systemic allergic reaction (e.g., to food, drugs, stings, allergen injection), subcutaneous adrenalin is generally part of the initial therapy, and antihistamines may be useful to combat the systemic manifestations. When a severe episode of bronchoconstriction is caused by a beta-adrenergic blocking drug, it is recommended that anticholinergic drugs (atropine, ipratropium) be part of the initial therapy. The more common causes of asthma exacerbations are inflammatory (allergen exposure, viral and *Mycoplasma* respiratory tract infections, noncompliance and/or tapering of anti-inflammatory drugs, and so forth), and the therapy for all these in the acute setting is the same. Antibiotics are indicated infrequently, and only when there is evidence of sinusitis (or otitis media) or bacterial pneumonia.

Objective assessment of expiratory flow rates is particularly helpful in determining the disposition of an asthmatic patient. This is important, since subjects recovering from an acute exacerbation of asthma often overestimate their well-being. Subjects with a post-treatment FEV_1 of 0.5 liters or less should probably be in the intensive care unit, those with post-treatment FEV_1 of 1 liter or less should be hospitalized. Those with an FEV_1 between 1 and 2 liters may require hospitalization, depending on their compliance, their distance from the hospital, and their wishes, as well as their past performance. Subjects with a post-treatment FEV_1 in excess of 2 liters can usually be discharged home. It is important to make sure that asthmatics discharged from the emergency department (or hospital) have appropriate arrangements for ongoing follow-up and management, as noted earlier.

ASTHMA IN CHILDREN

method of
DIRK K. GREINEDER, M.D., PH.D.
Harvard Medical School and Harvard Community Health Plan
Boston, Massachusetts

Asthma is one of the most common chronic diseases worldwide in children. The prevalence, morbidity, and mortality of asthma in children are increasing, and the reasons are poorly understood. The prevalence of asthma may be related to environmental factors, including exposure to allergens and pollutants, and it is more common in affluent than in nonaffluent countries. Asthma is the leading cause of time lost from school, amounting to more than 10 million days per year in the United States alone. In addition, children with asthma may suffer from increased academic failure and decreased levels of self-esteem. The economic cost of asthma in the United States exceeded $6 billion per year in 1990.

Although the specific definition of asthma remains elusive, an operational definition has recently been proposed by the International Consensus Report: "Asthma is a chronic inflammatory disorder of the airways in which many cells play a role, including mast cells and eosinophils. In susceptible individuals this inflammation causes symptoms which are usually associated with widespread but variable airflow obstruction that is often reversible either spontaneously or with treatment, and causes an associated increase in airway responsiveness to a variety of stimuli." Immunologic and nonimmunologic mechanisms are involved in the chronic airway inflammation, and neural control of the airways may also be involved in the regulation of airway inflammation and caliber. In addition to the cells mentioned above, the role of lymphocytes in the development of eosinophilic inflammation is now recognized. Many studies have emphasized the importance of environmental factors. Allergy has an important role in childhood asthma. The majority of children with severe or moderate asthma have positive skin tests, and the prevalence and severity of asthma are associated with exposure to indoor allergens such as dust mites, cockroaches, and pets. The prevalence of asthma is also correlated with elevations of serum IgE.

Asthma presents with cough, wheeze, and shortness of breath, in association with airway hyper-reactivity. The differential diagnosis of such symptoms includes foreign body, anatomic abnormalities, aspiration, cystic fibrosis, bronchopulmonary dysplasia, and congestive heart failure. History, physical examination, chest x-ray, sweat test, and barium swallow are usually adequate to rule out these diseases. The results of the physical examination and tests are often normal between exacerbations. Clues suggesting asthma typically include episodic exacerbations, particularly if triggered by viral respiratory infection, allergens, or night time, and asthma can usually be confirmed by responsiveness to bronchodilators. In patients who are old enough, objective measurements of lung function (peak flow, FVC, FEV_1, and FEF_{25-75}) before and after bronchodilator use can establish the diagnosis. In selected subtle cases, bronchoprovocation with methacholine (or other triggers) can be useful. In smaller children in whom objective tests cannot be performed, the diagnosis may need to be based on the examination at the time of a symptomatic exacerbation and the clinical response to bronchodilator. Most experts agree that the diagnosis of bronchiolitis should be limited to the first episode of wheezing in a child under the age of 1 year experiencing a viral respiratory infection; subsequent episodes of wheezing should be characterized as asthma.

In the past, asthma was principally classified according to etiology (extrinsic or intrinsic), but such classification is of limited usefulness, since the exacerbating triggers overlap. Classification according to severity, although somewhat arbitrary, has been useful. Figure 1 summarizes this classification but is based on assessment *before* treatment, which is not always feasible, particularly with sicker children. When possible, symptom patterns should be confirmed with objective measures of lung function to ensure accurate classification.

MANAGEMENT

Goals. The goals of asthma management are to improve the quality of patients' lives by achieving and maintaining control of symptoms; preventing asthma exacerbations and mortality; attaining normal lung function, to the extent possible; maintaining normal activity levels, including exercise; and avoiding adverse effects from asthma medications. It is hoped that achieving these goals will prevent the development of irreversible airway obstruction.

Prevention. Primary prevention (prevention of the initial development of asthma) has the potential to decrease the prevalence of asthma, and urgent investigation of appropriate strategies is required. Reducing exposure to indoor allergens, particularly mites (and roaches?), is promising, especially for the very young. Avoidance of passive smoking and outdoor pollutants such as vehicle emissions and industrial pollutants is likely to be beneficial. Prevention of viral respiratory infections (e.g., vaccination with respiratory syncytial virus) may be useful. Finally, prevention of food allergy reactions may be helpful, although data in this area are still very preliminary.

Six-Part Management Program. Various national and international consensus groups have suggested a comprehensive six-part asthma management program to achieve the goals listed earlier. Prevention of asthma mortality is one of the goals that deserves special attention. Certain factors that predispose to a high risk of mortality are listed in Table 1. In addition to providing a rational framework for asthma management, the six-part management program can diminish the impact of these risk factors.

1. PATIENT EDUCATION AND ESTABLISHMENT OF A

TABLE 1. **Factors Associated with Asthma Mortality**

History of previous life-threatening acute asthma exacerbation
Hospital admission for asthma within the last year
Inadequate general medical management
Psychosocial problems
Lack of access to medical care
History of intubation for asthma
Recent alterations in systemic corticosteroid dosage

PARTNERSHIP IN ASTHMA MANAGEMENT. Patients and families must be educated in at least in four domains: (1) information about the pathophysiology of asthma, including precipitating triggers (allergens, irritants, exercise, and infection) and ways to avoid them, early warning signs of exacerbation, and the nature of asthma attacks; (2) types, uses, and side effects of asthma medications; (3) types and uses of asthma devices such as inhalers, nebulizers, spacers, peak flow meters, and diary charts; and (4) expectations about asthma treatment and partnerships between families and medical providers. Detailed information in many of these domains is the subject of other parts of this six-part management program. The goal of this education is to establish trust and clear communication among patients, caregivers, and the medical team, with special attention to family needs and motivations. This process develops an effective partnership between the family and the medical care providers and provides the knowledge, confidence, and skills needed to take control of the asthma. Some of the education can be obtained from asthma support groups and asthma education sessions provided by local chapters of the American Lung Association, the Asthma and Allergy Foundation of America, and Mothers of Asthmatics. However, the principles learned in group sessions must be clarified and customized for each patient and family at regular visits with their individual physicians.

2. ASSESS AND MONITOR ASTHMA SEVERITY WITH MEASUREMENTS OF SYMPTOMS AND LUNG FUNCTION. Asthma severity can be judged by measurements of symptoms and signs, including frequency of limitations in activity and use of reliever medications. Presently, these methods are still crude, and the questionnaires used to elicit this information require validation, but they may be the only measurements available in small children who cannot perform objective lung function tests. Lung function studies are essential in children over 5 years old. Spirometry before and after bronchodilator use is helpful in diagnosing and assessing asthma severity and may provide an indirect measure of airway hyper-responsiveness, which may correlate with the degree of airway inflammation. Peak expiratory flow (PEF) measurements may be used for home monitoring and for assessment of the severity of exacerbations and response to therapy in the office and emergency department. Physical examination and subjective symptom assessment at baseline and during exacerbation are unreliable and may be a major factor causing delay in treatment, thereby contributing to

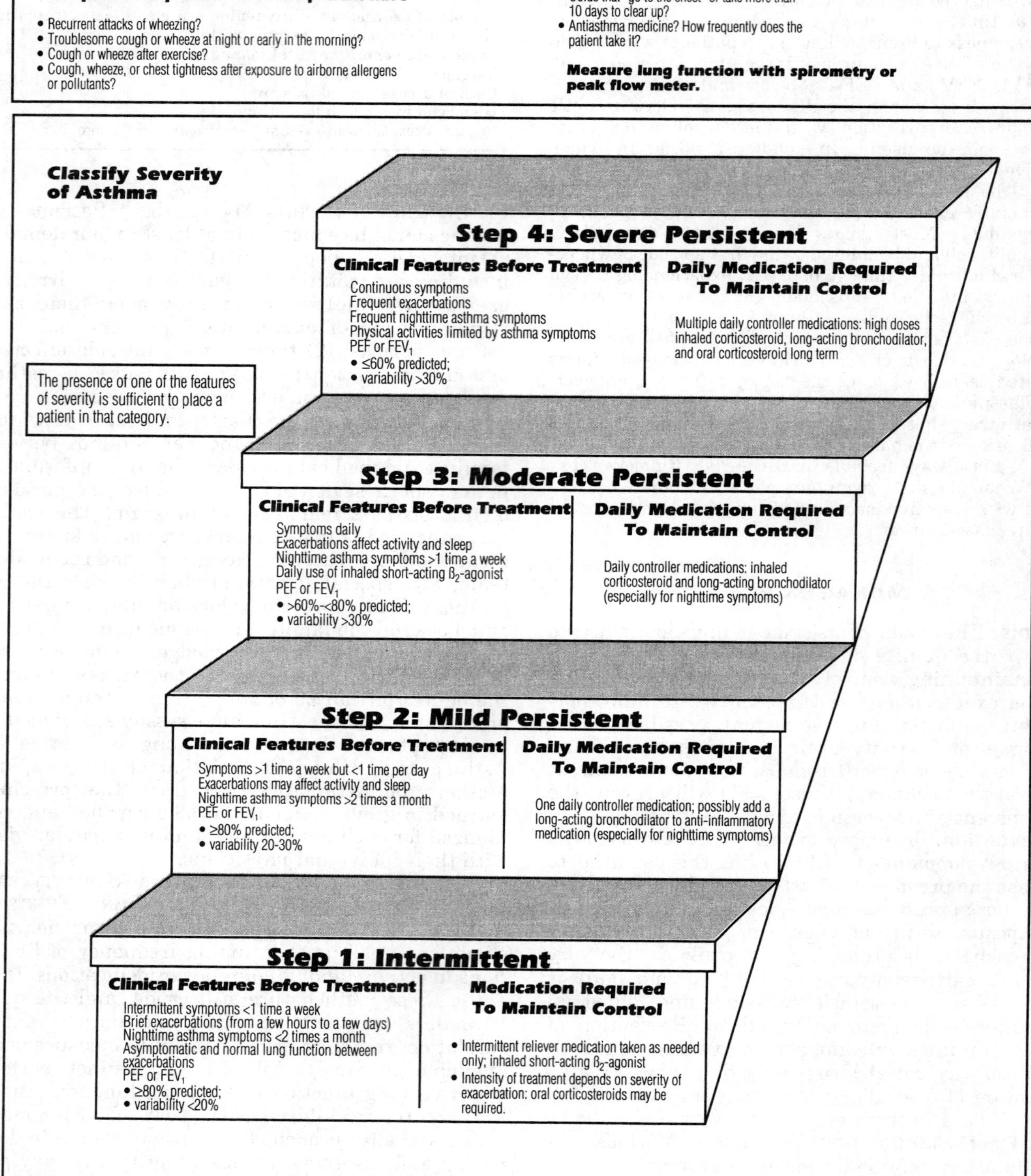

Figure 1. The long-term management of asthma: diagnose and classify severity. (From National Institutes of Health: Global Initiative for Asthma. NHLBI publication number 95-3659, January 1995, p. 89.)

increased morbidity and mortality from asthma. Home PEF monitoring and charting should be considered for patients who need to take medications daily. This can provide some level of quantification of the severity of asthma symptoms, guide home management plans for exacerbations (see later), and improve communication between family and physician during an acute exacerbation. Finally, assessment of daily variability in PEF can be an index of instability and severity (i.e., high degrees of variability correlate with poor control of asthma). Percentage of daily variability = (evening PEF − morning PEF)/ ½ (evening PEF + morning PEF) × 100. PEF measurements are optimally based on the patient's personal best value (often obtained only after aggressive treatment with bronchodilators and corticosteroids) rather than on predicted charts, which are much less reliable. Finally, PEF measurement is dependent on an accurately functioning meter and the patient effort used in obtaining the reading, so results should always be correlated with the patient's status. Additional objective measures of lung function include arterial blood gas determinations and pulse oximetry.

3. IDENTIFY AND CONTROL ASTHMA TRIGGERS. The discussion in this section focuses on controlling exposure to triggers that exacerbate asthma airway inflammation (allergens, pollutants, pharmacologic agents, and viral infections) rather than triggers that do not increase inflammation (exercise, cold air, and emotions) and are part of a normal lifestyle; asthma management needs to be adapted to allow these exposures to be tolerated without excessive symptoms. Avoidance of indoor allergens (domestic mites, animal allergens, cockroaches, and fungi) should be viewed as a primary anti-inflammatory therapy for asthma. The occurrence of asthma symptoms is closely related to the amount of environmental allergen, and reduction is important, even though it is rarely possible to achieve complete control. Measures to control house dust mite exposure are summarized in Table 2. Removal of warm-blooded animals from the patient's home environment is important, since all such animals produce potent allergens that circulate through the house. Cockroach exposure is difficult to avoid and may require professional extermination or moving to a roach-free environment. Fungi are best avoided by reducing humidity, providing adequate ventilation and light, and removing fabrics or wallpaper in areas prone to high humidity or condensation. Exposure to outdoor allergens (pollens and outdoor molds) can be reduced by keeping windows closed and running air conditioners during times of high prevalence. Avoidance of indoor air pollutants, including smoke, various gases (nitrogen oxides, carbon monoxide, formaldehyde, sulfur dioxide), and biologicals such as endotoxins, may be difficult and is of unknown value at present; however, adequate ventilation, maintenance of flues and ducts, and avoidance of wood stoves and household aerosols are recommended. Absolute avoidance of tobacco smoke (active and passive) should be enforced. Besides being a significant irritant, exposure to tobacco smoke increases the risk of allergic sensitization in children. Pharmacologic agents such as sulfites, nonsteroidal anti-inflammatory agents, and beta blockers can cause significant asthma exacerbations and should be avoided. Food allergies and food additive intolerances (tartrazine, benzoate, monosodium glutamate) may contribute to asthma, particularly in children, but the diagnosis is difficult and should be confirmed in specialty clinics with the ability to conduct double-blind challenges before these foods are eliminated from the diet. Reduction of viral respiratory infections is probably best achieved by vaccination. Influenza vaccines reduce the likelihood of infection and have been purified to reduce adverse reactions; in the future, a respiratory syncytial virus vaccine may offer some hope of reducing infection and the resultant airway inflammation.

The role of specific allergen immunotherapy is under investigation and should not replace patient education, avoidance measures, and pharmacologic therapy. Specific immunotherapy may be considered when avoiding the allergen is not possible and appropriate medication at reasonable doses fails to control symptoms. Specific immunotherapy has been shown to be effective in asthma caused by grass pollen, dust mites, animal dander (cat), and *Alternaria* allergy. This treatment is effective only when potent, standardized extracts are used under controlled and monitored situations by professionals trained to avoid potentially dangerous reactions.

4. ESTABLISH MEDICATION PLANS FOR LONG-TERM MANAGEMENT. A plan for chronic asthma management has three components: the medications, a stepwise approach to pharmacologic therapy, and an asthma zone management system. Asthma medications are now classified as controllers and relievers (Table 3). A medication plan based on the stepwise classification system (see Figure 1) is summarized in Figure 2 (for older children able to perform lung function tests) and Figure 3 (for infants and younger children).

Controllers are medications taken on a regular basis to keep persistent asthma under control. These include inhaled and systemic corticosteroids, sodium cromoglycate, nedocromil sodium, sustained-release theophylline, and long-acting inhaled or oral beta₂ agonists. Anti-inflammatory agents, particularly the inhaled corticosteroids, are presently the most effective controllers. Antiallergic agents (ketotifen,* other antihistaminic agents) and antimediator agents (zafirlukast,* zileuton,* other leukotriene antagonists) are currently not available in the United States, although they may soon become available. These agents have variable degrees of bronchodilator

TABLE 2. **House Dust Mite Control Measures**

Encase the mattress in an allergen-nonpermeable cover
Either encase the pillow or wash it weekly
Wash the bedding (including blankets, comforters, and
  stuffed animals) weekly in >55° C water
Avoid sleeping or lying on furniture upholstered with
  fabric
Remove carpets that are laid on concrete
Reduce indoor humidity to less than 50%
Remove carpets from patient's bedroom
Use chemical agents (acaricides) to kill mites in the house

From International Consensus Report on Diagnosis and Treatment of Asthma, Bethesda, Md., NHLBI, NIH, 1992.

*Not available in the United States.

TABLE 3. **Dosages for Therapy in Childhood Asthma**

RELIEVERS

Beta₂ agonists

Albuterol (Proventil, Ventolin), metaproterenol (Alupent), bitolterol (Tornalate), terbutaline (Brethine), pirbuterol (Maxair)

MDI	2 puffs q 4–6 h
Dry powder inhaler	1 capsule q 4–6 h
Nebulizer solution	Albuterol 5 mg/mL; 0.1–0.15 mg/kg in 3 mL saline q 4–6 h; maximum 5 mg
	Metaproterenol 50 mg/mL; 0.25–0.50 mg/kg in 3 mL saline q 4–6 h; maximum 15 mg
Liquids	
Albuterol	0.1–0.15 mg/kg q 4–6 h
Metaproterenol	0.3–0.5 mg/kg q 4–6 h
Tablets	
Albuterol (Proventil, Ventolin)	2–4 mg tablet q 4–6 h
Metaproterenol (Alupent)	10–20 mg tablet q 4–6 h
Terbutaline (Brethine)	2.5–5 mg tablet q 4–6 h

Anticholinergics

Ipratroprium bromide (Atrovent)	
MDI	2 puffs q 4–6 h
Nebulizer solution	1.25–2.5 mL q 4–6 h

Theophylline

Liquid, tablets, capsules	Dosage to achieve serum concentration 5–15 µg/mL

Corticosteroids

Oral liquid, tablets	
Prednisone	1–2 mg/kg/day for 3–5 days
Prednisolone	1–2 mg/kg/day for 3–5 days
Methylprednisolone	1–2 mg/kg/day for 3–5 days

CONTROLLERS

Beta₂ agonists

Albuterol	4-mg sustained release tablet q 12 h
Salmeterol MDI (Serevent)	21 µg/puff; 2 puffs bid

Cromolyn sodium (Intal)

MDI	1 mg/puff; 2 puffs qid
Nebulizer solution	20 mg/cap; 1 cap qid

Nedocromil sodium (Tilade)

MDI	2 mg/puff; 2 puffs bid–qid

Theophylline

Sustained-release tablets, capsules	Dosage to achieve serum concentration 5–15 µg/mL

Corticosteroids

Beclomethasone (Beclovent, Vanceril)	42 µg/puff; 2–4 puffs bid–qid
Triamcinolone (Azmacort)	100 µg/puff; 2–4 puffs bid–qid
Flunisolide (AeroBid)	250 µg/puff; 2–4 puffs bid–qid
Liquids	
Prednisone	For acute exacerbations, doses of 1–2 mg/kd/day in single or divided doses are
Prednisolone	used initially and are then modified; reassess in 3 days, as only a short burst
Tablets	may be needed; there is no need to taper a 3- to 5-day course of therapy; if
Prednisone	therapy extends beyond this period, it may be appropriate to taper the
Prednisolone	dosage
Methylprednisolone	

Abbreviation: MDI = metered-dose inhaler.

From National Institutes of Health, U.S. Department of Health and Human Services: Guidelines of the Diagnosis and Management of Asthma. Washington, D.C., U.S. Government Printing Office, 1991.

and anti-inflammatory activity, and their precise role in asthma management remains to be defined and is not discussed here. Other experimental controller agents include immune suppressive agents such as methotrexate and cyclosporine. These latter agents should be used only in selected patients under the supervision of an asthma specialist, as the steroid-sparing effects may not outweigh the risk of side effects.

The goal is to control asthma with the least possible medication. Control is achieved by increasing the number and frequency of medications and then stepping down to the least amount of medication that maintains asthma control. The clinician's judgment determines the initial level of medication required to control the asthma and the rate at which therapy can be reduced to maintain control. Children who experience episodic, predictable seasonal exacerbations (induced by pollen or infection) may need increased levels of medication during that season.

Reliever medications include short-acting inhaled or oral beta₂ agonists, anticholinergics, short-acting

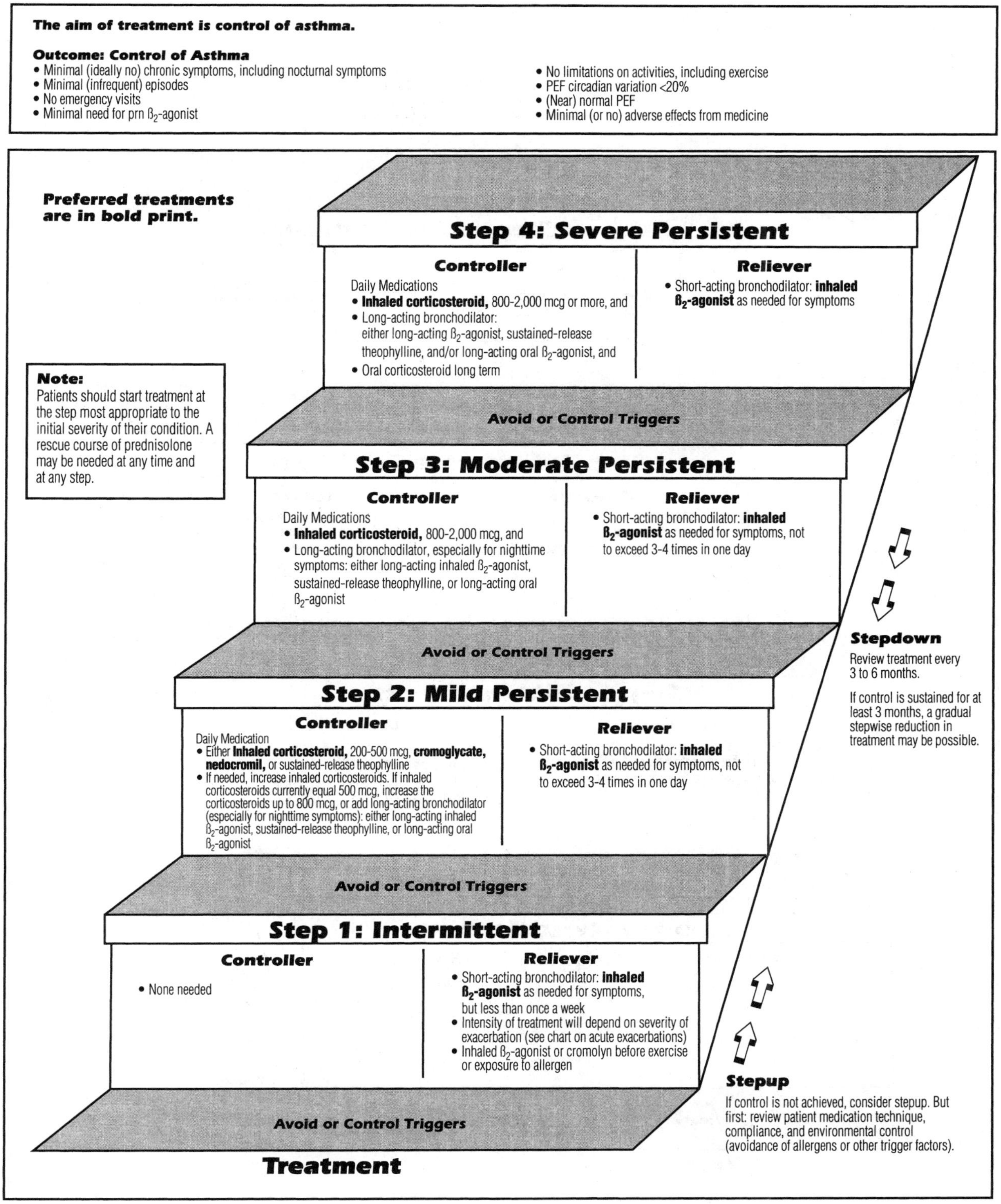

The aim of treatment is control of asthma.

Outcome: Control of Asthma
- Minimal (ideally no) chronic symptoms, including nocturnal symptoms
- Minimal (infrequent) episodes
- No emergency visits
- Minimal need for prn β_2-agonist
- No limitations on activities, including exercise
- PEF circadian variation <20%
- (Near) normal PEF
- Minimal (or no) adverse effects from medicine

Preferred treatments are in bold print.

Note:
Patients should start treatment at the step most appropriate to the initial severity of their condition. A rescue course of prednisolone may be needed at any time and at any step.

Step 4: Severe Persistent

Controller
Daily Medications
- **Inhaled corticosteroid,** 800-2,000 mcg or more, and
- Long-acting bronchodilator: either long-acting β_2-agonist, sustained-release theophylline, and/or long-acting oral β_2-agonist, and
- Oral corticosteroid long term

Reliever
- Short-acting bronchodilator: **inhaled β_2-agonist** as needed for symptoms

Avoid or Control Triggers

Step 3: Moderate Persistent

Controller
Daily Medications
- **Inhaled corticosteroid,** 800-2,000 mcg, and
- Long-acting bronchodilator, especially for nighttime symptoms: either long-acting inhaled β_2-agonist, sustained-release theophylline, or long-acting oral β_2-agonist

Reliever
- Short-acting bronchodilator: **inhaled β_2-agonist** as needed for symptoms, not to exceed 3-4 times in one day

Avoid or Control Triggers

Step 2: Mild Persistent

Controller
Daily Medication
- Either **Inhaled corticosteroid,** 200-500 mcg, **cromoglycate, nedocromil,** or sustained-release theophylline
- If needed, increase inhaled corticosteroids. If inhaled corticosteroids currently equal 500 mcg, increase the corticosteroids up to 800 mcg, or add long-acting bronchodilator (especially for nighttime symptoms): either long-acting inhaled β_2-agonist, sustained-release theophylline, or long-acting oral β_2-agonist

Reliever
- Short-acting bronchodilator: **inhaled β_2-agonist** as needed for symptoms, not to exceed 3-4 times in one day

Avoid or Control Triggers

Step 1: Intermittent

Controller
- None needed

Reliever
- Short-acting bronchodilator: **inhaled β_2-agonist** as needed for symptoms, but less than once a week
- Intensity of treatment will depend on severity of exacerbation (see chart on acute exacerbations)
- Inhaled β_2-agonist or cromolyn before exercise or exposure to allergen

Avoid or Control Triggers

Treatment

Stepdown
Review treatment every 3 to 6 months.

If control is sustained for at least 3 months, a gradual stepwise reduction in treatment may be possible.

Stepup
If control is not achieved, consider stepup. But first: review patient medication technique, compliance, and environmental control (avoidance of allergens or other trigger factors).

Figure 2. The long-term management of asthma: treatments in the stepwise approach. (From National Institutes of Health: Global Initiative for Asthma. NHLBI publication number 95-3659, January 1995, p. 90.)

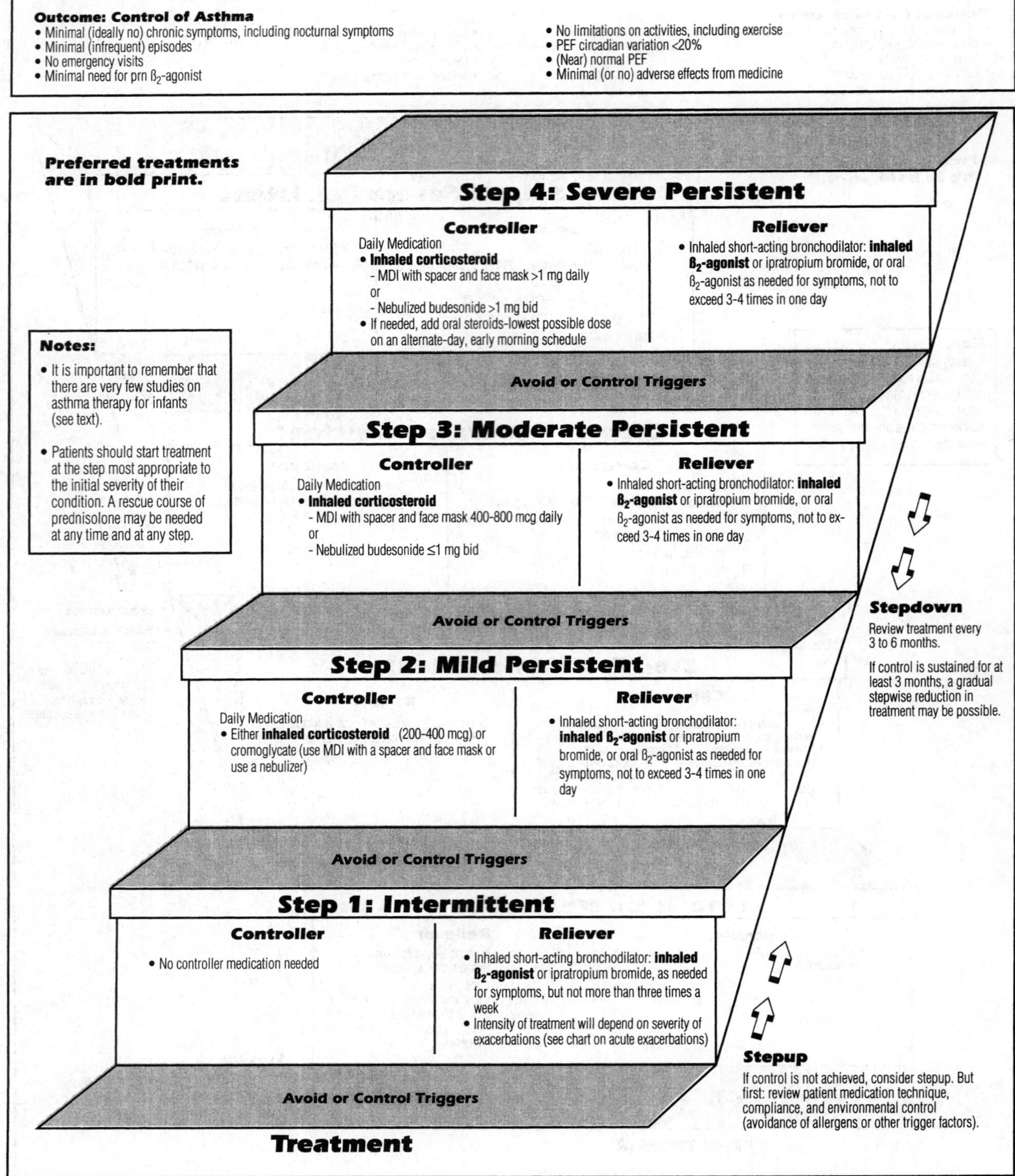

Figure 3. The long-term management of asthma: treatments in the stepwise approach for infants and young children. (From National Institutes of Health: Global Initiative for Asthma. NHLBI publication number 95-3659, January 1995, p. 92.)

theophylline, and systemic corticosteroids. Although the onset of action of the oral corticosteroids is usually 4 hours or more, they are important in the treatment of acute exacerbations, because they prevent the progression of the exacerbation and have been shown to decrease the need for emergency department visits and hospitalization. These agents are usually administered in short bursts for 3 to 10 days at a dose of 1 to 2 mg per kg per day, usually in divided doses. There is no need to taper bursts of 3 to 5 days duration, but longer courses may be tapered.

Children with mild, intermittent asthma are usually treated with a short-acting beta$_2$ agonist as needed for symptomatic or "reliever" therapy (step 1). Increasing use of short-acting beta$_2$ agonists indicates deteriorating control and a need to increase medication by adding a controller (step 2). Children with persistent asthma should receive inhaled anti-inflammatory therapy on a daily basis, using cromolyn (Intal), nedocromil (Tilade), or corticosteroids. Cromolyn is a nonsteroidal anti-inflammatory agent that is active in the management of chronic asthma. Its onset of action is slow, and a 4-week trial may be needed before concluding that the drug is not effective. Side effects are minimal, but the drug must be given three to four times a day to ensure efficacy. Nedocromil is a more potent nonsteroidal inhaled agent. Benefits may be seen sooner than with cromolyn, and the drug is probably effective when given twice a day. Inhaled corticosteroids are the most effective maintenance anti-inflammatory treatment for asthma. A spacer device reduces oropharyngeal adverse effects and systemic absorption. Currently available agents in the United States include beclomethasone (Beclovent, Vanceril), triamcinolone (Azmacort), and flunisolide (AeroBid); these agents are roughly equivalent in efficacy and safety. Budesonide* and fluticasone* are likely to become available soon and may offer somewhat more favorable topical to systemic efficacy, thereby increasing the safety for those children needing high-dose therapy. Patients not controlled by step 2 medications should receive additional controller medications (step 3). The dose of inhaled corticosteroid can be increased, although levels above 800 µg per day may produce adverse systemic side effects. Cromolyn or nedocromil may be added to control symptoms produced by exercise, cold air, or allergens and to minimize the need to increase inhaled corticosteroids. The addition of a sustained-release theophylline or the long-acting inhaled beta$_2$ agonist salmeterol (Serevent) may be useful to control frequent or nocturnal symptoms. At this point, consultation with an asthma specialist is indicated. If adequate control is still not achieved, step 4 interventions—consisting of multiple daily medicines and possibly maintenance oral corticosteroids—are needed. Ongoing consultation with an asthma specialist should be obtained for children with this level of severity.

---

*Not available in the United States.

5. ESTABLISH PLANS FOR MANAGING EXACERBATIONS. Exacerbations of asthma are episodes of worsening cough, wheeze, chest tightness, or shortness of breath. Exacerbations usually reflect failure of the maintenance management plan or exposure to an asthma trigger. Severity may range from mild to severe, and deterioration may occur gradually or precipitously. Although respiratory distress is common, PEF or FEV$_1$ measurements are more reliable indicators of the severity of airflow obstruction than symptoms, and objective measurements should be obtained whenever possible. Initial treatment of exacerbations depends on the availability of medications and the degree of knowledge that the patient has regarding their use. A written asthma management zone system can provide sensible initial guidance for patients and alert them when to call a health professional for assistance. Although several different zone systems have been proposed, the most generally accepted is based on the traffic light system.

The green zone indicates that asthma is under control. At this point, the patient should have no symptoms, and the PEF should be greater than 80% of personal best.

The yellow zone indicates caution, that asthma is not under adequate control. Asthma symptoms are present (nocturnal symptoms, cough, wheeze, or chest tightness with activity or at rest) and/or PEF is between 50 and 80% of personal best. Typically, doses of short-acting beta$_2$ agonists are given, up to three times over the first hour, to reduce symptoms and restore PEF to greater than 80%. If this is not readily achieved or if the patient experiences exacerbations more often than every 4 hours or repeatedly during the same day, additional medication should be given based on a prearranged plan written out by the physician. Usually, the patient either adds or increases inhaled corticosteroids by 8 inhalations per day for milder episodes or starts a short course of oral corticosteroids (3 to 5 days at 2 mg per kg per day) for more acute or severe episodes. If oral corticosteroids are started, the patient should consult the clinician urgently (the same day). Frequent exacerbations dipping into the yellow zone—more than once per day or more than twice per week—usually signal the need to increase baseline, maintenance medications by one step and should trigger a call to the health professional during the next working day. Severe exacerbations not reversed by the three treatments of beta$_2$ agonist over the first hour should be considered red zone exacerbations.

The red zone signals a medical alert. Asthma symptoms are present at rest, and the PEF is below 50% of personal best. An inhaled short-acting beta$_2$ agonist should be taken immediately, and if the PEF remains below 50 to 60%, immediate medical attention should be obtained. The dosage of short-acting beta$_2$ agonist may be higher than usual for red zone incursions (at the physician's discretion), and oral corticosteroids may be started automatically by some patients. If the PEF improves after bronchodilator treatment, the appropriate yellow zone plan should

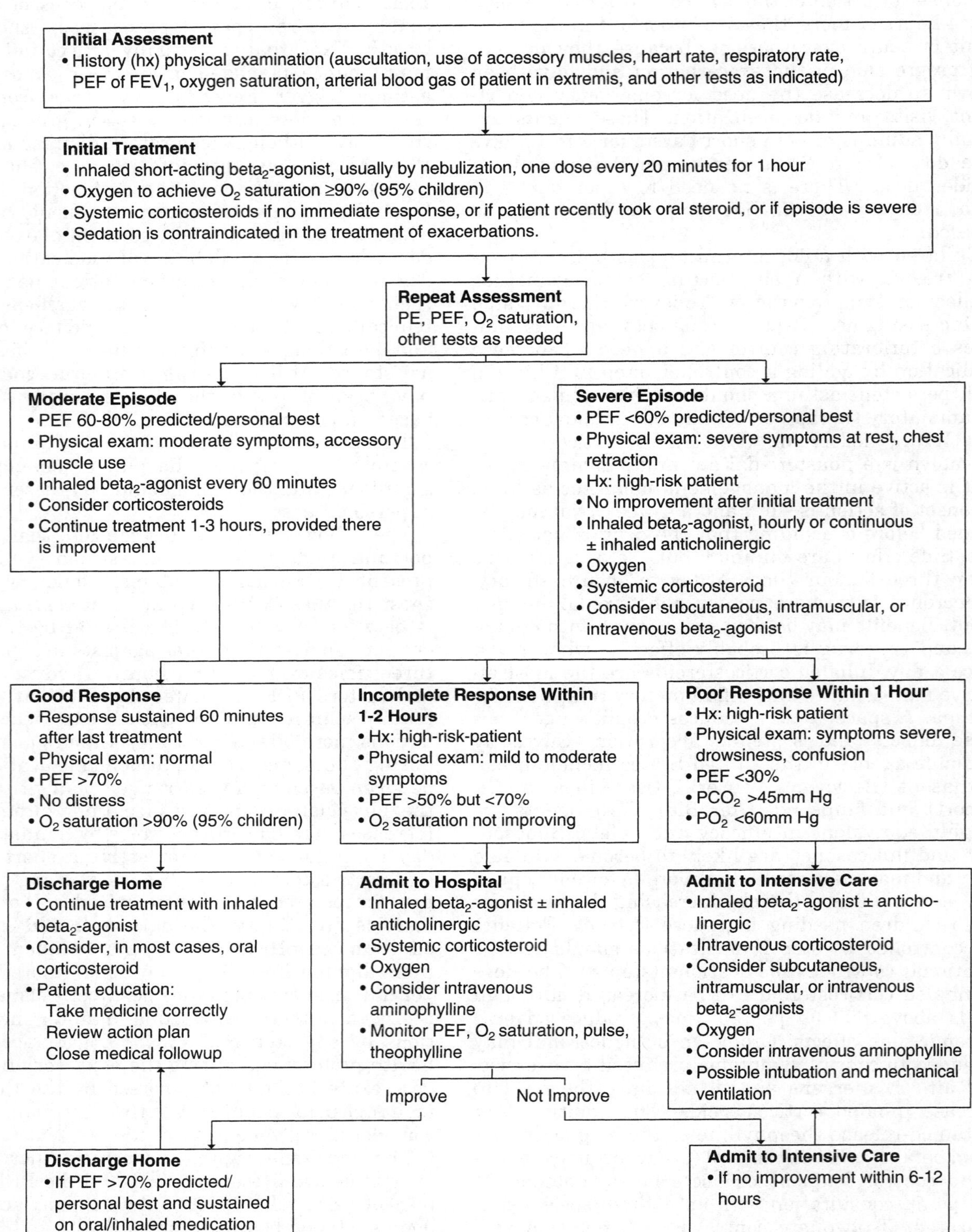

Figure 4. Management of exacerbations of asthma (see also Table 4). (From National Institutes of Health: Global Initiative for Asthma. NHLBI publication number 95-3659, January 1995, p. 103.)

TABLE 4. **Severity of Asthma Exacerbations**

	Mild	Moderate	Severe	Respiratory Arrest Imminent
Breathless	Walking	Talking Infant—softer, shorter cry; difficulty feeding	At rest Infant—stops feeding	
Talks in	Can lie down	Prefers sitting	Hunched forward	
Alertness	Sentences	Phrases	Words	
Respiratory rate*	May be agitated	Usually agitated	Usually agitated	Drowsy or confused
	Increased	Increased	Often >30/min	
Accessory muscles and suprasternal retractions	Usually not	Usually	Usually	Paradoxical thoracoabdominal movement
Wheeze	Moderate, often only end expiratory	Loud	Usually loud	Absence of wheeze
Pulse/min†	<100	100–120	>120	Bradycardia
Pulsus paradoxus	Absent <10 mmHg	May be present 10–25 mmHg	Often present >25 mmHg (adult) 20–40 mmHg (child)	Absence suggests respiratory muscle fatigue
PEF after initial bronchodilator (% predicted or % personal best)	Over 80%	Approx. 60–80%	<60% predicted or personal best (<100 L/min adults) or response lasts <2 h	
Pa_{O_2} (on air)‡	Normal Test not usually necessary	>60 mmHg	<60 mmHg Possible cyanosis	
and/or				
Pa_{CO_2}‡	<45 mmHg	<45 mmHg	>45 mmHg: possible respiratory failure (see text)	
SaO_2% (on air)‡§	>95%	91–95%	<90%	

*Guide to rates of breathing associated with respiratory distress in awake children:

Age	Normal rate
<2 months	<60/min
2–12 months	<50/min
1–5 years	<40/min
6–8 years	<30/min

The presence of several parameters, but not necessarily all, indicates the general classification of the exacerbation.

†Guide to limits of normal pulse rate in children:
  Infants (2–12 months): <160/min
  Preschool (1–2 years): <120/min
  School age (2–8 years): <110/min

‡Kilopascals are also used internationally; conversion would be appropriate in this regard.

§Hypercapnea (hypoventilation) develops more readily in young children than in adults and adolescents.

From National Institutes of Health: Global Initiative for Asthma. NHLBI publication number 95-3659, January 1995, p. 100.

be implemented, and the clinician consulted the same day.

The asthma zone management system permits initial home management of exacerbations and gives patients increased control over their asthma. It also provides a concrete framework to guide the patient's need to consult a clinician. When writing the home management plan, the clinician should take into consideration any high-risk factors (see Table 1) exhibited by the patient. When an exacerbation is severe or fails to respond to home management, the clinician needs to consider whether office- or hospital-based management is needed. Experienced patients may be permitted to add treatments that are otherwise limited to supervised office interventions, such as the use of nebulizers or higher-dose, short-acting beta₂ agonist metered-dose inhaler (MDI) therapy (4 to 10 puffs given with a spacer) and the addition of anticholinergics (4 to 6 puffs via MDI or nebulizer). In general, these increased levels of intervention are associated with the initiation of oral corticosteroid treatment.

Office, emergency department, and hospital management of acute exacerbations is summarized in Figure 4. The severity of exacerbations should be assessed as summarized in Table 4. Because these are only guidelines, not all the features in each category need to be present. If the patient fails to improve with initial therapy, if the deterioration has progressed rapidly, or if the patient is at high risk for death, a more severe grade should be given. In each situation, therapy is designed to relieve airway obstruction, relieve hypoxemia, and restore lung function to normal. Initial treatment consists of repeated use of reliever bronchodilators and early addition of oral glucocorticoids. Full recovery is usually gradual, and it may take days for lung function to return to normal and weeks for airway hyper-responsiveness to decrease. Symptoms are not always reliable, and whenever possible, treatment should be based on objective measurements.

Several differences place infants and young children at increased risk. Close monitoring and careful assessment using the parameters listed in Table 4 permit fairly accurate assessment. Infants are more likely to become hypoxemic than older children, and oxygen saturation measurements should be performed and should be maintained above 95% by the use of oxygen. Nebulizers may be driven with oxygen when pulse oximetry is not available or reveals hypoxemia. Infants and young children are at risk for dehydration as a result of increased respiratory rates and reduced intake.

6. PROVIDE REGULAR FOLLOW-UP CARE. Patients with asthma require regular supervision and support. Continual monitoring is needed to ensure that management goals are met. While the patient is initially establishing control of asthma, frequent follow-up visits are needed to adjust medications and to review treatment plans, diaries, home PEF and symptom records, and medication techniques. If an exacerbation results in emergency care or hospitalization, follow-up within 1 week should be obtained to ensure resolution of the exacerbation and to review the long-term management plan for adequacy.

Once control is established, regular follow-up visits (1- to 6-month intervals, based on severity and patient need) are essential. These visits should include review of the medication plan, PEF and symptom records, and medication and peak flow techniques. Consultation by an asthma specialist is indicated when the patient has had a life-threatening exacerbation, has poor self-management skills or difficult family dynamics, or is not responding adequately to asthma therapy. Consultation is also appropriate when signs and symptoms are atypical, there are difficulties with the differential diagnosis, there is a complicating illness (e.g., sinusitis, nasal polyps, aspergillosis, severe rhinitis), or additional testing is indicated (e.g., skin testing, pulmonary function testing, rhinoscopy, provocative studies). Since the majority (85 to 90%) of children with asthma have associated respiratory allergies, consultation with an allergist should be obtained if the patient is exposed to high levels of common allergens that cannot be removed or fails to respond optimally to asthma therapy.

CONCLUSION

The prognosis of asthma remains in doubt. Although asthma often improves during adolescence, many individuals redevelop asthma in adulthood. Adults with a history of allergy, rhinitis, eczema, hyper-reactive airways, or exposure to tobacco smoke have a higher incidence of adult asthma. Additional studies are needed to determine the best therapy for childhood asthma and the degree to which asthma during childhood may affect adult lung function. Delays in making the diagnosis of asthma in infancy and childhood may postpone appropriate interventions (allergen and tobacco avoidance, adequate access to controller medications), which may be associated with decreased functional status later.

Psychosocial aspects of asthma are significant and can affect compliance with asthma care and other important aspects of psychological development. Children with asthma, whether mild or severe, can have significant psychological dysfunction. Depression is seen more commonly in children with asthma. An awareness of these issues and the institution of optimal asthma therapy designed to minimize any intrusion into the life of the patient and family are likely to reduce these psychological manifestations.

ALLERGIC RHINITIS CAUSED BY INHALANT FACTORS

method of
IRAKLIS LIVAS, M.D., and
ALKIS TOGIAS, M.D.
*Johns Hopkins University School of Medicine at the Johns Hopkins Asthma and Allergy Center
Baltimore, Maryland*

Allergic rhinitis, the most common form of atopic disease, is also one of the most common chronic diseases, affecting between 15 and 20% of the U.S. population. Although the disease can occur at any age, two-thirds of patients develop symptoms before the age of 30, with peak incidence in childhood and adolescence. This disorder has a significant impact on public health because of missed days from work and school, reduced work and school performance, and the cost of treatment, which amounts to billions of dollars per year. The morbidity of allergic rhinitis results from the disease per se as well as from its complications, including chronic and recurrent sinusitis, chronic cough, otitis, nasal polyposis, and sleep disturbance. There is also convincing evidence that untreated allergic rhinosinusitis can result in worsening of asthma. Allergic rhinitis is associated with a genetic predisposition for atopic disease. Offspring with one atopic parent have a 30% chance of having allergic rhinitis. If both parents have allergies, this chance increases to 50%.

PATHOPHYSIOLOGY

Atopic patients produce excessive amounts of IgE antibodies against particular allergens, provided they have been adequately exposed. IgE binds to high-affinity receptors on the surface of mast cells and basophils, serving as an allergen receptor. With re-exposure, binding of the allergen to the mast cell surface IgE takes place in the nasal mucosa. The binding results in cross-linking of IgE molecules, triggering a cascade of cell activation. This is followed by the release of a number of inflammatory mediators, including histamine, prostaglandin D_2, and leukotriene C_4. The actions of these mediators on the nasal tissue (nerve endings, blood vessels, mucous glands) are responsible for the symptoms of sneezing, pruritus, congestion, and rhinorrhea, which occur promptly after allergen exposure.

The mast cell–dominated immediate reaction can be reproduced in the laboratory using nasal allergen challenge. Both the acute symptoms and the release of mediators subside after approximately half an hour. In about 50% of patients with allergic rhinitis, the acute response is followed by a late phase, 3 to 12 hours later. This is accompa-

TABLE 1. **Major Inhalant Allergens in Allergic Rhinitis**

Outdoor

Pollens
Trees (e.g., oak, birch, alder)
Grasses (e.g., timothy, orchard, bermuda)
Weeds (e.g., ragweed, plantain)
Molds (e.g., *Alternaria, Cladosporium*)

Indoor

Dust mites
Cats
Dogs
Cockroaches
Molds (e.g., *Aspergillus, Penicillium*)
Laboratory animals

nied by the release of most but not all of the acute-phase mediators as well as by the influx of eosinophils, neutrophils, lymphocytes, and basophils. Cellular activation results in a subacute inflammatory reaction, which can last for a longer period. Changes in the function of the nasal mucosa take place, the most important being the development of hyper-reactivity. This hyper-reactivity is of a nonspecific nature (reactivity against nonallergic environmental stimuli) and explains why patients with allergic rhinitis also complain of symptoms when exposed to irritants such as tobacco smoke, chemicals, and perfumes. Also, mucosal changes lower the threshold for subsequent allergen activation (priming effect), causing symptoms with much less allergen exposure. This may explain why patients continue to have symptoms at the end of the pollen season, when pollen counts are significantly decreased. The major allergens responsible for the symptoms of allergic rhinitis are shown in Table 1.

DIAGNOSIS

The diagnosis is usually established by a thorough history and can be confirmed with either skin or blood tests. Physical examination, although important in evaluating complications of allergic rhinitis, is rarely helpful in establishing the diagnosis. Table 2 shows a number of conditions that can produce symptoms that mimic allergic rhinitis.

History

The patient usually presents with nasal congestion, rhinorrhea, recurrent sneezing, and pruritus of the upper

TABLE 2. **Causes of Chronic Nasal and Sinus Symptoms**

Allergic rhinitis (seasonal, perennial)
Nonallergic, noninfectious, chronic rhinitis
Nonallergic rhinitis with eosinophilia syndrome (NARES)
Sinusitis
Infectious rhinitis (bacterial, fungal)
Rhinitis medicamentosa (caused by topical decongestants)
Drug-induced rhinitis (aspirin, oral contraceptives, beta blockers, reserpine)
Anatomic abnormalities (septal deviation, septal spurs, concha bullosa)
Obstructive lesions (polyps, hypertrophic adenoids, tumors)
Endocrine causes (hypothyroidism, pregnancy, menstruation)
Granulomatous diseases (Wegener's granulomatosis, sarcoidosis)

respiratory passages. Most of the patients also have associated ocular symptoms such as tearing, redness, and pruritus of the eyes. Less common symptoms include ear "popping," posterior nasal drainage, throat clearing, and chronic cough. In fact, rhinitis is considered the most common cause of chronic cough in adults. Chronic sufferers may complain of malaise and fatigue. Pruritus and sneezing are the most characteristic symptoms of allergic rhinitis and should be helpful in the differential diagnosis of other rhinitis syndromes.

The interviewer should clarify whether the patient's symptoms are perennial and/or seasonal and how they are affected by seasonal changes. In seasonal allergic rhinitis (hay fever or rose fever), there is a temporal relationship between exposure to particular antigens, usually pollen or molds, and the occurrence of symptoms. The age of onset, the severity and progression of symptoms are important elements of the history. Early onset of rhinitis indicates very high probability of allergic etiology. Of all patients whose chronic rhinitis begins at an age younger than 10, more than 90% have allergic disease. In contrast, of patients whose rhinitis begins at an age older than 40, a nonallergic etiology is diagnosed in close to 60%.

Exacerbating factors such as cutting grass, raking leaves, weather changes, animal contact, dust, and so forth should be identified. An assessment of the home and work environment—school environment for children—is also important in allergic diseases. The patient should be asked about his or her living conditions, the type and age of the mattress and pillow used, and the decor in the bedroom. The presence of pets in the house, and especially in the bedroom, should also be assessed. Exposure to animal material, indoor dust, and molds at the workplace can be important. It is of particular importance to be able to identify any temporary environmental changes related to the onset or worsening of symptoms. Frequently, however, especially when the problem is related to pets, the patient denies any symptomatic association. Although this may reflect the patient's psychology, it must also be recognized that continuous exposure to an allergen versus sudden exposure to a high dose may present with a different (more subtle, albeit chronic) clinical picture.

Past medical history as well as current medication use should be evaluated, as they can provide important diagnostic clues. Some forms of nonallergic rhinitis can be caused by pharmacologic agents (topical decongestant sprays, some antihypertensives) or by systemic illnesses, including autoimmune disease or vasculitis and granulomatous disorders. Family history of any atopic diseases should be elicited. This enhances the confidence of a history-based diagnosis. The most important historic elements for the differential diagnosis of allergic rhinitis are summarized in Table 3.

Diagnostic Testing

To confirm the diagnosis of allergic rhinitis, laboratory tests can be performed, with the goal of establishing the presence of specific IgE antibodies against suspected allergens on the patient's skin tissue or in the serum. Because serum IgE is in equilibrium with the clinically important mast cell and basophil-bound IgE, serum testing is a viable alternative to the "gold standard," which continues to be skin testing. When skin testing or serum testing is performed, careful selection of the material to be tested needs to be done to include all relevant allergens, depending on the geographic location and the patient's environment. The interpretation of allergy tests should take into account

TABLE 3. Diagnostic Clues to Differentiate Allergic from Nonallergic Rhinitis

Temporal relationship between symptom onset, duration, and seasonal or environmental changes (moving to a new location, acquiring a pet) is suggestive of allergic rhinitis
Sneezing, nasal pruritus, and associated conjunctival symptoms are characteristic of allergic rhinitis
Allergic triggers (pollen, dust, molds, pets) suggest allergic rhinitis; nonspecific irritants (perfumes, tobacco smoke, cold or dry air) suggest nonallergic disease
Age of onset: the earlier the onset, the more likely that allergies are involved
Personal or family history of rhinitis, asthma, or eczema: more likely to identify patients with allergic rhinitis

the patient's history. For example, if the patient does not complain of food-related symptoms, testing for food allergies is of no use.

There are two types of skin tests, puncture (prick) and intradermal. It is safer to start with puncture and then perform intradermal testing if the puncture tests give negative results. Negative skin test results in conjunction with a history of nonspecific aggravating factors such as tobacco, strong odors, paint, or solvents is diagnostic for nonallergic rhinitis. In a general practitioner's office, skin testing is not an option, and the patient must be referred to an allergy specialist. However, serum-specific IgE detection tests (in vitro allergy tests) can be used to partially fulfill the same purpose. The most common such test is the radioallergosorbent test (RAST). RASTs are less sensitive and also more expensive than skin tests. In addition, their results are delayed. However, a screen RAST panel including a major tree pollen (e.g., oak for the northeastern United States), a common grass (e.g., timothy), ragweed, a dust mite, cat and/or dog, cockroach, and possibly a mold (e.g., *Alternaria*) may offer a rough idea of the atopic status of the patient. Skin tests and, therefore, a referral to an allergy specialist may be required if, despite a negative or equivocal RAST panel, the suspicion of allergic rhinitis based on the patient's history is high, or if management with detailed environmental control and/or immunotherapy is indicated; in these cases, testing needs to be more extensive, and the sensitivity of the procedure should be optimal. Still, even in the allergist's practice, in vitro testing may be the only option in patients with skin diseases such as severe eczema or dermatographism, in those who are being treated with antihistamines and cannot discontinue treatment for the required 2- to 5-day period, or in those who have received astemizole for the prior 2 months (astemizole is a nonsedating antihistamine with a very long half-life).

Nasal smears have been used to detect local eosinophilia (greater than five eosinophils per high-power field). This test is suggestive but not diagnostic for allergic rhinitis, since eosinophils can be seen in a syndrome termed nonallergic rhinitis with eosinophilia (NARES). However, nasal eosinophilia predicts a favorable response to treatment with topical intranasal corticosteroids. The presence of neutrophilia without eosinophils in the nasal secretions should point away from allergic rhinitis, because it tends to be indicative of bacterial sinus infection. Blood eosinophilia and total serum IgE are not useful tests for the diagnosis of allergic rhinitis, since they are neither specific nor sensitive. Some patients may have significant levels of specific IgE to a particular allergen (or to a small group of allergens) with normal or even low total serum IgE.

Physical Examination

Physical examination is not very helpful in the diagnosis of allergic rhinitis. A normal examination does not preclude the diagnosis, and mucosal appearances that are different from those described later are frequently observed in allergic rhinitis. In classic cases, examination of the eyes shows mildly hyperemic conjunctivae, with tearing or the presence of a gelatinous exudate. By routine anterior rhinoscopy, the nasal mucosa typically has pale or slightly bluish discoloration, with boggy and edematous turbinates. Various amounts of watery, clear secretions can be observed. Erythematous mucosa with thick, yellow-appearing mucus should raise suspicion for other causes of rhinitis. Anterior rhinoscopy can offer further information regarding the presence of polyps or tumors, as well as anatomic lesions such as septal spurs or septal deviation. Topical decongestant sprays (Afrin, Neo-Synephrine) can be helpful to visualize the posterior structures if the mucosa is severely swollen, with the inferior turbinates touching the septum. Nasal endoscopy (using either a rigid or a flexible rhinopharyngoscope) can be even more helpful in this regard.

In children, darkening under the eyes due to chronic venous pooling can sometimes be observed (allergic shiners). Also, because of frequent rubbing of the nose upward (allergic salute), a characteristic nasal crease may be seen.

MANAGEMENT

Allergen Avoidance

After identification of the offending allergens, avoidance is the first step that should be initiated. It is difficult to completely avoid pollen exposure; however, avoidance of outdoor activities during the peak season of a particular allergen can be helpful. Air-conditioning and keeping the windows closed can effectively reduce pollen levels inside the house. High-efficiency particulate air (HEPA) filters in the main ventilation system can further reduce indoor pollen.

If the patient is allergic to pets, the obvious and most effective environmental control is to remove the pet from the indoor environment. If this is not an acceptable option (as is the case with a significant percentage of such patients) the pet should at least be kept out of the bedroom to minimize allergen accumulation on the bedding and the floors. Actually, removal of carpeting—a major reservoir for most indoor allergens—may be of significant help. Also, transfer of pet allergen into the bedroom can be minimized by removing shoes and possibly clothes prior to entering the room and by frequent carpet vacuuming using a vacuum cleaner equipped with HEPA filters. Obviously, any close contact between the patient and the pet should be minimized. The patient should also be informed that it takes from several weeks to several months after an animal is removed from the environment for the indoor allergens to fall to substantially low levels. This is well documented in the case of cat allergens but should be considered for other pets as well.

Both indoor and outdoor molds can be inducers and triggers of allergic rhinitis. Outdoor molds, most commonly *Alternaria* and *Cladosporium,* are higher in the fall, as the decaying leaves and rotting vegetation provide an excellent material for fungal growth. Patients should avoid activities such as raking leaves, cutting grass, and working in barns or with compost. If this is not feasible, wearing a paper mask or a scarf may provide some protection. *Penicillium* and *Aspergillus,* the most common indoor molds, are more prevalent in basements and damp areas. Indoor relative humidity of 50% or less is an effective way to decrease mold growth. Adequate ventilation and repair of water leaks, as well as care not to overwater indoor plants, help keep humidity under control. In very humid environments (such as in waterfront residences), dehumidifiers can be useful.

Dust mites constitute the most common source of indoor allergen for patients with perennial allergic rhinitis. The gastrointestinal tract of the two species of house dust mites, *Dermatophagoides farinae* and *Dermatophagoides pteronyssinus,* produces allergenic glycoproteins that are released in the environment through the fecal material. Since dust mites feed on the dead skin that humans continually shed, they tend to congregate in mattresses, pillows, carpets, and places where people generally sit or lie. Dust mites also thrive in high-humidity areas such as inside old organic materials. Placing plastic mite-proof covers over the mattresses, box springs, and pillows can result in a significant reduction in dust mite exposure. Patients should avoid using feather pillows and having upholstered furniture in their bedroom. Stuffed animals are a high dust mite reservoir in children's bedrooms and should be removed. Washing the bed sheets, blankets, pillowcases, and comforters in hot water (120° to 140° F) every week is an effective way to kill dust mites. Maintaining an indoor humidity of 50% or less can also slow dust mite growth. Acaricides (benzyl benzoate), substances that kill dust mites, and allergen denaturing chemicals (tannic acid) are relatively effective, but only temporarily. Air filtration devices are not particularly useful in eliminating dust mites, because the particles of decaying body parts and fecal material, where allergens are contained, are relatively heavy and settle quickly on the floor.

Cockroach sensitivity has been recognized as a significant problem in lower socioeconomic status populations who live in inner-city areas. The most common species in the United States are the German cockroach (*Blattella germanica*) and the American cockroach (*Periplaneta americana*). Although several studies have found a significant association between cockroach sensitivity and asthma, the relationship is less clear in allergic rhinitis. Since these conditions often coexist, an attempt to decrease exposure to cockroach allergens should be encouraged. Helpful measures include reducing access to food material and water sources, spraying cockroach runways with 0.5 to 1% diazinon or chlorpyrifos, blowing boric acid powder in nonaccessible areas, or placing bait stations containing hydramethylnon (Combat).

Pharmacologic Intervention

Antihistamines

Antihistamines compete with histamine for the H_1 receptors on specific target cells. They are effective in reducing pruritus, sneezing, tearing, and rhinorrhea, but not nasal congestion. They can be used on an as-needed basis, although they have a better effect if taken before symptoms develop or continuously. The use of the older compounds (first-generation antihistamines) has been limited because of unwanted side effects, mainly sedation. These agents, due to their lipophilic structure, are able to cross the blood-brain barrier and cause central nervous system (CNS) suppression (histamine is an excitatory CNS neurotransmitter). The sedative effect often decreases after continued use for 1 to 2 weeks. Another important side effect is the prolongation of voluntary reaction time, which affects the performance of motor tasks such as driving, job performance, and school work. These drugs also have side effects due to their anticholinergic action, including dry mouth, constipation, blurry vision, and difficulty in urination. They should be avoided in elderly people, especially those with symptomatic benign prostate hypertrophy, bladder neck obstruction, and narrow angle glaucoma.

A new generation of antihistamines was introduced about 10 years ago. These are relatively poor CNS penetrants, and the incidence of sedation is no different from that of placebo (Table 4). They also show no interference with the performance of motor tasks and have no anticholinergic side effects. There is evidence that these compounds have a broader mechanism of action. For some, the ability to inhibit the release of inflammatory mediators from a variety of cells has been documented. Several of the newer antihistamines have longer half-lives and active metabolites, which also prolong their action. This allows them to be administered once or twice daily, thus enhancing patient compliance. The active metabolite of astemizole, methylastemizole, has a half-life of 10 to 12 days. Astemizole (Hismanal), loratadine (Claritin), and terfenadine (Seldane) are metabolized by the

TABLE 4. **Old and New Antihistamines Used for Allergic Rhinitis**

Agent	Dosage
Old	
Chlorpheniramine (Chlor-Trimeton)	4 mg PO 4 to 6 times a day
	8 mg PO tid
	12 mg PO bid
Clemastine (Tavist)	1.34–2.68 mg PO bid
Diphenhydramine (Benadryl)	25–50 mg PO qid
Tripelennamine (PBZ)	25–50 mg PO qid
	100 mg PO bid
New	
Astemizole (Hismanal)	10 mg PO qd
Cetirizine (Zyrtec)	5–10 mg PO qd
Loratadine (Claritin)	10 mg PO qd
Terfenadine (Seldane)	60 mg PO bid

same P-450 hepatic cytochrome system as some antifungals (ketoconazole [Nizoral], fluconazole [Diflucan], itraconazole [Sporanox]) and macrolide antibiotics (erythromycin, clarithromycin [Biaxin], troleandomycin [Tao]); thus, concomitant administration of these agents may elevate serum levels of the antihistamine. This can result in side effects involving the cardiac muscle such as QT prolongation, which could then lead to more serious cardiac adverse effects, including ventricular tachyarrhythmias (torsades de pointes) and sudden death. Cardiovascular side effects have been reported with both astemizole and terfenadine but not with loratadine or cetirizine. Increased awareness of the potential interaction and patient education have been very successful in substantially controlling this problem. It is important to mention that the dose needs to be reduced in patients with hepatic dysfunction, in those who receive medications affecting the QT interval (procainamide), or in those with cardiac dysrhythmias affecting repolarization.

In conclusion, antihistamines are a reasonable choice for intermittent or mild symptoms of allergic rhinoconjunctivitis (first-line agents). In moderate or severe disease, they can be useful adjunct therapy to topical corticosteroids or cromolyn sodium.

Decongestants

Decongestants belong to the alpha-adrenergic agonist family and are effective in the treatment of mucosal congestion, as they can constrict the blood vessels and reduce blood flow to the nasal tissues. They have no significant effects on the other symptoms of rhinitis. Decongestants exist in topical preparations as well as oral forms.

Topical forms include oxymetazoline (Afrin, Nōstrilla), naphazoline (Privine), and phenylephrine (Neo-Synephrine) sprays. Patients should be cautioned not to use these preparations for more than a few (3 to 5) days, because prolonged use can cause rhinitis medicamentosa (tolerance, rebound nasal congestion, and hyperemic nasal mucosa). In the occasional patient who presents with severe nasal swelling, intranasal administration of a topical decongestant for the first few days can facilitate the administration of other sprays such as topical steroids and cromolyn. Topical decongestants are also used to allow visualization of the posterior nasal passages during diagnostic rhinoscopy and to help patients sleep when they experience severe nasal blockage.

Oral decongestants such as pseudoephedrine hydrochloride (Sudafed) and phenylpropanolamine hydrochloride (Entex) can be taken for longer periods than topical preparations, because they do not cause rhinitis medicamentosa. However, alpha-adrenergic agonists can stimulate the CNS and cause nervousness and insomnia. For some patients, it is advisable to avoid them at night. Decongestants can elevate blood pressure, and subjects with hypertension or borderline blood pressure should use them cautiously. Also, decongestants should be avoided in patients with coronary artery disease, with hyperthyroidism, on monoamine oxidase inhibitors, and with seizure disorders.

Oral decongestants are often combined with antihistamines. Given the ineffectiveness of antihistamines in relieving nasal congestion, these preparations are superior to the individual compounds. The usual dose of pseudoephedrine hydrochloride is 60 mg for adults taken every 6 hours. Children 6 to 12 years old should take half of this dose, and those between 2 and 5 years old should take only a quarter of the dose (15 mg) every 6 hours. Twice-a-day preparations (120 mg) also exist.

Guaifenesin

Guaifenesin (Humibid L.A.), originally an expectorant used in preparations aimed toward the lower respiratory tract, is currently an ingredient of numerous prescription and over-the-counter preparations for the treatment of rhinitis. It is formulated either as a single agent or in combination with antihistamines and decongestants. Its mode of action is believed to be the loosening of respiratory secretions by increasing their water content. It is therefore thought to facilitate mucociliary clearance of secretions from the sinus and the nasal mucosa.

The recommended dose of guaifenesin for upper respiratory tract therapy is 1200 mg twice a day. The clinical effect of this compound is quite subtle. It is not clear whether it is beneficial in allergic rhinitis, but it can be tried as adjuvant therapy to any other compound in patients whose rhinitis is complicated by chronic sinus complaints and by posterior nasal drainage of secretions that is refractory to other treatment. Guaifenesin has an excellent safety record.

Ipratropium Bromide

Intranasal ipratropium bromide (Atrovent Nasal Spray 0.03%) is now available for use in allergic rhinitis. This anticholinergic preparation is not absorbed into the circulation, and any atropine-like systemic side effects are minimal to nonexistent.

Ipratropium should be used mainly to control nasal secretions in selected cases in which rhinorrhea is not responding to other preparations. It does not affect the other symptoms of allergic rhinitis. The recommended dose is 2 sprays per nostril two to three times a day. Adjusting the dose can prevent nasal dryness, which is the main side effect.

Cromolyn Sodium

Cromolyn sodium (Nasalcrom) is used as a 4% topical spray for the treatment of allergic rhinitis. Its mode of action is claimed to be through the stabilization of mast cells in the nasal mucosa. However, studies on human mast cells do not strongly support this mechanism. When taken properly (1 to 2 sprays in each nostril four to six times a day), its efficacy is similar to or somewhat better than that of antihistamines. In addition to the symptomatic relief, cromolyn appears to have various anti-inflammatory properties that could be beneficial in the long term. This agent works better if used preventively a couple of weeks before seasonal symptoms begin. Because of its anti-inflammatory action, it takes some time for the effects of cromolyn to become obvious. Cromolyn is not very useful when taken on an as-needed basis. Nasal application is usually well tolerated, and except for mild, transient stinging, no side effects have been reported. Cromolyn is a pregnancy category B agent. Therefore, it is used frequently in pregnant or lactating women. An ophthalmic preparation of cromolyn (Crolom) is available to be used for the treatment of allergic conjunctivitis. This form also needs frequent dosing—1 to 2 drops in each eye four to six times per day.

Glucocorticosteroids

Glucocorticosteroids are the most effective agents for the treatment of allergic rhinitis. Because systemic administration causes a variety of side effects, topical preparations should be used. The use of systemic steroids should be limited to the occasional patient who presents with complete nasal obstruction. Since this condition can cause significant discomfort, with eustachian tube dysfunction and sleep disturbance, a short course of oral corticosteroids (e.g., 40 mg of prednisone for 5 days) is recommended. This type of management is meaningful, however, only when it is offered in parallel with the initiation of a topical steroid preparation. Oral steroids should not be used as a substitute for topical preparations.

The potency of topical corticosteroids is higher compared with all other treatment modalities. In fact, topical application is equally effective as, if not more effective than, systemic treatment and is not associated with systemic side effects because the dose is small and the absorption minimal. The number of available topical corticosteroids is increasing (Table 5), and their share of the allergic rhinitis prescription market has risen from 8 to 20% within the past 10 years. The mode of action of glucocorticoids at the cellular level is not fully understood. However, their anti-inflammatory activity in allergic rhinitis has been clearly demonstrated. Topical application of nasal steroids for 1 week inhibits not only the late inflammatory sequelae of acute exposure to allergen (cellular infiltration, increased nasal reactivity to nonallergic stimuli, nasal priming to allergen) but also, surprisingly, the symptoms and the release of

inflammatory mediators of the immediate allergic reaction. The latter effect is believed to be secondary to the ability of local glucocorticoids to reduce the number of mucosal mast cells. This effect is not obtained with systemic steroid treatment.

Patients should be informed that nasal corticosteroids do not result in the rapid responses seen with antihistamines or decongestants and that the drug must be used for at least a few days before significant effects are noticed. Patients should be instructed to place the tip of the apparatus in the middle of the nasal passages and to avoid aiming toward the septum or the inferior turbinate. After each puff is administered, they should sniff slightly to facilitate distribution in other parts of the nasal mucosa.

After a few weeks of treatment, these preparations should provide excellent results in the majority (>80%) of patients with allergic nasal symptoms. At that point, the dose can be adjusted according to the patient's clinical picture. Once-a-day dosing, even below insert recommendations, is often enough to control the disease.

Local side effects are minimal and usually involve irritation of the nasal mucosa. About 10% of patients using intranasal steroids may complain of burning or sneezing after local application. Epistaxis in the form of blood-tinged secretions and, quite rarely, in the form of hemorrhage has been observed in about 2% of patients. Discontinuing the medication for 2 to 3 days and applying a topical ointment such as boric acid (Borofax) on the nasal mucosa usually resolves this problem. Septal perforation has been rarely reported; although the mechanism for this adverse event is unknown, it is important that rhinoscopy be performed prior to the initiation of treatment to rule out the pre-existence of septal mucosal ulcerations that might contraindicate the application of steroids. Prolonged administration of topical steroids has been studied and appears to be a safe option. In one study, beclomethasone (Beconase, Vancenase) administration for 5 years did not cause nasal atrophy in mucosal biopsy specimens. In contrast to inhaled steroids, these compounds very rarely cause nasal or oral candidiasis.

The available preparations are in both aqueous and aerosol form. The decision to use one versus the other is more a matter of patient preference. Aerosol preparations, with the exception of budesonide (Rhinocort), seem to be more irritating to the nasal mucosa, whereas with aqueous preparations, the liquid may drip into the throat, resulting in reduced deposition of active medication in the nasal mucosa.

Some practitioners use intramuscular or intranasal injections of long-acting steroid preparations. Because of the prolonged half-life, these preparations can ameliorate the symptoms of allergic rhinitis during the entire pollen season. However, the risk of side effects—adrenal suppression in intramuscular injections and blindness in intranasal—makes these practices potentially hazardous.

Immunotherapy

Immunotherapy is the only therapy for allergic rhinitis that entails the theoretical potential for cure.

TABLE 5. **Nasal Glucocorticosteroid Preparations**

Drug	Dosage
Beclomethasone diproprionate (Vancenase, Beconase)	1–2 puffs/sprays bid
Budesonide (Rhinocort)	2–4 puffs qd
Dexamethasone sodium phosphate (Dexacort)	2 puffs bid to tid
Flunisolide (Nasalide)	2 sprays bid
Fluticasone (Flonase)	2 sprays qd
Triamcinolone acetonide (Nasacort)	2–4 puffs qd

This involves the administration of specific allergens in an escalated-dose fashion until a target dose (maintenance) is reached. Administration is usually subcutaneous. Approximately 80% of patients have symptomatic improvement with immunotherapy. It is not clear, however, what this percentage is among patients who have failed all other treatments.

The mechanism of action of immunotherapy is still unknown, although several immunologic changes have been observed. Increased serum-specific IgG antiallergen antibodies (which are thought to block the allergen's encounter with mast cell–bound IgE) and the generation of antigen-specific suppressor T cells have been reported. Recently, several studies reported a reduction in "pro-allergic" cytokine (interleukin-4 and interleukin-5) production by lymphocytes and other cells of the immune system and/or promotion of the "antiallergic" (TH$_1$) phenotype of T lymphocytes. TH$_1$ cells characteristically produce interferon-gamma and interleukin-2 upon activation.

Several placebo control trials have documented the efficacy of immunotherapy with a variety of allergens. However, although high doses of allergen extracts are considered better than antihistamines and decongestants and probably similar to topical steroids, low-dose immunotherapy is not better than placebo and should be avoided. Also, allergen immunotherapy is a proven treatment modality only by subcutaneous injections; other methods (oral or intranasal) have not been found to be efficacious or practical. Recently, it has been suggested that sublingual immunotherapy may be an effective form of treatment, but more studies are needed to confirm this. Usually, immunotherapy starts at extremely low concentrations of allergen; injections are given once or twice weekly for 4 to 6 months until a maintenance dose is reached, and then every 2 to 4 weeks. Therapy should be offered for 1 year before a firm evaluation of efficacy is performed. If therapy has been successful, at least 5 years of treatment are recommended. After that, a decision whether to discontinue treatment has to be made. Unfortunately, this decision can be based only on intuition rather than on scientific evidence, because there is no way to predict the outcome of immunotherapy discontinuation. The beneficial effects can be sustained for a long time in some patients, but in others, symptoms recur soon after discontinuation of the injections.

We tend to reserve immunotherapy for patients not responding to pharmacologic therapy or those who have significant side effects from the drugs. Also, some patients have a preference for immunotherapy because of its appealing "natural" form of treatment. The patient needs to be presented with the risks and benefits of this treatment. Although local reactions at the site of injection are frequent, they are easily controlled. Systemic reactions occur infrequently and may require the use of epinephrine and intravenous fluid support. Adjustment of the allergen dose in patients with even mild systemic reactions is important, and immunotherapy should

TABLE 6. **Summary of Recommended Therapeutic Regimens for Allergic Rhinitis**

Mild disease:	As-needed antihistamines and decongestants
Moderate disease:	Continuous cromolyn or topical steroids and as-needed antihistamines and decongestants
Severe disease:	Continuous topical steroids, immunotherapy, and as-needed antihistamines and decongestants
Difficult to control rhinorrhea:	Ipratropium bromide
Thick secretions:	Guaifenesin

be administered only by practitioners trained in the management of anaphylaxis.

Table 6 summarizes our recommendations with respect to available therapies in allergic rhinitis.

ALLERGIC REACTIONS TO DRUGS AND BIOLOGIC AGENTS

method of
RICHARD D. deSHAZO, M.D.
University of South Alabama
Mobile, Alabama

Allergic and other immunologic reactions to drugs are a major problem, as they account for 6 to 10% of all adverse drug reactions (ADRs). Estimates of hospitalizations resulting from ADRs range from less than 1 to 30% of nonsurgical inpatients. Success in the management of patients with ADRs depends on familiarity with several issues discussed in this article.

CLASSIFICATION OF DRUG REACTIONS AND THEIR PATTERNS

ADRs are conveniently divided into Type A, predictable adverse reactions that can occur in any patient, and Type B, unpredictable adverse reactions that occur only in susceptible patients (Table 1). Such predictable reactions are related to known pharmacologic actions of a drug, are frequently dose dependent, and account for 80% or more of ADRs. Overdosage is a characteristic but excessive pharmacologic effect of a drug caused by administration of larger than recommended doses. Side effects are excessive degrees of the known, usually primary effects of the drug, occurring at usual dosages. Secondary effects are pharmacologic effects that occur as an indirect consequence of the primary drug action but are not related to overdosage, idiosyncrasy, hypersensitivity, or intolerance. Interactions are unusual pharmacologic effects due to two or more drugs acting simultaneously. These reactions are special problems in older patient populations, in which pharmacokinetics and pharmacodynamics are naturally altered.

Unpredictable adverse reactions (Type B) include drug intolerance, idiosyncratic, and allergic or pseudoallergic reactions. Except for intolerance, these reactions are unrelated to a drug's pharmacologic actions and tend to be independent of dose. Intolerance occurs when a pharmacologic effect occurs at a much lower dose of the drug than is

TABLE 1. **Classification of Adverse Drug Reactions with Examples**

Type A: Common and Predictable Adverse Reactions

I. Effects of overdosage: seizures secondary to theophylline
II. Side effects—immediate or delayed: sedation with antihistamines
III. Secondary or indirect effects
    A. Related to drug alone: diarrhea from disturbance of bacterial flora
    B. Related to both disease and drug: maculopapular rash from ampicillin with viral infection
IV. Drug interactions: bleeding with simultaneous use of warfarin and cimetidine

Type B: Uncommon and Unpredictable Reactions

I. Intolerance: tinnitus due to small doses of aspirin
II. Idiosyncratic reaction: coumarin-induced skin necrosis with protein-C deficiency
III. Hypersensitivity (immunologic) reaction including allergic (anaphylaxis to penicillin) or pseudoallergic (anaphylactoid reaction to iodinated contrast dye) reactions

Adapted from Borda IT, Slone D, Jick H: Assessment of adverse reactions within a drug surveillance program. JAMA *205*:645–647, 1968, copyright 1968, American Medical Association; and Rawlins MD, Thompson W: Mechanisms of adverse drug reactions. *In* Davies DM (ed): Textbook of Adverse Drug Reactions. New York, Oxford University Press, 1991, pp 18–45, by permission of Oxford University Press.

usually the case. Idiosyncratic reactions are uncharacteristic responses to a drug that are unrelated to its pharmacologic actions. They may be difficult to separate from immunologic reactions to drugs.

Hypersensitivity reactions, also called immunologic and allergic reactions, are immunologically mediated and have special characteristics that are useful in their identification. They occur in small numbers of patients, require previous exposure to the same drug for sensitization, develop rapidly on re-exposure, and resemble common clinical patterns of hypersensitivity. The most common pattern of drug hypersensitivity is anaphylaxis, one of several patterns of ADR involving multiple organ systems (Table 2). Anaphylaxis is an acute allergic reaction, manifested by combinations of urticaria, angioedema, hypotension, bronchospasm, diarrhea, and cardiac arrhythmia, that reflects IgE-dependent (anaphylactic) or IgE-independent (anaphylactoid, pseudoallergic) mast cell mediator release. Other patterns of ADR may reflect only a single organ system, most often the skin.

APPROACH TO ADR IN A PATIENT ON MULTIPLE DRUGS

Management of a patient who experiences a drug reaction while receiving multiple drugs may be difficult. The most recently administered drug is frequently the culprit, but drugs administered more than 2 weeks previously can cause delayed-onset reactions, such as serum sickness. The clinical goal is to facilitate resolution of the reaction while determining the drug responsible and the type of reaction, if possible. The approach outlined in Figure 1 consists of discontinuing all but essential drugs and then postulating the most likely drug causing the reaction. The most likely drug is identified on the basis of the reaction pattern outlined in Table 2. For instance, the drugs most likely to cause multisystem reactions

are antibiotics (including antituberculosis and antifungal drugs), diuretics, anticonvulsants, allopurinol, coumarin, heparin, oral hypoglycemics, and antiarrhythmic agents. The occurrence of ADRs in patients on multiple drugs provides an opportunity to review the patient's therapy and eliminate nonessential drugs.

Diagnostic Testing and Desensitization for Drug Allergy

Eighty percent of anaphylactic reactions to drugs are to beta-lactam antibiotics. Most drugs that successfully pass through clinical trials either have molecular weights too low (<1000) to be effective antigens or have molecular structures that prevent their conjugation with the carrier molecules necessary to form antigenic hapten-carrier complexes. Beta-lactam antibiotics are an exception, as disruption of the beta-lactam ring produces reactive groups that readily haptenate to form complete antigens. Other drugs that cause hypersensitivity reactions often do so by generation of a metabolite that is a more effective hapten than the parent compound.

Clinical testing for drug hypersensitivity is limited due to the fact that most drugs are unable to function as antigens in diagnostic testing systems. However, immediate hypersensitivity skin tests and, in some cases, the in vitro surrogate of these skin tests, the radioallergosorbent test (RAST), have been used to detect the presence of IgE antibody to aid in risk assessment for allergic reactions to a few drugs and biologic agents. These drugs include penicillin, some other beta-lactam antibiotics, insulin, measles-mumps-rubella (MMR) vaccine, tetanus toxoid, heterologous sera (e.g., diphtheria antiserum, snake venom antiserum), chymopapain, streptokinase, protamine, and some quaternary ammonium muscle relaxants (e.g., suxamethonium). Skin testing is more sensitive, more specific, quicker, and less expensive than RAST for drug allergy. Allergy skin tests to drugs are read 15 minutes after the test is performed. When the prick skin test method is used, tests are read positive when wheal sizes are equal to or greater than those of the positive histamine control. Drug skin tests are performed by making epicutaneous needle pricks through drops of dilute concentrations of the drug of interest. Appropriate positive (histamine) and negative (diluent) controls are performed simultaneously.

"Desensitization" protocols may be useful in established cases of drug hypersensitivity to beta-lactam antibiotics, insulin, heterologous sera, MMR vaccine, and tetanus toxoid and in ADR to several other drugs when hypersensitivity has not been established as the operative mechanism (trimethoprim-sulfamethoxazole, furosemide, aspirin, and local anesthetics). Both diagnostic testing and desensitization for drug allergy are best accomplished in consultation with an allergist or other physician with expertise in this area. Informed consent and documentation of the risk/benefit considerations leading to these interven-

TABLE 2. **Representative Organ-Specific Patterns of Adverse Drugs Reactions**

I. Multiple Organ System Pattern

Anaphylactic/anaphylactoid: antimicrobials, proteins, iodinated contrast media, nonsteroidal anti-inflammatory drugs (NSAIDs), ethylene oxide, taxol
Stevens-Johnson syndrome/toxic epidermal necrolysis: sulfonamides, beta-lactam antibiotics, hydantoins, carbamazepine
Hypersensitivity syndrome: anticonvulsants, sulfonamides, allopurinol, dapsone
Serum sickness/vasculitis: proteins, antimicrobials, allopurinol, thiazides, pyrazolones, hydantoins, propylthiouracil
Drug fever: bleomycin, amphotericin B, sulfonamides, beta-lactams, methyldopa, quinidine, procainamide
Drug-induced lupus erythematosus: hydralazine, procainamide, isoniazid, methyldopa, chlorpromazine, quinidine, anticonvulsants

II. Dermatologic Patterns

Urticaria/angioedema: same as for anaphylactic reactions, plus opiates; isolated angioedema: angiotensin-converting enzyme (ACE) inhibitors
Pruritus without urticaria: gold, sulfonamides
Morbilliform rashes: penicillins, sulfonamides, barbiturates, antituberculosis drugs, anticonvulsants, quinidine
Fixed eruption: phenolphthalein, analgesic/antipyretics, barbiturates, beta-lactam antibiotics, sulfonamides, tetracycline
Photoallergic photosensitivity: phenothiazines, sulfonamides, griseofulvin
Phototoxic photosensitivity: tetracyclines, sulfanilamide, chlorpromazine, psoralen
Contact dermatitis: local anesthetics, neomycin, paraben esters, ethylenediamine, antihistamines, mercurials

III. Hepatic Patterns

Cholestasis: macrolides, phenothiazines, hypoglycemics, imipramine, nitrofurantoin
Hepatocellular: valproic acid, halothane, isoniazid, methyldopa, quinidine, nitrofurantoin, phenytoin, sulfonylureas
Granulomatous: quinidine, allopurinol, methyldopa, sulfonamides

IV. Renal Patterns

Nephrosis (membranous glomerulonephritis): gold, captopril, NSAIDs, penicillamine, probenecid, anticonvulsants
Acute interstitial nephritis: beta-lactams (especially methicillin), rifampin, NSAIDs, sulfonamides, captopril, allopurinol

V. Respiratory Patterns

Rhinitis: reserpine, hydralazine, alpha-receptor blockers, anticholinesterases, iodides, levodopa, triethanolamine
Asthma: inhaled proteins (pancreatic extract, psyllium), beta-lactam antibiotics, sulfites, NSAIDs, beta-receptor blockers
Cough: ACE inhibitors
Pulmonary infiltrates with eosinophilia: nitrofurantoin, methotrexate, NSAIDs, sulfonamides, tetracycline, isoniazid
Chronic fibrotic reactions: nitrofurantoin, cytotoxic chemotherapeutics

VI. Hematologic Patterns

Eosinophilia: gold, allopurinol, 5-acetylsalicylic acid, ampicillin, tricyclics, carbamazepine, digitalis, phenytoin
Thrombocytopenia: quinidine, sulfonamides, gold, heparin
Hemolytic anemia (Coombs' positive)
  Hapten-carrier mechanism: penicillin, cisplatin
  "Innocent bystander": sulfonamides, quinines, chlorpromazine, para-aminosalicylic acid
  Drug-induced autoimmune antibodies: methyldopa, penicillin
  Granulocytopenia: sulfasalazine, procainamide, penicillins, phenothiazines

Many but not all of these ADRs have been demonstrated to be immunologically mediated.
Adapted from DeSwarte RD: Drug allergy. *In* Patterson R (ed): Allergic Diseases: Diagnosis and Management, 4th ed. Philadelphia, JB Lippincott, 1993, p 395.

tions are essential because of the substantial risk for ADR during the testing and desensitization process. Personnel familiar with and equipped to treat anaphylaxis must be available throughout the procedure, which should not be undertaken unless the drug is absolutely necessary.

APPROACH TO A PATIENT WITH A HISTORY OF ADR WHO REQUIRES DRUG TREATMENT FOR THE SAME INDICATION

Physicians often see patients with histories of ADRs who require treatment with a drug or drug class to which they claim to have had previous reactions. A systematic approach based on the information discussed earlier is proposed in Figure 2.

First, determine what type of ADR the patient experienced. A detailed history may reveal a poorly characterized reaction without clinically serious features that occurred in the distant past. Such reactions are unlikely to recur. The physician should correct erroneous chart entries and stickers, educate the patient, and make an appropriate note in the medical record documenting the process. More often than not, a patient with a purported drug allergy has had a predictable drug reaction such as a side effect, a common problem in the elderly. In such a case, modification in dose or substitution of a drug within the same drug class may be all that is required. If, after review of the history, a serious reaction on readministration is considered highly unlikely and the patient requires further assurance, the patient may be given an initial small dose under observation. This is best accomplished in a setting where an acute ADR can be adequately treated.

Certain ADRs are not amenable to dose adjustment or immunologic manipulation, including intolerance and idiosyncratic or hypersensitivity reactions associated with dermal blistering (Stevens-Johnson syndrome, toxic epidermal necrolysis), drug fever, or serum sickness. These reactions require that further

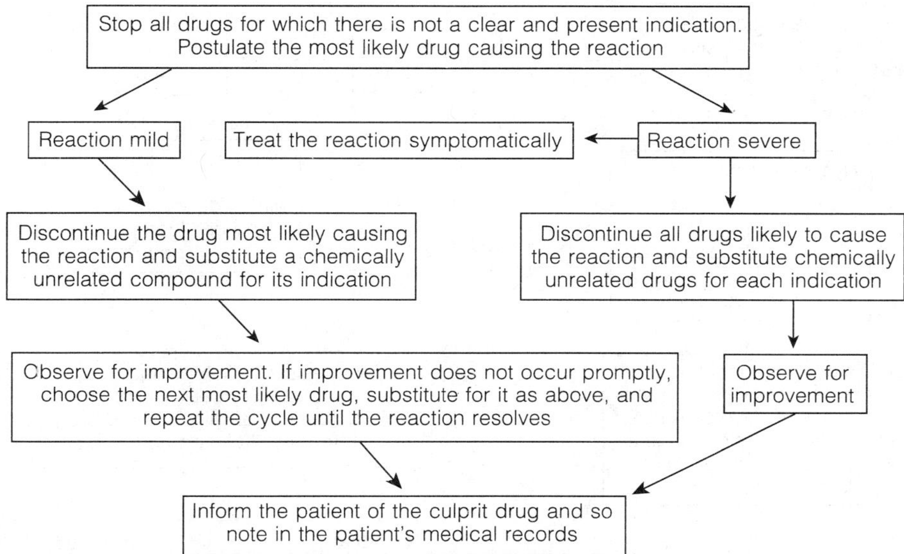

Figure 1. Approach to a patient with a drug reaction while on multiple drugs. (From Smith DL, deShazo RD: Drug reactions. *In* Lichtenstein LM, Fauci AS [eds]: Current Therapy in Allergy, Immunology, and Rheumatology, 5th ed. St. Louis, CV Mosby, 1996.)

administration of the responsible drug and others of the same chemical class be avoided.

As discussed earlier, the indications for skin testing and/or desensitization are limited, as these procedures may result in anaphylaxis. For instance, penicillin skin testing is not required if the patient does not immediately require the drug. A patient with a history of penicillin allergy should be assured that procedures are available to administer this drug, even if anaphylaxis occurred previously, if the drug is absolutely required in the future. If an alternative, structurally unrelated drug is available, that drug may be used without further evaluation. In the absence of a suitable alternative drug and in a patient with a history compatible with an allergic reaction, evaluation usually consists of skin testing for IgE-mediated hypersensitivity. Skin testing is most often followed immediately by a challenge procedure, if negative, or desensitization, if positive.

Skin Testing Followed by a Combination Skin Test–Challenge

Skin testing followed by graduated challenge (often an abbreviated desensitization) has been reported to

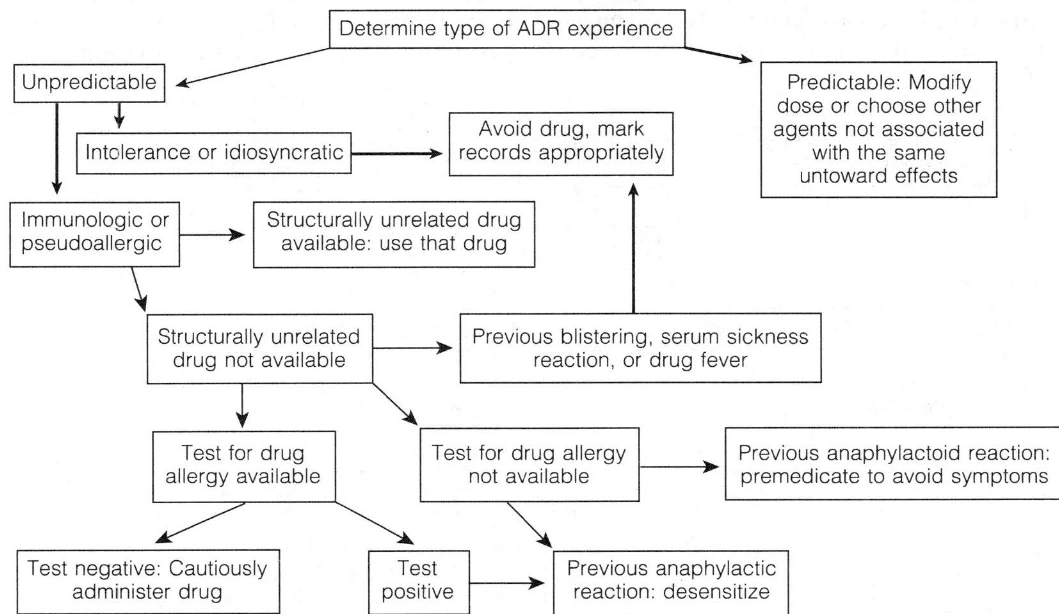

Figure 2. Approach to a patient with a previous adverse drug reaction (ADR) who requires treatment for the same indication. (From Smith DL, deShazo RD: Drug reactions. *In* Lichtenstein LM, Fauci AS [eds]: Current Therapy in Allergy, Immunology, and Rheumatology, 5th ed. St. Louis, CV Mosby, 1996.)

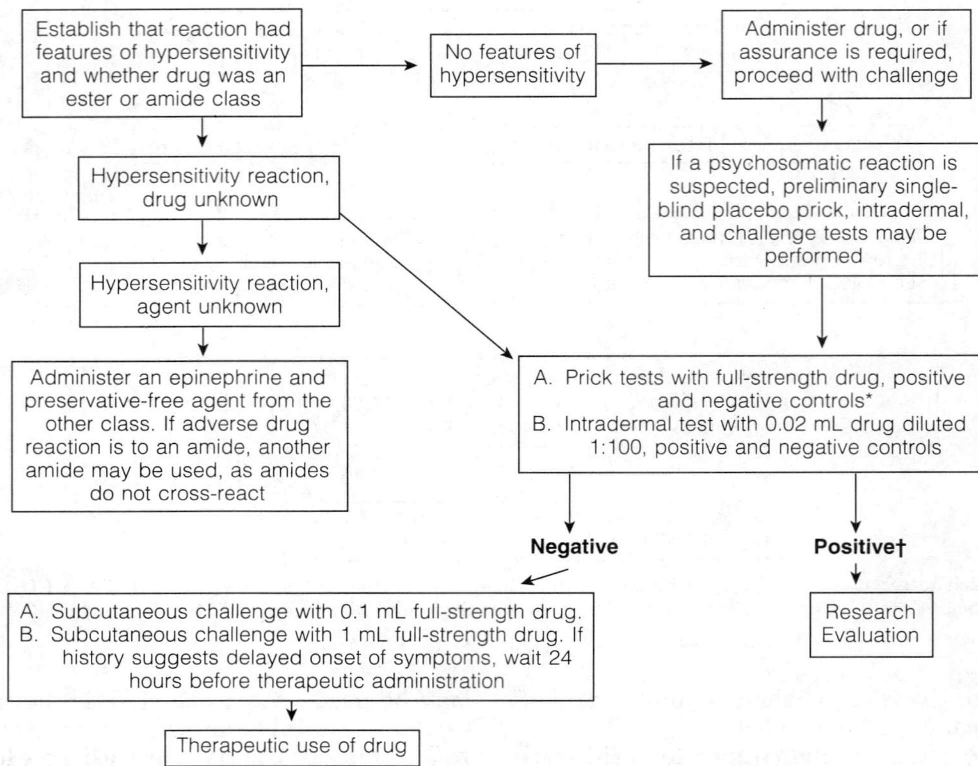

Figure 3. Method of skin testing and provocative dose challenge for local anesthetics. *Positive control is histamine phosphate 10 mg/mL; negative control is phosphate buffered saline. †Rarely occurs at this dilution. (Adapted from deShazo RD, Nelson HS: An approach to the patient with a history of local anesthetic hypersensitivity. Experience with 90 patients. J Allergy Clin Immunol *63:*387, 1979.)

be useful in the management of patients with purported reactions to local anesthetics (Figure 3), tetanus toxoid (Figure 4), and several other agents when administration of these agents is essential. Local anesthetic reactions are rarely, if ever, immunologically mediated and are usually easily identifiable as vasovagal or psychosomatic. Testing and challenge/desensitization to MMR, yellow fever, and influenza vaccines (Figure 5) may be undertaken in patients with clinical allergy to (unable to eat) eggs but is not required merely because of a positive skin test to egg. Recent reports suggest that children with severe egg allergy may safely receive MMR without such a procedure. Package inserts for heterologous serums

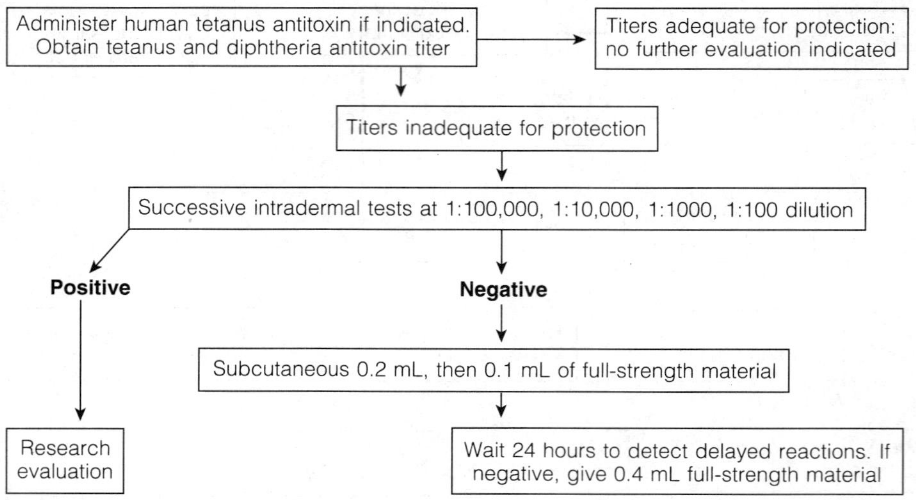

Figure 4. Skin test–challenge procedure for patients with possible hypersensitivity to tetanus-diphtheria toxoid. (Adapted from Jacobs RL, Lowe RS, Lanier BQ: Adverse reactions to tetanus toxoid. JAMA *247:*40–42, 1982. Copyright 1982, American Medical Association.)

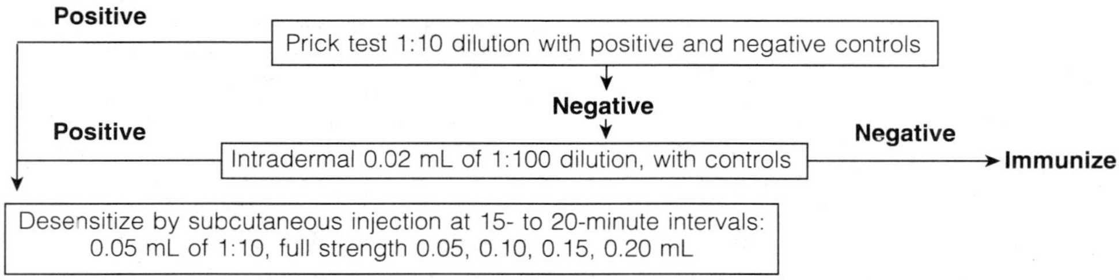

Figure 5. Skin test–challenge procedure for patients with possible sensitivity to measles-mumps-rubella (MMR), influenza, or yellow fever vaccines. (Adapted from Peter G [ed]: Report of the Committee on Infectious Diseases, 22d ed. Elk Grove Village, IL, American Academy of Pediatrics, 1994, pp 36–37.)

(antivenin) give appropriate procedures for skin testing and challenge with these agents. A positive skin test for beta-lactam antibiotics and proteins such as insulin is often followed by desensitization.

Desensitization When Skin Testing Is Not Informative

Desensitization to a limited number of drugs has been successful when skin testing is not available or is uninformative. Most regimens for the prevention of repeat anaphylactic reactions, such as that for aminoglycosides, give a doubling dose every 15 to 20 minutes so that a full therapeutic dose has been given after 3 to 8 hours. The patient usually remains desensitized as long as the drug is administered at least every 12 hours, but if therapy is interrupted, desensitization may have to be repeated. Trimethoprim-sulfamethoxazole (discussed later) is another drug in this category.

Nonsteroidal anti-inflammatory drugs (NSAIDs), including aspirin, may cause asthmatic or anaphylactoid reactions. An oral aspirin challenge and desensitization protocol has allowed the administration of NSAIDs to asthmatic patients, including those with rheumatoid arthritis who require these drugs. Desensitization for urticarial and anaphylactoid reactions to NSAIDs has not been successful.

Premedication Regimens

Premedication is not routinely used in desensitization procedures, because clinical evidence of a developing allergic reaction is used to determine the rate at which desensitization proceeds. However, if the original reaction was anaphylactoid in nature, premedication may minimize or prevent symptoms on readministration. For instance, premedication with corticosteroid and antihistamines has been shown to reduce the reaction rate to iodinated radiocontrast media to less than 5% (Figure 6) and may be similarly effective for other anaphylactoid reactions such as those to taxol.

SPECIAL PROBLEMS IN DRUG HYPERSENSITIVITY

Penicillin and Other Beta-Lactam Antibiotics

Although the majority of patients with histories of penicillin allergy do not experience reactions on subsequent penicillin administration, beta-lactam antibiotics are the most common cause of drug anaphylaxis, which occurs in 0.7 to 10% of individuals receiving them. Thus, if a patient claims to have penicillin allergy, it is prudent to assume that the patient is allergic until proved otherwise. It appears that the more distant the history of previous allergic reaction, the lower the risk for anaphylaxis on readministration. For instance, positive immediate hypersensitivity skin tests to penicillin decrease at a rate of 10% per year after an allergic reaction.

Ninety-five percent of penicillin is metabolized to the penicilloyl metabolite called the major haptenic

Prednisone 50 mg PO or hydrocortisone 200 mg IV 13, 7, and 1 hour before radiocontrast procedure

plus

Diphenhydramine 50 mg PO or IV, 1 hour before procedure

plus

Ephedrine 25 mg PO, 1 hour before procedure (may be withheld in patient with contraindication such as angina)

plus

Use lower osmolarity radiocontrast media, e.g., iopamidol or iohexol

Figure 6. Combination regimen to prevent reactions to radiocontrast agents in patients with previous reactions. (Adapted from Greenberger PA, Patterson R: The prevention of immediate generalized reactions to radiocontrast media in high-risk patients. J Allergy Clin Immunol 87:867, 1991.)

TABLE 3. **Beta-Lactam Antibiotic Skin Tests**

Skin Test Reagents	Route	Dilution	Dose
Penicilloyl-polylysine (Pre-Pen)	Prick	Full strength	1 drop
	Intradermal	Full strength	0.02 mL
Penicillin G potassium (fresh—1 wk old)	Prick	10,000 U/mL	1 drop
	Intradermal	10,000 U/mL	0.02 mL
	Serial (optional)	10, 100, 1000 U/mL	0.02 mL each
Penicillin minor determinant mix	Prick	10^{-2} mol/L	1 drop
	Intradermal	10^{-2} mol/L	0.02 mL
	Serial (optional)	10, 100, 1000 U/mL	0.02 mL each
Other penicillins or cephalosporins	Prick	0.05, 0.1, 0.5, 1.0 mg/mL (serial tests)	1 drop each
(optional and investigational)	Intradermal	0.1, 0.5, 1.0 mg/mL (serial tests)	0.02 mL each

Modified from Anderson JA: Allergic reactions to drugs and biological agents. JAMA *268*:2845–2857, 1992, Copyright 1992, American Medical Association.

determinant. This major determinant, bound to a polylysine carrier, is commercially available as Pre-Pen. Other metabolites, termed minor determinants, including penicilloate and penilloate, are also effective haptens but are not available commercially for diagnostic testing.

Reactions to penicillin are classified as immediate when they occur within 1 hour of administration (anaphylaxis), accelerated (usually urticaria) when they occur within 1 to 72 hours, and late when they occur after 72 hours. (Treatment of allergic reactions is discussed elsewhere in this text.) The probability of immediate or accelerated reactions on readministration of penicillin in patients with previous reactions can be determined by specialized skin testing with major determinant, minor determinant mixture (available in research centers), and penicillin G (Table 3). Positive immediate hypersensitivity skin tests to minor determinant are more closely associated with a risk for anaphylaxis, although these reactions may occur in the presence of IgE (positive skin test or RAST) only to the major determinant. The ability of these skin tests to predict immediate and accelerated allergic reactions to penicillin approaches 97% for major determinant plus penicillin G and 99% for major determinant plus minor determinant.

The great majority of patients who have no evidence of penicillin allergy fail to experience reactions to semisynthetic penicillins and cephalosporins. However, patients occasionally develop IgE antibody to non–beta-lactam side chain antigenic determinants of these antibiotics. In such cases, patients may have amoxicillin or cephalosporin allergy without concomitant allergy to penicillin G. These patients, as well as those with late reactions to penicillin, may not be identified by skin testing with penicillin major and minor determinants and penicillin G. Thus, administration of penicillin to patients with previous histories of allergic reactions to penicillin and negative skin tests must be done with caution and in a setting where anaphylaxis can be expeditiously and appropriately treated. Up to 16% of patients with histories of previous allergic reactions to penicillin, negative skin tests, and no reaction on penicillin administration convert to positive penicillin skin tests after a course of a beta-lactam antibi-

otic. Therefore, repeat skin testing of such patients after uncomplicated therapy with a beta-lactam antibiotic should be considered prior to readministration.

The true incidence of ADR to beta-lactam antibiotics in penicillin-allergic patients is not clear. All beta-lactam antibiotics (penicillins, cephalosporins, monobactams, carbapenems, oxacephems, and clavams) contain the characteristic four-member beta-lactam ring, which, except for monobactams, is fused to a second five- or six-member ring (Table 4). All except the clavams contain a side chain joined to the beta-lactam ring, and some cephalosporins, carbapenems, and oxacephems contain a side chain joined to the second ring. High levels of immunologic cross-reactivity exist between penicillin and the carbapenems (imipenem); lesser degrees of cross-reactivity exist with cephalosporins, and there is the least degree of cross-reactivity with monobactams (aztreonam). Estimates of cross-reactivity between penicillin and

TABLE 4. **Antibiotics Belonging to the Six Beta-Lactam-Containing Groups**

Penicillins	Cephalosporins
Penicillin G	Cephalothin (Keflin)
Penicillin V	Cefazolin (Ancef)
Methicillin (Staphcillin)	Cephaloridine*
Oxacillin (Prostaphlin)	Cephalexin (Keflex)
Cloxacillin (Tegopen)	Cephradine (Velosef)
Nafcillin (Unipen)	Cefadroxil (Duricef)
Ampicillin (Omnipen)	Cefamandole (Mandol)
Amoxicillin	Cefuroxime (Zinacef)
Carbenicillin (Geocillin)	Cefonicid (Monocid)
Ticarcillin (Ticar)	Cefotetan (Cefotan)
Azlocillin*	Ceforanide*
Mezlocillin (Mezlin)	Cefotaxime (Claforan)
Piperacillin (Pipracil)	Ceftixozime (Cefizox)
Propicillin*	Ceftriazone (Rocephin)
Monobactams	Cefoperazone (Cefobid)
Aztreonam (Azactam)	Ceftazidime (Fortaz)
Carbapenems	**Clavams**
Imipenem	Clavulanic acid
	Oxacephems
	Moxalactam (Moxam)

*Not available in the United States.
Adapted from Blanca M, Vega JM, Garcia J, et al: New aspects of allergic reactions to beta lactams: Crossreactions and unique specificities. Clin Exp Allergy *24*:407–415, 1994.

cephalosporins range from 10% for first-generation cephalosporins to 1 to 3% for third-generation cephalosporins.

Skin testing with cephalosporin antibiotics should be considered experimental, as the minor haptenic determinants of these drugs are unknown. Thus, penicillin-sensitive patients are not routinely skin tested with cephalosporins prior to administration. If cephalosporins are given to penicillin-allergic patients, the first dose is best given under observation. Figure 7 outlines an approach to managing a patient requiring antibiotic treatment with a beta-lactam drug who has had a previous allergic reaction to penicillin.

Insulin

Allergic reactions to insulin, although uncommon, require prompt attention. Local reactions that occur at the site of insulin injection are most common and may be immediate (within 1 hour of injection), late (6 to 12 hours after injection), or biphasic (immediate and late) in timing. They tend to resolve spontaneously with continued insulin usage. Since the size of these reactions appears to be related to the insulin dose, local reactions are usually attenuated by decreasing the dose or dividing the dose for administration at multiple sites. Local reactions may be harbingers of systemic (anaphylactic) reactions to insulin. For that reason, individuals with these reactions should be trained to use epinephrine (EpiPen auto-injector) in the event that symptoms of anaphylaxis occur.

Anaphylactic (systemic) insulin hypersensitivity is usually manifested by a large local reaction at the site of insulin injection followed by generalized urticaria and angioedema. Exclusion of other causes of anaphylaxis and demonstration of IgE to insulin are central to the diagnosis. A positive intradermal skin test (wheal and flare reaction within 15 minutes)

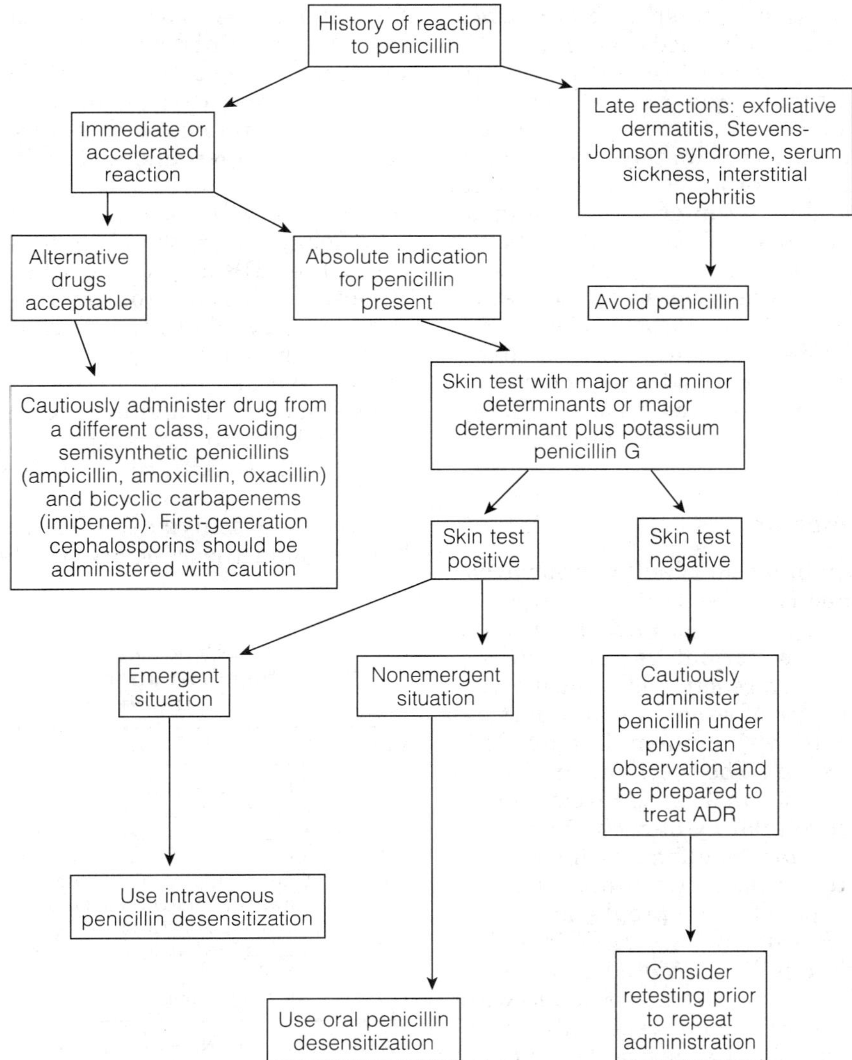

Figure 7. Approach to managing a patient requiring antibiotic treatment with a beta-lactam drug who has had a previous allergic reaction to penicillin.

TABLE 5. **Insulin Desensitization**

Day	Time	Route	Type*	Units†
1	A.M.	ID	Reg	0.00001
	Noon	ID	Reg	0.0001
	P.M.	ID	Reg	0.001
2	A.M.	ID	Reg	0.01
	Noon	ID	Reg	0.1
	P.M.	ID	Reg	1.0
3	A.M.	ID	Reg	2.0
	Noon	SC	Reg	4.0
	P.M.	SC	Reg	8.0
4	A.M.	SC	Reg	12.0
	Noon	SC	Reg	16.0
5	A.M.	SC	NPH/Lente	20.0
6	A.M.	SC	NPH/Lente	25.0
≥7	A.M.	SC	NPH/Lente	Increase 5 U/day until reaching therapeutic level

*Reg indicates regular crystalline zinc insulin; NPH/Lente, long-acting insulin.
†The starting dose may be modified by the patient's insulin sensitivity, based on skin testing, 24 to 48 hours after start of severe reaction.
Abbreviations: ID, intradermal; SC, subcutaneous.
Anderson JA, Adkinson NF Jr: Allergic reactions to drugs and biologic agents. JAMA *258*:2891–2899, 1987. Copyright 1987, American Medical Association.

with 1 U of insulin (0.02 cc of a 50 U/mL solution) is effective in demonstrating insulin-specific IgE. Once the diagnosis has been established, patients with urticaria alone frequently respond to cutting the insulin dose in half, with subsequent small increases in total dose on a daily basis. In urgent situations when insulin is required immediately, more rapid intravenous desensitization protocols may be utilized (Table 5). Since repeated interrupted courses of insulin increase the risk for anaphylaxis, insulin should not be discontinued for long intervals, and desensitization should be performed as soon as possible after insulin allergy develops. The syndrome of systemic insulin allergy and the desensitization process itself may be associated with severe allergic reactions. Therefore, patients with suspected insulin allergy are best hospitalized for diagnosis and treatment.

Sulfonamides

Co-trimoxazole, a combination of sulfamethoxazole and trimethoprim (Bactrim, Septra), is the most widely used sulfonamide antibiotic. Idiosyncratic reactions, including bullous dermatitis, preclude its further use. A more common reaction is a maculopapular rash occurring in 3.4% of recipients and in more than half of individuals with human immunodeficiency virus (HIV) infection. The mechanism of such maculopapular reactions is unclear. Hydroxylamine metabolites with direct cellular cytotoxicity and antibody responses to the sulfa N^4-sulfonamethoxyl moiety have been suggested to be contributory. The fact that co-trimoxazole is an effective prophylactic and therapeutic agent for *Pneumocystis carinii* infection in HIV-infected individuals has resulted in a series of attempts to readminister the drug to patients with previous maculopapular reactions, especially when dapsone is not an acceptable alternative treatment. One such desensitization protocol is outlined in

Table 6, and similar regimens have been suggested for sulfadiazine. When treatment with these drugs is essential, administration of corticosteroids and antihistamines may attenuate febrile and maculopapular eruptions that occur during desensitization.

Another sulfonamide, sulfasalazine (Azulfidine), contains sulfapyridine and aminosalicylic acid joined by a diazo bond. About 2% of patients treated for inflammatory bowel disease with this drug develop a maculopapular rash, drug fever, or both. In most cases, the ADR is caused by the sulfapyridine moiety. A desensitization protocol has been described for such patients. Since the therapeutic moiety in sulfasalazine is acetylsalicylic acid (ASA), treatment with one of several special preparations of ASA available allows successful administration in 90% of patients with ADRs to sulfasalazine. Individuals who develop ADRs to these ASA compounds are most likely ASA allergic.

Patients with hypersensitivity to sulfonamide antibiotics could theoretically be allergic to thiazide di-

TABLE 6. **Protocol for Desensitization to Trimethoprim-Sulfamethoxazole (TMP–SMX) (Bactrim, Septra)**

Day	Dose	TMP–SMX
1	1 mL of 1:20 pediatric suspension	0.4/2 mg
2	2 mL of 1:20 pediatric suspension	0.8/4 mg
3	4 mL of 1:20 pediatric suspension	1.6/8 mg
4	8 mL of 1:20 pediatric suspension	3.2/16 mg
5	1 mL of undiluted pediatric suspension	8/40 mg
6	2 mL of pediatric suspension	16/80 mg
7	4 mL of pediatric suspension	32/160 mg
8	8 mL of pediatric suspension	64/320 mg
9	1 tablet	80/400 mg
10	1 double-strength tablet	160/800 mg

Adapted from Absar N, Daneshvar H, Beall G: Desensitization to trimethoprim/sulfamethoxazole in HIV-infected patients. J Allergy Clin Immunol *93*:1001, 1994.

uretics, furosemide (Lasix), sulfonylurea, hypoglycemic agents, chlorthalidone (Hygroton), and diazoxide, all of which contain variants of the para-aminobenzoic acid ring. However, case reports of such cross-sensitivity are rare.

ACKNOWLEDGMENT

The author wishes to thank Mark Gillespie, Ph.D., for his review of this manuscript and Lesley R. Dupuy for editorial assistance.

ALLERGIC REACTIONS TO INSECT STINGS

method of
HOWARD J. SCHWARTZ, M.D.
Case Western Reserve University School of Medicine and University Suburban Health Center Cleveland, Ohio

An estimated 0.4 to 4% of the general population is believed to be allergic to the venom of stinging insects. These insects, of the order Hymenoptera, include bees, wasps, hornets, yellow jackets, and fire ants. They are widely distributed throughout the world and are responsible for an estimated 100 to 150 deaths in the United States each year as a result of insect sting anaphylaxis.

Hymenoptera insect venoms are complex mixtures of enzymes, peptides, and biogenic amines that have toxic effects on tissues due to their inherent biologic activities. Thus, the "normal" reaction at a sting site is local swelling, redness, pain, itching, and local heat. Normally, these signs and symptoms are localized to the sting site and resolve within a day. Local therapy, including cold compresses and soothing lotions, are ordinarily sufficient for patient comfort. This "normal" reaction is *not* the result of an immune response of the patient but is due to the local, toxic effects of the venom constituents on the local tissue. Although in rare instances, when a person is subjected to multiple stings simultaneously, a severe toxic reaction can occur that mimics anaphylaxis, these toxic reactions are not the result of an IgE-mediated allergy and can be distinguished from anaphylaxis by a careful history of the event. Having such localized toxic reactions does not predispose an individual to an allergic or anaphylactic reaction if the person is stung again at a later date.

Insect venom contains foreign proteins that are potent allergens and can cause sensitization in stung individuals, so that subsequent stings can cause allergic reactions. These can occur in anyone, and atopic individuals (i.e., those with allergic rhinitis, asthma, or allergic eczema) are not unusually predisposed to the later development of stinging insect venom allergy.

Although it is not known whether a specific number of stings is necessary before allergic sensitization occurs, it is generally believed that the protein constituents of venom are potent allergens that can sensitize, and in subsequent stings, an allergic reaction may occur. Allergic insect sting reactions, like all other allergic reactions, can involve both an immediate and a late phase. The immediate phase usually begins within a few minutes and peaks within the first hour. The late phase, or delayed phase, usually starts within 6 to 12 hours of the sting and can last for 24 to 48 hours. In some unusual situations, there can be recurrent late-phase events. The acute immediate reaction is more likely to be fatal than the late reaction, although the risks of late-phase reactions are severe and are not to be underestimated. Thus, drug treatment should be extended for several days in most patients.

Clinically, it is useful to separate immediate reactions into large local swellings and systemic reactions. The large local reactions can be quite disturbing to the patient but are not inherently dangerous unless complicated by local infection of the sting site, which can spread.

Systemic reactions are generally described as mild if they involve only pruritus, urticaria, or angioedema at sites remote from the sting site. Moderate systemic reactions involve both the skin and non-life-threatening symptoms of mild asthma and tachycardia, without a change in blood pressure. Severe systemic reactions are life-threatening and include a sense of impending doom, shock, hypotension, upper airway swelling, stridor and severe respiratory distress, uvular and/or upper airway edema, loss of consciousness, and severe gastrointestinal distress.

The treating physician must clarify the type of reaction, because this may predict the response to future stings. Patients with stinging insect venom allergy have a 50 to 60% chance of having an equally severe or perhaps worse reaction to a subsequent sting for as long as 10 years after the prior episode. A patient with a history of a large local reaction seldom has a systemic reaction to a later sting, or if it does occur, the incidence is not significantly greater than in patients with a negative history of a noticeable insect sting reaction.

The natural history of reactions is somewhat different in children than in adults. Children with a history of systemic reaction limited to skin have a 10% chance of anaphylaxis if stung again; these reactions are ordinarily mild and rarely life-threatening. However, adults with systemic reactions of all sorts, and children with systemic reactions involving organs in addition to (or other than) the skin, have up to a 50% chance of having anaphylaxis following another sting.

Other factors that influence the morbidity and chance of fatality from a sting reaction include the age of the adult, the presence of other medical conditions, and concomitant beta-blocker therapy.

Adults are substantially more likely to die from a systemic insect sting reaction than are children. The location of the sting is important, in that stings to the head or neck tend to be more severe. Underlying medical problems such as coronary artery disease and obstructive lung disease raise the morbidity of systemic insect sting reactions. Concomitant beta-blocker therapy is also a risk, because epinephrine and other beta agonists are less effective in reversing the symptoms of anaphylaxis immunopathogenesis in the presence of beta blockers. Insect venoms are complex chemical mixtures. They contain enzymes such as hyaluronidase, phospholipase A, and acid phosphatase. Phospholipase A can itself cause smooth muscle contraction, hypotension, increased vascular permeability, and the release of histamine from mast cells. Some of the peptides contained in venom are melittin, apamin, and a mast cell degranulating peptide. Melittin can cause erythrocyte hemolysis, local pain and inflammation, capillary permeability, hypotension, smooth muscle contraction, and direct histamine release. All these effects are pharmacologic events that explain the normal local reaction to an insect sting—pain, swelling, redness.

The major allergens in insect venom appear to vary, depending on the insect species. All honeybee and vespid (yellow jacket and hornet) venom contains the common antigen phospholipase A and hyaluronidase. Antigen 5 is present only in vespid venom, and melittin is present only in honeybee venom.

There tends to be a high degree of immunologic cross-reactivity between venoms from yellow jackets and hornets. There is less cross-reactivity between yellow jacket and wasp venom and very little cross-reactivity between yellow jacket and honeybee venom. Imported fire ant venom does not cross-react with any of the other venoms mentioned.

Allergic insect sting reactions are typical IgE hypersensitivity reactions; antivenom IgE antibodies in these patients can be demonstrated by either skin or blood tests utilizing in vitro assays for specific antivenom IgE antibodies. In the few cases that have been reported, no venom-specific IgE was detectable, despite the patients having had classic systemic sting reactions. In large local reactions, cell-mediated immunity is believed to play a significant role.

DIAGNOSIS

The diagnosis of systemic insect sting allergy is quite obvious in most cases. The physician should document the location of the sting, the number of stings suffered in the event, and both the entire complex of symptoms the patient is suffering and, if possible, the sequence and speed with which the symptoms developed. It is ordinarily not useful to probe the patient's memory for the name of the stinging insect; most people are unable to identify the specific species of insect responsible for the sting. Care must be taken to distinguish between a large local reaction, an anxiety reaction, and a mild, moderate, or severe systemic reaction. This information is helpful in determining the type of treatment the patient should be given.

All patients with systemic allergic reactions to insect stings should undergo skin testing with insect venom, but this is not necessary in patients with large local reactions. Skin testing detects the presence of specific IgE to insect venom, helps distinguish between a pharmacologic or toxic and a true IgE-mediated event, and is both less expensive and more reliable than in vitro tests in making the diagnosis of insect venom allergy. Of course, proper skin testing technique is essential, but details of this procedure are not immediately relevant here.

TREATMENT

Any discussion of the appropriate treatment of a patient allergic to insect venom involves staging. Anaphylaxis due to an insect sting is treated similarly to anaphylaxis from any other cause. Early and aggressive management is crucial. The first drug to be given is aqueous epinephrine; its immediate subcutaneous administration is the treatment of choice. The standard dosage in children 14 years and younger is 0.01 mL per kg, up to a maximum of 0.3 mL of the 1:1000 dilution, given subcutaneously every 15 minutes as necessary. For adults or children above age 14, the standard dosage is 0.3 to 0.5 mL of 1:1000 dilution given subcutaneously every 15 minutes as necessary. Higher dosages must be given with caution, especially in high-risk patients with underlying cardiovascular disease. The patient's air-

way must be immediately secured; maintaining a patent airway is essential, and endotracheal intubation should be done promptly if laryngeal edema, stridor, or severe bronchospasm occurs. An intravenous line should be established early; fluids may be critical if hypotension develops, and intravenous pressors may be needed.

An H_1 antihistamine can then be given; intravenous or intramuscular diphenhydramine (Benadryl) works quickly to relieve some of the patient's skin discomfort. Most authorities now recommend that an H_2 antihistamine such as ranitidine (Zantac)* be used as well. Although this is not yet approved by the Food and Drug Administration (FDA) for this indication, it is believed that H_1 and H_2 antihistamines together represent better therapy for patients suffering anaphylaxis. Ranitidine 50 mg intramuscularly or intravenously every 6 to 8 hours or cimetidine (Tagamet)* 150 to 300 mg orally or intravenously (given over a 15- to 20-minute period) is often used. It is currently accepted that every patient should also receive at least one dose of steroids (125 mg intravenous methylprednisolone or 40 to 80 mg oral prednisone). Although not first-line drugs, these steroids prevent or lessen the severity of late-phase reactions. Intravenous aminophylline or beta agonist by inhalation and oxygen may be necessary to deal with associated bronchospasm and hypoxia.

Patients with systemic allergic reactions should be kept under observation for 6 to 12 hours so that any late-phase reaction can be promptly treated.

The treatment of large local reactions consists of local application of cold compresses, oral antihistamines, and oral analgesics. If the local reaction is very uncomfortable, a short course of oral steroids can also be given.

Before being sent home after recovering from an acute reaction, every patient should be given a prescription for an injectable epinephrine device (ANA-Kit, EpiPen) for self-care. EpiPen Jr. is appropriate for younger patients. Patients should be instructed in the appropriate use of these devices and must be urged to carry them at all times, for immediate use in the event of a reaction to a later sting. They should also carry Medic Alert tags that identify them as insect-allergic. Finally, they should be referred to a certified allergist for consultation, skin testing, and immunotherapy if indicated.

AVOIDANCE

Patients should be instructed in several measures that can help them avoid stings. They should not wear brightly colored clothing or flower-scented cosmetics, perfumes, or hair sprays. They should have known insect nests exterminated, keep insecticides available, and be cautious near picnic areas, eaves, attics, trash containers, and rotting tree limbs. They should not walk outdoors in bare feet, and when working outdoors doing high-risk activities such as

---

*Not FDA-approved for this indication.

gardening, they should wear long-sleeved shirts, long pants, and gloves.

Venom immunotherapy is a highly successful means of preventing future systemic allergic reactions in venom-allergic patients and has been demonstrated to be 98% effective in preventing anaphylaxis from re-sting. Challenge in venom-allergic patients who are beginning venom immunotherapy can be dangerous and must be done in a controlled medical environment where trained personnel, equipment, and appropriate rescue medications are immediately available.

Venom immunotherapy should be limited to patients with a clear-cut history of a significant systemic reaction to a sting and proven venom-specific IgE as documented by positive skin tests or in vitro assay. Currently, the recommendation is that all adults who have had a systemic reaction (mild, moderate, or severe) and children with a moderate or severe systemic reaction should be treated with venom immunotherapy. Children with mild systemic reactions, limited only to skin manifestations (i.e., urticaria, angioedema), do not need venom immunotherapy, since fewer than 10% will have an anaphylactic reaction to a subsequent sting. Most patients can discontinue immunotherapy after 3 to 5 years after evaluation by a certified allergist that desensitization has been accomplished.

Patients with a history of a large local reaction do not need immunotherapy because they are at very low risk of anaphylaxis from future stings.

Venom immunotherapy clearly protects insect sting–allergic patients from future systemic allergic reactions; the peace of mind this affords venom-allergic patients is an important part of the therapy.

Diseases of the Skin

ACNE VULGARIS AND ROSACEA

method of
MARTI JILL ROTHE, M.D., and
JANE M. GRANT-KELS, M.D.
University of Connecticut Health Center
Farmington, Connecticut

ACNE

Acne vulgaris is one of the most common and emotionally disabling skin disorders. More than 80% of teenagers and nearly 5% of adults aged 25 to 44 years are affected.

Acne usually begins in puberty and affects the face, back, and upper chest. "Adult-onset acne," in contrast, affects women in their mid-twenties to late thirties, involves the chin and jawline, and often flares with the menstrual cycle.

Current acne therapy is generally very effective in treating active disease and in diminishing the risk of permanent scarring. Most patients with acne are treated with a combination of topical and oral medications that are directed toward the multiple factors implicated in the pathogenesis of acne. Therapies are also selected according to individual characteristics such as childbearing potential, concomitant medications, and tolerance of skin irritants. Patient education concerning the risks and benefits of therapy, the proper use of prescriptions, and the facts and fiction of acne is important in acne management.

Pathogenesis

Acne lesions are classified as noninflammatory and inflammatory. The noninflammatory lesions include the microcomedo, the closed comedo or whitehead, and the open comedo or blackhead. Inflammatory lesions include papules, pustules, nodules, and cysts.

Acne lesions develop as a consequence of multiple pathogenetic factors: androgen activity, sebum production, *Propionibacterium acnes,* follicular proliferation and keratinization, and inflammation.

Androgens stimulate sebaceous glands at the base of hair follicles to produce sebum; *P. acnes* within the follicle produces lipases that degrade the sebum into free fatty acids; free fatty acids irritate the lining of the follicle, stimulating hyperproliferation and abnormal keratinization and leading to the formation of a microscopic plugged follicle or microcomedo. Distention of the microcomedo results in the open and closed comedo. Papules and pustules develop when the follicular wall breaks and contents of the comedo are extruded into the dermis, resulting in a foreign body–type inflammatory reaction; deep inflammation leads to the development of nodules and cysts. The disruption of the follicular wall may be the consequence of multiple factors, including chemotactic factors and enzymes produced by *P. acnes.*

Pathogenesis-Directed Therapy

Most patients with acne are treated with a combination of topical and oral medications that affect the multiple pathogenetic factors described earlier. Antiandrogens, usually in the form of oral contraceptives and spironolactone, are generally reserved for women with treatment-resistant acne or adult-onset acne or those who intend to use oral contraceptives for birth control. Sebum production can be effectively inhibited by the oral retinoid isotretinoin (Accutane), which is usually considered a treatment of last resort for patients with refractory acne or rapidly scarring papulopustular or nodulocystic acne. *P. acnes* can be inhibited by topical and oral antibiotics, topical benzoyl peroxide, and isotretinoin. Both isotretinoin and the topical retinoid tretinoin (Retin-A) can inhibit follicular hyperproliferation and normalize keratinization. Tretinoin and benzoyl peroxide also have a comedolytic effect. Topical and oral antibiotics and isotretinoin have anti-inflammatory properties.

Therapy Directed by Clinical Severity

In general, predominantly comedonal acne is treated with tretinoin alone or in combination with benzoyl peroxide. Many experts believe that all grades of acne should be treated with tretinoin because it acts directly against the microcomedo, which is the precursor of all noninflammatory and inflammatory lesions.

Mild inflammatory acne is generally treated with tretinoin in combination with a topical antibiotic and/or benzoyl peroxide. In some instances, an oral antibiotic is used initially in combination with these topicals and then discontinued once remission is achieved.

Moderate and severe inflammatory acne is treated with a combination of tretinoin, topical antibiotic, benzoyl peroxide, and oral antibiotic. Again, once remission is achieved, the oral antibiotic is discontinued but topical therapy is maintained. Isotretinoin and antiandrogens are appropriate considerations for treatment-resistant acne.

Characteristics of Specific Therapies

Tretinoin (Retin-A) is manufactured in three formulations: cream, gel, and solution. The cream and gel are available in three strengths. All forms of tretinoin can be highly irritating, and it is the rare patient who can tolerate the solution. Whether the cream or the gel is selected for a particular patient depends largely on the patient's complexion—cream for dry skin and gel for oily skin—and the ambient temperature and humidity. Patients should be instructed to apply tretinoin to dry skin, at least 30 minutes after washing the face. Patients can become accustomed to tretinoin by first using it every third night for several applications, then every other night for 1 to 2 weeks, and then every night as tolerated. A flare of papulopustular acne can occur initially; a flare of comedonal acne in a patient using the cream formulation suggests that the gel may be preferable, in that it is less occlusive. If the patient tolerates the cream or gel but fails to have an adequate therapeutic response, the strength of tretinoin may be increased. When increasing the strength or switching from cream to gel, applications should again be intermittent until daily use is tolerated. Tretinoin is usually applied at bedtime. Patients should be advised that tretinoin may be photosensitizing, and some studies suggest that it may be a photocarcinogen. It is controversial whether tretinoin can be teratogenic; at this time, its use in pregnancy should be avoided.

Benzoyl peroxide is formulated as creams, gels, lotions, or washes in various strengths and in combination with erythromycin (Benzamycin). Benzoyl peroxide can cause both irritant and allergic contact dermatitis; it bleaches fabrics, cleaves tretinoin when used simultaneously (therefore benzoyl peroxide is used in the morning), and may act as a photocarcinogen in laboratory animals. Manufacturers may soon be required to alert patients to the risk of photocarcinogenesis on the package labeling. Benzamycin has the added advantage of improved compliance for patients who would benefit from concomitant use of a topical antibiotic.

Erythromycin and clindamycin (Cleocin T) are the most commonly prescribed topical antibiotics and are available in gel, solution, pledget, lotion, and ointment forms. A teenager might be more compliant with a roll-on solution, whereas a fastidious adult might not like repeated use of the applicator head. Lotions and ointments are particularly useful for patients with significant skin irritation from concomitant topicals. There is no particular advantage of one antibiotic over the other.

Tetracycline, minocycline (Minocin), doxycycline (Monodox, Vibramycin), and erythromycin are the most commonly prescribed oral antibiotics. First- and second-generation tetracyclines are generally more effective than erythromycin. Minocycline (50 to 200 mg per day) and doxycycline (50 to 200 mg per day) are generally more effective than tetracycline for more severe inflammatory acne; the second-generation tetracyclines are dosed once or twice daily and may be taken with food. All tetracyclines can be photosensitizing and should be avoided during pregnancy and in children younger than 8 years. Although the dermatology literature suggests that antibiotics for acne are unlikely to decrease the efficacy of oral contraceptives, patients should confer with their prescribing physicians regarding concomitant therapy. Long-term oral antibiotic therapy for acne has not been thought to pose significant risks or require laboratory monitoring, although a recent publication noted autoimmune arthritis and hepatitis in minocycline-treated acne patients.

Isotretinoin (Accutane), an extremely effective monotherapy for patients with severe inflammatory and scarring acne, is given for a 20-week course. Inflammatory flares can be seen during the first 1 to 2 months of therapy; these may be sufficiently severe to require treatment with prednisone. Concomitant treatment with erythromycin (tetracycline and isotretinoin both carry the risk for pseudotumor cerebri and are not prescribed simultaneously) and gradually increasing the dose of isotretinoin from 0.5 mg per kg per day to the optimal 1 mg per kg per day during the initial period of therapy may help prevent the flares. Numerous risks are associated with isotretinoin: dry skin and mucous membranes, chemical hepatitis, elevated triglycerides, and decreased high-density lipoprotein. The most significant risk is teratogenicity. Women treated with isotretinoin must not be pregnant when treatment is initiated and cannot become pregnant during therapy or for 1 month after therapy. Appropriate monitoring for pregnancy before and during treatment, two forms of effective birth control, and pregnancy prevention counseling are all essential when prescribing isotretinoin to women with childbearing potential. Even women who report surgical sterilization in themselves or their partners should be counseled, and pregnancy should be excluded by laboratory testing, except in the case of hysterectomy.

Spironolactone (Aldactone) 50 to 200 mg per day can be used alone, in combination with conventional therapy, or with oral contraceptives. Spironolactone may cause irregular menses and can feminize a male fetus; therefore, use with an oral contraceptive is recommended. Electrolyte and blood pressure disturbances are unlikely at these doses, but monitoring is appropriate after 1 month of therapy and then at 4- to 6-month intervals. Oral contraceptives for acne patients should have the least progestational (and therefore androgenic) activity possible.

Facts and Fiction

Patients, particularly teenagers and their parents, should be educated about acne myths. For example, with the exception of overingestion of halogens, food does not cause acne. Overly zealous washing with harsh soaps and sponges will not improve acne; in fact, such cleansing may heighten the irritation associated with prescriptions and cause the rupture of comedonal acne, promoting the development of more inflammatory lesions.

ROSACEA

Rosacea is an acne-like condition characterized by erythema and telangiectasia, acneform papules and pustules, and sebaceous hyperplasia. Rhinophyma is the consequence of sebaceous hyperplasia of the nose. Ocular rosacea may be an associated feature. Rosacea generally affects the central face of adults, is often associated with heightened tendency to cutaneous irritation, and can be triggered by a variety of stimuli, including caffeine, spicy foods, alcohol, hot drinks, and sun exposure. *Demodex folliculorum* and more recently *Helicobacter pylori* have been implicated in the pathogenesis of rosacea. Seborrheic dermatitis is often seen in association with rosacea.

Mild acneform changes are typically responsive to topical antibiotics, particularly topical metronidazole (MetroGel and the less irritating MetroCream) and nonirritating topical erythromycin or clindamycin formulations. Sulfur-containing products may act as anti-inflammatory agents and, when tinted, also act as concealers (Sulfacet-R). More severe acneform changes and erythema and telangiectasia respond best to a combination of topical therapy and oral antibiotics. Rarely, isotretinoin is prescribed for patients with severe acneform disease that is unresponsive to topical and oral therapy. Laser therapy, beta blockers, nonsteroidal anti-inflammatory agents, and avoidance of provocative factors may be of value in the treatment of the telangiectatic component of the disease. Some practitioners are treating patients with regimens that are effective against *H. pylori.* Gentle cleansers (Cetaphil, Aquanil) can be helpful in minimizing skin irritation and dryness and are preferable to using topical corticosteroids, which can cause a flare of rosacea when withdrawn. Associated seborrhea should ideally be treated with topical ketoconazole (Nizoral) rather than topical corticosteroids.

HAIR DISORDERS

method of
ELISE A. OLSEN, M.D.
Duke University Medical Center
Durham, North Carolina

The effective treatment of hair loss is totally dependent on the diagnostic acumen of the observing physician. Just as in cutaneous medicine in general, there are genetic, inflammatory, hormonally related, autoimmune-driven, infectious, and self-induced types of alopecia. Diagnosis can largely be made through history and physical examination, with the additional aids of a microscope and a few blood tests. Only occasionally is a scalp biopsy necessary to make a diagnosis of hair loss—usually this is merely confirmatory.

The most important parts of the evaluation of the scalp are (1) the determination of a patchy (or patterned) loss versus diffuse (evenly distributed or global) loss, (2) scarring versus nonscarring hair loss, (3) abnormal hair shedding versus breakage, and (4) inflammatory versus noninflammatory changes of the scalp. Mere observation of the scalp can determine the pattern of loss and whether scale, erythema, or induration exists. In nonscarring loss, the follicular openings are obvious on the scalp, even without hairs physically in the follicles. In scarring loss, this finding is absent, leaving slick areas where viable follicles once resided. To help establish whether an abnormal amount of shedding is occurring, a hair pull is performed. This is done by grasping clumps of 25 to 50 hairs close to the scalp and gently pulling to the distal ends. Normally, 6 to 8 such hair pulls should net no more than 2 to 5 telogen hairs. The proximal ends of the hair so collected should then be evaluated microscopically to confirm that they are indeed telogen and not anagen hairs. Anagen (or actively growing) hairs are pigmented at the base with attached inner root sheaths, and telogen (resting) hairs are nonpigmented with a "club" end and no attached inner root sheaths. Anagen shedding and telogen shedding stem from different etiologic factors and require different evaluations. The distal ends of the hairs obtained by a hair pull can also be evaluated to determine whether breakage is present and, if so, what type. This helps delineate the etiology of the hair loss.

Scalp biopsies are done primarily to confirm a scarring alopecia and to determine the subtype. Scalp biopsies may also be done to differentiate patchy alopecia areata from trichotillomania or, in cases of androgenetic alopecia in women, from diffuse alopecia areata and telogen effluvium. There are very few independently "diagnostic" scalp biopsies of alopecia. Because of this, scalp biopsies should be done only by those with a knowledge of the differential diagnosis involved and interpreted only by dermatopathologists experienced in the assessment of scalp pathology. To do less makes this an expensive and usually worthless exercise.

Most types of alopecia can be readily diagnosed and have effective therapeutic options for the control and/or reversal of the clinical abnormality (Table 1). The discussion that follows addresses only the most common forms of alopecia.

TELOGEN EFFLUVIUM

Abnormal shedding of scalp hair can occur as a result of an increase in the percentage of telogen hairs. This is a very common problem, probably accounting for 20 to 40% of women with hair loss presenting to physicians. Normally constituting 10% of the scalp hair, telogen (or resting) hairs are shed with usual daily traction (brushing, shampooing), secondary to their relative lack of anchoring in the scalp compared with anagen hairs. An increase in the percentage of telogen hairs, rarely beyond 50%

TABLE 1. **Differential Diagnosis of Hair Loss**

Nonscarring hair loss
 Diffuse
  Breakage
   Anagen effluvium
   Hair shaft disorder
   Physical or chemical processing
  Telogen effluvium
  Androgenetic alopecia (women)
  Alopecia totalis or universalis
  Loose anagen syndrome
  Failure of or abnormal production
 Focal
  Infection
  Traumatic
  Alopecia areata (patchy)
  Hair breakage
  Androgenetic alopecia (men and women)
  Developmental
Scarring hair loss

of the total, may occur as a reaction to a variety of medical or psychological insults or with certain drugs (notably beta blockers, anticoagulants, retinoids). The scalp is otherwise normal. The loss is diffuse or global on the scalp, an important differentiating point from androgenetic alopecia in women. Because the loss usually presents 3 to 4 months after the inciting event, and many stresses are of brief duration, the patient typically presents at the time of worst loss, and improvement generally follows over the next 6 to 12 months, unless the promoter of hair loss is still present. Treatment is generally directed at the underlying offender, not the hair loss itself.

ANDROGENETIC ALOPECIA

This androgen-dependent, genetically mediated (autosomal dominant with variable penetrance) type of alopecia occurs in 50% of both men and women, although with quite variable severity. The onset is usually in the third or fourth decade but can begin as early as puberty. Men develop a recession and resculpturing of the frontotemporal hair line, as well as loss of hair on the top and vertex of the scalp. This can proceed to frank baldness. Women do not develop baldness but rather a generalized thinning of the hair over the top of the scalp. The process is caused by progressive miniaturization of the involved hair follicles, so abnormal telogen shedding, if present, is generally only a transient part of the clinical picture. It is unnecessary to pursue any laboratory evaluation in men with this disorder or in women who do not have signs of hyperandrogenism. In women with irregular periods, acne, or hirsutism, however, it is reasonable to screen with dehydroepiandrosterone sulfate (DHEA-S) and free testosterone. If these are elevated, further work-up may be indicated.

Treatment for both men and women can be with either a hair-growth promoter or hair transplants. Currently, the only hair-growth promoter approved by the Food and Drug Administration (FDA) is 2%
topical minoxidil (Rogaine). This medication must be applied a minimum of twice a day to the scalp (less is subthreshold for response), with the earliest response seen at 6 months and a maximum response at 1 year. Only about 20 to 25% of subjects have notable regrowth, and generally these are the men and women whose involved hairs are finer than normal but not minuscule at treatment onset. Most patients experience at least a stabilization of hair loss. Higher concentrations of topical minoxidil work better but are not yet commercially available.

Surgical treatment for androgenetic alopecia has undergone dramatic improvements in recent years. Donor dominance allows continued growth of hair transferred from the portions of the scalp that are genetically immune to hereditary thinning to those areas exhibiting baldness. Cosmetic coverage is limited by the amount and thickness of available donor hair and the expertise of the surgeon. Male candidates for this procedure should be those whose balding process is no longer active. A combination of standard 4-mm plugs of donor hair and/or minigrafts (1.5- to 2.5-mm grafts) and micrografts (one to two hairs per graft) are used to fill in areas of baldness. The micrografts are particularly useful, as they do not require removal of a plug of tissue to insert the graft into; rather, a slit can be made to accommodate a few donor hairs. This is the surgical treatment of choice in women with androgenetic alopecia, who, unlike men, never have complete baldness and for whom the use of standard hair transplants means a loss of recipient tissue that still has hair.

For women with androgenetic alopecia, particularly those with androgen excess, the use of medications that block either the production or the cellular utilization of androgens can be helpful. Combination oral contraceptive pills that utilize a nonandrogenic progestin (such as norgestimate) decrease both ovarian and adrenal production of androgens. Systemic antiandrogens such as spironolactone (Aldactone)* in doses of ≥100 mg daily and flutamide (Eulexin)* in doses of 250 to 500 mg daily have shown effectiveness in small numbers of hirsute women with concomitant androgenetic alopecia. Spironolactone is a potassium-sparing diuretic whose main side effects are hyperkalemia, irregular menses, and breast tenderness or bloating. Flutamide users must be monitored for potential hepatotoxicity. Because both drugs can cause feminization of a male fetus, they should be used only in women of nonchildbearing potential or in those women who are using effective contraception, preferably combination oral contraceptives. Topical antiandrogens, which could theoretically be used in men also, are not commercially available at this time.

Drugs that block the enzyme 5-alpha-reductase, which is responsible for the transformation of testosterone to dihydrotestosterone, are currently being evaluated for use in androgenetic alopecia. Dihydrotestosterone appears to be the hormone that mediates the hair miniaturization process in androgenic

---

*Not FDA-approved for this indication.

alopecia. Because it does not block testosterone from direct action on other cells, men can be treated for androgenetic alopecia with a 5-alpha-reductase inhibitor without sacrificing libido and potency. Early studies suggest that finasteride* 1 to 5 mg a day can cause both regrowth and stabilization of hair loss in androgenic alopecia. No "head to head" comparison studies with topical minoxidil have yet been performed.

ALOPECIA AREATA

Alopecia areata presents as patches of hair loss on the scalp, with variable amounts of hair loss elsewhere. The scalp is otherwise normal. Telogen hair shedding is increased in areas of hair loss, with "exclamation point" hairs present in areas of active loss. The latter are short (less than a quarter of an inch) pigmented hairs that are broader at the tip than at the base (the opposite of normal new hair growth) and are pathognomonic of alopecia areata. Some cases of alopecia areata are more diffuse (global) rather than patchy and can mimic a telogen or anagen effluvium. In these cases, a biopsy can be useful. A peribulbar chronic inflammatory infiltrate with sparing of the "bulge" area near the sebaceous gland is confirmatory evidence of alopecia areata.

Current effective treatments can be divided into three major categories: steroids (or other immune suppressive agents), topical irritants or allergens, and psoralen plus long-wave ultraviolet light (PUVA). Those patients with patchy scalp alopecia areata (the vast majority) are usually best served by an externally directed approach first. Intralesional (intradermal) steroids are very effective in doses of 5 to 20 mg per mL of triamcinolone, usually showing subtle hair growth by 1 month following injection. Injections are painful, however, and must be repeated monthly until hair growth is complete. Intralesional steroids can lead to depressions in the scalp secondary to inadvertent injection into the subcutaneous tissue (this is generally reversible) or potential systemic effects when given repetitively over several months. Eyebrows can also be injected, but a lower concentration (≤ 5 mg per mL) of steroid must be used because of the greater risk of atrophy in these areas.

Topical steroids are easy to use and to tolerate and are very effective for patients with patchy alopecia that is limited or extensive in scope. The key to their effective use lies in consistent daily application of a mid- to high-potency steroid through complete regrowth *and beyond*. It is not necessary to use a high-potency steroid (Class 1 and 2) to induce hair growth, and high-potency steroids carry a greater risk of local side effects (adrenal suppression, cushingoid appearance). In my practice, I generally employ a mid-potency (Class 3–5) steroid in a solution or lotion vehicle, the latter to facilitate application to slick areas as well as areas with partial hair regrowth.

The first signs of regrowth are generally apparent 3 to 4 months following topical treatment. Application must be continued for 3 to 6 months after clearing to prevent fallout of newly regrown hair. Children can also use Class 5 potency steroids topically on the scalp (this represents only about 3% of body surface area) without the development of systemic side effects. Patients should be careful about letting the topical steroids drift down onto the face; this can lead to hair growth on the face and acne, both reversible conditions.

Systemic steroids are always more effective in alopecia areata than intralesional or topical steroids but have the risk of systemic side effects. Some cases of extensive or rapidly progressive alopecia areata, however, require systemic steroids for either curtailment of hair loss or induction of hair growth. Side effects can be minimized by tapering prednisone over 6 to 8 weeks, beginning at 40 mg or less daily. Patients *must* be on a concurrent topical regimen (not topical irritants or allergens) as the doses of prednisone fall below 10 to 20 mg per day and must be continued on this regimen well beyond the end of the systemic taper; without this, 50% of patients with systemic steroid–initiated hair growth will experience fallout of the newly regrown hair. Cyclosporine (Sandimmune)* is another systemic immunosuppressive agent that has been effective in inducing hair growth in alopecia areata, but its profile of side effects makes it even less desirable to use in this setting than systemic steroids.

The induction of contact dermatitis (irritant or allergic) in areas of alopecia often induces hair growth in alopecia areata. Agents that can be used to this end include the allergens topical dinitrochlorobenzene, diphencyprone, or *Rhus* antigen or irritants such as anthralin. Irritants require no prior induction of allergy and one (anthralin) is more readily available in the United States than the other aforementioned chemicals. Anthralin (Anthra-Derm, Drithrocreme)* is FDA-approved for the treatment of psoriasis and is irritating to nonpsoriatic skin in a dose-dependent fashion. It can be utilized very effectively in alopecia areata in 0.5 to 1% concentrations applied daily to the involved areas of hair loss. Hair growth can be effectively induced by a threshold minimal irritation so that the length of application is tailored to the time necessary to achieve this reaction versus a more blatant and debilitating dermatitis—a time that is variable in each patient. As with topical steroids, the first signs of regrowth with anthralin usually occur in 3 to 4 months. Patients should be warned that a purple discoloration can occur in treated areas where the medicine is incompletely removed and can persistently discolor nails that come in contact with the medicine. The concomitant use of topical steroids to ameliorate or modify irritation should be avoided, as these two therapies presumably work through diametrically opposed mechanisms, and co-treatment can be counterproductive.

---

*Not FDA-approved for this indication.

*Not FDA-approved for this indication.

PUVA may work in alopecia areata as an externally directed immune suppressive. It is an arduous treatment and is best used in extensive and/or treatment-refractory alopecia areata of the scalp or with concomitant body hair loss (alopecia totalis or universalis). The initiation of hair growth may take 40 to 80 treatments, and complete regrowth could take 1 to 2 years. However, PUVA is often effective when all else has failed. Potential side effects are acute erythema, PUVA lentigines, and skin cancer (nonmelanoma), the latter usually identified years later. Patients must be screened with an antinuclear antibody (phototoxicity is an issue here) and an eye examination (protective glasses must be worn for 24 hours following psoralen to protect the eye from the risk of cataracts or retinal damage).

A fourth possibility for the treatment of alopecia areata is the category of drugs known as hair-growth promoters, of which topical minoxidil is the prototype. Although data suggest that 5% topical minoxidil can be an effective agent in alopecia areata, the commercially available agent (2% topical minoxidil [Rogaine]) falls short of effectiveness as a single-agent therapy. Rogaine two to four times daily is useful, however, as an adjuvant to systemic steroid or topical anthralin use in the treatment of alopecia areata.

TINEA CAPITIS

Tinea capitis is a common problem in children, particularly in poor African American children, but it can occur in any age group. There are three usual clinical presentations: a seborrhea-like scale on the scalp, with thinning of the hair in the involved areas; areas of noninflammatory, nonscaly alopecia, with hairs broken off flush or near flush on the scalp (so called "black-dot" ringworm); and inflammation and induration of the scalp, with associated hair loss that can progress, in extreme cases, to a kerion. Each is best diagnosed with both a potassium hydroxide preparation and culture (the former may be negative). The most common causative agent in the United States is *Trichophyton tonsurans*.

Treatment must be systemic, although 2.5% selenium sulfide shampoo two to three times per week is an effective adjuvant that decreases shedding of viable spores. Griseofulvin in doses of 10 to 20 mg per kg of the microsize product (or 5 to 10 mg per kg of the ultra-microsize form) given with a fatty meal (glass of milk) for 6 to 8 weeks is effective in most cases. A fungal culture should be negative prior to discontinuation of treatment. Ketoconazole (Nizoral) is a much less effective drug for tinea capitis, and the best alternative treatment to griseofulvin is probably itraconazole (Sporanox) or terbinafine (Lamisil). Household and other close contacts should be checked for simultaneous infection and treated; to not do so invites incomplete eradication or recurrence of infection in the proband.

CANCER OF THE SKIN

method of
LEONARD SHVARTZMAN, M.D., and
R. STAN TAYLOR, M.D.
University of Texas, Southwestern Medical Center
Dallas, Texas

Basal cell carcinoma (BCC) is the most common malignancy in the United States. BCC and squamous cell carcinoma (SCC) of the skin have an annual incidence estimated to exceed 1 million. Squamous cell cancers tend to be the more aggressive of the two neoplasms but fortunately occur less commonly.

RISK FACTORS

The major risk factors for developing BCC or SCC are cumulative sun exposure, age, male sex, freckles, light or red hair, inability to tan (easily burned), light-colored eyes, and previous history of skin cancer. Several inheritable genetic conditions (xeroderma pigmentosum, basal cell nevus syndrome) are associated with the development of BCC and/or SCC. The pathogenesis of both tumors is linked to radiation exposure (x-rays and ultraviolet light). SCC is frequently associated with extrinsic factors such as cigarette smoke, arsenic, industrial chemicals (coal tar, oil), chronic immune suppression, scars, chronic ulcers, and certain viral infections. SCC can also be associated with albinism and chronic cutaneous autoimmune diseases.

BASAL CELL CARCINOMA

The classic presentation of BCC is a smooth-surfaced papule with a translucent "pearly" border and fine surface telangiectasias usually on sun-exposed skin. Sometimes, however, BCC can present as a bound-down scarring lesion, a pigmented or hyperkeratotic papule or plaque, or a scaly patch. It must be differentiated from a scar, malignant melanoma, and SCC, and to do so often requires a skin biopsy. BCC presents with a slow but relentless pattern of growth, expanding by direct extension into surrounding skin and adjacent structures. Although hardly ever metastatic (0.01 to 0.1% rate of metastasis), this tumor can cause significant morbidity by local extension into cosmetic and functional structures such as the eyelids, ear, lips, and nose. If treated inadequately, it can recur locally around the edges of the scar as well as invade deeply and perineurally. Several histologic presentations are recognized, including superficial spreading, nodular, and morpheaform. The morpheaform variety is the most aggressive but the least common.

SQUAMOUS CELL CARCINOMA

SCC often presents as a rough keratotic papule, a sharply demarcated scaly plaque, a large ulcerating tumor, or a warty growth. It is often induced by radiation. As mentioned, however, many chronic inflammatory conditions and other predisposing factors can lead to aggressive forms of this tumor. Precursor lesions for invasive SCC are actinic keratoses and Bowen's disease (SCC in situ), as well as some viral warts (human papillomavirus 16,18). The risk of metastasis depends on a variety of factors, including the location on the body (lower lip and vulva lesions metastasize at a 16% rate) and the etiology (actinically induced SCC metastasizes at a 0.5% rate, whereas SCC associated with chronic osteomyelitis metastasizes at a rate of 31%). The aggressiveness of SCC can also be assessed histologically by the proportion of poorly differentiated squamous cells.

DIAGNOSIS

Cutaneous examination and biopsy remain the most reliable tools for the accurate diagnosis of cutaneous malignancies and their differentiation from benign conditions. A shave biopsy that includes dermis for the evaluation of histology and invasion, or a punch biopsy of a nonulcerated area, is usually adequate to confirm the clinical diagnosis. An excisional biopsy is preferred for any lesion suspected of being malignant melanoma.

TREATMENT

Selection of therapy is based on the goals of minimizing recurrence and disability while maximizing the aesthetic result. Important considerations when selecting therapy include location, whether the lesion is recurrent, depth of invasion, tumor size, and quality of surrounding skin. Anatomic locations prone to high risk of recurrence are periauricular, periocular, scalp, and central face. Curettage and electrodesiccation (C&E), cryosurgery, radiation therapy, simple excision, and Mohs' micrographic surgery should all be considered. Each technique is effective, but the cure rates and cosmetic results are not identical. Review of 5-year recurrence rates for primary BCC found a rate of 1% for Mohs' micrographic surgery, 10.1% for surgical excision, 7.7% for C&E, 8.7% for radiation therapy, and 7.5% for cryosurgery. In a similar review comparing Mohs' surgery with all other modalities, the local recurrence of SCC was 3.1 to 36.6% versus 10.9 to 53.6%. The best cosmetic results are obtained with scalpel surgery, followed by sutured repair of defects. Ionizing radiation therapy can also produce good short-term cosmetic results, but the disfiguring changes of chronic radiation dermatitis eventually supervene. Cryosurgery with electrocautery leaves flat, coin-shaped depigmented scars that, on occasion, form keloids.

A regional lymph node examination is mandatory in patients with SCC. Palpable adenopathy necessitates microscopic evaluation of the node by either fine-needle aspirate or open biopsy. If SCC is present in the node, the patient's disease is staged by physical examination, radiographic studies, and a node dissection. If no adenopathy is detected, prophylactic radiation to regional lymph nodes is used in high-grade tumors.

Curettage and Electrodesiccation

C&E is a rapid, convenient method for treating small (<10 mm) BCCs. The tumor is scraped with a curet, and the base is electrodesiccated. The procedure is repeated three times. It is routinely utilized on the trunk, neck, shoulders, upper arms, and other cosmetically less sensitive areas. Since the wound must granulate by secondary intention, it often takes several weeks to fill in completely and heals with a depigmented flat scar. The area chosen for this therapy needs to be flat so that the scraping can be performed effectively, and the dermis should not have been previously breached with a punch biopsy, because this prevents adequate scraping. A 3-mm margin of normal-appearing tissue is also scraped as an attempt at margin control in this blind technique. This technique should not be used for (1) SCC, because the tumor cells are not easily cureted and there is the risk of disrupting cutaneous architectural defenses, leading to micrometastases; (2) recurrent cancer, due to the inability to use the curet effectively in scar from the previous procedure; (3) morpheaform BCC; (4) tumors greater than 20 mm; (5) tumors with indistinct margins; and (6) tumors located in areas with a high risk of recurrence, such as the central face.

Cryosurgery

Cryosurgery is the use of liquid nitrogen to freeze tumor cells. It is useful for patients who are not good surgical candidates and are not worried about cosmesis. The technique should not be used for tumors greater than 20 mm, morpheaform BCC, cancers with perineural invasion, tumors with indistinct margins, or tumors with fat involvement. A thermocouple is placed under the lesion to monitor the desired freezing temperature ($-50°$ C) at a measured depth. Liquid nitrogen is sprayed on the tumor until the desired temperature under the lesion is reached. This temperature is then maintained for 1 minute. The cycle is repeated two to three times. Since this is a blind technique, clinical margins of several millimeters need to be included in the frozen field. The technique first produces edema and blistering, then leaves a deep necrotic ulceration that heals by secondary intention.

Radiotherapy

Radiotherapy is effective and can, in the short run, leave the patient with a cosmetically excellent result. However, it should be used in younger patients with caution, because the changes of chronic radiodermatitis and the development of BCC and SCC can supervene. Radiotherapy should thus be used in poor surgical candidates or elderly patients. As with cryotherapy and C&E, x-ray therapy is a blind technique, and adequate margins of skin need to be irradiated.

Excision

Surgical excision can be used on almost any skin tumor. Three-millimeter margins of normal-appearing tissue are usually excised with some subcutaneous fat, and the specimen is sent for examination of surgical margins. It must be emphasized, however, that only representative margins are examined routinely, not the whole margin surface. Sometimes defects cannot be closed primarily and require flap or graft coverage. As with C&E, this technique should not be used for recurrent tumors, morpheaform BCC, or tumors in areas with a high risk of recurrence.

Mohs' Micrographic Surgery

Mohs' surgery is a technique that allows visualization of the entire outer surface of a dished-out specimen. This technique controls all tumor margins and is simultaneously tissue sparing. As soon as the outer layer of the specimen is tumor free, the patient is ready for closure. Technically, the tumor is first debulked up to its clinical margin, then a thin continuous slice of saucer-shaped tissue is cut out around and underneath the original wound. This saucer cannot lie flat on a slide, so it is sectioned into quadrants or multiple sections. Frozen tissue sections are then taken from the outer surface of each quadrant and examined under the microscope. If tumor is present in one quadrant, the surgeon takes a second margin in that quadrant and processes it in the same manner. This is done for each quadrant until the section is clear of tumor. All treatment is performed under local anesthesia as an outpatient. Indications for Mohs' surgery are tumor greater than 20 mm, recurrent tumor, morpheaform tumor, a cosmetically sensitive area where tissue preservation is paramount, tumor in areas with a high risk of recurrence, and cases of perineural invasion.

CUTANEOUS T CELL LYMPHOMA

method of
FRANCINE M. FOSS, M.D.
Boston University Medical Center
Boston, Massachusetts

The cutaneous T cell lymphomas constitute a spectrum of diseases, all of which are characterized by infiltration of the skin by neoplastic lymphocytes. Within this spectrum are several clinical entities, including more aggressive diseases such as acute T cell leukemia/lymphoma associated with human T cell lymphotropic virus Type I (HTLV I), peripheral T cell lymphomas, and the primary Ki-1+ large cell lymphomas of the skin, as well as more indolent disorders, including lymphomatoid granulomatosis, lymphomatoid papulosis, and T-gamma lymphoproliferative disorder (Table 1). The most common diseases falling into this category, however, are mycosis fungoides (MF) and Sézary's syndrome (SS), distinguished from other cutaneous T cell lymphomas by distinct histopathologic and clinical features. This article reviews the biology, etiology, and clinical management of MF and SS.

EPIDEMIOLOGY AND ETIOLOGY

MF and SS represent about 2% of all lymphomas in the United States. The overall incidence of MF and SS in the United States is 1000 cases per year. There has been a striking increase in incidence over the past few decades that parallels an overall increase in the incidence of non-

TABLE 1. **Cutaneous T Cell Lymphomas**

Low Grade	Intermediate or High Grade
Mycosis fungoides	HTLV-I–associated adult T cell leukemia/lymphoma
Sézary's syndrome	
Lymphomatoid papulosis	Peripheral T cell lymphoma
Pagetoid reticulosis	Primary cutaneous Ki-I+ large cell lymphoma
Granulomatous slack skin	
Lymphomatoid granulomatosis	
Large plaque parapsoriasis	
T-gamma lymphoproliferative disorder	

Hodgkin's lymphomas. Incidence increases with age, although childhood cases have been documented, and the disease occurs more frequently in men and in blacks.

Epidemiologic studies have not yielded definitive etiologic factors. An early study suggested a correlation with occupational exposure to industrial solvents, but these results could not be validated in recent case-control studies. Familial clustering has been reported, as has an association with certain histocompatibility loci (B8, BW35). Other possible etiologies examined in these studies include history of atopy or chronic dermatitis, allergies, and other forms of chronic antigen stimulation.

The similarity in the clinical manifestations of MF and HTLV I–associated leukemia/lymphoma has led to an extensive search for the virus in patients with MF and SS. Serologic tests for HTLV I have been negative, but recent studies using in situ hybridization and polymerase chain amplification have demonstrated the presence of portions of the HTLV I genome in a subset of patients with MF and SS. Further studies are under way to examine the frequency of these findings. Currently, there is no epidemiologic clustering of MF to support a horizontal or infectious transmission.

PATHOLOGY AND BIOLOGY

The diagnosis of MF and SS is based on characteristic light microscopic findings on skin biopsy, including the presence of a bandlike infiltrate of atypical lymphocytes with hyperconvoluted cerebriform nuclei in the upper dermis, epidermotropism or mononuclear exocytosis into the epidermis, and Pautrier's microabscesses or clusters of atypical "mycosis cells" in the epidermis. Although this constellation of findings is often seen in patients with advanced disease, the biopsies of earlier-stage patients often lack some of these criteria and are often confused with benign or reactive dermal infiltrates, including parapsoriasis and dermatitis. In some instances, large-plaque parapsoriasis or lymphomatoid papulosis may precede MF, and the diagnosis of a definitive neoplastic disorder in these patients is a clinicopathologic one, based on longitudinal evaluation of the disease process as well as evolution of the histopathologic findings. SS is a variant of the disease associated with circulating hyperconvoluted neoplastic lymphocytes, or Sézary cells, constituting at least 20% of the total lymphocytes. Review of a peripheral blood smear by an experienced hematopathologist is essential in all patients with MF or SS.

Several new techniques, including immunohistochemistry and molecular analysis for clonality of T cell receptor gene rearrangements, are now utilized to enhance diagnostic accuracy. In most cases of MF, the atypical lymphocytes in the skin express early T cell antigens, including CD2, CD3, CD5, and CD6. Most lack expression of CD7, thus

distinguishing them from normal T lymphocytes, which are CD7-expressing. The majority of cases of MF and SS are of a helper-inducer phenotype (CD4+, CD45RA−, CDw29+), although a suppressor phenotype (CD8+) is infrequently seen. About 50% of cases demonstrate expression of CD25, a component of the interleukin-2 (IL-2) receptor. Circulating Sézary cells typically bear the same immunophenotype as the skin infiltrate, but there may be antigen discordance, especially for the CD25 antigen, which is often absent from circulating Sézary cells.

T cell antigen receptor gene studies have provided a molecular tool to determine the clonality of lymphoid processes and have been particularly useful in the diagnosis of early-stage MF and SS. The T cell antigen receptor is a heterodimeric structure that complexes with other surface antigens, including CD3, and is important in antigen recognition and in intracellular signal transduction. Molecular genetic techniques, including Southern blotting, have demonstrated clonal rearrangements of the T cell receptor (TCR) beta chain in lymph nodes and peripheral blood from patients with MF. Newer techniques, including the polymerase chain reaction (PCR), allow for the detection of clonal gene rearrangements in tissues containing few atypical lymphocytes, where detection would be impossible at the level of sensitivity of conventional Southern blotting. PCR has been especially valuable in early-stage MF to establish clonality; however, it has recently been demonstrated that several non-neoplastic conditions that mimic MF, including lymphomatoid papulosis, can be associated with TCR clonality. These studies suggest that TCR rearrangements, although a useful diagnostic tool, are not pathognomonic for MF in the case of atypical histopathologic findings.

Other genetic analyses have been reported in MF and SS, including cytogenetics. Unlike chronic myelogenous leukemia, follicular B cell lymphomas, and other hematopoietic disorders, there have been no characteristic karyotypic findings identified in patients with MF and SS, although frequent abnormalities of chromosomes 1 and 6 have been reported. Mutations and functional loss of the p53 tumor suppressor oncogene have been reported in MF, along with overexpression or mutations of known oncogenes, including *myc, ras,* and *lck.*

CLINICAL FEATURES, STAGING, AND PROGNOSIS

Many patients with MF initially present with a history of skin lesions diagnosed as a nonspecific dermatitis. As the skin lesions evolve, they assume more characteristic features of patches (erythematous macular lesions) or plaques (erythematous and scaling, with raised margins). Cutaneous tumors may appear de novo or may represent an evolution from prior patch- or plaque-stage disease. Diffuse erythroderma most frequently occurs in the setting of circulating Sézary cells. Pruritus is often a feature of MF skin lesions at all stages. In addition, the lesions can be associated with skin fissuring and ulceration, leading to secondary infection. At diagnosis, 42% of patients have limited plaques covering 10% or less of their body surface, 30% have extensive plaques, 16% have cutaneous tumors, and 12% have generalized erythroderma. Palpable lymphadenopathy occurs infrequently in patients with limited plaque disease and in about 50% of patients with extensive plaques, tumors, or erythroderma.

Peripheral blood involvement can be demonstrated in patients at all stages of disease: 12% of patients with skin plaques, 16% with tumors, and the majority of patients with erythroderma. The circulating neoplastic lymphocytes may consist of small hyperconvoluted cells or may be a mixture of small and large cells. The absolute number of circulating neoplastic cells can be quantitated by light microscopic analysis of a peripheral smear or, with greater accuracy, of thick smears. Recently, methods have evolved to quantitate circulating cells by flow cytometry using aneuploidy or immunophenotypic analysis. The neoplastic lymphocytes can be identified by size or by brightness of fluorescence of certain antigens, including CD3. Other hematologic findings in MF and SS include absolute lymphopenia and varying degrees of eosinophilia. Both eosinophilia and the presence of large blastic cells in the peripheral blood are poor prognostic features.

Visceral involvement is seen more frequently in patients with advanced skin disease or blood involvement. The most common sites of involvement at autopsy are liver, lungs, and spleen. Bone marrow infiltration is most common in patients with blood involvement or extensive lymph node disease but can be found in up to 18% of patients with early plaque-stage disease.

The most important adverse prognostic factors in MF and SS are advanced skin stage, extensive lymph node involvement, and visceral involvement. The median survival for patients with limited skin plaques is 8 to 10 years; for those with tumors or erythroderma, it is 40 months. The median survival for patients with visceral involvement is 30 months. Although many patients with MF and SS manifest a slowly progressive course of the disease, the major cause of death is infection. Bacterial infections with *Staphylococcus aureus, Staphylococcus epidermidis,* and *Pseudomonas aeruginosa* are most common, perhaps due to poor skin integrity and the presence of intravenous catheter devices for chemotherapy. The defects in cell-mediated immunity inherent to MF and other lymphomas predispose patients to viral and fungal infections as well. Good skin care is of paramount importance in the management of these patients to decrease the incidence of life-threatening systemic infections.

STAGING

The staging system for MF and SS is based on both clinical and histopathologic criteria (Table 2). In this classification, skin disease is described as limited plaque covering 10% or less of the body surface (T1), extensive plaque covering greater than 10% of the body surface (T2), tumor (T3), or erythroderma (T4). Lymph node classification is defined by the extent of node involvement, with LN4 being a node in which the normal architecture is effaced by lymphomatous infiltrate, LN2 being a node with small clusters of atypical lymphocytes with preserved architecture, and LN3 being a node with large clusters of atypical lymphocytes and paracortical expansion but otherwise preserved architecture. Blood involvement is not included in this staging system.

Recently, Sausville and colleagues at the National Cancer Institute proposed a simplified version of this staging system that categorizes patients as low, intermediate, or high risk based on the results of a retrospective analysis of clinical and histopathologic prognostic factors. According to this system, low-risk patients have skin plaques with minimal or absent node involvement and no visceral disease, high-risk patients have histopathologically effaced lymph nodes or evidence of visceral involvement, and all other patients fall into the intermediate-risk group.

TABLE 2. Modified Staging System

Bunn and Lamberg	Sausville
IA: T1, LN0–2, Ad-, V-	Low risk: T1–2, LN0–2, V-, B-
IB: T2, LN0–2, Ad-, V-	
IIA: T1–2, Ad+, LN0–2, V-	
	Intermediate risk: T1–2, LN0–2, V-, B+
IIB: T3, Ad±, LN0–2, V-	T3–4, LN2, V-, B±
III: T4, Ad±, LN0–2, V-	T1–4, LN3, B±
IVA: T1–4, LN3–4, Ad±, V-	
IVB: T1–4, LN3–4, Ad±, V+	High risk: T1–4, LN4 and/or V+

V = Visceral involvement; B = blood smear; Ad = adenopathy; T1 = skin patch or plaque <10% body surface; T2 = skin plaque >10% body surface; T3 = tumor; T4 = erythroderma; LN0–2 = uninvolved or small clusters of atypical lymphocytes; LN3 = clusters of six or more atypical lymphocytes with preserved node architecture; LN4 = effaced node.

CLINICAL MANAGEMENT

The focus of treatment of MF and SS is control of the skin disease and, thus, palliation of symptoms. Multiple therapeutic modalities have been employed, including both topical and systemic therapies (Table 3). Therapies directed at control of symptoms include emollients, antipruritics, and topical steroids. Antineoplastic therapies include topical and systemic chemotherapies, ultraviolet light therapy, skin irradiation, extracorporeal photopheresis, and an expanding list of new, biologically oriented therapies. Many of these therapies induce a response in most patients, but long-term remissions are rare. There is probably a subset of patients with very early disease who may be cured using these modalities, but for the majority of incurable patients, therapies are directed at palliation of the disease.

Topical Chemotherapy

Topical steroids are often the first therapy for MF and SS, as they are often prescribed early in the disease, when a benign etiology for the skin rash is suspected. In the setting of known MF, steroids may also play a role in palliating the skin disease and decreasing pruritus. Patients with limited patch-stage disease may have complete clearing with steroid therapy, but the disease usually recurs.

Topical chemotherapeutic agents have been used for many years as primary therapy for MF. The two drugs with demonstrated efficacy are mechlorethamine hydrochloride (Mustargen) and bis-chloroethyl-nitrosourea (BCNU, carmustine). Both agents can be administered as an aqueous solution that is painted onto the involved skin areas or in an ointment base. The ointment preparations are preferred due to the ease of application and lower incidence of skin hypersensitivity reaction, although they require special compounding by a pharmacist. These agents are potential carcinogens, and patients and their families should be instructed on the proper use and disposal of the solutions at home. Complete remissions have been reported in 80%, 68%, and 61% of patients with limited plaque, extensive plaque, and tumor lesions, respectively, with response durations of 15, 5, and 12 months. The median time to complete remission with mechlorethamine ranged from 6 to 48 months and for BCNU from 8 to 28 months when the agent was applied daily. Many patients are maintained in remission on less frequent schedules of application.

Side effects include cutaneous hypersensitivity, consisting of erythema and pruritus or burning. The frequency of side effects is less with the ointment-based therapies. Patients can often be desensitized by injecting small doses of the agent intradermally over the course of several weeks, with gradual dose increments. Skin telangiectasias occur frequently with BCNU and usually resolve after therapy is discontinued. The most significant long-term toxicity of topical chemotherapy is secondary skin cancers (basal cell and squamous cell), which occur in up to 12% of treated patients. Systemic absorption has not been documented with mechlorethamine, but BCNU has been associated with mild neutropenia in 3 to 5% of patients, so blood counts are followed during treatment.

TABLE 3. Therapeutic Modalities for Mycosis Fungoides and Sézary's Syndrome

Topical Therapies	Systemic Therapies
Topical steroids	Single-agent chemotherapy
Topical chemotherapy	(methotrexate, chlorambucil
(mechlorethamine	[Leukeran])
[Mustargen], carmustine	Combination chemotherapy
[BiCNU])	Interferon-alfa* (Roferon-A,
PUVA	Intron A)
Electron beam or photon	Purine analogues (pentostatin
irradiation	[Nipent],* fludarabine
Extracorporeal photopheresis	[Fludara],* cladribine
	[Leustatin]*
	Retinoids (*cis*-retinoic acid
	[Accutane], all-*trans* retinoic
	acid)
	IL2 fusion toxin (DAB$_{389}$IL2)†
	Thymopentin†
	Monoclonal antibodies

*Not FDA-approved for this indication.
†Investigational drug in the United States.

Radiation and Phototherapy

Phototherapy with ultraviolet A (UVA) light and the photoactivated compound 8-methyl-psoralen

(PUVA) has been an effective therapy in early-stage MF. Psoralen acts to inhibit DNA and RNA synthesis through the formation of monofunctional or bifunctional thymidine adducts, gene mutations, or sister chromatid exchanges when the drug is exposed to UVA light. Initial PUVA exposure is between 1.5 and 3.0 joules per cm² and depends on the degree of skin pigmentation and ease in tanning. Therapy is given three times per week until clearing occurs, and then frequency is reduced. Up to 59% of early-stage patients with patch or plaque disease can be cured, but relapses often occur if therapy is stopped. The long-term cure rate with PUVA is 15 to 20%. Potential side effects include nausea due to psoralen ingestion, erythema, worsening pruritus, and chronic dry skin. Like the topical chemotherapy agents, PUVA is associated with an increased incidence of cutaneous carcinomas, especially squamous carcinomas of the skin and male genitalia.

Another form of phototherapy is extracorporeal photopheresis, in which patients ingest psoralen and then undergo leukapheresis with isolation of the mononuclear fraction. The cells are then exposed to UVA light ex vivo and reinfused into the patient. Therapy is administered every 2 to 4 weeks. The exact biologic mechanism at work in this form of therapy is still speculative, but it is believed that circulating neoplastic lymphocytes, damaged by the psoralen and UVA exposure, are reinfused into the patient and stimulate an immune-mediated antitumor response. About 15 to 30% of MF and SS patients respond to photopheresis with skin clearing, and most responses have been seen in patients with erythroderma and SS.

Radiation therapy has also been an important therapeutic modality in both early and advanced MF and SS. Total skin electron beam irradiation has been demonstrated to be a curative therapy in a subset of patients with early patch or plaque disease. Linear accelerator-generated electrons are scattered by a penetrable plate placed at a collimator site, and this reduces the energy of the electrons to 4 to 7 MeV, allowing for penetration of several millimeters to 1 cm into the dermis. Since there is no deep tissue penetration, there is no internal organ toxicity. Total doses of 3000 to 3600 cG are administered over a 10- to 12-week period. Although initially 80 to 90% of patients treated with total skin electron beam irradiation attain a clinical remission, only 50% of those with limited plaques and 25% with advanced plaques have durable remissions. Several studies have demonstrated prolonged remissions when topical mechlorethamine was used in the adjuvant setting after completion of electron beam therapy.

In patients with more advanced skin disease, cutaneous tumors, or erythroderma, electron beam irradiation can be palliative by reducing tumor burden and cutaneous symptoms, including skin ulceration and pruritus. Tumor-stage patients and patients with deep plaques may also be treated with spot photon radiation for palliation of refractory or disfiguring lesions.

Electron beam radiation is associated with both short- and long-term toxicities. During the course of therapy, skin erythema, dryness, scaling, or ulcerations may occur. After completion of therapy, skin thickening and tightness and telangiectasias are seen in many patients. The therapy is associated with hair and sweat gland atrophy, which may be permanent. Secondary skin cancers occur in about 10% of patients. Because of these effects and the availability of other topical therapies with similar response rates, electron beam irradiation has fallen out of favor as a front-line curative therapy and is used mostly in the palliative setting.

Systemic Therapies

Systemic therapies are used in MF and SS when patients become refractory to topical therapies or when they demonstrate signs of advanced systemic disease in the form of lymphadenopathy or visceral involvement. Single-agent alkylating agents and methotrexate have been used in many patients as the first systemic therapy. Methotrexate given twice weekly or as a weekly intravenous infusion is active in about 40% of patients. Toxicities include mouth ulcerations, diarrhea, and cytopenias. Chlorambucil (Leukeran) given as a single agent or in combination with prednisone has shown activity, especially in patients with SS.

Combination chemotherapy has been used in MF and SS, with response rates of 80 to 100% to standard non-Hodgkin's lymphoma regimens, including CHOP (cyclophosphamide [Cytoxan], doxorubicin [Adriamycin], vincristine [Oncovin], prednisone), CAPO (cyclophosphamide, Adriamycin, vincristine, etoposide), and COP-bleo (cyclophosphamide, vincristine, prednisone, bleomycin). Unfortunately, remission duration in these studies was measured in months. A large randomized study performed at the National Cancer Institute examined aggressive chemotherapy combined with total skin electron beam irradiation or conservative topical therapies in untreated MF patients. This study was unable to demonstrate a difference in overall survival or disease-free survival in the aggressively treated group. Combination chemotherapy is therefore reserved as a palliative modality for patients who have failed other therapeutic approaches or who require an immediate decrease in tumor burden.

There is little experience with bone marrow transplantation in MF and SS. In one small study, two of six patients treated with autologous transplantation are alive without disease recurrence. The increased susceptibility of MF patients to infection due to poor skin integrity and underlying immunologic defects makes them poor candidates for high-dose therapies associated with prolonged periods of granulocytopenia.

Interferon-alfa* (2a [Roferon-A] and 2b [Intron A]) remains one of the most active systemic therapies for

---

*Not FDA-approved for this indication.

MF and SS. Response rates vary from 25 to 30% in heavily pretreated patients to up to 90% in previously untreated patients. Doses and schedules vary, but the optimal starting dose is believed to be 3 million U three times per week, with dose escalation if no response is seen. Toxicity is dose-dependent and includes fevers, chills, myalgias, malaise, anorexia, and, at higher doses, cytopenias. Doses of up to 12 million U three times a week are usually well tolerated. The median time to optimal response with interferons is 4 to 6 months, and treatment is often continued in responding patients for years. Interferons have been combined with other therapies, including PUVA and photopheresis. The combination of PUVA plus low-dose interferon (3 to 9 million units) is associated with a complete response rate of up to 90%, and this combination is now widely implemented as first-line therapy in many patients.

A novel category of chemotherapeutic agents, the purine nucleoside analogues, has demonstrated significant activity in patients with advanced MF. Fludarabine (Fludara),* 2-chlorodeoxyadenosine (cladribine [Leustatin]),* and pentostatin (Nipent)* have all demonstrated response rates of 30 to 40% as single agents or, in the case of fludarabine and pentostatin, in combination with interferon-alfa. Toxicities of these agents include bone marrow suppression, immune suppression, and neurologic dysfunction, and these agents are generally used only in patients with advanced or refractory disease.

Other novel investigational agents, including retinoids, monoclonal antibodies, fusion toxins, and immunomodulators, have shown promise in MF and SS. Analogues of *cis*-retinoic acid given systemically have been associated with a 20% response rate in early-stage patients, and studies with *trans*-retinoic acid are under way.

One of the most promising novel therapies is the IL2 fusion toxin $DAB_{389}IL2$,† which consists of the active moiety of diphtheria toxin and the full-length sequence of the IL-2 gene. This chimeric protein targets cells bearing high-affinity IL2 receptor and liberates the active toxin fragment intracellularly after internalization of the ligand-receptor complex. Preliminary studies have demonstrated that up to 50% of MF patients express the IL2 receptor on their neoplastic cells, and 35 to 40% of these have responded to IL2 fusion toxin therapy. Further randomized phase III studies using this agent in MF and SS patients are under way.

Another agent that has shown promise is thymopentin,† a pentapeptide similar to the thymic hormone thymopoietin. In one study, up to 60% of patients with early SS responded to this therapy, but larger confirmatory studies have not yet been completed.

In conclusion, several therapies have been demonstrated to be effective in MF and SS, and cure is a possibility for patients at the earliest stages of these diseases. In this group of patients, the disease should be addressed aggressively in the hope that a cure will be attained. For most other patients, therapy is individualized. Because of the relatively indolent nature of the disease at its onset, therapies are directed at achieving maximum palliation without undue discomfort or inconvenience for the patient.

PAPULOSQUAMOUS DISEASES

method of
DAVID L. HURT, M.D., and
WARREN W. PIETTE, M.D.
University of Iowa College of Medicine
Iowa City, Iowa

Papulosquamous eruptions refer to a group of skin disorders that are characterized by scaling papules and plaques but are unrelated to one another. The classic papulosquamous eruptions include psoriasis, pityriasis rubra pilaris, pityriasis rosea, lichen planus, and secondary syphilis (Table 1). Seborrheic dermatitis, although not usually considered a papulosquamous eruption, is a frequent diagnostic consideration and is therefore also included. Secondary syphilis is discussed elsewhere in this volume.

PSORIASIS

Psoriasis is a common inflammatory dermatosis affecting 1.5 to 2% of the population in Western countries. Approximately one-third of the cases occur in patients younger than 20 years of age. Inheritance is multifactorial, and there is no gender predilection. Psoriasis can be divided into four groups: psoriasis vulgaris, generalized pustular psoriasis, localized pustular psoriasis, and erythrodermic psoriasis. Guttate and inverse psoriasis are variants of psoriasis vulgaris.

The lesions of psoriasis vulgaris consist of sharply demarcated erythematous, salmon-pink to red plaques and papules with a silvery-white scale. Removal of the scale may result in pinpoint bleeding called the Auspitz phenomenon. The sites of predilection are the extensor surfaces of the elbows and knees as well as the scalp, intergluteal cleft, and lumbar region of the back. Plaques may be present anywhere on the body. Patients may also present with plaques in the genital area, axilla, or under the breasts, referred to as inverse psoriasis, which can mimic intertrigo, candidiasis, or tinea cruris. Pruritus is a common symptom, especially in lesions on the scalp and in the anogenital area.

Guttate psoriasis is rare, constituting less than 2% of all psoriasis. The lesions are characterized by small pink droplike papules with a fine scale that usually appear rapidly in crops. Trunk and proximal extremity involvement predominates, but face and scalp may also be involved. Flares often follow streptococcal pharyngitis. This may be the initial appearance of psoriasis or an acute exacerbation of chronic

---

*Not FDA-approved for this indication.

†Investigational drug in the United States.

TABLE 1. **Classic Papulosquamous Eruptions**

	Characteristic Lesion	Location	Scale	Mucosal and Nail Involvement	Extracutaneous Manifestations
Psoriasis Vulgaris					
Plaque	Sharply marginated plaques	Knees, elbows, scalp, intergluteal cleft	Silvery-white	For all variants: Mucosa spared	Psoriatic arthritis can be seen with all skin variants, and in the absence of cutaneous disease
Guttate	Pink droplike papules <1 cm	Trunk proximal extremities	Fine silvery-white	Nail changes: Pitting Oil drop Leukonychia Onycholysis Splinter hemorrhage	
Inverse		Intertriginous areas	Often minimal		
Localized pustular	Pustules	Localized palms and soles	In addition to pustules, may retain more typical plaques		
Generalized pustular	Pustules	Generalized			Fever, chills, leukocytosis, rarely hypocalcemia
Erythrodermic	Total body erythema	Total body	Desquamative scale		Yes*
Secondary syphilis	Erythematous papules with scale	Generalized, frequently affect palms or soles	Psoriasiform to fine	Mucosa involved, alopecia	Lymphadenopathy, malaise
Pityriasis rosea	Erythematous round to oval patches; herald patch: initial lesion	Trunk, neck, proximal extremities	Marginal collarette of scale	Mucosa and nails spared	No
Pityriasis rubra pilaris	Salmon-colored patches with islands of sparing; palmoplantar keratoderma	Initially head, neck and trunk; spreads distally to palms and soles; rarely, erythroderma	Psoriasiform scale	Mucosa spared	No, unless there is erythroderma*
Lichen planus	Flat-topped purple or violaceous polyangular papules with a superficial network of fine white lines	Flexor wrists, forearms, shins, ankles, dorsal hands, lumbosacral area	Reticulate network of fine white lines (Wickham's striae)	Buccal mucosa, lips with superficial fine white lines, nail changes, alopecia	No
Seborrheic dermatitis†	Erythematous scaling patches	Scalp, eyebrows, malar area, nasolabial folds, presternal area, central back; rarely, erythroderma	Yellow flaky scale	Mucosa and nails spared	Not usually; Leiner's disease in pediatric patients*

*With any erythroderma, hypoalbuminemia, pedal edema, temperature dysregulation, and high-output cardiac failure may occur.
†Not a classic papulosquamous disease, but frequently enters the differential diagnosis.

plaque-type psoriasis. Guttate psoriasis most commonly affects children and young adults.

There are two forms of pustular psoriasis: generalized and localized. Generalized psoriasis, or von Zumbusch type, is a condition in which the patient needs to be admitted for intensive treatment. Generally the patient is ill, has a history of plaque-type psoriasis, and rapidly develops shallow pustules on an erythematous base that eventually coalesce into larger pools of pustules. It is often associated with fever, chills, arthralgias, hypocalcemia, and a leukocytosis. Frequently there are triggering events that cause the flare, such as the withdrawal of systemic corticosteroid treatment for plaque-type psoriasis. The localized form of pustular psoriasis may occur when there has been prolonged treatment of a given plaque occasionally with corticosteroids but usually with irritants such as tars or anthralin. Pustular acrodermatitis is another localized form of psoriasis characterized by a chronic, relapsing eruption limited to the palms and soles, with numerous sterile, yellow, deep-seated pustules. This condition is rare and more commonly affects females.

Erythrodermic psoriasis produces red skin with desquamative scale over much or most of the body surface. Generally, erythrodermic psoriasis arises in patients with widespread plaque-type psoriasis with a flaring of their disease. It can be associated with dysfunction of temperature regulation, hypoalbuminemia, pedal edema, and high-output cardiac failure due to inflammatory vasodilatation, as can occur in any erythroderma of any cause.

Nail changes are common, occurring in approximately 10 to 50% of patients. Nail changes include nail pitting, oil drop or salmon patches, leukonychia (nail whitening), onycholysis, and splinter hemorrhage. Psoriatic arthritis is relatively uncommon but occurs in about 3 to 4% of patients. The arthritis may occur with the cutaneous lesions, may precede the lesions, or may occur in the absence of cutaneous disease. The arthritis may present as an asymmetrical oligoarthropathy or affecting predominantly distal interphalangeal joints or as a mutilating type of arthritis.

The etiology of psoriasis is unknown. However, in areas of the psoriatic plaque there are abnormal cell kinetics characterized by an increased mitotic rate and a shortened transit time of 3 to 4 days from the basal cell layer to the stratum corneum, rather than the normal time of 28 days.

Therapy. Application of emollients is extremely important in the treatment of psoriasis, whether the degree of psoriasis is mild, moderate, or severe. Emollients alone can help decrease the amount of scale on the psoriatic plaques as well as the thickness of the plaque. White petrolatum or a hydrated ointment should be applied several times a day.

For minimal to moderate plaque-type psoriasis, topical corticosteroid preparations are the mainstays of therapy. Usually a midpotency topical corticosteroid is applied twice daily, followed by the application of an emollient. Moist vinyl occlusion (MVO) can also be used to help control an acute flare of psoriasis. MVO enhances the cutaneous penetration of the steroid and should be used sparingly. For areas on the face and on skin folds, only a low-potency steroid, such as 1% hydrocortisone, should be used twice daily.

For the treatment of moderate to severe psoriasis that is resistant to topical therapy, ultraviolet B (UVB) radiation is very helpful. PUVA therapy, ultraviolet A (UVA) combined with psoralen (a photosensitizing agent), may also be used if the patient fails UVB. These and other types of therapy, such as methotrexate, etretinate, or cyclosporine, should be administered by a physician skilled in their use.

Calcipotriene (Dovonex), a vitamin D_3 derivative, has been shown to inhibit the proliferation of keratinocytes and can be helpful in treating mild to moderate plaque-type psoriasis. It is used twice daily on the plaques. Calcipotriene is systemically absorbed, and if used in sufficient quantities, it can alter calcium metabolism. Since systemic absorption limits the total body surface area to which it can be applied, this treatment is generally avoided in extensive psoriasis.

Topical coal tar preparations and anthralin may be used for plaque-type psoriasis. The tar preparations (Estar gel, Fototar) are applied for 2 to 12 hours and then washed off. Anthralin creme (Drithocreme) is applied in concentrations of 0.1 to 1% to the plaques and left on for 5 to 30 minutes and then washed off. Both tar and anthralin tend to be messy and can stain clothing, and anthralin can stain normal skin as well. In addition, both tars and anthralin may cause an irritant dermatitis and should generally be administered by a physician experienced in the use of this therapy.

In guttate psoriasis patients, streptococcal infection may be a triggering factor. Therefore, if cultures or antibody titers are positive, systemic antibiotics should be considered. UVB can help accelerate the resolution of the lesions, as can lubrication and natural sunlight.

Localized pustular psoriasis on the palms and soles is treated with topical steroids or, in resistant cases, with localized hand-foot PUVA. Generalized pustular psoriasis is a potentially life-threatening disorder. These patients should be admitted to the hospital, with special attention paid to renal function and calcium metabolism. Etretinate or sometimes methotrexate is an appropriate therapeutic option in such patients.

SEBORRHEIC DERMATITIS

Seborrheic dermatitis is an extremely common chronic dermatosis. It can arise in any age group but is most common in those between 20 and 50 years of age. Males are more commonly affected, and the disease is most severe during the winter. Seborrheic dermatitis has a characteristic distribution seen in the scalp, eyebrows, malar area, nasolabial folds, retroauricular creases, beard, presternal area, and central back. It is less commonly seen in the axillae, groin, submammary areas, and umbilicus. It is also known as "cradle cap" in infants. The lesions are characterized by erythematous, scaling patches that may be fairly discrete on the face and the trunk and diffuse on the scalp. The scale may be either dry and powdery or oily. Other diseases in the differential diagnosis include psoriasis, atopic dermatitis, tinea corporis, tinea faciale, contact dermatitis, and lupus erythematosus.

The etiology of seborrheic dermatitis is unknown, but many believe *Pityrosporum ovale* to be the causative agent, as the number of organisms correlates best with the severity of the disease.

Therapy. Antiseborrheic shampoos are the standard therapy for the scalp. Most of the shampoos are over the counter and include 1% selenium sulfide suspension (Selsun Blue), zinc pyrithione (Head and Shoulders, Sebulon), and tar derivatives (T/Gel). These preparations all work well. In mild to moderate cases, the shampoos can be used one to three times a week, but control may require daily use. Two percent ketoconazole (Nizoral) may also be used two to three times a week for 4 to 6 weeks and thereafter once a week prophylactically. As tar products can discolor gray and blonde hair, selenium sulfide or zinc pyrithione may be more suitable for these patients. The shampoos should be left on for a minimum of 5 minutes before washing out. Topical steroids are also useful in reducing the erythema and work well in conjunction with the antiseborrheic shampoos. For the scalp and face, a 1% hydrocortisone lotion or cream can be applied once to twice daily. For more severe cases on the scalp, a stronger steroid can be used, such as 0.01% fluocinolone acetonide (Synalar) solution once to twice daily. In severe cases in which there is thick, adherent scale on the scalp, Baker's P & S Liquid applied to the scalp overnight under a shower cap is helpful in removing the scale. Severe irritation can result if this is not used properly. Use of antiseborrheic shampoos and topical steroids is still important.

Facial lesions are usually adequately controlled with 1% hydrocortisone lotions or creams applied once to twice daily. Two percent ketoconazole (Nizoral) cream may also be used on the face and body, but its use is generally reserved for patients in whom topical steroids have failed, because of the cost. For scaling along the eyelid margin, topical application of baby shampoo with a cotton-tipped applicator and warm compresses are usually effective.

PITYRIASIS ROSEA

Pityriasis rosea is a common eruption typically seen in children and young adults. It is clinically characterized by erythematous round to oval patches with a marginal collarette of scale. The first cutaneous manifestation is a "herald patch." This is the first lesion to appear, is usually larger than the rest of the lesions, and often occurs on the trunk, although it can appear anywhere on the body. Within 2 weeks of the onset of the herald patch, crops of similar but smaller lesions develop over the trunk, neck, and proximal extremities. The lesions tend to follow skin tension lines, forming a "Christmas tree" pattern on the trunk. Pruritus may or may not be present. Spontaneous remission usually occurs in 6 to 12 weeks. The etiology is not known but is suspected to be an otherwise asymptomatic infection. Second episodes of pityriasis rosea are rare.

Therapy. If pruritus is present, a midpotency topical steroid such as triamcinolone 0.025% ointment twice daily is reasonable therapy. A counterirritant such as Sarna lotion used on an as-needed basis may be helpful. Hydroxyzine (Atarax, Vistaril) 25 to 50 mg every 6 hours is also useful in controlling pruritus. For more severe cases, UVB may be effective.

PITYRIASIS RUBRA PILARIS (PRP)

PRP is an uncommon dermatosis characterized by salmon-colored patches with psoriasiform scale that generally appear first on the upper half of the body and spread distally. The scalp is rarely affected. A characteristic finding is patches of normal skin within large lesions, so-called islands of sparing. Also characteristic is a well-demarcated palmoplantar keratoderma. In the typical form, spontaneous remission occurs within 3 years, although there are cases of severe unremitting disease. PRP affects all ages. The cause is unknown.

Therapy. Treatment of patients with this disease is difficult and usually requires specialty management. Mild to moderate cases may be treated with topical steroids, emollients, and keratolytics for the palms and soles. Calcipotriene (Dovonex) has also been shown to be helpful. Appropriate longer-term treatment includes etretinate (Tegison), isotretinoin (Accutane), or methotrexate.*

LICHEN PLANUS

Lichen planus (LP) is characterized by flat-topped, purple or violaceous, polyangular pruritic papules with a reticulated superficial network of fine white lines. The lesions can occur at any age but most commonly are seen in patients between 30 and 60

years of age, with a slight female predominance. The sites of predilection include flexor wrists, forearms, shins, ankles, penis, dorsal surface of the hands, and lumbosacral area. LP can remain localized or may disseminate, usually within 1 month of onset. Linear lesions may result from Koebner's phenomenon, an isomorphic response to nonspecific trauma. Approximately 50% of patients with cutaneous LP have mucosal involvement, characterized by a reticulate network of fine white lines. Nail involvement is seen in about 10% of cutaneous cases. Most cases remit within 6 to 18 months; recurrence is seen in 10 to 20% of patients. This disease is less common than psoriasis, but patients frequently present to primary care physicians with this problem. The etiology is unknown. Lichenoid drug eruptions can mimic LP.

Therapy. Treatment of mild to moderate LP includes the use of high-potency topical steroids, such as fluocinonide (Lidex), twice daily. For more severe cases or for prolonged therapy, referral is probably indicated.

CONNECTIVE TISSUE DISEASE
(Systemic Lupus Erythematosus, Dermatomyositis, Other Myopathies, and Scleroderma)

method of
ALAN C. JACOBSON, M.D., and
DAVID G. BORENSTEIN, M.D.
The George Washington University Medical Center
Washington, D.C.

SYSTEMIC LUPUS ERYTHEMATOSUS

Systemic lupus erythematosus (SLE) is a complex, multisystem autoimmune disease. The disease affects young and middle-aged women, with a female to male ratio of 8:1. Criteria for the classification of SLE have been proposed by the American College of Rheumatology; they include involvement of cutaneous, musculoskeletal, genitourologic, neurologic, hematologic, and immunologic systems. The presence of at least 4 of the 11 criteria is required for the classification. These criteria should be used as aids in categorizing the range of abnormalities associated with the illness and therefore should be interpreted with flexibility. To understand how to treat SLE, one should be aware that each patient may present in his or her own manner of organ involvement, and that there are different degrees of disease activity. For example, certain skin changes are mild and require only hydroxychloroquine (Plaquenil), whereas other, more severe cutaneous abnormalities require prednisone (Deltasone). The spectrum of therapy corresponds to the severity of the clinical manifestations of SLE.

---

*Not FDA-approved for this indication.

Skin Manifestations

Cutaneous manifestations of SLE cause a variety of skin disorders. Approximately one third of patients have the classic butterfly malar rash. Photosensitivity is present in 10% to 60% of patients and may be in the form of a patchy rash. Cutaneous vasculitic lesions may also occur. Sunscreens with at least SPF 15 are recommended, but it is best to avoid ultraviolet light exposure. Subacute cutaneous lupus is characterized by symmetric, superficial lesions consisting of scaly and erythematous macules and papules. Discoid lupus lesions are often well circumscribed, erythematous plaques with scaling.

Topical steroids such as hydrocortisone (low potency Corticaine cream 0.5%), intermediate strength betamethasone valerate 0.1% (Valisone cream 0.1%), or high potency fluocinonide 0.05% (Lidex cream 0.05%) can be applied to affected areas. Low-potency steroids should be applied initially. Topical steroids can lead to skin atrophy with chronic use and should not be used on the face.

Hydroxychloroquine (Plaquenil) should be used for the treatment of lupus skin conditions with a dose of 200 to 400 mg daily. One must first check for glucose-6-phosphate dehydrogenase (G6PD) deficiency before initiating hydroxychloroquine to decrease the risk of hemolysis. Eye examinations should be done every 6 months to exclude retinal deposits of the drug. Chloroquine phosphate (Aralen),* 250 mg daily, may be substituted for hydroxychloroquine. Chloroquine has more adverse side effects: indigestion, rash, and retinopathy. In severe extensive skin disease, systemic steroids may be utilized at doses of 20 to 40 mg per day.

Arthritis

Arthritis is a common initial manifestation of SLE. It is usually nonerosive, episodic, and oligoarticular. The leukocyte count in synovial fluid, when present, is lower than in rheumatoid arthritis. Soft tissue structures are damaged to a greater extent than are articular cartilage and bone. Joint deformity occurs in the absence of bone erosion. Deformities in the hand may resemble those of patients with rheumatoid arthritis. This pattern of nonerosive deforming disease has been called Jaccoud's arthropathy. Early on, the deformities due to subluxation are reversible. With the onset of contractures, they may become fixed. Tendinitis is common. Arthritis and tendinitis can generally be controlled with nonsteroidal anti-inflammatory drugs (NSAIDs).

Individual trials of different NSAIDs at maximum therapeutic doses may be necessary. NSAIDs should be tried for periods of 2 to 4 weeks before switching to another NSAID. For example, diclofenac (Voltaren), 75 mg twice daily, or naproxen (Naprosyn), 500 mg twice daily, is an effective agent. Other NSAIDs used for lupus arthritis include oxaprozin

(Daypro), 600 mg, two tablets, one in the morning and one at night, nabumetone (Relafen), 500 mg, two tablets every 12 hours, or ketoprofen (Oruvail), 200 mg once a day. One should always be aware of the adverse effects of NSAIDs, particularly renal (decreased renal function, hyperkalemia) and gastrointestinal (ulcerations, bleeding). Antimalarial compounds are also used in treating musculoskeletal features. Hydroxychloroquine is given at 200 to 400 mg daily. If these medications fail, low-dose corticosteroids, such as oral prednisone, may be necessary in doses of 20 mg daily.

Renal Manifestations

Renal involvement in SLE occurs in a majority of patients and may vary from minimal change to diffuse proliferative glomerulonephritis. Treatment depends on the pathologic characteristics of the renal lesions. The World Health Organization (WHO) classification of lupus nephritis has generally been well accepted. It uses light microscopy, immunofluorescence, and electron microscopy to classify glomerular involvement. WHO class I is normal. WHO class II biopsy specimens have involvement restricted to mesangial areas, not requiring treatment. Class III biopsy specimens have focal proliferative changes associated with proteinuria. One half of patients with proliferative disease have an active urinary sediment. Transition to diffuse proliferative glomerulonephritis or membranous nephritis may occur. Class IV biopsies, diffuse proliferative nephritis, are lesions similar to those of class III, but they affect more than 50% of the glomerular surface. Proteinuria, greater than 3 grams over 24 hours in at least half, and hematuria are associated with this form of lupus nephritis. Hypertension is common. Renal insufficiency evolves in most patients.

Both active focal proliferative (FPLN) and diffuse proliferative lupus nephritis (DPLN) require aggressive treatment. Prednisone at 1 mg per kg per day for at least 6 weeks and up to 6 months, depending on clinical response, should be given. With clinical improvement, prednisone is tapered; however, a maintenance dose of 10 mg daily for 2 years is continued. Intravenous cyclophosphamide (Cytoxan)* is added at the onset of therapy, increasing the probability of improvement of kidney function. The patient is first treated with a test dose of 500 mg per m². Eight hours of prehydration and 10 hours of posthydration is given to reduce the occurrence of hemorrhagic cystitis. An antiemetic such as ondansetron hydrochloride (Zofran), 0.15 mg per kg, should be infused 30 minutes prior to cyclophosphamide and then at 4 and 8 hours after infusion. The antiemetic granisetron hydrochloride (Kytril) (0.7 mg if the patient is less than 70 kg, 1.0 mg if the patient is greater than 70 kg) can be given 30 minutes prior to cyclophosphamide. The infusion of antiemetic is a one-time dose. A complete blood count (CBC) and

---

*Not FDA-approved for this indication.

platelet count are obtained at the nadir point, 10 to 14 days after the infusion of cyclophosphamide. The cyclophosphamide is increased by 10% each subsequent dosing to obtain a nadir white count of 4000 cells per ml. This therapy is administered monthly for 6 months, then every 2 to 3 months for 2 years.

Class V lesions, membranous glomerulonephritis, have a slowly progressive course. Patients are treated with prednisone, 1 mg per kg per day for 6 to 12 weeks, then tapered to a maintenance dose of 10 to 20 mg daily. If protein excretion increases and/or creatinine clearance decreases, the prednisone dose should be increased. Cytotoxic agents have not been shown to benefit membranous lupus nephritis. A sixth class of lupus nephritis is that with advanced and sclerosing glomerulonephritis, an end-stage lesion. In deciding to treat lupus nephritis, one should know the pathologist's chronicity and activity assessment of the biopsy. A high chronicity assessment generally has a worse response to treatment.

Toxicities of cyclophosphamide including nausea, vomiting, hemorrhagic cystitis, gonadal failure, alopecia, pancytopenia, opportunistic infections, and the late occurrence of malignancy. Because of its serious toxicities, the use of cyclophosphamide requires careful clinical consideration. The treating physician must have a clear idea concerning the potential for response of the lupus patient and goals for therapy. If these goals cannot be achieved (reversal of severe renal failure), the lupus patient should receive dialysis and be considered for renal transplantation, as opposed to being exposed to the toxicities of cyclophosphamide.

Central Nervous System Manifestations

CNS disorders associated with SLE include stroke, seizures, movement disorders, meningitis, confusion, mood changes, psychosis, and headaches. Peripheral nervous system disorders are peripheral neuropathies that affect motor or sensory functions or both. Mononeuritis multiplex can occur associated with wrist drop or foot drop. The most consistent neurologic pathologic changes of CNS lupus are microinfarcts of the brain. Often there is diffuse vasculopathy and, sometimes, a vasculitis. Clotting causing strokes may be associated with antiphospholipid antibodies. Infection, drug side effects, hypertension, and electrolyte imbalance all need to be excluded as possible causes of neurologic dysfunction. A diagnostic work-up should include cerebrospinal fluid evaluation, including cultures and antiphospholipid antibodies. Magnetic resonance imaging (MRI) is more sensitive than computed tomography (CT) in identifying areas of CNS pathology. A cerebral angiogram may be necessary to identify vasculitic lesions. An MR angiogram can be substituted if a noninvasive test is preferred to document vessel lesions.

Therapy differs according to the type of presentation, its severity, and the underlying process. High-dose prednisone, 60 mg per day, is the first line of treatment. Patients with psychosis should be treated with psychotropic medications. Pulse methylprednisolone therapy, 1 gram per day for 3 days, may be needed in severe cases. Intravenous pulses of cyclophosphamide, as given for lupus nephritis, may be helpful in patients with severe disease including stroke, transverse myelitis, or organic brain syndrome. Plasmapheresis is utilized in combination with these other therapies when CNS patients fail to respond to corticosteroids and immunosuppressive agents.

Cardiac Disease

Cardiac manifestations include valvular lesions, Libman-Sacks endocarditis, pericardial effusions, pericarditis, myocarditis, and myocardial infarction. Valvular lesions include valve thickening, with or without regurgitation or stenosis. Many patients have asymptomatic pericardial effusions. Pericarditis may be treated with indomethacin (Indocin), up to 50 mg three times daily. Accelerated atherosclerosis secondary to the illness or as a toxicity of therapy (corticosteroids) is a significant cause of morbidity and mortality. Glucocorticoids induce dyslipoproteinemia; renal disease may lead to hyperlipidemia and hypertension. These cardiac risk factors should be treated as in nonlupus patients with similar disorders.

Pulmonary Manifestations

Acute pulmonary disease includes pneumonitis and alveolar hemorrhage; both are life-threatening syndromes. The symptoms of pneumonitis are abrupt onset of fevers, dyspnea, hypoxemia, and patchy alveolar infiltrates. The alveolar hemorrhage syndrome has symptoms like pneumonitis, with an associated decline of hemoglobin. Glucocorticoids, 60 mg per day, are considered as the first line of therapy. If pulse methylprednisolone is not effective, cyclophosphamide may need to be added.

Chronic pulmonary disease may also be primary or a consequence of pneumonitis. The differentiation between inflammatory alveolitis, a treatable lesion, and chronic fibrosis is difficult. In addition to lung biopsy, high-resolution CT helps distinguish the two disorders. Patients with pulmonary hypertension have a poor prognosis. There is no proven effective therapy. Other pulmonary disorders include shrinking lung syndrome, bronchiolitis obliterans, and pulmonary embolism.

Hematologic Disease

Hematologic disorders consist of leukopenia, lymphopenia, hemolytic anemia, and thrombocytopenia. Leukopenia—WBC less than 4000 cells per mm^3—is very common and does not require treatment. Patients also have anemia of chronic disease. About 10% of patients have an autoimmune hemolytic anemia. Autoimmune thrombocytopenia may occur in as many as 25% of patients; it requires no treatment unless bleeding occurs. Glucocorticoids are recommended as initial treatment for patients with severe hemolytic anemia or thrombocytopenia. Prednisone, at 1 mg per kg orally daily, is the initial therapy. For patients who fail glucocorticoid treatment, danazol (Danocrine),* 200 to 800 mg orally daily, may be given. Other alternative therapies include intravenous immunoglobulin, intermittent pulses of methylprednisolone, cyclophosphamide, vinca alkaloids, or in severe cases, surgical splenectomy.

Pregnancy and SLE

Only about one half of pregnant patients with lupus deliver full-term normal-weight babies. Complications include fetal death, prematurity, and intrauterine growth retardation. Pregnancy does not always induce SLE flares. It can be difficult to distinguish between a lupus flare and preeclampsia. Both may present with musculoskeletal pain, swelling, and headaches. Each can have an increased blood pressure and proteinuria. A distinguishing laboratory value is serum complement. Complement tends to decrease in active lupus and increase in pregnancy. The two conditions can coexist. Treatment needs to focus on both conditions. Therapy includes high-dose prednisone, 1 mg per kg per day, antihypertensive therapy, and delivery. The patient's care should include the input of a high-risk obstetrician.

Drug-Induced Disease

Many drugs have been known to cause a lupuslike syndrome. Procainamide, hydralazine, anticonvulsants, and chlorpromazine are the most commonly implicated drugs. Drug-induced SLE does not have associated renal and CNS disease. The antinuclear antibodies (ANA) are histone-dependent with a homogeneous pattern. Symptoms should resolve, after the drug has been discontinued, within 6 to 8 weeks. The positive ANA test can remain detectable up to a year after drug discontinuation.

Antiphospholipid Antibodies

Antiphospholipid antibodies are more prevalent in SLE patients than in the general population. Clinical features are arterial and venous thrombosis, thrombocytopenia, cerebral ischemia, GI and renal vein thrombosis, livedo reticularis, and fetal loss. Other obstetric complications include placental abruption and fetal growth retardation. If a lupus patient has no history of thrombi or miscarriages and is positive for antiphospholipid antibodies, either a baby aspirin daily or observation is recommended. A history of thrombi or recurrent fetal loss warrants more aggressive therapy.

There is no general agreement on effective treatment. Corticosteroids, prednisone 30 to 60 mg daily, and aspirin or subcutaneous heparin alone or subcutaneous heparin and aspirin in combination, may be beneficial. Heparin should be sufficient to increase the activated partial thromboplastin time (PTT) 1.5 to 2 times normal in those with an initial normal PTT. If the activated PTT is prolonged at the initiation of therapy, the dose should be sufficient to achieve a thrombin time of greater than 100 seconds. Heparin is more effective than corticosteroids and aspirin in the prevention of fetal loss.

MYOSITIS

Polymyositis and dermatomyositis are inflammatory myopathies. The symptoms are symmetrical weakness of the proximal muscles: trunk, neck, and limbs. Serious complications include dysphagia and dyspnea. Signs of muscle damage are reflected in elevation of creatine kinase (CK), aldolase, and lactate dehydrogenase (LDH). An electromyogram (EMG) classically demonstrates fibrillation potentials and increased insertional irritability. The definitive diagnosis is based on muscle biopsy findings. Characteristic features are inflammatory mononuclear cell infiltration, degenerating and regenerating muscle fibers, and centralization of muscle cell nuclei. Myopathy may be associated with other conditions: SLE, scleroderma, Sjögren's syndrome, hypothyroidism, and hypoparathyroidism. Viral infections such as hepatitis, influenza, and human immunodeficiency virus (HIV) and bacterial infections may cause muscle inflammation. Drugs, especially lovastatin, clofibrate, and cimetidine, can cause myositis and CK elevation.

Dermatologic features of dermatomyositis are purple discoloration of the eyelids (heliotrope), periorbital edema, erythema over the metacarpophalangeal and proximal interphalangeal joints (Gottron's papules), and an erythematous or scaly rash involving the extensor surfaces of the face, neck, back, and chest in a V-shaped pattern. The autoantibodies present in dermatomyositis and polymyositis are to transfer-RNA-synthetases (Jo-1). Anti-Jo-1 is positive in about 30% of patients with polymyositis.

High-dose corticosteroids—prednisone, 30 to 60 mg in divided doses per day—should be given to these patients. Serial muscle testing helps document therapeutic response. Serial determinations of CK and, if necessary, aldolase should be obtained to document improvement. If improvement occurs, steroids should be slowly tapered at 5-mg decrements every 2 to 3 weeks while monitoring muscle enzymes. Low-dose prednisone, 10 to 20 mg per day, should be maintained for 6 to 12 months. If a relapse occurs, high-dose corticosteroids should be reinstituted. If patients are steroid-resistant or if steroid-sparing agents are needed, immunosuppressive agents should be begun. Methotrexate has been successful in these cases. Doses vary from 7.5 to 30 mg* orally per week with daily prednisone. One must monitor blood counts and liver function tests. The risk of

---

*Not FDA-approved for this indication.

*Exceeds dosage recommended by the manufacturer.

malignancy associated with dermatomyositis is greater in those patients who remain weak with elevated muscle enzymes despite corticosteroid and immunosuppreseve therapy. Another more controversial drug for therapy of myositis is cyclosporine. Most patients develop decreased renal function when taking cyclosporine, limiting its utility. Hydroxychloroquine (Plaquenil), 200 to 400 mg daily, may improve the rash associated with dermatomyositis.

SYSTEMIC SCLEROSIS

Systemic sclerosis is a disorder characterized by microvascular damage and excessive accumulation of fibrous tissue in the skin, gastrointestinal tract, lung, heart, and kidneys. Patients with limited cutaneous involvement are said to have CREST (calcinosis, Raynaud's phenomenon, esophageal dysmotility, sclerodactyly, and telangiectasias). These patients have a lower incidence of renal and generalized skin involvement. Patients with diffuse scleroderma often present with arthritis or skin thickening. The skin thickening may involve the upper arms and trunk. A tendon friction rub may be present over the wrists and is a poor prognostic sign. Autoantibodies such as those against topoisomerase I (anti-scl 70) and the centromere can aid in distinguishing between systemic sclerosis and CREST, respectively. These antibodies have high specificity. Raynaud's phenomenon is characterized by reversible vasospasm of the arteries. This clinically results in triphasic color changes: white, blue, then red. Cold sensitivity results in the color changes. Nailfold microscopy reveals a decrease in the number of capillary loops and dilatation of the remaining loops.

Treatment should first be preventive. Patients should dress warmly, avoiding exposure to the cold of any part of the body, including the head. They should stop smoking. Calcium channel blockers, like nifedipine (Procardia), can decrease the frequency of attacks. For example, Procardia XL 30 mg may be given, titrating upward while following the blood pressure. Topical nitroglycerin has also been effective.

The gastrointestinal abnormalities, including dysphagia, esophageal reflux, diarrhea, and malabsorption, are most commonly seen. Up to 85% of patients have hypomotility of the esophagus that may lead to dysphagia and reflux. Bacterial overgrowth can lead to steatorrhea. Wide-mouthed diverticula of the colon may also occur. Metoclopramide hydrochloride (Reglan), 10 mg 30 minutes before each meal and at bedtime, or cisapride (Propulsid), initially 10 mg 30 minutes before each meal and at bedtime, which may be increased to 20 mg, may help with dysphagia and esophageal reflux. The symptoms of esophageal reflux can be reduced with H_2 blockers, such as ranitidine hydrochloride (Zantac), 150 mg twice daily and omeprazole (Prilosec), 20 mg daily. Strictures should be treated with esophagoscopy with dilation.

Renal involvement includes reduced creatinine clearance, azotemia, microscopic hematuria, and proteinuria. Patients should be evaluated for microangiopathy. Although patients are usually hypertensive, some may be normotensive. Renal crisis is characterized by hyperreninemia. Before the availability of angiotensin-converting enzyme inhibitors, the mortality rate was high, with scleroderma kidney and malignant hypertension. Captopril (Capoten), up to 400 mg daily in two or three divided doses, is the drug of choice to treat renal crisis. Aggressive control of blood pressure tends to preserve renal function.

Cardiopulmonary complications include pericarditis, arrhythmias, pulmonary hypertension, and fibrosis. Pericarditis can be treated with NSAIDs. Steroids are given if NSAIDs are not successful. Arryhthmias are managed with antiarrhythmic agents. There are no accepted therapies for pulmonary hypertension. Pulmonary function tests, including diffusing capacity of the lungs for carbon monoxide (DL_{CO}), should be obtained in patients with possible lung involvement. CT evaluation aids in assessing the degree of parenchyma and pleural disease. Bronchoalveolar lavage, to detect an increase in neutrophils that confirms an inflammatory alveolitis, is indicated if the choice of therapy will be based on the presence of characteristic inflammatory cells. Prednisone, in doses of 60 mg per day, is used to treat an inflammatory alveolitis. Prednisone is not likely to be helpful in a fibrotic lung. Intravenous cyclophosphamide added to prednisone may improve active lung disease. Pulmonary parameters, such as the forced vital capacity (FVC), have significantly improved with cyclophosphamide.

Musculoskeletal complaints should be treated with NSAIDs while monitoring kidney function. There is no acceptable treatment for skin disease.

VASCULITIS

Vasculitis is characterized by inflammation of blood vessels. Although there is overlap, the vasculitides can be classified by whether small, medium, or large vessels are involved. Three representative vasculitides will be discussed. *Hypersensitivity vasculitis* mainly involves postcapillary venules. *Polyarteritis nodosa* is a necrotizing vasculitis of medium arteries. *Temporal arteritis* involves inflammation of medium and large vessels.

Hypersensitivity vasculitis characteristically causes vasculitic skin lesions, palpable purpura, fever, and myalgias. Hyperpigmentation may occur during resolution of the vessel lesions. Other features are arthritis, renal dysfunction (hematuria) in one third of patients, and to a lesser extent, GI involvement and peripheral neuropathy. Treatment usually consists of supportive therapy, discontinuation of the sensitizing factor if known, and the possible addition of prednisone, 1 mg per kg per day.

Polyarteritis nodosa is a multiorgan system disorder. Clinical symptoms are related to vasculitis, which can lead to thrombosis and ischemia. Generalized malaise, arthralgias, and arthritis are common manifestations. Renal disease can lead to hypertension. GI involvement may lead to vomiting, abdominal pain, and bowel infarction. Mononeuritis multiplex occurs. Painful erythematous nodules and livedo reticularis are skin manifestations. Coronary artery involvement can result in myocardial infarcts. High-dose corticosteroids in the dose of 1 mg per kg daily is the initial treatment. If patients do not respond or have a fulminant course, oral cyclophosphamide, 1 to 2 mg per kg per day, or intravenous if the oral dose is not tolerated, should be added. Patients are maintained on oral cyclophosphamide for 1 to 2 years.

Temporal arteritis classically affects the temporal artery but can involve any medium or large artery with an elastic lamina. It characteristically occurs in patients greater than 55 years of age. Symptoms include temporal headaches, jaw claudication, and decreased vision leading to blindness. It is associated with polymyalgia rheumatica (PMR) in 80% of patients; PMR patients have proximal muscle stiffness and pain without weakness. In temporal arteritis, the erythrocyte sedimentation rate may be greater than 100 mm per hr.

Therapy should be initiated before a biopsy is obtained, at a prednisone dose of 1 mg per kg per day. Divided doses of corticosteroids may be needed for control of disease. A temporal artery biopsy is obtained to confirm the diagnosis. Therapy should be tapered after 4 to 6 weeks if symptoms abate. Maintenance steroids, 10 to 20 mg daily, are needed for at least a year. If a steroid-sparing agent is needed, methotrexate may be given. Prednisone, 1 mg per kg per day, needs to be given for a relapse, manifested by an elevation of sedimentation rate or recurrence of headache or visual symptoms.

CUTANEOUS VASCULITIS

method of
PEARON G. LANG, JR., M.D.
Medical University of South Carolina
Charleston, South Carolina

The most common form of cutaneous vasculitis is a necrotizing vasculitis of the venule characterized by recurrent crops of palpable purpuric lesions. These lesions most commonly occur on the lower extremities and other dependent areas, and over areas of pressure. The purpuric lesions may be preceded by erythematous macules and papules or urticarial lesions. This form of cutaneous vasculitis is usually referred to as a leukocytoclastic vasculitis; however, if a distinct set of clinical, pathologic, and immunopathologic findings are present, it may be more specifically designated, for example, Henoch-Schönlein purpura. Although leukocytoclastic vasculitis is often confined to the skin, systemic involvement may occur, with other organs such as the kidney, central nervous system, and gastrointestinal tract being affected. Often a cause for the leukocytoclastic vasculitis cannot be found. However, reported associations include infection (e.g., group A streptococci, *Mycobacterium leprae,* and hepatitis B and C viruses), drugs, chemicals, preservatives, foods, foreign proteins, complement defi-

ciency (C2), malignancy, cryoglobulinemia, and collagen-vascular disease.

The vasculitides are primarily classified on the basis of pathologic findings. However, because of overlap, they are further subdivided on the basis of clinical findings and variations in their histopathology. As an example, Wegener's granulomatosis and Churg-Strauss angiitis are both classified as granulomatous vasculitis; however, eosinophils are more prominent in the inflammatory infiltrate of the latter and renal involvement is more common in the former. Table 1 contains a classification of the major types of necrotizing vasculitis. Although palpable purpura is the most common presentation of cutaneous vasculitis, depending on the disease process and the size of the vessel(s) involved, other cutaneous lesions are possible—for example, subcutaneous nodules, ulcers, plaques, vesicles, or bullae; pustules; infarcts with eschar; livedo reticularis; and urticaria/angioedema. These lesions may be asymptomatic or associated with pruritus, burning, and pain. The presence of nodules and large areas of necrosis usually implies larger vessel involvement typical of polyarteritis nodosa, and the granulomatous vasculitides.

In contrast to cutaneous leukocytoclastic vasculitis, systemic involvement is the rule rather than the exception, when it comes to the vasculitides affecting larger vessels. A number of organ systems may be involved, including the lungs, heart, gastrointestinal tract, joints, muscles, sinuses, eye, and the central and peripheral nervous systems. However, even in the absence of significant systemic involvement, patients with cutaneous vasculitis often will have fever, arthralgias, myalgias, malaise, and edema.

PATHOGENESIS

The events involved in the generation of a vasculitic lesion have best been elucidated for leukocytoclastic vasculitis. However, it has been postulated that all the vasculitides share a similar pathogenesis. The vasculitides are believed to represent a hypersensitivity reaction to a known (e.g., hepatitis B virus) or unknown antigen, in which immune complexes are deposited in the vessel wall. This deposition then leads to the activation of the complement cascade, which in turn attracts polymorphonuclear leukocytes into the area. Lysosomal enzymes, released from the polymorphonuclear leukocytes, then damage the vessel, leading to the extravasation of erythrocytes. Although serving as a nice model, this explanation of the vasculitic process is probably an over-simplification. Platelets, mast cells, lymphocytes, and various other mediators of inflammation are also likely to be involved in this process.

EVALUATION

Although cutaneous vasculitides, especially leukocytoclastic vasculitis, can often be diagnosed clinically, it is

TABLE 1. **Major Types of Necrotizing Vasculitis**

Leukocytoclastic vasculitis
Polyarteritis nodosa
Classic
Cutaneous
Infantile (Kawasaki disease)
Granulomatous vasculitis
Allergic granulomatous angiitis (Churg-Strauss syndrome)
Wegener's granulomatosis
Lymphomatoid granulomatosis
Giant cell arteritis
Temporal arteritis
Takayasu's arteritis

best to confirm this by a biopsy. The lesion selected for biopsy should be at least 24 hours old, since younger lesions may not demonstrate the typical pathologic features of vasculitis. Purpura, livedo reticularis, cutaneous infarcts, and subcutaneous nodules may be due to other nonvasculitic processes, including superficial migratory thrombophlebitis, disseminated intravascular coagulopathy, hypercoagulable states (e.g., lupus anticoagulant, macroglobulinemia), thrombocytopenia, scurvy, atrial myxoma, atheromatous emboli, IV drug abuse, and calciphylaxis. On the lower extremities, because of hydrostatic forces, cutaneous eruptions, other than vasculitis, on occasion, may be associated with purpura.

In addition to confirming the diagnosis, it is important to identify any treatable precipitating factors and to determine if there is systemic involvement. In evaluating a patient with cutaneous vasculitis, it is always important to start with a thorough history and physical examination. These may allow the physician to detect extracutaneous disease, underlying disease processes, and precipitating factors. They may also aid in the selection of appropriate laboratory tests and may give a clue as to the correct diagnosis even before the results of the biopsy and other laboratory data are back. For example, in a patient with chronic urticaria, if the lesions last longer than 24 hours or are associated with purpura or hyperpigmentation, one is dealing with urticarial vasculitis, not ordinary urticaria. Subcutaneous nodules following the course of a vessel would be highly suggestive of polyarteritis nodosa, and an ulceration confined to the temple would be typical of temporal arteritis. A history of dry eyes and mouth and a positive Schirmer test would suggest a diagnosis of Sjögren's syndrome and an associated vasculitis. Prominent pulmonary symptoms would be most compatible with a diagnosis of Wegener's granulomatosis or allergic granulomatosis. Abdominal pain and neurologic findings would most likely be associated with polyarteritis nodosa.

Even in the absence of signs and symptoms of extracutaneous disease or underlying disease processes, the patient should have at a minimum a complete blood count with differential and platelet count, a chemistry profile that includes an assessment of hepatic and renal function, a urinalysis, a stool guaiac test for occult blood, and a chest x-ray. If clinical data warrant or in the absence of an etiology for the vasculitis, additional laboratory and radiologic studies may be needed. Such tests would include a hepatitis screening panel to detect hepatitis B and C infection, a serum protein electrophoresis, and immunoelectrophoresis, an antinuclear antibody determination, complement studies (e.g., CH50, C2 level), an antistreptolysin O titer, a throat culture (for group A streptococci), SSA(SSB) antibody determination, a cryoglobulin and cryofibrinogen screen, a rheumatoid factor determination, anticardiolipin antibody and antineutrophil cytoplasmic antibody screening, and an erythrocyte sedimentation rate. If polyarteritis nodosa is suspected, arteriography can be used both to confirm the diagnosis and assess systemic involvement, since 80% of patients have arterial aneurysms. Biopsies of extracutaneous sites (e.g., lung, kidney) at times may be required to diagnose extracutaneous involvement.

The erythrocyte sedimentation rate can be particularly helpful in diagnosing and managing several types of vasculitis. A patient with chronic urticaria and an elevated erythrocyte sedimentation rate most likely has urticarial vasculitis and not ordinary urticaria. In a patient with an ulceration of the temple, a markedly elevated erythrocyte sedimentation rate suggests a diagnosis of temporal arteritis. Monitoring of the erythrocyte sedimentation rate in such patients aids one in the tapering of these patients' corticosteroid dosage.

Although initially touted as being diagnostic for Wegener's granulomatosis, the indirect immunofluorescence test for antineutrophil cytoplasmic antibody (C-ANCA) has been found to be positive in other disease states and thus cannot be considered pathognomonic of Wegener's granulomatosis. However, in several studies of patients with Wegener's granulomatosis, a rise in titer or reappearance of this antibody has correlated with disease relapse. Thus it may be useful in monitoring some of these patients.

Direct immunofluorescence of a skin lesion has limited usefulness in the management of patients with cutaneous vasculitis. It is primarily used when a diagnosis of Henoch-Schönlein purpura is suspected. In this disease, IgA deposits are found in the skin. Biopsy specimens for immunofluorescence studies should be obtained on lesions less than 24 hours old.

TREATMENT

Treatment should be tailored to the severity and extent of the vasculitis. If an underlying disease is thought to be causally related, treatment should be directed at that disease. If a drug is thought responsible, it should be discontinued.

In patients with vasculitis in association with chronic hepatitis B and C infection, interferon alpha 2b (Intron A) is the treatment of choice. This may be combined with plasma exchange. The interferon is administered in a dosage of 3 million units thrice weekly for up to 1 year if necessary. However, treatment can be discontinued earlier if the virus is cleared from the circulation. The treatment is usually well tolerated, the major side effects being a mild leukopenia and fever and chills early in the course of treatment. The latter can be ameliorated by pretreating the patient with acetaminophen (Tylenol). Using the preceding regimen, a long-term survival rate of 80.5% has been reported. Corticosteroids and immunosuppressive agents should be avoided if possible because they promote viral replication, which can lead to a chronic hepatitis and cirrhosis. However, in life-threatening cases, a short course (2 weeks) of systemic corticosteroids may be required. In patients relapsing or not responding to interferon, long-term treatment with systemic corticosteroids with or without immunosuppressive agents may be required.

If the vasculitis is mild, self-limited, and confined to the skin, minimal treatment in the form of leg elevation, support stockings, antihistamines, and nonsteroidal anti-inflammatory agents may be all that is required. The antihistamines and nonsteroidal anti-inflammatory agents, in addition to improving the vasculitis, may also relieve the pruritus and burning and alleviate any accompanying myalgias and arthralgias.

Local measures for managing areas of cutaneous necrosis include soaks, whirlpool baths, gentle débridement, topical antibiotics, and nonadherent dressings.

There have been occasional reports of food preservatives (benzoates and tartrazine) and certain foods precipitating a vasculitis. This must be extremely rare. Most of these patients had urticarial vasculitis. Such cases are detected by an elimination diet and direct challenge.

A variety of agents have been employed to manage chronic cutaneous vasculitis in the absence of systemic involvement. These include H_1 and H_2 antihistamines; nonsteroidal anti-inflammatory agents, including indomethacin (Indocin)*; colchicine*; antimalarial agents such as hydroxychloroquine (Plaquenil)*; diaminodiphenylsulfone (dapsone)*; pentoxifylline (Trental)*; dipyridamole (Persantine)*; saturated solution of potassium iodide (SSKI)*; stanozolol (Winstrol)*; and gold (Myochrysine, Solganal, Ridaura).* There have been no large well-controlled studies that evaluated the overall usefulness of these drugs in the management of cutaneous vasculitis. Most reports have been anecdotal or consisted of a small series of cases. In general, these agents have primarily been employed in patients with mild to moderately severe disease. Patients with severe cutaneous leukocytoclastic vasculitis usually require oral corticosteroids alone or in combination with immunosuppressive agents.

Colchicine in doses of 0.6 mg, two to three times a day, has been reported to be effective when used alone or in combination with systemic corticosteroids in the management of some patients with urticarial vasculitis or more typical cutaneous leukocytoclastic vasculitis.

Although reported to be effective in doses of 100 to 300 mg per day, in some patients with classic cutaneous leukocytoclastic angiitis and urticarial vasculitis, diaminodiphenylsulfone (dapsone) has been shown to be most consistently effective in erythema elevatum diutinum. This is a rare, low-grade, chronic vasculitis of the skin characterized by purple, red-brown, or occasionally yellow papules and plaques occurring over joints and extensor surfaces. Side effects include agranulocytosis, anemia, methemoglobinemia, allergic reactions, peripheral neuropathy, psychoses, and aggravation of angina. Patients deficient in glucose-6-phosphate dehydrogenase are particularly susceptible to the hemolytic effect of this drug.

For severe, extensive, cutaneous leukocytoclastic vasculitis, with or without systemic involvement, oral corticosteroids in doses of 40 to 60 mg per day (prednisone) are the mainstay of treatment. If control cannot be achieved with oral corticosteroids alone or if the dosage cannot be significantly lowered or long-term treatment is necessary, an immunosuppressive agent should be added to spare the patient the inevitable side effects of long-term, high-dose corticosteroid administration. The two most commonly used immunosuppressive agents have been cyclophosphamide (Cytoxan)* and azathioprine (Imuran).* These are usually administered in doses of 1 to 2 mg per kg per day, but higher doses have been used. It may require a minimum of 3 to 4 weeks before the benefit of these agents can be appreciated and a taper of the corticosteroids begun. Although there has been less experience with methotrexate, oral or intramuscular doses of 7.5 mg up to 50 mg once a week have been reported to be effective in the management of vasculitis. The side effects of these immunosuppressive agents include bone marrow toxicity, hepatitis, cirrhosis, hemorrhagic cystitis, infertility, infection, and the possibility of therapy-associated malignancies. Thus, close monitoring is essential.

In severe, rapidly progressive vasculitis with systemic involvement, or in patients not responding to oral treatment, intravenous pulse therapy may be used. Methylprednisolone (Solu-Medrol), in doses of 1 gram per day for 3 to 5 days, or cyclophosphamide (Cytoxan),* in doses of 3 to 4 mg per kg per day for 3 days, has been used with success. However, pulse therapy is not without risks. Rapid electrolyte shifts may occur with pulsed corticosteroid therapy, resulting in cardiac arrhythmias, cardiac arrest, and death. Upon completion of pulsed therapy, the patient is usually placed on oral maintenance therapy using an oral corticosteroid (prednisone, 40 to 60 mg per day) and an immunosuppressive agent (Cytoxan, 2 mg per kg per day). Some patients, however, following pulse therapy with cyclophosphamide (Cytoxan), are maintained on intermittent pulse therapy with cyclophosphamide in doses of 0.5 to 1.0 gram per m^2 given at 1- to 3-month intervals. Hemorrhagic cystitis, with its possible sequelae of fibrosis and bladder cancer, is a major complication of the chronic oral administration of cyclophosphamide. This side effect can be ameliorated by intermittent pulse therapy, in combination with sodium 2-mercaptoethane-sulfonate (mesna [Mesnex]), which binds to and neutralizes the toxic metabolites that cause hemorrhagic cystitis.

Cyclophosphamide, in combination with oral corticosteroids (prednisone), is considered the treatment of choice for Wegener's granulomatosis. A combination of oral corticosteroids (prednisone) and immunosuppressive agents (Cytoxan, Imuran, methotrexate) is also often necessary in the management of classic polyarteritis nodosa and the granulomatous vasculitides. Although the advent of corticosteroids significantly improved survival in these diseases, the addition of immunosuppressive agents may have not. This is because of the high incidence of side effects, especially infection, which themselves may lead to death. However, these agents do have a corticosteroid-sparing effect and aid in the control of these diseases. Long-term follow-up, however, has shown that relapses are common in these patients (i.e., very few are cured by treatment). Because of the high incidence of hemorrhagic cystitis with the chronic oral administration of cyclophosphamide, and other potential side effects, many clinicians have either gone to intermittent pulse therapy or once a remission is obtained used azathioprine (Imuran)* in combination with oral corticosteroids (prednisone) to maintain the remission. If the patient is maintained

---

*Not FDA-approved for this indication.

on oral corticosteroids and cyclophosphamide, treatment should not extend beyond a year, if possible.

POLYARTERITIS NODOSA

method of
J. L. DÍAZ-PÉREZ, M.D., Ph.D., and
J. GARDEAZABAL, M.D.
*University of the Basque Country and Cruces
   Hospital*
Bilbao, Spain

Classic polyarteritis nodosa (PAN) is a multisystem disease characterized by inflammatory vasculitis of the medium and small arteries and arterioles. The clinical manifestations include fever, arthralgias, myalgias, peripheral neuropathy, and visceral involvement (kidneys, gut, and occasionally heart and lung). Renal vasculitis with or without infarcts is responsible for the renal insufficiency that frequently leads to renal failure. Cutaneous lesions are present in 20 to 30% of cases, and they usually consist of petechiae, hemorrhagic papules and blisters, ecchymosis, and infarction. High erythrocyte sedimentation rate, leukocytosis with or without eosinophilia, and proteinuria are the more frequent laboratory changes. Anticytoplasmic antibodies are found in a few patients (10 to 20%). Microaneurysms of the branches of the abdominal aorta are frequently found. Without treatment, most patients have a fatal course within a few months.

In the last few decades, the diagnosis and differentiation from other types of vasculitis have become more clearly defined, although there remains some confusion. Microscopic PAN is presently accepted as a subset of PAN. It is histopathologically characterized by small vessel vasculitis, glomerulonephritis (rare in classic PAN), frequent lung involvement, and absence of microaneurysms. Anticytoplasmic antibodies are more frequently found than in classic PAN (50%). In general, the clinical course is more severe and relapses are more frequent than in classic PAN. Distinguishing microscopic PAN from Wegener's granulomatosis and Churg-Strauss syndrome can be difficult in some cases.

Cutaneous PAN is a distinct entity, clinically characterized by nodules, livedo reticularis, and ulcers. It has a prolonged, relapsing course that does not compromise the life span of patients. In general, the skin findings in systemic PAN are clearly different from those of the benign cutaneous variety. Most patients with systemic PAN do not have cutaneous lesions, and if they do, inflammatory subcutaneous nodules are not usually found. In contrast, nodules are the hallmark of the cutaneous variety of PAN, and flares of small-sized nodules, isolated or in groups, with livedoid patches are characteristic. Some of the inflamed nodules may ulcerate during the course of the disease. There is little relationship between patients with the cutaneous and systemic varieties of PAN, although in a few cases, it may be difficult to differentiate them clearly. Patients with systemic PAN and prominent cutaneous lesions frequently have a prolonged benign course, similar to the course of pure cutaneous PAN. Cases of cutaneous PAN leading to systemic PAN have been reported only rarely. These few cases can be considered the exception that confirms the rule that cutaneous PAN remains confined to the skin. Histopathologically, the cutaneous lesions of systemic PAN show small vessel leukocytoclastic vasculitis, which contrasts with the arteritis found in the nodules of cutaneous PAN.

The concept of Kawasaki's disease as the childhood counterpart of adult periarteritis nodosa, maintained over the last 2 decades by some authors, has been completely abandoned.

Drugs, chemicals, and bacterial and viral infections have been implicated as possible etiologic factors in PAN. Hepatitis B and C virus (HBV and HCV), cytomegalovirus, human immunodeficiency virus, and parvovirus B19 are the viruses more frequently involved in human vasculitis. HBV has been implicated in systemic PAN for a long time. The recent discovery of HCV and its frequent finding in vasculitis and cryoglobulinemia suggest that cases previously related to HBV could also have involved HCV. It is estimated that 2 to 5% of the patients with HCV, with or without cryoglobulinemia, develop different types of vasculitis, including PAN. HBV has not been related to cutaneous PAN, but the possible implication of HCV is still not well known.

TREATMENT OF SYSTEMIC PAN

Prednisone plus cyclophosphamide has been the usual therapy for systemic PAN. A number of trials combining prednisone with plasma exchange and cytostatic drugs offer conflicting results. Although prednisone has proved to be useful, the beneficial effects of cytostatic drugs and plasma exchange are controversial. Most authors agree that plasma exchange is beneficial in patients with renal insufficiency, especially in advanced cases that require dialysis, and that cytostatic drugs decrease the number and intensity of exacerbations of the disease. Immune suppression has proved to have a deleterious effect in patients with virus-induced PAN, and cytostatic drugs are contraindicated in these cases. Despite its immune suppressive potential, prednisone has proved to be beneficial, probably because of its effect on the virus-related immune complex disease. Antiviral agents such as vidarabine and interferon-alfa have proved to be beneficial and even curative in some cases of HBV- and HCV-induced PAN.

TREATMENT OF CUTANEOUS PAN

General measures, including bed rest and nonsteroidal anti-inflammatory drugs, are useful for most patients. For some, this is the only treatment required. In general, short courses of prednisone (0.5 to 1 mg per kg per day for a few weeks) are required to control the acute flares of nodules. Sulfa drugs, antibiotics, and pentoxifylline (Trental)* can be useful in individual cases.

TREATMENT SCHEDULES

General Measures. Bed rest and nonsteroidal anti-inflammatory drugs are useful for most patients. Antibiotics and specific treatment of the visceral pathology are necessary in individual cases.

HBV-Induced PAN. Prednisone 1 mg per kg per

---

*Not FDA-approved for this indication.

day plus interferon-alfa* 4 to 6 million IU subcutaneously three times a week for 4 months. Some authors prefer plasma exchange plus interferon-alfa.

HCV-Induced PAN. Prednisone 1 mg per kg per day plus interferon-alfa* 3 million IU subcutaneously three times a week for 1 year. In the future, plasma exchange plus interferon-alfa may prove to be more beneficial. Other antiviral drugs such as lamivudine (Epivir) or ribavirin (Virazole) may prove to be useful in this group of patients in the near future. In general, patients develop PAN in the first 6 months of HBV infection. Delay in the diagnosis of the HBV infection and the use of previous immune suppressive therapy seem to worsen the prognosis.

Idiopathic PAN. Prednisone 1 to 2 mg per kg per day plus cyclophosphamide (Cytoxan)* 2 mg per kg per day plus plasma exchange (in some cases). Once the disease is under control, the treatment can be tapered but should be continued for at least 1 year. In general, the schedule of tapering and duration of treatment are individualized for each patient. Relapses are rare after 1 year of disease control. Sulfa drugs, colchicine, intravenous immune globulin, bolus prednisone, or cyclophosphamide can be useful in some cases.

DISEASES OF THE NAILS

method of
ECKART HANEKE, M.D.
Skin Hospital, Ferdinand-Sauerbruch-Klinikum Wuppertal, Germany

The nail apparatus is a complex structure made up of four different epithelial structures, periungual connective tissues, and the terminal bony phalanx of the digit. Disturbance of any of these components will have profound effects on the formation, shape, and quality of the nail. The nail plate is produced by the matrix, which is covered by the proximal nail fold, thereby forming the nail pocket. The free margin of the proximal nail fold forms the cuticle, which is a special structure to seal the nail pocket. Distal from the matrix is the nail bed; it has a particular epithelium firmly adhering to the nail plate. The border between the nail bed and the pulp skin is the hyponychium. It is critical for the adherence of the nail plate to the bed, and any injury to the hyponychium might therefore result in onycholysis. On both sides, the nail plate is surrounded by the lateral nail walls. The bone of the terminal phalanx is directly situated under the dermis of the matrix and nail bed without any cushioning fat tissue. The space between the nail plate and the bone is only 2 to 3 mm wide, and the proximal matrix epithelium is less than 1 mm from the bone and the tendon insertion.

The nail grows at about 0.1 mm per day on the dominant hand of a young adult; it takes two to three times longer for the toenails to grow. A number of physiologic conditions and diseases may interfere with normal nail growth.

INFECTIONS OF THE NAIL ORGAN

Onychomycoses

Onychomycoses are fungal infections of the nail organ. The term "tinea unguium" more specifically denotes dermatophyte nail infections. Onychomycoses are the most frequent nail diseases, making up 20% to 40% of all nail disorders. About 25% of all skin mycoses are fungal nail infections; they are the most difficult to treat of all mycotic infections of the skin. Onychomycoses are exceptional in children and rare in adolescents, but their frequency increases steadily with age. It appears that a healthy nail organ is not susceptible to a fungal infection and that predisposing factors such as nail damage from massive trauma or repeated microtrauma and even nail avulsion, impaired arterial blood supply, venous insufficiency, lymphatic obstruction, peripheral neuropathy, diabetes mellitus, or immune incompetence are a prerequisite for the development of an onychomycosis. It has also been suggested that the susceptibility to onychomycosis might be inherited as an autosomal dominant trait. Whenever a single nail is affected, an underlying trauma is a probable explanation.

Onychomycoses are different according to the etiologic agents and the clinicopathologic forms. *Trichophyton rubrum* accounts for about 80% to 85% of all infections, *T. mentagrophytes (interdigitale)* for 10% to 15%. Molds usually infect already damaged nails and hence are often seen in association with dermatophytes. Toenails are predominantly infected by *Scopulariopsis brevicaulis* that gives the infected nail a brownish-yellow color. *Scytalidium* species, however, are able to infect nails primarily. *Candida albicans* and other yeasts are mainly found in fingernails of persons performing wet work, such as housewives, cleaning personnel, barmen, fishmongers, brewers, and so on. However, *C. albicans* was found to be the main causative fungus for onychomycosis in Saudi Arabia. Onychomycoses must be differentiated also according their method of development.

Distal subungual onychomycosis is the most frequent type, with about 80% of all fungal nail infections. It develops from an infection of the pulp of the digit. The fungus invades the hyponychium and slowly grows proximally toward the nail bed. In response to the infection, it forms a subungual hyperkeratosis that harbors almost all the fungal pathogens. The undersurface of the nail plate is only secondarily invaded, and the nail plate acts rather like a barrier than the favorite site of infection. However, *T. soudanense* appears mostly to spare the nail bed and invade the nail plate, giving rise to endonyx onychomycosis. With the gradual proximal advancement of the fungus toward the matrix, the subungual hyperkeratosis becomes more pronounced, eventually lifting up the nail plate from the nail bed (mycotic onycholysis). Discoloration, brittleness, and finally nail plate destruction are late events.

Proximal subungual (white) onychomycosis develops from an infection of the proximal nail fold and

---

*Not FDA-approved for this indication.

the cuticle. The fungus grows along the undersurface of the proximal nail fold toward the matrix. When the matrix is reached, a considerable portion of the pathogen gets included into the growing nail plate. With further distal advancement of the fungus, all layers of the nail plate may contain large amounts of fungi. This is the reason for the white discoloration characteristically seen in this variant. Inflammatory symptoms are usually less pronounced. This type of onychomycosis is now frequently seen in acquired immunodeficiency syndrome (AIDS) patients in whom it may develop within 2 to 4 weeks, whereas it takes months or even years to develop in immunocompetent persons.

Superficial white onychomycosis, when seen in temperate climates, occurs on toenails as chalky white to yellowish, sharply delimited spots and is always due to *T. mentagrophytes*. Histopathology shows chains of regular, small spores in the splits of the nail plate surface; this pattern is consistent with a saprophytic form of *T. mentagrophytes*. Infection of the nail plate surface with *Scytalidium dimidiatum* may cause *black superficial onychomycosis*. Recently a clinically similar form has been observed in fingernails of AIDS patients due to *T. rubrum*. However, on close inspection it is seen that the white color is more cloudy and less sharply delimited.

Total dystrophic onychomycosis can develop from distal subungual or proximal white subungual onychomycoses when the entire matrix is involved. It is also the characteristic nail infection in chronic mucocutaneous candidiasis, where it develops primarily. Due to heavy inflammation with matrix and nail bed papillomatosis, a normal nail substance can no longer be formed, and only irregular keratinous masses are produced.

Diagnosis

Although onychomycoses are the most frequent nail diseases, the diagnosis must be confirmed before treatment. In distal subungual onychomycosis, the nonadherent portion of the nail plate is cut away to expose the infected nail bed. Hyperkeratotic material is taken from the most proximal portion for potassium hydroxide (KOH) wet mount and mycologic culture. Since cultures often remain negative despite obvious fungal infection, histopathology of the subungual hyperkeratosis and nail plate can prove the infection when stained with PAS or Grocott's stain. In proximal subungual onychomycosis, the fungal pathogens are in and under the proximal portion of the nail plate; superficial scrapings are therefore useless. After soaking the digit in warm water for about 10 minutes to soften the nail, a punch biopsy may be taken from the nail plate. This is usually painless because the infected nail plate does not adhere to the underlying matrix and nail bed. For the demonstration of fungi in superficial white onychomycosis, simply the surface is scraped and the material collected; for histopathologic examination, a surface layer of the nail is cut tangentially. Total dystrophic onychomycosis is usually heavily contaminated on its surface with bacteria or other airborne saprophytes that may overgrow the very pathogen. Cleansing of the nail with 70% alcohol and scraping away superficial layers of the dystrophic nail material prior to taking the specimen for culture is recommended.

KOH wet mounts are easy to perform. Scrapings of infected horny material are collected on a glass slide, two drops of 20% KOH are added and cover-slipped. The slide is put into a moist chamber for about 20 to 30 minutes; during this time the horny cells will be cleared, allowing the fungal elements to be seen under the microscope. The addition of Parker's ink makes it even easier to find fungi. For cultures, Sabouraud's and Kimmig's agar are recommended. For toenail samples, the addition of cycloheximide (Actidione)* is advisable to suppress molds that tend to overgrow dermatophytes.

Treatment

Superficial white onychomycosis is very easy to treat. As long as the white spot does not reach under the proximal nail fold, any topical antimycotic may be applied on the nail surface. A solution is preferred that is allowed to dry and covered with an antifungal cream. Softening of the nail plate surface with 40% urea cream and scraping off the diseased nail layer hastens healing.

All other types of onychomycoses are much more resistant to treatment. *Distal subungual onychomycosis* not exceeding 50% of the nail length and not reaching the matrix at any point may benefit from topical treatment. Forty percent urea paste containing 1% bifonazole has been marketed in many countries and proved to be effective in compliant patients. However, it is not feasible in persons with many nails affected since it takes a considerable time to apply the paste, cover the surrounding skin with a neutral tape and then the whole tip of the digit with an adhesive tape. After a few days, the infected portion of the nail plate is usually softened so that it can be pared down to the proximal border of the infection and the nail bed hyperkeratoses removed. The treatment is then continued with a potent topical antifungal product until the nail has grown out completely healthy. Quite often, the atraumatic removal of the nail plate has to be repeated. This treatment is demanding but has a good success rate.

Alternatives for the treatment of mild distal subungual onychomycosis are the new antifungal delivery systems such as amorolfine (Loceryl)* or ciclopirox (Batrafen)* nail lacquers. Nail lacquers deliver the drug continuously to the underlying nail plate and thus provide good drug concentrations also in the deep layers of the nail plate; however, most pathogens are in the nail bed hyperkeratosis, not in the nail plate. For penetration, the drugs need a homogeneous structure such as the nail plate, but the subungual keratosis is inhomogeneous and therefore a barrier for deep penetration. Amorolfine nail

---

*Not available in the United States.

varnish requires once or twice weekly applications and ciclopirox daily or every-other-day applications. The infected nail need not be cut. Response rates were reported at about 70%.

Systemic treatment is the most efficient and reliable therapy in onychomycosis. Griseofulvin, introduced 35 years ago, is safe but has low cure rates with about 50% to 60% in fingernails and 20% in toenails. Recurrence rates approach almost 100%. The recommended daily doses of 500 mg micronized (Grisactin) or 330 mg ultramicronized (Grisactin Ultra), respectively, of griseofulvin have to be doubled or even tripled for the treatment of toenail mycoses. Griseofulvin resorption is improved when given with a meal rich in fat. Although usually well-tolerated, headache and gastrointestinal complaints are relatively frequent but not serious. Pregnancy, lactation, and some rare diseases are contraindications. Griseofulvin is thought to be incorporated into the growing nail, and the griseofulvin-imbibed nail is not attacked by the fungus. How it reaches the subungual keratoses containing the fungi is not known. Treatment duration is a minimum of 6 to 8 months for fingernails and 12 to 18 months for toenails. Only dermatophyte infections respond. Success rates can be improved and treatment duration shortened with atraumatic removal of all infected nail plate and subungual horn material. Very slowly growing nails cannot respond.

Ketoconazole (Nizoral), the first orally active broad-spectrum antimycotic drug, was shown to be more active also in onychomycosis. It has been abandoned for this indication in many countries because of occasional idiosyncratic hepatic side effects. In chronic mucocutaneous candidiasis, 200 mg of ketoconazole daily was highly efficacious in eradicating oral, skin, and nail lesions alike. Higher doses than 200 mg daily may interfere with androgen biosynthesis. Itraconazole is a new *bis*-triazole antifungal drug. It is effective against dermatophytes, pathogenic yeasts, and many molds, especially *Aspergillus* species. It is strongly lipophilic and well absorbed from the gastrointestinal tract, in particular when taken with a meal. It is bound to plasma proteins and rapidly distributed to all organs, including the skin. Like all other azole derivatives, it inhibits fungal cell wall ergosterol synthesis in a cytochrome P450-dependent reaction; however it selectively binds to fungal P450 and is therefore better tolerated than ketoconazole. Significant drug levels in the free margin of the nail plate can be found as early as one to two weeks after the first application. Daily doses of 200 mg of itraconazole (Sporanox), give sevenfold higher nail concentrations than 100 mg, and relevant drug concentrations remain in fingernails for 6 and in toenails for 9 months. Six to 8 weeks of treatment for fingernail and 3 to 4 months for toenail mycoses were found to be sufficient for 80% to 90% cure rates. Clinical and mycologic clearance of the nails continues even after withdrawal of the drug. Recurrence rates were below 10%.

Due to the rapid distribution of itraconazole to the nails and its long persistence, pulse therapy with itraconazole was introduced. Two pulses of one week per month with 400 mg daily were given for fingernail and three to four pulses for toenail infections and were well tolerated. Despite reducing the overall drug amount to one half, cure rates were almost as good as with continuous daily treatment using 200 mg a day.

Fluconazole (Diflucan) is another *bis*-triazole antimycotic substance. It is water soluble and well absorbed independent from gastric acid. It is not metabolized by the liver, and almost 80% is excreted as the active drug by the kidney. It is very rapidly distributed in the body and appears within a few days in the nails. Persistence in the nail after withdrawal is, however, shorter than that of itraconazole. Although not FDA-approved for this indication, it is widely used in onychomycosis at a dose of 100 mg daily or 150 mg once weekly. Treatment duration is from 6 to 12 months.

Terbinafine (Lamisil)* is an orally active allyl amine derivative with high potency against dermatophytes. It is very lipophilic, well absorbed from the gastrointestinal tract, and metabolized in the liver. It inhibits the fungal squalene epoxidase, and its effect is cytochrome P450-independent. It is generally well tolerated, with occasional gastrointestinal side effects and taste loss. Recently, some cases of serious skin reactions were observed. Terbinafine is fungicidal, and treatment duration is 6 weeks for fingernail and 3 months for toenail infections. Recurrence rates are under 10%. *Proximal subungual* and *total dystrophic onychomycoses* always require systemic treatment. To enhance cure rates, atraumatic removal of as much infected nail and keratotic material as possible is feasible.

Nail Avulsion

Nail avulsion is performed far too often for onychomycosis. As has been stressed, any injury to the nail may render it more susceptible to fungal infections, and surgical nail avulsion is the most severe iatrogenic trauma. Atraumatic removal of diseased nail portions is, however, recommended to shorten treatment periods.

Paronychia

Paronychia is the inflammation of the periungual soft tissues. It may occur as an acute disease, mostly as a bacterial, less frequently as a viral infection, or as chronic paronychia with or without subacute exacerbations.

Chronic paronychia is frequently due to *C. albicans*, although this has recently been debated. Any irritation and damage to the nail fold may induce an inflammation — allergic, toxic, microbial — breaking the continuity of the cuticle and thus allowing foreign material such as carbohydrates, food particles, hairs, bristles, and so on to get entrapped under the proxi-

---

*Not available in the United States.

mal nail fold. The resulting chronic inflammation causes a thickening of the nail wall, which makes the cuticle disappear spontaneously and the nail plate detach from the proximal nail fold's undersurface. More and more foreign material will accumulate under the nail fold, giving excellent conditions for fungi and bacteria. Probing the nail pocket does not hurt and usually yields a creamy-gray material from which *C. albicans* and bacteria can be grown quite often. Because moisture and contact with carbohydrates are the most important predisposing factors, this condition is common among house cleaners, confectioners, chefs, brewers, and housewives. Treatment is often protracted, since patients often find it difficult to adhere strictly to the management regimen, which has to be nonmedical and medical. First, the space under the proximal nail fold is cleaned of foreign material by using the fine water jet of a mouth douche. Since moisture is the most important predisposing and aggravating factor, the hands must not be wet and must not be washed more than three times a day. After drying the fingers with a towel, a hair dryer should be used to further dry out the nail pocket. Any housework, such as dishwashing and preparing meals, is done using cotton gloves under heavy-duty rubber gloves. When the cotton gloves become moist from perspiration, they have to be changed for dry ones.

Medical treatment consists of topical application of broad-spectrum antimycotic substances with antibacterial activity (ciclopirox olamine [Loprox], fenticonazole [Lomexin]*). The solutions reach the most proximal part of the infection by capillary forces. They are applied several times a day with a soft nail- or handbrush. If *C. albicans* is repeatedly cultured from under the nail fold, a 10-day course of itraconazole, 100 mg daily, or ketoconazole, 200 mg daily, is given. Corticosteroid preparations have not been found to be necessary. A grayish-green discoloration of the margin of the nail plate is usually indicative of a secondary infection with *P. aeruginosa*. This is best treated using sodium hypochlorite or diluted acetic acid solutions.

Excessively chronic paronychia may result in a very hard swollen proximal nail fold not regressing even after prolonged treatment. A crescent excision of the redundant tissue is then necessary. Beveling the excision margin speeds up the healing time.

Bacterial Infections

The most common bacterial infection of periungual tissue is the *whitlow*. A particular type of *impetigo contagiosa* is called *bulla rodens* or *bulla repens*. It is usually a bullous impetigo due to staphylococci. Because the periungual epidermis has a resistant horny layer, the roof of the blister remains intact for several days, and the bulla may run around the proximal and lateral nail margins. Treatment consists of removing the entire blister roof and soaks

with antiseptic solution and antibiotic dressings twice daily. A short course of systemic antibiotics may be necessary. Impetigo on other skin sites should be looked for and treated accordingly.

When arising from a trauma, any whitlow may develop to a *felon*, extending in the tissue under the nail or connecting to the tendon sheath. Systemic staphylococcus-fast antibiotics should immediately be instituted, which may be changed to another drug according to culture-proved sensitivity. Pyogenic infections of the matrix lasting longer than 48 hours carry the risk of permanent nail damage, particularly in children. When pus is seen under the nail plate, this is cut away and a wick of gauze is placed under the proximal nail fold and changed twice daily and soaked with an antiseptic. The finger and hand should be splinted.

Viral Infections

Recurrent digital herpes simplex involving the nail region is not so rare, especially in dentists and personnel of intensive care units. These persons should always wear rubber gloves when contact with another person's saliva is inevitable. Being accompanied by severe pain, lymphangitis, and tender lymphadenitis from early onset, recurrent *herpetic whitlow* nail is quite often misdiagnosed as a bacterial felon and treated as such by surgeons with incisions, antibiotics, and splinting. Treatment is essentially conservative. Severe symptoms and inability to perform professional activities warrant systemic treatment with oral acyclovir (Zovirax), 200 mg five times daily, or valacyclovir (Valtrex), 500 mg three times daily.

Periungual warts are the most common type of viral infection. Human papillomavirus causing both common and plantar warts is found. The warts are easily diagnosed in children. Several benign tumors and Bowen's disease must be differentiated in adults. Treatment includes supportive and specific measures.

Since warts prefer cool skin, bathing the hand or foot in very hot water twice a day to increase blood supply has proved to be very valuable. Additional trauma from biting, picking, scratching, or tearing must be avoided. Especially in children, suggestion therapy may be tried: 1% gentian violet or 1% eosin painting plus ultraviolet radiation are impressive and will show stained lips when the child bites the warts. Since warts are benign, weakly contagious, self-limited fibroepithelial tumors, treatment should be conservative and must not leave disfiguring scars for the rest of the patient's life. X-irradiation is obsolete for the same reasons. Unfortunately, no antiviral substance is known against human papillomaviruses.

We prefer an aggressive but conservative keratolytic approach, but many doctors have their own tricks. Saturated monochloroacetic acid (80%) is applied sparingly on the wart, allowed to dry, and covered with 40% salicylic acid plaster held in place with adhesive tape. This is kept on the periungual

---

*Not available in the United States.

warts for about one week, during which time hot baths are also taken without removing this special dressing. Monochloroacetic acid slowly works its way down into the wart, necrosing its superficial portion. This is removed using a curette. The procedure is then repeated until all warts have disappeared. With time the procedure may become painful, requiring the monochloroacetic acid to be omitted. If pain becomes unbearable, the dressing is removed and the digit immersed in lukewarm or even cold water. *Subungual warts* require removal of the overlying portion of the nail plate prior to treatment.

Alternative conservative treatments include concentrated salicylic acid ointment or lacquers (Duo-Film) that may also contain lactic acid or cantharidin (Cantharone), which induces a blister, the roof of which contains the wart. Intralesional bleomycin is popular in the United States. Using a bifurcate vaccination needle, multiple punctures are made through a drop of bleomycin solution containing 1 U per mL. This treatment should not be done in pregnant women nor in subjects prone to acrocyanosis and Raynaud's phenomenon. Surgery is only the last resort and must not be mutilating. Electrosurgery produces considerable scarring and delayed healing and is therefore obsolete. Curettage may be performed under digital ring block anesthesia. Blood-clotting procedures such as ferric sulfate or Burow's solution or electrodesiccation cauterize the wound and delay healing. Therefore, a thick, padded dressing using antibiotic tulle gras is applied for the first 24 hours. The first change of the dressing is performed with a hand or foot bath to permit the adherent gauze to float off without pain. Cryosurgery, a safe and effective method in other locations of the body, carries the risk of important postcryotherapy edema and pain as well as damage to the matrix.

Infestations

Nail scabies may be seen in Norwegian scabies, severe immunodeficiency such as AIDS, malignant lymphoma, Langerhans' cell histiocytosis, during immune suppressive therapy, and occasionally in elderly people. Moderate subungual hyperkeratosis develops, harboring the mites. This particular site of scabies is usually not treated sufficiently with scabicides and may give rise to multiple recurrences. The scabicide must be applied to the fingers and toes with a "surgical hand wash" twice a day for at least 3 days.

Tungiasis is caused by the fertilized female sandflea, *Tunga penetrans*. It digs into plantar skin, particularly under and around the toenails, by entering the skin with its abdomen pointing outward. It can mimic a foreign body. Secondary infection is common. Cautious removal under digital block anesthesia is the first line of treatment.

THE NAIL IN DERMATOLOGIC DISEASE

Psoriasis is the dermatosis with the most frequent nail involvement. When first seen, about 50% of all psoriatic patients present nail lesions, but there is a 90% chance of developing nail changes over the lifetime. Pits are the most common signs of nail psoriasis. They are due to minute, short-term lesions in the most proximal portion of the nail matrix. Small psoriasis plaques in the nail bed give rise to salmon patches which, when reaching the hyponychium, may cause onycholysis. Severe matrix involvement leads to nail destruction.

Treatment of nail psoriasis is difficult. Pits are best left untreated but may be covered with a cosmetic nail varnish when producing cosmetic embarrassment. Salmon patches are also not amenable to treatment. High-potency corticosteroids (clobetasol [Temovate] and halometasone [Halovate]*) may be applied once daily as solutions that spread under the nail due to capillary forces. To prevent secondary yeast and bacterial infection, the fingers should be dipped twice daily in a disinfective solution, e.g., chlorhexidine, hexamidine, or a broad-spectrum antimycotic. Psoriasis of the nail folds responds to anthralin (dithranol, [Lasan]), but this causes discoloration that many patients find unacceptable. Calcipotriene (Dovonex) is a new and effective, cosmetically acceptable alternative. Long-term treatment with calcipotriol has also been shown to be effective in subungual lesions. A nearly 90% improvement was also achieved with twice-daily applications of 1% 5-fluorouracil cream (Efudex); however, nail dystrophy may rarely develop. Intralesional-subungual injections of triamcinolone acetonide crystal suspension, 10 mg per mL, are frequently effective. Under regional block anesthesia, about 0.1 mL is injected into the proximal nail fold on either side of the extensor tendon and/or under the nail. These injections have to be repeated at 4- to 6-week intervals. Relapses are frequent. X-irradiation may achieve rapid clearing but is not recommended because many patients find it tempting to repeat this "clean treatment without greasy and sticky ointments" and they often insist on further x-ray courses, risking chronic radiodermatitis, nail dystrophy, and cancer.

Any effective systemic psoriasis treatment is usually beneficial for the nails. This is true for photochemotherapy with ultraviolet light and psoralen and especially for cyclosporin A, less so for oral retinoids (acitretin [Neo-Tegison]*, isotretinoin [Accutane]). Pustular psoriasis of the nails, especially Hallopeau's *acrodermatitis continua suppurativa*, responds well to retinoid treatment. Methotrexate, very popular in the United States but not much used in Europe, slows down nail growth so that the nail lesions will hardly be seen changing.

Reiter's disease frequently affects the nails and is usually not distinguishable from ungual psoriasis. Systemic treatment with cyclosporin A, retinoids, or methotrexate will also improve the nails.

Eczematous dermatitis is mainly seen in allergic contact dermatitis (particularly in hairdressers), in

---

*Not available in the United States.

atopic hand dermatitis, and in immediate-type contact allergy to foods. In the acute stage, red, oozing papulovesicles predominate but gradually develop into chronic eczema with thickening of the proximal nail fold, disappearance of the cuticle, loss of the eponychium–nail plate adherence, nail plate deformations with irregular horizontal grooves and ridges, and discoloration, the latter mainly occurring at the lateral nail plate portion. Nail involvement of allergic contact and dyshidrotic atopic dermatitis of the nail region are not distinguishable on clinical grounds alone. The most important therapeutic measure is strict and consistent avoidance of allergens, moisture, and other irritants. Supportive treatment is identical to that of chronic paronychia. Specific therapy includes potent topical steroids applied as solutions for involvement of the eponychium and nail bed and as creams for the nail walls. Potency of the steroids is tapered gradually according to the resolution of the lesions. Recurrences may occur even under strict allergen avoidance, probably due to nonspecific primary irritation. A so-called two-phase eczema with specific sensitization subsequent to primary irritant dermatitis is not rare, especially when the patient wears rubber gloves and develops an allergy to rubber chemicals.

Nail involvement in *chronic atopic dermatitis* is more recalcitrant and may occasionally require intralesional or even systemic steroids.

Lichen planus of the nails occurs in about 10% of all lichen planus patients. It may pose differential diagnostic difficulties when occurring isolated in the nails. The proximal matrix and eponychium are most frequently attacked by this disease, explaining the loss of luster and nail sheen, the rough ridging of the plate, and thickening of the proximal nail fold. Ungual lichen planus is a scarring dermatosis leading to pterygium formation and permanent nail dystrophy. Treatment is usually unrewarding. High-potency topical steroids rubbed in twice daily with salicylic acid to enhance penetration may be of benefit in mild cases. Severe lichen planus requires intralesional steroid injections every month to avoid pterygium formation. Oral steroids are only effective in doses greater than the Cushing's threshold. Oral retinoids are not very helpful as is topical cyclosporin A.

Alopecia areata quite often also affects the nails; sometimes isolated alopecia areata of the nails may be observed. *Trachyonychia* (twenty-nail dystrophy) is thought by some authorities to be alopecia areata. The more severe the alopecia, the more likely is nail involvement. Histology shows a spongiotic dermatitis of the nail bed, matrix, and eponychium that does not permit a differentiation from other spongiotic dermatitides. Treatment is not very effective. High-potency steroids may be tried but usually only intralesional injections are helpful. Since permanent nail changes do not generally occur, the rough nails may as well be left untreated.

Autoimmune bullous dermatoses, such as pemphigus vulgaris, bullous pemphigoid, cicatricial pemphigoid, epidermolysis acquisita, as well as *Stevens-Johnson* and *Lyell's syndromes* may affect the nail region. Systemic steroids and topical antibiotics are usually necessary to suppress the disease activity. Scarring is a frequent sequel in Lyell's syndrome.

SPECIFIC NAIL DISORDERS

Twenty-nail dystrophy is typically seen in children—affecting one nail after the other until almost all nails are rough, gray, pitted, and ridged. The disease runs a benign course, with remission usually after several years. Scarring or nail loss is not observed. Reassurance is sufficient.

Onycholysis is the detachment of the nail bed from the plate. Most cases, especially those induced by overzealous manicure, start at the central portion of the hyponychium and slowly take the appearance of a half-moon (onycholysis semilunaris). The detachment area gradually progresses proximally and may eventually involve the entire nail. In the space under the nail, foreign particles, food, dirt, and microbes will accumulate, stimulating the patient to even more vigorously clean this space and injure the nail plate–nail bed attachment. Chromogenic bacteria such as *Pseudomonas aeruginosa*, *Klebsiella* spp, *Proteus* spp, and *Enterobacter* as well as *Candida* spp may be cultured from under the nail. Treatment is very similar to that of chronic paronychia. The detached nail has to be cut to abolish the dead space under the nail plate that offers a greenhouse microclimate for microbial agents, both pathogenic and saprophytic. The fingers have to be kept dry. Antiseptic solutions are used several times a day. At monthly intervals, the regrown but not attached nail portion is cut away. With avoidance of water and other irritants, this treatment is usually effective in "idiopathic" onycholysis, which is almost invariably found in fingers of women. A great variety of ungual and systemic diseases may also cause loss of nail attachment to the nail bed. A full check-up is therefore necessary in all onycholysis patients.

Brittle nails are a frequent complaint of women. Several clinical types must be differentiated. *Onychorrhexis* denotes a series of fine parallel longitudinal superficial furrows and splits; *onychoschisis* is the lamellar splitting of the nail plate at its free margin, transverse splitting and breaking of the lateral edge close to the distal free margin, and breaking resulting in a crenellated margin. A vast number of different causes have been offered; however, only repeated microtrauma from chronic immersion in water, detergents, organic solvents, mineral oils, alkalis, oxidizing agents, and concentrated salt solutions, and cosmetic hair and nail procedures are proven causes.

Nails in women are more susceptible to brittleness than those of men. Treatment includes strict avoidance of any possible cause. Topical therapy is rarely effective, although rubbing in of bland emollients is recommended by many workers; the action may well be mediated via an improved blood circulation. Soft nails may be hardened by applying a base coat, nail polish, and hard top coat. It is, however, the nail varnish removers that tend to dry out the nails and render them more susceptible to the harmful effects of hydration and dehydration. Other systemic treatments are biotin, 2.5 mg per day over many months, oral iron medication, evening primrose oil (40 mg gamma-linoleic acid six times daily), pyridoxine 30 mg, or ascorbic acid 2 to 3 grams daily, low-dose vitamin A, and gelatin. However, it takes many months for the nails to grow out, and any of these drugs must be taken for at least half a year before being evaluated. It is a common observation that a certain proportion of these patients claim better nails after only a few weeks, which gives strong evidence for psychological factors.

Hangnails are small triangular tags of hard keratotic epidermis of the proximal nail fold. They are painful and can be a portal of entry for bacterial infections. Hereditary susceptibility appears to be the major cause, aggravated by hydration and dehydration. Hangnails have to be cut with fine sharp scissors and not torn. Consistent use of bland emollients, under occlusion overnight, is beneficial.

Ingrown toenails are a common ailment, often limiting physical activities and causing a lot of discomfort. Five different types have to be differentiated: (1) neonatal form with an incompletely grown-out nail, (2) neonatal-infantile form due to a hypertrophic lateral nail fold (lip), (3) infantile form due to congenital malalignment of the hallux nail, (4) the most frequent adolescent type, mainly seen in tall youngsters with a very wide, often overcurved nail and hyperhidrosis of the feet, and (5) adult form due to a thick, hard, overcurved nail plate. *Neonatal ingrown toenails* are due to a distal nail fold and distally narrowing lateral nail folds. Massaging the nail folds in distal and distal-lateral directions with a bland emollient will gradually free the nail plate and permit it to grow out. Once the nail plate has completely grown out, no recurrence will be seen. Surgery is not indicated. The *hypertrophic lateral lip* is also treated conservatively with massage to free the nail wall from the nail plate. *Congenital malalignment of the great toenail* is a lateral deviation of the long axis of the nail. Due to repeated microtrauma from walking, transverse ridging and waving, partial nail shedding, onycholysis with permanent shrinking of the nail bed, discoloration, and eventually irreparable nail dystrophy may develop. Treatment of choice is the surgical correction of the long axis of the toenail that is best done before age 2 years. A crescentic wedge of tissue is excised from the tip of the toe under general anesthesia, and the entire nail apparatus is dissected from the bone and swung to achieve a correct axis. Healing is surprisingly fast and uneventful. However, when probing reveals a great area of onycholysis, treatment is usually too late.

Ingrown toenails are very common in schoolchildren and young adolescents. Whatever the precipitating factor, there is always a discrepancy between a wide nail plate and a narrow toe. It is therefore logical to leave the nail folds and nail bed intact and to narrow the nail plate permanently. The easiest way is the lateral selective matrix horn cautery using liquefied (90%) phenol. A digital ring block is performed; the offending lateral nail edge is freed from the nail bed and overlying proximal nail fold. The lateral nail edge is cut and removed. Digital anemia is produced using a tourniquet. The space under the proximal nail fold is cleaned and dried using a cotton-wool applicator, and liquefied phenol is then vigorously rubbed onto the matrix epithelium for about 3 minutes. Abundant granulation tissue in the lateral nail sulcus may also gently be cauterized. Tapered antibiotic tablets are put into the wound cavities, the tourniquet is released, and a thick padded dressing is applied. This is changed after 24 hours in a foot bath containing povidone-iodine soap. Postoperative pain is minimal, and infections are extremely rare because phenol has local anesthetic and disinfective actions. Toxicity from the minute amounts of phenol used has not been observed by us. Recurrences are exceedingly rare. Surgical dissection of the lateral matrix horns is an alternative; however, it requires some surgical skills and takes more time. Healing is, however, more rapid than with phenol cautery.

Pincer nails are characterized by a transverse nail plate overcurvature increasing distally. The lateral margins of the nail plate pinch the nail bed tissue and may dig deeply into the lateral furrows. Most cases are remarkably painless; however, sometimes pain is exceedingly intense. Four variants of pincer nails are to be differentiated: (1) a hereditary type with symmetrical involvement, lateral deviation of the great and medial deviation of the lesser toenails (this type is quite often seen in several members of the family); (2) an acquired form with asymmetrical involvement that is due to foot deformation and mainly seen in elderly people; (3) overcurvature due to nail involvement of psoriasis and some other chronic dermatoses; and (4) tubed fingernails due to degenerative osteoarthritis of the distal finger joints. In the most frequent hereditary type, x-ray examination always reveals very broad bases of the terminal phalanx with lateral osteophytes that are even more marked on the medial aspect, explaining the lateral deviation of the long axis of the nail. We therefore believe that conservative treatment, such as orthonyx braces, thinning the nail plate by filing in order to make it less resilient, and so on, cannot be successful. A successful treatment is to narrow the nail plate permanently by excision or cautery of the lateral matrix horns, dissecting the pinched nail bed from the bone to be able to spread it out after removal of the dorsal distal traction osteophyte, and to keep the nail bed flat using reversed tie-over sutures that are removed after 18 to 20 days.

Trauma

Subungual hematoma is the most frequent sequel of a substantial acute trauma to the nail unit. A blow of a hammer or a crush injury from a door are the most common types of injury. The extent of the subungual hematoma depends on the severity of the trauma and the site hit. Small hematomas not exceeding 40% to 50% of the nail area may be cautiously drained through a small hole burnt with a red-hot paper-clip or drilled with a pointed scalpel blade that is rotated with gentle pressure. Hematomas greater than 50% of the nail area usually are due to severe lacerations of the matrix and nail bed, quite often also involving a fracture of the terminal bone. A radiograph is therefore always necessary. Any step formations in the matrix and/or nail bed require meticulous repair in order to avoid permanent nail dystrophy.

Habits such as *picking, nail biting (onychophagia), excessive cutting and filing (onychotillomania)* are not rare. The most common abnormality due to chronic self-inflicted trauma is the *washboard nail*. It is usually seen on the thumb nail and due to chronic picking of the lunular area; the proximal nail fold is habitually pushed back, its free margin is thickened and lifted up from the nail, the cuticle is lost, and the nail appears unproportionally long. The condition is symmetrical when the thumb nail of the opposite hand is used, or unilateral when the index finger nail of the same hand is used for this habit. The most common misdiagnosis is Heller's median canaliform dystrophy. Full explanation of the pathogenesis is necessary for therapy; however, most patients with nail habits require some psychotherapy.

Tumors of the Nail Apparatus

Myxoid pseudocysts (dorsal finger cyst, mucinous cyst) are benign lesions usually seen in the proximal nail fold of fingers, far less frequently of toes. They present as ill-defined, elastic, flesh-colored to transparent tumors sparing the midline of the nail fold. Continuous pressure to the matrix gives rise to a longitudinal depression in the plate. Any puncture will reduce this pressure and cause transverse rims in the furrow. Myxoid pseudocysts are degenerative lesions, not true tumors. Repeated punctures and expression and injection of hyaluronidase, sclerosing agents, or steroid crystal suspension are rarely permanently successful. Cryosurgery in experienced hands gives cure rates of about 80%. Surgery performed under regional block anesthesia is our treatment of choice. Sterile methylene blue solution, 0.05 to 0.1 mL, is injected into the joint space via the volar aspect of the distal joint crease. This will stain the stalk that frequently develops and connects the pseudocyst with the joint, and will show the true extent of the degenerative lesion. An incision is made around the tumor, and a small transposition flap is incised. The stained lesion is meticulously dissected and the flap raised; this often shows more degenerative lesions. The stalk is followed, resected, and sutured with 6-0 resorbable sutures. The transposition flap is sutured to cover the primary defect; the secondary defect is allowed to granulate in. Both the

functional and cosmetic results are excellent. Recurrence rate is below 2%.

Periungual fibromas and *fibrokeratomas* are not rare. They are cut at their base down to the bone. The defect is usually so small that secondary epithelialization occurs rapidly without subsequent nail dystrophy. *Multiple periungual fibromas (Koenen's tumors)* in tuberous sclerosis are also sectioned at their base.

Subungual filamentous tumors appear as a longitudinal streak of whitish to yellowish to brown color, usually not wider than 1.5 mm. On close examination, a tiny rim of keratotic material is seen adhering to the nail plate's undersurface. It is probably an extremely thin subungual fibrokeratoma. It can be pared down painlessly.

The *glomus tumor* is the most characteristic subungual tumor. It is associated with radiating pain elicited by minor trauma or cold that can often be relieved by a tourniquet. Clinically, the tumor presents as a bluish-red to violaceous spot under the nail. Probing characteristically yields intense pain and allows the tumor to be more exactly localized. Small lesions are removed after punching a 6-mm hole into the nail plate, incising the nail bed, and dissecting the grayish glomus tumor. Lesions in a lateral position are excised via a lateral L-shaped incision allowing the nail bed to be dissected from the nail bed until the tumor is reached.

Giant cell synovialoma is one of the most common tumors of the hand and can be found in the proximal nail fold. It is a multilobulate, firm, subcutaneous tumor invading the overlying dermis and interfering with nail growth. It is removed by sharp dissection from the dermis and blunt dissection from the underlying surrounding tissues. Full-thickness skin grafts are used for larger defects.

Malignant Tumors

Bowen's disease of the nail organ is relatively frequent. It may mimic common warts, butcher's nodule, chronic paronychia, granulation tissue, fibrokeratoma, and even malignant melanoma. Rare variants may be pigmented. Its onset is insidious and it remains asymptomatic for years. Human papillomaviruses type 16, 18, 35, and others have been detected in a number of ungual Bowen's disease; they may be responsible for multiple Bowen's lesions. Treatment of choice is complete surgical excision, preferably with microscopic control of the wound margins. Depending on the size of the defect, flaps or grafts may be used to cover the defect. Serial and step sections are needed to rule out invasive squamous cell carcinoma histopathologically.

Squamous cell carcinoma of the nail is a slow-growing, low-grade malignancy developing de novo, in chronic radiodermatitis, after trauma and osteitis terminalis, as well as from Bowen's disease. Differential diagnosis includes paronychia, ingrown nail, pyogenic granuloma, warts, and amelanotic melanoma. Complete extirpation using Mohs' surgery is mandatory.

Melanonychia Striata and Melanoma

The nail apparatus contains melanocytes that are normally nonfunctional but may give rise to both benign and malignant melanocytic proliferations in the matrix, nail bed, and periungual tissues. Any melanocytic lesion continually producing melanin in larger quantities will result in a longitudinal brown to black streak. This may be a focus of active melanocytes, a lentigo, a melanocytic nevus, or a malignant melanoma. Multiple pigmented bands are seen physiologically in dark-skinned people; they may also be seen after PUVA treatment or in adrenal insufficiency, malnutrition, or acquired immune deficiency syndrome, or during or after therapy with zidovudine, cytotoxic drugs, antimalarials, or minocycline (Minocin). Any brown band in the nail of a fair-skinned individual is suspicious and should prompt a biopsy. Excisional biopsy is preferable to make the correct diagnosis and rule out technical errors. *Hutchinson's melanotic whitlow*, the spreading of pigment from under the nail to periungual skin, is usually associated with melanoma. Although malignant melanonychia striata is commonly dark brown, *subungual melanoma* may masquerade as a light-brown band, and 20 to 25% of ungual melanomas are nonpigmented, mimicking pyogenic granuloma, granulation tissue, or ingrown nail. Bands that are wider than 5 to 6 mm are highly suspicious of malignancy, and darkening and widening of a light-brown band in a black or Asian individual is suggestive of melanoma. Bleeding, ulceration, and onychodystrophy are signs of advanced melanoma.

Many patients present only after trauma to the nail, and a subungual hematoma or bacterial infection with nail discoloration may obscure the subungual melanoma. Pigmented material should therefore be scraped from the nail, boiled in a test tube, and tested for blood using a conventional Hemostix. Blood tends to grow out with the nail, presenting a proximal border parallel to the lunula. Microbial pigment may be seen on histologic slides as a diffuse brownish discoloration; melanin is finely granular and argentaffin-positive.

Confronted with a pigmented nail lesion, one has to consider that overtreatment of a benign alteration may cause unnecessary mutilation, but delay in diagnosis and treatment of ungual melanoma may favor dissemination. An individual approach is recommended: Narrow brown bands are diagnosed and treated by punch excision after reflection of the proximal nail fold and identification of the melanocytic lesion in the matrix. Lesions in lateral position are removed by a lateral longitudinal biopsy, eventually resulting in a somewhat narrower nail. Wider lesions are either biopsied or a transversally oriented fusiform excision of the matrix is performed. Periungual pigmentation has to be seen as widespread melanoma (in situ), requiring wide excision of the nail organ and plastic repair of the defect. Far advanced, deeply invasive melanoma may require amputation of the digit.

KELOIDS

method of
KEVIN C. CHUNG, M.D., and
DAVID J. SMITH, JR., M.D.
University of Michigan Medical Center
Ann Arbor, Michigan

Keloids, a word derived from Greek *kelis* (blemish) and *lidos* (form), are abnormal fibrous growths sometimes occurring after skin trauma. Any surgical or unintentional trauma to the skin of susceptible individuals incites an exuberant fibroblastic reaction. The resulting pendulous, tumor-like scars are disfiguring, although malignant transformation is quite rare. In contrast to hypertrophic scars, which are confined to the boundary of the original dermal injury, keloids extend beyond the border of the original tissue trauma. Differentiating keloids and hypertrophic scars may be important in devising appropriate treatments. Keloids and hypertrophic scars can often be distinguished by clinical examination, even though differentiating these two types of abnormal scars may be difficult under the light microscope. Histologically, both scars consist of dense irregular collagen bundles, but keloids may exhibit eosinophilic refractile hyaline-like collagen fibers and a paucity of fibroblasts in the dermis.

Keloids have the highest incidence in the African-American population, occurring on the ear lobes, shoulders, anterior chest, upper arms, and mandibular angles. Hypertrophic scars tend to occur weeks after trauma and regress slowly during the ensuing months. Local treatments such as steroid injections, compressive garments, and Silastic sheetings are generally effective against hypertrophic scars, but keloids usually do not respond to these local measures. Recurrences are common, and treatment outcomes are unpredictable.

TREATMENT

Currently, no ideal treatment is available for keloids. Since prevention is best, susceptible individuals should avoid any nonessential esthetic procedures. While promising new pharmacologic agents are being tested to alter the scar response in keloids, traditional treatment can be categorized into three types: surgical treatment, nonsurgical treatment, and combination treatment.

Surgical Treatment

Surgical excision appears to be simple and effective in treating keloids. Simple excision, however, merely recreates the original trauma and does not address the fundamental wound-healing abnormalities. The recurrence rate may be as low as 50% and as high as 80% to 100% after 2 years. Since tissue trauma stimulates keloidal scars, others have used carbon dioxide or argon lasers to excise keloids in an effort to minimize tissue injury. Recurrence is high when laser is used alone; surgical removal of keloids must be combined with some form of adjuvant therapy to reduce abnormal local tissue response to trauma.

Nonsurgical Treatment

Corticosteroids

The mechanism of corticosteroids in keloid treatment is not completely understood. Corticosteroids may enhance collagen degradation by inducing fibroblast production of collagenase. The commonly used corticosteroid is Kenalog-40 (triamcinolone acetonide). Intralesional injections of Kenalog-40 may not totally obliterate the keloid but they often flatten the nodularity and reduce redness and pruritus.

Kenalog-40 contains 40 mg of triamcinolone per mL and is often diluted with 1 mL of 2% plain lidocaine for keloid injection. Kenalog-40 is quite viscous; diluting with lidocaine in a 50:50 mixture provides easier and more comfortable injections. The mixture can be injected with either a 25- or a 27-gauge needle fitted with a tuberculin syringe. The small syringe generates the high pressure required to inject the mixture into the dense keloidal scar.

The thick, unyielding keloid scar makes injection quite difficult, and sometimes the solution may escape into normal surrounding tissues, causing permanent depigmentation. A spring-powered mechanical device called the Dermajet may provide easier and more controlled injections. It may be more comfortable for adolescents. The corticosteroid injections can be repeated every 4 weeks until no clinical improvement is observed.

The effectiveness of corticosteroid injections as an isolated therapy is variable. More than 90% of patients will see symptoms such as redness and pruritus alleviated. The data on resolution and recurrence of keloids are unclear. It is difficult to compare results from different reports because the definition of clinical response is different and the follow-up time is inconsistent. Since corticosteroid injection can be done quite readily in the clinic, it may be offered to patients as the first treatment option. Complications of corticosteroid injections consist of hypopigmentation and atrophy of the surrounding tissues. Systemic glucocorticoid effects of local steroid injections are quite rare.

Radiation

Radiation therapy as the primary treatment has not gained much acceptance according to medical literature, probably because of the required high radiation dose and the attendant risk for radiation burns and tumor induction. Radiation therapy may decrease keloid scars by destroying fibroblasts. By decreasing the fibroblast population, the scar is diminished as collagen degradation surpasses collagen synthesis. Although radiation is not used as a first-line therapy, low-dose radiation is promising as an adjuvant therapy after keloid excision.

Pressure

In hypertrophic scars, pressure is shown to be effective in reducing scar formation, but pressure is less effective in keloidal scars. For patients with earlobe keloids, compression ear clips may decrease the scar, and recurrent keloid formation is high when the device is not applied. In other keloidal sites such as the chest and the shoulder, a compression garment is less effective.

Combination Therapy

Surgery and Radiation

An effective treatment for keloid is surgical excision followed by adjuvant radiation therapy. Recurrence after this combination treatment has been reported to be less than 10% in most series. The optimal radiation dose ranges from 1000 cGy to 1500 cGy, and with modern shielding techniques, most radiation therapists reported minimal risks of developing radiation-induced malignancies. When patients with keloids fail or refuse corticosteroid injections, we use the combination therapy of surgery and radiation at our institution. We excise the keloids extramarginally and close the wound primarily. In wounds with a broad base, the excised skin may be used as a skin graft. Obtaining a skin graft from a different donor site poses the problem of new keloid formation. After scar excision, the wound is irradiated on the same day with 300 cGy of radiation. This same dose is administered on 3 successive days for a total dosage of 1200 cGy. The side effects of this combination therapy are minimal, typically local skin pigmentation changes. Young children with open epiphyses should not be irradiated, because the treatment may affect the growth plates and retard bone growth.

Surgery and Steroids

An alternative to combining surgery and radiation is to combine surgery and corticosteroid injections. For patients who object to radiation treatment, adjuvant steroid injections may be a second-best approach in recalcitrant keloids. After extralesional excision of keloids, the fresh wound edges are infiltrated with Kenalog-40 and 2% lidocaine in a 50:50 mixture. The wound is closed with nonabsorbable sutures to be removed at 2 weeks. Corticosteroid injections are repeated every 4 weeks for a minimum of 6 months. Since most keloid recurrence is evident within 2 years, these patients will need to be followed closely, and repeat steroid injections may be needed. This regimen is not well accepted by patients, and the drop-out rate is quite high because of the need for frequent clinic visits. Even with stringent adherence to this treatment regimen, reported recurrences may be over 50%.

SUMMARY

Despite intense research on wound healing, a successful treatment regimen for keloidal wounds still eludes us. Medications such as colchicine, penicillamine, and beta-aminopropionitrile have been used with little success in altering the wound-healing response of keloid scars. Until the mechanism of abnormal wound healing is understood, the results of the treatments will be unpredictable.

For patients with newly formed keloids, we recommend a trial of corticosteroid injections. For patients who do not respond to steroid injections, surgical excision and low-dose radiation therapy may be the best treatment option for keloid scars. Recent studies have shown that lymphokine interferon-gamma inhibits collagen synthesis. Understanding the role of these lymphokines in modulating collagen metabolism may provide the solution for this disfiguring disease.

WARTS
(Verruca Vulgaris)

method of
RONALD W. SWINFARD, M.D.
University of Missouri
Columbia, Missouri

Warts are extremely common, with a significant portion of the worldwide population having warts at some point in their lives. The ubiquitous nature of the papillomavirus means that the clinical presence of warts reflects more on the host's lack of immunity to this virus than the simple presence of the virus. Accordingly, warts are seen more frequently in those previously unexposed to the virus (children) and those with compromised immune systems (transplant patients on immunosuppressives, human immunodeficiency virus (HIV)-infected individuals, and so on). Of the more than 60 serotypes of human papillomavirus (HPV), few are oncogenic, with almost all the oncogenic types being found on the genitals (condyloma acuminata).

DIAGNOSIS

Rarely does a competent clinician have trouble distinguishing common warts from other skin neoplasms. The characteristic roughened surface, interruption of normal skin lines (dermatoglyphics), and the presence of black dots representing thrombosed capillaries (not "seeds") make this an easy diagnosis. Rarely the clinician may need to pare the wart and observe punctate bleeding from the capillaries in order to be fully convinced that the lesion is a wart. Other morphologic types may be more difficult to discriminate. For example, the threadlike spikes of filiform verrucae can simulate seborrheic keratoses. The pink, barely elevated papules of flat warts (verruca plana) can mimic seborrheic or stucco keratoses. Finally, plantar verrucae and plantar calluses (clavi) can be difficult to differentiate without paring the lesion to watch for the punctate bleeding points found in warts or the central spikelike keratin core found in clavi.

APPROACH TO TREATMENT

Every practitioner has her or his favorite method of treating warts. While each of us takes pride in our particular destructive procedure, ultimate success depends on the response of the patient's immune system. This is why, left untreated, a significant frac-tion of warts spontaneously regress. This may also be why the various methods of "charming" away warts are successful, e.g., "buying the wart," or rubbing with a potato and burying half the potato, and so on. So for all we do to warts, all we are probably accomplishing is exposing HPV antigens to the immune system with subsequent cell-mediated involution of the wart. This also confers lifelong immunity, explaining why many patients are never subsequently afflicted with warts after successful treatment as a child or young adult.

Listed here is the repertoire of treatments available, roughly in the order I use them.

Salicyclic/Lactic Acid Preparations

"Wart paints" have long been used as a mainstay of treatment. Preparations previously requiring a prescription (Duofilm, Occlusal, and so on) are now available over-the-counter (OTC). I use these particularly on children to avoid the trauma and pain of in-office destructive procedures. The patient soaks the affected area 5 to 10 minutes at bedtime (or takes a nightly shower or bath), then applies the compound. These preparations are in collodion and dry quickly. This results in superficial destruction, as evidenced by the development of a white, devitalized surface after several nights' use. Consequently, the patient is instructed to abrade the area every 3 to 7 nights using a callus file, pumice stone, or old nail file. This nightly application of weak acid should produce inflammation around the wart sufficient to provoke an immune response. If no reaction is occurring in about 3 weeks, then I recommend occluding the wart paint overnight, using adhesive tape (not a Band-Aid). If the wart is not showing involution in 6 to 8 weeks, a more destructive method may be necessary. For plantar warts, I use the same regimen but recommend OTC 40% salicylic acid plasters (Mediplast) instead of "paint." If no response is seen after 3 weeks, I have the patient keep the plaster in place a full 24 hours (rather than overnight) and observe for response in 6 to 8 weeks.

Cryosurgery

Liquid nitrogen freezing is the leading destructive method used in the dermatologist's office. The liquid nitrogen may be applied with a Q-tip or one of the commercially available spraying devices. For planar or filiform warts, the time from complete freezing to complete thawing (the so-called freeze-thaw time, or FTT) need be only 10 to 20 seconds. For most common warts, a FTT of 30 to 40 seconds is recommended, with large or recalcitrant lesions receiving two FTT cycles. If an FTT of greater than 40 seconds is desired, consider local anesthesia, as freezing to this depth can be quite painful. Paring the lesions is recommended prior to freezing, especially with plantar warts.

Freezing is moderately painful and results in a serous or hemorrhagic blister several hours after the procedure. The patient should be instructed in appropriate postoperative wound care. One should be particularly cautious about freezing superficial nerves, such as on the sides of the digits, as this can result in nerve injury lasting several weeks to months (if not permanent), with resulting anesthesia. Following freezing one can expect pigmentary alteration (rarely permanent) and occasional scar. Cryosurgery is contraindicated in patients with Raynaud's disease, cryoglobulinemia, or cold urticaria.

Periungual warts are particularly troublesome. I recommend light freezing (say 15 to 20 second FTT) every 3 to 4 weeks, instructing the patient to use a wart paint under adhesive tape occlusion overnight between office visits.

Electrodesiccation and Curettage

After local anesthesia, the wart is fulgurated, then a sharp curette (I recommend Acuderm disposable) is used to scrape out the wart. It is surprising that most warts will "shell out," with brisk bleeding expected. Hemostasis can be either by electrocoagulation or a liquid hemostatic agent (aluminum chloride or ferrous subsulfate). This procedure can, of course, result in a slight skin depression or area of hypopigmentation.

Surgical Excision

This is seldom necessary and rarely indicated, since one is ultimately attempting to provoke an immune response to the wart virus. In addition, warts on the hands and feet can be difficult to close and may result in a scar of a size comparable to the original wart. One may biopsy warts from immunocompromised hosts (especially transplant patients) in order to obtain a surgical specimen for pathologic examination for a suspected squamous cell carcinoma.

Bichloracetic Acid

A kit is available from Glenwood, Inc., which contains all one needs to use bichloracetic acid to treat small benign growths such as warts. It is much more potent than salicylic or lactic acid preparations and results in immediate devitalization of the tissue it touches. Hence, one sees immediate whitening of the treated tissue. It can burn or sting transiently (several minutes), and protecting the normal surrounding skin with petrolatum is recommended, which comes with the kit. Like podophyllin, bichloracetic acid can be used to treat condyloma acuminata; treatment of condyloma is discussed in a separate section of this text.

Tretinoin (Retin-A)*

For patients who present with a large number of flat warts, especially on the face, application of Retin-A gel, 0.01% to 0.025% at bedtime can be effective. This necessarily produces an irritant reaction manifested by erythema, flaking, and desquamation. This can also be used for flat warts on the lower legs, frequently seen in young women. Topical 5-fluoro-

uracil,* as 5% cream or 1% or 2% solution, has also been used for flat warts, but less effectively than Retin-A in my experience. Patients being treated for flat warts should also be instructed to avoid excessive sun exposure to the affected area, and women should try to discontinue leg shaving during treatment.

Bleomycin (Blenoxane)*

I have little experience using this modality, mostly because I seldom treat warts not responding to some combination of previously discussed modalities. I also am reluctant to use such a potent anticancer drug for a benign lesion, and bleomycin is not currently FDA-approved for treatment of warts. When used, it is injected into the base of the wart. One needs only a small volume (0.2 to 1.0 mL) of 0.5 to 1.0 U per mL. Excessive use or injection into normal adjacent tissue can be quite painful.

Lasers

The carbon dioxide laser is most frequently used to treat warts because it has been around the longest and is less expensive to purchase. Patients are enamored with the "high-tech" nature of this treatment, but its expense makes it a therapy of last resort among the destructive methods. When used, appropriate precautions should be observed, including eye protection and use of a smoke evacuator, since viral particles have been isolated from the plume.

Immunotherapy

Without pretense of destruction, immunotherapy uses a potent contact sensitizer to "bait" T lymphocytes to a wart, then exploits the sensitization arm of the contact response on the premise that another population of T cells develops immunity to the wart virus. Because it requires an average of 5 to 6 treatments at 3- to 4-week intervals, it is reserved for special circumstances. These include extensive number of warts (dozens) making other methods impractical, treatment failures by all other methods, or a patient who will not tolerate any destructive procedures. In addition, this is not approved by the FDA, so (at least) verbal informed consent is advised.

The ideal allergen for wart immunotherapy is that it is a potent sensitizer, preferably synthetic rather than naturally present in the environment so the patient is unlikely to encounter it later, and safe to use. This latter issue has been debated, since formal long-term studies have not been carried out on these chemicals. However, no late sequelae have been verified despite the use of these chemicals for at least 15 years.

The most common sensitizers used are dinitrochlorobenzene (DNCB), squaric acid dibutyl ester (SADBE), and diphenylcyclopropenone (DPC). A small quantity (usually 50 to 100 μL of a 1% to 2% solution, delivered with an Emendorf pipette) is placed on the skin between the warts and the suspected draining lymph glands. As warts are common

---

*Not FDA-approved for this indication.

*Not FDA-approved for this indication.

on the hands and feet, this is usually on the medial upper arm above the elbow or near the popliteal fossa, respectively. The application is painless and should be covered with a Band-Aid to prevent spread to other sites. The sensitizer should be left in place at least 4 hours before washing it off, although I usually leave it in place until bedtime of the day of application. After 5 to 10 days, the patient should develop a poison ivy–like rash that may blister. Management of a typical contact dermatitis is appropriate. This area frequently develops postinflammatory hyperpigmentation, and this site may reactivate when the warts are treated. At the next visit in 3 to 4 weeks, one ensures a sensitizing reaction, then applies a small quantity of 1% to 2% solution sufficient to saturate the wart and a 1- to 3-mm periphery. If, on the next visit in 3 to 4 weeks there is no local reaction, try adhesive tape occlusion to enhance penetration. This same technique can be used if the initial sensitizing dose failed to evoke a reaction. I will usually give five to six treatments before declaring a failure, even in the absence of or minimal reaction. If the area is reacting appropriately with a contact dermatitis, I will treat 10 to 12 times before giving up. If treating the patient for recalcitrance to all other therapies, I would switch sensitizers after 10 to 12 treatments, as failure with one does not necessarily imply failure to all.

GENITAL WARTS

method of
KARL R. BEUTNER, M.D., PH.D.
University of California, San Francisco
San Francisco, California

Genital warts are the most common clinical manifestation of infection of the genital area with the human papilloma virus (HPV). There are multiple genotypes of HPV, which have been further classified based on their association with cervical cancer as low-, intermediate-, and high-risk types. On the external genital area, the low-risk HPV type (predominantly types 6 and 11) causes genital warts. The high-risk HPV types are associated with squamous cell carcinoma in situ (also known as bowenoid papulosis) of the external genital skin and in situ and invasive squamous cell carcinoma of the cervix. In immunocompetent hosts, cutaneous in situ squamous cell carcinoma rarely, if ever, evolves into invasive squamous cell carcinoma. Genital skin appears not to be as susceptible to the oncogenic potential of HPV as is the transformation zone of the uterine cervix and the anal canal. Whereas 25% to 50% of sexually active adults may have genital HPV infection acquired by sexual contact with an infected partner, at any given time 1% have visible genital warts.

Three types of skin are found in the genital area: fully keratinized hair-bearing, fully keratinized nonhair-bearing, and partially keratinized nonhair-bearing. The latter are often mistakenly referred to as "mucous membranes," which they are not because there are no mucus glands in the underlying dermis. They are moist not because of mucus glands but because they are only partially keratinized.

Skin types influence wart morphology, which should be considered in selecting therapy. Warts occurring on moist surfaces respond better to a variety of topical therapies. The four morphologic types of genital warts are (1) hypertrophic or cauliflower-type, or condyloma acuminatum; (2) smooth papular type; (3) keratotic type, which may mimic seborrheic keratosis; and (4) flat type. The condyloma acuminatum type occurs essentially on moist, partially keratinized skin whereas the smooth papular and keratotic types are seen most frequently on fully keratinized areas; the flat type of warts is seen on both types of skin.

TREATMENT

It is important for the clinician to have and to communicate to the patient reasonable expectations of therapy. In general, rather than a treatment there is a course of therapy to achieve a wart-free state. Treatment will clearly alleviate the symptoms of HPV infection, i.e., warts, but it is not currently known whether elimination of warts will decrease or eliminate the patient's infectivity to current or future sexual partners. It is currently thought that once two individuals are infected they will not "Ping-Pong" the infection back and forth. In addition to treatment of their warts, it is important that women with external genital warts or whose male partners have external genital warts have a Papanicolaou smear and remain in the system for monitoring for cervical cancer.

The currently available treatments include cryotherapy, interferon, podophyllin resin, podofilox, surgery, and trichloroacetic acid (Table 1). The average patient has one to ten warts with an average wart area of 0.5 to 1.0 cm². If a patient fails to respond to treatment, has pigmented warts, or appears to worsen with treatment, biopsy is indicated to confirm the clinical diagnosis of genital warts. The major differential diagnosis of genital warts includes lichen planus, skin tags, seborrheic keratoses, molluscum contagiosum, condyloma latum, pearly penile papules, and squamous cell carcinoma in situ. While the latter is treated with the same modalities as warts, it is particularly important to caution the patient and the patient's current and future sexual contacts about the oncogenic potential of HPV types associated with bowenoid papulosis.

Cryotherapy

Cryotherapy is most often performed with liquid nitrogen applied by the spray technique; a large, loosely wound piece of cotton on a wooden stick; or with a cryoprobe. Cryotherapy cannot be effectively done with a small, tightly wound Q-tip that simply cannot hold adequate amounts of liquid nitrogen to effectively freeze a wart.

While freezing a few small warts without an anesthetic may not be unreasonable, patients with more than a few warts should at least be offered local anesthesia, either with injections of lidocaine or topical application of a eutectic mixture of lidocaine 2.5% and prilocaine 2.5% (Emla). How "hard" to freeze the warts can be learned with time and experience. Inadequate freezing will reduce efficacy, and over-

TABLE 1. **Currently Available Treatment for Genital Warts**

	Cryotherapy	Interferon	Podophyllin Resin	Podofilox	Surgery	Trichloroacetic Acid
Method of Action	Physical destruction	Antiwart/antiviral immunostimulator	Antimicrotubules	Antimicrotubules	Physical destruction	Caustic
Application	Liquid nitrogen spray cotton/stick cryoprobe	Intradermal injection below wart	Topical application in clinic	Patient application	Scissors, curettage, electrodesiccation, laser	30%–70% solution
Treatment Schedule	q 1–2 wk	3 × wk × 3 wk 2 × wk × 8 wk	q 1–2 wk	bid 3 d/wk × 4–6 wk	q 3–4 wk	q 1–2 wk
Effectiveness	+*	+†	+*	+†	+*	+*
Safety	100% local reaction; no systemic reaction	Flulike syndrome	Mild-to-moderate local reaction	Mild-to-moderate local reaction	Local wound	Local reaction variable
Limitations	Requires training	Expense	Preparation not standardized, stability unknown	Patient compliance	Requires training	Effective limited to small, moist warts

*Not established in well-controlled trials.
†Established in well-controlled trials.

freezing will greatly increase pain and the probability of scarring and other complications. In general, one wants the wart and a 1- to 2-mm border to be frozen solid. For other than small warts, two freeze-thaw cycles may improve efficacy.

Clinicians should not undertake cryotherapy without proper training and/or supervision. Although complications of cryotherapy are rare, inexperienced clinicians underfreeze more often than overfreezing, and this does not give the patient a good therapeutic outcome.

Interferon

The interferons represent the first drug approved for the treatment of genital warts. Currently, recombinant and natural alfa interferons (Alferon N, Roferon-A, and Intron A) are used to treat genital warts. Interferon is most commonly administered as an intradermal injection at the base of the wart. Because treatments are given either three times a week for 3 weeks or twice a week for 8 weeks, coupled with the high cost of the interferon and efficacy only comparable to that of other modalities, interferon cannot be considered a first-line treatment.

Podophyllin Resin

Podophyllin resin is a plant resin obtained from plant species *Podophyllum peltatum* or *Podophyllum emodii*. This resin contains several biologically active lignins that include podofilox (podophyllotoxin), 4-dimethylpodophyllotoxin, alpha-peltatum, and beta-peltatum. These lignins bind to tubulin at a site close to that of the colchicine-binding site, preventing polymerization of tubulin into microtubules and interfering with all cellular functions, such as mitoses, that are dependent upon intact microtubules.

Although podophyllin was one of the first treatments for genital warts, it suffers greatly from the lack of a readily available, standardized preparation with a known shelf life. Podophyllin resin is most commonly used as a 25% solution in tincture of ben-

zoin (Podofin, Podocon-25). Proper application is important; a small amount should be applied directly to the wart and allowed to air dry before the patient assumes a normal anatomic position. Medical tradition often advises patients to "wash it off" 2 to 4 hours after application. The reality is that benzoin is essentially water insoluble and cannot be removed simply with soap and water. Another ill-advised but not uncommon practice is to surround the wart with Vaseline, K-Y jelly, or other "barriers," then apply a moderate-to-large amount of podophyllin resin to the central wart. After application at body temperature the "barrier" becomes thinner, mixes with the podophyllin resin, and spreads over the genital area, often resulting in a rather impressive irritant reaction. I advise patients to leave the podophyllin resin on overnight and to avoid washing, bathing, and sexual contact while it is on. Podophyllin resin should be avoided in pregnancy.

Podofilox

The major active lignin in podophyllin resin is podofilox. This lignin is available as a 0.5% podofilox solution (Condylox) for patient applications. Patients apply this solution to the warts in treatment cycles of twice daily for 3 days followed by a 4-day treatment-free period. These weekly cycles can be repeated four to six times to achieve clearance of warts.

Surgery

The surgical approach to genital warts has the major advantage that the patient is rendered wart-free with a single visit. The only issue remaining is when and if the patient will experience a wart recurrence. In terms of external genital warts, there does not appear to be a clearly superior surgical modality. Selection of a surgical approach is most commonly dictated by the clinician's experience and availability of equipment. In experienced hands, good results can be achieved with simple tangential scis-

TABLE 2. Factors That Influence Selection of Therapy

Modality	Wart Morphology	Individual Wart Size	Total Wart Area	Wart Count
Cryotherapy	All	Small to average	Limiting*	Limiting*
Interferon	All	All	Limiting	Limiting
Surgery	All	All	All	All
Trichloroacetic acid	Nonkeratotic, moist	Small to average	Limiting*	Limiting*
Podophyllin resin	Nonkeratotic, moist	Most	<10 cm†	Not limiting
Podofilox	All	Most	<10 cm†	Not limiting

*Limited by extent of necrotic tissue and associated wound care.
†Limited by dose-related systemic reactions.

sor excision, electrodesiccation, hot cautery, curettage, and laser surgery.

Trichloroacetic Acid

Trichloroacetic acid (Tri-Chlor) is a caustic agent that chemically coagulates warts and adjacent skin. Although 30% to 70% solutions are employed, the optimal concentration has not been determined. With the higher concentrations extreme caution is important, for these can be highly caustic solutions.

Choice of Treatment

At the present time, without consideration of factors that may influence therapy, all treatments appear to be at least comparable in effectiveness. With any given treatment, there is a 40% to 75% chance of clearing and a 25% to 50% chance of recurrence. Recurrences are thought to be due to the existence of HPV in surrounding normal epidermis and not reinfection. The most common reason for outright treatment failure is improper selection of therapeutic modalities or improper use of a modality. Recurrence is the major cause of a prolonged course for the patient.

Several factors influence the selection of treatment. Immunosuppressed patients have a high recurrence rate, suggesting that immune responses may influence recurrence rates. Not all patients will respond equally well to all modalities. It is important to have a plan or set protocol, particularly when a limited number of modalities are available. If, after three to four treatments with a given therapy, a clinically significant response has not been seen, the treatment should be changed and the patient should be re-evaluated. Are these really genital warts? Factors to consider include selection of treatment, morphology (keratotic versus nonkeratotic), wart size, anatomic site, total wart area, wart count, clinician's experience, and patient preference (Table 2).

Proper matching of patient with modality will usually shorten the duration of therapy. In general, podophyllin resin and trichloroacetic acid are most effective for small warts on moist surfaces. Cryotherapy that induces necrosis followed by a slough and erosion is somewhat limited to the average case. Proper application of cryotherapy in large areas results in some wound care problems for the patient during the necrosis and sloughing stages. Podofilox will be effective in many patients but requires the patient to be able to visualize the warts.

ADDITIONAL NEEDS

Whereas treatment will alleviate the physical symptoms of the infection, the emotional impact of this sexually transmitted disease has the greatest long-term impact on patients' lives. A heavy emotional trauma is often associated with acquisition of a sexually transmitted disease. Patients often have significant fears of discovery, rejection, and guilt, and feel that someone has "done them wrong." They view themselves as less sexually desirable, enjoy sex less, and have concerns about transmission. It is important that patients be educated about transmission and the natural history of the infection. Patients should be taught to tell current and future sexual partners that they have had this infection. Teaching and educational materials are available from the American Social Health Association (1-919-361-8422).

NEVI

method of
RONALD P. RAPINI, M.D.
Texas Tech University
Lubbock, Texas

The term nevus (plural, nevi) refers to a variety of common benign neoplasms of the skin. Most of them are acquired in early childhood or young adulthood, but about 1% of them are congenital. About 99% of nevi are tumors of melanocytes, the pigment-producing cells in the skin, so when the term nevus is used by itself, the adjective melanocytic is presumed. However, as one can see from Table 1, not all melanocytic nevi are brown, and there are other types of nevi besides melanocytic ones. Table 1 is actually an oversimplification, as the clinical appearance can vary, and there are many other types of nevi that are beyond the scope of this discussion.

TREATMENT

Since nevi are benign, treatment is usually considered to be cosmetic or optional, unless they are suspi-

TABLE 1. **Nevi and Their Treatment**

Type	Usual Clinical Features	Usual Treatment
Junctional melanocytic	Brown macule	None, except (1)
Intradermal melanocytic	Flesh-colored papule	None, except (1)
Compound melanocytic	Brown papule	None, except (1)
Dysplastic melanocytic (= Clark's = nevus with architectural disorder = atypical)	Variegated brown, reddish, or black macule or papule, most common on trunk	Complex, depending upon how suspicious lesion is and family history of melanoma
Halo	White halo around nevus; usually on children, young adults	None, except (1)
Spitz's (= spindle and epithelioid)	Red, brown, or black papule, children or young adults; histology may resemble that of melanoma	Biopsy; completely excise suspicious ones when pathologist is not certain
Congenital melanocytic	Brown plaque larger than 1 cm	Controversial need for complete excision or surveillance because of increased risk of melanoma
Blue	Blue-black papule or nodule	None, except (1)
Nevus sebaceus	Congenital verrucous yellowish linear plaque on head or scalp	None, except some advocate excision to prevent basal carcinoma
Linear epidermal nevus	Congenital verrucous linear plaque on trunk or extremities	None, except (1)

(1) If suspicious, growing, changing, symptomatic, or irritated, or for cosmetic reasons, these can be (tangentially) shaved, excised without sutures, or excised to superficial adipose tissue and sutured. If melanoma is suspected, biopsy should extend below deepest portion.

cious-looking, growing, changing, symptomatic, or irritated. The main issue is to make certain that one is not dealing with malignant melanoma (see clinical description in next article). This can at times be difficult for both the clinician and the pathologist, and sometimes the expert assistance of a dermatologist or dermatopathologist is needed. Lesions with uncertain histologic diagnoses sometimes need to be more widely excised, with margins of 5 to 10 mm, depending upon the situation, to make sure that they are completely removed. It is not feasible to remove all nevi prophylactically to prevent melanomas, since the average person has about 20 nevi, and only about one third of all melanomas arise from previous nevi anyway.

Patients with more than 100 nevi, a family or personal history of melanoma, a history of fair skin and sun damage, or those with atypical-appearing nevi need to have close follow-up, and suspicious lesions ought to be biopsied. A biopsy can be of the tangential (shave) variety if care is taken to excise beneath the deepest portion of the lesion. Melanoma prognosis and subsequent treatment depend upon the depth of invasion, which is determined from the biopsy specimen by the pathologist. Hemostasis of shave biopsies is best accomplished by pressure alone, followed by the application of antibiotic ointment such as bacitracin or Polysporin. If necessary for hemostasis, light electrodesiccation can then be used, or topical aluminum chloride (Drysol) or ferrous subsulfate solution (Monsel's solution) can be applied with a cottontip applicator. All of these may produce more scarring and slower healing than pressure alone. Monsel's solution also has the added problem of occasionally leaving residual brown pigmentation at the biopsy site.

When melanoma is suspected, complete excision to adipose tissue is preferred. If the lesion is large, it is acceptable to punch-biopsy into the lesion, extending to adipose tissue. The shave method of removing nevi results in a recurrence rate of 10% to 30%, often resulting in a lesion that is well known clinically and histologically to resemble a melanoma (so-called recurrent melanocytic nevus or pseudomelanoma). Shave excisions can sometimes produce excellent cosmetic results for selected nevi, and they are quick and easy to perform. However, the complete cure rate is higher when nevi are excised to adipose tissue and sutured.

It is important to be able to distinguish clinically between nevi and other benign skin lesions. This is because many superficial growths, such as skin tags (acrochordons), seborrheic keratoses, and viral warts, can be treated by local destruction (only if the diagnosis is certain), without producing pathology specimens. As seen in Table 2, in the opinion of dermatologists nevi should not be treated in this way, largely because of their propensity to resemble melanomas clinically and histologically. Dermatologists generally always send pathology specimens when removing nevi. If ten nevi are removed, there should be ten separate bottles, each labeled according to site.

Most tangential excisions or excisions down to adipose tissue can be carried out under local anesthesia with 1% lidocaine with or without epinephrine. Topical anesthesia, such as a eutectic mixture of the local anesthetic agents lidocaine and prilocaine (EMLA

TABLE 2. **Treatments for Nevi That Are *Not* Recommended**

Destruction of any kind without pathology specimen:
    Cryotherapy with liquid nitrogen
    Topical acid application (trichloroacetic, salicylic, lactic, and so on)
    Topical podophyllin or cantharidin
    Electrosurgical destruction
    Carbon dioxide laser ablation (other than cutting)
    Curettage, even if fragments are sent to pathology
Superficial shave excision of lesions suspicious for melanoma

cream), is useful in children or frightened adults before or instead of injected anesthesia. A slow injection technique using a 1-mL syringe and a 30-gauge needle helps minimize pain. Contrary to popular teaching, it is not necessary to draw back on a syringe to avoid intravascular injection of minute amounts of anesthetic into the small dermal vessels while raising a dermal wheal beneath a superficial skin lesion. Often a long scar can be avoided by excising perilesionally all around the nevus with 1- or 2-mm margins, or by punch-excising the nevus, regardless of its shape. This is followed by 5-0 or 6-0 nylon or polypropylene suturing, followed by "dog-ear" repairs if necessary. This perilesional method avoids the creation of an elliptical specimen whose length is unfortunately often recommended to be at least three times the width of the nevus.

MALIGNANT MELANOMA

method of
DANIEL G. COIT, M.D.
Memorial Sloan Kettering Cancer Center and
    Cornell University Medical School
New York, New York

Malignant melanoma is increasing in incidence more rapidly than any other human malignancy, with an estimated 34,100 new cases anticipated in the United States in 1995. If in situ melanomas are included in this estimate, the incidence may be over 80,000 new cases per year. The rising incidence in melanoma does not simply reflect earlier diagnosis of highly curable cases, as the death rate from melanoma is increasing second only to lung cancer in the United States, with 7200 melanoma-related deaths anticipated in 1995. If the current trend continues, it is estimated that by the year 2000, 1 in 90 white Americans will develop melanoma. The reasons for this dramatic increase may be in part related to increased sun exposure. Although this is undoubtedly not the only factor responsible, it may be the only one over which we have some measure of control.

SIGNS AND SYMPTOMS

Melanoma often, although not invariably, arises within the context of a long-standing pre-existing nevus. Classically, melanoma is described using the ABCD paradigm: **a**symmetry, **b**order irregularity, variegated **c**olors, and **d**iameter greater than 8.0 mm. It is important to recognize, however, that melanomas need not conform to these descriptors and may present as nonpigmented dermal nodules. The most common presenting symptom is a change in a skin lesion, in appearance, itching, or bleeding.

DIAGNOSIS

In the setting of a suspicious pigmented lesion, excisional biopsy is the preferred method of diagnosis. This biopsy should be oriented with a definitive wide excision in mind. Shave biopsies of suspicious pigmented lesions are to be discouraged. They often yield incomplete information on the depth of invasion of the lesion and may compro-

mise definitive treatment planning. There are specialized sites (subungual, digital, plantar, auricular, or facial) where excisional biopsy prior to definitive therapy is not always possible. In those instances, a full thickness punch-biopsy of the thickest area of the lesion is recommended to establish a diagnosis.

STAGING

Treatment of localized primary melanoma depends on adequate microstaging of the primary lesion. Primary melanoma is staged both by its level of histologic invasion relative to defined layers in the dermis (Clark system), as well as its measured thickness (Breslow system). The American Joint Committee on Cancer has adopted the staging system shown in Table 1. It should be noted that when the Clark level and Breslow thickness are in conflict, the lesion is staged by the least favorable indicator.

TREATMENT

Management of the Primary. Once the diagnosis of primary malignant melanoma has been established, a definitive wide excision is indicated. Although historical and retrospective data had suggested that wider margins were necessary, more recent prospective randomized trials have defined appropriate margins yielding an irreducibly small rate of local recurrence. For premalignant or dysplastic lesions, a 2- to 3-mm margin is sufficient. For those lesions classified as melanoma in situ, a 0.5-cm margin is appropriate. For melanomas measuring less than or equal to 1.0 mm in thickness, a 1.0-cm margin is appropriate. For melanomas measuring 1.0 to 4.0 mm in thickness, a 2.0-cm margin is acceptable. For melanomas measuring greater than 4.0 mm

TABLE 1. **American Joint Committee on Cancer 1988 Melanoma Staging System**

Primary Tumor

Tx	Cannot be assessed
T0	No primary tumor
Tis	In situ melanoma, Clark I
T1	≤0.75 mm, Clark II
T2	0.76–1.5 mm, Clark III
T3	1.6–4.0 mm, Clark IV
T4	>4.0 mm, ± satellitosis, Clark V

Regional Nodes

Nx	Cannot be assessed
N0	No regional node metastases
N1	Regional node metastases <3 cm in diameter
N2	Regional node metastases >3 cm in diameter and/or in transit metastases

Distant Metastases

Mx	Cannot be assessed
M0	No distant metastases
M1	Distant metastases

Stage Grouping

Stage 0	Tis	N0	M0
Stage I	T1–2	N0	M0
Stage II	T3–4	N0	M0
Stage III	Tany	N1–2	M0
Stage IV	Tany	Nany	M1

in thickness, the appropriate margin is unknown, although intuitively a margin of at least 3.0 cm is recommended (Table 2). These margins should serve as guidelines and must occasionally be modified in cosmetically sensitive sites.

The technique of wide excision commonly involves an elliptical incision oriented along lines of skin tension, usually along the axis of an extremity. In general, this ellipse is at least three times as long as it is wide to avoid excessive "dog-ears" at the ends. If primary closure is not possible, local rotation flaps can minimize the need for split-thickness skin grafting, which is occasionally required in the absence of other alternatives. Free tissue transfer with microvascular anastomosis may be appropriate for extensive resections of the weight-bearing surface on the sole of the foot.

Elective Lymph Node Dissection. A great deal has been written about the controversy regarding elective lymph node dissection for patients with intermediate-thickness melanoma at risk to harbor micrometastatic disease in their regional lymph nodes. Retrospective studies have suggested a survival advantage in node-positive patients whose disease is dissected early before it becomes clinically apparent. Prospective randomized trials have failed to establish the role of elective lymph node dissection in improving long-term outcome. Recently, Morton and colleagues have described a technique of preoperative lymphatic mapping using lymphoscintigraphy, followed by intraoperative lymphatic mapping using a blue dye in combination with a hand-held gamma counter to localize the "sentinel" lymph node, the first draining lymph node of a given primary melanoma site. This sentinel node has proved to be extremely predictive of the presence or absence of regional nodal metastases. When the node is positive, completion lymph node dissection yields additional nodes in approximately one third of patients. When the node is negative, with high probability all nodes in that regional nodal basin will be negative. This method results in the ability to stage patients with melanoma at risk for regional nodal metastases with a relatively minor surgical procedure, thus helping define their long-term prognosis, as well as their eligibility for postoperative adjuvant immunotherapy trials (discussed later). The impact of this technique on survival compared with the standard approach of wide excision alone plus observation of the regional lymph node basin has yet to be proved and is the subject of an ongoing prospective randomized national trial.

In the absence of data from that trial, or in the absence of a need pathologically to stage a patient at risk for regional nodal metastases at the time of presentation, standard management of patients with primary localized melanoma should be wide excision and observation.

Therapeutic Lymph Node Dissection. In patients who present with clinically enlarged regional nodes in the setting of a concurrent or remote primary melanoma, in general, cytologic confirmation of the diagnosis of metastatic disease is recommended. Fine needle aspiration biopsy is an appropriate, minimally invasive, and reproducible procedure. If the node is inaccessible to needle biopsy, excisional biopsy is recommended prior to formal lymphadenectomy. Once the diagnosis of regional recurrence has been established, a thorough lymph node dissection of the affected nodal basin is recommended. Controversy exists as to what compromises a thorough and/or adequate lymph node dissection in all three anatomic subsites: neck, axilla, and groin.

Palliative Lymph Node Dissection. Even in the presence of established distant metastatic disease, regional lymphadenectomy may be indicated for clinical nodal metastases to achieve regional control, especially in patients with a reasonable life expectancy. Uncontrolled regional disease can be extremely debilitating and difficult to manage.

In Transit Metastasis. Of patients with recurrence following regional lymph node dissection, approximately 10% to 15% will recur with regional in transit metastases. If these metastases are solitary, the initial approach should be surgical excision, with the expectation of a high probability of further in transit metastases. If in transit metastases are multiple, dermal or subdermal, and less than 5.0 mm in diameter, injection therapy with dinitrochlorobenzene (DNCB) or CO_2 laser vaporization results in a high likelihood of resolution of treated lesions. For patients with in transit disease that is neither surgically resectable nor amenable to injection or CO_2 laser ablation, standard therapy involves hyperthermic isolation limb perfusion. The most commonly used drug in the perfusion circuit is phenylalanine mustard (melphalan [Alkeran]). This yields an overall response rate of approximately 80%, but only half of these responses are complete, and of the complete responses approximately half are durable. Reports of perfusion with melphalan combined with tumor necrosis factor have suggested a higher response rate. The long-term impact on overall survival of this potentially toxic combination, compared with melphalan alone, has not yet been shown in an ongoing prospective randomized trial.

Distant Metastatic Disease. Although patients who die with metastatic melanoma have metastases throughout all systems, patients who initially relapse following treatment of their primary melanoma usually do so with a solitary site, and of these solitary site recurrences, most of them are soft tissue or remote nodal recurrences, accessible to careful physical examination. In the absence of disseminated disease,

TABLE 2. **Suggested Surgical Margins for Primary Cutaneous Melanoma**

Thickness	Margin
In situ	0.5 cm
≤1 mm	1 cm
1–4 mm	2 cm
>4 mm	≥3 cm (?)

solitary nonvisceral or remote nodal metastases should be aggressively resected, with the expectation of long-term survival in approximately 20%. Solitary visceral metastases are much less common. Solitary pulmonary metastases may be resected, with the expectation of long-term cure in 5% to 20%. Metastases to the brain or gastrointestinal tract are usually not solitary, and resection in these sites is usually for palliation of identifiable symptoms.

Adjuvant Therapy. There has been a great deal of interest in the application of adjuvant immunotherapy to patients with metastatic melanoma to regional nodes, completely resected. One recent trial has suggested a small, but significant, improvement in both disease-free and overall survival after treatment with high-dose interferon in the adjuvant setting. The cost and toxicity of this treatment, however, are substantial, and these need to be weighed against the potential benefit. Other trials using lower-dose interferon, although showing less toxicity, have failed to show a survival benefit. Adjuvant chemotherapy has not proved effective in reducing the risk of relapse following surgical resection of metastatic melanoma. Adjuvant radiation therapy may be of benefit in highly selected patients at risk for regional recurrence, although this benefit has not been proved in prospective randomized trials.

Advanced Nonsurgically Resectable Metastatic Disease. Standard therapy for surgically unresectable advanced metastatic melanoma involves the use of single agent dacarbazine (DTIC). This is a relatively nontoxic regimen that can be administered on an outpatient basis with the expectation of a 10% to 20% response rate, depending on disease site. Combination chemotherapy with DTIC, carmustine (BCNU), cisplatin (Platinol), and tamoxifen (Nolvadex) has a reported response rate of up to 50%, at the expense of significantly increased toxicity. The impact of the more intensive regimen on survival when compared with the single agent DTIC has not yet been shown. A great deal of investigation is ongoing in the use of biologic therapy with interferon and interleukin, alone or in combination with chemotherapy. To date, none of these regimens has proved to be superior to the simpler regimens.

PROGNOSIS

The 5-year survival for patients with stage I localized melanoma is generally over 90%; for patients with stage II melanoma, the corresponding figure is 50% to 80%. Factors influencing the prognosis of patients with primary localized melanomas (stages I, II) include thickness, Clark level, anatomic site, patient gender and age, and, in some series, primary tumor ulceration. For stage III patients, approximately 30% to 40% of those undergoing complete surgical excision will be alive and free of disease in 5 years. Adjuvant immunotherapy with high-dose interferon may improve this figure slightly. In patients with stage IV melanoma, very few are cured with any therapeutic modality, and less than 5% can expect to be alive and free of disease in 5 years.

PREMALIGNANT SKIN LESIONS

method of
IRA DAVIS, M.D.
New York Medical College
Valhalla, New York

Premalignant lesions are lesions that have an increased likelihood of developing into a malignancy, but not all such lesions will do so. Observation and early treatment of premalignant lesions prevent the morbidity and mortality associated with their respective malignancies.

ACTINIC KERATOSIS

Actinic keratosis (AK), also called solar keratosis or senile keratosis, is the most common type of premalignant lesion. The rate of malignant transformation of these lesions is reported to range from 0.1 to 20%. The estimate that 1 per 1000 AK per year converts to squamous cell carcinoma is probably closer to the true rate of malignant transformation. Ten percent of AK may spontaneously remit.

AK develops on chronically sun-exposed skin. Fair-skinned persons who sunburn easily and tan poorly are most susceptible to developing AK. The prevalence of these lesions increases with age, and lesions are more commonly seen in patients with a history of excessive occupational or recreational sun exposure. However, younger patients may also have AK, and lesions may appear outside the classic sun-exposed areas. AK acts as a marker for patients who are at increased risk for skin cancer.

AK appears as a rough, scaly area that may be better noted by palpation than by inspection. Most patients have multiple lesions. Most commonly a red-brown to yellow color is noted. Lesions may vary in size from 1 to 2 mm to several centimeters in diameter. Although AK is usually asymptomatic, patients have reported associated pruritus, burning, or a splinter-like sensation.

AK can be diagnosed clinically. Biopsy is recommended for lesions in which a malignancy is suspected. Features that may predispose one to perform a biopsy include induration or a palpable dermal component, erosions, pain, and hyperkeratoses. Shave biopsy, including a portion of the dermis, is adequate to assess for the presence of malignancy. If melanoma is included in the differential diagnosis, an excisional biopsy should be chosen. If an excisional biopsy cannot be performed due to lesion size and anatomic constraints, an incisional biopsy may be done.

Multiple modalities are available for the treatment of AK, including chemical destruction, cryosurgery, curettage, electrosurgery, dermabrasion, laser, and combination therapies.

The most common type of chemical destruction is the use of 5-fluorouracil (5-FU [Efudex]) cream or solution. 5-FU is available in 1, 2, and 5% concentrations. Some clinicians prefer to use the 1 or 2% concentrations on the face and lips and the 5% concentration in other areas. The medication is used twice daily for 3 to 8 weeks. 5-FU is applied to the entire involved area in order to treat clinically inapparent lesions, which will become red and inflamed. Amelioration of the inflammatory response can be obtained with the use of a medium-strength topical corticosteroid. Some patients tend to stop the medication due to the irritation and inflammation before achieving an optimal response. Since sunlight can intensify the reaction, the treatment is reserved for the winter months. Topical tretinoin cream (Retin-A) has been used for pretreatment for 2 weeks and in conjunction with 5-FU. An alternative regimen using 5-FU twice a day on 1 day of each week for 6 to 9 weeks resulted in less patient discomfort and successful treatment of AK. A newer agent, 10% masoprocol cream (Actinex), is used twice a day for 4 weeks. Approximately 20% of patients have discontinued this drug due to local adverse effects (erythema, itching, flaking, burning, edema, and soreness).

Liquid nitrogen cryotherapy remains the mainstay of office treatment of AK. Individual lesions are treated with liquid nitrogen in a spray or on a dipped cotton swab for a total of 5 to 15 seconds. Overtreatment may result in hypopigmentation. A blister may form after treatment; this should not be removed, but the fluid may be drained. Crusted areas should be treated with a topical antibiotic (bacitracin or polymyxin B sulfate and bacitracin zinc [Polysporin]) two to three times daily until healed. Recently, medium-depth chemical peel with Jessner's solution and 35% trichloroacetic acid has been advocated as an alternative. The technique was preferred by patients over topical 5-FU for widespread AK in a recent study.

Other acceptable treatments include sharp curettage followed by electrodesiccation, and dermabrasion. Continuous-wave or superpulsed carbon dioxide laser is a useful alternative for the treatment of actinic cheilitis, diffuse AK of the lip.

Prevention of AK should be part of any treatment plan. This begins with adequate sun protection beginning in childhood. The threefold strategy consists of avoiding the sun from 10 A.M. to 3 P.M., wearing adequate sun-protective clothes, and using a sunscreen with a sun protection factor (SPF) of 15. Daily use of a high-SPF sunscreen reduces the number of lesions that develop.

BOWEN'S DISEASE

Bowen's disease (BD), or squamous cell carcinoma in situ, is a full-thickness intraepidermal neoplasm that manifests as a scaly, well-defined erythematous raised lesion (plaque). BD should be suspected in lesions that do not respond to topical corticosteroid therapy. A shave biopsy with some underlying dermis is needed to rule out squamous cell carcinoma. If left untreated, at least 5% of lesions progress to squamous cell carcinoma. BD is most common in sun-exposed skin in elderly patients. BD in non–sun-exposed skin may indicate prior exposure to inorganic arsenic from contaminated well water, agricultural products (insecticides, fungicides, herbicides, and defoliants), or medicaments (e.g., Fowler's solution and asiatic pill). BD related to arsenic exposure may be associated with an increased risk of internal malignancy. Erythroplasia of Queyrat is Bowen's disease of the penis. It occurs almost exclusively in uncircumcised males.

Treatment of BD includes excision, cryotherapy, curettage and electrodesiccation, 5-FU, radiotherapy, carbon dioxide laser surgery, and Mohs' micrographic surgery. Surgical excision allows for histologic confirmation that the lesion has been completely removed. Mohs' micrographic surgery should be reserved for extensive lesions in which preservation of tissue is paramount.

BOWENOID PAPULOSIS

Bowenoid papulosis (BP) lesions appear as multiple red, violaceous, or hyperpigmented papules in the genital area of young adults, usually during the third of fourth decade of life. Clinically, these lesions resemble warts. Histologic examination exhibits the features of squamous cell carcinoma in situ. These lesions rarely develop into invasive squamous cell carcinoma. Human papillomavirus types 16, 18, and 31 are most commonly found in BP lesions. An increase in cervical dysplasia may be seen in females with BP and in partners of males with BP.

Conservative ablative therapies are utilized in the treatment of these lesions. Although medical treatments such as trichloroacetic acid (Tri-Chlor), podophyllin (podophyllum resin [Podofin, Podocon-25]), or podofilox (Condylox) can be utilized, lesions may be resistant. Therefore, curettage and electrodesiccation, cryotherapy, excisional surgery, or carbon dioxide laser ablation is preferred.

MELANOCYTIC LESIONS

Atypical Nevi

The incidence of melanoma is increasing faster than that of any other cancer. The estimated lifetime risk for the general U.S. population is 1%. In contrast, patients with atypical nevi without a personal or family history of melanoma have a 6% 25-year risk of developing melanoma. This percentage increases to 50% for those patients with atypical moles who have more than one family member with melanoma.

Atypical moles show some or all of the features used to differentiate malignant melanoma from banal nevi. These features, known as the ABCD's, consist of asymmetry, border irregularity, color variation, and diameter greater than 6 mm. Atypical nevi are frequently found in covered areas of the body, such as the back, and in unusual locations (e.g., buttocks, breast, scalp). Although histologic criteria have been proposed for atypical nevi, lesions that are clinically atypical may not be histologically atypical.

Multiple syndromes have been described, with varying criteria based on family history of melanoma and presence of atypical moles or many nevi. The tenet of utmost importance is to realize that there is a spectrum of increased risk—from patients who have several atypical moles or many normal moles to those patients with atypical moles and a personal and/or family history of melanoma.

Controversy exists about whether most of these patients develop melanoma adjacent to atypical moles. Although these nevi may not be true premalignant lesions, they are markers for patients at increased risk for developing melanoma.

Management of patients includes physician examination, self-examination, and sun-avoidance strategies. Patients should be examined every 3 to 12 months. Those patients with only a few atypical moles and no family or personal history of melanoma need to be examined annually. A handheld hair dryer is useful for examining the scalp. Lesions suspicious for melanoma should be excised. Patients should begin to be screened at puberty. Regular ophthalmic examinations are needed. Total cutaneous photographs may be helpful in detecting the presence of new moles and changes in pre-existing lesions. Patients should be educated in self-examination of the skin and should do so every 2 to 3 months. Sun-avoidance or protection strategies as discussed for AK should be instituted. Special clothing made by Sun Precautions offers better protection than conventional clothes. Blood relatives should be screened for atypical moles and malignant melanoma.

Large Congenital Nevi

Large (or giant) congenital nevi are those that measure 20 cm or more in largest diameter. It is important to note that lesions less than 20 cm in infancy will increase in size during the child's development. Risk for the development of malignant melanoma ranges from 3.8 to 18%. Seventy percent of these melanomas are diagnosed before puberty. Only patients with xeroderma pigmentosum and those with atypical moles with a personal and/or family history of melanoma have a higher relative risk of developing melanoma.

Although efforts are made to remove as much of the large congenital nevus as surgically feasible, melanomas can develop in extracutaneous sites. In addition, melanoma may develop in sites where the nevi were not completely removed. Therefore, patients should be examined regularly for the development of cutaneous and extracutaneous melanoma. Some physicians propose magnetic resonance imaging with gadolinium contrast of the central nervous system to assess for neurocutaneous melanosis, since these patients have a poorer prognosis and extensive cutaneous surgery may not be indicated.

Small Congenital Nevi

Small congenital nevi are defined as lesions less than 1.5 cm in diameter. Controversy exists about whether patients with these lesions have an increased risk for developing melanoma. Clinicians differ in their recommendations regarding removal of these lesions. In any event, the risk for prepubertal development of melanoma is low, and those who advocate excision of these lesions generally wait until the patient reaches adolescence.

Management of medium-sized congenital lesions is similar to that for small congenital nevi.

Lentigo Maligna

Lentigo maligna is melanoma in situ involving sun-exposed areas. These lesions should be treated with surgical excision with a 5-mm margin or Mohs' micrographic surgery. Radiation may be an alternative treatment in patients with extensive lesions or those who cannot undergo extensive surgery.

PREMALIGNANT CONDITIONS

Some conditions are associated with an increased likelihood of developing skin cancer, including genodermatoses, immune suppression, and chronic radiodermatitis.

Genodermatoses associated with malignant neoplasms include albinism, xeroderma pigmentosum, nevoid basal cell carcinoma syndrome, and epidermodysplasia verruciformis.

Immune suppression, as occurs in organ transplant recipients and patients with underlying malignancies and human retroviral infection, increases the likelihood of developing skin neoplasms.

Patients treated with ionizing radiation are at increased risk of developing basal cell and squamous cell carcinoma, as well as melanoma, in the irradiated fields.

Chronic ulcerations as well as changes in burn scars should alert the clinician to the possible development of a malignancy at the site.

GENERAL CONSIDERATIONS

Patients with premalignant lesions or conditions should be examined on a regular basis at least every 6 to 12 months. These patients should be instructed to contact their physicians if they note persistence or recurrence of treated lesions or a change in an existing lesion. Close follow-up and early intervention minimize the treatment morbidity of premalignant lesions and allow for early detection of any associated malignancies.

BACTERIAL DISEASES OF THE SKIN

method of
NEIL S. SADICK, M.D.
Cornell University Medical College
New York, New York

Bacterial skin infection is the single most common diagnosis among patients with skin problems, accounting for 17% of clinic visits.

IMPETIGO

Impetigo is a highly communicable infection. It is predominantly noted in preschool-age children. The two classic forms of impetigo are nonbullous and bullous. Nonbullous impetigo accounts for more than 70% of cases. Lesions of nonbullous impetigo typically begin on the traumatized skin of the face or extremities. Intact skin is resistant to impetiginization. Chickenpox, arthropod reactions, abrasions, lacerations, and burns are common predisposing factors. Peak seasonal occurrence is in late summer and early fall.

Bullous impetigo presents as rapidly spreading flaccid bullae that may cover extensive areas of the torso. A tiny vesicle or pustule forms initially and rapidly develops a honey-colored crusted plaque that is most often less than 2 cm in diameter. The lesions dry, leaving fine crusts, and the intraepidermal nature of these lesions means no residual scarring. Nursery epidemics are most common. Lesions are usually minimally symptomatic with little pain and minimal surrounding erythema, although pruritus may occasionally be noted. Regional lymphadenopathy is found in 90% of cases, and leukocytosis is present in approximately 50% of patients. Without treatment, lesions may progress slowly for several weeks and occasionally may form a chronic ulcer, but in most cases spontaneous resolution without scarring occurs within approximately 2 weeks.

Crowding, poor hygiene, contact sports, and neglected minor skin trauma contribute to interfamily spread. Impetigo may also complicate other skin diseases such as scabies, varicella, and atopic dermatitis. Group A streptococcus has been the most common isolate from nonbullous impetigo in the United States; however, the bacteriologic spectrum of the disease is changing, with an increasing role for *Staphylococcus aureus*.

Bullous impetigo is primarily caused by group II *Staphylococcus aureus*, usually phage type 71. Mixtures of streptococcus 1 and *S. aureus* have been isolated in about 50% of patients with nonbullous impetigo; however, the pathogenic role of *S. aureus* in this setting is unclear. Finally, nongroup A (groups B, C, and G) streptococci may be responsible for rare cases of impetigo, and group B streptococci are associated with impetigo in the neonate. Group A streptococcal impetigo is rarely noted before age 2 years.

Ecthyma is a subtype of impetigo that extends more deeply and produces a shallow ulcer that heals with scarring. Lesions having a similar clinical appearance may be produced in the setting of *Pseudomonas* septicemia.

Ultimately, Gram stain and appropriate cultures help differentiate the specific bacterial pathogen. Histopathology reveals a subcorneal acantholytic blister with a mixed inflammatory infiltrate of the superficial dermal plexus. Anti-DNAase B is the test of choice for detecting preceding streptococcal infection of the skin.

Potential complications noted after nonbullous or bullous impetigo include osteomyelitis, septic arthritis, pneumonia, septicemia, and glomerulonephritis. Positive blood cultures are rare but are more common with skin than with respiratory infection with group A beta-hemolytic streptococcus (GABHS). Cellulitis has been reported in 10% of patients with nonbullous impetigo but rarely follows the bullous form. Lymphangitis, suppurative lymphadenitis, guttate psoriasis, and scarlet fever may follow streptococcal impetigo occasionally. Infection with nephritogenic strains of GABHS may result in acute poststreptococcal glomerulonephritis (APSGN). Impetigo-related nephritogenic strains are commonly M groups 2, 49, 53, 55, 56, 57, and 60. A latent period of 18 to 21 days from cutaneous infection to the development of glomerulonephritis has been noted, versus 10 days after pharyngitis. Treatment of nonbullous impetigo probably does not alter the incidence of development of glomerulonephritis but may be helpful in limiting epidemic spread.

Treatment

The treatment includes appropriate therapy against the associated pathogens as well as improvement of environmental factors and associated disease states (poor hygiene, crowding, atopic dermatitis, and so on). The latter should include crust débridement. This may be accomplished with mesh gauze sponge (type VIII) soaked in an antibacterial soap such as Lever 2000, chlorhexidine (Hibiclens), or povidone-iodine (Betadine). Pain from this maneuver may be lessened by utilizing a nontoxic surfactant like poloxamer 188 (Shur-Clens), or an antibacterial soak such as anhydrous aluminum acetate 5% (Domeboro's solution). Avoidance of crowded living conditions and the utilization of separate cleansing devices may also be helpful.

In localized disease, topical mupirocin ointment (Bactroban) is the treatment of choice. It is applied three times daily until clinical clearing. It has been shown to be as effective as oral erythromycin in the treatment of localized impetigo. It has not been shown to be as effective in treating the scalp and mouth areas. Widespread impetigo or ecthyma requires treatment with a beta-lactamase–resistant oral antibiotic. In areas with low prevalence of *S. aureus* erythromycin resistance, erythromycin ethyl succinate or erythromycin estolate are acceptable oral therapies. If there is widespread erythromycin resistance in the community, alternative antibiotics that have been shown to be more than 85% effective in children for treatment of impetigo include cloxacillin (Tegopen), amoxicillin plus clavulanic acid (Augmentin), clindamycin (Cleocin), or a cephalosporin such as cephalexin (Keflex), cefaclor (Ceclor), cefadroxil (Duricef, Ultracef), cefprozil (Cefzil), or cefpodoxime (Vantin). The choice among these various agents may be guided primarily by issues of cost, local availability, and compliance (Table 1).

Clarithromycin (Biaxin) may be advantageous primarily in cases of intolerance to erythromycin, but it does not produce cure rates superior to those of erythromycin in areas with high rates of *S. aureus* resistance to erythromycin.

Bullous impetigo produced by exfoliative toxin-producing *S. aureus* may require intravenous administration of a beta-lactamase–resistant penicillin such as oxacillin (Bactocill, Prostaphlin) or nafcillin (Nafcil, Unipen).

There is little evidence to suggest that a 10-day course of therapy is superior to a 7-day course. If a satisfactory clinical response is not achieved within 7 days, a repeat culture should be made; if a resistant organism is detected, an appropriate antibiotic should be given for an additional 7 days.

CELLULITIS/ERYSIPELAS

Cellulitis is an acute, spreading inflammation of the skin involving the deeper subcutaneous tissues. Erysipelas is a characteristic type of superficial cellulitis in which an edematous, brawny, infiltrated, sharply demarcated plaque develops and spreads peripherally. The lesions are usually hot and red, with distinct borders. The face and scalp are sites of predilection, followed by the hands and genitalia. A history of an antecedent process, such as tinea pedis, stasis ulcer, or a puncture wound, is often obtained. Within a day or two, brawny erythema and tenderness may follow, associated with malaise, fever, and chills. Erysipelas may be predated by puncture

injuries, ulcers, and fissures secondary to chronic eczematoid dermatitis. Both conditions occur with increased frequency in states that invite colonization by group A streptococci and *S. aureus,* which are the commonest etiologic agents. These include burns, diabetes, and malnutrition. Occasionally other organisms are implicated, such as *Haemophilus influenzae* type B, producing facial cellulitis in children, group B streptococci in neonates, and pneumococcal cellulitis in patients with underlying diabetes mellitus or other immunosuppressive states. *Staphylococcus epidermidis* as a pathogenic agent of cellulitis is also being recognized with increasing frequency.

After development of the initial inflammatory skin lesions, tender regional lymphadenopathy may occur. Superficial pustules and vesicles may occur, which may lead to localized exfoliation, particularly in the case of *S. aureus* as a pathogen. Finally, local abscesses may develop with necrosis of underlying skin. Gangrene may occur in the most severe cases, usually indicating the presence of a mixed bacterial infection.

The etiology of bacterial cellulitis may be determined by fine needle aspiration with Gram stain plus cultures. An associated polymorphonuclear leukocytosis is commonly present.

Because of their tendency to spread via the lymphatics and bloodstream, cellulitis and erysipelas may lead to septicemia if left untreated. Other complicating sequelae include thrombophlebitis or superinfection with gram-negative organisms.

Erysipelas must be distinguished from allergic contact dermatitis; erysipeloid, which occurs most commonly on the hands and fingers; or an "erysipeloid carcinoma" of the breast.

Treatment

Attacks of cellulitis and erysipelas may be quickly suppressed by appropriate antimicrobial therapy. Gram stain and culture sensitivity determinations remain the cornerstone of choosing the appropriate antibiotic. Cellulitis occurring secondary to group A streptococci is usually treated with penicillin G, 1 to 2 million units intravenously every 2 to 3 hours. Patients who are penicillin-allergic may be treated with a cephalosporin agent such as cefazolin (Ancef, Kefzol), 75 to 80 mg per kg of body weight per day, given intravenously in four divided doses. Vancomycin (Vancocin) may be administered as an alternative agent when cross-reactivity between penicillin and cephalosporin is of concern. If *Haemophilus influenzae* infection is suspected, then ampicillin, 200 to 250 mg per kg of body weight per day should be administered in six divided doses. With recent emergence of beta-lactamase–producing ampicillin-resistant strains, a cephalosporin (cefuroxime or cefotaxime) may be chosen. An alternative in the penicillin-allergic patient is trimethoprim/sulfamethoxazole (Bactrim, Septra). When Gram stain reveals gram-positive and gram-negative organisms, a combination of an aminoglycoside, cephalosporin, and clinda-

TABLE 1. **Cost of Antibiotics for Treatment of Impetigo**

	Dose (mg/kg/d)	Dosing Interval	Cost ($)
Amoxicillin/clavulanate (Augmentin)	20	tid	29.50
Cefaclor (Ceclor)	20	tid	31.05
Cefadroxil (Duricef)	30	bid	24.95
Cephalexin (Keflex)	40	tid	19.75
Cefpodoxime (Vantin)	10	bid	58.95
Cefprozil (Cefzil)	20	qd or bid	35.35
Clarithromycin (Biaxin)	15	bid	24.30
Clindamycin (Cleocin)	15	tid or qid	28.45
Dicloxacillin (Dynapen)	30	qid	25.95
Erythromycin estolate (Ilosone)	30	tid or qid	10.25
Erythromycin ethylsuccinate (EES)	40	tid or qid	15.40
Mupirocin (Bactroban)	15-gm tube	tid	18.25

mycin (Cleocin), may be utilized. Alternatively, imipenim-cilastatin (Primaxin), may be used as a single agent. In the case of penicillin allergy, vancomycin may be used with an aminoglycoside and clindamycin.

Mild erysipelas or cellulitis without systemic symptoms may be treated with oxacillin, 0.5 to 1.0 gram orally four times daily, or with erythromycin, 0.25 to 0.5 gram orally four times daily in penicillin-allergic patients. The newer macrolides clarithromycin (Biaxin) or azithromycin (Zithromax) may be chosen as therapeutic alternatives.

Care of the local lesions of erysipelas and cellulitis includes immobilization and elevation of the involved area in order to diminish local edema. Cool sterile saline or anhydrous aluminum acetate 5% (Domeboro's solution) wet-to-dry compresses may diminish pain and help dry up bullous and crusted lesions. In addition, moist heat may aid in localization of cellulitis. Drainage may be performed locally for areas of abscess formation, whereas extensive débridement and grafting may be required for necrotic areas of streptococcal gangrene.

FOLLICULITIS

Folliculitis is a pyoderma that originates within the hair follicle. These infections are most commonly divided into superficial and deep subdivisions. Usually infection is initiated by coagulase-positive staphylococcus; however, when host resistance is impaired, other organisms such as gram-negatives and saprophytic flora such as micrococci and *Pityrosporum* organisms may be causative.

Superficial folliculitis, also known as Bockhart's impetigo, is a superficial form of impetigo characterized by dome-shaped pustules situated at the ostia of the pilosebaceous unit. Rupture of the pustule may lead to crust formation. The scalp, beard, and extremities are the sites of predilection, with the former more common in children. Maceration and poor hygiene are precipitating factors.

Gram-negative folliculitis may occur as a superinfection of patients with acne vulgaris treated with antibiotic therapy. *Klebsiella, Enterobacter,* and *Proteus* species are the most common organisms. Pustular lesions commonly aggregate around the nose. Another form of superficial gram-negative folliculitis is "hot tub folliculitis" due to *Pseudomonas aeruginosa.* It begins 6 hours to 5 days after hot tub exposure. Pustulovesicular lesions on an erythematous base involving the trunk, buttocks, legs, and arms are characteristic. Organisms are readily cultured from pustules and infected water.

Infection in the deep aspects of the hair follicle may lead to several forms of deep-seated folliculitis. A furuncle either complicates a preceding folliculitis or develops as a deep-seated nodule around a hair follicle. Its deep location and containment by thickened dermis prevent surface drainage and contribute to the hard, nodular, painful characteristics of this lesion. Rupture may follow, with discharge of a core of necrotic tissue. Keratin plugs filling dilated follicular infundibula are characteristic features of furuncles. Furunculosis may be chronic and recurrent. Chronic carriers of *S. aureus* are especially prone to this process. The preferred sites are those that are unusually hairy or that are exposed to friction and maceration, such as the buttocks, neck, face, axillae, and areas underlying the belt.

Carbuncles are larger, more degenerated extensions of hair follicle infection, with spreading of the infective process under and in between fibrous tissue septa, forming a series of interconnected abscesses. Damage may occur on the skin through a number of necrotic points.

Furuncles may complicate secondarily infected dermatoses such as pediculosis, scabies, and excoriated dermatitis. Athletes who are exposed to excessive friction and perspiration are also highly susceptible. Systemic host factors that lower resistance also predispose individuals to these processes. These factors include diabetes, obesity, hematologic disorders, cachexia, malnutrition, immunoglobulin deficiency states, and long-term treatment with corticosteroids and cytotoxic agents.

Other less common deep-seated hair follicle infections include sycosis barbae (barber's itch), which commonly presents as deep-seated follicular nodules in the bearded areas of the face. If this condition is left untreated, a chronic cicatricial folliculitis called lupoid sycosis may ensue. Acne keloid is a chronic hypertrophic deep-seated folliculitis of the posterior neck and occipital scalp of young black men. Follicular papules coalesce into firm plaques and nodules that may be associated with scarring alopecia.

S. aureus is the common pathogen in all cases of hair follicle infection. Folliculitis around the lips and nose may spread retrograde, leading to cavernous sinus thrombosis.

Treatment

The emphasis in treating hair follicle infections is to find and treat any predisposing factors that may play a role in its etiologic development.

Semisynthetic penicillins are the drugs of choice and should be given parenterally in every case of carbuncles as well as in severe cases of furunculosis. Beta-lactamase–resistant antibiotics such as cloxacillin (Tegopen) or cephalosporins such as cefazolin (Ancef, Kefzol) are commonly employed. Hair plucking is contraindicated. Shaving should be performed with disposable razors. Antibacterial soap such as Lever 2000 or a chlorhexidine wash (Hibiclens) are commonly employed in daily usage. Hygroscopic powders such as Zeasorb may be helpful in minimizing excessive sweating in athletes.

Warm soaks are helpful. Squeezing or too early incision of furuncles may actually be harmful. Lesions should be allowed to "point," then be gently nicked with a No. 11 blade and drainage established. Antibiotic ointments such as mupirocin (Bactroban) may be applied after compressing, although the only effect may be in preventing new skin lesions. Deeper incision, particularly of the cruciate type, that was formerly recommended in the management of carbuncles may actually be harmful because it breaches the dike of reaction that has been built upon the site of infection. Areas of involvement of acne keloid may also be treated with intralesional injections of corticosteroids (triamcinolone diacetonide [Kenalog], 5 mg per mL intralesionally) or scarred regions of involvement may be surgically excised or vaporized and left to heal secondarily utilizing the carbon dioxide or ultrapulsed carbon dioxide laser.

PARONYCHIA

Paronychia is inflammation involving the folds of tissue surrounding the nail, which serves as excellent potential spaces for the development of infection. When caused by bacteria, it is often referred to as "pyonychia." Although streptococcal species and *S. aureus* are the most common pathogens, infection with *Candida* species and other bacteria such as *Pseudomonas* may also play a role, particularly in chronic infections. Painful erythema and localized swelling are the most common presentations. Purulent discharge may be noted, and chronic infection of the nail matrix may lead to deformity of the nail plate.

Predisposing factors include direct injury, hangnails, water immersion, caustic chemicals, and overzealous manicures.

Diagnostic and therapeutic interventions are best made by aspiration and subsequent Gram stain and culture techniques. Subungual abscesses are the major complications of bacterial paronychia. Bright light transillumination is helpful in detecting such occult abscesses. Co-infection with pyogenic bacteria and *Candida* species is common and in this setting, treatment must be directed toward both organisms.

Treatment

Acute bacterial paronychia due to staphylococci or streptococci species is treated by hot bland soaks with anhydrous aluminum acetate 5% (Domeboro's) soaks or 0.25% acetic acid compresses plus systemic antibiotic therapy. Dicloxacillin (Dynapen) orally, 1 to 2 grams per day; cephalexin (Cefanex, Keftab, Keflex) orally, 1 to 2 grams per day; cefadroxil (Duricef, Ultracef) orally, 1 gram per day; or erythromycin (ERYC, Ery-Tab, E-Mycin) orally, 1 to 2 grams for 7 to 10 days in penicillin-allergic patients are excellent choices. Other organisms are treated as indicated by culture sensitivities. Drainage is also a cornerstone of therapy, as the posterior nail fold must be freed from the underlying nail plate. Chronic cases may require long-term systemic antibiotic therapy or partial matrectomies in cases of recurrent paronychia secondary to recurrent ingrown nails.

LYMPHANGITIS

Acute lymphangitis is an infection involving the subcutaneous lymphatic channels. Group A streptococci are most commonly the pathogen responsible, although rarely other organisms such as *S. aureus* and *Pasteurella multocida* may be responsible. Common predisposing factors include puncture wounds on an extremity, infected blisters, or paronychia. Systemic symptoms or pain may predate the development of clinical erythema. Unusual infections leading to lymphangitis include interdigital web space infection of the hands or feet. Infections in the hands in particular can bypass elbow nodes and drain into axillary or subpectoral nodes and pleural lymphatics, leading to subpectoral abscesses and pleural effusions.

Red linear streaks extending from involved lesions to draining lymph nodes are characteristic. Usually tenderness is present. In late stages, skin breakdown with subsequent ulceration may occur if left untreated. Fever and leukocytosis are often accompanying manifestations. In cases refractory to conventional therapy, lymph node aspiration with appropriate culture and Gram stain techniques may be necessary.

Treatment

Parenteral antibiotic therapy with warm tepid soaks every 1 to 4 hours and immobilization and elevation of the affected extremity are the cornerstones of therapy. Lymphangitis secondary to *Streptococcus pyogenes* is treated with penicillin G, 1 to 2 million units intravenously every 2 to 3 hours. Penicillin-allergic patients may be treated with cefazolin (Ancef, Kefzol), 75 to 80 mg per kg of body weight per day, given intravenously in four divided doses. Vancomycin (Vancocin), 500 mg intravenously every 6 hours or 1 gram every 12 hours or clindamycin (Cleocin), 600 to 1200 mg per day in two, three, or four equal doses are alternative agents in select settings when primary therapeutic choices are contraindicated because of patient allergy or the culture sensitivity pattern.

NECROTIZING FASCIITIS

Necrotizing soft tissue infections (NSTIs) differ from other versions of cellulitis because of the associated tissue necrosis and lack of response to antimicrobial treatment alone, requiring surgical débridement of devitalized tissues. NSTIs are divided into three categories based on their depth of involvement: necrotizing cellulitis, necrotizing fasciitis (NF), and myonecrosis (Table 2). Because fascial necrosis can be determined only by surgical exploration of the identified site and confirmed by histologic examination, NSTIs cannot be diagnosed accurately on clinical findings alone. Rather, NF is a progression of necrotizing cellulitis, involvement of fascia (necrotizing fasciitis), or primary infection of muscle after trauma as an extension of NF to muscle—myonecrosis.

Middle-aged to older patients are more likely to develop NF, although cases have been reported in

TABLE 2. **Classification of Necrotizing Soft Tissue Infections**

Infection Type	Predisposing Factors	Onset: Progression	Clinical Findings	Systemic Toxicity	Bacteriology	Pathologic Findings	Tissue Involvement
Cellulitis							
Streptococcal necrotizing cellulitis	Usually arises in an epithelial break site, traumatic or surgical; GBS patients often elderly but otherwise healthy	Rapid; may progress to NF if not treated	Fever; overlying skin becomes dusky blue ± bullae; may progress to necrosis of tissue; initially very painful; gangrenous areas become anesthetic	Severe	Usually GAS, occasionally GBS, in wound ± blood	Vasculitis, fibrin thrombi, necrosis of epidermis and dermis; heavy infiltrate of neutrophils; gram-positive cocci	Skin through fascia
Synergistic necrotizing cellulitis	Diabetes, perineal involvement, peripheral vascular disease, renal disease, may extend to involve fascia and muscle	Days; rapid	"Dishwater" pus or edema, crepitus, fever, blebs, necrosis; begins as an ulcer that gradually enlarges	Severe	Microaerophilic or anaerobic streptococci from edematous margin; *Staphylococcus aureus* from central ulcer	Dense leukocytic infiltration and edema of dermis and superficial muscle	Skin through muscle
Pseudomonas aeruginosa cellulitis and ecthyma gangrenosum	Neutropenia	Days; severe	Cellulitis with central necrosis in axillae or anogenital regions; fever, sepsis	Moderate to severe	*P. aeruginosa*	Cellulitis with vasculitis	Subcutaneous tissues
Vibrio vulnificus cellulitis	Diabetes, alcoholism cirrhosis; ingestion of raw seafood; trauma in aquatic environment	Days; severe	Fever, blebs, edema, pain	Moderate to severe	*V. vulnificus* and other species	Neutrophilic cellulitis and fasciitis	Skin through muscle
Aeromonas hydrophila cellulitis	Trauma; most patients are immunocompetent; 80% of patients are male	Days; severe	Cellulitis, NF, or myonecrosis	Mild to severe	*A. hydrophila* may be polymicrobial	Neutrophilic cellulitis and fasciitis	Skin through muscle
Clostridial cellulitis	Trauma	3–5 d; moderate	Fever, crepitus, blebs, red-brown fluid, edema, extreme wound pain	Mild	*Clostridium,* mixed gram-positive and -negative organisms	Dense leukocytic dermal infiltrate with necrosis of vessels and sweat glands	Subcutaneous tissues
Mucormycosis (zygomycosis phycomycosis)	Diabetes with ketoacidosis; traumatic to soft tissue; immuno-compromised	Days; moderate to severe	May occur as primary cutaneous infection at site of injury or extension from deeper focus to overlying skin	Mild to severe	Mucoraceae	Large, branched, nonseptate hyphae invading blood vessel walls	Soft tissues ± deeper structures
Fasciitis							
Necrotizing	Diabetes, traumatic, peripheral vascular disease, decubitus ulcer, abdominal surgery, perirectal abscess, intestinal perforation, alcoholism, parenteral drug use	Hours, days; rapid	Red-purple color, blebs, edema, hypoesthesias, fever. Sites: lower extremities, abdominal wall, perineum, operative wounds ± Crepitus	Moderate to severe	GAS or GBS; mixed infection with at least one facultative anaerobe; gram-positive cocci ± gram-negative bacilli	Intense leukocytic infiltration, focal necrosis of fascia, thrombosis of microvasculature	Skin through muscle
Myonecrosis							
Clostridial myonecrosis	Trauma, wound contamination	Hours, days; rapid	"Bronze" erysipelas, sweet odor, fever, crepitus, necrosis, tan color	Severe	*Clostridium,* mixed gram-positive and -negative organisms	Dense leukocytic dermal infiltrate with hyaline necrosis of muscle and gas formation	Muscle to skin

Abbreviations: GAS = group A streptococcus; GBS = group B streptococcus; NF = necrotizing fasciitis.

neonates. NF can be caused by a single microorganism, such as group A streptococcus, *Vibrio* species, or Zygomycetes; however, the majority of cases are caused by polymicrobial infections with synergistic facultative aerobic (*Streptococcus* or *Enterobacter* species) and anaerobic (*Bacteroides* and *Peptostreptococcus*) gas-forming organisms.

Early cutaneous signs of bacterial NF include local erythema, marked edema, and moderate tenderness. Later, gangrenous skin changes evolve and a fasciitis spreads rapidly beyond the border of cutaneous necrosis. As a consequence of cutaneous nerve necrosis, local tenderness is replaced by anesthesia. Synergistic polymicrobial NF is marked by a characteristic "dishwater pus" and toxicity out of proportion to the skin changes, with or without crepitation. In order of decreasing frequency of anatomic sites involved, NF arises on the extremities, trunk, perineum, and head and neck. On the extremities, the most common predisposing conditions are trauma, drug injections, and burns. In the head and neck area, odontogenic infections and traumatic injuries are predisposing factors.

Regional variants of NF include Fournier's gangrene—necrotizing fasciitis of the penis with or without perineal involvement.

Early, deep incisional lesional biopsy and histopathologic examinations on frozen sections have been shown to improve mortality in NF by expediting treatment. For more rapid diagnosis, bacteriologic evaluation of wound exudate, bulla fluid, excised tissue, needle soft tissue aspirates, and blood is essential. The mortality rate for NF has been reported to be 39%. Early diagnosis and aggressive treatment are the most important factors in determining outcome. Risk factors that negatively affect outcome include age of more than 50 years, diabetes mellitus, malnutrition, hypertension, and intravenous drug abuse. Death is usually due to sepsis, multisystem organ failure, or invasion of major vessels.

Treatment

The main modality of treatment of NSTIs includes early and complete surgical débridement of necrotic tissue in combination with high-dose antibiotics. The accepted approach is broad coverage until cultures identify causative pathogens. Vancomycin (Vancocin), 500 mg intravenously every 6 hours or 1 gram every 12 hours, may be chosen. In addition, gentamicin sulfate (Garamycin) intravenously, 3 mg per kg per day in three divided doses, may be initiated. Metronidazole hydrochloride (Flagyl), loading dosage of 15 mg per kg infused over 1 hour followed by 7.5 mg per kg infused over 1 hour every 6 hours; and clindamycin (Cleocin), 600 to 1200 mg per day in two, three, or four equal divided doses, are part of the broad-spectrum coverage that may be employed as well. Although clostridia are susceptible to penicillin, clindamycin, and chloramphenicol, optimal treatment has not been established. High-dose penicillin G potassium (Pfizerpen), 10 million units per day in four divided doses, either alone or in combination with clindamycin (see aforementioned dosage schedule), or chloramphenicol (Chloromycetin) intravenously, 50 mg per kg per day in divided doses at 6-hour intervals, may be adequate.

Although prospective studies are lacking, retrospective data indicate that adjunctive hyperbaric oxygen therapy may reduce morbidity and mortality in both clostridial and nonclostridial necrotizing infections. Other important adjuvant maneuvers in these critically ill patients include nutritional support, fecal diversion, and surgical drains when serosa-lined cavities are involved. As a rule, débridement defects are not repaired primarily but rather should be allowed to heal by secondary intention or delayed closure. Plastic surgery is often necessary for correction of functional or cosmetic defects.

VIRAL DISEASES OF THE SKIN

method of
ELEN CASSO DONAHUE, M.D., and
RICHARD L. SPIELVOGEL, M.D.
Medical College of Pennsylvania and
* Hahnemann University*
Philadelphia, Pennsylvania

HERPESVIRUS

The Herpesviridae family is a ubiquitous group of large DNA viruses that includes herpes simplex virus type 1 (HSV-1), herpes simplex virus type 2 (HSV-2), varicella-zoster virus (VZV), Epstein-Barr virus (EBV), cytomegalovirus (CMV), and human herpesvirus type 6 (HHV-6).

Herpes Simplex Virus

Herpes simplex infections are caused by Herpesvirus hominis, which has two antigenic subtypes. Type 1 (HSV-1) is the most frequent cause of herpes labialis, whereas type 2 (HSV-2) is traditionally associated with genital herpes. However, HSV-1 is the cause of genital herpes in 15% to 30% of cases, and HSV-2 has been increasingly associated with orofacial disease.

Infections with HSV have two distinct phases, referred to as primary and recurrent. Primary infection is acquired by a direct exposure to the virus through mucocutaneous contact with an infected individual. This transmission may occur from active lesions or during periods of asymptomatic viral shedding. Following this initial infection, the virus travels to a sensory nerve ganglion where it becomes latent. Reactivation of the virus then elicits recurrent episodes of the disease.

Clinical Manifestations of Primary Infection

Primary infection with herpes simplex virus may be asymptomatic, mild, or severe. Primary orofacial HSV infection most commonly occurs in children and frequently goes unnoticed. However, the most common symptomatic presentation is gingivostomatitis, characterized by widespread painful vesicles and ulcers on an erythematous base on the oral mucosa, tongue, palate, gingiva, and lips. This is often accompanied by high fever, lymphadenopathy, and malaise. Symptoms usually begin 5 to 10 days after exposure and resolve in 1 to 2 weeks.

Primary genital herpes occurs approximately 3 to 14 days after a sexual exposure in 95% of cases. The eruption is characterized by small grouped vesicles that may evolve into pustules, erosions, or ulcerations, which eventually become crusted. In women, lesions typically occur on the labia majora or minora, perineum, perianal area, or vaginal or cervical mucosa. In men, the penile shaft, glans, urethra, and scrotum are often involved. Fever, malaise, regional lymphadenopathy, pain, pruritus, dysuria, and vaginal or urethral discharge are commonly present. Lesions may remain for 2 to 4 weeks, with approximately 11 days of viral shedding that spans from the onset of symptoms to the crusting over of lesions.

Neonatal herpes is another form of primary infection. It is caused by HSV-2 in 70% of cases and is acquired during delivery through an infected genital tract. Resultant disease may be localized or severe and disseminated. Alternatively, HSV can be contracted by the fetus in utero and can potentially cause anomalies of the neonate.

Primary herpes simplex infection may also occur elsewhere on the skin. Herpetic whitlow is a form of cutaneous herpesvirus infection that occurs most commonly on the fingers or hands of medical or dental personnel who are inoculated by infected patients actively shedding the virus. Herpes gladiatorum is a widespread primary inoculation infection occurring among participants of contact sports due to direct contact with active recurrent lesions.

Clinical Manifestations of Recurrent Infection

Recurrent HSV infections appear in previously infected patients in whom the latent herpesvirus becomes reactivated and causes lesions at the site of the primary infection. Triggering mechanisms responsible may include sunlight, febrile diseases, emotional stress, local trauma, chemical peels, or menstruation. Recurrences are usually characterized by smaller and fewer grouped localized lesions, the absence of constitutional symptoms, and a shorter course, with spontaneous healing usually within 1 week. Often, the appearance of recurrent lesions may be preceded by a prodrome of tingling, itching, or burning.

Recurrent facial-oral herpes simplex episodes occur in about 30% to 50% of infected patients. Commonly, lesions are seen at or near the vermilion border of the lip as grouped papules on a red base that rapidly become vesicular and then ulcerate and crust over. Genital herpes infections recur with much greater frequency than do oral episodes. Up to 80% of patients infected with HSV-2 and up to 55% of patients

with HSV-1 have recurrent episodes within the first year. Recurrences tend to be more common in men but are typically more painful in women.

In immunocompromised patients, herpetic infections may be localized and self-limited or may be more severe, with larger, more progressive ulcerations and a prolonged course. This may lead to viremia, dissemination, and significant morbidity and mortality.

Complications

Infection with herpes simplex virus may lead to a number of potential complications. In some cases, recurrent infection may be followed in 7 to 10 days by the development of erythema multiforme, possibly due to an immunologic response to herpes simplex antigens. HSV infection of the eye may cause herpetic keratoconjunctivitis as a result of recurrent erosions of the conjunctiva and cornea, followed by ulcerations and then keratitis. Eventually, blindness may ensue if early treatment is not instituted. In patients with pre-existing skin diseases, such as atopic dermatitis, severe seborrheic dermatitis, and Darier's disease, infection with HSV may lead to eczema herpeticum (Kaposi's varicelliform eruption) characterized by widespread cutaneous HSV infection throughout eczematous areas. This disease is usually self-limited in healthy patients but may be recurrent. HSV may also cause a necrotizing hemorrhagic encephalitis of the temporal lobes, which carries a mortality rate of greater than 70% if untreated.

Diagnosis

Several laboratory methods are available for aiding in the diagnosis of HSV infections. A viral culture is the most reliable method, providing results within 1 to 10 days. It has the highest sensitivity and specificity, especially when specimens are obtained from early lesions. The Tzanck smear is a relatively easy, inexpensive technique that allows for rapid diagnosis. Fluid from an early vesicle is smeared onto a slide, stained with Giemsa or Wright stain, and examined for the presence of multinucleated giant cells, and/or the characteristic cytologic changes of herpesvirus infection. This can confirm the diagnosis of a herpesvirus but cannot differentiate between HSV and varicella-zoster virus (VZV). A monoclonal antibody-based office test that can identify HSV within 15 minutes is available; however, it is costly and unable to subtype the HSV infection. Serologic tests are helpful in diagnosing primary HSV infection by documenting seroconversion; subtyping can be performed with Western blot analysis. HSV antigen detection through immunofluorescent techniques can also diagnose and subtype HSV infections. It is likely that molecular virology techniques, especially those using the rapid, sensitive, and specific polymerase chain reaction (PCR) amplification, will become the diagnostic methods of choice once widely available.

TABLE 1. **Treatment of Herpes Simplex Virus Infections with Acyclovir (Zovirax)***

Immune Status	Primary Infection	Recurrent Infections	Abortive Treatment	Suppressive Treatment
	Therapeutic Treatment	*Therapeutic Treatment*		
Immunocompetent	200 mg PO 5 ×/d × 10 d 5 mg/kg IV q 8 h × 5 d 5% ointment q 2 h × 7 d†	200 mg PO 5 ×/d × 5 d 5 mg/kg IV q 8 h × 5 d	200 mg PO 5 ×/d × 5 d 5 mg/kg IV q 8 h × 5 d	400 mg PO bid 200 mg PO 3 to 5 ×/d 5 mg/kg IV q 8 h × 5 d
Immunocompromised	200 mg PO 5 ×/d × 10 d 5 mg/kg IV q 8 h × 7 d 5% ointment q 2 h × 7 d†	400 mg PO 5 ×/d until healed 5 mg/kg IV q 8 h × 7 d 5% ointment q 2 h until healed†	400 mg PO 5 ×/d × 5 d 5 mg/kg IV q 8 h × 5 d	400 mg PO bid 5 mg/kg IV q 12 h

*Doses are for adults with normal renal function.
†For use in genital HSV only. Topical is not as effective as oral or intravenous therapy.

Treatment

In treating HSV infections, a number of different modalities exist, each with its own goals. When the clinical signs of infection are present, *therapeutic* treatment may be initiated in order to reduce the time of healing, viral shedding, and the duration of pain. *Abortive* therapy is started at the onset of prodromal symptoms with the purpose of preventing recurrent clinical disease. *Suppressive* therapy is administered during latent infection to prevent recurrences. With any of these methods, the treatment of choice for herpes simplex virus infections is acyclovir (Zovirax).

In primary HSV infections, treatment is intended to be therapeutic, and dosing is determined primarily by the immune status of the patient (Table 1). In the case of neonatal HSV, also a primary infection, treatment is typically with acyclovir,* 10 mg per kg or 500 mg per square meter of body surface area intravenously every 8 hours for 10 to 14 days. Alternatively, vidarabine (Vira-A), 15 to 30 mg per kg per day for 10 days, has a similar efficacy but has significantly more side effects.

Recurrent HSV episodes that are self-limited and mild do not necessarily require treatment. However, if either therapeutic or abortive treatment is desired, then acyclovir can be administered orally or intravenously (Table 1). Topical acyclovir is not usually indicated for recurrent disease in immunocompetent patients. Suppressive therapy with acyclovir during latent periods is indicated in patients who have six or more episodes of HSV per year or who experience recurrences that involve structures such as the eyes (Table 1). Suppression may also be initiated in patients who have been or will be exposed to known triggers of HSV such as sunlight, chemical peels, or local trauma.

In immunocompromised patients with recurrent disease, many of the acyclovir doses and schedules differ (Table 1). In the specific case of a recurrent episode occurring after a previous outbreak of acyclovir-resistant HSV, acyclovir, 10 mg per kg intravenously every 8 hours for 7 days, may be effective.

With any of these treatment regimens, the dosing of acyclovir must be adjusted in patients with impaired renal function since the drug is eliminated by the kidney. No serious side effects have been associated with oral acyclovir therapy. Intravenous infusions may result in a reversible nephropathy, usually when accompanied by rapid infusion of less than 1 hour, dehydration, and renal dysfunction. The safety of acyclovir has not been established in pregnancy or in children younger than 2 years of age.

Other pharmacologic agents may also be used for the treatment of HSV infections. Subcutaneous interferon-alfa* may aid in suppressing and decreasing the duration of HSV infection in patients with frequent recurrences. Local application of interferon-alfa* or -beta ointment may reduce recurrences and the duration of labial and genital herpes. Currently, these are not FDA-approved uses. Valacyclovir (Valtrex), a valine ester of acyclovir, is a new antiviral agent that has been shown to have higher plasma concentrations than acyclovir. Valacyclovir, 500 mg orally twice daily for 5 days, is an effective alternative treatment for recurrent genital herpes in immunocompetent adults. For acyclovir-resistant HSV in acquired immunodeficiency syndrome (AIDS), foscarnet (Foscavir) is the drug of choice. Foscarnet, 40 mg per kg intravenously every 8 to 12 hours, is prescribed for 2 to 3 weeks or until healed. Intravenous acyclovir as a continuous infusion at 2 mg per kg per hour for 6 weeks may also be effective. Zidovudine (Retrovir) in combination with acyclovir may be beneficial in the treatment of chronic HSV infection in HIV-positive patients.

Prevention

To prevent transmission, intimate contact with an infected individual should be avoided from the time prodromal symptoms begin to the time lesions are re-epithelialized. However, asymptomatic shedding can occur and is probably responsible for the transmission of many infections. Therefore, in genital HSV,

*Not FDA-approved for this indication.

the regular use of condoms with spermicides is recommended to reduce the risk of spread. Prevention of recurrences may be aided by the avoidance of known triggering mechanisms such as sunlight, emotional stress, and local trauma.

Varicella-Zoster Virus

Herpes Zoster

The varicella-zoster virus (VZV) is the etiologic agent in both varicella (chickenpox) and herpes zoster (shingles). Primary infection with VZV causes varicella, after which the virus travels to sensory nerve ganglia and becomes latent. Reactivation of VZV produces the eruption of herpes zoster. The mechanisms of reactivation are not fully understood, but they appear to involve certain triggers such as local trauma, surgery, or immunosuppression due to HIV infection, malignancy, or various medications. Recurrences of herpes zoster are rare. Although both diseases are caused by VZV, herpes zoster is less contagious than varicella. However, an individual without a prior history of varicella infection can acquire chickenpox after being exposed to a patient with active herpes zoster. In contrast, herpes zoster is not usually transmitted between individuals.

Clinically, herpes zoster is characterized by grouped vesicles on an erythematous base within the distribution of a single sensory ganglion. The eruption may extend into nearby dermatomes but typically remains unilateral. The onset of the eruption is rapid and may be accompanied by fever and varying degrees of neuralgic pain. The initial vesicles progress to pustules and possibly ulcers before becoming crusted in 7 to 10 days. Lesions usually resolve within 2 to 3 weeks, and atrophic scarring may result. In some cases, this acute eruption may be preceded by a prodrome characterized by itching, tenderness, tingling, or severe pain localized to the involved dermatome. Herpes zoster occurs most frequently and with increased severity in patients who are either over the age of 50 years or immunocompromised.

Complications

One of the most feared complications of herpes zoster is postherpetic neuralgia. This is manifested as severe, intractable pain in the affected dermatome that may persist for months to years after the acute eruption has resolved. It occurs in 10% to 15% of patients and is most commonly seen in elderly patients over the age of 60 years. Complications such as conjunctivitis, uveitis, keratitis, oculomotor palsies, and blindness can result from involvement of the ophthalmic division of the trigeminal nerve. Other potential complications include cutaneous dissemination, secondary superinfection, scarring, granulomatous arteritis, motor paralysis of involved areas, visceral dissemination, and meningoencephalitis. In a healthy individual, herpes zoster usually follows a self-limited course. Complications are most often encountered in patients who are immunosuppressed.

Diagnosis

The characteristic clinical presentation of herpes zoster is usually diagnostic. To confirm this diagnosis, laboratory methods may be employed. The Tzanck smear, as previously described, allows for the rapid diagnosis of a herpesvirus infection but cannot differentiate between VZV and HSV. In contrast, a viral culture performed on vesicular fluid can reliably isolate VZV and clearly distinguish it from HSV. This distinction may be important, especially in cases of zosteriform HSV, which may be clinically indistinguishable from herpes zoster.

Treatment

The goals in the treatment of herpes zoster are to limit the extent, duration, and severity of the acute eruption and to prevent potential complications, including postherpetic neuralgia (PHN). These goals are of particular importance in immunocompromised and elderly patients in whom the risk of developing cutaneous or visceral dissemination of PHN is greatest. Currently, the drug of choice for the treatment of herpes zoster is acyclovir (Zovirax). It has been shown to hasten healing, shorten the duration of viral shedding and new lesion formation, and reduce the duration and severity of acute pain as well as the risk of dissemination. Some studies have shown that it may also reduce the duration and severity of PHN. In order to achieve these benefits, however, treatment should be initiated within 48 to 72 hours of the appearance of vesicles. Depending on the extent and location of the eruption, acyclovir is administered as 800 mg orally five times per day or 10 mg per kg intravenously every 8 hours for 7 to 10 days. In immunocompromised patients, the intravenous route is preferred. The dosing of acyclovir must be adjusted in patients with impaired renal function, and caution must be taken to avoid renal damage with the use of intravenous infusions.

Vidarabine (Vira-A) is also an effective treatment, although it does have more potentially adverse side effects than does acyclovir. Intravenous doses of 10 mg per kg per day may be used alone or in combination with acyclovir to treat immunocompromised hosts. Alternatively, vidarabine can be used when acyclovir resistance develops during cutaneous or visceral dissemination in these patients. Famciclovir (Famvir) is another effective antiviral medication with essentially the same therapeutic benefits as acyclovir, including a reduction in the duration of PHN. In addition, the oral dosing of 500 mg three times per day for 7 days is more convenient than that of acyclovir. As with acyclovir, these doses must be adjusted in patients with impaired renal function. At this time, famciclovir is indicated only for acute uncomplicated herpes zoster in immunocompetent patients. Foscarnet (Foscavir) appears to be effective in the treatment of HIV-positive patients with acyclovir-resistant herpes zoster, although it is not yet FDA-approved for this indication. It is administered intravenously at doses of 60 mg per kg twice per day or 40 mg per kg three times per day for 10 days or until healed. Valacyclovir (Valtrex) is a newer agent that may shorten the duration of both acute pain and PHN more effectively than acyclovir. The oral dosing of 1 gram three times per day is also more convenient. In addition, a number of experimental anti-VZV drugs are currently under investigation.

Variable intramuscular doses of interferon-alfa,* ranging from 1.7 to 5.1 times 10^5 IU per kg per day, may reduce the acute pain, cutaneous dissemination, and severity of PHN associated with herpes zoster. However, this drug is costly, potentially toxic, and not FDA-approved for this use. The role of systemic steroids in the treatment of herpes zoster remains controversial with regard to its effects on PHN. Studies examining oral and intramuscular modes of administration have given varying results, and further investigations are needed to clarify its potential indications.

During the acute phase of herpes zoster, pain may be controlled with analgesics such as acetaminophen and codeine or nonsteroidal anti-inflammatory drugs (NSAIDs). In addition, the application of cool compresses with 5% aluminum acetate (Burow's solution) may serve to decrease local symptoms and hasten the drying of vesicular lesions.

Once the complication of postherpetic neuralgia occurs, treatment is usually unsatisfactory and essentially symptomatic. Specific treatment guidelines have not been clearly defined, although numerous modes of treatment exist. Conventional analgesics such as NSAIDs are often tried first but usually fail. Opioids are another option, although long-term use is controversial and carries a risk of resulting in drug dependence. Capsaicin cream (Zostrix) applied locally three to four times per day may provide some pain relief. However, these effects may not occur until 14 to 42 days after beginning treatment, and topical use may cause symptoms of local burning, stinging, or redness. Other topical therapies such as 10% lidocaine (Xylocaine) gel, a eutectic mixture of local anesthetics (Emla) cream, aspirin mixed with chloroform or diethyl ether, and ethyl chloride have all been reported to decrease PHN in some cases. Antidepressants have also been shown to reduce pain in selected patients with PHN. Amitriptyline (Elavil)* or nortriptyline (Pamelor)* may be initiated at 25 mg orally daily in patients less than 65 years old or at 10 mg orally daily in patients older than 65. Doses are usually titrated upward weekly until pain relief is achieved or side effects are encountered. Desipramine (Norpramin)* may produce less sedation and fewer anticholinergic side effects. The combined use of these antidepressants with phenothiazines such as perphenazine* (Trilafon), thioridazine (Mellaril),* or fluphenazine (Prolixin)* has been advocated. Other studies have found no benefit with their addi-

tion. Combination therapy with nortriptyline and various anticonvulsant medications has also been used with some success. The use of steroids, either intramuscularly or intralesionally, has been shown to have some benefits, although this is not widely accepted. Transcutaneous electrical stimulation performed three or four times per day may afford some patients a degree of pain reduction. A 1- to 2-week trial may be necessary in order to assess the response. In patients with very severe persistent pain unresponsive to other therapies, neurosurgical intervention may be a desired option.

Cytomegalovirus

Cytomegalic Inclusion Disease

Cytomegalic inclusion disease, caused by cytomegalovirus (CMV) infection, is a common viral infection of the neonate. Transmission occurs from mother to fetus either during gestation or at the time of delivery through an infected genital tract. Contaminated blood transfusions can also be a source of infection. Congenital infection is usually asymptomatic. In approximately 10% of cases, however, clinical manifestations range from mild to severe, and the disease may often be fatal if involvement is extensive. Some of the many manifestations include jaundice, hepatosplenomegaly, hematologic abnormalities, neurologic defects, and respiratory disorders. Cutaneous involvement is rare and may be related to associated anemia and thrombocytopenia, resulting in petechiae, purpura, or a generalized bluish-red papulonodular eruption with a characteristic "blueberry muffin" appearance. Vesicles or ulcerations may occasionally be seen.

Symptomatic and cutaneous acquired CMV infection in adults is uncommon. Perianal ulcerations are the most specific cutaneous manifestations. Also, a rubelliform eruption may occur in adults as part of a CMV mononucleosis-like illness. A variety of other types of CMV infections may be seen commonly in immunocompromised patients.

Currently, there is no known effective treatment for CMV in the neonate. Ganciclovir (Cytovene) and foscarnet (Foscavir) have been used for treatment, and acyclovir (Zovirax), interferon-alfa, and hyperimmune globulin have been used for partial prevention of certain CMV infections in immunocompromised or transplant patients. However, the potential benefits of these medications, especially ganciclovir, in treating congenital CMV infection are currently under investigation.

Herpesvirus Type 6

Exanthem Subitum (Roseola Infantum, Sixth Disease)

Exanthem subitum, caused by herpesvirus-6, is the most common exanthem in children between the ages of 6 months and 3 years. The disease is characterized by the sudden onset of a high fever lasting 3 to 5

---

*Not FDA-approved for this indication.

days, followed by a rapid defervescence and a cutaneous eruption of rose-colored macules on the trunk and neck, and occasionally on the extremities or face. Periorbital edema may also be seen. Febrile seizures are a potential complication. Treatment is usually symptom-directed since the course of exanthem subitum is self-limited; the rash typically resolves within 1 to 2 days without sequelae. If seizures occur, appropriate therapy with anticonvulsants should be instituted.

Parvovirus

Erythema Infectiosum (Fifth Disease)

Erythema infectiosum, a mildly contagious exanthem that primarily affects children, is caused by parvovirus B19. Initially, it is characterized by a malar erythema with a "slapped cheek" appearance. This is followed by a reticulated erythematous eruption on the extremities and trunk that lasts about 10 days and tends to recur. Low-grade fever, malaise, pharyngitis, cough, diarrhea, and arthralgias may occur. Adults, especially women, may experience a temporary symmetric polyarthritis. Potential complications of parvovirus B19 infection include the induction of aplastic crisis in patients with increased red blood cell turnover, chronic anemia in immunocompromised patients, and midtrimester spontaneous abortions in pregnant women. In healthy patients, erythema infectiosum is self-limited and follows an uncomplicated course. Treatment, other than supportive measures, is not usually necessary.

Enterovirus

Hand-Foot-and-Mouth Disease

Hand-foot-and-mouth disease is a highly contagious viral infection that primarily affects children. It can be caused by a variety of enteroviruses, most commonly coxsackievirus A16. The fever and vesicular eruption that characterize the disease are occasionally preceded by a prodrome consisting of a low-grade fever, malaise, abdominal pain, and a sore mouth. One to two days later, oral lesions appear as small red macules that develop into vesicles on an erythematous base and then evolve into painful ulcerations. Cutaneous lesions may also occur, most commonly on the hands and feet. These begin as red papules that become grayish vesicles with an erythematous areola. Symptoms of malaise, diarrhea, joint pains, and adenopathy may occasionally occur. Rarely, recurrences, myocarditis, or pneumonia may result. Serious neurologic complications have also been reported, particularly in association with enterovirus 71. Diagnosis may be aided by the recovery of the virus from rectal, pharyngeal, or vesicular fluid swabs. Rising antibody titers may also be detected. Spontaneous resolution typically occurs within 7 to 10 days, making treatment primarily symptomatic, including adequate hydration and acet-

aminophen for fever. Topical applications of lidocaine (Xylocaine) ointment or viscous solution, or diphenhydramine (Benadryl) elixir may reduce the discomfort of oral ulcerations.

Poxvirus

Molluscum Contagiosum

Molluscum contagiosum is a common cutaneous poxvirus infection characterized by multiple, asymptomatic, 2- to 5-mm white, flesh-colored, or translucent dome-shaped umbilicated papules. Transmission of this infection occurs through intimate skin-to-skin contact, fomites, or autoinoculation. Molluscum are most prevalent in children, in whom lesions are typically distributed over the face, trunk, and extremities. In adults, molluscum are usually sexually transmitted and therefore are primarily seen in the genital region and on the lower abdomen. In HIV-infected and other immunocompromised patients, molluscum contagiosum often has an atypical presentation and a more aggressive course. Lesions may be giant (up to 1.5 cm), numerous, and disseminated.

The diagnosis of molluscum contagiosum can usually be made by the characteristic clinical appearance. Microscopic confirmation is often possible by expressing the soft core of an individual papule, crushing it between two slides, and staining the material with toluidine blue, Wright, Giemsa, or Gram stain. Visualization of large, rounded, homogeneous molluscum bodies confirms the diagnosis.

Treatment

In healthy individuals, untreated lesions may spontaneously involute within several months. However, treatment may be warranted to prevent autoinoculation and transmission to others. Available therapies primarily involve local destructive methods. Curettage of individual lesions is simple and effective and provides material for histologic examination. Light electrodesiccation may be used either alone or following curettage. To minimize any discomfort produced by these methods, pretreatment with a topical anesthetic agent may be beneficial. Two effective agents are ethyl chloride spray or a mixture of 2.5% lidocaine and 2.5% prilocaine available as Emla cream (eutectic mixture of local anesthetics), which is applied under occlusion for 1 hour prior to treatment. Another relatively easy and efficient treatment for molluscum is light cryotherapy with liquid nitrogen at 1- to 4-week intervals. Chemical destructive agents may also be used by applying the particular agent either to individual intact lesions or to the base of lesions after expressing the contents. The application of cantharidin (Cantharone) solution to lesions may be effective after one to three treatments but is usually too irritating to be used in genital areas and should not be used around the eyes. Variable results have been obtained with topical tretinoin (Retin-A), which should be applied in the highest concentration tolerated once to twice daily in order to induce an inflammatory response in the skin. Other chemical agents include 1% tincture of iodine, silver nitrate, phenol, salicylic acid, and podophyllin. Some success has been reported with the use of 0.5% podophyllotoxin cream, which is self-administered by the patient. Laser ablation is another destructive method available. Systemic therapy with griseofulvin (Gris-PEG) or methisazone (Marboran) has not shown consistent results.

In HIV-infected patients, molluscum contagiosum lesions are usually recalcitrant to therapy. Locally destructive methods are not as effective and usually are followed by a slow recurrence of lesions. Adjuvant therapy with trichloroacetic acid peels in concentrations of 35% or less have been reported to reduce the numbers of lesions with no serious complications. Combination therapies such as the application of cantharidin, followed by curettage and tretinoin cream, have also been reported to have some success. No effective systemic therapy is available, although zidovudine (Retrovir) has been thought possibly to affect the disease course of molluscum.

Due to the fact that the molluscum contagiosum virus has an incubation period of 14 to 50 days, all patients should be re-examined approximately 6 weeks after treatment to check for the appearance of new lesions. This is necessary regardless of the immune status of the patient and the method of treatment employed.

Orf (Ecthyma Contagiosum)

Orf is a parapox virus infection endemic among sheep and goats that can be transmitted to humans. After an incubation period of 3 to 6 days, one or several cutaneous lesions appear at the site of inoculation, most commonly on the dorsal fingers, hands, wrists, or face. Lesions begin as papules and progress to target lesions with a red center surrounded by a white ring and a peripheral red halo. Next, weeping nodules develop that soon become papillomatous before flattening and becoming crusted prior to healing. Regional lymphadenopathy, lymphangitis, fever, and secondary infection may occur. Complications such as ocular involvement, erythema multiforme, toxic erythema, or widespread papulovesicular eruptions are rare. Orf is a self-limited disease with spontaneous resolution of lesions within 6 to 10 weeks. Treatment therefore is primarily symptomatic. In immunosuppressed patients, however, lesions may be progressive, and early shave excision may reduce the healing time and the risk of complications.

Milker's Nodules

Milker's nodules are characterized by one or few 1- to 2-cm brown-red dome-shaped nodules usually localized to the fingers, hands, or forearms. They are caused by the paravaccinia virus, a poxvirus, acquired from the udders of infected cows. The primary lesion is an erythematous macule that develops into a papule and then a targetoid papulovesicle with a red center, a white ring, and a surrounding red halo. Next, the lesion weeps, erodes, forms crusts, and becomes papillomatous before darkening, sloughing, and healing without scar formation. Potential complications include lymphadenopathy, lymphangitis, erythema multiforme, and secondary infection. Treatment is generally not necessary due to the self-limited course of milker's nodules, which undergo spontaneous involution in 4 to 6 weeks. Infection in humans typically induces a lasting immunity.

PARASITIC DISEASES OF THE SKIN

method of
JAMES S. McCARTHY, M.B.B.S, and
THOMAS B. NUTMAN, M.D.
National Institutes of Health
Bethesda, Maryland

A wide variety of parasitic diseases have dermatologic manifestations (Table 1). Most are confined to tropical regions of the world and thus are rarely encountered in the United States. For this reason, a carefully taken exposure history is a crucial component of the diagnostic evaluation of parasitic causes of skin disease. Of equal importance to evaluation of the skin findings is the search for the infectious organism in organs other than the skin (intestinal amebiasis, helminthiasis, the presence of microfilariae in the blood or skin, and so on).

PROTOZOA

Cutaneous Leishmaniasis

Of the parasitic infections of the skin, leishmaniasis (caused by several species of the protozoan parasite *Leishmania*) is an important cause of chronic non-healing skin ulcers following travel to Asia, the Middle East, Africa, or Latin America. Diagnosis can be generally made by visualization of amastigotes from a touch preparation of a skin biopsy. The disease may follow a benign course with self-healing or healing following local treatment (heat, cryotherapy, or local chemotherapy with paromomycin), but systemic therapy with intravenous pentavalent antimony (sodium stibogluconate,* Pentostam*), at a dose of 20 mg of antimony (Sb) per kg per day intravenously for 20 days, may be required for chronic, nonhealing lesions and is absolutely indicated if the infecting species is *Leishmania braziliense* (acquired in Central and South America). Without treatment, individuals may later develop disfiguring and refractory mucocutaneous infection.

HELMINTHS

Cutaneous Larva Migrans

Individuals with a history of exposure to soil or sand contaminated with dog or cat feces may develop cutaneous larva migrans, an acutely painful in-

---

*Investigational drug in the United States.

TABLE 1. **Dermatologic Manifestations of Parasitic Diseases and Their Treatment**

Class	Causative Organism	Predominant Clinical Manifestations	Dermatologic Manifestations	Treatment
Protozoa	*Entamoeba histolytica*	Amebic dysentery, liver abscess	Amebiasis cutis	Metronidazole (Flagyl), 750 mg q 8 h PO for 5–10 d and diloxanide furoate, 500 mg tid × 10 d
	Leishmania spp	Cutaneous, mucocutaneous, and visceral leishmaniasis	Cutaneous, mucocutaneous, and post kala-azar dermal leishmaniasis	Observation, local measures, pentavalent antimony (Pentostam† or Glucantime*), 20 mg Sb/kg/d IV × 20 d
Helminths	*Ancylostoma duodenale*	Hookworm	Ground itch	Mebendazole (Vermox), 100 mg PO each 12 h for 3 d
	Ancylostoma braziliense, Necator americanus		Cutaneous larva migrans	Topical 10% thiabendazole (Mintezol) ointment bid for 2 d
	Brugia malayi, Wuchereria bancrofti	Lymphatic filariasis	Lymphedema	Diethylcarbamazine (DEC, Hetrazan), 6 mg/kg/d PO for 14 d
	Dracunculus medinensis	Dracunculiasis	Guinea worm	Symptomatic care, surgical removal
	Loa loa	Loiasis	Migratory angioedema (Calabar swellings)	Diethylcarbamazine (DEC, Hetrazan), 6 mg/kg/d PO for 21 d; use escalating dosage regimen
	Onchocerca volvulus	Onchocerciasis (river blindness)	Onchodermatitis	Ivermectin† 150 µg/kg PO as a single dose each 6 mon for up to 15 yr
	Schistosoma spp	Schistosomiasis	Cercarial dermatitis (swimmer's itch)	Symptomatic, praziquantel
	Strongyloides stercoralis	Strongyloidiasis	Urticaria, larva currens	Thiabendazole (Mintezol) 25 mg/kg each 12 h for 2 d, ivermectin (Mectizan)*
Ectoparasites	*Sarcoptes scabiei*	Scabies	Scabies	5% permethrin cream (Nix, Elimite), 10% crotamiton (Eurax), ivermectin (Mectizan)*
	Pediculus humanus var. *capitis* var. *corporis* *Phthirus pubis*	Head lice Body lice Pubic lice		1% permethrin (Nix, Elimite), pyrethrin (RID), 0.5% malathion (Prioderm),* γ-benzene hexachloride (lindane)
	Other	Myiasis	Furuncle, creeping eruption	Débridement, occlusive dressing (petroleum jelly)
		Mites	Chiggers	Symptomatic
		Ticks	Ticks, paralysis	Removal, antisera

*Not available in the United States.
†Available from the Centers for Disease Control and Prevention.
Abbreviations: Sb = antimony.

flammatory condition of the skin surface exposed to the ground, caused by the arrested migration of the larval hookworm. This condition can respond to topical thiabendazole (Mintezol) formulated in a 10% cream or ointment and applied twice daily for 2 days.

Strongyloidiasis

Individuals infected with the intestinal nematode parasite *Strongyloides stercoralis* may complain of an intermittent and transient urticarial rash, beginning at the anus and extending onto the buttocks, thighs, or abdomen, so-called larva currens. Infection may persist for many years following exposure because of the autoinfective cycle, and it may be difficult to diagnose because of the intermittent shedding of larvae in the stool. A clue to the diagnosis is an unexplained eosinophilia. Treatment is by oral thiabendazole (Mintezol) in a dose of 50 mg per kg per day orally in two doses (maximum dose, 3 grams per day) for 2 days. Although ivermectin and albendazole appear to be as effective and are better tolerated, both are unavailable for this indication in the United States.

Onchocerciasis

Individuals complaining of chronic pruritus and dermatitis following travel to or residence in West Africa or Central or South America should be evaluated for infection with *Onchocerca volvulus,* the cause of onchocerciasis (river blindness). The diagnosis is made by finding microfilariae by skin snip examination or by positive serology. Symptoms respond to treatment with ivermectin (Mectizan)* in a dose of 150 µg per kg orally as a single dose. Treatment is effective against the larval stage of the parasite but must be given yearly or semiannually, as the adult worms are unaffected by ivermectin therapy and continue to produce microfilariae for their lifespan (up to 15 years).

Many of the drugs used in treatment of parasitic

---

*Investigational drug in the United States.

infections are not readily available. Advice on their availability may be obtained from the Centers for Disease Control and Prevention Drug Information Service (404-639-3670).

ECTOPARASITES

Ectoparasites (parasites living exclusively on the skin) have a worldwide distribution, with scabies and pediculosis being a significant problem in daycare, school, and institutional settings as well as in situations in which personal hygiene is reduced.

Scabies

Infection is generally transmitted by intimate personal contact. Transmission through casual contact or fomites may occur occasionally. Clinical manifestations vary with the intensity and duration of infection, as well as host factors, including hypersensitivity to mite antigens (leading to an eczematous eruption or nodular scabies), or with underlying immunosuppression (leading to the development of *crusted* [Norwegian] scabies in individuals with Down syndrome, human immunodeficiency virus (HIV) infection, or other chronic debilitating conditions).

The principal manifestation of infection is severe pruritus, which is usually worse at night. Erythematous, pruritic papules and burrows appear characteristically in the interdigital web spaces of the fingers and toes, wrists, axillae, umbilicus, waist, groin, penis, and ankles. In infants, small children, and subjects with crusted scabies, infection may involve any epidermal surface, including the face and scalp. Crusted scabies appears as widespread hyperkeratotic crusted nodules and plaques. Secondary pyoderma may develop and obscure the underlying condition. In suspected cases of scabies, the diagnosis can be confirmed by the microscopic demonstration of mites in skin scrapings.

Treatment

Topical treatment of all skin surfaces from chin to toes should be applied, best timed for a single overnight application. In infants and patients with crusted scabies, the head, including scalp and face, should be treated as well.

Permethrin 5% cream (Elimite) has replaced γ-benzene hexachloride 1% (lindane) as the treatment of choice, as it is both more effective and poorly absorbed through the skin and thus less likely to cause systemic effects. If lindane is used, it should not be applied after a hot bath and should not be left on children for more than 6 to 8 hours, to avoid possible systemic absorption and neurotoxicity. A safe alternative in pregnant women and infants is 5% to 10% precipitated sulfur in petrolatum applied daily for 3 days. Alternative topical agents include malathion 0.5% to 1.0% lotion (Ovide), crotamiton (Eurax), and benzyl benzoate 20% to 50%. The macrolide antibiotic ivermectin (Mectizan),* which is used in treatment of onchocerciasis, has been shown to be highly effective as an oral agent for treatment of scabies (particularly in crusted scabies, which may be difficult to treat due to the intensity of infection and hyperkeratosis). Both ivermectin and malathion lotion, however, are not readily available in the United States.

The patient's fingernails should be trimmed and all bedclothes and clothes should be laundered and dried in the hot cycle of the dryer. In addition, all household and close personal contacts should also be treated. Secondary bacterial infections should be appropriately treated, and therapy with calamine lotion, antihistamines, and topical corticosteroids may provide symptomatic relief. Further, patients should be warned that lesions and pruritus may take some time to resolve completely because of persisting hypersensitivity to remaining mite antigens.

Individuals with crusted scabies are highly contagious and require contact isolation. They should be bathed prior to application of the scabicide and treated with keratolytic agents. They may require recurrent treatment.

Pediculosis

Pediculosis Capitis

Pediculus humanus var. *capitis* is the cause of head lice. Infection is transmitted by close personal contact and by sharing hats, combs, and brushes. Eggs laid by an adult female louse are glued to the hair shafts and appear as small ovoid excrescences, or nits. The intense pruritus that accompanies infestation is caused by hypersensitivity to the saliva of the feeding lice. Infestation is more common in children than in adults. The diagnosis is confirmed by microscopic examination of the nits.

TREATMENT

Several topical lotions, shampoos, and liquids are available for treatment. One percent γ-benzene hexachloride (now lindane [Kwell]) is widely used but is not ovicidal, so repeat application after 1 week is usually advised. Systemic toxicity from use in treatment of head lice is unlikely. However, there are increasing reports of lindane resistance. Pyrethrin combined with piperonyl butoxide (RID) is an effective agent and has the advantage of having some activity against the ova. Other active compounds include permethrin 1% cream (Nix, Elimite) rinse and malathion lotion 0.5% (Prioderm). The latter compound is no longer marketed in the United States despite its excellent ovicidal activity. Nits should be removed from the hair by combing with a fine-toothed comb that has been dipped in vinegar.

Pediculosis Corporis

Infection with *Pediculus humanus* var. *corporis* is found predominantly in individuals with poor per-

---

*Not available in the United States.

sonal hygiene, such as the homeless and refugees. Infestation results in pruritic, erythematous macules, papules, and excoriations that are mainly confined to the trunk, particularly at the upper back and neckline. Secondary impetigo may occur; subjects with long-standing untreated infestation may develop generalized hyperpigmentation and lichenification. The louse is found only on the clothing; thus discarding the clothes, washing them in hot water, or treatment with 1% malathion powder or 10% DDT powder is sufficient to eradicate infection. The body louse is an important vector of several infectious diseases, including epidemic typhus (*Rickettsia prowazekii*), trench fever (*Rochalimaea quintana*), and relapsing fever (*Borrelia recurrentis*).

Pediculosis Pubis

Infestation with the pubic louse (*Phthirus pubis*) generally results from sexual contact. Though it is generally confined to the pubic hair, the eyelashes, axillary hair, coarse truncal hair, beard, and rarely the scalp may be involved. Clinical manifestations include pruritus, an erythematous maculopapular rash, and maculae ceruleae (blue spots), which appear as small gray-to-blue nonpruritic lesions on the trunk, thighs, and upper arms. Nits and occasionally adult lice may be visible at the base of affected hairs.

The pediculocides used for treatment of scabies are effective for treatment of pubic lice. However, the safest treatment of eyelid infestation requires application of a thick layer of petrolatum twice a day for 8 days, or 1% yellow oxide of mercury four times a day for 2 weeks. Subjects should be evaluated for other sexually transmitted infections, and sexual partners should also be treated.

SUPERFICIAL FUNGAL INFECTIONS OF THE SKIN

method of
JAMES B. STEWART, JR., M.D.
University of Oklahoma
Oklahoma City, Oklahoma

Superficial fungal infections of the skin are a frequent cause of outpatient visits to physicians. The most common infections are tinea caused by dermatophytes, candidiasis caused by *Candida albicans* and pityriasis versicolor caused by *Malassezia furfur*. These organisms invade the outer layer of the epidermis, the stratum corneum, with varying amounts of inflammation that can simulate other cutaneous inflammatory conditions. Accurate diagnosis is therefore confirmed by potassium hydroxide (KOH) preparation or culture or both.

DERMATOPHYTES

Dermatophytes are a class of fungi whose natural environment or reservoir is animal (zoophilic), the soil (geophilic), or humans (anthropophilic). Three genera make up the class: *Trichophyton, Microsporum,* and *Epidermophyton.* Five species account for most dermatophyte disease in the United States: *Trichophyton rubrum, Trichophyton mentagrophytes, Trichophyton tonsurans, Microsporum canis,* and *Epidermophyton floccosum.* The site of infection, the causative organism, and the host response make the clinical presentation. To designate a dermatophyte location, use the term "tinea" followed by the anatomic site term: tinea capitis (scalp), tinea corporis (body), tinea unguium (nails), and tinea cruris (inguinal area).

Tinea capitis is the most common fungal infection of children and has three clinical presentations: (1) a mild scaling inflammation like seborrheic dermatitis, (2) annular scaling plaques with central hair loss leaving short, broken hair shafts (black dots), or (3) a boggy edema and exudate called kerion. Microscopic examination of an infected hair shaft reveals spores in the shaft (endothrix) or outside the shaft (ectothrix). *T. tonsurans,* the most common cause of tinea capitis in the United States, is an endothrix and does not fluoresce on Wood's light (black light) examination. *Microsporum canis,* the second most common cause of tinea capitis in the United States, typically shows more inflammation and fluoresces on Wood's light examination (ectothrix). Tinea capitis is treated with oral ultramicronized griseofulvin (Gris-PEG, Fulvicin, Grisactin), 10 to 15 mg per kg per day in divided doses for 8 weeks, or ketoconazole (Nizoral), 200 mg per day for 8 weeks. Itraconazole (Sporanox), 100 mg per day for 30 days, is effective but has not been FDA-approved for tinea capitis. While the oral form is not approved for use in the United States at this time, terbinafine, 250 mg per day for 2 to 4 weeks, may eventually become the drug of choice because of its fungicidal activity and low adverse effect profile. Family members may harbor this disease and should be treated if infected. Shampoos such as selenium sulfide (Selsun, Exsel) or ketoconazole (Nizoral) decrease the spread by reducing infectious spores, allowing children to return to school sooner. However, selenium sulfide or ketoconazole shampoos are not effective therapy.

Tinea corporis typically presents as scaling plaques with sharp borders. *Microsporum canis* and *Trichophyton rubrum* are the most common etiologic agents. Inflammatory plaques are usually due to *Microsporum canis* whereas extensive noninflammatory infections are most likely due to *Trichophyton rubrum.* Tinea cruris is caused by *Trichophyton rubrum* and *Epidermophyton floccosum.* Solitary tinea corporis and tinea cruris are treated with any of the several topical imidazoles (ketoconazole [Nizoral], clotrimazole [Lotrimin, Mycelex], oxiconazole [Oxistat], sulconazole [Exelderm], miconazole [Micatin, Monistat], and econazole [Spectazole]) or the allylamines (terbinafine [Lamisil], naftifine [Naftin]), or cyclopirox olamine [Loprox]. Extensive or resistant lesions should be treated with griseofulvin, 500 mg twice per day for 6 weeks, or ketoconazole, 200 to 400 mg per day for 6 weeks. Terbinafine, 250 mg per day for 2 weeks, is effective for tinea corporis and tinea cruris but has not been approved for American sale by the Food and Drug Administration.

Tinea pedis shows three clinical variants: (1) inflammatory type with vesicles (due to *Trichophyton mentagrophytes*), (2) interdigital scaling and itching (*T. rubrum*), and (3) hyperkeratotic type (*T. rubrum*). Tinea pedis usually responds to topical therapy of imidazole, allylamine, or cyclopirox olamine. However, griseofulvin, 250 mg twice per day for 4 weeks; ketoconazole, 200 mg per day for 4 weeks; or itraconazole, 200 mg twice daily for 1 week, is effective. Recurrences are frequent but may be reduced by prophylactic use of an antifungal powder such as tolnaftate (Tinactin) or undecylenic acid (Desenex).

Onychomycosis (tinea unguium) is very common. Distal subungual onychomycosis is diagnosed by cutting the nail at the area of separation and culturing there. Culture most frequently reveals *T. rubrum.* High recurrence rates have been reported despite oral therapy. New studies indicate that flluconazole, itraconazole, and the not yet approved terbinafine have low recurrences. Itraconazole (Sporanox) is given at 200 mg per day for 3 months; fluconazole (Diflucan) is given at 150 to 450 mg one time per week pulsed for 8 to 12 weeks. Terbinafine,* 250 mg per day for 6 weeks for fingernails and 12 weeks for toenails is awaiting FDA approval.

Proximal subungual onychomycosis reveals white discoloration of the proximal nail. It is most frequently seen in immunosuppressed persons and people with human immunodeficiency virus (HIV). It clears with griseofulvin, 250 mg twice per day, or ketoconazole, 200 mg per day till clinically clear. White superficial onychomycosis is caused by *T. mentagrophytes* or nondermatophytes and responds to topical imidazole or allylamine or cyclopirox olamine.

Pityriasis Versicolor

Pityriasis versicolor, previously called tinea versicolor, is caused by the lipophilic yeast *Malassezia furfur.* The name tinea versicolor has been dropped as this condition is not due to a dermatophyte. Overgrowth of this normal skin inhabitant is reflected as slightly scaling hypopigmented skin lesion and/or hyperpigmented patches of the trunk and proximal extremities. Potassium hydroxide (KOH) preparation reveals "spaghetti and meatball" hyphae on microscopic examination. The simplest, most effective treatment is daily application of selenium sulfide 2.5% suspension to the scalp and neck to knees for 10 minutes, then showered off, for 2 weeks. Recurrences may be thwarted by a 10-minute reapplication once every 2 weeks after the initial 2 weeks. Resistant cases respond to a one-time dose of ketoconazole (Nizoral), 400 mg. Patients should be warned that dyspigmentation will take months to return to normal despite adequate treatment.

---

*Not available in the United States.

Candidiasis

Cutaneous candidiasis is due to the yeast *Candida albicans,* a normal gastrointestinal inhabitant. Excessive moisture in athletes and workers predisposes to candidiasis. Obesity, diabetes mellitus, immunosuppression, oral contraceptives, steroids, and antibiotic usage are predisposing factors. The folds of the inguinal, perineal, perianal, and vaginal areas are most susceptible. Red superficial scaling plaques with satellite pustules are typical. Treatment consists of correcting the underlying problem when feasible. Topical nystatin applied three times per day or an imidazole applied twice per day is effective. Oral ketoconazole (Nizoral), 200 mg per day, should be used for refractory or severe cases and for patients with mucocutaneous candidiasis. Griseofulvin is ineffective against *Candida.*

DISEASES OF THE MOUTH

method of
GRANVIL L. HAYS, D.D.S., M.S.
University of Texas—Houston
Houston, Texas

A number of mucocutaneous diseases manifest singularly within the oral cavity or in association with skin lesions. The oral cavity may also exhibit reactions to medications used to treat systemic diseases. The clinical appearance of the lesions is perhaps the best way to categorize lesions when discussing diagnosis and treatment. In many cases a biopsy is required to establish a definitive diagnosis. Discussion here concerns generalized conditions; white, vesicular/ulcerative, and pigmented lesions; and exophytic growths. Only the most common or significant conditions will be covered.

GENERALIZED ORAL INVOLVEMENT

Xerostomia

Reduced salivary flow may result from drug therapy, dehydration, emotional stress, mechanical blockage, infections of the salivary glands, local surgery or radiation, avitaminosis, anemia, diabetes, and autoimmune disorders. Some secretion reduction is also involved with the aging process. Medications used by elderly people aggravate this natural process. Medications implicated as causes of dry mouth include antidepressants, antiparkinsonism drugs, antihistamines, antihypertensives, antispasmodics and anticholinergics, and antipsychotic agents.

Symptoms of xerostomia may be subjective, ranging from thick, ropy saliva (mucositis) to total dryness. Conservative management of patients, particularly those with medication-induced relative xerostomia, includes

Stopping caffeinated beverages, alcoholic beverages, and mouthwash containing alcohol;

Drinking lots of water and fruit juices;

Using unsweetened lemon drops and sugar-free gum to stimulate salivary flow.

Patients report they like Biotene Dry Mouth toothpaste and Biotene chewing gum. Oralbalance moisturizing gel also gives some relief. The degree of dryness dictates the next steps. Some patients obtain relief sipping water throughout the day and letting ice chips melt in the mouth. A number of commercial saliva substitutes (Xero-Lube, Salivart) are available, or the patient can get a 0.5% aqueous solution of sodium carboxymethyl cellulose without a prescription with which to rinse the mouth as frequently as needed. Use of a humidifier in the bedroom reduces nighttime oral dryness.

Lack of saliva can lead to difficulty in plaque control and increased dental caries without appropriate preventive measures. Daily self-applied fluoride treatment is indicated. A number of 0.4% stannous fluoride gels are available (Gel-Kam, Thera-Flur). When the patient has ceramic restorations, a neutal pH sodium fluoride gel (Thera-Flur-N) should be used. The patient puts about 10 drops of fluoride gel in a specially prepared plastic carrier, then places the carrier in the mouth for a minimum of 5 minutes. The patient should avoid rinsing or eating for 30 minutes following treatment.

The antiplaque agent chlorhexidine gluconate helps in plaque control. The patient rinses with 0.5 ounce of chlorhexidine gluconate 0.12% (Peridex) for 30 seconds twice a day. In xerostomic patients, use Peridex concurrently with an artificial saliva to increase substantivity. Peridex is 11.6% alcohol and may be irritating to dry, soft tissues. Pharmacists can prepare a chlorhexidine using a low- or nonalcohol mouthwash as a flavoring agent. Peridex* also acts as an antifungal agent and can be used to prevent the development of the erythematous form of oral candidiasis, frequently seen in the xerostomic patient. If candidiasis occurs, it can be treated with a number of antifungal agents. Most of the oral troches and pastilles have high sucrose concentrations. If cost is a factor or sugar is a problem, the patient can use clotrimazole (Gyne-Lotrimin)* vaginal suppositories as troches.

Sjögren's Syndrome. This autoimmune disorder results in xerostomia. A definitive diagnosis may require a biopsy removing four to five accessory salivary glands from the inneraspect of the lower lip. Oral management is the same as that for other xerostomic patients.

Radiation to the Head and Neck

Because salivary glands are very sensitive to ionizing radiation, radiation therapy to the head and neck region results in their destruction. Patients requiring radiation to the head and neck need a complete dental work-up. Periodontally involved teeth, impacted teeth, and teeth with extensive caries should be ex-

tracted prior to the start of radiotherapy. Diseased teeth in the field of radiation that have to be removed later are prone to the development of osteoradial necrosis following radiation. This does not mean that sound teeth must be removed prior to radiation, but preventive care and maintenance must be ensured.

Dry oral tissues are susceptible to traumatic ulceration. Although this makes the wearing of prosthetic appliances difficult for patients with xerostomia, if ulcerations expose bone in the radiated patient, osteoradial necrosis can develop.

During radiation therapy, frequent rinsing with a dilute solution of sodium bicarbonate and salt provides some comfort for the patient. This alkaline saline mouth rinse consists of 0.5 teaspoon each of salt and baking soda dissolved in a large glass of water. If the patient experiences pain when eating, recommend rinsing with one of the following:

Diphenhydramine HC1 (Benadryl) elixir, 12.5 mg per 5 mL, 1 teaspoonful,

Diphenhydramine HC1 (Benadryl) elixir, 12.5 mg per 5 mL, mixed with Kaopectate or unflavored Maalox, 50% mixture by volume, 1 teaspoonful,

Lidocaine HC1 (Xylocaine Viscous) 2%, 1 tablespoonful, or

Dyclonine HC1 (Dyclone) 0.5%, 1 teaspoonful

prior to meals, taking care to avoid choking due to numbness.

Frequently check patients receiving radiation for the development of an oral fungal infection. Recommend the use of soft toothbrushes and a bland toothpaste containing fluoride. Arm and Hammer Dental Care toothpaste, which is bicarbonate-based, is excellent. Preventive care during radiation is the same as for any xerostomia.

Burning Mouth Syndrome

Burning mouth syndrome (BMS) includes pain from the gingiva, buccal mucosa, tongue, and lips. Possible etiologies of this disorder include allergy, candidiasis, chronic infection, habits, hormonal imbalances, immunologic abnormalities, inflammation, medications, nutritional deficiencies, referred pain, reflux of gastric acid, sensory neuropathies, trauma xerostomia, psychogenic factors, and idiopathy. All these factors must be taken into account when investigating BMS. Baseline blood studies include complete blood count, glucose, Hb A_{1c}, Fe^{++}, ferritin, serum folate, B_{12}, rheumatoid factor, SS-A and SS-B antigens, antinuclear antibody titer, and erythrocyte sedimentation rate. Predilection of women to men is at least 3:1. Female patients' estrogen levels should be evaluated. Intraoral mucosal disorders with symptomatology described as "burning" are found in patients with candidiasis, contact mucositis, lichen planus, pemphigus, and cicatricial pemphigoid.

For symptomatic relief, use one of the topical agents recommended for xerostomia. A diphenhydramine (Benadryl) elixir with Kaopectate clings to the tissues and gives longer-term relief. The patient can rinse with 1 teaspoonful every 2 hours and spit out.

---

*Not FDA-approved for this indication.

Locating the underlying cause of BMS is difficult. Patients with idiopathic or psychogenic causes frequently experience a reduction or elimination of symptoms while taking amitriptyline.* Adjust dosage according to clinical symptoms and patient reaction. Successful results are reported from the use of clonazepam (Klonopin)* 0.25 mg, 1 tablet three times daily.

I have seen several patients with burning lips. When the lip is folded out and dried for approximately 60 seconds, the salivary gland fluid fails to bead up around the ducts. Placing fluocinonide (Lidex) gel in the burning area three times a day and at bedtime results in elimination of symptoms and increased function of the glands.

WHITE LESIONS

Candidiasis

Oral candidiasis classically appears as white lesions that can be removed by wiping and leave a erythematous base. They may be curdlike in appearance or, in the hypertrophic form, plaquelike and quite adherent. In the atrophic or erythematous form the lesions may appear as a generalized erythema. This erythematous form is frequently found under prosthetic appliances. Predisposing conditions for candidiasis include poor oral hygiene, prosthetic appliances, diabetes mellitus, xerostomia, broadspectrum antibiotics, corticosteroids, and cytotoxic agents. When the clinical diagnosis is questionable, it is advisable to make a cytologic smear concurrent with starting therapy. One clotrimazole (Mycelex) 10-mg troche dissolved in the mouth five times a day is an effective topical agent. Chlorhexidine gluconate (Peridex)* 0.12% also has antifungal properties and can be used as a preventive agent with susceptible patients.

When topical therapies are ineffective, one ketoconazole (Nizoral) 200-mg tablet taken daily with a meal is an effective, well-tolerated therapy. Liver function tests should be performed initially and monthly while a patient is taking this medication.

The erythematous form is frequently found under prosthetic appliances, particularly those worn nearly continuously, and may be found in tissue that is erythematous and smooth or granular. If there are no other problems with the denture, the cause is usually candidiasis, which is usually asymptomatic. The patient should use clotrimazole troches with the dentures out of the mouth. The prosthesis is soaked overnight in a denture cup in a solution of 1 teaspoon of sodium hypochlorite (Clorox) to 8 ounces of water. If the prosthesis has a metal base, substitute a teaspoon of nystatin oral suspension, 100,000 units per mL, for the Clorox.

Angular Cheilitis

In this condition, the commissure of the mouth may appear cracked and fissured. The creases may be white, red, or crusted. This may be caused by decreased intermaxillary space, drooling, nutritional deficiency, or extension of oral infections. Despite the cause, *Candida* is usually found in these lesions. First, correct the predisposing factors. The secondary infection is best treated with Mycolog-II (nystatin-triamcinolone acetonide) ointment, applied after each meal and at bedtime. When lesions recur, intraoral antifungal treatment may be required.

Dry, Cracked Lips

This condition may be treated for a short time with betamethasone valerate (Valisone) ointment 0.1%, applied after meals and at bedtime. Use of the ointment for an extended period of time results in thinning of the tissue. Lanolin-based ointments are better than Vaseline or other petroleum-based creams or sticks that coat nicely but draw moisture from the tissues.

Lichen Planus

This common dermatologic condition occurs more frequently in the mouth than on the skin. Many patients with oral lichen planus never develop skin lesions.

The classic reticular form of oral lichen planus appears as white, lacy lesions found bilaterally on the buccal mucosa. Lesions may also be on the tongue, lips, gingiva, or any of the oral mucosa. The cause is unknown but lichen planus has been initiated by a number of factors, including emotional stress, hypersensitivity, infection, and debilitation. The reticular form is asymptomatic. It requires only recognition and evaluation at a future appointment. If the lesions are not bilateral, it is prudent to biopsy.

Three other forms of lichen planus exist: erosive lichen planus, the plaque-type variant, and the atrophic variant. Erosive lichen planus is seen on the buccal mucosa as erythematous ulcers surrounded by radiating white striae. The patient will complain of a burning sensation from spicy foods and acidic fruits and juices. This variant can be confused with erythroplakic premalignant lesions. It should be biopsied.

The plaque-type variant mimics leukoplakia, and a biopsy should be performed. Once diagnosed as lichen planus, the lesions are treated symptomatically.

The atrophic variant is seen as erythematous and raw, with free and attached gingiva. It may also involve other oral sites. Atrophic lichen planus is extremely painful, causing difficulty in eating. This variant may be mistaken for pemphigus, pemphigoid, desquamative gingivitis, or oral lesions of discoid or systemic lupus.

Exhibiting more than one variant is not unusual in a severe case of lichen planus. Patients get symptomatic relief using the topical anesthetics listed for xerostomia.

If the areas of involvement are small and localized, fluocinonide (Lidex) gel may be applied to the area four to five times a day. If the areas of involvement

---

*Not FDA-approved for this indication.

are extensive and multiple, use dexamethasone (Decadron) elixir, 0.5 mg per 5 mL. Have the patient rinse with 1 teaspoonful for 2 to 4 minutes and spit out, after each meal and before retiring.

If the lesions are confined to the gingiva, a medication delivery tray may be fabricated. This is very similar to a mouth guard and nearly identical to fluoride trays, except the vinyl extends over the soft tissue. Fluocinonide (Lidex) gel is placed in the tray and the tray is placed over the teeth and gums for 15 to 30 minutes.

Severe cases may require systemic steroids. The following regimen from the American Academy of Oral Medicine (Clinicians Guide to Treatment of Common Oral Conditions, Fall 1990) has been very successful:

Rx: Dexamethasone (Decadron) elixir, 0.5 mg per 5 mL
Disp: 237 mL
Sig: (1) For 3 days, rinse with 1 tablespoonful (15 mL) four times a day and swallow. Then,
(2) For 3 days, rinse with 1 teaspoonful (5 mL) four times a day and swallow. Then,
(3) For 3 days, rinse with 1 teaspoonful (5 mL) four times a day and swallow every other time. Then,
(4) Rinse with 1 teaspoonful four times a day and spit out. Discontinue medication when mouth becomes comfortable

Very severe cases may require systemic steroids and immunosuppressants. Prescribe prednisone in a dosage appropriate to the severity of the symptoms. Concomitantly, the patient takes one azathioprine (Imuran)* 50-mg tablet twice daily. In many of the lichen planus patients candidiasis is also present and should be treated with an antifungal agent.

The severity of the gingival lesions can be reduced by removing plaque and other local irritants. Good oral hygiene with frequent professional prophylaxis can reduce symptomatology.

Lichenoid reactions may be precipitated by flavoring agents in candy, toothpastes, and mouthwashes (cinnamic acid, cinnamon aldehyde). Nickel in the gold alloy used in many porcelain or metal crowns has caused lichenoid reactions. If the patient has trouble wearing metal watch blanks or inexpensive cosmetic jewelry, the nickel in dental restorations may be the problem. Some patients also have problems with tartar control toothpastes. These lichenoid conditions have little response to medication until the precipitating agent is removed.

Medications also can cause lichenoid drug reactions. Some of the drugs implicated are the thiazides, meprobamate, methyldopa, chloroquine, para-aminosalicylic acid, and gold salts. If patients show no improvement on systemic steroids, changes in their medications should be considered.

---

*Not FDA-approved for this indication.

Desquamative Gingivitis

The condition manifests as multiple white areas on the free and attached gingiva that desquamates, leaving red, inflamed mucous membrane. In many cases there is a positive Nikolsky's sign. The cause may be traced to a change in dentifrice or mouthwash, flavoring agents in candy (especially cinnamon), or medication reaction. Treatment is the same as that for lichen planus. Medication trays are particularly advantageous since lesions are confined to the gingiva.

Linea Alba

This is a normal finding, seen as a white line of moderately thick epithelium on the buccal mucosa along the line of occlusion.

Cheek Chewing

In this harmless chronic habit, buccal mucosa along the line of occlusion has a white shaggy appearance.

Benign Migratory Glossitis

This frequently seen tongue condition is identified by well-delineated zones of papilla atrophy surrounded at least partially by a white linear border. The areas resolve only to reappear in another place. This is a benign condition, treated only when symptomatic. Patients who complain of sensitivity to acidic fruit or spicy foods may require treatment. With severe symptoms, have the patient rinse with dexamethasone elixir (Decadron) three or four times a day.

White Hairy Tongue

This is seen on the dorsum of the tongue as elongated filamentous strands that resemble hairs. The whitish appearance results from the accumulation of keratin on the filiform papillae. In patients who smoke, these papillae may take on a brown or black coloration. This is not a fungal infection. If appearance is a problem, tongue brushing or use of a tongue scraper is recommended.

Hairy Leukoplakia

These white, vertically corrugated hyperkeratotic lesions, usually found on the lateral border of the tongue, are asymptomatic. Caused by the Epstein-Barr virus, this leukoplakia may be an early sign of immune suppression. No treatment is necessary. Patients with unknown human immunodeficiency virus (HIV) status should be tested.

Leukoedema

This is observed as a filmy, opalescent, whitish cast to the buccal mucosa. When the mucosa is stretched, the tissue takes on a normal or near-normal appearance. While this condition appears to occur mostly in smokers, it is benign and no treatment is indicated.

Benign Hyperkeratosis

These white lesions, flat or elevated, rough or smooth, are primarily asymptomatic calluses. The hyperkeratotic lesion associated with spitting tobacco usually has a washboard texture. Tissues return to normal when the irritation is removed. If tissue does not return to normal, a biopsy is indicated to evaluate the underlying tissue for dyskeratosis and to rule out verrucous leukoplakia. Lesions, particularly those with a red component, erythroplasia, may be severely dysplastic, a carcinoma in situ, or a squamous cell carcinoma. When possible, hyperkeratotic lesions should be removed by total excision. When total excision is not practical, stain the area with toluidine blue. First apply the dye to the entire lesion. After waiting a few seconds for the dye to be taken up, decolor the area with 1% acetic acid. The dye will remain in the area with the most cellular proliferative activity and thus identify the area or areas to biopsy. Once the diagnosis is established, large hyperkeratotic lesions can be removed with a laser. When total removal is not practical, good results have been found in reducing the size of hyperkeratotic oral lesions with chemoprevention. The chemoprevention used with the greatest success is systemic 13-*cis*-retinoic acid (isotretinoin [Accutane]*).

Carcinoma in Situ

These lesions are diagnosed histologically and treated by surgical excision and frequent follow-up. Stopping the use of cancer-causing irritants is necessary. Patients should be evaluated for enrollment in a cancer chemopreventive study, if available.

Squamous Cell Carcinoma

Squamous cell carcinoma accounts for approximately 91% of all oral malignancies. The tongue is the most common site for oral cancer, and the most frequent location is the posterior third along the lateral borders. Oral cancer is usually seen as an ulcer or erythematous lesion within or associated with a white plaque. Nearly three fourths of all oral cancers are caused by excessive smoking and heavy consumption of alcohol. These co-carcinogens affect the entire upper aerodigestive tract and may result in "field cancerization." When an oral cancer is found, there is a nearly one in four incidence of a synchronous second primary cancer within the upper aerodigestive tract.

Prior to beginning radiation or chemotherapy, patients need a complete dental work-up. Oral infections need to be treated before therapy begins. Patients receiving chemotherapy will benefit from many of the measures described for the mucositis and xerostomia caused by radiation therapy.

Pigmented Lesions

Amalgam Tattoo. These smooth, flat, black or bluish pigmented areas are usually found in the vicinity of amalgam fillings or an edentulous ridge where restored teeth were extracted. The discoloration is caused by microscopic granules of amalgam filling material under the epithelium. Pieces of amalgam may be seen on radiographs. No treatment is required. Biopsy only if necessary to rule out melanoma.

Melanotic Macule, Nevus, and Melanoma. These are primarily skin lesions that are discussed in other sections. They do occur in the oral cavity. One and a half percent of all melanomas occur in the mouth.

Kaposi's Sarcoma. Before acquired immunodeficiency syndrome (AIDS), these were rare oral tumors. The tumors usually are seen in the palate and may be flat or raised. The lesions are nontender and of bluish or purple pigmentation; they may resemble a bruise or vascular growth. Treatment until recently consisted of radiation therapy and surgical excision. Intralesional injection of chemotherapeutic agents has shown excellent results. Because of the pain produced by these injections, first anesthetize the lesion with the local anesthetic Marcaine Hydrochloride with Epinephrine 1:200,000. Then inject vinblastine sulfate (Velban), 0.2 to 0.4 mg per mL for each square centimeter of lesion.

VESICULAR/ULCERATIVE LESIONS

Traumatic Ulcer

Frequently associated with prosthetic appliances, these lesions also may be associated with broken teeth, broken restorations, or thin epithelium irritated by hard food. The first step is to remove the source of irritation. Treat the ulcers symptomatically. Benzocaine in Orabase gives relief for easy-to-reach ulcers in the buccal mucosa. For ulcers on the tongue, use the previously described Benadryl and Maalox rinse. Nonpainful ulcers should increase the suspicion of malignancy. If healing does not occur within 2 weeks, a biopsy is recommended to rule out malignancy. About 60% of squamous cell carcinomas present as a solitary, indurated ulcer of long duration.

Recurrent Aphthous Stomatitis

The most common form of aphthous ulcers is classified as minor aphthae. These ulcers present as 1- to 10-mm ulcers with a smooth, erythematous border. They are extremely painful and covered with a gray membrane. They usually occur singly on nonkeratinized (movable) oral mucosa.

Herpetiform aphthous ulcers are crops of small, shallow, painful ulcers resembling recurrent intraoral herpes simplex. These ulcers can occur on any oral mucosal surface.

Single ulcers in the buccal gutters respond well to triamcinolone acetonide (Kenalog) in Orabase. Coat the lesion after each meal and at bedtime. When the lesions are multiple or on the tongue, use dexamethasone (Decadron) elixir; rinse as described for lichen planus.

Major aphthae present as large, painful ulcers. They may last for weeks or months and heal leaving a scar. These ulcers may need a stronger topical

---

*Not FDA-approved for this indication.

steroid. Have a pharmacist mix clobetasol propionate 0.05% (Temovate) ointment with an equal amount of Orabase. The patient should be advised to dry the ulcer site lightly and to place sufficient paste to cover the lesion on a washed finger or Q-tip. The paste should be applied gently into the center of the ulcer. As the body temperature melts the paste, the medication is spread to cover the margins of the ulcer. Applications vary from three to six times daily, depending on the size, distribution, and symptomatology of the lesions. Where the paste is impractical or systemic steroids are desired, try the dexamethasone (Decadron) elixir, rinse and swallow. In very severe cases you may have to resort to prednisone, or prednisone with azathioprine.* See severe lichen planus.

Major aphthous-like ulcers in the HIV-positive patient may be the result of cytomegalovirus. Although many of these ulcers can be resolved with Temovate in Orabase, they need histologic confirmation. The presence of these cytomegalovirus-induced ulcers indicates systemic viral involvement.

Primary Herpes Simplex

This condition usually occurs in children between 1 and 3 years of age. The first lesions are yellowish vesicles that rupture quickly, leaving a shallow, painful ulcer. Lesions may be oral or paraoral. The patients may exhibit systemic signs and symptoms, including fever and regional lymphadenitis. To relieve symptoms, use one of the topical anesthetics and coating agents described earlier. Force fluid to avoid dehydration and prescribe an antibiotic for secondary infections. Systemic acyclovir (Zovirax) is not currently recommended by the FDA for oral herpes. The exception is the immunocompromised patient.

Recurrent Herpes Simplex

These lesions start with an itching, followed by reddening and formation of vesicles that rupture. Intraorally, vesicles and then ulcers occur in the hard palate adjacent to the first molar or on the keratinized gingiva. An isolated cluster of ulcers may be covered with benzocaine in Orabase for symptomatic relief.

On the lips, the vesicles become crusted after rupture. The latent virus residing in the sensory ganglia of the trigeminal nerve usually manifests itself as lesions after trauma, stress, fever, or hormonal alteration. Recurrences on the lips are frequently precipitated by exposure to sunlight. Sunscreen with an SPF of 15 or greater should be applied to the lips prior to exposure.

Acute Necrotizing Ulcerative Gingivitis

This condition manifests as ulceration of the interdental papillae. There are a "cupped-out" destruction of the papillae, necrosis, fetid odor, pain, and malaise. Treatment is débridement of the areas with hand or ultrasonic cleaning devices and a soothing mouthwash (Benadryl and Maalox). If the patient is feverish, prescribe an antibiotic and encourage fluids. After the acute phase, prescribe an antibacterial mouthwash, chlorhexidine gluconate 0.12% (Peridex). Concurrent systemic conditions may include HIV and diabetes.

Pemphigus

These oral lesions consist of multiple bullae that rupture rapidly, leaving painful ulcers. There is a positive Nikolsky's sign. Oral lesions may precede skin lesions. If the bullae are not evident, the erythematous, ulcerative areas can be mistaken for erythematous lichen planus, erythema multiforme, cicatricial pemphigoid, or the oral lesions of systemic or discoid lupus. Biopsy of chronic oral ulcerations is required. Diagnosis of pemphigus is based on histologic and immunofluorescent characteristics of a biopsy of a new lesion.

The oral lesions of pemphigus, pemphigoid, and lupus are treated very similarly to severe lichen planus. Even when the patient is already on systemic steroids, topical steroids may be needed for symptomatic control of oral lesions. Isolated ulceration in an otherwise well-controlled patient may be treated with intralesional injection with methylprednisolone acetate (Depo-Medrol). Prior to injection of the steroid, anesthetize the lesion with lidocaine. This procedure has largely been replaced with the more potent topical steroids clobetasol propionate 0.05% (Temovate) and halobetasol 0.05% (Ultravate).

EXOPHYTIC GROWTHS

Exostosis

These hard, nodular bony enlargements are most frequently seen on the tongue side of the mandible in the premolar area (mandibular tori). They may occur in the midline of the palate (torus platinus) and are seen less frequently on the outer aspects of the maxilla and mandible. The enlargements will slowly increase in size over time but need to be removed only if they become a problem for the patient or interfere with construction of prosthetic appliances.

FIBROMAS AND GRANULOMAS

These all appear to represent an overzealous response of tissues to local trauma—and with pregnancy, to hormonal factors.

Irritation Fibroma

These occur most frequently in buccal mucosa along the line of occlusion but can occur on the tongue. They are seen as sessile, smooth-surfaced, dome-shaped nodules and are associated with local mild, persistent trauma. The lesions consist of dense connective tissue covered with normal epithelium, and they should be removed if there is any question about diagnosis or if they are a source of irritation to the patient.

---

*Not FDA-approved for this indication.

Peripheral Fibroma

These are very similiar in appearance to an irritation fibroma but occur on gingiva and may have a more erythematous surfaces. Within the connective tissue there are sometimes foci of calcification. These may in fact be the residual of pyogenic granulomas. Treatment is excision, with care not to create a gingival defect.

Peripheral Giant Cell Granuloma

Usually located on interdental papillae of gingiva, these lesions may be pedunculated or broad-based, smooth or lobulated. They are always hemorrhagic and red in appearance. The tissue is made up of small blood vessels, abundant fibroblasts, and many giant cells. These lesions may represent a healing pyogenic granuloma.

Pyogenic Granuloma

Pyogenic granulomas are very similar to peripheral giant cell granulomas but may bleed easier and are more likely to show a bloody crust. Some resemble a raspberry. They are found primarily on the gingiva and tongue but can occur on any oral mucosa. These lesions are only partly covered by stratified squamous epithelium and are composed primarily of granulation tissue.

Pregnancy Tumors

Clinical and microscopic features are the same as those of pyogenic granuloma. They may begin about the third month of pregnancy and may resolve after delivery. It is best to wait until after parturition, but they can be removed earlier if they become unsightly or interfere with function.

Epulis Fissurata

In their advanced state, these are red, hemorrhoid-like folds of tissue in the buccal gutters associated with the periphery of ill-fitting dentures. They are composed of connective tissue with dense infiltration of plasma cells and lymphocytes. When these lesions are small they may resolve with the removal of the irritation. Surgical excision prior to fabrication of a new appliance is required.

Parulis

This erythematous papule appears at the drainage site of a tract originating from a periapical abscess. Pain usually stops once the tract is established. The offending tooth needs either endodontic therapy or extraction.

MISCELLANEOUS LESIONS

Papilloma

Most frequently found in the palate, these are pedunculated, filiform epithelial growths. They can range in color from pink to white. With a confident clinical diagnosis and an asymptomatic patient, periodic observation may be appropriate. Otherwise removal, including the base of the lesion, is recommended.

Condyloma Acuminatum

In the oral cavity, these growths resemble papillomas but are more cauliflower-like in appearance.

Focal Epithelial Hyperplasia (Heck's Disease)

Seen as painless, multiple papules of the oral mucosa, these lesions occur primarily in children and usually undergo spontaneous regression. Human papillomaviruses 13 and 32 (HPV-13 and HPV-32) are used as "markers" for these lesions. The papules are mentioned here because they have been mistaken for condylomas. In adults, the lesions have a more fibrous component, indicating that they remain because of trauma.

Drug-Induced Gingival Enlargement

Thirty to fifty percent of patients receiving calcium channel–blocking agents, phenytoin (Dilantin), or cyclosporine (Sandimmune) exhibit gingival enlargement. Tissue is dense, resilient, and insensitive but of normal color. Plaque and calculus contribute to the hyperplastic process. Good oral hygiene greatly reduces the problem. Use of chlorhexidine gluconate 0.12% (Peridex) helps with plaque control. Specific drugs may deplete serum folate levels and result in compromised tissue integrity. Folic acid supplement may help if the serum folate level is low. Gingivoplasty will need to be performed when indicated.

Mucocele

These arise as solitary, compressible, translucent, sometimes bluish lesions usually found in the mucosa of the lower lip. There is usually a history of occurrence, rupture with discharge of mucoid material, and then recurrence. Treatment is local excision with removal of the associated accessory salivary glands.

Sialadenitis

Patients with this condition relate a history of pain and swelling associated with eating. This can involve any major salivary gland, but the submandibular glands are the most frequently involved. Diagnosis is by history and palpation of stones in the salivary duct. Small stones may be removed by cannulating the duct. Larger stones are removed surgically with proximal repositioning of the salivary duct opening.

Accessory Salivary Gland Tumor

These tumors are found most frequently in the palate, presenting as rubbery, firm, nontender masses. Their clinical appearance does not distinguish the benign from the malignant tumors. The malignant lesions, however, are more likely to be ulcerated and may have a history of slow growth with sudden rapid activity. The pleomorphic adenoma accounts for about 50% of the accessory salivary gland tumors. Although benign, the tumor cells may be extracapsular. Treatment is by wide excision, including the overlying mucosa and underlying periosteum. The malignancies need to be treated even more aggressively.

VENOUS STASIS ULCERS

method of
TANIA J. PHILLIPS, M.D., and
MICHELLE CHOUCAIR, M.D.
Boston University School of Medicine
Boston, Massachusetts

Venous ulcers are a growing problem in the United States, especially in a population with increased longevity. Large-scale studies in the United Kingdom and Europe suggest that 1% to 2% of the population have lower extremity ulcers at some point in their lives: venous ulcers account for 80% to 90%. It is important for internists, dermatologists, and vascular surgeons to be familiar with venous ulcers and their presentation, because the majority of cases respond to conservative therapy.

In a patient presenting with a complaint of leg ulcer, causes other than venous insufficiency should be excluded. A detailed medical history, including personal habits (smoking, alcohol), medications, and family medical history, should be recorded.

Typically, a venous ulcer arises over the medial malleolar region, never above the knee or on the plantar aspect of the foot. The majority are shallow, with irregular borders. Hemosiderin pigmentation, lipodermatosclerosis, varicosities, lower extremity edema, and lymphedema are physical findings sometimes associated with venous ulcers.

A small initial ulcer area, short duration of ulceration, young age, and absence of deep vein thrombosis signify a good prognosis.

Arterial disease should always be excluded. In nondiabetic patients, a simple, noninvasive measurement performed at the clinic is the ankle/brachial index (ABI). It is calculated by dividing the systolic pressure in the ankle by that in the arm. An ABI of less than 0.7 indicates moderate-to-severe arterial disease. These patients should have further vascular evaluation.

TREATMENT

Once arterial disease is excluded, the treatment of venous disease aims to improve calf muscle pump function. Compression and elevation are the cornerstone of therapy. A variety of compression devices are available, including compression stockings, bandages, and compression pumps. One commonly used compression bandage is the zinc paste bandage (Unna's boot). It is applied, with the foot dorsiflexed, from the base of the toes to below the knee. A modified boot is provided by multilayer bandages with an outer elastic wrap, which has the additional advantage of an evenly distributed pressure to the limb. For patients with lipodermatosclerosis, a legging orthosis using Velcro tape (Circaid) is advised. The intermittent pneumatic compression pump is helpful to patients with lower extremity edema uncontrolled by the aforementioned methods. Once the ulcer has

TABLE 1. **Types of Dressings for Venous Stasis Ulcers**

Products	Properties	Indications
Hydrogel	Semitransparent	Minimal-to-moderate wound exudate
Vigilon	Nonadherent	Second-degree burns
IntraSite Gel	Absorbent	Split-thickness skin graft donor sites
2nd Skin Dressing	Permeable to water vapor and oxygen	
Biofilm		
Cutinova Gel		
Hydrocolloid	Adherent	Minimal-to-moderate wound exudate
Comfeel	Absorbent	Shallow pressure ulcers
DuoDerm	Opaque	Minor burns
3M Tegasorb	Moisture-retentive	Donor sites
Restore		Diabetic foot ulcers
Actiderm		
Alginate	Nonadherent	Moderate-to-heavy exudate
Algosteril	Nonocclusive	Deep wounds
Curasorb	Moisture-retentive	Slough necrotic tissue
Kaltostat	Absorbent	Pressure ulcers
Sorbsan		Donor sites
Foam	Absorbent	Minimal-to-heavy exudate
Allevyn	Moisture-retentive	Necrotic wounds
Flexzan	Nonadherent	Pressure ulcers
Lyofoam		
Cutinova Plus		
Ulcer Care		
Film	Transparent	Minimally exuding wounds
Opsite	Adherent	Donor sites
Polyskin II	Nonabsorbent	Pressure ulcers
Tegaderm	Permeable to water vapor and oxygen	Abrasions or burns
Bioclusive		Diabetic foot ulcers
Omiderm		Surgical incisions
Opraflex		Wounds with eschar and slough tissue

healed, compression stockings should be worn for the rest of the patient's life.

A leg ulcer of 3 months' duration failing to respond to therapy is an indication for a skin biopsy to rule out other causes of lower extremity ulceration, including skin malignancy.

Moist, occlusive dressings are helpful in chronic wound management. Table 1 lists the different types of dressings with their characteristics. The choice of a dressing is dictated by the nature of the wound bed, surrounding skin, and amount of exudate. Occlusive dressings and compression bandages are usually changed weekly. More frequent changing may be necessary in highly exudative wounds.

Healing of venous ulcers is slow. Some require further treatment, which might include skin grafting (pinch grafts or split-thickness skin grafts) or perhaps in the future laboratory-grown skin replacements.

PRESSURE ULCERS

method of
GARY M. YARKONY, M.D.
Schwab Rehabilitation Hospital
Chicago, Illinois

Pressure ulcers are commonly known as ischemic ulcers, bed sores, pressure sores, and decubitus ulcers. Since pressure is the major causative factor that results in sloughing of necrotic tissue resulting in an ulceration of skin, subcutaneous tissues, and muscle, the preferred term is pressure ulcer. Pressure ulcers still occur commonly in hospitals, in nursing homes, and in disabled individuals. A recent systematic study in an acute care hospital showed an incidence of approximately 13%. Studies in nursing homes indicate an incidence at 1 year of residence of 9.5%, and at 2 years, of 21.6%, with a prevalence at time of admission of 17.4%.

PERSONS AT RISK

Impaired mobility is the key risk factor for pressure ulcer development. Any immobilized person with nonblanchable erythema of intact skin is at particular risk. Although the skin is intact, nonblanchable erythema should be considered a pressure ulcer. Other risk factors include lymphopenia, dry skin, and decreased body weight. In an acute hospital, fracture patients who are not quickly mobilized are at high risk. Fecal incontinence, which is often associated with immobility, may increase the risk of pressure ulcers as well. Physically disabled individuals with conditions such as spinal cord injury and other forms of paralysis remain at risk throughout their lifetimes. Factors that may affect pressure ulcer development in these people include the availability of caregivers, proper equipment, and psychological factors.

ETIOLOGY

Pressure and shear are the key etiologic factors in pressure ulcer development. The longer the duration of the pressure, the less pressure that is needed to result in an ulcer; the more intense the pressure, the time for ulcer development is diminished. Shearing forces are the second most significant factor in ulcer development. The term "presshear ulcer" has been proposed as a new term to describe pressure ulcers and highlight the two key etiologic factors.

Pressure is exerted on bony prominences such as the sacrum, trochanters, ischium, and coccyx. It is more highly concentrated in the muscle and fat adjacent to bone, and these areas will become damaged prior to the presence of a visible skin lesion. Intermittent pressures above capillary pressure from repetitive trauma can damage the tissue as well, resulting in ulceration. Other factors include friction, skin maceration from incontinence, and cigarette smoking. Atrophied, scarred, or infected tissue is at increased risk.

PREVENTION

Adequate nursing care and nutrition are the cornerstones of pressure ulcer prevention. Hospitalized patients should be turned every 2 hours. Erythema should resolve in 30 minutes, and nonblanchable erythema should be considered a Grade I ulceration. No pressure should be placed on these areas until the erythema resolves.

Turning schedules should be individualized, if necessary, based on the person's response as well as changing the support surface if needed. Friction and shear should be avoided during turns and transfers. If possible, persons at risk should be encouraged to be prone. Four-inch foam pads are the minimum amount of basic padding to give pressure relief. Minimal air loss beds can be used if basic nursing care is not adequate or effective. These beds are commonly available and are helpful in both preventing and treating ulcers. Air-fluidized beds are more expensive and are used in special circumstances such as following surgical repair of ulcers. Wheelchair users should be provided with wheelchair cushions and mattresses with proper support. They should do pressure reliefs regularly and inspect their skin daily. Moisturizers should be applied to dry skin, and nonalkaline soap should be used. Doughnut-shaped devices cut off circulation and should not be used.

DESCRIPTION OF PRESSURE ULCERS

Pressure ulcers must be described adequately to monitor healing or deterioration and allow for appropriate communication between caregivers. Several systems are used to grade ulcers, and two are described in Table 1. The National Pressure Ulcer Advisory Panel (NPUAP) classification is more commonly used than the Yarkony-Kirk classification, although the latter's utility has been studied and documented whereas that of the NPUAP has not. The Yarkony-Kirk classification has the advantage of using the base of the wound as the method of grading and has a pressure sore healed (PSH) classification to indicate a potential area of scarred tissue where breakdown may occur.

Necrotic tissue or eschar must be débrided prior to grading an ulcer. In addition, the location of the ulcer and its size, shape, and depth should be indicated. The presence of undermining, if present, should be indicated. The color of any necrotic tissue (black eschar, yellow slough) should be indicated, and drainage described. The surrounding tissue should be inspected and described and any redness or induration indicated.

PATHOLOGY

Initial damage occurs in deep muscle, with progression toward the skin. Skin may remain intact, with muscle

TABLE 1. **Pressure Ulcer Grading Systems**

National Pressure Ulcer Advisory Panel		Yarkony-Kirk Classification

Stage I	Nonblanchable erythema of intact skin: the heralding lesion of skin ulceration	1. Red area
		  A. Present longer than 30 minutes but less than 24 hours
		  B. Present longer than 24 hours

Stage II	Partial thickness skin loss involving epidermis and/or dermis. The ulcer is superficial and presents clinically as an abrasion, blister, or shallow crater	2. Epidermis and/or dermis ulcerated with no subcutaneous fat observed 3. Subcutaneous fat observed, no muscle observed
Stage III	Full-thickness skin loss involving damage or necrosis of subcutaneous tissue, which may extend down to, but not through, underlying fascia. The ulcer presents clinically as a deep crater with or without undermining of adjacent tissue	4. Muscle/fascia observed, but no bone observed 5. Bone is observed, but no involvement of joint space
Stage IV	Full-thickness skin loss with extensive destruction, tissue necrosis, or damage to muscle, bone, or supporting structures (e.g., tendon, joint capsule, etc.)	6. Involvement of the joint space PSH-Pressure sore healed*

*Indicates a potential recurrence.

damage occurring at high pressures of short duration or low pressures of long duration. This will extend to subcutaneous tissues next, with an increase in time or pressure, until skin damage is eventually visible. Bacteria in septic patients can localize in areas of pressure and cause breakdown at lower pressures. Skin changes begin with capillary and venule dilatation. This is followed by edema at the papillary dermis and perivascular infiltrate. Red blood cell engorgement and perivascular hemorrhage follow. Sweat glands and subcutaneous fat show signs of necrosis, and finally epidermal necrosis occurs.

COMPLICATIONS

Pressure ulcers should not be considered benign localized lesions. They can lead to complications such as localized abscesses, osteomyelitis, and septicemia. Infection is recognized by surrounding inflammation, induration, purulent drainage, and fever. Anaerobic infections are indicated by a foul odor. Swab cultures are not useful and should not be done. Quantitative tissue cultures or the irrigation aspiration technique should be used. Osteomyelitis should be suspected in nonhealing lesions. Although bone biopsy is the definitive diagnostic technique, pressure ulcers can be suspected with a plain x-ray that is positive, a white cell count of 15,000 mm³ or greater, or a sedimentation rate greater than 120 mm per hour. Chronic ulcers of longer than 20 years' duration may undergo malignant degeneration. This is known as Marjolin's ulcer. Clinical signs include pain, odor, bleeding, increasing discharge, and verrucous hyperplasia.

DIFFERENTIAL DIAGNOSIS

Pressure ulcers are often confused with lesions from venous stasis or peripheral vascular disease. Individuals with healed ulcers should have their arterial circulation assessed. Other considerations include tinea cruris or other nonpressure-related skin lesions.

TREATMENT

Treatment should consider the medical, nutritional, psychological, and other predisposing conditions in the person with a spinal cord injury. Adequate nutrition and treatment of anemias are essential. Vitamin C is required for collagen synthesis, and 1 gram per day of supplements is routinely given. A multivitamin with minerals is given routinely as well. If zinc levels are low, supplements are given. This should not be done routinely, since levels greater than 400 mg per dL can interfere with macrophage function.

The first step is removal of pressure from the ulcer. This is critical, as the ulcers will not heal without elimination of the primary etiologic factor. The next step is removal of necrotic tissue. Surgical débridement is the quickest and most effective method. Wet to dry dressings can remove small amounts of necrotic tissue but should be discontinued once the wound is clean. Enzymatic débridement is expensive and slow. If this method is chosen, collagenase is used and discontinued when necrotic tissue has been removed. If the ulcer is causing septicemia, it should be débrided as soon as possible to remove the source of infection and allow for resolution of the sepsis with appropriate antibiotics.

After necrotic tissue has been removed, a myriad of dressings are available. No single dressing has been proved to be the treatment of choice or more effective than others. Certain agents should not be used. Povidone-iodine can be absorbed and result in metabolic acidosis, hypernatremia, hyperosmolarity, and renal failure. It is toxic to fibroblasts. Other toxic substances that should not be used include hydrogen peroxide, sodium hypochlorite (Dakin's solution), and acetic acid.

Topical antibiotics, including silver sulfadiazine (Silvadene), bacitracin, and combinations of neomycin, bacitracin, and polymyxin B, may enhance epidermal healing and can be used with nonadherent gauze on superficial ulcers.

Wound healing in a moist environment is the principal technique to be used. Ulcers should not be dried out. This can be accomplished with occlusive dressings, moistened gauze that is not allowed to dry, or nonadherent gauze covered by a dry sterile gauze. Occlusive dressing can remain in place for up to a week if the wound is not draining, and the infrequent dressing changes are an advantage. Dressings should not be placed over a surrounding dermatitis or infected lesions. They may not be more effective than gauze when muscle is exposed. Hydrocolloid occlusive dressings are not traumatic to healing tissue if removed after several days of treatment; but, if they are removed in less than 24 hours, they can damage healing tissue. Antibiotics are not used routinely. They are indicated if there is evidence of surrounding cellulitis or septicemia.

Surgical management is indicated to repair large ulcers that will not heal and chronic ulcers not healing with pressure removal and appropriate dressings. Surgical repair requires excision of the ulcer, underlying scar tissue, and bursas. The underlying bony prominence is resected, and the area is covered with a myocutaneous flap. The person must be prepared to slowly build up skin tolerance after surgery, because the healed surgical site has minimal skin tolerance initially. Since there is a high recurrence rate after pressure ulcer surgery, an educational program is required.

Growth factors are currently under study as a means of healing pressure ulcers. At the current time, prevention is still the most desirable treatment.

ATOPIC DERMATITIS

method of
JULIE S. PRENDIVILLE, M.B.
University of British Columbia
Vancouver, British Columbia, Canada

Atopic dermatitis (eczema) is a common disease characterized by dry, sensitive skin, pruritus, and a chronic or recurrent skin eruption. It is genetically determined and associated with a personal or family history of other atopic disorders such as asthma and allergic rhinitis. The prevalence of atopic dermatitis has risen in recent decades. It is currently estimated to affect 10 to 20% of children in the urban industrialized countries of Europe and North America.

Atopic dermatitis usually becomes manifest in infancy and early childhood. The morphology and distribution of the disease tend to alter with age. In infants, there is a characteristic erythematous, scaling eruption on the scalp and face that subsequently spreads to involve the trunk and extensor limbs. The diaper area may be spared. In older children, atopic dermatitis has a predilection for the popliteal and antecubital fossae, neck, infragluteal creases, wrists, and ankles. Chronic inflammation and excoriation lead to lichenification and postinflammatory skin changes. Secondary infection with *Staphylococcus aureus* is common in all age groups; superinfection with group A beta-hemolytic streptococcus (GABHS) and herpes simplex may also occur.

The differential diagnosis of atopic dermatitis includes seborrheic dermatitis, scabies, allergic contact dermatitis, and dermatophyte infections. Skin eruptions associated with nutritional or metabolic disease and immunodeficiency may also have an eczematous morphology.

Atopic dermatitis tends to improve with age, although it can persist into adulthood. There is a lifelong tendency to sensitive, dry skin.

MANAGEMENT

Informative discussion, reassurance, and empathy with the patient and/or parents are essential. It is important to explain the nature of the disease and to emphasize that although there is no cure, good control can be obtained by treatment. Parents must also understand that there is no single "cause" for atopic dermatitis and that attempts to find one are fruitless. In particular, overzealous food restriction should be discouraged. Unsupervised dietary manipulation may adversely affect a child's nutrition, and such restrictions can be a source of unnecessary stress and anxiety for both parents and child. Infants in whom atopic dermatitis appears to be exacerbated by cow's milk or soy protein may benefit from a change to a hypoallergenic casein hydrosylate formula; reported exacerbations of eczema by foodstuffs in older children should be carefully evaluated. Similarly, children with atopic dermatitis should not be kept indoors to avoid contact with potential environmental allergens, nor should they be prevented from participating in sports they enjoy, such as swimming. Insofar as possible, they should be allowed and encouraged to have a normal childhood without undue restrictions.

Standard treatment of atopic dermatitis involves a combination of skin care, judicious use of topical corticosteroids, treatment of secondary infection, if present, and control of pruritus.

Skin Care

Patients with atopic dermatitis should avoid irritants such as bubble baths, detergents, perfumed soap and skin care products, and alcohol-containing "baby wipes." Skin care products designed for babies are often heavily scented and not suitable for infants with eczema. Soft cotton clothing should be worn next to the skin, and irritating fabrics such as wool or nylon should be avoided. Adequate rinsing of clothing to remove detergent or soap residue is recommended, and the use of fabric softeners is discouraged. Furry or feathered pets must be banished from the child's sleeping environment. Parents should be discouraged from smoking in the home.

Lubrication of the skin is best achieved by daily baths (not showers) followed by application of a bland emollient. A superfatted, unscented soap such as White Dove is recommended; soap substitutes such as Cetophil are also satisfactory, although more expensive. Addition of bath oils (nonperfumed) is optional; if these are used, a mat must be placed in the bathtub to prevent slipping. For patients with severely crusted, infected eczema, twice-daily saline baths are beneficial. For optimal lubrication, the emollient should be applied immediately after the bath while the skin is still damp. Ointments and creams are preferable to lotions except in very humid weather. There are a wide variety of emollients available, and patient preference differs. Unscented petroleum jelly, Aquaphor, "creamy" Vaseline and Eucerin cream are examples of suitable preparations. Products containing urea, lactic acid, or other alpha-hydroxy acids have a tendency to sting and are best avoided in children with inflamed skin.

Topical Steroids

Topical corticosteroid preparations are the mainstay of treatment in atopic dermatitis. They serve to both reduce skin inflammation and control pruritus. The more lubricating ointment-based preparations are preferable to creams or lotions, except in hot, humid weather. Cutaneous absorption of corticosteroid is more efficient from an ointment base, and because ointments do not contain preservatives, they are less likely to sting when applied to inflamed skin or to induce allergic contact dermatitis. Topical steroid creams are necessary for the occasional patient who cannot tolerate ointments and for older children, adolescents, and adults if compliance with application of ointments is poor for cosmetic reasons. Lotions and creams are suitable for treating scalp dermatitis, in conjunction with a bland or tar shampoo.

Potent topical corticosteroids should not be applied to the face, diaper area, genitalia, or axillae. Twice-daily application of 1% hydrocortisone or 0.05% desonide (DesOwen, Desocort) ointment is appropriate for these areas. A moderately potent topical corticosteroid is often necessary for control of atopic dermatitis on the trunk, limbs, and scalp. Commonly used preparations include betamethasone valerate (Valisone), fluocinolone acetonide (Synalar), and triamcinolone (Kenalog). For chronic lichenified eczematous plaques, it may be necessary to utilize a more potent topical steroid such as mometasone furoate (Elocon) or fluocinonide (Lidex). The patient or parents should be instructed to apply topical corticosteroids only to inflamed pruritic areas. Once the dermatitis is in remission, an emollient alone should be sufficient. Topical steroid preparations are best applied before general emollients.

Treatment of Infection

Severe, excoriated, and weeping eczema is almost invariably superinfected with *Staphylococcus aureus* and sometimes with GABHS. Secondary infection should also be considered in less severely affected patients with recalcitrant lesions. Except for localized disease, where a topical agent such as mupirocin (Bactroban) may suffice, an oral antistaphylococcal antibiotic, such as cephalexin (Keflex) 25 to 50 mg per kg per day, is the treatment of choice.

Superinfection with the herpes simplex virus (eczema herpeticum) requires treatment with oral or intravenous acyclovir (Zovirax), depending on the extent and severity of the herpetic lesions.

Control of Pruritus

Avoidance of irritants, lubrication of the skin, and topical corticosteroid therapy are the most effective means of controlling pruritus associated with atopic dermatitis. An oral antihistamine, such as hydroxyzine (Atarax) 2 mg per kg per day, may help reduce symptoms, particularly at nighttime. The newer nonsedating antihistamines are less effective in atopic dermatitis. It is also important to recognize and address psychological factors that may exacerbate scratching behavior, such as stress, anxiety, frustration, boredom, or secondary gain.

Advanced Therapy

Tar preparations are useful for the treatment of chronic lichenified atopic dermatitis. These are often used as bath oils or topical application of liquor carbonis detergens (LCD) 5 or 10%. Prolonged oral antibiotic therapy for several months is sometimes necessary for patients with frequently recurrent superinfection. Environmental modification, such as a humidifier or measures to reduce house dust mite concentrations, can be helpful in some cases. Psychological factors should be evaluated when poor compliance, high stress levels, or altered family psychodynamics contribute to a lack of response to standard therapy.

Phototherapy with ultraviolet A and/or B or PUVA (psoralen plus ultraviolet A) can be beneficial in adolescents and adults with chronic recalcitrant disease. Systemic corticosteroids are indicated only rarely and are often associated with a severe rebound effect once they are discontinued. New experimental therapies for severe atopic dermatitis include cyclosporine (Sandimmune),* interferon-gamma (Actimmune),* and decoctions of Chinese medicinal herbs.

ERYTHEMA MULTIFORME

method of
F. M. TATNALL, M.D.
Mount Vernon and Watford Hospitals Trust
Watford, United Kingdom

and

I. M. LEIGH, M.D.
The London Hospital Medical College and the
Medical College of St. Bartholomew's Hospital
London, United Kingdom

Erythema multiforme (EM) is a self-limiting inflammatory condition of the skin and mucous membranes. Attacks may be single, recurrent, or rarely continuous. This condition is an immunologically mediated reaction to a number of triggers in genetically susceptible individuals. Although usually mild and self-limiting, EM may progress to a toxic epidermal necrolysis–like illness. Different names are

---

*Not FDA-approved for this indication.

given to different degrees of severity for the same pathologic process: EM minor has been used to describe less severe forms of the disease and EM major, or Stevens-Johnson syndrome (SJS), describes the severe bullous form.

ETIOLOGY

EM probably represents a cell-mediated immune response directed against relevant antigens. Histologically, EM is characterized by necrosis of epidermal keratinocytes and an inflammatory infiltrate within the dermis and epidermis that consists of monocytes/macrophages and T lymphocytes, consistent with a delayed-type hypersensitivity reaction.

Triggering agents can often be identified, the commonest being drugs and infections. More unusual causes include systemic lupus erythematosus, lymphomas, leukemia, radiotherapy, and reactions to vaccinations such as hepatitis B. In some cases no obvious trigger can be identified. The drugs that frequently cause EM are phenytoin (Dilantin), carbamazepine (Tegretol), sulfonamides, other antibiotics, particularly cephalosporins, nonsteroidal anti-inflammatory drugs, and allopurinol (Zyloprim). Recently it has been suggested that drugs rather than infections are more likely to trigger the more severe bullous forms of EM.

Infections that trigger EM are herpes simplex, mycoplasmal pneumonia, chickenpox, hepatitis B, and infectious mononucleosis. The commonest and most important infective cause is herpes simplex virus (HSV). The attack of EM usually occurs 7 to 10 days after the onset of the herpes infection, which may easily be overlooked. The relationship between herpes simplex and EM has been extensively studied. HSV cannot be cultured from cutaneous lesions, but studies using polymerase chain reaction (PCR) have shown the presence of herpes simplex DNA within cutaneous lesions, suggesting that the virus is more widely located within the skin. In recurrent erythema multiforme, it is clinically apparent that 60% to 70% of cases are triggered by HSV. Even in those cases that appear to be idiopathic, HSV seems to be the likely trigger, and it is presumed the herpes simplex episode is subclinical. Using PCR, herpes simplex virus DNA has been shown to be present in lesional skin in cases that are not obviously HSV-associated.

Continuous EM is associated with systemic lupus erythematosus, underlying malignancy, and Epstein-Barr virus infection.

CLINICAL FEATURES

Erythema multiforme may affect the skin and mucous membranes or the skin alone. Attacks are self-limiting and may last from 1 to 3 weeks. The clinical lesions are characteristic, with erythematous papules acrally distributed and evolving into concentric target lesions. The rash may be both painful and itchy. Lesions may progress to become bullous. The rash affects the dorsa of the hands, palms, knees, elbows, and feet. Oral involvement starts with blisters that progress to erosions, which may affect the entire oral mucosa and lips. The eyes may be affected by conjunctivitis. Sequelae of eye involvement include synechiae and corneal opacities. The genital mucosae may be involved, and mucosal adhesions may be seen as a long-term complication.

In severe cases of SJS there may be clinical overlap with toxic epidermal necrolysis (TEN). In these cases, the characteristic cutaneous target lesions, the hallmark of EM, are found to be atypical, and the lesions are centrally rather than acrally distributed. This gray area, in which cases of severe erythema multiforme merge with TEN, has been reclassified into five categories: (1) bullous erythema multiforme with less than 10% total body surface area blistered and either typical target lesions or raised atypical target lesions; (2) SJS with less than 10% body surface area blistered with atypical target lesions or purpuric or erythematous macules; (3) overlap SJS-TEN with 10% to 30% body surface area blistered and atypical target lesions or purpuric macules; (4) TEN with spots in which there is greater than 30% body surface area blistered and atypical target lesions or purpuric macules; and (5) TEN without spots with greater than 10% body surface area blistered in sheets without other cutaneous lesions. Patients with severe forms of EM may have constitutional symptoms of fever and malaise. Internal organ involvement may occur.

In classic erythema multiforme, the diagnosis is usually straightforward because of the presence of target lesions and the symmetrical, acral distribution of the rash. An EM-like rash may be seen in systemic lupus erythematosus. Atypical erythema multiforme may be confused with drug eruptions, urticarial vasculitis, and Kawasaki disease.

TREATMENT

Single Attack Erythema Multiforme. For a single attack of EM, it is generally agreed that there is no specific treatment. Any suspected trigger such as a drug should be discontinued. In those cases with limited cutaneous involvement, only symptomatic treatment is required. However, such treatment is unsatisfactory, and perhaps the most helpful aspect of management is an explanation of the self-limiting nature of the condition. A potent topical steroid such as clobetasol propionate may relieve itching and burning to some degree. Sedating antihistamines (hydroxyzine [Atarax], chlorpheniramine) may also be helpful. Systemic steroids may provide some symptomatic relief but tend to prolong attacks. Even in EM that is obviously triggered by HSV, acyclovir (Zovirax) is of no benefit once the rash has appeared.

Oral involvement is the most debilitating aspect of the disease. Treatment of the mouth requires attention to oral hygiene, with the regular use of an antiseptic mouth wash. Oral lesions in EM have been reported to improve with the use of both fluocinonide and clobetasol propionate in Orabase. Patients with severe eye and oral involvement need to be treated as inpatients. The advice of an ophthalmologist should be sought to prevent long-term eye complications.

The Severe Bullous Forms of Erythema Multiforme or Stevens-Johnson Syndrome. Severe bullous forms of EM require hospital admission where good nursing care and symptomatic treatment can be provided. If there is doubt about the clinical diagnosis of EM, a skin biopsy may be indicated to distinguish EM from other blistering disorders. Those cases with extensive blistering and erosions should be treated as burn patients and managed in the intensive care unit. Patients with extensive oral erosions are unable to eat or drink, and fluid or calories should then be given intravenously or through a nasogastric tube. Appropriate dressings should be applied to wounds and secondary bacterial infection treated. Care must be taken in the choice of antibacterial antibiotic, as severe cases of EM are usually triggered by drugs. Systemic steroids are frequently given to patients with severe EM. These drugs may help symptomatically and reduce fever, but there is no evidence to suggest that they reduce morbidity or mortality. The cutaneous damage is done early in the attack, but the erosions may take weeks to heal, and this process is unlikely to be enhanced by systemic steroids. In certain cases, e.g., elderly persons, the risks of the side effects of steroids may far outweigh any possible benefit. Cyclosporine has been reported to be of benefit in severe EM.

Recurrent Erythema Multiforme. This is usually HSV-associated. In most series, in 60% to 70% of cases there is clinical evidence of the disease being triggered by HSV. However, as previously discussed, there are data that suggest that most, if not all, cases are HSV-associated. This knowledge has important implications for treatment (Table 1). For patients whose disease is sufficiently frequent and disabling to warrant treatment, acyclovir is the first choice. If there is a clear-cut relationship between the HSV attack and the EM, acyclovir (Zovirax), 200 mg five times per day for 5 days, can be given. This must be given at the earliest sign of the HSV attack or it will not abort the EM. In a significant number of patients with recurrent EM, short-course acyclovir is not a suitable treatment option. This is particularly so in patients whose EM may appear to be coincident with the onset of the HSV attack and in those whose attacks are very frequent. In these cases, continuous acyclovir, 400 mg twice daily for a 6- to 12-month period, is the treatment of choice. If this fails, the dose can be increased to 800 mg twice daily. Following a period of continuous treatment with acyclovir, recurrent EM may go into remission, but the HSV attacks can continue. Failure to respond to continuous acyclovir treatment may be attributed to resistance of the herpes simplex virus to acyclovir.

In patients who fail to respond to acyclovir, continuous treatment with dapsone* or the antimalarial drugs (hydroxychloroquine [Plaquenil],* quinacrine,† chloroquine [Aralen]*) can be effective. Azathioprine (Imuran),* is the final treatment choice and is usually effective in completely suppressing attacks. If the attacks of EM are very severe yet infrequent and unsuitable for short-course acyclovir, decisions about continuous treatment with any systemic therapy are difficult. Isolated reports describe successful treatment of recurrent EM with cimetidine (Tagamet),* intravenous immunoglobulins, levamisole (Ergamisol),* potassium iodide, and thalidomide.‡ Systemic steroids should be avoided in the treatment of recurrent EM because they prolong attacks and make them more frequent.

BULLOUS DISEASES

method of
JO-DAVID FINE, M.D., M.P.H.
The University of North Carolina at Chapel Hill and National Epidermolysis Bullosa Registry Chapel Hill, North Carolina

Many diseases are associated with blistering of the skin. These include systemic diseases (the porphyrias; amyloidosis; renal failure; diabetes mellitus), as well as endogenous (the autoimmune bullous and mechanobullous dermatoses) and exogenous disorders (allergic and irritant contact dermatitis) of the skin. This discussion is limited to the treatment of those primary blistering diseases of endogenous origin. A brief summary of the salient features of each is included.

PEMPHIGUS

Pemphigus encompasses several related autoimmune diseases that are the result of tissue injury induced by circulating autoantibodies, which bind to specific structural proteins within the epidermis. Two major types of pemphigus exist. One, typified by pemphigus vulgaris and pemphigus vegetans, is characterized by intraepidermal blister formation that occurs just above the level of the stratum basalis. Patients with pemphigus vulgaris have mechanically fragile ("Nikolsky's sign–positive") skin, resulting in the development of flaccid blisters, crusts, and erosions, often over widespread areas of the skin. In addition, other mucosal sites may be involved, including the oral cavity and, to a lesser extent, other selected tissues (e.g., urethra, vagina, esophagus, conjunctiva). Healing is commonly associated with postinflammatory hyperpigmentation, whereas scar formation is rare. Patients with pemphigus vegetans develop thick, malodorous, verrucous plaques, most commonly within body folds. The autoimmune target

TABLE 1. **Treatment of Recurrent Erythema Multiforme**

(1) EM with a clear-cut relationship to HSV	Attack-initiated acyclovir (Zovirax), 200 mg 5 times/d for 5 d
(2) a. Failed short-course acyclovir b. Very frequent EM attacks c. No clear-cut relationship between HSV and EM d. Non-HSV–associated EM	Continuous acyclovir, 400 mg bid for 6–12 mon
(3) Recurrent EM failing to respond to acyclovir	Trial of dapsone* followed by a trial of antimalarial drugs and, finally, azathioprine (Imuran)*

*Not FDA-approved for this indication.

*Not FDA-approved for this indication.
†Not available in the United States.
‡Investigational drug in the United States.

in pemphigus vulgaris, and presumably also in pemphigus vegetans, is desmoglein-3, a 130-kD cadherin, previously referred to as the pemphigus vulgaris antigen, which is present along the keratinocyte cell membrane. As in all forms of pemphigus, this disease process is autoantibody-dependent but inflammatory cell- and complement-independent, although damage is facilitated by secondary complement fixation.

The second major type of pemphigus, best typified by pemphigus foliaceus, is characterized by the presence of blisters within the stratum granulosum. Since the latter location is much more superficial than the site of blistering observed in pemphigus vulgaris, intact blisters are infrequently seen. Instead, most patients present with recurrent crusts and erosions, particularly over the head and neck regions. The target of autoimmunity in pemphigus foliaceus is desmoglein-1, a 160-kD component of the keratinocyte cell membrane associated with desmosomes.

Other rare forms of pemphigus include pemphigus erythematosus (a disease sharing some features of both pemphigus foliaceus and lupus erythematosus), pemphigus paraneoplastica (a disease associated with internal malignancy and characterized by the presence of autoantibodies to at least five different structural proteins within skin), and drug-induced pemphigus.

Untreated, the prognosis for the more generalized forms of pemphigus is grave. Indeed, death, usually secondary to sepsis, was the norm for patients with pemphigus vulgaris prior to the introduction of systemic corticosteroids. Mortality is now uncommon in pemphigus, with the exception of pemphigus paraneoplastica, owing to the availability of prednisone and several other immunosuppressant drugs. Unfortunately, development of pemphigus paraneoplastica usually is associated with death as a result of the underlying malignancy.

Systemic corticosteroids are the mainstay of therapy in all forms of generalized pemphigus. Although dosage may vary, depending on the extent of disease activity, the rapidity of its onset and spread, patient age, and the presence or absence of other potentially conflicting medical problems (insulin-dependent diabetes mellitus, secondary infection, other), most patients are begun on 1 mg per kg of body weight of prednisone daily, given as a single morning dosage. In adults, this equates to 60 to 80 mg of prednisone per day. In the absence of significant response within 2 to 3 days, the daily dosage is sequentially increased by about 0.25 mg per kg every several days until either remission is achieved or a final dosage of 2.0 to 2.5 mg per kg per day is being employed. Secondary impetiginization, when present, is treated concurrently with a broad-spectrum systemic antibiotic (chosen on the basis of the results of skin cultures) and with astringent wet-to-damp wraps or compresses (with either isotonic saline or 1:40 aluminum acetate [Burow's] solution, applied for 15 to 20 minutes three to four times daily). Erosions are covered with a thin layer of an antibiotic cream or ointment,

such as silver sulfadiazine (Silvadene), and a nonadherent sterile pad, such as Telfa. In patients with sulfa allergies, a bacitracin- and polymyxin B–containing ointment (Polysporin) may be substituted for Silvadene. This topical medication and any adherent dressings can be gently removed from the skin by brief soaks with tap water. With rare exceptions, the labor-intensive nature of such topical care, especially when it is to be performed over widespread areas of the skin, is best done while the patient is hospitalized on a ward familiar with such nursing practices.

Regardless of whether partial or complete remission is achieved with high-dosage prednisone, most pemphigus patients experience relapses when this drug is tapered, and all will predictably develop one or more side effects of corticosteroids if prednisone is required at high dosages for prolonged periods of time. A second corticosteroid-sparing drug will therefore be required in all but a few pemphigus patients. The choice of such a drug and the time when it is initiated varies considerably among authorities and is influenced by the general medical status of each patient and the presence or absence of relative or absolute contraindications to the use of specific drugs (e.g., history of drug allergy, evidence of significant hematologic or hepatic abnormalities, other).

As a general rule, I usually choose azathioprine (Imuran)* as my preferred corticosteroid-sparing drug, and begin it within the first 7 days of starting high-dosage prednisone therapy. After an oral test dosage of 25 mg, I sequentially administer this drug in the following manner: 25 mg twice daily for 2 weeks, 50 mg twice daily for 2 weeks, then 50 mg every morning and 75 mg every evening. This dosage is continued for about 6 to 8 weeks, at which time I attempt to assess its efficacy as a corticosteroid-sparing agent by slowly tapering the prednisone dosage. I usually do not exceed 125 mg of azathioprine per day, since only rarely have I found additional benefit from a total daily dosage of 150 mg. Laboratory studies (hematologic, chemistry) are obtained every 2 weeks initially; later these may be checked every 4 to 6 weeks once it is clear that the drug is not causing any predictable adverse side effects (to include neutropenia, thrombocytopenia, significant anemia, or hepatocellular dysfunction). It has recently been suggested that the determination of thiopurine S-methyltransferase in erythrocyte lysates may be helpful in predicting drug-induced myelosuppression and in choosing optimal therapeutic dosages of azathioprine; unfortunately, this particular test is as yet unavailable in most diagnostic laboratories.

Although some patients show clinical evidence of benefit from a combination of prednisone and azathioprine within the first 4 to 6 weeks of the latter's implementation, I prefer not to deem azathioprine ineffective or attempt to taper the prednisone dosage until usually about 10 to 12 weeks into azathioprine therapy, since longer use of azathioprine may result

---

*Not FDA-approved for this indication.

in complete remission. If azathioprine appears to be ineffective after this lengthy clinical trial, then it is discontinued and another immunosuppressant agent is immediately begun. If, however, azathioprine has resulted in complete remission, then the prednisone dosage is slowly tapered, usually by about 5 mg every 2 weeks, until either none is required or low-dosage alternate-day prednisone therapy can be substituted. Reduction in azathioprine dosage should be attempted only after at least several more months of complete remission can be documented following the complete elimination of prednisone.

An excellent alternative to azathioprine is cyclophosphamide (Cytoxan).* In the setting of most autoimmune bullous diseases, I prefer to employ cyclophosphamide in the following manner every morning as an undivided dosage, but only after administration of an oral test dosage of 25 mg has proven to be safe: 50 mg daily for 1 week, then 75 mg daily for 2 weeks, and then 100 mg daily for 2 weeks. If blistering is still occurring, then the dosage is increased to 125 mg daily for 2 weeks and then, if necessary, to 150 mg daily. In an effort to minimize the risk of hemorrhagic cystitis, patients must be told to void just prior to taking cyclophosphamide, to drink at least 16 ounces of water during the 2 hours immediately after taking this drug, and to empty their bladders every 20 minutes during this 2-hour period. Laboratory tests, including microscopic examination of urine sediment, are carefully monitored in a manner identical to that described for azathioprine. Subsequent tapering of prednisone and, later, of cyclophosphamide, is done like that previously described for azathioprine.

Some other therapeutic options are available for those rare pemphigus patients who fail to respond adequately to one of the previous described multidrug approaches. Cyclosporine (Sandimmune)* may prove to be a suitable alternative to azathioprine or cyclophosphamide, although both relative cost and potential nephrotoxicity make cyclosporine less appealing as a first-line corticosteroid-sparing agent. Weekly intramuscular gold sodium thiomalate (Myochrysine)* has been shown to be beneficial in the management of some patients with pemphigus vulgaris. It is only rarely employed, however, owing to its frequent association with side effects (microscopic hematuria, hematologic rash) and the prolonged course often required before any clinical efficacy can be expected. There is no evidence that oral gold therapy has any role in the management of patients with pemphigus.

Rare patients having widespread involvement with pemphigus vulgaris and high-titer autoantibodies to desmoglein-3 may benefit by serial plasmapheresis (usually 6 cycles given over a 2 to 3-week period of hospitalization). To avoid a marked rebound, both in autoantibody titer and in disease activity, patients are begun on both prednisone (usually at 1 mg per kg per day) and a corticosteroid-sparing immunosup-

pressant drug (such as azathioprine) immediately following completion of plasmapheresis. In addition, just prior to plasmapheresis, such patients may be put into rapid remission if given intravenous pulse corticosteroid therapy (1 gram of methylprednisolone daily for 5 days, given over 60 minutes by a mechanical pump in association with continuous cardiac monitoring). Several other immunosuppressant drugs have been reported to be beneficial in small numbers of pemphigus patients, although confirmatory data on efficacy are lacking from controlled clinical trials.

In contrast, patients with mild, localized forms of pemphigus may sometimes respond to intralesional corticosteroids, dapsone, or, in the case of rare patients with pemphigus foliaceus, to a course with a broad-spectrum systemic antibiotic.

BULLOUS PEMPHIGOID

Bullous pemphigoid is a chronic autoimmune bullous disease that usually occurs in elderly people. This disease is characterized by the presence of subepidermal blister formation, in association with a predominantly or exclusively eosinophilic dermal infiltrate. Direct immunofluorescence reveals the presence of IgG and/or C3 in linear, homogeneous array along the dermoepidermal junction; at the ultrastructural level, these deposits are present within the lamina lucida of the skin basement membrane zone. About 80% of bullous pemphigoid patients also have circulating antiskin basement membrane autoantibodies, which can be shown to bind primarily or exclusively to the epidermal half of normal human skin when the latter has been previously exposed to 1.0 M of sodium chloride (so-called "salt-split skin indirect immunofluorescence" study). It is now known that there are two target proteins for this autoimmune response in bullous pemphigoid. Most patients develop autoantibodies against a 230-kD noncollagenous, proteinaceous component of the hemidesmosome, which has been named bullous pemphigoid antigen-1. Less commonly, autoantibodies may be directed against bullous pemphigoid antigen-2 (also known as type XVII collagen), a 180-kD hemidesmosome-associated collagenous protein. There appear to be no differences in the clinical appearance of these patients, regardless of which of these two proteins is the autoimmune target.

Most patients with bullous pemphigoid develop tense, pruritic blisters of variable size over widespread surfaces of the skin; oral involvement occurs in only a minority and is usually localized or relatively asymptomatic. When less generalized in distribution, lesions tend to predominate in flexural areas and may infrequently be associated with adjacent erythema or urticaria-like dermal edema. Lesions usually heal without milia, scarring, or significant pigmentary changes, although the latter may be seen in more darkly pigmented patients. Mechanical fragility is absent in bullous pemphigoid, in contrast to that observed in pemphigus. Untreated, patients with bullous pemphigoid usually experience severe

---

*Not FDA-approved for this indication.

pruritus; secondary impetiginization may occur if this symptom is uncontrolled. Unfortunately, some bullous pemphigoid patients requiring chronic treatment with high-dosage prednisone eventually develop many of this drug's worst side effects, to include cataracts, accelerated osteoporosis (leading, in some, to vertebral fractures and collapse), hypertension, and diabetes mellitus. In contrast to pemphigus, however, untreated bullous pemphigoid is usually unassociated with mortality.

In the absence of contraindications to its use, high-dosage prednisone remains the mainstay of therapy for bullous pemphigoid. Most patients respond to 1 to 1.25 mg per kg per day of prednisone, given as a single dosage every morning. Slow tapering (by about 5 mg every 1 to 2 weeks) is attempted only after complete remission is achieved and maintained for several weeks. A corticosteroid-sparing immunosuppressant drug, analogous to that chosen for the treatment of pemphigus, is begun in those bullous pemphigoid patients who cannot be slowly tapered off significant dosages of prednisone. My preference is to begin with azathioprine and switch to cyclophosphamide only if the former drug fails or leads to adverse side effects.

Alternative systemic therapies have been described for the treatment of bullous pemphigoid. These appear to be most effective in those patients who experience more localized disease activity. Dapsone,* for example, in dosages of 50 to 150 mg per day, may prove to be highly effective, either as an initial therapy or as an adjunct to prednisone and/or a second immunosuppressant drug; as will be discussed later, careful laboratory monitoring is necessary whenever dapsone is employed. There are now several reports of patients with bullous pemphigoid achieving good-to-excellent responses following treatment with a combination of tetracycline* (1.5 to 2.0 grams daily) and niacinamide* (1.5 grams daily). Unfortunately, I have not personally seen lasting remissions with this regimen, although my less-than-optimal results may simply reflect a selection bias in the manner in which patients were chosen for this treatment. There are also reports of complete remission in some patients with bullous pemphigoid who have been treated with plasmapheresis, even in the absence of detectable circulating autoantibodies within their sera. Considering the many logistic problems with the performance of plasmapheresis, as well as the risk of complications, this latter, rather aggressive, approach should be reserved for those patients unresponsive to other, more conventional therapeutic regimens.

CICATRICIAL PEMPHIGOID

Cicatricial pemphigoid is a rare, autoimmune blistering disease that primarily involves mucous membranes, most notably external eye and oral cavity, although skin and other organs infrequently can also be affected. Cicatricial pemphigoid may occur at any age, although it most commonly occurs in or after middle-age. Cicatricial pemphigoid is histologically indistinguishable from bullous pemphigoid. Direct immunofluorescence may be similarly indistinguishable, although additional tissue-bound immunoreactants, most notably IgA, are usually present along the dermoepidermal junction. In contrast to bullous pemphigoid, only rare patients with cicatricial pemphigoid have circulating antibasement membrane autoantibodies detectable within their serum. Apparently any of several basement membrane components, including bullous pemphigoid antigen-2 and laminin-5, may be the target of autoimmune response in this particular disease.

The approach to therapy in cicatricial pemphigoid is highly dependent on the severity of disease activity and the organ(s) involved. Conjunctival and/or corneal involvement, for example, are particularly concerning findings, since blindness may result if the disease is progressive and untreated. Systemic treatment in more severely affected patients, especially those with ocular disease, is identical to that described for bullous pemphigoid—that is, prednisone (1 to 1.25 mg per kg per day), followed by a corticosteroid-sparing immunosuppressant such as azathioprine* or cyclophosphamide.* Unfortunately, some patients with severe cicatricial pemphigoid experience only partial benefit from such combined therapy.

Dapsone* (in a dosage of 50 to 150 mg daily) may prove beneficial in some patients with cicatricial pemphigoid, although its use is usually reserved for those patients who have exclusively intraoral disease activity. Patients with mild-to-moderate involvement confined to the gingival sulci may respond to the application of a high-potency fluorinated corticosteroid ointment or gel when applied two or three times daily to affected tissue under an occlusive acrylic dental mold. For patients with only very localized intraoral disease, pain may be at least partially controlled with swish-and-spit administration of diphenhydramine (Benadryl) elixir* or 1% dyclonine HCl (Dyclone) solution.

HERPES GESTATIONIS

Herpes gestationis is a rare, autoimmune, subepidermal bullous disease that is confined to pregnancy and the postpartum period. Patients experience intermittently severe pruritus, in association with tense blisters, vesicles, and polycyclic urticarial plaques. Although the eruption may be widespread, it often is most dense on the abdomen. Herpes gestationis is characteristically cyclic or episodic in its severity, usually worsening just before, during, or immediately following delivery and subsiding weeks to a few months postpartum. Additional pregnancies or the use of oral contraceptives may be associated with recurrences. The findings of routine histology and direct immunofluorescence are usually indistin-

---

*Not FDA-approved for this indication.

*Not FDA-approved for this indication.

guishable from those of bullous pemphigoid. Although routine indirect immunofluorescence is only rarely positive, the majority of patients have a circulating complement-fixing, antibasement membrane autoantibody (so-called "herpes gestationis factor") detectable within their sera. The target autoantigen in herpes gestationis is bullous pemphigoid antigen-2.

Prednisone (at a dosage of 1 mg per kg per day) is the initial drug of choice and may, if necessary, be safely used throughout the remainder of pregnancy. The dosage is altered as necessary to control blistering and pruritus. Dapsone* (usually in the range of 125 to 150 mg per day) may be used in those patients intolerant of prednisone. If necessary, a systemic antihistamine may be added for more complete control of pruritus, although this is rarely required.

EPIDERMOLYSIS BULLOSA ACQUISITA

Epidermolysis bullosa acquisita (EBA) is an uncommon, autoimmune, subepidermal bullous disorder. It may occur at any age, although it usually first arises during or after mid-adulthood. There are many different phenotypic presentations for EBA, including a "classic" form that clinically mimics dominant dystrophic epidermolysis bullosa (with mechanical fragility of the skin, scarring, milia, and nail dystrophy present), a generalized inflammatory form that may be indistinguishable from bullous pemphigoid, and two more localized forms that morphologically mimic porphyria cutanea tarda and cicatricial pemphigoid. Histologically, EBA is characterized by subepidermal blister formation and the presence of neutrophils, the latter aligned linearly along the dermoepidermal junction. Direct immunofluorescence reveals linear, homogeneous deposits of IgG, IgA, C3, fibrin, and/or IgM along the dermoepidermal junction; immunoelectron microscopy confirms their localization to the lamina densa and sublamina densa regions of the skin basement membrane zone. Most EBA patients have IgG-class antibasement membrane autoantibodies detectable within their sera; when split-skin indirect immunofluorescence technique is employed, EBA autoantibodies can be shown to bind exclusively to the dermal half of the tissue substrate, permitting ready differentiation from those autoantibodies associated with bullous pemphigoid. Type VII collagen, the major component of the anchoring fibril, is the exclusive target of autoimmunity in EBA.

Prednisone is the initial drug of choice for EBA. Usually begun at a dosage of 1.0 to 1.25 mg per kg per day, very high dosages, equal to those used in severe pemphigus vulgaris, may be required in some severely affected EBA patients. Most require a second drug, such as azathioprine* or cyclophosphamide,* either to achieve complete remission or to permit partial tapering of the prednisone dosage. Small numbers of EBA patients who have failed such multidrug regimens have been reported to benefit from cyclosporine, photopheresis, or dapsone. Unfortunately, only partial remission is observed in some more severely affected EBA patients, regardless of the therapy employed. Neither plasmapheresis nor gold therapy appears to be beneficial in this disease.

BULLOUS ERUPTION OF SYSTEMIC LUPUS ERYTHEMATOSUS

The bullous eruption of systemic lupus erythematosus may be morphologically as protean as that of EBA. At times it may present as sparse numbers of tiny vesicles, similar to those seen in dermatitis herpetiformis, whereas at other times it may even be confused with erythema multiforme or bullous pemphigoid. It is histologically and immunohistochemically indistinguishable from EBA and is also characterized by autoimmunity to type VII collagen.

Typically, patients with the bullous eruption of systemic lupus erythematosus develop blisters in the setting of often high-dosage prednisone and antimalarials that have been given for control of other aspects of their systemic lupus erythematosus. Most patients respond quickly to dapsone,* usually in the range of 125 to 175 mg per day, although higher dosages are occasionally required. Once remission is achieved, subsequent alterations in dapsone dosage are dictated by clinical need.

DERMATITIS HERPETIFORMIS

Dermatitis herpetiformis is an autoimmune blistering disease that usually occurs in young adults. It is characterized by recurrent subepidermal vesicles that occur symmetrically over the elbows, knees, buttocks, lumbosacral area, and scalp. It is associated with intense pruritus or a burning sensation of the skin. A minority of patients have concurrent thyroid disease and/or symptoms consistent with mild celiac sprue. Disease activity in dermatitis herpetiformis is characteristically exacerbated by ingestion of gluten; in some patients, consumption of shellfish, such as shrimp, which are rich in iodine, may also lead to a rapid flare. Biopsy of lesional skin reveals collections of neutrophils within the uppermost papillary dermis (so-called "papillary microabscesses"). Direct immunofluorescence reveals focal granular deposits of IgA within the papillary dermal tufts. Routine indirect immunofluorescence is invariably negative. Some patients have detectable IgA-class antibodies against gliadin, reticulin, or endomysium, although their pathophysiologic significance is uncertain. The actual target of autoimmunity in dermatitis herpetiformis is as yet unknown.

Dapsone,* usually in a daily dosage of 50 to 150 mg, is the treatment of choice for dermatitis herpetiformis. When sufficient dapsone is administered, the clinical response is rapid; blistering can cease within as little as 72 hours. Absolute contraindications to

---

*Not FDA-approved for this indication.

*Not FDA-approved for this indication.

dapsone include glucose-6-phosphate dehydrogenase (G6PD) deficiency and allergies to sulfa drugs. Patients given dapsone should be carefully monitored serially, initially every 2 weeks, for potential systemic injury, most notably to the bloodstream and liver. Higher dosages may lead to peripheral motor neuropathy. Useful alternatives to dapsone include sulfapyridine* and sulfoxone* sodium (Diasone), although both are now difficult to obtain. Dapsone-induced methemoglobinemia may be partially offset by the co-administration of cimetidine.

It is well known that strict adherence to a gluten-free diet may control blistering in many dermatitis herpetiformis patients in the absence of dapsone therapy. Unfortunately, this diet must be implemented for 12 to 18 months before an excellent response can be expected. Owing to the stringency of this diet, most patients with dermatitis herpetiformis choose dapsone therapy instead and attempt to reduce rather than fully eliminate gluten from their diets.

LINEAR IgA DERMATOSIS

Linear IgA dermatosis encompasses at least two clinically identical autoimmune bullous diseases that are characterized by the presence of subepidermal blisters and linear homogeneous deposits of IgA along the dermoepidermal junction. Ultrastructurally, these immune deposits may be present either within the lamina lucida or beneath the lamina densa of the skin basement membrane zone, suggesting possible heterogeneity of disease. Some patients also have IgA-class antiskin basement membrane autoantibodies present within their sera. It has been suggested that an as yet only partially characterized 97-kD component (ladinin, LAD-1) of the dermoepidermal junction is the target of autoimmunity in this group of diseases. Adult patients with linear IgA dermatosis often clinically resemble those with dermatitis herpetiformis, whereas affected children usually have a more characteristic collection of larger blisters in strikingly arcuate array on the abdomen, upper thighs, and groin areas. Dapsone is the treatment of choice for linear IgA dermatosis. Infrequently, some patients also partially benefit by the addition of prednisone (at 1 mg per kg per day). The gluten-free diet is unfortunately ineffective in this disease.

INHERITED EPIDERMOLYSIS BULLOSA

Inherited epidermolysis bullosa (EB) comprises a group of at least 23 phenotypic variants of markedly variable severity, which are all characterized by the presence of mechanically fragile skin and blisters. Ultimately at least some forms of EB may be treatable with gene therapy. At present, however, therapy for inherited EB remains primarily supportive and requires a multidisciplinary approach, particularly since many organs, including the external eye, oral cavity, gastrointestinal and genitourinary tracts, and musculoskeletal system may be involved. Open skin wounds are usually first covered with a thin layer of an antibiotic ointment or cream (i.e., silver sulfadiazine, mupirocin [Bactroban], bacitracin–polymyxin B), followed by a nonadhesive sterile pad and a thick dressing of sterile gauze. Alternatively, a nonadhesive, synthetic, hydrocolloid sheet (such as Vigilon) may be applied to the surface of the wound. Adhesive tapes and tightly applied dressings are to be avoided, since they will mechanically precipitate further blistering. Chronic nonhealing ulcerations may eventually require placement of split-thickness skin grafts, local flaps, or autologous cultured keratinocyte sheets, once the possibility of a squamous cell carcinoma arising in a chronic ulcer has been excluded by skin biopsy. Mixed success has been noted with the use of cultured keratinocyte allografts.

Despite favorable reports in the past, it is now clear that phenytoin is of long-term benefit in only rare patients with recessive dystrophic and junctional forms of EB. It is thus only rarely employed any more in the management of this disease. No other systemically administered drugs (e.g., retinoids, corticosteroids) have proven efficacy in any form of EB.

CONTACT DERMATITIS

method of
CHRISTOPHER J. GALLANT, M.D.
Dalhousie University Faculty of Medicine
Halifax, Nova Scotia, Canada

Our skin is in daily contact with a surprisingly large number of chemicals under varying conditions of temperature, humidity, and trauma. These chemical/physical interactions can cause urticaria, acne, pigmentary changes, atrophy, and dermatitis.

Contact dermatitis is one of the most commonly acquired skin diseases in adults. Large surveys suggest a prevalence of up to 10% in the general population. There are a myriad of precipitating factors, which may be found in any worksite, home, school, or play area. No one, regardless of occupation, age, sex, or lifestyle, is immune to this common problem.

Contact dermatitis is an inflammatory process that occurs as the result of interactions between the skin and substances in the environment. Simplistically, these reactions can be divided into either irritant or allergic, depending on whether the inflammatory response was caused by direct injury to the skin (irritation) or via an immunologic trigger (allergic). Once the inflammatory process has been initiated, the end pathways for both allergic and irritant dermatitis are very similar, and thus the microscopic and clinical findings are often identical.

Almost any chemical can act as an irritant under the proper circumstances. The chemical nature of the contactant, concentration of the contactant, duration of exposure, site of exposure, hydration of the skin, degree of occlusion, and local trauma are all factors that may influ-

---

*Investigational drug in the United States.

ence the severity of both irritant and allergic reactions. There are about 3000 known contact allergens; however, relatively few chemicals are potent sensitizers. As a result, over 75% of all contact dermatitis cases are diagnosed as irritant reactions.

Contact dermatitis can occur on any mucous membrane or skin surface on the body. However, the majority of reported cases occur on the hands. The importance of contact dermatitis as a cause of significant morbidity is often overlooked. Minor cases of contact dermatitis can alter normal skin function for months. Prolonged episodes can result in permanent damage to the skin. Chronic dermatitis or skin fragility may continue even after all causative agents have been eliminated. Many of those who develop contact dermatitis related to their daily work will go on to develop chronic debilitating skin disease. Millions of dollars are lost on wages, treatment, and decreased productivity directly related to contact dermatitis.

Early diagnosis and treatment of contact dermatitis are two of the most important factors in preventing long-term morbidity.

Dermatitic eruptions can be broadly classified as acute and chronic, although there is no sharp delineation between the two. The acute phase is marked by edema, vesiculation, and occasionally bullae and crusting. Patients usually complain of pruritus or burning discomfort. The chronic phase has less vesiculation and more scaling, hyperkeratosis, fissuring, and lichenification of the affected skin.

Contact urticaria reactions are now recognized as an important subtype of allergic contact reactions. The reported incidence of contact urticaria has increased rapidly in the past few years, with many of the new cases caused by natural rubber latex proteins. Health care workers, atopic patients, and patients with a history of multiple surgeries (more than five) or multiple invasive medical procedures, as in spina bifida patients, are all at increased risk to develop natural rubber latex sensitivity. Although the immediate response is urticarial, patients may also have a superimposed nonspecific dermatitis that complicates the clinical picture. Patients with Type 1 hypersensitivities may also develop life-threatening anaphylaxis; 16 fatalities have been reported due to natural rubber latex reactions.

Clinically, it is often impossible for even the most experienced physician to differentiate between irritant and allergic eruptions, especially after they have become chronic.

The distribution of the eruption often provides the best clue in determining the cause of contact reactions. In most cases the contact dermatitis reaction is localized and most pronounced in the area of maximum contact. However, in instances of severe irritation, strong allergic reactions, antibody-mediated reactions, or systemic exposure to some allergens, a widespread eruption can develop.

Contactants carried as dust or aerosols frequently affect the ears, eyelids, face, neck, and other exposed areas, whereas liquid contactants often leave a characteristic drip or smear pattern on exposed skin. Cosmetics, skin care products, and medications, which are common causes of contact allergy, often trigger reactions in areas where they have been applied or inadvertently spread. Work-related exposure is most often seen on the hands.

Severe acute irritant contact reactions, caused by potent irritants like acids, are similar to burns, so the patient is often able to identify the offending agent because the eruption develops rapidly. Irritant reactions seem to cause more pain and burning than itching. In most instances, however, contact irritant dermatitis develops gradually after re-

peated exposures as a cumulative response, making the link less obvious. It is often very helpful for the patient to keep a detailed diary of day-to-day activities to aid in identifying patterns of exposure.

Contact allergic reactions often flare 24 to 48 hours after exposure to the offending allergen, which can help in identifying the source of exposure. Most patients complain of pruritus. Unfortunately, continued repeated exposure, as is often found in the workplace, frequently blurs the pattern of response.

Proper evaluation and management of contact dermatitis requires a detailed history, a careful examination of the skin, and an inquisitive physician. Diagnosis is usually based on a compilation of history, distribution of the eruption, and testing.

The course and appearance of contact dermatitis may be altered or mimicked by endogenous dermatoses such as atopic dermatitis and psoriasis, fungal infections, and xerosis. It is essential for the examining clinician to look for evidence of these other disorders in order to determine the part they may play in the overall picture. Contact allergic or irritant eruptions may take on an atypical appearance if superimposed upon a patient's pre-existing dermatosis.

MANAGEMENT

There are two main steps in the management of contact dermatitis. The first is treatment of the active dermatitis, and the second is to prevent recurrence of the eruption through re-exposure to the offending agent.

Acute vesicular/bullous eruptions usually require open wet compresses with tap water, saline, or Burow solution, followed by topical application of a corticosteroid cream. Secondary infection, if present, should be treated with appropriate antibiotics. In severe cases, oral corticosteroids tapered over 14 days may be warranted, but in most cases liberal use of medium-to-high-potency topical steroids is sufficient. Topical corticosteroid therapy should be tapered as the eruption clears and replaced with bland emollients. Prolonged use of corticosteroids can lead to atrophy and other complications.

In chronic cases, more prolonged, aggressive topical corticosteroid treatment, sometimes under occlusion, may be needed. Close follow-up is important to avoid the complications of steroid use. Liberal use of emollients is essential to protect the recovering skin. Recalcitrant cases may require adjuvant therapy with PUVA (psoralen and ultraviolet A).

Patch testing can be used to help identify or confirm most suspected Type 4 contact allergens. Proper patient selection, correct choice of allergens at appropriate test concentrations, and interpretation of results require experience and a detailed knowledge of proper test procedures. A natural rubber latex IgE-specific radioallergosorbent test (RAST) is available but has a low sensitivity. Because of the risk of anaphylaxis, use and prick testing for latex sensitivity should be undertaken only by physicians trained to perform these tests and prepared to deal with potential complications.

Once the offending product has been identified, avoidance through product substitution, task redesign, or appropriate personal protective equipment is important. Protection of the skin from even minor irritants is needed for up to 12 months after the active dermatitis clears, as the skin slowly returns to normal function.

SPECIFIC DERMATOSES OF PREGNANCY

method of
M. JOYCE RICO, M.D.
New York University
New York, New York

and

BARBARA R. REED, M.D.
University of Colorado
Denver, Colorado

The nosology of specific dermatoses of pregnancy continues to undergo change as attempts are made to categorize appropriately those cutaneous disorders associated with pregnancy and the puerperium. Disorders to be covered in this review include herpes gestationis and pruritic urticarial papules and plaques of pregnancy, two cutaneous diseases specific to pregnancy and the puerperium (Table 1).

HERPES GESTATIONIS

Herpes gestationis (HG), which is known as pemphigoid gestationis in the United Kingdom, is a rare, autoimmune, blistering disease that typically arises during the second or third trimester but may develop at any time during pregnancy or the puerperium. Patients typically present with extremely pruritic, hivelike papules and plaques surmounted by tense, clear vesicles and bullae. The lesions characteristically begin periumbilically and involve the trunk and extremities. The face or mucosa is rarely involved. Spontaneous decrease in disease activity late in pregnancy, and flares during the puerperium, are not uncommon. Patients with this disease usually remit after delivery; however, recurrence in subsequent pregnancies is common. Patients may also experience exacerbation with menstruation or the use of oral contraceptives. Infants born to affected mothers may be small for gestational age (SGA) or premature.

Herpes gestationis is a rare disease with an estimated incidence of 1:1700 to 1:60,000 pregnancies. The frequency of disease may depend on the HLA haplotype of the population at risk. HG is associated with specific HLA (HLA DR3, DR4) and complement haplotypes.

Histologic examination of lesional skin from a patient with HG reveals a subepidermal blister with an inflammatory infiltrate marked by the presence of numerous eosinophils. By direct immunofluorescence (DIF), perilesional skin biopsies from patients with HG demonstrate complement (C3) (100% of patients) and IgG (25% of patients) deposits in a linear band at the dermal-epidermal junction (DEJ). Serum from approximately half the patients with HG demonstrates IgG, which binds to the DEJ by complement fixation (HG factor) by indirect immunofluorescence (IDIF). This circulating antibody is directed at a 180-kD hemidesmosomal protein, BPAG2, which is critical in normal epidermal-dermal adhesion.

Treatment

Corticosteroids are the mainstay of therapy for patients with this disease. Patients with mild disease may be treated with midpotency topical steroids [triamcinolone 0.1% cream or ointment (Aristocort, Kenalog)] up to three times daily. Patients with extensive disease should be treated with oral prednisone in initial doses ranging from 20 to 40 mg per day as a single oral dose. Patient response should be monitored by assessing pruritus and new blister formation. If patients do not respond to this dose of prednisone, then the dose should be increased by 50% every 3 to 5 days until disease control occurs. After the majority of lesions have healed, the dose of prednisone should be gradually tapered by 5 to 10 mg every week to determine the minimum dose necessary to alleviate symptoms and control blister formation. The goal of therapy is not to remain totally disease-free, and patients may develop occasional blisters during treatment. As noted, HG often improves late in pregnancy and may flare immediately after parturition; therefore, the dose of prednisone should be adjusted based on each patient's clinical course. It has been reported that women with HG who breast-

TABLE 1. **Dermatoses of Pregnancy**

	Herpes Gestationis	PUPP
Onset	3rd trimester, puerperium	Late 3rd trimester, primigravida
Clinical Presentation	Urticarial papules, vesicles, bullae	Urticarial papules, plaques
Diagnosis	DIF: linear C3 and IgG at DEJ	DIF: negative
	IDIF: HG factor	
Recurrence in Subsequent Pregnancies	Common	Rare
Treatment	May require systemic steroids	Symptomatic, topical antipruritics, antihistamines, steroids
Complications	SGA, premature infants	None

Abbreviations: PUPP = pruritic urticarial papules and plaques of pregnancy; DIF = direct immunofluorescence; IDIF = indirect immunofluorescence; DEJ = dermal-epidermal junction; SGA = small for gestational age.

feed their infants remit more rapidly than women who do not nurse, although controlled studies are lacking.

The use of topical steroids during late pregnancy is thought to be of minimal risk to mother or fetus, although manufacturers of Class I steroids such as clobetasol (Temovate) or halobetasol propionate (Ultravate) generally issue a warning against their use in pregnancy. During lactation, topical steroids should be avoided on the areola as infantile hypertension has been reported. In general, oral steroids in the dose range used to manage HG are relatively well tolerated, although hypertension and gestational diabetes may be unmasked by prednisone and it should be used with caution during late pregnancy and lactation. During lactation, some investigators recommend that if the dose of prednisone is more than 25 mg per day (20 mg per day of prednisolone), mothers wait at least 4 hours after taking prednisone before nursing. Prednisone is excreted in breast milk, albeit such small amounts that significant effects to the fetus are unlikely, even at a dose of 80 mg per day of prednisone in lactating women.

For patients with severe, unremitting disease during pregnancy, not controlled by corticosteroids alone, therapeutic options are limited. Antihistamines may be added to the therapeutic regimen for symptomatic management of pruritus, with the concerns noted later. Plasmapheresis has been reported to be effective and is relatively safe for mother and fetus. Following parturition, immunosuppressants such as azathioprine (Imuran),* cyclophosphamide (Cytoxan),* or cyclosporine (Sandimmune)* may be added as adjuvants; however, nursing is contraindicated because of the risk to the neonate. The luteinizing hormone–releasing analogue goserelin (Zoladex)* has also been used postpartum in patients with recalcitrant HG, although neonatal risk is unknown. Neither dapsone, gold (aurothioglucose, [Solganal]), nor methotrexate has demonstrated efficacy as an adjuvant in managing patients with HG, and their use in this condition should be discouraged.

PRURITIC URTICARIAL PAPULES AND PLAQUES OF PREGNANCY

Pruritic urticarial papules and plaques of pregnancy (PUPP), also known as polymorphic eruption of pregnancy, is fairly common, with an incidence estimated at 1:160 pregnancies. PUPP is more common in primigravidas. It usually appears during the last trimester of pregnancy, after 36 weeks' gestation, or immediately postpartum but has been reported as early as the 4th week of gestation. PUPP lasts up to 6 weeks and remits spontaneously. No adverse effects on infants or mothers have been reported. In contrast to HG, PUPP does not tend to recur with subsequent pregnancies, with menstruation, or with oral contraceptive use.

Patients typically present with urticarial papules

*Not FDA-approved for this indication.

and plaques, although vesicles can develop in up to 40% of patients. Some patients may develop targetoid lesions, as seen in erythema multiforme, or concentric wheals. Patients may develop lesions in areas of the skin that have been injured (Koebner's phenomenon). The rash becomes scaly with resolution and may clinically resemble eczema. Lesions begin in striae on the lower abdomen, with relative sparing of periumbilical skin, and subsequently spread to involve the trunk and extremities. PUPP typically spares the face, palms, soles, scalp, and mucous membranes. The differential diagnosis includes drug eruption, erythema multiforme, scabies, and herpes gestationis, particularly in those patients with significant blistering. The etiology of PUPP is unknown. Because the rash is frequently found in striae, some workers have speculated that PUPP arises as a consequence of abdominal stretching.

A skin biopsy from affected skin of a patient with PUPP demonstrates a superficial perivascular and interstitial lymphohistiocytic infiltrate with eosinophils. Epidermal and dermal edema are prominent in urticarial lesions. Vesicular lesions show intense focal spongiosis, and eosinophilic spongiosis may be noted. In contrast to HG, DIF is negative.

Treatment

The treatment of PUPP is symptomatic. Emollient creams, especially those with menthol (Sarna), or cool baths with 1 cup of table vinegar or colloidal oatmeal (Aveeno) are helpful. For patients with persistent itch, antihistamines may be indicated. Topical antihistamines include topical doxepin (Zonalon Cream) and diphenhydramine (Caladryl) cream and lotion. The use of topical doxepin during lactation is contraindicated by the manufacturer; significant absorption of topical doxepin occurs, and the use of oral doxepin during lactation has been associated with apnea in an infant. Topical diphenhydramine should not be used as it is not effective in relieving pruritus in this situation and is a known contact sensitizer.

Oral antihistamines have been widely used for control of itching. However, recently concerns have emerged about the effect of antihistamines on the cardiovascular response to stress in a newborn infant. Many antihistamines also exert an anticholinergic effect, resulting in decreased milk production by the mother. If benefits of oral antihistamines are judged by the physician to outweigh the risks to the fetus, diphenhydramine (Benadryl), 25 to 50 mg orally, or hydroxyzine (Atarax), 10 to 30 mg every 6 hours, may be helpful. Nonsedating antihistamines usually have little effect in severe pruritus. If oral antihistamines are used, it is recommended that the time between drug administration and nursing be maximized. For patients unresponsive to symptomatic treatment, topical steroids for mild cases and systemic steroids for severe cases may be useful, with the caveats described earlier.

PRURITUS ANI AND VULVAE

method of
LIBBY EDWARDS, M.D.
Carolinas Medical Center
Charlotte, North Carolina

Anogenital skin is especially prone to irritation, not only from specific dermatoses and infections but also from exposure to perspiration, heat, and body secretions. Some patients are likely to perceive sensations produced by irritation as an itch. Scratching exacerbates irritation and intensifies itching. Therefore, the management of pruritus vulvae and pruritus ani requires the identification and elimination of irritation and interruption of the itch-scratch cycle.

Anogenital pruritus of sudden onset is most often due to an infection. Candidiasis and trichomoniasis are the most common infections producing vulvo-vaginal pruritus, whereas pinworms is a classic cause of anal pruritus. Other infections, including herpes simplex virus (HSV) infection, bacterial superinfection, and multiple genital warts that trap feces and keratin debris cause or complicate itching in some patients.

Chronic itching is usually associated with skin disease, especially eczema (also called atopic dermatitis, neurodermatitis, and lichen simplex chronicus). Sometimes referred to as the itch that rashes, eczema generally begins as itching in response to an irritant and is perpetuated by the irritation of scratching. Vulvar and perianal pruritus in women is sometimes caused by lichen sclerosus (et atrophicus), which is characterized by white, thin, crinkled, plaques of fragile skin. Superimposed irritant or allergic contact dermatitis to medications, cleansers, and overuse of water often complicate itching.

Less common but extremely recalcitrant causes of anogenital pruritus are depression and anxiety. These patients generally exhibit normal-appearing skin and are often visibly depressed or anxious in the physician's office.

The identification of causes and exacerbating factors for pruritus requires a careful history that includes the names and frequency of cleansers and medications that are applied to the area. Specific dermatoses can be identified by the clinical appearance, with a biopsy when needed either for diagnosis or, for refractory red, scaling anogenital skin, to rule out Paget's or Bowen's disease. Clear cellophane tape applied sticky side down to the perianal area before arising in the morning can then be affixed to a microscope slide and examined for ova of pinworms. A microscopic examination of vaginal secretions should be performed to identify any irritating discharge.

THERAPY

There are five specific issues to be addressed in each patient with anogenital pruritus.

First is the identification and elimination of any infection. Even when specific testing fails to yield the presence of an infection, empiric therapy is reasonable in the face of a high index of suspicion. For *Candida albicans*, any standard anticandidal therapy can be used. Those patients with extremely inflammatory or fissured skin are best treated with oral fluconazole (Diflucan), 150 mg once, since creams contain irritating alcohol. For those with crusting of the skin, or pustules suggestive of bacte-

rial folliculitis, an oral antistaphylococcal/antistreptococcal antibiotic should be prescribed and continued until the pruritus is controlled. The patient whose anogenital pruritus is driven or exacerbated by frequent recurrences of HSV infections should be maintained on suppressive oral acyclovir (Zovirax) at 400 mg twice a day. The treatment of bulky anogenital warts that produce itching due to retention of secretions and keratin debris often relieves itching.

Once infections have been addressed, the second specific intervention is the application of topical corticosteroids, which should be tried in virtually every patient. Even those with minimal skin findings often respond well to hydrocortisone cream 1% (over-the-counter) or 2.5% (by prescription) applied twice daily. Immediate itching is often improved by the addition of a local anesthetic, pramoxine, to hydrocortisone (Pramosone 1% or 2.5%). Patients with more significant inflammation, lichenification, or unresponsiveness to hydrocortisone can be given a trial of a midpotency corticosteroid such as triamcinolone (Kenalog, Aristocort) 0.1% on a short-term basis. Rarely, such as with extreme lichenification or lichen sclerosus, a higher-potency topical corticosteroid can be used for a limited time and with frequent follow-up. Those patients with very inflamed or excoriated skin tolerate ointment bases better than cream because of the alcohol contained in creams.

Third, careful local care is crucial to minimize ongoing irritation. A very common factor in anogenital pruritus is overwashing, so harsh soaps, antiseptics, deodorants, and even very frequent exposure to water should be eliminated. Some patients experience irritation from feces trapped between the perianal skin folds. Scrubbing with toilet paper often only serves to cause more irritation and leaves bits of paper in skin folds. However, gentle flushing of the skin with tepid water often removes remaining feces, and the skin can then be gently patted dry. In addition, Tucks pads can also gently remove remaining body secretions from the perianal area. Patients should be specifically instructed to avoid all topical agents to the area except for twice a day (at most) water and specifically prescribed medications. Some physicians believe that the avoidance of spicy foods and caffeine can improve itching by removing irritating remnants eliminated in feces.

Fourth, nighttime sedation is important. Although daytime itching cannot be controlled with medication, the patient can be sedated at night so that at least nighttime scratching does not perpetuate irritation. This can be achieved with sedating doses of antihistamines such as hydroxyzine HCl (Atarax), diphenhydramine (Benadryl), or the longer-acting amitriptyline (Elavil).

Finally, those patients with a prominent component of anxiety or depression should have that aspect specifically addressed. Most patients will have already noticed that minor itching escalates into a major problem in the presence of anxiety, depression, or stressful situations. Some patients require only a sympathetic ear and nighttime oral amitriptyline as an antidepressant and nighttime sedative. Other patients may require professional intervention.

Inadequate response to therapy is usually due to the failure of the physician to address all the above issues concomitantly or the failure to advise the patient of the tendency for recurrence with future irritants.

URTICARIA

method of
CHARLES D. KENNARD, M.D.
Wilford Hall Medical Center
Lackland AFB, Texas

Urticaria, which is recognized by wheals in the dermis, is a common affliction with a lifetime incidence of 15% to 20%. Angioedema is a similar condition, with acute edema involving the dermis and subcutaneous tissues, often of the perioral or genital regions or upper aerodigestive mucosa. Identification and avoidance of causative agents that directly or indirectly precipitate the whealing eruption is the most direct and effective therapy. This therapeutic approach is most applicable in cases of acute urticaria. Unfortunately, in most cases of long-standing urticaria, it is not possible to determine the triggering factors. Nevertheless, the treatment of urticaria may be guided by an understanding of the various pathophysiologic mechanisms involved even when clearly identifiable causes have not been identified. In this manner, trials of various medications, guided by the clinical response within the limits of acceptable side effects, may be necessary to find the optimal therapy.

EVALUATION: ACUTE URTICARIA

Urticaria is recognized by the appearance of variably pruritic wheals. The individual lesions persist for up to 24 hours, and crops of wheals may recur sporadically. Urticaria usually resolves spontaneously within a few months. Cases that resolve within 6 to 12 weeks have been termed acute urticaria; cases lasting longer are considered chronic. Food and medication exposures are the most common causes of acute urticaria. The patient is often suspicious of a possible offending agent, and the history alone may be sufficient to suggest the culprit. Elimination and addition diets may be useful in the evaluation of some cases. However, a period of 2 to 3 days between additions or deletions of a dietary item must be observed in order to differentiate true sensitivity from the normal variations in disease activity. Intracutaneous skin testing can rule out IgE-dependent food sensitivity, such as is seen with nuts, fish, and eggs. Other urticaria-inducing foods include shellfish and strawberries. Substances in food, such as salicylates, tartrazine, and benzoic acid derivatives (PABA), can cause urticaria. Cross-reaction to *Candida* and food yeasts may be manifested as urticaria; such patients may be helped by anticandidal therapy and a low yeast diet.

A detailed medication history should be obtained. Penicillin is the medication most commonly causing urticaria, which it does through IgE-dependent mechanisms. Radiocontrast media, opiates, and other medications can produce urticaria by directly causing mast cell degranulation without IgE mediation. Aspirin, perhaps through interactions

with the arachidonic acid metabolic pathways and inhibition of prostaglandin synthesis, can produce urticaria and/or angioedema. In some patients, aspirin-induced urticaria is seen in association with nasal polyps and asthma, often with a familial pattern.

Contact urticaria is, in my opinion, an unusual form of urticaria. The most frequent source of contact urticaria is probably latex. Patients with an IgE-mediated hypersensitivity to latex are often medical workers or patients with frequent contact with catheters or other latex-containing medical equipment. Reactions may be severe, with rapid anaphylaxis and collapse. Thus, testing for such possible latex allergic responses must be performed in controlled settings with appropriate supportive equipment and trained personnel immediately available.

Hereditary angioedema is an autosomal dominant trait having a deficiency of serum inhibitor of the activated first component of complement. It is manifested by acute isolated *painful*, rather than pruritic, edema. Angioedema can potentially cause fatal upper airway obstruction, precipitated by trauma or other stress. A frequently noted presentation is laryngeal edema following dental procedures. The biochemical marker is usually a lack of C1 esterase inhibitor, although functional deficiency of the inhibitor with normal levels of the inhibitor by immunoassay is seen in 15% of cases. Evaluation should include assay of C4 levels, which are chronically low, C1 inhibitor immunoassay, and possibly a functional assay if the immunoassay levels are normal.

EVALUATION: CHRONIC URTICARIA

In an uncertain proportion of patients, initially episodic urticaria progresses to a continuous, chronic form of the disorder. This chronic urticaria remits in about 50% of cases within one year, but 20% of patients continue to have urticaria for more than 20 years. Diagnostic testing is relevant to this subgroup of chronic urticaria. Efficacious, and cost-effective, evaluations require an individualized approach to the patient's clinical condition and often to the patient's emotional need to know a "cause" of the urticaria.

Unfortunately, the etiology of chronic urticaria is determined in less than 25% of cases. Again, the medical history may be most helpful: patients may have an opinion about the triggering of their urticaria, or they may have symptoms of sinusitis, arthralgias, urinary symptoms, or constitutional symptoms pointing to an underlying etiology. Such symptoms may direct the physical examination to the indicated areas, with laboratory examinations as indicated from the findings. A "shotgun" approach to laboratory studies rarely uncovers an infection or connective tissue disease as the cause of urticaria that was not suggested by the history or physical examination. However, some studies have indicated that occult sinus infections may be a treatable cause of urticaria. Thus, a useful screening protocol of laboratory examinations for patients with chronic urticaria may be those confirmatory tests for conditions specifically suggested by the patient's history or physical examination, with a sinus roentgenogram series for all other patients.

For extreme cases, when the initial evaluation is negative and symptoms have persisted for several months, more in-depth laboratory testing could include the erythrocyte sedimentation rate (ESR) to screen for inflammatory or occult neoplastic processes. A complete blood count (CBC) with differential might show an elevated white blood cell count as an indication of an infection, with eosinophilia possibly implicating a helminthic disease, atopy, or drug eruption. Hepatitis B and infectious mononucleosis may both be associated with urticaria and have abnormal serum transaminase levels and abnormal liver function values. Abnormal renal function tests and urinalysis may indicate nephritis or urinary tract infection. Antinuclear antibodies, rheumatoid factor, serum complement (C3 and C4), and/or cryoglobulins may point to autoimmune disease or cold-induced urticaria. Cold urticaria may also be detected by simple testing with an ice cube applied to the forearm. Cholinergic urticaria can be diagnosed when very small urticarial papules appear on a large background flare following a provocative challenge of perspiration-inducing exercise. Pressure urticaria and other forms of physical urticarias may be confirmed through appropriate stimulatory challenges. Stool guaiac testing and chest roentgenogram may reveal occult malignancies that rarely present through urticaria. Urticarial vasculitis, an uncommon whealing eruption, is characterized by individual lesions that persist for greater than the 24 hours of duration specified in the diagnosis of other urticarial disorders. Urticarial vasculitis is often associated with hepatitis B or C, mononucleosis, and autoimmune disorders.

THERAPEUTIC APPROACH

Acute Urticaria

Since the cause of acute urticaria is most likely to be an ingested food or medication, avoidance of the offending substance may be all that is required for relief. Symptoms of whealing and pruritus are usually controllable with oral antihistamines of the H_1 class. Hydroxyzine (Atarax), 10 to 50 mg three or four times daily, is my choice for urticaria since it appears to have less "hangover" from bedtime doses, and tolerance to side effects often develops early in treatment. Diphenhydramine (Benadryl), 25 to 100 mg three to four times daily, is effective but is often overly sedating for daytime use. Cyproheptadine (Periactin), 4 mg four times daily, is especially useful for cold-induced urticaria. Chlorpheniramine (Chlortrimeton), 8 to 12 mg twice daily, or triprolidine (Actidil), 2.5 mg four times daily, may produce less drowsiness but central nervous system (CNS) stimulation or irritability is seen in some patients; sustained-release forms are available. To lessen these side effects, newer, nonsedating antihistamines have been produced; see the discussion in the Chronic Urticaria section. When these methods are ineffective, oral prednisone, 40 mg each morning tapering over 10 to 14 days, should give relief.

In the case of hereditary angioedema, long-term prophylaxis can be achieved with oral androgens. Stanozolol (Winstrol),* 2 mg three times daily, and then reduction of dose to the lowest possible is effective. Short-term prophylaxis in a previously untreated patient can be achieved with 2 U of fresh-frozen plasma.

Severe urticaria or angioedema that is accompanied by signs of compromised respiration or the potential of circulatory collapse may require subcutaneous injection of epinephrine, 0.3 to 0.5 mL of 1:1000. Supplemental oxygen should be given in accordance

with the patient's clinical picture, and pulse oximetry readings and intravenous access should be established in such cases and intubation/tracheostomy should be immediately available. Intravenous diphenhydramine, 50 to 100 mg, may be a useful supplement. In cases of severe reactions, systemic corticosteroids and hospitalization for observation and airway management are indicated.

Chronic Urticaria

Unfortunately, the vast majority of chronic urticaria cases do not have an easily identifiable cause, but the end result is the same: histamine that has been released from mast cells interacts with the H_1 receptor on dermal vasculature, producing edema. Thus, antihistamines are the therapeutic cornerstone in chronic urticaria. Other general, non-specific treatment should include the avoidance of possible triggering factors such as opiates, aspirin, heat, exercise, and alcohol if these factors are present.

Side effects are common in traditional H_1 antihistamine therapy; sedation occurs regularly with all classes of traditional H_1 antihistamines. The sedation at bedtime may provide relief from the exacerbation of pruritus that plagues many patients as they attempt to fall asleep. Tachyphylaxis to this hypnotic effect may develop with continued use. Additional side effects that may be seen with this class of medication include dizziness, incoordination, blurred vision, diplopia, and paradoxical symptoms of CNS stimulation, particularly in young children and elderly people. Seizure activity may be induced in patients with focal lesions in the CNS. Anticholinergic effects such as dryness of mucous membranes, urinary retention, palpitations, agitation, and increased intraocular pressure may be seen. Phenothiazine-class antihistamines can produce a cholestatic jaundice. Since traditional H_1 antihistamines can induce hepatic microsomal enzymes, medications such as warfarin (Coumadin), griseofulvin (Gris-PEG), and phenytoin (Dilantin) that are metabolized by this route may have decreased effectiveness.

A new generation of antihistamines has been developed that do not significantly cross the blood-brain barrier, have little anticholinergic activity, and are nonsedating. Most of these second-generation antihistamines have a prolonged half-life, permitting once daily dosing. For these reasons, nonsedating antihistamines are the treatment of choice for chronic, idiopathic urticaria. Terfenadine (Seldane), 60 mg twice daily or 120 mg once a day, astemizole (Hismanal), 10 mg once daily, loratadine (Claritin), 10 mg daily, and cetirizine (Zyrtec), 10 mg daily, are all effective with little or no sedation. With cetirizine, the incidence of sedation is slightly higher than in placebo. Astemizole may produce increased appetite with or without weight gain. Astemizole and loratidine should be taken on an empty stomach. Terfenadine and astemizole can cause torsades de pointes, a potentially fatal ventricular arrhythmia, when these medications are taken in overdosage. This can also

---

*Not FDA-approved for this indication.

occur when they are taken concomitantly with medications that would compromise their hepatic metabolism by the cytochrome P450 enzyme system or in the face of medical conditions limiting the liver's metabolic capacity or predisposing to a prolonged electrocardiographic QT interval.

ALTERNATIVE THERAPIES

For some patients who do not respond to H_1 antihistamines alone, the addition of an H_2 antagonist such as cimetidine (Tagamet),* 400 mg four times daily, may aid in the control of their symptoms. Beta-agonists such as terbutaline (Brethine),* 2.5 mg orally three times daily, and other agents that raise mast cell intracellular cAMP levels may have a small effect on controlling chronic urticaria in some patients, but they cannot be relied upon as first-line medications for this disorder. The calcium channel blocker nifedipine (Procardia),* 10 mg up to three times daily, can rarely improve the control of chronic, idiopathic urticaria when added to a regimen of traditional or nonsedating H_1 and H_2 antihistamines. Tricyclic antidepressants are potent antagonists of H_1 histamine receptors. Doxepin is 700 times more potent on a molar basis than diphenhydramine as an in vitro H_1 blocker, and doxepin (Sinequan),* 10 mg three times daily, can be more effective than diphenhydramine in controlling symptoms. Doxepin has been formulated in a topical form (Zonalon cream), but unless urticarial symptoms are restricted to a specific area of skin, it would offer no benefit in the treatment of chronic urticaria. Systemic corticosteroids may give temporary respite from an overwhelming bout with chronic urticaria. However, the severe side effects associated with the prolonged use of corticosteroids, such as adrenal suppression and exacerbation of hypertension and diabetes, prevent their regular or sustained use in chronic urticaria. Oral cyclosporine (Sandimmune),* 6 mg per kg per day, can produce rapid resolution of severe, chronic urticaria and angioedema. Cost and systemic immune suppression limit its use. Recent studies have shown evidence for a circulating histamine-releasing factor, perhaps an IgG autoantibody to IgE, and patients with severe, chronic idiopathic urticaria can be significantly improved for up to 2 months by a week-long course of plasmapheresis.

PIGMENTARY ALTERATIONS

method of
DEREK B. WOOLNER, M.D., and
KEYOUMARS SOLTANI, M.D.
University of Chicago
Chicago, Illinois

LOCALIZED HYPERPIGMENTATION

Melanin within the epidermis produces shades of tan, brown, or black. When melanin is situated in the dermis, it may appear gray or blue because of light scattering from dermal collagen. Making this distinction on examination may predict responsiveness to therapy. Conditions in which the pigmentation is epidermal are more amenable to topical therapy than are those conditions in which melanin is situated in the dermis.

The most frequent cause of acquired pigmentary abnormalities, both hypo- and hyperpigmentation, is cutaneous injury or inflammation. The spectrum of inflammatory skin diseases that eventuate in pigmentary disturbance is broad, from acne to psoriasis, eczema, or lichen planus. The darker an individual's skin color, the more likely that postinflammatory pigmentary change will develop after cutaneous injury. Therapy begins with adequately treating the underlying disease process, if possible, to prevent or limit injury. Further therapy may include hydroquinone preparations, which are available in a 2% strength over the counter and by prescription at 3% and 4%, applied to the hyperpigmented skin twice a day. An unusual but notable complication of hydroquinone preparations is paradoxical darkening of the skin with prolonged application. If hydroquinone preparations have not produced results in 3 months, they should be discontinued as it is unlikely that more extended therapy will succeed. The use of topical tretinoin (Retin-A)* at bedtime has also proved effective in treating postinflammatory pigmentation, beginning with the 0.025% cream and progressing to 0.1% cream or 0.05% gel as tolerated. Tretinoin and hydroquinone may have an additive effect when used together. Unfortunately, in many cases of postinflammatory pigmentation, the melanin is situated in the dermis and is poorly responsive to therapy.

Melasma or chloasma is characterized by tan-to-brown pigmentation of the sun-exposed face, especially the forehead, temples, and malar cheeks. Melasma occurs much more frequently in women, and estrogen appears to be important in causation, whether in the setting of pregnancy or with the oral contraceptive pill. In treatment, exogenous estrogen should be discontinued when possible. The most important aspect of therapy must be a focus on sun protection. The areas of hyperpigmentation are more responsive to ultraviolet light than adjacent skin, and sun exposure accentuates contrast with the normal skin. Women should be encouraged to apply a sunscreen of at least SPF 15 daily throughout the year.

Hydroquinone preparations twice a day or tretinoin at bedtime is useful in many women and as noted, a combination of these products enhances efficacy. However, tretinoin may prove irritating to many women, especially at higher concentrations of 0.1%. To overcome this irritancy, 5% hydroquinone and 0.1% tretinoin can be compounded by a pharmacist in 0.1% dexamethasone* ointment; this combination is applied twice a day. More recently, alpha-hydroxy acid preparations such as lactic and glycolic

---

*Not FDA-approved for this indication.

*Not FDA-approved for this indication.

acids have been promoted for melasma. Despite cosmetic company claims and anecdotal reports, the value of these products for this indication remains to be proved. Chemical peeling has been reported to be of value in at least some patients whose melasma is unresponsive to other topical therapy. More recently, lasers have been used for a variety of pigment disorders.

GENERALIZED HYPERPIGMENTATION

Addison's disease is the endocrinopathy classically associated with hyperpigmentation, but acromegaly and hyperthyroidism can also be characterized by generalized darkening of the skin. Among metabolic diseases, hemochromatosis produces hyperpigmentation in up to 90% of patients.

Drugs are an important cause of generalized pigment change. Drug eruptions (and indeed erythroderma of any cause) may resolve with widespread postinflammatory change. Prolonged use of chlorpromazine can result in blue-gray pigmentation over sun-exposed skin of the face, neck, chest, and hands. Phenytoin and the antimalarials chloroquine and hydroxychloroquine are also important causes of drug-induced hyperpigmentation. The antineoplastic agents busulfan (Myleran), cyclophosphamide (Cytoxan), bleomycin (Blenoxane), and doxorubicin (Adriamycin) figure prominently in the differential diagnosis of drug-induced hyperpigmentation.

LOCALIZED HYPOPIGMENTATION

Diminution of pigment is properly called hypopigmentation, and complete absence of melanin pigmentation is referred to as depigmentation. The clinical distinction between hypopigmented and depigmented skin can be difficult. The use of an ultraviolet light source, a Wood's lamp, can aid in the identification of hypopigmented lesions and may also allow distinction between hypomelanosis and depigmentation. The distinction between true depigmentation and hypopigmentation is necessary if one is to separate vitiligo (characterized by depigmentation) from most other diseases of hypopigmentation in which some shades of tan or brown persist. Strictly speaking, depigmented skin is not white, but rather pink. Those disorders that produce truly white areas of skin are characterized by scarring with evidence of dermal sclerosis or epidermal change, such as atrophy. Thus, the lesions of morphea or lichen sclerosus et atrophicus or the healed lesions of discoid lupus erythematosus may be white, but on careful examination it will be appreciated that the pigmentary change is not the primary cutaneous abnormality.

Vitiligo features prominently in the differential diagnosis of any local loss of skin pigment. It affects about 1% of the population but is most disabling in individuals of darker skin tones. Melanocytes in affected skin have been destroyed, and the areas are therefore truly depigmented. Facial skin, especially perioral and periocular skin, is frequently involved, as are the hands and feet. There is sharp delineation of normal skin from depigmented skin, and the patches lack scaling or dermal change. In darker skin types, the borders of vitiliginous patches may be transiently hypomelanotic in the process of evolving to depigmentation. Vitiligo appears to result from the autoimmune destruction of melanocytes and is associated with autoimmune endocrine disease, especially thyroid disease. Although a high level of suspicion must be maintained for endocrine disease in these patients, testing of thyroid indices or other endocrinologic investigation should be guided by clinical findings and not performed as screening investigations.

When counseling patients, remember that the depigmented skin of vitiligo sunburns easily and that tanning emphasizes the contrast between normal and diseased skin; these patients need to use high SPF sunscreens daily. Camouflage with makeup is a technique that can be used in a variety of pigmentary abnormalities, especially vitiligo. Brands like Covermark and Dermablend are available in many shades suitable for blending with normal skin tones, and with careful application they can effectively disguise either hypo- or hyperpigmentation.

Topical corticosteroids are effective as initial therapy of vitiligo in 40% of cases. Higher-potency steroids produce the best responses, but atrophy and other local side effects limit their use, especially on the face. The young age of many patients demands caution in choice of steroids, and a preparation like 2.5% hydrocortisone may be appropriate on the face of a child as initial therapy. Use of even "weak" steroid preparations around the eyes may be associated with cataracts and glaucoma, and therapy of periocular vitiligo must be closely monitored. Midpotency preparations such as 0.1% triamcinolone acetonide may be reasonable initial therapy in adults. The potent (e.g., 0.05% fluocinonide) and superpotent agents (e.g., 0.05% betamethasone dipropionate or 0.05% clobetasol) may be necessary on the hands or arms. If no improvement is evident after 6 weeks of therapy, consider alternatives.

The single most efficacious therapeutic modality in vitiligo is the PUVA (psoralen and ultraviolet A). PUVA involves ultraviolet A exposure after administration of psoralen, which is a photosensitizing compound. The psoralen can be administered topically for very limited disease, although more typically it is given orally. Therapy with PUVA is often prolonged and may require a year or more for good response. An evolving therapy for vitiligo is the grafting of melanocytes to repigment diseased skin.

When entertaining the diagnosis of vitiligo, it is important to consider the possible role of chemicals in producing the depigmentation. Phenolic compounds are used as germicides but can also be toxic to melanocytes. When incorporated in cleaning agents, these substituted phenols can produce occupational depigmentation, usually of the hands but also at sites not directly contacted. Careful inquiry must be made into the job description of persons presenting with "vitiligo" of the hands. The role of hydroquinones as bleaching agents has been discussed earlier, but any discussion of chemical depigmentation merits inclusion of the compound monobenzylether of hydroquinone (Benoquin), which acts to depigment skin permanently. Use of this compound should be reserved for cases of widespread vitiligo that are unresponsive to therapy and when the decision has been made to achieve uniformity of pigment by destroying remaining melanocytes. Monobenzylether of hydroquinone should not be used for lightening any form of hyperpigmentation.

Cutaneous inflammation can resolve with hypopigmentation as well as with hyperpigmentation, as discussed earlier. The history should clearly identify antecedent injury or eruption. Eczematous eruptions, especially in darker skin types, are frequently followed by hypopigmentation. Pityriasis alba is an eczematous eruption of childhood in which hypopigmentation is the prominent feature of the clinical presentation. The process is characterized by ill-defined, hypomelanotic macules, usually on the face. Faint scaling may be observed. These individuals are frequently, but not always, atopic. Itch is not a prominent symptom. Therapy for pityriasis alba should focus on moisturization and mild steroids. The condition will resolve without residual pigmentary change, but the skin can be slow to repigment, often requiring many months to improve.

A discussion of the diagnosis and treatment of tinea versicolor is available in the article on superficial fungal infections. However, it is worthy of note that tinea versicolor regularly presents with hyperpigmented truncal lesions in light-skinned individuals and hypopigmented patches in darker-skinned patients. Even after the fungal overgrowth is treated and scaling has subsided, return to normal skin color may require months.

In darker-skinned individuals, sarcoidosis may present as hypopigmented patches. In much of the world, the strongest and perhaps most feared association with hypopigmented patches is leprosy. The finding of hypopigmented patches or plaques that demonstrate decreased sensation, especially temperature sensation, should suggest the diagnosis.

GENERALIZED HYPOPIGMENTATION

Much of this category is occupied by congenital diseases. Albinism is characterized by profound pigmentary dilution secondary to absent or defective tyrosinase, a key enzyme in melanogenesis. Other diseases of pigment dilution are largely congenital and beyond the scope of this discussion.

SUNBURN

method of
DAVID R. BICKERS, M.D., and
MARY GAIL MERCURIO, M.D.
Columbia-Presbyterian Medical Center
New York, New York

From ancient times through the early part of this century, men and women of affluence carefully protected themselves from sunlight exposure so as to distinguish themselves from outdoor, manual laborers. This theme has been reversed in modern times, in which a suntan has come to symbolize leisure, wealth, and beauty. Despite the media's zealous attempts to publicize the adverse effects of sunlight, getting a tan remains highly desirable. Perhaps this phenomenon is best exemplified by the increasing popularity of maintaining a year-round suntan through the use of tanning salons.

Sunlight is a form of transmitted energy and a component of the broad spectrum of electromagnetic radiation, which also includes higher-energy cosmic, gamma, and x-rays, as well as lower-energy infrared, microwave, and radio waves. Each component of the electromagnetic spectrum has specific and unique properties, including characteristic wavelength, frequency, and photon energy. The photon energy is the product of the frequency and Planck's constant. Wavelength and frequency are inversely proportional and their product is a constant, the speed of light. Shorter wavelength radiation has greater photon energy— i.e., 400-nm radiation has twice as much energy per photon as 800-nm radiation.

The sunlight portion of the electromagnetic spectrum including ultraviolet and visible light is most relevant to dermatology. Visible light ranges from 400 to 750 nm, with red having the longest wavelength and lowest energy and violet having the shortest wavelength and highest energy. Adjacent to the visible red light is the infra*red* region and adjacent to the violet visible light is the ultra*violet* region. Ultraviolet radiation (UVR) possesses higher-energy photons than visible light and thus has greater tendency toward photochemical reactions and photobiologic responses. UVR encompasses the wavelengths from 200 to 400 nm and is divided into three segments: UVA (320 to 400 nm), UVB (290 to 320 nm), and UVC (200 to 290 nm).

UVA penetrates window glass and interacts with a variety of systemic medications. It causes immediate and delayed tanning, while contributing minimally to sunburn erythema. UVB is absorbed by window glass and is principally responsible for erythema (sunburn), suntanning, and cutaneous carcinogenesis. UVC is completely absorbed by stratospheric ozone and does not reach the earth's surface. The varying effects of these wavelengths of ultraviolet light form the basis for the arbitrary division into UVA, UVB, and UVC (Table 1).

Light imparts important detrimental biologic effects on the skin. Exposure to certain wavelengths of light is essential to the pathogenesis of a variety of dermatologic disorders and critical to the exacerbation of others. The role of this ubiquitous environmental carcinogen in the pathogenesis of skin cancer is a subject of great concern. Molecular biologic advances have provided much insight on the role of oncogenes and tumor suppressor genes in ultraviolet carcinogenesis. Epidemiologic evidence strongly sug-

TABLE 1. **Characteristics of UV and Visible Light**

Light Type	% of Solar Radiation Reaching Earth's Surface	Wavelength (nm)	Depth of Penetrance	Window Glass Penetrance	Ozone Layer Absorption (%)	Erythrogenicity	Carcinogenicity	Delayed Tanning
UVC	0	200–290	Epidermis	—	100	+ + +	+ + +	—
UVB	1.7	290–320	Papillary dermis	—	90	+ +	+ +	+ +
UVA	6.3	320–400	Reticular dermis	+	0	+	+	+
Visible	92	400–800	Subcutis	+	0	—	—	+

—, Little to no effect; +, mild effect; + +, moderate effect; + + +, great effect.

gests that UVB is preferentially responsible for sunburn and skin cancer induction. The UVA region, on the other hand, is most frequently implicated in photosensitivity reactions in which chemical photosensitizers and UVA radiation interact to cause biologic phenomena. UVB is essential for vitamin D photosynthesis, and this appears to be the only useful interaction between the skin and sunlight. The therapeutic application of UVA and UVB is effective in several dermatologic diseases, including psoriasis, cutaneous T cell lymphoma, vitiligo, atopic dermatitis, and pruritus associated with renal failure and human immunodeficiency virus (HIV) infection.

Ozone depletion is a significant concern because stratospheric ozone is the primary agent responsible for limiting biologically damaging solar UVC radiation from reaching the earth. Ozone is created by the absorption of high-energy solar radiation, which splits doublet oxygen molecules. The resultant singlet oxygen species recombine with other doublets to form triplet oxygen, the ozone molecule. Ultraviolet radiation makes up only 8% of the solar energy that reaches the earth's surface (6.3% UVA and 1.7% UVB). All UVC and 90% of UVB radiation are blocked by ozone, whereas UVA is unaffected by the ozone barrier. Most of the increased transmission of UVR as a result of ozone depletion will be in the shorter wavelength, more energetic UVB. Mathematical models suggest that ozone depletion will result in increased skin cancer incidence, including basal cell carcinoma, squamous cell carcinoma, and malignant melanomas. The skin is the most relevant organ implicated in UVR-induced damage; with the exception of the minimal amount of radiation absorbed through the eye, all radiant energy absorbed by the human body requires transmission through the skin, where virtually all of it is absorbed in the epidermis and the dermis. Specifically, about 90% of incident UVB and 50% of incident UVA is absorbed by the epidermis and attenuated within the uppermost papillary dermis. Melanin strongly absorbs both visible and ultraviolet light and is a major absorbing entity (chromophore) in the skin.

Erythema is the most obvious result of the sunburn reaction. The intensity of UVA or UVB reaching the skin is referred to as irradiance and is subject to numerous variables, including time of day, geographic latitude, season, altitude, and interference by atmospheric pollution. The minimum erythema dose (MED) is defined as the minimum dose of UVR producing clearly marginated erythema at the site of exposure. The human population varies widely in its susceptibility to sunburn erythema. Individuals who are fair-skinned and tend to sunburn easily demonstrate MEDs of 20 to 40 mJ per cm^2, as compared with the MED for individuals of darker color in whom the MED may exceed 200 mJ per cm^2.

UVB, often referred to as the "erythema range of UV light," readily produces painful redness, and severe blistering sunburn can occur in susceptible individuals with as little as five to eight times the MED. UVB is 1000 times more efficient at causing erythema than UVA. UVA's contribution is, however, quite relevant because much more UVA than UVB is present in the solar spectrum; i.e., UVA irradiance far exceeds that of UVB. Throughout the day, more UVA reaches the earth's surface, and this discrepancy is greatest in the morning and evening. UVB irradiance is maximal during midday when the sun is directly overhead, because with increasing solar zenith angle, the atmospheric attenuation of UVB exceeds that of UVA. UVA exposure favors the development of a sun*tan* over a sun*burn*, but this concept has been greatly exploited by the tanning salon industry touting misleading claims such as, "the *healthy* tan without the harmful effects of UVB radiation."

One approach to defining individual variability in responding to sunlight is known as skin typing and this can be ascertained by asking: Do you always, sometimes, or never burn and tan? (Table 2).

The increased pigmentation evident following UVR exposure is bimodal. Immediate pigment darkening (IPD), first described by Meirowsky, causes a transient blue-gray hue and is induced by UVA or visible light. It begins during or minutes after irradiation,

TABLE 2. **Skin Typing in Tanning Ability**

Skin Type	Tanning Ability	Complexion
I	Always burns, never tans	Very fair
II	Often burns, tans minimally	Fair
III	Burns moderately, tans gradually	Lightly pigmented
IV	Burns minimally, tans easily	Moderately pigmented
V	Rarely burns, tans profusely	Darkly pigmented
VI	Never burns	Very darkly pigmented

fades within a few hours, and can be prevented by rendering the skin hypoxic. The proposed mechanism is photo-oxidation of existing melanin and its transfer from melanocytes to keratinocytes. It is most easily seen in whites with darker complexions (skin types IV to VI). There is no associated increase in melanosomes or melanocytes, and IPD does not appear to provide protection against subsequent UVR.

Delayed tanning (DT) is primarily a response to UVB, although it also follows UVA and UVC irradiation. After UVB irradiation, erythema begins in 3 to 5 hours and reaches a maximum at about 15 hours. Erythema fades over several days to be replaced by tanning and desquamation. This process is associated with increases in tyrosinase activity, size and number of melanocytes, and synthesis and transfer of melanosomes—all of which result in darker skin color. The function of DT is to protect basal cells and underlying structures from subsequent UVR.

Melanin pigmentation of human skin can be divided into two categories: (1) constitutive or intrinsic skin color, and (2) facultative or inducible skin color. Constitutive skin color is the genetically programmed level of melanin pigmentation that defines an individual's skin type. Facultative skin color characterizes the UVR-induced increase in melanin pigmentation beyond the constitutive level and is commonly referred to as a suntan. Melanin pigment is a superb filter reflecting, scattering, and absorbing incident UVR and visible light. Thus constitutive pigmentation in Type V and Type VI individuals affords substantial protection from UVR. Resistance to the induction of erythema by UVR is conferred by both constitutive and facultative pigmentation. The mechanism of UVR-induced melanocyte activation is unknown; the importance of other methods to diminish the injurious effects of melanogenesis through intermediates such as antioxidants and enhancers of DNA repair is a major focus of current research.

Melanin is not the only photoprotective component in the skin. Another consequence of UVR is to stimulate keratinocyte proliferation with resulting hyperplasia. The preferential thickening of the stratum corneum confers a greater optical barrier to subsequent UVR, thereby shielding the vulnerable cells of the basal and suprabasal layers. Albino skin, despite its lack of melanin, can tolerate some degree of UVR, owing to decreased transmission through thickened skin. It has been suggested that epidermal ornithine decarboxylase (ODC), the rate-limiting step in the polyamine biosynthetic pathway, may be involved in this stimulation of epidermal proliferation.

Following skin exposure to UVR, there is a transient depression in DNA, RNA, and protein synthesis, reaching a nadir after 1 to 6 hours, followed by a sustained increase in mitotic activity peaking at 24 to 48 hours. Absorption of UVR leads to cellular damage, with resultant disruption of tissue function and inflammation clinically manifested as erythema, pain, heat, and swelling. Normal skin responds acutely to UV light exposure with complex inflammatory mechanisms. Eicosanoids play an important role as soluble mediators in immunologic suppression as well as the delayed erythema response and in DT. This is evidenced by the fact that their production parallels erythema onset, and eicosanoid inhibition decreases UVB erythema. Arachidonic acid metabolites—prostaglandin E_2 (PGE_2), PGD_2, $PGF_{2\alpha}$ and 12-hydroxyeicosatetraenoic acid (12-HETE)—are increased in suction blister aspirates immediately following exposure to UVB, with peak concentrations at 18 to 24 hours. UVB erythema is suppressed up to 50% by administration of cyclo-oxygenase inhibitors within 24 hours after injury. Following UVB irradiation, there is also increased cytokine elaboration, including epidermal interleukin-1, interleukin-6, and tumor necrosis factor production, and keratinocyte intercellular adhesion molecule (ICAM-1) expression. Increased histamine levels and mast cell degranulation also occur at the onset of UVB erythema in human skin.

Topical corticosteroids and cool compresses provide some relief in the management of moderate sunburn. Oral nonsteroidal agents are also helpful in suppressing prostaglandin formation in the skin. Severe sunburn can be improved by administration of a rapidly tapered course of oral corticosteroids, at a dose of 1 mg per kg of prednisone, within a few hours of sun exposure. A severe blistering sunburn is not unlike a second-degree thermal burn in which fluid management and meticulous wound care to prevent infection are critical. However, the best way to treat sunburn is to prevent it in the first place. This can be achieved by appropriate clothing and by the application of sunscreen preparations.

Sunscreens are increasingly being used with the growing awareness of the harmful effects of sunlight exposure, particularly the increasing incidence of skin cancer. Sunscreens were initially categorized as cosmetics until 1978, when the United States Food and Drug Administration reclassified these agents as drugs intended to protect "the structure and function of human integument against actinic damage." Topical sunscreens can be divided into two broad categories: chemical and physical agents. The great majority of sunscreens function as artificial chromophores by absorbing incident radiation, thereby preventing UVR from reaching the skin. Sunscreen absorbers are generally aromatic compounds, and conjugation of this aromatic ring by UVR enables conversion of high-energy UVR through resonance localization into harmless long-wave radiation that is re-emitted as insignificant quantities of heat. Chemical sunscreens can be further divided into UVA and UVB absorbers.

The most common categories of UVB sunscreens include para-aminobenzoic acid (PABA) and PABA esters (padimate O), salicylates (octyl salicylate), and cinnamates. These substances absorb little in the UVA or visible range; consequently, they are not protective in patients with UVA or visible light sensitivities—i.e., porphyria, polymorphous drug eruption, phytotoxicity, photoallergy, or solar urticaria. Sunscreen efficacy can be quantified as sun protection factor (SPF), which defines UVB protection afforded by the preparation. It is defined by the ratio of UVB required to produce an MED in sunscreen-protected skin compared with nonprotected skin.

The recent accumulation of data implicating the contribution of UVA to the deleterious effects of UVR has enhanced awareness of the need for broader-spectrum sun protection. Benzophenones and anthranilates absorb to a limited extent in the short UVA range. The dibenzoylmethanes, including avobenzone (e.g., Parsol 1789), are sunscreens capable of absorbing energy across the entire UVA range. No standardized test for assessing UVA protection similar to the SPF for UVB has been defined. One approach to measuring UVA photo protection is based on the amount of UVA needed to produce a phototoxic response in sunscreen-protected photosensitized skin compared with unprotected photosensitized skin. The agents most commonly employed as photosensitizers are psoralens and fluoranthene.

Chemical sunscreens have varying substantivity (ability to adhere to skin) and potential for inducing sensitization. Reactions to sunscreens are quite common, and all sunscreen groups have been reported to cause allergic reactions—either contact (irritant or allergic) or photocontact in nature. Patch testing of suspected ingredients can identify the causative agent and allow for selection of a nonreactive sunscreen. PABA is responsible for more sensitization reactions than any other sunscreen compound. Cross-sensitization is also a factor in the case of PABA, which is chemically similar to several drugs, including thiazide diuretics and sulfonamides.

The second major category of sunscreens is physical blocking agents. They protect by reflecting the sun's rays from a film of inert metal particles. Examples include zinc oxide and titanium dioxide. They block the broadest spectrum of light, including ultraviolet and visible. Because they do not rely on a chemical reaction to photoprotect, they are appropriate for individuals sensitive to chemical sunscreens. In the past, use of these agents was limited by their cosmetic unacceptability owing to their high visibility and occlusiveness. Recent advances in micronization into smaller particles has yielded products with much greater cosmetic acceptability.

The use of sunscreens is the most effective means of preventing the adverse sequelae of excessive sun exposure. Although more research is needed to clarify the potential effects of sunscreens, most agree that the benefits of sunscreen use far outweigh the risks. In the meantime, other photoprotective practices, in addition to sunscreens, must be encouraged, such as avoidance of peak midday exposure and the use of protective clothing. Chemoprevention with retinoids, beta carotene, and other substances may also play important roles in the future, although current evidence is insufficient to justify their widespread use at this time.

The Nervous System

BRAIN ABSCESS

method of
MAURICE MURPHY, M.B., and
DONALD ARMSTRONG, M.D.
Memorial Sloan-Kettering Cancer Center
New York, New York

Brain abscess is a focal suppurative process of the brain parenchyma. Although uncommon, it remains a serious and life-threatening condition. More effective antimicrobial agents and, in particular, improved diagnostic modalities of computed tomography (CT) scanning and magnetic resonance imaging (MRI) have led to a significant lowering of mortality rates from brain abscess in the past 2 decades. Although mortality had decreased, morbidity and neurologic sequelae remain considerable.

PATHOGENESIS AND MICROBIOLOGY

Brain abscess can arise from direct spread of infection from a contiguous site (e.g., middle ear, paranasal sinus, dental infection), hematogenous spread from a remote site of infection, and by direct inoculation of microorganisms into brain parenchyma from a penetrating injury or surgery. In many instances no obvious source of infection can be identified. Such cryptogenic abcesses account for 15% to 20% of all cases. Suppurative processes of the paranasal sinuses and middle ear are the most common sources of underlying infection, accounting for almost half of reported cases. Contiguous spread of infection from an extracranial site occurs through direct extension of osteomyelitis or by retrograde thrombophlebitis of the diploic veins.

The distribution of brain abscesses frequently reflects the contiguous focus of infection from paranasal sinuses or middle ear/mastoid. Frontal and temporal lobes are most commonly involved, followed by the parietal lobe, cerebellum, and occipital lobe. Brain abscesses that result from hematogenous spread of infection occur most commonly in the distribution of the middle cerebral artery (predominantly the parietal and temporal lobes). Less common sites such as thalamus and brain stem are usually the result of metastatic infection. Metastatic abscesses tend to be poorly encapsulated and are often multiple. Typically they manifest in the watershed area of the corticomedullary junction where blood flow is slowest and collateral circulation least. Congenital cyanotic heart disease is one of the common predisposing factors for hematogenously derived brain abscess. Patients with hereditary telangiectasia (Osler-Weber-Rendu disease) or other conditions with arteriovenous shunts also have an increased lifetime risk of developing brain abscess. Right-to-left shunting allows blood-borne bacteria to bypass filtering by the pulmonary capillary bed. In addition, long-standing hypoxemia leads to polycythemia and hyperviscosity predisposing to microinfarcts that act as a nidus for infection. Brain abscess following pene-

trative cranial trauma is well recognized. Brain abscess following intracranial surgical procedures fortunately occurs less frequently than local wound infections, osteomyelitis of the flap, subdural empyema, or meningitis.

Histopathologically, brain abscess formation is divided into four stages: early cerebritis (days 1 to 3), late cerebritis (days 4 to 9), early capsule formation (days 10 to 13), and finally late capsule formation (day 14 on). This sequence is influenced by the predisposing condition, the type and virulence of the infecting microorganism(s), and the host immune response. Less extensive capsule formation occurs in brain abscesses that arise from hematogenous spread of infection than from a contiguous focus of infection. In experimental models, *Staphylococcus aureus* and aerobic streptococci promote the formation of a thick capsule, whereas anaerobic organisms—e.g., *Bacteroides* spp—tend to retard encapsulation. In immunocompromised hosts, particularly those on corticosteroids, the early inflammatory response and resulting edema may be decreased and capsule formation impeded.

Brain abscesses are caused by a wide variety of bacteria, fungi, and parasites. The causative organisms are determined largely by the origin of the infection and the immune status of the patient (Table 1). Pathogens can be isolated from the majority of lesions at surgery even after empiric antibiotic therapy has been commenced. Streptococci—aerobic, anaerobic, and microaerophilic—are isolated in up to 70% of cases. These include α-streptococci, viridans streptococci, group A β-streptococci, and enterococci. Strains of the *Streptococcus intermedius* subgroup of α-hemolytic streptococci are the most common streptococci isolated from brain abscess. A relative increase in the incidence of anaerobic streptococci, including *Peptostreptococcus* and *Peptococcus* spp and *Bacteroides* spp (*B. melaninogenicus*, *B. oralis*, and *B. fragilis* are found in 40% of cases), has been observed, partly due to improved methods of isolation and identification. Anaerobic organisms predominate in abscesses of otogenic and dental origin. Since the antibiotic era, staphylococci have declined as a cause of brain abscess but are still important etiologic agents following trauma. Aerobic gram-negative bacteria causing brain abscess are often found in mixed culture. *Proteus* spp are particularly associated with otogenic and neonatal brain abscess. Other gram-negative isolates include *Escherichia coli*, *Klebsiella*, *Enterobacter*, and *Pseudomonas* spp. *Pseudomonas* spp, especially *P. aeruginosa*, are associated with chronic middle ear infections. Bacteria associated with pyogenic meningitis, such as *Streptococcus pneumoniae* and *Haemophilus influenzae* are uncommon causes of brain abscess.

The epidemiology, presentation, and etiology of brain abscess have been altered in recent years by the increasing numbers of immunocompromised patients. *Listeria monocytogenes* and *Nocardia asteroides* can cause brain abscess in individuals with T cell or mononuclear phagocytic defects and in patients taking corticosteroids. The majority of fungal brain abscesses occur in immunocompromised

TABLE 1. **Predisposing Conditions, Microbiologic Isolates, and Suggested Initial Antimicrobial Chemotherapeutic Regimens* for Brain Abscess**

Underlying Condition/Source	Site of Abscess	Frequent Pathogenic Isolates	Suggested Empirical Therapy
Paranasal sinus infection/dental infection	Frontal, temporal lobe	Streptococci (aerobic and anaerobic), *Fusobacterium* spp, *Bacteroides* spp, *Staphylococcus aureus*	Penicillin G or 3rd-generation cephalosporin† + metronidazole ± oxacillin
Otitis media/mastoiditis	Temporal lobe, cerebellum	Streptococci, *Bacteroides* spp, Enterobacteriaceae, *Proteus* spp, *Pseudomonas aeruginosa*	Penicillin G + metronidazole + ceftazidime ± aminoglycoside
Trauma/surgery	Variable	*S. aureus*, Enterobacteriaceae, *Clostridium* spp, *Bacillus* spp, *Staphylococcus epidermidis, Propionibacterium acnes*	Oxacillin (or vancomycin) + 3rd-generation cephalosporin ± metronidazole
Hematogenous source (pulmonary, intra-abdominal, genitourinary tract, endocarditis)	Parietal, temporal, and occipital lobe, cerebellum, thalamus, brain stem	Streptococci (aerobic and anaerobic), Enterobacteriaceae, *Fusobacterium, S. aureus,* enterococci, *Nocardia* spp	Penicillin G + metronidazole + 3rd-generation cephalosporin (ceftazidime)
Immunosuppression (neutropenia, cell-mediated/T cell defects, corticosteroids, immunoglobulin deficiency/B cell defects)	All lobes, cerebellum, thalamus, brain stem	Enterobacteriaceae, *Listeria monocytogenes, Nocardia* spp, *Candida* spp, *Aspergillus* spp, *Mucor, Cryptococcus neoformans, Toxoplasma gondii,* mycobacteria	Ceftazidime + aminoglycoside + metronidazole + oxacillin (or vancomycin) ± amphotericin B
Acquired immune deficiency syndrome	All lobes, cerebellum, brain stem	*Toxoplasma gondii*	Sulfadiazine + pyrimethamine

*Recommended dosages for 70-kg patient with normal renal function: penicillin G, 20–24 million units/d; cefotaxime, 2 gm q 4 h; ceftriaxone, 2–3 gm q 12 h; ceftazidime, 2–4 gm q 8 h; metronidazole, 7.5 mg/kg q 6 h; oxacillin, 2 gm q 4 h; vancomycin, 1 gm q 12 h; amphotericin B, 0.7–1.5 mg/kg/d.
†Cefotaxime, ceftriaxone, and ceftazidime.

patients. Systemic *Candida albicans* and *Aspergillus* infections can disseminate to the brain. Other fungal causes include *Cryptococcus neoformans, Blastomyces dermatitidis, Histoplasma capsulatum,* and the Mucorales, among others. The parasite *Toxoplasma gondii* is the commonest cause of brain abscess in patients with acquired immune deficiency syndrome (AIDS). Various protozoa and helminths may cause brain abscesses. *Entamoeba histolytica* is the most common cause of amebic brain abscess, and cysticercosis is a major cause of brain abscess in the developing world.

CLINICAL FEATURES AND DIAGNOSIS

The clinical manifestations of brain abscess depend on the size, number, and location of the lesion, the virulence of the causative organism(s), the inflammatory response, and the immune status of the host. The clinical course can be insidious, but the majority of abscesses are recognized within 2 weeks of the onset of symptoms. The prominent symptoms of brain abscess are those of an expanding intracranial mass. The classic triad of fever, headache, and focal neurologic deficit is present in less than half of all cases. Headache, the most frequent symptom (70% to 97%) is usually constant, progressive, and refractory to symptomatic treatment. Nausea and vomiting occur in 25% to 50% of patients, and approximately 50% will have fever, usually low grade. Altered mental status is prominent in up to two thirds of cases and ranges from mild lethargy to coma. Focal neurologic deficits are common and depend on the location of the abscess(es). Seizures occur in up to 30% to 50% of cases preoperatively. Physical findings include meningismus, papilledema, and focal neurologic deficits. Rupture of an abscess into the ventricles or the subarachnoid space is an acute and often catastrophic event.

Laboratory findings are frequently nonspecific and are of little value in diagnosing brain abscess. A moderate peripheral leukocytosis may be present but exceeds 20,000 per mm³ in only approximately 10% of cases. The erythrocyte sedimentation rate is usually elevated but is a nonspecific test. Blood cultures are usually negative unless the brain abscess derives from an intravascular source. Lumbar puncture is contraindicated in patients with suspected brain abscess owing to the risk of brain stem herniation. Cerebrospinal fluid (CSF) examination is usually nonspecific. There is generally a mild-to-moderate pleocytosis (<500 cells per mm³) in 60% to 70% of cases, with a predominant mononuclear lymphocytosis. An elevated protein is seen in up to 80% and hypoglycorrhachia in only 10% to 25% of patients. CSF cultures are usually negative unless the abscess has ruptured into the ventricle or communicates with the subarachnoid space.

The advent of CT and MRI has revolutionized the management of brain abscess and contributed to a significant lowering of mortality from this condition. The characteristic features of a brain abscess on CT scan are a mass lesion with a hypodense center, surrounded by a uniform ring of enhancement following intravenous contrast, and a hypodense region of parenchymal edema outside of this area of enhancement. The features of a brain abscess are differentiated more accurately on gadolinium-enhanced MRI than on contrast-enhanced CT, and MRI appears to be more sensitive than CT in detecting early cerebritis. With inconclusive CT or MRI scans, radionucleotide scanning with [111]indium-labeled leukocytes may help clarify the diagnosis.

MANAGEMENT AND ANTIMICROBIAL THERAPY

The optimal management of brain abscess generally requires a combined neurosurgical and medical approach. Appropriate treatment strategies need to be individualized for each patient. Prior to the advent of effective antimicrobial agents, surgery was the only treatment, and it continues to be the mainstay of therapy. Current operative management includes aspiration and excision. Neither method has been shown to be superior by prospective studies. Aspiration using stereotactic CT guidance is perhaps the procedure of first choice because of the reduced potential for direct brain tissue damage and a lower incidence of postoperative neurologic sequelae. It is particularly useful in the management of the patient with multiple abscesses or inaccessible or deep-seated lesions, including brain stem abscesses. The technique is sufficient to establish a microbiologic diagnosis in the majority of cases. Excision is a more definitive treatment and is indicated if there is neurologic deterioration from a mass effect or incomplete drainage of a multiloculated abscess. Excision is also required when the etiologic organisms are drug-resistant or when effective agents penetrate brain tissue poorly. Fungal abscesses usually require excision.

Since the early 1970s, antimicrobial therapy alone has been used successfully for the treatment of some brain abscesses. However, this approach should be reserved for the treatment of small (<2.5 cm) lesions in the early cerebritis stage rather than well-formed abscesses. The patient should be neurologically stable and conscious, with no evidence of increased intracranial pressure. Medical therapy alone may be the only option in patients with multiple or deep-seated abscesses in vital structures.

Antimicrobial Regimens

Whenever possible, antibiotic therapy should be directed against specific organisms based on Gram stain, culture, and sensitivity testing. Until culture results are available, empirical broad-spectrum therapy should be used based on an assessment of the likely source of infection, the most frequently encountered pathogens, and the immune status of the patient (see Table 1). Preferably, the antimicrobial agents should be bactericidal and administered parenterally at dosages that achieve therapeutic concentrations within brain tissue. However, no controlled trials of antimicrobial regimens for brain abscess have been performed. Until relatively recently, penicillin G and chloramphenicol (Chloromycetin) was the combination of choice for suspected bacterial brain abscess, particularly if the abscess originated from the paranasal sinuses or a dental source. Penicillin penetrates well into abscesses and is bactericidal for most streptococci and most anaerobes other than *Bacteroides fragilis*. Metronidazole (Flagyl) has replaced chloramphenicol in recent years because of its excellent anaerobic activity, the achievement of tissue levels often in excess of serum levels, and a possible survival benefit compared with chloramphenicol. The frequent isolation of Enterobacteriaceae as part of the mixed flora in brain abscess of

middle ear or mastoid origin should prompt the addition of a third-generation cephalosporin.

Cefotaxime (Claforan), ceftriaxone (Rocephin), and ceftazidime (Fortaz), which penetrate the CSF in therapeutic concentrations, have broad gram-negative coverage and are active against the majority of streptococcal isolates. Cefotaxime has shown good penetration into brain abscess tissue and is an alternative to penicillin in empirical regimens. Ceftazidime, with its added antipseudomonal activity, should be considered as part of the initial regimen for treating brain abscesses that result from chronic middle ear infections. Aminoglycosides, whose penetration into the CNS and brain tissue is unpredictable, may be useful adjuncts for the prevention of emergence of resistance to beta-lactam antibiotics used to treat gram-negative organisms such as *Serratia* and *Enterobacter* species. *S. aureus* brain abscesses that may occur following penetrating trauma or bacteremia are best treated with a semisynthetic penicillinase-resistant penicillin such as oxacillin (Bactocill, Prostaphlin). Vancomycin (Vancocin), which achieves brain tissue concentrations of 60% to 80% of serum levels, should be substituted if methicillin-resistant *S. aureus* is suspected or the patient is allergic to penicillins. It is also the drug of choice for coagulase-negative staphylococcus infections (e.g., *S. epidermidis*), which are more frequent following neurosurgical procedures.

In immunocompromised patients, such as those with neutropenia, defects in cell-mediated immunity, and B cell deficits, the range of possible etiologic agents causing brain abscess is wide. In addition to an increased incidence of pyogenic abscess due to Enterobacteriaceae and *P. aeruginosa*, these patients are at risk from opportunistic infections with *Listeria monocytogenes, Nocardia* spp, *Aspergillus* spp, *Candida* spp, *Mucor, Cryptococcus neoformans,* mycobacteria, *Toxoplasma gondii,* and a variety of other microorganisms. The diversity of potential etiologic agents precludes practical empirical regimens, and in general early surgical intervention is indicated to establish an accurate diagnosis. Patients with AIDS are an exception to this. The commonest cause of a focal intracerebral lesion in patients with AIDS is cerebral toxoplasmosis, which develops in 20% to 47% of patients who are seropositive for *Toxoplasma gondii.* AIDS patients with ring-enhancing lesions on contrast CT or MRI scans should be treated empirically with sulfadiazine, 4 grams daily orally (or clindamycin [Cleocin], IV/PO, 600 mg every 6 hours if sulfa-allergic), and pyrimethamine (Daraprim), 50 to 75 mg daily orally. Failure to show clinical and/or radiologic improvement by CT or MRI scan after 10 to 14 days should prompt biopsy of the lesion to establish a definitive diagnosis.

Although no clear guidelines exist, bacterial brain abscess should be treated for at least 4 to 6 weeks with parenteral antibiotics. Four weeks may be adequate if there has been complete excision of the lesion. Fungal abscess, particularly due to *Aspergillus* infection, often requires excision and prolonged antifungal therapy with intravenous amphotericin B (Fungizone), 0.7 to 1.5 mg per kg per day, alone or in combination with flucytosine (Ancobon) or rifampin (Rifadin). Oral therapy is usually not recommended for brain abscess, with the exception of cerebral toxoplasmosis in AIDS patients.

The use of adjunctive corticorsteroids in brain abscess is controversial. They clearly have a role in the management of patients with raised intracranial pressure resulting from associated intracerebral edema. However, there is evidence to suggest that steroids may impair penetration of antibiotics into the central nervous system (CNS) and therefore may hinder sterilization of lesions.

PROGNOSIS AND OUTCOME

Advances in diagnosis and treatment have resulted in a dramatic reduction in mortality from brain abscess, which in recent series is less than 10%. Factors associated with an adverse outcome include rapidity of progression of symptoms before hospitalization; alteration in the patient's mental status and neurologic impairment prior to admission; multiple, deep, or multiloculated abscesses; ventricular rupture; fungal etiology; and delay in diagnosis. Although mortality has decreased, the incidence of neurologic sequelae and disability is high, ranging between 30% and 50%. Long-term morbidity is most frequently related to seizures, cognitive dysfunction, and focal neurologic deficits. Factors influencing neurologic outcome are the location of the abscess and the age of the patient. Children may be less prone to epilepsy than adults but are more likely to suffer from intellectual impairment, learning disabilities, and behavioral changes.

ALZHEIMER'S DISEASE

method of
CHRISTOPHER M. CLARK, M.D., and
STEVEN E. ARNOLD, M.D.

University of Pennsylvania Medical Center
Philadelphia, Pennsylvania

Dementia is a nonspecific term encompassing a variety of clinical disorders characterized by progressive memory loss, impaired judgment and decision making, changes in personality and behavior, confusion, reduced attention, and loss of language skills. It is distinct from delirium or encephalopathy. These latter terms describe a clinical condition of cognitive impairment with altered level of consciousness that is typically associated with infections, metabolic derangements, or toxicity.

Alzheimer's disease (AD) is a specific type of neurodegenerative dementia characterized clinically by a progressive loss of memory and other aspects of cognition and pathologically by the presence of neurofibrillary tangles, amyloid plaques, and neuronal cell death (Table 1). It is an etiologically heterogeneous disease that in some instances is due to a single cause, such as a genetic mutation, whereas in

TABLE 1. Clinical Features of Alzheimer's Disease

Memory loss
Inconsistent ability to hold on to new information
Mild difficulty with expressive language
Impaired insight about cognitive and functional problems
Difficulty performing complicated motor skills (apraxia)

other instances it is due to a confluence of risk factors that combine to produce the characteristic pathology.

The development of consensus criteria for definite, probable, and possible AD has greatly facilitated the diagnostic exercise (Table 2). However, given the protean nature of the clinical features, the variable completeness of the history from a knowledgeable caregiver, and the lack of a diagnostic marker with adequate specificity and sensitivity, arriving at a clinical diagnosis of AD can sometimes seem closer to an art than a science. Even in the hands of dementia specialists, a clinical diagnosis of AD is only validated at autopsy about 90% of the time. Most of the 10% who are misdiagnosed have pathologic evidence of another neurodegenerative condition. Rarely is a treatable condition missed if patients undergo a complete evaluation and are re-examined periodically to preclude unexpected changes in the clinical course that would suggest an alternative diagnosis. Table 3 lists the most frequent autopsy findings in patients with a clinical diagnosis of AD.

ESTABLISHING A CLINICAL DIAGNOSIS

A clinical diagnosis of Alzheimer's disease requires memory loss of sufficient magnitude to interfere with normal function and impairment in at least one other area of cognition. Frequently there are also personality and behavioral changes. All changes should be verified by a knowledgeable informant as the patient can rarely present an adequate description of the symptoms. Cognitive impairment should be confirmed by a brief standard psychometric test battery.

There are considerable variations in the age of onset, rate of progression, degree of language impairment, presence of extrapyramidal signs, and psychotic features. The majority of patients have their first symptoms between the ages of 70 and 85 years, and the disease generally runs a relentlessly progressive course, terminating in death within 5 to 12 years. Many patients have some evidence of a mild anomia early in their course and occasionally expressive language is severely affected. Extrapyramidal signs usually do not appear until the terminal phase of the

TABLE 2. Consensus Criteria for Alzheimer's Disease

Probable AD

Memory loss sufficient to disrupt daily function
Cognitive impairment documented by psychometric testing
Onset of symptoms between age 40 and 90 years
Absence of an alternative explanation for the dementia

Possible AD

Clinical picture of AD but with a coexisting condition that could contribute to the dementia, or in the presence of one or more atypical features

Definite AD

Clinical and pathologic features of AD

Condensed from National Institute of Neurological and Communicative Disorders and Stroke—Alzheimer's Disease and Related Disorders Association.

TABLE 3. **Pathologic Diagnosis in 176 Patients with a Clinical Diagnosis of Alzheimer's Disease**

Pathologic Diagnosis	Number	Percent
Alzheimer's disease	147	83.0
Alzheimer's/Parkinson's combination	10	5.6
Lewy body variant of Alzheimer's disease	8	4.5
Stroke	3	1.7
Diffuse Lewy body disease	1	0.6
Alcoholic dementia	1	0.6
Pick's disease	1	0.6
Lobar atrophy	1	0.6
Progressive supranuclear palsy	1	0.6
Cortical degeneration	1	0.6
Corticonigral degeneration	1	0.6
Normal brain	1	0.6

illness, but about 20% of patients develop rigidity, postural instability, and other manifestations of parkinsonism at a time when their cognitive impairment is relatively mild.

It is important to be sure the patient is not taking medications capable of causing or contributing to mental confusion. A general physical examination should be done to identify the presence of major organ failure (heart, lung, kidney, liver) that could compromise brain function. Blood studies (complete blood count [CBC], electrolytes, biochemical profile, rapid plasma reagin (RPR) test, thyroid function tests, B_{12} and folate levels) and an anatomic imaging study (computed tomography or magnetic resonance imaging) will help identify any potentially treatable conditions.

At present there are no specific diagnostic markers. However, several recent studies indicate that the presence of an elevated cerebrospinal fluid tau level is highly correlated with the clinical diagnosis of AD (specificity = 98%). However, in almost half of the AD patients tested the level was normal, giving the test a low sensitivity (51%). Therefore, while an elevated level would lead to a high suspicion, a normal level does not exclude the diagnosis of AD.

Risk Factors

Autosomal dominant gene mutations on chromosomes 21, 14, and 1 have been identified, each of which is capable of independently causing AD. These genetic forms account for less than 10% of all cases. The 90% of patients with nongenetic AD can be divided into those who have a history of two or more first-degree family members with an AD-like dementia (familial AD) and those without a strong familial history (sporadic AD). Members of a familial AD family have about a fourfold increased risk to develop AD. Other well-established risk factors include increasing age, female gender, and ApoE ε4 genotype (Table 4). Less well-established risk factors include low education, a history of head trauma, and coexisting thyroid disease.

Behavioral Disturbances

At some point during the illness a majority of patients will exhibit one or more of the following: agitation, sundowning (acute nocturnal disorientation and agitation), wandering, psychosis, emotional lability and depression, sleep disturbance, and altered sexuality. These behavioral disturbances can cause significant distress for caregivers and patients alike. They are the most common reasons for placement in a long-term care facility. Assessing the na-

ture, causes, and severity of these behavioral symptoms requires careful observation and explicit questioning of the caregiver. Alternative explanations for these psychiatric symptoms, especially drug toxicity or intercurrent medical illness with delirium, or even complex partial seizures, must be considered.

Agitation is the most common behavioral symptom associated with AD, occurring in up to 70% of nursing home residents and half of AD patients cared for at home. It is characterized by psychomotor restlessness, irritability, and verbal and/or physical aggression. Physical aggression is the most disturbing agitated behavior and typically takes the form of hitting, biting, grabbing, and pushing as the patient resists assistance with personal care needs. It is frequently seen in association with psychotic symptoms but may also be a manifestation of an intercurrent medical illness or physical discomfort. Less disturbing manifestations of behavioral agitation include wandering, akathisia, pacing, and orneriness.

Delusions, hallucinations, and misperception syndromes occur in up to 78% of AD patients. Delusions often take the form of paranoid misbeliefs about theft, infidelity, danger, or strangers. Hallucinations are less common than delusions, occurring in approximately 30% of patients, and are more commonly visual than auditory or olfactory.

The coexistence of depression occurring as a treatable component of AD remains controversial. Evaluating mood is especially difficult in the AD patient because many symptoms, such as the loss of interest, loss of insight, sleep and appetite changes, could be due to either dementia or depression. Nonetheless, recognition and treatment of depression are important, as depression can significantly worsen cognition and function.

Sleep disturbances in AD include frequent nocturnal awakenings, diminished slow wave sleep, delayed and decreased REM sleep, and sleep fragmentation. Sundowning, manifest by acute nocturnal disorientation and agitation, can be especially troublesome.

Sexual activity is usually decreased in AD, although occasional increased sexual interest and socially inappropriate sexual behavior are seen. Sexual aggression is rare.

TREATMENT

General Principles

A number of general environmental and behavioral management principles can optimize safety, enhance function, and thus delay institutionalization. Disorientation can be reduced by maintaining familiar physical surroundings with adequate nighttime lighting. The daily routine should be as simple and

TABLE 4. **Risk Factors for Alzheimer's Disease**

Variable	Risk
Established	
Old age (prevalence at age 75–84 years)	18.7%
Sex (female:male ratio)	1:2
Family history of dementia	3.23 (odds ratio)
ApoE ε4 allele (in nonfamilial AD)	2.84 (odds ratio)
Potential	
Education less than 7 years	4.65 (odds ratio)
Head trauma with loss of consciousness	1.82 (odds ratio)
Thyroid dysfunction	1.53 (odds ratio)

constant as possible, since variations and surprises may produce unnecessary anxiety and confusion. Door locks to prevent wandering, protection against hot stove surfaces, gas stove turn-off valves, and secure storage of toxic substances are all important safety measures.

Helpful communication techniques include using concrete language, avoiding open-ended questions or abstract/metaphoric phrases, maintaining social greetings and rituals, using a soft tone of voice, using more gestures along with verbal communication, simplifying and repeating instructions frequently, orienting the patient repeatedly to situations ahead of time, and sometimes using posted written messages. In addition, avoiding sensory overstimulation by maintaining a calm, predictable environment and not placing unreasonable expectations for a patient in social settings can help avoid agitated or aggressive reactions.

Nondrug Management of Behavior Problems

When behavioral difficulties arise, it is important for the caregiver to see if there is anything that could have caused or exacerbated the problem. Physical conditions that can precipitate behavioral problems include constipation, hunger, pain, vision and hearing impairment, drug toxicity, or intercurrent illness. Identifying, characterizing, and documenting the circumstances in which a behavioral problem occurs frequently lead to a specific intervention and resolution of the problem. It is also important to recognize that some behavioral symptoms may not need intervention. For instance, if a delusion or hallucination is not distressing to a patient and is otherwise harmless, no intervention is necessary.

Medication for Behavior Problems

There are few controlled studies assessing the efficacy and safety of psychotropic medications in AD. Nonetheless, the use of medication for the management of behavioral disturbance can be quite effective. A number of general principles should be followed: (1) medication should be instituted only after environmental and behavioral strategies have proved inadequate; (2) clear goals or target symptoms should be defined; (3) start with the lowest possible dosage and titrate carefully; (4) monitor for untoward effects; and (5) reassess the need for continued use at regular intervals.

Agitation and aggression are the most disturbing and potentially dangerous behavioral manifestations of AD, and a wide variety of medications have been used in their management. The most common are neuroleptics. In an attempt to increase the quality of care in nursing homes and reduce the use of "chemical restraints," neuroleptic use is now regulated by the Omnibus Budget Reconciliation Act passed by Congress in 1987. These regulations stipulate that neuroleptics for nursing home residents can be used

only for behaviors or psychotic symptoms that cause functional impairment or constitute a danger to the patient. They may not be used for staff convenience or to punish a particular behavior (e.g., screaming, hitting, biting). The frequency with which the medication is used must be documented and the need for continuation periodically reassessed.

Neuroleptics are modestly effective for acute and chronic management of agitation, especially when the agitation is associated with psychotic symptoms, such as paranoia, delusions, or hallucinations, emotional lability, and hostility. Traditional neuroleptic medications with demonstrated efficacy include haloperidol (Haldol), 0.5 to 5 mg per day in divided doses, trifluoperazine (Stelazine), 1 to 20 mg, loxapine (Loxitane), 5 to 100 mg, and thioridazine (Mellaril), 10 to 200 mg. Side effects common to all the traditional neuroleptics include extrapyramidal signs such as parkinsonism, acute dystonic reactions, akathisia (which itself can cause agitation), and the possibility of developing tardive dyskinesia. Because extrapyramidal signs may also be an inherent feature of AD, even low doses of neuroleptics may produce troublesome side effects. The new, "atypical" neuroleptics risperidone (Risperdal)* and clozapine (Clozaril)* have a lower incidence of extrapyramidal side effects. Because of the need for weekly CBCs to monitor for agranulocytosis in patients on clozapine and its significant lowering of seizure threshold, it is rarely used in AD. Other side effects that may limit the use of the neuroleptics include orthostatic hypotension, sedation, increased confusion, falls, a lowered seizure threshold, and anticholinergic effects (especially constipation and urinary retention).

Benzodiazepines can also reduce agitation and are especially effective when there is an associated anxiety component. Short- and intermediate-duration agents such as lorazepam (Ativan), 0.5 to 2 mg, alprazolam (Xanax), 0.25 to 1 mg, or oxazepam (Serax), 10 to 30 mg, can be used to manage acute episodes of agitation or anxiety. For more chronic problems, a longer half-life agent such as clonazepam (Klonopin),* 0.5 to 1 mg twice daily, may be more appropriate. Side effects associated with benzodiazepines include sedation and falls. Also, a paradoxical increase in agitation or aggression may occur as a disinhibitory effect of the medication.

Anecdotal reports of other drugs that have been used successfully to help control agitation exist. Although not useful for acute management, they can be quite effective when used as maintenance therapy. This is particularly important in AD as agitated behaviors are frequently chronic, and inadequate efficacy, side effects, and the misuse potential of neuroleptics and benzodiazepines limit their use. These medications include the anticonvulsants carbamazepine (Tegretol),* 100 to 1200 mg per day in divided doses, and valproic acid (Depakote),* 250 to 1500 mg; lithium carbonate,* 300 to 1800 mg; antidepressants such as trazodone (Desyrel),* 50 to 400 mg, or fluox-

---

*Not FDA-approved for this indication.

etine (Prozac),* 10 to 40 mg; the beta-blocker propranolol (Inderal),* 20 to 560 mg; the anxiolytic buspirone (Buspar),* 5 to 60 mg; and for highly refractory, physically aggressive men, estrogen therapy with conjugated estrogen (Premarin)* or diethylstilbestrol.*

Depressive symptoms exacerbate cognitive impairments in AD, and so the recognition and treatment of mood disturbance represent an opportunity to optimize function as well as alleviate suffering. The selective serotonin reuptake inhibitor (SSRI) agents such as paroxetine (Paxil), 10 to 40 mg per day, sertraline (Zoloft), 25 to 200 mg, or fluoxetine (Prozac), 10 to 40 mg, are first-line agents as they are effective, safe, and usually well tolerated. A newer serotonergic agent, nefazodone (Serzone), 50 to 400 mg, may also be effective as it is well tolerated and has notable anxiolytic properties. Tricyclic antidepressants, especially nortriptyline (Pamelor), 10 to 100 mg, or desipramine (Norpramin), 25 to 250 mg, are also useful, although the anticholinergic side effects of dry mouth, constipation, urinary retention, atrioventricular conduction delay, and orthostatic hypotension must be monitored.

Hypnotic medications are often necessary for patients with difficulty initiating and maintaining sleep. Prior to their use, caregivers should try non-pharmacologic techniques for good sleep hygiene. These include maintaining a regular schedule of activity during the day, minimizing daytime naps, adhering to a regular bedtime, and avoiding excess fluid intake in the evening. Useful bedtime medications to induce sleep include trazodone (Desyrel),* 50 to 150 mg, zolpidem (Ambien), 5 to 20 mg, chloral hydrate, 250 to 1000 mg, or intermediate-acting benzodiazepines such as temazepam (Restoril), 15 to 30 mg.

Antidementia Treatment

Tacrine (Cognex)

Acetylcholine is one of several neurotransmitters reduced in AD, and it is particularly relevant because of its involvement in the classic memory pathways. This fact, as well as the observation that scopolamine, an acetylcholine receptor blocker, could induce memory loss similar to that seen in AD, led to an assessment of the ability of various acetylcholinesterase inhibitors to improve the symptoms of AD. However, because of the complex array of pathologic changes manifest by patients with AD, and the fact that the illness is associated with extensive neuron and synaptic loss as well as reductions in a number of different neurotransmitters, many investigators felt that the benefit of this therapeutic strategy might be quite modest. This has proved to be the case. Nevertheless, there is evidence that this class of medication provides measurable efficacy in a subset of patients with AD. Unfortunately, it has not been possible to identify ahead of time who will re-

spond, who will develop medication-associated toxicity, and who will fail to respond. As of January 1996, tacrine (Cognex) remains the only antidementia drug that has received FDA approval for use in the United States in the past 10 years.

Efficacy Data. The efficacy of tacrine is based on several short-term (12- to 30-week) double-blind placebo-controlled trials using a variety of randomization and dose exposure designs. Primary end points included both performance-based cognitive testing (the cognitive component of the Alzheimer's Disease Assessment psychometric test) and a subjective rating by the investigators of the overall change associated with treatment. The results of most trials demonstrated a small dose-related efficacy with a consistent side effect and organ toxicity profile. Overall, very modest improvement could be detected in about 40% of the patients treated. Although the magnitude was measurable, it was often less than the physicians and caregivers had hoped for.

Nevertheless, it may be the best that can be expected from a first-generation symptomatic drug in a complex, relentlessly progressive disease. Among the changes reported by caregivers were improved attention, a better ability to accomplish tasks, greater spontaneity, more self-initiation, and in general, a very modest reversion of the personality toward what it had been before the illness began.

Tacrine was studied only in AD patients who were otherwise healthy. It is unclear how beneficial it will be in patients with coexisting medical problems who are taking multiple medications. It is also unclear how effective it will be in more complex dementias such as the Lewy body variant of AD or patients who have both Parkinson's disease and Alzheimer's disease. It has no effect on the pathophysiology of the illness and thus does not prolong survival. However, patients who respond may enjoy a slightly higher level of function for a period of time.

Initiation of Treatment, Maintenance, and Efficacy Monitoring. Tacrine is available in capsules of 10, 20, 30, and 40 mg. After verifying that the patient's alanine aminotransferase (ALT) level is normal, patients are usually started on 10 mg four times daily. If given with food, the absorption may be decreased by as much as 30% to 40%. The initial dose should be maintained for a minimum of 6 weeks and serum ALT levels checked every other week. It is helpful to establish realistic goals to use as measures of efficacy, which, in turn, can guide treatment decisions. Using a brief psychometric battery that will assess memory, language, and praxis skills, such as the one developed by the Consortium to Establish a Registry for Alzheimer's Disease (CERAD) and a caregiver functional report questionnaire (such as the Dementia Severity Rating Scale), can provide a measure of objectivity to the results of treatment. The Folstein Mini Mental State Examination is generally not sensitive enough when used on its own.

Generally the daily dose can be increased by 40 mg every 6 weeks until a satisfactory response is

---

*Not FDA-approved for this indication.

seen, unacceptable side effects occur, or liver toxicity develops. The maximum daily dose is 160 mg per day.

With standard doses, no clinically meaningful cardiovascular effects were seen. Most side effects involved the gastrointestinal system. Mild nausea, usually without vomiting, occurred in about 28% of the patients, diarrhea in 16%, and anorexia in 9%.

Tacrine-Induced Organ Toxicity. A greater than threefold elevation in serum ALT levels occurred in 29% of all patients exposed to tacrine. Overall, 8% of all patients started on the drug had to discontinue because of liver toxicity. Ninety-five percent of the ALT elevations occurred within the first 8 weeks of treatment. Once the drug was stopped, the ALT level often continued to rise for an additional 2 weeks before gradually falling back to normal over the subsequent 6 weeks.

Because the liver toxicity is potentially life-threatening, it is imperative to continue to check ALT levels every 2 weeks for a minimum of 18 weeks after the patient reaches a stable dose. Monitoring can then be reduced to once every 3 months.

Safety. Patients with a current or past history of liver disease probably should not take tacrine. It should be used with caution in patients who have a history of peptic ulcers or are taking medication that may lower the threshold for ulcers. Tacrine may lower the threshold for seizures and should be used with caution in patients with a past or current history of epilepsy. It may exacerbate pre-existing orthostatic hypotension. Tacrine is associated with a twofold increase in half-life of theophylline and may exaggerate succinylcholine-type muscle relaxants given during anesthesia.

Second-Generation Acetylcholinesterase Inhibitors

Donepezil (Aricept),* a product of Eisai Pharmaceutical that will be marketed in the United States in collaboration with Pfizer, is a second-generation acetylcholinesterase inhibitor whose efficacy is similar to that of tacrine. However, it has the added advantage of once-a-day dosing and no liver toxicity at the doses tested. Combining the results of a 15-week and 30-week treatment trial, study investigators (who were blinded to treatment status) labeled about 30% of the patients taking donepezil as at least

*Investigational drug in the United States.

TABLE 5. Sources of Information for Healthcare Providers and Caregivers

Organization	Phone
Alzheimer's Association	1-800-272-3900
Alzheimer's Disease Education & Referral Center	1-800-438-4380
National Caregiving Foundation	1-800-930-1357
National Institute on Aging	1-800-222-2225
Eldercare Locator	1-800-677-1116

minimally improved compared with 16% of those taking placebo. As with tacrine, there is no information relating the probability of improvement to the severity of dementia, duration of disease, or presence of specific clinical characteristics. It should be available by the second half of 1996.

Other Drugs Nearing End of Phase III Clinical Trials

Other drugs are under development that have novel (or poorly understood) mechanisms of cognitive enhancement or are designed to slow the rate of progression of Alzheimer's disease. They include both newly developed compounds such as Sebeluzole* (Janssen) and SKB202026* (SmithKline-Beecham) as well as drugs such as selegiline (Eldepryl)† and estrogen, which are currently used in other situations.

Caregiver Support and Life Planning

No matter what the treatment strategy, the most important goal is to maximize the patient's capacity to function and preserve the ability to live in familiar surroundings as long as possible. Maintaining the well-being of the primary caregiver is a key factor for success. Caregivers who can not get enough sleep or are frustrated, anxious, or angry cannot maintain an environment in which patients can function at their maximum capacity. Caregivers must learn how to handle behavior problems before they get out of hand and the importance of planning for the future before it arrives. They should be encouraged to discuss issues such as advance directives, obtaining power of attorney for the patient, and planning for long-term care.

*Investigational drug in the United States.
†Not FDA-approved for this indication.

TABLE 6. Internet Resources

Location	Web Home Page Address
Alzheimer's Disease Education & Referral Center	http://www.alzheimers.org/adear
Alzheimer's Disease Review	http://www.coa.uky.edu/ADReview
Michigan Alzheimer's Research Center	http://www.med.umich.edu/madrc/MADRC.html
Case Western Reserve Alzheimer's Center	http://www.cwru.edu/orgs/adsc/intro.html
Institute for Brain Aging & Dementia	http://www.alz.uci.edu
Alzheimer's Web	http://werple.mira.net.au/dhs/ad.html

One of the best ways of obtaining information about these matters is through the Alzheimer Caregiver Support groups sponsored by the local chapters of the Alzheimer's Association (1-800-272-3900 for information about local chapters). In addition, there is a large number of brochures, videos, caregiving manuals, and information about services for patients with dementia that can be obtained from the Alzheimer's Association as well as organizations such as the National Institute on Aging's Alzheimer's Disease Education and Referral Center (ADEAR), The National Caregiving Foundation, and the Eldercare Locator. Phone numbers for these organizations are listed in Table 5. The ADEAR program can also provide information and phone numbers for the 27 National Institute on Aging–sponsored Alzheimer Disease Centers. Books, such as *The Thirty-Six-Hour Day*, by Mace and Rabins, can also be helpful. A number of informative internet sources of information can provide very useful and timely information to both physicians and caregivers. They are listed in Table 6.

Specialized daycare programs for patients with dementia, as well as respite care programs, are becoming more available and can delay the need for nursing home placement. Both Eldercare Locator and the local chapter of the Alzheimer's Association can usually provide a list of programs available in specific areas of the country.

INTRACEREBRAL HEMORRHAGE

method of
JOSÉ BILLER, M.D., and
MITESH V. SHAH, M.D.
Indiana University School of Medicine
Indianapolis, Indiana

Intracerebral hemorrhage (ICH) is a common neurologic cause of disability or death. It is one of the most deadly stroke subtypes and accounts for about 10% to 15% of all strokes. Proper diagnosis, evaluation, and treatment of patients with ICH remain important components of the clinical practice of neurology.

ETIOLOGY

The most common causes of spontaneous ICH are those related to arterial hypertension. Hypertensive hemorrhages tend to occur in specific sites (putamen, thalamus, subcortical white matter, cerebellum, and pons). Hemorrhage in any area of the brain, but especially lobar, may be due to a specific etiologic factor. Other major causes include cerebral aneurysms, vascular malformations, bleeding diatheses, cerebral amyloid angiopathy, brain tumors, vasculitis, and drug abuse. Brain hemorrhages associated with cerebral venous occlusive disease, infectious disorders, or following surgical procedures are less frequent but well recognized (Table 1).

CLINICAL FEATURES

ICH may vary from a relatively mild to a rapidly fatal disease. The observed neurologic manifestations depend on the location, size, direction of spread, and rate of development of the bleeding. Depending on the location and size, approximately half the patients complain of headaches, nausea, and vomiting. Patients may have a variable level of alertness. Seizures are common with lobar hemorrhages. The structures most likely to be involved by spontaneous ICH are the putamen, the lobar subcortical white matter, the thalamus, the pons, cerebellum, and caudate nucleus.

Putaminal Hemorrhage

The putamen is the most common site for hypertensive ICH; approximately 33% of ICH occur in the putamen. Fibrinoid necrosis of the small penetrating vessels at the base of the brain leads to hemorrhages that may remain localized to the putamen or may enlarge to involve the internal capsule, corona radiata, centrum semiovale, or temporal lobe, or may rupture into the ventricular system. The classic picture is characterized by contralateral hemiparesis or hemiplegia, accompanied by conjugate gaze preference to the side of the hematoma. There may be less severe contralateral hemisensory loss. Left putaminal hemorrhages result in aphasia; right putaminal hemorrhages produce apractagnosia, left visual neglect, and constructional apraxia. Homonymous hemianopsia may be present.

Lobar Hemorrhage

About 23% of ICHs occur in the subcortical white matter. The clinical syndromes often resemble those seen with

TABLE 1. **Etiologies of Spontaneous Intracerebral Hemorrhage**

Arterial Hypertension	**Drug-Related**
Aneurysms	Amphetamines
Saccular	Cocaine
Infective	Phenylpropanolamine
Traumatic	Talwin-pyribenzamine
Neoplastic	Phencyclidine
Vascular Malformations	Heroin
Arteriovenous malformations	MAOI
Capillary telangiectases	**Intracranial Tumors**
Cavernous angiomas	Primary malignant or benign
Venous malformations	Metastatic
Bleeding Diatheses	**Cerebral Venous Occlusive Disease**
Leukemia	
Thrombocytopenia	**Miscellaneous**
Disseminated intravascular coagulation	After carotid endarterectomy
Polycythemia	After selective neurosurgical procedures
Hyperviscosity syndromes	After spinal anesthesia
Hemophilia	Postmyelography
Hypoprothrombinemia	Cold-related
Afibrinogenemia	Lightning stroke
Selective factor deficiencies	Heat stroke
von Willebrand's disease	Fat embolism
Sickle cell anemia	After painful dental procedures
Anticoagulant therapy	Protracted migraine
Thrombolytic therapy	Methanol intoxication
Cerebral Amyloid Angiopathy	
Arteritis/Arteriopathies	
Infectious vasculitis	
Multisystem vasculitis	
Isolated CNS angiitis	
Moyamoya disease	

Abbreviations: CNS = central nervous system; MAOI = monoamine oxidase inhibitors.

thromboembolic cerebral infarctions. Frontal lobe hemorrhages may result in contralateral hemiparesis and abulia; conjugate gaze deviation toward the hematoma may be found. Parietal hemorrhages may cause contralateral hemisensory loss and neglect of the contralateral visual field. Dominant temporal lobe hemorrhages can result in Wernicke's aphasia. Intracerebral hematomas involving the left temporoparietal area can also cause conduction or global aphasia. Right temporal hematomas may result in variable degrees of visual field deficits. Occipital lobe hemorrhages are characterized by ipsilateral orbital pain and contralateral homonymous hemianopia.

Thalamic Hemorrhage

About 20% of ICHs occur in the thalamus. They are usually hypertensive but may be secondary to an underlying structural lesion. Thalamic hemorrhages may be confined to the thalamus or extend laterally to involve the internal capsule, inferomedially to compromise the subthalamus and midbrain, or medially to involve the third ventricle. Thalamic hemorrhages are characterized by hemisensory loss affecting all modalities. Hemiparesis develops if the internal capsule becomes involved. Depression of the reticular activating system may account for decreased level of consciousness and hypersomnolence. Inferomedial extension accounts for the development of restriction of vertical gaze, convergence retraction nystagmoid movements, pupillary light-near dissociation, and disconjugate gaze with impaired abduction of one or both eyes. The eyes become tonically deviated down and slightly abducted. The eyes may be tonically deviated away from the thalamic hematoma, or there may be a conjugate gaze deviation as seen in putaminal hemorrhages. Pathologic lid retraction occurs with damage to the posterior commissure. Left thalamic hemorrhages can cause an evanescent aphasia. Right thalamic hematomas have been associated with visuospatial abnormalities and anosognosia.

Cerebellar Hemorrhage

About 8% of ICHs occur in the cerebellum, and untreated patients have a high mortality. These hemorrhages most frequently occur in the region of the dentate nucleus and less often in the vermis. Variations in location, size, and development of the hematoma, brain stem compression, fourth ventricular penetration, and development of hydrocephalus result in variations in the mode of presentation of cerebellar hemorrhage. The history is typically that of a sudden onset of inability to stand, occipital or frontal headaches, nausea, vomiting, and dizziness or vertigo. The most frequently observed signs are truncal or limb ataxia, ipsilateral gaze palsy, and small, reactive pupils. Horizontal gaze paretic nystagmus and facial weakness are often seen. Frank hemiparesis is absent. Progression can occur because of development of hydrocephalus or edema. Since the advent of computed tomography (CT), it has now been found that not all patients with cerebellar hemorrhage present such a dramatic picture. Those with small (usually less than 3 cm in diameter) cerebellar hemorrhage may present only with vomiting without headaches, gait instability, and limb ataxia. Cerebellar infarcts can produce an identical syndrome.

Pontine Hemorrhage

Approximately 7% of ICHs occur in the pons. Signs and symptoms of pontine hematomas depend on size, location, and presence or absence of ventricular rupture or hydrocephalus. Primary pontine hematomas tend to occur at the junction of the basis pontis and tegmentum and to be symmetrically placed. Massive pontine hematomas cause coma, decerebrate rigidity, quadriparesis, absent horizontal eye movements, and miotic pupils reactive to light until later in the course. Ocular bobbing, characterized by rapid conjugate downward movements of the eyes followed by a slow upward drive to primary position, may be present. Partial damage to the lateral basis pontis may cause pure motor hemiparesis. Hemorrhages originating in the lateral pontine tegmentum may account for an ipsilateral conjugate gaze paresis, ipsilateral internuclear ophthalmoplegia, the "one-and-a-half" syndrome, and ocular bobbing. Laterally situated tegmental hemorrhages may cause ipsilateral hemiataxia with contralateral hemiparesis and hemisensory deficits.

Caudate Hemorrhage

Caudate hemorrhages account for approximately 4% of ICHs. Hemorrhages in the region of the caudate nucleus cause headache, vomiting, neck stiffness, confusion, and decreased short-term memory. Variable findings include a transient contralateral conjugate gaze paresis, contralateral hemiparesis, transient hemisensory deficits, and rarely, an ipsilateral oculosympathetic palsy.

DIAGNOSTIC TECHNIQUES

Because many conditions can cause ICH, patients suspected of it deserve a thorough evaluation. In all patients, initial history and cardiopulmonary and neurologic assessment are obtained prior to proceeding with imaging techniques. Specific information regarding hypertension and its control, drug or alcohol ingestion, and systemic diseases is sought. CT is mandatory. Unenhanced CT is still the safest, most effective method currently available to identify accurately the location, site, direction of its extension, and type of an acute ICH. CT also shows the degree of hydrocephalus, indicates ventricular shift or compression, and indicates degree of edema.

Since the first objective is to exclude hemorrhage, magnetic resonance imaging (MRI) is not the imaging modality of choice for initial evaluation of the patient with an acute ICH. MRI becomes an important diagnostic tool for identifying bleeding lesions such as vascular malformations and/or tumors. Cerebral angiography continues to play an important role in the evaluation. Angiography is of importance when there is reason to suspect an aneurysm, arteriovenous malformation (AVM), vasculitis, or moyamoya disease. Angiography is performed in patients who have an atypical location for hypertensive hemorrhage or in the young patient who is not hypertensive. We routinely perform cerebral angiography in ICHs among cocaine users, as there is a high frequency of associated vascular malformations and aneurysms. There is almost no indication for lumbar puncture in patients suspected of having ICH. Paraclinical investigations recommended as part of the evaluation of patients with ICH are listed in Table 2.

TREATMENT

All patients with ICH should be admitted to the hospital for emergency evaluation and treatment. This is better accomplished in a stroke unit, intensive care unit, or other advanced care unit, where

TABLE 2. **Paraclinical Evaluation in Intracerebral Hemorrhage**

All Patients

1. Complete blood count with platelet count
2. Prothrombin time (INR), partial thromboplastin time
3. Erythrocyte sedimentation rate
4. Blood glucose
5. Serum alkaline phosphatase, serum glutamic oxaloacetic transaminase, serum calcium, blood urea nitrogen, serum creatinine
6. Urinalysis
7. Chest roentgenogram
8. Electrocardiogram
9. Unenhanced cranial computed tomography (CT)

Selected Patients

1. Blood cultures
2. Drug screen
3. Antinuclear antibodies assay
4. Sickle cell screen
5. Hemoglobin electrophoresis
6. Serum fibrinogen, fibrinogen split products, serum viscosity
7. Thrombin time, reptilase time, bleeding time
8. Type and screen
9. HIV titer
10. Enhanced computed tomography
11. Magnetic resonance imaging of the brain
12. Cerebral angiography

INR = international normalized ratio; HIV = human immunodeficiency virus.

close nursing and medical observation are possible. Before the patient with a presumed ICH arrives at a critical care unit, a basic medical and neurologic evaluation and, if necessary, stabilization should be performed in the emergency department. Management of the airway and maintenance of adequate ventilation and oxygenation should be accomplished immediately. Supportive respiratory care is provided to all patients, and ventilatory assistance if needed. The airway of an obtunded patient should be protected. Dysphagia increases the risk of aspiration. Standardized evaluation by a trained specialist should be done. Tube feedings may be needed for some patients.

If there are signs of respiratory depression (Glasgow Coma score of less than 8) or raised intracranial pressure and herniation, intubation, hyperventilation, and intravenous osmotherapy are indicated (Table 3). The patient's head is elevated to 15 to 30 degrees to promote venous drainage. Intravenous mannitol, 20% solution for infusion, is initially used in a dose of 1 gram per kg body weight given in 20 to 30 minutes, followed by a dose of 0.25 to 0.5 gram per kg body weight every 4 to 6 hours depending on clinical findings, serum osmolality, and intracranial pressure values if available. Furosemide is often used in conjunction with mannitol. Corticosteroids have not been proved effective in treating cerebral edema associated with ICH, and we do not routinely use them. Hyposmolar fluids raise intracranial pressure and should be avoided. An intravenous line is used for administration of fluids in the form of normal saline, and for the administration of emergency drugs if needed.

The blood pressure should be measured frequently or continuously monitored in these patients during the first 72 hours after ICH. If the mean arterial blood pressure is higher than 130 torr, it should be cautiously lowered but not to hypotensive levels, and we favor the use of labetalol (Normadyne, Trandate) for this purpose. Labetalol is contraindicated in patients with asthma, congestive heart failure, severe bradycardia, and greater than first-degree heart block. Although no data have shown significant benefits for the hyperacute use of antihypertensive treatment in patients with ICH, we feel that markedly elevated blood pressures (systolic blood pressures > 170 to 180) should be controlled but not overcompensated. A cerebral perfusion pressure of at least 70 mmHg should be maintained.

We use prophylactic anticonvulsants in cases of lobar hemorrhages or metastatic melanoma. Phenytoin (Dilantin) is used for seizure control. Due to its effect on platelets, divalproex sodium (Depakote) should be avoided. Because of limb paresis, immobilization, and corticosteroid therapy, ICH patients have an increased risk of deep venous thrombosis (DVT).

TABLE 3. **Medical Management Guidelines of Elevated Intracranial Pressure and Arterial Hypertension in Intracerebral Hemorrhage**

Correction of Factors Exacerbating Increased ICP

Hypercarbia
Hypoxia
Hyperthermia
Acidosis
Hypotension
Hypovolemia

Positional

Avoid head and neck positions compressing jugular veins
Avoid flat supine position; elevate head of bed 15–30 degrees

Medical Therapy

Endotracheal intubation and mechanical ventilation, if Glasgow Coma Scale < 8
Hyperventilate to Pa_{CO_2} of 25 mmHg (if herniating); gradual withdrawal
Hyperosmolar therapy with mannitol (20% solution), 1 gm/kg over 30 min
Maintenance dose: 0.25–0.5 gm/kg over 30–60 min q 4–6 h, depending on clinical course, serum osmolality, and ICP measurements

Fluid Restriction

Avoid glucose solutions; use normal saline; maintain euvolemia
Replace urinary losses with normal saline in patients receiving mannitol

Blood Pressure Control

Maintain mean arterial blood pressure around 100–110 mmHg. Labetalol (Normodyne, Trandate), 20 mg IV bolus (0.25 mg/kg), then 20-mg boluses IV q 10–15 min, titrated to desired blood pressure (max 300 mg/d), or infusion of 0.5–2 mg/min (max 300 mg/d); **OR**
Nitroprusside sodium (Nipride, Nitropress), 0.25–10 µg/kg/min IV (50 mg in 250 mL of D_5W), titrated to desired blood pressure*

*Since nitroprusside reduces venous return and causes peripheral vasodilation, it is not the drug of choice in patients with increased intracranial pressure.

We use pneumatic compression stockings for DVT prophylaxis. We avoid indwelling bladder catheters, if possible, to limit the risk of urosepsis. Decubitus ulcers are prevented by frequent turning and by the use of variable pressure mattresses.

Hemostatic defects, if present, should be corrected. Adequate factor replacement should be initiated immediately in hemophiliacs. Immediate neurosurgical consultation is required. Therapy with factor VIII should be brought to about 80% to 100% before surgery, in patients with classic hemophilia, and then be maintained above 30% for approximately 2 weeks after craniectomy. Oral anticoagulant-related hemorrhages require discontinuation of the offending drug and administration of vitamin K (phytonadione), 10 mg subcutaneously (or 10 to 20 mg in 50 to 100 mL of intravenous fluids over 30 to 60 minutes), and fresh-frozen plasma, 20 mL per kg. If a life-threatening ICH occurs in a patient receiving heparin, the drug should be immediately stopped and slow (over 10 to 20 minutes) infusion of intravenous protamine sulfate (1% solution) given. Each milligram of protamine sulfate neutralizes approximately 100 USP heparin units. Protamine sulfate is given 1 mg intravenously for the amount of heparin infused in the previous 2 hours, but no more than 50 mg in a 10-minute period.

Thrombolytic therapy–associated bleeding requires discontinuation of thrombolytics and the administration of 10 units of intravenous cryoprecipitate; fresh-frozen plasma, 20 mL per kg, may also be needed. Aminocaproic acid (Amicar) may be required if bleeding persists. We use a 5-gram loading dose of Amicar in 250 mL of normal saline or 5% dextrose and water over 30 to 60 minutes, followed by 1 gram per hour in a continuing intravenous infusion until bleeding is controlled. Patients with profound thrombocytopenia who develop ICH should be treated immediately with platelet transfusion therapy. Additional measures in patients with ICH complicating idiopathic thrombocytopenic purpura may include administration of systemic corticosteroids, plasmapheresis, emergency splenectomy, and possible evacuation of the intracranial hematoma.

Surgery

The indications for surgical treatment of spontaneous ICH have been debated for decades. The current indications for surgery are uncertain. There is no definitive randomized prospective study to show whether surgical evacuation is better than medical therapy alone. Despite the continuous controversy, there appears to be general agreement that (1) surgery is of no benefit in patients with massive hemorrhage who are deeply comatose, with loss of pupillary reactivity and impaired brain stem function at the time they are seen; and (2) patients with small intracerebral hematomas, regardless of location, who are fully conscious, rarely need surgical therapy. The more critical issue, and the most frequently argued, is whether patients with medium-size hemorrhages (3 cm) are better managed with surgical or medical modes of therapy.

A review of the recent literature suggests that putaminal hemorrhages less than 3 cm in diameter without ventricular rupture do reasonably well without surgery. Patients with large putaminal hemorrhages with ventricular rupture do poorly, no matter what therapy is used. Management of moderate-sized putaminal hemorrhages may require surgery if there is progression. Surgery is rarely indicated for thalamic hemorrhages and is restricted to management of hydrocephalus. Surgery appears rarely indicated in cases of brain stem hemorrhages. Lobar hemorrhages are the most favorable location for surgical evacuation. Advantages of surgery include the opportunity to remove the source of the hematoma, to provide a reduction in intracranial hypertension by quick removal, and to obtain pathologic confirmation of the cause of the hemorrhage. However, the functional deficit is not influenced by removal of the hematoma, and unless there is a progressive course despite medical therapy, it appears that lobar hemorrhages less than 2 to 3 cm in diameter may be managed medically. Whether surgical evacuation leads to a more cost-effective means of reaching a rehabilitative status needs to be determined.

Particular emphasis must be placed on the patient with cerebellar hemorrhage for whom emergency surgery may be indicated. Cerebellar hemorrhage is a potentially lethal but often completely reversible condition when compression on the brain stem is released promptly. Patients with acute cerebellar hemorrhages greater than 3 cm in diameter, even if fully conscious, are referred for surgery. Since the advent of CT, medical management under strict and careful observation has been recommended for small (<3 cm in diameter) cerebellar hemorrhages. However, if there is any evidence of deterioration, surgery should be undertaken immediately. Thus, factors that are crucial to determining the best therapeutic approach include (1) size and location of hematoma, (2) etiology of ICH, and (3) temporal profile of clinical presentation and course.

Timing of surgery has also been debated among the proponents of surgical therapy for ICH. Benefits of very early (<7 hours) or early (<24 hours) operation have been proposed by some investigators. Stereotactic aspiration of the hematoma has been found to be a useful tool that may provide certain advantages over standard surgical methods. Endoscopic surgical techniques for evacuation of intracerebral hematomas are being investigated. Stereotactic irrigation with thrombolytic agents is being evaluated. The indications for these agents in ICH have not been established.

ISCHEMIC CEREBROVASCULAR DISEASE

method of
LEWIS B. MORGENSTERN, M.D., and
JAMES C. GROTTA, M.D.
University of Texas Medical School
Houston, Texas

The decade of the brain is little more than half over and we are in the midst of a treatment revolution for ischemic cerebrovascular disease. Gone are the days when a stroke patient was relegated to the recesses of the Emergency Department (ED) and all we could do is scratch our heads and wish we could do something. Now, we have a tremendous fund of knowledge in the fight against stroke. Our ability to treat modifiable risk factors has led to a decline in stroke mortality for decades. Treatment of carotid artery disease and cardiac sources of embolization also put the primary care physician in the front lines of the war against this devastating disease. Thrombolytic and possibly neuroprotective therapy given within the first few hours after acute stroke has radically changed the concept of stroke treatment. Our message is that "time is brain." There is much we can do right now to prevent and treat stroke patients.

STROKE PREVENTION

The diagnosis and management of transient ischemic attacks (TIAs) and stroke are considered together here since they reflect the same pathophysiology. TIAs imply a tenfold increase risk of major stroke, the majority of which occur soon after the initial symptoms. By definition, these patients are neurologically normal. They frequently ignore their symptoms or are given little credence by their physician. We believe these patients have the most to gain from a thorough, expeditious evaluation. We ask our patients carefully about these transient symptoms and tell them to come to the Emergency Department immediately should they occur. We suggest admitting these patients unless a rapid outpatient work-up and social support are guaranteed.

The modifiable risk factors for TIA and stroke include hypertension, diabetes, smoking, atrial fibrillation, coronary heart disease, and hyperlipidemia (indirectly). There is no better way to treat a stroke than by preventing it (Table 1). For example, studies have shown that decreasing cholesterol and tobacco use result in decreased stroke risk, and optimal control of blood pressure can prevent up to half of all

TABLE 1. **Stroke Risk Factors**

	Relative Risk
Hypertension	6×
Smoking	2×
Diabetes mellitus	2–4×
Atrial fibrillation	3×
Coronary artery disease	2–6×
Recent TIA	10×

strokes in the United States. In addition, we strive to prevent the complications of acute stroke. Aspiration precautions and deep venous thrombosis prophylaxis with pneumatic compression stockings and/or subcutaneous heparin should be standard treatments. Early feeding, if necessary by dobhoff tube, has been shown to benefit patients. Finally, we recognize that patients with stroke are most likely to die from myocardial disease. Patients who present with a stroke or TIA should have a thorough assessment of their cardiac status individualized to the patient. At the least, a careful history, examination, and electrocardiogram (ECG) are mandatory. In other patients, radionuclide stress test or cardiac catheterization may be necessary.

Pharmacotherapy is important in stroke prevention. Aspirin (ASA) is the first line of therapy to prevent vascular events (Table 2), and should be used in all high-risk patients and those with any symptoms of ischemic stroke or TIA. It has mild side effects and is inexpensive. Debate still rages as to the proper doses. Although 1300 mg *may* be more effective than 325 mg, the side effects are much greater and compliance diminishes. We use 325 mg daily but rarely increase this dose in patients who have vascular events while on this dose.

A better alternative to increasing the aspirin dose is ticlopidine (Ticlid), 250 mg twice a day with meals. In a placebo-controlled, double-blinded randomized study, patients who received ticlopidine did slightly better (12%) than those who received aspirin. Ticlopidine has several drawbacks. Side effects include gastrointestinal distress, usually easily overcome with patients taking the medicine with food. A rash is common, necessitating at least temporary drug discontinuation. The most serious adverse event is neutropenia, which is rare but requires biweekly complete blood counts (CBCs) for the initial 3 months. The neutropenia is potentially reversible with discontinuation of the drug. Roche-Syntex will run the CBCs free if you contact them. It takes ticlopidine 7 to 10 days to reach maximal efficacy, so ASA should be continued during this time. Ticlopidine is a good agent, however, and should be used for patients who are aspirin intolerant or who have vascular events while taking aspirin ("aspirin failures"). A post hoc analysis of the Ticlopidine-Aspirin Stroke Study suggested that certain subgroups, especially women, diabetics, and those with intracranial atherosclerosis or posterior circulation symptoms, profited most from ticlopidine.

The decision to employ other therapeutic approaches like anticoagulation or carotid endarterectomy depends on the results of the diagnostic evaluation.

EVALUATION OF STROKE AND TIA PATIENTS

Deciphering the etiology of stroke or TIA is critical to proper treatment. The first step is to localize the

TABLE 2. **Medical Therapy for Stroke**

Drug	Indication	Dose	Adverse Reaction
Aspirin (ASA)	Ischemic stroke or TIA	325 mg STAT and qd; 650 bid in peri-CEA	GI distress and bleed Caution in renal disease
Ticlopidine (Ticlid)	Ischemic stroke or TIA in ASA failure or intolerance	250 mg bid with meals	Neutropenia GI upset Rash Takes 10 days to work (continue ASA)
IV heparin	Embolic source *and* TIA/minor stroke Postcirc. thrombus Progressing Sx	No bolus PTT goal 1.5–2.0 × control	Cerebral bleed Systemic bleed Death
Warfarin	Cardioembolism Intracranial stenosis	INR goal 3.0 Consider 2 mg plus ASA in elderly	Cerebral bleed Systemic bleed Death
rtPA (Activase)	Ischemic stroke within 3 h of onset	0.9 mg/kg IV over 1 h, 10% given over first min (max 90 mg)	Cerebral bleed Systemic bleed Death

Abbreviations: CEA = carotid endarterectomy; PTT = partial thromboplastin time; INR = international normalized ratio.

lesion to the anterior or posterior circulation (Table 3).

The determination of etiology of patients with cerebrovascular disease proceeds from lesion localization. Patients with anterior circulation lesions should have carotid duplex ultrasonography. The North American Symptomatic Carotid Endarterectomy Trial (NASCET) has convincingly established that patients with a symptomatic, greater than 70% ipsilateral carotid stenosis benefit from carotid endarterectomy. This study showed that without surgery about a quarter of patients in the very-high-risk group had a stroke in the year following TIA. The risk was reduced to approximately 10% with endarterectomy. The benefit occurs with surgeons who have a documented low complication rate (<3%). If ultrasound suggests a significant stenosis, a cerebral angiogram is ordered to confirm stenosis, describe collateral circulation, and ensure that other pathology does not exist that would preclude surgery, e.g., a distal intracranial carotid occlusion.

NASCET has demonstrated benefit from carotid endarterectomy (CEA) in symptomatic arteries that have a greater than 70% *diameter* stenosis by angiography. Stenosis is measured as the ratio of the diameter at the tightest point of stenosis over the diameter at a distal, disease-free location of the internal carotid. The perioperative treatment is ASA, 650 mg twice a day. Patients should have a cardiac evaluation done expeditiously prior to CEA. If concomitant surgical cardiac and carotid disease is found, then the clinically most severe lesion is attended to first. There is little evidence to support simultaneous cardiac and carotid surgery.

The Asymptomatic Carotid Atherosclerosis Study (ACAS) actually demonstrated little more than a 1% risk for CEA in patients randomized in their trial. This study projected a modest 5-year risk reduction of stroke from 10% to 5% in those receiving CEA for greater than 60% *asymptomatic* stenosis. The critics of this study point to the fact that the benefit was not as great for major stroke as it was for minor, nondisabling stroke.

Our policy is to refer patients for CEA who are good operative candidates and either (1) have a greater than 70% symptomatic carotid artery stenosis, or (2) have a hemodynamically significant asymptomatic stenosis in a relatively young, healthy patient who is expected to live at least 5 years. We know from NASCET that patients with stenoses of less than 30% do not benefit from CEA. NASCET will soon report whether the 30% to 70% group benefits from surgery.

Although carotid angiography is the "gold standard," it is an invasive test. In the recent Asymptomatic Carotid Atherosclerosis Study, the risk of angiography almost equaled the risk of CEA. It is an important test but should be done only when necessary. The advent of magnetic resonance angiography (MRA) provides useful information that in some institutions rivals that of conventional angiography. With advanced technology and experience over the next few years, perhaps the combination of carotid ultrasound and MRA will obviate the need for conventional angiography.

Cardiac sources of emboli causing stroke or TIA are screened for by obtaining a history of arrhythmia or coronary heart disease (CAD), by examination, and by ECG. If all three of these are "negative," it is

TABLE 3. **Anterior and Posterior Circulation Symptoms**

Anterior	Posterior
Hemiparesis	Hemiparesis
Hemisensory loss	Hemisensory loss
Dysarthria	Dysarthria
Aphasia	Diplopia
Monocular visual loss	Ataxia
Lower face weakness	Upper and lower face weakness
	Severe vertigo
	Inability to walk
	Perioral numbness
	Tinnitus and hearing loss

very unlikely that a cardiac source of emboli is the culprit. A transthoracic echocardiogram (TTE) is a good screening tool for cardioembolism. Keys to potential emboli are regional wall motion abnormalities, global hypokinesis with poor ejection fraction, mural thrombus, a positive "bubble study" suggesting a right-to-left cardiac shunt, valvular abnormalities, and enlarged left atrium. TTE, however, is not as sensitive as transesophageal echocardiography (TEE) in detecting some cardiac sources of emboli, including the left atrial appendage and also the aortic arch. In general, when any suspicion remains of cardioembolism in a patient with a "negative" TTE, then a TEE should be obtained. This is particularly true in younger patients and those with no other defined etiology (cryptogenic stroke), or in patients with multiple infarcts in more than one vascular territory. Similarly, a Holter monitor can be useful in documenting paroxysmal arrhythmias such as atrial fibrillation.

Several large trials have been completed or are underway comparing warfarin (Coumadin) with aspirin for secondary stroke prevention in patients with atrial fibrillation and intracranial cerebrovascular disease. Since warfarin is more likely to cause major bleeding than aspirin, we currently reserve warfarin use to a few circumstances. The Stroke Prevention in Atrial Fibrillation (SPAF) trial has shown that warfarin is better than aspirin in preventing stroke in patients with this condition. This is especially true in patients older than 60 years who have either hypertension, congestive heart failure, or previous cerebrovascular symptoms. The goal of warfarin therapy is to keep the international normalized ratio (INR) close to 3.0. Unfortunately, although older patients benefit the most from warfarin, they also have the most serious bleeding complications.

Cardiac mural thrombus and clot in the left atrium should be managed the same way as atrial fibrillation. We also manage patients with high-grade vertebrobasilar stenosis with warfarin. The INR goal is again 3.0. Symptoms of vertebrobasilar stenosis seem to be especially amenable to hemodynamic influences. We have obtained successful benefit from removing antihypertensive treatment or adding fluorocortisone to raise blood pressure. Since the vertebrobasilar circulation is not surgically accessible, researchers interested in endovascular neuroradiology have targeted this area for trials of intra-arterial thrombolysis and angioplasty.

If strokes are not caused by extracranial carotid or cardiac sources, we look to the intracranial circulation. Disease of the intracranial internal carotid or its branches can result in thromboembolic disease. MRA is a good way to screen for such abnormalities.

Patients with hypertension and diabetes are prone to develop large artery disease as we have discussed, but also "small vessel disease." Small vessel disease results from chronic damage to small arteries and arterioles. Previously, the term "lipohyalinosis" was used to describe the pathologic changes. Small vessel disease results in small infarcts in the deep white matter, so-called "lacunes." Recent studies, however, suggest that some subcortical infarcts may be caused by emboli and therefore should be evaluated with the same rigor as larger infarctions. The lacunar syndromes—pure motor hemiparesis, ataxic hemiparesis, and clumsy-hand dysarthria—are caused by infarcts in the periventricular white matter and pons. In these cases, when an evaluation for an embolic source is negative and the patient has a history of diabetes and/or hypertension, small vessel disease can be presumed as a diagnosis of exclusion. These patients are treated with aspirin or ticlopidine and rigorous risk factor reduction.

As we discussed previously, treatment requires knowing the etiology. The concept of "cryptogenic" stroke implies cerebrovascular disease without a clear etiology. We submit that this term should be invoked *only* after an exhaustive search is made for possible mechanisms. Patients, especially young, who do not have a cardiac, aortic arch, carotid, or intracranial source for stroke deserve an evaluation for rarer mechanisms. These include arteriopathy, including vascular dissection and moyamoya disease; coagulopathy, including the antiphospholipid syndrome; and genetic diseases, such as sickle cell disease and mitochondrial disease. The evaluation of these conditions is expensive and of low yield. However, these rarer diseases benefit from specific treatments, including long-term anticoagulation with warfarin for specific coagulopathies and arterial dissection, and surgery for moyamoya disease. A more cost-effective strategy may be to refer these rare patients to a stroke center.

TREATMENT OF ACUTE ISCHEMIC STROKE

When a patient presents to the Emergency Department with focal neurologic signs, it is first important to exclude other possible mechanisms (Table 4). A patient with stroke risk factors who has the acute onset of anterior or posterior circulation symptoms is most likely to have ischemic cerebrovascular disease as the etiology. However, certain diseases can rarely masquerade as stroke. Brain tumor and intracerebral hemorrhage are excluded by CT. Recent studies have suggested that it is impossible to distinguish hemorrhage from ischemic infarction at the bedside. Endocarditis, mycotic aneurysm, and abscess forma-

TABLE 4. **Conditions that Mimic Ischemic Stroke**

Intracerebral hemorrhage
Brain tumor
Endocarditis, mycotic aneurysm
Cerebral abscess
Migraine
Postseizure (Todd's) paralysis
Metabolic disorder exacerbating prior structural lesion
Hypoglycemia
Drug or toxin
Conversion disorder

tion are usually distinguished on history and examination as well as imaging. Coagulopathy is detected by laboratory analysis. Postseizure (Todd's) paralysis should be suspected from history. Drug and metabolic effects can frequently mimic focal deficits by exacerbating a previous structural deficit. Certain illicit drugs such as cocaine have been implicated as a cause of stroke.

Patients with atherosclerotic ischemic stroke frequently fluctuate. This reflects the fact that the core of an infarction is surrounded by a territory that has borderline perfusion, the so-called penumbra. In order to keep the penumbra alive, we seek to maintain perfusion. It is our position that, in acute ischemic stroke during the first 24 to 48 hours, blood pressure should not be lowered pharmacologically unless there is evidence of acute end-organ damage. Although chronic high blood pressure is a cause of stroke, in the acute stroke patient blood pressure is a friend, not a foe. The brains of patients with chronic hypertension have autoregulated so that a higher blood pressure is required to maintain normal cerebral blood flow. Usually blood pressure will fall spontaneously by at least 10% in the first 24 hours. Active reduction of blood pressure in the acute stroke patient deprives the brain of perfusion at the time it is most needed. Certainly, drugs such as nifedipine (Procardia) that precipitously lower blood pressure are contraindicated. If we need to lower blood pressure (e.g., in acute myocardial ischemia), we monitor the pressure by intra-arterial monitoring and use carefully titrated intravenous labetalol, enalapril, or nicardipine for precise control.

Keeping the penumbra perfused requires adequate blood volume. We use isotonic saline to establish normovolemia. Hypotonic fluids leak into the extravascular space and contribute to edema formation.

The use of heparin anticoagulation in acute ischemic stroke, in doses larger than subcutaneous deep venous thrombosis (DVT) prophylaxis, is controversial (see Table 2). In December 1995, researchers from Hong Kong reported a study on low-molecular-weight heparin in *The New England Journal of Medicine*. This double-blind, randomized, placebo-controlled study using 312 Chinese patients found that the use of low-molecular-weight heparin as nadroparin,* 4100 antifactor Xa IU subcutaneously twice daily for 10 days, was safe. They also concluded that use of this agent resulted in better outcome when assessed at 6 months after the stroke. A global assessment labeled "all poor outcomes," which included recurrent stroke, death, and incomplete recovery, was reduced from 65% to 45% in the patients receiving the drug. This exciting result suggests that this new anti-thrombotic agent has fewer bleeding complications than conventional heparin and may aid recovery. We hope that ongoing studies in the United States will soon follow to see if the results can be generalized.

Conventional heparin is a different story. It has never been shown to be effective in acute ischemic stroke. In fact, heparin can be dangerous. Patients with large, particularly cortical, embolic strokes are at risk to undergo hemorrhagic transformation. Heparin increases this risk. We recommend that in large strokes, conventional heparin should not be used in the first 48 hours and perhaps the first 5 days.

We will need to continually re-evaluate whether low-molecular-weight heparin is not a better alternative to conventional heparin. We have used conventional heparin in two circumstances. The first is in a patient with a known embolic source, i.e., the heart or carotid arteries, who has had a minor stroke or transient ischemic attack (TIA). A good example would be a patient with atrial fibrillation and a TIA, or intraluminal thrombus, due to atherosclerosis or dissection of the extracranial carotid or vertebral arteries proved by arteriography. The other situation in which heparin may be useful is in vertebrobasilar thrombosis. This condition results in brain stem infarction and usually very ill patients. Heparin anticoagulation or consideration of thrombolysis at a stroke center should be made early, when the patient first presents with brain stem signs and symptoms, since the morbidity and mortality are frequently quite high.

When conventional heparin is used, a bolus is avoided owing to the risk of hemorrhagic conversion, unless the patient has had a TIA or basilar artery thrombosis is suspected. A partial thromboplastin time (PTT) goal of 1.5 to 2.0 times control is sought. In all cases when heparin or antiplatelet therapy is used, a head CT should be performed prior to the initiation of therapy to exclude intracerebral hemorrhage. Any neurologic worsening while the patient is on anticoagulation should prompt emergency CT and consideration of reversing heparin with protamine. If heparin is not used, patients with ischemic stroke or TIA should be treated with aspirin, 325 mg, in the Emergency Department and then daily.

The recombinant Tissue Plasminogen Activator (rtPA) Study results from the National Institute of Neurological Diseases and Stroke, released in December 1995, provided data on the first agent shown to help patients with acute ischemic stroke. Use of this agent resulted in an approximately 10% absolute increase in the percent of patients who returned to completely independent function following a stroke. rtPA (Activase)* was given in a dose of 0.9 mg per kg, with 10% of this given as a loading bolus over 1 minute and the rest over 1 hour up to a maximum of 90 mg. Although beneficial in carefully selected patients, thrombolytic therapy is potentially dangerous and must be approached with caution. Treatment must commence within 3 hours from the onset of symptoms. A head CT prior to treatment is mandatory to exclude intracerebral hemorrhage (ICH). Systolic blood pressure must be below 185, but extreme caution should be used in lowering blood pressure,

---

*Not available in the United States.

*Approved by the FDA for acute ischemic stroke when treatment has begun within 3 hours of symptom onset.

as already discussed. Patients must not receive any form of anticoagulation, including ASA, within 24 hours following treatment. Use of warfarin or heparin immediately preceding treatment is a contraindication. Close monitoring of neurologic status is crucial and should be carried out in an ICU for at least 24 hours. ICH was increased in patients who received tPA, but this was predominantly in the group who would have been left seriously disabled or dead regardless of treatment.

The European tPA trial (ECASS) supports the notion that patients with large strokes already apparent on CT scan are least likely to benefit from rtPA and are at the highest risk of ICH and should not be treated with intravenous rtPA. Studies with streptokinase have shown an unacceptable rate of brain hemorrhage and mortality. Intra-arterial administration of thrombolytics is under evaluation.

The data with thrombolytic drugs, in particular intravenous rtPA given within 3 hours, have conclusively demonstrated that ischemic stroke is a treatable disease. The challenge to the medical community is now to reorganize and educate paramedics and emergency services to assess, select, and treat patients within a very narrow time window. *This can be done,* since data demonstrate that at best a third of stroke patients in the United States currently reach the Emergency Department within 3 hours. Patient education on the warning symptoms of stroke is also critical. Assuming that we can treat 20% of ischemic stroke patients within 3 hours, we estimate we will save over 10,000 Americans from disabling stroke each year.

The other challenge to the medical community is to use the results with rtPA to stimulate further development in stroke therapy. Other agents are far along in the process of development and testing. Neuroprotective agents, including glutamate antagonists and Lubeluzole, an agent whose precise mechanism of action is unknown, are in their final stages of testing in the United States. Both agents have had success in phase II studies and are quite promising. Other agents with a variety of actions from free radical scavengers to white blood cell inhibitors are also being investigated.

REHABILITATION OF THE STROKE PATIENT

method of
RICHARD L. HARVEY, M.D.
The Rehabilitation Institute of Chicago
Chicago, Illinois

There are 500,000 new cases of acute stroke per year in the United States, as reported by the Framingham Heart Study. Although stroke remains the third leading cause of death, behind cardiovascular disease and cancer, many more people are surviving stroke and leading active and productive lives despite residual neurologic impairment and disability. The prevalence of stroke is now just over 3 million people, and many of those who survive have benefited from rehabilitation care.

The purpose of stroke rehabilitation as stated by Kottke in 1974 is to "restore optimal physical function and psychosocial vocational restoration; to enable the patient to become a productive participant in the community." Although ongoing research efforts medically to restore neurologic impairment are showing some promise, effective therapy remains lacking. The focus of rehabilitation, therefore, is to maximize a person's functional ability despite neurologic impairment and to retrain individual skills aggressively as spontaneous recovery emerges. Fortunately, the majority of patients with acute stroke experience natural recovery. However, without the use of therapeutic interventions, including physical therapy, occupational therapy, and speech therapy, patients will develop a "learned disuse" and dependence leading to long-term complications, such as reduced mobility, contractures, pain, decubitus ulcers, and impaired communication. Above all, a central focus of rehabilitation care is to educate both patient and family in order to make them "experts" in their own care, so that maintaining optimal functional ability becomes a lifelong practice.

COMMON STROKE SYNDROMES

A precise understanding of the impairments resulting from an acute stroke that lead to disability is a critical part of designing a comprehensive rehabilitation program. Ischemic cerebral infarctions typically occur in cerebrovascular distributions that result in predictable stroke syndromes (Table 1). In addition, other physical impairments that have an impact on functional recovery, such as cardiovascular disease, peripheral vascular disease, pulmonary disease, diabetes mellitus, renal insufficiency, orthopedic and rheumatologic disease, and malnutrition, need to be considered. Thus a thorough medical history is necessary, including premorbid functional ability and a physical examination with special attention to the neurologic status. The rehabilitation program is tailored to the patient's impairment profile and disability, as determined by a comprehensive functional evaluation. For example, a patient with cardiomyopathy who has an embolic stroke to the lower branch of the left middle cerebral artery will commonly have only language and cognitive impairments without hemiplegia. The rehabilitation program will require speech therapy for treatment of Wernicke's aphasia; occupational therapy for independence in self-care, focusing especially on problem solving, safety awareness, judgment, and family education; and physical therapy, focusing on increasing physical endurance during functional activities, with special attention to the patient's cardiac response to exercise.

REHABILITATION SETTING

The setting in which rehabilitation services are most appropriately delivered after acute stroke depends on several factors: degree of disability, medical

TABLE 1. **Physical and Cognitive Impairments Associated with Common Stroke Syndromes**

Stroke Syndrome	Impairment
Middle cerebral artery (main stem)	Contralateral hemiplegia
	Contralateral hemianesthesia
	Contralateral homonymous hemianopsia
	Head and eye turning toward lesion
	Dysphagia
	Uninhibited bowel and bladder
Dominant hemisphere	Global aphasia
	Ideomotor apraxia
Nondominant hemisphere	Aprosodic speech
	Affective agnosia
	Visuospatial disorder
	Hemi-inattention
Middle cerebral artery (upper branch)	Contralateral hemiplegia (hand/face > leg)
	Contralateral hemianesthesia
	Contralateral homonymous hemianopsia
	Head and eye turning toward lesion
	Dysphagia
	Uninhibited bowel and bladder
Dominant hemisphere	Broca's aphasia
	Ideomotor apraxia
Nondominant hemisphere	Aprosodic speech
	Visuospatial disorder
	Hemi-inattention
Middle cerebral artery (lower branch)	Contralateral homonymous hemianopsia
Dominant hemisphere	Wernicke's aphasia
Nondominant hemisphere	Affective agnosia
Anterior cerebral artery	Contralateral hemiplegia (shoulder/foot > arm/face)
	Contralateral hemianesthesia
	Head and eye turning toward lesion
	Grasp and groping reflex
	Ideomotor apraxia
	Akinetic mutism
Lacunar stroke syndromes	
Posterior limb internal capsule or pyramids	Pure contralateral hemiplegia
Thalamus	Pure hemianesthesia
Junction of thalamus and internal capsule	Contralateral hemiplegia and hemianesthesia
Anterior limb internal capsule or pons	Dysarthria and clumsy hand
Cerebellum or tegmentum of brain stem	Hemiataxia

stability, need for rehabilitation nursing, tolerance for physical activity, and level of social support. Comprehensive rehabilitation services can be provided within the inpatient, outpatient, and home settings (Table 2). Acute inpatient rehabilitation is appropriate for patients who require 24-hour skilled rehabilitation nursing and daily medical physiatric assessment, and who can tolerate and learn from an intensive daily rehabilitation program. Subacute inpatient rehabilitation is designed for patients with limited impairment and disability who do not require an intense rehabilitation program, skilled rehabilitation nursing, or daily physician visits. Some subacute rehabilitation units will also accommodate patients

TABLE 2. **Appropriate Settings for Stroke Rehabilitation**

Acute inpatient rehabilitation
Subacute inpatient rehabilitation
Acute outpatient day rehabilitation
Outpatient rehabilitation
Home-based rehabilitation

with more complicated medical issues or severe neurologic impairment who can benefit from rehabilitation but cannot tolerate an intense program.

For patients to enter the outpatient setting for rehabilitation care, they must be safe in the home setting with or without family supervision. Their homes must be accessible, and transportation to the outpatient facility must be available. Comprehensive day rehabilitation treatment programs provide the same daily therapeutic intensity as acute inpatient rehabilitation, with a special focus on vocational and community reintegration. Traditional outpatient rehabilitation provides specialized rehabilitation therapies, one to three times per week.

Home rehabilitation services are ideal for stroke survivors who have limited accessibility to the community. Rehabilitation therapies can be provided one to five times a week, with a focus on basic self-care and household mobility.

THE REHABILITATION TEAM

Regardless of the setting, comprehensive rehabilitation is best provided using a goal-oriented interdis-

TABLE 3. **The Stroke Rehabilitation Team**

Physiatrist	Recreational therapist
Rehabilitation nurse	Rehabilitation engineer
Occupational therapist	Orthotist
Physical therapist	Dietitian
Speech and language pathologist	Respiratory therapist
Psychologist	Clergy

ciplinary approach. Realistic interdisciplinary goals are developed through regular and frequent team conferences, at which functional data shared by individual team members are integrated to form a practical treatment plan that can be uniformly implemented by all care providers. Members of the rehabilitation team can include a variety of professions (Table 3), but each member must be familiar with the rehabilitation method, philosophy, and terminology. Typically, team conferences are held on a weekly or biweekly basis, but ongoing communication among team members is beneficial for efficient and effective care.

New functional goals are added or previous goals adjusted to match a patient's potential as neurologic recovery, endurance, medical stability, and skill allow. When functional skills are achieved, they are reinforced by all team members and integrated into daily activities. Early in rehabilitation, goals are focused in areas of basic self-care, mobility, communication, and cognition (Table 4). Later, more complex psychosocial and vocational goals are added as patients begin to reintegrate into family and community life. Family education and caregiver training by all team members is also an integral part of the total rehabilitation process.

MEDICAL COMPLICATIONS FOLLOWING STROKE

Intercurrent medical complications frequently encountered after stroke can impede the rehabilitation

TABLE 4. **Basic Functional Skill Areas in Stroke Rehabilitation**

Feeding and mastication
Grooming
Oral and facial hygiene
Upper and lower body dressing
Toileting and toilet hygiene
Bathing
Bladder management
Bowel management
Transfers between even level surfaces
Transfers between uneven surfaces
Toilet, tub, and shower transfers
Wheelchair propulsion
Floor-to-chair transfers
Ambulation
Stair climbing
Verbal expression
Auditory comprehension
Reading and writing
Calculations
Interpersonal socialization
Memory and problem solving

process, impair functional improvement, and result in further morbidity or mortality. A key role of the physiatrist on the rehabilitation team is to anticipate and prevent such complications to maximize outcome and facilitate recovery. A detailed discussion of some of the complications listed in Table 5 follows.

Deep vein thrombosis (DVT) can develop insidiously, beginning between 4 and 14 days after stroke, and is often difficult to detect clinically. The incidence ranges from 23% to 75%. Pulmonary embolism is the most common cause of sudden death during acute stroke rehabilitation. Immobility, degree of hemiplegia, and severity of acute illness enhance the risk for venous thromboembolism. Early prophylaxis, preferably with subcutaneously injected heparin (100 U per kg twice daily) for nonambulatory patients after cerebral infarction is recommended. Patients with intracerebral hemorrhage can usually tolerate heparin injections if the risk for rebleed is low and blood pressure is under control. Graded compression stockings and pneumatic compression boots are safe prophylactic alternatives.

Aspiration pneumonia can prolong acute hospitalization, delay initiation of rehabilitation care, and cause between 7% and 34% of stroke-related deaths. Pneumonia can often be prevented if a careful swallowing evaluation is performed prior to initiation of oral feeding and if attention is paid to the proper positioning of patients who have a reduced level of consciousness. Frequently patients with dysphagia can be fed safely using modified diets and strategies that reduce the risk of aspiration. Modified videofluoroscopic swallow studies can be extremely helpful for prescribing a safe diet. Speech therapists can train and reinforce the use of appropriate dietary strategies and modifications. Patients with severe dysphagia will benefit from enteral feeding. Fortunately, 80% of patients with dysphagia resulting from acute stroke will recover safe swallowing ability such that frequent re-evaluation is indicated.

Malnutrition can be avoided after stroke if dietary needs are addressed immediately. Patients with depressed consciousness, dysphagia, perceptual or motor deficits, depression, or bowel impaction may not be able to eat or drink sufficiently to supply daily needs. Inadequate hydration and malnutrition predict poor rehabilitation outcome. Use of enteral feeding, including temporary placement of a gastric tube, can prevent dehydration and malnourishment. In the

TABLE 5. **Medical Complications After Stroke**

Venous thromboembolism
Aspiration pneumonia
Cardiac disease (congestive heart failure, angina, and
    myocardial infarction)
Sleep apnea and atelectasis
Urinary tract infection and incontinence
Constipation and stool impaction
Bacterial enterocolitis
Pressure sores
Depression
Musculoskeletal injury

rehabilitation setting, gastric tubes are preferred over nasogastric tubes when prolonged enteral feeding is required because they are more durable and can be safely used for intermittent or "bolus" feeding, making it easier for the patient to participate in rehabilitation therapies.

Sleep apnea and other ventilatory dysfunction occurs in 50% of those with stroke and can lead to excessive fatigue and daytime sleepiness. Use of supplemental oxygen or continuous positive airway pressure (CPAP) in those patients with obstructive sleep apnea is often therapeutic. Physical therapy to treat and prevent restrictive changes within the hemiplegic chest wall can also be beneficial.

Seventy-five percent of stroke survivors have some variant of heart disease, including hypertension (53%), coronary artery disease (32%), and congestive heart failure (18%). Heart disease is the leading cause of long-term mortality after stroke and the second leading cause of early death. Monitoring of vital signs in all patients who are at risk for heart disease as they begin a comprehensive rehabilitation program is prudent. Symptoms of dyspnea on exertion, lightheadedness, or a reduction in heart rate and blood pressure during exercise are indicators of cardiac ischemia. Attentive management of cardiac disease in the rehabilitation setting can reduce morbidity and improve functional outcome.

Stroke survivors universally have disruption in their usual bowel and bladder elimination patterns. Immobility, dehydration, communication deficits, and change in nutrition can lead to constipation. Early mobilization and provision of appropriate diet and fluids are preventive. Foley catheters should be used only if necessary for skin protection or monitoring of urinary volumes. Infections of the urinary tract are common and can be reduced if bladder instrumentation is minimized. Urinary incontinence typically results from a loss of voluntary inhibition over normal reflex voiding due to brain injury above the pontine micturition center. These patients experience urgency of urination, and communication impairment, perceptual deficits, and poor mobility also contribute to incontinence. Appropriate management includes treatment of urinary tract infection and use of "timed voiding," by offering to toilet a patient every 2 hours before urgency leads to incontinence.

POSTSTROKE SHOULDER DYSFUNCTION

Shoulder pain and mechanical dysfunction in stroke hemiplegia is arguably the most difficult and frustrating management problem in stroke rehabilitation. Limited useful research has been published in this area, and the biomechanical issues remain poorly understood. The primary cause of shoulder dysfunction after stroke is loss of mechanical integrity in the shoulder, arm, and hand, enhancing the risk of traumatic injury, inflammation, and soft tissue contracture. Both autonomic and somatic neuropathic changes occur as well and can work in combi-

nation with orthopedic problems to cause pain and dysfunction (Table 6).

Shoulder pain is uncommon during the initial flaccid stage of hemiplegia. When pain is present, stretch injury of soft tissue or nerve is likely. Care must be taken to protect the arm from injury and yet maintain normal range of motion both in the glenohumeral and scapulothoracic articulations. Positioning is critical and should include shoulder abduction (90 degrees) and external rotation in the early stages. Use of resting hand splints and wheelchair arm support is important. Daily passive range of motion should be performed and taught to family members. All health care staff and family members need to carefully monitor the positioning of the upper limb in patients with hemi-inattention, who often don't notice when the affected arm is malpositioned.

When muscle tone, spasticity, and voluntary movement return to the hemiplegic arm, 80% of patients will experience pain. Spastic tone will cause scapular retraction and downward rotation, leading to shoulder impingement with passive abduction of the humerus. Careful attention to maintaining scapular mobility can help reduce the risk of subacromial impingement, but it cannot usually be eliminated. It is more important to maintain *functional* shoulder range (0 to 100 degrees) rather then to obtain normal range of motion. Subacromial bursitis, bicipital tendinitis, and joint inflammation can be managed using local heat and cold modalities or, if necessary, steroid injections, without neglecting daily ranging of joints. Management of spasticity may also help reduce shoulder dysfunction.

Reflex sympathetic dystrophy (shoulder-hand syndrome) is a poorly understood phenomenon that can appear from 2 weeks to 3 months after onset of hemiplegia. It will typically present with hand swelling, hand and shoulder joint pain, skin temperature dysregulation, and allodynia (skin hypersensitivity). Daily range of motion and control of edema is the first line of treatment, followed by use of nonsteroidal anti-inflammatory medications or stellate ganglion blockade in more severe cases. Aggressive treatment of this disorder is necessary to prevent severe joint contractures and pain that can interfere with upper limb flexibility, positioning, and functional use.

SPASTICITY

Muscle spasticity due to upper motor neuron injury after stroke hemiplegia can impair functional im-

TABLE 6. **Etiology of Shoulder Pain and Dysfunction After Stroke**

Glenohumeral subluxation
Impingement syndrome
Frozen shoulder
Shoulder spasticity
Brachial plexus and nerve stretch injury
Trigger point
Central poststroke pain
Reflex sympathetic dystrophy
Bicipital tendinitis
Subacromial bursitis

provement, cause muscle and joint contracture, make hygiene difficult, and result in skin breakdown. Upper limb spasticity can impair voluntary skilled movement, positioning, and stretching. Lower limb spasticity can result in energy-inefficient gait and difficult fitting of orthotic devices and shoes. Clinical use of common antispasticity medications such as baclofen (Lioresal), diazepam (Valium), and dantrolene sodium (Dantrium) have been largely unsuccessful due to a lack of a significant reduction of muscle tone at moderate doses and their negative effect on cognition in brain-injured patients. Twenty-five to 50 mg of dantrolene sodium or 0.5 to 1 mg of clonazepam (Klonopin) at bedtime can be useful for patients with painful night spasms that impair sleep. Liver function tests must be monitored every 2 weeks for the first 3 months of treatment with dantrolene.

Local intramuscular injections of botulinum toxin A (Botox)* or a 3% solution of phenol are much more effective for management of spasticity after stroke (Table 7). Botulinum toxin is a safe and easy medication to use; it has a dose-related effect that is superior to that of phenol, but it is far more expensive. Botulinum toxin acts by impairing release of acetylcholine from intramuscular nerve endings. Precise localization of the neuromuscular junction (motorpoint) is unnecessary because the toxin diffuses through a 5-cm radius from the injection site, but injections at two to three sites along the length of muscles improve response to the medication. In contrast, phenol destroys cell microstructure through chemical lysis and requires careful motorpoint localization. Dose response with phenol can vary depending on the number of motorpoints treated and the precision with which the clinician localizes the intramuscular nerve. Thus, phenol injections are more technically difficult to perform. The initial effect of phenol is noted within 6 to 12 hours after injection and lasts 3 to 12 months, whereas botulinum toxin takes 3 to 7 days for initial effect and lasts 3 to 6 months. The total dose of botulinum toxin must be limited to 400 units per 3-month period due

*Investigational drug in the United States.

TABLE 7. **Botulinum Toxin A* Dosing for Stroke-Related Spasticity**

Muscle	Dose (Units)
Pectoralis major	100–200
Biceps brachii	80–180
Brachialis	50–150
Brachioradialis	50–100
Flexor carpi radialis	30–80
Flexor carpi ulnaris	30–80
Pronator teres	25–50
Flexor digitorum superficialis	50–100
Flexor digitorum profundus	50–100
Medial or lateral gastrocnemius	100–200
Soleus	75–150
Posterior tibialis	75–130

*Investigational drug in the United States.

to risk of antibody formation that can render further injections ineffective. Phenol has no total dose limitations, but patients frequently complain of local burning during injection.

Muscle localization for botulinum toxin injection can be safely performed by needle electromyography (EMG) in larger superficial muscles of the upper and lower limb, using a Teflon-coated injector needle. Confirmation of appropriate needle location is achieved by noting increased EMG activity during gentle stretch of the muscle along the line of its origin and insertion, while keeping other muscles slack (e.g., needle insertion in the flexor carpi radialis can be confirmed by passive extension and ulnar deviation of the wrist with the fingers flexed and the elbow extended). For thin and deep muscles such as the posterior tibialis, use of needle electrical stimulation (NES) is superior to EMG. The principle behind NES is to deliver pulsed low-ampere current through the needle tip to stimulate muscle contraction. The needle is adjusted until a maximal contraction of the muscle is stimulated with a low current (<3 milliamperes); however, when injecting botulinum toxin, noting a contraction that is appropriate for the muscle of interest is most important for confirming location. Only NES can be used for phenol injection, because the motorpoint must be carefully identified to ensure that the needle tip is near the intramuscular nerve. Thus for phenol, finding a strong contraction with low current before injection is critical for an effective response to treatment.

EPILEPSY IN ADOLESCENTS AND ADULTS

method of
LORI A. SCHUH, M.D., and
IVO DRURY, M.B., B.Ch.
*University of Michigan Medical School
Ann Arbor, Michigan*

Approximately 1 percent of the population has epilepsy. The incidence is bimodal, being higher in children and elderly people. Eighty percent of patients will be well-controlled on anticonvulsants, with the remainder refractory to currently available medical treatment.

Epilepsy is defined as the tendency to recurrent, unprovoked seizures. Seizures may be provoked by a systemic derangement or medical illness (Table 1) and not represent epilepsy. In these instances, treatment of the underlying disorder should prevent further seizures.

DIAGNOSIS

The diagnosis of epilepsy is made by history. First, determine whether the events in question are consistent with epileptic seizures, or another condition such as syncope, pseudoseizures, confusional migraine, panic attacks, transient ischemic attacks (TIAs), or movement disorders. Syncope is a common cause of loss of consciousness, usually preceded by feelings of lightheadedness, nausea, diaphore-

TABLE 1. **Etiologies of Provoked Seizures**

I. Toxic/Metabolic

  A. Electrolyte abnormalities
    Hyponatremia
    Hypomagnesemia
    Hypocalcemia
  B. Drugs (major causes)
    Cocaine
    Theophylline
    Phenothiazines and atypical antipsychotic agents
    Lithium
    Tricyclic antidepressants
    Anticholinesterases
    Imipenem and penicillins
    Isoniazid
  C. Acute drug withdrawal
    Alcohol
    Benzodiazepines
    Barbiturates
    Cocaine
  D. Metabolic
    Hypoglycemia
    Uremia
    Hepatic encephalopathy
    Anoxia
    Porphyria

II. Associated with Other Systemic Conditions
(incomplete list)

  A. Eclampsia
  B. Cardiac disease
    Syncope
    Arrhythmias
  C. Hyperthermia
  D. Infections
    Shigella and cholera
    Infections leading to shock or hypoxia

sis, or changes in skin color. After a syncopal attack, patients are at most briefly confused, whereas prolonged confusion is more characteristic of an epileptic seizure. Incontinence is more common in seizures but may occur with syncope. TIAs and migraine, like seizures, may cause transient neurologic symptoms. The symptoms of these disorders tend to be "negative"—i.e., numbness or weakness, as opposed to the "positive" symptoms of seizures, i.e., paresthesias or jerking movements. Migraine and TIAs only rarely result in loss of consciousness. The presence of a headache may aid in the diagnosis of migraine; however, some patients with seizures have postictal headache. The duration of migraine symptoms is usually longer (minutes to hours) than that of seizure or TIAs (seconds to minutes). Movement disorders may superficially resemble seizures, but do not result in loss of consciousness. Panic attacks may be very difficult to differentiate from limbic epileptic seizures; both may consist of fear with prominent autonomic symptoms. The duration of panic attacks is usually longer than seizures and may involve feelings of derealization but not usually frank loss of consciousness. Pseudoseizures (or psychogenic seizures or nonepileptic seizures) should be considered when there is much variability in the manifestation of a patient's events. Video-electroencephalographic monitoring of events may be necessary to make this diagnosis.

It is vital to obtain an accurate description of the events, and speaking to witnesses is superior to simply asking the patient, who may be amnestic for these events. Helpful laboratory evaluations include imaging studies of the brain (magnetic resonance imaging is preferred) and electroen-

cephalography (EEG). In the interictal (between seizures) state, the EEG may show epileptiform activity or other abnormalities (focal slowing, temporal intermittent rhythmic delta activity, and so on). The diagnostic yield of epileptiform activity on a single interictal EEG is about 50%, which increases to about 90% after three recordings. Despite this, a small proportion of individuals will have consistently normal interictal EEGs and have epilepsy. The "gold standard" of prolonged concurrent video-EEG recording to monitor suspected seizures (ictal recordings rather than interictal) is occasionally necessary, especially when atypical seizure features are present or when appropriate treatment fails. In the case of certain rare forms of epilepsy, such as progressive myoclonic epilepsy, other diagnostic tests may be helpful, but these individuals should be under the care of an epileptologist.

The most common risk factors in developing epilepsy are atypical febrile convulsions (febrile convulsions lasting at least 30 minutes or those with focal postictal neurologic deficits), a prior history of meningitis or encephalitis, tumor or vascular anomalies, and closed head injury, especially if loss of consciousness lasts more than 30 minutes. Genetic predisposition plays an important role in the development of certain epilepsies.

CLASSIFICATION

The aim in classifying epilepsy is to guide medical therapy and determine prognosis. Seizure type, or classification, is distinct from the epilepsy type, or epilepsy diagnosis. Individuals with partial epilepsies and generalized epilepsies may have both grand mal or generalized tonic clonic seizures (being secondarily generalized in the partial epilepsies); however, first-line anticonvulsants may be different for each. The International League Against Epilepsy has proposals for both the classification of seizures and of the epilepsies (Tables 2 and 3). The manifestations of a partial seizure may be protean and are a function of the spread of the ictal discharge in the brain. Seizures of the primary motor strip consist of progressive clonic or jerking movements of the contralateral body. Seizures of the primary sensory cortex consist of progressive sensory symptoms (paresthesias). Olfactory hallucinations may occur with seizures involving the medial temporal cortex, and more complex experiences such as déjà vu occur with seizures involving the limbic cortex. A simple partial seizure is not associated with loss of awareness or consciousness. A complex partial seizure is characterized by loss of awareness or consciousness, frequently with a blank stare and stereotyped motor behaviors called automatisms. Complex partial seizures usually last no longer than 2 or 3 minutes. Partial seizures may also evolve into tonic-clonic or grand mal seizures.

Of the generalized seizures, absence seizures consist of unresponsive staring, cessation of ongoing activity, and occasionally eye flutter lasting less than 20 seconds. Generalized tonic-clonic seizures begin without warning and usually manifest with axial and appendicular rigid extension, followed by rhythmic jerking of the extremities, head, and trunk. Apnea occurs during generalized tonic-clonic seizures and may result in cyanosis. The seizure usually lasts no longer than 1 to 2 minutes. Myoclonic seizures consist of rapid jerking movements of muscles, which may be focal or widespread. Not all myoclonus is epileptic. Atonic seizures manifest with brief loss of muscle tone that may result in a fall, or simply a head drop.

TABLE 2. **International Classification of Epileptic Seizures**

I. Partial Seizures
  A. Simple partial seizures (consciousness not impaired)
     1. With motor symptoms
     2. With somatosensory or special sensory symptoms
     3. With autonomic symptoms or signs
     4. With psychic symptoms
  B. Complex partial seizures (with impairment of consciousness)
     1. Beginning as simple partial seizures and followed by impairment of consciousness
        a. with no other features
        b. with features as in A.1 through A.4
        c. with automatisms
     2. With impairment of consciousness at onset
        a. with no other features
        b. with features as in A.1 through A.4
        c. with automatisms
  C. Partial seizures evolving to secondarily generalized seizures

II. Generalized Seizures (Bilaterally Symmetrical and Without Local Onset)
  A. Absence seizures
  B. Myoclonic seizures
  C. Clonic seizures
  D. Tonic seizures
  E. Tonic-clonic seizures
  F. Atonic seizures

III. Unclassified Epileptic Seizures (Inadequate or Incomplete Data)

Modified from International League Against Epilepsy: Proposal for revised classification of epilepsies and epileptic seizures. Epilepsia 22:489–501, 1981.

PRINCIPLES OF MEDICAL TREATMENT

After establishing the diagnosis of a seizure disorder, the next decision is when to initiate treatment. Most neurologists do not initiate therapy for those who have had a single seizure and who have a normal EEG. Most will initiate therapy after a second unprovoked seizure. The goal of therapy is to control all seizures completely with the lowest dose of a drug possible, avoiding side effects and long-term adverse effects. In some individuals with medically refractory epilepsies who are not candidates for other therapies, such as surgery, the goal of treatment is maximal seizure control with an acceptable level of adverse side effects, such that the individual can function as normally as possible.

Treatment should begin with a single drug, indicated for the patient's seizure type or epilepsy diagnosis. Other factors should be taken into consideration when choosing an anticonvulsant. These include cost, half-life (less frequent dosing will increase compliance), frequently encountered adverse effects (e.g., sedation with phenobarbital), long-term adverse effects (e.g., coarsening of facial features with long-term phenytoin use), and consideration of teratogenic effects in a woman of childbearing age. Although there is no single correct means to start anticonvulsant medications for an outpatient, we typically begin with a low dose of anticonvulsant and slowly increase the dose over days or weeks until reaching the lower end of the "therapeutic range." Clearly, one will encounter instances when a loading dose or rapid increase is indicated, but if there is no clear urgency, increasing the dose slowly will mitigate adverse effects and may increase compliance. Subsequent dose adjustments are made according to clinical response—that is, with continued seizures the anticonvulsant dose is increased in small increments to the point of complete seizure control or unacceptable side effects. Most epileptologists do not stop in the upper therapeutic range, unless the patient is experiencing unacceptable side effects, or a significant laboratory abnormality is detected (e.g., aspartate aminotransferase [AST] or alanine aminotransferase [ALT] elevated more than twice baseline, neutropenia, and so on). In some patients, maximal seizure control is attained only at "supratherapeutic levels" but without unacceptable side effects. The therapeutic range is only a guide to adjusting anti-

TABLE 3. **International Classification of Epilepsies and Epileptic Syndromes**

I. Localization-Related (Focal, Local, Partial) Epilepsies and Syndromes
  A. Idiopathic (age-related onset)
     1. Benign epilepsy of childhood with centrotemporal spikes
     2. Benign epilepsy of childhood with occipital paroxysms
  B. Symptomatic
     1. Temporal lobe epilepsies
     2. Frontal lobe epilepsies
     3. Parietal lobe epilepsies
     4. Occipital lobe epilepsies

II. Generalized Epilepsies and Syndromes
  A. Idiopathic (age-related onset)
     1. Benign neonatal familial convulsions
     2. Benign neonatal convulsions
     3. Benign myoclonic epilepsy in infancy
     4. Childhood absence epilepsy
     5. Juvenile absence epilepsy
     6. Juvenile myoclonic epilepsy
     7. Epilepsy with grand mal seizures on awakening
  B. Idiopathic or symptomatic
     1. West's syndrome
     2. Lennox-Gastaut syndrome
     3. Epilepsy with myoclonic-astatic seizures
     4. Epilepsy with myoclonic absences
  C. Symptomatic
     1. Specific syndromes may complicate many disease states: e.g., Lafora's disease resulting in myoclonic, generalized clonic, generalized tonic-clonic, and partial seizures

III. Epilepsies and Syndromes, Undetermined Whether Focal or Generalized
  A. With both generalized and focal seizures
     1. Neonatal seizures
     2. Severe myoclonic epilepsy in infancy
     3. Epilepsy with continuous spike-waves during slow wave sleep
     4. Acquired epileptic aphasia

Modified from Proposal for Revised Classification of Epilepsies and Epileptic Syndromes. Commission on Classification and Terminology of the International League Against Epilepsy. Epilepsia 30:389–399, 1989.

convulsant dosage. It is usually a mistake to discontinue or lower anticonvulsant doses in an asymptomatic, seizure-free individual with a mildly elevated anticonvulsant level. If a patient fails a monotherapy trial, cross-over to a second agent effective for the individual's seizure or epilepsy type is indicated.

Currently it is in vogue to speak of "rational polytherapy," i.e., using anticonvulsants with different mechanisms of action in combination. Despite this there are several advantages to monotherapy treatment, including fewer side effects, lack of drug interactions, less teratogenic potential, increased compliance, and lower cost. Despite our increasing arsenal of anticonvulsants and increased knowledge of their actions, the issue of compliance remains paramount. Studies show that as many as one-third to one-half of persons with epilepsy are noncompliant to the point of adverse effect on seizure control.

One may initiate treatment on the basis of epilepsy diagnosis or seizure type. Table 4 is an incomplete list of treatment of seizure types. Table 5 lists the pharmacokinetic properties, dosage information, common side effects, and cost of the most commonly used anticonvulsants.

Seizure Flurries

Patients who are prone to seizure flurries or clusters, which may result in emergency department visits, should be considered for home treatment with oral or rectal benzodiazepines to abort these flurries.

TABLE 4. **First-Line Treatment of Epilepsy**

Partial-Onset Seizures

Simple partial and complex partial seizures
   Carbamazepine (Tegretol)
   Phenytoin (Dilantin)
Secondarily generalized seizures
   Carbamazepine
   Phenytoin
Alternate treatment of partial-onset seizures
   Valproic acid (Depakote, Depakene)
   Lamotrigine (Lamictal)*
   Gabapentin (Neurontin)*
   Phenobarbital
   Primidone (Mysoline)
   Felbamate (Felbatol)†

Generalized Onset Seizures

Absence seizures
   Ethosuximide (Zarontin)
   Valproic acid
   Alternative: clonazepam (Klonopin)
Myoclonic seizures
   Valproic acid
   Alternative: clonazepam
Generalized tonic-clonic seizures
   Valproic acid
   Alternatives: phenytoin, carbamazepine, lamotrigine,*‡
      phenobarbital, primidone, felbamate†‡

---

*FDA-approved as adjunctive therapy only.

†High relative risk of aplastic anemia and fatal hepatotoxicity; FDA warning in effect.

‡There is no FDA-approved use of these drugs for these seizure types; however, clinical experience argues in favor of their utility.

Various techniques have been used effectively, but the one we favor utilizes a 1-mL disposable insulin syringe without a needle or catheter attachment. With the patient lying on the left side, the insulin syringe containing 5 mg of intravenous diazepam (Valium) is introduced 4 to 5 cm into the rectum and instilled. "Therapeutic" concentrations of benzodiazepines are more quickly attained with rectal administration, but an oral route using oral preparations may also be used. Studies show that significant systemic complications such as respiratory depression or arrest are rare, but nonetheless, a patient must be monitored closely for respiratory depression or arrest following administration.

PREVENTION

Prevention of epilepsy may be considered on several levels: preventing acquired epilepsy, preventing epileptic seizures, and preventing the consequences of epilepsy. Risk factors for developing epilepsy include head trauma, central nervous system infection, febrile convulsions—especially atypical febrile convulsions, and premature, low-birthweight infants. Preventive measures for head injury include helmet use when riding a bicycle or motorcycle, avoiding sports such as boxing, and obeying speed limits. Immunization against *Haemophilus influenzae,* measles, and rubella will prevent these sources of meningitis and encephalitis. Worldwide, parasitic infection remains the largest source of epilepsy. It should be possible to eliminate cysticercosis and echinococcosis with public health measures.

It may be possible to identify provocative factors leading to seizures in individual patients (e.g., video games) and by eliminating these factors, improve seizure control. General recommendations for all individuals with epilepsy, especially those with primary generalized epilepsy, include avoiding sleep deprivation, avoiding excessive alcohol and recreational drugs, and avoiding certain medications that may lower the seizure threshold. Preventing the consequences of epilepsy include the psychosocial consequences and physical consequences. Teratogenicity and safety issues will be discussed later. The psychosocial impact of epilepsy is one of the most frustrating aspects of this disorder. Myths about epilepsy still abound despite the efforts of the American Epilepsy Society and other organizations to educate the public. Limitations in occupation, obtaining health care or life insurance, mobility (driving), and participation in social, educational, and sporting activities vital for development leave their mark on an individual.

PREGNANCY, TERATOGENICITY, AND CHILD CARE ISSUES

In women of childbearing years, the issues of pregnancy prevention, the teratogenic effects of anticonvulsants, and child care must be addressed. Prepregnancy counseling is paramount. The effectiveness of oral contraceptives may be reduced in women taking the following anticonvulsants: phenytoin, carbamazepine, phenobarbital, primidone, and possibly ethosuximide. Breakthrough midcycle bleeding is one warning of such a risk. These failures may be prevented with a higher-dose estrogen oral contraceptive.

Long before conception, physician and patient should discuss whether an attempt to taper anticonvulsants should be made (see later section). If continued treatment is necessary, a woman should be on the lowest dose of preferably a single anticonvulsant necessary to control her seizures (a low serum level with complete seizure control does not justify increasing the dose).

Children born to mothers with epilepsy have about twice the risk of a malformation (4% to 6%) compared with the general population (2% to 3%). This risk is higher in women on more than one anticonvulsant, but it has not been proved that multiple medications are causative, as there may be other differences between these groups. The risk of malformations in women with epilepsy is increased over the general population even if they are taking no anticonvulsants during pregnancy. The most common malformations include cleft lip/palate, cardiac defects, unusual facial features, and digit anomalies. Neural tube defects (i.e., spina bifida) have been associated with valproic acid (1% to 2% risk) and carbamazepine (1%). These anomalies may be detected by ultrasound at 16 to 18 weeks' gestation. Folic acid may reduce the risk of malformations and should be a part of therapy in all women of childbearing potential before conception. Some advocate checking serum folate levels in women planning a pregnancy. Generalized convulsions pose clear risks of injury to the mother and increased fetal loss. Excluding ethosuximide and phenobarbital, free anticonvulsant levels should be checked during pregnancy, especially the third trimester. The free level of a drug is the active portion. In the third trimester, total levels of carbamazepine and phenytoin may drop significantly while free levels remain relatively stable, obviating the need to increase drug dose if seizure control remains optimal. Valproic acid total levels may decrease while free levels increase in the third trimester of pregnancy. Oral vitamin K should be administered in the last 1 to 4 weeks of pregnancy to prevent hemorrhagic complications caused by competition between vitamin K and anticonvulsants at the level of the placenta.

Only about one-third of women with epilepsy have an increase in seizure frequency during pregnancy. The cause of this increase is probably multifactorial, including poor sleep and noncompliance with regimen. At least one study showed that the postpartum period was the most likely time for worsened seizure control.

Following delivery, family or friends should be encouraged to assist with child care in an attempt to avoid sleep deprivation in the mother. The more protein-bound an anticonvulsant, the less likely it will be transmitted into breast milk. Sedation may occur in infants breast-fed by mothers on anticonvulsants, especially phenobarbital, primidone, and benzodiazepines. The transmission rates of anticonvulsants into breast milk are valproic acid, 5% to 10%; phenytoin, 30%; phenobarbital, 40%; carbamazepine, 45%; primidone, 60%; and ethosuximide, 90%. Gabapentin (Neurontin) and lamotrigine (Lamictal) are known to be transmitted into breast milk in animal studies, but human transmission rates are unknown. A withdrawal syndrome may be seen postpartum or after discontinuing breast-feedings in the infants of women taking barbiturates or benzodiazepines. Safety precautions should be discussed with mothers to reduce the risk of potential harm to their infant, should a seizure occur when unsupervised. These include changing diapers on the floor or strapping the baby if using a changing table, never bathing the baby alone, and not holding the baby while cooking or ironing.

THE ELDERLY PATIENT

Incidence rates of afebrile seizures increase after the age of 60 years. An etiology is frequently not identified; however, some of this increase is due to cerebrovascular disease, dementia, or tumor. Challenges in treating elderly people include polypharmacy with drug interactions, altered pharmacokinetics and pharmacodynamics, and concomitant diseases. A variable 1% decline in P-450 function in the liver, altering hepatic metabolism, and in renal function, altering renal clearance, begins around age 40 years. Carbamazepine clearance is approximately 40% less, phenytoin metabolism is reduced by approximately 20%, free valproic acid levels are 50% greater, but free clearance is 40% less in elderly than in young people. In general, elderly patients require smaller doses of anticonvulsants given less frequently to maintain "therapeutic" free anticonvulsant levels. Pharmacodynamic changes in elderly patients include increased sensitivity to sedating anticonvulsants, namely barbiturates and benzodiazepines. There is a fourfold increased risk of hyponatremia in elderly patients taking carbamazepine. Other considerations in elderly people, especially when unexpected medical failure or side effects are seen, include incorrect medication use due to visual loss or dementia and medication "stretching" caused by living on a low fixed income.

SAFETY

Safety issues should be discussed with patients who have epilepsy. The most important to many individuals are driving restrictions. These vary according to state and country of residence. Six states in the United States (California, Delaware, Nevada, New Jersey, Oregon, and Pennsylvania) have mandatory physician-reporting to the Division of Motor Vehicles. Patients who do not live in a mandatory reporting state should be cautioned with regard to driving and

TABLE 5. **Commonly Used Anticonvulsants**

Drug	Unit Quantity	Half-Life	Time to Steady State	Usual Daily Dose	"Therapeutic" Level	Common Side Effects	Idiosyncratic Reactions	Elimination	Estimated Retail Cost of Month Supply	Common Drug Interactions		Mechanism of Action
										Affect Anticonvulsant	*Drugs* Affected	
Carbamazepine (CBZ) (Tegretol)	100 mg chewable 200 mg tablets 100 mg per 5 mL suspension	Initial: 8–72 h Chronic: 12–17 h	3–5 d (auto-induction lasts up to 1 mon)	10–20 mg/kg bid, tid, or qid	6–14 µg per mL	Diplopia Dizziness Sedation Nausea Ataxia	Blood dyscrasias (very rare: 2-fold risk) Rash	>90% hepatic	(1000 mg/d) $54.08	↑ CBZ: erythromycin, cimetidine, propoxy-phene, fluoxetine ↓ CBZ: PHT, PB, FBM	Oral contraceptives, warfarin, theophylline, doxycycline, FBM	Sodium channels
Ethosuximide (ETX) (Zarontin)	250 mg capsule 250 mg/5 mL solution	30–60 h	4–10 d	500–2000 mg/d qd or bid	40–100 µg/mL	Nausea Vomiting Fatigue Dizziness	Rash Psychiatric disturbances Blood dyscrasias (very rare)	50% hepatic 20% renal	(1000 mg/d) $86.06	VPA may ↑ or ↓ level	May have effect on PHT, CBZ, oral contraceptives	T-calcium channels
Gabapentin (GBP) (Neurontin)	100 mg capsule 300 mg capsule 400 mg capsule	Normal renal function: 5–7 h Up to 132 h in anuric patient	1–2 d	1200–3600 mg/d tid or qid	Not established	Sedation Dizziness Ataxia	Weight gain	100% renal	(2400 mg/d) $218.57	Aluminum hydroxide and magnesium hydroxide may ↓ level	None reported	? Sodium channels ? GABA-A receptors
Lamotrigine (LMT) (Lamictal)	25 mg tablets 100 mg tablets 150 mg tablets 200 mg tablets	Monotherapy: 25.4 h with EIAED: 13.5–15 h with VPA: 59 h (Please see package insert for recommen-dations on starting and increasing dose of this medication)	Monotherapy: 4–5 d with EIAED: 3 d with VPA: 10–12 d	200–500 mg/d (with VPA less) qd or bid	Not established	Headache Dizziness Ataxia Nausea Blurred vision Diplopia	Rash Stevens-Johnson syndrome (increased with VPA, rapid dose increases)	90% hepatic	(400 mg/d) $198.60	PHT & CBZ ↓ level VPA ↑ level VPA + EIAED: no change	May ↑ CBZ epoxide ↓ VPA	Sodium channels ? Other
Phenobarbital (PB) (Various brand names)	Elixir: 20 mg/5 mL Tablets: 15 mg, 30 mg, 60 mg, 100 mg Parenteral: 30 mg/mL, 60 mg/mL, 65 mg/mL, 130 mg/mL	24–110 h	2–3 wk	2–3 mg/kg qd	10–40 µg/mL	Sedation Impaired cognition	Rash Paradoxical hyper-activity	75% hepatic 25% renal	(120 mg/d) $3.90	↑ PB: VPA, acetazolamide PHT may ↑ or ↓ level	CBZ cyclosporine, haloperidol, oral contraceptives, PHT, steroids, theophylline, tricyclic anti-depressants, VPA, warfarin	Sodium channels GABA-A receptors

Drug	Preparations	Half-life	Time to steady state	Dose	Therapeutic level	Side effects (dose-related)	Side effects (idiosyncratic)	Metabolism	Cost	Drug interactions (level affected)	Affects	Mechanism
Phenytoin (PHT) (Dilantin)	50 mg chewable 30 mg & 100 mg capsule 125 mg/5 mL suspension Parenteral: 50 mg/mL	7–42 h (average, 22 h)	5–7 d	5–7 mg/kg qd, bid, or tid	10–25 µg/mL	Nystagmus Ataxia Slurred speech Nausea	Rash Hypertrichosis Gingival hypertrophy Osteomalacia Lymphadenopathy Blood dyscrasias very rare	>90% hepatic	(300 mg/d) $17.33	↑ PHT: FBM, cimetidine, PB, acute alcohol use, warfarin, fluconazole, isoniazid ↓ PHT: CBZ, PB, chronic alcohol use, antacids, VPA	Oral contraceptives, quinidine, vitamin D, folic acid	Sodium channels
Primidone (PRM) (Mysoline)	Suspension: 250 mg/5 mL 50 mg tablet 250 mg tablet	PRM: 10–21 h PEMA: 24–48 h PB: 24–168 h	PRM: 3–7 d PB: 2–3 wk	10–15 mg/kg bid or tid	PRM: 5–12 µg/mL PB: 10–40 µg/mL	Nausea Sedation Dizziness Ataxia	Rash Paradoxical hyperactivity	20% metabolized to PB 20% renal 60% metabolized to PEMA	(500 mg/d) $56.92	↑ PRM and ↑ PB: VPA ↑ PRM, ↓ PB: isoniazid, nicotinamide ↓ PRM and ↑ PB: PHT, CBZ	CBZ, cyclosporine, haloperidol, PHT, oral contraceptives, steroids, theophylline, tricyclic antidepressants, VPA, warfarin	Sodium channels
Valproic acid (VPA) (Depakote, Depakene)	Solution: 250 mg/5 mL Depakene: 250 mg capsule Depakote: 125, 250, & 500 mg tablets 125 mg sprinkles	5–20 h (average: 10.6 h)	2–3 d	15–60 mg/kg bid, tid, or qid	50–100 µg/mL	Tremor Nausea Vomiting Diarrhea Thrombocytopenia	Hepatic dysfunction Hepatic failure Alopecia Weight gain	>90% hepatic	(2000 mg/d) $138.52	↑ VPA: cimetidine, salicylates ↓ VPA: PB, PHT, CBZ, LMT	PB, FBM, LMT	Sodium channels GABA-A receptors T-calcium channels
Felbamate (FBM) (Felbatol)	400 & 600 mg tablets Suspension: 600 mg/5 mL	20–23 h	5–7 d	1800–3600 mg/d tid or qid	Not established	Anorexia Vomiting Weight loss Headache Insomnia	Aplastic anemia: 100-fold risk Hepatic failure	50% renal 50% hepatic	(3600 mg/d) $118.80 plus the cost of bimonthly lab exam	↑ FBM: VPA ↓ FBM: PHT, CBZ	↑ PHT, VPA, & CBZ Epoxide ↓ total CBZ	?

Abbreviations: See Drug column, and: GABA = gamma-aminobutyric acid; EIAED = enzyme-inducing antiepileptic drug; PEMA = phenylethylmalonamide.

potential side effects from anticonvulsants. In a study from a French epilepsy center, approximately one-fifth of patients with epilepsy admitted to having seizures while driving, with over half of these resulting in an accident and one-third avoiding accidents due to good fortune. In people with complex partial seizures, those without an aura were twice as likely to have an accident as those with. It is surprising that even in those with only simple partial seizures when driving, 3 of 11 seizures resulted in accidents. Other safety concerns include swimming; bathing (as opposed to showering); cooking; ironing; working at heights, with heavy machinery, around open flames, or with sharp implements; and other potentially dangerous activities. Individuals with epilepsy should be closely supervised in such activities or not participate.

DISCONTINUING ANTICONVULSANTS

After being 2 to 4 years free of seizures, with the exclusion of the primary generalized myoclonic epilepsies (e.g., juvenile myoclonic epilepsy), it is reasonable to attempt an anticonvulsant taper. Certain factors correlate with a better chance of successful anticonvulsant taper: a normal IQ, normal neurologic examination, and normalization of interictal EEG. Despite this, there are no absolute indices that discontinuance will be successful. A frank discussion between patient and physician regarding the uncertainty of success, potential risks (recurrent seizures, losing driving privileges, job-related concerns, and so on), and benefits (long-term toxicity of anticonvulsants, potential teratogenic effects, perception of not having a chronic disorder) is in order. Controversy also exists over the rate of tapering drugs. Although it is imperative that barbiturates and benzodiazepines be tapered slowly because of the risk of withdrawal seizures, and no clear documentation exists for withdrawal seizures from discontinuing other anticonvulsants, most patients will feel more comfortable with a slow taper.

TREATMENT OF MEDICALLY REFRACTORY EPILEPSY

Patients refractory to medical treatment should be considered for other treatments such as epilepsy surgery or experimental drug protocols with novel anticonvulsants. Each requires referral to an epilepsy center. The most common surgical procedure is an anterior temporal lobectomy. In carefully selected patients, the success rate in terms of seizure resolution may be as high as 80%.

TREATMENT OF STATUS EPILEPTICUS

Convulsive status epilepticus is a medical emergency requiring prompt treatment. Other forms of

---

TABLE 6. **Status Epilepticus Protocol**

I. Basic Life Support—Elapsed Time 3 Minutes
- A. Airway
  1. Head position
  2. Suctioning
  3. Intubation—if orotracheal intubation necessary, use short-acting agent such as succinylcholine for neuromuscular blockade so that clinical assessment is possible
- B. Cardiovascular
  1. Hypotension is not a direct consequence of status epilepticus; determine and treat etiology
  2. Hypertension will be reversed with appropriate treatment of status epilepticus
- C. Venous access. Start IV line with normal saline
- D. Administer thiamine (1 mg/kg IV), and if immediate accurate glucose detection is not available, glucose (1 gm/kg IV)
- E. Monitoring: continuous ECG, frequent BP and respiratory monitoring during drug administration (about q 2 min)

II. Terminate Status Epilepticus
- A. Administer lorazepam (Ativan), 0.05–0.2 mg/kg IV at 2 mg/min. Maximal suggested dose for adults is 8 mg
- B. Administer phenytoin (Dilantin), 20 mg/kg IV at no faster than 50 mg per min in normal saline; slow rate of administration if hypotension develops
- C. If phenytoin fails—**Elapsed Time 40 Minutes**
  1. Intubate patient if not already done; consider:
     a. Midazolam, 0.2 mg/kg IV loading dose followed by a continuous infusion of 0.1–0.4 mg/kg/h. End-point seizure control as documented by EEG, not burst-suppression
     b. Phenobarbital, 10–20 mg/kg IV at <100 mg/min
     c. Paraldehyde, 0.1–0.2 mg/kg/rectum mixed in oil (if no IV access)
  2. Institute EEG monitoring
- D. If status epilepticus continues—**Elapsed Time 80 Minutes:** Begin pentobarbital, 12 mg/kg loading dose with an initial maintenance infusion rate of 5 mg/kg/h; titrate infusion rate to complete seizure control and burst-suppression EEG. Slow rate of infusion after this control has been maintained for approximately 12 h

III. Prevent Recurrences
- A. Etiology. Determine whether etiology indicates longer-term therapy (e.g., it may not be necessary to treat status epilepticus due to alcohol withdrawal with chronic anticonvulsants)
- B. Are anticonvulsants needed? If yes, treat with an appropriate agent as described earlier. In many individuals, phenytoin is used as they have already received a loading dose. In individuals who experience status epilepticus due to medication noncompliance, restarting the previous anticonvulsant is an option, unless some side effect or dosing interval of that medication warrants changing regimen

---

status epilepticus, such as absence status epilepticus and epilepsia partialis continua (simple partial status epilepticus), do not seem to have the serious consequences of convulsive status epilepticus and should not be treated with a protocol such as the one that follows. Complex partial status epilepticus may require an aggressive approach as listed in Table 6. The treatment of convulsive status epilepticus is threefold: basic life support, terminating status epilepticus, and preventing recurrence. The most common etiologies of status epilepticus are noncompliance with anticonvulsant treatment, alcohol withdrawal, anoxia, tumor, metabolic disturbance, cerebrovascular disease, head trauma, and central nervous system infection.

EPILEPSY IN INFANTS AND CHILDREN

method of
EILEEN P. G. VINING, M.D.
The Johns Hopkins Medical Institutions
Baltimore, Maryland

A seizure is a sudden, paroxysmal electrical discharge of neurons in the brain. For us to make the clinical diagnosis, this electrical discharge must recruit sufficient surrounding neurons to alter the child's function or behavior. Epilepsy is generally defined as recurring, unprovoked seizures. In recent years, careful attention has been paid to classification of seizures (Table 1) and to the classification of epilepsy syndromes (Table 2). The genetic basis of some of these syndromes is now being recognized; etiology, therapy, and prognosis are greatly influenced by the type of epilepsy syndrome that is present.

TABLE 1. Seizure Classification

International Classification	"Old Terms"
I. Partial Seizures	Focal or local seizures
A. Simple partial seizures (consciousness not impaired)	Focal motor
1. With motor symptoms	Jacksonian seizures
2. With somatosensory or special sensory symptoms	Focal sensory
3. With autonomic symptoms	
4. With psychic symptoms	
B. Complex partial seizures (with impairment of consciousness)	Psychomotor seizures
1. Simple partial onset	Temporal lobe seizures
2. With impairment of consciousness at onset	
C. Partial seizures that secondarily generalize	
II. Generalized Seizures (convulsive or nonconvulsive)	
A. Absence	Petit mal
1. Classic absence	
2. Atypical absence	
B. Myoclonic	Minor motor
C. Clonic seizures	Grand mal
D. Tonic seizures	Grand mal
E. Tonic-clonic seizures	Grand mal
F. Atonic seizures (astatic)	Akinetic, drop attacks

TABLE 2. Classification of the Epilepsies

1. Localization-related epilepsies
   Benign rolandic
   Benign occipital
2. Generalized epilepsies
   Age-related (benign neonatal convulsion, West's syndrome, childhood absence, benign juvenile myoclonic epilepsy of Janz)
3. Undetermined (? focal or generalized)
4. Special syndromes
   Febrile seizures
   Chronic progressive epilepsia partialis continua in children (Rasmussen's syndrome)

DIAGNOSIS/EVALUATION OF SEIZURES

Seizures are diagnosed on the basis of the history of the event. Efforts are made to differentiate a seizure from other paroxysmal but nonepileptogenic events that are shown in Table 3. Other diagnostic evaluations are dependent upon this process. Hematologic and biochemical measurements should be obtained if the clinical situation warrants, particularly in the acute setting of a currently occurring or just witnessed seizure in a child with no previous history of seizures. An electroencephalogram (EEG) is usually helpful in providing additional prognostic information but generally should be deferred until 7 to 10 days after the event. It should be done with the child both awake and asleep. Imaging studies are generally not necessary in children with a first seizure unless trauma and ongoing concern about the neurologic examination warrant it. If seizures persist, particularly if partial, then magnetic resonance imaging (MRI) is the best imaging technique.

WHY SEIZURES ARE TREATED

Prophylactic medication is prescribed because of fear of the consequences of seizure recurrence. These fears include the fear of neurologic and physical injury. There are no data to support the concept that a few seizures are linked to any form of intellectual deterioration or any other form of neurologic damage, nor is there convincing evidence of kindling or seizures begetting seizures in humans. Although sudden unexplained death is somewhat more frequent in persons with epilepsy, there are no data to suggest that therapy reduces this occurrence. Obviously, there is a risk of physical injury if a seizure should recur in a dangerous or unsupervised setting. The greatest motivation for treatment is the fear of the psychosocial consequences of seizure recurrence. These risks must be appreciated, but more than medication is required to minimize

TABLE 3. Paroxysmal Nonepileptic Episodes in Children

Anoxic-ischemic events	Paroxysmal movement
Cyanotic breath holding	disorders
Pallid breath holding	Tics
Syncope	Spasmus nutans
Autonomic dysfunction	Paroxysmal choreoathetosis
Migraine	and dystonia
Basilar	Toxins and drugs
Sleep disorders	Psychological problems
Night terrors (pavor nocturnus)	Stress/anxiety/panic
Sleepwalking	Other problems
Narcolepsy	Gastroesophageal reflux
	(Sandifer's)
	Shuddering attacks

them. Counseling concerning the nature of seizures, the minimal risk of physical or neurologic consequences, and the problems associated with overprotection must be provided.

A seizure should be treated when the risk of recurrence and the consequences of that recurrence are clearly greater than the risk of treatment and the consequences of daily prophylactic therapy.

Recent data suggest that a child with a single seizure has a 30% to 40% chance of having a second seizure. Children with absence seizures, myoclonic seizures, or atonic seizures routinely have had multiple seizures prior to consultation with the physician and will continue to do so unless treated. There is increasing evidence that in children who have had a generalized, idiopathic tonic-clonic seizure with an abnormal EEG, the recurrence rate is as low as 20% to 25%. Children who are known to have had damage to the central nervous system earlier in life, described as remote symptomatic, and those who have an abnormal EEG, have a 50% to 60% chance of recurrence. The recurrence rate after a second seizure is much higher, ranging from 60% to 90%.

THE TREATMENT PLAN

The decision to treat should be made *after* a discussion of the risk/benefit ratio with the patient and family. This includes the risks of seizure recurrence, considering the probability of it happening again and the impact that a recurrence would have on the life of the child. It also includes the information that prophylaxis is successful in only 70% to 80% of individuals and that there are possible side effects of the medications. The treatment plan must be described to the patient and family to ensure their understanding and knowledgeable participation (Table 4). The type of seizure and epilepsy should be determined since the choice of antiepileptic medication is based primarily on the type of seizure or epilepsy syndrome (Table 5). This choice also is influenced by possible side effects. In some children, the possible cosmetic side effects of phenytoin (Dilantin) would not be a concern, whereas in others it would be very undesirable.

Many medications—carbamazepine (Tegretol), gabapentin (Neurontin),* lamotrigine (Lamictal),† primidone (Mysoline), and valproic acid (Depakene, Depakote)—must be started at suboptimal doses to avoid immediate and unpleasant side effects that might lead the family to want to abandon therapy prematurely. The amount of medication is then increased until the desired goal is achieved. That goal is the control of seizures without toxicity. Toxicity means evidence of clinical dysfunction, not simply high serum levels. If the medication is not effective, the medication of second choice should be added. When the second drug is in therapeutic range, the first drug should be tapered and discontinued. This is obviously problematic if the second drug has brought control of seizures, and no one can be certain whether the first medication is vital to that process. However, the benefits of monotherapy are multiple. Increasing data indicate that monotherapy has many advantages, including equal efficacy, fewer side effects, and easier monitoring. Also, it frequently permits less costly treatment of seizures.

Once the medication regimen has been established, monitoring of the patient is essential. This includes being certain that the seizures are controlled. More importantly, it includes ascertaining that there are no unwanted side effects. This requires going beyond the traditional monitoring of hematologic and hepatic side effects to ensure that appearance, motor coordination, learning, and behavior are not being adversely affected. Frequently, physicians will need information from other sources and cannot rely solely on their observation of the patient. They will need to question carefully both parents and teachers regarding changes they may be perceive in the child as medications are introduced or increased. The children also should be asked how they feel the medication is affecting them.

The therapeutic plan must also include an awareness that seizures may not be forever. Probably 70% to 75% of children will ultimately have their seizures completely controlled. Once the seizures have been controlled for 2 or more years, it is reasonable to consider discontinuation of medication. Recent studies show that children who have been seizure-free for 2 or more years have a 75% chance of remaining seizure-free when medication is discontinued. The children who appear to have the greatest likelihood of nonrecurrence are those who have a recent normal EEG and who were younger than 12 years of age when the seizures began.

A therapeutic plan is not complete without dealing with the informational, psychosocial, and emotional needs of the child and the family. This may require considerable counseling that can be augmented by the family reading one of the several books available and by requesting information from the Epilepsy Foundation of America (1-800-EFA-1000) or from the local affiliate.

TABLE 4. **Treatment Plan for Childhood Epilepsy**

1. Discuss the risk/benefit ratio with the child and family.
2. Discuss the treatment plan with child and/or family.
3. Be sure of diagnosis and classification.
4. Choose the most appropriate drug; consider seizure type and possible side effects.
5. Increase the drug dose until control of seizures is achieved or until there is clinical toxicity (not just high serum levels).
6. If the drug is not effective (i.e., if there is not control of seizures without side effects), add a second drug. When it is in therapeutic range, slowly discontinue first drug. **TRY TO ACHIEVE MONOTHERAPY.**
7. **MONITOR THOROUGHLY.**
8. Provide support, counseling, and education to child and family.
9. If seizures are controlled for 2 years, consider tapering off drug.

---

*Licensed as adjunctive therapy for children over age 12 years.
†Licensed as adjunctive therapy over age 16 years.

TABLE 5. **Antiepileptic Therapy in Children**

Drug	Seizure Types*	Usual Dose (mg/kg/d)	Half-Life (h)	Usual Dosing	Side Effects	Usual Range (mg/L)
Carbamazepine (Tegretol)	P, C, G	10–40	12	bid–qid	Headache, drowsiness, dizziness, diplopia, blood dyscrasias, hepatotoxicity, arrhythmia	5–14
Clonazepam (Klonopin)	M, A	0.05–0.3	24–36	bid–qid	Drowsiness, ataxia, secretions, hypotonia, behavior problem	
Ethosuximide (Zarontin)	A (? C, M)	20–40	30	qd–bid	GI distress, rash, drowsiness, dizziness, SLE, blood dyscrasias	40–100
Gabapentin (Neurontin)	P, C	15–45	5–7	tid–qid	GI distress, dizziness, anxiety-change BP, drowiness	
Ketogenic diet	All	4:1 ratio			Behavior problem, renal stones, dehydration	
Lamotrigine (Lamictal)	P, C (? other)	1–5 (on VPA) 5–15 (off VPA)	15–60	qd–bid	Rash, dizziness, diplopia, GI distress	
Phenobarbital	P, C, G, S	2–8	48–100	qd–bid	Drowsiness, rash, ataxia, cognitive change in behavior	10–25
Phenytoin (Dilantin)	P, C, G, S	4–8	6–30	qd–bid	Drowsiness, rash, gums, hirsutism, anemia, ataxia	10–20
Primidone (Mysoline)	P, C, G	12–25	6–12	bid–qid	Drowsiness, dizziness, rash, anemia, ataxia, diplopia	6–12
Valproic acid (Depakene, Depakote)	P, C, G, M, A	10–60	6–18	bid–qid	GI distress, hepatitis, alopecia, drowsiness, ataxia, pancreatitis, tremor, weight gain	50–100

*P = partial (simple partial); C = complex partial; G = generalized (tonic-clonic); A = absence; M = minor motor (akinetic, atonic, myoclonic); S = status epilepticus.
VPA = valproic acid.

SEIZURE TYPES AND EPILEPSIES

Generalized Tonic-Clonic Seizures

The four most prescribed (and often described as primary) antiepileptic medications are phenobarbital, phenytoin (Dilantin), carbamazepine (Tegretol), and valproic acid (Depakene, Depakote). Phenobarbital is inexpensive and well known to pediatricians and family practitioners. It has a very long half-life and can be given once a day. However, its major disadvantages are hyperactivity, behavioral disorders, cognitive difficulties, and sleep disorders in at least 30% to 40% of children. Data indicate that many more experience more subtle alterations in learning and behavior. If phenobarbital is used, it is mandatory that the physician pay careful attention to any adverse changes in the child's function. This may be particularly pertinent to adolescents, in whom depression may be seen.

Phenytoin is also an effective antiepileptic medication, but changes in appearance and gingival hyperplasia may occur in up to 90% of children. One also must recall that phenytoin has nonlinear kinetics. As the therapeutic range is approached, small increases in dosage may cause dramatic increases in drug levels, leading to toxicity.

Carbamazepine appears to have fewer adverse effects on neuropsychologic function than many other medications. This drug has a fairly short half-life and may need to be given as frequently as four times a day in order to smooth the peak and trough levels. Aplastic anemia associated with carbamazepine use is extremely rare and apparently cannot be predicted by routine hematologic monitoring. On the other hand, neutropenia is more frequent, but rarely produces clinical problems.

Valproic acid is useful in generalized seizures and also appears to have minimal adverse effect on neuropsychologic function or behavior. It also has a short half-life. The hepatic side effects of valproic acid are quite rare but are more frequent in children under 2 years of age who are receiving polytherapy. Children over 11 years and on monotherapy have virtually no risk of hepatic failure from the medication.

Partial Seizures

Both simple and complex partial seizures can be effectively treated by phenobarbital, phenytoin, carbamazepine, valproic acid, and primidone. Primidone is rapidly converted to phenobarbital. Prior to conversion, primidone and another active metabolite (PEMA) are also active antiepileptic medications. It has many of the side effects of phenobarbital and, in addition, has significant initial toxicity, requiring that it be introduced at very low doses and be increased in small increments. Valproic acid is also effective in treating complex partial seizures. In addition, if the partial seizures secondarily generalize, valproic acid would be a useful medication.

Two new medications have become available recently as adjunctive therapy. These are gabapentin (Neurontin) and lamotrigine (Lamictal). Gabapentin is a particularly important addition to the armamentarium since it is not metabolized by the liver but rather is cleared by the kidneys. This is important because it means that few drug interactions are to be expected. Lamotrigine is effective in treating complex partial seizures and may also be effective in some generalized seizures. It is somewhat complicated to use if added to valproic acid, by which its half-life is greatly increased. The dose must be markedly decreased to avoid toxicity and the development of drug-related rash.

Absence Seizures

Absence seizures are best treated with either succinamides or valproic acid. Valproic acid is probably more effective in atypical absence seizures and would certainly be preferred when both absence and tonic-clonic seizures occur in the same patient. Ethosuximide (Zarontin) is effective in classic absence seizures. Side effects include headaches and nausea. In addition, benzodiazepines are frequently used as adjunctive drugs. These medications include clonazepam (Klonopin), clorazepate (Tranxene), and lorazepam (Ativan). It is discouraging that the benzodiazepines are often effective initially but decrease in efficacy over time. Side effects may also be quite intolerable and include sedation, behavior changes, and sometimes difficulty in handling secretions.

Myoclonic and Atonic Seizures

Valproic acid is the medication of choice for these seizures. The benzodiazepines may also be effective, and recently lamotrigine has shown significant efficacy. The ketogenic diet also can play an important role in controlling these seizures. The diet involves fasting the child into ketosis and maintaining this ketosis in a chronic fashion by using a diet with a high proportion of ketogenic food (fats). The diet usually consists of a ratio of 4 grams of fat to 1 gram of protein plus carbohydrate (36 calories of fats: 4 calories of protein + carbohydrate). Children require 60 to 75 calories per kg per day and at least 1 gram per kg per day of protein. Fluids are traditionally restricted to 600 to 1200 mL per day, but this can be liberalized depending on the child's actual needs. The diet is deficient in calcium and fat-soluble vitamins and requires supplementation with calcium and multivitamins with minerals and iron. The child is monitored for ketosis by examining urinary ketones that should be large, especially late in the afternoon.

Febrile Seizures

Febrile seizures occur in 3% to 4% of all children, most commonly between 9 and 20 months of age. Children are at greater risk if they are in day care, experienced a prolonged hospital stay as a neonate, have delayed development, or have a family history of febrile seizures. Thirty to 40% of children will experience a recurrence after the first seizure. This is more likely if the child is under a year of age, had the febrile seizure at a temperature of less than 38.4°C (101°F), or had the febrile seizure within the first hour of illness. Even when there is recurrence of febrile seizures, there is no increased risk of mental retardation, cerebral palsy, or other significant neurologic sequelae. Only children with two or more risk factors (atypical febrile seizure—lasting longer than 15 minutes, recurring within 24 hours, or focal in nature; a first-degree relative with a history of epilepsy or abnormal neurodevelopmental status prior to the first febrile seizure) are at a significantly increased risk for epilepsy. Even with two or more of these risk factors, the risk of afebrile seizures did not exceed 13% in one study.

Therefore, the use of prophylactic therapy should be *considered* only in the face of these risk factors or multiple recurrences. Daily phenobarbital, maintaining blood levels of greater than 15 mg per liter, will reduce recurrence. However, this therapy frequently produces the previously mentioned behavioral changes and may have a negative impact on intellectual function. Valproic acid is apparently effective but potentially too toxic to consider for use in these young children in whom the risk from recurring febrile seizures is virtually zero. Rectal or oral diazepam (Valium), in a dose of 0.5 mg per kg every 8 hours for temperatures greater than 38.4°C, is also moderately effective. However, a significant number of children will have side effects, and it is frequently impossible for parents or other caretakers to recognize that the child is ill before the febrile seizure occurs. *Normally we do not recommend prophylactic therapy for children with febrile seizures.*

Neonatal Seizures

Neonatal seizures remain the most reliable clinical predictor of later neurologic deficit. However, the majority of infants with neonatal seizures who survive do well. The most important therapy is the search for the cause of the seizures and the appropriate treatment. If the neonatal seizures are recurrent or appear significantly to threaten or interfere with the child's well-being, therapy with antiepileptic medication is undertaken. Phenobarbital is the drug of choice, with a loading dose of 20 mg per kg intravenously as a slow bolus or in divided doses over a short period of time. Phenytoin can also be used, again with a loading dose of 20 mg per kg. Diazepam is a useful agent in its rapidity of action; however, it has a short half-life. It can be used at a dose of 0.2 to 0.5 mg per kg. Frequently, we will treat an infant with a single loading dose of phenobarbital. If this is effective and ongoing insult to the brain does not appear to be occurring, we will not place the child on maintenance phenobarbital. The long half-life (approximately 100 hours) can be expected to protect the infant over the period of recovery from such problems as asphyxia.

Infantile Spasms

These seizures classically consist of sudden flexion of the head, abduction and extension of the arms, and simultaneous flexion of knees. These are the only type of seizure that occurs in series or clusters.

Frequently, the EEG pattern will be that of hypsarrhythmia. Prognosis is generally poor for this group of children, especially in the two thirds who are considered to be symptomatic and experiencing these seizures due to a definable underlying pathology. Treatment should begin promptly, usually with ACTH (adrenocorticotropic hormone) gel,* given intramuscularly, 150 U per m². This dose is gradually tapered over a period of 6 to 9 weeks. The child needs to be followed closely for side effects such as infection and hypertension. Behavioral disturbances, including severe irritability and transient decrease in psychomotor performance, are not uncommon. Prednisone, given at 2 mg per kg or 75 mg per m² may be equally effective, but it is not used as the first therapy in our center. Valproic acid and benzodiazepines may also be effective. Vigabatrin (Sabril)† has been used with considerable efficacy in Europe where it has been available for a number of years.

Lennox-Gastaut Syndrome

The Lennox-Gastaut syndrome consists of an EEG pattern of slow spike-waves and rapid spikes, two or more types of seizures (one of which is usually myoclonic or atonic), and mental retardation. Onset is usually between 1 and 6 years of age, and it may frequently be seen as part of an evolution from infantile spasms. Valproic acid is the treatment of choice but often must be used with additional antiepileptic medications. Recently, lamotrigine has also been shown to be a potentially effective therapy. A slightly older therapy, felbamate (Felbatol), has shown some significant efficacy, but the recently reported cases of aplastic anemia and hepatic failure have led to virtual cessation of its use except in very desperate cases and only after careful explanation of the risks to the family. We find the ketogenic diet particularly helpful in controlling the varied seizures seen in this seizure disorder.

Benign Rolandic Epilepsy

This benign form of epilepsy generally begins at between 3 and 13 years of age, consisting of seizures characterized by facial movements, grimacing, and vocalization, followed by a tonic-clonic component. The EEG frequently shows characteristic repetitive spikes in the midtemporal or centroparietal area. This activity is generally much worse in non-REM sleep. Seizures are quite benign and often occur only at night. Frequently antiepileptic medication is not necessary. When it is necessary, carbamazepine appears to be the drug of choice.

Juvenile Myoclonic Epilepsy

This disorder begins in late childhood or early adulthood with mild myoclonic seizures, often experienced on awakening. These may then progress to tonic-clonic seizures. Absence seizures can be seen also. This seizure disorder appears to have a genetic basis and generally needs to be treated throughout life. It appears to respond particularly well to valproic acid.

Status Epilepticus

Although brief tonic-clonic seizures almost certainly do not cause brain damage, there is fear that status epilepticus, or seizures lasting more than 30 minutes, may be a threat to the integrity of the central nervous system as well as to life itself. In treating status, there is a fine line between aggressive therapy to stop the seizures and the production of iatrogenic problems requiring intubation and ventilation, and the potential morbidity associated with this. Before medications are given, maintenance of vital function should be established. This includes adequate ventilation, maintenance of perfusion, and monitoring of vital signs. An intravenous line should be placed to obtain appropriate blood work and to administer both glucose (as necessary) as well an antiepileptic medication. Diazepam is usually the initial drug of choice because of low toxicity and rapid onset of action. It is given as 0.2 to 0.5 mg per kg over a 2-minute period with a 10-mg maximum single dose. The dose may be repeated in 10 minutes if status persists. This can also be done using rectal diazepam. Lorazepam (Ativan)* at a dose of 0.05 to 0.1 mg per kg, is increasingly being utilized as an alternative because of its longer duration of action. Because diazepam is effective for only a short time, the child also should be treated with an intravenous loading dose of phenytoin or phenobarbital. A loading dose of 15 to 20 mg per kg of phenytoin is infused at a rate not to exceed 25 mg per minute. Simultaneous ECG and monitoring of blood pressure are mandatory. Maintenance dosages should be begun within 6 to 8 hours. Phenobarbital can be given in a loading dose of 15 to 20 mg per kg.

SURGICAL THERAPY

Medical therapy is effective in perhaps 75% of children. However, there are individuals whose seizures are intractable and/or who are experiencing life-altering side effects from the medicine. In these individuals, the search for identifiably abnormal tissue and the potential for surgical remediation should be considered. This frequently requires intensive monitoring to determine the exact focus or source of the seizure activity. Sometimes a subdural electrode grid is placed directly on the brain, enabling the clinician to identify the source of the seizure as well as areas that should be spared to preserve important neurologic functions (movement and speech). In addition, there is a group of youngsters with severe or progressive disease of a single hemisphere, either

---

*Not FDA-approved for this indication.
†Not licensed in the United States. Licensed in Canada.

---

*Not FDA-approved for this indication.

due to developmental abnormalities, trauma, or Rasmussen's syndrome. These youngsters should be considered for removal of the entire hemisphere (hemispherectomy). Embarking on seizure surgery requires a team approach in the evaluation, counseling, and management of these patients.

ATTENTION DEFICIT HYPERACTIVITY DISORDER (ADHD)

method of
JUDITH A. OWENS-STIVELY, M.D., M.P.H.
Hasbro Children's Hospital and Brown
  University School of Medicine
Providence, Rhode Island

Attention deficit hyperactivity disorder (ADHD) is one of the most commonly diagnosed behavioral problems in childhood, affecting some 3 to 5% of school-aged children in the United States, and one of the most extensively studied in terms of its etiology, evaluation, and treatment. The changes in nomenclature for this disorder over the past 50 years, from "minimal brain damage" (MBD) to "hyperkinesis" to attention deficit disorder (ADD), reflect an increased understanding of its neurochemical and neuropathologic basis, as well as the development of a more sophisticated and rigorous set of criteria for diagnosis and classification. Despite this increased body knowledge, however, the consistent application of strict evaluation criteria and the use of appropriate multimodal treatment by clinicians remain problematic. In recent years, this has led to controversial allegations by some groups of widespread overdiagnosis and overmedication of ADHD.

Recent studies strongly support a neurobiologic basis for this disorder. Highly sophisticated neuroimaging techniques such as positron emission tomography (PET) scanning have demonstrated altered functioning in individuals with ADHD in areas of the cerebral cortex known to be linked to arousal and activity control. Multiple neurotransmitters are likely involved, including dopamine, norepinephrine, and serotonin. This provides a direct rationale for the use of certain classes of psychopharmacologic agents that affect these neurotransmitters in the treatment of ADHD. Increased understanding of the differential effects of individual neurotransmitter dysfunction, such as the link between norepinephrine dysregulation and inattention, has already led to a more specific approach to matching target symptoms with psychopharmacologic agents.

EPIDEMIOLOGY AND RISK FACTORS

Multiple family, twin, and adoption studies have demonstrated a genetic link in the etiology of ADHD. Symptoms of ADHD are clearly more common in first-degree biologic relatives of children diagnosed with the disorder, and some authors have postulated a single autosomal major dominant gene mode of inheritance. Not all individuals with ADHD have a positive family history (estimates range from 30 to 50%), but there is a suggestion that the familial type of ADHD may carry an increased risk of co-morbid learning disabilities. Girls may need a higher genetic loading to express ADHD symptoms. Many other mental health diagnoses, including depression and anxiety disorders, sub-

stance abuse, and antisocial behavior or conduct disorder, are also more prevalent in family members of children with ADHD.

Many authors emphasize, however, that a variety of psychosocial risk factors may be as important as heredity in the pathogenesis of ADHD. These include lower socioeconomic class, marital discord and domestic violence, and sexual and physical abuse, among others. It is, in particular, the cumulative effect of multiple psychosocial stressors that may make an individual child more vulnerable to the expression of ADHD symptoms. Parents of children with ADHD may themselves have residual symptoms of the disorder, such as disorganization and impulsivity, which may create compliance problems in carrying out behavioral treatment plans.

Finally, certain biologic risk factors may contribute to the development of ADHD symptoms. These include prenatal alcohol and substance abuse, prematurity and birth complications, and significant head trauma and central nervous system infections. Even low levels of lead exposure (venous lead in the 10 to 20 mg per dL range), especially if it occurs during the period of most rapid neuronal development (12 to 36 months), may later be manifested in symptoms of ADHD and subtle learning deficits. Recently, a strong association has been demonstrated between the syndrome of General Resistance to Thyroid Hormone and ADHD, although this familial disorder is rare. The behavioral side effects of certain medications used for chronic conditions in childhood, such as phenobarbital for seizures and theophylline preparations for reactive airway disease, may mimic symptoms of ADHD. Obstructive sleep apnea, usually related in childhood to adenotonsillar hypertrophy, may present with ADHD-like symptoms of inattentiveness and hyperactivity secondary to chronic sleep deprivation.

CLINICAL FEATURES

The hallmark of ADHD in children is the clinical constellation of inattention, distractibility, impulsivity, and physical or motor hyperactivity, often described as restlessness, fidgetiness, and the inability to sit still. Inattention refers to difficulty in focusing, sustaining, and redirecting attention appropriately, and in children with ADHD, it is often highly dependent on motivation and interest. Distractibility may result from internal preoccupation and daydreaming and/or the inability to screen out external stimuli. Impulsivity or acting without thinking, can be verbal or physical and often results in a multitude of secondary behavioral concerns, such as aggressiveness with peers and disruptiveness in the classroom setting.

The most recent DSM IV classification (Table 1) further subdivides ADHD into three subtypes—hyperactive/impulsive, inattentive, and combined—according to the relative prominence of more "externalizing" versus "internalizing" target symptoms. Children with predominantly inattentive ADHD usually do not have pronounced hyperactivity and, in fact, may be described as "sluggish" and "spacey."

The number and severity of symptoms of ADHD can vary widely and can differ with age (younger children tend to be more physically active than adolescents), the setting (structured vs. unstructured), gender (ADHD is 3 to 10 times more commonly diagnosed in boys, and boys are far more likely than girls to have the hyperactive/impulsive subtype), and the presence or absence of co-morbid conditions. The chronicity, persistence, pervasiveness, and developmental inappropriateness of symptoms all help distinguish a child with ADHD from a behaviorally disordered child who may be responding to an acute stress or whose

TABLE 1. **Diagnostic Criteria for Attention Deficit Hyperactivity Disorder**

A. Either 1 or 2:
  1. Six (or more) of the following symptoms of inattention have persisted for at least 6 months to a degree that is maladaptive and inconsistent with developmental level:
     a. Often fails to give close attention to details or makes careless mistakes in schoolwork, work, or other activities
     b. Often has difficulty sustaining attention in tasks or play activities
     c. Often does not seem to listen when spoken to directly
     d. Often does not follow through on instructions and fails to finish schoolwork, chores, or duties in the workplace (not due to oppositional behavior or failure to understand instructions)
     e. Often has difficulty organizing tasks and activities
     f. Often avoids, dislikes, or is reluctant to engage in tasks that require sustained mental effort (such as schoolwork or homework)
     g. Often loses things necessary for tasks or activities (e.g., toys, school assignments, pencils, books, or tools)
     h. Is often easily distracted by extraneous stimuli
     i. Is often forgetful in daily activities
  2. Six (or more) of the following symptoms of hyperactivity-impulsivity have persisted for a least 6 months to a degree that is maladaptive and inconsistent with developmental level:
     Hyperactivity
     a. Often fidgets with hands or feet or squirms in seat
     b. Often leaves seat in classroom or in other situations in which remaining seated is expected
     c. Often runs about or climbs excessively in situations in which it is inappropriate (in adolescents or adults, may be limited to subjective feelings of restlessness)
     d. Often has difficulty playing or engaging in leisure activities quietly
     e. Is often "on the go" or often acts as if "driven by a motor"
     f. Often talks excessively
     Impulsivity
     g. Often blurts out answers before questions have been completed
     h. Often has difficulty awaiting turn
     i. Often interrupts or intrudes on others (e.g., butts into conversations or games)
B. Some hyperactive-impulsive or inattentive symptoms that caused impairment were present before age 7 years.
C. Some impairment from the symptoms is present in two or more settings (e.g., at school [or work] and at home)
D. There must be clear evidence of clinically significant impairment in social, academic, or occupational functioning
E. The symptoms do not occur exclusively during the course of a pervasive developmental disorder, schizophrenia, or other psychotic disorder and are not better accounted for by another mental disorder (e.g., mood disorder, anxiety disorder, dissociative disorder, or personality disorder)
Code based on type:
314.01 Attention deficit hyperactivity disorder, combined type: if both criteria A1 and A2 are met for the past 6 months
314.00 Attention deficit hyperactivity disorder, predominantly inattentive type: if criterion A1 is met but criterion A2 is not met for the past 6 months
314.01 Attention deficit hyperactivity disorder, predominantly hyperactive-impulse type: if criterion A2 is met but criterion A1 is not met for the past 6 months
Coding note: For individuals (especially adolescents and adults) who currently have symptoms that no longer meet full criteria, "in partial remission"

From Diagnostic and Statistical Manual of Mental Disorders, 4th ed. Washington, DC, American Psychiatric Association, 1994.

behavioral problems are a reflection of inconsistent parental limit setting.

Additional associated features of ADHD include low frustration tolerance, difficulty initiating and impersistence in completing tasks, relative resistance to rewards and punishment, and the failure to learn from one's mistakes. The failure to recognize and respond appropriately to social cues and social immaturity, in addition to the impulsivity and intrusiveness, can often lead to problems with peer relations. ADHD children are often highly inconsistent in their behavior from day to day and even hour to hour, and they are disorganized in their approach to tasks. Understandably, these symptoms often lead to academic failure, especially when coupled with learning disabilities, behavior problems in school and at home, and low self-esteem.

Most children with ADHD develop symptoms, at least in retrospect, before the age of 7 years. More severely affected youngsters, especially those with the hyperactive/impulsive subtype, may be recognized as preschoolers. The persistence of at least some symptoms into adolescence, occurring in up to 70% of children with ADHD, and even into adulthood is now well recognized. ADHD, particularly the inattentive type, occasionally goes unrecognized until adolescence, when previously successful compensatory strategies become inadequate to meet the increased academic and social demands of junior and senior high school.

ADHD in adolescence is characterized by a disorganized approach, variability in academic performance, mental fatigue (often interpreted as laziness or boredom), excessive dependence on motivation, and difficulty in distinguishing between salient and irrelevant material ("the forest for the trees" phenomenon). Social interactions with peers are particularly problematic because of failure to attend and respond appropriately to social cues, verbal impulsivity, and difficulty in delaying gratification. The subgroup of adolescents with co-morbid conduct disorders is at especially high risk for antisocial behavior, delinquency, truancy, and substance abuse.

CO–MORBID CONDITIONS

The issue of co-morbidity in ADHD is a complex one because of the frequent coexistence of a variety of psychiatric problems in children and adolescents with ADHD and because the behavioral manifestations of many of these psychiatric problems may overlap. For example, aggression in a preschooler may be part of the ADHD symptom constellation, or it may result from post-traumatic stress disorder associated with a history of sexual abuse, reflect exposure to and modeling of domestic violence in the home setting, or be a transient behavioral response to an acute stressor, such as divorce. In addition, the symptoms of the most common co-morbid conditions often show a typical developmental progression and may become evident only over time. ADHD symptoms often develop first (in preschoolers), followed by signs of oppositional defiant disorder (age 4 to 5 years), anxiety and depression disorders (often by 5 to 7 years of age), conduct disorder (8 to 9 years of age), and finally substance abuse problems (adolescence).

Oppositional behavior, characterized by defiance, noncompliance, negativity, and difficulty in following rules, is the most common (60%) co-morbid psychiatric disorder with ADHD. Conduct disorder, occurring in up to 45% of older children with ADHD, has as its central feature a basic disregard for the rights of others and is behaviorally manifested by lying, stealing, and physical aggression. Recognition and treatment of a conduct disorder are especially important because of the high risk for later development of serious problems such as substance abuse and delinquency. Depression and anxiety disorders, including separation anxiety and school phobia, eventually develop in up to one-third of ADHD youngsters.

Several other co-morbid conditions deserve comment. The prevalence of specific learning disabilities in ADHD is estimated at 10 to 35%, and their presence may add significantly to the risk of academic failure. ADHD is also diagnosed in 20 to 50% of individuals with Tourette syndrome, which is characterized by the presence of both vocal and motor tics and is often accompanied by additional symptoms such as coprolalia (involuntary utterance of profanity) and obsessive-compulsive behavior.

Although a large percentage of children presenting with ADHD in a primary care setting do not develop serious psychiatric problems, the presence of additional mental health concerns in ADHD has important implications for treatment and prognosis and should be appropriately evaluated and tracked. Referral to a child psychiatrist, psychologist, or other mental health professional may be warranted.

EVALUATION

The evaluation of children with possible ADHD may be performed by a variety of health professionals, including child and adult psychiatrists, neurologists, psychologists, and neuropsychologists. It is most often the primary care physician, however, whom the parent or school first approaches about making the diagnosis. There is no single reliable diagnostic test for ADHD; rather, the diagnosis is based on a comprehensive clinical assessment that should include the following.

History of the Problem. This includes onset, type, and severity of ADHD symptoms; associated symptoms; behavior in different settings (school, home, office); and current and previous attempts at behavioral management. Description of the child's typical behavior in situations that are likely to be problematic (mealtimes, chores, bedtime) may be particularly helpful.

Assessment of Common Co-Morbid Conditions. Symptoms of depression or anxiety (including separation anxiety, school avoidance, and school phobia), oppositional behaviors and conduct problems, and motor and vocal tics should be noted.

School History. This includes previous and current academic and behavioral difficulties, history of grade retention, current educational program and setting (classroom size and child's placement in the classroom, special education services or resource help, individualized education plan [IEP]), recent report card results, academic strengths and weaknesses, homework management, and peer relationships.

Assessment for Learning Disabilities. The results of any previous educational or achievement tests and neuropsychological evaluations (IQ or language, cognitive, or processing abilities) should be reviewed. Because of the high incidence of learning disabilities in ADHD (up to 35%) and the fact that some learning disabilities (such as auditory processing deficits) can mimic symptoms of ADHD, any child in whom learning problems are suspected should have a neuropsychological assessment.

Although a neuropsychological evaluation cannot make the diagnosis of ADHD, certain tests, as well as trained observation of the child's testing behavior, may be helpful in substantiating the clinical impression. The Freedom from Distractibility Factors subscale on the WISC-R IQ test, as well as the Continous Performance Test (CPT) and various cancellation tests that assess for errors of commission and omission, may underscore problems with inattention and distractibility. The description of a child who needs to be constantly "refocused," is easily frustrated, rushes through work without checking it, fails to follow directions, and is easily distracted during a one-on-one testing session also strongly suggests the diagnosis of ADHD.

Family History. Note the presence of other family members with ADHD, academic problems or learning disabilties, mood or anxiety disorders, substance or alcohol abuse, or thyroid disease.

Social History. Determine the educational levels of parents and siblings, family constellation, marital history, history of domestic violence or sexual or physical abuse, recent or ongoing stressors in the home, and family response to the child's behavior and academic problems.

Developmental History. Note major milestones and the results of previous developmental evaluations.

Medical History. This includes a description of the pregnancy and birth, significant or chronic illnesses, lead poisoning, significant head trauma, allergies, and medications.

Physical Examination. Note growth parameters and baseline vital signs and perform a brief neurologic examination. Although ADHD may be associated with neurologic "soft signs" (e.g., clumsiness, poor fine motor coordination), their significance is unclear. In general, unless specific signs or symptoms emerge, laboratory testing, neuroimaging, and electroencephalograms (EEGs) are not indicated in the general evaluation of ADHD.

Sleep History. This includes sleep onset difficulties, night waking, quality and duration of sleep (restless), early awakening, symptoms of obstructive sleep apnea (disruptive snoring, gasping), and enuresis.

Child Interview. Observe ADHD target symptoms in the office setting, oppositional or defiant behavior, general cognitive and language levels, child's understanding of behavioral concerns, and parent-child interactions. The interview with the parents and child should generally last 60 to 90 minutes.

Standard ADHD Questionnaires. Connor's Parent Questionnaire and Teacher Questionnaire (Table 2) provide information about diagnosis and allow for a standardized measure of treatment efficacy. The Achenbach Child Behavior Checklist (CBCL), which has parent, teacher, and self-report forms, is also an excellent screening tool for many behavioral problems, including ADHD.

TREATMENT

It cannot be overemphasized that a successful treatment plan for children with ADHD involves a comprehensive approach to the behavioral, academic, social, family, and self-esteem issues that may be operative in each individual case. The primary care physician's role should be one of a case manager, coordinating medical intervention, education services, and mental health treatment components. Es-

TABLE 2. **Connor's Teacher Questionnaire (Abbreviated Form)**

TEACHER'S QUESTIONNAIRE

Name of the Child ____ Grade ______________

Date of Evaluation ________________________________

Please answer all questions. Beside each item indicate the degree of the problem by a check mark ($\checkmark$).

	Score 0	1	2	3
	Not at all	Just a little	Pretty much	Very much
1. Restless in the "squirmy" sense.				
2. Demands must be met immediately.				
3. Distractibility or attention span a problem.				
4. Disturbs other children.				
5. Restless, always "up and on the go."				
6. Excitable, impulsive.				
7. Fails to finish things that he starts.				
8. Childish and immature.				
9. Easily frustrated in efforts.				
10. Difficulty in learning.				

Possible range: 0 to 30
Cut-off point: 15

sential case management components include facilitating communication and feedback among the different treatment providers; supplying education about ADHD to patients, families, and schools; making appropriate referrals for additional services; supporting the family; and serving as an advocate for the child. This last point underscores the need to ensure the child's understanding of and cooperation with the treatment plan as an essential factor in treatment compliance.

Educational intervention by the school involves both diagnosing and addressing any specific coexisting learning disabilities and designing programs for classroom management. Parents should be strongly encouraged to become active participants in their child's educational plan. They need to be made aware of federally mandated special education services for children with significant ADHD-related academic impairment under the 1990 Individuals with Disabilities Education Act, as well as provisions for classroom modification under Section 504 of the Rehabilitation Act of 1973. The IEP, which operationalizes the stated educational goals, should be part of the patient's medical record and should be reviewed periodically by the primary care physician and the parents.

Classroom management consists of age- and child-specific modifications to improve attention and impulse control, enhance organizational skills and self-esteem, and increase productivity. Examples include breaking work down into smaller components; avoiding multistep directions; using a cue (such as a pat on the shoulder) to refocus attention; seating the child in the front of the classroom, providing frequent "stand up and stretch breaks" during seated work; reinforcing orally presented material with visual aids, and vice versa; establishing clear expectations and consequences for behavior, and tracking these with a daily report form; allowing the child to dictate written assignments; and using a daily communication notebook to track homework assignments. Positive reinforcement and focusing on academic and extracurricular strengths are also key variables.

Behavioral management of an ADHD child in the home involves some of the same principles: using sticker or star charts or a token-reward system for specific target behaviors, engaging the child's attention before giving directions, anticipating and structuring problematic situations in which the child is likely to be overstimulated (e.g., holiday gatherings), and providing safe outlets for excess energy. Parents may benefit from referral to parent-training workshops or individual parent-child behavior therapy to learn these skills.

Children who have particular problems with peer relationships often benefit from social skills training groups, which many schools are developing for behaviorally disordered youngsters. Individual psychotherapy referral may be necessary for children with significant self-esteem concerns and co-morbid depression or anxiety. Family therapy can be extremely helpful in dealing with problematic family relationships. The primary care physician can also provide information about adult mental health referral for the identification and treatment of a parent's ADHD symptoms. Finally, parent support groups such as Children with Attention Deficit Disorder (Ch.A.D.D.) are often extremely helpful in providing emotional support, practical management techniques, and information to parents (Table 3).

Many parents question the role of dietary factors, including sugar consumption, food additives and dyes, and food allergies, in the exacerbation of ADHD symptoms. Multiple well-controlled, double-blind studies have failed to demonstrate a consistent benefit from sugar-free, allergen-free, oligoantigenic, or additive-free diets for the vast majority of ADHD children. Most of these special diets are nutritionally adequate (although some, like the Feingold diet, can be very restrictive and expensive). Therefore, diets that restrict sugar or preservatives generally do not result in harm to the child. Care should be taken, however, not to make the child feel singled out from siblings and peers by such dietary restrictions.

Two other controversial treatments for ADHD deserve mention: motor therapies, which focus on sensory integration skills or eye movement training, and EEG biofeedback, in which children are taught to "normalize" their EEG patterns. Proponents' claims of increased concentration, improved academic performance, and even increased IQ thus far remain unsubstantiated, but these therapies do not appear to be harmful.

PSYCHOPHARMACOLOGY OF ADHD

General Considerations

Since the first documented use of dextroamphetamine to treat hyperactivity in the late 1930s, the use of psychopharmacologic agents to treat symptoms of ADHD has risen dramatically—as much as sixfold over the past 5 years, according to Drug Enforcement Agency statistics. Approximately 2 million Americans, nearly 1 in every 30 children between the ages of 5 and 18 years old, are currently being medicated for ADHD, and psychostimulants are the most widely prescribed psychotropic medication. Despite concern about overuse, the rationale for the use of drug treatment in ADHD remains sound as part of a multimodal, integrated treatment plan. For many children and adolescents with ADHD, successful amelioration of symptoms by medications such as methylphenidate (Ritalin) and dextroamphetamine (Dexedrine) allows them to make full use of other treatment modalities, such as educational modifications, and represents the difference between academic success and failure.

Several general principles of medication management deserve comment. First, medication should be selected on the basis of specific target symptoms, and treatment success should be measured on the basis of remission of, or at least improvement in, these symptoms. Target symptoms should be well defined and measurable whenever possible (e.g., percentage of schoolwork completed, number of times out of seat) and prioritized according to the degree to which they interfere with the child's daily functioning. Standardized questionnaires such as the Connor or daily behavioral rating charts may be especially helpful in documenting treatment success over time.

Second, age and developmental stage should be a prime consideration in drug selection. For example, preschool-aged children tend to metabolize psychostimulants faster and may need a more frequent dosing schedule, and they tend to have more unpredictable behavioral effects from these medications. Because of the risk for cardiac dysrhythmia, tricyclic antidepressants should be used with caution in prepubertal children.

Third, any medication should be started at the lower end of the dosage range and gradually titrated up at a pace commensurate with the behavioral half-life. In general, the shorter-acting medications such as methylphenidate may be increased more quickly.

Fourth, medications should always be titrated to maximize the cognitive and behavioral benefits while minimizing the development of both short- and long-term side effects.

Fifth, different medications in the same class should be tried before moving on to another class of drug. For example, some individuals respond well to

---

TABLE 3. **References About ADHD for Parents**

Children and Adults with Attention Deficit Disorders (Ch.A.D.D.)
499 Northwest 70th Avenue
Suite 308
Plantation, Florida 33317
(305) 587-3700

Books for Parents and Teachers

Barkely, R. (1985). *Taking Charge of ADHD: The Complete Authoritative Guide for Parents.* New York: Guilford.

Fowler, Mary Cahill. (1990). *Maybe You Know My Kid: A Parent's Guide to Identifying, Understanding, and Helping Your Child with Attention-Deficit Hyperactivity Disorder.* Birch Lane, 600 Madison Ave., New York, NY 10022.

Ingersoll, B., and M. Goldstein. (1993). *Attention Deficit Disorder and Learning Disabilities: Realities, Myths, and Controversial Treatments.* New York: Doubleday.

Parker, Harvey. (1988). *Attention Deficit Disorders: A Parent and Teacher Workbook.* Ch.A.D.D., 1859 Pine Island Road, Suite 185, Plantation, FL 33322.

Silver, Larry. (1993). *Dr. Larry Silver's Advice to Parents on Attention Deficit Hyperactivity Disorder.* American Psychiatric Press, Inc., 1400 K Street NW, Washington, DC 20005.

Wodrich, David. (1994). *What Every Parent Wants to Know: Attention Deficit Hyperactivity Disorder.* Baltimore: Paul H. Brookes Publishing Co.

Books for Children

Galvin, Matthew. (1988). *Otto Learns About His Medicine.* New York: Magination Press (5–8 years old).

Gordon, Michael. (1922). *I Would If I Could.* GSI Publications, PO Box 746, DeWitt, NY 13214 (siblings).

Moss, Deborah. (1989). *Shelly the Hyperactive Turtle.* Bethesda, Maryland: Woodbine House (5–8 years old).

Parker, Roberta. (1992). *Making the Grade.* Impact Publications, 300 NW 70th Avenue, Plantation, FL 33317 (or call the ADD Warehouse at 800-233-9273 to order) (8–12 years old).

Quinn, Patricia. (1992). *Putting on the Brakes.* New York: Magination Press (8–12 years old).

Quinn, Patricia. (1994). *ADD and the College Student.* New York: Magination Press.

methylphenidate but not to dextroamphetamine, and vice versa. If an individual child does not respond to several different adequate medication trials, the possibility of alternative or additional diagnoses should be strongly considered.

Sixth, medications should be initiated one at a time and their effectiveness documented before combination therapy is considered in the treatment of resistant or complicated cases. Special consideration should also be given to possible drug interactions when using combination regimens. Consultation with a child psychiatrist or neurologist before initiating additional medication may be appropriate.

Finally, every child on medication for ADHD should be followed for continued medication efficacy and side effects at regular intervals (at a minimum, every 4 to 6 months) once a stable dose has been reached. Some children develop tolerance to a previously effective medication or dose. Each child deserves a yearly trial off medication, preferably timed at a few weeks into the new school year, to assess the continued need for drug therapy.

Psychostimulants

The psychostimulants methylphenidate (Ritalin), amphetamines (Dexedrine, Dextrostat, Desoxyn, Adderall), and pemoline (Cylert) are generally considered to be the first-line medications in the treatment of children and adolescents with ADHD (Table 4). The stimulants, at least partially through their indirect effects on the intrasynaptic availability of norepinephrine and dopamine, exert their major neurobehavioral effects by decreasing excessive variability in arousal and reactivity. Inattention, distractibility, motor hyperactivity, and behavioral intensity are all reduced by stimulants. Secondary beneficial effects include improved accuracy and speed in completing academic tasks, decreased off-task behavior, and a reduction of excessive motivation dependency. Stimulant use often results in a decrease in oppositional, aggressive, and noncompliant behavior and an improvement in peer and family relationships.

Stimulants result in improvement or remission of ADHD symptoms in approximately 70 to 80% of individuals for whom they are appropriately prescribed. Gender does not appear to affect stimulant response, but there may be differences in individual responsiveness to the different psychostimulants. The response rate may be lower in very young children (the lower age limit for stimulant use is generally 3 years old) and in adolescents and children with the inattentive type of ADHD. However, because stimulants also improve attention and reduce distractibility in non-ADHD individuals, a positive clinical response should not be taken as confirmation of the diagnosis of ADHD.

Sympathomimetic agents, including pseudoephedrine, can potentiate the effects of stimulants, and antihistamines may diminish their effectiveness. Stimulants should be used with caution in children with seizure disorders, as they may both delay ab-

sorption and increase levels of anticonvulsants. Methylphenidate can inhibit tricyclic antidepressant metabolism and result in elevated serum levels. Recently, concern has been raised about the possible role of methylphenidate and the alpha$_2$ agonist clonidine (Catapres) in the sudden deaths of several children on this combination regimen for ADHD. Although the investigation of these cases did not substantiate drug interaction as the cause of death, theoretical considerations about the possibility of hyper- or hypotensive events suggest that caution should be exercised when prescribing stimulants and clonidine together; dosage and timing are important variables.

The short-term side effects of the psychostimulants include mild headaches and abdominal discomfort (which usually disappear within the first 1 to 2 weeks), irritability or depression, mild increases in blood pressure and pulse (usually clinically insignificant), appetite suppression, and sleep problems. The appetite suppression can result in significant weight loss in some children, especially initially, and may necessitate adjustment of the dosage schedule (during or after meals) and the institution of additional snack times. The relationship between psychostimulants and sleep is a complex one. Some children appear to be very sensitive to the stimulant effect and may experience increased sleep difficulties on medication, necessitating a reduction or earlier timing of a second daily dose. Many children with ADHD are described by their parents as having significant baseline sleep difficulties, especially bedtime struggles and delayed sleep onset, which may actually be improved by the addition of stimulant therapy. Other children on a morning and noon dosing regimen of the shorter-acting stimulants experience a "rebound" phenomenon in which behavioral symptoms of hyperactivity and impulsivity actually increase over baseline when the noon dose wears off. If this rebound coincides with bedtime, sleep onset problems may result. These can be addressed by adding a third, smaller dose of medication late in the day to "piggyback" into bedtime. Finally, the addition of a bedtime dose of clonidine* (0.025 to 0.1 mg), with its sedative effects, is becoming increasingly more common in the management of ADHD-related sleep difficulties.

Recent longitudinal studies that showed no significant compromise in adult height suggest that concerns about long-term growth suppression by psychostimulants are largely unfounded. Some clinicians continue to advocate the use of "drug holidays" on weekends and school and summer vacations to allow for "catch-up" growth, but this strategy may be problematic for children who feel particularly "out of control" when they are off medication during these typically less-structured periods. Concerns about stimulant therapy and later substance abuse have also not been substantiated by long-term studies, although clearly ADHD itself and its co-morbid con-

---

*Not FDA-approved for this indication.

TABLE 4. **Common Psychostimulants Used for ADHD in Children and Adolescents**

Generic Name	Brand Name	Preparations	Usual Dosing Range to Maximum	Onset of Action/ Duration of Action	Usual Dosing Schedule	Additional Comments
Methylphenidate	Ritalin	5-, 10-, 20-mg tablets	0.3–0.6 mg/kg/day up to 2 mg/kg/day Max 60–75 mg/day	30–60 min/3–6 h	bid–tid; increase weekly	May combine short- and long-acting forms; possible recreational abuse
Methylphenidate slow release	Ritalin-SR	20-mg tablets	Equivalent to 10 mg bid	30–60 min/up to 8 h	Once a day in A.M.	*Advantages*—avoids need for in-school dose, decreased rebound *Disadvantages*—may not be as effective as bid dose; may develop tolerance; more expense; may be toxic if chewed
Dextroamphetamine	Dexedrine	5-, 10-mg tablets 5-, 10-, 25-mg spansule 5 mg/5 mL elixir	0.1–1 mg/kg/day Max 30–40 mg/day	30 min/3–6 h (tablet) 7–8 h (spansule)	Once a day–bid	May combine short- and long-acting forms; abuse potential with all amphetamines
Dextroamphetamine	Dextrostat	5-, 10-mg tablets	Max 40 mg/day		Starting dose: 3–5 years—2.5 mg in A.M. Over 6 years—5 mg 1–2 times a day	Less expensive; scored tablet
Methamphetamine	Desoxyn	5-, 10-, 15-mg tablets	20–25 mg/day	4–6 h	5 mg 1–2 times a day; may increase by 5 mg weekly	
Pemoline	Cylert	18.75-, 37.5-, 75-mg tablets 37.5-mg chewable tablets	0.5–3 mg/kg/day	60 min/8–12 h	Once a day in A.M.	*Advantages*—24-h coverage; decreased sympathomimetic/cardiovascular side effects *Disadvantages*—baseline and liver function tests every 6 months, 2% incidence of clinical hepatitis; some immediate benefit but may be 3–4 weeks before full effects noted
Dextroamphetamine sulfate Dextroamphetamine saccharate Amphetamine aspartate Amphetamine sulfate	Adderall	10-, 20-mg tablets	Max 40 mg/day	6–8 h	3–5 years—2.5 mg in A.M.; may increase by 2.5 mg weekly Over 6 years—5 mg 1–2 times a day; may increase by 5 mg weekly	*Advantages*—longer duration of action; question of more predictable medication release; crushable

ditions (especially conduct disorder) are risk factors for later drug and alcohol abuse. However, there have been reports of recreational use of methylphenidate—usually "snorting" of the crushed pills by non-ADHD adolescents. Methylphenidate, although structurally similar to cocaine, does not appear to share its addictive pharmacokinetics. Clinicians should be alert, however, to the potential street value of stimulants and monitor prescription practices accordingly. Finally, recent reports (January 1996) suggest a possible weak carcinogenic potential (an increase in hepatoblastomas in mice) for methylphenidate, which appears at this point not to be clinically significant.

The relationship between tic disorders, including Tourette syndrome, and psychostimulants is somewhat controversial. Currently available information suggests that tics do not generally appear de novo in a nonsusceptible individual who is placed on psychostimulants. Motor tics, when they do occur, are frequently reversible after medication discontinuation. However, psychostimulants are relatively contraindicated in children and adolescents with a previous history of motor or vocal tics or a family history of tics or Tourette syndrome, because stimulant therapy may precipitate or exacerbate tics in these individuals.

Clinical wisdom about the duration of psychostimulant therapy for childhood ADHD has been modified in the past few years. Many adolescents and adults with ADHD continue to benefit substantially from ongoing pharmacotherapy, although target symptoms may change, and the class of drug used, dose, and dosing intervals may require modification over time. Clear evidence of long-term significant improvement in academic achievement from psychostimulant treatment, however, has been disappointingly lacking so far. Although certain academic areas (arithmetic, language skills, likelihood of staying in school) do show long-term improvement, the most consistently identified benefits of chronic psychostimulant therapy have been in the areas of social and life skills and self-esteem.

Because of the high prevalence of co-morbid behavior problems in children with developmental disabilities, including fragile X syndrome, the use of psychostimulants to treat ADHD symptoms in mental retardation deserves special mention. Methylphenidate has been demonstrated to result in substantial clinical improvement in ADHD symptoms, especially in higher cognitively functioning children. Although the side effects of stimulant therapy, especially social withdrawal and motor tics, tend to be more prominent and more problematic in developmentally delayed children, the higher-functioning children appear to be at lower risk.

Antidepressants

Antidepressants, tricyclic antidepressants (TCAs), selective serotonin reuptake inhibitors (SSRIs), monoamine oxidase inhibitors (MAOIs), and several newer antidepressants are generally considered to be second-line pharmacotherapy for the treatment of ADHD in children (Table 5). TCAs such as imipramine (Tofranil),* desipramine (Norpramin),* nortriptyline (Pamelor),* and amitriptyline (Elavil)* appear to exert their effect by blocking presynaptic uptake of neurotransmitters, including norepinephrine and serotonin. They are used clinically in ADHD in a variety of situations:

Failure to respond to adequate stimulant trial or intolerance of stimulant side effects

High risk of stimulant abuse

Patient or family history of tic disorder or Tourette syndrome (although there have been reports of tics emerging during TCA therapy as well)

Co-morbid depressive or anxiety disorder

Strong family history of affective disorders or alcohol abuse

Co-morbid enuresis

Preference for continuous coverage of ADHD symptoms without rebound

Clinician preference for availability of serum drug level monitoring (compliance issues)

Preference for once-daily dosing and/or avoidance of in-school medication administration

Low risk of intentional or accidental overdose by patient or family member

Patient at low risk for cardiotoxicity (negative patient and family history of significant cardiac disease, sudden death)

The last two points emphasize the potential for TCAs to cause cardiac conduction abnormalities and dysrhythmias. Recent reports of sudden death in several children under 12 years old who were being treated with desipramine, in particular, have raised concerns about its safety. Most clinicians adhere to a conservative approach, including obtaining baseline electrocardiograms (ECGs) and repeat ECGs with significant dose changes (baseline ECG limits: PR intervals no > 0.20 second, QRS no > 0.12 second; ECG on medication: QRS interval no $> 30\%$ over baseline, QTC no > 0.44 to 0.46), monitoring systolic (>80 mmHg and <140 mmHg) and diastolic (>50 mmHg and <85 mmHg) blood pressures and pulse (<130 beats per minute) and cautioning patients to avoid excessive exercise. Dosing should not exceed 5 mg per kg per day, and serum drug levels should be monitored at the initiation of therapy and 5 days after significant dose changes. Although serum drug levels do not correlate well with clinical efficacy, they identify the 5 to 10% of the population who are "slow metabolizers" of TCAs.

TCAs may cause anticholinergic side effects (dry mouth, constipation, blurred vision) in children as well as sedation, cognitive impairment, weight gain or loss, insomnia, nightmares, and lowering of the seizure threshold. Abrupt discontinuation of TCAs or too infrequent dosing schedules (twice- to thrice-a-day dosing may be needed in younger children) may

---

*Not FDA-approved for this indication.

TABLE 5. **Common Antidepressants for ADHD in Children and Adolescents**

Generic Name	Brand Name	Preparations	Dosing Range
Tricyclic Antidepressants			
Desipramine*	Norpramin	10-, 25-, 50-, 75-, 100-, 150-mg tablets	2–5 mg/kg/day daily or bid; may increase every 3–5 days
Imipramine*	Tofranil	10-, 25-, 50-mg tablets	2.5 mg/kg/day
Nortriptyline*	Pamelor	10-, 25-, 50-, 75-mg capsules 10 mg/5 mL liquid	0.5–2.5 mg/kg/day; dose limit 150 mg/day
Amitriptyline*	Elavil	10-, 25-, 50-, 75-, 100-, 150-mg tablets	1–5 mg/kg/day; dose limit 300 mg/day
Selective Serotonin Reuptake Inhibitors			
Fluoxetine*	Prozac	10-, 20-mg pulvules 20 mg/5 mL liquid	*Younger children:* 5 mg/day or 10 mg every other day *Older children and adolescents:* 20 mg/day
Paroxetine*	Paxil	20-, 30-mg tablets	10 mg qhs to 50 mg/day; increase by 10 mg every 1–2 weeks
Sertraline*	Zoloft	50-, 100-mg tablets	25 mg in A.M. to 75–100 mg/day; may increase every 1–2 weeks; dose limit 200 mg/day
Bupropion*	Wellbutrin	75-, 100-mg tablets	3–6 mg/kg/day in tid schedule; dose limit 450 mg/day

*Not FDA-approved for this indication.

lead to flulike withdrawal symptoms with gastrointestinal distress, agitation, and sleep disturbances.

Although not extensively studied in children, other antidepressants, especially the SSRIs, fluoxetine (Prozac),* sertraline (Zoloft),* and paroxetine HCl (Paxil),* appear to be promising in the treatment of resistant or complex cases of ADHD. SSRIs have been successfully and safely used in children as young as 4 years old and generally have fewer side effects than the TCAs. Bupropion (Wellbutrin),* a relatively new antidepressant, blocks norepinephrine and serotonin uptake and has been successfully used in children and adolescents to treat ADHD at a dose of 3 to 6 mg per kg per day. Its major side effects include dermatitis, pruritus, edema, gastrointestinal symptoms, agitation, lowering of the seizure threshold, and possible exacerbation of underlying tic disorders. Most of the antidepressants can be used in combination with stimulants, especially for co-morbid ADHD and mood or anxiety disorders, often allowing a reduction in the dose of both drugs. MAOIs have also been used to treat childhood ADHD, but their utility is limited by the need for dietary restrictions and by possible drug interactions and side effects.

Alpha₂ Agonists

Among the most recent additions to the ADHD psychopharmacologic armamentarium are the alpha₂-agonists, namely clonidine (Catapres)* and guanfacine (Tenex).* The alpha₂ agonists decrease the endogenous release of norepinephrine and bind postsynaptic receptors in the central nervous system arousal center, the locus ceruleus. They may have indirect effects on serotonin and dopamine as well.

Clonidine and guanfacine appear to be particularly effective in decreasing arousal levels in ADHD without significantly altering distractibility and attention. They are clinically most useful in the treatment of highly active, impulsive, and aggressive ADHD children who have an early onset of symptoms and co-morbid oppositional and conduct disorders. The alpha₂ agonists may also be particularly helpful in treating ADHD children with a personal or family history of motor tics.

Clonidine was originally used as an antihypertensive, and one of its principal side effects is mild, usually clinically insignificant, hypotension and orthostatic hypotension, occasionally leading to subjective symptoms of dizziness and lightheadedness. Sedation, which may limit its effectiveness in the school setting, is the other major side effect associated with clonidine. Guanfacine generally appears to be both less apt to cause hypotensive symptoms and less sedating than clonidine. Other side effects of clonidine include headaches, vivid dreams and night waking, gastrointestinal symptoms, and dry mouth. Depression may occur in about 5% of patients, who usually have a positive family history for affective disorders. Abrupt discontinuation of alpha₂ agonists, especially clonidine, may lead to rebound hypertension, and all patients being taken off the medication should be tapered in 0.05-mg increments at 1- to 3-day intervals. The patch form of clonidine may cause a local hypersensitivity reaction.

Clonidine is effective within 30 to 45 minutes and has a behavioral half-life of 3 to 6 hours, with sedation peaking at 30 to 90 minutes and the hypotensive effects at 2 to 4 hours. The usual daily dose range is 3 to 6 μg per kg per day in a three- to four-times-daily schedule. Treatment is usually initiated with a bedtime dose, and the daily dose is increased every 3 days (Table 6). Clinical effects may not be evident until 2 to 4 weeks into treatment, and the maximum effect may not be reached for 2 to 3 months. Cloni-

*Not FDA-approved for this indication.

TABLE 6. **Guidelines for Starting ADHD Treatment with Oral Clonidine**

Time	Day											
	1	2	3	4	5	6	7	8	9	10	11	12
A.M.	—	—	—	X	X	X	X	X	X	X	X	X
Noon	—	—	—	—	—	—	X	X	X	X	X	X
P.M.	—	—	—	—	—	—	—	—	—	X	X	X
Night	X	X	X	X	X	X	X	X	X	X	X	X

The schedule calls for increasing the dose by half a 0.1-mg tablet every third day.
X = 0.05 mg.
From Journal of Child and Adolescent Psychopharmacology, Vol *1:* No 1, Spring 1990.

dine is available in 0.1-, 0.2-, and 0.3-mg strengths in oral form as well as in a transcutaneous patch (Catapres-TTS-1, 2, 3). The patch should be used only after an appropriate oral dose has been titrated. Advantages of the patch include considerable convenience (replaced every 5 days) and less sedation. Guanfacine is usually given in 0.5- to 1-mg doses twice to three times a day. Tolerance may develop, necessitating an increase in dose.

The combination regimen of methylphenidate and clonidine may be useful in treating children with both severe hyperactivity/impulsivity and significant inattentiveness, allowing for up to a 40% reduction in the methylphenidate dose used. This combination may be particularly useful in reducing methylphenidate side effects, including rebound symptoms. The addition of methylphenidate may also diminish the sedative effect of clonidine. As noted earlier, clonidine has increasingly been used as a bedtime adjunct to methylphenidate in children with prolonged sleep onset delay. However, caution should be exercised in response to recent reports of possible severe hypo- or hypertensive episodes in patients on this combination regimen. Clonidine should never be used in conjunction with beta blockers.

ADULT ADHD

Both longitudinal studies and clinical experience suggest that 30 to 50% of children diagnosed with ADHD continue to have mild symptoms, including cognitive dysfunction, inattention, distractibility, impatience, and irritability, into adulthood. It is estimated that an additional 10 to 20% have functional impairment significant enough to warrant a diagnosis of adult ADHD. Adult ADHD, as defined by the Utah criteria (Table 7), may result in a host of diffi-

TABLE 7. **Utah Criteria (Revised) for Adult ADHD**

Includes four symptoms of seven and at least (1) or (2)
1. Inattention persisting from childhood
2. Hyperactivity persisting from childhood
3. Inability to complete tasks
4. Impaired interpersonal relationships or inability to sustain relationships over time
5. Affective lability
6. Hot or explosive temper
7. Stress intolerance

culties in such diverse areas as school achievement, job performance, success in intimate relationships, drug and alcohol abuse, motor vehicle accidents, and personal satisfaction and self-esteem. Many of the same medications used in childhood ADHD, including methylphenidate, TCAs, SSRIs, and bupropion have been successfully used to treat adult ADHD, in conjunction with behavior therapy or psychotherapy. As might be expected, co-morbid conditions such as depression and anxiety are especially common in adult ADHD and may necessitate combination drug therapy.

GILLES DE LA TOURETTE SYNDROME

method of
RUTH DOWLING BRUUN, M.D., and
CATHY BUDMAN, M.D.
North Shore University Hospital
Manhasset, New York

Gilles de la Tourette syndrome, now more commonly known simply as Tourette('s) syndrome (TS) or Tourette's disorder, is a genetically transmitted, heterogenous, neuropsychiatric disorder consisting of a spectrum of tic disorders, obsessive-compulsive symptoms, attention disorders, and other behaviors linked to deficits of impulse control. As such, TS truly bridges the fields of psychiatry and neurology.

As more physicians have become aware of TS, it has been diagnosed far more frequently. Still, confusion about the diagnostic criteria, a typically fluctuating symptomatology, and the lack of a biologic marker have led to wide variations in estimates of its prevalence (from 1 case per 2500 to 1 per 200).

Genetic studies have indicated that TS is transmitted as a sexually influenced, autosomal dominant gene with variable penetrance. While affected males are more likely to have motor and vocal tics, the phenotypic expression of the gene in females may more often be expressed by obsessive-compulsive symptoms. A relatively small percentage of cases appear to be caused by perinatal stressors (e.g., low birthweight or CNS trauma). While the majority of individuals who inherit the genetic defect have mild symptoms that do not require medical intervention, there are a variety of symptoms on the severe end of the spectrum that may require a sophisticated knowledge of pharmacologic treatment.

DIAGNOSIS

There is, as yet, no biologic marker for TS and no test that can be performed to confirm the diagnosis. Therefore, physicians must still rely on criteria set forth in the *Diagnostic and Statistical Manual of Mental Disorders* published by the American Psychiatric Association (DSM-IV). These criteria are as follows: (1) Both multiple motor and one or more vocal tics have been present at some time during the illness, although not necessarily concurrently. (2) The tics occur many times a day (usually in bouts) nearly every day or intermittently throughout a period of more than 1 year, and during this period there was never a tic-free period of more than 3 consecutive months. (3) The disturbance causes marked distress or significant impairment in social, occupational, or other areas of functioning. (4) The onset is before the age of 18 years. (5) The disturbance is not due to the direct physiologic effects of a substance (e.g., stimulants) or a general medical condition (e.g., Huntington's disease or postviral encephalitis). Unfortunately, these criteria draw what now appears to be an artificial line between TS and milder tic disorders and do not include any mention of associated problems such as obsessive-compulsive disorder (OCD) and attention-deficit hyperactivity disorder (ADHD). Nevertheless, when OCD and/or ADHD are present, they may be more debilitating than tics and thus may constitute the focus of treatment.

Tics are defined as sudden, rapid, repetitive, nonrhythmic, meaningless, stereotyped movements or vocalizations. Some TS patients also exhibit slower, dystonic-like movements as well as conventional tics. Tics are divided into categories of simple and complex, motor and vocal. Simple motor tics include such actions as blinking, nose twitching, and jerking of the head, arms, or legs. Complex motor tics appear more purposeful, involve more than one muscle group, and include such complex actions as twirling around, squatting, and hopping. Simple vocal tics include noises such as sniffing, coughing, squeaking, and meaningless sounds ("eh," "ooh," "boo," etc). Complex vocal tics are somewhat more curious, consisting of words or phrases blurted out involuntarily. Coprolalia, the involuntary utterance of socially unacceptable words, a TS symptom that has attracted much attention, is nevertheless a relatively rare symptom, occurring in less than 25% of patients at some time during the course of the disorder. Many TS patients describe localized, often poorly defined, somatic sensations that are relieved by a tic in that part of the body. These have been termed "sensory tics." Other symptoms include echolalia (echoing sounds or words heard); palilalia (repetition of ones own sounds or words); echopraxia (imitation of gestures seen); and copropraxia (involuntary obscene gestures).

In actuality, the term "involuntary" is not completely accurate because tics can usually be suppressed for minutes to hours at a time. Because of this, the term "unvoluntary" has been suggested as more accurate.

Over a period of time, tic symptoms typically change in nature and wax and wane, either spontaneously or in response to external factors. Stress, physical or psychic, often causes an exacerbation of tics while relaxation brings about an amelioration. However, after suppressing tics for a period of time, there is often an outpouring of excessive ticcing when the patient reaches a comfortable place such as home. In addition to suppressing tics, many patients will try to disguise them by making them look intentional (e.g., an arm movement will be turned into brushing back hair).

Because tics may be suppressed or altered to appear purposeful, it is often difficult to make a diagnosis during a visit to a physician's office. It may be necessary to accept a description of the tics or, if in doubt, to ask for videotapes that document them. It may also be helpful to observe these patients while they are in the waiting room and do not necessarily know they are being watched. Some patients inhibit their tics in public situations with little conscious effort. Others do this only with great effort.

Though tics may begin anywhere from age 2 to 18 (and some later onsets have been reported), onset occurs most commonly at age 6 or 7. Usually simple tics will be manifested first, facial tics being the most common of these. However, in individual cases, any type of tic may constitute the initial symptom. Tics may progress rapidly in frequency and/or severity or may develop slowly, with remissions and recurrences, over a period of several years. Approximately two-thirds of TS patients will experience a remission or a marked lessening of tics when they reach maturity. Associated ADHD will typically begin before the emergence of tics, while OCD usually has a later onset and may increase in adult years.

When evaluating a patient with TS, it is important to inquire about possible symptoms of hyperactivity, distractibility, impulsivity, and obsessions and compulsions. Many patients do not connect these problems with their tics and may omit mention of them. Obsessive-compulsive symptoms are often deliberately concealed because they are perceived as strange and cause embarrassment.

The differential diagnosis of TS includes Sydenham's and Huntington's chorea, postencephalitic syndromes, Wilson's disease, drug toxicity, heavy metal poisoning, seizures, brain tumors, tardive dyskinesia, and chronic or transient tic disorder. Radiologic tests, blood tests, and EEGs are indicated only if there is sufficient reason to suspect another condition.

TREATMENT

There is no cure for TS, only the possibility that distressing symptoms may be ameliorated, usually by pharmacologic means. In many cases, however, medical treatment is not necessary. An understanding of the nature of the disorder may be enough to relieve the patient and/or family. Since complex tic symptoms or associated disorders may be easily misunderstood, not only it is important that the person with TS and the family receive appropriate information, but also it may be necessary to educate teachers, employers, neighbors, and others. Many informative pamphlets and other educational materials are available from the Tourette Syndrome Association. The headquarters of this organization is in New York City (42-40 Bell Boulevard, Bayside, NY 11361).

Pharmacologic treatment should be undertaken when tics are interfering enough in a person's life to cause significant distress. With all pharmacologic agents used for TS, there are a number of guidelines that will be helpful to follow:

1. Always start with the smallest dose that can reasonably be given considering the patient and the symptoms.

2. Increase the dose gradually, checking for positive effects and side effects with each increment. When (1) and (2) are adhered to, the chance of devel-

oping severe side effects will be considerably diminished.

3. Maintain the patient on the lowest dosage possible. Almost all drugs used for tics are primarily used for other indications, yet effective doses are usually less than would be ordinarily recommended (e.g., treatment with neuroleptics does not require the same doses that are used for psychotic disorders).

4. If symptoms are controlled on a certain dose but then recur, a slight increase of dosage may be indicated. However, if one continues to increase the dose in order to "catch up," the patient will almost certainly be overmedicated. Some drugs may actually worsen tics at higher doses. It is best to try to "ride out" a symptom increase for a certain length of time, since it may merely represent a natural waxing phase of the disorder.

5. If using more than one medication, make changes only in one medication at a time.

6. When discontinuing medications, be careful to follow recommendations. Rapid withdrawal may cause adverse reactions and may worsen the tics. This is particularly true for drugs such as clonidine, clonazepam, and neuroleptics.

There is no scientific evidence indicating that any medication is better for motor tics as opposed to vocal tics or vice versa. Neither is there any way to predict ahead of time what medication will be more successful for an individual patient. Therefore, the authors' method of treatment is based on the principle of first trying the medication with the least possibility of side effects. Even though haloperidol (Haldol) is the best known TS medication and has been proven effective, the authors believe that it is better to avoid using a neuroleptic if possible. TS is a chronic condition, and it is likely that the patient will be on a medication for years. The chances of developing tardive dyskinesia from neuroleptic treatment increase with time.

Clonidine (Catapres),* though often less effective for tic suppression than haloperidol, has beneficial effects on attentional problems, impulsivity, temper outbursts, anxiety, and oppositional behavior, which may make it particularly suitable for certain patients and worthwhile as a first-choice medication. While not documented, it is the authors' impression that clonidine is generally more effective for the treatment of children than for adults. Although not FDA-approved for any indication other than hypertension, clonidine has been used as a treatment for TS since 1980. Side effects are few, consisting mostly of sedation, which abates after days to weeks. Occasional irritability and/or insomnia may also occur. Serious hypotension is rare when the drug is started at a low dose and increased slowly. Nevertheless, blood pressure should be monitored with each increase of dosage and an ECG before treatment and after a therapeutic dose has been attained may be prudent.

Clonidine is started at a dose of 0.05 mg per day

(0.025 for very young children) and increased slowly, over a period of several weeks, to a total daily dosage between 0.1 mg and 0.5 mg per day. It is unlikely to be effective in doses above 0.5 mg per day. Since clonidine has a short half-life, it is necessary to give it in 3 or 4 small doses, leaving about 4 hours between doses. While sedation may appear in the beginning of treatment, this should wear off and the full therapeutic benefit may not be achieved for several weeks.

Clonidine is also available in the form of a transdermal patch (Catapres-TTS) that provides a steady flow of medication over the course of a week at a 0.1, 0.2, or 0.3 mg per day rate. The consistency of dosage provided by the patch is often more effective than frequent daily doses. The disadvantages of the patch lie in the difficulty in keeping it on for a whole week, the development of localized allergic reactions, and a higher cost.

If clonidine is to be discontinued, it is important to do this slowly. A rate of 0.05 mg less per day, every 3 days, is considered safe. Abrupt cessation of the drug, though unlikely to cause rebound hypertension in a normotensive patient, will be likely to cause increased ticcing, anxiety, irritability, nightmares, and insomnia.

Haloperidol (Haldol) was the first medication found to be effective for the treatment of TS. Although it is still considered one of the most effective drugs, the number and nature of its side effects have made it a less popular choice in recent years. Nevertheless, when used judiciously, haloperidol can be a most effective drug.

Haloperidol may be started at 0.25 to 0.5 mg per day. Increases should not be made sooner than every fifth day, and the most effective daily dose is usually less than 5 mg per day. At low levels, there is a good chance that tics will be significantly alleviated with few or no side effects. Although rare patients require doses as high as 15 mg per day, they seldom do as well as those who respond to less medication.

Side effects that may appear early in treatment, such as dystonic reactions, parkinsonian symptoms, blurring of vision, and slurring of speech, may be effectively treated by the addition of an anticholinergic medication such as benztropine (Cogentin) or trihexyphenidyl (Artane). The adverse effects that are usually the most distressing to patients are those that tend to appear more insidiously. These include weight gain, dysphoria, apathy, cognitive dulling, memory loss, akathisia, personality changes, school and work phobias, loss of libido, and diminished sexual function. These will usually respond to a decrease in dosage. Tardive dyskinesia, the only potentially permanent side effect, should always be a concern of the treating physician.

Discontinuation of haloperidol should be gradual. A decrease of 0.5 mg per day, made every week, is not unreasonable. Reactions due to rapid withdrawal include increased ticcing, anxiety, irritability, and even withdrawal dyskinesias.

Pimozide (Orap) is a neuroleptic with potent dopa-

---

*Not FDA-approved for this indication.

mine blocking effects similar to those of haloperidol. Although the side effect profile is also similar to that of haloperidol, many patients tolerate pimozide better. Concerns about pimozide's potential for cardiotoxicity were raised when it was introduced in the United States in 1984. Since then, studies have indicated that these concerns are probably not justified. However, routine ECGs (with attention to possible prolongation of the Q-T interval) are still advised before treatment and periodically while the patient is on the drug.

Pimozide treatment may be initiated at a dose of 1 mg per day and raised slowly as with haloperidol. Decreases should also be gradual. A decrease of 1 mg per day every week usually is safe in so far as avoiding potential withdrawal reactions.

In the authors' experience, *fluphenazine* (Prolixin) and *thiothixene* (Navane) are the only other conventional neuroleptics that are effective in the treatment of TS. Some patients do better on these medications and/or experience fewer side effects than they do on haloperidol or pimozide.

These medications also must be started at a low dose, raised slowly, and decreased slowly. Side effects are essentially the same as those of haloperidol.

Risperidone (Risperdal)* is a "novel neuroleptic" that has only recently been introduced in the United States for treatment of schizophrenia. It has been shown to have less risk of causing extrapyramidal side effects. The hope is that it will also have less risk of causing tardive dyskinesia. At this time, only a few studies have been conducted on TS patients, but the results have been encouraging. Tic reduction has been achieved on low doses (most often on 1 to 4 mg per day). Though extrapyramidal side effects do occur, they are less frequent than with conventional neuroleptics. The most bothersome side effects appear to be weight gain and sedation.

Clonazepam (Klonopin),* an antiepileptic drug in the benzodiazepine class, is sometimes effective in controlling relatively mild tics. It may also be used as an adjunct to treatment with other medications. Its disadvantage lies in its potential to cause addiction. Clonazepam is usually started at a dose of 0.25 to 0.5 mg twice daily and raised by this amount weekly. Side effects include sedation, depression, memory loss, ataxia, and behavioral changes. Withdrawal of the drug may be difficult.

Treatment of Obsessive-Compulsive Symptomatology

As mentioned earlier, many TS patients suffer from obsessive-compulsive symptoms or obsessive-compulsive disorder (OCD). These symptoms may need treatment as well as the tics or may be more severe than tics and thus the primary target of treatment.

Sometimes a physician and a patient are both unable to be sure if a certain persistent tic is truly a tic (therefore likely to respond to anti-tic medications) or is, perhaps, more a compulsion (therefore likely to respond to treatment with medications used for OCD).

While mild OC symptoms may be helped by clonidine, this is probably due mainly to its antianxiety effect. However, because of its low side effect profile, clonidine may be worth trying for OC symptoms in young children.

Clomipramine (Anafranil) is a tricyclic antidepressant and a serotonin reuptake inhibitor. It was available in Europe and elsewhere for many years before its introduction in the United States and has been well studied for both adults and children. Treatment with clomipramine may be started with a dose of 25 mg per day (12.5 mg for younger children) and raised no more often than every 7 to 10 days by the same amount to a maximum dose of 250 mg per day (3 mg per kg in children). Anti-OC effects may not be noted until a dose of at least 75 mg per day has been attained and administered for 2 to 3 weeks. Rare patients may feel relief sooner and on less medication.

Side effects that may be bothersome consist of sedation, dizziness, dry mouth, constipation, and sexual dysfunction. Clomipramine also lowers the seizure threshold.

Fluoxetine (Prozac) was the first of a group of selective serotonin reuptake inhibitor medications (SSRIs) that are effective as antidepressants and have fewer side effects than those previously available (e.g., tricyclics and MAO inhibitors). Fluoxetine has also recently been approved as an anti-OCD medication.

Fluoxetine treatment is usually initiated at a dose of 10 mg per day. The dose may be increased, if well tolerated, at a rate of 10 mg every 10 to 14 days to a maximum of 80 mg per day. The anti-OCD effect may be attained only after several weeks on a dose of at least 20 mg per day.

Side effects consist of gastrointestinal complaints (nausea, dyspepsia, diarrhea), agitation, insomnia, and tremors. They often abate with time if the drug is raised very slowly.

Fluoxetine is available in a liquid concentrate as well as in capsule form. The liquid may be useful when smaller doses are desired. Children may start at a dose of 5 mg or less per day.

Sertraline (Zoloft)* and *paroxetine* (Paxil)* are SSRIs, similar in their chemistry to fluoxetine. Though not now approved for the treatment of OCD, they have this capacity. Sertraline may be started at 25 mg per day and raised to a maximum of 200 mg per day. Paroxetine may be started at 10 mg per day and raised to 50 mg per day. The side effects of these two drugs are essentially the same as those of fluoxetine, but they may have less tendency to cause excitatory effects. Paroxetine is often especially effective for temper outbursts, which are sometimes associated with TS and its associated disorders.

---

*Not FDA-approved for this indication.

*Not FDA-approved for this indication.

Fluvoxamine (Luvox) has only recently been introduced in the United States. It is an SSRI medication that is approved specifically for the treatment of OCD. Side effects may be somewhat less than those of other SSRIs. A starting dose of 25 to 50 mg per day can be raised slowly to a maximum of 300 mg per day.

Treatment of Attention-Deficit Disorder with TS

Stimulant medications are the conventional medications of choice for treatment of ADHD and ADD. In many cases, however, these medications will worsen tics. Therefore, when treating a child who has tics or TS and ADHD (as well as those who have TS in their family), it may be judicious to try clonidine first. The method for the use of clonidine is described previously.

Tricyclics such as *imipramine* (Tofranil),* *desipramine* (Norpramin),* and *nortriptyline* (Pamelor)* have been used for a long time as second-line medications for attention disorders. They usually do not have any adverse effect on tics. Treatment with these medications should start at a dose of 10 to 25 mg per day. They rarely have more effect on ADHD in doses above 150 mg per day. Possible prolongation of the Q-T interval should be monitored with ECGs. Side effects are the same as those described for clomipramine.

Another medication that has only recently been studied for the treatment of ADHD is *guanfacine* (Tenex). Although very closely related to clonidine, guanfacine is somewhat less sedating and may be more effective for improving attention. It appears to have very little effect on tics. Guanfacine may be started at 0.5 mg per day and raised to a level of 3 mg per day in 2 or 3 divided doses. Blood pressure measurements and ECGs are recommended as with clonidine.

Treatment of Other Associated Behavior Problems

Other behavior problems that cause difficulty for TS patients and their families are rage outbursts, oppositional behavior, depression, and anxiety. These problems and their relationship to TS are as yet poorly understood, and treatment is purely symptomatic. As mentioned, paroxetine is sometimes quite effective for rage outbursts. This and the other serotonin reuptake inhibitors may also be effective in moderating anxiety.

---

*Not FDA-approved for this indication.

HEADACHE

method of
GLEN D. SOLOMON, M.D.
Cleveland Clinic Foundation
Cleveland, Ohio

Headache is considered the most common pain complaint of humankind. Headache may be simply categorized as benign (primary headache disorder) or organic (secondary). Organic headaches present as a symptom of an underlying disease (e.g., giant cell arteritis, meningitis), whereas benign headaches are further classified based on temporal patterns and accompanying symptoms (e.g., migraine, cluster).

HISTORY

The headache history is the key to determining whether a headache is migraine, cluster, or tension type or whether it represents a symptom of underlying disease. Evaluating factors such as age at onset, temporal pattern, quality and location of pain, and trigger factors allows the physician to make a presumptive diagnosis, which can then be confirmed by physical examination and laboratory or radiographic studies.

The duration of the headache problem is often a key indicator of probable underlying cause. Severe headache of sudden onset, especially if associated with focal neurologic signs or changes in level of consciousness, suggests serious illness, such as intracerebral hemorrhage or meningitis (which must be immediately ruled out by physical examination and laboratory evaluation). Recurrent episodic headaches dating back many years more likely reflect a type of vascular headache—migraine or cluster. A patient's initial migraine headache, unless preceded by a characteristic aura, may be confused with serious neurologic problems, such as meningitis or intracerebral hemorrhage. A long history of daily headaches without associated symptoms suggests chronic tension-type headache.

The most difficult headaches to evaluate are those developing over weeks or months. These may be benign or can arise from conditions as diverse as sinusitis, ocular disease, subdural hematoma, mass lesion, hydrocephalus, or—in a patient over age 60—giant cell arteritis.

After establishing the frequency and duration of the headache, the timing with respect to other physiologic events can be crucial to correctly diagnosing recurrent headache. One should inquire as to the time of day the headache occurs and its relationship to puberty, menses, pregnancy, menopause, or the use of hormones.

Migraine often begins at puberty and may resolve following menopause. It may occur irregularly for months to years, or it may follow a regular pattern occurring with menses. An acute migraine attack can last from 4 to 72 hours, with headache-free intervals between attacks.

Episodic cluster headache follows a pattern of cyclic bouts of attacks, lasting from 2 weeks to several months, often in the spring and fall. These bouts are separated by headache-free periods lasting from months to years. During the cluster period, severe headaches occur from one to four times a day, often awakening the patient from sleep at night. Cluster headaches are of short duration, lasting from 15 minutes to 3 hours. The duration of the cluster headache attack distinguishes it from trigeminal neuralgia, which presents with recurrent jabs of pain lasting less than a minute. Cluster variant headaches, such as chronic paroxysmal hemicrania, show a pain pattern similar to cluster headache, but attacks are more frequent and occur predominantly during the day.

Chronic tension-type headaches show no periodicity, and there are few headache-free intervals. The patient typically describes a daily, unrelenting headache. Patients often have both chronic tension-type headache and migraine (mixed headache syndrome, chronic daily headache). This is characterized by intermittent paroxysms of severe, throbbing, "sick" (migraine) headaches superimposed on a constant daily headache.

Location of the head pain can sometimes aid in diagnosis, such as in cluster headache or trigeminal neuralgia. Migraine is unilateral two-thirds of the time and bilateral one-third of the time. Chronic tension-type headache is usually bitemporal, occipital, or holocranial but may be unilateral. Cluster headache, trigeminal neuralgia, and headaches linked to local disease of the eye, nose, sinuses, or scalp are always unilateral. Headaches arising from hemorrhage or space-occupying lesions may begin unilaterally but usually become bilateral. Migraine usually alternates sides with different attacks but may be predominantly unilateral throughout life. Cluster headache is invariably unilateral and affects only one side during a series of attacks.

The patient's description of the quality of the pain can be valuable. Migraine is usually throbbing or pulsatile, whereas a constant ache suggests tension-type headache, and a deep, boring intense pain points to cluster headache. Trigeminal neuralgia is marked by short, intense, shock-like jabs.

The intensity of pain in cluster headache and trigeminal neuralgia is invariably described as severe, so much so that cluster headache patients usually cannot remain still. The migraine sufferer, by contrast, often seeks to rest in the stillness of a darkened room.

If the patient tells of an aura preceding the headache, this generally means migraine with aura (classic migraine), the only type of headache with a recognizable warning. Visual or neurologic symptoms commonly precede the headache by 10 to 60 minutes (usually 20 minutes). Premonitory symptoms, which can include euphoria, fatigue, yawning, and craving for sweets, may occur 12 to 24 hours before an attack.

Associated symptoms that may accompany migraine include photophobia, phonophobia, anorexia, nausea, vomiting, and focal neurologic signs. Seen with cluster headache are partial Horner's syndrome, constricted pupils, injected conjunctiva, and unilateral lacrimation and rhinorrhea. Rhinorrhea and nasal congestion are also common in sinusitis. Neck stiffness or other signs of meningeal irritation can signal meningitis, encephalitis, or intracerebral hemorrhage. A mass lesion, hydrocephalus, or encephalitis may be suggested by decreased level of consciousness or obtundation. Seizures can reflect cortical irritation resulting from a mass lesion or arteriovenous malformation.

One should also consider precipitating factors. Fatigue, particularly loss of sleep, may trigger either migraine or tension-type headache. Stress may exacerbate tension-type headache, whereas migraine may occur after a period of stress, often on weekends or vacations. Migraine sufferers may associate their headaches with menses, missing meals, or imbibing foods rich in tyramine, such as red wine or aged cheese. Alcohol triggers a cluster attack during a cluster cycle but has no effect during a quiescent period. Weather changes can be associated with migraine or exacerbation of sinusitis. Symptoms commonly associated with chronic tension-type headache include sleep and appetite disturbances, poor memory or concentration, chronic fatigue, and fibromyalgia.

One should also assess possible exposure to occupational toxins, chemicals, or infectious agents. Carbon monoxide poisoning, for example, often manifests as headache. Certain chemicals such as nitrates induce withdrawal and reintroduction headache. It should be emphasized that exposure to infectious agents in immune suppressed or AIDS patients may induce encephalitis or meningitis unaccompanied by classic fever and stiff neck.

Reviewing the patient's family history may prove rewarding. Migraine is a familial disorder, with a positive family history in two-thirds of cases. Cluster headache is familial in only about 3% of patients. In tension-type headache, a family history of depression or alcohol abuse is common.

The patient's medical-surgical history and history of current and previous medications can aid in diagnosis. Head trauma, for instance, may suggest subdural hematoma or skull fracture. Certain medications can trigger the onset of headache or exacerbate headache in patients with an underlying headache disorder. Medication-induced headache has been commonly reported with the following medications: indomethacin (Indocin), nifedipine (Procardia, Adalat), cimetidine (Tagamet), atenolol (Tenormin), trimethoprim-sulfamethoxazole (Bactrim, Septra), nitroglycerin, isosorbide dinitrate (Isordil), ranitidine (Zantac), retinoin (Retin-A), captopril (Capoten), piroxicam (Feldene), granisetron (Kytril), erythropoietin (Epogen, Procrit), metoprolol (Lopressor, Toprol), and diclofenac (Voltaren). Medications that may aggravate existing migraine include vitamin A, its retinoic acid derivatives, and hormonal therapy, such as oral contraceptives, clomiphene, and postmenopausal estrogens. Migraine and cluster headaches may be exacerbated by vasodilators such as nitrates, hydralazine (Apresoline), minoxidil (Loniten), nifedipine (Procardia, Adalat), and prazosin (Minipress).

Reserpine can cause depression, migraine, and tension-type headaches. Indomethacin, although useful in treating cluster variant headaches, can cause a generalized headache. Frequent or chronic use of some prescription and over-the-counter medications used to treat headache, including opioids, barbiturates, caffeine, and ergots, can lead to rebound or withdrawal headaches.

The following symptoms should lead to a strong consideration of headache of organic etiology:

1. Newly developed, massive, or gradually increasing headache.
2. Alterations in personality.
3. Constant headache, worsening in horizontal position.
4. Headache in the late nights or morning.
5. Headaches precipitated by coughing or exertion.
6. Epileptic attacks.
7. Diplopia.
8. Start of headache after age 50.

DIFFERENTIAL CONSIDERATIONS

In medical practice, most headaches are benign and are not caused by underlying disease. It is important to recognize, however, that headache can be the presenting symptom of several diseases. Fever, regardless of etiology, is probably the most common medical problem that causes headache. Less common causes include pheochromocytoma, chronic renal failure, hyperthyroidism, organ transplantation, and malignant hypertension. Pheochromocytoma may present with a pounding headache associated with hypertension, diaphoresis, tachycardia, and palpitations.

Rheumatologic diseases may have headache as an early manifestation. Headache is common in systemic lupus erythematosus, polyarteritis nodosa, and giant cell arteritis. About two-thirds of patients with either fibromyalgia or chronic fatigue syndrome report headache, usually tension-type headache. Many types of vasculitis can also present with headache.

Headache upon awakening may be the initial symptom of sleep apnea syndrome. The headache often improves as the day progresses. Sleep apnea is most commonly observed in obese, middle-aged males. Associated symptoms include snoring, daytime somnolence, hypertension, and arrhythmias.

PHYSICAL EXAMINATION

After evaluating the headache history, the physician should perform a targeted physical examination. This should include a mental status examination (often performed as part of obtaining the history), blood pressure and pulse measurement, examination of the cranial nerves, funduscopic examination, palpation of the head and neck, auscultation of the carotid arteries and heart, evaluation of motor and balance, and palpation of peripheral pulses (particularly if vasoconstrictor medications are to be prescribed).

The following signs should lead to a strong consideration of headache of organic etiology:

1. Fever plus rigidity of the neck.
2. Papilledema.
3. Tender temporal arteries.
4. Loss of local neurologic function, including loss of sight.

DIAGNOSTIC TESTING

Diagnostic testing of a headache patient should be determined by the results of the history and physical examination. In a patient with a typical headache history of several years duration and a normal neurologic examination, no further evaluation may be needed. All patients older than 60 with new onset headache or a change in the headache pattern should have a sedimentation rate or C-reactive protein measurement to evaluate for giant cell arteritis. If elevated, a temporal artery biopsy should be obtained to confirm the diagnosis.

Several commonly ordered tests have little or no value in the headache evaluation. "Routine" laboratory screening with complete blood count, urinalysis, and chemistry profile adds little diagnostic information. Electroencephalography (EEG) may be abnormal in some migraine patients, but EEG changes are neither specific for nor diagnostic of migraine. As a screening test to localize organic lesions, EEG has been supplanted by more specific computed tomography (CT) and magnetic resonance imaging (MRI). Evoked potentials (visual, auditory, and somatosensory) fail to show specific findings in migraine. Like EEG, evoked potentials have no utility as a screening test for headache. Review of the medical literature fails to support the use of thermography in generating a diagnosis, in guiding therapy, or in determining prognosis for headache disorders. The use of thermography in headache should be discouraged. The use of cervical spine x-rays is rarely useful in the diagnosis and management of headache patients.

Neuroradiology has little role in the diagnosis of headache beyond ruling out occult lesions such as neoplasm, hemorrhage, vascular malformations, brain abscesses, hydrocephalus, or congenital malformations (e.g., Arnold-Chiari malformations). MRI and CT will not pick up other organic etiologies of headache, such as idiopathic intracranial hypertension (pseudotumor cerebri), meningitis or other infections, glaucoma or eye disease, and metabolic or toxic causes of headache. It is critical that the physician obtain a complete history and examination and not rely solely on the MRI or CT to eliminate organic causes of headache.

Most patients suffering from acute severe headaches should undergo imaging with CT or MRI to rule out the organic causes listed above. Because organic causes of headache are rare (estimated at less than 1% in headache clinics), these tests are generally unrevealing. The benefits of a normal CT or MRI in reassuring the patient and doctor should not be overlooked, however. Some patients (and physicians) may be unwilling to embark on a course of therapy for a benign headache disorder without the reassurance of a normal scan.

In summary, the appropriate screening for an outpatient with recurrent headaches includes (1) obtaining a complete headache history, (2) performing physical and neurologic examinations, (3) or ordering lab tests only if indicated from the history and physical, and (4) performing CT or MRI if the headaches are of recent onset or associated with abnormalities on the neurologic examination, or if indicated by troubling neurologic symptoms in the history.

TYPES OF HEADACHE AND THEIR TREATMENT

Migraine

Migraine is a hereditary disorder of neurovascular instability marked by intermittent headaches of moderate to severe intensity lasting from 4 to 72 hours. The headaches are typically unilateral, throbbing in quality, and associated with nausea or vomiting and sensitivity to light and/or noise. Aura, usually scintillating scotomata or fortification spectra, precedes the headache in about 15% of patients. The prevalence of migraine in the United States is 20% in women and 8% in men.

Most migraines are precipitated only when several triggers occur in close temporal proximity, usually in the 12 hours preceding the migraine onset. The simultaneous elimination of multiple headache triggers has an additive effect in decreasing the probability that the migraine threshold will be crossed. Migraines are rarely induced 100% of the time upon exposure to individual triggers.

The most common migraine trigger factors are alcohol and four food substances—tyramine (found in aged cheese and fermented foods), aspartame (found in many diet soft drinks), monosodium glutamate (MSG, found in Chinese restaurant food and flavor enhancers), and phenylethylamine (found in chocolate). Additional common trigger factors are hormonal changes (menses, climacteric), alterations in sleep patterns (shift changes, jet lag, sleeping late on weekends), fasting, weather changes, and letdown after stress (weekends, vacations).

A wide variety of medications have been utilized in the prophylaxis of migraine, including methysergide (Sansert), beta blockers, calcium channel blockers, nonsteroidal anti-inflammatory drugs (NSAIDs), tricyclic antidepressants, divalproex (Depakote), and cyproheptadine (Periactin),* (Table 1). Methysergide is less commonly used today for migraine prophylaxis

---

*Not FDA-approved for this indication.

TABLE 1. **Prophylactic Medications for Migraine**

Beta Blockers

Propranolol	(FDA approved)	60–160 mg/day
Timolol	(FDA approved)	10–20 mg/day
Nadolol*		20–120 mg/day
Metoprolol*		50–200 mg/day
Atenolol*		25–100 mg/day

Side effects may include fatigue, depression, sleep disorders, diarrhea, exacerbation of asthma, Raynaud's syndrome, and congestive heart failure.

Calcium Entry Blockers

Verapamil	120–480 mg/day
Diltiazem*	90–360 mg/day
Nicardipine	40–90 mg/day
Nimodipine	60–120 mg/day
Flunarizine†	10 mg/day

Side effects may include constipation with verapamil; sedation, weight gain, and parkinsonism with flunarizine; flushing and edema with nicardipine; and gastrointestinal upset with diltiazem. Verapamil and flunarizine are the best studied calcium channel blockers in migraine.

NSAIDs

Aspirin	325 mg/day
Fenoprofen	600 mg tid
Flurbiprofen	100 mg bid
Ketoprofen	75 mg tid
Naproxen	250–500 mg bid

Side effects may include dyspepsia, heartburn, upper gastrointestinal bleeding, diarrhea, constipation, nausea, and vomiting. Renal effects may include decreased glomerular filtration rate and analgesic nephropathy.

Others

Antidepressants (see Table 2)
Methysergide
Divalproex (see Table 2)
Cyproheptadine

*Not FDA-approved for this indication.
†Investigational drug in the United States.

due to the risk of serious complications such as retroperitoneal fibrosis. Cyproheptadine is generally used for migraine prophylaxis in children. Adults often find the side effects of fatigue and weight gain from this antihistamine-antiserotonin drug to be intolerable.

Beta blockers, calcium channel blockers, and NSAIDs are valued as first-line drugs for the prophylaxis of migraine. Several beta blockers have been shown to be effective in migraine prophylaxis, including propranolol (Inderal) and timolol (Blocadren)—(the only beta blockers currently approved by the U.S. Food and Drug Administration (FDA) for migraine prophylaxis—and nadolol (Corgard),* metoprolol (Lopressor, Toprol),* and atenolol (Tenormin).* Beta blockers with intrinsic sympathomimetic activity, such as pindolol (Visken)* and acebutolol (Sectral),* have not been found to be useful in migraine prophylaxis.

Although generally well tolerated, beta blockers are contraindicated in patients with congestive heart failure, bronchospastic disease (e.g., asthma, emphysema, chronic bronchitis), diabetes mellitus, and

Wolff-Parkinson-White syndrome. Beta blockers may also exacerbate Raynaud's phenomenon, a condition found more commonly in migraine sufferers. Side effects of beta blockers include fatigue and sleep disorders. Depression is more commonly reported with propranolol than with other beta blockers.

Calcium entry blockers are useful in the prophylaxis of migraine and cluster headache. Several calcium entry blockers have been shown to be effective in migraine prophylaxis, including verapamil (Isoptin, Calan, Verelan), diltiazem (Cardizem),* flunarizine (Sibelium),† nimodipine (Nimotop), and nicardipine (Cardene).* Nifedipine (Procardia, Adalat) is either weakly effective or ineffective for migraine prophylaxis and can exacerbate migraine in some patients because of profound vasodilatation. In the United States, verapamil is considered the calcium channel blocker of choice for migraine and cluster prophylaxis.

The calcium entry blockers constitute a diverse group of drugs with varying effects on the heart and peripheral vasculature. Verapamil and diltiazem* have negative inotropic effects and slow conduction through the atrioventricular node. Therefore, these agents should be avoided in patients with congestive heart failure, advanced heart block, or sick sinus syndrome. The dihydropyradine calcium entry blocker nifedipine, nicardipine, and nimodipine have no effect on cardiac conduction but can cause marked vasodilatation.

Adverse effects of calcium entry blockers include constipation with verapamil; sedation, weight gain, and parkinsonism with flunarizine; flushing and edema with nifedipine; and gastrointestinal upset and parkinsonism with diltiazem.

NSAIDs are valuable both in the prophylaxis of migraine headache and as adjunctive therapy for tension-type headache. This dual effect on migraine and tension-type headache allows NSAIDs to be used as single-drug therapy in some patients with the mixed headache syndrome.

Several NSAIDs have been reported to have prophylactic activity in migraine. Among these are aspirin, naproxen (Naprosyn), flurbiprofen (Ansaid), ketoprofen (Orudis), and fenoprofen (Nalfon).

Adverse effects from NSAIDs are relatively common and may include gastrointestinal symptoms such as dyspepsia, heartburn, nausea, vomiting, diarrhea, constipation, and generalized abdominal pain. Most NSAIDs can cause bleeding of the upper gastrointestinal tract. Renal effects of NSAIDs may include decreased glomerular filtration rate with sodium, chloride, and water retention. Renal problems are most likely to occur in patients who are elderly, are hypertensive, have renovascular or advanced atherosclerotic disease, or take diuretics. Indomethacin and fenoprofen appear to be more nephrotoxic than other NSAIDs. Analgesic nephropathy, the most common cause of drug-induced renal failure, has

---

*Not FDA-approved for this indication.

*Not FDA-approved for this indication.
†Investigational drug in the United States.

been associated with excessive use of NSAIDs along with phenacetin or acetaminophen (Tylenol).

For a patient who has failed conventional therapy, alternatives include the monoamine oxidase inhibitor phenelzine (Nardil)* or divalproex (Depakote). Because of their potential for serious toxicity, these agents should be prescribed only by physicians experienced in their use.

For the abortive (acute) treatment of migraine headaches, an NSAID or isometheptene compound (Midrin) is generally prescribed initially. The most effective NSAIDs to abort migraine attacks are naproxen sodium (Anaprox, Aleve), flurbiprofen (Ansaid), and meclofenamate (Meclomen). Generally, a dose is given at the onset of the headache (naproxen sodium 550 mg, flurbiprofen 100 mg, meclofenamate 200 mg) and repeated in 1 hour if the headache is still present. Isometheptene compound is prescribed as 2 capsules initially, followed by 1 capsule every hour, as needed, with a limit of 5 per day and 15 per week.

When initial therapy is ineffective or the migraine is associated with significant disability, serotonin agonist agents should be considered. Sumatriptan (Imitrex), a serotonin 1-D agonist, is effective in about 60% (oral formulation) to 80% (subcutaneous formulation) of migraine attacks. When given subcutaneously (6 mg), it acts rapidly, often within 20 minutes. Both subcutaneous and oral (25 to 50 mg) formulations are generally well tolerated, with chest pressure and sensations of heaviness being common adverse reactions. Limitations to its use include expense and the problem of recurrent headache in up to 40% of patients. Dihydroergotamine (DHE-45) can be given intramuscularly (1 mg), subcutaneously (1 mg), or intranasally (2 mg). Repetitive doses of intravenous DHE-45 may be given to abort prolonged (status) migraine. Parenteral DHE-45 usually induces nausea; pretreatment with an antiemetic is recommended. Several other serotonin agonist drugs are under development for the acute treatment of migraine.

Ergotamine tartrate (Wigraine, Cafergot) is often effective for the acute treatment of migraine. The usual oral dose is 2 mg initially, followed by 1 mg every 30 minutes, as needed, with a maximum of 6 mg daily and 10 mg per week. Rectal absorption of ergotamine is greater than oral absorption. To reduce the likelihood of nausea, a 2-mg rectal suppository should be cut into thirds, with one-third given as the initial dose and additional thirds every hour as needed, up to the maximum of 6 mg per day. When ergotamine is prescribed, it should be given no more often than every 4 days to prevent rebound headaches. Vasoconstrictors, such as ergotamine preparations, sumatriptan, and isometheptene products, should be avoided in patients with coronary artery disease, peripheral vascular disease, or poorly controlled hypertension.

Chronic Tension-Type Headache

Chronic tension-type headache is a syndrome of frequent (greater than 15 days per month) or constant pressure headache of mild to moderate intensity. The headache is often described as bandlike and is commonly located in both temples, across the forehead, or in the occiput and neck. There are no associated symptoms such as nausea or photophobia with tension-type headache. Chronic tension-type headache has a population prevalence of 3% and is somewhat more common in women than men.

Antidepressants are the drugs of choice for chronic tension-type headache, and several of these agents are also effective in migraine prophylaxis. Of the antidepressants, the tricyclic drugs and the newer serotonin reuptake inhibitors are usually the agents of first choice, because of the lower incidence of side effects and less serious drug interactions compared with the monoamine oxidase inhibitors (MAOIs).

The selection of a specific antidepressant drug should be based primarily on whether the patient has a sleep disturbance. Patients who initiate and maintain sleep easily generally tolerate nonsedating drugs better than sedating agents. Those patients who have difficulty initiating or maintaining sleep respond better to sedating drugs. Patients often note improvement in headaches within 1 or 2 weeks after their sleep disturbance is corrected.

The nonsedating antidepressants include fluoxetine (Prozac),* sertraline (Zoloft),* bupropion (Wellbutrin),* paroxetine (Paxil),* nefazodone (Serzone),* venlafaxine (Effexor),* protriptyline (Vivactil),* and desipramine (Norpramin)* (Table 2). The MAOIs are nonsedating and may induce insomnia.

The sedating antidepressants include amitriptyline (Elavil, Endep),* doxepin (Sinequan),* nortriptyline (Pamelor),* imipramine (Tofranil),* trimipramine (Surmontil),* and trazodone (Desyrel).* Of these drugs, nortriptyline appears to cause the least amount of morning sedation.

The second consideration, after effect on sleep, is whether the patient is likely to be intolerant of anticholinergic side effects. The common anticholinergic side effects seen with tricyclic antidepressants are urinary retention (primarily in men with prostatic hypertrophy), dry mouth, blurred vision, and constipation.

All tricyclic antidepressants have anticholinergic side effects. Of the tricyclics, doxepin appears to cause the least anticholinergic side effects. Serotonin reuptake inhibitors and newer antidepressants such as fluoxetine, sertraline, bupropion, paroxetine, nefazodone,* and venlafaxine are generally free of anticholinergic effects.

Treatment of daily tension-type headaches with abortive medications is difficult. Muscle relaxants such as chlorzoxazone (Parafon Forte),* metaxalone (Skelaxin),* and orphenadrine citrate (Norflex),* either alone or in combination with aspirin and caffeine (Norgesic Forte), are generally helpful. NSAIDs are also useful as analgesics for daily headache. The prescription of benzodiazepines, butalbital combinations (Fiorinal, Fioricet, Esgic, Axotal, Phrenelin),

---

*Not FDA-approved for this indication.

TABLE 2. Prophylactic Medications for Tension-Type Headache

Tricyclic Antidepressants

Nonsedating		*Sedating*	
Protriptyline*	5–30 mg/day	Amitriptyline*	10–150 mg/day
Desipramine*	25–150 mg/day	Doxepin*	10–150 mg/day
		Nortriptyline*	10–150 mg/day
		Imipramine*	10–150 mg/day

Side effects may include constipation, dry mouth, weight gain, blurred vision, and urinary retention. Nortriptyline causes the least morning sedation in its group.

Serotonin Reuptake Inhibitors (Antidepressants)

Nonsedating		*Sedating*	
Fluoxetine*	10–80 mg/day	Trazodone*	50–300 mg/day
Sertraline*	50–200 mg/day		
Paroxetine*	20–60 mg/day		

Side effects may include insomnia, agitation, sexual dysfunction, diarrhea, and nausea. Adverse effects are less common compared with tricyclic drugs. Fluoxetine is associated with cytochrome P-450 enzyme induction and multiple drug interactions.

Other Antidepressants

Phenelzine*	15–60 mg/day
Bupropion*	200–300 mg/day
Nefazodone*	200–600 mg/day
Venlafaxine*	75–225 mg/day

NSAIDs (see Table 1)

Others

Divalproex	250–2000 mg/day (adult dose)

Side effects may include hepatic dysfunction, gastrointestinal upset, weight gain, and hair loss.

*Not FDA-approved for this indication.

and opiates should be carefully controlled or avoided because of the risk of habituation and rebound headache.

Prophylactic therapy of the mixed headache syndrome generally consists of treatment of both the daily tension-type headache and the migraine component. This often requires the use of more than one daily preventive medication. Treatment of acute headache attacks is a major challenge in patients with the mixed headache syndrome. Because headaches occur daily, with intermittent severe attacks, the patient may use abortive drugs quite frequently. Avoidance of habituating medications is critical.

Nonpharmacologic therapy also has an important role in the management of chronic headache syndromes. Biofeedback can help patients change vasomotor tone and relax tight muscles. Physical therapy is used to train patients to strengthen neck muscles, improve mobility, and correct poor posture. Physical therapy should not be limited to heat and massage. Although heat and massage provide short-term pain relief, only strengthening exercises provide long-term benefit.

Cluster Headache

Cluster headache is an uncommon headache disorder with a prevalence of about 1 in 1000, and a male/female ratio of 6:1. Cluster headache is marked by cycles of headache lasting 1 to 4 months, separated by remissions of 6 to 24 months. Ten to 15% of cluster patients suffer with chronic cluster headache that lasts more than 1 year without remission. The cluster headache attacks are always unilateral, located around the eye, temple, or upper jaw. Associated symptoms include reddening and tearing of the eye, drooping of the eyelid, nasal stuffiness, and rhinorrhea. The attacks generally last from 15 minutes to 2 hours, occur one to four times daily, and often awaken the patient after 90 to 120 minutes of sleep. The pain is excruciating in severity, and the patient commonly paces the floor during an attack.

Medications used in the prophylaxis of cluster headache include ergotamine, glucocorticoids, methysergide (Sansert), verapamil (Isoptin, Calan, Verelan),* and lithium carbonate (Eskalith, Lithobid).* Verapamil 240 to 480 mg daily is useful in both episodic and chronic cluster headache and is generally considered the drug of choice for cluster prophylaxis. Prednisone (Deltasone) 40 mg every morning for 1 week, tapering by 10 mg every week, or methysergide is used only in episodic cluster headache because of the potential adverse effects with long-term use. Verapamil may be combined with either prednisone or ergotamine tartrate (Wigraine), 1 mg at bedtime, if ineffective as monotherapy. Lithium carbonate 300 mg three times daily is generally reserved for patients with chronic cluster headache because of its slow onset of activity (Table 3).

For the acute treatment of cluster headache, the drug of choice is oxygen, given at 8 to 10 liters per minute by mask for 10 minutes. Other useful abortive medications include ergotamine, DHE-45, sumatriptan, and lidocaine (Xylocaine) nose drops.

Chronic Paroxysmal Hemicrania and Hemicrania Continua

Chronic paroxysmal hemicrania (CPH) is a rare headache syndrome that resembles cluster headache but is seen most commonly in women. The pain is intense and unilateral, lasts 10 to 30 minutes, and occurs 10 to 30 times daily. Autonomic signs similar to cluster headache may be seen. The headaches may be provoked by neck movement or pressure on the upper neck. Unlike cluster headache, attacks rarely awaken the patient from sleep.

Hemicrania continua (HC) is a unilateral headache without change of sides. Each episode of pain lasts up to 24 hours, with moderate to severe intensity, and with or without autonomic signs.

*Not FDA-approved for this indication.

TABLE 3. Prophylactic Medications for Cluster Headache

Verapamil*	240–480 mg/day
Prednisone*	20–60 mg/day
Lithium carbonate*	300–900 mg/day
Methysergide	2–8 mg/day

*Not FDA-approved for this indication.

Both CPH and HC are defined by a complete response to indomethacin. It is prescribed for 3 or 4 days in doses up to 150 to 200 mg per day, in divided doses. Maintenance doses generally range between 25 and 150 mg per day.

Giant Cell Arteritis

Giant cell arteritis should be considered in any patient older than 60 who presents with a new onset headache. Symptoms may include constitutional symptoms, shoulder and hip girdle aching, neck or ear pain, and jaw claudication. Patients often present with a swollen and tender scalp artery and have an elevated sedimentation rate.

Because giant cell arteritis can affect the ophthalmic arteries, leading to partial or complete blindness due to retinal ischemia, treatment should begin as early as possible. Treatment is with glucocorticoids, often given over a period of months to years. The headache invariably disappears within 48 hours of glucocorticoid therapy.

Drug Habituation and Detoxification

Because drug habituation is a common accompaniment of many chronic headache syndromes, this is often the first issue that must be considered in patient management. Medications that are known to cause habituation and rebound headaches include opioids, barbiturates, ergotamine tartrate compounds, and benzodiazepines. Although adjuvant therapy with caffeine may improve the efficacy of analgesics when used for acute pain, chronic use of caffeine-containing analgesic preparations (Anacin, Excedrin, Vanquish, and others) may also lead to rebound headaches. There is no evidence that simple analgesics such as aspirin, acetaminophen, or NSAIDs cause rebound headaches with daily use.

Detoxification from habituating drugs is the initial step in the treatment of patients who are taking excessive pain medications (i.e., using daily or almost daily habituating pain medication or taking ergotamine more than twice weekly). Prophylactic medication is ineffective in patients suffering from rebound or withdrawal headaches. Frequently patients say that they "would stop taking pain medication if only the preventive medication prevented the headaches." Patients must be instructed that the "pain medication" is part of the cause of the headaches, and that headache therapy is futile until the rebound-habituation cycle is resolved.

Management of a habituated patient can be difficult, and the medical literature offers little insight into proper techniques of detoxification. Patients who are habituated to opioids can benefit from clonidine (Catapres)* to prevent physical signs and symptoms of withdrawal. Glucocorticoids and phenothiazines may be prescribed for outpatient detoxification from butalbital, ergotamine, or low doses of opioids. Gen-

---

*Not FDA-approved for this indication.

erally, a 6- to 14-day tapering course of glucocorticoid is given, with chlorpromazine (Thorazine) suppositories prescribed for severe withdrawal headaches associated with vomiting. For patients with concomitant medical problems, a history of seizures, or prior unsuccessful outpatient detoxification, inpatient detoxification is often required.

The management of chronic headache disorders requires close follow-up and frequent physician visits until therapy is successful with a minimum of adverse effects. Although this takes commitment on the part of both the practitioner and the patient, good results should be expected in the vast majority of cases.

EPISODIC VERTIGO

method of
MARIANNE DIETERICH, M.D.
University of Munich
Munich, Germany

Vertigo is an erroneous perception of self- or object-motion or an unpleasant distortion of static gravitational orientation, which is due to a mismatch between the three sensory systems: the vestibular, visual, and somatosensory. These systems are mutually interactive and redundant in that orientation and balance are guided by simultaneous reafferent cues. The functional ranges of the three systems overlap so that they are able to compensate in part for each other's deficiencies. Thus, vertigo is not a well-defined disease entity, but rather a multisensory syndrome induced either by stimulation of the intact sensorimotor system by motion (e.g., as in motion sickness or height vertigo), or by pathologic dysfunction of any of the stabilizing sensory systems (e.g., as in vestibular neuritis).

The reflexes that provide postural and ocular motor responses to head motion are mediated from the semicircular canals and otoliths via the vestibular nuclei in the medullary brain stem to the ocular motor nuclei in the mesencephalic brain stem (i.e., the vestibulo-ocular reflex that allows compensatory eye movements during head movements). The paired vestibular nuclei receive neural input from all three sensory systems and transmit this information to the spinal cord (for postural stabilization), the vestibular thalamus and cortex (for motion perception and spatial orientation), and the upper brain stem and cerebellum (for the vestibulo-ocular reflex). Lesions along these pathways can induce vertigo, which manifests in a combination of phenomena that are dependent on the site within these vestibular pathways. Clinical phenomena—characteristic for both physiologic as well as clinical vertigo syndromes—include postural, perceptual, oculomotor, and vegetative syndromes, which manifest with ataxia, nystagmus, vertigo, and nausea. These four manifestations correlate with different aspects of vestibular function: postural imbalance and vestibular ataxia are due to an abnormal activation or dysfunction of vestibulospinal pathways; nystagmus is due to a direction-specific imbalance in the vestibulo-ocular reflex activating brain stem neuronal circuitry; vertigo itself is due to a disturbance of cortical spatial orientation; and the unpleasant vegetative effects—nausea and vomiting—are due to an activation of the reticular formation, the vomiting center, in the medullary brain stem.

The differential diagnosis of peripheral labyrinthine and central vestibular vertigo syndromes is guided by manifestations of ear signs (Meniere's disease, perilymphatic fistula, neurovascular cross-compression) or brain stem signs (central positional vertigo, vertebrobasilar ischemia, basilar artery migraine, paroxysmal ataxia/dysarthria), certain provoking factors such as head motion (benign paroxysmal positioning vertigo, central positional vertigo, neurovascular cross-compression, bilateral vestibulopathy), or family history (congenital vertigo).

GENERAL TREATMENT

Since the central nervous system has a strong impulse to compensate for, or habituate to, a persisting sensory mismatch, all therapy for vertigo should avoid disturbing these naturally compensatory mechanisms, a center of which is within the vestibular nuclei. It must be stressed that the central nervous system needs the stimulus of the sensory mismatch for habituation and compensation. Adequate therapy for vertigo must consider that antivertiginous drugs will suppress such mechanisms, because most of these drugs are vestibular sedatives. Therefore, vestibular suppressants should be applied only when vertigo is accompanied by distressing nausea and vomiting, i.e., in acute peripheral vestibulopathy and in acute brain stem and cerebellar lesions (near the vestibular nuclei), or to prevent motion sickness. These drugs are not indicated in patients suffering from chronic dizziness or positioning vertigo. If possible, specific therapies directed at the underlying cause should be chosen. In some cases it is best to recommend rehabilitation, since the central nervous system compensates by itself over time. Vestibular rehabilitation is often needed to speed recovery and central compensation.

If nausea is a prominent symptom of a vestibular vertigo syndrome, vestibular sedatives should be administered for symptomatic relief, despite the major side effect of general sedation. The most commonly used antivertiginous drugs are the antihistamines, anticholinergic drugs, phenothiazines, benzodiazepines, and butyrophenones (Table 1). Anticholinergic drugs, e.g., scopolamine, have been given in combination with noradrenergic substances, e.g., ephedrine, but double-blind, placebo-controlled studies have reported no significant difference when scopolamine was given alone or in combination with ephedrine. The only known similarity among the drugs used to counter labyrinthine vertigo and motion sickness is their capacity to act as acetylcholine antagonists by competitive inhibition. The most probable sites of their primary action are the synapses of the vestibular nuclei, which exhibit reduced discharges and diminished neuronal responses to body rotation.

PERIPHERAL LABYRINTHINE VERTIGO SYNDROMES

Benign Paroxysmal Positioning Vertigo (BPPV)

BPPV is a mechanical disorder of the inner ear in which precipitating positioning of the head causes

TABLE 1. **Antivertiginous Drugs**

| Substance | Action | | Dosage | Side Effects | Precautions |
	Antiemetic	Sedative			
Antihistamines					
Dimenhydrinate (Dramamine)	+	+	PO: 50 mg q 4–6 h Supp: 100 mg q 12 h	Dry mouth, blurred vision	Glaucoma, asthma, prostate enlargement
Meclizine (Bonine, Antivert)	+	±	PO: 25 mg q 12 h Supp: 50 mg qd		Glaucoma, asthma, prostate enlargement
Promethazine (Phenergan)	+	+ +	PO: 25 mg q 8 h Supp: 50 mg q 12 h IM: 25 mg q 6 h	Extrapyramidal symptoms	Glaucoma, asthma, prostate enlargement
Anticholinergics					
Scopolamine (Transderm Scōp)	+	±	Transdermal: 0.5 mg q 3 d	Dry mouth, disturbed accommodation, tachycardia, mental disturbances	Glaucoma, tachyarrhythmia, prostate enlargement
Phenothiazine					
Prochlorperazine (Compazine)	+ + +	+	PO: 5–10 mg q 8 h Supp: 25 mg q 12 h IM: 5–10 mg q 6–8 h	Extrapyramidal symptoms (dystonia, dyskinesia, parkinsonism)	Known hypersensitivity
Butyrophenone					
Droperidol (Inapsine)	+ +	+ + +	IM/IV: 2.5–5 mg q 12 h	Extrapyramidal symptoms, tachycardia	Extrapyramidal disorders, asthma, glaucoma
Benzodiazepine					
Diazepam (Valium)	+	+ + +	PO: 2,5,10 mg qd IM: 5–10 mg q 6–8 h IV: 5–10 mg q 6 h (slow)	Drug dependency, respiratory depression	Glaucoma

Abbreviations: PO = oral; Supp = suppository; IM = intramuscular; IV = intravenous.

an abnormal stimulation, usually of the posterior semicircular canal of the undermost ear. Patients with this most common form of vertigo develop brief attacks of rotational vertigo and concomitant rotatory nystagmus precipitated by rapid head tilt toward the affected ear or by head extension—typically when turning over in bed, extending the neck to look up, or lifting the head after bending over. The clinician can induce the symptoms by rapid position changes from the sitting to the head-hanging-to-the-right or -left positions (Hallpike's maneuver). Rotatory nystagmus starts after a few seconds latency and beats with a crescendo-decrescendo rate, reaching a maximum within a few seconds and lasting 10 to 60 seconds. When the patient returns to the sitting position, nystagmus is in the opposite direction. The typical nystagmus pattern and the characteristics of short latency, limited duration, reversal on returning to the upright position, and fatigability on repeated provocation are sufficient to establish the diagnosis. This strong correlation between vertigo and rotatory nystagmus makes the diagnosis unlikely if a patient reports intense vertigo but no nystagmus. The most common causes are idiopathic (50%), head injury (17%), viral neurolabyrinthitis (15%), and long bed confinement. Whereas a striking preponderance of females (female:male = 2:1) was found in the idiopathic group, the two sexes were equally distributed among post-traumatic and postviral groups. In general, it is a disease of elderly people, with a peak of occurrence between the ages of 50 and 70 years.

In 1969, Schuknecht hypothesized that heavy debris settles on the cupula ("cupulolithiasis") of the canal, transforming it from a transducer of angular acceleration into a transducer of linear acceleration. It is now generally accepted that the debris in most cases floats freely within the endolymph of the canal ("canalolithiasis"). The debris (possibly particles detached from the otoliths) gravitates to the most dependent part of the semicircular canal during head-position changes (Figure 1).

Therapy. In 1980, the first effective physical therapy—the positional exercises after Brandt and Daroff—was proposed. These exercises consist of a sequence of rapid lateral head-trunk tilts repeated serially. Meanwhile, single liberatory maneuvers have been introduced by Semont and coworkers (1988), as well as Epley (1992). If performed properly, all forms of physical therapy—the Brandt-Daroff exercises and the Semont and Epley liberatory maneuvers—are effective in BPPV patients. Since the liberatory maneuvers often require only a single session (Figure 1), they should be preferred in case of canalolithiasis of the posterior semicircular canal.

In case of the rare anterior canal BPPV, spontaneous symptoms occur when the affected ear is uppermost. The Brandt-Daroff exercises, with repeated lateral head-trunk tilts to both sides from a sitting position, seem to be more effective than liberatory maneuvers in patients with the equally rare horizontal canal BPPV. All maneuvers should be performed serially until vertigo and rotatory nystagmus have completely disappeared.

Surgical transection of the posterior ampular nerve via a middle ear approach can be considered in the very few patients with intense BPPV over many years who do not respond completely to physical therapy. However, sensorineural hearing loss is a possible complication, and it is difficult to locate surgically the particular semicircular canal nerve.

Acute Peripheral Vestibulopathy

An acute episode of severe rotational vertigo with horizontal-rotatory spontaneous nystagmus toward the affected side, a falling tendency to the normal side, and severe nausea and vomiting gradually resolving over days to weeks results from an acute peripheral vestibulopathy, the second most common cause of vertigo. The etiology may be bacterial labyrinthitis (otitis media), stroke, or trauma, but in most cases viral involvement of the vestibular nerve is the common cause (vestibular neuritis is its idiopathic form). Concomitant auditory dysfunction is absent in vestibular neuritis, which is characterized by a partial rather than a complete vestibular paresis. This condition mainly affects patients 30 to 60 years old. Caloric testing shows ipsilateral hypo- (33%) or non-responsiveness (66%) of the horizontal semicircular canal function, which resolves in 70% to 80% of the patients over months. Relief of the symptoms over 2 to 3 weeks (rarely up to 6 weeks) is due to the central compensation of the lesional vestibular tone imbalance. Later, a restoration of peripheral function takes place, which may lead to a mild spontaneous nystagmus beating in the opposite direction. In the few cases of no or only minor peripheral restoration of labyrinthine function, oscillopsia may persist *during* rapid head movements. This is caused by a persisting deficit of the vestibulo-ocular reflex in the higher frequency range, which cannot be compensated for centrally.

Therapy. Vestibular sedatives (see Table 1) should be administered parenterally on days 1 to 3, when nausea and vomiting are severe, for symptomatic relief while the patients rest in bed and avoid head movements. These drugs should be given only as long as nausea lasts, because antivertiginous drugs suppress the mechanisms of central compensation. Treatment with steroids (methylprednisolone sodium succinate) should be considered in cases of viral vestibular neuritis, since it may accelerate the process of central compensation as well as peripheral restoration. Further management includes physical therapy, doing the first exercises in bed (days 3 to 5) to suppress nystagmus by visual fixation: voluntary saccades and eccentric gaze-holding should be performed, as well as sitting freely. During days 5 to 7 approximately, when the spontaneous nystagmus is suppressed by fixation but there is continued gaze nystagmus in the direction of fast phase, upright stance and then head oscillations during free stance should be trained. Afterward, during weeks 2 to 3

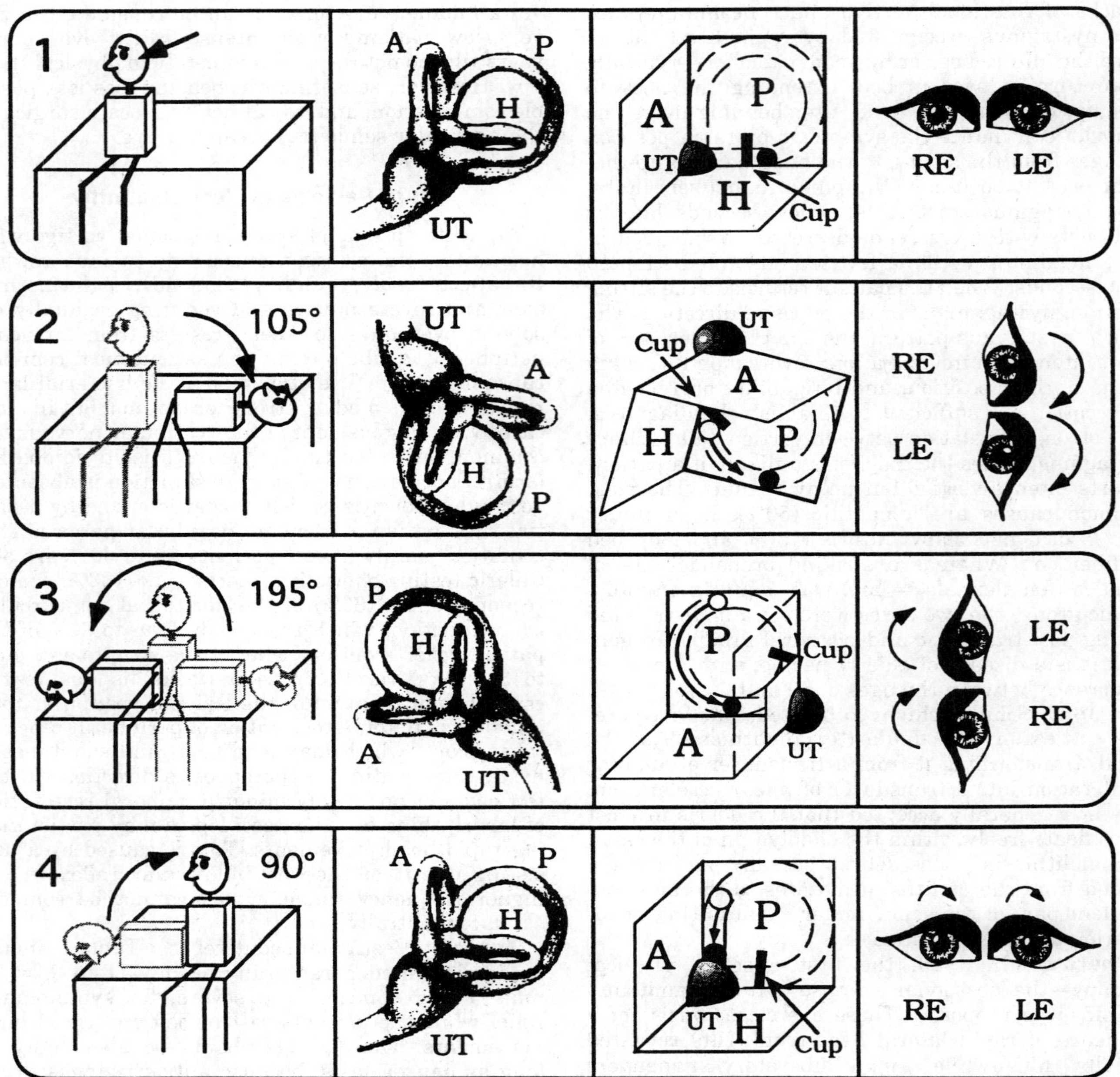

Figure 1. Schematic drawing of the liberatory maneuver in a patient with typical benign paroxysmal positioning vertigo (BPPV) of the left ear. Boxes from left to right: position of body and head, position of labyrinth in space, position and movement of the clot in the posterior semicircular canal and resulting cupula deflection, and direction of the rotatory nystagmus. The clot is depicted as an open circle within the canal; a black circle represents the final resting position of the clot. (1) In the sitting position, the head is turned horizontally 45° to the unaffected ear. The clot, which is heavier than endolymph, settles at the base of the left posterior semicircular canal. (2) The patient is tilted approximately 105° toward the left (affected) ear. The head position change, relative to gravity, causes the clot to gravitate to the lowermost part of the canal and the cupula to deflect downward, inducing BPPV with rotatory nystagmus beating toward the undermost ear. The patient maintains this position for 3 minutes. (3) The patient is turned approximately 195° with the nose down, causing the clot to move toward the exit of the canal. The endolymphatic flow again deflects the cupula such that the nystagmus beats toward the left ear, now uppermost. The patient remains in this position for 3 minutes. (4) The patient is slowly moved to the sitting position; this causes the clot to enter the utricular cavity. *Abbreviations:* A, P, and H = anterior, posterior, and horizontal semicircular canals; Cup = cupula; UT = utricular cavity; RE = right eye; and LE = left eye. (Reprinted from Brandt T, Steddin S, Daroff RB: Therapy for benign paroxysmal positioning vertigo, revisited. Neurology 44:796–800, 1994. By permission of Little, Brown and Company, Inc.)

and later, balance exercises should become more complex, gradually increasing in difficulty (e.g., during active head oscillations with increasing frequencies) to reach a level above the demands for postural control under daily life conditions. All these exercises are used to recalibrate the vestibulo-ocular reflex in its three major planes of action—the yaw, pitch, and roll planes—for a perfect eye-head coordination.

Meniere's Disease

See the article "Meniere's Disease."

Vestibular Paroxysmia (Neurovascular Cross-Compression of the Eighth Nerve)

In analogy to trigeminal neuralgia, the diagnosis of vestibular paroxysmia (also termed "disabling positional vertigo") is based on a few characteristic features. Due to neurovascular cross-compression of the eighth cranial nerve close to the brain stem, short vertigo attacks are characterized by a rotational or to-and-fro vertigo lasting from seconds to minutes in combination with hypoacusis or tinnitus (permanently or during the attack) and auditory or vestibular deficits measurable by neurophysiologic methods. Frequently, attacks are dependent on the particular head position, and their duration can be modified by changing it.

Therapy. Since this disorder has not yet been well defined and surgery entails a craniotomy of the posterior fossa for microvascular decompression of the eighth nerve at its root-entry zone (mortality up to 1%, neurologic complications up to 10%), carbamazepine should be recommended as first-choice therapy of suspected vestibular paroxysmia before an operation is contemplated. Carbamazepine (Tegretol), the drug of first choice in trigeminal neuralgia, phenytoin (Dilantin),* and pimozide (Orap),* have been effective in several patients with vestibular paroxysmia.

Perilymphatic Fistula

Perilymphatic fistulas may lead to episodic vertigo and sensorineural hearing loss. The clinical picture ranges from no symptoms to pure vestibular symptoms, pure hearing loss, or combinations of both. Vestibular dysfunction is more frequent than hearing loss and often begins after barotrauma, heavy lifting, or surgery. The symptoms are caused by a pathologic elasticity of the otic capsule, usually at the oval and round windows, which permits abnormal transfer of pressure changes to the receptors of the maculae and cupulae. Thus, symptoms are exacerbated by sneezing, pressing, and lifting of heavy weights. Despite the availability of clinical fistula tests (pressure fistula test, vascular fistula test), a definite diagnosis

---

*Not FDA-approved for this indication.

can be made only by exploratory tympanotomy with inspection of the round and oval windows.

Therapy. Since most fistulas heal spontaneously, conservative therapy is useful in the acute phase. Conservative therapy consists of bedrest with the head elevated for 2 to 3 weeks and avoidance of sneezing, coughing, pressing, and head-hanging positions. Mild tranquilizers and stool softeners may be helpful. Physical activity should be limited, and heavy lifting or straining should be avoided for several weeks.

When symptoms persist over 4 weeks or hearing loss worsens, surgical exploration via a posterior tympanotomy should be considered, even though the results of the surgical intervention are not encouraging (improvement rate of hearing deficit, 25% to 50%; of vestibular symptoms, 50% to 70%). The recurrence rate of symptoms exceeds 10%.

CENTRAL VESTIBULAR VERTIGO SYNDROMES

Vertebrobasilar Ischemia

Basilar insufficiency due to vertebrobasilar ischemia is a disease of elderly people, who present most often with transient attacks of rotational or to-and-fro vertigo as an early symptom. Over time, additional brain stem symptoms (e.g., dysarthria, double vision, numbness, drop attacks) may occur in varying combinations and to different extents. This syndrome is based on the steep pressure gradient from the aorta to the long circumferential terminal pontine arteries, which provide a highly vulnerable blood supply to the vestibular nuclei in the pontomedullary brain stem. In addition to arteriosclerosis of the small arteries, there is often found a functional compression of the vertebral artery secondary to atheromas, cervical spondylosis, or osteophytes that narrow the transverse foramina. In such cases, vertigo, postural imbalance, and nystagmus are induced when the head is maximally rotated or extended while standing. Since the blood supply to the inner ear (labyrinthine artery) originates from the anterior inferior cerebellar artery, it is also possible that a transient ischemia of a labyrinth can cause these transient attacks of vertigo.

Therapy. Antiplatelet agents or anticoagulants may be effective.

Basilar Artery Migraine

Basilar artery migraine is characterized by transient attacks of variable combinations of vertigo, nausea, vomiting, ataxia, visual disturbances, and other brain stem signs, followed by headache, which is more commonly occipital than hemicranial. Impairment and loss of consciousness are rare facultative symptoms. The acute onset of the syndrome, the sequence of events, the occurrence of other more common migraine attacks at other times, the short duration of the single attack (minutes to hours), and a family history of migraine confirm the diagnosis. In some cases, the syndrome is monosymptomatic—presenting only with rotational or to-and-fro vertigo—and not accompanied by headache; in such cases the diagnosis is difficult to differentiate from transient ischemic brain stem attacks. Diagnosis is then supported by a longer sequence of identical attacks, complete recovery from the symptoms, and mild central-vestibular oculomotor signs even during the symptom-free interval. There are two forms of basilar artery migraine: a more severe form characterized by various symptoms, which typically starts in childhood or early adolescence and predominantly affects girls (female:male = 3:1), and a monosymptomatic form (female:male = 1.5:1). The latter presents with vertigo as the leading symptom, has a more continuous disease onset between the 1st and 7th decades and shows a broad-based plateau of occurrence between ages 35 and 55 years. Attacks occur irregularly and infrequently, sometimes in clusters, but most often they spontaneously improve with age.

Benign paroxysmal vertigo of childhood (BPV), which has an onset in the first 4 years of life, is probably related to migraine. These sudden attacks last seconds to minutes and do not require drug therapy. They have a natural history of spontaneous relief within months or years. *Benign recurrent vertigo* may be an equivalent to migraine in adults; it is also characterized by short rotational vertigo attacks without headache.

Therapy. Pharmacologic management of the acute migraine attack is identical to that of other migraine attacks. They can be suppressed by ergotamines, sumatriptan (Imitrex), acetylsalicylic acid, or acetaminophen. In most cases it is not possible to abort an acute basilar migraine attack because of its sudden onset and spontaneous recovery within a short time. In such cases and when the attacks occur at least twice a month or present with significant brain stem deficits, a preventive medication with a beta blocker (metoprolol,* propranolol) should be tried for a period of 9 to 12 months. Other preventive medications are flunarizine† and serotonin antagonists (see "Migraine," page 917).

Central Positional Vertigo

There are a variety of *central positional vertigo* syndromes in which rotational vertigo, nystagmus, postural imbalance, nausea, and vomiting may be abrupt and more violent than in acute labyrinthine disease. In this severe form of central positional vertigo, during which the patient must lie in bed without moving the head, the lesion is located dorsolaterally of the fourth ventricle or near the vestibular nuclei. Causes are most often hemorrhages, tumor, or plaques in multiple sclerosis.

Therapy. The symptoms gradually improve over a few days or weeks, during which a treatment with vestibular suppressants may be necessary. These antivertiginous drugs should be reduced in parallel with improvement of symptoms, because they interfere with mechanisms of central compensation.

Central positional nystagmus without major vertigo is indicative of a posterior fossa lesion within the caudal brain stem and the vestibulocerebellum. A more precise location is to date not possible, because the lesions are mostly so small that MRI is unable to determine the site. This fits with clinical experience that central positional nystagmus frequently occurs in elderly people (lacunar ischemia?) and often resolves spontaneously.

Positional downbeating nystagmus presents with slight vertigo in the head-hanging position and may be related to the downbeat nystagmus syndrome (downbeating nystagmus in the primary position of gaze increasing on lateral gaze and accompanied by oscillopsia and postural instability). It is also activated with head extension and is indicative of a vestibulocerebellar lesion that may be caused by multiple sclerosis, ischemia, intoxication, craniocervical malformation, or cerebellar degeneration.

In permanent downbeat nystagmus due to structural lesions in the posterior fossa, baclofen (Lioresal),* or clonazepam (Klonopin)† can be recommended.

Paroxysmal Central Vertigo

Nonepileptic paroxysmal attacks of vertigo, ataxia, and dysarthria are well known in multiple sclerosis, possibly as the initial symptom. The attacks last a few seconds to a few minutes and occur with varying frequency of a few to 200 per day. They are sometimes provoked by hyperventilation or when arising. The character of the vertigo is sometimes rotational, but there is more often to-and-fro vertigo or an absence of postural coordination with ataxia and broad-based gait, associated with nystagmus and other central ocular motor signs. The mechanism of the attacks is suggested to be a transversally spreading ephaptic activation of adjacent axons within a partially demyelinated lesion in fiber tracts of the pontine tegmentum and involvement of the brachium conjunctivum.

Therapy. Carbamazepine (Tegretol)* is highly effective, causing complete disappearance of the attacks, which otherwise may persist for months if untreated.

Downbeat, Upbeat, and Periodic Alternating Nystagmus

All three types of nystagmus are central vestibular disorders with a nystagmus in the primary position of gaze, accompanied with oscillopsia and postural instability, and presenting as a clinical syndrome. Patients with downbeat nystagmus have structural

---

*Not FDA-approved for this indication.
†Investigational drug in the United States.

*Not FDA-approved for this indication.
†Investigational drug in the United States.

or functional lesions involving either the pontine brain stem between the vestibular nuclei at the floor of the fourth ventricle or the flocculus bilaterally. The two most common causes are cerebellar ectopia (25%) and cerebellar degeneration (25%), including alcoholic cerebellar degeneration; other conditions are multiple sclerosis, intoxication, ischemia, hematoma, vitamin B_{12} deficiency, and magnesium depletion. Upbeat nystagmus presents with lesions of the pontomesencephalic or pontomedullary brain stem, which may be due to brain stem infarctions, hematomas, tumors, cavernomas, plaques in multiple sclerosis, abscess, alcoholic degeneration, and drug intoxication. In contrast to downbeat nystagmus and periodically alternating nystagmus, upbeat nystagmus starts more often dramatically with nausea, vomiting, and severe oscillopsia, but ceases spontaneously over weeks. Lesions in the cerebellar nodulus and uvula can induce the periodic alternating nystagmus, which shows a horizontal spontaneous nystagmus with reversing directions periodically after 60 to 300 seconds.

Therapy. The treatment depends on the etiology, of course. At first one should try to eliminate the underlying cause, e.g., remove the drugs in intoxications, substitute vitamins, surgically remove the tumor, and treat the multiple sclerosis with corticoids. Surgical suboccipital decompression may be discussed in patients with Arnold-Chiari malformation to improve the compression of the herniating cerebellum against the caudal brain stem. This can gradually reduce nystagmus. Medical treatment with baclofen,* clonazepam,* and scopolamine* in upbeat/downbeat nystagmus and baclofen in periodic alternating nystagmus may be helpful for patients with persistent syndromes due to brain defects or degeneration. The GABA-ergic baclofen,* given 5 to 15 mg three times a day, suppresses nystagmus and oscillopsia in about half of the patients.

Familial Periodic Ataxia

Recurrent attacks of unsteady stance and gait or vertigo and nystagmus among several members of a family characterize the rare condition called familial periodic ataxia, which may last from minutes to days. Attacks may occur daily or may be separated by longer intervals—years in some cases. During the attack as well as in the symptom-free intervals, these patients often show central vestibular ocular motor disorders (especially downbeat nystagmus) and ataxia, although MRI cannot demonstrate a structural deficit. In view of the slowly progressive course of the disease in some families, a kind of hereditary spinovestibulocerebellar degeneration (e.g., olivopontocerebellar form) is under discussion.

Therapy. Acetazolamide (Diamox)* is a potent drug for preventing periodic ataxia/vertigo. Alprazolam (Xanax)* or the calcium-entry blocker flunarizine† can also be tried.

PSYCHOGENIC VERTIGO

The sensation of vertigo, a subjective complaint, is a frequent symptom of psychiatric illness, in particular in anxiety, depression, and personality disorders, less frequently in psychosis. The two most frequent episodic forms are acrophobia and phobic postural vertigo.

Acrophobia

Neurotic acrophobia results when physiologic height vertigo induces a conditioned phobic reaction characterized by a dissociation between the objective and subjective risks of falling. Although the acrophobic patients are normally aware of this dissociation, they cannot overcome their avoidance behavior. The long-term course of untreated anxiety neurosis indicates that during a 5- to 6-year interval, most children's phobias and 40% to 60% of adults' phobias either resolve or improve substantially.

Therapy. Psychotherapy is dominated by behavioral approaches, which can be classified as either systematic or in vivo desensitization procedures. Drugs used for symptomatic relief from panic attacks are either tranquilizers or antidepressants, such as imipramine (Tofranil).*

Phobic Postural Vertigo

The syndrome of phobic postural vertigo attacks—the third most common cause of vertigo and distinguishable from agoraphobia and acrophobia—is characterized by a combination of dizziness and subjective disturbance of balance in an upright static position as well as during motion in the form of postural vertigo attacks. These attacks occur both spontaneously and in association with particular constellations of perceptual stimuli (e.g., bridges, staircases, empty rooms, streets, driving a car) or social situations (e.g., store, restaurant, cinema, concert, meeting, reception), from which the patient has difficulty withdrawing and which are recognized as provoking factors. There is a tendency for rapid conditioning, generalization, and avoidance behavior to develop. Anxiety and distressing vegetative symptoms often (57%), but not always, accompany the vertigo attack, the symptoms of which have to be elicited by direct questioning. Most patients experience vertigo attacks both with and without excess anxiety. A recent neurologic and psychiatric follow-up study of 42 patients with phobic postural vertigo found that although an association with anxiety disorders was evident, not all patients presented with symptoms of anxiety or panic during attacks of vertigo. Rather, 42% developed a disabling phobic-avoid-

---

*Not FDA-approved for this indication.

*Not FDA-approved for this indication.
†Investigational drug in the United States.

ance pattern with recurrent vertigo attacks without anxiety disorder.

Typically, an obsessive-compulsive type of personality is often found to have affective lability and mild reactive (to the subjective vertigo) depression. The onset of the condition frequently occurs after the patient has experienced an illness (37%), usually a vestibular disorder (21%), or after important psychosocial stress and psychodynamic conflicts. The course of illness varies depending on the neurologic syndrome of vertigo, on the one hand, and the concomitant psychopathologic syndromes, on the other. Despite a considerable rate of improvement (79%) in vertigo complaints, the group of patients with phobic postural vertigo as a whole presented with significant psychopathologic problems at follow-up term (74%), requiring specific psychiatric and/or psychotherapeutic interventions. Dependent or avoidant personality traits, a pronounced somatic concept of illness, and hypochondria were prognostic of a more negative course of illness.

Therapy. The therapeutic regime consists mainly of relieving the patients of their fear of an occult organic disease and of giving a detailed explanation of the causative mechanism and factors provoking phobic reactions. Then we recommend a controlled self-desensitization (by repeated exposure to situations that evoke the condition) within the context of behavioral therapy.

PHYSIOLOGIC VERTIGO

Physiologic Height Vertigo

Physiologic height vertigo is a visually induced subjective instability of stance and gait coupled with a fear of falling and vegetative symptoms. It is commonly experienced atop high buildings. Although height vertigo may be part of a phobic syndrome, there is a geometric explanation for physiologic postural instability under height vertigo conditions. When the distance of the observer to the nearest stationary contrasts in the environment becomes critically large, a visually induced postural imbalance occurs, based on a perceptual conflict. The vestibular and somatosensory receptors sense a body shift that the visual system cannot detect (visual-vestibular conflict = mismatch). There is a spontaneous remission after the inducing stimulus is terminated.

Prevention. Susceptible subjects should avoid the free upright stance in critical situations at high altitudes—for example, by leaning against a wall or grasping for a support. When looking down, one should obtain stationary cues from nearby contrasts in the peripheral visual field. Unfamiliar head positions, which bring the otoliths out of their optimal working range, should be avoided. Looking through binoculars can be very dangerous, because the binoculars restrict the visual field and introduce an unadapted magnification factor of the visual surroundings.

Motion Sickness

Autonomic symptoms of motion sickness develop such as dizziness, physical discomfort, tiredness, periodic yawning, and pallor when an unadapted person is exposed to prolonged motion. Subsequently, nausea, vomiting, sensitization to odors, weariness, and salivation occur in about 60% of the cases. Motion sickness is induced during passive locomotion in vehicles and is generated either by unfamiliar accelerations to which a person has not yet adapted or by an intersensory mismatch involving conflicting visual and vestibular stimuli. Thus, reading or sitting in an enclosed space while in motion in a car or a boat elicits this mismatch. Most people experience motion sickness, e.g., on a rough sea, but there is a great interindividual variability of susceptibility. The susceptibility is greater in children (peak at 10 to 13 years) and females than in adults and males; infants below the age of 2 years are highly resistant. Only persons with defects of both labyrinths do not develop motion sickness. Spontaneous recovery occurs with ongoing stimulation by central habituation—readjustment of expectation to actual stimulation—within 3 to 6 days.

Therapy. Physical prevention of motion sickness involves vestibular training to promote central habituation, as well as head fixation and head position during stimulation to avoid head movements. Adequate visual control of body motion to avoid a visual-vestibular conflict stimulation can reduce the condition, because the vestibular signals of acceleration are contradicted by visual information of a seemingly stationary environment. For susceptible persons, the use of antivertiginous drugs (see Table 1) with moderate sedating action, such as transdermal scopolamine (Transderm Scōp, for longer trips) or dimenhydrinate (Dramamine, for short exposures) is effective, preventing both vestibular and optokinetic motion sickness. Transdermal scopolamine must be affixed for several hours before exposure to motion.

MENIERE'S DISEASE

method of
ANTONIO DE LA CRUZ, M.D.
*University of Southern California School of
Medicine and House Ear Clinic, Inc.*
Los Angeles, California

and

DONALD D. ROBERTSON, M.D.
McMaster University
Hamilton, Ontario, Canada

Meniere's disease (syndrome) is an uncommon form of true vertigo. In our experience, approximately two-thirds of patients who have been told they have Meniere's do not. Specifically, *idiopathic* endolymphatic hydrops, or Meniere's disease, occurs when normal fluid and electrolyte control mechanisms within the inner ear are disrupted.

The diagnosis of the syndrome *must* include four things: episodic true vertigo, fluctuating low-tone sensorineural hearing loss (often accompanied by hyperacusis), low-pitched roaring tinnitus, and aural fullness or pressure feeling in the involved ear. If any of these is missing, the diagnosis should be cochlear hydrops (low-pitched roaring tinnitus and hearing loss only) or vestibular hydrops (true episodic vertigo and pressure sensation only), but not Meniere's disease.

PATHOGENESIS

Meniere's disease by definition is idiopathic. The underlying pathology is endolymphatic hydrops: distention and temporary rupture of the membranous labyrinth secondary to increased endolymphatic pressure, altered endolymphatic sac function, a relative overproduction of endolymph, a defect in endolymph absorption, or a combination of these factors. Membranous labyrinth rupture causes a disruption of endolymph-perilymph sodium and potassium barriers, leading to paralysis of the surrounding vestibular or auditory hair cells and neural structures. The estimated time required for an endolymph-perilymph rupture to close and for fluid and electrolyte balances to re-equilibrate is thought to be about 2 to 3 hours, the approximate duration of a classic Meniere's attack.

NATURAL HISTORY

The prevalence of Meniere's disease in the United States is approximately 40 per 100,000 per year. Men and women are equally affected. The disease is most frequently seen in adults less than 60 years of age, with a peak age distribution in the fourth decade. It can also occur in children. Meniere's usually begins in one ear but may ultimately involve both ears in 10% to 78% of cases. Patients with Meniere's have a positive family history in 9% of cases. Women with prominent premenstrual fluid retention may find an exacerbation in symptoms during their menstrual cycle.

SIGNS AND SYMPTOMS

Meniere's is characterized by an episodic triad of vertigo, tinnitus, and fluctuating sensorineural hearing loss (SNHL). The typical prodrome of tinnitus, aural fullness, and hearing loss heralds an acute vertigo attack. Initially, 95% of patients will experience episodic vertigo associated with nausea, vomiting, and ataxia, with 75% of the episodes lasting less than 2 hours. Disequilibrium and imbalance may last a further 1 to 2 days. Later in the course of the disorder, vegetative symptoms may last hours to days, and vertigo attacks, although less intense, occur with less warning, which becomes more disabling to the patient. In the early stages of Meniere's, patients are generally asymptomatic between episodes, but after several years, recovery between attacks is often incomplete, and the patient may be left with constant tinnitus, a permanent moderate-to-severe hearing loss, and longer-lasting unsteadiness.

DIAGNOSIS

A thorough history is the most important part of the neuro-otologic diagnosis. Questioning should be directed to onset and duration of symptoms, in particular the association between hearing loss, tinnitus, and vertigo. Examination during an acute attack typically shows spontaneous nystagmus directed toward the affected ear. When the patient is assessed between attacks, examination of the eyes, ears, cranial nerves, gait, and postural control (Romberg and tandem Romberg testing) is generally normal. However, the individual with long-term Meniere's who has sustained significant loss of vestibular function may have difficulty with tandem eyes-closed Romberg testing.

Once the diagnosis is suspected, the patient should be referred to an otolaryngologist for more specific testing and initial therapy.

Audiometric testing is essential in the diagnosis of Meniere's. Common abnormalities in early-stage disease include a low-frequency hearing loss or a peaked audiogram with both low- and high-frequency losses. Advanced disease is often associated with a flat sensorineural loss. Hydrops can be demonstrated by fluctuating bone conduction pure tone thresholds on serial audiograms. Speech discrimination may initially be normal. As the disease progresses, low-frequency hearing loss increases, with deterioration of intelligibility. In late-stage Meniere's, the thresholds flatten to result in a moderate-to-severe hearing loss with intelligibility scores profoundly compromised.

Some clinical research centers using electrocochleography (ECoG), glycerol, and urea testing are finding that these tests may provide diagnostic information in hydrops. ECoG is a graphic recording of the electrical potentials of the cochlea and auditory nerve. When performed on subjects with Meniere's, ECoG results may be abnormal in half the patients who satisfy diagnostic criteria for Meniere's. We do not perform these tests because we do not find that they are in themselves helpful except from a research standpoint.

In the early stages of Meniere's disease, vestibular function tests, such as electronystagmography (ENG), are usually normal. After several years of repeated Meniere's episodes, vestibular deficits become more diverse, with gradual damage to the vestibular sensorimotor structures. This may cause a positional nystagmus, unilateral or bilateral caloric weaknesses, or abnormal vestibulospinal responses. A typical patient with end-stage Meniere's disease is likely to show a reduced or absent caloric in the affected ear(s).

At the House Ear Clinic, we perform screening blood tests for occult autoimmune, collagen-vascular, or infectious disorders that might cause otic capsule softening and secondary endolymphatic hydrops. This battery includes a complete blood count, erythrocyte sedimentation rate, fluorescent treponemal antibody, antinuclear antibody, rheumatoid factor antibody, and serum protein electrophoresis. If progressive unilateral hearing loss occurs, either gadolinium-enhanced magnetic resonance imaging (MRI) or T2 fast spin echo MRI should be considered to rule out an acoustic neuroma.

DIFFERENTIAL DIAGNOSIS

The diagnosis of Meniere's may be established only by exclusion. Conditions with sensorineural hearing loss and dizziness to be considered in the differential diagnosis include autoimmune disorders, syphilis, acoustic neuromas, vertebrobasilar insufficiency, allergies, and metabolic disorders such as diabetes, hypercholesterolemia, and hypothyroidism.

MANAGEMENT OF THE ACUTE ATTACK

Even though there is no known specific cure for Meniere's, most patients can be controlled with medication. Management is aimed at patient reassurance and symptom control, with the most problematic symptoms usually arising from the vestibular system.

During an acute vertiginous episode, patients should be reassured that it is a self-limited event. We recommend that they loosen tight clothing, lie down on a firm surface, close their eyes (some patients may be more comfortable with their eyes fixated on a target), and remain in that position until the acute vertigo stops, usually 30 minutes to 2 hours. If the patient is vomiting, we recommend taking nothing by mouth until the vomiting stops, then starting with sips of water or ice chips. Antiemetic drugs such as promethazine (Phenergan), dimenhydrinate (Dramamine), prochlorperazine (Compazine), or trimethobenzamide (Tigan) (Table 1) are all appropriate and may be used if needed. If vomiting is prolonged (>6 to 8 hours in children or 10 to 12 hours in adults), intravenous fluids and electrolytes and parenteral or rectal antiemetics may be required. Useful vestibular suppressants in the acute phase include intravenous diazepam (Valium), oral meclizine, or sublingual atropine (Table 1).

Preventive Therapy

Once the diagnosis has been made by the otolaryngologist, patients may be counseled in preventive therapies. Treatment of the Meniere's patient includes reassurance, dietary control, diuretic therapy, intermittent use of vestibular suppressants, and vestibular exercises to improve balance system adaptation. Among the most convincing mechanisms proposed to date for endolymphatic hydrops is failure of the inner ear fluid mechanisms to protect the inner ear fluid compartments from osmotic fluctuations. The goal of initial treatment recommendations for

Meniere's is the reduction of secondary osmotic effects on the inner ear. Initially, this may be achieved through a low-salt diet and diuretic therapy. Patients are advised to distribute food and fluid intake evenly throughout the day, to eat meals and snacks at the same time from one day to the next, and not to skip meals. They are cautioned to have a moderation diet, with avoidance of excess salt, sugar, alcohol, caffeine, or monosodium glutamate. It is the regularity of meals and even distribution of foods and fluid intake that is helpful, and, in many patients, the dietary changes alone may result in marked improvement. As a dietary supplement, a lemon bioflavonoid vitamin complex has been shown to be helpful in inner ear symptom control, and we use it empirically.

In addition to dietary suggestions, a diuretic is added. The aim of diuretic therapy is to drive the kidney to maintain a relatively constant urine output throughout the day, thereby minimizing rapid shifts in systemic fluid and electrolyte balance. In our practice, hydrochlorothiazide (25 to 50 mg by mouth once daily) or triamterene (37.5 mg) plus hydrochlorothiazide (25 mg) (Dyazide) is the diuretic of choice.

Patients with long-term Meniere's and spontaneously fluctuating, asymmetric vestibular function are more apt to experience constant dizziness and frank motion sickness–like symptoms. They may benefit from oral vestibular suppressants such as meclizine hydrochloride, recognizing that these central suppressants can slow recovery. To be most effective, these drugs must be taken continuously (not only when symptoms are experienced) and at relatively high doses for a limited time, usually titrated to just below individual side effect levels. We begin with a dose of meclizine, 25 mg by mouth every 8 hours. Drowsiness is the most common patient complaint; if this occurs, we initially reduce the dose to 12.5 mg every 8 hours. Once the initial dosing is tolerated, we will increase the dose, if needed, by 12.5 to 25 mg every other day until either a maximum dosage of up to 150 mg per day is reached or the patient experiences side effects (drowsiness, dry mouth, double or blurred vision). Once the effective dose has been reached, the medication is continued for no less than 3 weeks at dosages below side effect levels. Other useful medications are included in Table 1. Prednisone (60 mg daily for 10 days, then tapered) may be helpful in those patients experiencing sudden hearing loss.

In regard to activity restrictions, a patient with active Meniere's should be cautioned not to climb on chairs or stepstools, ladders, roofs, or other high places from which he or she could fall and be injured. Patients should not operate dangerous machinery (e.g., lawn mowers, construction equipment) and should be cautioned not to drive a car until balance and coordination have stabilized and symptoms have subsided completely after an attack. Patients should avoid swimming underwater, because the loss of somatosensory references induced by the water's buoyancy could cause them to lose orientation.

TABLE 1. **Useful Medications in Symptomatic Treatment of Vestibular Dysfunction**

Class	Drug	Dosage
Anticholinergic	Scopolamine	0.6 mg PO q 4–6 h or 0.5 mg transdermally q 3 d
	Atropine	0.4–0.6 mg sublingually q 4–6 h
Antihistamine	Meclizine (Antivert)	25 mg PO q 4–6 h
	Dimenhydrinate (Dramamine)	50 mg PO/IM/PR q 4–6 h
	Promethazine (Phenergan)	25–50 mg PO/IM/PR q 4–6 h
Phenothiazine	Prochlorperazine (Compazine)	5–10 mg PO/IM q 6 h or 25–50 mg PR q 12 h
Benzodiazepine	Diazepam (Valium)	2–10 mg PO/IM/IV q 6 h
Butyrophenone	Haloperidol (Haldol)	1–2 mg PO/IM q 8–12 h
Calcium channel blocker	Flunarizine (Sibelium)*	10 mg PO daily
Histamine	Betahistine (Serc)*	8 mg PO q 8 h
Miscellaneous	Trimethobenzamide (Tigan)	250 mg PO tid/qid or 200 mg PR/IM q 6–8 h

*Investigational drug in the United States.

Surgical Therapy

Medical treatment is ineffective in approximately 10% to 15% of patients. When disabling vertigo continues, surgical therapy is indicated. For patients with unilateral disease, the procedures of choice are endolymphatic mastoid shunt and vestibular nerve section. These procedures are preferred over labyrinthectomy because cochlear nerve integrity is preserved, leaving open the possibility of future cochlear implantation should bilateral profound hearing loss develop.

Telischi and Luxford (Oto Head Neck Surg, 1993) published good long-term results in endolymphatic sac surgery from the House Ear Clinic. This is recommended as the surgical procedure of first choice. Eighty percent of patients undergoing sac surgery do not require further surgical procedures, and 93% report no further dizziness or mild to no disability. The sac procedure has only a 2% chance of hearing loss or hearing worsening. Patients who fail sac procedures or who are severely symptomatic, show a 90% vertigo cure rate to vestibular neurectomy.

In other clinical centers, patients with bilateral Meniere's or an only hearing ear are treated by pharmacologic ablation with titrated ototoxic drugs (gentamicin* or streptomycin*). We do not perform intratympanic injections of ototoxic drugs in patients with serviceable hearing in the involved ear, although intramuscular streptomycin may be considered for bilateral disease.

Hearing aids play an important role in the management of patients with stable moderate-to-severe hearing loss. Assistive listening devices such as infrared TV amplifiers, telephone amplifiers, or wire loop systems play an important role in maintaining quality of life for the patient and the family. Speech reading lessons can be beneficial.

---

*Not FDA-approved for this indication.

VIRAL MENINGITIS AND ENCEPHALITIS

method of
ROBERT S. RUST, M.D.
University of Wisconsin
Madison, Wisconsin

Most central nervous system (CNS) diseases that are ascribed to viruses are secondary processes: (1) secondary invasion of the CNS leading to CNS cell death, or (2) induction of a dysregulated immune response that injures CNS cells or fiber pathways. In the first case, diseases are termed "aseptic" meningitis, encephalitis, or meningoencephalitis, depending on the predominant location in which the virus is found or produces dysfunction. Although certain viruses tend to produce meningitis (e.g., enteroviruses) and others encephalitis (e.g., La Crosse virus), there is only limited clinical usefulness of distinguishing viruses

by their preferred site of invasion. On the other hand, fairly specific clinical features (e.g., exposure, time of year, features of the primary viral illness, cerebrospinal fluid [CSF] or electroencephalographic [EEG] findings) may designate a particular virus as the most likely etiologic agent. Invasive viral disease may be acute, subacute, or chronic; viruses that may produce invasive CNS disease are shown in Table 1.

In the second case, a poorly understood collection of postviral illnesses is known to occur, designated variously as acute disseminated encephalomyelitis (ADEM), acute hemorrhagic leukoencephalitis (AHLE), a wide variety of focal postinfectious CNS syndromes, and overlap syndromes involving the combination of CNS and peripheral nervous system (PNS) dysfunction. These immunodysregulatory processes may be acute, subacute, or chronic and are often difficult to distinguish from invasive CNS viral disease. Furthermore, some CNS viral diseases involve a contribution from both mechanisms. Herpes simplex encephalitis and subacute sclerosing panencephalitis (SSPE) are excellent examples. Some other forms of CNS dysfunction (e.g., acute cerebellar ataxia) remain so poorly understood that they cannot as yet be classified.

The critical clinical problems posed by a patient presenting with possible viral-related CNS dysfunction are (1) to exclude nonviral etiologies, and (2) to determine whether drug therapy is indicated. Nonviral processes that may produce meningeal and/or focal neurologic signs are noted in Tables 2 and 3. Therapy for diseases related to viral invasion and/or immune dysregulation may be treated with specific (antiviral) or nonspecific (anti-inflammatory) medications or both. Thus, specific determinations as to etiologic agent are important in therapeutic planning as well as to anticipate complications (e.g., syndrome of inappropriate antidiuretic hormone [SIADH], increased intracranial pressure [ICP]); to estimate prognosis; and to assure that appropriate public health measures are undertaken.

Viruses generally produce disease of other organ systems prior to achieving CNS invasion. Viral etiology for CNS dysfunction is suspected when such dysfunction is preceded by a "viral" prodrome. This may involve fever, malaise, irritability, and signs or symptoms referable to the skin as well as to the respiratory, gastrointestinal, renal, hepatic, reproductive, or other organ systems. Highly successful public health measures have rendered certain distinctive prodromatic clinical syndromes (e.g., polio, varicella, mumps, or measles) infrequent in immunized nations, but these illnesses and their associated encephalitides remain all too common in developing countries. Recognition of more subtle evidence of viral infection or of risk factors, in combination with CSF analysis, serology, and neuroimaging, permits most patients to be diagnosed and treated in a rapid and appropriate fashion.

VIRAL MENINGITIS

Viral meningitis is usually, but not always, a benign and self-limited illness. It is characterized by the acute onset of the combination of headache, fever, and meningeal signs. Headache is generally the most prominent clinical feature and may be severe. Pain location and quality are variable and are often exacerbated by eye movements, neck flexion, or bright light. Fever is variable, ranging from low-grade to very high. Meningeal signs are generally obvious, but some patients exhibit only subtle manifestations. Irritability and malaise are common, but, typically,

TABLE 1. **Viruses That Cause Meningitis or Encephalitis**

	Region	Men	Enc	TOY	VEC	Risk Grp	Mrbd	Mrtl
Adenoviruses various	Tmp/WW	+	+	W	Hm	Chld/ImmCx	M	L
*Alphaviruses**								
Eastern equine	N/SAmer	+	+ + +	S	Mq	Infants	H	H
Venezuelan	C/SAmer	+	+ + +	S	Mq	Children	L	L
Western equine	N/CAmer	+	+ + +	S	Mq	Infants	M	L
Arenaviruses								
Lymphocytic choriomeningitis	WW	+ +	+	W	R		L	L
Bunyaviruses								
Bwamba	Afr	+ +		S	Mq		L	L
Inkoo	Scand	+	+	S	Mq		L	L
La Crosse/snowshoe hare	NAmer	+	+ + +	S	Mq	Children	L	L
Jamestown Canyon	NAmer	+	+	S	Mq	Adults	L	L
Tahyna/Lumbo	Afr/Eur/As	+	+	S	Mq		L	L
*Enteroviruses***								
Coxsackie	WW	+ + +	+	S	Hm	Children	L	L
Echovirus	WW	+ + +	+	S	Hm	Children	L	L
Enterovirus	WW	+ + +	+	S	Hm	Children	L	L
Poliovirus	WW	+ + +	+ +	S	Hm	Children	H	L
Flaviviruses								
Central Europe EV	Eur	+	+ +	S	T		L	L
Japanese EV	Rus/As	+ +	+ + +	S	Mq	Chld/Eld	H	M
Kyasanur Forest	India	+	+ +	S	T		M	M
Murray Valley	Aus/NZ	+	+ +	S	Mq		M	H
Omsk hem fever	Rus	+	+	S	T		L	L
Powassan	NAmer	+	+	S	T		L	L
Rocio	SAmer	+	+ + +	S	Mq	YAdult	M	M
Russian spring-summer virus	Rus/As	+ +	+ +	S	T		L	L
St. Louis EV	NAmer	+	+ + +	S	Mq	Adult	M	M
Wesselsbron	SAfr		+ +	S	Mq		L	L
West Nile EV	Afr/As	+	+	S	Mq	Chld/Eld	L	L
Herpesviruses								
Cytomegalovirus	WW	+	+		Hm	Nbn/ImmCx	M	L
Epstein-Barr	WW	+	+ +		Hm		M	L
Human herpes-6	WW	+	+		Hm	ImmCx	L	L
Herpes simplex-1	WW	+ +	+ + +		Hm	YAdult	H	M
Herpes simplex-2	WW	+	+ + +		Hm	Nbn/ImmCx	H	H
Varicella	WW	+	+		Hm	ImmCx	H	H
Orthomyxoviruses								
Influenza A, B	Tmp	+	+	W	Hm		M	L
Paramyxoviruses								
Measles	WW	+	+ +		Hm	YAdult	H	H
Mumps	Tmp	+ +	+ +		Hm			
Parainfluenza	Tmp			W	Hm		L	L
Reoviruses								
Orbivirus	NAmer	+	+	S	T	Adult	L	L
Togaviruses								
Rubivirus	Tmp	+	+	W	Hm	Children	L	L

Abbreviations: + = modest incidence; + + = intermediate incidence; + + + = high incidence; Afr = Africa; As = Asia; Aus = Australia; CAmer = Central America; Chld = children; Eld = elderly; Eur = Europe; EV = encephalitis virus; Grp = group; H = high; Hm = human; ImmCx = immunocompromised; L = low; M = medium; Men = meningitis; Mq = mosquito; Mrbd = morbidity; Mrtl = mortality; NAmer = North America; Nbn = newborn; NZ = New Zealand; R = rodents; Rus = Russia; S = summer; SAfr = South Africa; SAmer = South America; Scand = Scandinavia; T = ticks; Tmp = temperate regions; TOY = time of year; VEC = vector; W = winter; WW = worldwide; YAdult = young adult.
*Togavirus family.
**Picornavirus family.

mental status is intact and there are no other focal neurologic signs.

Evaluation is aimed at determining (1) whether this combination of findings is the result of some treatable cause other than virus and (2) whether CNS parenchymal tissues are directly involved, either by viral invasion or virus-induced inflammatory disease. CSF analysis is central to such determinations, but lumbar puncture should not be performed until after potential risks for herniation are calculated. If a clinical possibility of bacterial meningitis or HSV encephalitis exists and lumbar puncture is for some reason temporarily deferred, administration of appropriate intravenous treatments for these agents should be undertaken without associated delay.

Classically, the CSF opening pressure and glucose are normal, CSF protein is normal or mildly elevated, and microscopy shows no red blood cells, bacteria, or fungi. Lymphocytic pleocytosis is typical of most cases of viral meningitis; granulocytic predominance may occur early in the course and prior to achieve-

TABLE 2. Differential Diagnosis of Viral Meningitis

Viral meningoencephalitis
Presumed viral (see Table 5)
Nonviral CNS infectious processes
    Bacterial/spirochetal (particularly tuberculosis, *Mycoplasma*,
      syphilis, leptospirosis, borreliosis, ehrlichiosis, brucellosis,
      sporotrichosis, listeriosis, *Rickettsia*, cat-scratch disease,
      legionnaires' disease, toxic shock syndrome)
    Fungal (cryptococcosis, coccidioidomycosis, candidiasis,
      histoplasmosis, blastomycosis)
    Parasitic (echinococcosis, toxicariasis, angiostrongyliasis,
      paragonimiasis, toxoplasmosis, *Acanthamoeba, Naegleria*,
      malaria, schistosomiasis)
Non-CNS infectious
    Parameningeal (viral, bacterial, fungal infections of cranium,
      epidural space, sinuses, eye, ear, oropharynx)
    Remote (whooping cough encephalitis, shigellosis)
Noninfectious
    Cervical disk herniation/cervical stenosis
    Complicated migraine, low-pressure headache
    Chemical irritants (contrast material, lead, mercury)
    Drugs (azathioprine, cytosine arabinoside, isoniazid, penicillin,
      trimethoprim, NSAIDs, caffeine withdrawal, amantidine,
      rimantidine, vidarabine)
    Immune-mediated (IVIG, OKT3, serum sickness, graft-versus-
      host, post–cardiac transplant syndrome)
    Impending herniation (acute hydrocephalus, mass lesion)
    Malignancy (meningeal carcinomatosis)
    Post–lumbar puncture syndrome
    Subarachnoid or subdural hemorrhage
    Venous sinus thrombophlebitis
    Vasculitis (Kawasaki's disease, polyarteritis nodosa, primary
      CNS vasculitis, rheumatoid arthritis, systemic lupus
      erythematosus, temporal arteritis)

ment of maximal pleocytosis. Mixed cellular pleocytosis may occur; granulocytic predominance is rare in viral meningitis. Low glucose suggests the possibility of tuberculous or fungal meningitis, meningeal carcinomatosis, lymphoma, or sarcoidosis, which must then be excluded. Highly elevated protein suggests the possibility of tuberculous meningitis, various processes with spinal block, or connective tissue diseases.

Decisions about the value of various specific antimicrobial therapies depend upon the clinical syndrome and CSF results; when uncertainty exists, appropriate broad-spectrum therapy should certainly be started while awaiting cultures and serologic results. Decisions concerning duration of therapy in patients who are treated with antibiotics prior to lumbar puncture must depend on availability of reliable cultures from other sites, the clinical appearance of the patient, and serologic evaluation. In some cases, repeat sampling of CSF may be worthwhile; in uncomplicated aseptic meningitis, CSF pleocytosis may persist for several months. Particular care must be taken in making therapeutic decisions about patients treated with antibiotics prior to obtaining any cultures; in some cases a full course of broad-spectrum antibiotics will be necessary if "partially treated" bacterial meningitis cannot be excluded.

Consideration from among the other possible explanations for meningeal irritation (see Table 2) should be based on the particular features of a given case (exposures, susceptibilities, physical findings),

recent community history of epidemic aseptic meningitis, and so forth. Once the diagnosis of probable viral meningitis is accepted, therapeutic goals are usually limited to supportive care. This should include appropriate fluid and dietary management, provision of analgesics, and information about the probable outlook. Potentially treatable viral causes of meningitis include influenza and human immunodeficiency virus-1 (HIV-1).

VIRAL ENCEPHALITIS

The term "encephalitis" implies direct viral invasion of the substance of brain or spinal cord. As noted, most cases arise as secondary CNS infection after establishment of viral infection elsewhere in the body. Clinical determination of such a diagnosis is based on evidence of focal CNS dysfunction. Typical signs and symptoms include changes in mental status, occurrence of seizures, and new onset of motor or sensory deficits. Motor signs may be referable to cranial nerves, cerebellum, pyramidal or extrapyramidal upper motor neuron systems, or the anterior horn cells. Signs typical of meningeal inflammation (fever, headache, meningismus) are quite common.

A primary viral "prodrome" is also suggestive of viral encephalitis (or of ADEM) and often provides important clues as to the probable etiologic diagnosis. As with viral meningitis, such features as time of year, history of viral inoculation (e.g., mosquito, tick, or rabid mammal bite), presence of respiratory or gastrointestinal signs, history of recent epidemics, exposure to an endemic region, and the age of the patient may provide important diagnostic clues. Some sporadic forms of viral encephalitis may arise suddenly without a prodrome (e.g., herpes simplex

TABLE 3. Differential Diagnosis of Viral Encephalitis

CNS infectious
    Bacterial/spirochetal (see Table 2)
    Brain abscess/gumma (bacterial, tuberculoma, fungal)
    Basilar/brain stem meningitis (borreliosis, *Mycoplasma*,
      disease, syphilis, *M. tuberculosis, Nocardia*)
    Fungal/parasitic (see Table 2)
    Presumed viral (see Table 5)
    Whipple's disease
Non-CNS infectious
    Parameningeal or remote (see Table 2)
Noninfectious
    Complicated migraine
    Head trauma
    Inflammatory (sarcoidosis)
    Metabolic (Reye's syndrome, mitochondrial cytopathy,
      amino and organic acidurias, Menkes' disease, hereditary
      fructose intolerance, deficiencies of adenosine deaminase,
      purine nucleotide phosphorylase, or glycogen synthetase)
    Parainfectious/postviral syndromes (ADEM, ACA, etc.)
    Stroke (septic embolus, Moyamoya, dissection)
    Tumor (meningeal carcinomatosis, CNS lymphoma, other
      primary or metastatic malignancies)
    Vasculitis (see Table 2)

Abbreviations: ADEM = acute disseminated encephalomyelitis; ACA = adenocarcinoma.

virus [HSV] encephalitis) or subacutely (e.g., subacute sclerosing panencephalitis [SSPE]).

Laboratory testing should be selected in order to exclude other nonviral etiologic possibilities as well as to support the diagnosis of viral encephalitis; the selection of tests will vary depending on the age and exposures of the patient and other factors, as determined from the history and examination. CSF should be obtained in virtually every case, although caution must be shown when elevated intracranial pressure is a possibility. CSF findings are similar to those of viral meningitis, typically showing lymphocytic pleocytosis with normal glucose. Polymorphonuclear predominance may be found early in the course of viral encephalitis; glucose is occasionally low, but (as in La Crosse encephalitis) it may be high. The presence of CSF red blood cells after a nontraumatic tap suggests HSV-1 encephalitis. Microscopy should be reviewed for bacteria, tumor cells, acid-fast bacilli, and fungi.

Brain imaging is usually indicated; the magnetic resonance (MR) scan is generally more suited to the detection of viral encephalitis and of the relevant differential conditions. Electroencephalography may be helpful in diagnosis (HSV-1 encephalitis) and management of electrographic seizure activity. Specific acute and convalescent titers for appropriate viruses should be obtained from CSF and serum; special studies (IgM antigen capture enzyme-linked immunosorbent assay [ELISA], polymerase chain reaction studies) should be considered where appropriate. Positive specific titer rise is rare, and when detected may be too late to influence acute management, thus clinical judgment is at a premium.

Blood, CSF, stool, and nasopharyngeal swab specimens should be submitted, as indicated, for viral, bacterial, acid-fast bacilli, and fungal cultures. Isolation of virus is rare, except in the case of enteroviruses; if obtained from sources other than CSF, it may not be the causative agent. Brain biopsy may be necessary in particularly difficult cases, with sampling of leptomeninges as well as carefully selected areas of neuropil. Biopsy is particularly valuable in ruling out nonviral causes of brain injury. Serologic studies for illnesses indicated in the differential diagnosis (Table 3) may be indicated in individual cases; jejunal biopsy may be helpful if Whipple's disease is considered. Metabolic conditions (e.g., Leigh's disease) may occasionally need to be excluded by appropriate metabolic assessment.

The most commonly diagnosed cause of sporadic encephalitis is HSV-1, and it should be treated without delay by the administration of acyclovir (Zovirax) (Table 4). The recommended intravenous dose is 10 mg per kg every 8 hours for 10 days (adjusted in the case of renal disease). Treatment can be discontinued earlier when another specific diagnosis is made, or reliable serologic tests for HSV-1 are negative and the clinical appearance is not suggestive. Bright signals on T-2 weighted MRI imaging located in the orbitofrontal or mesiotemporal lobes of brain are highly suggestive, especially if there is evidence for necrosis. Subsequent worsening of MRI with associated clinical relapse may represent relapsing viral illness or postviral demyelinative changes and may require treatment with a combination of acyclovir and high-dose intravenous steroids (e.g., 20 mg per kg per day of methylprednisone).

The most common cause of *endemic* encephalitis in North America is La Crosse, a mosquito-borne virus that generally afflicts children. Japanese encephalitis virus, another arbovirus, is the most important agent in much of the rest of the world. *Epidemic* encephalitis may be caused by any of a great number of regionally or seasonally distinctive viruses. In North America, the most common agent is the mosquito-borne St. Louis encephalitis virus. Acute retroviral encephalitis is of increasing importance. In the rest of the world, poliovirus has been the most common epidemic agent. None of these viruses are specifically treatable, but supportive care is of great importance.

Intracranial hypertension may complicate HSV and many other forms of encephalitis, often representing the most serious cause of morbidity and mortality. Careful attention should be paid to the detection of signs of elevated ICP elevation; when detected, treatment should be prompt and aggressive. Initial management involves elevation of the head of the bed, sedation, and hyperventilation (PCO_2 22 to 26). Treatment with mannitol (1 gram per kg intravenously) and dexamethasone (initial dose 0.3 mg per kg; thereafter, 0.1 mg per kg IV each 6 hours as needed; maximal dose: 10 mg).

Supportive therapy for encephalitis involves detection and treatment of seizures, careful attention to nutrition and skin care, detection and treatment of electrolyte imbalances, adequate sedation and sleep management, and treatment of headache. Postencephalitic weakness, spasticity, ataxia, and move-

TABLE 4. **Drug Treatment of Viral Encephalitis**

Drug	Virus	Dose (mg/kg)	Toxicity
Acyclovir (Zovirax)	Herpes simplex	10–15 IV q 8 h	Renal
Amantidine (Symmetrel)	Influenza A	2.2–4.2 PO q 12 h	CNS
Ganciclovir (Cytovene)	Cytomegalovirus	2.5 IV q 8 h	Bone marrow
Ribavirin (Virazole)	Myxovirus	? qd	Bone marrow
Rimantidine (Flumadine)	Influenza A	3.3 PO q 12 h	CNS
Vidarabine (Vira-A)	Herpes simplex	15–10 IV qd*	CNS

*Not available in the United States—the intravenous preparation has been discontinued—the ophthalmic form is still available.

ment disorders require an appropriate combination of physical, occupational, and pharmacologic therapy.

POSTVIRAL ENCEPHALITIDES
(Table 5)

A wide variety of viruses may produce postinfectious CNS dysfunction, mediated either by vasculitis or by direct immunodysregulative effects on blood-brain barrier or brain tissues or both. In many cases it is not known whether a given "encephalitis" is produced by direct viral effects or these indirect mechanisms. In many cases the pathophysiologic substrate, particularly in children, is perivenular demyelination. Illnesses are named for the specific site of injury (e.g., optic neuritis), or when multiple sites are involved, the term "acute disseminated encephalomyelitis" (ADEM) is applied. With more intense antigenic stimulus, hemorrhage may occur (acute hemorrhagic leukoencephalopathy). In other cases, the exact substrate for postviral CNS dysfunction is unknown (e.g., acute cerebellar ataxia, opsoclonus-myoclonus, postviral parkinsonism).

The signs and symptoms of these postviral conditions vary, but fever, lethargy, headache, and mild transient meningismus are common; electroencephalographic (EEG) slowing, CSF pleocytosis with abnormalities of IgG and myelin basic protein, and T-2 bright signal abnormalities on MRI are all common. Treatment is generic and consists of support. Immunotherapy may be justified. Although efficacy of steroids, intravenous immune globulin (IVIg), and adrenocorticotropic hormone (ACTH) is unproved, there is an emerging consensus that such treatment short-ens the period of illness. There is no proof that ultimate outcome, which is generally good despite the severity of acute illness, is improved. As noted, immunotherapy may play a particularly important role in treatment of HSV encephalitis.

Treatment protocols vary significantly; one approach is the administration of 10 to 20 mg per kg of methylprednisolone as a single morning dose for periods ranging from 5 days to several weeks (depending on response). Patients treated for longer than 5 days require a switch to oral dosage (e.g., 2 mg per kg of prednisone daily) with subsequent taper. Some patients will require extended taper, as relapse during taper may be seen in as many as 15% of patients. There is a slight and poorly understood risk that steroid therapy may produce a relapsing form of illness or that steroid dependency may develop. Intravenous human immune globulin (IgIV) and ACTH (corticotropin [Acthar]) have also been successfully used for various forms of postinfectious encephalitis.

REYE'S SYNDROME

method of
CHING-SHIANG CHI, M.D.
Taichung Veterans General Hospital
Taichung, Taiwan, Republic of China

Reye's syndrome (RS) is a disease of unknown etiology characterized by acute encephalopathy accompanied with fatty infiltration of the liver. Unless recognized early and treated properly, it often has a high fatality rate or severe neurologic sequelae. The outcome of the disease is closely related to the intensity and duration of the increased intracranial pressure (ICP) or cerebral edema. In the past, many specific therapeutic regimens have been applied. These include exchange transfusion, peritoneal dialysis, hypothermic asanguineous total body washout, ornithine, citrulline, arginine, carnitine, bowel sterilization, and intensive supportive care with or without intracranial pressure monitoring. However, the most favorable results seem to be related to intensive supportive care under intracranial pressure monitoring. Over the past 12 years, we have developed a standardized form, which is a modified De Vivo's method of intensive medical management for patients with RS. Recently, the incidence of RS has decreased worldwide, but physicians still need to keep it in mind to make an early diagnosis and provide appropriate management.

DIAGNOSIS

Early diagnosis is crucial to satisfactory outcome. Although there is a bimodal distribution of RS, with highest frequencies under the age of 3 years and between 7 and 15 years, most patients present a stereotypical clinical and laboratory profile. Confirmatory diagnosis of RS is based on an electron microscopic examination of the liver cells, but the advisability of a liver biopsy has been challenged, especially in patients with increased intracranial pressure. We thus categorize RS into clinical Reye's syndrome (CRS) and pathologic Reye's syndrome (PRS). The diagnostic cri-

TABLE 5. **Chronic Encephalitides
(Viral or Presumed Viral)**

Known viral
  Encephalopathy of X-linked hypogammaglobulinemia
    (Coxsackie)
  Human immunodeficiency virus encephalopathy (HIV-1)
  Progressive multifocal leukoencephalopathy (JC virus, simian
    virus 40)
  Progressive rubella panencephalitis
  Subacute encephalitis of immunosuppression (Epstein-Barr
    virus [EBV], adenovirus, poliovirus, cytomegalovirus
    [CMV], measles, varicella-zoster)
  Subacute sclerosing panencephalitis (SSPE)
  Tropical spastic paraparesis (human T cell leukemia virus-1)
Prion diseases
  Creutzfeldt-Jakob
  Gerstmann-Straeussler
  Kuru
Presumed/possible viral
  Behçet syndrome
  Chronic encephalitis with basal ganglia calcification
  Chronic fatigue syndrome (Akureyri/Icelandic/Royal Free
    Hospital "diseases")
  Epidemic encephalitis lethargica
  Harada-Vogt-Koyanagi disease
  Idiopathic hemorrhagic shock–encephalopathy syndrome
  Mollaret's meningitis
  Postasthmatic poliomyelitis syndrome
  Rasmussen's encephalitis
  X-linked lymphoproliferative syndrome (EBV)

teria are shown in Table 1. In recent years, it has been reported that mitochondrial diseases, organic acid disorders, acute encephalopathy with centrolobular necrosis of the liver, hemorrhagic shock encephalopathy, and so on, may present as a Reye's-like syndrome. Therefore, differential diagnosis is essential for physicians to perform further work-up in order to make an accurate diagnosis (Table 2).

TREATMENT

All patients with RS should be hospitalized immediately. Management of RS should always be carried out in the intensive care unit, because early vigorous treatment and close observation will limit the progression of the syndrome. Management of the individual patient is determined by the neurologic stage at time of admission to hospital (Table 3), and degree of increased intracranial pressure (Table 4). Patients in stage I are managed by intravenous hydration with 10% to 15% hypertonic glucose multielectrolyte solution at a rate of 1600 to 1800 mL per square meter per day. Vitamin K_1 is administered intravenously every 24 hours at a dose of 1 mg. Monitor blood glucose, electrolytes, and gases every 4 hours; ammonia and osmolality every 8 hours; transaminase, amylase, creatine, prothrombin time, creatine phosphokinase, phosphate, blood urea nitrogen, and creatinine every day. Patients at or beyond stage II are given a dose of 50% glucose in water, 1 mL per kg, immediately. Then, under anesthesia, the patient is intubated and receives hyperventilation therapy to maintain a state of mild hyperoxia and hypocapnia with Pa_{O_2} values of 110 to 150 mmHg and Pa_{CO_2} values of 15 to 25 mmHg. In the meantime, the patient is also subjected to placement of a nasogastric tube, radial artery catheter, urinary catheter, and central venous catheter through the superficial

---

TABLE 1. **Diagnostic Criteria for Reye's Syndrome**

Clinical Reye's Syndrome (CRS)

History of an antecedent viral illness
A latent interval of a few days before the onset of symptoms
The development of an acute, diffuse encephalopathy
No other obvious explanation for the encephalopathy
A threefold or greater elevation of serum transaminase without
   jaundice
Prolongation of the prothrombin time
Hyperammonemia
Normal cerebrospinal fluid examination except for elevation of
   pressure
Blood amino acid, urinary amino acid, and organic acid assays
   show no evidence of inborn errors of metabolism, especially in
   infants and toddlers

Pathologic Reye's Syndrome (PRS)

Liver biopsy consistent with the following:
1. Microscopic examination of the liver cells shows diffuse
   microvesicular fatty infiltration with central nuclei, no
   necrosis or fibrosis, no remarkable inflammatory cell
   infiltration
2. Electron microscopic examination of the liver cells shows
   microvesicular steatosis, glycogen depletion, depleted Golgi
   membranes, proliferation of peroxisomes, and distorted
   mitochondrial organelles

TABLE 2. **Differential Diagnosis of Reye's Syndrome**

Disorders	Clues
Inborn errors	Recurrent, possible positive family history, abnormal neurologic findings, dysmorphism may be present
(1) Urea cycle defects	No hypoglycemia, no metabolic acidosis
(2) Mitochondrial diseases Fatty acid oxidation defects	Normal or mild elevation of blood ammonia, abnormal mitochondrial structure, mild liver function impairment
Pyruvate, Krebs cycle, or electron transfer defects	Abnormal mitochondrial structure, presence of ragged red fibers, elevation of lactic acid, abnormal oral glucose lactate stimulation test, hypertrophic cardiomyopathy, ventriculomegaly of the brain
(3) Organic acid disorders	Mild elevation of the serum transaminase, remarkable ketoacidosis, abnormal urine odor
Herpes simplex encephalitis	Normal blood ammonia, normal liver function, no progressive hepatomegaly, presence of red blood cells in the cerebrospinal fluid, abnormal brain imaging
Acute encephalopathy with centrolobular necrosis of the liver	Remarkable or severe elevation of the serum transaminase, normal intracranial pressure, distinguishable liver pathology
Hemorrhagic shock encephalopathy	Shock, bleeding tendency, usually normal blood ammonia
Toxic encephalopathy	Positive contact history, positive blood and urine toxin screening
Sepsis	Leukocytosis or leukopenia, no hyperammonemia, mild liver function impairment, elevation of C-reactive protein, positive blood culture
Fulminant hepatitis	Jaundice, no obvious metabolic acidosis, gradual shrinkage of liver size, distinguishable liver pathology

---

saphenous vein or the femoral vein into the inferior vena cava for delivery of hypertonic solutions of glucose or mannitol, and for monitoring central venous pressure. Intravenous fluid is given as a 20% glucose multielectrolyte solution, containing 40 mEq of sodium chloride, 15 mEq of potassium acetate, and 15 mEq of potassium phosphate per liter. One ampule (10 mL) of multiple vitamins is added per liter of the solution; this solution is infused at a daily rate of 1600 to 1800 mL per square meter to keep blood glucose at 200 mg/dL and serum osmolality not over 320 mOsm. Adequate fluid volume is mandatory to permit gradual rehydration according to the central venous pressure and intracranial pressure. Vitamin K_1 therapy is the same as for stage I. In addition, elevation of the head of the bed by 20 to 30 degrees and maintenance of the head and neck in a neutral

TABLE 3. **Stages of Reye's Syndrome**

I	Vomiting; responds to verbal stimuli; subtle behavior disturbance including inattention, inappropriateness, mild irritability; lethargy
II	Combative, delirious, confused, appropriate responses to pain stimuli
III	Stupor or coma, decorticate posturing, intact papillary reflex, overactivity of the sympathetic nervous system, including hyperpnea, diaphoresis, tachycardia, dilated pupils
IV	Coma, decerebrate posturing, intermittently forced into downward gaze, pupils sluggish
V	Coma, flaccid, loss of brain stem function

midline position are required. Fever is managed by the use of a cooling pillow. If the patient has seizures, phenobarbital is administered intravenously, with an initial dose of 15 to 20 mg per kg and a maintenance dose of 3 to 7 mg per kg per day. Then the advice of a pediatric neurosurgeon or neurosurgeon is sought to place a Ladd epidural intracranial pressure monitor.

During intracranial pressure (ICP) monitoring, nursing care plays an important part. Maintenance of normal blood pressure, an ICP lower than 15 mmHg, and a cerebral perfusion pressure (CPP) above 50 mmHg are essential. If the patient's ICP is

TABLE 4. **Management of Reye's Syndrome According to Intracranial Pressure**

Stage I

10%–15% glucose multielectrolyte solution, 1600–1800 mL/m²/d
Vitamin K₁, 1 mg IV qd
Multiple vitamins added in solution
Correct metabolic derangement
L-Carnitine, 50 mg/kg q 6 h
Check blood glucose, gases, electrolytes q 4 h
Check blood ammonia, osmolality q 8 h
Check blood transaminase, amylase, blood urea nitrogen, creatinine, phosphate, creatine phosphokinase, prothrombin time qd

Stages II–V

Intubation under anesthesia
Therapy as in Stage I, except 20% glucose multielectrolyte solution instead
Hyperventilation (PaCO₂ 15–25 mmHg, PaO₂ 110–150 mmHg)
Control seizures and fever
Keep head of bed elevation 20–30°
Blood exchange transfusion if hyperammonemia
Avoid unnecessary stimulation and manipulation
Intracranial pressure (ICP) monitoring:
  ICP less than 15 mmHg: Patient remains in a state of hyperventilation; calm down patient by sedation or muscle relaxant
  ICP between 16 and 20 mmHg: Check and eliminate inducing factors, manual hyperventilation to lower PaCO₂, control seizures, give thiopental sodium (Pentothal), 2–4 mg/kg/dose, give a dose of 20% mannitol (Osmitrol), 0.25–1 gm/kg, if ICP does not drop
  ICP between 20 and 30 mmHg: Intermittent IV 20% mannitol, 0.25–0.5 gm/kg q 6–8 h for 24–36 h
  ICP higher than 30 mmHg for 30 min: Consider craniectomy
  If the patient's condition is stable and ICP is less than 15 mmHg for 36 hours, wean hyperventilation gradually by increasing PaCO₂ 2–3 mmHg q 4 h

less than 15 mmHg and the CPP above 50 mmHg, keep the patient under a state of hyperventilation. Intermittent pancuronium (Pavulon), 0.01 mg per kg per dose; thiopental sodium, 2 to 4 mg per kg per dose; or 10% chloral hydrate, 0.5 mL per kg per dose, may be given to calm the patient. If the ICP is between 16 and 20 mmHg, hyperventilate the patient manually and check and correct inducing factors such as seizures, airway obstruction, respiratory dysfunction, movement, and so on. Suctioning of the airway is carried out carefully and coordinated with the administration of thiopental sodium. If the ICP still does not drop, give 20% mannitol (Osmitrol) intravenously in a dose of 0.25 to 1 gram per kg. If the ICP is between 21 and 30 mmHg, intermittently give mannitol every 6 to 8 hours for 24 to 36 hours. If the ICP is higher than 30 mmHg and persists for 30 minutes, craniectomy is considered. Patients who have hyperammonemia need to receive blood exchange transfusion (BET) until a normal level of the blood ammonia is obtained; the patient usually needs double-volume BET at least. During the second or third day of hospitalization, a percutaneous needle liver biopsy should be performed after correction of coagulopathy as well as stabilized ICP. If the patient's condition stabilizes, and the ICP is under 15 mmHg for 36 hours, start to wean hyperventilation gradually. After discharge, patients need to have a follow-up evaluation of psychomotor development, including auditory evoked potential and electroencephalography.

OUTCOME

Patients with blood ammonia levels higher than 500 to 700 μg/dL, persistent ICP of above 35 to 40 mmHg, and stage V have a bad prognosis. Overall mortality is around 5% to 20%; some survivors may have language impairment, attention deficit, hyperactivity, learning disability, seizures, and/or psychomotor retardation at long-term follow-up period. Some cases, however, may have an uneventful recovery under the intensive supportive care, with intracranial pressure monitoring and blood exchange transfusion.

MULTIPLE SCLEROSIS

method of
DENNIS BOURDETTE, M.D.
Oregon Health Sciences University and
* Department of Veterans Affairs Medical Center*
Portland, Oregon

Multiple sclerosis (MS) is a common, often disabling disease of the central nervous system. Although the cause of MS remains uncertain, considerable evidence suggests that MS has an immunopathogenesis. T lymphocytes, inflammatory cytokines, and macrophages appear to cause demyelination in MS. The targets of this T cell–mediated attack are uncertain but may be myelin proteins or viral antigens.

MS usually begins between the ages of 20 and 55 years, affects women more often than men, and has its highest prevalence among whites. In the United States, the prevalence of MS is about 50 to 100 per 100,000. In North America and Europe, MS occurs more commonly in northern latitudes, and epidemiologic studies suggest that the latitudinal gradient reflects an environmental exposure during the first two decades of life. A family history of MS significantly increases the risk of MS, with first-degree relatives typically having a tenfold increased risk and identical twins having a 25% concordance for MS. Multiple genes influence the risk for disease, although the only genes thus far to be clearly identified are major histocompatibility class II genes. MS thus appears to be an immune-mediated disease induced in genetically susceptible individuals by an environmental exposure, which most likely is a virus.

MS is rarely fatal but is a chronic illness that patients must contend with for decades. Patients do not necessarily become severely disabled from MS, and about 60% of patients are still ambulatory 20 years after onset. However, no more than 30% of patients have a truly benign course, with the remainder eventually developing varying levels of permanent disability. Male sex, age of initial symptoms after 40 years, progressive disease, and motor impairment at onset are all associated with a less favorable outcome. However, there is no reliable way of predicting who will have a benign course and who will become disabled from the illness.

DIAGNOSIS

MS is a clinical diagnosis. There is no laboratory test or imaging study that makes the diagnosis. Diagnosis depends on a knowledgeable physician taking a history, performing a neurologic examination, and, when indicated, obtaining appropriate tests. Diagnosis rests on objectively demonstrating white matter lesions within the central nervous system that are disseminated in time and space. Patients must have had two or more white matter lesions objectively demonstrated by either neurologic examination, magnetic resonance imaging, or evoked potentials. Patients also must have had at least two discrete episodes, or relapses, or have had a progressive deterioration extending over at least 6 months. Finally, patients must not have another condition, such as cerebrovascular disease, that can explain their neurologic problems. Making a correct diagnosis depends on the physician having considerable experience with MS and other neurologic conditions that can masquerade as MS; usually only a neurologist has sufficient experience to make the diagnosis of MS confidently.

GENERAL PRINCIPLES OF TREATMENT

1. *MS patients and their families need to be well educated about MS*. Patients who are well educated about their illness tend to adapt to MS better than those who are not. Unfortunately, there is considerable misinformation available about MS, and misinformed patients may make ill-advised decisions about their health care. I urge patients to join the local chapter of the National MS Society and to obtain information about MS from the National MS Society.

I also recommend that they read Lechtenberg's *Multiple Sclerosis Fact Book* (Davis) or Rosner and Ross's *Multiple Sclerosis: New Hope and Practical Advice for People with MS and Their Families* (Prentice-Hall). Schapiro's *Symptom Management in MS* (Demos) is an excellent resource for information on symptomatic management. I also warn them that they will hear about many unproved treatments for MS from the news media, friends, and family members. These unproved treatments are quite varied and even imaginative, ranging from special diets to bee stings. Many of these therapies are benign, some are frankly dangerous, and most are expensive. Physicians should warn their patients that they need to protect their pocketbooks and health. The National MS Society is an excellent source of information about the latest fad therapies, and I recommend that physicians and patients refer to Sibley's *Therapeutic Claims in Multiple Sclerosis* (Demos) for objective information about putative therapies for MS.

2. *MS patients should take positive steps to improve their health*. I recommend that MS patients follow a low-fat diet, exercise regularly, reduce stress, and avoid harmful habits. In my experience, patients who act on these recommendations adjust to their MS better than those who do not. Patients derive a psychological benefit in taking active steps to improve their health and combat their illness, and they may be directly influencing their MS. Stress in particular seems to activate MS in at least some patients, and lowering stress can be beneficial. For several decades some physicians have advocated a low-fat diet as a specific treatment for MS. Although claims about the beneficial effects of diet may have been overstated in the past, a low-fat diet may have some positive influences on the immune system in MS. Finally, MS patients who smoke, drink alcohol excessively, or use illicit drugs, particularly cocaine and amphetamines, tend to have more disabling disease than those who do not. Following these general health measures does not guarantee that MS patients will do well, but patients who take positive measures to improve their health feel more in control of their lives and may well be improving their chances of having a more benign course.

3. *MS patients need to have individualized management plans*. MS is a highly variable illness, and physicians cannot simply follow formulas or "clinical pathways" in managing patients. Patients vary both in the course and severity of their illness and in the types of problems MS creates for them. Physicians must individualize treatment plans and involve patients and their families in devising the plans. In addition, disabled patients can have a large number of problems, and it can be difficult to devise a treatment plan efficiently. When first assessing patients, I ask them to list the top three problems MS causes for them and then seek to find solutions for these problems.

4. *MS patients have a treatable illness*. Patients sometimes mistakenly believe that MS is "untreatable," and this can lead patients and their physicians

to become therapeutic nihilists. However, although not curable, MS is treatable. A variety of therapies are available to help patients manage the symptoms of MS, and symptomatic therapy is appropriate for all patients with MS. In addition, we now have a number of treatments that can favorably alter the course of MS, and these disease-altering therapies are becoming increasingly important in the management of MS patients. Both physicians and patients need to think of MS as a chronic yet treatable illness.

DISEASE–ALTERING THERAPIES

The type of MS that patients have determines which disease-altering therapy might be appropriate for them (Figure 1). About 90% of patients initially have relapsing remitting disease in which periods of disease activity, or relapses, punctuate periods of disease inactivity, or remissions. The frequency of relapses varies considerably. In the first few years of illness, patients typically have one relapse every 2 years, but relapses may occur much more or less frequently. During relapses patients develop new neurologic problems or worsening of existing difficulties. These neurologic changes usually evolve over days to weeks, following which patients stabilize and then improve. Some neurologic improvement nearly always follows relapses, and patients may recover completely or be left with varying degrees of permanent impairment. Typically, recovery is complete or nearly so with the initial relapses but, as more relapses occur, patients make less complete recoveries. However, up to 30% of patients with relapsing remitting MS never develop significant permanent disability and have "benign MS."

Up to half of patients with relapsing remitting MS will eventually develop secondary progressive MS in which there is progressive worsening of the disease. Patients with secondary progressive MS may or may not continue to have relapses superimposed on their progressive deterioration in neurologic function. About 10% of patients have primary progressive MS in which there is steady progression of the illness from its onset without a preceding period of relapsing remitting disease. The rate of neurologic deterioration varies considerably for both primary and secondary progressive MS, but generally patients with progressive MS note that each year their function is worse than that of the preceding year. Most MS patients who become severely disabled do so after developing progressive disease.

Disease-altering treatments include those that treat relapses, prevent relapses, or slow progressive disease.

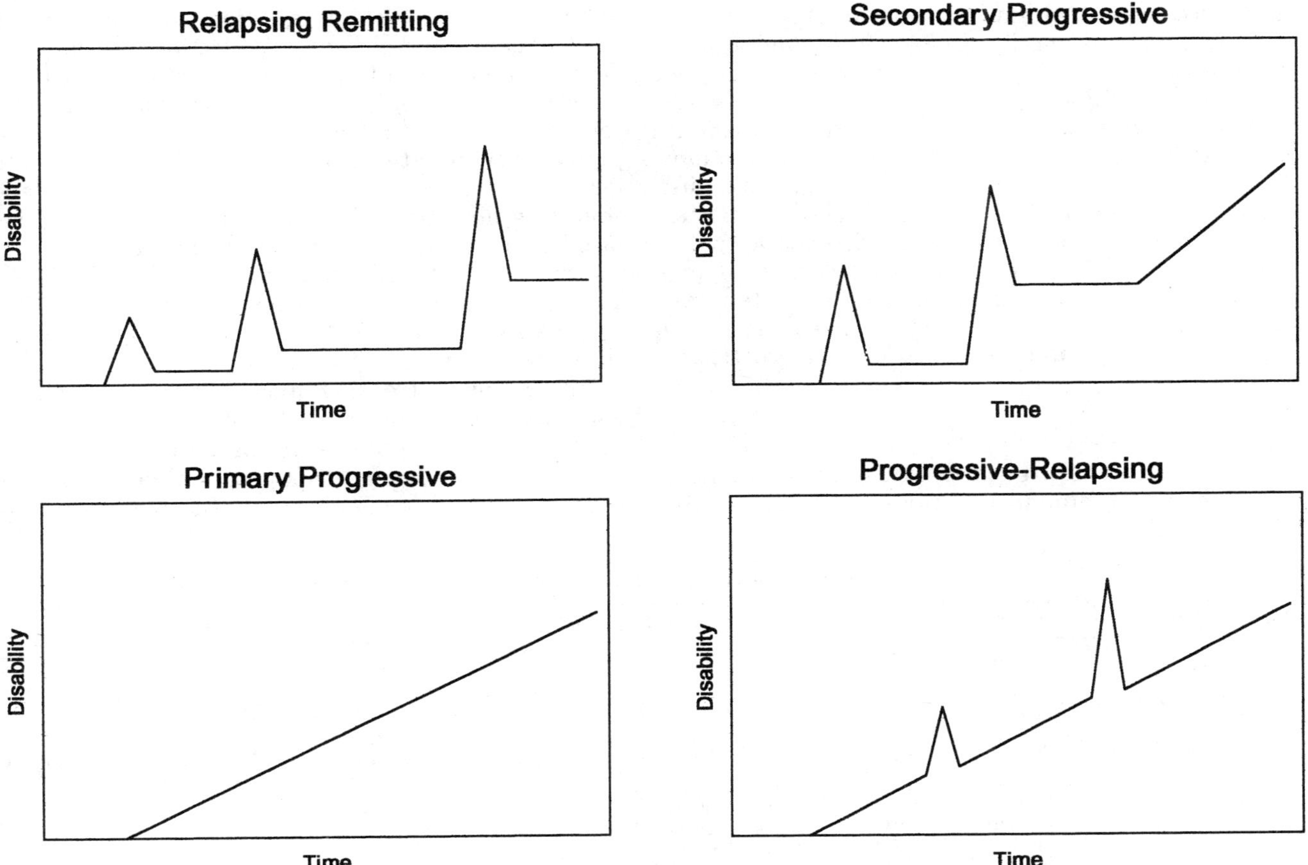

Figure 1. Classifications of MS.

Treatment of Relapses

Treatment with corticosteroids can significantly shorten the duration of MS relapses. Corticosteroids thus can benefit patients by returning them to work and their usual daily activities sooner than if they are not used. However, treatment does not affect the extent of recovery from relapses. Following recovery, treated and untreated patients have similar levels of residual disability; it just takes untreated patients longer to recover. Neither physicians nor patients thus should feel obligated to treat relapses with corticosteroids. My approach is not to treat mild, nondisabling relapses, such as those consisting only of sensory symptoms and fatigue; to recommend strongly treatment of severe, disabling relapses; and to individualize the decision for relapses that fall in-between.

When I treat with corticosteroids, I always use high-dose therapy, typically giving methylprednisolone (Solu-Medrol), 1 gram per day by intravenous infusion for 3 to 5 consecutive days (Table 1). I usually administer this in a single dose given over 30 to 60 minutes as an outpatient. I alter the schedule for patients who require hospitalization and give methylprednisolone, 250 mg every 6 hours for 3 to 5 days. I follow the methylprednisolone with a short prednisone taper. Although some neurologists do not use prednisone after methylprednisolone therapy, I have found that patients have fewer early recurrences of relapses if I use a short tapering course of prednisone. An occasional patient will have an allergic reaction to intravenous methylprednisolone, and I will then substitute intravenous dexamethasone (Decadron) at a dose of 200 mg per day.

I do not treat relapses with low-dose prednisone therapy without a high-dose corticosteroid induction phase. Low-dose prednisone is not as effective in shortening the course of relapses as high-dose methylprednisolone and may exacerbate disease activity in some patients. I do not use adrenocorticotropin, which was the first corticoid shown to shorten relapses of MS, since it is not more efficacious than methylprednisolone and has more mineralocorticoid side effects.

Prevention of Relapses

The first treatment proved to reduce the frequency of relapses of MS, human recombinant interferon β-1b (Betaseron), became available in 1993. Interferon β-1b appears to work by inhibiting interferon γ-induced expression of major histocompatibility class II molecules needed for T lymphocyte activation within the central nervous system and by stimulating T suppressor cells. Interferon β-1b has biologic activity similar to that of natural human interferon β, although it is not glycosylated like natural interferon and has a single amino acid substitution. Treatment of ambulatory patients with relapsing remitting MS with 8 MIU (0.25 mg) of interferon β-1b subcutaneously every other day reduces the frequency of relapses of MS by 30% to 50%. Importantly, interferon β-1b significantly reduces the development of new MS lesions within the brain, as demonstrated by magnetic resonance imaging (MRI). Since MS disease burden on MRI correlates, albeit imperfectly, with disability, it is likely that interferon β-1b decreases long-term disability, even though this has yet to be objectively demonstrated.

Interferon β-1b is generally well tolerated. The most common side effects are "flulike" symptoms and injection site reactions. The flulike symptoms, consisting of fever, myalgias, and malaise, can generally be managed by using acetaminophen or ibuprofen. This side effect generally disappears after patients have been on therapy for several months, but it persists in some. Injection site reactions generally consist of erythema, but large, painful reactions and occasionally skin necrosis can occur. Use of proper technique and rotating injection sites may reduce the frequency and severity of injection site reactions. Occasionally, patients will develop mild elevations of liver enzymes or mild leukopenia, and complete blood counts and liver function tests should be performed periodically in patients taking interferon β-1b. Interferon β-1b may cause depression. In my experience, this does not occur often and is most likely to be a problem in patients with significant, untreated depression prior to initiating therapy. Finally, 30% to 40% of treated patients develop neutralizing antibodies against interferon β-1b, which may reduce its clinical efficacy.

I recommend treating most ambulatory patients who have relapsing remitting MS with interferon β-1b. The major exceptions are patients who have had only mild, nondisabling relapses without permanent neurologic residua, particularly if they have had MS

TABLE 1. **Treatment of Acute Relapses of Multiple Sclerosis**

Medication	Dose	Route	Frequency/Duration	Comment
Methylprednisolone	1 gm	IV	qd/3–5 d	Standard outpatient regimen
or				
Methylprednisolone	250 mg	IV	q 6 h/3–5 d	Standard inpatient regimen
or				
Dexamethasone	200 mg	IV	qd/3–5 d	For patients who are allergic to methylprednisolone
Followed by:				
Prednisone	80 mg	PO	qA.M./3 d	
then	60 mg	PO	qA.M./3 d	
then	40 mg	PO	qA.M./3 d	
then	20 mg	PO	qA.M./3 d	

for many years and appear to have benign MS. When instituting therapy, it is very important that patients have realistic expectations for interferon β-1b. Patients should not expect improvement in their symptoms; interferon β-1b will not repair any damage that has already occurred. They also should expect to have relapses again, although the relapses will occur less frequently and less severely. I also warn patients regarding potential side effects and specifically warn them and family members about depression. I do not initiate treatment until I am assured that patients have realistic expectations and are not significantly depressed. I have a nurse instruct patients in how to administer the drug; patients self-administer the first dose in the presence of the nurse.

Some patients have frequent, disabling relapses and either do not tolerate interferon β-1b or continue to have active disease despite interferon treatment. I currently treat these patients as I do those with progressive MS (see later).

Another form of human recombinant interferon β, interferon β-1a (Avonex), also decreases the frequency of relapses of MS. More importantly, it has been demonstrated that interferon β-1a significantly slows the development of disability in patients with relapsing remitting MS in comparison with placebo. Although not presently available outside of clinical trials, it appears likely that the Food and Drug Administration will release interferon β-1a in 1996. Unlike interferon β-1b, it has the same amino acid sequence as natural human interferon β and is glycosylated. It is given in a dose of 6 MIU (30 μg) by intramuscular injection once a week. Interferon β-1a seems to have a lower incidence of side effects than interferon β-1b, with flulike symptoms being the most common. Antibodies to interferon β-1a may occur less frequently in treated patients than occurs in patients treated with interferon β-1b, and this may be an important advantage.

An entirely different drug, copolymer 1 (Copaxone), also decreases the frequency of relapses of MS. Copolymer 1 is a random polymer of four amino acids that suppresses a MS-like disease in animals by inhibiting myelin-reactive T lymphocytes. Copolymer 1, given subcutaneously in a dose of 20 mg a day, has fewer side effects than the interferon β products. Copolymer 1 is currently available only as an investigational drug, but the Food and Drug Administration is considering whether or not to release it for the treatment of MS.

Treatment of Progressive MS

A large multicenter placebo-controlled trial of interferon β-1b for ambulatory patients with secondary progressive MS is currently underway. Until this trial is completed, we will not know whether interferon β-1b favorably alters the course of progressive MS. Interferon β-1b was released only for the treatment of relapsing remitting MS, and third-party payers are reluctant to cover this expensive treatment for patients with progressive MS. Until there are good data supporting its use for progressive MS, I will use only interferon β-1b for patients with secondary progressive MS who continue to have relapses. I consider treating other patients with progressive MS with chronic immunosuppressive therapy.

Chronic immunosuppressive therapy is not indicated for all patients with progressive MS and must be used with caution. Three criteria need to be met. First, the patients should be ambulatory with or without aids. Nonambulatory patients have a greater risk of having serious side effects from immunosuppressants and have less to gain from therapy than ambulatory patients. (However, I occasionally treat nonambulatory patients who are rapidly losing upper extremity function.) Second, patients must be objectively worsening year-to-year. Many patients with progressive MS change very slowly, and immunosuppressive therapy in these patients is not warranted. Third, patients must be reliable so that they follow through with needed monitoring, and their physicians must be experienced in using the immunosuppressive regimen. The medications that I use are reasonably safe as long as there is careful monitoring of patients for toxicity. If patients cannot be reliably monitored, immunosuppressive therapy should not be instituted.

My first choice of immunosuppressive therapy for progressive MS is pulse intermittent methylprednisolone. I initially give patients intravenous methylprednisolone as for a relapse of MS and then give them 1 gram of methylprednisolone intravenously every 4 weeks. I continue this treatment for a minimum of 1 to 2 years. For patients who cease progressing, I attempt to slowly taper them off therapy by giving them methylprednisolone, 1 gram every 8 weeks for 6 months, then every 12 weeks for 6 months, and then discontinuing therapy. Some patients are able to come off methylprednisolone and will remain stable for several years thereafter. However, others begin progressing again once the methylprednisolone is stopped; I keep these patients on pulse methylprednisolone indefinitely. This treatment is generally well tolerated. Occasionally patients are allergic to intravenous methylprednisolone, and I then substitute intravenous dexamethasone at a dose of 200 mg. Patients may have symptoms of reflux esophagitis or insomnia for a day or two after treatment, and I treat these symptomatically. I have patients undergo bone densitometry at the start of therapy and every year thereafter to monitor for osteoporosis. An endocrinologist evaluates and treats patients with osteoporosis. I also have patients undergo an ophthalmologic examination at the start of therapy and yearly thereafter to monitor for cataract formation and glaucoma.

For patients who continue to worsen despite treatment with pulse methylprednisolone, I will add azathioprine (Imuran),* 2 mg per kg per day orally. Female patients should not become pregnant while taking azathioprine. To monitor for hepatotoxicity

---

*Not FDA-approved for this indication.

and dose-dependent bone marrow depression, I perform a complete blood count and liver function tests every 2 weeks for 2 months while initiating therapy and then obtain complete blood counts monthly and liver function tests every 3 months thereafter. I lower the dose if the total white blood cell count drops below 3000 cells per mm³ or the absolute neutrophil count goes below 1500 cells per mm³. Occasionally hepatotoxicity or an allergic reaction manifesting as fever, arthalgias, and rash will necessitate stopping azathioprine. I continue therapy for at least 1 year since azathioprine works slowly. If patients tolerate azathioprine and they cease worsening, I continue azathioprine indefinitely and try to taper them off methylprednisolone, although patients often require both medications.

For patients who continue to worsen despite an adequate trial of azathioprine or who do not tolerate azathioprine, I add methotrexate* to the pulse methylprednisolone at a dose of 7.5 mg orally once a week. Methotrexate is generally well tolerated. Potential side effects include anemia, dose-dependent suppression of hematopoiesis, stomatitis, acute and chronic hepatotoxicity, and pulmonary fibrosis. Patients should take folic acid (1 mg per day) while on methotrexate to prevent anemia and should avoid alcohol to reduce the risk of hepatotoxicity. Female patients should not become pregnant while on therapy. A chest radiograph is obtained at the start of therapy and yearly thereafter. When initiating treatment, patients should have complete blood counts and liver function tests every 2 weeks for 2 months and then once a month. Methotrexate should be stopped after 2 to 4 years to reduce the risk of chronic hepatotoxicity and pulmonary fibrosis.

Occasionally I will use azathioprine or methotrexate alone, generally in patients who have not tolerated pulse methylprednisolone or have problems with intravenous access.

Aside from patients in experimental treatment protocols, I do not use any other immunosuppressive therapies for progressive MS. Cyclophosphamide (Cytoxan),* cyclosporine (Sandimmune),* and total lymphoid irradiation may have some benefit for progressive MS, but I believe the risks of these treatments outweigh any potential benefits. Plasmapheresis and intravenous immunoglobulins are relatively safe and may be beneficial for progressive MS. However, I do not use them for MS because they are expensive, and third-party payers in my community generally will not cover them for MS. Finally, cladribine (Leustatin),* which is used for hairy cell leukemia, may slow progression of MS. While it is well tolerated, cladribine causes long-term bone marrow suppression. A large multicenter placebo-controlled trial currently underway should determine whether cladribine slows progression of MS and answer questions about safety. Until the results of this trial are known, I recommend that cladribine not be used for progressive MS outside of research protocols because

of concerns about potential long-term toxicity and uncertainty about efficacy.

SYMPTOMATIC THERAPIES

Symptomatic therapy is an important and often neglected part of the management of MS patients. Symptomatic therapy encompasses not only medications but also rehabilitative interventions and counseling. Management of MS may require referral of patients to urologists; physical, occupational, and speech therapists; physiatrists; social workers; and psychologists or psychiatrists to help manage the various problems created by MS.

Aids to Ambulation and Mobility

MS very commonly affects the mobility of patients, often with enormous social consequences. The principal problems that interfere with ambulation and mobility are leg weakness, gait imbalance, and spasticity. Useful ambulation aids for MS patients include lightweight ankle-foot orthoses for foot drop and canes, forearm crutches, and walkers for gait imbalance and leg weakness. Useful mobility aids include motorized scooters, lightweight wheelchairs, and motorized wheelchairs. In trying to determine whether an aid to ambulation or mobility is appropriate for patients, I remember a few principles. First, patients are usually functionally worse outside of my office than inside it. Because demyelinated nerve fibers fatigue easily, patients often worsen as the day goes on, and while they may do well walking into my examination room, their gait can deteriorate significantly after sustained walking. Second, the time to use ambulation or mobility aids is when the aids will help patients do things they otherwise would not do. Because of mobility impairment, patients may experience difficulty getting to and from work or stop going on family outings or shopping. Using ambulation or mobility aids can solve these problems and allow patients to resume more normal activities. Third, patients often are reluctant to use an ambulation or mobility aid. They often feel that using aids indicates to society that they are "disabled" or that they are "giving up." Physicians may need to encourage patients strongly to use aids. Finally, patients must be fitted for the appropriate aid and taught how to use it. I do not merely give prescriptions for aids to patients and send them to a medical supply store. I refer them to a physical therapist or rehabilitation medicine specialist who can help them choose the right aid and teach them to use it.

Spasticity

Spasticity commonly occurs in MS. It may interfere with the ability of patients to walk or transfer. Muscle spasms at night may interrupt sleep, and spasticity can even be painful. Regularly performed stretching exercises often can control mild spasticity. A physical therapist should teach patients these ex-

---

*Not FDA-approved for this indication.

ercises. Stretching exercises are also important to use in conjunction with antispasticity medicines in the management of moderate and severe spasticity. I prescribe baclofen (Lioresal) initially for spasticity when stretching exercises are not sufficient, starting at a low dose and increasing as tolerated and needed. I begin with 5 mg twice a day. After 3 days I increase the dose to 5 mg three times a day and then increase the total daily dose by 5 mg per day every 3 days. Patients with nocturnal spasms should take one of their doses at bedtime. Patients typically require 5 to 20 mg three or four times a day. The appropriate dose varies widely. Some patients have symptoms controlled with only 5 or 10 mg a day, whereas others require 80 to 120 mg a day. In addition, baclofen may increase the weakness of patients, often limiting its effectiveness.

Diazepam (Valium) and clonazepam (Klonopin) are also effective for spasticity. For diazepam, a dose of 2 to 5 mg one to three times a day usually suffices. I will use diazepam as an adjunct to baclofen or alone in patients who do not tolerate baclofen. Clonazepam in a dose of 0.5 to 2.0 mg at bedtime often helps manage nocturnal spasms that interfere with sleep. Clonazepam also can be used in conjunction with baclofen or alone. I do not use dantrolene (Dantrium) for spasticity.

For severe spasticity, particularly in nonambulatory patients, that does not respond to oral medications, intrathecal baclofen administered through a programmable subcutaneous pump is highly effective. Adductor spasms of the legs that interfere with walking or perineal care can be treated with motor point ablation with phenol or botulinum toxin.* Specialized circumstances necessitate these modalities, and a rehabilitation specialist can often help determine when these treatment approaches are indicated.

Management of the Neurogenic Bladder

Most patients with MS develop bladder problems during the course of their MS. I rarely see MS patients with significant leg weakness or spasticity who do not also have significant problems with their bladders. Symptoms include urinary urgency, urge incon-

tinence, hesitancy, nocturia, and recurrent urinary tract infections. Bladder symptoms often are quite disabling for patients. Some patients stop leaving their homes because they fear "having an accident." Fortunately, physicians can help most MS patients with urinary symptoms with appropriate interventions. However, successful management requires knowing what type of neurogenic bladder patients have. Three types of neurogenic bladders occur in MS: detrusor hyperreflexia, detrusor hyporeflexia, and detrusor-sphincter dyssynergia; the management of each type differs (Table 2).

Detrusor hyperreflexia, or "spastic bladder," occurs in about 40% of MS patients with bladder symptoms. With this pattern, there are uninhibited bladder contractions, a reduced bladder capacity, and no urinary retention. Anticholinergic medications usually control the symptoms of detrusor hyperreflexia. I generally use oxybutynin (Ditropan) in a dose of 2.5 to 5 mg two or three times a day. I include a dose at bedtime if the patient has significant nocturia. Alternatives include hyoscyamine (Levsinex), given as a timed-release capsule in a dose of 0.375 to 0.75 mg once or twice a day, or propantheline bromide (Pro-Banthine), in a dose of 7.5 to 15 mg three or four times a day.

About 20% of MS patients with urinary problems have detrusor hypotonia, or a "flaccid bladder." With detrusor hypotonia, weak detrusor contractions result in incomplete urinary emptying, urinary retention, and recurrent bladder infections. In my experience, patients with clinically significant urinary retention due to detrusor hypotonia are not symptomatically controlled with cholinergic medications such as bethanechol, and those with minor symptoms generally prefer not to take a medication. Significant retention, particularly when associated with recurrent urinary tract infections or incontinence, requires treatment with intermittent self-catheterization three to four times a day. Although many patients balk at the idea of self-catheterization, most learn the technique easily and adjust to performing self-catheterization. Patients use a "clean" technique, and an experienced nurse should instruct patients in the procedure. Caregivers can learn to catheterize patients who are unable to perform self-catheterization. Patients with recurrent urinary tract infections despite good catheterization technique may require

*Investigational drug in the United States.

TABLE 2. **Management of Neurogenic Bladder in Multiple Sclerosis**

Type of Dysfunction	PVR*	Treatment
Detrusor hyperreflexia	<100 mL	Oxybutynin, 5 mg bid–tid *or* hyoscyamine timed-release capsules, 0.375–0.75 mg qd–bid *or* propantheline bromide, 15 mg tid–qid
Detrusor hyporeflexia	>100 mL	Intermittent catheterization
Detrusor-sphincter dyssynergia	>100 mL	Intermittent catheterization ± oxybutinin, hyoscyamine, or propantheline bromide

*Refer patients with postvoid residuals (PVR) of over 100 mL to a urologist for evaluation.

treatment with prophylactic antibiotics, typically trimethoprim/sulfamethoxazole (Bactrim), ½ to 1 double-strength tablet a day, or nitrofurantoin (Macrodantin), 50 to 100 mg per day. I avoid placing indwelling urinary catheters, but occasionally these are appropriate for severely disabled patients.

Detrusor-sphincter dyssynergia occurs in about 40% of MS patients with neurogenic bladders. With this pattern, there is failure of relaxation of the external sphincter on initiation of urination with resultant incomplete emptying of the bladder. Most patients with detrusor-sphincter dyssynergia also have detrusor hyperreflexia with uninhibited bladder contractions. Patients with significant urinary retention due to detrusor-sphincter dyssynergia usually do not respond to α-adrenergic blockers to relax the urinary sphincter, such as prazosin (Minipress). I recommend treating patients with significant urinary retention with intermittent self-catheterization as for detrusor hyporeflexia. These patients also usually require treatment with an anticholinergic medication because of coexistent detrusor hyperreflexia.

Although the treatment of each type of bladder dysfunction varies, one cannot reliably predict the type of bladder dysfunction patients have from their symptoms. Prior to initiating treatment, I perform some evaluations to help predict the type of bladder dysfunction. For patients with significant urinary problems, I check a postvoid urinary residual and a urinalysis. If there are signs of infection, I treat the infection and then reassess the postvoid urinary residual. If the urinary residual is less than 100 mL and the urinalysis is normal, I treat patients for presumed detrusor hyperreflexia. If the urinary residual exceeds 100 mL, I refer patients to a urologist to exclude another cause of the urinary retention, such as tumor, and to determine whether patients have detrusor-sphincter dyssynergia or detrusor hyporeflexia. I also refer patients for urologic evaluation when they have low urinary residuals and significant symptoms, despite treatment with anticholinergic medications, recurrent urinary tract infections, or persistently abnormal urinalysis.

Management of Fatigue

Most MS patients complain of fatigue, and it is often one of their most troubling symptoms. Several types of fatigue affect MS patients, and successful management requires determining what patients mean when they complain of fatigue. The three most common types of fatigue in MS are nerve fiber fatigue, the fatigue of depression, and generalized fatigue or lassitude of MS.

Nerve fiber fatigue results from the increased energy demands and sensitivity to metabolic changes of demyelinated axons. Nerve fiber fatigue most commonly manifests as weakness brought on by repetitive motor activities, such as walking or writing. Currently no approved medications help nerve fiber fatigue, but an experimental agent, 4-aminopyridine, appears to be beneficial and may eventually be available outside of clinical trials. I refer patients with significant nerve fiber fatigue for physical and occupational therapy evaluations because these patients often benefit from mobility aids and instruction in energy conservation.

Depression affects up to 60% of patients with MS. Many patients with MS who complain of fatigue are depressed. These patients often say they awaken feeling tired and their fatigue worsens as the day progresses. They often also complain of insomnia but may or may not admit to feeling sad or depressed. These patients are excellent candidates for treatment with an antidepressant that inhibits serotonin uptake, and I will usually use fluoxetine (Prozac) at a dose of 20 to 40 mg per day.

Finally, generalized fatigue or lassitude commonly affects patients with MS. Typically, patients report feeling refreshed on awakening in the morning, but they develop excessive fatigue as the day progresses. Their energy usually is at its lowest in the afternoon. For generalized fatigue of MS, I recommend that patients take a brief nap in the early afternoon if practical. I also will try amantadine (Symmetrel),* taken as either 200 mg in the late morning or 100 mg on arising and 100 mg at lunch. An alternative is pemoline (Cylert),* given at a dose of 18.75 to 37.5 mg once a day. Insomnia and dysphoria may be complications of either medication and may require lowering the dose or adjusting the timing of doses. Finally, a referral to an occupational therapist for energy conservation can also help in the management of generalized fatigue.

Management of Depression and Emotional Lability

Depression commonly occurs in MS and usually responds to antidepressant medications. There are pitfalls in the management of depression in MS patients. First, patients, their families, and even their physicians often overlook depression. There is a tendency to attribute mood changes as "expected" and "understandable" in patients with a disabling disease. Second, because of cerebral involvement with MS, patients often are sensitive to side effects from antidepressants, and physicians should initiate antidepressants, particularly tricyclics, with a low dose and slowly increase the dose as tolerated. Finally, physicians often undertreat patients; failure to respond to antidepressants often results from using inadequate doses.

In MS patients in whom fatigue is a prominent associated symptom, I start with an antidepressant that inhibits serotonin uptake, such as fluoxetine (Prozac), beginning with 20 mg a day, or sertraline (Zoloft), starting with 50 mg a day. If emotional lability, neuropathic pain, or insomnia coexists with depression, I begin with a tricyclic antidepressant, such as amitriptyline (Elavil), 10 to 25 mg at bedtime, or nortriptyline (Pamelor), starting with 10 mg at

---

*Not FDA-approved for this indication.

bedtime. Doses for amitriptyline and nortriptyline need to be gradually increased as tolerated, and plasma levels should be monitored. Other tricyclic antidepressants I have found useful for MS patients with depression include imipramine (Tofranil) and desipramine (Norpramin). I refer patients who do not respond to a trial of two or three different antidepressants to a psychiatrist for further management.

Occasionally patients develop socially disabling emotional lability as a result of cerebral MS. Most commonly this manifests as difficulty with temper outbursts or easy crying. Less commonly, patients develop pathologic laughter and weeping in which there is uncontrollable laughter or crying without an appropriate affective experience. These forms of emotional discontrol often respond to low doses of tricyclic antidepressants. I prescribe amitriptyline, beginning with 10 to 25 mg at bedtime, gradually increasing the dose as tolerated to 50 to 100 mg. I use nortriptyline in a dose of 25 to 50 mg as an alternative.

Management of Cognitive Disturbance

The first and most important step in managing cognitive changes in MS is for physicians to acknowledge the problem. Most patients with MS eventually notice some changes in their mental efficiency. Cognitive changes typically are mild but can be severe. Importantly, cognitive changes in MS reflect white matter changes within the brain and do not correlate well with motor impairment, which largely results from spinal cord damage. Thus patients may have significant cognitive abnormalities but minimal problems walking or using their hands, whereas other patients may be wheelchair-bound from spinal MS but cognitively intact. I suspect cognitive dysfunction in patients who have widespread cerebral involvement on their MRI scans, difficulty in working, particularly when they have only mild motor impairment, chaotic social situations, or depressions that fail to respond to antidepressant medications.

The most common complaint among patients is that they can no longer do two tasks at once. Typically patients find that they must perform one task at a time without any distractions. Patients may find that they are committing errors at work when there is too much noise or when they are interrupted. Generalized fatigue often increases their difficulties. Other patients may develop more serious cognitive deficits manifesting as problems with short-term memory, learning, planning, organization, and judgment.

For patients with mild symptoms, merely acknowledging that the symptoms are real and secondary to their MS can allay much anxiety. Other patients may need formal neuropsychological testing. This is particularly helpful in documenting problems for patients who are no longer able to work partly or entirely because of cognitive difficulties. The formal documentation may be quite important in their successful application for Social Security disability bene-

fits. Referral to an occupational therapist, speech therapist, or psychologist to counsel patients and their families and to devise successful coping strategies may be helpful.

Management of Cerebellar Tremor

Cerebellar tremor affecting the upper extremities can be very disabling and difficult to manage. I refer patients with significant cerebellar tremor of their upper extremities to an occupational therapist. Adaptive aids, such as handles on feeding utensils, may be beneficial. I will also recommend a trial of clonazepam (Klonopin), starting with a dose of 0.5 mg twice a day and gradually increasing the dose as tolerated to 1 to 2 mg two or three times a day. Some patients respond quite well to this, while others either develop unacceptable sedation or derive no benefit.

Management of Pain

Pain affects many patients with MS. Trigeminal neuralgia occurs in about 5% of MS patients and can be severely disabling. Patients may also develop burning, dysesthetic pain, particularly in the lower extremities, from spinal cord lesions. Severe spasticity at times will also be painful. Finally, low back pain commonly afflicts MS patients who spend considerable time in wheelchairs or motorized scooters.

Carbamazepine (Tegretol) controls trigeminal neuralgia in most patients. I start with 100 mg twice a day and then increase the total daily dose by 100 mg every 3 days until reaching 200 mg three times a day. This or a lower dose usually controls the pain of most patients. However, before deciding that carbamazepine does not work, I adjust the dose so that serum levels reach a high therapeutic range (8 to 12 μg per mL). Carbamazepine, even in low doses, can worsen the balance of some MS patients, and this often limits the dose they can tolerate. I try phenytoin (Dilantin),* 100 to 300 mg per day, as an alternative for patients who fail to respond to or cannot tolerate carbamazepine. I refer patients with chronic trigeminal neuralgia who do not respond to medications to an experienced neurosurgeon for percutaneous trigeminal ganglioneurolysis. In my opinion, posterior fossa neurosurgical procedures are rarely, if ever, indicated in the treatment of trigeminal neuralgia in MS.

Burning, dysesthetic pain due to MS involvement of the spinal cord generally responds to treatment with tricyclic antidepressants. I start with amitriptyline* at a dose of 10 to 25 mg at bedtime and gradually increase the dose as tolerated. I substitute nortriptyline for patients who do not tolerate amitriptyline. Carbamazepine can be tried in those who do not respond to tricyclic medications. Occasionally patients continue to have severe pain despite treatment with tricyclic antidepressants or carba-

---

*Not FDA-approved for this indication.

mazepine. I refer these patients to pain specialists for management, and sometimes these patients are successfully managed only with chronic narcotics.

Management of pain secondary to spasticity should be directed at controlling spasticity (see earlier).

Low back pain often occurs in MS patients who spend much of their time sitting in wheelchairs or motorized scooters. Degenerative disease of the lumbosacral spine and weakness and spasticity of the paraspinal muscles often contribute to their low back pain. I evaluate the lumbosacral spine with computed tomography or magnetic resonance imaging to exclude the presence of a significant herniated disk, which can be difficult to diagnose in patients with impaired sensation secondary to MS. Usually, however, low back pain is musculoskeletal in origin, and nonsteroidal anti-inflammatory medications can be of some benefit. Even more important is to have a physical therapist or rehabilitation medicine specialist evaluate these patients. Often improper cushioning or support on their wheelchairs or motorized scooters aggravates their low back pain, and improvement in their seating can significantly help their back pain.

MYASTHENIA GRAVIS

method of
ALAN ZACHARIAS, M.D., and
LINTON C. HOPKINS, M.D.
Emory University School of Medicine
Atlanta, Georgia

Myasthenia gravis (MG) is an autoimmune disease characterized by fatigable weakness due to antibodies directed against acetylcholine receptors on the postsynaptic membrane of the neuromuscular junction. The true incidence is not well established but is estimated at 0.2 to 0.4 per 100,000 population. The data on prevalence have varied over the years, but recent estimates are as high as 14 per 100,000 population. As patients live longer, the number will likely increase. Men and women are affected to a similar degree after age 50 years but before then, more women are affected. The disease typically affects men in their sixth or seventh decade and women in their third or fourth decade, with broad ranges for each sex. There is no definitely established genetic transmission of the autoimmune form of the disease. Through dramatic improvements in intensive care, the disease is rarely fatal. Life expectancy is not statistically shortened, but pharyngeal and respiratory muscle weakness, if untreated, may be fatal, especially in an elderly patient or in one with coexisting heart and lung disease.

Purely ocular myasthenia gravis represents 10% to 25% of patients. Most patients who start with ocular symptoms will proceed to a generalized form within 1 or 2 years. If progression does not occur during this time, the disease is likely to remain ocular.

CLINICAL SIGNS AND SYMPTOMS

The hallmark of MG is fatigable skeletal muscle weakness. The most common clinical presentation is ptosis and diplopia. Additional symptoms may include decreased energy, dysphagia, choking, nasal regurgitation, slurred speech, neck weakness, or generalized weakness. Weakness is, of course, a common complaint. By asking detailed questions about the nature of the weakness, the physician should attempt to differentiate fixed or fluctuating weakness from simple lack of energy. One should determine whether the weakness occurs in the morning, afternoon, or evening and whether strength decreases during the day. Patients should be asked if specific daily activities are altered, such as fixing hair, shampooing, reading, long conversations, chewing meat, typing, or climbing stairs. If there is not fluctuation in the weakness, then one should consider alternative diagnoses. There should be no complaints of autonomic or sphincter disturbances.

A thorough physical and neurologic examination serves primarily as an opportunity to demonstrate an objective strength deficit that is exacerbated by repetitive testing. Having the patient sustain upgaze or forward arm elevation for 30 seconds to 1 minute to look for fatigue is an effective test. Other tests include having the patient cough or count to 100 while listening for changes in the voice or the duration of counting before taking a breath. Evaluation of eye movements may elicit dysconjugate movements or produce a complaint of diplopia with sustained gaze in any direction. Pupillary abnormalities are not seen in MG. Checking the patient's ability to sustain strength against repetitive resistance is essential, particularly the neck extensors and muscles of the shoulder and hip girdle. An objective sensory deficit is inconsistent with MG. Coordination testing is normal unless weakness is severe enough to simulate a problem. Reflexes are usually normal. Absence of reflexes should trigger thoughts of Lambert-Eaton myasthenic syndrome (LEMS).

The patient who fits the typical profile most likely has MG. Two important differential considerations are hyperthyroidism and LEMS. The former may coexist with MG, and its treatment may improve the weakness. The latter is commonly associated with occult malignancy, especially small cell carcinoma. Other conditions occasionally confused with MG are motor neuron disease, Guillain-Barré syndrome, chronic inflammatory demyelinating neuropathy, muscular dystrophies (especially facioscapulohumeral dystrophy), inflammatory myopathies, mitochondrial myopathies, brain stem disease (multiple sclerosis or stroke), or cranial nerve palsies. The differential diagnosis for the most common presentation (ptosis and diplopia) includes third nerve palsy, Horner's syndrome, oculopharyngeal muscular dystrophy, myotonic dystrophy, and mitochondrial myopathy.

PATHOPHYSIOLOGY

Acquired myasthenia gravis is an autoimmune disease in which there is a defect in neuromuscular transmission. Release of acetylcholine from the presynaptic terminal is normal, but transmission is impaired due to postsynaptic abnormalities that include (1) alteration in the postsynaptic membrane, (2) a decrease in the number of acetylcholine receptors, and (3) impaired binding of acetylcholine to its receptor. These abnormalities are due to an antibody against the acetylcholine receptor that is present in approximately 65% of patients with ocular myasthenia and 90% with generalized disease.

DIAGNOSTIC TESTING

The confirmation of the clinical diagnosis of MG does not always require a full battery of diagnostic studies. If the specific antibody to acetylcholine receptor (AChR) is present, the patient has MG. Many cases, however, require extensive and sometimes repeat testing before establishing a diagnosis. The most common nonserologic tests utilize edrophonium chloride (Tensilon), nerve conduction studies (NCSs) with repetitive nerve stimulation (RNS), electromyography (EMG), and single-fiber electromyography (SFEMG). Choosing additional tests depends on the clinical concerns, but thyroid function studies are essential since coexisting hyperthyroidism will be found in 5% to 15% of patients with MG.

Antiacetylcholine Receptor Antibodies

Of the several different types of antibodies to the acetylcholine receptor (AChR), the most common is known as binding antibody. It is present in the serum in about 65% of patients with ocular MG and 90% of those with generalized MG. Slightly higher sensitivity is reported by testing additionally for blocking as well as modulating antibodies, but these are not tested for in many laboratories. Although antibody testing is highly specific, false-positive results may occur in thymoma without muscle weakness, systemic lupus erythematosus, primary biliary cirrhosis, first-degree relatives of patients with MG, and autoimmune thyroiditis. Also, a group of amyotrophic lateral sclerosis (ALS) patients who received cobra venom had positive AChR antibodies, and there is one report of slightly elevated AChR antibodies in a group of tardive dyskinesia patients. We recommend testing all patients for the antibodies because they are specific, easy to obtain, and relatively cheap. When there is high clinical suspicion for disease and the need for a rapid diagnosis is low, a positive test confirms the diagnosis and further testing is rarely indicated. We also obtain antistriated muscle antibodies on all patients. These antibodies are found in approximately 50% of patients over 60 years of age and are more common in patients with thymoma.

Electrophysiologic Testing—Repetitive Nerve Stimulation and Single-Fiber Electromyography

As with all tests, the sensitivity of repetitive nerve stimulation (RNS) is greater in generalized MG (80%) than in ocular MG (40%). It is less specific than anti-AChR antibodies, as it may also be positive in motor neuron disease, peripheral neuropathy, and other defects of neuromuscular transmission. There is greater sensitivity in testing proximal versus distal muscles. A 10% drop in the amplitude of the compound muscle action potential is considered a positive test when supramaximal stimulation is applied at 2 to 3 Hz. The test is performed at rest and after 10 seconds of isometric exercise at 1-minute intervals up to 5 minutes. A weak muscle should be chosen for testing when available. The advantage of this test over antibody testing is that the results are immediately available, which is helpful in the clinic. Combining this test with anti-AChR antibody testing provides laboratory confirmation of the diagnosis in the majority of patients.

Single-fiber electromyography (SFEMG) is the most sensitive test for confirming the clinical diagnosis of MG (80% for ocular and 90% to 100% for generalized). The drawbacks are that the technical expertise needed to perform the test is not available in every hospital, it is expensive, and it requires an alert and cooperative patient. False-positive results occur in the same conditions as for RNS. We perform this test when the AChR and RNS are negative and occasionally use it to increase our confidence that new "weakness" is actually due to MG. The combination of antibody testing, RNS, and SFEMG should confirm the diagnosis of MG in nearly all cases. However, repeat testing may be necessary.

Tensilon Test

The intravenous injection of edrophonium (Tensilon) is an important diagnostic test since the drug is available readily and the results are instantly available. Tensilon is a short-acting acetylcholinesterase inhibitor that prevents the destruction of acetylcholine in the neuromuscular junction, thus prolonging its action. The major problems are that (1) the drug is dangerous and life-threatening, particularly in elderly people, those with heart disease, and those with obstructive lung disease; and (2) the results of the test are commonly difficult to interpret and to tell from placebo response, especially when the issue is a mild degree of ptosis.

The test should be performed only when there is an objective deficit to measure. Subjective improvement is not a positive test. An injection of saline prior to the Tensilon with simulation of the full testing maneuver is an excellent idea as it gives the physician a measure of the effect of placebo on the sign being observed. Sometimes it is useful also to blind the physician. However, we prefer that only the patient be blinded so we can know when a potentially harmful drug is being injected and can be prepared to handle the consequences. The test should be described in detail in the record so that a physician coming later will not be confused by what was done. If we need to, we sometimes do Tensilon tests at different times of the day and on different occasions. Also it is useful to produce a deficit at the bedside by sustained upgaze or prolonged counting before the injection. If the weakness is more obvious, its reversal will be easier to appreciate. We prepare three tuberculin syringes—one with Tensilon, one with saline to use as placebo, which we give first, and the third with atropine. The total dose for adults is 10 mg and 0.15 mg per kg per day for children. For adults, we begin with a test dose of 2 mg (0.2 mL) and observe the patient for 1 minute. If there is no response or bradycardia, then further incremental doses of 2 or 3 mg can be given with 2 to 3 minutes of observation between doses. If bradycardia occurs to 2 mg, we abort the test. An objective improvement in the observed deficit is a positive response, and testing should stop at that point. A positive Tensilon test is not specific for MG. A positive response may also occur in motor neuron disease and even in lesions of the oculomotor nerves. Life-threatening side effects are bradycardia, bronchospasm, and hypotension. Others are excessive sweating or salivation, lacrimation, fasciculations, diarrhea, abdominal cramps or nausea, urinary or stool incontinence, and small pupils. Atropine (0.4 to 1.0 mg) and an Ambu bag must be available to treat severe reactions.

Chest Computed Tomography

Adult patients with a confirmed diagnosis of MG should have a chest computed tomography (CT) scan to search for a thymoma. Children rarely have thymoma, and the scan may be deferred. Thymoma is present in about 10% of patients. The remaining 90% will have either thymic hyperplasia (70%) or atrophy (20%). The decision to recommend thymectomy, whether or not a thymoma is present, is discussed later.

Additional Laboratory Testing

The clinical situation should dictate the extent of laboratory testing in each patient, but thyroid tests are essential. Hyperthyroidism is the most commonly associated thyroid abnormality. Abnormalities are found in nearly 10% of cases. A sedimentation rate, rheumatoid factor, and antinuclear antibody are good screens for other autoimmune disease.

PATIENT MANAGEMENT

Reassurance and Education

All patients with newly diagnosed MG are frightened. They usually have no knowledge of the disease and will require some time to interact and ask questions of a doctor or nurse, preferably both, who are experienced in its management. Every patient with MG should be given information about the wide variety of treatments available and be given the expectation of response to treatment. They should be told that it is important to learn that simply resting the weak muscle gives improvement. If their voice becomes weak, they should stop talking; if chewing and swallowing is a problem, they should stop trying for a few minutes, then try again. Each symptom can be related to a specific muscle, and they can be made to understand how to relax it.

Drug Therapy
(Table 1)

Cholinesterase Inhibitors

Pyridostigmine (Mestinon) is the most commonly prescribed cholinesterase inhibitor and is considered first-line therapy for most patients. It produces reversible inhibition of acetylcholinesterase, which increases the availability of acetylcholine and allows improved neuromuscular transmission and muscle strength. After oral administration, the onset of action is 10 to 30 minutes, with peak effect in 2 hours. The benefit then declines over the next 2 hours. Most patients benefit from taking Mestinon, but only a minority attain complete relief of symptoms. This is particularly true with ocular symptoms such as diplopia. We start with a dose of 30 mg three times

per day (on awakening and every 6 hours times two) and ask the patient to decide about a dose increase in 3 days. If there are no side effects and the symptoms remain, we suggest increasing the dosage to 60, 90, or 120 mg every 4 to 6 hours, and teach the patient how to assess the response and evaluate side effects. Higher and more frequent dosing may be required. We advise reliable patients to adjust the dose to the amount and frequency that provides the greatest benefit. The common side effects are abdominal pain and cramping, nausea, diarrhea, increased sweating and lacrimation, and fasciculations. Diarrhea can be helped by hyoscyamine sulfate (Levsin), propantheline bromide (Pro-Banthine), diphenoxylate hydrochloride with atropine (Lomotil), or glycopyrrolate (Robinul). Atropine tablets are difficult to find, but one brand available is Sal-Tropine 0.4-mg tablets. However, we usually treat diarrhea due to Mestinon with dose reduction. Chronic obstructive pulmonary disease with asthma and cardiac conduction abnormalities are relative contraindications to the administration of Mestinon.

Physicians and patients must be careful to avoid excessive doses of pyridostigmine since weakness may develop. The best way to avoid overdoses is to be sure the effects are wearing off before the next dose. A long-acting preparation is available (Mestinon Timespan). We recommend that Timespan be taken only at bedtime by patients who have problems with weakness during the night or early morning. An intravenous preparation is also available, which is 30 times more potent than the oral form (2 mg IV = 60 mg orally).

Neostigmine bromide (Prostigmin) is available for oral or parenteral administration, but a shorter half-life makes it less attractive in most cases. Mestinon syrup is available for children or for nasogastric tube administration. Mestinon and neostigmine for intranasal administration or in a nebulized form might be helpful for patients who cannot tolerate other forms, but we have no experience with them.

Corticosteroids

Prednisone is first-line therapy for immunotherapy. The precise mechanism of action in MG is unknown. There are likely many different effects on the lymphocytes, cell-to-cell interaction, and macrocyte function, and there may be direct effects at the neuromuscular junction. Seventy percent to 90% of patients stabilize or improve on the drug. During the first 3 weeks of steroid therapy, weakness may get worse, so those with bulbar or respiratory weakness will need to be hospitalized and closely monitored during this period. Some will need more aggressive immunotherapy with therapeutic plasma exchange (TPE) or high-dose intravenous immunoglobulin (IVIg).* Once improvement begins, outpatient monitoring is continued. A response will usually occur during the first 2 to 6 weeks. There is no single right way to start prednisone. The goal is to attain the

TABLE 1. **Medications That May Produce Weakness in Myasthenia Gravis***

Aminoglycoside antibiotics	Tetracyclines
Quinine	Fluoroquinolones
Quinidine	Phenytoin (Dilantin)
Procainamide (Pronestyl)	Trimethadione (Tridione)
Bretylium	Trimethaphan
Beta blockers	Phenothiazines
Neuromuscular blocking agents	Lithium
Calcium channel blockers	Chloroquine (Aralen)
Lidocaine	D-Penicillamine (Cuprimine)
Penicillins	Iodinated contrast agents

**When considering a new medication in a myasthenic, the clinician should look for specific information and be suspicious of any agent that has sedation, muscle weakness or tingling, or numbness listed as side effects.*

**Not FDA-approved for this indication.*

maximum benefit as soon as possible and minimize side effects. We start with a daily dose of 1 mg per kg per day (50 to 100 mg) orally. This dose is given on awakening to coincide with the diurnal release of endogenous steroids. We begin some less severely affected patients on 20 mg per day as outpatients and increase by 10 to 20 mg per week. Occasionally we start with lower doses and increase more slowly.

Once a plateau in improvement occurs, we ask patients to taper the alternate-day dose. This usually maintains control of the disease and minimizes the side effects. The change is achieved by a weekly decrease of 10 mg on the alternate day until every-other-day dosing is established. We continue the full every-other-day dose as long as the patient is improving, then begin a reduction when a satisfactory plateau is reached. The dose is then tapered by 10 mg every month down to 20 or 30 mg every other day. We then slow the descent and use smaller decreases of 5 or 2.5 mg every 1 to 2 months. This continues until 5 to 20 mg every other day or until the lowest effective dose is established. A cautious approach is needed in tapering prednisone because when the weakness returns, reinstitution of higher doses will not always produce the same benefits.

When a patient has been asymptomatic on low-dose prednisone for a year, the decision to discontinue therapy arises. This decision depends on side effects and the overall benefits of therapy. Because the disease may be suppressed only by therapy, we generally recommend maintaining the lowest effective dose indefinitely. However, discontinuation is a reasonable option in those patients who no longer have any symptoms and signs of MG, as long as they understand the potential for return of symptoms.

In our patients, the two most disabling side effects of prednisone are severe depression with suicidal ideation and severe osteoporosis with compression fractures. Other side effects of prednisone therapy include immunosuppression, hyperglycemia, weight gain, electrolyte imbalance, hirsutism, coarsening of facial features, euphoria, skin fragility, cataracts, hypertension, and gastrointestinal ulceration. Growth retardation may occur in children. Steroids may be relatively contraindicated in diabetics, and some hyperglycemia should be anticipated. Most side effects are dose dependent, however, and can be minimized by every-other-day dosing, regular follow-up, and dietary guidelines. Supplemental calcium and vitamin D are important for postmenopausal women. The patient and family should be counseled to watch for changes in mood. Significant depression should be treated by prompt dosage reduction, antidepressants, and psychiatry consultation if needed.

Prednisone is effective in about 70% of patients, easy to administer and monitor, and is inexpensive and has a relatively rapid onset of action. For these reasons, we consider it to be first-line therapy for patients uncontrolled by cholinesterase inhibitors alone. However, since the long-term side effects may cause significant morbidity, we consider alternative therapies in certain patients.

Immunotherapy Other Than Prednisone

The immunosuppressant actions of chemotherapeutic agents are utilized to treat MG when patients with generalized or bulbar disease are unable to tolerate prednisone, have not had an adequate response, or are dependent on too large a dose of prednisone and are experiencing side effects. The most commonly used agent is azathioprine (Imuran).* Cyclosporine (Sandimmune)* has been shown to be effective; cyclophosphamide (Cytoxan)* is rarely used. Chronic immunosuppression is expensive, requires frequent monitoring, introduces the risk of potentially life-threatening infection, and raises the possibility of an increased incidence of malignancy. The benefits include ease of administration and long-term disease control with reduced prednisone side effects.

Azathioprine (Imuran)*

Imuran inhibits DNA and RNA synthesis to produce immunosuppression. Response rates vary from 30% to 90%. The main indications are for patients who are failing steroid monotherapy or to allow a reduction in steroid dosage. It is also a potential first-line immunotherapy for patients who are already depressed, diabetics, elderly people, or patients with osteoporosis. The onset of action is approximately 2 to 4 months, but maximum benefit may not be reached for 12 to 36 months. A starting dose of 50 mg per day is given for 1 week. If a complete cell count and liver enzyme study are normal, then further dose escalation can be safely undertaken. Increases of 25 to 50 mg per week are made until the target dose of 2 to 3 mg per kg is reached. A complete blood count and liver enzyme study are obtained on a weekly basis until the target dose is reached and then at regular intervals during therapy (every 6 to 8 weeks). The mean corpuscular volume (MCV) is expected to rise to greater that 100 fL and does not require a dose reduction. A total white blood cell count of 3000 to 4000 per mm^3 is a reasonable target. If the total white blood cell count falls below 2500 per mm^3 or the absolute neutrophil count is less than 1000 per mm^3, the dose should be discontinued until the cell count has risen again. The medication can then be restarted at a lower dose. Since corticosteroids produce leukocytosis, a target of 5% to 10% absolute lymphocyte count is reasonable for patients on both medications.

For patients on prednisone and Imuran, the steroid dose may be tapered slowly once the azathioprine maintenance dose is established. Some patients may be able to stop the steroids completely or reach a low maintenance dose. The Imuran dose may also eventually be reduced. We usually attempt to taper and discontinue these potentially harmful drugs if patients have been asymptomatic for a year. We explain to patients that it is possible that weakness, even severe weakness, may appear in the future, but

---

*Not FDA-approved for this indication.

we assure them that modern treatment of MG will be effective if it is required in the future.

Known side effects of Imuran include increased risk for infections, leukopenia, anemia, thrombocytopenia, hepatitis, nausea, vomiting, anorexia, and pancreatitis. A rash and alopecia are rare. The effect of Imuran on the risk of malignancy is not known, although kidney transplant patients on the drug seem to have an increased risk of lymphoma. We think that the drug does increase the risk, but we do not know how much.

An important drug interaction is with allopurinol (Xyloprim), which inhibits the catabolism of Imuran. The dose of Imuran may need to be lowered by as much as 75% to avoid toxicity during allopurinol use. A flu-like syndrome of fever, malaise, myalgia, and diarrhea may occur early in therapy at low doses. This is felt to represent a hypersensitivity reaction and would likely preclude continued therapy. Most symptoms respond to a dose reduction. Regular follow-up evaluation is mandatory for patients on Imuran to assess toxicity and benefits.

Cyclosporine (Sandimmune)*

Cyclosporine is a fungus-derived cyclic peptide that selectively impairs T cell function. It has not been as extensively used as azathioprine but has been shown in a controlled trial to be effective. Like azathioprine, its main indication is failure of prednisone therapy. The response to cyclosporine is more rapid than to azathioprine. Onset of improvement usually begins in a few weeks, with maximum improvement in 3 to 4 months. We begin with 5 mg per kg per day in two to three divided doses. Maintenance therapy is determined by plasma trough levels and by the monitoring of side effects. Blood levels should be obtained before the morning dose every 2 weeks until stable, and then every month unless the dosage changes or potential toxicity is suspected. A serum creatinine level determination is needed at the same intervals. The target trough level varies for different laboratory techniques, and we recommend consulting with the laboratory directly to determine the normal trough values. In our laboratory, the goal is a trough level of 100 to 150 ng/mL. Dosage adjustments should be by no more than 1 mg per kg per day once a month unless otherwise dictated by toxicity. Assuming stable trough levels, 6 to 9 nine months is an adequate trial. Once a stable dose and response are established, we then consider tapering the dose to the lowest possible level. An appropriate guideline is tapering by no more than 0.5 mg per kg per day every 2 to 3 months. The drug should be abruptly stopped if renal insufficiency is noted. MG can always be managed in other ways; no single drug is essential.

There are many potential drug interactions with cyclosporine, but the two absolute contraindications are nonsteroidal anti-inflammatory drugs and amphotericin B. The physician may consult a pharmacist or appropriate resource for further detail. There are many side effects of cyclosporine that may limit therapy. Nephrotoxicity and hypertension are the ones to monitor closely, but patients may also develop seizures, infections, hirsutism, headache, gingival hyperplasia, nausea, edema, cramps, paresthesias, and hepatotoxicity. It does not produce bone marrow suppression.

Cyclophosphamide (Cytoxan)*

Cyclophosphamide (CP) is an alkylating agent that exerts its effects on the proliferation of B cells and T cells. We have little experience with the drug in MG. We believe that it should be considered only for patients who have failed other, more traditional regimens. The response rates are reported as high as 80% to 90%, but the data are confounded by concomitant use of other immunosuppressants. The recommended dose range is 2.5 to 3.0 mg per kg per day, adjusted to maintain a WBC count of 2500 to 4000 per mm^3 and a relative lymphocyte count of less than 10%. An alternative with potentially fewer side effects is intravenous pulse injections of 200 mg per day for 5 days.

Toxicity is the main factor limiting the use of CP. The side effects include increased risk for malignancy, alopecia, myelosuppression, nausea, vomiting, skin discoloration, anorexia, hemorrhagic cystitis, dysuria, and arthralgias. Direct cardiac toxicity is rare, but monitoring of the electrocardiogram is recommended. Frequent urinalyses are needed to monitor for hemorrhagic cystitis, and adequate hydration must be maintained.

Intravenous Immunoglobulin (IVIg)

IVIg (Gamimune N, Gammagard) is prepared from pooled human plasma and has now become our first-line parenteral therapy for severe MG (impending or full-blown crisis). The precise mechanism of action is unknown but likely involves modulation of the immune system. Antibody titers are not decreased in the majority of patients. The benefit is seen within days of initiating therapy and generally lasts for 2 to 3 months. The standard regimen is 400 mg per kg per day for 5 days (shorter regimens are also utilized). Some of the advantages of IVIg over therapeutic plasma exchange (TPE) are ease of administration, shorter duration of therapy, and potential outpatient application. We recommend that any patient with weakness that requires urgent administration of IVIg be monitored in the hospital, but home infusion or outpatient hospital or clinic infusion is commonly employed when the patient is stabilized.

The cost of IVIg is comparable to that of TPE. Acute renal failure is our major concern, and we obtain a serum creatinine level before infusion. Other side effects include a flulike reaction, hypotension, headache, nausea during the infusion, fever, aseptic meningitis, fluid overload, and stroke. There is a potential for an anaphylactic reaction in the rare

---

*Not FDA-approved for this indication.

*Not FDA-approved for this indication.

patients with IgA deficiency. Screening for IgA antibodies should be considered prior to administration. Although there have been previously reported cases of transmission of hepatitis C following IVIg treatment, human immunodeficiency virus (HIV) and hepatitis B and C transmission are prevented by the current preparation process.

Therapeutic Plasma Exchange

TPE is still considered by many to be standard therapy for rapid reversal of life-threatening exacerbations of MG. Most patients will respond. Before the emergence of IVIg, we also commonly used it prior to surgery to maximize function. Some unusual patients require regular TPE to maintain function. Retrospective and uncontrolled trials have shown a clear benefit. Although further comparison trials are needed before it will be known whether IVIg is comparable to TPE, our experience suggests that the two have similar benefits. The process involves the removal of circulating antibodies as well as other plasma constituents. The subsequent improvement is rapid but of short duration. Patients may respond within 24 hours of an exchange but generally reach a peak benefit after a series of exchanges in 1 to 2 weeks. Sustained improvement rarely lasts beyond 2 to 3 months. A typical regimen involves the removal via intravenous cannulation of 3 to 4 liters of plasma on an every-other-day schedule for a total of 5 to 7 exchanges. Albumin (5%) with saline solution is used as replacement solution. Most patients tolerate the procedure well. Poor venous access may require the placement of a large venous catheter, which has risks of infection, pneumothorax, air embolism, and hemorrhage. Other potential side effects include hypotension, local thrombosis, cardiac arrhythmias, electrolyte imbalance (particularly hypocalcemia), disseminated intravascular coagulation, stroke, infections, and thrombocytopenia.

Either TPE or IVIg should be used for treatment of a myasthenic crisis. There is a general correlation of antibody titer and response to treatment, but monitoring of the antibody levels during therapy is not indicated. Patients who are seronegative still respond to TPE and IVIg.

Immunoadsorption (IA)

Selective adsorption columns are utilized with IA in an attempt selectively to remove pathogenic plasma proteins in MG. This technology holds promise of equal efficacy to TPE with fewer complications. It is not widely available, and comparison trials are needed before it becomes standard therapy.

Thymectomy

Although it has still not been proved to help, thymectomy for the treatment of MG has become accepted as standard practice for younger patients with the generalized form of disease. It began after patients with thymoma were noted to have improvement in their myasthenic symptoms following thymectomy. The precise pathogenic role of the thymus in MG is not established. Although rare patients obtain a rapid improvement in symptoms following thymectomy, most of the benefit is delayed.

The pathologic changes in the thymus in MG support the idea that it plays some role in the disease. Lymphoid follicular hyperplasia is the rule, and thymoma is present in about 10% of patients. The presence of anti–striated muscle antibodies increases the probability of thymoma. Most thymomas are benign neoplasms, but invasive tumors do occur and they require aggressive treatment. Not all patients with MG require thymectomy. Most physicians do not recommend the surgery for those with purely ocular disease unless a thymoma is present. Even for bulbar and generalized disease, individual circumstances determine whether therapeutic thymectomy should be performed. Many physicians believe that patients under age 50 years who are otherwise in good health should have a thymectomy for the potential long-term benefit even if there is no thymoma, but there is still controversy on this issue. We do not recommend the surgery over age 60 years unless a thymoma is found.

We do not recommend thymectomy for the short-term reversal of weakness. The operation is a significant physiologic stress and frequently makes the patient weaker in the short term. For this reason, our practice is to use IVIg, plasma exchange, prednisone, or other immunotherapy to get the patient as strong as possible before thymectomy, or any other surgery. Since the modern physician has effective, less invasive treatment to improve strength, we take the position that thymectomy is always elective. It slowly reduces the population of T cells and seems to improve the chance of long-term remission.

There are several possible surgical approaches, but we recommend that all patients undergo transthoracic (sternal splitting) thymectomy to allow the greatest chance for removal of all thymic tissue. If strength is maximized by IVIg or TPE and immunosuppressants prior to surgery, patients usually tolerate the procedure well and do not usually require extra time intubated or prolonged intensive care. Despite the lower surgical morbidity of transcervical and endoscopic methods, we believe that there is the potential for incomplete resection and decreased response. We have not needed to recommend repeat thymectomy but would consider it if we thought there had been an incomplete resection in a patient with generalized symptoms. Although there are reports of patients who were unresponsive to modern immunotherapy and could not be removed from artificial ventilation until they had the surgery, we have not encountered this situation.

Miscellaneous Therapies

A variety of other treatments have been tried with variable success. The role for these therapies is to treat patients who have failed traditional approaches. Treatments include total body irradiation, splenic radiation, splenectomy, methotrexate,* chlorambucil,* ephedrine,* anti-CD4 antibody, and 3,4-diaminopyridine, which is an investigational drug in the United States.

PATIENT MANAGEMENT PROBLEMS

Management decisions require the application of certain general principles to the specific situation presented by every patient. There is no rigid blueprint.

1. Mestinon may provide temporary symptomatic benefit, but it has no action against the disordered immune process. The effect of Mestinon lasts only a few hours.
2. Prednisone is effective treatment for generalized MG but is limited by the usual side effects.
3. Thymectomy is indicated whenever a thymoma is present, but the operation is always elective. There is time to reverse significant weakness prior to surgery.
4. Immunosuppressant therapy should be considered when significant weakness persists after several months of prednisone treatment, or when the prednisone dose cannot be tapered to a level that controls side effects.
5. When immunosuppression is used, the dose should be adequate, but when the weakness is reversed, control should be maintained on the lowest effective dose.
6. Weakness of life-sustaining bulbar and respiratory muscles should not be tolerated in this treatable condition, and we do not hesitate to start high-dose intravenous gamma globulin (IVIg) infusion or plasma exchange in this situation.

UNIQUE CONDITIONS

Neonatal Myasthenia Gravis

This transient condition is characterized by the onset, 12 to 48 hours after birth, of hypotonia, poor sucking and crying, and respiratory distress in 10% to 20% of neonates born to myasthenic mothers. The mean duration of symptoms has been estimated at 21 days but may last up to 12 weeks. The condition is due to the passive transfer of maternal antibodies to the fetus. Some physicians recommend treating mothers who are known to have MG 2 weeks before the expected delivery with plasma exchange. This usually prevents neonatal MG. If the condition does occur, treatment with supportive care is usually adequate. Neostigmine may also be used. For refractory cases, exchange transfusion may be considered. Neonatal MG does not predispose to the development of idiopathic MG later in life.

---

*Not FDA-approved for this indication.

Congenital Myasthenic Syndromes

These genetic disorders are characterized by a variety of pre- and postsynaptic defects in neuromuscular transmission. Autoimmunity does not play a role, and the patients do not respond to immunosuppressant therapy. These patients usually present in the neonatal or early childhood period with hypotonia, oculobulbar weakness, and respiratory distress. Rarely, the presentation is in early adulthood. The diagnosis is suspected based on electrophysiologic testing and the response to Tensilon. Specific defects are established in specialized laboratories. Patients may respond to cholinesterase inhibitors and rarely steroids. Some patients seem to benefit from a medication (3,4-diaminopyridine*) that is not available for general prescription in the United States.

Penicillamine-Induced Myasthenia Gravis

D-Penicillamine is used in the treatment of rheumatoid arthritis, Wilson's disease, and cystinuria. It may induce autoimmune myasthenia gravis. The clinical condition is indistinguishable from idiopathic forms, though it is typically milder and frequently restricted to the extraocular muscles. Repetitive nerve stimulation produces the characteristic decremental response of myasthenia. Antibodies to the acetylcholine receptor are usually present. Discontinuation of the medication is essential and improves symptoms, which usually resolve within 1 year. The same treatment guidelines apply as in idiopathic myasthenia except that thymectomy is not indicated.

---

*Investigational drug in the United States.

TRIGEMINAL NEURALGIA

method of
ROBERT H. WILKINS, M.D.
Duke University Medical Center
Durham, North Carolina

Trigeminal neuralgia (tic douloureux) is a symptom, not a disease. These two terms are applied to a type of facial pain that can be caused by several disease processes. Characteristically, the pain is sudden in onset; it is confined to some portion of the distribution of the right or left trigeminal nerve; is sharp, lancinating, or electrical in quality; lasts for some seconds; and subsides quickly only to return a short time later. It often can be triggered by a nonpainful stimulus such as touching the same side of the face, speaking, or eating. After a series of paroxysms of lancinating pain, a more long-lasting aching pain may occur in the same area of the face. In the natural history of the disorder, the pain may disappear for months at a time, but successive cycles tend to occur more frequently and to become more severe. The lower part of the face is more often affected than the upper part, the right side is more often involved than the left, and women are more often affected than men. Most patients with trigeminal neuralgia are over 50 years old. Because the pain frequently is felt in the region of one or more teeth and feels like an exposed nerve, the patient may initially see a dentist rather than a physician.

The diagnosis of trigeminal neuralgia as a symptom is made by the history. It must be differentiated from glossopharyngeal neuralgia, postherpetic neuralgia, cluster headaches, pain from dental or sinus infection, and other disorders.

Approximately 5% to 8% of patients with trigeminal neuralgia will have a structural lesion adjacent to some portion of the ipsilateral trigeminal nerve, such as a tumor in the cerebellopontine angle (e.g., a meningioma, acoustic neuroma, or epidermoid tumor). On physical examination, a patient with such a lesion will usually show evidence of dysfunction of the trigeminal nerve and perhaps of adjacent cranial nerves as well. A magnetic resonance imaging (MRI) scan or a computed tomography (CT) scan of the head is a useful screening test for patients with trigeminal neuralgia, not only to identify a structural lesion external to the brain but also to identify the plaques of multiple sclerosis. About 2% to 3% of patients with trigeminal neuralgia have multiple sclerosis, which often may be suspected by the history and physical findings and confirmed by appropriate testing. Among those patients without evidence of multiple sclerosis or a structural lesion adjacent to the trigeminal nerve, many have compression of the trigeminal nerve at the pons by an adjacent vessel (most often the superior cerebellar artery). Such patients usually demonstrate no abnormalities on neurologic examination, CT scanning, or MRI scanning.

If a structural lesion adjacent to the trigeminal nerve is identified, treatment is directed toward eradicating the lesion; relief of the trigeminal neuralgia usually occurs as a result of this treatment. If such a structural lesion is not present, the trigeminal neuralgia is ordinarily treated medically. A variety of drugs have been used to treat trigeminal neuralgia, but the most effective have been carbamazepine (Tegretol), phenytoin (Dilantin), and baclofen (Lioresal).

TREATMENT

Medical Treatment

Carbamazepine is ordinarily begun at a dosage of 200 mg per day and is increased to as much as 400 mg three times a day (maximum, 1200 mg per day). The occasional side effects of nausea, unsteadiness, and drowsiness can sometimes be avoided by starting at a low dosage and increasing gradually. The lowest dose that provides adequate pain relief should be used for maintenance. Because carbamazepine can (rarely) cause aplastic anemia, agranulocytosis, thrombocytopenia, or leukopenia, the complete blood count should be monitored periodically while a patient is receiving this medication. Similarly, because liver function may be altered, liver function tests should also be monitored. If bone marrow depression, hepatic dysfunction, or dermatitis develops, the drug should be discontinued.

If carbamazepine does not give pain relief or if it causes side effects that cannot be tolerated, phenytoin* can be given instead. Phenytoin is ordinarily used at a dosage of 300 to 400 mg per day in divided doses. In general, it is better tolerated than carbamazepine but is less effective in the treatment of trigeminal neuralgia. Phenytoin may have to be stopped if it causes dermatitis; dose-related ataxia, dysarthria, and confusion can usually be reversed by reducing the phenytoin dosage.

If carbamazepine and phenytoin are ineffective alone, they can be tried in combination. If the combination also does not provide relief, baclofen* can be given, starting at a dosage of 5 to 10 mg three times a day, and gradually increasing to as much as 15 to 20 mg four times a day.

Surgical Treatment

In the event that medical therapy proves to be insufficient for adequate pain relief, a number of operative alternatives can be considered that are aimed at the peripheral branches or trunk of the trigeminal nerve or at central trigeminal pathways.

The injection with alcohol or the avulsion of a trigeminal division or branch can ordinarily be done with little risk. However, the nerve will eventually grow back and the pain will return. The average times for pain relief from alcohol injection (using local anesthesia) are about 8.5 months for the supraorbital nerve, 12 months for the infraorbital nerve or second trigeminal division, and 16 months for the third trigeminal division. After surgical avulsion of a trigeminal branch (under local or general anesthesia), the pain relief is a little longer, averaging 2 to 3 years.

The trigeminal nerve can be partially destroyed at the gasserian ganglion or just central to it by the heat produced by an inserted radiofrequency electrode or by an injected substance (e.g., glycerol). Both procedures are done percutaneously under local anesthesia supplemented by intravenous medication. Since both produce pain relief by partial destruction of neural tissue, there is usually some resulting facial numbness, and there may be weakness of the muscles of mastication. More annoying side effects may also occur, such as facial paresthesia and corneal anesthesia. A review of 989 cases from three reported series of patients treated by percutaneous trigeminal radiofrequency coagulation showed that between 91 and 98% of patients were relieved of pain, with a mortality rate of 0%. The recurrence rate varied from 14% over 4 years in one series to 80% over 12 years in another. The incidence of trigeminal motor palsy in the three series was 22%, 43%, and 50%, respectively; the incidence of postoperative paresthesia was 19%, 2%, and 93%. In general, glycerol injection is less precise than radiofrequency coagulation and is more often followed by annoying facial paresthesia.

Another approach to gasserian ganglion/trigeminal nerve root injury involves compressing these structures with a percutaneously inserted Fogarty catheter balloon that is inflated through the foramen ovale for a short period. This is done with general anesthe-

---

*Not FDA-approved for this indication.

*Not FDA-approved for this indication.

sia; it does not require that the patient's facial sensation be tested during the procedure. In one series of 100 patients so treated, relief persisted at 5 years in 80%; 4% of the patients reported paresthesia; virtually all patients experienced ipsilateral trigeminal motor weakness but this resolved within 3 months.

The other major area where the trigeminal nerve is attacked surgically is at its entry into the pons. At the nerve root entry zone, the axons that carry pain sensation are located within the main sensory root, whereas the motor axons are located within one or more accessory rootlets. Therefore, trigeminal neuralgia can be treated at this site without interference with the muscles of mastication.

When the trigeminal nerve root entry zone is exposed surgically through a retromastoid craniectomy (performed with general anesthesia), the surgeon frequently (i.e., about 70% to 80% of the time) can identify compression of the trigeminal nerve at that point by an adjacent vessel or vessels. If this is the case, the surgeon, with the help of the operating microscope, can then separate the aberrant vessel(s) from the nerve root entry zone and coagulate and divide the vessel (if it is a vein) or insert a pad such as a sponge of polyvinyl alcohol foam (Ivalon) to maintain the separation of the aberrant vessel from the entry zone (if it is an artery). Such an approach ordinarily provides excellent or good pain relief without facial numbness or paresthesia. About 75% of patients so treated will still have excellent or good relief after 5 years; 25% will have insufficient initial relief or will experience recurrence of pain during that time.

If the surgeon explores the trigeminal nerve root entry zone and does not find vascular compression, he or she can cut about half of the cross-sectional diameter of the main trigeminal sensory root. This also frequently provides excellent or good pain relief but does cause some degree of facial hypesthesia, most often consisting of partial sensory loss on the side of the tongue and on the face adjacent to the mouth on the affected side. In one series, the failure rate was 17% for the first year, and the recurrence rate averaged 2.6% each year thereafter.

The operation of retromastoid craniectomy is a major one. The patient spends about a week in the hospital, with another month of recovery at home before the resumption of full-time work. With the use of intraoperative monitoring of auditory nerve function (evoked potential monitoring), the incidence of significant ipsilateral hearing loss has been reduced from about 8% to almost nil. The operative mortality rate is less than 1%.

A Plan of Treatment

My approach is as follows: If there is no evidence of a posterior fossa tumor, the patient should be tried on medical therapy. If this fails, the choice of subsequent treatment is based on the location of the tic and the age and general health of the patient. In an elderly patient or a patient in poor health, with

tic restricted to the forehead, supraorbital/supratrochlear nerve avulsion or balloon compression of the gasserian ganglion would be my next choice of treatment. In a similar patient with tic restricted to the cheek, I recommend alcohol injection or avulsion of the infraorbital nerve or one of the three percutaneous procedures (but favoring balloon compression to reduce the risk of corneal denervation). Finally, in an elderly or infirm patient with tic in the region of the eye, in the third division, or in multiple divisions, I recommend percutaneous trigeminal balloon compression, radiofrequency coagulation, or glycerol injection. These same recommendations apply to the patient of any age whose tic is related to multiple sclerosis.

If the patient is younger, is in good health, and has not been helped or is no longer helped by medication, I believe that microvascular decompression is the treatment of choice, especially if the pain involves the area of the eye (less possibility of producing corneal anesthesia than with a percutaneous procedure) or the mandible (less likelihood of producing weakness of the muscles of mastication than with a percutaneous procedure). Intraoperative monitoring of brain stem auditory evoked potentials is used to minimize the risk of ipsilateral deafness. If definite vascular compression is not identified at the time of operation, the caudal one-half or two-thirds of the main sensory root of the trigeminal nerve should be divided adjacent to the pons. An alternative approach (which is actually the preferred choice of many authorities) in the healthy patient who has pain despite an adequate trial of medical therapy is percutaneous trigeminal balloon compression, radiofrequency thermocoagulation, or glycerol injection.

If pain recurs after any of these procedures, it should be approached therapeutically as a new event, beginning with a trial of medication. Alcohol injection, nerve avulsion, balloon compression, radiofrequency coagulation, and glycerol injection can be repeated, but recurrence after microvascular decompression is probably best approached by a percutaneous technique or by partial division of the sensory root at the pons rather than by a second microvascular decompression.

GLOSSOPHARYNGEAL AND GENICULATE NEURALGIA

Glossopharyngeal neuralgia is a sharp, lancinating, paroxysmal pain, similar to trigeminal neuralgia, that is felt in the side of the throat, centered about the tonsil. During a severe attack the patient may develop bradycardia and even asystole, with resulting syncope. The treatment of glossopharyngeal neuralgia is analogous to the treatment of trigeminal neuralgia. The same medications are tried. If medical therapy fails, the glossopharyngeal and vagus nerves can be exposed through a retromastoid craniectomy. Vascular decompression of these nerves at the medulla can be performed if an offending vessel is found; otherwise the glossopharyngeal nerve and upper vagus rootlets can be divided to provide pain relief.

Geniculate neuralgia refers to pain felt in the sensory distribution of the facial nerve, especially in the region of the ear. In cases of postherpetic geniculate neuralgia, there may be herpetic lesions in this area as well as the oropharynx at the onset of the illness. The pain of geniculate neuralgia is more variable than the stereotyped pain of trigeminal neuralgia and glossopharyngeal neuralgia. If the patient with geniculate neuralgia is not helped by carbamazepine or phenytoin, amitriptyline* can be tried, starting at 25 mg at bedtime with a gradual increase to as much as 150 mg. If such a medical approach does not provide significant pain relief, the nervus intermedius portion of the facial nerve can be cut intracranially through a retromastoid craniectomy.

---

*Not FDA-approved for this indication.

OPTIC NEURITIS

method of
EDSEL ING, M.D.
Allegheny General Hospital
Pittsburgh, Pennsylvania

and

JAMES GARRITY, M.D.
Mayo Clinic
Rochester, Minnesota

Idiopathic optic neuritis is an immune-mediated inflammation of the optic nerve characterized by acute or subacute visual loss, with gradual recovery of vision over the ensuing months. It is one of the most frequent causes of neurogenic visual loss in patients less than 50 years old. Optic neuritis, like multiple sclerosis, is a clinical diagnosis. Laboratory and radiologic studies are supportive but not diagnostic. Much of the recent information on optic neuritis is derived from the Optic Neuritis Treatment Trial (ONTT). The reader is encouraged to follow the results of the ongoing Longitudinal Optic Neuritis Study (LONS).

SYMPTOMS

Optic neuritis characteristically occurs in young women (age 20 to 45 years). Visual loss, usually monocular, occurring over 1 day to 2 weeks, followed by gradual visual recovery, is typical. Ocular pain, especially with eye movement, is reported by over 90% of patients. Transient visual deterioration may occur with increased body temperature (Uhthoff's phenomenon). Colored or flashing lights are noted by a third of patients. Objects traveling in straight lines may appear to have a curved trajectory (Pulfrich's phenomenon) owing to asymmetric conduction in the two optic nerves. In patients with optic neuritis, features suggestive of multiple sclerosis, such as weakness, numbness, paresthesia, Lhermitte's sign, or bladder difficulties, should be asked for.

SIGNS

The presenting visual acuity in patients with optic neuritis ranges from 20/20 or better in 10% of patients, to finger counting or worse in 15% of patients. An ipsilateral relative afferent pupillary defect (swinging flashlight test) provides important objective confirmation of suspected optic neuritis. A relative afferent pupillary defect may not be seen if the contralateral eye has coincident or previous optic neuritis. Altered color vision (dyschromatopsia) is seen in 88% of patients. Loss of contrast sensitivity is common. Various visual field defects may be noted on confrontation field testing or Amsler grid testing and are best documented with formal perimetry. Altitudinal defects, arcuate defects, and nasal steps are more common findings than central or centrocecal scotomas. Optic disk edema (papillitis) is seen in 35% of patients with optic neuritis. In the remainder, the inflammation is behind the globe (retrobulbar), and the optic nerve may initially appear normal. Optic disk pallor is not seen until at least 4 weeks after the onset of visual loss.

Periphlebitis (inflammatory venous sheathing) or, less commonly, a vitritis of the pars plana may be seen. Infrequently neuroretinitis (a "macular star" of retinal inflammatory exudate secondary to optic disk edema) occurs. Although an internuclear ophthalmoplegia is not pathognomonic of multiple sclerosis, it should be looked for in every optic neuritis suspect.

DIFFERENTIAL DIAGNOSIS

Compressive lesions, ischemia, collagen vascular disease, infections, toxins, nutritional deficiencies, hereditary optic neuropathies, retinal diseases such as cone dystrophies, and malingering should be considered in the differential diagnosis of optic neuritis. Compressive lesions usually are associated with a longer course of visual loss (months to years) and may show repeated worsening of vision with attempts at steroid withdrawal. Examples of compressive lesions include meningiomas, optic nerve glioma, various orbital tumors, Graves' ophthalmopathy, sphenoid sinus mucoceles, craniopharyngiomas, and pituitary tumors. Since neuroimaging of the brain is presently recommended for cases of presumed optic neuritis, it is unlikely that a compressive lesion will be missed.

Optic neuritis is rare in patients older than age 50 years. Ischemic optic neuropathies, including temporal arteritis, must always be excluded in these older patients. Temporal arteritis occurs in elderly patients and is characterized by headache, scalp pain, polymyalgia rheumatica, jaw claudication, and an increased erythrocyte sedimentation rate. Nonarteritic ischemic optic neuropathy (NAION) should be distinguished from temporal arteritis. NAION generally occurs in middle-aged patients, and classically shows a small cup-disk ratio, sectoral disk pallor, and an altitudinal visual field defect.

Systemic inflammatory diseases such as sarcoidosis and systemic lupus erythematosus may present with optic nerve involvement. Syphilis, Lyme disease, Epstein-Barr virus, and human immunodeficiency virus (HIV) are some of the infectious causes of optic neuritis.

Two eye disorders that can mimic optic neuritis, especially in male patients, are central serous retinopathy and Leber's hereditary optic neuropathy. Central serous retinopathy (CSR) is a relatively benign serous separation of the macula that characteristically occurs in anxious young men. CSR is best diagnosed with a dilated stereoscopic fundus examination by the ophthalmologist, and it can be confirmed by fluorescein angiography. Leber's hereditary optic neuropathy (LHON) is a rare mitochondrial cytopathy that presents initially with unilateral, painless visual loss in young men. A history of visual loss in maternal uncles is highly suggestive. Women are rarely affected. Testing for mitochondrial deoxyribonucleic acid mutations should be considered in any patient with presumed optic neuritis whose vision does not improve.

One of the hallmarks of optic neuritis is recovery of visual acuity, usually by 1 month. This is in contrast to the ischemic optic neuropathies, in which there is typically little if any visual amelioration, and compressive optic neuropathies, in which vision continues to decline, especially upon cessation of steroid treatment.

INVESTIGATIONS

Since optic neuritis is a clinical diagnosis, the physician must distinguish idiopathic optic neuritis from a treatable optic neuropathy. However, laboratory studies are not routinely performed in patients with optic neuritis, unless the presentation is atypical (e.g., bilateral visual loss, visual loss progressing after 1 week, lack of visual recovery after 2 months, marked vitritis). In black patients or those with prominent uveitis, sarcoidosis should be considered, and an angiotensin-converting enzyme study and chest radiograph may be indicated. Syphilis remains the great imitator, and if suspected, both a fluorescent treponemal antibody absorption (FTA-ABS) test and a rapid plasma reagin (RDR) test should be performed. Lyme disease is an uncommon cause of optic neuritis, and we do not routinely order Lyme serology unless the patient comes from an endemic area or has findings such as erythema chronicum migrans. Lumbar punctures and oligoclonal banding may be performed at the discretion of the neurologist.

Magnetic resonance imaging (MRI) is not required to make the diagnosis of optic neuritis. However, MRI of the head is recommended in patients with suspected optic neuritis to assess the risk of future neurologic events of multiple sclerosis (see Treatment section). In half of the patients with optic neuritis, high-signal intensity lesions on T2-weighted images may be seen in the cerebral white matter, especially in the periventricular areas.

Formal perimetry can characterize and document the progression of optic neuritis. On automated perimetry, diffuse visual field loss is the most common pattern of visual loss. Arcuate and altitudinal field defects are also seen. Central scotomas were previously regarded as characterisitic of optic neuritis but were seen in only 8% of patients in the ONTT study. Subtle visual field defects are often noted in the fellow, clinically uninvolved eye.

Contrast sensitivity testing and color vision testing are other helpful adjuncts in the diagnosis and monitoring of patients with optic neuritis. Many neurologists order visual evoked potentials (VEPs) to confirm the clinical impression of optic neuritis. Most ophthalmologists find that the test provides little additional information to a thorough eye examination.

TREATMENT

Consultations with an opthalmologist and a neurologist are invaluable. Antibiotics may greatly benefit cases of infectious optic neuropathy. The early and aggressive use of steroids in patients with systemic inflammatory diseases such as sarcoidosis or systemic lupus erythematosus may avert profound, irreversible visual loss. Proper identification of central serous retinopathy or retinal cone dystrophy averts the potential morbidity of steroid therapy.

The ONTT has established that oral steroids in standard doses (prednisone, 1 mg per kg daily) should not be used *alone,* since they do not improve visual outcome and increase the risk of subsequent optic neuritis in both eyes. The benefit of intravenous steroids in patients with multiple sclerosis who later develop optic neuritis is unknown. However, in patients without prior multiple sclerosis and with new-onset optic neuritis with cerebral white matter plaques on MRI, treatment with high-dose intravenous steroids, followed by oral steroids, reduces the 2-year risk of progression to multiple sclerosis by half. Unfortunately, the 3- and 4-year follow-up results of the ONTT show that this protective benefit subsides. Because the rate of development of multiple sclerosis was so low in patients with optic neuritis and normal MRI scans, the value of steroid treatment in this group is difficult to assess.

The ONTT steroid regimen was 250 mg intravenous methylprednisolone (Solu-Medrol) every 6 hours for 3 days, followed by oral prednisone (Deltasone), 1 mg per kg daily for 11 days. Some practitioners now administer the intravenous methylprednisolone as a single daily dose in the outpatient or home setting. Others consider the oral prednisone taper as optional. It should be understood that patients with optic neuritis who are not treated with steroids have the same long-term *visual* outcome as patients who receive steroid treatments. However, intravenous steroids hasten the time to visual recovery. Immunoglobulin therapy to promote remyelination and potassium channel blocking agents (derived from the plant *Ruta graveolens*) may be of benefit in the future treatment of optic neuritis.

Thirteen percent of patients in the ONTT presenting with optic neuritis had probable or definite multiple sclerosis. Such patients should be considered for subcutaneous interferon-beta-1b (Betaseron) therapy.

PROGNOSIS

In most patients with idiopathic optic neuritis, recovery of visual acuity is almost complete in 30 days. The severity of the initial visual loss is the only predictor of final visual outcome. In the ONTT study, at 12-month follow-up, visual acuity was 20/40 or better in 93% of the patients, better than 20/20 in 69%, and 20/200 or worse in 3%. Even if patients recover 20/20 vision on the Snellen eye chart, they frequently complain of visuospatial disorientation or dimness in the affected eye. These complaints correspond with persistent deficits in motion perception, color vision, and contrast sensitivity. Such visual irregularities may compromise the patient's ability to perform tasks such as driving on foggy days.

At 3- to 5-year follow-up, a repeat episode of optic neuritis occurs in the same or opposite eye in up to a quarter of patients.

Isolated optic neuritis may be regarded as a forme

fruste of multiple sclerosis. The risk of progression to multiple sclerosis is significantly higher in patients with white matter abnormalities on MRI, previous optic neuritis, white race, previous neurologic symptoms, or family history of multiple sclerosis. Children may develop a postviral optic neuritis, which is often bilateral, but rarely develop multiple sclerosis. Patients with neuroretinitis rarely develop multiple sclerosis.

GLAUCOMA

method of
MICHAEL V. DRAKE, M.D.
University of California, San Francisco
San Francisco, California

Glaucoma is a common disease characterized by progressive cavernous optic atrophy and visual loss. It is the third leading cause of blindness in the United States overall and the leading cause of blindness among African Americans. Glaucoma occurs in two relatively distinct forms—chronic open angle glaucoma (85 to 90% of cases in the United States) and acute angle closure glaucoma. Each of these categories is further divided into primary and secondary forms of glaucoma based on etiology. In both types of glaucoma, the overwhelming majority of cases are primary or idiopathic.

Elevated intraocular pressure is the most important risk factor for developing glaucoma, and once glaucoma has developed, intraocular pressure is the leading prognostic indicator. Lowering the intraocular pressure is the central focus of glaucoma therapy. In contrast to the management of systemic hypertension, mildly elevated pressure alone is not necessarily an indication for treatment. The statistically normal intraocular pressure range is between 10 and 20 mmHg.

The decision of when and how to treat glaucoma depends first on the type of glaucoma the patient suffers from. Acute angle closure glaucoma warrants emergency treatment, because glaucomatous visual loss can occur within a few days. Chronic open angle glaucoma progresses more slowly and is treated in a more deliberate fashion.

ACUTE ANGLE CLOSURE GLAUCOMA

In acute angle closure glaucoma, the eye is red and painful. Symptoms generally arise over a period of a few hours as the pressure rises from normal levels to 60 to 80 mmHg or higher. Acute corneal edema causes rapid and profound visual loss. Nausea and vomiting are common and may be so severe that the patient complains more about the gastrointestinal symptoms than the ocular symptoms. There have been anecdotal reports of angle closure glaucoma being misdiagnosed as an acute abdomen. Although acute angle closure glaucoma can be bilateral, it is usually unilateral. Advancing age, farsightedness, and Asian heritage are all risk factors for angle closure glaucoma. In fact, in some Asian populations, the prevalence of angle closure glaucoma exceeds that of open angle glaucoma.

The treatment of choice for angle closure glaucoma is iridotomy, a procedure in which a small hole is created in the peripheral iris to allow for communication of aqueous humor between the anterior and posterior chambers of the eye. Currently, most iridotomies are performed by laser. The most popular is the yttrium, aluminum, garnet (YAG) laser, although other types of laser sources and delivery systems are available.

Medical therapy for angle closure glaucoma is essentially limited to initial emergency room treatment. This therapy is continued only until an iridotomy can be performed. Medical therapy to lower the intraocular pressure in angle closure glaucoma has three goals: to protect the optic nerve from serious permanent damage, to relieve pain, and to reverse pressure-induced corneal edema (which interferes with the ability to perform laser iridotomy). Medical therapy is routinely successful in lowering the intraocular pressure or "breaking" the attack of angle closure glaucoma. Depending on the circumstances, laser iridotomy is usually performed within 1 to 24 hours of the initiation of medical therapy.

Initial medical therapy consists of a combination of topical and oral agents. Therapy is initiated with pilocarpine (Pilocar) 2%, 1 drop to the affected eye every 15 minutes for 1 hour. Pilocarpine is an important drug in this setting because it lowers intraocular pressure and constricts the pupil. Constricting the pupil helps break the pathophysiologic block of aqueous humor flow within the eye and makes subsequent iridotomy easier.

The second topical agent used is a nonselective beta blocker such as timolol maleate (Timoptic) 0.5%, 1 or 2 drops to the affected eye every 30 minutes for 1 hour. The beta-blocker drops are applied roughly 5 minutes after the pilocarpine drops are administered.

At the same time as the initial eye drops are being applied, the patient is given acetazolamide (Diamox) 250 mg orally. The acetazolamide can also be given prior to the initial eye drops, but the initial treatment should be started as rapidly as possible.

The fourth agent used is a hyperosmolar agent, given orally or intravenously. Oral treatment consists of glycerin (Osmoglyn) 50% solution 2 mL per kg. This agent is often chilled or given over crushed ice to make it more palatable. Diabetic patients are given isosorbide (Ismotic) solution 2 mL per kg instead, to minimize treatment-induced hyperglycemia.

The oral agents are quite effective but are generally not given until 10 or 15 minutes after the acetazolamide, because they frequently exacerbate nausea and vomiting. It is preferable to have at least some of the acetazolamide absorbed before the patient vomits. Some patients are too nauseated to tolerate any of the oral agents. If this is the case, mannitol 1 mg per kg is given intravenously. This is given as rapidly as the patient's general health permits—usually at a rate of 500 mL over 15 to 20 minutes.

In addition, topical dorzolamide (Trusopt) 2% is given 1 drop every 30 minutes. Other topical agents have been used as well, but there is no evidence that they outperform the ones listed earlier. Many ophthalmologists use apraclonidine (Iopidine) 0.5 or 1%, 1 drop every 30 minutes for 1 hour. The attack is usually breaking by the time this fifth line of therapy can be instituted, or the patient is being prepared for emergency surgery.

Over the past 10 years, the author has treated dozens of patients with this medical regimen followed by laser iridotomy. In 95% of cases, medical therapy was successful in breaking the attack, and in 95% of those cases, laser iridotomy was successful. All the laser failures occurred in eyes that had secondary angle closure due to inflammatory disease or trauma.

CHRONIC OPEN ANGLE GLAUCOMA

Medical treatment for open angle glaucoma is initiated with one of several topical medications. The specific medication and dosage depend on a complex series of factors such as the patient's general medical condition and the severity of the disease process. Initiating therapy can be difficult for patients for a variety of reasons. As with many chronic diseases, the benefits of treatment are not immediately apparent. Further, because chronic open angle glaucoma causes few if any symptoms until a very advanced state, patients do not feel any different from day to day whether they take their medicines or not. Finally, for many patients, eye drops are more difficult and inconvenient to use than pills. Instillation requires dexterity, and if multiple drops are needed, they must be taken several minutes apart to give full effect. All these factors combine to make compliance a major problem.

Several questions are important when the decision to begin treatment is made. What is the patient's current intraocular pressure, and what is the target pressure? Does the patient have concurrent medical conditions that will prevent her from using certain medications? Does he have a history of drug sensitivity? Does her mental and physical condition allow her to use eye drops successfully?

Because there is no strict normal or abnormal pressure, it is not easy to guarantee a "safe" pressure for each glaucoma patient. Some patients have progressive damage with pressures in the upper teens; others tolerate pressures in the low thirties for decades. A reasonable approach is to establish a target pressure for each patient and then follow the patient at that pressure until there are signs of further progression. If progression occurs, a new, lower target pressure is chosen. Current practice varies widely among experts, but target pressures of roughly 20 to 30% below the presenting pressure, or below an absolute value of 18 to 20 mmHg, are commonplace. In the past, 20 mmHg was the most widely sought target pressure, but recent information has shown that this is not low enough in many cases and is lower than necessary in others. The vigor with which a target pressure is pursued depends largely on the patient's glaucoma. Advanced glaucoma in a young person is treated more aggressively than early glaucoma in an elderly person.

Once the target pressure has been established, there are several primary medications to choose from (Table 1). Primary medications tend to be effective and well tolerated and have a relatively long duration of action. The goal is to lower the intraocular pressure to the target level with an agent that the patient will be able to use on a daily basis indefinitely. The most popular primary drugs are beta-adrenergic blocking agents, such as timolol (Timoptic) or betaxolol (Betoptic). Beta blockers are popular because they lower the intraocular pressure effectively—usually about 25% for patients who present with pressures in the mid-20s. They cause few if any local side effects, and some patients even report that the drops are soothing. Systemic side effects are also uncommon but may be significant enough to force discontinuation. This is especially true for patients with marginally compensated chronic obstructive pulmonary disease or asthma. These patients can have serious exacerbations of their disease soon after beginning beta-blocker eye drops. Rare patients with a remote history of asthma have required emergency room treatment of an acute asthmatic attack within 48 hours of starting beta-blocker drops. Other patients have reported extreme fatigue, to the point that they could not get out of bed for several days after first beginning beta-blocker drops. This occurs most often in elderly patients (ninth or tenth decade). Finally, endurance athletes have reported a diminished capacity to reach or maintain near-maximum heart rate.

Systemic beta-blocker side effects are reportedly more severe and common with nonselective agents such as timolol or levobunolol (Betagan). Betaxolol is a selective beta$_1$ blocker and seems to cause less systemic compromise. In clinical practice, betaxolol is less effective at lowering intraocular pressure as well.

The usual dosage for beta-blocker eye drops is 1 drop in the affected eye once or twice per day. One drop a day in the morning is often successful, but care must be taken to ensure that the intraocular pressure has not risen above the target pressure by the next morning dose. Most patients require twice-daily treatment.

Another primary drug is dipivefrin (Propine). This adrenergic agent is metabolized to epinephrine in the eye. It is an interesting and poorly understood paradox that both beta-blocking agents and adrenergic (sympathomimetic) agents lower the intraocular pressure. Like the beta blockers, dipivefrin lowers the pressure by about 25% in patients whose presenting pressures are in the mid-20s. Studies have shown very slight differences in the pressure-lowering potency of these agents. In contrast to beta blockers, however, dipivefrin causes local side effects

TABLE 1. **Glaucoma Medications**

Drug	Strength	Dosage
Primary Agents		
Beta-adrenergic antagonists		
Nonselective		
Timolol maleate (Timoptic)	0.25%, 0.5%	qd, bid
Levobunolol hydrochloride (Betagan)	0.25%, 0.5%	qd, bid
Metipranolol (OptiPranolol)	0.3%	qd, bid
Carteolol hydrochloride (Ocupress)	1%	qd, bid
Selective		
Betaxolol hydrochloride (Betoptic)	0.25%, 0.5%	qd, bid
Adrenergic agents		
Epinephrine hydrochloride (Epifrin)	0.1%, 0.5%, 1%, 2%	qd, bid
(Glaucon)	1%, 2%	qd, bid
Epinephryl borate (Epinal)	0.5%, 1%, 2%	qd, bid
(Eppy/N)	1%, 2%	qd, bid
Epinephrine bitartrate (Epitrate)	2%	qd, bid
Dipivefrin (Propine)	0.1%	qd, bid
Cholinergic agents		
Pilocarpine hydrochloride (Isopto Carpine)	0.25% to 10%	bid to qid
(Pilocar)	2.5%, 1%, 2%, 3%, 4%, 6%	bid to qid
(Other generic)	0.5%, 1%, 2%, 3%, 4%, 6%	bid to qid
(Pilopine HS gel)	4%	qd at bedtime
(Ocusert Pilo)	20 or 40 µg/h	Weekly
Pilocarpine nitrate (Pilagan)	1%, 2%, 4%	bid to qid
Secondary Agents		
Alpha-adrenergic agonist		
Apraclonidine (Iopidine)	0.5%, 1%	s/p laser Rx, tid
Carbonic anhydrase inhibitors (topical)	2%	tid
Dorzolamide (Trusopt)		
Parasympathomimetic (mitotic)		

with significant frequency. Perhaps as many as 25% of patients treated chronically with dipivefrin must discontinue treatment due to local inflammation and irritation. Systemic side effects are rare. Dipivefrin, 1 drop, is administered twice daily to the affected eye.

The third first-line drug is pilocarpine. Pilocarpine has been in continuous use for glaucoma treatment for nearly 125 years. It was the first-line drug of choice for over a century before falling to the popularity of beta blockers in the 1980s. Pilocarpine was popular because it causes a significant drop in intraocular pressure (again, about 25% for patients with pressures in the mid-20s), with very few systemic side effects. Unfortunately, pilocarpine causes significant and prolonged miosis and accommodative spasm. These combine to dim vision in elderly patients, particularly those with some degree of cataract, and to cause an unstable myopic shift in younger (under age 50) patients. The accommodative ciliary spasm can be associated with a prolonged headache or brow ache. Pilocarpine's pressure-lowering effect lasts only about 6 hours, so it is usually taken four times a day. For these reasons, pilocarpine is not tolerated as well as beta blockers or adrenergics in most patients. It is used as a first-line drug only when there is some reason not to use a beta blocker or an adrenergic agent.

Pilocarpine is supplied in wide variety of concentrations, from 0.5 to 10%, but its use in glaucoma is usually limited to concentrations of 1 to 4%. The lower concentration works well for initial therapy or for prolonged therapy in some patients with lightly pigmented irides. Higher concentrations are needed for patients with heavily pigmented irides, because significant pigment binding occurs with topical pilocarpine.

Although pilocarpine often causes local side effects, most patients tolerate the medication well. It has the advantages of being the least expensive antiglaucoma medication and one of the most stable. It can be carried in a pocket or purse for months without losing potency.

Many glaucoma patients are treated successfully with single agents, but many others require multiple agents. The Ocular Hypertension Treatment Study, sponsored by the National Eye Institute, has provided a formula for determining when to use combinations of primary drugs and when to move on to second-line therapy (Figure 1). In that study, the target pressure was defined as 20% below the baseline pressure. If a patient meets the target pressure on a single medication, therapy is continued with that medication alone. If the pressure reduction does not reach the target pressure but achieves more than 50% of the desired reduction, a second medication is added to the first. If the initial agent yields a pressure reduction of less than half the desired goal, it is discontinued and an alternative drug is started. For example, if the target pressure is 20% below baseline and the first medication yields a drop that is less than 20% but more than 10% below baseline, a second agent is added. If the initial agent gives a drop of less than 10%, it is stopped and therapy is started with a new agent alone. This stepped approach to

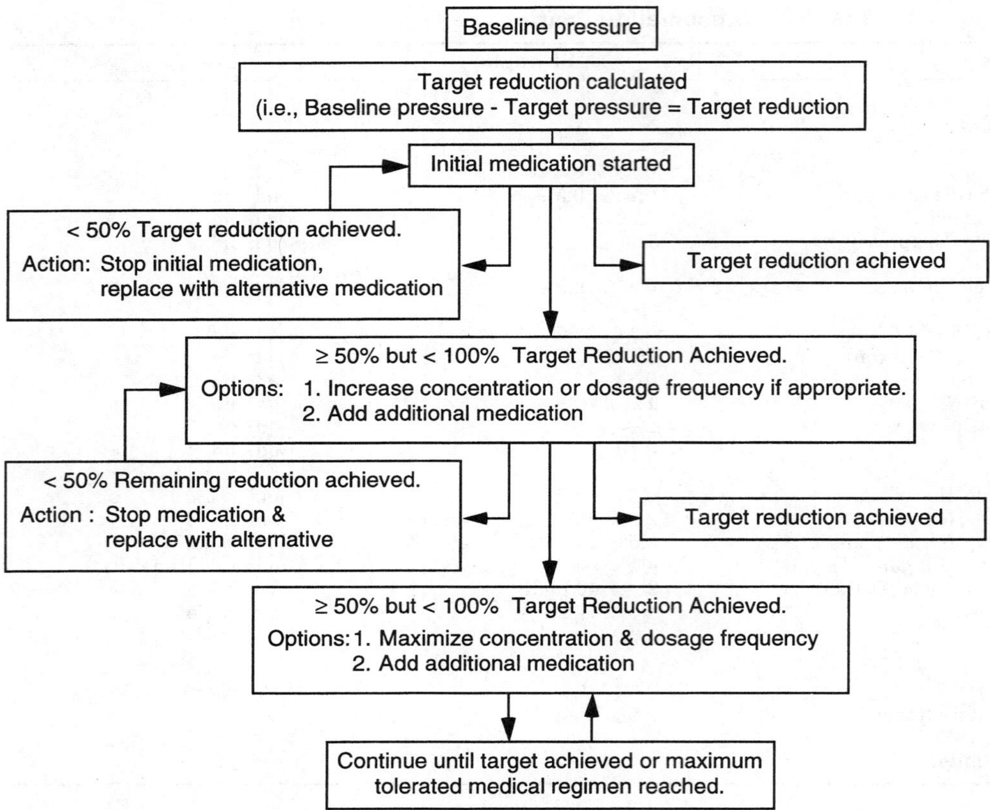

Figure 1. Treatment of glaucoma, using combinations of primary drugs or second-line drugs.

adding or substituting medication simplifies instructions to patients and provides a more rational approach to choosing medication regimens for patients.

When one first-line drug has failed to provide a reduction of at least 50% of the goal, a different first-line drug is tried. Similarly, a second first-line drug is added when single-agent therapy is only partially successful. The same guidelines are used when evaluating the efficacy of multiple-drug therapy.

Secondary drugs are used when first-line drugs fail. Secondary drugs differ from first-line drugs in a variety of subtle ways. Some tend to be less well tolerated or to have a shorter duration of action. Others are considered second-line drugs simply because they are so new that the larger community has not yet gained widespread clinical experience with them. Current second-line agents of choice include apraclonidine 0.5% (Iopidine) and dorzolamide 2% (Trusopt). Both of these are taken three times daily.

If a combination of first- and second-line drugs fails to achieve satisfactory pressure reduction or does so at the expense of intolerable side effects, tertiary agents or laser or surgical intervention should be considered. Tertiary agents include acetazolamide (Diamox) or methazolamide (Neptazane) pills and phospholine iodide or carbachol drops. Tertiary agents are very effective in lowering intraocular pressure, but local and systemic side effects limit their use.

Argon laser trabeculoplasty is a straightforward and easily tolerated procedure that lowers intraocular pressure approximately the same amount as many of the first-line agents. It is used when topical medications are ineffective or poorly tolerated. Argon laser therapy may be used in conjunction with or instead of any of the previously mentioned drugs or combinations of drugs. In practice, this means that some patients have argon laser trabeculoplasty and subsequently take no topical or systemic medicines. Others may have argon laser trabeculoplasty performed and still must take three topical medications plus an oral carbonic anhydrase inhibitor.

Surgical therapy is offered when the patient's glaucoma cannot be controlled effectively by nonsurgical means. The most frequently performed operation today, trabeculectomy, has a success rate of approximately 80%, depending on patient risk factors and the specific definition of success employed. As with other glaucoma treatments, surgical therapy is offered at different points in the therapeutic cascade, depending on a complex array of patient factors. In some cases, surgery is offered very early—even before medications. This is particularly true in Great Britain and Western Europe. In other cases, surgery is offered only after progressive visual loss has been demonstrated in patients who have been offered the full range of medication and laser therapy.

Using a combination of medications, laser, and conventional surgery, the vast majority of glaucoma patients can achieve satisfactory pressure reduction. The importance of simplifying the treatment regimen for a given patient and helping patients to achieve compliance is obvious.

ACUTE PERIPHERAL FACIAL PARALYSIS
(Bell's Palsy)

method of
EBERHARD STENNERT, M.D., and
CHRISTIAN SITTEL, M.D.

University of Cologne
Cologne, Germany

Paralysis of the facial nerve is the most frequent of all peripheral nerve lesions. In the vast majority of cases, the etiology remains unknown and is labeled idiopathic (Bell's palsy). Insufficient treatment may result in severe stigmatization of the patient.

Bell's palsy is a disease of sudden onset occurring in all age groups, regardless of race and sex. It appears as a partial or complete paresis of one or, rarely, both sides. Usually, there is only one occurrence in a lifetime, although the possibility of recurrence cannot be ruled out. Diagnosis is made by excluding traumatic injuries, tumors, and inflammation of the surrounding tissue.

CLINICAL COURSE

In typical cases, the paralysis appears suddenly. The full extent of paralysis is normally reached within 1 to 3 days, and the degree varies from slight to complete. There is usually no change in the patient's general condition. There is often a mixed lesion, with simultaneous manifestation of blocked and denervated fibers. The involvement of different fiber types may also vary, since motor, sensory, and secretory neurites react in distinct ways to hypoxia and compression. Additional symptoms may be a positive Schirmer's test, hyperacusis, and taste disorder. The severity of pain in the ear region does not necessarily correlate with the clinical course of the paresis.

The length of time that the paresis lasts and its final outcome are solely dependent on the extent of morphologic damage. In counseling patients as to the expected recovery time, one can assume as a general rule that the fibers suffering from neurapraxia will need 3 to 6 weeks, whereas denervated axons will need 3 to 6 months for regeneration. If a patient shows no or insufficient functional recovery within 6 months, the diagnosis of Bell's palsy must be questioned and a second, more thorough work-up, including neurologic and serologic testing and imaging of the complete course of the facial nerve (by ultrasound and magnetic resonance imaging [MRI] or computed tomography [CT]), is mandatory. If the results are still negative, careful monitoring of the whole mimetic musculature by needle electromyelography should be continued for about 4 months. If no reinnervation potentials are detectable, a surgical exposure of the whole nerve should be performed. If there is no pathologic finding, decisions about procedures such as hypoglossal-facial nerve anastomosis and dynamic muscle transposition must be made on an individual basis.

PROGNOSIS

Although a complete recovery rate of about 80% is widely accepted, a critical analysis of the literature demonstrates that the average rate of complete clinical recovery in patients who seek treatment is actually only 60%.

LATE SEQUELAE

Patients may experience residual paresis, synkinesia, contractures, disturbances of tear secretion, dysacusis, dysgeusia, and pain. The extent of such sequelae can vary widely, and the possibility of a complete lack of functional recovery cannot be ruled out. The majority of these secondary defects are due to false sprouting of regenerating axons. Their development can be neither influenced nor avoided once the endoneural tubes, and especially the perineurium, are disturbed, resulting in heteromorphous reneurotization.

PATHOPHYSIOLOGY

Although it has been suggested that Bell's palsy is caused by various factors, the damaging action always affects the connective tissue of the nerve and its supplying vessels. Damage to the neurites develops as a consequence of hypoxia and, to a lesser extent, compression. Figure 1 shows a simplified model of the pathophysiology of Bell's palsy. It represents a vicious circle as an organism's main pattern of reaction. This circle can never be interrupted surgically, but only by drug therapy.

There is also a hypothesis that Bell's palsy may represent an autoimmune disease related to entities such as acute polyneuritis or mononeuritis multiplex. Acute viral infections are suspected of playing a key role as a precondition for immunopathologic phenomena. Escalating inflammation leads to edema of the nerve, followed by ischemia due to compression. Effective therapy must counteract both these mechanisms.

THERAPY

Therapeutic Nihilism

Neurologists and internists tend not to treat Bell's palsy at all, arguing that there is a complete recovery in almost all cases. This attitude should be rejected vigorously. Defective healing can be expected in 40% of cases. Although not a life-threatening condition, Bell's palsy may lead to a lifelong stigma that cannot be concealed.

Surgical Decompression

Decompression of the facial nerve was in wide use for decades, with the idea of interrupting the vicious circle by mechanical pressure relief. Later, the importance of the "bottleneck" at the transition of the fundus of the internal auditory channel to the facial nerve's labyrinthine segment was stressed. The arguments against any kind of decompression procedure are as follows:

1. Surgery is not indicated for an inflammatory tissue reaction. Compared with metabolic changes within the nerve, suspected mechanical pressure in the bony channel is of minor relevance.

2. There is broad consensus that Bell's palsy is an emergency. Surgical intervention is risky and time-consuming, making a delay more likely.

3. Decompression via a middle fossa approach requires great skill and experience, and there is a risk of causing additional damage to the nerve. This is

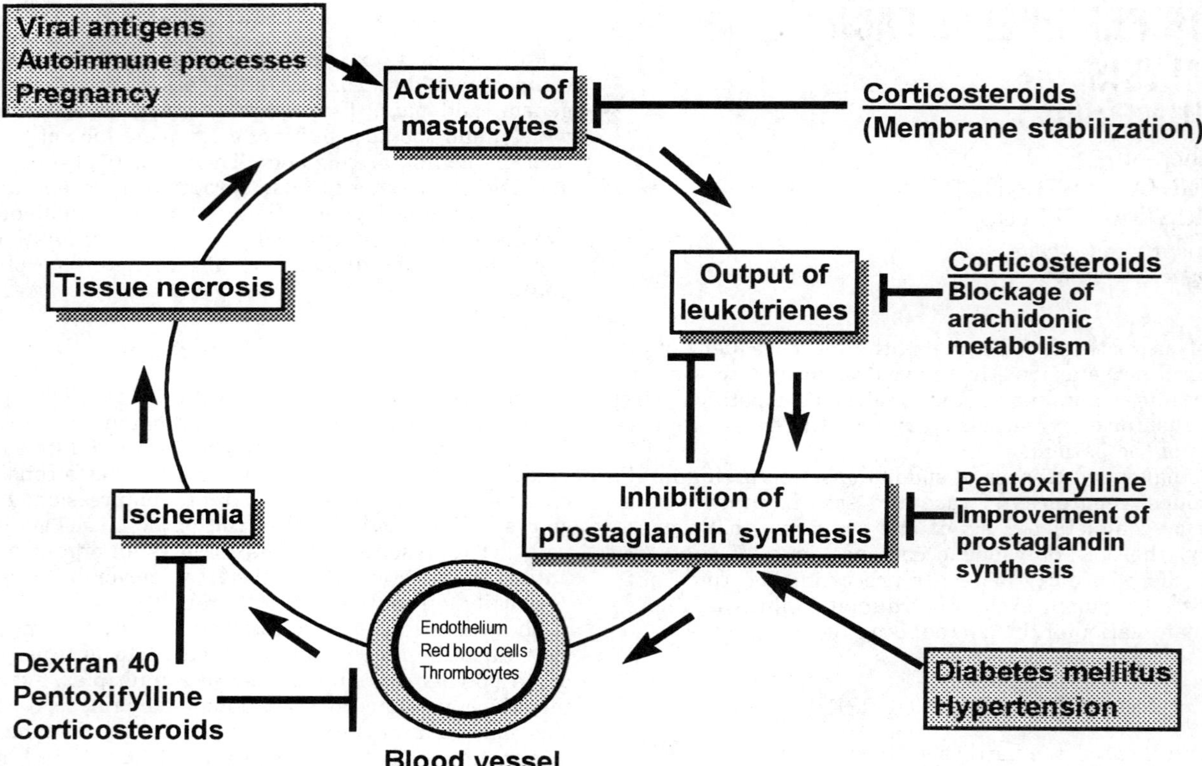

Figure 1. Bell's palsy—vicious circle and therapy rationale.

especially true for the critical bottleneck, where the nerve is covered by only a thin epineural sheath and is in close contact with the surrounding bone.

4. Because of the risks, pitfalls, and technical difficulties of the middle fossa approach, surgeons and patients tend to watch and wait. However, only early therapy can be successful.

5. Few surgeons are capable of performing such an operation. Taking into account the high incidence of Bell's palsy, it is clear that this therapy would not be available in all places, not even in industrialized Western countries.

Drug Therapy

Nonsteroidal Anti-inflammatory Drugs (NSAIDs; e.g., diclofenac [Voltaren], flufenamic acid,* ibuprofen). Synthesis of inflammation- and pain-mediating prostaglandin E_2 is blocked. To compensate, the production of other mediators of inflammation, such as leukotrienes, increases. In contrast, glucocorticoids block the arachidonic acid metabolism, affecting the production of all mediators of inflammation. Clinically, the anti-inflammatory potential of NSAIDs is inferior to that of glucocorticoids. As a consequence, single therapy with an NSAID is not acceptable.

Vitamin B Group. From the available data, there

---

*Not available in the United States.

is no evidence of any therapeutic value of these substances.

Acyclovir (Zovirax). This drug is active primarily against herpesvirus infection, acting as a competitive substrate for viral DNA polymerase. There is a growing conviction that herpesviruses play an important role in Bell's palsy etiology. Although there are no clinical studies documenting efficacy, clinical use of acyclovir in an early stage is justified.

Glucocorticoids. The debate about the efficacy of glucocorticoids for the treatment of Bell's palsy has been going on for a while. The world literature contains strong support for the use of cortisone, although a definitive study proving the statistical value of steroids has not yet been done. The question is not if but how steroids should be administered. The popular dosage of 40 to 80 mg of oral prednisone seems to be insufficient.

Anti-Inflammatory Rheologic Infusion Therapy. Steroids are the most potent anti-inflammatory agents. Additionally, microcirculation must be optimized to fight vascular ischemia. Based on these considerations, an infusion therapy was designed (Table 1); it has been in use since 1979, with convincing success. The following factors should be regarded as contraindications: left heart failure, renal insufficiency, recent history of peptic ulcer, bacterial infections, and coagulation defects. In pregnant patients, the attending gynecologist should be consulted, although objections are unlikely.

Compared with surgical decompression, this ther-

TABLE 1. **Anti-Inflammatory Rheologic Therapy Following Stennert**

Day of Treatment	Dextran 40/10% (mL/day IV)*	Pentoxifylline (mL/day IV)*†	Prednisolone (mg/day IV)*	Add
1	2 × 500/16 h	15	250	
2	2 × 500/16 h	15	250	
3	2 × 500/16 h	15	150	**1. Potassium**
4	500/8 h	15	150	
5	500/8 h	15	100	
6	500/8 h	15	100	
7	500/8 h	15	75	
8	500/8 h	15	50	**2. Fluid** IV or
9	500/8 h	15	PO: 40	PO (about
10	500/8 h	15	20	1000 mL/day)
11		May be prolonged with	15	
12		PO medication for	12.5	
13		another week	10	
14			7.5	
15			5	
16			2.5	
17			2.5	
18			2.5	

*All three drugs are administered simultaneously as a mixture.

†Not available for IV infusion in some countries. In this case, pentoxifylline can be administered orally in a dose of 400 mg tid.

apy has the great advantage of being applicable anywhere and anytime. The sooner the therapy is begun, the less the risk of morphologic damage to the nerve fibers. There are no negative consequences if it turns out that the facial paralysis is not Bell's palsy (except for acute intracranial hemorrhage with traumatic facial paralysis). Additional testing to rule out other diagnoses can take place while the therapy is under way.

Physical Therapy

Electrical stimulation for peripheral nerve lesions must be used with caution. It can lead to irreversible facial contractures in a higher percentage of patients and greater severity. However, facial exercises, combined with massage, may be helpful following the acute phase. Generally, more severe, prolonged cases benefit from such therapy.

PARKINSON'S DISEASE

method of
RONALD F. PFEIFFER, M.D.
University of Tennessee, Memphis
Memphis, Tennessee

BACKGROUND

The astounding advances that have taken place in medicine during the past century, with the consequent increase in life expectancy, have dramatically changed the complexion of medical practice. Care for elderly people and treatment of disease processes primarily affecting them are assuming ever-greater importance. The neurodegenerative diseases, such as Parkinson's disease, loom as increasingly important challenges for physicians and other health care professionals.

Parkinson's disease is a common neurodegenerative process that carries a prevalence in the general population of approximately 100 per 100,000. If, however, attention is directed to those individuals over the age of 65 years, a strikingly different picture emerges: a prevalence of 1000 to 2000 per 100,000. Some epidemiologic studies have suggested a slight male preponderance and some, but not all, suggest that Parkinson's disease may occur more frequently in white compared with black populations.

Despite exhaustive attention and study, the etiology of Parkinson's disease remains a mystery. Some investigators favor a genetic origin, and ever-increasing numbers of kindreds with familial parkinsonism have been reported. These kindreds usually display an autosomal dominant inheritance pattern, but atypical clinical and pathologic features are also usually evident. Other investigators have focused on potential neurotoxic explanations for Parkinson's disease. Both externally encountered and internally generated toxic mechanisms have been proposed. Indeed, cerebrospinal fluid from individuals with Parkinson's disease has been reported to be toxic to cultured dopaminergic neurons. Although the specific toxic factor has not been identified, these findings bolster the idea of a neurotoxic mechanism for Parkinson's disease. The possibility that a toxic substance, whether endogenously generated or exogenously encountered, might produce neuronal damage via oxidative stress mechanisms through free radical formation has received extensive scrutiny but remains speculative. It is also possible that both genetic and neurotoxic mechanisms are important in Parkinson's disease and that genetic susceptibility must be combined with toxin exposure for the disease to become clinically evident.

Parkinson's disease is characterized pathologically by progressive destruction of dopaminergic neurons. The dopaminergic neurons that originate in the substantia nigra and send their axons to the caudate and putamen, forming the striatonigral tract, are most prominently involved in Parkinson's disease, but other dopaminergic pathways are also affected. Moreover, the neurochemical changes as a consequence of neuronal loss are not limited to dopamine depletion, and other neurotransmitters are also altered in Parkinson's disease. This may explain why not all clinical features of Parkinson's disease respond equally well to our current therapy, which is primarily directed at compensating for the dopamine deficiency. A characteristic microscopic pathologic feature of Parkinson's disease is the development of Lewy bodies in surviving dopaminergic neurons. Lewy bodies are a cytoplasmic inclusion consisting of neurofilament-derived material; their significance is unknown, but it has been suggested that they may reflect a process in which damage to neurofilaments results in impaired cellular transport mechanisms and, ultimately, cell death.

CLINICAL FEATURES

Parkinson's disease is characterized by a tetrad of cardinal features: tremor, rigidity, bradykinesia, and postural abnormalities. A rather wide variety of additional secondary features may also be present. Individuals with Parkinson's disease need not display all four cardinal features, and the number of secondary features present in any individual varies widely.

Tremor is the most frequent presenting, or initial, clinical feature noted by the individual with Parkinson's disease. It is the initial feature in approximately 70% of patients. The tremor classically is present when the involved portion of the body is at rest, and it disappears with movement. The tremor most frequently first appears in one arm, subsequently spreading into the leg on the same side and later to the contralateral limbs. The jaw may also be involved. Some individuals with Parkinson's disease will also display a postural tremor when a position is maintained against gravity, but this type of tremor more typically is seen in essential tremor. Head bobbing, or titubation, actually represents a postural tremor of cervical muscles as they hold the head erect and is generally not seen in Parkinson's disease. Its presence should suggest a diagnosis of essential tremor. The resting tremor of Parkinson's disease is accentuated by stress; it disappears during sleep.

Rigidity is ultimately the most common clinical feature of Parkinson's disease, eventually developing in virtually everyone with the illness. It is characterized by a persistent resistance to passive joint movement. A cogwheeling, or ratchety, quality to the rigidity may be present, but is not invariably demonstrable and is not essential for diagnosis. The rigidity may be mistaken for arthritis or bursitis, especially if some pain is also present, as may occur in Parkinson's disease. In the office examination of the individual with Parkinson's disease, mild rigidity can be accentuated by reinforcement maneuvers, such as having the patient open and close the opposite hand or tap the opposite foot while testing the ipsilateral limb.

Bradykinesia is the quintessential symptom of Parkinson's disease. It entails not only slowness of movement, as implied by the name, but also impaired ability to initiate or modify movement and to perform repetitive or simultaneous motor tasks. There may also be difficulty in terminating motor actions, leading to the phenomena of propulsion and festination. These difficulties have been attributed to an inability to carry out ingrained "motor programs" correctly and efficiently—actions that are performed so routinely that it is not necessary to employ conscious thought processes in implementing the movement. Bradykinesia seems to entail difficulty integrating both motor and mental plans. Although bradykinesia is a very complex phenomenon neurophysiologically, patients in the office often simply interpret bradykinesia as weakness, even though actual weakness is not present.

Postural abnormalities are, perhaps, the least specific of the cardinal features of Parkinson's disease and tend to develop only later in the course of the illness. Difficulty maintaining postural fixation and impairment of righting reflexes both develop. Falling is a dangerous consequence of the righting reflex impairment and is especially prone to occur when the individual with Parkinson's disease is turning or when unexpectedly bumped.

A rather extensive array of secondary signs may also occur in Parkinson's disease. Handwriting may become smaller in size. Facial expression is diminished, with a staring or masklike quality produced by a combination of diminished facial muscle mobility and decreased blink rate. The voice becomes soft and dysarthric. Walking often becomes characterized by small, shuffling steps with reduced armswing, which is typically asymmetric, at least initially. A variety of symptoms indicative of autonomic dysfunction may develop, including abnormalities of perspiration, orthostatic hypotension, urinary difficulties, and impotence. Gastrointestinal dysfunction, which may include problems such as dysphagia, excessive saliva due to diminished swallowing frequency, impaired gastric emptying, and constipation as a result of both slowed colon transit and defecatory dysfunction, is surprisingly common in Parkinson's disease. Difficulty with vision, especially reading, is frequent, as is microsomia. Mental status changes are also common in Parkinson's disease: depression is seen in approximately 40% of individuals, sometimes even antedating motor symptoms, while cognitive impairment is more typically seen in the advanced stages of the disease.

Parkinson's disease is a slowly progressive neurodegenerative process, and the various clinical features reflect this as they gradually progress and accumulate with the passage of time. Therapy may ameliorate symptoms for a time but cannot prevent their ultimate appearance and progression.

DIFFERENTIAL DIAGNOSIS

The diagnosis of Parkinson's disease can be a challenging exercise since no specific diagnostic test is available. A number of other conditions may display parkinsonian features and, therefore, be confused with Parkinson's disease.

A rather extensive variety of medications may produce parkinsonism, including virtually all antipsychotic drugs, various antiemetic medications (especially metoclopramide [Reglan]), calcium channel blockers, certain antidepressant medications (amoxapine [Asendin], trazodone [Desyrel], Triavil), several older antihypertensive drugs (reserpine, methyldopa [Aldomet]), and still others.

Several toxins, such as carbon disulfide, cyanide, carbon monoxide, manganese, and methanol, may produce parkinsonism along with other neurologic features. Metabolic disorders, such as hypothyroidism, parathyroid dysfunction, and Wilson's disease, may also display parkinsonism as part of their clinical picture. Viral infections of the central nervous system (CNS) may rarely produce parkinsonism. Multiple lacunar infarctions, repeated head trauma, and normal pressure hydrocephalus may also feature parkinsonism or pseudoparkinsonism as part of their clinical picture.

Perhaps the most difficult conditions to separate from Parkinson's disease, however, are the group of neurodegenerative processes in which parkinsonism, usually without tremor, develops but is eventually accompanied by other distinguishing signs. In progressive supranuclear palsy, paresis of vertical and, later, horizontal gaze develops. The term "multiple system atrophy" (MSA) is now commonly used to encompass a trio of previously described conditions: Shy-Drager syndrome, olivopontocerebellar atrophy (OPCA), and striatonigral degeneration. In the Shy-Drager syndrome variant of MSA, progressive autonomic failure accompanies akinetic-rigid parkinsonism, whereas in OPCA cerebellar dysfunction is the distinguishing feature. The striatonigral degeneration variant of MSA has no clearly distinguishing clinical feature from Parkinson's disease, except for its lack of responsiveness to levodopa, an attribute shared by the other variants as well.

One other entity that is important to differentiate from Parkinson's disease is essential, or familial, tremor. This condition is characterized by a postural, rather than resting, tremor that most commonly involves the arms but may also involve the cervical muscles, producing head bobbing, or titubation. Vocal tremor may also occur. Other features of Parkinson's disease do not develop, and treatment is with either propranolol (Inderal) or primidone (Mysoline) rather than antiparkinson medications.

PHARMACOTHERAPY

The pharmacologic management of Parkinson's disease may be divided into two approaches: protective therapy and symptomatic therapy. The latter approach is firmly grounded and widely accepted, while the former approach remains a source of controversy.

Protective Therapy

The term "protective therapy" refers to the idea that the actual progressive neurodegenerative process that constitutes Parkinson's disease might be slowed, if not halted altogether, by pharmacologic therapy. This idea currently revolves largely around the hypothesis that free radical formation is responsible for or potentiates dopaminergic neuronal damage and that inhibition of free radical formation would, then, slow or halt the destructive process.

Considerable evidence has accumulated that free radicals play a role in the development and progression of Parkinson's disease. Free radicals are atoms or molecules with an unpaired electron. As such, they are highly reactive and capable of damaging cell membranes by seizing electrons from other molecules with which they come into contact, producing lipid peroxidation. To protect against free radical–induced damage, a number of protective mechanisms have evolved. Thus, protective enzymes, such as superoxide dismutase, catalase, and glutathione peroxidase, and free radical scavengers, such as vitamins E and C, may inhibit free radical formation and serve as a "damage control" system. There is increasing evidence that Parkinson's disease is characterized both by increased free radical production and a reduction in protective mechanisms.

Selegiline

Selegiline (Eldepryl) is a monoamine oxidase (MAO) inhibitor that at low doses selectively inhibits MAO Type B (MAO-B). Although originally introduced as a symptomatic therapy agent (see later), selegiline has received most attention for its possible neuroprotective effects. Multiple studies have demonstrated that with selegiline it is possible to delay the introduction of levodopa therapy, but the issue of whether or not this is because of actual neuroprotection has been clouded by symptomatic benefits that occur when selegiline is introduced. Although it has been assumed that any neuroprotective effects of selegiline occur via inhibition of MAO-B, there have been suggestions based upon basic laboratory work that such effects might actually occur via other mechanisms.

Selegiline is typically utilized at a dosage of 5 mg twice daily and at this dosage demonstrates selective MAO-B inhibition. In fact, selegiline doses of only 5 mg daily inhibit 90% to 100% of platelet MAO-B and so may be adequate, although they have not been systematically studied. At daily dosages of 30 mg or higher, selegiline begins to lose its specificity for MAO-B and also begins to inhibit MAO-A. Moreover, doses higher than 10 mg daily have not been shown to provide any additional symptomatic benefit and have not been evaluated with regard to neuroprotective effects.

When used by itself as possible neuroprotective therapy, selegiline is generally well tolerated. However, some individuals experience insomnia, and some describe a "buzz" with selegiline, similar to the effect of too much caffeine. These effects may be a consequence of selegiline's metabolism to amphetamine-related metabolites.

Drug interactions are a potential problem with selegiline, and life-threatening complications have been reported when selegiline and meperidine have been given concomitantly. Dextromethorphan, a common ingredient in many cough syrups, may provoke a similar reaction. A "central serotonergic syndrome" has been described when selegiline and the selective serotonin reuptake inhibitor fluoxetine (Prozac) have been administered together. This has led to a manufacturer's warning against coadministration of fluoxetine and similar drugs (sertraline [Zoloft], paroxetine [Paxil]) with selegiline. Use of tricyclic antidepressant medications in conjunction with selegiline has also been discouraged. However, these recommendations are somewhat controversial, and some investigators suggest that cautious coadministration of these medications with selegiline is acceptable.

It has recently been reported that individuals with Parkinson's disease receiving selegiline for its potential neuroprotective effects have a higher mortality after 5 years of administration. The significance and reproducibility of this observation are currently unclear. These investigators also reported that the combination of levodopa and selegiline did not improve functional outcome at 5 years compared with treatment with levodopa alone. The British investigators who reported these findings have advocated discontinuing selegiline, but other investigators feel this recommendation may be premature.

Vitamins E and C

Because they are free radical scavengers, both vitamin E and vitamin C have been proposed as potential neuroprotective agents in Parkinson's disease. It has been suggested that early-life consumption of foods with high vitamin E content may provide protection against the development of Parkinson's disease. However, in a large double-blind, placebo-controlled study (the DATATOP trial), vitamin E in a daily dosage of 2000 IU provided no neuroprotection. Vitamin C has not been adequately studied. Therefore, currently no role for either vitamin E or vitamin C in the treatment of Parkinson's disease has yet been identified.

Symptomatic Therapy

Anticholinergic Drugs

The anticholinergic drugs have long been used in the treatment of Parkinson's disease and for many years were the only effective therapy available. As newer agents have been developed, however, the use and usefulness of the anticholinergic drugs has waned. The two most frequently employed anticholinergic antiparkinson drugs are trihexyphenidyl (Artane) and benztropine (Cogentin). A third agent, ethopropazine (Parsidol), is no longer available in the United States.

The reason for the diminishing use of anticholinergic drugs in the treatment of Parkinson's disease is twofold. These medications are modestly effective at best, providing some reduction in tremor and, perhaps, in rigidity but no improvement in bradykinesia or postural instability. Moreover, elderly individuals, in particular, are very sensitive to these medications, and both peripheral and central anticholinergic toxic effects are prone to develop. Peripheral adverse effects include blurred vision, dry mouth, anhidrosis, constipation, and urinary retention; central toxicity may include impaired memory, confusion, and even psychosis.

Anticholinergic agents may be used advantageously in the younger individual who presents with tremor as the principal Parkinson's disease symptom, but they should probably be avoided in individuals above age 65 years. There is no real rationale for anticholinergic administration in persons who do not have tremor, whatever their age.

Amantadine

Amantadine (Symmetrel) is another "veteran" antiparkinson medication that was initially introduced and still is utilized as an antiviral agent. Its mechanism of action in Parkinson's disease remains enigmatic.

Amantadine is, like the anticholinergic drugs, capable of diminishing tremor but also able to reduce rigidity and improve bradykinesia. Its beneficial effects, however, are usually modest. Amantadine has the somewhat peculiar tendency to display waning or even vanishing effectiveness rather quickly following its introduction, sometimes within weeks. The reason for this rapid tachyphylaxis is uncertain. In some individuals, however, this loss of benefit does not develop and prolonged benefit is experienced. In those in whom amantadine efficacy wanes, the medication can sometimes be discontinued and later "recycled" with renewed efficacy.

Amantadine is generally very well tolerated. It is not, however, without potential toxicity that may include pedal edema, nightmares, confusion, and livedo reticularis, a purplish, mottled skin discoloration that may be frightening to the patient but is a benign process. It is not necessary to discontinue amantadine because of livedo reticularis.

Amantadine dosage is straightforward—200 to 300 mg daily is utilized. Titration is not necessary in most instances, and dosages above 300 mg daily provide no additional benefit. Although appealing because of its safety and ease of use, the role of amantadine in the treatment of Parkinson's disease is somewhat limited. It can be used as a first-line agent in individuals with mild Parkinson's disease; there is also an occasional patient who shows a clinically useful response when amantadine is added to levodopa as adjunctive therapy for more advanced parkinsonism.

Levodopa

Since its successful introduction into clinical use in the late 1960s, levodopa has become firmly ensconced as the single most effective therapeutic agent for Parkinson's disease. Once it was identified in the late 1950s that Parkinson's disease is characterized by striatal dopamine deficiency, dopamine replacement therapy became a logical therapeutic goal. However, dopamine itself cannot cross the blood-brain barrier and, therefore, cannot replenish depleted striatal dopamine. Levodopa, the immediate precursor of dopamine, is transported across the blood-brain barrier by the large neutral amino acid carrier system and, thus, can serve as a source for dopamine replacement in the brain.

It was recognized quite rapidly that when given by itself the bulk of administered levodopa was rapidly converted into dopamine by the ubiquitous enzyme dopa decarboxylase before it ever was able to cross the blood-brain barrier and gain access to the CNS. This had two consequences: massive doses of levodopa were necessary to achieve effective elevations of CNS dopamine concentrations while adverse effects due to peripheral dopamine formation—such as nausea, orthostatic hypotension, cardiac arrhythmia, and glaucoma—were distressingly common.

This quite rapidly prompted the development of drugs capable of inhibiting dopa decarboxylase but incapable of crossing the blood-brain barrier, thus allowing much more efficient and safer delivery of dopamine to the intended striatal sites. Several such peripheral decarboxylase inhibitors were developed in the 1970s but only carbidopa, combined with levodopa and marketed as Sinemet, has ever been approved for use in the United States. With the carbidopa/levodopa (CD/LD) combination, levodopa dosages of several hundred milligrams instead of several thousand milligrams daily can be employed. Sinemet has recently become available in generic form.

A more recent innovation with CD/LD has been the introduction of a controlled-release preparation, Sinemet CR. This preparation, because of its slow dissolution, allows for less frequent administration, although not a once-daily regimen. Sinemet CR can be effective in dealing with mild end-of-dose wearing off of levodopa efficacy (discussed later). It has also been proposed that using Sinemet CR right from the very beginning when levodopa becomes necessary may delay the appearance of motor fluctuations such as wearing off because of the more constant, and presumably more physiologic, dopamine receptor stimulation a controlled-release preparation allows. This theory is currently being tested in a large clinical trial.

The appropriate CD/LD dosage for initiation of therapy may vary with the age and frailty of the individual. An ideal starting dosage is CD/LD 25/100, one tablet three times daily. This dosage provides 75 mg of carbidopa, which comes close to delivering the 75 to 100/mg of carbidopa daily that is necessary to block effectively the peripheral conversion of levodopa to dopamine. Therefore, an individual is less likely to experience nausea when CD/LD 25/100 is utilized to initiate therapy than if CD/LD 10/100 were employed. After a person has been taking CD/LD for a number of months, the proclivity of levodopa to produce nausea diminishes in most persons, and it is possible to switch to CD/LD 10/100 to take advantage of its cheaper cost. If one chooses to initiate therapy with Sinemet CR 50/200, an initial dosage of one half or one tablet twice daily is typically employed. In elderly or otherwise especially sensitive patients, it may be preferable to initiate therapy with lower CD/LD dosage. Occasionally it is necessary to begin with the subtherapeutic dosage of one half tablet daily and slowly build dosage from there.

There is often considerable confusion among patients (and perhaps also physicians) about whether CD/LD should be taken with or without food. Whereas absorption is more thorough and more predictable if CD/LD is taken without food, the incidence of nausea, especially when the drug is first being introduced, is higher. In light of this, a practical approach is to initiate therapy with CD/LD being taken at mealtimes to minimize the likelihood of nausea; after several months of therapy, the timing of CD/LD administration can be adjusted to precede mealtimes by 30 to 60 minutes.

The initial response to CD/LD therapy is generally quite gratifying and unmistakable. In fact, absence of CD/LD responsiveness may presage an alternative diagnosis. Individuals typically find during the early stages of CD/LD therapy that they derive prolonged benefit from individual doses of medication and may actually miss several doses of CD/LD without experiencing any noticeable loss of therapeutic benefit. This prolonged benefit has been labeled the "long-duration levodopa response" and is presumed to occur because sufficient dopaminergic nigrostriatal neurons still remain to manufacture, store, release, and reutilize the supplemental dopamine in a fashion approximating the normal state. At this stage in therapy individuals can be less precise in the timing of medication administration, although it may be good "training" for the later stages of therapy, when timing of administration becomes more critical, to have patients utilize a set, strictly timed dosage schedule right from the outset.

In the early stages of therapy, individuals with Parkinson's disease characteristically awaken in the morning feeling refreshed and with good motor function, as if their dopamine stores had been replenished during the nighttime hours. The physiologic explanation for this "sleep benefit" is not precisely known, but because of its presence it is typically unnecessary to administer CD/LD at bedtime in the initial stages of CD/LD therapy. This changes with time as "sleep benefit" disappears with disease progression.

Titration of CD/LD dosage must be individualized. Both dosage requirements and tolerance may vary widely among individuals. It is also important to remember that not all parkinsonian symptoms respond equally well to antiparkinson medication and that it is usually not realistic (on the part of either physician or patient) to expect CD/LD therapy to obliterate all traces of the parkinsonism completely. Failure to address this fact at the beginning of therapy may lead to inappropriate expectations, dashed hopes, and both frustration and anger from patient and family.

Although careful introduction and titration of CD/LD therapy may reduce the chances of adverse effects from and intolerance to the medication, problems with CD/LD still may occur and can be divided into two categories: those that may occur at initiation of (or actually at any time during) therapy and those that develop only after extended use of the medication.

ADVERSE EFFECTS OF EARLY LEVODOPA THERAPY

Nausea. The most frequently encountered complication of early CD/LD therapy is gastrointestinal dysfunction, which may range from mild anorexia to severe nausea and vomiting. Levodopa-induced nausea has been attributed to stimulation of dopamine receptors in the chemoreceptor trigger zone of the area postrema in the brain stem, which is not protected by the blood-brain barrier. As detailed earlier, the introduction of carbidopa into use with levodopa, especially utilizing the 25/100 dosage form, has dramatically reduced the incidence of this complication but has not totally eliminated it. In some individuals, 75 to 100 mg of carbidopa is insufficient to prevent levodopa-induced nausea, and it is not uncommon for levodopa to be inappropriately abandoned as a therapeutic option in these individuals. With persistence and ingenuity, however, a "pathway" around the nausea can usually be charted. One method to circumvent the nausea entails the use of additional carbidopa, which is not marketed but can be obtained from the manufacturer (without charge) as 25-mg tablets. Individuals can be placed on carbidopa alone, 25 mg three times daily, for 2 weeks, at which time CD/LD is very gingerly reintroduced while the supplementary carbidopa is continued. Starting with a dose of one half tablet daily, the daily CD/LD dosage can be slowly increased at a rate of one half tablet weekly until therapeutic levels are achieved. This approach is generally successful, but when it is not, an alternative is to add domperidone to the treatment regimen. Domperidone is a dopamine receptor antagonist that does not cross the blood-brain barrier and, thus, blocks only peripheral dopamine receptors, including those in the area postrema and in the enteric plexi of the gastrointestinal tract. Unfortunately, domperidone has never been introduced into use in the United States, but it is available in and can be obtained from Canada.

Although it is tempting to utilize antiemetic medications to control nausea, this is an approach that should be avoided in the individual with Parkinson's disease. Conventional antiemetic drugs, including metoclopramide (Reglan), prochlorperazine (Compazine), and promethazine (Phenergan), function as dopamine receptor antagonists in both the CNS and the periphery and, thus, can exacerbate parkinsonism in individuals with Parkinson's disease.

PSYCHIATRIC TOXICITY

Psychiatric symptoms in the form of hallucinations, delusions, and paranoia are a dramatic and distressing complication of levodopa therapy. Although they are most prone to develop in individuals with advanced Parkinson's disease who have been on long-term levodopa therapy and display some degree of dementia, psychiatric symptoms may also occur early in the course of levodopa therapy. Levodopa-induced hallucinations are virtually always visual, rather than auditory. Full-blown hallucinations may be preceded by other phenomena, such as vivid dreaming, anwesenheit (illusions of presence in which images are sensed in the visual periphery but disappear when gaze is directed toward them), and hallucinations with a clear sensorium in which fully formed hallucinations occur but the individual recognizes that the image is false. Generally, these hallucinatory "fragments" do not require specific therapy; only when the hallucinations assume reality and become accompanied by delusions and paranoia does corrective treatment become necessary. It has traditionally been assumed that levodopa-induced psychiatric toxicity is the consequence of excessive dopaminergic stimulation at limbic dopamine receptors. Recent conjecture, however, has also suggested that serotonergic mechanisms may be active.

When full-blown levodopa-induced psychosis develops, the first response should be to look for any possible precipitating factor, such as a urinary tract infection. Attention may then turn to possible offending medications that may precipitate psychosis. Both antiparkinson and all other medications the patient is taking should be exposed to scrutiny. Over-the-counter medications should not be forgotten. Expendable medications should be eliminated and then antiparkinson medications should be serially withdrawn, beginning with the least essential. Anticholinergic drugs might be withdrawn first, followed by selegiline, amantadine, and dopamine agonists. If the hallucinations still persist at that point, CD/LD dosage can be progressively reduced. It is possible at any point along this pathway that an unacceptable exacerbation of parkinsonism may appear, precluding further dosage reductions. Occasionally the psychiatric symptoms may be so severe and disruptive that it is necessary to immediately discontinue all antiparkinson medications, including CD/LD. This, however, exposes the patient to the risk of development of a potentially fatal neuroleptic malignant-like syndrome characterized by fever, increased tremor and rigidity, rising muscle enzymes, and autonomic dysfunction.

If withdrawal of medication or dosage reduction does not eliminate the psychosis, the institution of antipsychotic drug therapy must then be considered. Conventional neuroleptics such as haloperidol (Haldol) and chlorpromazine (Thorazine) should be studiously avoided because they block both limbic and striatal dopamine receptors and very predictably will aggravate parkinsonism. Several less potent neuroleptics, thioridazine (Mellaril) and molindone (Moban), have been suggested as alternatives, but these drugs typically will also produce deterioration in motor function. Even newer drugs, such as risperidone (Risperdal), have been disappointing in this situation and will often cause unacceptable deterioration in parkinsonism when used in dosages sufficient to ameliorate the hallucinations.

Clozapine (Clozaril) is an "atypical" neuroleptic that appears to block limbic dopamine (possibly D4) receptors preferentially and produces little effect on the nigrostriatal dopaminergic pathway and thus on extrapyramidal function. Because of this pharmacologic profile, clozapine has been the subject of numerous small, nonblinded clinical trials in patients with Parkinson's disease and levodopa-induced psychosis. Experience in these studies seems to indicate that clozapine is a very effective antipsychotic agent in this setting and that it rarely aggravates parkinsonism. However, individuals with Parkinson's disease are exquisitely sensitive to clozapine, and dosages far lower than those used in patients with schizophrenia are appropriate. Initial dosage should be 6.25 mg (0.25 tablet) at bedtime with subsequent upward titration. It is rare for a maximum dosage to exceed 100 mg daily and dosages around 50 mg are common. Even at these minuscule dosages, adverse effects such as drowsiness, orthostatic lightheadedness, and increased salivation may occur, but they are usually manageable and do not necessitate discontinuation of the drug. Bone marrow suppression remains a small but real potential risk even at these low dosages and mandates that weekly blood counts be obtained. Despite this, clozapine remains the drug of choice in treating levodopa-induced psychosis if simple elimination or dosage reduction of other medications fails.

Recently, ondansetron (Zofran)* has been reported to relieve levodopa-induced psychosis very effectively, presumably via serotonergic mechanisms. This potentially is a very appealing alternative to clozapine, but further study is warranted before unqualified recommendation of the drug in this setting can be made.

ORTHOSTATIC HYPOTENSION

Orthostatic hypotension with postural lightheadedness is a complication of levodopa therapy that may develop upon initiation of therapy or in the more advanced stages of Parkinson's disease, following prolonged therapy. It is felt to be mediated by both central and peripheral mechanisms. If CD/LD dosage reduction alone is not sufficient or if it cannot be tolerated because of increasing parkinsonism, treatment with the mineralocorticoid fludrocortisone (Florinef)* is the next line of therapy. The efficacy of fludrocortisone, however, is inconsistent and frequently insufficient. Indomethacin (Indocin)* is sometimes effective as an alternative to fludrocortisone. The most effective treatment modality for levodopa-induced orthostatic hypotension, however, may be nonpharmacologic. Jobst stockings, preferably waist-high, can very effectively ameliorate orthostatic lightheadedness even when medications have failed, but the stockings also have their drawbacks. They are difficult to put on, uncomfortable to wear, and are expensive, especially since they must be replaced approximately every 3 months because of stretching.

SLEEP DISTURBANCES

Sleep disturbances may be a part of Parkinson's disease itself but may also be a result of CD/LD therapy. Excessive daytime drowsiness can be a persistent CD/LD-induced problem, and may occur in up to 20% of individuals on the medication. Effective treatment can be elusive, but sometimes stimulant medications like methylphenidate (Ritalin), pemoline (Cylert), methamphetamine (Desoxyn), or dextroamphetamine (Dexedrine) can be useful. Levodopa can also produce nocturnal myoclonus, which may not always disturb the patient but may awaken the spouse instead. If myoclonus is sufficiently severe to warrant therapy, clonazepam (Klonopin) may significantly reduce the symptom. While CD/LD may occasionally cause insomnia, this more commonly is a consequence of Parkinson's disease itself. Bedtime Sinemet CR or administration of CD/LD during the nighttime hours may be necessary to combat insomnia of this type.

ADVERSE EFFECTS OF PROLONGED LEVODOPA THERAPY

As noted earlier, when individuals are first placed on CD/LD therapy they generally enjoy prolonged

---

*Not FDA-approved for this indication.

benefit from individual CD/LD doses, resulting in a smooth response termed the "long-duration levodopa response." As Parkinson's disease progresses, however, this prolonged, smooth response begins to fragment, and a more clear-cut pattern of responsiveness to individual CD/LD doses emerges. As this "short-duration levodopa response" appears, it is initially characterized by a mild, often vague, loss of medication benefit as the time for the next dose of CD/LD approaches. With time, this "wearing off" becomes more prominent and begins to occur earlier in the dosage interval. At the same time individuals will begin to note a progressive loss of the "sleep benefit" they had previously enjoyed and will find themselves "off" in the morning until they take their first dose of CD/LD.

Another phenomenon may also make its appearance at this time. Involuntary movements, perhaps consisting of facial grimacing or squirming, fidgety movements of limbs or trunk, may develop. These involuntary movements, or dyskinesia, are typically choreiform in character. Initially the individual with Parkinson's disease may be totally unaware of the involuntary movements until attention is drawn to them by spouse, family, or physician. Dyskinesia may first appear when the individual is concentrating on a task, such as writing or tying a shoelace, or when the person is under stress. The dyskinesia reflects excessive stimulation of dopamine receptors in the striatum and tends to occur at the time of peak clinical efficacy of a CD/LD dosage. Rarely, a different pattern of dyskinesia develops, the "diphasic dyskinesia" pattern, in which involuntary movements appear as the effect of a CD/LD dose is emerging and then disappear, only to re-emerge as the effectiveness of the dose is wearing off. The pathophysiology of this type of response is poorly understood.

Initially the pattern of peak-dose dyskinesia followed by end of dose wearing off is quite predictable. Eventually, however, this predictability is lost and more unpredictable, chaotic fluctuations in motor performance become apparent. Moreover, sometimes patients may experience a delayed response to a dose of levodopa; on other occasions, no response at all to a dose will occur. The term "on-off" motor fluctuations is utilized to describe these unpredictable responses to CD/LD.

Treatment of motor fluctuations can be challenging. Mild end of dose wearing off of CD/LD efficacy can be managed initially by several maneuvers. CD/LD can be given more frequently, with a shorter dosage interval. Alternatively, Sinemet CR may be employed very effectively to ameliorate the wearing off, since the slow dissolution of the tablet provides a more prolonged response to an individual dose. Studies have shown that a reduction of dose frequency in the range of 33% can be achieved with Sinemet CR, but, because of decreased levodopa bioavailability, it is also necessary to increase daily levodopa dosage by approximately 25%. Sinemet CR is most effectively employed in individuals with mild-to-moderate end of dose wearing off. It is much less effective in individuals with advanced disease. Adjunctive medications, such as selegiline, bromocriptine, pergolide, and even amantadine may also be of value in treating end of dose wearing off of CD/LD efficacy. The treatment of peak dose dyskinesia usually requires a reduction in individual CD/LD dosage strength.

The net result of therapeutic manipulations undertaken to deal with motor fluctuations is an increasingly complex dosage regimen with multiple therapeutic agents. In spite of this, ideal control of motor fluctuations becomes increasingly elusive as disease severity relentlessly progresses.

Dopamine Agonists

Because the primary pathologic feature of Parkinson's disease is the loss of nigrostriatal dopaminergic neurons, the very neurons responsible for the synthesis, storage, and release of dopamine in the striatum under normal circumstances, it is understandable that the efficacy of levodopa will be increasingly compromised as Parkinson's disease progresses (though by no means eliminated since administered levodopa can apparently be "adopted" by other neurons, such as serotonergic, and converted to dopamine there). This has led pharmaceutical companies to develop and test drugs that do not rely on presynaptic function or integrity, but rather stimulate the postsynaptic dopamine receptor directly. An impressive array of such drugs has been tested, but only two, bromocriptine and pergolide, have been approved for use in the United States. Several additional dopamine agonist drugs are currently undergoing experimental trials also. The initial hopes that dopamine agonists would be as or more potent than dopamine itself and that their effectiveness would continue undiminished in the advanced stages of Parkinson's disease have not been borne out by experience, but dopamine agonists nevertheless have assumed a valuable position as adjunctive therapy that can be useful in ameliorating levodopa-related motor fluctuations. For reasons that are not entirely clear but presumed to be related to their pharmacologic profile as predominantly D_2 receptor agonists, dopamine agonists such as bromocriptine and pergolide are less likely to provoke dyskinesia than is levodopa.

BROMOCRIPTINE

Bromocriptine (Parlodel) is an ergot derivative with selective dopamine D_2 receptor agonist properties and modest D_1 receptor antagonist activity. When introduced into use in the early 1970s by Calne, bromocriptine was utilized in high doses—up to 100 mg daily or more—with the intent of replacing levodopa in individuals with advanced Parkinson's disease. At such doses bromocriptine was effective but also produced toxicity in many individuals.

In lower dosages bromocriptine has also been utilized as initial monotherapy in Parkinson's disease, with the goal of delaying introduction of levodopa and, thus, postponing the appearance of motor fluctuations. This approach has met with only limited success since in most individuals bromocriptine alone in low dosages is not sufficiently effective for more than 6 to 12 months. Where bromocriptine has found a role is as adjunctive therapy, in which it is added to CD/LD when fluctuations in motor performance have developed in an effort to reduce end of dose wearing off. In this setting, dosages of at least 10 to 30 mg daily are usually necessary. The idea of adding bromocriptine even earlier—before motor fluctuations have developed—as a levodopa-sparing strategy in which it is hoped that motor fluctuations will be postponed has received both approbation and repudiation.

Bromocriptine is capable of producing adverse effects that largely mirror those of levodopa. Orthostatic lightheadedness and nausea are the most common adverse effects. Psychiatric toxicity with hallucinations and outright psychosis may also develop. Rarely, recurrent episodes of hallucinations can occur long after bromocriptine has been discontinued, a phenomenon reminiscent of the flashbacks seen after the use use of another ergot derivative, LSD.

Digital vasospasm and increased angina, probably additional reflections of bromocriptine's ergot roots, are rare complications of bromocriptine; even classic ergotism has been described. Pleural effusion and pleural thickening are two additional rare complications of bromocriptine therapy.

PERGOLIDE

Pergolide (Permax) is a semisynthetic ergoline derivative that has both D_1 and D_2 agonist properties, although its principal effect, like that of bromocriptine, is on the D_2 receptor. The pharmacologic characteristics that separate pergolide from bromocriptine, especially the D_1-stimulating properties of pergolide, have received much attention, but the similarities between the two medications far outweigh their differences.

Pergolide, like bromocriptine, is used primarily as adjunctive therapy with levodopa. It is a significantly more potent substance than bromocriptine, and daily dosages are correspondingly lower. A conversion ratio of 10:1 is used for comparing bromocriptine to pergolide; thus, 30 mg of bromocriptine daily is roughly equivalent to 3 mg of pergolide. The efficacy of pergolide is generally similar to that of bromocriptine. Individuals who are no longer responding well to bromocriptine may show improvement when switched to pergolide; whether the converse is also true has not been systematically evaluated. Choosing between pergolide and bromocriptine may be largely a matter of personal preference, although pergolide is currently less expensive than bromocriptine in comparable doses.

Adverse effects encountered with pergolide are virtually identical to those seen with bromocriptine. Initial concerns about cardiac toxicity have not proved to be justified.

SELEGILINE

The effectiveness of selegiline (Eldepryl) in ameliorating levodopa-induced motor fluctuations, specifically end of dose wearing off, was first reported over 20 years ago, in 1975, and multiple subsequent studies have confirmed this symptomatic benefit of selegiline. Selegiline is most effective in reducing CD/LD-related end of dose deterioration in individuals with mild or moderate disease and provides little benefit to those with advanced disease and severe, unpredictable motor fluctuations.

As noted earlier, adverse effects of selegiline itself are generally infrequent and mild. When selegiline is added to CD/LD, however, levodopa-generated adverse effects may appear because of the reduction in levodopa metabolism as a result of MAO-B inhibition. If dopaminergic adverse effects occur, a reduction in CD/LD dosage of 10% to 30% may eliminate the problem. Although it is generally not necessary to reduce CD/LD dosage automatically when selegiline is introduced, it is prudent to begin selegiline at a reduced dose of 5 mg daily, increasing to 10 mg daily in 1 to 2 weeks, if necessary.

Dietary Therapy

Several nutritional and dietary issues have received attention in the management of Parkinson's disease. Administration of the dietary amino acid precursors of levodopa, specifically phenylalanine and tyrosine, has not proved to be of any therapeutic benefit for the individual with Parkinson's disease.

When levodopa was first introduced into clinical use, prior to the advent of carbidopa coadministration, it was discovered that pyridoxine (vitamin B_6) could nullify the effectiveness of the administered levodopa. However, when levodopa is administered with carbidopa this antagonism does not occur, and it is not necessary for the individual with Parkinson's disease to avoid pyridoxine.

Competition between administered levodopa and other dietary large neutral amino acids (LNAA) can assume clinical importance in some, but by no means all, individuals. Levodopa and other LNAAs share a common transport system both at the level of the intestinal mucosa and at the blood-brain barrier. High-protein meals have been shown to reduce the response to a dose of levodopa, presumably via competition for absorption between the dietary-derived LNAAs and the levodopa. This is usually not clinically apparent in individuals with mild Parkinson's disease, but it may become a significant problem in individuals with more advanced disease who are already experiencing troublesome fluctuations in motor performance. In this setting, employment of dietary protein restriction and redistribution of protein primarily to the evening hours has been effective in ameliorating some of the response inconsistency. However, it should be clearly communicated to patients and family that not everyone—and in fact only a minority of patients—requires this type of dietary manipulation and that if it is utilized, it should be done under the guidance of dietitian.

Surgical Therapy

Surgical therapy has a long history in the treatment of Parkinson's disease. During the past 30 years surgical approaches have been eclipsed by pharmacologic advances, but recently there has been a resurgence of interest in these procedures. Advances in technology have made stereotaxic surgery both safer and more precise, making surgery a more appealing therapeutic option than in the past. Two stereotaxic surgical approaches are currently utilized in the treatment of Parkinson's disease.

Thalamotomy has long been an accepted treatment approach for tremor that has not responded satisfactorily to medical management. With current surgical techniques it is a very safe, although certainly not risk-free, procedure. However, thalamotomy has no significant effect on clinical features of Parkinson's disease beyond tremor, a fact that limits its usefulness since for most individuals with Parkinson's disease tremor is not the primary disabling feature.

There has been a flurry (maybe blizzard is a more accurate term) of publicity and interest within the past 1 to 2 years about stereotaxic pallidotomy for the treatment of Parkinson's disease. Pallidotomy is certainly not a new procedure, but technical refinements such as microelectrode guidance have led to more precise, effective, and safe lesion placement and, consequently, improved outcome. Although pallidotomy may reduce tremor also, its primary usefulness is in individuals who are experiencing uncontrollable fluctuations in motor performance with severe dyskinesia and prominent "off" periods. Pallidotomy may less consistently ameliorate gait difficulties and freezing (a sudden inability to move), but this is somewhat controversial.

Both thalamotomy and pallidotomy should be considered as part of the therapeutic arsenal available for the treatment of Parkinson's disease, especially in individuals who are no longer responding adequately to medical management alone. It should be made clear to patients and family, however, that these surgical procedures do not cure Parkinson's disease and will not eliminate the need for ongoing medical therapy for their malady.

SUMMARY

Tremendous advances have been made in the past 30 years in the treatment of Parkinson's disease, but many challenges and obstacles remain. The etiology of Parkinson's disease remains elusive and the ideal therapy—prevention—probably awaits its identification. Nevertheless, the future is full of exciting prospects for more effective symptomatic and protective therapy of Parkinson's disease. More potent and longer-acting dopamine agonists are being tested, as are inhibitors of MAO-B and the other metabolic enzyme of levodopa, COMT. New routes of administration—transdermal, sublingual, subcutaneous, and others—are being explored. The role of growth factors is being investigated and gene therapy for Parkinson's disease may be on the horizon.

In the midst of all this excitement, however, it is important to remember that the day-to-day management of Parkinson's disease demands the type of close patient-physician relationship that is becoming increasingly difficult to maintain in the current medical environment. Effective manipulation of the medications and other treatment modalities available for Parkinson's disease requires that the physician know the patient and the nuances of the patient's disease symptoms well and that frequent interactions between physician and patient take place. Returning a telephone call and simply listening to a problem may be as important a therapeutic maneuver as adding a new medication. Although we cannot currently cure Parkinson's disease or even halt its progression, it is possible with judicious use of medication and meticulous attention to detail to provide most individuals with Parkinson's disease a quality of life that, while far from ideal, is certainly both meaningful and manageable.

PERIPHERAL NEUROPATHIES

method of
MICHAEL E. SHY, M.D.
Wayne State University
Detroit, Michigan

The peripheral nervous system (PNS) consists of motor, sensory, and autonomic neurons that extend outside the central nervous system (CNS) and are associated with Schwann cells or ganglionic satellite cells. The PNS includes the dorsal and ventral spinal roots, spinal and cranial nerves, sensory and motor terminals, and the bulk of the autonomic nervous system. Motor neurons extend from their cell body in the ventral horn of the spinal cord to the neuromuscular junctions at the muscle they innervate. The cell bodies of primary sensory neurons lie outside the spinal cord in the dorsal root ganglia (DRG) where they extend peripherally to specialized sensory end organs including nociceptors, thermoreceptors, and mechanoreceptors. Central projections from DRG enter the spinal cord through the dorsal roots. At each spinal segment the ventral roots, carrying motor axons, and the dorsal roots, carrying sensory axons, join to form mixed sensorimotor nerves. In the cervical, brachial, and lumbosacral areas, the mixed spinal nerves form plexuses from which the major anatomically defined limb nerves emanate. Each mixed nerve is composed of large numbers of myelinated and nonmyelinated nerves of varying diameter. The large, myelinated axons include motor neurons and large-fiber sensory nerves, which subserve position and vibration senses. Small, thinly myelinated or nonmyelinated axons primarily subserve nociception and autonomic modalities. Preganglionic sympathetic autonomic fibers begin in the intermediolateral column of the spinal cord and synapse in the sympathetic trunk with sympathetic ganglia. Preganglionic parasympathetic fibers travel long distances from their cell bodies in the brain stem or sacral spinal cord to reach terminal ganglia that are near the organs the parasympathetic fibers innervate. The sympathetic and parasympathetic divisions work synergistically to mediate motivational and emotional states as well as in monitoring

the body's basic physiology. Peripheral neuropathy is a general term for disorders affecting peripheral nerves. These disorders can be genetic, toxic, immunologic, or metabolic. Some or all populations of peripheral nerves can be affected. Since in many cases mixed sensorimotor nerves are affected, the majority of peripheral neuropathies are sensorimotor, although isolated motor or sensory neuropathies do exist (see later).

The key element in evaluating a patient with peripheral nerve disease is to take a systematic approach. A multitude of laboratory abnormalities, toxins, and hereditary and acquired disorders can cause peripheral neuropathy. A "shotgun" approach in which every conceivable cause of neuropathy is excluded is expensive, may not identify the cause of the neuropathy, and is therefore not in the patient's best interests. The approach suggested here is to use the history and physical examination to demonstrate peripheral nerve disease, utilize electroneuromyography (ENMG) to characterize the demyelinating or axonal nature of the process, and then order the relevant tests to diagnose the neuropathy. This work-up is outlined in Figure 1, which is modified from a figure by Arthur Asbury, and forms the structure for the remainder of this article.

HISTORY AND PHYSICAL EXAMINATION

The first goal of the history and physical examination is to identify the problem as a peripheral neuropathy. This is based on characteristic motor, sensory, and autonomic features discussed later. Secondly, it is important to determine whether the onset is acute (< 1 month), subacute (< 6 months), or chronic (> 6 months). The third goal is to determine whether or not the disorder is symmetrical or asymmetrical.

Motor. Weakness in peripheral nerve disease is often distal and more severe in the legs than the arms. Extensor muscles tend to be more affected than flexors. Therefore, the extensors of the great toe and of the foot in the lower extremity, and the wrist or finger extensors in the upper extremity, are particularly useful muscles to test. When the weakness is caused by axonal destruction, there is wasting of muscle that is more severe than when weakness is caused by central nervous system disease, such as occurs following a stroke. Wasting in the lower extremity is frequently detected on the anterior calf and, in the upper extremity, on the dorsal hand between the index finger and the thumb. Cramps, the painful knotting of a muscle, frequently occur in motor or sensorimotor neuropathies. Fasciculations appear as small twitches of the muscle. They represent the random firing of a motor unit, which consists of a motor neuron and all the muscle fibers it innervates. When fasciculations are associated with weakness and wasting of muscle, they suggest the diagnosis of

TABLE 1. **Predominantly Motor Neuropathies**

Immune mediated
  Guillain-Barré syndrome
  Chronic inflammatory demyelinating polyneuropathy (CIDP)
  Pure motor neuropathy (PMN) (often with conduction block)
Toxic
  Lead
  Dapsone
Paraneoplastic
  Motor neuropathy associated with lymphoma
Hereditary
  Porphyria
  Hexosaminidase A deficiency

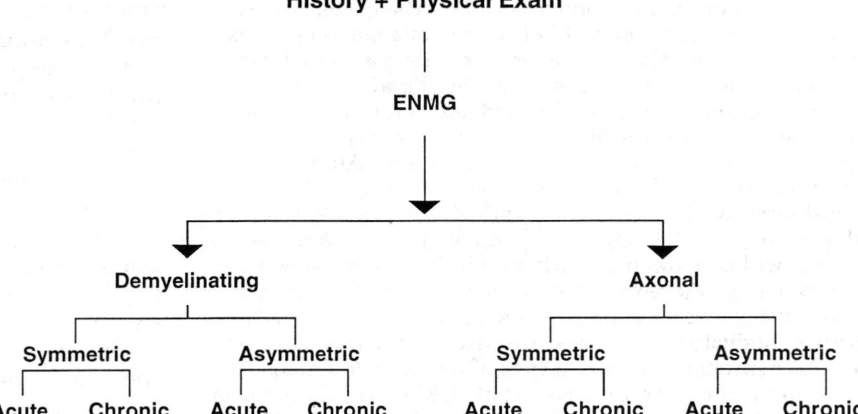

Figure 1. Work-up for the evaluation of a patient with peripheral nerve disease. ENMG = electroneuromyography.

motor neuron disease or amyotrophic lateral sclerosis (ALS). However, fasciculations are also present in many normal people, particularly when they are tired or have ingested too much caffeine. Their presence, in the absence of weakness and muscle wasting, is not likely to be significant. Reflexes in motor neuropathies, as in sensorimotor or sensory neuropathies, are usually reduced. Although the majority of neuropathies are sensorimotor, a group of predominantly motor neuropathies is listed in Table 1.

Sensory. Sensory loss in peripheral nerve disease is also predominantly distal and can be separated into sensory modalities of large fibers (position and vibration) and small fibers (pain and temperature). Large fibers are usually ensheathed by myelin whereas small fibers are only thinly myelinated or not myelinated at all. Small fiber neuropathies are often accompanied by burning or stabbing pain as well as by loss of sensation to pain and temperature.

The predominantly sensory neuropathies are listed in Table 2.

Autonomic. Autonomic abnormalities frequently accompany neuropathies with small-fiber sensory predominance. These abnormalities include orthostatic hypotension, urinary retention or incontinence, impotence, gastric motility dysfunction, pupillary dysfunction, heat intolerance, and disorders of sweating. Examples of neuropathies with predominant autonomic features are listed in Table 3.

ELECTRONEUROMYOGRAPHY

The next step is to obtain an electroneurogram (ENMG) on the patient. The ENMG permits determination of whether a neuropathy is demyelinating or axonal. If the neuropathy is demyelinating, the ENMG allows one to distinguish between what is likely to be a hereditary or an acquired demyelinating neuropathy. If the neuropathy is axonal, the ENMG can help distinguish between uniform axonal neuropathies or the asymmetrical mononeuritis multiplex. The ENMG can also help identify whether the neuropathy is chronic. These distinctions are important because they identify potentially treatable neuropathies. Acquired demyelinating neuropathies virtually all respond to therapy directed at suppressing the immune response, as do many axonal forms of mononeuritis multiplex. On the other hand, few effective treatments are available for the hereditary or chronic axonal neuropathies. Once neuropathies have been classified by ENMG, intelligent decisions can be made about which laboratory tests may be useful to further characterize the neuropathy.

The ENMG is typically divided into two sections: nerve conduction velocities and the needle electromyogram (EMG). Nerve conduction velocities measure conduction along the fastest conducting, myelinating, motor and sensory nerves. Slowed conduction velocities (70% of normal) suggest the neuropathy is demyelinating. For technical

TABLE 2. **Predominantly Sensory Neuropathies**

Large Fiber Neuropathies

Immune mediated
   Sensory neuropathy associated with Sjögren's syndrome
Toxic/metabolic
   Cisplatin
   Paclitaxel
   Vitamin E deficiency
   Vitamin B_{12} deficiency
Paraneoplastic
   Sensory neuropathy with "anti-Hu" antibodies
Hereditary
   Hereditary sensory neuropathy
   Abetalipoproteinemia

Small Fiber Neuropathies

Associated with systemic disease
   Diabetes mellitus
   Amyloidosis
   Human immunodeficiency virus
Toxins
   Metronidazole
   Misonidazole
   Vacor
Hereditary
   Hereditary sensory neuropathy
   Fabry's disease
   Tangier disease

Modified from Bird SJ, Brown MJ: Peripheral neuropathies. *In* Conn RB (ed): Current Diagnosis 8. Philadelphia, WB Saunders, 1991, pp 992–1004.

TABLE 3. **Neuropathies with Autonomic Features**

Associated with systemic disease
   Diabetes mellitus
   Amyloidosis
Toxins
   Vacor
Hereditary
   Riley-Day syndrome
   Shy-Drager syndrome

reasons, motor nerve conduction velocities measure conduction over the main body of nerves but not their proximal or distal portion. Distal motor latencies and F-wave latencies measure velocities over the distal and proximal portions of the nerves. In inherited demyelinating neuropathies, such as Charcot-Marie-Tooth disease type 1, conduction velocities tend to be uniformly slowed. Alternatively, in acquired demyelinating neuropathies such as the Guillain-Barré syndrome, nerve conductions are likely to be slowed asymmetrically. In asymmetrical slowing, some nerves will be slowed but others will have normal conduction velocity. Moreover, some regions of the same nerve may have slow conductions while other regions are normal. Nerve conduction velocities are also useful in diagnosing axonal neuropathies. In the case of motor conductions, the compound muscle action potential (CMAP) is the sum of action potentials of the individual muscle fibers that have been stimulated to fire by individual axons. The sensory nerve action potential (SNAP) is a summation of action potential from individual sensory axons. In axonal neuropathies axons are lost, so the summated potentials are reduced in amplitude. Therefore, in axonal neuropathies the size of the CMAP, SNAP, or both are reduced.

The needle EMG is also important in analyzing axonal neuropathies. At rest the muscle is electrically silent. However, when axons are acutely damaged, the muscle they innervate develops "spontaneous" activity characterized by fibrillations and positive sharp waves. If nerves are transected from trauma, portions of the axon distal to the lesion degenerate in a process called wallerian degeneration. In this setting fibrillations and positive sharp waves develop within 2 to 3 weeks of the injury. In an axonal neuropathy, if the process is acute or subacute, one is also likely to see fibrillations or positive waves although they may disappear in a chronic axonal neuropathy. Fasciculations, the random, spontaneous firing of motor units, also appear when the muscle is at rest. When healthy axons attempt to reinnervate denervated muscle fibers, the waveform of their motor units becomes more complex or polyphasic. Thus in chronic axonal neuropathies, there is a higher percentage than normal of polyphasic potentials in early recruited motor units. Recruitment of motor units is also reduced in patients with axonal neuropathies since there are fewer axons, and therefore fewer motor units available for recruitment.

DEMYELINATING PERIPHERAL NEUROPATHIES

Evaluation of Demyelinating Neuropathies

When the history, physical examination, and ENMG suggest the presence of a demyelinating neuropathy, appropriate laboratory testing can be obtained to categorize and clarify the disorder further. If the demyelination is uniform, particularly if there is a family history of neuropathy, the patient is likely to suffer from a form of Charcot-Marie-Tooth disease, summarized later. These neuropathies are usually chronic, progressing slowly over years. The appropriate testing for these patients is genetic screening of DNA from blood, for abnormalities in the genes encoding myelin proteins PMP-22, PO, or the myelin-related protein, connexin 32.

When the history, physical examination, and electrophysiology suggest an asymmetrical process, without a family history, the evaluation should include a cerebrospinal fluid (CSF) examination. Spinal fluid examination is important in characterizing demyelinating neuropathies. Many of the acquired demyelinating neuropathies such as the Guillain-Barré syndrome (GBS) or chronic inflammatory demyelinating polyneuropathy (CIDP) have high spinal fluid proteins with only a few white blood cells (cytoalbumino dissociation). The work-up for acquired demyelinating neuropathies should also include serum protein electrophoresis (SPEP) and an immunoelectrophoresis (IPEP) to detect monoclonal gammopathy.

The question of when to screen for the presence of specific autoantibodies in demyelinating (or axonal) neuropathies is controversial. Several commercial firms provide antibody testing for patients with neuropathy. Although detection of these antibodies (particularly anti-MAG, anti-Hu and anti-GM$_1$) can be useful in certain circumstances (see later), they are expensive to obtain and, if ordered indiscriminately, can actually confuse the patient's management. In fact, the antibodies, although associated with certain neuropathies, are not completely specific for them. Thus, treatment decisions based solely on the presence of autoantibodies will lead to treatment of some patients who should not be treated. In addition, many patients with treatable neuropathies do not have antibodies to MAG or GM$_1$. In this case, not treating patients because they lack these antibodies will lead to the lack of treatment to patients who should be treated. A good rule of thumb is to look hard for evidence of an acquired demyelinating neuropathy. If this is present, the patient is likely to be a candidate for immunosuppressive therapy. Then, if the information will be clinically useful, a screen for antibodies to MAG or GM$_1$ can be considered.

Sural nerve biopsy is useful when it can answer a specific question about the neuropathy. It is rarely useful when ordered as part of a "fishing expedition" in which one does not know the cause of a neuropathy and is just hoping to find something helpful. Appropriate use of sural nerve biopsy in demyelinating neuropathies is to document CIDP (see later) or detect IgM deposits on nerve suspected to be damaged by monoclonal IgM M-proteins. An outline to follow in evaluating demyelinating neuropathies is included in Table 4 prior to discussion of individual types of demyelinating neuropathies.

Inherited Demyelinating Neuropathies

The inherited neuropathies are listed in Table 5 and, in many cases, can now be diagnosed with certainty by DNA analysis. The most frequent is Charcot-Marie-Tooth disease type 1A (CMT1A), which is inherited as an autosomal dominant disorder. CMT1A is very frequent, with an incidence of up to 1 in 2500, and typically presents around 12 years of age with difficulties in running, climbing, or jumping. Calf muscles, in particular, may appear atrophied ("storklike legs"), and high arches or flat feet are frequent. Nerve conduction velocities are uniformly

TABLE 4. **Laboratory Evaluation of Acquired Demyelinating Neuropathies**

Necessary Studies

Electroneuromyography (ENMG)
Cerebral spinal fluid (CSF) evaluation
(protein, cells, glucose)
Serum protein electrophoresis (SPEP),
immunoelectrophoresis (IPEP),
urine protein electrophoresis (UPEP)

Useful Studies

Thyroid function studies
Human immunodeficiency virus (HIV)
Sural nerve biopsy

slowed, with rates as slow as 10 to 20 meters per sec (normals, 40 to 50 meters per sec). The disease is slowly progressive, with many patients needing ambulatory aid as they grow older. However, the disease frequently has a variable expression, and an affected family member may have only high-arched feet, for example, making an accurate family history difficult to obtain. Sural nerve biopsies of patients with CMT1A show uniform demyelination, little if any inflammation, and many "onion bulbs," which are thought to represent concentric rings of Schwann cells trying to remyelinate axons. CMT1A is caused by a 1.5-megabase duplication on chromosome 17 in the region that contains the Schwann cell myelin-specific gene PMP-22. Point mutations in PMP-22 may also cause a phenotype that resembles CMT1A, suggesting that it is the abnormality of PMP-22 that causes CMT1A. Certain point mutations in PMP-22 lead to very severe, autosomal dominant, demyelinating neuropathies that appear before the age of 5 years. Typically, severe demyelinating neuropathies presenting in young childhood are called Dejerine-Sottas disease. Since Dejerine-Sottas is often autosomal recessive, the relationship between PMP-22 mutations and all cases of Dejerine-Sottas disease is unknown.

When patients have a deletion of PMP-22 instead of a duplication or point mutation, they develop a distinct neuropathy termed "hereditary neuropathy with liability to pressure palsies" (HNPP). These patients have an increased tendency to develop entrapment syndromes such as the carpal tunnel or tarsal tunnel syndrome but tend not to develop clinical evidence of diffuse neuropathy.

Charcot-Marie-Tooth disease type 1B is much less

frequent than CMT1A, with only rare cases reported. It is also an autosomal dominant neuropathy and is caused by various point mutations in the gene encoding the major PNS myelin protein, PO. Only a few families have been characterized and, at the time of this article, there is little to distinguish CMT1B from CMT1A with the possible exception that CMT1B may have larger numbers of onion bulbs on sural nerve biopsy, and very thickened nerve roots that are apparent on MRI examination of the spinal cord. These associations are not certain, however, and neither sural nerve biopsy or MRI need be part of the routine work-up of patients with CMT.

The X-linked form of Charcot-Marie-Tooth disease (CMTX) is more frequent than CMT1B but less frequent than CMT1A. Clinically it is distinguished from CMT1A and CMT1B by the X-linked pattern (males get the neuropathy) of inheritance. CMTX is caused by point mutations in the Schwann cell gene connexin 32. The diagnosis of CMT1A, CMT1B, and CMTX can be made by analyzing DNA obtained from blood cells.

There is also a small group of inherited disorders that have demyelinating neuropathies as a component of the disease but not necessarily as the main feature. These include Refsum's disease (phytanic acid accumulation with associated retinitis pigmentosa and cerebellar ataxia), metachromatic leukodystrophy (galactosyl-3-sulfate accumulation with associated CNS dysmyelination), adrenoleukodystrophy (long chain fatty acid accumulation induced by mutations in the ALD gene on the X-chromosome, with associated CNS dysmyelination and adrenal failure), Krabbe's disease (galactocerebroside abnormalities associated with CNS dysmyelination), and Pelizaeus-Merzbacher disease (mutations in the myelin gene proteolipid protein [PLP] with associated CNS dysmyelination).

Acquired Demyelinating Neuropathies
(Table 6)

Acquired demyelinating neuropathies tend to be distinguished from inherited neuropathies by the lack of a family history and by the fact that they are asymmetric in nature. Moreover, in some types, the rapid nature of their onset is not consistent with the diagnosis of CMT. Acquired demyelinating neuropa-

TABLE 5. **Gene Defects in Inherited Demyelinating Neuropathies**

Charcot-Marie-Tooth 1A	Duplication on chromosome 17 (region containing PMP-22 gene)
Charcot-Marie-Tooth 1B	Point mutations in P0 gene
Hereditary neuropathy with liability to pressure palsies (HNPP)	Deletion of PMP-22 allele
Charcot-Marie-Tooth X	Point mutations in connexin 32

TABLE 6. **Acquired Demyelinating Neuropathies**

Guillain-Barré syndrome	Rapid onset
Chronic inflammatory demyelinating polyneuropathy (CIDP)	Subacute to chronic onset
Associated with plasma cell dyscrasia	
IgM anti-MAG (myelin-associated glycoprotein)	Subacute to chronic onset
IgG with POEMS (*peripheral neuropathy, organomegaly, endocrinopathy, myeloma, skin changes*)	Subacute to chronic onset
MMN with conduction block	Subacute to chronic onset

thies are critical neuropathies to identify since virtually all of them are treatable.

Guillain-Barré Syndrome

The most frequent acquired demyelinating neuropathy is the Guillain-Barré syndrome (GBS). In two thirds of the cases its onset is about 2 weeks following an upper respiratory infection or other viral illness. Patients develop the rapid onset of weakness often in an ascending pattern from their legs to arms and face. Breathing is often affected, and respiratory distress can be a life-threatening component of GBS. Approximately 50% of patients reach their nadir within 2 weeks, 75% within 3 weeks, and over 90% within 4 weeks of the onset of weakness. After a short period of stabilization, patients tend to improve spontaneously at the rate at which they became weak. Over two thirds of patients recover spontaneously. Sensation is also lost in GBS but usually to a lesser extent than strength. Because plasmapheresis and intravenous gamma globulin (IVIg) have been shown to be efficacious in the treatment of GBS, they are often given to improve the rate and extent of recovery. The diagnosis of GBS is based on a triad: patchy demyelination on nerve conduction velocities, arreflexia, and an elevated protein in the absence of an elevated cell count on spinal fluid elevation. The amplitude of the compound muscle action potential on nerve conduction studies is thought to be the best prognostic indicator for recovery: the more normal the compound muscle action potential (CMAP), the better the chance for recovery. Typically there should be fewer than 5 to 10 white blood cells in the CSF and the protein may run higher than 100 mg per dL. One condition in which a high CSF cell count is associated with GBS is when there is HIV infection. GBS in this setting often occurs around the time of seroconversion and should lead to suspicion of HIV. The cause of GBS is not known. Some cases, however, appear to be associated with prior infection by the enteropathogenic gram-negative rod *Campylobacter jejuni*. This bacterium contains the Gal(β1-3)GalNAc carbohydrate, which is also a part of the ganglioside GM_1. Since some patients with GBS contain antibodies to GM_1, it is thought that an autoimmune process related to *Campylobacter* may play a role in the pathogenesis of some cases of GBS.

Two variants of GBS deserve mention. The first is the Miller-Fischer variant and consists of ophthalmoplegia, ataxia, and arreflexia. The time course is similar to that of GBS. It is interesting that the ataxia occurs in the absence of any obvious cerebellar lesion or extensive large fiber sensory loss. Why typical GBS patients do not develop ophthalmoplegia and these patients do is unknown. Nerve conduction velocities are either normal or mildly slowed in the Miller-Fischer variant. Recently, patients with the Miller-Fischer variant have been shown to have autoantibodies to the ganglioside GQ1b, which may be involved in the pathogenesis of the disease.

A second variant is an acute axonal form of GBS called the acute motor axonal neuropathy (AMAN) syndrome that has recently been discovered in northern China. AMAN patients are particularly likely to have preceding *Campylobacter jejuni* infections and antibodies to GM_1, implicating the *Campylobacter jejuni* infection in the cause of the disease. Cases of the AMAN syndrome are now being reported in North America.

The differential diagnosis of GBS is usually not difficult with the acute onset of a patchy demyelinating neuropathy. However, two rarer disorders can mimic GBS. The first is diphtheria, in which the toxin can induce an acute demyelinating neuropathy. The second is ingestion of buckthorn berries, which are located in temperate regions of the United States.

Chronic Inflammatory Demyelinating Polyneuropathy (CIDP)

Unlike GBS, which is acute, CIDP progresses more slowly, by definition over at least 4 months. Occasionally CIDP cases remit and exacerbate on their own (relapsing CIDP), but most often patients steadily become weaker. Like GBS, CIDP also is associated with asymmetrical slowing on nerve conduction velocities, increased protein with few cells in the CSF, and arreflexia. Unlike GBS, usually a viral illness does not precede CIDP.

Neuropathies Associated with Plasma Cell Dyscrasia

Plasma cell dyscrasia (PCD) is associated with both axonal and acquired demyelinating neuropathies. However, the treatable forms are the demylinating neuropathies. The others will be discussed in the section discussing axonal neuropathies. PCD consists of monoclonal antibodies produced by individual clones of B lymphocytes. These monoclonal antibodies, or M-proteins, are detected by serum protein electrophoresis (SPEP), immunoelectrophoresis (IPEP), and urine protein electrophoresis (UPEP). In some cases the M-proteins invade and damage tissue, causing multiple myeloma or Waldenström's macroglobulinemia. In many other cases, however, the plasma cell dyscrasia is associated with no disease aside from the neuropathy and is termed monoclonal gammopathy of uncertain significance (MGUS). The presence of PCD with neuropathy does not by itself implicate the antibody in the disease. Over 1% of the population older than 50 years have monoclonal gammopathy, frequently with no associated disorder.

NEUROPATHY AND IgM MONOCLONAL GAMMOPATHY (IgM M-PROTEINS)

IgM M-proteins that bind to carbohydrate determinants shared by the myelin-associated glycoprotein (MAG), PO, PMP-22, and a glycolipid termed SGPG are associated with an acquired sensorimotor demyelinating neuropathy that has many features in common with CIDP. The neuropathies are chronic and usually develop over years, beginning with the loss of large and small fiber sensory abnormalities. Weakness does occur and eventually can become debilitating. The IgM M-protein can be shown by Western blot or enzyme-linked immunosorbent assay (ELISA) to bind to the carbohydrate moiety mentioned earlier. The M-protein has also been shown to bind to peripheral nerve by immunohistochemistry and has caused neuropathy when injected into cat nerve or when passively transferred into chicken.

Rare patients with IgM M-proteins have a motor neuropathy that resembles a lower motor neuron form of amyotrophic lateral sclerosis (ALS). These IgM patients have weakness and wasting of muscle and may have fasciculations but have decreased rather than the increased reflexes associated with ALS. The M-protein from these patients binds to GM_1 in ELISA or immuno thin-layer chromatography assays. Some of these patients have been shown to improve following immunotherapy. Other patients with this clinical syndrome but no M-protein have been identified who have polyclonal IgM antibodies that bind to GM_1. Many of these patients have also improved with immunotherapy. Careful multisegment nerve conduction analysis reveals that many, but not all, of the patients have conduction block, suggesting focal demyelination. These cases are usually known as multifocal motor neuropathy (MMN) associated with conduction block, may exist in the absence of antibodies to GM_1, and are worth identifying because they represent a treatable disorder, unlike the ALS they resemble.

Some IgM M-proteins associated with demyelinating neuropathies do not bind to any known antigen in peripheral nerve. Nevertheless these patients may improve when treated with immunotherapy.

NEUROPATHY AND IgG MONOCLONAL GAMMOPATHY (IgG M-PROTEINS)

Most neuropathies with IgG M-proteins are axonal, but there is one important exception; patients with osteosclerotic multiple myeloma and the related POEMS syndrome. About 3% of myeloma patients have sclerotic lesions in bone, and over 50% of these patients have a demyelinating neuropathy that may respond to immunotherapy. When the peripheral neuropathy (P) and myeloma (M) are associated with organomegaly (O), endocrinopathy (E), and skin changes (S), the disorder is called the POEMS syndrome.

Treatment of Demyelinating Neuropathies

In terms of improving the neuropathy, treatment is primarily for the acquired neuropathies, since gene therapy for the inherited neuropathies is not yet a reality.

Guillain-Barré Syndrome

Therapy for the GBS initially is to ensure that respiration is adequate. A vital capacity of less than 1 liter, a negative inspiratory force of less than 30 cm H_2O or the inability to clear pharyngeal secretions is a sign to place a patient in an intensive care unit and consider endotracheal intubation. Because autonomic instability can also be a feature of the disease, cardiac and blood pressure monitoring should also be performed in severely affected patients. Care should be taken to diagnose the syndrome of inappropriate antidiuretic hormone (SIADH). Subcutaneous heparin, pneumatic boots, and other supportive care should be considered in immobilized patients to prevent pulmonary emboli, bed sores, or other complications of immobilization. It is worth remembering that the prognosis for GBS is good, with more than two thirds of patients making a good recovery in the absence of anything more than supportive treatment.

Several multicenter trials in the United States and Europe have shown that plasmapheresis or intravenous gamma globulin (IVIg)* improves the rate and extent of recovery in GBS, particularly when either is given in the first 2 weeks of the disease. Plasmapheresis consists of 5 to 6 exchanges of 3 to 3.5 liters per session over a 10-day period. IVIg is given at a total of 2 grams per kg over 2 to 5 days, depending on the ability of the patient to handle the accompanying fluid load. One cycle of plasma exchange or IVIg is usually enough to treat the patient adequately. About 10% of patients slightly regress after their last treatment and need one more day of exchange or IVIg.

CIDP

The standard treatment for CIDP is corticosteroids, usually oral prednisone. A typical approach is to start the patient on 80 mg per day for 3 months and monitor the patient's strength. If it improves, a gradual taper of 5 mg per week, reducing at first only on alternate days, can be undertaken. Alternate approaches include a trial of low-dose prednisone at 20 mg per day for a few weeks to see if there is improvement, or the use of high-dose intravenous methylprednisolone (Solu-Medrol) pulses, as with multiple sclerosis exacerbations. Cases that are refractory to prednisone are usually treated with stronger immunosuppressive medication, including azathioprine (Imuran),* 2 mg per kg per day, or methotrexate,* 7.5 mg per week. Plasma exchange and IVIg* are not routinely used in treating CIDP, in part because they are expensive, are short lived (need to be repeated every month to 6 weeks), and have not been shown clearly to be effective.

Monoclonal Gammopathy

The demyelinating neuropathies associated with PCD are treated like CIDP. Patients with IgM M-proteins and demyelinating neuropathy, particularly when the M-protein binds to MAG, may not respond to steroids and may need azathioprine (Imuran),* methotrexate, or cyclophosphamide (Cytoxan).* The approach I take, if the symptoms are mild, is to limit the treatment to occupational or physical therapy and be more aggressive if the neuropathy becomes more severe.

In patients with POEMS syndrome, treatments have included prednisone, melphalan,* cyclophos-

---

*Not FDA-approved for this indication.

phamide (Cytoxan),* azathioprine (Imuran),* and radiation of solitary plasmacytomas. In many cases therapy has only halted progression rather than improving the neuropathy.

AXONAL NEUROPATHIES

Symmetrical axonal neuropathies can also be divided into acute, subacute, and chronic forms. Acute axonal neuropathies are unusual. The axonal variant of GBS, the AMAN syndrome, has been discussed. In addition, the acute ingestion of arsenic or thallium can lead to acute neuropathic pain although the resultant neuropathy is more slowly progressive. Axonal neuropathies of acute onset can also occur with porphyria and tick bite paralysis.

The great majority of neuropathies associated with systemic disease caused by metabolic abnormalities, medications, or toxins are axonal neuropathies that occur over months to years. When an axonal neuropathy progresses over more than 5 years, it is more likely to be inherited, although some of the axonal neuropathies associated with systemic disease can progress over this period as well.

Evaluation of Axonal Neuropathies

When the axonal neuropathy is uniform, much of the initial screening is a natural outcome of the patient's initial history, physical examination, and laboratory evaluation (Table 7). For example, it should be clear if the patient is diabetic, has renal failure, or abuses alcohol or other drugs, all of which can lead to neuropathy. It should also be known whether he or she is taking chemotherapeutic agents that can cause neuropathy. SPEP, IPEP, and UPEP are also helpful in diagnosing some cases of axonal neuropathy associated with M-proteins, but these

---

*Not FDA-approved for this indication.

TABLE 7. **Laboratory Evaluation of Axonal Neuropathies**

Necessary Studies
Electroneuromyography (ENMG)
Knowledge of medications and drugs ingested
Routine fasting electrolytes (glucose, creatinine, BUN especially)
Urinalysis
Liver function tests
Sedimentation rate
Antinuclear antibodies
Rheumatoid factor
Useful Studies
Lyme titers
SPEP, IPEP, UPEP, cryoglobulins (see Table 4)
B$_{12}$ assay (consider Schilling's test)
Nerve biopsy (looking for specific abnormalities only)
Urine for porphyrins
Hair sample for arsenic

Modified from Bird SJ, Brown MJ: Peripheral neuropathies. *In* Conn RB (ed): Current Diagnosis 8. Philadelphia, WB Saunders, 1991, pp 992–1004.

cases tend to respond much more poorly to treatment than the demyelinating neuropathies associated with PCD. Sural nerve biopsy can be useful in diagnosing amyloidosis, vasculitis, sarcoidosis, leprosy, or giant axonal neuropathy. However, it should not be used as part of a fishing expedition when there is nothing else that suggests one of these disorders in the patient's evaluation.

Inherited Axonal Neuropathies

Charcot-Marie-Tooth disease type II is an axonal sensorimotor neuropathy that is inherited as an autosomal dominant disorder. Although not as frequent as CMT1A, it is not rare. The clinical presentation is similar to that of CMT1A, with progressive difficulties in running, climbing, or jumping. However, CMT II is likely to come on later in life and may be milder. Patients may not even realize they have a neuropathy but develop many foot and ankle problems in their middle years. The axonal nature of the process is illustrated by normal nerve conduction velocities with reduced CMAP and SNAP amplitudes. Sural nerve biopsy typically reveals axonal loss but not demyelination. The genetic abnormality causing CMT II has not yet been identified so the diagnosis remains clinical. It is often necessary to examine family members carefully to demonstrate the autosomal dominant inheritance pattern.

Axonal neuropathies are associated with other inherited diseases that affect multiple systems. Predominantly sensory axonal neuropathies are a component of Friedreich's ataxia and Fabry's disease. There are also rare hereditary sensory neuropathies that affect both large and small sensory fibers. Familial dysautonomia, known as the Riley-Day syndrome, leads to a degeneration of unmyelinated autonomic and sensory fibers. The Shy-Drager syndrome is a multisystem disorder in which there is autonomic dysfunction secondary to the degeneration of autonomic neurons.

Acquired Axonal Neuropathies

Neuropathies Associated with Systemic Disease

DIABETES MELLITUS

Patients with Type I (insulin dependent) and type II (noninsulin dependent) diabetes frequently develop neuropathies in middle age although the neuropathy can occur earlier. The neuropathies are similar in both Type I and Type II. By far the most frequent is the symmetrical predominantly sensory form that occurs in up to 50% of diabetics. Typically the neuropathy begins with paresthesias and loss of sensation in the feet. In some cases the neuropathy progresses in an ascending fashion. When symptoms or signs reach the knees, problems begin to occur in the fingers. By this time autonomic abnormalities, including orthostatic hypotension, diarrhea, impotence, incontinence, and anhidrosis, may occur. Although weakness is a minor component of the neuropathy, nerve conduction velocities show abnormalities of both sensory and motor nerves. Interpretation of the conduction velocities can be confusing because there is often evidence of both demyelinating and axonal damage. Pathologically, however, the neuropathy appears axonal. The cause of the symmetrical sensory neuropathy is not known but likely involves a combination of vascular and metabolic abnormalities. Speculation on the etiology involves abnormalities of myoinositol or sorbitol pathways, but this remains controversial. Usually, but not always, the more severe neuropathies are associated with poor glucose control.

Diabetic patients may also develop acute mononeuropathies, including mononeuropathy multiplex (see later), although the incidence is much less than with the symmetrical sensory neuropathy. The basis for these mononeuropathies is probably nerve infarction. Typical clinical presentations of these focal neuropathies are ophthalmoplegia (third, fourth, or sixth nerve palsies), proximal leg weakness (femoral neuropathy or "diabetic amyotrophy"), and thoracic pseudoradiculopathy (intercostal neuropathies). The mononeuropathies usually present with pain followed by loss of function of the nerve involved. Thus symptoms may be motor or sensory, depending on the nerve. Gradual recovery of function may occur over a period of months.

Patients with diabetes also are more likely to develop compression neuropathies, such as the carpal tunnel syndrome, tarsal tunnel syndrome, or ulnar neuropathy.

MALIGNANCY

Sensorimotor axonal neuropathies occur in the presence of malignancy, but the association between the two is not always clear. There are, however, cases in which the neuropathy is clearly associated with the malignancy. We have previously discussed the pure sensory neuropathy associated with "anti-Hu" antibodies. This is a paraneoplastic syndrome associated predominantly with small cell carcinoma of the lung. The anti-Hu neuropathy is predominantly large fiber with severely decreased vibration and position sense and has preceded the malignancy by up to 2 years. The osteolytic form of multiple myeloma is associated with neuropathy in over 10% of patients, and this neuropathy is usually axonal. Up to 25% of Waldenström's macroglobulinemia patients have neuropathy, and many of these are axonal. These neuropathies can be sensory or sensorimotor, involve large as well as small fibers, and respond poorly to treatment. Rare lymphoma patients have predominantly motor axonal neuropathies.

Several medications used to treat malignancy are associated with neuropathy. Vincristine (Oncovin) and vinblastine (Velban) cause a neuropathy that begins with paresthesias before evolving into a predominantly motor axonal neuropathy. Cisplatin (Platinol) and paclitaxel (Taxol) cause predominantly large fiber sensory neuropathy.

COLLAGEN VASCULAR DISEASE

Collagen vascular diseases also cause mononeuritis multiplex, which will be discussed separately. However, up to 50% of patients with polyarteritis nodosa (PAN) have axonal neuropathy, which can be the presenting system. Wegener's granulomatosis, Churg-Strauss vasculitis, and hypersensitivity vasculitis can be associated with axonal neuropathies. Approximately 10% of patients with systemic lupus erythematosus (SLE) have neuropathy. Rheumatoid arthritis is associated with an increased frequency of entrapment syndromes. Sjögren's syndrome may be accompanied by a large fiber sensory neuropathy. Although not classically a collagen vascular disease, the inflammatory disorder sarcoidosis may be associated with a sensorimotor axonal neuropathy or polyradiculopathy.

AMYLOIDOSIS

Primary amyloidosis is caused by mutations in the transthyretin gene. Acquired amyloidosis is associated with deposits of monoclonal antibodies. Both are associated with small fiber sensory and autonomic neuropathies. Predominant symptoms are painful dysesthesias accompanied by impotence.

INFECTION

Virtually every patient with HIV infection will develop a peripheral neuropathy in the course of the disease. At the time of seroconversion, there is susceptibility to develop the Guillain-Barré syndrome. However, after the CD4 count has dropped below 400, all patients develop a predominantly small fiber sensory axonal neuropathy associated with painful dysesthesias and decreased sensation to pain and temperature. The cause of the neuropathy is unknown. Some patients with acquired immunodeficiency syndrome (AIDS) develop a painful lumbosacral polyradiculopathy caused by cytomegalovirus (CMV) infection. The medications ddI (2'3' dideoxyinosine), ddC (2'3' dideoxycytidine), and d4T (2'3' didehydro-2'3' dideoxythymidine) used to treat AIDS all induce dose-dependent, painful sensory neuropathies that mimic the small fiber sensory neuropathy associated with the disease itself.

Lyme disease, caused by infection with the tick-borne spirochete *Borrelia burgdorferi,* can give rise to multiple cranial neuropathies and mononeuritis multiplex. Axonal sensorimotor neuropathies have been reported in occasional patients.

Leprosy is the most common cause of neuropathy in the world and is increasingly present in the United States. The neuropathy is axonal, occurs in the lepromatous form of the disease, and is caused by direct infection of the nerve by *Mycobacterium leprae.* Since the bacteria grow best at 36° C, the neuropathy predominantly affects the cooler (distal) portion of the extremities.

METABOLIC DISEASES

The predominant metabolic disorders associated with neuropathy are renal, hepatic, and thyroid diseases. Patients with renal failure are likely to develop an axonal sensorimotor neuropathy that is painful and may progress to involve large fiber sensory modalities and even weakness. The chances for neuropathy are increased if the renal failure progresses to the point at which the patient needs dialysis or transplantation. However, patients with long-standing elevations of creatinine (>2) are susceptible to develop these neuropathies.

The porphyrias (acute intermittent, variegate, and coproporphyric) are associated with predominantly motor axonal neuropathies that may affect the arms more than the legs. Barbiturates, anesthesia, or other drugs may precipitate the neuropathy.

Hypothyroidism may be associated with axonal neuropathy, although increased frequencies of entrapment syndromes are more likely sequelae.

Neuropathies Associated with Toxins

ALCOHOLIC NEUROPATHY

Ethanol is the predominant toxin causing neuropathy. It is associated with chronic alcohol abuse, and most patients have ingested at least 100 mL of ethanol for at least 3 years. The neuropathy is symmetrical and predominantly sensory in early stages, affecting both small and large fibers. Eventually weakness also occurs. Both sensory and motor loss are length dependent, with initial symptoms occurring in the feet. Painful paresthesias are a frequent early feature of the neuropathy. Whether the neuropathy is caused by the alcohol itself or by associated vitamin deficiencies remains unclear.

VITAMIN DEFICIENCIES

Sensorimotor axonal neuropathies occur with thiamine, pyridoxine, folate, and pantothenic acid deficiencies. These neuropathies frequently present with painful dysesthesias. They are rare in the United States unless associated with alcoholism, malabsorption, or fad diets. Vitamin B_6 deficiency can occur when isoniazid therapy is given without supplementation of the vitamin. Vitamin B_{12} deficiency can induce a large fiber sensory neuropathy as part of a combined system degeneration. Vitamin E deficiency, usually from malabsorption, results in a large fiber sensory neuropathy associated with ataxia.

HEAVY METAL INGESTION

Lead ingestion induces a motor neuropathy that appears axonal in adults, who are likely to present with bilateral wrist drops. It is interesting that in children and laboratory animals, lead appears to induce a demyelinating neuropathy. Patients who survive acute arsenic or thallium ingestion develop a painful, predominantly sensory axonal neuropathy. Organic mercury poisoning may cause axonal sensorimotor neuropathy in addition to CNS damage. In all these situations, neuropathy rarely occurs without intensive exposure and involvement of other systems besides the PNS.

MEDICATIONS

We have previously discussed axonal neuropathies associated with medications used to treat HIV and malignancy. Other medications are also associated with axonal neuropathy. The antibiotics or antifungal agents amphotericin, ethambutol, and chloroquine cause axonal neuropathies. Chronic metronidazole treatment for Crohn's disease may cause sensory neuropathy. Dapsone, used in the treatment of leprosy or skin diseases, can cause a pure motor neuropathy. Sulfonamide or nitrofurantoin may cause axonal neuropathies. Phenytoin (Dilantin) leads to a sensorimotor axonal neuropathy after many years of usage. Seafood (usually large tropical fish like grouper) containing ciguatera toxin may cause a painful sensory axonal neuropathy. Ingestion of the rat poison vacor leads to a severe small fiber sensory and autonomic neuropathy with orthostatic hypotension as a predominant feature.

Mononeuritis Multiplex

Asymmetric neuropathies in which some peripheral nerves are spared and others damaged are called mononeuritis multiplex. Most of these are axonal and will be discussed in this section. The demyelinating forms, like the GBS or CIDP, have been discussed in the section on acquired demyelinating neuropathies. The most frequent causes of axonal mononeuritis multiplex are diabetes mellitus and the collagen vascular diseases, which have also been discussed earlier. Other causes of mononeuritis multiplex include mixed cryoglobulinemia and inflammatory diseases such as sarcoid and leprosy. Causes of mononeuritis multiplex are listed in Table 8.

Treatment of Axonal Neuropathies

Treatment of many axonal neuropathies consists of reversing the problem that caused the neuropathy. For example, neuropathies associated with diabetes are often less severe if the blood glucose is well controlled, and alcoholic neuropathies may arrest if ethanol abuse is discontinued and the diet improves. Similarly, if medications, drugs, or vitamin deficiencies that cause neuropathies can be discontinued or

TABLE 8. **Axonal Causes of Mononeuritis Multiplex**

Diabetes mellitus
Vasculitis
    Polyneuritis nodosa (PAN)
    Wegener's granulomatosis
    Allergic granulomatous angiitis (Churg-Strauss)
    Rheumatoid arthritis
Chronic inflammatory
    Sarcoidosis
Infectious
    HIV (cytomegalovirus)
    Leprosy
Cryoglobulinemia
Amphetamine abuse
Tumors (myeloma, neurofibromatosis)

reversed, it is likely that the neuropathy will at least stabilize. In collagen vascular diseases with multisystem involvement (e.g., SLE, rheumatoid arthritis), the treatment of the neuropathy is the treatment of the collagen vascular disease itself. In cases of vasculitis that affect only peripheral nerve, treatment approaches have included corticosteroids, azathioprine (Imuran),* and cyclophosphamide (Cytoxan).

The treatment of painful dysesthesias in axonal neuropathies deserves special mention. A group of medications has been used to treat these dysesthesias, and few have been studied carefully. Amitriptyline (Elavil)* is probably the drug of choice to begin treatment. Usually doses begin at 10 mg at bedtime and are increased every few days until the pain disappears or side effects are reached. Typical side effects are drowsiness or difficulty starting a stream when urinating. Heart block and difficulty urinating are contraindications. Nortriptyline (Pamelor)* has also been used effectively. Mexiletine (Mexitil),* an oral form of lidocaine, is being increasingly used to treat dysesthetic neuropathy. A cardiac history can be a contraindication. Tremulousness, gastrointestinal discomfort, and confusion are side effects. Other medications that help some people are phenytoin (Dilantin),* carbamazepine (Tegretol),* and topical capsaicin (Zostrix). Transcutaneous electrical nerve stimulators (TENS units) also are occasionally helpful. Which of these treatments will be effective is difficult to predict in an individual patient, and management of dysesthetic pain often involves trial and error.

Rehabilitation in Patients with Neuropathy

Physical and rehabilitation medicine, with accompanying occupational and physical therapy, is often an essential component of therapy. Ankle and foot orthoses, canes, walkers, and wheelchairs can keep patients ambulatory or independent. Debilitated patients can be helped to dress, write, or feed themselves with assistance from occupational therapy. If proper rehabilitation facilities are not available or not staffed with professionals who are used to seeing neuromuscular disease, it is difficult to give proper care to many patients with neuropathy.

---

*Not FDA-approved for this indication.

ACUTE HEAD INJURIES IN ADULTS

method of
RICHARD F. CODY, Jr., M.D., and
M. SEAN GRADY, M.D.
University of Washington
Seattle, Washington

Trauma is the leading cause of death for the 15- to 40-year-old age group, with traumatic brain injury (TBI) comprising a significant portion of morbidity and mortality.

TBI is classified into three categories: mild, moderate, and severe, based on the Glasgow Coma Scale (GCS), a simple, neurologically based scoring system (Table 1). In addition, a large portion of patients with TBI may be placed in a "trivial" category. Correlation of predicted outcome with degree of acute injury may be difficult: some patients with altered mental status (MS) but minimal intracranial injury on computed tomography (CT) scan may fare quite poorly, whereas some patients whose initial CT scans show apparent dramatic injury may recover fully. Rapid diagnosis and appropriate treatment can help minimize pathophysiologic events, and they yield the greatest probability for a favorable outcome for any given level of TBI.

INITIAL ASSESSMENT AND DIAGNOSIS

When evaluating a patient with either isolated head trauma or multiple trauma, immediate attention must focus on "ABCs"—Airway, Breathing, and Circulation—critical to basic life support. In addition, the spinal column should be protected *and treated as though it were injured* until clinically and (if necessary) radiographically cleared. Initial protection is usually accomplished by emergency medical technicians at the injury scene by applying a "Philadelphia" hard cervical collar and placing the patient on a rigid board.

Once ABCs and spinal precautions have been addressed, assessment of the GCS should be performed. Sometimes verbal and/or eye-opening responses are unobtainable, e.g., intubation, massive facial trauma, or pharmacologic paralysis. In these situations, the motor component of the GCS is an accurate descriptor of the severity of injury and may be used alone to provide a clear description of the injury. For example, if a patient with isolated facial trauma is intubated and his eyes are swollen shut but he is alert and following commands briskly, his GCS would be $V_1E_1M_6 = 8$. By separating and recording the GCS into its individual components, as well as its sum, the most accurate picture of a patient's neurologic status will be recorded.

Emergency department (ED) radiographic assessment should include a lateral cervical spine radiograph (with visualization from the occiput down to the first thoracic vertebra) and, if the patient has been intubated, an anteroposterior (AP) chest radiograph. In cases of penetrating trauma to the head or suspected skull fracture, AP and lateral skull films may be obtained, but head CT remains the best diagnostic test for bone or parenchymal damage. Head CT scans (without intravenous contrast dye) should be obtained in cases of decreased mental status, or if the patient's examination is clouded by psychoactive drugs (including alcohol). Brain, blood, and bone windows can be obtained from the same CT scan protocol and provide needed information for adequately visualizing the cranial vault structures.

TRIVIAL HEAD TRAUMA

Diagnosis. Patients classified with trivial TBI should have no loss of consciousness (LOC), score a GCS of 15, and be alert, oriented, and following commands briskly for the examiner. No visible or palpable skull fracture should be present. CT scans are not usually obtained unless the mechanism of injury suggests a strong possibility of delayed intracranial contusion (e.g., high-speed motor vehicle accident with ejection of patient from vehicle, or blow to head with significant swelling/hematoma). Other indications for CT scans in trivial TBI include elderly

TABLE 1. **The Glasgow Coma Scale**

Points Awarded	Verbal Response	Eye Opening	Motor Response
1	Unresponsive	Unresponsive	Unresponsive
2	Incomprehensible sounds	Opens to painful stimuli	Extensor posturing (to pain)
3	Scattered or inappropriate words	Opens to voice	Flexor posturing (to pain)
4	Speech fluent but confused	Opens spontaneously	Withdraws nonpurposefully (to pain)
5	Alert, fluent speech		Purposeful response; localizes pain (e.g., clearly reaches to grab examiner's hand)
6			Follows commands
GCS score = SUM	Verbal Score (1–5)	Eye Score (1–4)	Motor Score (1–6)

Points are assigned in each category for the patient's best response to stimuli (e.g., sternal rub in the apparently comatose patient). The minimum score is 3 (completely unresponsive); the maximum is 15 (no apparent mental status deficits).

From Teasdale G, Jennett B: Assessment of coma and impaired consciousness. Lancet 2:81–84, 1974. © by The Lancet Ltd., 1974.

patients, alcoholics, and patients on blood thinners such as warfarin (Coumadin) or with bleeding disorders.

Treatment. These patients may usually be discharged to home if they have responsible individuals with them who can watch them for the first 6 hours after injury. They do not need further observation or nighttime periodic awakenings if this period passes uneventfully. If any signs of MS decline are present, they should immediately return to the ED.

Major or complicated scalp lacerations with good hemostasis may be referred to plastic surgery for ideal cosmetic closure. If emergency hemostasis is needed, several vertical mattress skin stitches with 0 to 2-0 monofilament nylon (Ethicon) may be inserted.

If repair is attempted, the wound margins should be anesthetized with bupivacaine (Marcaine) 0.5% with epinephrine, and/or lidocaine 1% with epinephrine (if the patient is not allergic to these substances) and the wound thoroughly irrigated with sterile normal saline solution. The wound should be explored and foreign bodies removed. If the galea (the tough fascia overlying the skull) is torn, it should be repaired in a sterile fashion with 3-0 braided polyglycolic acid suture (Vicryl, Dexon) in interrupted, inverted vertical mattress stitches. Large lacerations should be approximated with subcutaneous interrupted, inverted vertical mattress stitches using the same suture material. Skin should be closed with 3-0 monofilament nylon in either simple interrupted stitches or a running, locked stitch. Instruct the patient to return for a wound check in 2 days and to return for skin suture removal in 7 to 10 days. The patient should not immerse the head in water for 2 days and should keep the wound area clean and dry. Prophylactic antibiotics may be administered (e.g., cephalexin [Keflex], 500 mg orally every 6 hours for 7 days) in notably dirty wounds; in addition, parenteral antibiotics (e.g., cefazolin [Ancef], 1 gram intramuscularly or intravenously) may be given prior to wound closure. Tetanus immunization status should be checked and a booster administered if more than 5 years has elapsed since the patient's last immunization.

MILD HEAD INJURY

Diagnosis. Patients with mild head injury should have a presenting GCS of 13 to 15 and no longer than 30 minutes total of postinjury amnesia or LOC. The patient should be able to follow commands. Guidelines for obtaining CT scans are similar to those just described for trivial head injury; if one is obtained, it should be entirely normal.

Treatment. The patients may be discharged to home if there are responsible people with them who can diligently assess their MS every 1 to 2 hours for the first 24 hours after injury, including waking them up at night for MS checks. If no such individuals are present, if probable compliance with discharge instructions is in question, or if the patient is impaired by psychoactive drugs, she or he should be admitted overnight for observation. If discharged, patients and families should be educated to the signs and symptoms of increased intracranial pressure and the need to return to the ED immediately in case of MS decline.

MODERATE TRAUMATIC BRAIN INJURY

Diagnosis. These patients have a presenting GCS of 9 to 12 and a combined LOC/postinjury amnesia of between 30 minutes and 6 hours. A skull fracture may be present. An emergency CT is standard; if any intracranial bleeding exists, the patient is then classified as having severe TBI.

Treatment. In the ED, a wide-bore peripheral intravenous line (intravenously) should be inserted. If the patient's MS deteriorates from initial presentation, there is a decrease of 2 or more points in the GCS, and/or abnormal pupillary dilation occurs, mannitol (Osmitrol) 20% solution, 200 mL intravenous bolus, may be administered, and a new CT scan immediately obtained. If an epidural hematoma (EDH) is suspected—the classic presentation is a patient with a lucid interval following a significant application of force to the head, with acute neurologic decline and pupillary anisocoria (dilated ipsilateral to injury)—an immediate CT scan is indicated, likely followed by an emergency burr hole and/or craniotomy for decompression. Patients with EDH may do very well if timely drainage is provided; however, due to their rapidly expanding nature (they are usually due to arterial rupture), they may induce uncal herniation and irreversible brain damage within 15 to 30 minutes if untreated.

SEVERE TRAUMATIC BRAIN INJURY

Diagnosis. Severe head injury is manifested by a presenting GCS of 8 or less, or a combined LOC/postinjury amnesia of more than 6 hours. Many of these patients may be intubated by paramedics en route to the ED; if not, they should be intubated on arrival at the ED. Multiple injuries are often present, and a team approach involving trauma surgeons, orthopedic surgeons, and neurosurgeons is frequently applied; a rapid, emergency diagnostic peritoneal lavage (DPL) may be performed by the trauma surgeon if gross intra-abdominal blood loss is suspected. Multiple large-bore peripheral intravenous lines and a urethral (Foley) catheter may be quickly inserted. Once the patient is hemodynamically stabilized, an emergency CT scan is obtained.

The initial neurologic evaluation in the ED of a patient with severe TBI includes GCS, brain stem reflexes (pupillary, corneal, and gag), and assessment of motor and reflex function in extremities, if possible. If patients have been given paralytic agents (e.g., pancuronium [Pavulon]), pupillary reactivity will be the only objective index available until the paralytics are metabolized. In entirely unreactive patients (GCS = 3) without paralytic agents, one should consider the possibility of a high spinal cord injury. Absence of a bulbocavernosus reflex should heighten this suspicion in this situation. Because of the greatly increased yield of information, patients who require administration of paralytic agents should be first examined by the consulting neurosurgeon before these agents are given, if possible.

Treatment. If an acute subdural hematoma (SDH) or EDH is present, the patient may need an emergency craniotomy for evacuation of these blood clots in the operating room (OR). Intracranial operations may be performed simultaneously with any life-saving operative procedures by other specialties (e.g., emergency laparotomy for a positive diagnostic peritoneal lavage).

ED goals in severe TBI include maximizing the patient's cerebral perfusion pressure (CPP), or the amount of blood available to the brain. The CPP is the patient's mean arterial pressure (MAP) minus the intracranial pressure (ICP). Insertion of an arterial line and an intraparenchymal ICP monitor (Camino monitor) may be done quickly at the ED bedside to obtain these values. Normal ICP is 20 mmHg or less. Sustained ICP above 20 may lead to reduced CPP and, if high enough, cerebral ischemia and/or uncal herniation. ICP may be controlled by three main methods:

1. *Head elevation*: The head of the bed should be elevated at least 30 to 45 degrees (more if needed and if the patient's blood pressure tolerates it). This helps increase venous return from the brain owing to increased gravitational force.

2. *Hyperventilation*: Hyperventilation (to Pa_{CO_2} of 30% to 35%) induces vasoconstriction and helps reduce cerebral edema.

3. *Osmotic therapy*: Bolus intravenous administration of mannitol 20% solution (up to 1 gram per kg initially) helps reduce parenchymal water, drawing it into the blood vessels, thus reducing edema. Mannitol may be given every 2 to 4 hours if needed, 100 to 200 mL per dose, to maintain ICP at 20 or less. Mannitol should be held if the systolic blood pressure (SBP) is less than 100, serum sodium 152 or greater, or serum osmolality 310 or less. A Foley catheter *must* be inserted into the patient's bladder prior to initiating mannitol therapy.

Several other treatments that have been previously used by some to treat high ICPs are discussed:

1. *Barbiturates*: Barbiturates play no role in the management of acute head injury. (They are rarely used in tertiary care neurosurgical settings and then only when a patient's ICP remains elevated despite all medical and surgical attempts to normalize ICP.)

2. *Steroids*: Steroids (e.g., glucocorticoids) are not indicated in the management of TBI. They do not improve outcome or reduce ICP.

Disposition of the TBI Patient

Who to transfer to tertiary care facilities?

1. All patients with moderate or severe TBI, unless a neurosurgeon and critical care facilities are available.

2. Any patient, regardless of severity, with signs or symptoms suggestive of acute or delayed TBI, and evaluated in a hospital without definitive imaging or neurosurgical care.

When to transfer?

As soon as possible, once the need for experienced neurosurgical care has been established. Patients with suspected expanding intracranial bleeding should be transported with the utmost haste; the neurosurgeon or trauma surgeon at the destination hospital may assist in rapid deployment of helicopters, fixed-wing aircraft, or other appropriate means of transportation.

Recent Advances in TBI Treatment

1. *New drugs*: Multicenter, randomized controlled trials of tirilazad and PEG SOD (polyethylene glycol succinate/conjugated superoxide dismutase) have shown these substances to be ineffective in reducing damage or improving outcome after TBI. Trials are currently under way for Selfotel, an *N*-methyl D-aspartate (NMDA) channel blocker.

2. *Hypothermia*: Trials are being conducted examining the effect of induced hypothermia in patients with TBI.

3. *Guidelines for the Management of Severe Head Injury*, published by the Brain Trauma Foundation, provides an accurate and up-to-date synopsis of the applicable standards, guidelines, and treatment options for managing TBI. This text, scheduled to be

published in 1996, is the source of many of our recommendations in this chapter.

PEDIATRIC HEAD INJURY

method of
A. LOREN AMACHER, M.D., and
GARY R. SIMONDS, M.D.
Geisinger Medical Center
Danville, Pennsylvania

Fully 25,000 American children sustain mortal or crippling head injuries every year, and this figure does not include homicide and suicide statistics. Despite the age of the victim, the neurons of a child's brain are just as irreplaceable as those of an adult. No medical treatment, and no surgical intervention to date, have been successful in reanimating or replacing dead neurons. Nerve cell loss at the time of initial impact is known as *primary cerebral injury*. The only effective measure presently known to limit this type of injury is *prevention*. Through more aggressive education, public health policies, and enforcement, the devastating swath cut by this disease through the young of our society could be reduced significantly. Simple measures such as the routine use of child car seats and seat belts in automobile travel, and protective helmets in biking, roller skating, and sledding, should be actively promoted by all physicians. The scourges of child abuse and violent crime must also be aggressively addressed.

Clinical manifestations of primary injury include cortical contusions, brain laceration, brain stem contusion, and diffuse axonal shear injuries. Too often, the effects of these injuries are compounded by progressive neuronal loss, known as *secondary cerebral injury*, resulting from factors such as hypoxia, hypoperfusion, increased intracranial pressure (ICP), expansile masses (hematomas and contusions), infection, hydrocephalus, seizures, fever, hyperglycemia, and oxygen-species free radical formation. Currently the principal goal of therapy in pediatric head injury is the prevention and management of this secondary loss of nerve cells. To this end, treatment must begin in the field and continue throughout the course of care. All teams involved in the treatment of the head-injured child must understand this goal. Aggressive treatment to limit secondary injury will ensure the maximum functional return of surviving neurons and allow the child to achieve as optimal a recovery as possible.

Pediatric head injury is not necessarily a miniature version of the disease in adults. Pathophysiologic factors such as head to body weight ratio, skull thickness, white matter myelination, cerebral water content, functional plasticity, and regional blood flow are different from those of adults. Deterioration from good neurologic status and surgical mass lesions may occur less frequently in children, but post-traumatic seizures and diffuse cerebral edema seem to be more common. Therefore, head-injured children should be cared for by teams experienced in pediatric trauma evaluation, resuscitation, and treatment. Furthermore, special consideration must be given to factors such as the understanding, fear, and cooperation level of a young child and the involvement and support of the parent.

SEVERE CLOSED-HEAD INJURY

Closed-head injury is generally categorized as mild (Glasgow Coma Scale 13 to 15), moderate (GCS 9 to 12), or severe (GCS 3 to 8). A child with a severe closed-head injury is a medical, and potentially surgical, emergency. The airway must be secured, and the child must be resuscitated. Assessment for and immediate treatment of shock is critical. Shock is as devastating to the brain as it is to the other organs and must be corrected as the first priority. Hypoperfusion and hypo-oxygenation of the contused brain extend primary injury. Elevated cerebral lactate levels are toxic to neurons. Good oxygenation and perfusion should be the goal, starting in the field whenever possible.

On arrival at the trauma center, the trauma team must evaluate the child for associated multiple injuries. Although associated spine injuries may be uncommon in the very young, the neck should be stabilized in all cases and "cleared" appropriately.

Neurologic examination should include the Glasgow Coma Scale (especially the motor responses), evaluation of the pupil and corneal reflexes, and inspection of the head. The head should be examined for open wounds, bleeding sources, cerebrospinal fluid (CSF) leak, and Battle's (periauricular/mastoidal ecchymosis) and raccoon (periorbital ecchymosis) signs. Active scalp bleeding can lead to exsanguination with alarming rapidity in the young.

Protective intubation and hyperventilation to a Pa_{CO_2} of 30 should be initiated. If there is a history of rapid decline in sensorium, progressive focal deficit, or a dilated pupil (i.e., suspicion of expansile focal lesion), intravenous (IV) mannitol (Osmitrol), 0.25 to 0.5 gram per kg with or without IV furosemide (Lasix), 0.25 mg per kg (1/4 mg/kg) should be administered if the patient is hemodynamically stable. Emergency computed tomography (CT) of the head without contrast should be obtained at the earliest possible time. Magnetic resonance imaging (MRI) has no role in the initial imaging of the brain-injured child. A patient must not be transported for tests or imaging prior to airway access and resuscitation.

If CT scan of the head reveals a traumatic lesion with mass effect and shift (epidural hematoma, subdural hematoma, intercerebral hematoma, large contusion), a neurosurgeon should be consulted immediately, and mannitol, 0.25 to 0.5 gram per kg, and furosemide, 0.25 mg per kg, should be administered IV. Generally these types of lesions will be evacuated unless timing and examination suggest a hopeless situation. Small extra-axial hematomas or intraparenchymal contusions or clots may be treated conservatively if felt by the neurosurgeon to be a minor factor in the overall picture. Often these are simply signs of associated severe pulping or tearing of the parenchyma at the time of the primary injury, and their removal will be of no benefit to the patient.

The original CT may show only cerebral swelling with scattered deep white matter contusions. With a low GCS, this is the hallmark of a diffuse axonal shear injury. This is a severe injury to thousands of axons across wide neuronal fields, caused by the nature and violence of the initial trauma. Prognosis in this category is guarded at best.

Severe closed-head injury often is complicated by increased intracranial pressure (ICP). Increased ICP results from uncompensated expansion of the intracranial volume. The brain originally buffers the addition of blood or edema to the intracranial contents by expelling intravascular venous volume or CSF. When the buffering capacity is overcome, the pressure in the cranial vault rises sharply. Depending on the rate and degree of rise, elevated ICP is poorly tolerated and can result in irreversible secondary brain injury, cerebral herniation, and death.

In a child with a severe brain injury and CT evidence of significant cerebral edema (e.g., diffuse edema, loss of basilar cisterns), an ICP monitor should be placed to aid in ICP control. The goal of management is to keep the cerebral perfusion pressure (mean arterial pressure minus ICP) over 50, and the ICP below 20. Maintenance of the cerebral perfusion pressure (CPP) is paramount. ICP may be monitored using fiberoptic intraparenchymal systems (e.g., the Camino system), ventriculostomy, or subarachnoid "bolts." Ventriculostomy allows ICP measurement as well as a degree of control via CSF drainage, although this effect may be short-lived, with progressive obliteration of the ventricles by tissue edema.

Methods of ICP control include the following measures, often instituted serially: (1) head of bed raised and head kept straight with no cervical restrictions, to increase venous outflow. (2) Intubation, sedation, muscle paralysis must be reversed periodically to assess neurologic level. Generally this is an effective ICP control measure in patients with reversible injuries. (3) Hyperventilation to Pa_{CO_2} of 28 to 30. There is evidence that prolonged hyperventilation (24 hours) may be detrimental due to a vasoconstrictive effect in cerebral capillaries and arterioles; thus once ICP is under control the Pa_{CO_2} should be allowed gradually to rise toward 40. (4) Mannitol and furosemide boluses or drip. The patient, however, should not be "dried out." Hypovolemia will depress cerebral perfusion and may lead to P_{CO_2} elevation from A-V pulmonary shunting. Fluids should be replaced to maintain intravascular volume while keeping the serum osmolarity between 300 and 310 and sodium between 140 and 146. (5) Intermittent CSF drainage via ventriculostomy.

If the ICP remains poorly controlled, the use of pressors to raise the CPP may have a role. Finally, the use of metabolic coma may be considered as a last resort. This involves the administration of etomidate (Amidate) or pentobarbital to a serum level that results in the electroencephalographic (EEG) pattern of burst-suppression. If ICP is not controlled at EEG burst-suppression, higher concentrations of barbiturate will be ineffective. Barbiturate coma, once deemed a panacea, carries the threat of hemodynamic instability, loss of pulmonary and cerebral vascular autoregulation, and interference with white cell function.

When all of the preceding measures fail to control ICP, the child is unlikely to survive. Some authorities favor hypothermia in refractory ICP cases, but the purported benefits of such therapy remain unproved. Complications include cardiovascular instability, pulmonary compromise, and infection. Fever, however, should be aggressively treated with acetaminophen and cooling blankets. Steroids have no role in the acutely head-injured child. They offer no proven benefit, and their use can be complicated by hyperglycemic neuronal injury, depression of white cell function, and gastric ulceration.

ICP monitoring can be a two-edged sword. Many children remain intubated and sedated for unnecessarily long periods. ICPs creep up as children begin to awaken and struggle against the ventilator or restraints, resulting in further sedation and ICP monitoring rather than reassessment of neurologic function. Generally, a child who is awake enough to grab at and pull out a monitor no longer needs it. Similarly, an increase in ICP when a patient is turned or suctioned should not send care givers into a panic of barbiturate administration. ICP can be very sensitive to patient manipulations. Boluses of lidocaine,* 1.5 mg per kg IV, or a short-acting barbiturate given prior to required patient care activities will usually prevent the ICP pressure spikes.

Throughout the pediatric intensive care unit course of a child with a severe closed-head injury, perhaps the most important factors involved in the eventual outcome involve the supportive care provided. A multisystem approach must be maintained. Nutrition should be started within the first 48 hours. A schedule of frequent turning, when tolerated, prevents skin breakdown. Pulmonary toilet and rotation of lines are extremely important. Fevers are common but are seldom "central" and thus must be pursued aggressively with specific cultures and antibiotic therapy when indicated. Physical and occupational therapy is begun early to help preserve flexibility and prevent contractures.

Prophylactic administration of anticonvulsants is generally reserved for children exhibiting repetitive seizure activity. Their administration has not been shown to reduce long-term incidence of post-traumatic epilepsy and may cause drug-related fevers, rashes, and elevated liver enzyme levels. Persistent or repetitive seizures, however, can result in secondary injury and must be vigorously pursued and treated. EEG should be obtained with any suspicion of seizure activity.

CT scans should be repeated 24 to 48 hours after the initial injury, then at day 4 or 5, then weekly until the patient is improving or completely stabilized. CT is repeated promptly with any sudden unexplained rise in ICP or deterioration in neurologic status. Delayed hemorrhage may occur in the first week or later following the initial injury, and hydrocephalus may develop at any time. Diffuse cerebral contusion may induce coagulopathy, probably through the arachidonic acid cascade.

EEG or somatosensory evoked potential (SSEP)

---

*Not FDA-approved for this indication.

evaluation may be useful for prognosis, especially in children whose examinations remain compromised despite normalizing ICPs. However, no single test or test battery can predict functional outcome consistently and accurately. The strongest predictors still remain the child's original neurologic status and pupillary function. Children with low GCSs and pupillary abnormalities are at high risk of poor outcomes. Children with unmanageable or poorly controlled ICPs also fare poorly. When the injury is too severe for recovery, the family of the child should be prepared and supported with the assistance of all available ancillary services. They must understand that children who survive severe closed-head injuries may make excellent motor recoveries but usually have significant intellectual and psychosocial deficits on long-term testing.

MODERATE CLOSED-HEAD INJURY

Head-injured children who are neurologically compromised and are not in coma deserve aggressive evaluation and care. These children should survive their injuries but are at distinct risk of early or late deterioration from expansile lesions, increased cerebral swelling, or sequelae of associated injuries. Full trauma team involvement is paramount. A neurosurgeon must be involved. After initial evaluation and stabilization, a child in this category should be transferred to a trauma center with the resources to handle potential serious sequelae.

After establishment of airway access and resuscitation, a CT scan of the head must be obtained at the earliest juncture. Significant cerebral lesions should trigger early neurosurgical consultation. If the initial CT scan shows no operative lesion, the child should be admitted to an intensive care unit and monitored closely. Heavy sedation or paralyzing agents should be avoided. These agents deprive the clinician of the all-important neurologic examination. If at any time during the course of the child's illness progressive neurologic deficits develop, a space-occupying lesion (hematoma) should be assumed. Mannitol and furosemide should be administered, strong consideration given to intubation and hyperventilation (especially if the level of consciousness is diminished), and an emergency CT scan obtained. Persistent neurologic deficit in the face of a normal CT scan may be an indication for MRI imaging or other studies (such as arteriography to look for carotid dissection). MRI provides superior information regarding the extent and severity of tissue injury.

Children who recover from moderate closed-head injury (CHI) have a significant risk of long-term neuropsychological dysfunction. Aggressive neuropsychological evaluation should be pursued throughout the admission and follow-up. Appropriate rehabilitation services should be enlisted.

MILD CLOSED-HEAD INJURY

The phenomenon of the patient who "talks and dies" is rare in children. Nonetheless there is no such thing as a "trivial head injury" in a child. Mild head injury in children is too often taken very lightly in our society, especially in the sports arena. A child who has had his "bell rung" or is "dinged" has sustained a concussion or worse, and may suffer long-term sequelae. Thus all mild head injuries deserve the full attention of the treating physician.

A "hair-trigger" on ordering a CT scan in evaluation is recommended. A child who is neurologically normal may still be harboring an expanding extra-axial hematoma. It is prudent to CT scan all children who have sustained a loss of consciousness, who have a neurologic deficit, or whose mechanism of injury is significant (e.g., fall from bicycle to pavement on head). Children with a neurologic deficit or a history of a loss of consciousness longer than 20 seconds should be admitted for observation despite normal CT scan findings. CT scan windows should be adjusted to look for acute extra-axial hematomas that can be "averaged" (obscured) by the adjacent bone. Skull radiographs need not be routinely obtained.

Parents should be instructed thoroughly in the phenomenon of pediatric response to mild closed-head injury (i.e., headache, lethargy, and vomiting), and postconcussive syndrome (poor concentration, headaches, blurred vision, mood swings, sleepiness, potentially for several weeks). Follow-up is mandatory.

A concussion is a traumatically induced alteration in consciousness, usually a temporary loss of consciousness or confusion. No child should be sent back into a sporting event immediately after a concussion. At least six weeks for recovery is required. A second concussion within six weeks has a more deleterious effect on memory and learning than does the first. Any child who has sustained two or more concussions in any sport should give up that sport.

PENETRATING INJURIES

Sadly, penetrating head injuries have become more common in our pediatric population. Primary brain injury in gunshot wounds (GSW) is related to the velocity and spin of the projectile, less so to its mass. Higher velocity missiles may invoke tremendous damage remote from their tracts through the brain. A grim prognosis generally accompanies primary injuries that involve high velocity missiles (assault rifles), multilobe damage, transventricular missile tracts, bihemispheric tracts, or diencephalic or brain stem tracts. The focus of therapy lies in the prevention and management of secondary cerebral injury. Secondary injury typically occurs from hypoxia, hypoperfusion, expansile hematomas, diffuse intravascular coagulopathy (DIC), diffuse edema, raised ICP, seizure activity, abscess formation, meningitis, and rarely traumatic aneurysms.

Gunshot wounds must be treated at a trauma center. Full trauma and neurosurgery team evaluation must be initiated immediately. An adequate airway is essential. Those with depressed levels of consciousness should be intubated. Resuscitation must be initiated promptly and aggressively. Children can lose an alarming amount of blood from scalp and brain injuries. The entry and exit sites should be dressed to discourage blood loss and infection. A CT scan of the head must be obtained and should include brain and bone "windows."

Salvageable patients who are deteriorating from expansile hematomas require emergency decompression. Blood products, including platelets, fresh-frozen plasma, and cryoprecipitate must be available in the event of associated DIC. Stable patients undergo urgent débridement of the entry and exit sites with the goal of removal of as much superficial in-driven bone and necrotic brain as safely possible, and dural repair. Débridement of deep injury or the entire tract is seldom beneficial. In compromised patients, placement of an ICP monitor is wise. In patients who are conscious prior to surgery, it is better to awaken them immediately after the procedure and follow their neurologic examination. ICP is managed in the same fashion as discussed earlier.

Steroid administration is not an effective adjunct and may indeed be deleterious. Prophylactic administration of phenytoin (Dilantin), 15 mg per kg load, 4 to 7 mg per kg per day maintenance, antibiotics (5-day course of nafcillin [Unipen], cefazolin [Ancef], or ceftazidime [Fortaz], and so on), and H_2 blockers famotidine (Pepcid), ranitidine (Zantac), cimetidine (Tagamet) is recommended by many workers.

Patients with a GCS of 3 or 4, fixed and dilated pupils, or absent brain stem reflexes (corneals, doll's eyes, gag, oculovestibular) are treated expectantly. Patients with delayed hemorrhage or tracts that course through regions of great cerebral vessels should undergo angiography for traumatic aneurysms. Knife wounds and other penetrating head wounds are treated in a fashion similar to GSWs. No attempt should be made to remove residual penetrating materials (knife blade, arrow point) in the field or the emergency department.

SKULL FRACTURES

Skull fractures in children deserve special consideration. Linear skull fractures picked up on skull radiograph or CT are generally benign but indicate a significant mechanism of injury that may warrant admission and further study. For a child who has sustained concussion only, linear skull fracture contributes marginally to the risk of delayed trouble (1% vs. 0.5%). Fractures that cross the middle meningeal, however, deserve respect. Small epidural hematomas (20 mL or less) are common in such cases; most do not require evacuation, but all demand close attention. In younger children, linear skull fractures must be followed up in the ensuing 3 to 6 months to rule out a "growing fracture of childhood." In this entity, the fracture is associated with an undetected dural tear. Over time, the water-hammer effect of the leptomeninges through the dura can result in expansion of the fracture and the dural defect with leptomenin-

geal cyst formation, porencephaly, and secondary cerebral injury. Knowledgeable palpation, x-ray, or CT can rule out the entity.

Depressed skull fractures usually can be treated conservatively if the depression is less than the thickness of the skull. In-driven fragments with possible dural laceration warrant elective repair. Diagnosis can be made only radiographically. Subperiosteal hematomas are frequently misdiagnosed as depressed skull fractures in the emergency room. Open depressed skull fracture should be débrided by a neurosurgeon urgently with dural repair. "Dirty" wounds may necessitate delayed cranioplasty. Open depressed skull fractures are covered with a short course of prophylactic broad-spectrum, antistaphylococcal antibiotics. Use of prophylactic anticonvulsants is case-specific.

Basilar skull fractures are diagnosed from Battle's or raccoon signs, hemotympanum, CSF otorrhea or rhinorrhea, or CT scan. Most are self-limited injuries, although they signify significant traumatic force and may result in persistent CSF leaks. Patients with basilar skull fracture should be admitted to the hospital and observed. Prophylactic antibiotics are favored by many but carry the risk of selecting out resistant strains of bacteria. The risk of any CSF leak is meningitis. Parents must be counseled on the presentation of CSF leaks and meningitis. CSF otorrhea is almost always self-limited. CSF rhinorrhea may require lumbar CSF drainage or surgery when persistent.

CHILD ABUSE

Some investigators state that one tenth of all children treated for "accidental" head injury are the victims of child abuse. A high index of suspicion must be maintained when evaluating children with substantial head injuries, especially babies. Parental perpetrators of even the most savage beatings usually deny vehemently any hint of abuse and may appear distraught at their child's lot. The phenomenon is known to cross all socioeconomic boundaries.

Hallmarks of abuse include chronic or mixed-age subdural hematomas, new or chronic cerebral injuries, interhemispheric subdural hematomas, retinal hemorrhage, long bone fractures, multiple rib fractures, cigarette burns, and so on. Retinal hemorrhage and subdural hematomas in infants are due to abuse or shaking until proved otherwise. Child abuse evaluation teams should be enlisted early and without shame or embarrassment on the part of the clinician.

Treatment of abuse-related head injuries follows the protocols outlined in the previous sections. Victims of the "shaken baby syndrome" often have dreadful courses secondary to uncontrollable cerebral edema and vascular disautoregulation.

Chronic subdural hematomas in young children will generally respond to serial percutaneous taps. An emergency tap may be indicated in the rapidly deteriorating child. A 20-gauge intravenous catheter needle can be passed into the subdural space at the lateralmost aspect of the anterior fontanelle (coronal suture) under sterile conditions. The stylet is withdrawn and the hematoma allowed to drain spontaneously. The catheter should not be aspirated. This maneuver should be reserved for clinicians with experience in the procedure.

BRAIN TUMORS

method of
N. SCOTT LITOFSKY, M.D., and
LAWRENCE D. RECHT, M.D.
University of Massachusetts Medical Center
Worcester, Massachusetts

Brain tumors represent a heterogeneous group of neoplasms that has different presentations, prognoses, and treatments. Defining a single approach to these lesions can therefore be difficult. To facilitate decision making, we have noted that management issues for all brain tumor patients generally are classifiable into one of three possible categories: (1) symptoms arising from tumor or treatment effects on normal brain, (2) issues concerning correct diagnosis of the lesion, and (3) specific therapeutics of the particular brain tumors. The management of brain tumor symptoms spans the patient's entire clinical course; management decisions here are for the most part histology-independent, depending more on tumor location, the presence of mass effect, patient age, and the particular symptoms encountered. Decisions concerning making the proper diagnosis—specifically, when to operate and how much tumor to remove—are also for the most part histology-independent, being affected mainly by such issues as location and patient age. Only the specific therapy of brain tumor is crucially dependent on tumor histology.

We have found that dealing with brain tumors is much easier if treatment issues are first classified and dealt with. Such an approach facilitates management by non-neuro-oncologists, because most treatment decisions are related to symptoms and therefore are largely histology-independent. Furthermore, it emphasizes the importance of attending to patient symptoms, the effective treatment of which can markedly improve quality (and sometimes quantity) of life.

SYMPTOMATIC ISSUES

Seizures

Seizures are an important cause of morbidity in the brain tumor patient. In approximately 40% of patients with gliomas, seizure is the earliest manifestation of the disease, and 55% have had at least one spell by the time the tumor is diagnosed. Seizure frequency and pattern may vary as tumor size and pathology change. Status epilepticus is a frequent occurrence and may be a presenting symptom. In addition to the morbidities commonly associated with idiopathic epilepsy, seizures in tumor patients are particularly dangerous because of their propensity to increase intracranial pressure (ICP) in a patient with impaired compliance; this can result in sudden death due to cerebral herniation.

Although surgical resection can provide effective relief in patients with persistent refractory seizures secondary to infiltrative tumors in the temporal or frontal lobes, pharmacologic therapy remains the mainstay of treatment. Pharmacotherapy is unique for brain tumor patients in a number of aspects: (1) Brain tumor patients are frequently receiving other medications that may interact with anticonvulsants. For example, patients on phenytoin (Dilantin) frequently require higher doses of drug when they are on dexamethasone; conversely, when steroids are tapered, serum phenytoin levels may rise to toxic levels. (2) Brain tumor patients frequently receive cranial irradiation therapy (RT), which may predispose to Stevens-Johnson syndrome and erythema multiforme reactions; this is especially common with phenytoin. (3) Patients frequently have other neurologic impairments that can make anticonvulsant side effects more distressing. For example, brain tumor patients are particularly prone to develop shoulder-hand syndrome and diffuse arthralgias that can be discomforting enough to warrant withdrawal of the medication.

Despite these complications, phenytoin is generally the first-line drug. If breakthrough seizures develop or allergic reactions occur, carbamazepine (Tegretol), phenobarbital, or valproate (Depakote) can be substituted. In lower-grade neoplasms, tumor resections can be performed specifically to relieve epilepsy when medical management is ineffective. Patients with brain tumors are prone to develop seizures after intravenous contrast medium for computed tomography (CT) examinations. This tendency can be minimized by preprocedural administration of 5 to 10 mg of diazepam intravenously.

Mass Effect

Patients frequently present with symptoms related to mass effect from the tumor. These symptoms can be subdivided into symptoms of elevated ICP and those of focal neurologic deficits.

Brain tumors raise ICP either by the local effects of tumor mass coupled with vasogenic edema or by producing obstruction of cerebrospinal fluid (CSF) pathways leading to the development of hydrocephalus. Elevated ICP may therefore manifest itself in a variety of ways. *Headache* results from distortion of the dural membranes and intracranial blood vessels. The headache typically is described as holocranial and occurs on arising, because recumbency at night decreases venous drainage of the brain, and mild hypoventilation as the patient is sleeping causes cerebral vasodilatation. Patients may also experience *vomiting*, which is a result of pressure on the area postrema. Nausea may not be present, and the vomiting occurs most often in the morning (along with a headache) and is frequently projectile in nature. Chronically elevated ICP may also produce progressive cognitive abnormalities with resultant changes in personality and behavior or, alternatively, progressive diminution in the level of consciousness.

Medical and mechanical therapies are available that can treat both mechanisms responsible for causing elevated ICP. Patients with brain masses and symptoms or signs of elevated ICP should have the head of the bed elevated at least 30 degrees to increase cerebral venous drainage and reduce intracranial volume. Additionally, limiting fluid intake to 1.5 liters per day may help reduce the amount of edema fluid produced.

Analgesics may make the patient more comfortable. However, patients with large intracranial masses who hypoventilate even mildly may rapidly decompensate because of their limited cerebral compliance; therefore, sedation, with its attendant hypoventilation, should be avoided. Codeine is thus preferable to other narcotic analgesics because it is less sedating. Antiemetics are also helpful to reduce vomiting and improve patient comfort. Trimethobenzamide (Tigan) at a dose of 250 mg every 6 hours orally or 200 mg every 6 hours rectally is preferable to prochlorperazine (Compazine) or promethazine (Phenergan). Phenothiazine agents, while good antiemetics, can reduce the seizure threshold, an effect that should be avoided.

The most serious effect of elevated ICP is cerebral herniation. Management of this neurologic emergency includes patient hyperventilation and the administration of osmotic diuretics and steroids. Hyperventilation requires patient intubation and its effect rapidly attenuates; however, lowering PCO_2 will immediately cause cerebral vasoconstriction and decreased intravascular blood volume, effectively reducing ICP and potentially reversing the herniation syndrome. PCO_2 should not be lowered to below 25 torr, which may cause cerebral ischemia. Osmotic diuretics such as mannitol are also useful; their onset of action is slower than hyperventilation. An initial dose of 1 gram per kg, followed by 0.25 gm per kg every 4 to 6 hours, reduces the extracellular brain water volume and can control elevated ICP for several days. An initial dose of furosemide (Lasix) at 1 mg per kg can also hasten the response by its vasodilatative effect on the peripheral vasculature.

Glucocorticoids such as dexamethasone (Decadron) or methylprednisolone (Medrol) stabilize cell membranes and reduce vasogenic edema. Since their onset of action requires at least 30 to 60 minutes, they should be used only in conjunction with other modalities if the situation is an emergency. They are particularly useful, however, in the chronic management of elevated ICP. Dexamethasone is most commonly utilized. The initial dose is 10 mg, followed by 4 mg every 6 hours. It may be given either orally or intravenously, the latter route being necessary in urgent cases when the patient is unable to take oral medication.

Mechanical therapy can also be provided by placement of a ventriculostomy. This surgical procedure can be performed relatively rapidly by a neurosurgeon to divert CSF. Such intervention may rapidly reduce ICP and reverse a herniation syndrome, making it the treatment of choice for the deteriorating patient with hydrocephalus. The ventricular catheter can be removed once the CSF pathway is opened by reduction of edema, or by surgical decompression of tumor bulk. If continued CSF diversion is required following these maneuvers, then placement of a permanent ventriculoperitoneal shunt may be necessary.

Patients may develop focal neurologic deficits from mass effect, as well. These symptoms and signs may include hemiparesis from frontal, parietal, or thalamic masses, aphasia from dominant temporal lobe masses, hearing loss from vestibular schwannomas, visual loss from parasellar masses (such as pituitary adenomas, optic nerve and hypothalamic gliomas, and dorsum sella meningiomas), and hypothalamic-pituitary insufficiency from sellar and suprasellar masses.

Treatment for these symptomatic issues is similar to that described for elevated ICP. Dexamethasone is very effective in reducing neural compression by reducing edema and may significantly improve the symptoms. Often, however, surgical decompression of the affected structure by removal of the offending mass is required for improvement. If the symptoms are related to endocrine insufficiency, replacement therapy is the most effective method of improving the clinical condition. In the specific instance of visual loss from a sellar/suprasellar mass with an elevated prolactin level (usually a pituitary prolactinoma), treatment with bromocriptine (Parlodel) may rapidly shrink the tumor and improve vision.

Immediate and Long-Term Symptoms Related to Treatment

In recent years the treatment of patients with brain tumors has become more intensive, resulting in better response and survival rates. These more aggressive therapies are also associated with morbidities that must be distinguished from tumor progression.

Although operative mortality has decreased significantly in recent years, medical and neurologic morbidities of neurosurgical procedures remain problematic. Postoperative infections, including subdural empyema and meningitis, can be significantly reduced by the administration of prophylactic antibiotics. Abscesses are particularly difficult to differentiate from tumor both radiographically and clinically. Fever and high leukocyte count may suggest infection, but they are not invariably present in the patients who are on steroids. Abscess should therefore be a consideration in any patient developing signs of neurologic deterioration postoperatively, especially if imaging studies reveal an enlarging concentric ring lesion.

Shunt malfunctions can also produce symptoms and signs mimicking tumor recurrence; correction will reverse symptoms and afford effective palliation. Therefore, a high index of suspicion for malfunction is required in tumor patients with shunts, and appropriate imaging studies must be performed before attributing clinical worsening to tumor progression.

Radiation and chemotherapy, although mainstays of neuro-oncologic treatment, also may result in early and delayed neurologic side effects that may either mimic tumor recurrence or impair quality of life. External beam irradiation may result in symptomatic worsening either during its acute administration or as a delayed effect occurring from weeks to months after its completion. The early reactions are related to cerebral edema and usually respond to steroid administration. The delayed effects are more serious and usually represent a form of cerebral radionecrosis. This latter development is often indistinguishable in conventional imaging studies and clinical manifestations from tumor recurrence and represents a difficult diagnostic and therapeutic problem. We have found thallium-201, single photon emission computed tomography (SPECT) scans particularly useful in helping differentiate necrosis from recurrence; if decreased uptake in the area of imaging abnormality is noted, then necrosis is the more likely diagnosis. Often, however, biopsy is the only way to make the diagnosis. Surgical excision is sometimes required for symptomatic relief. No medical treatments are very effective, although recent reports of improvement after therapeutic anticoagulation are promising.

A number of more subtle long-term complications also arise in irradiated patients. Endocrine deficiency is a common occurrence. This generally results from the effects of irradiation (and possibly chemotherapy) on the hypothalamus and pituitary. A decrease in gonadotropin hormones is most common, and patients will frequently develop either amenorrhea or impotence. Thyroid dysfunction is also a common occurrence, and patients should be periodically screened for this problem.

A more vexing long-term complication of treatment is a deterioration in cognitive capabilities. Both very young and very old patients are particularly vulnerable to this development. Furthermore, the effects occur more frequently with higher total and fractionated doses of radiation and are probably aggravated by the addition of chemotherapy. The underlying pathologic process probably represents a leukoencephalopathy that is reflected by increased white matter abnormalities on magnetic resonance imaging (MRI). A gradual deterioration in cognitive abilities coupled with other signs of white matter dysfunction, especially gait dysfunction, characterize the disorder. Unfortunately, no effective treatments exist for this problem.

Deep Venous Thrombosis and Pulmonary Embolism

Deep venous thrombosis (DVT) and pulmonary embolism (PE) occur frequently in the brain tumor patient and present a difficult management problem. Patient immobilization and release of tissue thromboplastin from the brain tumor make peripheral venous thrombosis especially common in brain tumor patients, with incidence figures as high as 33%. Thrombosis can occur at any time of the disease, although it is more likely to develop in the first 6 weeks after craniotomy.

Patients with brain tumors who develop leg swelling or pain should be screened for DVT with impedance plethysmography. Patients who develop sudden shortness of breath or an encephalopathy of uncertain etiology should be evaluated for PE with radionuclide lung scanning. In those in whom DVT or PE is documented, treatment is indicated. The optimal therapy remains uncertain because of the risk of anticoagulating a patient with a brain tumor who has recently undergone craniotomy. Placement of a Greenfield filter or other type of vena caval interruption procedure has been advocated as a safer alternative to anticoagulation in the immediate postoperative period (i.e., within 4 weeks). However, the documented long-term morbidities of this procedure make it a less desirable choice for other patients, especially since anticoagulation is relatively safe with a very low incidence of intracranial hemorrhage.

Although they are liberally used in patients with malignant brain tumors, steroids are not without serious long-term complications. Myopathy, glucose intolerance, osteoporosis, avascular necrosis of the hips, and mental status changes can all result from their usage. Unfortunately, these problems often develop in a patient who needs the symptomatic benefit that steroids can provide. In these situations, *oral glycerol* (Osmoglyn), a potent osmotic diuretic that can achieve the same benefits as mannitol, can be substituted. Although the medication may be quite unpalatable for many patients, most patients will tolerate it when it is mixed with orange juice. Frequently, its addition will allow a reduction in or even discontinuation of glucocorticoid dosage.

DIAGNOSTIC ISSUES

Sometimes a definitive diagnosis of a brain lesion can be made on imaging and clinical criteria alone, such as when a cancer patient develops multiple enhancing lesions in the setting of progressive systemic disease. Often, however, establishing a definitive diagnosis is essential for planning specific therapy. Since tissue is required for a definitive diagnosis, a surgical procedure can be designed to make a tissue diagnosis as well as to decompress the lesion and improve symptoms. In some instances, however, diagnosis should be made by biopsy only, without specific therapeutic benefit to the patient.

Obviously, an adequate diagnostic work-up must be done before an appropriate surgical procedure can be performed. Patients between 20 and 40 years of age with parenchymal lesions are at risk for human immunodeficiency virus (HIV) related central nervous system (CNS) masses. If the patient is HIV-positive, stereotactic biopsy can establish whether the lesion(s) is related to an opportunistic infection or CNS lymphoma. Conversely, patients over the age of 40 years are more likely to have metastatic lesions. Therefore, screening tests consisting of a rectal examination with stool guaiac, urinalysis, skin and breast examinations, complete blood count (CBC), and chest radiograph may suggest a primary focus. If a primary lesion is identified, resection of a single parenchymal metastatic lesion will result in an improved prognosis. For multiple lesions, empiric radiation therapy is usual if a primary lesion is identified, and stereotactic biopsy can confirm the pathology if no primary lesion is found.

Most patients with newly diagnosed mass lesions do undergo some type of surgical procedure for either diagnostic or therapeutic purposes. Open craniotomy is necessary if therapeutic decompression (and acquisition of pathologic material) is desired. In most instances, this operation requires administration of general anesthesia. Some masses, such as meningiomas and metastatic neoplasms, have well-defined planes between themselves and the brain; these lesions can often be grossly totally removed. Other lesions, such as anaplastic astrocytoma and glioblastoma multiforme, send macro- or microscopic infiltrating fingers of tumor out from their tumor bulk; they can never be completely resected, but they can be significantly decompressed to reduce mass effect. If craniotomy is not felt to be indicated, then stereotactic biopsy is the preferable means of acquiring tissue for diagnostic purposes. This procedure can be performed under local anesthetic using CT or MRI guidance with minimal risk.

The choice of which surgical approach to use depends on a number of factors, including neuroimaging appearance, whether symptoms of mass effect are present, and patient age. Extra-axial lesions are well suited for surgical excision since these can often be totally removed. Lesions that are exerting significant mass effect on imaging studies are also suitable for surgical decompression if they do not involve eloquent cortical or subcortical structures. Stereotactic approaches are usually not appropriate for hemorrhagic lesions, which are probably better handled by craniotomy. On the other hand, those lesions involving the deep nuclear structures of the thalamus, basal ganglia, and brain stem are usually not amenable to surgical decompression, even if they have significant mass effect. If multiple lesions are present, stereotactic biopsy is likewise preferred.

The patient's age is an important determinant of surgical approach. For many childhood tumors, children have a more favorable prognosis with more radical excision of the mass. Therefore, if the lesion is in a surgically accessible location, craniotomy for resection is preferable. On the other hand, very elderly patients may not tolerate craniotomy well. Unless the lesion has significant mass effect, stereotactic biopsy is indicated.

SPECIFIC THERAPEUTIC ISSUES

A tumor's histology becomes particularly important when considering specific therapies such as radiation, chemo-, immune, and endocrine therapies that are administered specifically to eradicate tumor or control its growth. Even in this particular area of treatment, however, other factors must be taken into account. For example, in making the decision whether to administer radiation therapy, patient age must be taken into account because of the high incidence of deleterious effects that occur in the very young and very old patients.

The following brief survey will orient the physician to some of the more common brain tumors encountered. Since these are relatively rare events for which many clinical investigations are ongoing, we advise that whenever possible patients should be evaluated in settings where multidisciplinary (i.e., neurosurgery, radiation therapy, oncology) input is available.

Brain Metastasis

In patients older than 40 years, brain metastasis is the most common cause of brain tumor. Lung and breast cancers are the most frequent primary tumors; although most brain metastases develop late in the clinical course when systemic cancer is obvious, they may also be evident at time of presentation and not uncommonly may herald the diagnosis. For this reason, newly diagnosed brain tumor patients should have at least a chest radiograph (CT scan of the chest in patients with a smoking history), mammogram, urinalysis, and CT scan of the abdomen in patients in whom there is a suspicion of an intra-abdominal or retroperitoneal lesion prior to neurosurgical intervention.

The prognosis of patients with intracranial metastasis from systemic cancer is poor, with median survivals being less than 6 months. However, certain patients, especially those with no evidence of systemic disease at the time of neurologic presentation, may do much better.

From a therapeutic standpoint, brain metastases are approached differently depending on whether they are single or multiple. MRI most accurately determines the number of intracranial lesions. In patients with two or more lesions, whole brain radiation therapy, generally consisting of 10 fractions of 300 cGy per fraction, is the treatment of choice. Because of the long-term neurologic side effects of this high fractionation scheme, it has been our practice to administer an equivalent total dosage using only 200 cGy per dose in those patients who are deemed to be capable of a longer-term survival. In addition, if one larger lesion, especially in the posterior fossa, is causing significant neurologic deficits unresponsive to dexamethasone, surgical decompression may rapidly improve symptoms.

Management of single intracranial metastatic lesions depends on their location and the patient's symptoms. If the patient has a lesion in noneloquent brain or has significant symptoms of mass effect, then surgical resection followed by radiation therapy provides the best long-term care. On the other hand, if the patient has minimal neurologic signs and the lesion is in or adjacent to eloquent brain, radiation therapy alone will eliminate possible neurologic deficits related to surgery. Considering many recent studies documenting better outcomes in surgically treated patients, it has been our approach to consider all patients with single lesions, stable or inactive systemic disease, and reasonable performance status for surgical resection unless a contraindication exists.

High-Grade Gliomas

High-grade or malignant gliomas are the most commonly encountered primary brain tumors. They affect mostly middle-aged adults although they can occur at any age. The most malignant tumor of this group is the glioblastoma multiforme (GBM), characterized pathologically by the presence of endothelial proliferation and tissue necrosis. Anaplastic astrocytomas are distinguished from glioblastomas by the absence of necrosis. A number of factors affect prognosis: patient age (younger most favorable), the presence of necrosis on pathologic section (unfavorable), and postoperative performance status are the most frequently associated ones.

Unfortunately, these tumors are incurable, and treatment is geared toward maximal palliation. Debulking of as much tumor as deemed safe, combined with postoperative external beam radiation therapy to maximal brain tolerance (approximately 60 Gy), is associated with median time to tumor progression in patients with GBM of less than a year. Increasing the radiation dosage has minimal added effect and increases toxicity, as do newer radiation therapy modalities such as sterotactic radiosurgery. The addition of chemotherapy, administered either as a single agent or in combination, modestly increases survival, mainly by increasing the number of longer-term survivors. Patients with anaplastic astrocytomas have slightly better prognoses, and 5-year survivals, although uncommon, do occur.

Although chemotherapy is generally associated with at best a modest efficacy, recent reports indicate that a particular subtype of malignant glioma, the aggressive oligodendroglioma, may be particularly chemosensitive to a combination of procarbazine (Matulane), CCNU (lomustine [CeeNu]), and vincristine (Oncovin). A number of other experimental chemo- and immune therapies are currently being evaluated, but none so far has proved superior to the standard conventional approach of surgery, external beam irradiation, and single-agent chemotherapy.

Low-Grade Gliomas

Although gliomas represent a continuum of tumor types, it has been clinically useful to separate them into higher (i.e., malignant) and lower grades; however, it is important to remember that although clinically less aggressive, the low-grade tumors also are often incurable and represent low-grade malignancies rather than benign tumors. The most common tumor type is the diffuse fibrillary astrocytoma; oligodendroglioma and mixed tumor types are other important tumor types.

These tumors tend to occur at younger ages, usually between 20 and 50 years. They tend to arise in the cerebral hemispheres and present with a seizure or seizures. They pose a particularly difficult clinical problem when they produce an isolated seizure in an otherwise young, healthy patient whose imaging studies reveal an unenhancing supratentorial lesion without mass effect, since it is unclear whether early intervention results in improved patient outcome.

Unfortunately, although at the outset these tumors frequently behave very indolently, at some point (usually within 7 to 8 years), they begin to behave more like their malignant counterparts. It is not clear whether early irradiation postpones this event or prolongs survival, although a number of retrospective series suggest this. It has been our practice to approach each case individually and make clinical decisions based on the potential for complete resection, patient age (the older the patient, the sooner the tumor will become more aggressive so we tend not to postpone treatment), and patient and physician preference.

Central Nervous System Lymphomas

Primary CNS lymphomas were once considered rare, but their incidence is increasing, especially in the acquired immune deficiency syndrome (AIDS) population but also in the elderly. These tumors are identical in histology to non-Hodgkin's lymphomas that occur systemically. They tend to be multifocal and occur in deep periventricular locations; however, it is impossible to distinguish these tumors from GBM preoperatively.

Owing to their oncolytic actions versus lymphomas, the administration of glucocorticoids may result in a complete disappearance of the lesion; when this occurs, it strongly suggests lymphoma as a diagnosis. On the other hand, because it obscures the ability to make the diagnosis, it is recommended that at least a biopsy be obtained if possible before the long-term administration of steroids in patients in whom lymphoma is suspected.

Stereotactic biopsy is indicated to make the diagnosis; retrospective data indicate that more extensive surgery may be associated with a poorer outcome. Radiotherapy affords long-term palliation, but the median survival of these patients is still only slightly greater than a year. A number of reports demonstrate that these tumors are sensitive to chemotherapy; effective regimens include high-dose methotrexate and more intensive therapies. We thus routinely administer chemotherapy preirradiation to newly diagnosed, nonimmune suppressed patients with CNS lymphoma.

In patients with AIDS and CNS lymphoma, irradiation offers effective palliation; although survival is not appreciably increased, the pattern of disease is changed, and patients generally succumb to other complications of their disease. Chemotherapy has not proved particularly effective in this cohort of patients, although ongoing studies continue.

Meningiomas

Meningiomas are extraparenchymal tumors that arise from leptomeningeal tissue and produce symptoms by compressing contiguous neural structures. They are benign in the sense that they can be cured if totally removed; if this is not possible, however, further tumor growth can occur, which can produce further neurologic deficits or death. Thus, the goal of surgery is total resection of the tumor and its dural attachment without damaging surrounding neural and vascular structures. This may not be possible if the tumor has invaded the skull base or is attached to neural or vascular structures that would cause unacceptable neurologic morbidity if the tumor were completely removed. In these instances, the goal of surgery should be to remove as much of the tumor bulk as possible.

If a complete resection can be performed, no further therapy is necessary. When only partial removals are accomplished, radiation therapy focused on the residual component of tumor can be just as effective in preventing recurrence as "complete" excision in the long term. By using a focused form of radiation, the complications of radiation therapy on normal brain can be minimized. No truly effective chemotherapeutic agent has been identified for adjuvant therapy. RU486 (mifepristone) the "birth control" pill, has been shown to have some efficacy in some cases, but further study is necessary before this agent or others become part of the standard care.

Not all meningiomas require therapy. In many patients, lesions are discovered incidentally during evaluation of unrelated symptoms. In these cases, close follow-up with serial imaging every 6 months to a year can establish a growth pattern of the lesion. Surgical removal is indicated when progressive growth is documented or symptoms or signs develop.

Medulloblastomas

Medulloblastomas are primitive neuroectodermal tumors that arise most frequently in the cerebellum. They represent the most common malignant brain tumor of childhood. They affect mainly young children or adolescents; occurrence after 20 years of age is much less frequent. Until the early 1970s, fewer than one-third of patients with medulloblastomas survived 5 years after treatment. Owing to several factors including earlier diagnosis, safer anesthesia, advances in surgical techniques, improved postoperative care, and more effective use of radiotherapy, 5-year disease-free survival rates approaching 50% are common.

Generally, patients can be characterized into those of average risk (no disseminated disease, no marked hydrocephalus, total or near-total resection, and age greater than 4 years); and poor risk (some combination of disseminated disease, hydrocephalus or tumor infiltration of the brain stem, a less than total resection, or age less than 4 years). Medulloblastomas, unlike most other brain tumors, have a high likelihood of disseminating to other CNS sites early in the course of illness, and over 30% of patients will have either CSF cytologic or imaging evidence of leptomeningeal disease at diagnosis (which can be asymptomatic). Therefore, every newly diagnosed patient should have MRI of the spine, lumbar puncture for cytology, and bone marrow examination as part of the staging work-up.

Since many patients develop tumor outside the primary tumor site after local radiotherapy, the entire neuraxis is usually irradiated to improve long-term disease control. Conventionally, 36 cGy are given to brain and spine and an additional 20 cGy administered to the local disease site. Children with poor risk indicators may benefit from chemotherapy; other children do not. The optimal chemotherapy regimens for both initial and recurrent disease are currently being studied in prospective trials.

The Locomotor System

RHEUMATOID ARTHRITIS

method of
JOSEPH GOLBUS, M.D.
Evanston Hospital
Evanston, Illinois

Rheumatoid arthritis (RA) is a chronic, systemic inflammatory disease of unknown etiology. It is characterized by an inflammatory, progressive, often destructive arthritis. Extra-articular disease is common and can contribute to disability. Although most commonly beginning in the third to fifth decades of life, it can affect all age groups. It afflicts approximately 1 to 2% of the adult population worldwide; prevalence increases with age, with two to three times as many woman as men affected. By age 55, nearly 5% of women and 2% of men have the disease. Once considered benign, RA is now known to have a long-term outlook that is far worse than previously believed, with a high incidence of disability and accelerated mortality as well, particularly in those with more advanced disease and extra-articular features.

For many years, RA has been managed according to the traditional "pyramid of treatment" concept. This approach involved an orderly progression of therapies, beginning with simple interventions and progressing over years to more potent medications. Typically, treatment would begin with physical therapy and salicylates or a nonsteroidal anti-inflammatory drug (NSAID). Progression of the disease would prompt the addition of corticosteroids or a single disease-modifying antirheumatic drug (DMARD) such as gold, hydroxychloroquine, or penicillamine and cytotoxic agents such as azathioprine, methotrexate, or cyclophosphamide. These agents were used sequentially for a period of months to a few years until the development of toxicity or until the response was considered inadequate. Although this approach decreased pain and inflammation in the short term, it did not significantly alter the long-term outcome in terms of functional status and mortality. Further contributing to the inadequacy of this approach was the common practice of withholding the more toxic but potentially more effective therapies until after joint damage and disability had occurred.

Based on these past shortcomings and the new understanding of the true morbidity and mortality of RA, many authors advocate discarding the traditional pyramid in favor of a more aggressive approach designed to totally suppress inflammation before the development of irreversible bony erosions.

These strategies, in one form or another, suggest "inverting the pyramid," or using the more potent agents much earlier in the disease course. Very often, the more potent DMARDs need to be instituted within a few months of disease onset rather than waiting for the appearance of bony erosions and deformities 2 to 3 years later.

An increasingly popular approach is to use numerous medications analogous to cancer chemotherapy, whereby combinations of DMARDs and cytotoxic drugs are used simultaneously very early in the disease course in an attempt to induce a remission. The more toxic drugs are dropped as the disease comes under better control, maintaining the remission with safer agents. Similar to the rationale for cancer chemotherapy, combinations of drugs are used to overcome cellular resistance to drugs and, at the same time, reduce toxicity. This more aggressive approach implies accepting greater costs and risks in the short term in the hope of achieving far greater long-term benefits, with improved functional outcomes and survival rates. Although it is still unknown which combinations of drugs offer the greatest benefit and safest toxicity profile, numerous ongoing clinical trials are utilizing the traditional DMARDs in combination with cytotoxic agents.

On a cautionary note, due to their potential toxicities, the use of multiple agents simultaneously requires oversight by a rheumatologist or physician experienced in the use of these potent medications. Furthermore, not all patients with rheumatoid arthritis have disease sufficiently severe to justify the aggressive treatment schemes outlined in this article. Some individuals, for example, are well managed with an NSAID and a judicious balance of rest and exercise. Accordingly, it is important that we not only devise better treatment strategies but also identify more accurate predictors of erosive disease and poor outcome. Such prognostic information could identify patients who require earlier intervention with the more potent drugs.

GENERAL PRINCIPLES OF MANAGEMENT

The main goals in treating individuals with RA include relief of symptoms, prevention of joint destruction, maintenance of joint function, and, most important, preservation of a style and quality of life. These goals are accomplished through a variety of interventions that include both nonpharmacologic and pharmacologic therapies. Extensive patient education, early occupational and physical therapy, and the use of anti-inflammatory agents make up the early steps of most treatment programs. Given the long-term physical, emotional, and economic consequences of the disease, patient education is essential. Understanding the disease prognosis and the realistic expectations of therapy leads to an improved outcome, with less frustration and disillusionment. This education should provide basic information about the disease and reinforce the importance of compliance with all aspects of the treatment plan. Enlisting the support of family members can be very beneficial in ensuring compliance and providing emotional support.

A balanced program of rest and exercise is a key component of the treatment plan. There is good evidence that rest diminishes the signs and symptoms of synovitis. At the same time, a sufficient exercise program devised by a physical therapist is important to maintain joint mobility, periarticular muscle strength, and, ultimately, joint function. Exercise can also promote an improved sense of well-being. Assistive devices and splints can enhance comfort and improve functional status within the limits of pre-existing deformities.

In patients who have severely affected or damaged joints and disability, surgical intervention can restore or improve function. Procedures that are often successful in RA patients include total hip and total knee arthroplasties and several procedures for the hands and feet. For severe hand and wrist involvement, a combination of tendon transposition, bone resection, and joint fusion may be necessary, requiring the skills of an experienced orthopedic surgeon. Synovectomy, especially in the wrists or knees, may be helpful if the disease is limited to a small number of joints that do not respond well to medical therapy. A common complication of wrist synovitis is rupture of the fourth and fifth extensor tendons. Early splinting and synovectomy can help prevent this problem. When considering surgery that requires intubation, one must pay particular attention to the integrity of the cervical spine, assessing for C1–2 instability and the risk of subluxation, with resultant cervical myelopathy and paraplegia.

When used in combination with medications and aggressive physical and occupational therapy, surgical procedures can dramatically improve functional status and quality of life.

PHARMACOLOGIC THERAPY

NSAIDs

NSAIDs, including salicylates, have been the mainstay of early therapy for RA for many years. NSAIDs modify the inflammatory process through the inhibition of prostaglandin synthetase, although other mechanisms of action are being uncovered. Although helpful in reducing the degree of inflammation and discomfort, NSAIDs are not considered "disease modifying" (antierosive) and are often insuf-

ficient alone for the treatment of RA. The response to these agents is idiosyncratic, so the choice of agent is empirical. To accurately evaluate a response, a 2- to 3-week trial in full doses is necessary. Factors influencing the selection of NSAIDs include cost, drug potency, toxicity profile and tolerability, and dosing frequency.

The newer NSAIDs have an improved therapeutic profile over plain aspirin with respect to major gastrointestinal (GI) toxicity. In addition, patient compliance is generally enhanced because of easier dosing schedules. On the downside, NSAIDs more commonly cause certain side effects such as hypertension, congestive heart failure, edema, and renal insufficiency than does aspirin.

The major side effects of salicylates and NSAIDs occur in the GI tract and include dyspepsia, gastritis, gastric ulceration, and hemorrhage. Dyspeptic symptoms respond well to the addition of an H_2 blocker or sulcralfate (Carafate). Only misoprostol (Cytotec) has been shown conclusively to reduce the incidence of gastric ulcers and serious gastric hemorrhage. The use of misoprostol should be considered in individuals at high risk for those GI complications, including the elderly, smokers, those on concomitant steroid therapy, and those with a previous history of ulcer disease. Less common side effects from NSAIDs include renal dysfunction, platelet dysfunction, reversible elevations of liver transaminases, and central nervous system reactions, including headaches, dizziness, and confusion.

Recent data suggest that there are two isoenzymes of prostaglandin synthetase. One isoform (COX-1) is constitutively expressed in most tissues by a "housekeeping" gene that regulates normal cellular functions such as gastric cytoprotection, kidney function, and platelet aggregation. Another isoenzyme (COX-2) appears to be expressed by inflammatory cells and to be responsible for the production of inflammatory prostaglandins. Although several factors contribute to NSAID toxicity, more selective inhibition of COX-2 may provide anti-inflammatory activity, with less risk for gastric and renal toxicity. The significance of these isoenzymes is under active investigation.

As with all medications, the importance of monitoring for drug toxicity cannot be overstated. The American College of Rheumatology recommends that all individuals starting therapy with NSAIDs obtain a baseline blood count, blood urea nitrogen, creatinine, liver enzymes, potassium, and urinalysis. These initial studies should be repeated in 1 to 3 months and then at 3- to 12-month intervals thereafter, depending on an individual's risk factors for NSAID toxicity.

Corticosteroids

The proper role of corticosteroids in the treatment of RA remains controversial. According to the classic pyramid approach, low-dose steroid therapy has been used as a "bridge" to control inflammation that is resistant to NSAIDs until the DMARD exerts its effects. In recent years, as the risks of NSAIDs have become more apparent, many rheumatologists have come to favor the early use of low doses of prednisone (5 to 7.5 mg per day) in place of NSAIDs, especially in the elderly. Steroids have a favorable side-effect profile when used in these low doses and can be very effective in controlling inflammation in RA patients at high risk for NSAID-induced toxicity. Severe extra-articular manifestations of RA, such as vasculitis, serositis, or debilitating constitutional symptoms with weight loss, may require higher doses of corticosteroids, with an accompanying higher risk of side effects.

Common side effects in steroid-treated RA patients include osteoporosis, purpura, and accelerated cataract formation, although a number of other toxicities may also occur. Supplemental calcium, 1200 to 1500 mg per day, and vitamin D may be beneficial in minimizing bone loss. Whether an antiresorptive such as calcitonin (Calcimar, Miacalcin) or a bisphosphonate (etidronate disodium [Didronel], alendronate [Fosamax]) can prevent steroid-induced osteoporosis is uncertain. Of course, care should also be taken to use the smallest dose of steroid possible.

In addition to oral corticosteroids, injections of steroids into problematic joints benefit many RA patients. The side effects associated with oral steroids are rarely encountered with intra-articular injections. As a general rule, more than three injections in a given year into the same joint should be avoided.

DMARDs

Although the efficacy of DMARDs in preventing erosions and disease progression remains somewhat controversial, most rheumatologists believe that these drugs are essential in the treatment of RA. As discussed earlier, these agents are now used much earlier in the disease course to preserve joint function and improve overall prognosis. They often take many weeks to months to achieve their anti-inflammatory effects. A response to therapy can be measured by reductions in pain, morning stiffness, and the objective signs of inflammation, as well as improvement in the hematologic manifestations of chronic inflammation, such as anemia and thrombocytosis. The response to one agent does not predict the response to another agent. It is important to individualize therapy when picking a DMARD based on patient characteristics and the side-effect profiles of each agent. The recommended dosing schedules and features of these medications that may influence drug selection are outlined in Table 1.

The current standards in the treatment of RA include much earlier intervention with DMARDs or cytotoxic agents to prevent erosions, deformities, and functional loss. Furthermore, DMARD therapy should be additive, not sequential, utilizing combinations of drugs. For example, if a patient has shown a beneficial but incomplete response to hydroxychloroquine, a second agent such as methotrexate should be added to the regimen, building on the partial response already achieved. It is the physician's challenge to match the level of aggressive treatment to the expected level of outcome. In a chronic, slowly progressive illness such as RA, therapy must be tailored to prognosis. One must treat with an eye toward what is *going to happen,* not merely what one sees today.

Methotrexate

Although methotrexate was first shown to be beneficial in the early 1950s, the drug has been widely prescribed by rheumatologists for RA only in the last decade. During this period, numerous controlled prospective trials and extensive clinical experience have convincingly demonstrated the superior efficacy and safety of methotrexate compared with other DMARDs and cytotoxic agents. One distinct advantage of methotrexate is its rapid onset of action, despite the surprisingly small doses required. Because of these advantages, most rheumatologists now opt for a regimen that includes methotrexate, either as a single agent or in combination with other DMARDs or cytotoxic drugs. Whether methotrexate retards or stops bony erosions, however, remains to be proved.

The standard dosage of methotrexate ranges from 5 to 15 mg per week. Therapy is usually begun with a single dose of 7.5 to 10 mg orally once a week or divided into two doses taken 12 hours apart. The dose is increased every 4 to 6 weeks, as the clinical situation dictates. For patients in whom the oral form is not tolerated or in whom poor drug absorption is suspected, methotrexate can be given parenterally

TABLE 1. **Disease-Modifying Antirheumatic Drugs**

Medication	Dosage	Comments
Methotrexate (Rheumatrex)	7.5–25 mg/wk	? Most effective drug in RA; liver and lung toxicity
Gold thioglucose (Solganal)	50 mg/wk IM	Significant skin, renal, and bone marrow toxicity
Gold sodium thiomalate (Myochrysine)	50 mg/wk IM	As above, plus may cause nitritoid reactions
Auranofin (Ridaura)	3 mg bid PO	Less toxic than IM gold; modest efficacy
Hydroxychloroquine (Plaquenil)	200–400 mg/day PO	Low toxicity; often used with other DMARDs
Sulfasalazine (Azulfidine)	1000–1500 mg bid	For mild disease; may have quicker onset of action
Azathioprine (Imuran)	1–2.5 mg/kg/day PO	GI, liver, and bone marrow toxicity; ? carcinogenic
Penicillamine (Depen, Cuprimine)	250–1000 mg/day PO	High toxicity (skin, kidney, platelets)
Cyclophosphamide (Cytoxan)	1–2 mg/kg/day PO	Used in severe RA vasculitis; carcinogenic

Modified from Cohen MD: Rheumatoid arthritis. *In* Rakel RE (ed): Conn's Current Therapy 1995. Philadelphia, WB Saunders Co, 1995, p 904.

TABLE 2. **Frequency of Adverse Effects
of Cytotoxic Agents**

Toxicity	Methotrexate	Azathioprine	Cyclophosphamide
Leukopenia	+	+ +	+ +/+ + +
Thrombocytopenia	+	+/+ +	+
Gastrointestinal intolerance	+ +	+ + +	+ +
Hepatic damage	+/+ +	+	+
Pulmonary	+/+ +	Rare	Rare
Cystitis	0	0	+ +
Alopecia	+/+ +	+	+ + +
Susceptibility to infection	+	+	+ +
Azospermia	+	0	+ + +
Teratogenesis	+ +	Rare	+
Neoplasia	0	Rare	+ +

0 = not known to occur; rare = may occur rarely; + = occurs in <5% of patients; + + = occurs in 5–30% of patients; + + + = occurs in 30–40% of patients.

Modified from Clements PJ, Davis J: Semin Arthritis Rheum 15:231–254, 1986.

in doses of 10 to 25 mg once a week. Initial subjective improvement may occur as early as 3 to 4 weeks into therapy, with objective improvement in the synovitis often apparent in 6 to 8 weeks.

Several potential toxicities of low-dose weekly methotrexate therapy are recognized (Table 2). The most common adverse reactions include nausea, diarrhea, and stomatitis. These are thought to be due to the direct effects of the drug on the proliferating epithelial cells of the GI mucosa. In general, these effects are dose dependent and most apparent in the first 24 to 48 hours after taking the drug. Reducing the dose or adding folic acid, 1 mg per day, usually alleviates the problem.

A substantial percentage of individuals on methotrexate develop a subclinical chemical hepatitis, with increases in the liver enzymes alanine aminotransferase, aspartate aminotransferase, and lactate dehydrogenase. Elevation of these enzymes to two and one-half times the upper limit of normal is an indication to withhold the drug temporarily. Once the enzyme levels have returned to normal, the drug can be restarted at a lower dose. If the levels remain elevated several weeks after withholding the drug, the methotrexate should be discounted and other causes for the hepatitis should be considered. The relationship between biochemical hepatitis and the development of more serious liver damage, such as severe hepatic fibrosis and cirrhosis, is uncertain. Cases of severe end-stage liver disease secondary to methotrexate therapy in RA are rare. Although baseline liver biopsies and follow-up biopsies after 1.5 grams of cumulative methotrexate therapy were suggested in the past, most rheumatologists today do not believe that this is necessary. Current practice is to check the liver enzymes initially at 2-week intervals, and then at 4- to 12-week intervals thereafter. Liver biopsy is recommended if transaminase levels are elevated in five of nine or six of 12 yearly readings or if there is a fall in serum albumin. Risk

factors for the development of methotrexate liver toxicity include alcohol use, diabetes, obesity, and older age.

Low-dose methotrexate has been associated with two forms of pulmonary toxicity: a diffuse alveolar fibrosis, and a more acute hypersensitivity pneumonitis with granuloma formation and bronchiolitis. The clinical course of the latter condition may be fulminant, with a rapid onset of fever, nonproductive cough, and dyspnea. Left unchecked, it can quickly progress to severe respiratory distress requiring ventilatory support. In addition to stopping the drug, high-dose corticosteroids are often given to suppress the inflammatory response. Finally, patients taking methotrexate may have an increased vulnerability to pulmonary infections due to opportunistic organisms such as *Pneumocystis carinii, Aspergillus,* and *Cryptococcus.* Since methotrexate pneumonitis produces a clinical course indistinguishable from infection, bronchoalveolar lavage, biopsy, or both are often required to establish the correct diagnosis. Severely ill patients should receive broad-spectrum antibiotics along with high-dose corticosteroids during the evaluation.

Less common side effects associated with methotrexate include pancytopenia, skin rashes, gynecomastia, and subcutaneous nodule formation. These nodules often occur in unusual locations such as the fingers, toes, and ears. Methotrexate is teratogenic and should not be used in pregnancy. Since many RA patients are women in their childbearing years, this issue warrants close attention. In men, methotrexate may cause oligospermia, although sperm counts return to normal after cessation of the drug. There is no evidence that methotrexate is carcinogenic at either low or high doses.

Most of the drug is bound to serum proteins and slowly dissipates in cells and third-space fluids. For this reason, methotrexate must be used with caution in patients with ascites or large pleural effusions. The main route of excretion is the kidney. In patients with impaired renal function, therefore, adjustments in dose must be made, or the drug should be avoided altogether. Commonly used drugs that may influence the risk of methotrexate toxicity are listed in Table 3.

Gold

The use of gold compounds to treat RA was first proposed over 50 years ago. Because of the belief that

TABLE 3. **Drugs That May Influence
Methotrexate Toxicity**

Drugs That May Increase Toxicity	Drugs That May Reduce Toxicity
Barbiturates	Hydrocortisone
Colchicine	Tetracycline
Diphenylhydantoin	Trimethoprim
Oral contraceptives	
Phenylbutazone	
Probenecid	
Salicylates	

gold compounds possessed antimicrobial properties, they were used to treat a variety of chronic infectious diseases, including *Mycobacterium tuberculosis.* Although RA is no longer thought to be caused by tuberculosis, controlled prospective trials over the last 30 years have demonstrated the efficacy of parenteral gold in improving the symptoms and, in some patients, delaying or preventing the progression of bony erosions. The two gold compounds most commonly used in the United States are gold thioglucose (Solganal), a water-soluble organic compound in an oil suspension, and gold sodium thiomalate (Myochrysine), a soluble crystalline compound prepared in an aqueous solution. Both preparations contain 50% gold and are given intramuscularly. Auranofin (Ridaura), an oral absorbable gold preparation, was approved in the 1980s. Although it offers greater patient convenience and less toxicity, it is less effective than parenteral gold salts.

Intramuscular gold treatment usually begins with test doses of 10 and 25 mg 1 week apart. If these are well tolerated, the maintenance regimen of 50 mg a week is instituted for a period of 4 months until a total loading dose of 1000 mg is achieved. A favorable response may permit an increase in the dosage interval to 2 to 4 weeks. The usual auranofin regimen is 3 mg orally twice a day, although many clinicians begin therapy once a day for the first several weeks to reduce the incidence of diarrhea. For some patients, three-times-a-day dosing offers improved efficacy but also increased risk of diarrhea.

Drug reactions are fairly common, particularly with the parenteral forms of gold. Skin rashes are the most common side effect, with an incidence of 15 to 30% in most reported series. Pruritus precedes the skin lesions most of the time. Fortunately, the majority of skin reactions due to gold are mild and self-limited, although rarely they can cause a serious exfoliative dermatitis. Other forms of mucocutaneous toxicity include stomatitis with painful aphthous ulcers, glossitis, and gingivitis.

Mild proteinuria is seen in 5 to 7% of patients receiving gold salts. Low levels of proteinuria are rarely clinically significant, and protein excretions of less than 500 mg per 24 hours can be tolerated. In patients with larger protein losses, nephrotic syndrome can develop as a result of membranous nephropathy. Withdrawal of gold therapy results in a gradual resolution of proteinuria in most cases. Renal insufficiency as a result of gold salt therapy is extremely rare. Thrombocytopenia occurs in 1 to 3% of patients. It is unpredictable, is unrelated to dose, and can appear at any time in the course of therapy. Leukopenia and pancytopenia are much less common, although there are reported cases of fatal aplastic anemia. Gold sodium thiomalate, unlike gold thioglucose, may cause a nitritoid reaction characterized by sweating, dizziness, weakness, nausea, and, occasionally, hypotension. In general, all the adverse effects of gold are more common with the parenteral forms, except for diarrhea, which can occur in up to 50% of individuals taking auranofin.

To properly monitor for toxicity, it is recommended that individuals on parenteral gold obtain a complete blood count, platelet count, and urinalysis before every gold injection; individuals taking oral gold should obtain these studies once a month.

Hydroxychloroquine (Plaquenil)

Antimalarials have been used since the 1950s to treat RA. Hydroxychloroquine is now the most widely used antimalarial because of its lower toxicity and equivalent efficacy compared with other drugs in this class. However, relatively few RA patients treated with hydroxychloroquine achieve adequate long-term control of symptoms. It is generally employed in patients with early disease (with no or minimal radiographic erosions), in whom symptoms are refractory to NSAIDs alone, or in addition to other DMARDs to improve the therapeutic response. There is preliminary evidence that therapy with hydroxychloroquine may reduce the incidence of hepatic toxicity in individuals taking salicylates or methotrexate.

The usual dosage range of hydroxychloroquine is 200 to 400 mg per day. Three to 6 months of therapy may be required before the onset of therapeutic effect. Hydroxychloroquine is generally extremely well tolerated. Occasional patients develop skin rashes or GI intolerance. Corneal deposits may cause blurred vision but are reversible with drug discontinuation. The most serious potential long-term adverse effect is retinal toxicity, manifested by visual-field defects, central scotomata, and, ultimately, dense vision loss. Fortunately, this complication appears to be rare at doses of 400 mg per day or less. Because presymptomatic macular pigmentation can be detected during ophthalmic screening examinations, it is mandatory for all patients to have thorough eye examinations at baseline and at 6-month intervals for the duration of therapy.

Sulfasalazine*

Recently, interest in sulfasalazine (Azulfidine) has grown, perhaps motivated by its relatively favorable safety profile and newly proposed mechanisms of action, including inhibition of the pro-inflammatory 5-lipoxygenase pathway of arachidonic acid metabolism. A number of controlled trials have demonstrated efficacy in a percentage of patients with RA, although lack of benefit may be more common than with other second-line agents.

The usual starting dose is 0.5 gram twice a day, increasing by 0.5 gram weekly to a maintenance dose of 2 to 3 grams daily taken in two to three divided doses. Sulfapyridine appears to be the active moiety in RA, as serum salicylate levels are usually very low. Common adverse effects include GI intolerance, rash, dizziness, and headache. These symptoms necessitate withdrawal of therapy in one-third of patients. Patients must be monitored with periodic complete blood counts because of the rare occurrence of neutropenia. In general, serious side effects are

---

*Not FDA-approved for this indication.

less common than those seen with other disease-modifying drugs for RA.

D-penicillamine

The use of D-penicillamine (Cuprimine) has declined in recent years, largely due to the emergence of methotrexate as a more effective and less toxic alternative. It is usually reserved for patients in whom the other DMARDs have either caused toxicity or failed to control the disease. A "go low, go slow" approach to D-penicillamine therapy is essential to avoid heightening the already substantial risks of toxicity. The recommended initial dose is 250 mg per day, with subsequent 125- to 250-mg dose increments every 2 to 3 months, up to a maximum of 750 to 1000 mg per day. It should be taken between meals because its absorption is impaired by food. Careful clinical and laboratory monitoring is mandatory. Penicillamine's toxicity profile resembles that of gold, including skin rashes, stomatitis, proteinuria, and cytopenias. In addition, the drug may cause a severe taste disturbance (dysgeusia) and, rarely, severe autoimmune syndromes such as polymyositis, Goodpasture's syndrome, pemphigus, and bronchiolitis obliterans.

Azathioprine

Azathioprine (Imuran), a structural analogue of adenine and hypoxanthine, is a cell-cycle–specific antimetabolite. It rapidly undergoes hepatic metabolism to 6-mercaptopurine and then to a false purine analogue, thiouric acid. In doing so, it acts as a purine antagonist and suppresses the synthesis of adenine and guanine. Although the exact mechanism of action of azathioprine is unknown, it has been shown to act as an immune suppressant. Doses of 1.0 to 2.5 mg per kg per day are used, although lower doses have been shown to be as efficacious as higher doses in some studies, with less withdrawal due to adverse drug effects. Like other DMARDs, azathioprine has a gradual onset of action. It is unusual to observe a clinical response in less than 6 weeks, and frequently, a maximal response takes 4 to 6 months to be achieved. Therapy with azathioprine should begin at 1.0 mg per kg per day for a period of 6 to 8 weeks. The dosage may be increased by 0.5 mg per kg per day until an adequate response is obtained or the patient receives 2.5 mg per kg per day.

In general, azathioprine is a well-tolerated drug. The major side effects, in order of decreasing frequency, are GI disturbances (abdominal cramping, nausea, vomiting, and diarrhea being the most common), a mild reversible leukopenia, and elevation of the liver enzymes. Two forms of a rare hypersensitivity reaction have been described: an acute allergic hepatitis, and a systemic illness with fever, rash, polyarthritis, and sometimes meningismus. Although with long-term use in renal transplant recipients there is a risk of malignancy, many clinicians believe that the risk of azathioprine-induced cancer in RA patients is minimal or none. Due to this potential risk, however, some prefer to use the drug only in the elderly or in those in whom other agents have failed.

Cyclophosphamide*

Numerous trials have demonstrated cyclophosphamide (Cytoxan) to be an extremely efficacious drug in suppressing synovitis and retarding bony erosions. However, due to its toxicity profile, particularly the risk of cancer, its use is restricted to a very small subset of patients who have severe, advanced disease that is unresponsive to other agents or to those individuals with life-threatening extra-articular features of RA, such as rheumatoid vasculitis.

The short-term toxicities of cyclophosphamide include GI intolerance, bone marrow suppression (most commonly leukopenia), hair loss, and hemorrhagic cystitis. The long-term use of cyclophosphamide may lead to bladder fibrosis and carcinoma, serious infections, irreversible sterility, and hematologic malignancies. Although the disease usually flares after discontinuation of the drug, it is recommended that therapy with cyclophosphamide be limited to 1 to 2 years. The dosage is 1 to 2 mg per kg per day orally. When using cyclophosphamide in those with severe RA, monthly monitoring of blood counts and urine is recommended. Patients should be encouraged to drink large volumes of fluid to ensure frequent emptying of the bladder.

EXPERIMENTAL THERAPIES

A number of experimental therapies are being investigated at selected academic medical centers for patients who have not responded to the more conventional medications outlined earlier. Agents under study include cytokines and cytokine antagonists, including interferon-gamma, tumor necrosis factor (TNF), and interleukin-1 receptor antagonists; cyclosporine (Sandimmune); antibiotics such as minocycline (Minocin); and a number of monoclonal antibodies directed against T lymphocyte antigens or integrins. Clearly, these agents should be used with great care until their efficacy and safety have been established.

Fish oil supplements have been shown to provide in vitro anti-inflammatory activity but only modest clinical benefits. Studies of vitamins and other dietary supplements, including shark cartilage, snake or bee venom, aloe vera, and "gin-soaked" white raisins, have not demonstrated any advantage beyond basic and balanced nutritional principles, even though several of these compounds may have a theoretical rationale for use. Individuals with chronic diseases such as RA are particularly susceptible to anecdotes and claims of "cure." Education can play an important role in helping these individuals avoid expensive and potentially harmful remedies.

---

*Not FDA-approved for this indication.

JUVENILE RHEUMATOID ARTHRITIS

method of
TERRY L. MOORE, M.D.
*Saint Louis University Health Sciences Center
and Cardinal Glennon Children's Hospital
St. Louis, Missouri*

Juvenile rheumatoid arthritis (JRA) is a chronic arthritic disease of childhood of unknown etiology. It is a protean disorder with different modes of onset and patterns of disease accompanied by diverse signs, symptoms, and manifestations. JRA affects approximately 100,000 children in the United States, with a prevalence rate of 1 in every 2000 children. Diagnostic criteria for JRA include children less than 18 years of age having persistent synovitis of one or more joints for a least 6 weeks.

There are five basic onset types of JRA. The polyarticular-onset, rheumatoid factor (RF)–positive type is characterized by arthritis in five or more joints in the first 6 months of disease, associated with the presence of 19S IgM RF in the peripheral blood. Classically, peripheral non-weight-bearing joints are involved, including the metacarpophalangeal and proximal interphalangeal joints of the hands, wrists, knees, ankles, and metatarsophalangeal joints of the feet. All synovial joints can be involved. About 7% of children with JRA are in this category, and there is a female predominance. The second type, polyarticular-onset, RF-negative, is also characterized by arthritis in five or more joints, but RF testing is negative. These patients have a similar joint distribution as the aforementioned group and account for approximately 30% of cases, also with a female predominance. The third type, pauciarticular-onset with iridocyclitis (inflammation of the iris and ciliary body in the posterior uveal tract of the eye), is manifested by arthritis in one to four joints in the first 6 months of disease. About 50% of children with JRA are in this group; again, they are predominantly female. The majority have antinuclear antibodies (ANA) present, and 95% of those that will develop chronic iridocyclitis are ANA-positive. This group has a very good prognosis, with little residual joint damage. However, permanent eye damage can occur. The eyes require regular slit-lamp examinations, with follow-up by an ophthalmologist. The fourth type, pauciarticular-late onset, is found primarily in young males. Five or fewer joints develop synovitis in the first 6 months. Large joints such as the knees, ankles, and hips are most commonly involved. Low back pain may develop. Patients with this type of JRA may develop sacroiliitis and ankylosing spondylitis. Eighty to 95% of the latter carry the HLA-B27 marker. The last type, systemic-onset, is often the most difficult to diagnose. Initially, there may be daily temperature elevations to 103° to 106° F, occurring in an intermittent, spiking pattern. Usually, the fever persists for more than 2 weeks. It is usually associated with a rash, lymphadenopathy, splenomegaly, hepatomegaly, or other systemic manifestations. Joint involvement may develop subsequently. Approximately 20% of children with JRA have this type of onset.

JRA may present a difficult diagnostic problem because of a lack of specific laboratory abnormalities. It has to be differentiated from other diseases that may mimic JRA, including other connective tissue diseases, seronegative spondyloarthropathies such as psoriatic arthritis, Lyme disease, and other systemic illnesses.

The overall course and outcome of JRA are generally good. Treatment of JRA has several main elements: (1) to reduce inflammation and symptoms of JRA; (2) to suppress joint activity to decrease the possibility of long-term erosive changes, making a remission possible; (3) to prevent disability; and (4) to establish a team-oriented approach that includes a rheumatologist, physical and occupational therapists, ophthalmologist, and other paramedical personnel (Table 1).

The team approach includes first making a correct diagnosis. Once the diagnosis has been established, the rheumatologist must work with the pediatrician or primary care physician in considering the best drug therapy regimen. Baseline therapy of patients with JRA includes prescribing a nonsteroidal anti-inflammatory drug (NSAID), beginning recommended physical therapy procedures, and starting occupational therapy instructions for joint protection. Educating the parents and the patient about the disease is important, and it should be stressed that JRA is not a crippling disease in most cases. Approximately 75% of children with JRA do well over the long term. Those with a pauciarticular onset rarely having any residual damage. About 15%, usually from the polyarticular-onset and systemic-onset groups, develop chronic arthritis, but only about 5 to 10% develop any long-term disabling disease. Each step of the treatment plan should be discussed with the patient and the parents, describing the risks associated with the disease and the benefits as well as disadvantages of treatment.

When the disease is initially diagnosed, the physician should monitor the patient at least monthly, depending on the therapy employed and the activity of the disease. At each visit, it is important to note what joint manifestations are occurring, how long the morning stiffness is lasting, and whether there are any new joint complaints. Questions about problems with physical and occupational therapy modalities, school activities, and possible drug side effects are also required. At each examination, the physician should examine all joints to be sure that there are

TABLE 1. **Treatment Program for Juvenile
Rheumatoid Arthritis**

Reduce inflammation and symptoms
Suppress joint activity and erosions
Prevent disability
Establish a team-oriented approach

no new systemic manifestations. The detailed joint examination includes an evaluation for joint swelling, warmth, redness, pain, tenderness, and limitation of motion. Close monitoring of the side effects of medications should be performed, including laboratory testing. With NSAID therapy, a complete blood count (CBC), electrolytes, creatinine, liver function tests (aspartate aminotransferase [AST], alanine aminotransferase [ALT]), and urinalysis are performed at least every 3 to 4 months. The erythrocyte sedimentation rate (ESR) should be performed every few months. Baseline radiographs and then selected films at 6- to 12-month intervals are important to monitor the child for joint destruction. A progression of erosive disease suggests that additional therapy may be indicated. Slit-lamp examinations at 3- to 6-month intervals are needed.

DRUG THERAPY

NSAIDs

Current medical practice is to try to bring the disease under control with medications that offer the best therapeutic benefit with the least side effects (Table 2). Children with pauciarticular-onset JRA often go into remission with only the use of an NSAID, whereas polyarticular-onset and systemic-onset JRA may require remittive agents in addition to NSAIDs. For patients with mild arthritis, NSAIDs are often satisfactory by themselves. Four NSAIDs are approved by the Food and Drug Administration (FDA) for use in children: naproxen (Naprosyn), tolmetin sodium (Tolectin), ibuprofen (Motrin, Advil), and aspirin (ASA). Other NSAIDs have been evaluated in children but have not yet been approved. NSAIDs may cause significant gastrointestinal and/or renal toxicity. More than one NSAID should not be given simultaneously, because this doubles the toxicity. ASA used to be the NSAID of choice, but this is no longer true because of the risk of Reye's syndrome. Most pediatric rheumatologists in the United States now use naproxen or tolmetin sodium as their drug of choice, particularly naproxen.

Naproxen is an excellent first-line drug used in dosages of 10 to 20 mg per kg per day in two divided doses. Naproxen's advantage over other NSAIDs is that it is available as a liquid or tablet preparation and can be given just twice a day. The liquid prepara-

tion contains 125 mg per 5 mL. Tablets are available in sizes of 250, 375, and 500 mg. Monitoring for gastrointestinal toxicity is always indicated with naproxen. Occasionally it causes a pseudoporphyria-like rash located particularly on the face and appearing after sun exposure.

Tolmetin sodium is useful in a dosing schedule of three or four times per day. The dosage is usually 20 to 30 mg per kg per day. Tablets are available in sizes of 200, 400, and 600 mg. This drug also produces gastrointestinal irritation, but gastrointestinal toxicity is decreased if the medication is taken with skimmed milk or low-fat foods.

Ibuprofen comes in a liquid form (Children's Advil, Children's Motrin) at 100 mg per 5 mL. Tablet sizes are 200, 300, 400, 600, and 800 mg. The dosage is 30 to 40 mg per kg three to four times per day.

Other NSAIDs have undergone preliminary testing by the Pediatric Rheumatology Collaborative Study Group but have not been approved by the FDA for general use in children. These include sulindac (Clinoril)* 4 to 6 mg per kg twice daily, fenoprofen calcium (Nalfon)* 40 to 50 mg per kg three to four times a day, meclofenamate sodium (Meclomen)* 4 to 7 mg per kg three times daily, ketoprofen (Orudis)* 2 to 4 mg per kg three times daily, piroxicam (Feldene)* 0.2 to 0.3 mg per kg once a day, diclofenac sodium (Voltaren)* 2 to 3 mg per kg two to three times daily, flurbiprofen (Ansaid)* 4 mg per kg twice daily, and nabumetone (Relafen)* 20 to 40 mg per kg twice daily.

Remittive Therapy

Fifty percent of children with JRA, usually those with polyarticular onset or systemic onset, do not respond to NSAIDs or do not tolerate them, necessitating more aggressive therapy. Indications for further remittive therapy include poor clinical response to NSAIDs over at least a 3-month period, uncontrolled arthritis or evidence of erosive changes on radiographs, systemic manifestations, or steroid dependency or toxicity. Remittive drugs should be used with discretion; each has its own potential benefits and toxicities. Remittive drugs are ordinarily given in combination with an NSAID, and both the child and the parents should be advised about toxicities. Aggressive therapy in the first 2 years is very important in bringing the disease under control, since more erosions and pathology may occur during that time.

The remittive drug of choice is methotrexate (MTX) [Rheumatrex] administered orally. It is the most satisfactory medication of this type for children with JRA. A response appears as early as 3 to 4 weeks after starting therapy, but it may take longer. This response is much faster than that seen with the other remittive agents, including intramuscular gold or hydroxychloroquine (Plaquenil) therapy. MTX may reverse radiographic joint damage. It is given once

TABLE 2. **Drug Therapy in Juvenile Rheumatoid Arthritis**

NSAIDs	Remittive Agents
Naproxen (Naprosyn)	Methotrexate (Rheumatrex)
Tolmetin sodium (Tolectin)	Hydroxychloroquine (Plaquenil)
Ibuprofen (Motrin, Advil)	Gold salts (intramuscular)
Aspirin	(Myochrysine, Solganal)
	Sulfasalazine (Azulfidine)*
	Immune suppressives
	Combination therapy

*Not FDA-approved for this indication.

*Not FDA-approved for this indication.

weekly, usually in a dosage of 10 mg per m² of body surface area. The initial dose should usually be low, 2.5 to 5 mg once per week. Baseline tests include a CBC, urinalysis, and liver function tests. Potential toxicity of MTX includes hematologic (monitoring for a decrease in hemoglobin, white cell count, or platelet count); hepatic (testing for increasing ALT or AST or decreasing albumin levels); gastrointestinal, including nausea and abdominal pain; and pulmonary (nonspecific pneumonitis with associated cough) abnormalities. Laboratory tests should be repeated after 2 weeks and then every 4 weeks for the first 16 weeks of therapy. If the patient stays on a stable dosage, laboratory studies are checked monthly to every 6 weeks. If the dosage is raised, rechecking in 2 weeks is recommended, and then tests are repeated at monthly to 6-week intervals. The maximum dose per week is usually less than 15 mg, but infrequently, doses of 20 mg or higher are tried. MTX is available as a liquid or tablet and for intravenous and intramuscular injection. Nausea can sometimes be avoided by using the intramuscular route of administration. The liquid preparation, 2.5 mg per 0.1 mL solution, is potentially useful for small children. It can also be given by injection into the mouth with a small tuberculin syringe. If compliance is poor or if there is a possibility that nonrecommended dosages are being taken, the child can receive an intramuscular injection once weekly, given by medical personnel.

A major toxic effect of MTX is liver damage. If the ALT or AST level reaches more than twice the baseline level, the medication should be stopped for a week or two and then restarted if the levels normalize. If the liver enzymes remain abnormal, the medication should be discontinued. MTX can cause chronic liver damage with potential fibrosis and cirrhosis, but recent studies in JRA patients indicate that it is much less toxic in children than in adults. Total doses over 3 grams require close monitoring. The duration of MTX therapy may be 2 to 4 years. If the disease remits, MTX can be tapered slowly, usually in 2.5-mg decrements, and possibly switching later to every-other-week administration. If the child stays in remission, the medication may be discontinued after 6 months. The maximum duration of therapy is not known at this time. MTX is a good steroid-sparing drug.

A second remittive drug that works well in combination with an NSAID and/or MTX is hydroxychloroquine. It is a good anti-inflammatory medication for mild to moderate arthritis. Toxicity is low. The initial dose is usually 5 to 7 mg per kg per day administered once or twice daily. A baseline ophthalmic examination for color vision and peripheral field should be performed and repeated every 4 to 6 months to monitor the drug's eye toxicity.

Gold salts (Myochrysine, Solganal) are injected intramuscularly. Gold is the oldest remittive agent and has been used for both adults and children. A test dose of 2.5 to 5 mg is administered initially; the dose is increased gradually to 1 mg per kg per week to a maximum of 50 mg. The dose of gold is administered

weekly for 20 weeks, then every 2 weeks for eight injections, followed by every 3 weeks for a like period, followed by every 4 weeks if the patient is responding and doing well. Before each injection, a CBC, urinalysis, and platelet count should be performed. Monitoring the child for mouth ulcers and skin rash is necessary. If side effects develop, gold can be withheld for a week and the patient re-evaluated. If there is resolution of toxicity, gold at half the dosage is indicated. The medication must be discontinued if persistent side effects continue.

Other remittive agents have been used occasionally. Sulfasalazine (Azulfidine)* at 30 mg per kg per day is gaining wider acceptance. Penicillamine (Cuprimine, Depen) is often an effective remittive agent, but its toxicities include bone marrow suppression and proteinuria. The frequency of side effects limits its use in children.

Immune suppressive agents, such as azathioprine (Imuran), chlorambucil (Leukeran), and cyclophosphamide (Cytoxan), can be an alternative therapy to MTX in some cases, especially if results are poor or if toxicity occurs. In those patients with severe polyarticular-onset disease or multiple systemic manifestations, these medications can be tried. They also serve as steroid-sparing agents.

Different combinations of remittive drugs have been tried in some children with unrelenting disease. The combination therapy may result in a reduction of the overall total dosage of the separate medications, and decreased toxicity may follow. The synergistic effect of the agents may result in the desired improvement. The combinations of MTX and hydroxychloroquine and MTX and azathioprine have been used in severe JRA. These medications have also been used in combination with steroids, such as oral prednisone in 5- to 10-mg doses per day, or in combination with intramuscular or intravenous methylprednisolone (Solu-Medrol).

Low-dose cyclosporine (Sandimmune)* in dosages of 3 to 5 mg per kg per day may be used in the future. However, close monitoring of renal toxicity, hypertension, and weight gain is essential. The use of this drug in JRA remains experimental.

Mild flares of disease are usually managed by increasing the dose of medication, switching to another NSAID preparation, or increasing the MTX dosage. Predisone in doses of 1 to 2 mg per kg per day is usually administered for moderate to severe exacerbations manifested by marked swelling, warmth, and redness in the joints of children with polyarticular-onset and systemic-onset disease or if there are systemic manifestations such as fever, skin rash, hepatosplenomegaly, and pleural or pericardial effusions. Severe arthritis flares in children with polyarthritis are usually treated with 1 mg per kg per day in divided doses. The higher dosage of prednisone is often necessary in flare-ups of systemic-onset JRA. The dosage should be maintained for 2 to 4 weeks or until the disease becomes quiescent, and then ta-

---

*Not FDA-approved for this indication.

pered appropriately, trying to lower the dosage to the smallest maintenance level possible. The multiple side effects of steroids, including weight gain, growth retardation, glucose intolerance, and acneiform eruptions, emphasize the need to reduce the dose with long-term therapy. Occasionally, intravenous pulses of methylprednisolone can be given for severe flare-ups, usually over 3 days with doses at 30 mg per kg per day, to a maximum of 1 gram. Impressive therapeutic effects within 24 hours may result. Intravenous steroid therapy is usually reserved for patients with severe systemic manifestations.

Intra-articular injections of corticosteroids may prove beneficial if one or a few joints are causing difficulty. This is especially helpful in a pauciarticular-onset patient with one to two joints involved or a polyarticular patient with a few active joints. A dosage of 20 mg of triamcinolone acetonide preparation (Kenalog, Aristospan) in large joints such as the knee, or lower dosages in smaller joints, may be helpful. Any one joint should not be injected more often than every 3 to 4 months. This treatment does not produce systemic side effects if it is not used excessively.

TEAM THERAPY

A patient with JRA not only needs a rheumatologist but also requires the participation of other medical personnel. All children being evaluated for JRA should have a slit-lamp examination by an ophthalmologist for screening and follow-up. If the child is less than 7 years old at onset, has pauciarticular or polyarticular onset, and is ANA-positive, slit-lamp examinations should occur every 3 months for the first 4 years of disease and every 6 months thereafter into adulthood. These groups have the highest incidence of developing iritis, and eye symptoms are usually not present. Those who are ANA-negative and/or older than 7 at onset need evaluations at 6-month intervals. If mild iritis is present, local use of dilating eye drops with or without steroid drops is often adequate therapy. Occasionally, if the inflammation is unresponsive, local subtenon injections of steroids, oral prednisone, or immune suppressives may be indicated.

On first evaluation, a JRA patient should be seen by a physical therapist to evaluate joint involvement, muscle strength, and range of motion. The physical therapist will provide a daily or twice-daily home exercise program that parents can monitor; the goal is to avoid or reduce muscle atrophy and preserve range of motion. The importance of physical therapy cannot be overestimated. It is also necessary for maintaining good muscle tone and decreasing the impact loading on the joints, thus reducing flexion contractures and other range-of-motion problems.

An occupational therapist is also important in following the patient, observing the range of motion, muscle-strengthening exercises, fine motor abilities, and activities of daily living. The occupational therapist can teach the child and parent home exercise programs and modify them as indicated. Adaptive devices can be developed that may help the child have a better quality of life. Providing resting night splints, fabricating finger splints to preserve range of motion and prevent deformities, and working out a school program are part of their services.

A social worker may also be helpful in dealing with any denial problems, school adjustments, and monetary issues that may develop during the course of the disease. The social worker can advise families about eligibility for different state and federal programs and can provide local or outside counseling opportunities.

Occasionally, patients with JRA may also develop temporomandibular joint (TMJ) disease and may need close monitoring and early referral to an oral surgeon or orthodontist who is trained in the evaluation of TMJ problems and micrognathia.

Long-term problems may develop, and an orthopedist can be helpful in evaluating and treating severe hip or knee disease, cervical spine arthritis, peripheral joint arthritis, finger deformities, soft tissue contractures, and severely damaged joints requiring joint replacement.

The rheumatologist has to cooperate with the occupational and physical therapists and the orthopedist to solve difficult rehabilitation problems. Overall, the long-term prognosis for JRA is very good. Seventy-five percent of children usually enter into remission and do not have any long-term disabilities. Fifteen to 25% may have major long-term problems and should be monitored more closely, even into adulthood. The use of the team approach has reduced morbidity in these groups over the last few years, and this should only improve in the future.

ANKYLOSING SPONDYLITIS

method of
V. WRIGHT, M.D., and
P. S. HELLIWELL, D.M., PH.D.
Rheumatology and Rehabilitation Research Unit
University of Leeds, United Kingdom

Ankylosing spondylitis (AS) is an inflammatory disease that predominantly affects the spines of young men, but peripheral arthritis can be present. Its hallmark is sacroiliitis. The sites of tendon and ligament attachment to bone are affected with enthesopathy, as well as synovial and cartilaginous articulations. Most patients have the genetic marker HLA-B27, and AS is sometimes associated with psoriasis, Reiter's syndrome, or chronic inflammatory bowel disease.

CLINICAL FEATURES

The disease commonly begins as backache or buttock ache in young men in their late teens and twenties. The pain frequently disturbs their sleep. Women are believed to have milder disease than men, although a series of 123 matched patients in our clinic did not support that contention. The onset is usually insidious and may be accompanied by fatigue. Ten percent of patients have sciatica, and their condition is often confused with a prolapsed intervertebral disk. In the active phase, early-morning stiffness is prominent. Rest aggravates the symptoms, whereas exercise alleviates them. The patient often finds it difficult to get out of bed in the morning. Pain is frequently experienced in the dorsolumbar region, in the neck, and in the chest. This pain, which radiates from the back and is aggravated by coughing, is caused by costovertebral joint involvement. A small number of patients are virtually asymptomatic throughout their disease. It may come to light either by a flare precipitated by injury or by chance during some other investigation.

Back movements are restricted in all directions. As the disease progresses, the lumbar lordosis is obliterated, chest expansion is limited, a dorsal kyphosis develops, and cervical spine movements may be severely restricted. The last is often the bitterest complaint of the patient. Enthesopathy at costosternal junctions, spinous processes, iliac crests, and ischial tuberosities may produce tender areas. The hips and shoulders are commonly involved, but the knees and other peripheral joints may also be affected. Indeed, synovitis of the knees may be the presenting complaint.

In our clinic, we have found it useful to monitor progress with a functional index specifically designed for AS. The Leeds Disability Index is structured similarly to the Stanford Health Assessment Questionnaire and explores four areas: mobility, bending down, neck movements, and posture. Short-term improvement with physiotherapy can be demonstrated, although the scores tend to rise with disease duration.

If the spine becomes rigid, a pseudofracture may develop at one or more sites, particularly in the dorsolumbar region. The resulting pain is different from normal spondylitic pain in that it is alleviated by rest and aggravated by exercise. In a quarter of patients, anterior uveitis occurs at some stage; it may be severe, requiring vigorous treatment. It is typically unilateral and begins acutely. Symptoms include pain, increased lacrimation, photophobia, and blurred vision.

As kyphosis progresses, compensatory flexion of hips and knees may be necessary. Hip involvement, which is usually bilateral, results in flexion contractures, further exaggerating flexion at the knees to preserve an upright posture. Involvement of other peripheral joints seldom produces permanent damage. Ballooning of the abdomen occurs due to diaphragmatic breathing, occasioned by a rigid chest wall. Rarer complications include cardiac conduction abnormalities, aortic valve incompetence, apical pulmonary fibrosis and cavitation, amyloidosis, and IgA glomerulonephropathy.

DIAGNOSIS

AS is first a clinical diagnosis. Important features of the history are gender (male predominance), age of onset (usually before 40), aggravating and alleviating factors (rest and exercise, respectively), and pronounced spinal stiffness that is particularly prominent in the morning. Diagnostic criteria are given in Table 1.

Examination reveals limitation of thoracolumbar movement in all directions—in contrast to mechanical back problems, in which movements in one plane are usually satisfactory—and restricted chest expansion. Iritis may be the presenting feature, and ophthalmologists need to be alert to this possibility. Similarly, synovitis of the knees

TABLE 1. Modified New York Diagnostic Criteria for Ankylosing Spondylitis (AS)

Clinical Criteria

Low back pain for >3 months improved by exercise and not relieved by rest

Limitation of lumbar spine movement in the frontal and sagittal planes

Reduced chest expansion (corrected for age)

Radiologic Criteria

Bilateral sacroiliitis, Grade 2–4

Unilateral sacroiliitis, Grade 3–4

AS is diagnosed if either radiologic criterion plus any clinical criterion is present.

may usher in the disease; in a young man, this should always raise the possibility of AS. Radiologic sacroiliitis seen on an anteroposterior x-ray is mandatory for a definite diagnosis. It comprises bilateral symmetrical blurring of the subchondral bone plate, followed by erosions and sclerosis of the adjacent bone. Computed tomography (CT) and magnetic resonance imaging (MRI) may show changes before abnormalities are visible on plain x-ray. In adolescents, before the epiphyses are fused, it is very difficult to make a diagnosis of sacroiliitis on plain x-ray. Osteitis condensans ilii should not be confused with sacroiliitis. CT or MRI may help resolve doubts in both these contexts. The erythrocyte sedimentation rate is often mildly raised—up to 30 mm in the first hour—and serum IgA is elevated (although the latter is seldom used diagnostically). Rheumatoid factor is negative. Occasionally, HLA-B27 may be used to exclude the diagnosis of AS, but this is an expensive test that should not be used routinely. It has good sensitivity but poor specificity. Synovial fluid has inflammatory characteristics and is unhelpful diagnostically.

NATURAL HISTORY

Early diagnosis and vigorous treatment have altered the course of AS. The course is highly variable, with spontaneous remissions and exacerbations, but is generally favorable (85% of patients are still employed 10 years after initial diagnosis). Trauma may exacerbate the condition, and most serious is a fracture of a rigid spine with neurologic complications. Patients with hip involvement or a completely ankylosed cervical spine with kyphosis are more likely to be disabled.

MANAGEMENT

In patients with AS, *exercises are vital*. Ideally, they should be demonstrated by a physiotherapist and then reinforced by the physician as care continues. The patient should walk erect, do back extension exercises regularly, and sleep on a firm mattress with a pillow, if possible. It is better to sleep on the back or in a prone position with an extended and stretched back and to avoid sleeping curled on one side. Regular deep-breathing exercises are also important, and the patient must stop smoking, since this is liable to reduce diaphragmatic excursion and minimize the diaphragm's compensatory role. Swimming in a warm pool should be encouraged, but diving should

TABLE 2. **NSAID Therapy in Ankylosing Spondylitis**

Indomethacin (Indocin), diclofenac (Voltaren), or naproxen (Naprosyn) in a full dose is usually most effective, although any tolerated NSAID will help

Avoid combinations of NSAIDs

Slow-release preparations give better overall control and are effective in relieving morning stiffness

Co-prescribe a gastroprotective agent if there is a history of dyspepsia or peptic ulcer

Provide information on mode of action and potential side effects of drugs

be avoided, particularly if the neck is involved. The only situation in which rest may be encouraged is when spondylodiskitis and/or fracture necessitates a corset. Devices for helping the activities of daily living may be useful. If the hips are involved, a pickup stick, a long-handled shoehorn, and elastic laces often prove useful. When neck rotation is limited, as it frequently is, a wide-angle rearview mirror in the car is recommended. In the less usual cases of kyphosis impairing forward vision, prismatic spectacles overcome this difficulty.

Nonsteroidal anti-inflammatory drugs reduce pain and stiffness and enable the patient to exercise effectively (see Table 2). Phenylbutazone (Butazolidin)* is one of the most effective of this class of drugs but has a poor therapeutic ratio due to bone marrow toxicity.

The only second-line drug of proven worth is sulfasalazine (Azulfidine), which may be particularly helpful in patients with peripheral arthritis and/or those with concomitant inflammatory bowel disease. The optimal therapeutic dose is 40 mg per kg in two divided doses; this dose should be achieved by starting at 500 mg per day for a week and increasing weekly by 500-mg increments to the target dose. Nausea may occur and is minimized by using an enteric coated preparation and by employing the dosage schedule given previously. Initial monthly blood monitoring is necessary to detect the 2 to 3% of patients who develop neutropenia. After the first 3 months, a blood count, liver function tests, and urinalysis for protein should be carried out every 3 months. If therapy is successful, the full dose should be maintained for at least 12 months, after which the dose may be tapered but not discontinued.

Systemic steroids should be avoided, except for severe eye disease. Intralesional steroids may, however, be helpful in controlling local enthesopathy or synovitis. Spinal radiotherapy was used in the past (and was effective) but is not employed today because of the increased risk of leukemia and aplastic anemia. Local radiotherapy is still used in resistant cases of enthesopathy, particularly around the ankle. Radiation synovectomy may be of benefit in the knee, particularly for cases unresponsive to intrasynovial corticosteroids.

Acute anterior uveitis is treated with dilatation of the pupil and corticosteroid eye drops. Total hip

*Not available in the United States.

arthroplasty is worthwhile if the patient is having considerable pain and the quality of life is markedly diminished by restriction of movement, despite the patient's relative youth. Cardiac complications may require aortic valve replacement or pacemaker implantation.

TEMPOROMANDIBULAR DISORDERS

method of
SAMUEL F. DWORKIN, D.D.S., Ph.D., and
EDMOND L. TRUELOVE, D.D.S., M.S.D.
University of Washington
Seattle, Washington

Temporomandibular disorders (TMDs) are musculoskeletal conditions affecting primarily the muscles of mastication and/or the temporomandibular joint. Overwhelmingly, the most common presenting symptom for which treatment is sought is persistent pain, located predominately in the preauricular area or masticatory muscles and, to a lesser extent, the ear, temples, and muscles of the neck. In addition to pain, other common presenting symptoms accompanying pain include limitations in vertical range of motion of the jaw and noises in the temporomandibular joint during function. A small minority of patients present with complaints of stiffness or discomfort in the jaws or with intermittent but disturbing patterns of closed jaw locking, which prevents opening the jaw more than a few millimeters. Occasionally, otherwise asymptomatic patients present with complaints of clicking or popping noises in the temporomandibular joint; at present, no treatment for these pain-free noises of the joint is recommended.

TMD is best understood as a recurrent, chronic musculoskeletal pain condition that is self-limiting and is only rarely associated with significant physical disease progression. Thus, for the most part, procedures such as surgery or repositioning of the teeth or jaw, and "conservative" (i.e., noninvasive) treatment approaches that emphasize self-management are almost universally recommended. Finally, it is now well accepted that TMD involves both physical disease and subjective illness processes so that integrated *biomedical* and *biobehavioral* approaches to diagnosis and assessment as well as to management of TMD are required.

EPIDEMIOLOGY

TMD is a common disorder, and the 6-month prevalence of TMD-related pain is estimated at about 12% in the U.S. population. The presence of any one of the three major clinical indicators of TMD (pain, limitations in jaw opening, and joint noises) is estimated to be present in 5% to 50% of the population at any one time, although treatment seeking seems only poorly correlated with the presence of TMD signs and symptoms. Intensity of TMD-related pain seems the most reliable predictor of treatment seeking. Modal TMD patients are women in the child-bearing years. The rate at which women seek treatment for TMD is four to seven times greater than that for men, although the prevalence of TMD pain in the population is only about twice as high for women. The condition is most prevalent in the 18- to 45-year age group and falls off sharply with advancing middle age. Other than age and gender, there are no known risk factors for TMD that emerge with any reliability.

CLINICAL ASSESSMENT AND DIAGNOSIS

Biomedical Assessment and Diagnosis

Although a large number of pathologic states and diseases affect the tissues of the face and jaws, the term "temporomandibular disorder" (TMD) is generally restricted to painful and dysfunctional conditions affecting the muscles of mastication and the temporomandibular joint, leaving to more traditional categorizations pathologic conditions such as tumors, vascular pain syndromes, and generalized pathologic states affecting other organ systems and tissues. The predominate clinical subtypes of TMD are classified as masticatory muscle disorders, derangements (e.g., displacements) of the articular disk of the temporomandibular joint, and degenerative joint changes typically classified as arthralgia, arthritis, and arthroses of the joint.

Biomedical assessment should include evaluation of jaw symptoms and function. The location of pain is an important indicator of the type of condition. Pain reported in the muscles of mastication suggests the presence of myofascial pain, whereas pain reported by pointing directly at the joint suggests capsulitis, osteoarthritis, or disk derangements. The report of past or present joint sounds may also provide clues as to the type of pathology. Clicking is frequently a benign finding and is reported in about one third of otherwise asymptomatic adults. A history of clicking can be important if recent changes have occurred, such as a past history of clicking that has now stopped but is replaced with pain in the joint and limitation on opening. The progressive development of crepitus can signify either osteoarthritis or arthrosis. Jaw function also provides important keys to diagnosis and is assessed effectively by observing the opening pattern (straight, deviated, deviated with correction), measuring passive and active jaw opening, jaw excursions in lateral and protrusive directions, and pain intensity and location during these movements.

Deviations on opening may indicate variation that is normal or may suggest the presence of restriction caused by muscular tightness, joint dysfunction, or pain. Significant reduction in opening, while frequently seen in painful muscular disorders such as myofascial pain, is also suggestive of a displacement of the articular disk. Joint sounds are potential indicators of pathology and therefore should be assessed. Clicking is usually classified as either single (detected only on opening or closing) or reciprocal (detected during opening and closing). Reciprocal clicking frequently suggests that the articular disk is displaced on closing, and, while single clicks can indicate disk displacements, they also occur from irregularities within the tissue components of the joint or during movement of the condyle over the eminence of the articular process. Crepitus detected during joint movement may suggest osteoarthritis if the joint is also painful during function or movement, or indicate osteoarthrosis if no pain is present. In general, joint clicking or crepitus is not a finding that requires further extensive assessment unless the joint itself is painful, opening is restricted, or the patient reports changes in the bite, such as the development of an open bite in the anterior teeth.

Palpation of the muscles of mastication and the temporomandibular joint (TMJ) is an important component of assessment of patients with facial pain. Palpation must be carried out in a standardized manner or the diagnosis may be inaccurate. Studies have demonstrated that palpation of the muscles of mastication extraorally should be performed using approximately 2 pounds of pressure and that the joint should be palpated with no more than 1 pound of pressure. Use of greater force results in overdiagnosis of muscle and joint problems. Intraoral palpation should be restricted to 1 pound of force. Palpation of placebo sites is also useful in providing information about the relative value of the information received from the patient during these palpations.

Changes in occlusion should be assessed by question and observation. Progressive open bite in the anterior leading to inability to bite into foods suggests continued osteoarthritis or arthrosis. Severe wear on the occlusal surfaces of the teeth indicates a history of significant bruxism or jaw parafunction unless the patient's diet has been high in abrasive foods. Other dental defects, including malocclusion, although important to assess, have not been found to be highly associated with TMD, and epidemiologic studies have shown prevalence rates of malocclusion in TMD patients to be no higher than in normal populations. Obviously, very major malocclusions caused by skeletal discrepancies may, on an individual basis, contribute to TMD symptoms, especially if they result in increased rates of parafunction. Specific research diagnostic criteria for TMD have been developed by an expert team and are in use widely as clinical and research tools. Diagnostic criteria for the most prevalent forms of TMD are listed in Table 1.

Differential Diagnosis of Related and Other Conditions

A number of conditions can either present with symptoms confused as TMD or exist concurrently with TMD and contribute to increased TMD symptoms. Facial migraines in the region of the TMJ can be confused with transient joint dysfunction, and in elderly patients, temporal arteritis is difficult to distinguish initially from TMD. Since TMD is uncommon in elderly people, other conditions should be ruled out before considering TMD as the pain source. Cervical musculoskeletal pains can be referred into the face and TMJ region, thus confusing the diagnosis. Since cervical myofascial pain dysfunction and TMD are common and often concurrent, failure to resolve facial pain in such patients should trigger exploration for muscle trigger point referral sites in the muscles of the neck. Odontogenic pain from dental infections can cause changes in jaw function and provoke muscle or joint symptoms; therefore percussion of all teeth is wise to rule out such complications. Emerging dyskinesia may manifest as TMD because of jaw fatigue that occurs from dyskinesia-induced muscle hyperactivity. If trauma preceded the onset of TMD symptoms, it is essential to rule out a condylar fracture by use of imaging modalities, and great attention is needed to assure that a traumatic disk displacement or perforation is not present. Most traumatic injuries to the joint result in a sprain or capsulitis, but more severe damage can occur even in injuries such as whiplash in which no direct trauma is delivered to the mandible. In patients with rheumatoid arthritis or other immune-based inflammatory conditions, the TMJ is rarely the only joint involved, but patients can develop either concurrent TMJ involvement or initiate TMD symptoms while engaging in jaw tensing to cope with pain in other joints.

Biobehavioral Assessment

TMD bears many similarities to other common chronic pain conditions, such as back pain and headache, in its behavioral manifestations and personal impact. Behav-

TABLE 1. **Research Diagnostic Criteria for Temporomandibular Disorders**

Group I: Muscle Disorders

Ia. Myofascial Pain (pain in the muscles of mastication)

1. Pain or ache in the jaw, temples, face, preauricular area, or inside the ear at rest or during jaw function; plus
2. Palpation pain of 3 or more of 20 muscle sites (posterior, middle, or anterior temporalis; origin, body, or insertion of the masseter; stylohyoid, digastric, lateral pterygoid, and tendon of the temporalis). Palpation pain must be on same side as pain complaint for at least one site.

Ib. Myofascial Pain with Limited Opening

1. Myofascial pain as defined above; plus
2. Pain-free unassisted mandibular opening of less than 40 mm; plus
3. Maximum assisted opening of 5 mm more or greater than #2.

Group II: Disk Displacements

IIa. Disk Displacement with Reduction (anterior, lateral, or medial displacement)

1. Reciprocal clicking in the TMJ (click on both opening and closing, or a click on either opening or closing and click during lateral or protrusive excursions

IIb. Disk Displacement Without Reduction, with Limited Opening

1. Report of a significant reduction in opening; plus
2. Maximum unassisted opening ≤35 mm; plus
3. Passive stretch increases opening 4 mm or less over unassisted opening; plus
4. Contralateral excursion <7 mm and/or uncorrected deviation to the ipsilateral side on opening; plus
5. Absence of joint sounds, or presence of joint sounds not meeting criteria for disk displacement with reduction

IIc. Disk Displacement Without Reduction, Without Limited Opening

1. Report of significant limitation of mandibular opening; plus
2. Maximum unassisted opening >35 mm; plus
3. Passive stretch increases opening by 5 mm or more
4. Contralateral excursion ≥7 mm; plus
5. Presence of joint sounds not meeting criteria for disk displacement with reduction
6. If joint imaging is requested it should image the disk in closed and open mouth positions. The imaging modalities of value are arthrography and MRI.

Group III: Arthralgia, Arthritis, Arthrosis

IIIa. Arthralgia (pain in the joint)

1. Pain in one or both joint sites during palpation; plus
2. One or more self-reports of pain in the region of the joint, pain in joint during maximum unassisted or assisted opening, or lateral excursions
3. Absence of coarse crepitus

IIIb. Osteoarthritis of the TMJ (inflammatory changes in the joint)

1. Arthralgia (see above); plus
2. Coarse crepitus in the joint or joint imaging showing erosions, sclerosis of condylar head or articular eminence, or flattening of the joint surfaces

IIIc. Osteoarthrosis of the TMJ (remodeling of the articulating surfaces)

1. Absence of arthralgia; plus
2. Coarse crepitus or joint imaging showing joint changes

Abbreviations: TMJ = temporomandibular joint.

---

ioral, psychological, and psychosocial factors play an important role and require attention when diagnosing and planning treatment for TMD patients. Characteristics of TMD found in common with other chronic pain conditions include

Poor correspondence between the nature or extent of pathophysiologic change and global severity of pain and suffering;

Dysfunctional behaviors that directly affect the pain condition, such as oral parafunctional habits;

Transient psychological distress;

The potential for clinically meaningful depression, anxiety, and somatization;

Interference with ability to perform usual activities at home, work, or school; and

Frequent use of the health care system, with potential for excessive treatment-seeking and abuse of medications.

Four domains of biobehavioral assessment are recommended. When assessing for biobehavioral variables, attention is directed to subjective and psychological factors, as they may reveal the presence of psychological disturbance and inadequate coping with the chronic pain condition. For the most part, assessment of these biobehavioral domains is possible through routine history and examination methods and requires no special measuring instruments or questionnaires; when specialized measures may be useful, they are indicated.

1. **Patient's self-assessment.** Included here are recording of *pain complaint* (with special attention to consistency of subjective report with relevant anatomy and physiology); *treatment history* (with attention to record of prior successful and unsuccessful treatments and/or experiences with health professionals); the patient's *explanatory model* for the condition (with attention to physical vs. behavioral factors, such as stress) in perceived etiology, maintenance, and exacerbation of the condition. Patients with a rigidly held physical or biomedical model of their condition will

be more resistant to consideration of behavioral change strategies that may help them cope more adequately with their chronic pain problem.

2. **Jaw Disability and Oral Parafunction.** Included here is assessment of *oral parafunction* symptoms and habits such as jaw clenching or tooth grinding, which may both be reflections of stress and represent masticatory muscle abuse and dysfunction.

3. **Psychological Status.** Included here is assessment of *depression, anxiety*, and *somatization*. Formal assessment of psychological status requires specialized measurement instruments and/or diagnostic interview schedules. However, the inclusion of relatively straightforward measures in a clinical data base, such as the SCL-90-R, used routinely with all patients minimizes resistance to the perception that attention is being unduly given to psychological factors while the patient feels a physical pain problem is being presented. Such measures are more appropriate as screening aids and allow clinical impressions to be formed concerning the need for more specialized psychological assessment, generally achieved through referral to a psychiatrist or clinical psychologist. Depression commonly coexists with chronic pain conditions and has been documented in TMD clinic populations. Similarly, somatization is present in a significant minority of TMD patients, and there is ample evidence that even moderately elevated levels of long-standing somatization represent an important obstacle to successful treatment outcome.

4. **Psychosocial Status.** Included here is assessment of current level of psychosocial function, generally reflected for chronic pain patients in terms of extent of interference with activities of daily living attributed to TMD and extent of health care utilization. Prognosis is more guarded when self-reported activity limitations due to TMD are high and when pain interferes appreciably with ability to discharge responsibilities at home, school, or work and/or limits socializing activities. The assessment of both psychological status and level of psychosocial function are viewed as essential to allowing rational clinical decisions concerning management of TMD.

TREATMENT

Biomedical Treatments

Most patients with TMD experience a remission of symptoms over time and can be treated conservatively. Treatment modalities include most of the same strategies employed for other chronic musculoskeletal conditions; in general, aggressive approaches such as surgical interventions or costly dental therapies can be avoided. Since a small number of TMD cases become chronic, there is also the need to consider management of them using the same principles of chronic pain management as would be considered for other chronic pains. Initial management should include careful instructions for elimination of habitual jaw activities, including clenching, jaw posturing, bruxism, fingernail biting, and jaw tensing, which occurs when the teeth are held together even without actual clenching. TMD resulting from trauma or other events can be sustained through dysfunctional jaw function patterns. Stress often increases existing patterns of jaw parafunction; therefore attention to physical reactions to stressors is essential. Applications of ice or heat packs to tender muscles is very

effective symptomatic therapy and often provides transient relief of pain.

Once it is clear that a disk displacement without reduction is not present, passive jaw opening exercises are also of benefit and have been found to improve pain-free mandibular opening. Usually, the only opening exercise needed is passive vertical opening—lateral or protrusive exercises are unnecessary. Professional physical therapy is not usually necessary in the treatment of TMD except after surgical treatment of the joint, and most patients can provide the needed physical therapy themselves at home.

In the early stages, medications can be of value, but use of narcotic analgesics should be limited to 1 or 2 weeks except in cases of clear physical damage to the joint or capsule. Normally, 30 mg of codeine or the equivalent is adequate to control pain, and often nonsteroidal anti-inflammatory drugs (NSAIDs) are as effective as codeine while providing the added benefit of reducing joint inflammation if the joint is tender. Controversy exists as to the value of muscle relaxants in TMD, but patients do frequently report that such agents, including carisoprodol (Soma), cyclobenzaprine (Flexeril), and others seem to reduce symptoms, whether from actual muscle relaxation or secondary sedative properties. Care is needed, however, in prescribing muscle relaxants for other than the acute phase of TMD, since some potential for dependency exists. Use of muscle relaxants for periods greater than 3 to 4 weeks is not generally advised. When TMD is accompanied by significant anxiety or situational stress, transient use of an anxiolytic agent such as diazepam (Valium) or similar agents can be of value. Long-term use is not advised for most patients unless the medication is being used to treat the anxiety state rather than the pain.

When significant joint inflammation or disk displacement is present, use of NSAIDs may reduce symptoms, and in severe cases, use of systemic or intracapsular steroids is indicated. Prednisolone orally at dosages of 20 to 30 mg per day or as 4 to 8 mg injected into the joint can reduce persistent joint pain. More recently, antidepressants have been used increasingly to provide relief in chronic TMD. They improve sleep, which is frequently disturbed in chronic TMD, and may offer analgesic effects. Trazodone (Desyrel) is effective if the direction in therapy is sleep improvement, and amitriptyline (Elavil) has proved of benefit when pain and sleep dysfunction are significant.

Another common treatment for TMD involves the construction of jaw habit appliances. For most cases of TMD, a simple night guard made of acrylic and designed not to reposition the jaw is useful in assisting the patient to control jaw parafunction during times when conscious control is difficult (sleep, driving, concentration). About 40% of TMD patients may require such splints, and a much smaller percentage require more aggressive dental treatments such as orthodontics, expensive jaw repositioning therapy splints, or restorative care. Bite adjustment has not been shown to be much more effective than placebo treatments and therefore is not indicated unless the dentist finds severe bite problems.

For patients diagnosed as having disk displacements without reduction, TMJ surgery may be necessary to restore normal jaw opening. Currently, arthroscopic surgery is the most common approach but should be considered only after a clear diagnosis has been established via imaging and after a reasonable period of conservative therapy has failed to resolve pain. A small percentage of patients with progressive degenerative osteoarthritis may also require surgical intervention if films show large osteophytes in the joint, and pain is triggered in the joint with normal movement. Often patients with osteoarthritis have concurrent myofascial pain, and resolution of the muscle dysfunction and use of an NSAID result in significant reduction of joint symptoms to the point that surgical intervention becomes unnecessary. When the pain becomes chronic and persistent, assessment by a pain clinic or regional center devoted to TMD problems may be wise.

Biobehavioral Treatment

The treatment of all chronic pain conditions, including TMD, emphasizes a rehabilitation approach to treatment rather than a cure model. Consistent with such an approach, reliance is placed on the patient acquiring a useful set of self-management strategies that facilitate more adaptive pain-coping behaviors, emotional responses, and thought patterns.

General agreement has emerged that behavioral and educational modalities are useful and effective in the management of chronic pain conditions, although gains achieved are often modest, and factors contributing to the efficacy of such modalities remain to be more precisely defined. Behavioral and educational treatment modalities constitute a component of virtually every reported chronic pain treatment program, and management of temporomandibular disorders has benefited from such behavioral interventions as well.

Biobehavioral treatment approaches derive from applying behavioral science theory and methods to changing the perception of pain and ameliorating or eliminating the personal suffering and psychosocial dysfunction that often accompanies persistent pain conditions. These biobehavioral interventions are viewed as safe, reversible, and noninvasive and for the most part emphasize strategies under the patient's control. A large collection of treatment modalities is subsumed under the label of biobehavioral treatments; the most commonly used of these include biofeedback, relaxation, hypnosis, and cognitive-behavior treatment and education. These biobehavioral pain management modalities are drawn largely from cognitive-behavioral and behavioral psychotherapeutic approaches; the efficacy of psychodynamic and psychoanalytic treatment approaches for management of chronic pain has not yet been as scientifically validated.

Although the use of educational approaches to modifying TMD-related pain and dysfunction has not been extensively studied, there is evidence that a single psychoeducational group session early in treatment for TMD will modestly reduce TMD pain–related interference in psychosocial function compared with usual treatment, and the benefits gained continued to be present at 1-year follow-up. Educational methods have been demonstrated to be efficacious in the self-management of headache and back pain, using both group and individual approaches to deliver the educational interventions.

By and large, when biobehavioral treatments are employed in the management of TMD, effects are positive and in the hypothesized beneficial direction, though often effects are moderate in size. However, these biobehavioral methods, especially those subsumed under the label "cognitive-behavioral," appear to have the potential for producing long-lasting benefits when compared with usual clinical treatment for TMD. Increasingly, as noted, conservative, noninvasive approaches to TMD management are being advocated as the preferred overall treatment approach for this hard-to-understand chronic pain problem. These so-called "conservative treatments" generally incorporate many of the same elements (e.g., relaxation, stress-education, habit behavior modification, and so on) found in cognitive-behavioral and behavioral therapies for TMD. Thus, both usual clinical treatment for TMD and biobehavioral treatment employ multimodal approaches, and it does not yet appear possible to determine which of the multiple therapeutic components are most efficacious. If one method had to be singled out, relaxation seems to emerge consistently as an effective method for chronic pain management across a wide range of pain conditions and over a wide variety of clinical settings. In any event, the combined biobehavioral methods commonly used in clinical practice have as yet failed to establish one modality as superior to another. It is important to note that much the same situation obtains with regard to biomedical-based TMD treatments. Little is known about the superiority of any one of the multiple methods commonly employed to biomedically manage TMD—there is no strong scientific evidence to substantiate invasive vs. noninvasive treatments or pharmacologic treatments emphasizing analgesics vs. those stressing antidepressants or muscle relaxants. It is the absence of compelling evidence to the contrary that has compelled many clinical researchers to advocate conservative, reversible therapies for the largest majority of TMD patients.

A great deal more research is needed before it is possible to evaluate adequately how biobehavioral interventions achieve their desired effects and which components of the multi-modal approaches now in common use are most potent. Perhaps of greatest interest is the need to develop treatment approaches tailored to both the physical and the behavioral status of the patient. Typically, treatment of TMD seems currently driven largely by the physical diagnosis alone, without addressing the personal or psychosocial impact of TMD pain or the patterns of coping with TMD used by patients. Although TMD is regarded by many as a condition in which psychosocial factors influence the course of the condition, in fact little attention has been paid to assessing how psychological or psychosocial factors influence treatment outcome and whether successful clinical outcome is associated with improved psychosocial function. It seems fair to say that outcome assessment for TMD, except for assessing self-report of pain, is focused almost exclusively on assessment of physical factors (range of jaw motion, joint sounds, and so on).

Most recently, biobehavioral treatment approaches have been advocated that differ according to the differing levels of psychosocial functioning and/or level of cognitive or emotional disturbance exhibited by specific TMD patients or by groups of TMD patients. Such approaches give at least equal emphasis to biobehavioral assessment as to biomedical assessment for deriving treatment modalities tailored not only to the individual patient's biomedical status but also to their biobehavioral status. Future clinical research will determine whether such an approach is indeed effective in the management of TMD, in which chronic pain plays such a dominant role.

SOFT TISSUE PAIN SYNDROMES

method of
I. JON RUSSELL, M.D., PH.D.
University of Texas Health Science Center
San Antonio, Texas

The term "soft tissue pain syndromes" refers to a group of painful conditions that affect tendons, bursae, muscles, and nerves. Pain in mechanical soft tissue structures can interfere with volitional activities just as readily as painful arthritic disorders do. The Arthritis Foundation has listed over 100 arthritic disorders and a comparable number of distinct soft tissue pain syndromes.

The relevance of these conditions to clinical practice is illustrated by a British general practice study of 644 elderly outpatients. Twenty-one percent of those surveyed suffered from shoulder area pain. In 70% of affected individuals, the principal cause of the symptoms was found to be a soft tissue pain syndrome rather than arthritis. A recent U.S. community survey documented that 64% of the general public had no pain, 5% had transient pain, 21% had chronic regional pain, and 11% had chronic widespread pain. Of course, articular and soft tissue pain syndromes are not mutually exclusive, nor does their coexistence in the same patient necessarily define one as being due (secondary) to the other.

When a patient presents complaining of musculoskeletal pain or dysfunction, it is critical to establish the correct diagnosis. This can be accomplished by careful history taking and physical examination. First determine whether synovial joints, soft tissue structures, or both are involved, based on the nature, location, and duration of symptoms. Laboratory tests can then be used to seek support for the diagnostic impressions.

A laboratory database should be established if tests have not been done within the prior 12 months. It should include a complete blood count, erythrocyte sedimentation rate (ESR), multichannel chemistry panel, thyroid function tests, and urinalysis. The use of more sophisticated tests depends on the differential diagnosis. For example, antinuclear antibodies (ANAs) or rheumatoid factor (RF) should be measured only if historic and examination findings suggest an autoimmune rheumatic disease.

Table 1 provides a working classification of soft tissue pain syndromes divided into three broad categories: local, regional, and widespread pain. Each of these categories is further subdivided to accommodate anatomically and clinically distinct syndromes. Almost any structure around a joint can become painful if it is repeatedly stretched, contused, or compressed. A few injuries are clinically observed with sufficient frequency to deserve mention by name.

LOCAL PAIN SYNDROMES

Tenosynovitis (tendinitis) refers to a tender, painful inflammation of the tenovaginum that surrounds a tendon. Acute trauma or unaccustomed, repetitive use can cause swelling, pain, and impaired function. The diagnosis should be suspected from the pattern of pain and limitation. It is confirmed when digital palpation (pressure in a rolling motion across the tendon) reproduces the clinical symptoms.

Most of the common clinical syndromes are named anatomically. For example, biceps tendinitis involves the long head of the biceps tendon anterior to the shoulder, supraspinatus tendinitis involves the tendon that traverses the coracoacromial groove at the

TABLE 1. **Classification of Soft Tissue Pain Syndromes**

Local Pain Syndromes	
Tenosynovitis	Enthesopathies
Biceps	Epicondylitis
Supraspinatus	Plantar fasciitis
de Quervain's	Costochondritis
Achilles	Pellegrini-Stieda
Trigger fingers	Osgood-Schlatter
Bursitis	Entrapment syndromes
Subacromial	Carpal tunnel
Olecranon	Ulnar tunnel
Trochanteric	Tarsal tunnel
Prepatellar	Morton's neuroma
Pes anserine	Referred pain
Achilles	Diaphragm–shoulder
Last	Heart–left elbow
	Hip–knee
Regional Pain Syndromes	
Myofascial pain syndrome	Masticatory myofascial pain syndrome
Generalized (Widespread) Pain Syndromes	
Polymyalgia rheumatica	Chronic fatigue syndrome
Hypermobility syndrome	Fibromyalgia syndrome

Supported by the RGK Foundation of Austin, Texas.

Adapted from Russell I: J Musculoskel Pain *1*:1–7, 1995.

shoulder and attaches to the enthesis on the proximal humerus, and Achilles tendinitis involves the heel. Other names are less revealing, such as de Quervain's tenosynovitis, which affects the adductor pollicus longus and extensor pollicus brevis tendons at the radial side of the wrist, and trigger fingers, in which nodules on the flexor tendons at the metacarpophalangeal (MCP) joints cause the tendons to pop or hang up as they pull through the palmar fascia, giving the appearance of the finger resting on a trigger.

The initial interventions should be conservative. Immobilization of the moving structure, local heat, and oral nonsteroidal anti-inflammatory drugs (NSAIDs) often prove adequate. More resistant cases may benefit from local injection of an anesthetic agent (e.g., 1% lidocaine without vasoconstrictors) and a corticosteroid such as 10 mg of triamcinolone (Aristospan) into the tendon sheath. Careful skin cleansing reduces the risk of iatrogenic infection. Care must be taken not to enter the tendon itself, because that could predispose to tendon rupture.

Bursitis is an inflammatory swelling of a bursa, which normally contains only a small amount of viscous fluid within a highly innervated membrane. When the bursa is swollen or inflamed, there is tenderness to palpation and pain with movement of the overlying connective tissue structures. Bursitis can develop because of localized trauma or repetitive motion–related injury from an unaccustomed activity. But bursitis can also result from bacterial or fungal infection.

Most bursitis-related syndromes are named anatomically: subacromial bursitis (a bursa that lies below the shoulder acromion), olecranon bursitis (overlies the extensor surface of the elbow), trochanteric bursitis (overlies the greater trochanter of the proximal femur), and Achilles bursitis (beneath the Achilles tendon at the calcaneus). The names of other syndromes are not so anatomically obvious: pes anserine bursitis (distal to the medial aspect of the knee, beneath the conjoined tendon of the adductor muscles) and last bursitis (anterior medial or lateral aspect of the ankle after prolonged pressure from a shoe-strap last).

The most conservative approach to the treatment of bursitis is temporary splint immobilization of the joint that moves the affected bursa. Heat and NSAIDs should be administered in full anti-inflammatory dosages. If symptoms persist, an intrabursal injection of an anesthetic agent (e.g., 1 cc of 1% lidocaine) and a corticosteroid (10 mg triamcinolone) often eliminates the symptoms. Careful skin antisepsis is important.

Evidence suggesting infection in a painful bursa includes unusually severe pain, increased skin temperature, and fluctuance of the bursa. Early aspiration of bursal fluid for Gram's stain, culture, and polarized microscopy for crystals is indicated. The white cell count of infected bursal fluid is generally lower than would be expected for a comparably infected synovial joint. Specific antibiotic treatment

should be accompanied by repeated aspirations of bursal fluid as often as it reaccumulates.

An *enthesopathy* is a painful, tender inflammation of an enthesis, where ligament or tendon attaches to bone. Some enthesopathies result from local stretching injuries, including medial epicondylitis (golfer's elbow with microavulsions from the enthesis at the medial side of the elbow), lateral epicondylitis (tennis elbow), Osgood-Schlatter disease (infrapatellar ligament at the proximal tibia), Pellegrini-Stieda syndrome (dystrophic calcification of the medial collateral ligament of the knee), plantar fasciitis (longitudinal arch ligament of the foot), and costochondritis (anterior chest wall pain with tenderness at costochondral junctions). The seronegative spondyloarthropathy syndromes are systemic autoimmune enthesopathies occurring in individuals predisposed by their HLA-B27 genetic background. They are mentioned here because they can present as a local enthesopathy.

Treatment involves immobilization of the affected extremity, NSAIDs (especially indomethacin), and local injection (as with tendinitis). Avoidance of the exacerbating activity may be necessary.

Entrapment syndromes result from compression of a peripheral nerve as it traverses a closed compartment accompanied by other structures that can swell and compress the delicate nerve fibers. The diagnosis of each disorder depends on recognition of a characteristic clinical pattern coupled with a knowledge of the relevant neuroanatomy.

The *carpal tunnel syndrome* results from compression of the median nerve at the wrist. It is characterized by pain that awakens the patient 1 to 2 hours after going to sleep. There is painful dysesthesia in the palmar surface of the thumb, index finger, long finger, and radial side of the fourth finger. With chronicity, there can be atrophy of the thenar eminence and weakness of the opponens pollicus muscle (which opposes the tip of the thumb to the tip of the fifth finger). The Phalen test (full flexion of the wrist for 1 minute to exacerbate the symptoms) can be performed for supportive evidence. In severe cases, electrodiagnostic examination demonstrates slowing of nerve conduction across the wrist. Medical causes include hypothyroidism, rheumatoid arthritis, fluid retention, and amyloidosis.

The *ulnar tunnel syndrome* is caused by compression of the ulnar nerve at the elbow. It is characterized by pain or numbness in the fifth finger and the ulnar half of the fourth finger. There is weakness of the intrinsic muscles of the fingers (demonstrated by testing the strength of lateral spreading of the fingers). It can result from elbow arthritis or from excessive leaning on the elbows, as occurs among patients with chronic obstructive lung disease.

The *tarsal tunnel syndrome*, compression of the medial tibial nerve at the medial malleolus, is characterized by pain in the great toe. *Morton's neuroma*, a pathologic swelling of the second or third digital nerve in the forefoot, apparently occurs because of repeated weight-bearing trauma from shoes that are too narrow.

Management of compressive neuropathies is aimed at decreasing the pressure on the involved nerve, but that is accomplished differently for each clinical disorder. Patients with carpal tunnel syndrome benefit from a cock-up wrist splint to maximize the space in the carpal tunnel. When worn at night, it prevents flexion of the wrist, which narrows the tunnel and precipitates nocturnal pain. A full anti-inflammatory dose of an NSAID and perhaps a mild diuretic may reduce local swelling. If symptoms persist, an intra-tunnel injection of anesthetic (1% lidocaine without vasoconstrictors) and corticosteroid (5 to 10 mg triamcinolone) antiseptically reduces symptom severity. Patients with ulnar tunnel syndrome should use a large soft pillow under their elbows when resting on them. Patients with tarsal tunnel syndrome may benefit from a wedge in the shoe that inverts the foot and opens up the tarsal tunnel. Patients with Morton's neuroma should wear flat, wide shoes. Surgical resection of the neuroma is sometimes necessary but can predispose to recurrent neuroma.

Pain experienced in the area of a joint can have its origin in a visceral organ (called *referred pain*). Failure to consider this possibility can lead to inappropriate treatment of a normal joint while missing the visceral process. Examples include referral of pain from an irritated left hemidiaphragm (subphrenic abscess, pulmonary embolus, lobar pneumonia) to the left shoulder, referral from the heart (ischemia, pericarditis) to the left shoulder or elbow, and referral from a diseased hip to just above the ipsilateral knee.

Management must be directed at the underlying visceral problem, which is beyond the scope of this article. The understanding of pain radiation from the hip toward the knee can expedite proper management of hip arthritis.

REGIONAL PAIN SYNDROMES

The term "myofascial pain syndrome" (MPS) refers to a collection of muscle pain disorders thought to result from unaccustomed use of a muscle group. In its simplest form, this disorder is characterized by pain in a region of the body (e.g., near the shoulder, elbow, or low back) that can be reproduced by palpation of a more centrally located tender spot in a skeletal muscle. The tender muscle spot, of which patients are often unaware, is called a "trigger point." The location of the spontaneous discomfort, at a site distal to the trigger point, is called the "zone of reference."

Although MPS has been recognized clinically for 500 years, it is still poorly understood. Published criteria for the diagnosis of MPS include a muscle trigger point; a "taut band," which can exhibit a "twitch response" to firm stroking by the examiner's thumb or by needle penetration; and a zone of reference, which is the area of discomfort prompting the patient to seek care. There are two main problems

with the diagnosis of MPS. One is that clinicians who considered themselves skilled in its diagnosis failed to agree with one another when challenged with blinded cases of MPS and normal controls. A recent study showed that careful standardization of examiner technique can remedy that problem. Second, many clinicians believed that MPS could spread and cause "widespread pain" and were probably confusing such cases with the fibromyalgia syndrome (see the later discussion). These two issues raise concern about the accuracy of past literature concerning the clinical features of MPS and its pathogenesis.

There is growing consensus regarding the importance of spontaneous electrical activity at trigger point sites found in humans with MPS and in a rabbit model. The original study was unnecessarily complicated, however, by the choice of fibromyalgia patients for the study of MPS trigger points.

Since there are nearly as many MPSs as there are skeletal muscles, it is impossible in the space allotted to describe each pattern. For details regarding specific body regions, the reader is referred to the two-volume *Trigger Point Manual* by Travell and Simons or *Myofascial Pain and Fibromyalgia* by Rachlin. Briefly, the patient presents with unilateral pain involving an area of the shoulder, trunk, or extremity. A trigger point that might cause referral to that symptomatic region is sought in a reference text. The clinician then examines the predicted muscle area in search of a trigger point. With experience, the predicted patterns can become as familiar as the sensory dermatomes.

The principles of MPS treatment are similar irrespective of the trigger point site. The use of counterstimulation in its many forms such as massage, heat, and cold sprays has been advocated. A highly volatile liquid is sprayed lengthwise along the axis of the muscle containing the trigger point and toward the zone of reference, with passive stretching of both regions. Another approach (counterstrain) involves active contraction of an opposing muscle, so the affected muscle is placed at complete physiologically inhibited rest.

For cases in which the progress is slow or the pain is severe, injection of the trigger point may be helpful. Most clinicians who treat MPS prefer to inject an anesthetic agent, but saline injections and even "dry needling" reminiscent of acupuncture have their advocates. When the needle penetrates a trigger point, it can induce a twitch response. Several passes are made to the same general area, because the trigger point may be spread over the space of a few millimeters. Follow-up therapy should include local heat, stretching exercises, counterstrain exercises, and adherence to proper posture principles. Repeat trigger point needling may be required on a weekly basis for several weeks. Psychological problems should be addressed when present.

Masticatory myofascial pain (MMP), also referred to as the temporomandibular joint syndrome, temporomandibular dysfunction (TMD), or myofascial pain dysfunction syndrome, is usually treated by dental specialists. As with MPS, the cause is unknown. It has been associated with poor sleep, ear area pain, fatigue, and a variety of constitutional symptoms. In some patients there may be an associated click in the temporomandibular joint with excursion of the jaw. Some patients are recognized to have associated nocturnal bruxism and benefit from use of a bite plate prosthesis.

The current theory regarding the pathogenesis of this condition is that it parallels MPS as the head and neck presentation of that disorder. Based on that understanding, trigger points are sought in the temporalis, masseter, or pterygoid muscles, depending on the location of the spontaneous pain pattern. Suggested treatment is similar to that of MPS, except that the details of management are modified to accommodate the location of the involved muscles and their unique functions.

GENERALIZED (WIDESPREAD) PAIN SYNDROMES

Polymyalgia rheumatica (PMR) is included among the soft tissue pain syndromes because it is characterized by severe pain, aching, and stiffness in the shoulder and pelvic girdles. It occurs in elderly individuals with high sedimentation rates (ESR >50 mm per hour). Giant cell arteritis can be associated in 10 to 20% of patients. A destructive, inflammatory arthritis can also accompany PMR.

Hypermobility syndrome is a relatively benign variant of the Ehlers-Danlos syndrome, with increased elasticity of connective tissues. The diagnosis is characterized by hyperextensible joints, such as the metacarpophalangeal (painless extension >90 degrees) and wrist. Other hypermobile joints can include elbows, shoulders, knees, and ankles. It may be the most common cause of back pain in women and of recurrent ankle injuries due to instability. Hypermobility is more common in grade-school children (>30%) than in adults (<5%).

The *chronic fatigue syndrome* was initially recognized as an epidemic disorder that spread by unknown route through members of a community to a prevalence of about 0.001% of the general population. It was characterized by stringent criteria, including severe physical fatigue that reduced activity for at least 6 months to less than 50% of premorbid activity. Other common manifestations included low-grade fever, painful swollen lymph nodes, pharyngitis, myalgias, insomnia, headaches, and depression. Initial theories of an infectious etiology, such as Epstein-Barr virus, are no longer widely held. Neuroendocrine explanations, especially those involving dysfunction of the hypothalamic-pituitary-adrenal axis, are now in vogue. Table 2 provides an abbreviated summary of the new, substantially liberalized criteria. They greatly resemble the criteria for fibromyalgia.

Treatment for the chronic fatigue syndrome is nearly as unsure as the diagnosis. Conservative measures have probably been as successful as any of the dramatically touted interventions such as parenteral administration of gamma globulin or orally administered nutritional supplements.

The *fibromyalgia syndrome* (FS) is now recognized to be a chronic (lasting more than 3 months) disorder characterized by subjective widespread musculoskeletal pain and tenderness to palpation at anatomically defined, somatic tender points. Until recently, a prevalent belief had been that FS patients exhibited no objective abnormalities. As a result, the disorder was either accepted or rejected on the basis of the subjective symptoms, which were often rather dramatically portrayed by the patients. Initially, the most convincing evidence for an integrated syndrome was the relative consistency of the symptoms from one patient to another.

The American College of Rheumatology (ACR) criteria for the classification of FS have provided a highly sensitive and specific means of identifying affected individuals (Table 3). Systemic manifesta-

TABLE 2. 1995 Revised Criteria for Diagnosis of Chronic Fatigue Syndrome

Major criteria: Severe unexplained fatigue that is unrelieved by rest and reduces physical activity to less than 50% of usual activity

Minor criteria: Any four of the following:
Cognitive dysfunction
Sore throat
Tender lymphadenopathy
Arthralgia
Myalgia
Headaches
Nonrestorative sleep
Postexertional malaise

Exclusions: Active medical condition (e.g., untreated hyperthyroidism, major depression) that might explain any of the above (especially fatigue); fibromyalgia is not an exclusion

TABLE 3. 1990 ACR Criteria for Classification of Fibromyalgia Syndrome

History: Musculoskeletal pain in four quadrants
Examination: Reproducible tenderness with 4 kg of palpation pressure at 11 of 18 anatomically defined tender points

Anatomic Definition of Bilateral Tender Point Sites

Occiput: near the greater occipital nerve foramen
Cervical: anterior aspect of intertransverse spaces at C5–7
Trapezius: midpoint of upper trapezius border
Scapular: above scapular spine, over origin of supraspinatus muscle
Second rib: upper rib surface, lateral to second costochondral junction
Epicondyle: extensor fascia, 2 cm distal to lateral epicondyle
Gluteal: gluteus maximus muscle, near posterior ileal origin of gluteus medius
Trochanter: posterior margin of greater trochanter
Medial knee: soft tissue fascia just proximal to medial femoral condyle

Adapted from Wolfe F, et al.: Arthritis Rheum *33*:160–172, 1990.

tions that are common in FS (though not universal and not required by the ACR criteria) include persistent muscle contraction headaches, insomnia, fatigue, weakness, irritable bowel, interstitial cystitis, distal extremity dysesthesias, and, in some cases, a reactive depression.

Three important advances facilitated by reliable diagnostic criteria have included the determination of its prevalence, research into its biochemical pathogenesis, and its recognition in association with other medical conditions. FS occurs in about 10% of outpatients in medical clinics and in 2% of the general population, with adult women being affected seven to nine times more often than men. The peak age is the mid-fifties, but any age is possible. Five million persons in the United States have FS, resulting in an annual cost to the U.S. economy of more than $9.2 billion.

The pathogenesis of FS was at first thought to reside in the skeletal muscles near where the pain was felt, but ultrastructural studies have failed to identify a specific lesion. Confirmed abnormal biochemical findings in the research laboratory now include a persistently elevated cerebrospinal fluid substance P, a lower than normal serum (from platelets) serotonin, a lower than normal plasma insulin-like growth factor, and abnormal functions of the hypothalamic-pituitary-adrenal axis. A number of other abnormalities await confirmation by a second laboratory. These observations represent a major departure from the early perceptions that there were no objective abnormalities in FS. It should not be long before some of these tests are available clinically.

Table 4 summarizes a variety of medical conditions

TABLE 4. Clinical Illnesses That May Accompany Fibromyalgia and Tests That May Aid Assessment

Illness	Tests
Rheumatic disease	
Systemic lupus erythematosus	ANA + ESR
Rheumatoid arthritis	RF + ESR
Polymyositis	CPK
Sjögren's syndrome	ANA, RF, SS-A
Chronic infection/inflammation	
Tuberculosis	PPD + ESR
Chronic syphilis	VDRL + MHATP
Subacute bacterial endocarditis	Culture, ESR
Lyme disease	Serology
AIDS	Serology, CD4
Breast implant	? Serology
Myofascial pain syndrome	Trigger points
Endocrine disorders	
Hypothyroidism	T_4 + TSH
Hypopituitary	Serum prolactin

Abbreviations: ANA = antinuclear antibody; ESR = erythrocyte sedimentation rate; RF = rheumatoid factor; CPK = creatine phosphokinase; SS-A = Sjögren's syndrome antigen A; PPD = purified protein derivative; VDRL = test for syphilis; MHATP = microhemagglutination assay—*Treponema pallidum*; CD4 = T lymphocyte count; T_4 = thyroxine; TSH = thyroid-stimulating hormone.

Adapted from Russell I: *In* The Clinical and Scientific Basis of Myalgic Encephalomyelitis: Chronic Fatigue Syndrome. Ottawa, Nightingale Research Foundation, 1992.

TABLE 5. An Approach to Medical Management of Fibromyalgia Syndrome

Make a confident, accurate diagnosis of fibromyalgia
Identify and treat associated medical illnesses
Provide reassurance, explanation, instruction
Evaluate the role of domestic and emotional factors
Prescribe analgesic, propionic acid, NSAIDs, ? others
Provide physical therapy (3 wk outpatient course)
  Local heat for 30 minutes to neck, back, and shoulders (hydrocollater packs or infrared lamp)
  Deep sedative massage for 10 minutes to most symptomatic areas, as tolerated
  Instruction in relaxation therapy maneuvers
  Gradually progressive, active, aerobic, isotonic exercise (pool therapy or walking outside)
Give soft tissue injection occasionally for severely tender sites
Prescribe sedative-anxiolytic-antidepressant medications such as amitriptyline 10–35 mg hs or cyclobenzaprine 2.5–10 mg hs, alternating with alprazolam 0.25–1.5 mg hs
Schedule frequent, regular return visits

with which FS seems to coexist at a rate that may exceed the probability of chance. It is useful to recognize these "concomitant conditions" so that both they and FS can be managed appropriately. The laboratory profile outlined in the table is offered as an adjunct to a thoughtful medical history and physical examination.

There is little doubt that fibromyalgia patients experience considerable discomfort, but they also exhibit limitations of physical function comparable to that of rheumatoid arthritis. Nevertheless, there has been extensive debate about the extent to which FS is disabling. It is true that there is no progressive loss of articular structure in FS and no apparent reduction in longevity, such as occurs with inflammatory arthritic disorders and myopathic processes. Yet 30 to 45% of FS patients have accepted work changes that resulted in decreased job status and/or income. Two surveys disclosed that about 10% of FS patients were receiving social security disability payments. In many such cases, however, the basis for awarding the disability income was a concomitant condition such as osteoarthritis, even when careful assessment revealed that the most troublesome symptoms were actually due to the FS.

The other issue has been the extent to which FS is a disorder of personality, mood, or affective pathology. Indeed, the frequency of depression is elevated to about 30 to 40% in patients with fibromyalgia, but that value is nearly identical to the prevalence of depression in rheumatoid arthritis patients. Since depression is present in less than half of FS patients, it is less likely to be the cause of the disorder and more likely to be a consequence of chronic pain, insomnia, and dysfunction.

Table 5 summarizes the author's approach to the treatment of fibromyalgia. Most of the items listed are self-evident, so they are not discussed in detail. Clearly, the correct diagnosis must be made, and concomitant illness must be treated appropriately. Education about the disorder is critical to enlisting the patient's participation in self-care. The attitude of the clinician toward the disorder greatly influences the outcome of treatment. The author has prepared an inexpensive brochure, a book, and a video documentary to assist health care providers with this task. Spousal battery is an example of a domestic problem that should be addressed to help an abused patient focus fully on treatment of the FS.

Analgesic dosages of non-narcotic agents can be helpful as adjunctive therapy, even though they are usually inadequate as sole therapy. Despite the recognized abnormalities in the diurnal rhythm of cortisol production, the one study that addressed steroid treatment of FS failed to detect a benefit.

Physical therapy maneuvers have been advocated for FS patients, but the benefits they provide seem to be temporary. Heat is extremely helpful and can be achieved at home in a hot bath or shower. Aerobic exercise represents a long-term investment toward lasting benefit. The ideal program may be a progressive 20-minute session walking in place in chest-high water 3 days per week. Good alternatives include progressive power walking outside, walking on treadmills, or pedaling a stationary bicycle. The patient should start slow and increase the expended energy gradually as conditioning occurs.

Soft tissue injection should be reserved for rare occasions when a single area is tender out of proportion to other sites. Thus, injection therapy in FS would be subject to the same criteria used for healthy individuals with tendinitis or bursitis from unaccustomed exertion.

The use of low-dose tricyclic sedative hypnotic drugs in FS is advocated by many clinical studies, but these agents may be subject to tachyphylaxis after 2 or 3 months of continuous use. This central nervous system adaptation may result from an increase in the numbers of cell surface reuptake receptors for serotonin and norepinephrine. The author's approach is to discontinue the tricyclic drug after 3 months of continuous use and substitute low-dose alprazolam for 1 month. Then the cycle is repeated three times per year.

Follow-up visits at 2- to 3-month intervals provide the patient an opportunity to ask questions. At the same time, it allows the physician to assess responses to treatment and to screen for adverse effects from administered medications.

OSTEOARTHRITIS

method of
GARY L. CRAIG, M.D., and
REX T. HOFFMEISTER, M.D.
Rockwood Clinic
Spokane, Washington

Osteoarthritis, also termed degenerative arthritis, eventually affects the majority of our patients (and colleagues). Incidence rises with age, but predisposing genetic factors exist for hand and knee involvement. Obesity and preceding trauma are significant predictors for knee involvement, and even minor alignment abnormalities predispose to weight-bearing joint disease. Primary osteoarthritis can involve any joint but classically hits the knees, hips, and spine and the hand distal or proximal interphalangeal and carpal metacarpal joints (metacarpal phalangeal joint pain should raise suspicion of inflammatory joint disease or hemachromatosis). Osteoarthritis can be secondary to other joint processes, confusing the diagnosis. Shoulder, wrist, or ankle osteoarthritis may be triggered by calcium pyrophosphate deposition disease, and shoulder osteoarthritis is often a manifestation of rotator cuff arthropathy.

Recognition is based on history, distribution of joint involvement, and exclusion of other diseases, especially those with significantly different therapies. Inflammatory diseases generally occur in a younger age group, produce more intense morning stiffness and joint inflammation, and often have extra-articular features. Distal interphalangeal joint involvement similar to osteoarthritis is seen in spondyloarthropathies, including psoriatic arthritis. Shoulder and/or hip pain in an older patient forces consideration of polymyalgia rheumatica. Calcium pyrophosphate arthritis should be suspected with atypical large joint involvement or with quick deterioration of a previously stable osteoarthritic joint, even without radiologic evidence of chondrocalcinosis. The differential diagnosis for sudden worsening of pain in an osteoarthritic joint includes infections; other crystalline diseases (gout, hydroxyapatite disease); internal derangement; periarticular tendon, ligament, or bursa problems; knee trabecular microfractures (which clinically have marked tenderness above or below the joint line and can be revealed only by magnetic resonance imaging); and subcapital hip fractures. Likewise, rapid worsening of back pain or radicular symptoms in a patient with spinal degenerative disease has to lead to thoughts of new disk prolapse, compression fracture, or tumor.

Patients present with pain, joint swelling, loss of function, and periarticular bony bumps (osteophytes) or, in the case of the spine, with back pain, radicular pain or neurologic symptoms due to root irritation, or claudication-like pain that is eased more by sitting than by stopping and standing, indicative of spinal stenosis (often without back pain). Joint effusions, crepitus, and range loss may be highly variable and correlate poorly with pain, and x-rays may not correlate with symptoms. Pain commonly radiates proximally or distally; thus the joints above and below the source of complaint should always be examined (for hips, this includes the low back, and for shoulders, the neck). Investigations should be appropriate for the differential diagnosis, but the incidence of falsely positive rheumatoid or antinuclear factor tests rises with age. X-ray evidence of osteoarthritis does not exclude other causes of joint pain in an older patient. Elevation in the erythrocyte sedimentation rate indicates another diagnosis or other coincidental diseases (e.g., myeloma).

Treatment options include education to help patients recognize realistic capabilities, use of adaptive modalities, exercise programs, medications, and surgery. The latter is particularly appropriate for knee or hip involvement—joint replacement gives dramatic improvement. Arthroplasty is also appropriate for shoulder osteoarthritis but is better for pain relief than range restoration. Many patients need no further therapy than an explanation of what is going on, reassurance about the lack of other disease, and education about the appropriate use of affected joints. For example, it is unrealistic for a patient with patellar osteoarthritis to expect to kneel or squat while gardening, but use of a garden stool may accomplish functional gains that are unreachable with drugs or surgery. Other effective aids include enlarged grips for golfers with hand-range loss and utensils with larger handles and mechanical jar openers for chefs with similar problems. Walking programs on flat surfaces and swimming have been shown to reduce knee and back pain, and isometric quadriceps exercise benefits patellar pain. Weight control helps knee, hip, and back pain. Simple analgesics (acetaminophen) and nonsteroidal anti-inflammatory drugs (NSAIDs), preferably used intermittently, can reduce pain but do not slow disease progression. Side effects of NSAIDs include ulcer and, less frequently, fluid retention and renal and hepatic risks, all of which rise with age and the presence of other diseases. Co-administration of misoprostol reduces ulcer risk. Intra-articular corticosteroid injections can provide substantial short-term relief. Drugs to reduce osteoarthritis progression, such as novel anti-inflammatories (e.g., tenidap)* and metalloproteinase inhibitors (including tetracyclines),† are now being studied.

---

*Not yet approved for use in the United States.
†Not FDA-approved for this indication.

POLYMYALGIA RHEUMATICA AND GIANT CELL ARTERITIS

method of
JEFFREY R. LISSE, M.D.
University of Texas Medical Branch
Galveston, Texas

POLYMYALGIA RHEUMATICA

Polymyalgia rheumatica (PMR) is a syndrome that occurs in adults over 50 years of age and becomes more prevalent with advancing age. Incidence rates range from 3 per 100,000 per year for ages 50 to 59 to 45 per 100,000 per year for ages greater than 79. It is rare before the sixth decade of life. The goals of treatment in these patients are relief of symptoms and avoidance of the complications of giant cell arteritis (GCA) (discussed later).

Originally described in 1957, PMR involves proximal muscle aching in the hips, neck, and shoulders. Fatigue, weight loss, mild abnormalities in liver function tests, mild synovitis, and normochromic normocytic anemia may be accompanying features. There is no known cause, but the inflammatory nature of this syndrome is reflected in the elevated erythrocyte sedimentation rate (ESR), as well as prominent morning stiffness. The Westergren ESR is usually above 40 mm per hour.

One of the most difficult diagnostic challenges involves the exclusion of other potential causes for an elevated ESR and the symptoms noted earlier. The presence of chronic infection, rheumatoid arthritis, neoplasm, inflammatory muscle disease, endocrine disorders, or other neuromuscular disorders makes the diagnosis of PMR unlikely.

The physical examination may be relatively normal. Patients with PMR usually have normal muscle strength and bulk, and they give way during the musculoskeletal examination due to pain rather than weakness. Serum creatine phosphokinase (CPK) levels are normal in this syndrome, reflecting the lack of muscle destruction, as opposed to polymyositis and muscular dystrophy.

The clinician is often left with a patient with very little evidence of a definitive disease. The elevation in the ESR and the other associated findings suggest an inflammatory, systemic illness.

Treatment of this disorder consists of empirical therapy with 10 to 20 mg of prednisone per day. Most patients respond dramatically, symptoms may disappear, and the ESR normalizes within weeks. Patients who do not respond in 2 weeks should be re-evaluated for other potential illnesses. After a month, prednisone may be tapered, but probably no more rapidly than 1 to 2.5 mg per month. Symptoms and the ESR are monitored to evaluate efficacy. Prednisone therapy may be discontinued after 1 year in some patients, but many require treatment for up to 5 years after diagnosis. During this period, patients should be watched carefully for any of the signs and symptoms of GCA (see the following section). Overlap between the two syndromes is not viewed as common in North America, although it does occur. The potential risks from the higher doses of corticosteroids required to treat GCA outweigh the benefits of putting all patients with PMR on those doses.

GIANT CELL ARTERITIS

GCA is a large-vessel vasculitis that is often associated with PMR. It is also called temporal arteritis because of the propensity for involvement of the extracranial arteries of the head and neck, but similar changes have been described in a number of other vessels in the body.

It is estimated that 15 to 20% of patients with PMR also have GCA. GCA can also occur independently. Patients may complain of temporal headache, jaw or tongue claudication, altered mental status, cranial neuropathies, and transient ischemic attacks. The most feared complication is ophthalmic involvement. Amaurosis fugax and ischemic optic neuropathy are the findings usually associated with GCA and are two of the sequelae of vasculitic involvement of the ophthalmic arteries.

Physical examination may be normal, or there may be localized findings, such as tenderness or nodules over the temporal artery. The evaluation of GCA must include a biopsy of the temporal artery, usually ipsilateral to the symptomatic area. The typical biopsy should be at least 3 cm in length, and due to the possibility of skip lesions, careful examination of multiple sections is recommended. A strong suspicion and a negative initial biopsy should lead one to sample the contralateral temporal artery. Pathologically, giant cells and destruction of the internal elastic lamina are characteristic.

Treatment consists of 1 mg per kg per day of prednisone (40 to 60 mg per day) or its equivalent. This should be maintained for at least 1 month, after which the ESR can be followed, along with recurrence of symptoms. Prednisone doses can then be tapered: by 10 mg per month until a dose of 30 mg per day is reached, by 5 mg per month to 20 mg per day, by 2.5 mg per month to 10 mg per day, and then as slowly as 1 mg every 3 to 4 weeks. Duration of treatment is at least 1 year, and several years may be required to wean patients off corticosteroids completely. During this period, attention must be paid to the side effects of corticosteroids in the geriatric population, such as osteoporosis, hypertension, and hyperglycemia. Medications to treat these conditions in patients on corticosteroids can often be tapered and even discontinued as the glucocorticoid doses decrease.

OSTEOMYELITIS

method of
DEAN T. TSUKAYAMA, M.D.
Hennepin County Medical Center
Minneapolis, Minnesota

Osteomyelitis is one of the most difficult infections to treat effectively, especially when the infection is chronic. Many factors contribute to the chronicity of infection. The initial infection and inflammatory reaction are contained within the rigid structure of the bone, resulting in increased pressure that impairs the vascular supply and leads to necrosis. Abscess may also form within the bone (Brodie's abscess). Detachment of the periosteum from the bone cortex occurs when the mounting pressure forces the inflammatory exudate to work its way to the surface of the bone. When the periosteum is stripped away from bone, the periosteal blood supply to the cortex is lost, and the avascular cortical bone dies and becomes a sequestrum. The sequestrum acts as a foreign body, providing a nidus for colonization by bacteria. New bone, called the involucrum, may then form directly under the elevated perios-

teum, further isolating the sequestrum. The infection can extend beyond the bone to include adjacent soft tissue abscesses and sinus tracts leading to the skin. Necrotic bone, areas of fibrous scarring, and localized abscess are poorly vascularized, making the site of infection an inhospitable environment for both host defense cells and antibiotics. Bacterial virulence factors also play a role in the recalcitrant nature of this infection. Bacteria adhering to necrotic bone can live as microcolonies under a biofilm that protects them by preventing penetration of antibiotics and host defense cells. Management of osteomyelitis is difficult, often requiring multiple surgical débridements and prolonged, and sometimes repeated, courses of antibiotic therapy. An understanding of the pathogenesis of osteomyelitis and a systematic approach to management are essential for developing a strategy leading to the successful treatment of this infection.

Bacteria are introduced into the bone from the blood, by extension from a contiguous focus of soft tissue infection, or by direct inoculation from the environment in trauma-related injury. Hematogenous osteomyelitis is acute in presentation and usually involves the metaphyses of long bones. It is an infection seen predominantly in children. Vertebral osteomyelitis is also hematogenous in origin but has a more indolent clinical course. Elderly patients are predisposed to vertebral osteomyelitis, but it can also occur among users of illicit intravenous drugs. Extension from a contiguous soft tissue infection occurs most commonly under conditions of vascular insufficiency. Infected pressure ulcers, ulcers of vascular insufficiency that are secondarily infected, and diabetic foot infections are the usual clinical settings. Infections of this type are often polymicrobial, with gram-positive cocci, gram-negative bacilli, and anaerobes all isolated and all requiring antibiotic treatment. Open fracture is probably the most common predisposing factor leading to chronic osteomyelitis in adults. The risk of bone infection is related to the degree of soft tissue infection that accompanies the fracture. In fractures with soft tissue damage so severe that closure of the wound over the fracture is not possible (Gustilo Type 3 open fracture), the incidence of infection may exceed 30%.

DIAGNOSIS

Diagnosis of osteomyelitis is usually straightforward. Acute osteomyelitis presents with fever and severe bone pain, accompanied by leukocytosis and an increased erythrocyte sedimentation rate (ESR) and elevated C-reactive protein. Evaluation of acute osteomyelitis should include examination for septic arthritis in the adjacent joint. In chronic osteomyelitis, bone pain is less intense and may be intermittent. After a period of time, there may also be abscesses or sinus tracts leading from the infected bone to the skin. The ESR is increased in chronic osteomyelitis, but the white blood cell count is usually normal.

The goals in the assessment of osteomyelitis are to identify the pathogen or pathogens responsible for the infection and to determine the location and extent of disease. In acute hematogenous osteomyelitis, the pathogen can sometimes be isolated from the blood. Blood cultures are almost always negative in chronic osteomyelitis, and a culture from the infected bone must be obtained. This specimen can be obtained either by needle aspiration or by open biopsy at the time of surgery. Cultures taken from sinus tracts are unreliable in identifying the pathogens responsible for the bone infection. *Staphylococcus aureus* is the most frequently recovered pathogen. However, both aerobic and anaerobic cultures should be performed to recover other bacterial pathogens, such as facultative gram-negative bacilli or anaerobes, which may also be found. In selected cases, cultures for *Mycobacteria,* fungi, or other unusual pathogens may also be indicated.

Determining the location of osteomyelitis is first guided by the clinical manifestations. Radiographic evidence of bone infection should then be sought, but radiographs may be normal in early (less than 2 to 4 weeks) infection. Findings suggesting infection include osteopenia, osteolysis, disruption of the cortex, periosteal elevation, and sequestration. Technetium bone scans are very sensitive in detecting early osteomyelitis, but they lack specificity. Bone scans are useful when early osteomyelitis is strongly suspected but cannot be seen on radiographs. Imaging studies with gallium or indium-labeled white blood cells might also be considered in selected cases but have not proved to be of value in the routine evaluation of osteomyelitis.

Determining the extent of disease may be difficult. There may be more than one site of bone involvement, especially in vertebral osteomyelitis. The infection may extend within the intramedullary canal or to an adjacent joint. Soft tissue involvement can be extensive. Computed tomography (CT) provides excellent visualization of cortical abnormalities. Magnetic resonance imaging (MRI) can be helpful in identifying the extent of intramedullary involvement and in showing soft tissue abnormalities such as sinus tracts and abscesses. The role of CT and MRI in the evaluation of osteomyelitis is not well defined. However, one of these tests should always be performed in the evaluation of vertebral osteomyelitis to determine the extent of vertebral disease and to assess for epidural or paravertebral abscess.

TREATMENT

After the diagnostic evaluation is complete, the bacterial pathogens should be identified and the extent of infection known. Based on this knowledge,

there are four objectives that guide the treatment of osteomyelitis: adequate surgical débridement, appropriate antibiotic therapy, stabilization of bone if there is a fracture, and soft tissue coverage over the involved bone.

Surgical Débridement

The first, and most important, objective is to obtain adequate surgical débridement. Necrotic bone, infected tissue, sinus tracts, and nonviable tissue must be removed. The goal is to convert the site of infection into an area of viable tissue with adequate vascularity. Failure to achieve this goal compromises the effectiveness of any subsequent antibiotic therapy. However, thorough débridement is not always easily accomplished. Attempting to débride all the involved bone and soft tissue may threaten the stability and function of the limb. Intramedullary reaming permits débridement without sacrificing bone stability when the infection has propagated within the intramedullary canal. In some cases, segmental resection is the only option to adequately débride extensively involved bone. The Ilizarov method of external fixation permits this level of aggressive débridement by allowing bone lengthening after control of the infection. The only case in which débridedment may not be necessary is acute hematogenous osteomyelitis without necrotic bone or subperiosteal purulence. In this instance, osteomyelitis can be successfully treated with antibiotics alone.

Antibiotic Therapy

The second objective is to administer an effective course of antibiotic therapy (Table 1). Antibiotic ther-

TABLE 1. **Antimicrobial Activity of Selected Antibiotics Against Common Orthopedic Pathogens**

	S-MS	S-MR	Strep	EC	HF	E-GNB	PsA	A-GPC	Bact
Penicillin	1	0	3	3	0	0	0	3	1
Ampicillin	0	0	3	3	2	1	0	3	1
Oxacillin (Prostaphlin)	3	0	3	0	0	0	0	2	0
Piperacillin (Pipracil)	0	0	3	2	3	3	3	3	3
Ampicillin-sulbactam (Unasyn)	3	0	3	3	3	2	0	3	3
Ticarcillin-clavulanate (Timentin)	3	0	3	1	3	3	2	3	3
Piperacillin-tazobactam (Zosyn)	3	0	3	2	3	3	3	3	3
Cefazolin (Ancef)	3	0	3	0	1	1	0	2	0
Cefuroxime (Zinacef)	2	0	3	0	3	2	0	2	0
Ceftizoxime (Cefizox)	2	0	3	0	3	3	1	2	2
Ceftriaxone (Rocephin)	2	0	3	0	3	3	1	2	1
Ceftazidime (Fortaz)	1	0	2	0	3	3	3	0	0
Aztreonam (Azactam)	0	0	0	0	3	3	3	0	0
Ciprofloxacin (Cipro)	2	2	1	1	3	3	2	1	0
Clindamycin (Cleocin)	3	0	3	0	0	0	0	3	3
Gentamicin (Garamycin)	0	0	0	0	2	3	2	0	0
Imipenem (Primaxin)	3	0	3	2	3	3	3	3	3
Metronidazole (Flagyl)	0	0	0	0	0	0	0	2	3
Trimethoprim-sulfamethoxazole (Bactrim, Septra)	2	2	2	1	3	2	0	0	0
Vancomycin (Vancocin)	3	3	3	3	0	0	0	2	0

Abbreviations: S-MS = methicillin-sensitive staphylococci; S-MR = methicillin-resistant staphylococci; Strep = streptococci; EC = enterococci; HF = *Hemophilus influenzae;* E-GNB = enteric gram-negative bacilli; PsA = *Pseudomonas aeruginosa;* A-GPC = anaerobic gram-positive cocci; Bact = *Bacteroides. Clinical efficacy:* 0 = none; 1 = minimal; 2 = moderate; 3 = good.

apy should not be initiated before cultures are obtained, especially for chronic osteomyelitis in which the systemic component of disease is minimal. In acute osteomyelitis, presumptive antibiotic therapy is sometimes appropriate after blood cultures have been obtained. Infected bone has a poor blood supply, which means that a relatively small proportion of the antibiotic given systemically to the patient is actually delivered to the site of infection. The maximum recommended dose of the antibiotic should be given to ensure that adequate concentrations reach the infection site (Table 2). Measurements of the serum concentrations of antibiotics are not generally available to confirm that an effective dose of drug has been given. One method of indirectly confirming that the antibiotic dose is adequate is to measure the serum bactericidal titer (SBT) in the patient. The SBT is a measure of the ability of the antibiotic that is present in the serum (along with other serum factors) to kill the isolated pathogen. This method is especially useful when the patient is taking oral antibiotics, since the systemic absorption of an oral dose is variable, and the dose required is often higher than is customarily given. The required duration of antibiotic therapy has not been clearly defined. It is likely that the duration of antibiotic therapy required is inversely proportional to the adequacy of débridement; i.e., if the débridement completely eliminates the infection, no antibiotic therapy is needed. However, in almost all cases it must be assumed that some focus of infection remains, and experience has taught us that pathogens in osteomyelitis can be extremely difficult to eradicate. A prolonged duration of antibiotic administration, usually 4 to 6 weeks, remains the standard of treatment.

In an attempt to control the cost of medical care, more patients are receiving their intravenous antibiotic treatment at home after early discharge from the hospital. Patients with osteomyelitis are ideal candidates for this method of therapy because they are generally at low risk for complications that would require emergency treatment. Another cost-saving alternative to hospitalization and intravenous antibiotics is oral antibiotic therapy. In theory, if adequate antibiotic levels can be attained, the route of administration should make no difference. However, compliance with therapy can be a major issue, as can patients' inability to tolerate the high doses of drug that may be required. Agents with excellent properties of absorption that can be considered for oral therapy include amoxicillin, clindamycin, metronidazole, quinolones, and trimethoprim-sulfamethoxazole. There is good clinical experience with the use of dicloxacillin, other antistaphylococcal penicillins, and oral first-generation cephalosporins in the treatment of osteomyelitis.

In some patients, eradication of infection is not a realistic goal. The extent of surgical débridement required or the general medical and immune status of the patient may not permit definitive treatment. In these cases, suppressive antibiotic therapy with oral agents may keep clinical manifestations of the disease at an acceptable level. Malignancy and amyloidosis have been reported as long-term complications of ongoing osteomyelitis that has been present for many years.

Coagulase-positive staphylococci (almost always *S. aureus*) are the most common pathogens recovered in osteomyelitis. Coagulase-negative staphylococci are found in device-associated infections. Antibiotic treatment for staphylococcal infections, whether the organism is coagulase-positive or coagulase-negative, depends on the susceptibility of the pathogen to beta-lactam antibiotics. For bacteria that are susceptible, the antibiotic of choice is an antistaphylococcal penicillin such as nafcillin or oxacillin. A first-generation

TABLE 2. **Typical Adult Doses of Antibiotics for the Treatment of Osteomyelitis**

Generic Name	Brand Name	Usual Dose
Amoxicillin	Amoxil	500 mg tid to qid PO
Ampicillin	Omnipen, Principen	1–2 gm q 4–6 h IV
Ampicillin-sulbactam	Unasyn	3 gm q 6 h IV
Aztreonam	Azactam	1–2 gm q 6–8 h IV
Cefazolin	Ancef, Kefzol	1–2 gm q 8 h IV
Ceftazidime	Fortaz, Tazicef, Tazidime	2 gm q 8 h IV
Ceftizoxime	Cefizox	2 gm q 8 h IV
Ceftriaxone	Rocephin	2 gm q 24 h IV
Cefuroxime	Zinacef	1.5 gm q 8 h IV
Ciprofloxacin	Cipro	750 mg bid PO
Clindamycin	Cleocin	900 mg q 8 h IV
		300–450 mg tid to qid PO
Dicloxacillin	Dynapen	500–1000 mg tid to qid PO
Gentamicin	Garamycin	5 mg/kg/day in 1–3 divided doses IV
Imipenem	Primaxin	500 mg q 6–8 h IV
Metronidazole	Flagyl	500 mg q 6–8 IV or PO
Penicillin G	—	3–4 million U q 4–6 h IV
Piperacillin	Pipracil	3 gm q 4–6 h IV
Piperacillin-tazobactam	Zosyn	3.375 gm q 6 h IV
Ticarcillin-clavulanate	Timentin	3.1 gm q 6 h IV
Trimethoprim-sulfamethoxazole	Bactrim, Septra	10 mg/kg/day in 2–3 divided doses IV or PO
Vancomycin	Vancocin	1 gm q 12 h IV

cephalosporin such as cefazolin can also be used in this situation. Another alternative is clindamycin. Methicillin-resistant staphylococci, which are in fact resistant not only to methicillin but also to all penicillins and cephalosporins, are treated with vancomycin. If vancomycin cannot be used, quinolones or trimethoprim-sulfamethoxazole can sometimes be used as alternative agents.

Streptococcal organisms can be found as a single pathogen or as part of a polymicrobial infection of the bone. Included in this group are beta-hemolytic streptococci such as group A, group B, or group G streptococci, alpha-hemolytic streptococci, and *Streptococcus pneumoniae*. The antibiotic of choice for streptococcal infections is penicillin G. Effective alternative agents include other penicillins, cephalosporins, vancomycin, and clindamycin. Recent reports show that some strains of *S. pneumoniae* and alpha-hemolytic streptococci are now resistant to penicillin and must be treated with antibiotics such as vancomycin or third-generation cephalosporins.

Enterococci, formerly classified as streptococcal bacteria, are now classified in their own genus. The major species are *Enterococcus faecalis* and *Enterococcus faecium*. Enterococci are occasional pathogens in osteomyelitis, but when present, they can be difficult to treat. In general, enterococci are more resistant to antibiotics than are streptococci, and *E. faecium* is more resistant than *E. faecalis*. Ampicillin, penicillin G, piperacillin, mezlocillin, and imipenem are the most active agents in the penicillin class of antibiotics, but *E. faecium* is often resistant to these agents. Vancomycin has been a reliable antibiotic for penicillin-resistant enterococci, but disturbingly, recent isolates have been described that are vancomycin-resistant and, in fact, resistant to all currently available antimicrobial agents. In addition, bactericidal (killing of organisms) rather than bacteriostatic (preventing growth of organisms) activity requires the combination of an aminoglycoside and either a penicillin or vancomycin. Bactericidal activity is thought to be necessary in some enterococcal infections such as endocarditis, but there is no evidence to indicate that bactericidal activity is needed in the treatment of osteomyelitis.

Facultative gram-negative bacilli (GNB) are commonly found in osteomyelitis associated with open fractures, diabetic foot infections, pressure ulcers, and peripheral vascular disease. They are also pathogens in hematogenous osteomyelitis associated with intravenous drug abuse. Extended-spectrum penicillins and third-generation cephalosporins, because of their effectiveness and lower incidence of serious side effects, have supplanted aminoglycosides as the antibiotics of choice in the management of osteomyelitis involving GNB. Quinolone antibiotics are also potent anti-GNB agents and have the advantage of oral administration. Trimethoprim-sulfamethoxazole, although usually not considered a first-line choice, is another agent that can be given orally. Among GNB, *Pseudomonas aeruginosa* is a particularly difficult pathogen to treat. It is resistant to antibiotics that are active against other GNB. Ceftazidime is the only third-generation cephalosporin that is reliably active against *Pseudomonas. P. aeruginosa* is also more likely than other GNB to develop resistance to an antibiotic during therapy.

Anaerobic organisms are usually recovered as one of several pathogens in a polymicrobial infection. *Peptostreptococcus* and *Bacteroides* species are the most common isolates. Penicillin, clindamycin, and metronidazole are the most frequently used antibiotics in the treatment of anaerobic infections. Several other agents also have excellent anaerobic activity. These include imipenem, some second-generation cephalosporins (cefoxitin, cefotetan, cefmetazole), and beta-lactams that have been combined with beta-lactamase inhibitors (ticarcillin-clavulanate, ampicillin-sulbactam, piperacillin-tazobactam).

Stabilization of Fractures

Many cases of osteomyelitis in adults are associated with trauma, especially open fractures of the lower extremities. Stabilization of the fracture is as important as treatment of the infection. These two objectives often cannot be accomplished concurrently. The presence of the fixation device impedes the clearance of the infection, but if the fixation device is removed, the infection will not resolve in the face of an unstable fracture. The fracture often unites in the presence of infection, however. The solution, then, is to stabilize the bone and allow the fracture to heal, even if the infection persists. Suppressive antibiotic therapy can be given to keep the manifestations of infection under control. Once the fracture is healed, the fixation device can be removed and the infection definitively treated. One cannot use this strategy of management, however, if the patient shows evidence of significant systemic toxicity from infection. In such a case, the device must be removed, at least temporarily, until the infection is brought under control. The converse approach—first eradicating infection—may also be successful in some circumstances. Infected bone is radically débrided initially, and the bone is stabilized by external fixation by the method of Ilizarov. Function and bone length are restored over a period of time by bone transport. This method is reserved for cases in which extensive involvement of bone requires segmental resection.

Soft Tissue Coverage

One of the most significant recent advances in the treatment of osteomyelitis was the realization that soft tissue coverage over the area of bone infection was crucial to successful management. The importance of soft tissue injury is reflected in the observation that open fractures associated with extensive soft tissue damage are at higher risk for infection. Fractures associated with soft tissue injury that is so extensive that direct closure is not possible are at the highest risk of infection. A defect in soft tissue leaves a poor environment for healing and promotes superinfection by bacterial pathogens that are often resistant to the antibiotics that the patient has been treated with. Adequate soft tissue coverage negates these detrimental factors. Options include direct wound closure, skin grafts, musculocutaneous flaps, fasciocutaneous flaps, and muscle flaps. Muscle flaps not only protect the infected bone from the outside environment but also increase the blood supply to the area, bringing needed nutrients for wound healing, and white blood cells and antibiotics to fight the infection.

COMMON SPORTS INJURIES

method of
WALTER L. CALMBACH, M.D.
*University of Texas Health Science Center at
   San Antonio
San Antonio, Texas*

SHOULDER PAIN

Impingement syndrome is a common cause of shoulder pain in athletes. The patient reports a dull, achy, nocturnal pain and pain with certain movements such as dressing or reaching above the horizontal level of the shoulder. There is usually a history of recent trauma or unaccustomed activity, such as gardening, heavy lifting, or sporting activity. On examination, the patient may be point tender just under the lateral aspect of the acromion. On range-of-motion (ROM) testing, the patient may display a positive "drop arm" test while lowering the abducted arm. On rotator cuff muscle testing, the patient has give-way weakness of the supraspinatus muscle and possibly of the infraspinatus as well (see Table 1). Treatment requires rest from aggravating activity, nonsteroidal anti-inflammatory drugs (NSAIDs), and ice packs (15 minutes, three times daily and after activity). The rehabilitation process should begin with early ROM exercises, starting with Codman's pendulum exercises, and progressing through for-

TABLE 1. Rotator Cuff Muscle Testing

Muscle	Positioning
Supraspinatus	Arms forward-flexed 90 degrees Arms at 45-degree angle to coronal plan Forearms pronated Patient elevates arms against resistance
Infraspinatus	Arms at sides Elbows flexed 90 degrees Forearms in neutral Patient externally rotates arms against resistance
Subscapularis	Arms at sides Elbows flexed 90 degrees Forearms in neutral Patient internally rotates arms against resistance

TABLE 2. Shoulder Examination for Instability

Tests for Anterior Instability

Anterior drawer test	Patient supine, arm abducted 80–120 degrees; examiner grasps humeral head and subluxes it anteriorly
Apprehension test	Patient supine, arm abducted 90 degrees; arm is externally rotated to point of discomfort
Relocation test	Patient supine, arm abducted 90 degrees and externally rotated; examiner applies pressure at anterior humeral head as arm is fully externally rotated

Tests for Posterior Instability

Posterior drawer test	Patient supine, arm slightly flexed and medially rotated; examiner grasps humeral head and subluxes it posteriorly
Jerk test	Patient seated, arm abducted 90 degrees; an axial load is placed on the arm as it is medially rotated
Push-pull test	Patient supine, arm abducted 90 degrees; forward flexed 30 degrees; examiner grasps wrist with one hand and places other hand over proximal humerus; as the wrist is elevated, the humeral head is pushed posteriorly

Test for Multidirectional Instability

Sulcus sign	Patient seated, arm at side; examiner sits behind patient, stabilizes scapula with one hand, grasps distal humerus with other hand and pulls inferiorly

ward flexion, abduction, and extension. Once the pain has resolved and ROM is returned, rotator cuff muscle strengthening exercises should be started, especially for the supraspinatus and infraspinatus muscles.

Shoulder instability is a common cause of symptoms similar to impingement syndrome, especially in athletes less than 30 years old. The patient presents with a dull, achy, nocturnal pain but may also have a sharp, disabling "dead arm" pain that occurs during sports activity (e.g., during ball release and follow-through in throwing sports). In addition to physical findings suggestive of impingement syndrome, the athlete displays one or more signs of instability: anterior laxity, posterior laxity, or multidirectional instability (see Table 2). As with impingement syndrome, treatment starts with relative rest, NSAIDs, and ice, followed by ROM exercises and finally rotator cuff strengthening exercises. Only rarely is surgery indicated to correct multidirectional shoulder instability. Indications for surgery include recurrent dislocation, traumatic recurrent instability, nerve injury with muscle atrophy, or a patient who is a professional athlete.

Biceps tendinitis frequently causes vague anterior shoulder pain because the long head of the biceps originates at the superior aspect of the glenoid labrum, and the proximal portion of the tendon is intracapsular. The patient reports a history of repetitive biceps contraction and insidious onset of vague anterior shoulder pain. On examination, the long head of the biceps is tender, and the point of tenderness moves as the shoulder is flexed, abducted, and externally rotated (the "tenderness in motion" sign). Speed's test (resisted forward flexion of the arm) and Yergason's test (resisted supination of the flexed and pronated forearm) may demonstrate tenderness at the biceps tendon. Treatment consists of relative rest, NSAIDs, and ice packs. Steroid injection of the shoulder joint is usually not necessary and should be reserved for patients who have failed conservative therapy.

The differential diagnosis of shoulder pain should include bursitis, cervical radiculopathy, referred pain, and adhesive capsulitis. Bursitis causes a vague, constant, achy shoulder pain similar to impingement syndrome and mildly limited ROM, but rotator cuff muscle strength remains intact. Cervical radiculopathy may cause shoulder pain and can be diagnosed by neck tenderness on examination or extending the flexed, laterally bent neck (Spurling's maneuver). Referred pain to the shoulder is seen with heart disease, spontaneous pneumothorax, and diaphragmatic irritation (peritoneal free air, subphrenic abscess, Fitzhugh-Curtis syndrome). Adhesive capsulitis is sometimes seen in older athletes and presents with insidious onset of vague shoulder pain and significant loss of ROM; it may be distinguished from impingement syndrome in that passive ROM and active ROM are equal.

ELBOW PAIN

Lateral Elbow Pain

Lateral epicondylitis is a common cause of lateral elbow pain among athletes of all ages. The patient reports sharp pain at the lateral aspect of the elbow, especially with activity, such as a tennis backhand. This is usually a repetitive strain–chronic overuse injury, although in some cases the pain may start with a traumatic contusion or a single severe strain. On examination, the patient is point tender at the lateral epicondyle, has pain with passive wrist flexion and resisted wrist extension, and may be unable to lift a full coffee cup (Conrad's test). Radiographs are usually not necessary. Treatment consists of relative rest, NSAIDs, and ice packs (15 minutes, three times daily and after activity). As the pain subsides, stretching exercises are begun (e.g., wrist flexion, with the elbow extended), followed by wrist strengthening exercises (wrist curls, reverse curls). A fitted compression strap over the extensor-supinator muscle mass can reduce strain on the epicondyle by preventing full contraction of the extensors. Adequate conditioning, warm-up, and stretching can prevent recurrences. Technique and equipment should be reviewed as possible contributors to the problem. Steroid injection is rarely indicated for lateral epicondylitis and should be reserved for patients who have failed conservative therapy. Betamethasone (Cele-

stone), 0.5 mL in 1 to 2% lidocaine (Xylocaine) 2.0 mL, may be injected at the point of maximal tenderness, just off the bone, not entering the substance of the tendon. No more than three injections should be given over a 12-month period. Repeated injections are associated with tendon rupture.

The differential diagnosis of lateral elbow pain includes osteochondrosis, osteochondritis dissecans, radial nerve neuropathy, and bony tumor. Osteochondrosis of the humeral capitellum is an overuse injury seen in skeletally immature athletes and is caused by repetitive compression at the radiocapitellar joint. Plain radiographs show areas of sclerosis and rarefaction at the capitellum, and relative rest allows healing without significant sequelae. Osteochondritis dissecans is also a repetitive compressive stress injury, causing separation of subchondral bone and its adjacent cartilage. Plain films may be negative early on, but tomograms or magnetic resonance imaging (MRI) can demonstrate this disabling lesion. Radial nerve neuropathy can be caused by compression of the distal portion of the nerve, most commonly at the arcade of Frohse. The point of maximal tenderness is 4 cm distal to the lateral epicondyle. Bony tumor, though rare, is more commonly associated with night pain and pain at rest and can be diagnosed on plain radiographs.

Medial Elbow Pain

Medial epicondylitis is a common cause of medial elbow pain, especially among athletes in throwing sports or racket sports, where repetitive valgus stress places tension on the tendons of the flexor-pronator muscle group. Patients report a dull, achy pain at the medial elbow, especially with activity; a weak grip due to a painful elbow; and sometimes ulnar nerve paresthesias as well. On examination, the patient is tender at the medial epicondyle, has pain with passive wrist extension and resisted wrist flexion, and is unable to fully extend the elbow. Radiographs are usually negative in an adult with closed physes. Treatment consists of relative rest, NSAIDs, and ice packs (15 minutes, three times daily and after activity). As the pain subsides, elbow and wrist ROM exercises are begun, followed by strengthening exercises for the wrist flexors and forearm pronators. The patient may return to play when full painless ROM has been restored, and a counterforce brace or neutral wrist splint may help prevent recurrences. Adequate conditioning, warm-up, stretches, and proper technique are also important in preventing further symptoms.

The differential diagnosis of medial elbow pain includes ulnar collateral ligament sprain, medial apophysitis, ulnar neuritis, and cervical radiculopathy. Ulnar collateral ligament sprain is caused by repetitive valgus stress on the elbow, such as with throwing sports, and can be diagnosed by reproducing the patient's symptoms by applying a valgus stress to the slightly flexed, supinated elbow. Medial apophysitis is caused by chronic, repetitive traction on the medial apophysis in a young athlete with open physes. Plain radiographs may show widening of the physis or avulsion-fragmentation of the apophysis. Ulnar neuritis is a common cause of medial elbow pain, due to the subcutaneous position of the ulnar nerve as it passes through the cubital tunnel. Physical examination shows a positive Tinel's sign between the olecranon and the medial epicondyle, and ulnar paresthesias are present when the wrist is extended and the elbow hyperflexed. Cervical radiculopathy can cause vague medial elbow pain and can mimic ulnar neuritis. Physical examination shows midline posterior neck pain and reproduction of paresthesias by extending the flexed and laterally bent neck (Spurling's maneuver).

HIP PAIN

Muscle strain is a common cause of hip pain. The patient reports feeling a "pop" during a sudden burst of speed or, more likely, during a sudden deceleration. Tests of muscles that can cause hip pain are shown in Table 3. Treatment of most muscle strains consists of relative rest, including the use of crutches, until hip pain is reduced. As the pain subsides, ROM exercises (hip flexion, extension, abduction, adduction, external rotation, internal rotation) are begun, followed by physical therapy for muscle strengthening exercises. Return to play should not be expected for 8 to 12 weeks, and premature activity only delays the healing process.

Avulsion fractures may present as hip pain and may initially be misdiagnosed as muscle strains. The sartorius may avulse the anterior superior iliac spine, the rectus femoris may avulse the anterior inferior iliac spine, the iliopsoas may avulse the lesser trochanter, and the abdominal oblique muscles may avulse the iliac crest. The presenting history and physical examination are similar to those for the corresponding muscle strain, and the diagnosis is made in a young athlete with open physes by a high index of suspicion and plain radiographs showing an avulsion fracture at the site of tenderness. Treatment consists of rest from aggravating activity and use of crutches until the pain subsides. Only rarely is surgery required to reduce a displaced avulsion fracture or correct a nonunion.

Stress fracture of the femur is a particularly dangerous cause of hip pain in running athletes. Patients present with vague hip pain that is worsened by activity. In the early stages, the pain is present only during activity, but as the injury progresses, the pain begins earlier in activity and finally is present even at rest. Physical examination of the hip reveals full ROM, and plain radiographs are usually negative. Technetium 99m bone scan demonstrates the lesion, usually at the femoral neck or proximal femoral shaft. Absolute rest from aggravating activity is essential to prevent further progression of the fracture. Crutches are used until weight bearing is painless, and running is restricted for 8 to 12 weeks. Aerobic fitness may be maintained by swimming, leg kicks, or "water walking" in a life vest. When running is resumed, mileage, foot gear, technique, terrain, fitness, and biomechanics must be reviewed to prevent a recurrence of the stress fracture.

The differential diagnosis of hip pain includes bursitis, lumbosacral radiculopathy, slipped capital femoral epiphysis, and referred pain. Bursitis usually presents with a history of contusion to the lateral aspect of the hip; on examination, hip ROM is full, and there is point tenderness at the greater trochanter. Lumbosacral radiculopathy is diagnosed by midline or paraspinous back tenderness, nerve root paresthesias, a positive straight-leg raising test, and possibly loss of deep tendon reflexes at the knee (L4) or ankle (S1). Slipped capital femoral epiphysis causes groin pain and an antalgic gait in young patients with open physes and is diagnosed by painful limited ROM and radiographic evidence of a displaced epiphysis. Referred pain to the hip can be caused by lumbosacral pathology, abdominal or pelvic mass, or abdominal aortic aneurysm.

KNEE PAIN

Osgood-Schlatter disease is a common cause of anterior knee pain in teenagers. It is a periostitis caused by repetitive traction of the patellar tendon on the apophysis of the tibial tuberosity. The patient presents with a months-long history of vague anterior knee pain that is worsened with kneeling, walking down stairs, or active extension (e.g., hurdles). On examination, the tibial tuberosity is tender and swollen, and the patient has pain with knee hyperflexion or resisted knee extension. Radiographs are usually negative, although the apophysis may be mistakenly diagnosed as an avulsion fracture. Treatment consists of relative rest from aggravating activity (e.g., hurdles, basketball), a short course of NSAIDs, and ice packs (15 minutes, three times daily and after activity). As the pain subsides, gentle stretches are begun, as well as quadriceps strengthening exercises, especially straight-leg raises. The long-term prognosis for Osgood-Schlatter disease is very good, although some patients may have residual prominence of the tibial tuberosity.

Patellar subluxation is a common cause of anterior knee pain in teenagers, especially teenage girls. Patients present with a history of vague anterior knee

TABLE 3. **Muscle Testing in Hip Pain**

Muscle	Attachment	Pain with
Sartorius	Anterior superior iliac spine	Passive abduction, resisted adduction
Rectus femoris	Anterior inferior iliac spine	Passive extension, resisted flexion
Gluteus medius	Greater trochanter	Passive adduction, resisted abduction
Iliopsoas	Lesser trochanter	Passive abduction, external rotation; resisted adduction, internal rotation

pain, recurrent knee effusion, and a sensation of the knee "giving way." On examination, the patient may have a Q angle greater than 15 degrees (the Q angle is the angle measured between two lines—the first between the anterior superior iliac spine and the center of the patella, and the second between the center of the patella and the tibial tuberosity). The increased Q angle, generalized ligamentous laxity, and weak vastus medialis femoris muscle in some teenage girls predispose them to patellar subluxation. The patient demonstrates discomfort if the relaxed patella is displaced laterally (positive patellar apprehension sign) and has tenderness at the medial retinaculum of the patella. Radiographs are not indicated unless there is suspicion of a patellar fracture or an effusion is present. Treatment consists of quadriceps strengthening exercises, especially straight-leg raises, hamstring stretches, and a patellar cut-out knee brace.

Patellofemoral pain syndrome is a common cause of vague anterior knee pain, especially in young adults. The patient reports pain with prolonged sitting (positive "theater sign") and pain with activities such as climbing up or down stairs, jumping, or squatting. On examination, the patient usually has a mild effusion and pain with compression of the patella against the femur in the slightly flexed knee. Radiographs are usually negative. Treatment consists of relative rest from aggravating activities, NSAIDs, and ice packs as needed. Hamstring stretching exercises and quadriceps and hamstring strengthening exercises are begun, especially straight-leg raising exercises. A patellar cut-out knee brace may also be useful.

The differential diagnosis of knee pain includes medial collateral ligament sprain, anterior cruciate ligament sprain, meniscal injury, and hip pathology. Medial collateral ligament (MCL) sprain is usually caused by a direct blow to the lateral aspect of the knee and is diagnosed by tenderness at the MCL and increased pain with valgus stress to the slightly flexed knee. Anterior cruciate ligament (ACL) sprain is usually caused by deceleration forces, such as when a runner plants a foot and turns in the opposite direction. It is diagnosed by immediate swelling of the injured knee due to hemarthrosis and anterior joint laxity demonstrated by anterior drawer testing (patient supine, knee flexed 90 degrees, foot in neutral position) and/or by Lachman's maneuver (patient supine, knee flexed 25 degrees, examiner stabilizes distal femur and subluxes proximal tibia anteriorly). Meniscal injury is often seen in conjunction with MCL or ACL injuries and may not be apparent at the time of acute injury. Over the ensuing 6 months, the patient notes recurrent knee effusion with activity and a sensation of "locking" of the knee. On examination, the patient demonstrates relative atrophy of the vastus medialis and shows locking or catching of the knee during repeated flexion and extension of the hyperflexed knee (McMurray's test). Hip pathology should be suspected in all cases of knee pain, because

a branch of the obturator nerve, if inflamed, can cause referred pain to the knee.

FOOT PAIN

Plantar fasciitis is a common cause of foot pain in athletes, especially runners. Predisposing factors include flat foot, high arched foot, hyperpronation of foot at heel strike, and poor biomechanics, such as external rotation of the lower limb or leg length discrepancy. The patient reports sharp heel pain with walking or running, especially the first step in the morning. On examination, the patient has point tenderness at the plantar aspect of the heel and pain with passive dorsiflexion of the toes or with active heel raises. Radiographs are usually not necessary, and the presence of a calcaneal bone spur on x-ray does not change management. Treatment consists of relative rest, NSAIDs, and ice packs as needed. As the pain subsides, stretching exercises are begun, focusing on stretching the plantar fascia and Achilles tendon through foot and ankle dorsiflexion. Orthotics are used to correct abnormal biomechanics, appropriate foot gear is introduced (adequate heel pad, good arch support, straight last, good hindfoot control, flexibility at ball of foot), and a heel cup may be used in the shoe. Return to activity resumes when the patient is pain free, and intensity and duration of activity are adjusted to prevent recurrences.

Achilles tendinitis is a common cause of posterior heel pain. On examination, the patient has tenderness at the posterior aspect of the calcaneus, and pain is worsened with passive dorsiflexion of the foot. Treatment consists of relative rest, NSAIDs, and ice packs as needed. Steroid injection is contraindicated, as it predisposes the athlete to rupture of the Achilles tendon. As the pain subsides, Achilles tendon stretching exercises are begun, followed by strengthening of the gastrocnemius-soleus complex. A heel cup may alleviate symptoms, and a V-shaped cut-out at the posterior aspect of the athletic shoe prevents chronic irritation of the tendon. Achilles tendinitis must be distinguished from calcaneal apophysitis (Sever's disease) in a young patient with open physes and from retrocalcaneal bursitis (tenderness on squeezing the soft tissues medially and laterally just anterior to the Achilles tendon).

Metatarsal stress fracture can cause foot pain, especially in athletes who suddenly increase their weekly running mileage. The patient reports moderate gnawing pain at the plantar aspect of the forefoot, initially during heavy exertion; as the injury progresses, pain may be present at rest as well. On examination, the patient has tenderness at the plantar aspect of the second or third metatarsal. Early radiographs may be negative, but technetium 99m bone scan confirms the diagnosis. Treatment consists of absolute rest from running activities until healing has occurred; crutches may be required until the pain has subsided. Return to full activity may resume when the patient is pain free, and a carefully graduated program is necessary to prevent recurrences.

Other causes of foot pain in athletes include "turf toe," flexor hallucis longus (FHL) tendinitis, navicular stress fracture, and tarsal tunnel syndrome. Turf toe is caused by repetitive stress on the plantar aspect of the first metatarsophalangeal (MTP) joint and is diagnosed by point tenderness there and by increased pain with passive dorsiflexion of the first MTP. FHL tendinitis is caused by repeated forceful extreme plantar flexion of the foot and is diagnosed by tenderness and swelling posterior to the medial malleolus and reproduction of symptoms by forceful plantar flexion of the foot. Navicular stress fracture is caused by repetitive stress along the medial arch of the foot and is diagnosed by point tenderness anterior and inferior to the medial malleolus and a positive bone scan. Tarsal tunnel syndrome is caused by chronic compression of the posterior tibial nerve and is diagnosed by typical burning dysesthesias of the medial foot, nocturnal pain, and positive Tinel's sign just posterior to the medial malleolus.

Obstetrics and Gynecology

ANTEPARTUM CARE

method of
IFFATH ABBASI HOSKINS, M.D., and
JORGE L. GOMEZ, M.D.
New York University Medical Center
New York, New York

The objective of antepartum care is to ensure that every pregnancy is a planned, desired event that occurs in a healthy mother and results in the birth of a healthy baby. Many significant but reversible anatomic and physiologic changes occur in the mother starting from conception onward. These are the result of maternal-fetal interactions caused by the growth and development of the fetus and should not be considered as major disease processes.

Traditionally, antepartum care was thought to begin as soon as a pregnancy was identified. However, the new recommendation is that every woman of childbearing age who has the potential to become pregnant undergo preconception counseling and that this be considered the start of antepartum care.

PRECONCEPTION CARE

This intervention is one of the most essential aspects of all antepartum care delivered to the mother. At this time, the clinician can not only evaluate the patient's nutritional and psychosocial needs but also assess any medical problems or chronic diseases. Treating or correcting any abnormalities is infinitely easier and safer prior to pregnancy.

The components of a preconception counseling session are outlined in Table 1.

INITIAL ANTEPARTUM VISIT

The first visit is an important intervention because it establishes the tone for all subsequent interactions between the patient and the clinician. A detailed history and review of systems should be taken or updated. The components of the initial prenatal visit (in addition to the information obtained from Table 1), are outlined in Table 2.

SUBSEQUENT ANTEPARTUM VISITS

The traditional plan in an uncomplicated pregnancy is for an additional 14 to 15 visits. These include monthly visits up to 28 to 30 weeks, biweekly visits up to 36 weeks, and then weekly visits until delivery. However, this is controversial and has not been shown to have much benefit.

Regardless of the frequency and number of antepartum visits, there is universal agreement that certain properly timed visits and tests are crucial. These include a visit for prenatal diagnosis, if indicated, at 10 to 12 weeks for chorionic villus sampling, at 13 to 15 weeks for early amniocentesis, or at 16 to 20 weeks for a regular amniocentesis. At the 16- to 20-week visit, a maternal serum alpha-fetoprotein (MSAFP) screen and an anomaly scan are also performed. Another important visit is at 26 to 28 weeks. At this time, the diabetes screen, complete blood count (CBC), platelets, and Rh screen are repeated. The next important visit is at 36 weeks to reaffirm that fundal size matches gestational dates.

Optional interventions are a vaginal screening culture at 22 to 24 weeks for bacterial vaginosis (which has been associated with increased risk of preterm delivery) and a growth scan at 32 to 34 weeks to ensure adequate fetal growth.

The steps taken to confirm maternal and fetal well-being at each return visit are outlined in Table 3.

TABLE 1. **Components of a Preconception Counseling Session**

Medical history: inquire about any problems for which the patient seeks care on an ongoing basis.
Surgical history: inquire about any bleeding or anesthetic problems.
Current medications: inquire about indications for treatments. Assess whether any medications are teratogenic and whether they can be substituted.
Occupational and environmental exposures: inquire about the workplace (noise, pollution, ventilation, and so forth) and home (location, proximity to pollutants or toxins, ventilation, structural hazards, and so forth).
Family history: inquire about cardiovascular disease, cancer, and so forth.
Genetic history: inquire about the patient and her partner's ethnic origin (to assess risks for cystic fibrosis, Gaucher's disease, Tay-Sachs disease, thalassemia, sickle cell anemia). Inquire about mental retardation, metabolic abnormalities, chromosomal abnormalities, or multifactorial abnormalities (e.g., spina bifida, cleft lip/cleft palate).
Psychological issues: inquire about any fears, apprehensions, or folklore relating to pregnancy. Evaluate the relationship between the patient and her partner.
Social history: inquire about current and past use of tobacco, alcohol, recreational drugs. Encourage discontinuation of these substances prior to conception.
Obstetric history: inquire about previous pregnancies and their outcomes, including complications.

TABLE 2. **Components of the Initial Prenatal Visit**

Menstrual history: inquire about the triad (onset of menarche, duration of cycle and flow, presence of dysmenorrhea). What was the contraceptive used? Were there any associated complications?

Obstetric history: document the number, duration, and outcomes of prior pregnancies. Record neonatal weights and outcomes. Obtain copies of any cesarean sections to document the type of uterine scar so that a subsequent vaginal birth can be attempted.

Physical examination: include evaluation of the teeth and gums and the lower extremities, including feet. A pelvic examination should include measurement of uterine size, evaluation of the adnexa, and a Pap smear.

Dating the pregnancy: the estimated date of conception can be calculated from the last menstrual period if the menstrual history was regular, normal, on time, and not preceded by use of oral contraceptives in the past 3 months. Otherwise, sonographic dating is utilized.

Laboratory tests: all patients should have a complete blood count with platelets, blood type and Rh, indirect Coombs, antibody screen, serology for syphilis, rubella titer, hepatitis B antigen, and urine culture and sensitivity of midstream sample. Voluntary HIV antibody testing with follow-up counseling should be provided to all women. Selected populations should also receive a purified protein derivative test, diabetes screen, chlamydia and gonorrhea screening, G6PD, and sickle cell screening.

Additional instructions: address diet, relaxation, sleep, bowel habits, exercise, intercourse, and recreation.

GENERAL GUIDELINES DURING PREGNANCY

Nutrition. The patient should be counseled to eat healthy foods by choosing from the four basic food groups: Group I: vegetables and cereals; Group II: grains, breads, cereals; Group III: milk and milk products; Group IV: meat, poultry, fish. The daily caloric intake should be increased by 15% (300 to 500 kcal per day) over nonpregnant values. In addition, the recommended daily allowances for most vitamins and nutrients should increase during pregnancy. Pregnant women should take 30 mg of iron per day to replenish their iron stores. Maternal folate intake should be increased during pregnancy, and especially during the periconception period. Several investigators have associated maternal folate deficiency with an increased frequency of fetal neural tube defects. The Centers for Disease Control and Prevention (CDC) now recommends folic acid supplementation, 0.4 mg per day for 1 month before and 3 months after conception for all women contemplating pregnancy.

Weight Gain. The total maternal weight gain in pregnancy is between 20 and 40 pounds. Usually mothers gain 0.7 pound per week in the first trimester and 1 pound per week in the remaining two trimesters. Inadequate weight gain and intentional weight loss during pregnancy are causes for concern and should be strongly discouraged.

Rest. Most pregnant women complain of a sense of increased fatigue and should therefore be encouraged to have additional rest periods to promote well-being.

Exercise. In general, pregnant women can maintain their usual state of exercise and activity, provided they avoid excessive fatigue and exertion, which would entail conversion to anaerobic metabolism and lactic acid production.

Work. Healthy pregnant women may continue to work throughout pregnancy, provided they avoid strenuous physical exertion, prolonged standing, and exposure to potentially harmful toxins and gases.

Travel. Pregnant women need not be restricted from travel at any time during pregnancy, provided they have access to quality medical (and neonatal) care. If traveling by road, a pregnant woman should wear a three-point seat-belt restraint and should stop every 2 hours for 10 minutes to stretch her legs to encourage venous return and avoid stasis in the lower extremities.

Immunizations. Most vaccines are contraindicated during pregnancy because of the potential teratogenic risks. Live attenuated virus vaccines should be avoided. There is no evidence of fetal risk from inactivated virus vaccines or toxoids, and these can be given as needed.

Gastrointestinal System. Most women complain of nausea and vomiting early in the first trimester. Usually, this is not a cause for concern and is self-limited. Occasionally, patients may require anti-emetic drug therapy for relief. These drugs should be administered with caution, even though no teratogenicity has ever been attributed to them. The patient should be counseled regarding dietary adjustments—avoiding spicy, greasy foods and eating frequent small meals. Heartburn is a common complaint during pregnancy because of relaxation of the esophageal sphincter. This is usually relieved by maternal positional changes, but occasionally, antacid therapy may be indicated.

During pregnancy, bowel function usually becomes irregular. Constipation can be avoided by increasing consumption of liquids and eating a high-fiber diet. Occasionally, stool softeners such as Metamucil or Colace may be useful. Laxatives are rarely indicated.

Coitus. There are no restrictions on sexual activity

TABLE 3. **Steps Taken to Ensure Maternal and Fetal Well-Being at Each Return Visit**

Maternal

Blood pressure
Weight gain
Signs and symptoms of headaches, blurred vision, low back pain, vaginal discharge, bleeding, leaking of fluid
Fundal height

Fetal

Fetal heart rate
Fetal lie
Fetal presentation
Estimated fetal weight

Additional

Fetal kick counts to assess fetal activity, from 28 weeks onward
Pelvic examination for cervical effacement, dilatation, and position at term (38–42 weeks)
Non–stress test and amniotic fluid index measurements for testing fetal well-being twice a week from 41 weeks onward

during pregnancy, provided the patient maintains her comfort and safety. Often, there is a transient increase in uterine activity after intercourse; this is not a cause for concern.

Caffeine Intake. There is no evidence that caffeine increases the risk of pregnancy wastage or teratogenicity. However, it is prudent to restrict the daily intake of caffeine to a minimal comfortable level for the patient.

PRENATAL DIAGNOSIS

Prenatal diagnosis should be offered to all pregnant women identified as being at risk for fetal malformations. Approximately 3% of all pregnant women (regardless of risk factors) deliver newborns with major structural abnormalities. The risk of delivering a newborn with a minor abnormality is 10%. These background risks can be neither prevented nor lessened. Indications for offering prenatal diagnosis are outlined in Table 4. Of these, advanced maternal age is the most common. Traditionally, mothers who would be 35 years old at delivery were considered candidates for prenatal diagnosis, because the approximate risk of having a child with *any* chromosomal abnormality was 1 in 270, and this approximated the risk of pregnancy loss associated with amniocentesis. With advances in technology (using continuous, directed ultrasound guidance), the pregnancy loss rate after amniocentesis has dropped to 0.2 to 0.3%. Thus, prenatal diagnosis for chromosomal abnormalities is now offered to mothers who would be 33 years old at delivery.

Many inborn errors of metabolism can now be detected prenatally, including Tay-Sachs disease, cystic fibrosis, and Gaucher's disease. Prenatal detection of these diseases may help families avoid having children with seriously debilitating and life-threatening illnesses. Cystic fibrosis occurs in 1 in 2000 Caucasian babies. Approximately 1 in 25 Caucasian persons is a carrier. Tay-Sachs and Gaucher's diseases are more rare and are confined to Jewish populations. Thus, carrier testing for these diseases should be offered to the appropriate groups.

Screening for neural tube defects (NTDs) by determining the MSAFP level is routinely performed between 16 and 20 weeks gestation. An elevated (>2.5 MOM) MSAFP level requires repeat testing. If the second sample is also elevated, the patient should undergo an ultrasound examination to assess the accuracy of gestational age, the viability of the fetus, and whether it is a singleton pregnancy. If this fails to explain the elevated MSAFP level, the mother is counseled for further work-up. This includes a targeted anomaly scan (to rule out NTDs, ventral wall defects, placental abnormalities, and so forth) and an amniocentesis for amniotic fluid alpha-fetoprotein and acetyl cholinesterase levels. If these are elevated, the mother is counseled accordingly and offered pregnancy termination. If these are normal, this is considered an unexplained, elevated MSAFP value. These patients are followed in a high-risk clinic because they are at increased risk for developing preeclampsia, intrauterine growth retardation (IUGR), placental abruption, and fetal demise during the pregnancy.

A low (<0.5 MOM) MSAFP value denotes a one-third chance of having a fetus with a chromosome abnormality. A repeat sample is *not* obtained. Rather, the patient is counseled and offered an amniocentesis. The addition of two other biochemical markers (elevated human chorionic gonadotropin and low unconjugated estriol) to the MSAFP screen increases the detection rate for chromosome abnormalities to approximately two-thirds.

The techniques for prenatal diagnosis are outlined in Table 5.

DRUGS AND MEDICATIONS IN PREGNANCY

Many drugs are known to cross the placental barrier and therefore can potentially affect the fetus. Lipid-soluble, low-molecular-weight substances readily cross the placenta. Water-soluble, high-molecular-weight, highly protein bound substances do not cross as well.

Drugs should be used cautiously in pregnancy, and whenever possible, the lowest possible dose of the drug should be utilized. Any benefits derived from use of the drug should clearly outweigh the associated risks.

The Food and Drug Administration (FDA) has categorized drugs into five classes for use in pregnancy.

Class A. No known fetal risk exists as a result of human studies.

Class B. There are no human studies, and animal studies do not indicate fetal risk; or animal studies indicate fetal risk, but human studies refute that.

Class C. Animal studies demonstrate teratogenicity and no human studies are available, or no studies are available in animals or humans.

Class D. Risk for fetal teratogenicity exists, but the benefits outweigh the risks.

Class E. The risk for fetal teratogenicity exists, and the risks outweigh the benefits.

The critical period for teratogenesis is the embryonic period (conception to 7 to 9 weeks). During this time, major structures such as the heart, gut, and spinal cord are developing and are therefore prime targets for teratogenic exposure. Either the insult by

TABLE 4. **Indications for Prenatal Diagnosis**

Advanced maternal age
Prior first-degree relative (sibling or parent) with a chromosomal abnormality
Prior first-degree relative with a multifactorial abnormality
Prior first-degree relative affected with or a carrier for a genetic metabolic disease
Parental anxiety
Abnormal biochemical screen (MSAFP)
Sonographically detected fetal abnormality
Prior first-degree relative affected with or a carrier for hemoglobinopathy

TABLE 5. **Techniques for Prenatal Diagnosis**

Test	Timing	Technique	Indication	Results	Complications
Chorionic villus sampling (CVS)	10–12 weeks	Transvaginal: 0.3-mm diameter catheter inserted through cervix into placenta; under ultrasound guidance, 10–30 mg tissue obtained from analysis. Transabdominal: 20-gauge needle inserted into placenta; 5–10 mg tissue obtained for analysis.	Advanced maternal age chromosome abnormalities Metabolic disease Hemoglobinopathies Cannot detect neural tube defect	3–5 days	Limb reduction defects, midline defects, pregnancy loss 1–2%
Early amniocentesis	13–15 weeks	20–22-gauge needle inserted into pocket of amniotic fluid under ultrasound guidance; 1 cc of amniotic fluid per week of gestational age aspirated for analysis	Same as CVS and neural tube defect	7–10 days	Pregnancy loss approximately 2%
Regular amniocentesis	16–22 weeks	Same as early amniocentesis; 20–25 cc fluid aspirated for analysis	Same as early amniocentesis	7–10 days	Pregnancy loss 0.2–0.3%
Percutaneous umbilical sampling (PUBS)	20–40 weeks	20–22-gauge needle inserted under ultrasound guidance into umbilical vein; 0.5–3 cc blood aspirated for analysis	Chromosome analysis R/O infections (toxoplasmosis, cytomegalovirus, parvovirus) Hemoglobinopathies Acid-base analyses Blood transfusion Selective reduction (injection of KCl)	Varies with indication— 1 hour to 3 days	Pregnancy loss 1–3%
Fetoscopy	20–40 weeks	1-mm fetoscope (fiberoptic cannula) inserted through cervix for visualization and/or biopsy	Fetal visualization and/or biopsy Structural abnormalities Dermatologic diseases	1 hour to 3 days	Pregnancy loss 10–15%

the drug destroys the totipotential cells completely (and the pregnancy is lost), or any damage is overcome by other unaffected totipotential cells so that the embryo develops with minimal or no structural damage. This is called the "all or none phenomenon" of possible teratogenic damage to a pregnancy.

INTRAUTERINE GROWTH RETARDATION (IUGR)

IUGR occurs in less than 10% of pregnancies and is associated with significant perinatal morbidity and mortality. These babies have increased rates of neonatal asphyxia, hypoglycemia, hypocalcemia, and hypothermia. It is defined as a birthweight below the tenth percentile for gestational age. IUGR must be distinguished from small for gestational age (SGA) babies. Babies with IUGR exhibit fetal growth along the normal growth curves until the point at which they demonstrate a falling off or plateauing of weight and size from the growth curves. SGA babies, in contrast, continue to exhibit fetal growth along their own defined growth curves until term. IUGR may be symmetrical (secondary to chromosomal abnormalities) or asymmetrical—also called head sparing (secondary to maternal vascular disease).

The usual treatment is delivery if fetal lung maturity exists. If the fetus is immature, aggressive antepartum testing is utilized until delivery can be accomplished.

POST-DATE PREGNANCY

Post-date pregnancy is defined as a gestational age of 294 days or 42 weeks. It occurs in approximately 10% of pregnancies. Only 5% of all patients deliver on the estimated date of delivery. Another 5% deliver after 43 weeks. Most post-date pregnancies are erroneously classified as such because of inaccurate dates.

The associated perinatal morbidity and mortality are cause for concern. They are twofold higher than baseline at 42 weeks and sixfold higher at 44 weeks. These risks can be minimized by aggressive antepartum fetal testing beginning at 41 weeks, utilizing a regimen of twice-weekly non–stress tests (a reactive non–stress test being defined as one with two fetal heart rate accelerations over 20 minutes) and assessment of the amniotic fluid index (AFI ≥6 being considered adequate). If the patient has a favorable cervix (Bishop score ≥6) at any time after 38 weeks, labor should be induced. If the cervix is unfavorable, the twice-weekly antepartum fetal testing should be continued until 42 weeks, when a ripening agent such as prostaglandin gel can be used prior to inducing labor with oxytocin.

HYPERTENSION DISORDERS IN PREGNANCY

Hypertension complicates 6 to 8% of all pregnancies in the United States and is one of the leading causes of maternal mortality. Hypertensive disorders encountered in pregnant patients are classified as chronic hypertension and pregnancy-induced hypertension (PIH).

Chronic hypertension in pregnancy is defined as a blood pressure of 140/90 mmHg or greater and includes a history of hypertension preceding pregnancy, persistent high blood pressure ($\geq$140/90 mmHg) prior to 20 weeks of gestation not associated with a molar pregnancy, or evidence of persistent hypertension after 6 weeks post partum. It is classified as mild hypertension if the diastolic blood pressure is between 90 and 109 mmHg or the systolic blood pressure is between 140 and 159 mmHg. Severe hypertension is diagnosed when the diastolic blood pressure is greater than 109 mmHg or the systolic blood pressure is greater than 159 mmHg. A detailed medical history and physical examination are crucial for identifying secondary causes of chronic hypertension. Complete laboratory evaluation of these patients includes CBC and platelet count, serum creatinine, blood urea nitrogen, uric acid, electrolytes, glucose screen, electrocardiogram (ECG), urinalysis, and 24-hour urine collection for creatinine clearance and total protein.

The primary nonpharmacologic approaches to the treatment of hypertension in nonpregnant patients are relatively contraindicated in pregnancy. After 20 weeks of gestation, patients with persistent hypertension should be placed on modified bed rest. Serial sonographic and antepartum fetal heart rate assessment may be helpful in monitoring fetal well-being because of an increased risk of IUGR and fetal death in these pregnancies. Consideration of labor induction at term is appropriate to decrease the maternal and perinatal morbidity.

Serial blood pressure and urine protein analysis are important in identifying those patients who develop superimposed PIH. There is no evidence of increased maternal or fetal morbidity and mortality if the diastolic blood pressure remains below 100 mmHg. However, in a pregnant patient with persistent diastolic blood pressure greater than 100 mmHg, pharmacologic therapy should be instituted. Table 6 is a list of antihypertensive medications used as a

TABLE 7. Criteria for Diagnosis of Severe Preeclampsia

Systolic blood pressure >160
Proteinuria >5 gm/day
Elevated serum creatinine
Oliguria <500 mL/day
Thrombocytopenia
Elevated liver enzymes
Hyperbilirubinemia
Fetal growth retardation
Convulsions (eclampsia)
Hemolysis
Headaches
Visual disturbances
Upper abdominal pain
HELLP (hemolysis, elevated liver enzymes, low platelets
Pulmonary edema

first line of treatment. Angiotensin-converting enzyme inhibitors are strictly contraindicated in pregnancy, since they can cause fetal anuria, oligohydramnios, discrete fetal malformations, intrauterine growth restriction, neonatal renal failure, and death.

PIH has its onset after the twentieth week of gestation, except in patients with trophoblastic disease. Preeclampsia is defined as PIH with renal involvement, characterized by proteinuria. Preeclampsia is subdivided into mild and severe forms. Table 7 describes manifestations of severe preeclampsia. The only definitive treatment is delivery. At term, delivery is generally indicated. In women with signs and symptoms of severe preeclampsia at 32 to 34 weeks, delivery should also be considered, because the risks of continuing the pregnancy outweigh any potential benefits. However, at less than 32 weeks of gestation, some patients benefit from close observation, bed rest, and antihypertensive medications. If symptoms of severe preeclampsia persist or recur, delivery is recommended. If complications such as maternal oliguria, maternal renal failure, or HELLP syndrome (hemolysis, elevated liver enzymes, low platelets) occur, delivery is advised regardless of gestational age. Those patients who are selected for conservative management should have their blood pressure, proteinuria, renal and liver function, and platelet count closely monitored. Also, close fetal monitoring with serial sonography is essential to avoid serious perinatal morbidity. At the time of delivery, IV magnesium sulfate is indicated for seizure prophylaxis. The usual dose is 4 grams as a loading dose given parenterally over 20 minutes, followed by 2 grams per hour as a maintenance dose. Urine output and serum creatinine should be serially monitored to avoid toxicity. Vaginal birth is preferred in women with preeclampsia; however, the mode of delivery must be based on the individual circumstances, such as maternal complications or fetal jeopardy.

DIABETES

Diabetes mellitus complicates 2 to 3% of pregnancies. It is classified as Type I (insulin dependent)

TABLE 6. Antihypertensive Medications Used in Pregnancy

Type of Agent	Drug and Dose
Central acting agents	Clonidine (Catapres) 0.1–0.4 mg bid
	Methyldopa (Aldomet) 250–500 mg bid
Calcium channel blockers	Verapamil (Calan) 60–120 mg tid or qid
	Nifedipine (Procardia) 10–30 mg tid or qid
Beta-adrenergic blockers	Atenolol (Tenormin) 50–100 mg qd
	Labetalol (Normodyne) 200–300 mg q 6–8 h

TABLE 8. **Common Congenital Malformations in Infants of Pregestational Insulin-Dependent Diabetics**

Neural tube defects
Congenital heart defects
   Ventricular septal defect
   Transposition of the great vessels
Caudal regression syndrome (sacral agenesis)

or Type II (non–insulin dependent). Patients first diagnosed during the current pregnancy, whether or not they require insulin, are classified as gestational diabetics. Major congenital malformations associated with diabetes are listed in Table 8. These are the leading causes of perinatal morbidity and mortality in infants of pregestational diabetic mothers. They occur with a frequency of 6% in infants of insulin-dependent diabetic mothers. For this reason, preconception counseling and maintenance of euglycemia prior to conception are necessary for these patients. Glycosylated hemoglobin (Hgb A1C) levels in the first trimester are predictive of the risk of any fetal anomaly. Elevated values ($\geq$7.5 mg per dL) in the first trimester correlate with an increased risk of abnormalities. All patients at risk for diabetes should undergo glucose screening at the time of their first prenatal visit. If the results are normal, the test should be repeated at 24 to 28 weeks gestation. For those patients without risk factors, screening can be performed at 24 to 28 weeks. A glucose challenge test is performed. This involves a 50-gram glucose load followed by serum glucose determination 1 hour later. The patient need not be fasting. A value of less than 135 mg per dL is considered normal. A value equal to or greater than 135 mg per dL is considered abnormal and requires a 3-hour glucose tolerance test. Any two plasma values greater than or equal to those listed in Table 9 constitute an abnormal result.

Gestational diabetics are started on an American Diabetic Association diet of 30 to 35 kcal per kg per day, as determined by the patient's ideal body weight. They are instructed in home glucose monitoring using visually read Chemstrips. Fasting as well as 1-hour postprandial sugars are monitored. Insulin therapy is indicated if fasting glucose values are greater than 90 mg per dL or if 1-hour postprandial glucose values are greater than 120 mg per dL. Insulin therapy should be given in a combination of NPH and regular or human insulin. The dosage depends on the patient's weight and levels of serum glucose.

Patients first diagnosed as diabetics in the first trimester of pregnancy should have Hgb A1C monitored. Those with an elevated first-trimester value should be treated as preconceptional diabetics. Management of these patients includes 24-hour urine collection for total protein and creatinine clearance, ophthalmology consultation, ECG, fetal anomaly scan at 18 to 20 weeks of gestation, and a fetal echocardiogram at 20 to 22 weeks. A fetal sonogram should be repeated in the early third trimester to assess the adequacy of fetal growth. Antenatal fetal heart rate testing should be started at 32 to 36 weeks. Patients with good metabolic control can be allowed to go to term if all fetal surveillance studies are reassuring. Patients with pregestational diabetes and possible end-organ damage should be delivered by 40 weeks gestation. All gestational diabetic patients should undergo a standard, nonpregnancy, adult 2-hour glucose tolerance test (75-gram glucose load) at 6 weeks post partum.

PRETERM LABOR

Preterm deliveries are a leading cause of neonatal morbidity and mortality. Approximately 8 to 10% of all live births are preterm. Approximately 45% of preterm deliveries are associated with intact membranes, 30% are accompanied by premature rupture of the membranes, and the rest (25%) are delivered secondary to deteriorating maternal or fetal health. The pathophysiology of preterm labor is poorly understood but is thought to include cervical-decidual-amniochorionic activation. Causes related to this activation include maternal-fetal stress, ascending genital tract infection, and decidual hemorrhage. Risk factors associated with preterm labor are listed in Table 10.

Programs created to identify patients at risk for delivering prematurely have not been successful. Several risk scoring systems have been developed, but none has shown any degree of success; the sensitivity of all these systems is less than 50%. Routine cervical examinations have no predictive advantage. Other preventive approaches have been promoted, but none is clearly effective. These include patient education, self-palpation for uterine contractions, prophylactic oral tocolytics, reduced activity and bed rest, and home uterine activity monitoring (HUAM). The latter was approved by the FDA for use as an early warning device for women who had a history of preterm birth. However, several studies failed to show any significant benefit in reducing the preterm

TABLE 9. **Limit Values for Glucose Tolerance Test**

	Plasma Glucose (mg/dL)
Fasting	95
1 hour	180
2 hour	155
3 hour	140

TABLE 10. **Predisposing Factors for Preterm Labor**

Low socioeconomic status
Nonwhite race
Maternal age 18 years or younger or 40 years or older
Low pregnancy weight gain
Multiple gestation
One or more second-trimester spontaneous abortions
Maternal smoking
Alcohol or cocaine use
No prenatal care

birth rate. Other indicators to identify women who will develop preterm labor are being investigated. Of those, fetal fibronectin levels collected from cervico-vaginal secretions of patients with intact membranes who are at risk of delivering prematurely seem to be most promising, but the procedure is still not widely available.

Management of patients with preterm labor includes a complete history and physical examination to try to identify an underlying cause. If there are clinical signs or symptoms of chorioamnionitis, treatment with antibiotics and prompt delivery are indicated. In the absence of infection, initial therapy includes bed rest and hydration. If the symptoms are refractory to initial treatment, a tocolytic agent is administered. However, the effectiveness of tocolytic therapy in prolonging a pregnancy for more than 48 hours is questionable. All patients at risk for preterm delivery are candidates for corticosteroid therapy to enhance fetal lung maturation. Premature rupture of the membranes is not a contraindication for the use of steroids, provided the mother and baby can be closely monitored for evidence of infection.

ECTOPIC PREGNANCY

method of
EKKEHARD KEMMANN, M.D.
UMD–Robert Wood Johnson Medical School
New Brunswick, New Jersey

Ectopic pregnancy refers to the development of a pregnancy outside of its normal intrauterine location. The vast majority (97%) of ectopic pregnancies occur in the fallopian tube; other locations (cervix, ovary, peritoneum) are rare. The incidence has been rising over the last few decades, to some degree related to delayed childbearing and the impact of sexually transmitted diseases, but also to improved diagnosis. Approximately 1 of 70 pregnancies develops in an ectopic location. The clinical presentation ranges from an unrecognized state with gradual absorption, to various stages of abdominal pain and uterine bleeding, to an acute abdomen with tubal rupture and hemoperitoneum. Death from ectopic pregnancy remains one of the leading causes of maternal mortality.

Recent developments have improved the early diagnosis of ectopic pregnancy with the use of serial serum measurements of the beta subunit of human chorionic gonadotropin (beta hCG) and transvaginal sonography, utilizing the concept of the discriminatory zone. The traditional surgical approach of laparotomy and salpingectomy has largely been replaced by laparoscopic approaches, procedures that preserve the tube (salpingostomy), and, increasingly, nonsurgical therapy.

Tubal damage from infection, often clinically unrecognized chlamydia infection, is the main culprit in the etiology of tubal pregnancy. A second major cause is pelvic surgery. Patients with a previous ectopic pregnancy have about a 10-fold higher risk of recurrence. Infertility patients are also considered at increased risk.

DIAGNOSIS

Patients present with the signs or symptoms of pregnancy, bleeding, and various degrees of abdominal or pelvic pain. Patients with risk factors for ectopic pregnancy should be carefully assessed in early pregnancy. Symptoms of ectopic pregnancy typically develop between 6 and 8 weeks gestation (4 to 6 weeks after conception). A positive pregnancy test is essential to pursue the diagnosis.

Patients in the first trimester who present with an acute surgical abdomen or are suspected of having intra-abdominal hemorrhage should be considered to have a ruptured ectopic pregnancy and require surgery for diagnosis and treatment.

In patients with minimal or mild symptoms, a more expectant course can be pursued, utilizing serial quantitative hCG measurements. The mean hCG doubling time in early pregnancy is 2 to 3 days with a normal intrauterine pregnancy. A less than 66% increase over 48 hours is consistent with an abnormal pregnancy—either ectopic or intrauterine. Here the concept of the discriminatory zone becomes important.

The primary role for sonography is to investigate the presence or absence of an intrauterine pregnancy. Transvaginal sonography is useful because of early detection of the gestational sac. Failure to image a gestational sac 24 days after conception or later is presumptive evidence of an ectopic pregnancy. Typically, at that time, serum hCG levels are greater than 3000 IU per liter (Third International Standard). Sonography may also identify a gestational sac and/or a fetus with cardiovascular activity outside the uterine cavity.

Less than 24 days after conception, sonography may not identify a gestational sac. In these patients, an approach consisting of close monitoring is appropriate, unless there are significant symptoms of acute abdomen or pelvic pain. These patients with minimal or no symptoms can be followed by measuring hCG levels every 2 to 3 days. If hCG increases appropriately, patients are brought into the discriminatory zone where sonography becomes diagnostic. If hCG levels decline and the patient remains asymptomatic, continuous monitoring of hCG levels is required until the pregnancy becomes undetectable. If hCG levels plateau or fluctuate, the patient may have a pregnancy of "unknown site," in which sonography is unable to pinpoint its location. Rather than entering a protracted course of expectant management to reach a diagnostic conclusion as to the site of the pregnancy, methotrexate can be used to solve this medical dilemma.

MANAGEMENT

Surgery

Tait introduced salpingectomy by laparotomy in 1884, which became the treatment of choice for a century. This approach has largely been replaced by the use of laparoscopy, which has major advantages in terms of cost, patient recovery time, and possibly adhesion formation. Laparoscopy can be used for either salpingectomy or salpingostomy. The latter is often preferable when it is important to preserve the reproductive potential of the patient.

A patient whose ectopic pregnancy is removed with preservation of the fallopian tube has a 5 to 10% risk for "persistent ectopic pregnancy." Residual trophoblastic tissue in the preserved tube continues to grow and leads to symptoms and the risk of a recurring ectopic pregnancy about 10 to 20 days after the original surgery. Biweekly postoperative monitoring has to be instituted to identify these patients early, as patients at risk fail to show a continuous drop in hCG levels postoperatively. Methotrexate* therapy can be used to treat patients with persistent ectopic pregnancy. Alternatively, laparoscopic salpingectomy can be used.

Expectant Management

An asymptomatic patient with continual falling beta hCG levels can be managed expectantly with biweekly evaluations as long as she is reliable and has been apprised of the signs and symptoms of tubal bleeding and rupture. If the beta hCG level fails to fall or pelvic pain develops, either medical or surgical intervention is necessary.

Medical Therapy

Significant experience has been gained with the use of methotrexate (MTX),* a competitive inhibitor of dihydrofolic acid reductase that affects DNA, RNA, and protein synthesis. As a chemotherapeutic agent, its side effects are well known. Initial protocols for the treatment of ectopic pregnancy were adapted from oncology. Subsequent efforts have tried to reduce the dosage and toxicity, and a single-dose protocol without the use of leucovorin rescue has been shown to be effective and well tolerated in properly selected patients.

MTX is useful for the treatment of specific situations in which surgery may be dangerous (e.g., cervical or interstitial pregnancy). In addition, MTX is increasingly used as an alternative to surgery in those patients without pain when tubal gestation is detected early. A recently published study suggests that either hCG levels should be less than 1500 IU per liter or progesterone levels should be less than 7.0 ng per mL to achieve a better than 90% success rate. If both these levels are exceeded, patients have a significant risk of failing MTX therapy. Patients with contraindications to MTX, abnormal liver or kidney function, or difficulty in follow-up are not candidates for such therapy. Currently, approval for this use of MTX has not been obtained from the Food and Drug Administration. A written, informed consent is signed by the patient prior to medical therapy.

---

*Not FDA-approved for this indication.

TABLE 1. **Methotrexate (MTX)* Treatment Protocol for Ectopic Pregnancy**

Before treatment
CBC, SGOT, BUN, creatinine need to be normal
Beta hCG level
Progesterone level
Dosage
1 mg MTX/m² IM
Follow-up
Monitor closely for pain and side effects
CBC, SGOT in 1 week
Beta hCG biweekly until resolved
Repeat MTX dosage in 10 days if beta hCG level has not declined by 15%
Avoid
Intercourse until resolved
Vitamins until resolved
Pregnancy for 3 months

*Not FDA-approved for this indication.
Abbreviations: CBC = complete blood count; SGOT = serum glutamic-oxaloacetic transaminase; BUN = blood urea nitrogen; hCG = human chorionic gonadotropin.

The treatment protocol is listed in Table 1. Treatment failures are recognized by a failure of hCG levels to decline after a second MTX injection, or the development of significant abdominal pain. About 10% of appropriately selected patients can be expected to fail MTX therapy and require surgery.

VAGINAL BLEEDING IN LATE PREGNANCY

method of
CATHERINE Y. SPONG, M.D., and
GARY S. EGLINTON, M.D.
*Georgetown University School of Medicine
Washington, D.C.*

The presence of vaginal bleeding in pregnancy, especially in the second and third trimesters, is unexpected and worrisome and warrants evaluation by a physician. Vaginal bleeding occurring after 22 weeks gestation is "late bleeding" and complicates 2 to 5% of all pregnancies. The presence of bleeding increases the risk for preterm delivery, perinatal morbidity and mortality, hypovolemia, and transfusion. Significant bleeding requires immediate evaluation by a physician, with observation in a hospital, fetal assessment, stabilization (hydration, possible transfusion), and preparation for possible delivery. Patients remote from term require hospitalization at a perinatal center with adequate facilities and resources to care for a premature neonate.

Major identifiable causes of vaginal bleeding in late pregnancy include placenta previa, abruptio placentae, and other (marginal lake rupture, "bloody show," cervicitis, trauma, vulvar or vaginal varicosities, genital tumors, genital infections, hematuria, and vasa previa). Maternal mortality has improved significantly with the ready availability of cross-matched blood and blood products. Since the onset of vaginal bleeding is unpredictable and the patient and fetus may deteriorate rapidly, the physician managing this condition must understand the causes, initial steps of management, and indications for delivery.

The initial assessment of a patient presenting with vaginal bleeding includes a focused history, physical examination, and fetal and laboratory assessments. The initial history should define potential initiating factors, characterization of the bleeding, presence of abdominal pain and/or uterine contractions, leakage of amniotic fluid, estimated gestational age, prior bleeding episodes, and exposure to medications, smoking, alcohol, and illicit drugs. If medical records are available, a reliable last menstrual period recorded in early pregnancy and an early (<24 weeks) ultrasound estimate of gestational age and placental location are vitally important. The initial brief physical examination includes assessment of maternal pulse, blood pressure, respiratory rate, capillary refill, and absence of acute mental impairment from hypoperfusion. The abdominal examination should evaluate tenderness, contractions, and fetal presentation, and the fundal height should be marked with an indelible marker. Fundal height compatible or not compatible with the estimated gestational age and increasing fundal height from intrauterine blood distention are important findings. A vaginal examination should not be performed during the initial evaluation unless some unique feature of the history or medical record strongly suggests an intravaginal or cervical etiology. No vaginal examination should occur until the location of the placenta is certain. If placenta previa or low-lying placenta is possible, a premature vaginal examination contributes nothing to the patient's management but risks life-threatening hemorrhage. The amount and briskness of vaginal bleeding should be observed. After ruling out placenta previa, a speculum examination can be performed to evaluate the vagina and cervix for lesions or polyps and to obtain a blood specimen for the Apt test. To perform the Apt test, mix equal volumes of blood with 0.25% sodium hydroxide. Fetal hemoglobin is stable and remains pink. Adult hemoglobin denatures, turning a light brown color. A cervical examination is then permissible if there is an indication (suspected labor or incompetent cervix).

Immediate management includes a large-bore intravenous catheter (14 to 16 gauge) for fluid resuscitation, blood for laboratory evaluation of hematocrit (spun), complete blood count, blood type and screen (crossmatch 2 to 4 units if bleeding is significant), and Kleihauer-Betke test. The Kleihauer-Betke test identifies fetal red blood cells in the maternal circulation. If disseminated intravascular coagulation (DIC) is suspected, a blood sample should be obtained in a tube without anticoagulant to observe for clot formation and retraction. If the specimen does not clot or the clot undergoes prompt lysis, coagulation tests should be ordered, including prothrombin time, partial thromboplastin time, fibrinogen, and fibrin split products. If abruption seems possible, tests of blood urea, liver enzymes, and electrolytes and a toxicology screen for substances of abuse should be ordered. Intravenous fluid is infused for resuscitation and to replace blood loss. With a risk of hypoperfusion, a Foley catheter can be used to measure urine output accurately. An ultrasound examination shows placental location, gestational age, estimated fetal weight and presentation, evidence of abruption (often not visible in an acute bleed), major congenital malformations, and cervical length and effacement.

After narrowing the range of possibilities for the etiology of the vaginal bleeding, maternal and fetal conditions determine the management. Guidelines for the management of all cases of vaginal bleeding late in pregnancy include stabilization of the gravida, immediate delivery in the presence of uncontrolled bleeding, and expectant management of stable patients in an attempt to achieve greater gestational age in the face of prematurity. General goals are to maintain maternal hematocrit above 30% and urinary output above 30 cc per hour. Because fetomaternal bleeding may occur in the presence of vaginal bleeding in late pregnancy, all Rh-negative, unsensitized mothers should receive Rh_o (D) immune globulin (RhoGAM, Gamulin, HypoRho-D). In each vial, the 300 μg of Rh_o (D) immune globulin protects against sensitization from exposure to 15 mL or less of Rh-positive fetal red blood cells. The Kleihauer-Betke stain of peripheral maternal blood assists in the estimation of the number of vials required to prevent sensitization.

The presence of significant vaginal bleeding mandates continuous fetal heart rate monitoring in labor. Significant bleeding may cause loss of fetal heart rate variability, fetal tachycardia, and a sinusoidal fetal heart rhythm. With a stable parturient and fetus and the absence of placenta previa, attempted vaginal delivery is permissible.

PLACENTA PREVIA

Placenta previa is the implantation of the placenta in the lower uterine segment, between the fetal presenting part and the internal cervical os. Risk factors for placenta previa include advanced maternal age, multiparity, prior cesarean, history of placenta previa (recurrence risk 4 to 8%), and maternal smoking. Patients with placenta previa often present with painless vaginal bleeding that may occur unprovoked or after sexual intercourse or pelvic examination. The peak incidence is over 34 weeks gestational age, and over 50% of patients present before 36 weeks gestation. Ten percent of patients with placenta previa have a coexisting placental abruption. Maternal risks with placenta previa include maternal mortality (0.1 to 5%), postpartum hemorrhage (due to inefficient occlusion of venous sinuses in the lower uterine segment following delivery), anesthesia or surgery complications, air embolism (due to tearing of sinuses in the placental bed), postpartum sepsis (from ascending infection of the raw placental bed), and placenta accreta (occurring in up to 15% of patients with placenta previa). Fetal risks associated with placenta previa are prematurity, intrauterine growth restriction (IUGR—occurring in up to 16% of patients with placenta previa and more frequently in the presence of antepartum hemorrhage), congenital malformations (the risk of serious malformations is doubled in women with placenta previa; most involve the central nervous, cardiovascular, respiratory, and gastrointestinal systems), malpresentations, umbilical cord compression, fetal anemia, and intrauterine death.

Management options for patients with placenta previa include immediate delivery or expectant management. Immediate delivery is appropriate for patients with continued bleeding and gestational age greater than 36 weeks or uncontrolled bleeding at any gestational age. The goal of expectant management is to optimize perinatal outcome while minimizing maternal morbidity. If the patient and fetus are stable and the bleeding subsides, the patient remains in the hospital until no further bleeding occurs. If a patient has had more than one episode of bleeding, hospitalization until delivery may be the safest course. Patients managed expectantly commonly have episodes of preterm labor; beta-mimetic tocolytic drug therapy is controversial, because the side effects mimic some of the clinical signs of placental abruption. When maturity is likely (usually by 36 weeks gestation), an amniocentesis to document fetal pulmonary maturity before cesarean delivery is a common approach. Patients with prior cesarean and placenta previa have a 15% risk of placenta accreta, often requiring emergency hysterectomy and blood transfusions because of significant intrapartum hemorrhage. Vaginal delivery is possible for some patients with an anterior marginal placenta previa or a low-lying placenta, if a double set-up examination finds that the placental edge will permit safe vaginal delivery. The double set-up examination takes place in the operating room with all preparations completed for cesarean delivery, anesthesia personnel standing by in the room, and the surgeons gowned and gloved for possible emergency cesarean.

PLACENTAL ABRUPTION

Placental abruption is a premature separation of a normally implanted placenta before the third stage of labor and occurs in 0.49 to 1.8% of pregnancies. The abruption is occult in 20 to 35% of patients. The etiology may be trauma, history of abruption (recurrence rate is 8.3 to 16.7%), multiparity, maternal smoking, sudden decompression of uterus (amniotomy), external version, and placental abnormalities. Patients with placental abruption commonly present with some or all of the following: vaginal bleeding, abdominal pain, uterine contractions, and abdominal tenderness. Vaginal bleeding occurs in 65 to 80% of abruption cases and is typically nonclotting and dark in color. Over 50% of placental abruptions occur after 36 weeks gestation, and 25% of patients

have laboratory evidence of a coagulopathy. Maternal risks associated with placental abruption include hypovolemic shock, acute renal failure (as a complication of hypovolemia or DIC), maternal hemorrhage (because of coagulation failure or intramyometrial hemorrhage in the uterus), fetomaternal hemorrhage, and maternal mortality (1%). Fetal risks with placental abruption include IUGR (80% <26 weeks gestation), congenital malformations (up to 4.4%, twice the background rate), major malformations (up to three times the background rate, commonly involving the central nervous system), abnormal neonatal hematology (anemia from fetal bleeding, transient neonatal coagulopathies), and perinatal mortality (14.4 to 67.3%). Over 50% of perinatal deaths are stillbirths. Among liveborn infants, there is a 16% mortality within 4 weeks.

Management of placental abruption depends on the status of the mother and fetus and the gestational age of the fetus. If the fetus is dead, vaginal delivery is desirable after stabilization of the patient. If the fetus is alive, viable, and in distress, cesarean delivery as soon as practicable is desirable. If the fetus is alive, viable, and not in distress but there are signs of maternal or fetal deterioration, final delivery planning begins urgently. Attempted vaginal delivery requires continuous intensive maternal and fetal monitoring and the availability of immediate emergency cesarean delivery. If the fetus is alive, abruption is mild, patient and fetus are both stable, and gestational age is less than 37 weeks, expectant management is usually appropriate. This approach requires close monitoring of fetal growth and behavior and maternal hematologic and coagulation parameters. Delivery is indicated for deterioration of maternal or fetal status or documented fetal pulmonary maturity. Patients with more severe abruption require management of the resultant complications, including hemorrhagic shock, ischemic necrosis of distal organs, and major hemorrhage.

OTHER

Other causes of vaginal bleeding include marginal lake rupture (60%), "bloody show" (20%), cervicitis (18%), trauma (5%), vulvar or vaginal varicosities (2%), and genital tumors, hematuria, genital infections, and vasa previa (0.5% each). Rupture of a prior uterine scar may be a cause of vaginal bleeding, commonly presenting in the third trimester. All these conditions may cause painless vaginal bleeding. After ruling out placenta previa, the examiner may perform visual and digital examinations to identify cervicitis, varicosities, genital tumors, and infections. Some patients require microbiologic cultures or biopsies. Marginal lake rupture and vasa previa might be identifiable with color-flow two-dimensional sonography and Doppler interrogation for flow patterns, but these conditions are usually diagnoses of exclusion.

HYPERTENSIVE DISORDERS OF PREGNANCY

method of
WILLIAM M. BARRON, M.D.
Loyola University Medical Center
Maywood, Illinois

Elevated blood pressure during pregnancy is a challenging clinical problem that necessitates an approach to diagnosis and therapy differing from that employed in nonpregnant patients. First, the diagnostic spectrum is broader, since in addition to various forms of chronic hypertension, the patient may have a short-lived, pregnancy-specific form of hypertension, i.e., preeclampsia. Second, when considering treatment the physician must be aware of the likely benefits and risks, both acute and long-term, to the mother and a second patient, the fetus. Unfortunately, a paucity of well-performed studies addressing key management issues makes an evidence-based approach to many recommendations difficult, if not impossible.

BLOOD PRESSURE IN NORMAL PREGNANCY

Shortly after conception blood pressure begins to fall, reaching a nadir at 16 to 20 weeks at which time systolic and diastolic pressures average 3 to 5 mmHg and 5 to 10 mmHg, respectively, below pregestational values. Thereafter, values rise progressively such that at term, blood pressure is similar to levels measured prior to pregnancy. Appreciation of these changes is important because (1) The anticipated fall in blood pressure in midpregnancy may influence the decision to initiate antihypertensive medication during early pregnancy in the gravida with known chronic hypertension. (2) Chronic hypertension may be masked by the physiologic decrement in blood pressure if the patient is first seen in midgestation. (3) Since blood pressure normally increases during later pregnancy, the diagnosis of preeclampsia may be erroneous if made solely on the basis of increments in blood pressure.

CLASSIFICATION AND CLINICAL FEATURES

Although there are many published schemes for classifying hypertension in gestation, the preferred approach is that suggested in 1972 by the American College of Obstetricians and Gynecologists and endorsed in 1990 by the U.S. National High Blood Pressure Education Program since it remains the most concise and practical (Table 1).

PREECLAMPSIA-ECLAMPSIA

Preeclampsia, a disorder unique to pregnancy, occurs in 5% to 10% of all pregnancies, primarily in primigravidas after the 20th gestational week, and most frequently near term. It is associated with substantial maternal and perinatal morbidity and mortality.

Preeclampsia may be viewed as a multisystem disorder characterized by vasospasm, platelet and coagulation system activation, and as a consequence, reduced organ perfusion. The clinical diagnosis traditionally rests on the triad of hypertension, proteinuria, and edema; however, as noted later, important pathophysiologic disturbances may be present in other key organ systems.

Hypertension is defined as a blood pressure of 140/90 mmHg or greater or an increase in systolic and/or diastolic

TABLE 1. **Classification of Hypertension in Pregnancy**

I. Disorder unique to pregnancy: preeclampsia-eclampsia

Disease of 1st pregnancy, typically after 20 wk gestation
Multisystem disorder characterized by hypertension, proteinuria, and varying degrees of ↓ platelets, hemolytic anemia, abnormal liver function tests, reduced renal function, and ↑ uric acid
Edema not a reliable sign

II. Disorders unrelated to pregnancy: chronic hypertension of whatever etiology

Most common is uncomplicated, essential hypertension
Pheochromocytoma, collagen, vascular disease and/or moderate-to-severe renal insufficiency present most serious risks to mother and fetus

III. Preeclampsia-eclampsia superimposed upon chronic hypertension

Diagnosis frequently incorrect; should not be based solely upon increases in blood pressure. Criteria should include new-onset marked proteinuria, increased uric acid, thrombocytopenia, and/or abnormal liver function tests
Associated with substantially increased risk to mother and fetus

IV. Transient or late hypertension

Increased blood pressure near term without other evidence of preeclampsia
Rapid resolution postpartum
Generally manage as preeclampsia as diagnosis established definitively only postpartum

levels of 30 or more and 15 or more mmHg, respectively. However, because of the physiologic decrease in blood pressure during pregnancy, increased vigilance is advisable for patients with diastolic pressures of 75 or greater mmHg and 85 or greater mmHg during the second and third trimesters, respectively. *Proteinuria* is present when a semiquantitative dipstick is 2+ (1+ values may occur in healthy patients and require repeat testing) or greater or there is more than 300 mg of protein in a 24-hr urine collection. The third major traditional criterion, *edema*, must be interpreted with caution since most healthy gravidas develop dependent edema and patients with severe disease may have no edema.

Preeclampsia may progress rapidly, without warning, to the convulsive phase termed *eclampsia*. Most seizures occur antepartum, but a substantial number also develop during labor or within 48 hours following delivery. Other central nervous system abnormalities include cortical blindness and intracerebral hemorrhage, the leading cause of maternal mortality in the hypertensive disorders complicating gestation.

Markers of other organ system involvement in preeclampsia include

1. Liver: epigastric or right upper quadrant pain, elevated serum transaminases (aspartate aminotransferase, AST; alanine aminotransferase, ALT) or lactate dehydrogenase (LDH)

2. Hematologic: increased hematocrit due to loss of plasma volume from the intravascular into the interstitial space, thrombocytopenia, microangiopathic hemolytic anemia (fragmented red cells), and/or increased serum levels of AST or LDH from damaged red cells. Preeclampsia with prominent hepatic and hematologic involvement has been

referred to as the HELLP syndrome, for *h*emolytic anemia, *el*evated *l*iver enzymes, and *l*ow *p*latelets.

CHRONIC HYPERTENSION OF WHATEVER CAUSE

This diagnosis rests on the presence of sustained hypertension prior to or following pregnancy. In addition, levels of 140/90 or more mmHg prior to the 20th gestational week may be taken as presumptive evidence of chronic hypertension, although preeclampsia may rarely present at this early stage, especially when gestation is complicated by hydatidiform mole or nonimmune hydrops fetalis.

Most women with chronically elevated blood pressure will have mild-to-moderate, uncomplicated essential hypertension, and most will have a benign course during pregnancy, blood pressure often falling into the normal range. Poorer prognoses are also associated with severe hypertension (diastolic pressure 110 or greater mmHg); certain secondary causes of hypertension, especially pheochromocytoma; and moderate or severe renal functional impairment (serum creatinine level 1.4 or more mg per dL).

CHRONIC HYPERTENSION WITH SUPERIMPOSED PREECLAMPSIA

Superimposed preeclampsia, which complicates approximately 15% of pregnancies of women with chronic hypertension, is a difficult, often erroneous, diagnosis, especially in patients with proteinuric chronic renal disease. The classic criteria, increments of 30 or greater mmHg systolic pressure or 15 or greater mmHg diastolic pressure, cannot be relied upon since the blood pressure of many chronically hypertensive gravidas will increase substantially at the end of pregnancy in the absence of other evidence of preeclampsia. Therefore, it appears preferable to rely upon criteria such as new onset of abundant proteinuria, hyperuricemia, thrombocytopenia, and/or elevated serum transaminase levels. Of the four categories of hypertension complicating gestation, superimposed preeclampsia is associated with the poorest maternal and perinatal outcomes.

LATE OR TRANSIENT HYPERTENSION

This disorder is characterized by development of hypertension alone during the latter stages of pregnancy or in the early puerperium, followed by a return to normal blood pressure within 10 days postpartum. Maternal and fetal outcomes are similar to those of healthy gravidas. Included in this category are women who may have had early preeclampsia but fail to manifest other evidence of the disease. For this reason, gravidas with isolated elevation of blood pressure in late gestation should be considered to have preeclampsia until proved otherwise.

PREVENTION

Several approaches to the prevention of preeclampsia have been proposed. There is little evidence that diuretics or antihypertensives reduce the risk of preeclampsia even in individuals with chronic hypertension. Although results of some studies suggest that oral calcium supplementation may reduce the incidence of preeclampsia, further evidence is required before this practice can be recommended.

The most promising strategy for the prevention of preeclampsia involves administration of low-dose aspirin. The premise is that aspirin in small amounts (30 to 100 mg per day) inhibits synthesis of platelet thromboxane (a potent vasoconstrictor) to a greater degree than it does that of endothelial prostacyclin (a potent vasodilator). This effect, which has been demonstrated in both pregnant women and their fetuses, may prevent or reverse the vasodilator-vasoconstrictor imbalance considered to underlie much of the pathophysiology of preeclampsia.

The efficacy of low-dose aspirin in preventing preeclampsia has been evaluated in numerous trials. In the 1980s, a number of smaller trials suggested an approximately 75% reduction in the incidence of preeclampsia; however, in several more recent, larger trials, only modest or no improvement in outcomes was observed in aspirin-treated subjects. A meta-analysis of studies available in early 1994 indicates that prophylactic aspirin therapy reduces the incidence of preeclampsia by about 25% (absolute reduction 7.3% to 5.5%), has a modest positive effect on the incidence of preterm delivery (absolute reduction 19.8% to 18.3%), and reduces low birthweight (absolute reduction 8.7% to 7.9%). Despite these benefits, low-dose aspirin does not appear to reduce perinatal mortality. The safety record of low-dose aspirin during pregnancy has been excellent. No significant increase in fetal/neonatal or maternal bleeding has been observed even in women undergoing epidural anesthesia.

In summary, prophylactic low-dose aspirin appears to be safe and reasonably effective in reducing the incidence of preeclampsia in at-risk women. Unfortunately, it is difficult to identify accurately those high-risk patients most likely to benefit. As of late 1995, it is reasonable to employ daily aspirin (60 to 100 mg) from gestational week 12 through 36 in women with chronic hypertension and in those with a history of severe or early onset preeclampsia (prior to 34 weeks), since the risk of recurrent disease in these groups is substantial (>15%).

Finally, it should be noted that there is no evidence that aspirin is beneficial once preeclampsia is clinically evident. On the contrary, such treatment might increase the risk of maternal hemorrhage, particularly in those patients with thrombocytopenia and/or severe elevations of blood pressure.

MANAGEMENT OF PREECLAMPSIA—GENERAL APPROACH

In general, patients with preeclampsia should be managed in a hospital setting because eclamptic convulsions cannot be predicted accurately on clinical grounds and because life-threatening elevations in blood pressure may occur with alarming rapidity. Some centers have reported excellent results with home management of selected patients with very mild disease; however, success depends upon a well-organized program in which patients can be monitored on a daily basis.

Delivery is the only definitive treatment for preeclampsia—all else is palliation. Ending the pregnancy is always in the medical interest of the mother; however, this may or may not be the case for the fetus. If preeclampsia or severe hypertension occurs beyond the 36th gestational week, a point at which fetal pulmonary maturity has generally occurred, delivery is the therapy of choice following control of elevated blood pressure. Delivery is also generally indicated regardless of gestational age if there is evidence of advanced disease or impending eclampsia, since progression is virtually inevitable unless the uterus is evacuated. Particularly worrisome symptoms and signs include headache, blurred vision, scotomata, epigastric pain, systolic or diastolic blood pressure greater than 160 or 110 mmHg, respectively, after 24 hours of hospitalization, retinal hemorrhage, papilledema, clonus, rising serum creatinine level, platelet count less than 100×10^3 per mm^3, microangiopathic hemolytic anemia, abnormal liver function tests, or pulmonary edema. Some centers have reported favorable results, prolonging pregnancy by an average of 2 weeks, with an "expectant" approach to the care of selected patients with severe disease at 24 to 32 weeks' gestation. Such management should be undertaken only at tertiary care centers with the required high-risk obstetric and neonatal intensive care expertise.

Nonpharmacologic approaches in patients with suspected or documented preeclampsia remain of uncertain benefit. Bed rest is a standard part of the regimen in most institutions, but there is little evidence to support its value, and in theory it could increase the risk of venous thromboembolism. Given these ambiguities, strict enforcement of recumbency is not recommended. Finally, sodium restriction, more common in the past, has not been demonstrated to alter favorably the course of preeclampsia and may compromise an already reduced intravascular volume.

DRUG THERAPY OF ACUTE HYPERTENSION
(Table 2)

In the absence of controlled treatment trials to guide decision making, the U.S. High Blood Pressure Education Working Group has suggested initiating drug therapy for acute hypertension when the Korotkoff phase V (disappearance of sounds) diastolic pressure exceeds 105 mmHg with a goal blood pressure of 90 to 100 mmHg, levels at which the risk of cerebrovascular hemorrhage is extremely low. Nonetheless, it is important to individualize therapy; women with much lower blood pressures earlier in pregnancy should be treated at lower levels since the magnitude and rate of increase may be more closely related to adverse events than the absolute level of arterial pressure.

Hydralazine (Apresoline) has been the traditional agent of first choice for acute reductions of blood pressure and was endorsed by the U.S. High Blood Pressure Education Working Group; however, manufacturing difficulties have limited its availability. Labetalol (Normodyne, Trandate), administered intravenously, and nifedipine (Procardia), administered

TABLE 2. **Drug Therapy of Acute, Severe Hypertension in Pregnancy***

	Dose/Route	Onset of Action	Adverse Effects†	Comments
Hydralazine (Apresoline)	5 mg IV/IM, then 5–10 mg q 20–40 min	IV: 10 min IM: 10–30 min	Headache, flushing, tachycardia, nausea, vomiting; possible increase in ventricular arrhythmia	Drug of choice according to U.S. Working Party; broad experience of safety and efficacy
Labetalol (Normodyne, Trandate)	20 mg IV, then 20–80 mg q 20–30 min, up to 300 mg	5–10 min	Flushing, nausea, vomiting, tingling of scalp	Efficacy and safety equal to hydralazine
Nifedipine (Procardia)	5–10 mg PO; repeat in 30 min if necessary, then 10–20 mg PO q 3–6 h	10–15 min	Flushing, headache, tachycardia, nausea, inhibition of labor	Appears to have efficacy and safety similar to hydralazine; may have synergistic interaction with $MgSO_4$
Diazoxide (Hyperstat IV)	30–50 mg IV q 5–15 min	2–5 min	Inhibition of labor; hyperglycemia, fluid retention with repeated doses	Rarely required; doses of 150–300 mg may cause severe hypotension; may displace phenytoin from serum protein-binding sites
Relative Contraindication:				
Nitroprusside (Nipride)	0.5–10 µg/kg/min by constant IV infusion	Instantaneous	Cyanide toxicity, nausea, vomiting	Use only in critical care unit at low doses for briefest time feasible; may cause fetal cyanide toxicity

*Indicated for acute elevation of Korotkoff phase V diastolic blood pressure to >105 mmHg; goal is gradual reduction to 90–100 mmHg.
†All agents may cause marked hypotension, especially in severe preeclampsia.
Abbreviations: IV = intravenously; IM = intramuscularly; PO = orally.

sublingually or orally, have been demonstrated to be equally safe and effective.

DIAGNOSIS, PREVENTION, AND TREATMENT OF ECLAMPSIA

The most common cause of peripartum seizures is eclampsia; however, the physician should also consider other potential causes of fits such as epilepsy, subarachnoid hemorrhage, cerebral vein thrombosis, local anesthetic toxicity, water intoxication, amniotic fluid embolus, and cocaine intoxication. Diagnostic tests of neurologic function (electroencephalogram, computed tomography [CT] scan or magnetic resonance imaging [MRI]) in eclamptic gravidas are often normal or reveal nonspecific abnormalities and rarely alter management. Such neurodiagnostic tests are best restricted to evaluation of patients with atypical features, including focal neurologic deficits, persistent abnormalities of mental status, or late postpartum onset of seizures.

Magnesium sulfate (MgSO$_4$) has been the agent of choice in the United States for the prevention and treatment of eclampsia. Its use was criticized as archaic, associated with excessive risk, and irrational on the grounds that it is not a proven anticonvulsant. However, two recently published large, randomized controlled trials have demonstrated convincingly that, as a preventive agent, magnesium sulfate is superior to phenytoin, and in the setting of eclampsia magnesium sulfate is superior to either phenytoin or diazepam. The optimal regimen for dosing of MgSO$_4$ has not been determined. One reasonable approach is to administer 4 grams intravenously over 10 minutes, followed by a constant infusion of 1 to 2 grams per hour. Which preeclamptic patients should receive magnesium sulfate is uncertain. In the United States, many experts initiate magnesium sulfate in all patients in labor suspected of having preeclampsia. In other countries, therapy is given only to patients with severe disease or following the occurrence of eclampsia.

VOLUME EXPANSION AND CENTRAL HEMODYNAMIC MONITORING

Hemoconcentration and decrements in plasma volume are a fundamental pathophysiologic disturbance in preeclampsia. Acute volume expansion has been shown to increase cardiac output, decrease systemic vascular resistance, and in some cases reduce arterial pressure. Despite such transient salutary hemodynamic effects, no studies demonstrate that this approach reduces maternal or fetal morbidity or mortality in preeclampsia. On the contrary, such an approach may increase the risk of pulmonary and/or cerebral edema, and thus I caution against the use of volume expansion therapy in preeclamptic patients. Administration of 75 to 125 mL per hour of dextrose containing crystalloid is satisfactory fluid administration.

Central hemodynamic monitoring has a very limited role in preeclampsia. Indications include the unusual circumstance of severe oliguria combined with rapidly worsening azotemia, congestive heart failure, or pulmonary edema of unclear etiology.

CHRONIC HYPERTENSION

Evaluation

The initial history, physical examination, and laboratory testing of the pregnant patient with chronic hypertension is similar to that employed in nonpregnant subjects and is directed at answering three questions:

(1) *Does the patient have primary or secondary hypertension?*
(2) *Is end-organ disease present?*
(3) *Are cardiovascular risk factors present in addition to elevated blood pressure, i.e., smoking, glucose intolerance, hyperlipidemia?*

The minimal laboratory testing required to address these questions (i.e., urinalysis, serum creatinine, potassium, calcium, glucose) is similar in pregnant and nonpregnant patients, with the exception that it may be worthwhile to obtain baseline determinations of platelet count and uric acid as changes in these parameters may be helpful in distinguishing between superimposed preeclampsia and exacerbation of chronic hypertension in the gravida with rising blood pressure late in pregnancy.

Approach to Pharmacologic Treatment of Chronic Hypertension

The major risk of severe hypertension to the pregnant patient is cerebral hemorrhage. Therefore, the rationale used to treat elevated blood pressure in nonpregnant populations, i.e., prevention of vascular pathology that requires years to develop, cannot reasonably be applied during gestation. On the other hand, there is some evidence that treatment of mild-to-moderately elevated blood pressure during pregnancy reduces the progression to severe hypertension and/or the need for hospitalization. Although there appear to be fetal risks (e.g., growth retardation) associated with even minimally elevated blood pressure during pregnancy, whether or not this can be altered by drug therapy remains to be established.

Given the ill-defined benefits and risks of drug therapy of chronic hypertension during pregnancy, it is not surprising that current literature contains divergent recommendations. My practice is consonant with that of the U.S. High Blood Pressure Education Program. In the chronically hypertensive gravida, treatment is initiated when diastolic blood pressure is 100 or greater mmHg. This approach is also applied to patients not known to be chronically hypertensive who have isolated elevations in blood pressure without other evidence of preeclampsia. There are few data or recommendations concerning levels of systolic pressure that warrant therapy; my

TABLE 3. **Drug Therapy of Chronic Hypertension in Pregnancy***

	Daily Dose	Adverse Effects and Comments
Agent of Choice		
Methyldopa (Aldomet)	500–3000 mg in 2–4 divided doses	Drug of choice according to U.S. Working Party; safety for mother and fetus (after 1st trimester) is well documented
Second Line Agents		
Labetalol (Normodyne, Trandate)	200–1200 mg in 2–3 divided doses	Less experience than methyldopa; efficacy and short-term safety appear equal to methyldopa
Nifedipine	30–120 mg in 1–4 divided doses depending on preparation used	Limited data; may inhibit labor; may have synergistic action with $MgSO_4$
Beta-adrenergic inhibitors	Dependent on specific agent used	May cause fetal bradycardia and impair fetal responses to hypoxia. Risk of intrauterine growth retardation when begun in 1st/2nd trimester. Appears safe after 26th wk
Hydralazine (Apresoline)	50–300 mg in 2–4 divided doses	Appears best when combined with methyldopa or beta blocker. Few controlled trials but extensive experience with few serious adverse effects documented; several reports of neonatal thrombocytopenia
Clonidine (Catapres)	0.1–0.8 mg in 2 divided doses	Limited data
Prazosin (Minipress)	1–30 mg in 2–3 divided doses	Limited data
Thiazide diuretics	Dependent on agent used	Most controlled studies in normotensive gravidas; few data in hypertensive gestation. Implicated in volume depletion, electrolyte imbalance, pancreatitis, and thrombocytopenia
Contraindicated		
Angiotensin-converting enzyme inhibitors	Dependent on agent used	High rates of fetal loss in animals. Many cases of oligohydramnios, intrauterine growth retardation, neonatal anuric renal failure, occasionally fatal. Use only when absolutely necessary to preserve maternal well-being and other agents are unsuccessful
Angiotensin II receptor antagonist (losartan [Cozaar])	25–100 mg in 1–2 doses	No human data; however, similarity of action to ACE inhibitors raises concern that adverse effects will be similar

*Note that safety during the first trimester has not been established for any antihypertensive agent.

Drug therapy indicated for uncomplicated chronic hypertension when phase V diastolic BP ≥100 mmHg. Treatment at lower levels may be indicated for patients with renal disease.

practice is to initiate therapy when values reach 160 mmHg in the chronically hypertensive gravida.

Specific agents for the treatment of chronic hypertension are listed in Table 3. Methyldopa (Aldomet) remains our drug of choice because of the favorable results of both short- and long-term studies. Labetalol and nifedipine, although less well-studied, are employed by some experts as first-line agents. Because of the adverse effect on plasma volume, diuretics or sodium restriction or both are avoided except in the unusual patient with refractory hypertension and/or congestive heart failure. Concern remains about the association of beta blockers and intrauterine growth retardation, especially when initiated prior to the third trimester. Angiotensin-converting enzyme (ACE) inhibitors are contraindicated because of adverse effects on fetal and neonatal renal function and blood pressure. The recently released angiotensin II receptor antagonist (losartan [Cozaar]) should also be avoided because of theoretical concern that adverse effects may be similar to those produced by ACE inhibitors.

If a patient receiving medication for mild, uncomplicated hypertension is counseled prior to pregnancy or in the first trimester, an attempt is made to stop all drugs since little is known about the teratogenicity of antihypertensive agents. In addition, the hypotensive effect of early gestation will often lower blood pressure below levels requiring drug treatment. In the patient in whom continued drug therapy is deemed necessary (e.g., severe hypertension when untreated or the presence of renal disease), current medication may be continued (except ACE inhibitors or angiotensin II receptor antagonists), or methyldopa may be substituted.

OBSTETRIC ANESTHESIA

method of
MARIE E. MINNICH, M.D.
Geisinger Clinic
Danville, Pennsylvania

Physiologic changes of pregnancy influence the risks and benefits of various anesthetic techniques applicable to both vaginal and cesarean deliveries. These physiologic changes expose the parturient to potentially serious complications from anesthesia. For example, increased gastric acid production, decreased gastric emptying, and decreased lower esophageal sphincter tone result in an increased risk of pulmonary aspiration of gastric contents. Anesthesia-related maternal mortality has decreased from 2.7 per 100,000 to approximately 0.6 per 100,000, with many of these deaths related to pulmonary aspiration and/or inability to secure the airway during administration of general anesthesia. For this reason it is necessary to have qualified and experienced anesthesia personnel available for the care of the parturient. It must be emphasized that while not risk-free, current obstetric analgesic and anesthetic techniques are safe and effective, and can enable the parturient to participate in her delivery to a much greater extent than the use of heavy sedation and general anesthesia as was common in the past.

PHYSIOLOGIC CHANGES OF PREGNANCY

Several major changes occur during pregnancy that have influence on anesthetic technique and outcomes. Mucosal swelling of the upper airway and trachea, as well as increase in the breast mass and the anteroposterior diameter of the chest wall result in an increased risk of obstructed airway, bleeding, and inability to intubate the trachea. These factors in conjunction with the increase in O_2 consumption and a decrease in functional residual capacity (FRC) place the patient at risk of rapidly developing hypoxemia when apnea occurs. Early in pregnancy, arterial CO_2 drops to 30 to 32 mmHg with concurrent decreases in bicarbonate stores, which allows the normal parturient to maintain a pH of 7.4. The pregnant patient, therefore, has substantially less buffering capacity when presented with an acid load.

Intravascular volume is increased by approximately 40% at term. There is a larger increase in plasma volume than in cellular components, which results in a physiologic anemia. This increase in blood volume allows the normal parturient to tolerate the blood loss of vaginal or cesarean delivery without developing symptoms of hypovolemia. Cardiac output increases throughout pregnancy to peak after the third stage of labor. Due to the expanding size of the uterus during late second and third trimesters, patients at more than 24 weeks' gestational age are at risk of developing aortocaval compression (supine hypotension) syndrome. This can result in decreased placental perfusion and fetal heart rate changes with or without maternal hypotension.

Approximately 10% of term patients will develop overt hypotension and symptoms of inadequate central nervous system (CNS) perfusion (e.g., dizziness, faintness, nausea) when placed in the supine position. These symptoms are worsened during hemorrhage or other hypovolemic states and during sympathetic blockade. In order to prevent or ameliorate symptoms associated with aortocaval compression, all pregnant patients beyond 24 weeks' gestational age should be encouraged to avoid lying supine. This is especially critical during labor and following initiation of any sympathetic blockade.

The gastrointestinal system also undergoes major changes during pregnancy. Acid and volume production in the stomach are increased, and gastric emptying is delayed. Gastroesophageal reflux is a common finding in the pregnant patient. These factors place the pregnant patient at risk for passive regurgitation of stomach contents and potential pulmonary aspiration at any time that the protective airway reflexes are depressed (e.g., induction of general anesthesia, heavy sedation, high spinal blockade). Labor and administration of narcotics further delay emptying of stomach contents.

Changes in the central and peripheral nervous system result in greater sensitivity to general and local anesthetics, sedatives, and narcotics. Sensitivity to the toxic effects of these agents is increased. This is especially important with the local anesthetic bupivacaine (Marcaine or Sensorcaine), which is known to have greater cardiac toxicity than other commonly used local anesthetics.

LABOR ANALGESIA

Nonpharmacologic Techniques

Several nonpharmacologic techniques can be beneficial to patients, either alone or in combination with pharmacologic interventions. These techniques include psychoprophylaxis, breathing exercises, and hypnosis. Patients who attend childbirth preparation classes are exposed to and encouraged to practice these techniques. Interventions such as acupuncture and transcutaneous electrical nerve stimulation (TENS) have been used with varying degrees of success but are not usually included in routine childbirth education and preparation. These techniques require specialized training and equipment not readily available. None of these techniques can provide the level of analgesia comparable to regional anesthesia. However, the techniques may provide adequate control for some patients and are certainly a useful adjunct to regional analgesia.

Intravenous Sedatives and Narcotics

Agents such as barbiturates, phenothiazines, and benzodiazepines do not possess analgesic properties but are sometimes used in early labor to decrease anxiety. These agents may be used to augment the effectiveness of intravenous narcotics. Sedatives and narcotics have been shown to depress newborn respiration and should not be used in the latter stages of labor. In addition, dosages sufficient to control the pain of labor are likely to depress maternal respiratory drive and airway reflexes. Other side effects of narcotics include decreases in gastric emptying and nausea. The most commonly used narcotics are fentanyl (Sublimaze), meperidine (Demerol), and morphine. The agonist-antagonist nalbuphine (Nubain) is also used.

REGIONAL TECHNIQUES

Spinal (Intrathecal)

Spinal anesthesia for vaginal delivery (saddle block) is not a commonly used technique currently. It has lost favor for several reasons. When used alone with local anesthetics, this technique is of limited duration (unless one is willing to do repeated spinal punctures), is associated with significant motor blockade making expulsive efforts difficult, and is associated with a significant risk for development of spinal headache.

However, new developments in regional anesthesia utilize a single intrathecal injection preceding the placement of an epidural catheter for continuation of labor analgesia. The agents most commonly used to initiate labor analgesia in this manner are highly lipid-soluble narcotics such as fentanyl (Sublimaze) and sufentanil (Sufenta). These agents by themselves provide excellent analgesia for the visceral pain associated with the first stage but are not sufficient for the somatic pain of the second stage of labor. The onset of action is very rapid, usually less than 5 minutes. The duration of action, however, is limited, with a range of 60 to 100 minutes. If a patient has a rapidly progressing labor, these agents can be combined with a pudendal block for the second stage of labor.

Currently the use of intrathecal narcotics is most commonly applied in conjunction with the placement of an epidural catheter to provide continuous analgesia as the effects of the intrathecal narcotic wane. This will be discussed in depth in the next section.

Epidural (Peridural)

This is perhaps the most commonly utilized regional technique to provide labor analgesia. The extent of blockade may range from analgesia without motor blockade to an anesthetic level sufficient to proceed with a surgical delivery. This is easily accomplished by changing the local anesthetic and/or its concentration. The level of analgesia or anesthesia can be varied as labor progresses.

Epidural analgesia for labor is usually provided by placing an epidural catheter in the lumbar region. Analgesia is most often maintained by continuous infusion of local anesthetics, with or without lipid-soluble narcotics. The concentration of local anesthetic used is sufficiently dilute to prevent marked motor blockade in most individuals. If the pain of labor is not controlled with dilute local anesthetics, one can either increase the rate of infusion or provide boluses of a more concentrated local anesthetic or both.

The agents most commonly used to establish epidural blockade are bupivacaine (Marcaine, Sensorcaine), lidocaine (Xylocaine), and 2-chloroprocaine (Nesacaine). The pharmacologic profile of bupivacaine is favorable for labor analgesia as it provides sensory blockade to a greater extent than motor blockade. One of the most common infusions for maintenance of labor analgesia is bupivacaine 0.125%, often in combination with small amounts of lipid-soluble narcotics (e.g., fentanyl, 1 to 2 μg per mL). At this concentration, bupivacaine provides analgesia with minimal motor blockade. During second stage and especially at the expulsive stage, a bolus of a more concentrated local anesthetic may be required to provide adequate perineal anesthesia. This is especially true for repair of an episiotomy or laceration. If necessary, anesthesia can be rapidly established to provide for comfortable placement of vacuum or forceps for an assisted vaginal delivery.

While bupivacaine 0.125% does not cause marked motor blockade, the patient must be restricted to bed upon establishing blockade with this solution. Recently, investigators have studied the effectiveness of solutions of bupivacaine in the range of 0.04% to 0.06% in combination with lipid-soluble narcotics (e.g., fentanyl, 1 μg per mL) and/or epinephrine, 1.25 μg per mL. These solutions are usually provided by pumps allowing patient-controlled analgesia—that is, programmed continuous infusions plus patient-administered boluses. Ultradilute concentrations such as these provide substantial (though not always complete) analgesia for most patients without any demonstrable motor blockade. This will allow the patient to maintain her mobility for an extended period during labor despite having epidural analgesia. Many anesthesiologists prefer to establish these blocks with an initial injection of intrathecal or epidural narcotics without local anesthetic, followed by continuous infusion as noted. Many patients are sufficiently comfortable, prefer the sense of control, and can be maintained on the ultradilute solution until delivery. Others may require more concentrated solutions that necessitate restriction to bed during the latter portion of labor. Patient acceptance of the ultradilute solutions and patient-controlled analgesia is high. Many patients prefer the more active role that these solutions provide. Expulsive efforts are not inhibited with these solutions.

Most practitioners prefer to establish epidural analgesia in a nonaugmented labor after the cervix is dilated 5 cm, as blockade established in the latent phase may slow labor. In induced or augmented labors, however, epidural analgesia may be established earlier if the patient's comfort is not adequately maintained by other techniques. The technique for establishing epidural blockade requires aseptic preparation of the lumbar area, a specially designed epidural needle, and a catheter if continuous infusion is planned. After the catheter is placed, it is important to determine that it has not been placed in either a blood vessel or the intrathecal space to prevent untoward effects. Prior to injection, one should aspirate the catheter and then inject only small amounts of local anesthetic at a time. Between injections, one must assess for symptoms of intravenous or subarachnoid injections prior to the next bolus or establishment of a continuous infusion. It is important to note that a catheter may "migrate" into a vessel or the subarachnoid space during the maintenance phase of epidural analgesia. It is important that experienced anesthesia providers be available to assess for adequacy of blockade and misadventures of the epidural catheter.

ANESTHESIA FOR CESAREAN SECTION

Regional Anesthesia Techniques

Both epidural and spinal anesthesia are excellent techniques to provide anesthesia for cesarean delivery. Each can be used for elective or urgent delivery. These techniques provide for an alert mother who has a greater sense of participation in the birth of her infant. They also decrease pulmonary aspiration risk to the mother. These techniques are contraindicated in patients with active hemorrhage, coagulopathy, infection at the site of intended needle placement, sepsis, and in cases of maternal refusal. As previously discussed in the labor analgesia section, establishment of regional anesthesia is associated with increased risk of aortocaval compression syndrome due to sympathetic blockade.

Epidural Anesthesia

Epidural anesthesia for cesarean section may be established immediately prior to surgery or with an indwelling catheter that has been placed previously for labor analgesia. If a catheter is present, local anesthetic of sufficient concentration for surgical anesthesia (e.g., lidocaine 1.5% or 2% with epinephrine 1:200,000, bupivacaine 0.5%, or 2-chloroprocaine 3%) is injected to establish surgical anesthesia to a dermatomal level of at least T6. Surgical anesthesia can be obtained within 15 minutes in an urgent situation if labor analgesia has been maintained by continuous lumbar epidural analgesia.

Establishing a surgical anesthetic level in a patient who has not had epidural analgesia maintained for labor will require additional time. The time required will depend on the local anesthetic chosen and ranges from 25 to 50 minutes. The technique of placing an epidural catheter for cesarean section is similar to that of placing an epidural catheter for labor. It is essential to have an indwelling intravenous catheter of sufficient gauge (preferably a 16 gauge) to provide the ability to hydrate the patient rapidly, and uterine displacement must be maintained prior to delivery of the infant.

Spinal Anesthesia

Spinal anesthesia provides the ability to establish excellent surgical anesthesia in rapid fashion. It is associated with less risk of local anesthetic toxicity as the dosages used are much smaller than those required to establish epidural anesthesia. Spinal anesthesia is established by placement of a spinal needle into the subarachnoid space in the lumbar region. The most commonly used local anesthetics are bupivacaine 0.75% in D8.25W, tetracaine 1% in D10W, and lidocaine 5% in D7.5W. The duration of effective surgical anesthesia depends upon the agent chosen. As with epidural anesthesia, a large-bore intravenous catheter is mandatory.

With both regional techniques the patient may perceive pulling or pressure despite an adequate level of anesthesia. These sensations tend to be less with spinal anesthesia and can be lessened further with the administration of intraspinal (subarachnoid or epidural) fentanyl when either technique is used. If these sensations are unpleasant for the mother, intravenous sedative or analgesic agents in small amounts may be administered. However, the anesthesia practitioner must be extremely vigilant as these agents may cause respiratory depression and loss of airway reflexes. If small quantities of intravenous agents are not sufficient to provide adequate analgesia, general anesthesia with endotracheal intubation should be established.

General Anesthesia

General anesthesia should be used only when regional anesthesia is contraindicated. Maternal risk of major morbidity is higher with general anesthesia than with regional anesthesia. As discussed earlier, much of the risk of general anesthesia lies in difficulty establishing the airway and aspiration pneumonia. Although these risks are not eliminated with regional anesthesia, they are lessened substantially. It should be noted that the infant born following induction of general anesthesia will tend to have a lower Apgar score at 1 minute compared with those infants born to mothers undergoing regional anesthesia. However, by 5 minutes the effects of general anesthesia have dissipated and the Apgar scores of infants are equivalent. The lower Apgar score at 1 minute does not represent asphyxia but rather the effects of general anesthesia on the newborn infant.

The anesthesiologist should examine the parturient's airway prior to induction of any anesthesia, and this is especially important prior to the induction of general anesthesia. If there is evidence that intubation of the trachea will be difficult, either general anesthesia should be avoided or the airway should be secured prior to induction of general anesthesia. In addition, techniques to reduce the likelihood of aspiration pneumonia should be used. These include the oral administration of the nonparticulate antacid sodium citrate, preoxygenation of the mother prior to intravenous induction of anesthesia, and maintenance of cricoid pressure until endotracheal intubation has been assured. As with regional anesthesia, one must assure that aortocaval compression is minimized by left uterine displacement.

Numerous intravenous induction agents may be used, but the most common agent to establish general anesthesia is thiopental (Pentothal). Thiopental is used in conjunction with a muscle relaxant to facilitate intubation of the trachea. Most anesthesiologists use succinylcholine to establish rapid muscle paralysis. As noted, cricoid pressure should be maintained until endotracheal intubation has been assured. This pressure must be maintained by someone other than the anesthetist performing the intubation. General anesthesia is then maintained by use of inhaled agents until the infant(s) is delivered. Some anesthesiologists elect to use nitrous oxide 50% and oxygen 50%, whereas others will administer low concentrations of more potent inhaled anesthetics such as isoflurane (Forane), enflurane (Ethrane), or halothane. After delivery of the infant(s) is complete, the level of anesthesia is deepened with intravenous and/ or inhaled agents as necessary. After completion of the surgery, the patient is allowed to awaken until airway reflexes and consciousness have returned sufficiently prior to removal of the endotracheal tube.

Postoperative Analgesic Techniques

Administration of preservative-free morphine in the epidural or subarachnoid space provides 18 to 24 hours of good analgesia following cesarean section delivery under regional anesthesia. The dosage used in the epidural space ranges from 2.5 to 5 mg compared with a range of 0.2 to 0.3 mg in the subarachnoid space. The common side effects of morphine administered in this manner include pruritus, nausea, vomiting, and urinary retention. An uncommon, but potentially harmful, side effect is central respiratory depression, which occurs 10 to 14 hours after administration of the morphine. For this reason, it is important that vital signs, including respiratory rate, be checked hourly for 24 hours after neuraxially administered morphine.

For patients requiring general anesthesia, postoperative analgesia is best maintained by intravenous patient-controlled analgesia. This technique is associated with good analgesia, high patient satisfaction, and lower total doses of narcotics than intermittent intramuscular or intravenous narcotic administration.

COMPLICATIONS ASSOCIATED WITH ANESTHESIA

Complications of Regional Techniques

The most frequent complication of regional anesthesia is hypotension. The development of hypotension can be ameliorated or prevented by hydration of the parturient prior to the placement of spinal or epidural anesthesia and maintenance of left uterine displacement following the placement of the regional block. If hypotension persists despite these maneuvers, intravenous ephedrine is used to return blood pressure to adequate level while hydration is continued.

The local anesthetics are agents that reversibly inhibit action potentials from being propagated in any excitable tissue, including cardiac and central nervous tissues, as well as the peripheral nerves. Local anesthetic toxicity, including seizures and cardiac arrest, can occur if doses of local anesthetic intended for the epidural space are inadvertently administered into any vessel, e.g., an epidural vein. High or "total" spinal anesthesia may occur when local anesthetic doses intended for the epidural space are actually placed in the subarachnoid space. This may result in profound hypotension, circulatory collapse, and central respiratory inhibition. Any of these may occur during initial establishment of the epidural anesthesia, or the catheter may "migrate" to the subarachnoid space during the maintenance phase. All bolus doses of local anesthetics should be administered in a fractionated manner while eliciting signs of intravenous or subarachnoid administration of local anesthetics to decrease both the likelihood and severity of these complications. Should either intravenous or subarachnoid injection of local anesthetics result in any of these complications, maintenance of respiration (usually requiring endotracheal intubation) and circulation (with hydration, vasopressors, and cardiopulmonary resuscitation as necessary) is critically important. Avoidance of these complications is preferable to treatment of them.

Partial or complete failure of epidural or spinal anesthesia is an infrequent complication. This can be the result of inability to locate the needle properly into the epidural or spinal space, too small a dosage of local anesthetic, or, in the case of epidural anesthesia, a laterally placed epidural catheter. These complications may require repeating the procedure or proceeding to a general anesthetic, depending upon circumstances.

Postdural puncture headache can be associated with spinal anesthesia or with inadvertent dural puncture during attempted epidural placement. Recent advancements in spinal needle design and the increased use of smaller-gauge needles has decreased the frequency and severity of headache following spinal anesthesia. Postdural puncture headache is much more frequent following inadvertent dural puncture during epidural catheter placement. The incidence of this is uncommon (1% to 5%, depending on the skill of the anesthetist). However, postdural puncture headache associated with inadvertent dural puncture approaches 85% and frequently requires treatment other than hydration. The most common and effective treatment is an epidural blood patch using aseptically obtained autologous blood.

Nerve injury is uncommonly caused by regional anesthesia techniques. Most nerve injuries are position or birth related but are falsely associated with regional anesthesia.

Complications of General Anesthesia

Hypoxic injury due to inability to secure the maternal airway and pulmonary aspiration of gastric contents are the two most feared complications of general anesthesia. Either of these complications can be associated with severe morbidity or mortality. Prevention or amelioration of these complications was discussed in the section on general anesthesia. Other complications that can occur during general anesthesia include dental damage and recall of events during surgery due to maintenance of light levels of anesthesia, especially prior to delivery of the infant(s).

POSTPARTUM CARE

method of
TRACY COWLES, M.D.
Midwest Perinatal Associates
Overland Park, Kansas

The postpartum period, or the puerperium, begins with the delivery of the placenta and ends, by convention, after 6 weeks following delivery. At this time, most of the anatomic and physiologic changes associated with pregnancy have resolved, and ovulation has resumed in most non-breast-feeding women. Immediate care and subsequent postpartum care are usually provided in a hospital setting, with follow-up care administered in the outpatient setting. Early discharge from the hospital following either vaginal delivery or cesarean section has become increasingly common. Criteria for such discharge will be discussed.

IMMEDIATE POSTPARTUM CARE

Maternal blood pressure and pulse should be taken and recorded every 15 minutes following delivery unless the clinical condition warrants more frequent evaluations. The uterine fundus should be palpated often to ensure that it is well contracted, and the amount of vaginal bleeding should be assessed.

Intravenous infusion of a dilute solution of oxytocin is typically administered in the first few hours following delivery to prevent uterine atony and subsequent postpartum hemorrhage. If uterine atony unresponsive to fundal massage and oxytocin persists, an ergot preparation such as ergonovine maleate (Ergotrate Maleate) or methylergonovine (Methergine) at 0.2 mg intramuscularly may be given. Ergot drugs cause sustained uterine contractions beginning shortly after administration and lasting several hours. These medications may also cause a rapid increase in blood pressure and should be avoided in patients with cardiac disease or pre-existing hypertension. Intramuscular injection of prostaglandin 15-methyl-F2-alpha (carboprost tromethamine [Hemabate]), may provoke contractions in an atonic uterus that has not responded to oxytocin or an ergot preparation. Although 75% of patients with refractory uterine atony will respond to one dose, repeated doses every 15 to 90 minutes may be administered for up to 8 doses.

Excessive blood loss in the face of a well-contracted uterus suggests undiagnosed laceration of the genital tract. Careful examination of the cervix, vaginal walls, and perineum should be undertaken and hemostasis established. Retention of blood and placental fragments within the intrauterine cavity may cause the loss of a large amount of blood with little loss of blood from the vagina. This is detectable by the identification of an enlarging uterus on fundal palpation. Curettage may be necessary to remove the uterine contents and allow proper contraction.

Substantial perineal pain with or without unstable vital signs may be indicative of hematoma formation. Perineal examination, along with careful pelvic examination, may identify an expanding hematoma. These need to be explored surgically with bleeding points ligated. The use of pressure may be very helpful in controlling the bleeding.

Following major regional or general anesthesia for either vaginal or cesarean delivery, the patient should remain in an appropriately equipped area until she has adequately recovered. This setting should include complete cardiopulmonary resuscitation equipment and a staff trained to operate it.

Tubal sterilization in the immediate postpartum period is a possibility when the patient's condition is stable and there is no contraindication to the continuation of her anesthetic. If there is any question regarding the maternal or neonatal condition or if major regional anesthesia would have to be initiated at this point, the timing of this elective procedure should be re-evaluated.

SUBSEQUENT POSTPARTUM CARE

The remainder of the postpartum care provided in the hospital setting is directed at caring for the patient's physical condition, assessing psychosocial needs, and providing education regarding the patient's recovery and care of the newborn infant.

Bed rest is recommended only until the patient regains her strength and can recover from the effects of her analgesia or anesthesia. Following vaginal delivery, this may be a few hours; following cesarean delivery, it may be 8 to 12 hours. In either case, assistance during the first few times the patient is up will help prevent injury should she become syncopal. Early ambulation has been shown to prevent atelectasis, constipation, bladder dysfunction, and venous thrombosis. Diet should be advanced as tolerated, and the patient may shower as soon as she can ambulate.

Following vaginal delivery, the patient should be taught care of the vulva. An ice pack and oral analgesics should provide pain relief in the first 24 hours. Following this, moist heat will reduce discomfort and promote healing of the episiotomy. Patients undergoing cesarean delivery need to be instructed on care of the incision. Showering after 48 hours is not harmful to the incision. Skin sutures or staples may be removed on the third or fourth day postpartum.

Many women have difficulty in emptying their bladder following delivery and overdistention of the bladder is not uncommon. The liberal infusion of intravenous fluids and the cessation of oxytocin administration (an antidiuretic) contribute to the rapid filling of the bladder. Bladder sensation and the capability of the bladder to empty spontaneously may be hindered by regional anesthesia and painful genital lesions. The patient should be checked frequently; an overdistended bladder may be palpated as a suprapubic cystic mass. If attempts to have the patient void spontaneously are unsuccessful, single or indwelling catheterization may be necessary. Following cesarean delivery, the bladder catheter may be removed in 8 to 12 hours. Similar attention to bladder function is important.

The patient desiring to breast-feed her infant should receive encouragement and assistance during this period. Although initially it may appear that milk production is inadequate, persistence will stimulate an appropriate supply. The nipples should be cleaned and dried following each feeding. Contraindications to breast feeding include primary cytomegalovirus infection, chronic hepatitis B infection, and human immunodeficiency virus (HIV) infection. Many drugs are secreted in small amounts in breast milk; women taking medication should consult with their physician.

An unsensitized Rh(D)-negative patient who delivers an Rh(D or Du)-positive infant should receive 300 μg of RhIg in the first 72 hours postpartum. Certain clinical situations such as placenta previa or abruptio placentae, multifetal gestation, or the need for intrauterine manipulation may potentiate a fetal-maternal hemorrhage. Laboratory evaluation will quantify the additional fetal blood in the maternal circulation and help determine the additional amount of RhIg needed. The rubella-susceptible patient should receive the rubella vaccination prior to discharge from the hospital, even if she is breast-feeding.

DISCHARGE FROM THE HOSPITAL

Due to economic considerations facing third-party payers, the trend in the past decade in the United States has been toward shorter and shorter hospital stays for patients undergoing either uncomplicated vaginal delivery or cesarean section. For some patients, the hospital stay is as short as 12 to 24 hours following a vaginal delivery and less than 48 to 72 hours following cesarean section. Many times the shortened hospital stay is followed by a visit to the patient's home by a nurse or health care provider on the following day. Most studies comparing the carefully selected early-discharge patients with those who have a more traditional postpartum hospitalization do not show an increase in adverse maternal or neonatal outcomes or an increase in readmission rates. However, to ensure an optimal postpartum course in the face of pressures to discharge patients soon after delivery, certain criteria must be met.

Discharge from the hospital within 24 hours of delivery should occur following a normal antepartum course and an uncomplicated vaginal delivery. The patient should be observed for a sufficient time to ensure that her vital signs are stable and she has recovered from her analgesia. ABO blood group and Rh typing should be available, and the postpartum hemoglobin and hematocrit should indicate hemodynamic stability. RhIg and rubella vaccine should be administered if indicated.

Family members or other support persons should be available to the patient for the first few days following discharge. The patient should have clear, written instructions on normal physiologic changes that should be anticipated and on abnormal symptoms that should prompt contact with her physician. Fever, excessive vaginal bleeding, leg pain or swelling, shortness of breath, or chest pain warrant immediate evaluation. The patient should also understand which symptoms call for immediate neonatal evaluation and know the schedule for the routine neonatal follow-up.

Early discharge (<48 to 72 hours) following cesarean section may reasonably occur in patients who have had an uncomplicated pregnancy, a Pfannenstiel's incision that is free of inflammation and discharge, a lack of intraoperative complications (blood loss >1200 mL, bowel or bladder injury), and an afebrile postoperative course. The patient should be able to void and ambulate without assistance and have bowel sounds that can be auscultated. The remaining criteria for early discharge from the hospital are similar to those for the patient who has had a vaginal delivery. In the healthy patient with an adequate support system, early postpartum discharge from the hospital may be a reasonable option. Appropriate medical services should be provided to those whose clinical condition warrants additional care in the hospital setting.

FOLLOW–UP CARE

Follow-up care should occur 4 to 6 weeks after an uncomplicated vaginal or cesarean birth. In pregnancies that have been complicated by medical or obstetric conditions, this time interval may be shortened. An interval history is obtained at the first postpartum visit, including review of the patient's physical and emotional status, as well as her adaptation to caring for her newborn infant. Physical examination should include evaluation of blood pressure, weight, breast, abdomen, and pelvic structures. Episiotomy or cesarean incision should be checked for adequate healing. Counseling regarding birth control methods is important.

At this visit, patients whose pregnancies have been complicated may have questions regarding their own health or ability to reproduce in the future. Issues that affect patients who have experienced fetal anomalies, prematurity, gestational diabetes, growth retardation, or hypertension may be addressed at this time. The discussion regarding vaginal birth after cesarean section may be initiated.

The patient may have complaints that should be addressed. Severe anemia or hypothyroidism may cause excessive lethargy and fatigue. Probably over half of women experience some transient depression or *postpartum blues* following delivery. This may well be explained by the emotional letdown following the excitement and anxiety surrounding labor and delivery, and the associated lack of sleep and physical discomfort. This period of restlessness and moodiness usually lasts for 2 to 3 days, possibly up to 10 days, and resolves spontaneously. More severe or persistent depression is uncommon but warrants prompt psychiatric evaluation.

Papanicolaou's smear should be obtained during this examination. The patient should be encouraged to return for subsequent periodic examinations.

RESUSCITATION OF THE NEWBORN INFANT

method of
NEAL P. SIMON, M.D.
Emory University School of Medicine
Atlanta, Georgia

With the first active breaths after birth, a newborn infant sets into motion a cascade of hemodynamic events that ends with the successful physiologic transition from an intrauterine to an extrauterine existence. Most importantly, the placenta is replaced by the lungs as the organ of respiration. As the lungs inflate with air, alveolar PO_2 increases and pulmonary vascular resistance falls, accompanied by an increase in pulmonary blood flow. The removal of the placenta, a low-resistance organ, from the fetal circulation results in an increase in systemic vascular resistance. These hemodynamic changes, facilitated by chemical mediators, subsequently lead to the closure of the foramen ovale, the ductus venosus, and the ductus arteriosus. This process of converting from a fetal circulatory pattern to a more distinctive adult circulatory pattern is known as the transition period and generally takes from a few to several hours to complete.

Most newborn infants have no difficulty in establishing the first effective breaths that trigger this sequence of cardiopulmonary changes. Resuscitation is required for any neonate who cannot initiate and establish effective ventilation to exchange respiratory gases adequately, or whose cardiac function is inadequate to maintain sufficient perfusion to the vital organs. If successful resuscitation cannot be performed in the first few minutes following birth, a combination of hypoxemia, hypercapnia, metabolic acidosis, and ineffective perfusion, called perinatal asphyxia, will result. An asphyxial episode may quickly lead to organ damage and dysfunction, most importantly to the brain. Estimates suggest that 2 to 4 per 1000 full-term infants and as many as 60% of premature infants suffer some degree of hypoxic-ischemic brain damage prior to or during birth. Depending upon gestational age, between 10% and 60% of these infants will die. Of those who survive, approximately 25% will experience permanent brain damage resulting in lifelong neurologic disabilities, including cerebral palsy, mental retardation, learning disabilities, and epilepsy.

Resuscitation is required more often in the first few minutes of life than at any other time. Even when asphyxia is severe, the prognosis for recovery is good if the duration is short and the resuscitation precise and timely. Approximately 80% of very low-birthweight (birthweight <1500 grams) infants require resuscitation and stabilization, as do 6% of neonates born by cesarean section, 2% delivered vaginally, and 60% of meconium-stained infants. Ninety percent of hospitals where deliveries occur have only Level I nurseries in which on-site expertise in neonatal resuscitation may be limited or not readily available. The American Heart Association and the American Academy of Pediatrics jointly have developed the Neonatal Resuscitation Program, an instructional course that provides a systematic and rational approach to the assessment and resuscitation of all newborn infants. The neonatal resuscitation course is designed to be easily taught to all health care professionals involved in newborn care. The following text presents an abbreviated summary of the course. The reader is referred to the *Textbook of Neonatal Resuscitation* for details.

PREPARATION

Two major factors in determining the prompt and effective resuscitation of a newborn infant are anticipation of the need for resuscitation and the adequate preparation of equipment and personnel. In spite of the early recognition of high-risk deliveries, asphyxia at birth is predictable only 60% of the time. Although the majority of neonates born depressed may be unexpected, resuscitation can still be promptly and effectively initiated by well-trained, readily available personnel.

At all deliveries, there should be at least one person who has the skills required to perform a complete and appropriate neonatal resuscitation. Often, this may be the individual delivering the baby. If this individual is busy with the mother, another person capable of performing newborn resuscitation must be present in the delivery room. A recognized high-risk delivery demands two skilled people working together as a team in the delivery room who will be responsible only for the potential resuscitation of the baby. The most experienced person should manage the airway and ventilation and be capable of endotracheal intubation if required. The second person should monitor the baby's heart rate, perform chest compressions, administer medications, and assist in other resuscitative responsibilities as needed. If prolonged resuscitation is required, a third skilled person should assist.

The delivery room must be prepared for immediate resuscitation of an infant at all times. Resuscitation equipment and medications must be readily available and checked daily as a routine (Table 1). When a resuscitation is expected, appropriate resuscitation equipment should be unpacked and ready for use. Each piece of equipment that may be needed must be rechecked as present and properly functioning. The cost of resterilizing or repurchasing resuscitation equipment not used is far less than the lifelong cost of caring for a brain-damaged infant.

INITIAL STEPS

The very first step in newborn resuscitation is temperature regulation. All neonates have difficulty in tolerating a cold environment. Infants who have experienced asphyxia are particularly vulnerable to cold stress, resulting in an increased metabolic rate

TABLE 1. **Neonatal Resuscitation Supplies**

Equipment	Medications
Radiant warmer	Epinephrine 1:10,000
Warmed towels and blankets	Naloxone hydrochloride (Narcan) 0.4 mg/mL or 1.0 mg/mL
Stethoscope	
Clock with sweep second hand	Sodium bicarbonate 4.2% (0.5 mEq/mL)
Bulb syringe	Sterile water, 30 mL
Mechanical wall suction	Normal saline, 30 mL
Suction catheters (5F or 6F, 8F, 10F, 12F)	Volume expanders 5% albumin
8F orogastric tube	normal saline
Meconium aspirator	Ringer's lactate
Wall oxygen with flowmeter and tubing	**Other**
Oral airways for neonates	Umbilical catheters (3.5F, 5F)
Resuscitation bag with manometer or pressure-release valve	Umbilical catheterization tray
Masks, newborn and premature sizes	Syringes, 1, 3, 5, 10, 20, 50 mL
Laryngoscope with No. 0 and 1 straight blades	Needles and IV catheters
Extra laryngoscope bulbs and batteries	Three-way stopcocks
Endotracheal tubes (diameters of 2.5, 3.0, 3.5, 4.0 mm)	Adhesive tape, 1/2 or 3/4 inch
	Umbilical tape
	Suture
	Scissors
	Gloves and masks with eye shields

contributing to further oxygen demand and acidosis. Immediately after birth, the infant is placed under a preheated radiant warmer covered with prewarmed towels or blankets. The head and body are dried quickly with prewarmed towels to minimize evaporative heat losses. A hat should be placed on the infant's head, as the head is a major source of heat loss in infants. All of these activities should take only a few seconds. If the baby requires suctioning for meconium, drying is delayed until after the infant has been completely suctioned. Drying an infant stimulates breathing and increases the risk for meconium aspiration.

Premature infants are especially vulnerable to cold stress. Extra precaution should be exercised for prematures to minimize heat loss, including raising the temperature of the normally cool delivery room prior to the delivery.

Once an infant has been placed under a radiant warmer and dried, the steps involved in newborn resuscitation follow the classic ABCs of resuscitation:

A: Establish an open *airway.*
B: Initiate *breathing.*
C: Maintain *circulation.*

MANAGING THE AIRWAY

An open airway is established and secured by placing the newborn infant on his or her back with the neck slightly extended. A rolled blanket or towel may be placed under the infant's shoulders, raising them approximately 3/4 to 1 inch off the mattress, to main-

tain the correct position for a patent airway. If no meconium is present, a bulb syringe or mechanical suction is used to clear the airway quickly. If mechanical suction is used, the negative pressure should not exceed 100 mmHg when the suction tubing is occluded. The mouth is suctioned first, then the nose, to lessen the chances of the infant gasping and aspirating. Aggressive and deep suctioning is avoided as it may cause vagal stimulation and reflex bradycardia. If the infant does not cry following this initial stimulation, a brief period of tactile stimulation may be tried involving one or two slaps or flicks to the feet or rubbing the back. If there is no respiratory response to tactile stimulation after a few seconds, positive-pressure ventilation (PPV) should be started.

MANAGING MECONIUM

It is critical that the airway be cleared in all infants with evidence of meconium. This is accomplished initially on the perineum as soon as the infant's head is delivered and before spontaneous respirations begin. Thorough suctioning of the mouth, pharynx, and nose is performed by the person delivering the infant using a No. 10 French or larger suction catheter. When to suction meconium from below the cord relies upon clinical judgment. If the meconium is thin and watery and the infant is actively crying, suctioning on the perineum with further suctioning of only the mouth and nose after delivery is probably sufficient. If the infant is depressed or the meconium is thick and particulate, endotracheal suctioning under direct vision should be performed immediately after the infant is placed upon the radiant warmer (and before drying). In an infant who is severely depressed, it may be necessary to begin PPV before the airway has been completely cleared of meconium. If the infant is vigorously crying and has thick meconium, one must decide whether the potential difficulty and trauma in intubating an active baby poses greater risks than not completely suctioning the meconium from the airway.

Endotracheal (ET) suctioning for meconium should be done with a meconium aspirator attached to the ET tube or a large suction catheter (at least a No. 12 French) inserted directly into the trachea. A suction catheter should not be inserted through the ET tube, as the catheter size needed to fit through an ET tube is too small to remove meconium efficiently from the airway. Free-flow oxygen should be provided through oxygen tubing to prevent further hypoxia while performing endotracheal suctioning for meconium.

POSITIVE-PRESSURE VENTILATION (PPV)

The next step in resuscitation is evaluating the effectiveness of the infant's respirations. If the infant is apneic or has poor respiratory effort following the initial resuscitative steps, or if the heart rate is less than 100 beats per minute, PPV must be started. If the infant is severely depressed at birth, PPV may be initiated without first attempting tactile stimulation.

The majority of infants who require PPV can be adequately ventilated using only a bag and mask. Either an anesthesia (flow-inflating) bag or a self-inflating bag may be used. An anesthesia bag requires a continuous flow of compressed gas for inflation between breaths. There is frequently a flow-control valve that adjusts the inflation of the bag by regulating the amount of gas escaping the system. There may also be a pressure gauge site to which a manometer can be attached and a pressure release "pop-off" valve that prevents excessive pressure from developing in the system. All attachment sites must be connected or occluded for the anesthesia bag to inflate properly. The anesthesia bag is attached to a flowmeter adjusted to deliver 5 to 8 liters per minute of oxygen. A patient will receive the same concentration of oxygen as enters the bag.

A self-inflating bag automatically reinflates following a compression whether or not gas flow is directed into the bag. There is an oxygen inlet to which tubing from an oxygen source is attached. Some self-inflating bags also have a pressure gauge site and a pop-off valve. Although the bag will still inflate between breaths, all attachment sites must be connected or occluded to prevent positive pressure needed for resuscitation from escaping the system. Self-inflating bags normally deliver only 40% oxygen even when attached to a 100% oxygen source. An oxygen reservoir attached to the air inlet is needed to ensure that 90% to 100% oxygen will be delivered from the bag.

Face masks are selected to ensure a proper fit and seal against the infant's face. The mask should cover and seal the chin, mouth, and nose while avoiding the eyes. A cushioned mask is preferred as it conforms more easily to the infant's face, requiring less pressure to obtain an effective seal while reducing the chance of trauma to the face. Masks of various sizes suitable for premature infants as well as larger infants should be readily available.

The resuscitator handling the PPV should stand at the side or head of the warmer and have a clear view of the infant's chest and abdomen. Before beginning PPV, quickly recheck the infant's head position to assure that the airway is patent. The mask is placed over the baby's face and gentle pressure applied to establish a seal. Constant re-evaluation of the position of the mask will ensure that the seal is maintained.

PPV should be performed at a rate of 40 to 60 breaths per minute. The pressure needed to inflate the lungs will vary according to the size of the infant and the presence of lung disease. If the infant has not initiated the first breaths, the first assisted breaths may require pressures of 30 to 40 cm H_2O. Successive assisted breaths with pressures of 15 to 20 cm H_2O are usually sufficient. If lung disease affecting compliance is present, pressures of 20 to 40 cm H_2O may be required for adequate lung inflation. With severe lung disease, even higher inflation pressures may be required. The resuscitator must continually evaluate the adequacy of the assisted ventilation by observing the chest rise. If adequate chest expansion cannot be established with bag and mask ventilation, endotracheal intubation is required.

CHEST COMPRESSIONS

Only after adequate ventilation has been established and maintained for 15 to 30 seconds is the heart rate determined and further resuscitation decisions made. The heart rate is determined by palpating the pulse in the umbilical cord or brachial artery, or by direct auscultation of the heart. To minimize interference with the resuscitation, the heart rate is counted for 6 seconds and multiplied by 10. If the heart rate is greater than 100 beats per minute and the infant has regular, effective breaths, PPV can be discontinued and free-flow oxygen provided. If the infant shows poor or no spontaneous respirations, PPV is continued. If the heart rate is between 60 and 100 and increasing, PPV is continued. If the heart rate is between 60 and 100 and not increasing, the airway and adequacy of ventilation are rechecked and appropriate responses taken. If the heart rate fails to rise above 80, chest compressions are initiated. If the heart rate falls below 60, chest compressions are begun immediately and the airway and adequacy of ventilation are again rechecked. It is imperative that PPV continue with 100% oxygen during chest compressions. Once the heart rate is above 80, chest compressions may be stopped. Infants requiring PPV with a bag and mask for longer than 2 minutes should have an orogastric tube inserted and secured with tape to minimize gastric distention during the resuscitation.

The resuscitator responsible for chest compressions should be positioned either at the foot or side of the bed so as not to hinder the person performing the ventilation. When chest compressions are performed on a newborn infant, pressure is applied to the lower third of the sternum, just below an imaginary line drawn between the nipples. Either the thumb technique or the two-finger technique may be used. With the thumb technique, both hands encircle the torso with the thumbs placed either side-by-side or on top of one another on the sternum and the fingers under the infant for support. With the two-finger technique, the tips of the middle finger and either the index or ring finger are placed perpendicularly on the sternum and the free hand placed behind the infant for added support. With both techniques, pressure should be exerted directly downward on the sternum and not on the ribs so as to avoid fracturing the ribs or causing a pneumothorax. The depth of the compressions should be 1/2 to 3/4 inch.

Chest compressions should be interposed with ventilations at a rate of 90 compressions and 30 ventilations per minute (3:1 ratio), or three compressions and one ventilation every 2 seconds. The rate of ventilation with chest compressions is less than if no chest compressions were being delivered. The heart rate is re-evaluated every 30 seconds for the first few minutes of resuscitation. Heart rate checks may be performed less frequently in infants requiring prolonged resuscitation.

ENDOTRACHEAL INTUBATION

Endotracheal intubation is indicated when (1) prolonged PPV is required; (2) bag and mask ventilation is ineffective; (3) tracheal suctioning is required such as with meconium; (4) congenital diaphragmatic hernia is suspected; or (5) the infant is extremely premature. It should be performed by the person most experienced and comfortable in newborn resuscitation.

The size of the ET tube needed depends upon the estimated weight or gestational age of the infant. A 2.5-mm (internal diameter) tube should be appropriate for an infant with a birthweight less than 1000 grams or gestational age less than 28 weeks; a 3.0-mm tube for an infant between 1000 and 2000 grams or 28 and 34 weeks; a 3.5-mm tube for an infant between 2000 and 3000 grams or 34 and 38 weeks; and a 3.5- to 4.0-mm tube for an infant over 3000 grams or 38 weeks. The use of a stylet is optional. A No. 0 laryngoscope blade is used for premature infants and a No. 0 or No. 1 blade for term infants. After attaching the blade to the laryngoscope, make certain that the bulb is screwed in tightly and the light source is consistent and bright. There should be appropriate-sized suction catheters for each size of ET tube and oxygen tubing connected to a source delivering 100% free-flow oxygen.

The correct position of the infant for intubation is the same as for bag and mask ventilation. The laryngoscope is held in the left hand and the infant's head held and stabilized with the right hand. The blade is inserted midline between the tongue and palate and gently advanced until the tip rests in the vallecula. The entire blade is lifted by pulling up in the direction that the laryngoscope handle is pointing. The glottis (the opening between the vocal cords) is identified, and the ET tube, held by the right hand, is introduced into the right side of the mouth. Do not advance the ET tube down the laryngoscope channel as this will obstruct the view of the glottis. The tube is inserted through the glottis under direct and constant visualization until the vocal cord guide on the ET tube is at the level of the cords. This will position the tip of the ET tube in the trachea approximately halfway between the carina and vocal cords. The tube is held firmly, but not so much as to occlude the lumen, and the laryngoscope is carefully withdrawn. The correct position of the ET tube in the trachea may be further approximated by adding 6 to the infant's weight in kilograms, which corresponds to the centimeter mark on the ET tube that should be even with the infant's lips. After securing the ET tube with tape, the correct placement is confirmed by observing for a symmetrical chest rise, hearing equal breath sounds on auscultation, and obtaining a chest radiograph.

During the intubation procedure, hypoxia is minimized by administering continuous 100% free-flow oxygen, strictly limiting the time allotted for each intubation attempt to 20 seconds, and ventilating with bag, mask, and 100% oxygen between attempts.

MEDICATIONS

Most newborn resuscitations respond to ventilation and oxygenation. Few require cardiac compressions and only rarely are resuscitation medications necessary. Medications should be administered during resuscitation if an infant's heart rate remains below 80 beats per minute for more than 30 seconds in spite of adequate ventilation with 100% oxygen and chest compressions, or if the heart rate is 0.

The initial medication administered is epinephrine. Epinephrine increases heart rate and contractility and causes peripheral vasoconstriction, resulting in increased systemic blood pressure. It is available in a 1:10,000 concentration and is administered in a dose of 0.1 to 0.3 mL per kg. It may be given rapidly either intravenously or by ET tube. Epinephrine may be readministered every 3 to 5 minutes as long as the heart rate remains below 100 and is not rising. With severe asphyxia requiring prolonged resuscitation, metabolic acidosis may develop and contribute to the ineffectiveness of epinephrine. In suspected or documented metabolic acidosis, sodium bicarbonate may be used but only if the infant is adequately ventilated. The dose is 2 mEq per kg intravenously of a 4.2% solution (0.5 mEq per mL), administered slowly over at least 2 minutes to minimize the risk of intracranial hemorrhage, especially in premature infants. If the infant does not respond with an immediate increase in heart rate after giving sodium bicarbonate, consider another dose of epinephrine.

Hypovolemia should be considered in any infant requiring resuscitation with a history of a cord accident or placental hemorrhage. The clinical signs of hypovolemia in an infant are not always obvious but include pallor, weak pulses despite a good heart rate, and poor perfusion. Volume expanders may be administered in a dose of 10 mL per kg. The choice of volume expander will depend upon the urgency of the need for volume and how rapidly a specific volume expander can be obtained. Type O-negative whole blood, 5% albumin, normal saline, and Ringer's lactate are volume expanders commonly used in neonates. All volume expanders must be given intravenously over 5 to 10 minutes. Administration time should be prolonged in premature infants to reduce the risk of intracranial hemorrhage.

Naloxone hydrochloride (Narcan) is indicated for the reversal of respiratory depression in the neonate induced by a variety of narcotics given to the mother prior to delivery. Respiratory depression in the newborn infant may occur when a narcotic has been administered to the mother within 4 hours of delivery. Naloxone hydrochloride is available in a concentration of 0.4 mg per mL or 1.0 mg per mL, and it is given rapidly at a dose of 0.1 mg per kg. The intravenous route is preferred, but it may also be given intramuscularly, subcutaneously, or by endotracheal tube. Naloxone has a rapid onset of action, with a duration of action of 1 to 4 hours. Since the duration of action of the narcotic may be longer than that of naloxone, continued monitoring of the infant is necessary. Naloxone may be repeated as often as needed every 2 to 3 minutes. If a history of narcotic addiction is identified or suspected in the mother, naloxone should not be given to the depressed infant as it may precipitate seizures.

Ventilation and circulation must be supported in all infants until the appropriate resuscitation medications can be administered. All volume expanders and resuscitation medications should be administered intravenously. Epinephrine and naloxone are the possible exceptions. Unfortunately, intravenous access in infants has usually not been established when the need for medications becomes obvious. The umbilical vein can be easily accessed by cutting the umbilical cord to a length of approximately 1 to 2 cm with a scalpel. After identifying the umbilical vein, a No. 3.5 or 5 French umbilical artery catheter previously flushed with heparinized saline is inserted until good blood return is established. The catheter is secured with tape while umbilical ties are used around the base of the umbilicus to reduce bleeding. All newborn resuscitation medications and volume expanders can be safely given by this route.

CARE OF THE HIGH-RISK NEONATE

method of
ARUN K. PRAMANIK, M.D., and
RICHARD W. KROUSKOP, M.D.
Louisiana State University Medical Center
Shreveport, Louisiana

ANTICIPATION OF HIGH-RISK PREGNANCY AND DELIVERY

Anticipation and early recognition of problems have greatly aided our ability to respond to neonatal emergencies, and even to abort their onset. As it is generally accepted that the subsequent course and prognosis of an infant (especially the smaller prematures) correlate best with the events encountered in the first few minutes and hours of life, a significant impact on morbidity and mortality can be made by the timely recognition and treatment of antenatal and parturient complications. For instance, prenatal transfer of a high-risk mother to a tertiary center for delivery has improved the outcome of high-risk fetuses. We have found it much more effective to be able to resuscitate and begin therapy for a newborn infant immediately after birth, rather than delivering in outlying hospitals before transporting the sick infant. Such timely transfer requires early identification of pregnancies that are high risk (Table 1), thus enabling pregnancy monitoring, intervention, and preparation for delivery.

Prematurity itself remains the most frequent condition producing high-risk infants. In the United States, the prematurity rate has remained constant at 10%, while premature births account for 75% of perinatal mortality. Table 2 describes several risk factors for prematurity, for which

TABLE 1. **Maternal and Fetal Factors Contributing to High-Risk Neonates**

Maternal	Fetal
Pregnancy-associated hypertension	Growth abnormalities (SGA, LGA)
Diabetes	Chromosomal anomalies
Previous stillbirth or neonatal death	Other fetal anomalies
Maternal age <18 or >34 years	Poly- or oligohydramnios
	Hydrops
Anemia or abnormal hemoglobin	Elevated alpha-fetoproteins
	Abnormal stress or nonstress test
Rh sensitization	Multiple gestation
Maternal infection	Low biophysical profile score
Malnutrition or poor weight gain	Reduced fetal movement
Antepartum hemorrhage	Immature L/S ratio
Collagen vascular disorders	Cardiac dysrhythmias
Drug therapy	
Maternal drug or alcohol abuse	

Abbreviations: SGA = small for gestational age; LGA = large for gestational age; L/S ratio = lecithin-sphingomyelin ratio.

early identification and subsequent close monitoring reduced the prematurity rate from 6.75 to 2.4% in one obstetric service. Intrapartum complications that may potentially cause significant problems at birth are listed in Table 3. Delivery of infants with fetal anomalies requiring surgical intervention should be coordinated with a tertiary center equipped to manage such fetuses and infants.

Thus, implicit in the anticipation and planning for a high-risk delivery is the need for close communication between the obstetrician and neonatologist. Decisions such as the best time to intervene in a pregnancy to deliver a premature infant can best be made jointly. The pediatrician is in the best position to coordinate ancillary services with the anticipated resuscitation and stabilization needed following delivery (e.g., pediatric medical and surgical subspecialists or blood bank). Some pregnancies can be predicted to result in an ill or abnormal infant. Pediatrician contact with the family at that point, perhaps including an introduction and visit to the neonatal intensive care unit (NICU) will help ease anxieties when the birth occurs.

DELIVERY ROOM MANAGEMENT

Transition Physiology

An understanding of the physiologic and anatomic changes that occur in transition from life as a fetus to life as a neonate provides a background for the anticipation of problems and their prevention or cure.

Pulmonary Adaptation

At birth, one third of total lung fluid (different from, but contributing to, amniotic fluid) is squeezed from the alveoli and bronchi. Residual alveolar fluid is resorbed into the blood and lymphatics surrounding the lungs. Spontaneous respiratory effort at birth produces 30 to 50 cm H_2O negative pressure in the airway that opens the alveoli. Once an air-fluid interface is established, the surfactant within the fluid layer stabilizes the alveoli by reducing sur-

TABLE 2. **Scoring System for Risk of Preterm Delivery**

Points*	Socioeconomic Status	Past History	Daily Habits	Current Pregnancy
1	Two children at home Low socioeconomic status	One abortion <1 yr since last birth	Works outside home	Unusual fatigue
2	<20 years >40 years Single parent	Two abortions	>10 cigarettes per day	<13 lb gain by 32 weeks Albuminuria Hypertension Bacteriuria
3	Very low socioeconomic status, <150 cm, <45 kg	Three abortions	Heavy work; long, tiring trip	Breech at 32 wk Weight loss of 2 kg Head engaged Febrile illness
4	<18 years	Pyelonephritis		Metrorrhagia after 12 wk gestation Effacement Dilatation Uterine irritability
5		Uterine anomaly Second-trimester abortion DES exposure		Placenta previa Hydramnios
10		Premature delivery Repeated second-trimester abortion		Twins Abdominal surgery

*Score is computed by addition of number of points given any item. 0–5 = low risk; 6–9 = medium risk; ≥10 = high risk.
Abbreviation: DES = diethylstilbestrol.
Adapted from Creasy R, Gummer B, Liggins G: System for predicting spontaneous preterm birth. Obstet Gynecol 55:692, 1980. Reprinted with permission of the American College of Obstetricians and Gynecologists.

face tension, the lungs remain inflated during expiration, and subsequent breaths become easier.

Alterations to this process occur, for instance, when delivery by cesarean section or inadequate respiratory effort by a depressed infant results in delayed resorption of lung fluid, culminating in transient tachypnea of the newborn. Mucus or meconium plugging during the first few breaths, perhaps enhanced by high pressures during bagging, may lead to pneumothorax. Surfactant deficiency in the premature infant is the underlying pathophysiology of hyaline membrane disease.

TABLE 3. **Intrapartum Complications Contributing to High-Risk Neonates**

Prematurity or postmaturity
Premature or prolonged rupture of membranes
Placenta previa or abruptio placentae
Abnormal presentation
Prolapsed cord
Maternal fever or chorioamnionitis
Abnormal labor pattern
Prolonged labor >24 hr
Prolonged second stage of labor (>2 hr)
Persistent fetal tachycardia
Persistent abnormal FHR pattern
Loss of beat-to-beat variability in FHR
Meconium-stained amniotic fluid
Fetal acidosis
General anesthesia
Narcotic administered to mother <4 hr before delivery
Cesarean delivery
Difficult delivery

Abbreviation: FHR = fetal heart rate.

Cardiovascular Adaptation

Prior to birth, the lungs were nonfunctioning as the placenta provided oxygen and CO_2 scavenge. Coincident with the first breaths, the coiled arterioles of the lungs uncoil and vasodilate under the influence of oxygen. As right ventricular pressures drop, so does right atrial pressure, until it is less than left atrial pressure, thereby functionally closing the foramen ovale. At birth, the patent ductus arteriosus (which up until now has shunted blood away from the lungs) goes into spasm under oxygen and neurologic stimulus combined with diminution in circulating prostaglandin, redirecting right ventricular blood into the pulmonary arteries.

A major problem associated with this adaptation can occur in term or near-term infants when intrauterine hypoxia has sensitized the pulmonary vasculature (and in some instances has led to hypertrophied pulmonary arteriolar smooth muscle), resulting in poor or negligible vasodilatation and perfusion of the lungs. This leads to an extreme right-to-left shunt that in the past has been named "persistent fetal circulation," or more recently "persistent pulmonary hypertension." Premature infants are subject to incomplete closure (and later reopening) of the ductus arteriosus, initially producing a right-to-left shunt, then reversing to left-to-right after a few days when the right ventricular pressures drop further.

Neurologic Adaptation

The stimuli of labor and birth produce a massive sympathetic response, exhibited by alertness, labile tachycardia, crying, startle and Moro's reactions, sucking, chewing, grimacing, and tremors. This period of initial reactivity lasts 10 to 60 minutes, following which the infant enters a second stage of quiet and inactivity. This stage is characterized by slowing of heart and respiratory rate, sleep, irregular breathing and short periods of apnea, and general unresponsiveness. At 2 to 6 hours of age, the infant characteristically enters a second period of activity during which vital signs remain unstable. During this entire transitional period, it is important to recognize and differentiate normal variants from abnormal signs. For instance, an infant at 2 hours of age would be expected to be lethargic and have much less tone than after 6 hours of age.

Assessment and Apgar Score

The primary assessment parameters at birth (breathing, heart rate, and color) are described in the previous article on resuscitation. The Apgar score, performed at 1 and 5 minutes (Table 4) is an integral part of the early assessment of the newborn infant but is not intended to supplant or replace any of the steps described in neonatal resuscitation. A normal Apgar score is 7 or greater, a moderately depressed infant's score is 3 to 6, and a severely depressed infant's score is 2 or less. The Apgar score should be used to document the response (or lack of it) to resuscitation, and to predict the infant's need for observation or treatment in a transitional or intensive care nursery. The Apgar score at 5 minutes and thereafter also correlates with long-term prognosis.

NEONATAL TRANSPORT

Assessment of current and anticipated problems in a newborn infant may make maternal or neonatal transfer to a more specialized center desirable. The earlier the possibility is considered, the smoother, less complicated, and less dangerous the actual transport will be. Most secondary and tertiary NICUs that are referral centers can provide phone consultation or advice prior to the decision to transfer, and throughout the transport process.

Often the referral hospital can provide a transport team, equipment, and transportation. Personnel for a transport should be tailored to the particular needs of the infant and/or mother. Transport personnel include a nurse for a stable infant with an impending problem such as hyperbilirubinemia, a nurse and respiratory therapist for a stable ventilated baby, or a nurse or respiratory therapist plus a physician or nurse practitioner for unstable infants. Transport of infants requires appropriate equipment and ambulance to provide a "miniature NICU environment" throughout the transport. Everything must fit within the confined space of vehicles, yet provide good access to the infant and be battery operable. The vehicle used must be matched to the anchoring, power, and oxygen needs of the transport equipment.

Specialized regional transport centers are beginning to develop the ability to provide sophisticated neonatal care during transport, including high-frequency ventilation and extracorporeal membrane oxygenation (ECMO). However, in all cases, it would be beneficial to attempt to identify the high-risk infant early enough before delivery to permit safe transport in the mother's womb (safer, cheaper, and results in improved outcome).

CARE OF THE PARENTS

Bonding and Parental Involvement

Parent-infant bonding following delivery has important considerations for the infant's health and development after discharge. Disruptions to the normal bonding process by separation, usually beginning in the delivery room, have been associated with later failure to thrive and even child abuse. Parents relate that even minor separation, such as use of an incubator for phototherapy, has a negative effect on bonding. Although the normal bonding process is disrupted by the need to care for a high-risk infant in the NICU, most parents go through a delayed and more prolonged bonding process that is an effective substitute. Providing a way for the parents to maintain an active role in their infant's course and care over the prolonged hospitalization greatly aids this process.

Early, when the infant is unstable, the parent is dealing with shock, fear, and guilt. Daily (or more often) contact between the parent and nursery staff does much to alleviate the anxiety they feel, and reinforces explanations that often take several repeatings to be understood because of that same anxiety. Parent involvement at this stage might be limited to providing get-well cards, mementos, and symbolic toys. After the infant is more stable, even while still on a respirator, parents should be encouraged to provide simple caretaking tasks such as changing diapers and taking axillary temperatures. As soon as practical and safe, the infant can be held

TABLE 4. **Apgar Score**

Component	0	1	2
Heart rate	Absent	<100 beats/min	>100 beats/min
Respiratory effort	Apneic	Weak, irregular, gasping	Vigorous cry
Reflex irritability	Absent	Grimace	Active avoidance
Muscle tone	Flaccid	Weak, some flexion	Active movement, well flexed
Skin color	Pale, blue	Acrocyanotic	Pink

in a parent's arms for short periods. Older infants can be gavage-fed and bottle-fed by the parents as well. Instant photographs provide a means of contact for parents who live a distance away. Formal and informal contact with the health care team (especially nurses, social worker, and physician) gives needed support and an environment for expressing feelings about their infant's care, needs, and outlook.

Grieving

When an infant dies, parents must deal with stages of shock, denial, guilt, anger, and depression. Helping parents through the grieving process is begun by the NICU team through support and empathy. When an infant is very ill and dies soon after birth, the parent may resist even visiting at all. However, visiting both before and after death, although immediately painful, does much to alleviate denial and smooth the later adaptation process. Holding the infant before, during, or after dying is appropriate. A follow-up visit with the parents in a month or so provides a time to review autopsy findings and answer any outstanding questions, as well as to assess their adaptation to the loss. Medical (and clergy) long-term relationships can be instrumental in helping the parents with their own recovery over the ensuing months.

NEWBORN ASSESSMENT

A thorough evaluation of the newborn infant should be performed as soon after birth as possible. This includes the following:

History

A thorough review of history of pregnancy, labor, and delivery, along with medical histories of the parents and their families, is taken. This information is obtained by talking to the mother and her physician and reviewing the obstetric record (Hollister sheets), which are routinely sent to the nursery. Table 5 lists data that should be routinely collected.

Intrauterine Growth

Disturbances in normal fetal growth can give valuable guidelines for the anticipation, diagnosis, and

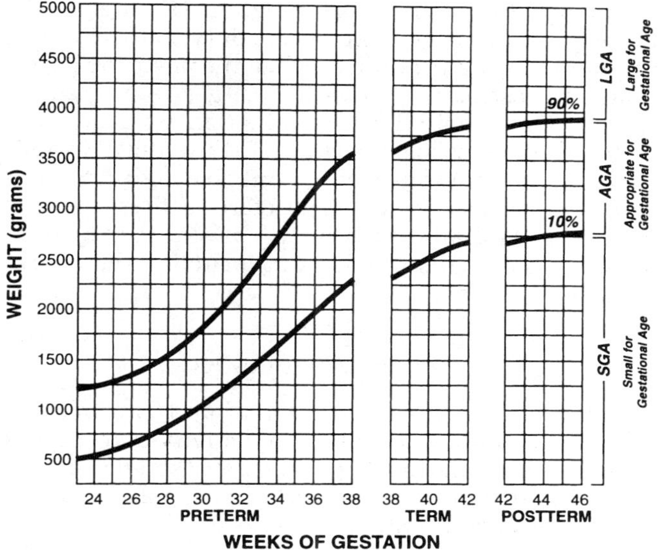

Term LGA	Preterm LGA	Post-term LGA
Birth trauma Hypoglycemia Transposition of the great vessels	Hypoglycemia Hyperbilirubinemia Birth injury Infant of diabetic mother Hypocalcemia Hyperviscosity Congenital anomalies	Birth trauma Polycythemia Hypoglycemia Meconium aspiration Pneumothorax
Term AGA Lowest Risk	**Preterm AGA** Respiratory distress syndrome Hypothermia Hypoglycemia Hyperglycemia Hyperbilirubinemia Hyponatremia Hypocalcemia Apnea Infection CNS hemorrhage	**Post-term AGA** Pneumothorax Meconium aspiration Hypoglycemia
Term SGA Hypothermia Hypoglycemia Meconium aspiration Polycythemia Malnutrition Congenital infection Congenital anomalies Maternal addiction	**Preterm SGA** Hypothermia Hypoglycemia Anemia Asphyxia Hyperbilirubinemia Hypocalcemia Malnutrition Congenital infection Congenital anomalies	**Post-term SGA** Polycythemia Hypoglycemia Congenital anomalies Dysmaturity

Figure 1. Neonatal morbidity risk. (Adapted from Lubchenco LO, et al: Neonatal mortality rate: Relationship to birthweight and gestational age. J Pediatr *81*:818, 1972; reprinted with permission from Coen RW, Koffler H: Primary Care of the Newborn. Published by Little, Brown and Company, Boston, 1987, p 60.)

TABLE 5. **Important History for Neonatal Evaluation**

Ages of mother and father
Obstetric history with gravidity and outcome
Prenatal care during current pregnancy
Medications (prescription and nonprescription)
Habits (drugs, alcohol, smoking)
Maternal blood type
Mode of feeding (breast or bottle)
Marital status
Last menstrual period and expected date of delivery
Prepregnant weight and pregnancy weight gain
Exposure to infectious diseases
Family and genetic diseases
Hepatitis and serologic tests

treatment of neonatal conditions. Based on the 90th and 10th percentiles, neonates are categorized as appropriate for gestational age (AGA), large for gestational age (LGA), or small for gestational age (SGA). Each category has an expected incidence of specific classes of problems (Figure 1). To classify an infant properly, an accurate assessment of gestational age at the time of birth must be made. Often menstrual history plus early fetal ultrasound will produce an accurate estimate, but these data may be missing or inaccurate. A combination neurologic and physical scoring system was devised by Dubowitz and refined by Ballard as a way to estimate gestational age by physical examination (Figure 2). As there is about a 1.5-week uncertainty to the Ballard examination, we generally utilize the obstetric gestational age estimate, unless it diverges from that obtained from the Ballard examination by 2 or more weeks. The neurologic portion of the Ballard examination may be influenced by maternal drugs, or a depressed or sick infant. Therefore, a first approximation of the Ballard score may be obtained by doubling the physical score without including the neurologic examination.

Physical Examination

A thorough physical examination that includes color, breathing pattern, level of activity and responsiveness, and morphologic features should be recorded. Listed next are areas of particular interest in the newborn infant.

Head. Shape and contour abnormalities at birth are largely a product of vaginal delivery. Particular attention should be paid to bruises, lacerations, separated sutures, and cephalhematomas. A caput is edema from pressure around the "presenting part" and has no significance other than to be differentiated from the cephalhematoma, which is a true hemorrhage. The cephalhematoma may be darker and firmer; it is subperiosteal and does not cross suture lines; however, two separate hemorrhages can rarely occur on adjacent cranial bones. Complications of cephalhematomas include jaundice, infection (if due to a scalp probe), and calcification and rarely may be associated with linear skull fracture.

Eyes. Eye examination may be difficult in some neonates. However, an attempt must be made to look for the red reflex. The presence of cataracts suggests metabolic or infectious etiology. Conjunctival hemorrhages are extremely common in vaginal deliveries and are usually of no consequence.

Ears. Anterior skin tags are common and usually isolated. Posterior rotation of the ears, causing them to be low set, may be part of complex anomalies. To determine low set, draw an imaginary line from the corner of the eye to the occipital prominence. If the upper attachment (not the tip of the ear) is below that line, the ears are low set.

Nose. Choanal atresia or stenosis is usually detected in the delivery room, as newborn infants are

Neuromuscular Maturity

	-1	0	1	2	3	4	5
Posture							
Square Window (wrist)	>90°	90°	60°	45°	30°	0°	
Arm Recoil		180°	140°-180°	110°-140°	90-110°	<90°	
Popliteal Angle	180°	160°	140°	120°	100°	90°	<90°
Scarf Sign							
Heel to Ear							

Physical Maturity

Skin	sticky friable transparent	gelatinous red, translucent	smooth pink, visible veins	superficial peeling &/or rash. few veins	cracking pale areas rare veins	parchment deep cracking no vessels	leathery cracked wrinkled
Lanugo	none	sparse	abundant	thinning	bald areas	mostly bald	
Plantar Surface	heel-toe 40-50mm: -1 <40mm: -2	>50mm no crease	faint red marks	anterior transverse crease only	creases ant. 2/3	creases over entire sole	
Breast	imperceptible	barely perceptible	flat areola no bud	stippled areola 1-2mm bud	raised areola 3-4mm bud	full areola 5-10mm bud	
Eye/Ear	lids fused loosely:-1 tightly:-2	lids open pinna flat stays folded	sl. curved pinna; soft; slow recoil	well-curved pinna; soft but ready recoil	formed &firm instant recoil	thick cartilage ear stiff	
Genitals male	scrotum flat, smooth	scrotum empty faint rugae	testes in upper canal rare rugae	testes descending few rugae	testes down good rugae	testes pendulous deep rugae	
Genitals female	clitoris prominent labia flat	prominent clitoris small labia minora	prominent clitoris enlarging minora	majora & minora equally prominent	majora large minora small	majora cover clitoris & minora	

Maturity Rating

score	weeks
-10	20
-5	22
0	24
5	26
10	28
15	30
20	32
25	34
30	36
35	38
40	40
45	42
50	44

Figure 2. Expanded new Ballard Score. (Adapted from Ballard JL, et al: New Ballard Score, expanded to include extremely premature infants. J Pediatr 119[3]:417–423, 1991.)

obligatory nose breathers. The passage of a feeding catheter through both nares into the pharynx is a routine test for unilateral choanal atresia in the delivery room. In the absence of respiratory distress, this should be delayed at least until after the 5-minute Apgar score to guard against vagal reflex bradycardia. A deformed nose may indicate a dislocated nasal septum, which should be corrected soon after birth. Flaring of the alae nasae is often the first sign of increased respiratory effort. However, during the first 6 hours of life, some nasal flaring will be normally seen in infants. This can be easily differentiated from respiratory distress as it is generally not coincident with inspiration but will occur variably during the breathing cycle.

Mouth. An asymmetrical mouth, especially when the neonate is crying, should raise the possibility of forceps compression of the seventh cranial nerve. In contrast to older children and adults, the side that appears to droop during crying is actually the intact side. The side that does not open completely is damaged. The inability to close the ipsilateral eye should be seen in addition to mouth droop to confirm facial nerve compression, as isolated hypoplasia of orbicularis oris muscles may give the same oral palsy.

Neck. Birth injury to the sternocleidomastoid muscle may present as a mass or limitation of spontaneous motion. The base of the neck should also be palpated to detect clavicular fractures.

Chest. Since the neonate's rib cage is cartilaginous and flexible, substernal retractions are an early indication of respiratory distress, in addition to sub- and intracostal retractions. One should look for widely spaced nipples and other rib cage or vertebral anomalies. Immediately following birth, some rales from unreabsorbed fluid may be heard transiently. Murmurs should be noted if present. Because of the rapid heart rate, it may be difficult to characterize a murmur, or even place it in diastole or systole. A murmur in a cyanotic infant should always be pursued aggressively. A low-pitched murmur in an otherwise healthy infant may be caused by delayed closure of the ductus arteriosus and can be expected to disappear by the next day.

Abdomen. The liver is usually palpable in normal infants (0.5 to 1 cm). When the infant is quiet during the first hours of life is an ideal time to palpate the kidneys, both of which should be detectable but not enlarged. They should feel about the size of the distal phalanx of your thumb. Masses in the abdomen are most frequently of renal (including collecting system) origin.

Genitalia. The degree of descent of the testes is related to maturity (see the Ballard examination earlier). Unilateral descent should be documented for follow-up. A small amount of mucoid vaginal discharge is normal.

Anus. Examine externally for patency and position.

Extremities. Examine for dislocatable or dislocated hips. Dislocatable hips are common in breech deliveries. Due to intrauterine positioning, a newborn infant's legs are usually bowed (internal tibial torsion), and the feet will exhibit pronation. As a general rule, if the ankle and forefoot can be moved to a neutral (normal) position with the gentle pressure of one finger, they are probably normal.

Neurologic. The neurologic examination in the newborn infant depends greatly on the infant's state of alertness. Subtle abnormalities need to be confirmed on several occasions before being labeled as abnormal. For instance, in an irritated infant, nonsustained clonus may be normal, and in a sleepy infant, the absence of reflexes may also be normal.

Use of Laboratory Tests

Laboratory studies are commonly performed following birth to provide screening data. A complete blood count (CBC), serum electrolytes, blood urea nitrogen (BUN), creatinine, glucose, and calcium levels are important parameters in the first day of life if maternal history is abnormal or in high-risk infants admitted for close observation. As infants are born with whatever electrolyte status their mother had at delivery, blood chemistries are usually delayed a few hours to reflect the infant's status more closely. In some infants, it may be critical to obtain certain laboratory tests immediately, such as serum glucose (in prematures, intrauterine growth retardation [IUGR], asphyxiated infants, or infants of diabetics), magnesium (if administered to the mother prenatally), or total bilirubin (prematures or suspected hemolytic conditions). A spun hematocrit should be performed soon after delivery for infants at risk for hemolysis, polycythemia, or blood loss.

GENERAL MANAGEMENT OF THE HIGH-RISK INFANT

Fluid and Electrolyte Management

Water

The daily intake of water must equal net losses plus any increase in body mass (cell growth). In an infant in water homeostasis, there is a balance between ingested water and water released by metabolism, on the one hand, with obligatory waste products and cell growth on the other hand. Obligatory water losses due to heat dissipation (through the skin and lungs) and renal function (excretion of solutes, urea, and acids) are directly related to energy metabolism.

Water requirements vary greatly, both daily and according to gestational age. The two major organs that determine obligatory losses, the kidneys and skin, function inversely to maturation and directly with postdelivery age. A term infant may require 75 mL per kg per day of free water, whereas a premature infant might require 100 mL per kg per day or more owing to porous skin that increases the insensible water losses. In addition to increased skin permeability, the premature infant also has a larger surface area compared with body weight, increased skin vascularity, and decreased renal concentrating ability.

Table 6 gives daily water requirements for infants with appropriate growth for gestational age. Other conditions that produce greater water losses include use of radiant warmers (20 mL per kg), phototherapy (10 to 20 mL per kg), elevated environmental or body temperature, high renal osmotic load (hyperglycemia, uremia, or bicarbonate administration), diarrhea or "ostomy" loss, hyperactivity, and low-humidity environment. Conditions requiring a reduction in water requirements include renal failure, congenital heart disease, syndrome of inappropriate antidiuretic hormone (SIADH) secretion, and mechanical ventilation.

Sodium and Potassium

Both the concentrating and diluting abilities of the kidneys are limited in the newborn infant and more so with decreasing gestational age. Under the best circumstances, renal function will be limited to between 40 and 700 mOsm per liter. In order to refrain from exceeding an infant's renal function, it is desirable to provide a renal solute load necessitating urine concentrations near the middle of that range. For a 1-kg infant on a standard oral or intravenous electrolyte intake providing 3 mEq of sodium, 2 mEq of potassium, and 5 mEq of chloride, an additional 10 mOsm is released through metabolism for a total of a 20-mOsm solute load. This would require a 220 mOsm per liter urine at 2.3 mL per kg per hour. Clinical assessment of hydration (synonymous with total body sodium content) includes weight or hematocrit change, urine output (normally 1 to 4 mL per kg per hour), and skin turgor. As renal function is often impaired in sick newborn infants, potassium is added to the intravenous fluids after 12 to 24 hours of life with demonstration of normal urine output and serum potassium.

Hypernatremia is a disturbance in electrolyte balance commonly encountered in small premature infants. It occurs at a few days of age when there has been a deficiency in water administration to keep pace with skin losses. Diabetes insipidus, adrenal hyperplasia, or steroid administration can also lead to hypernatremia. Hypernatremia is treated primarily with increases in free water. In severe or rapidly developing hypernatremia, remove sodium from the intravenous line and monitor electrolytes every 4 to 6 hours increasing water administration at a daily rate of 40 mL per kg at each determination until the sodium level starts to fall.

Conversely, hyponatremia is often seen in the second week of life when sodium restriction to treat hypernatremia has resulted in a sodium deficit, perhaps exacerbated by previous losses, growth, theophylline administration, decreased renal reabsorption, SIADH, diuretic administration, or sepsis. Factitious hyponatremia may be seen in states of high serum lipids, hyperglycemia, uremia, and mannitol administration. The therapy of hyponatremia requires careful correction (usually over at least 8 hours) to prevent iatrogenic seizures from too-rapid correction. Based on a "sodium space" of two thirds of weight, administer added sodium for the first 8 hours to raise the serum sodium to 130 mEq per liter, then provide the remainder of the correction over the remaining 24 hours.

Hypocalcemia

Hypocalcemia is frequently encountered in premature infants. It is also occasionally seen in term infants who are asphyxiated, have diabetic mothers, or otherwise are severely stressed. Normal serum calcium values are greater than 8 mg per dL for term and greater than 7 mg per dL for premature infants. Infants at risk should receive 20 to 30 mg per kg per day of calcium (300 mg per kg per day of calcium gluconate added to the maintenance intravenous fluid intake is a standard order). Infants with serum calcium levels of less than 6 mg per dL or who are symptomatic can be treated with 200 mg per kg of calcium gluconate, given by slow push with careful monitoring of the ECG.

Glucose

Conditions leading to hypoglycemia include prematurity, intrauterine growth retardation, diabetic mother, asphyxia, and adrenal insufficiency. As hypoglycemia may also be caused by rebound from withdrawal of intravenous glucose administration, emergency therapy should generally be limited to a 2 to 4 mL per kg bolus of 10% dextrose when the serum glucose is less than 20 mg%. Often, administration of IV fluids providing 6 to 8 mg of glucose per kg per min is all that is required when the serum glucose is between 20 and 40 mg%. Infants at risk should have frequent bedside "Stix" blood glucose determinations (e.g., Dextrostix), with laboratory confirmation when levels below 40 are first encountered. The Stix are accurate enough on which to base therapy, which should not be delayed for return of the laboratory

TABLE 6. **Daily Water Requirements for Healthy Infants**

Weight (grams)	Day					
	1	2	3	4	5–7	>7
<600	110–120	140–180	170–240	170–240	140–180	up to 150
<1000	90–110	110–130	130–160	130–170	140–160	up to 150
1000–1500	70–90	90–110	110–130	120–140	130–150	up to 150
>1500	60–80	80–100	100–120	100–130	120–130	up to 150
Full term	50–60	70–80	90–100	100–120	120–130	up to 150

report. To avoid rebound hypoglycemia, a bolus infusion of glucose should be followed by intravenous maintenance and slow weaning of the intravenous glucose.

Hyperglycemia is frequently encountered as an iatrogenic side effect of the very high rates of intravenous fluids (containing glucose) necessary to provide adequate free water to the smallest prematures. Hyperglycemia is also seen in sepsis, intraventricular hemorrhage, and inefficient metabolism secondary to stress and extreme prematurity. Medications such as steroids, theophylline, and diazoxide can produce hyperglycemia. Transient neonatal diabetes is an uncommonly encountered phenomenon. In an attempt to provide calories, a modest elevation of serum glucose may be tolerated (less than 160 mg% with no significant glucosuria). The intravenous glucose concentration may be reduced, remembering that less than 4.7 is hypotonic and may produce hemolysis. In some refractory cases, intravenous insulin (0.05–0.2 U per kg per hr) may be necessary.

Acid-Base

Metabolic acidosis is sometimes seen during recovery from asphyxia, hypoxia, and hypotension, when reperfusion releases accumulated lactic acid from tissue stores. However, it also may be a sign of current or new problems, such as the onset of sepsis or the opening of a ductus arteriosus. Persistent acidosis in small premature infants may also result from bicarbonate loss due to renal immaturity. Metabolic acidosis is occasionally encountered as protein intolerance in a premature infant and is suspected when there is a cessation in weight gain. This is termed "late acidosis of prematurity." Transient acidosis is corrected by bolus sodium bicarbonate administration (0.5 mEq per minute or slower, and less than 10 mEq per kg per day to avoid intracranial hemorrhage in prematures). To prevent overcorrection, it is generally advisable to administer bicarbonate corrections based on half the expected volume of distribution: base deficit · kg/3. Severe and persistent acidosis is sometimes treated by continuous infusion of bicarbonate, but it should be remembered that bicarbonate and calcium are not compatible in intravenous solutions.

Blood Pressure Support

Hypotension is common in sick neonates. Normal blood pressure varies with gestational age and postnatal age. A mean blood pressure of 25 mmHg may be adequate for a 500-gram, 25-weeks' gestation infant, whereas 40 mmHg is minimal for a full-term infant on the first day of life. Often hypotension is associated with hypovolemia, although other causes should be ruled out. Premature infants with hyaline membrane disease are usually hypovolemic by an average 10 mL per kg. Perinatal causes of hypovolemia include placenta previa, abruptio placentae or trauma, twin-to-twin or fetal-maternal transfusion,

and erythroblastosis fetalis. Vasoconstriction in an asphyxiated infant may shift blood volume to the placenta at birth. Generally, 5% albumin is the best blood volume expander in an emergency. It is readily available and stays in the circulation longer than normal saline. A volume of 15 to 20 mL per kg can be given rapidly and repeated as needed. A major part of the effectiveness of sodium bicarbonate has been shown to be volume expansion. Fresh-frozen plasma is useful if hypovolemia is associated with coagulopathy, and red cells should be given if acute blood loss is certain. O-negative blood can be obtained from most blood banks on an emergency basis within 15 to 20 minutes.

Following volume expansion, inotropic therapy may be instituted to raise the blood pressure. The most commonly used drug is dopamine, administered at a rate of 5 to 30 µg per kg per min. Dobutamine (same rate) can be added if reduction in afterload would help, while epinephrine (0.1 to 1.5 mg per kg per minute) is useful when myocardial contractility is impaired.

Hypertension is generally only seen in hyperrenin states as a result of renal injury from umbilical artery catheters, and also as a side effect of steroid therapy. The rare infant with hyperthyroidism may also be hypertensive. Captopril (Capoten), and hydralazine (Apresoline) are effective drugs.

Hematocrit

Polycythemia

Abnormally elevated hematocrit (HCT) is occasionally seen at birth. The consequent increase in viscosity and resulting decrease in tissue perfusion have been associated with neurologic signs ranging from irritability and poor feeding to apnea, seizures, and infarcts. Plethora, hematuria and proteinuria, pulmonary hypertension, jaundice, necrotizing enterocolitis (NEC), and priapism are also seen. The increased load of short-lived fetal red cells produces or exacerbates hyperbilirubinemia. Our practice is to reduce the HCT of any newborn infant with a central HCT of 70% or greater and any symptomatic infant with a central HCT of less than 65 (determined at 4 to 6 hours of age). HCTs should be determined by microcentrifuge, because when calculated by a Coulter Counter, the HCT is underestimated by approximately 6%. When polycythemia (or hyperviscosity) is present, 5% albumin, normal saline, or fresh-frozen plasma may be used to perform a partial exchange transfusion (using umbilical catheters and 10 to 15 mL aliquots) to lower the central HCT according to the following formula: (Observed HCT − 50) · kg · 90 / observed HCT.

Anemia

Anemia at birth may be due to fetomaternal transfusion, twin-twin transfusion, placental blood loss (placenta previa, abruption, tears), cord rupture, infant-to-placenta transfusion, hemolysis, or bone marrow suppression (Blackfan-Diamond, parvovirus). If severe anemia is known or strongly suspected prenatally, O-negative blood should be available in the delivery room. Otherwise, 5% albumin, Plasmanate, or normal saline can be administered to maintain cardiac output until blood is available.

Principles of Respiratory Support

Oxygen administered via hood or flooded into an incubator may be sufficient in some infants with mild respiratory distress. However, apnea or severe lung disease may require ventilator support. Assisted ventilation is generally required in infants with persistent apnea, Pa_{CO_2} greater than 60 torr, or FI_{O_2} greater than 0.80. In some cases, intubation is indicated much earlier, such as in an infant with hyaline membrane disease or persistent pulmonary hypertension.

Whatever the reason for needing ventilator support, whether central depression or severe hyaline membrane disease, the goal is the same: to provide oxygen and extract carbon dioxide at adequate rates while minimizing oxygen toxicity and barotrauma to the lungs. The standard ventilators used in neonates are constant flow, time cycled, and pressure limited. High-frequency oscillators and jet ventilators have special application in hyaline membrane disease, pulmonary air leaks, and any condition requiring very high mean airway pressures. Volume-cycled, and newer, more sensitive and responsive patient-triggering assist modes have been found useful primarily in management of larger infants and chronically ventilated infants.

Selection of endotracheal tube size is important, especially as cuffed tubes are not easily obtained below 4.5 mm. Table 7 gives appropriate sizes based on weight. Airway resistance is a problem with the smaller-diameter tubes (e.g., a 2.5-mm tube has twice the airway resistance of a 3.0-mm tube). The smaller tubes are also more difficult to suction adequately. To aid in proper placement, the tubes are generally marked near the tip to indicate where the vocal cords should lie. On chest radiograph, the tip of the endotracheal tube should lie between the carina and the level of the clavicles.

Although ventilator management is complex, a few general guidelines help in managing the standard respirator: to normalize Pa_{CO_2} (normally kept at 45 to 50 torr), make changes in peak pressure (normal settings: 15 to 20 cmH$_2$O) and rate (normally 20 to 40 per minute). High pressures are generally more injurious to the lungs than high rates. To increase

Pa_{O_2} (normally kept between 50 and 90 torr), one can increase the FI_{O_2}, PEEP (positive end-expiratory pressure), and inspiratory time. The chance of lung injury increases with ventilator parameter changes in that same order. Mean airway pressures greater than 8 cmH$_2$O are considered high; over 11 cmH$_2$O is an indication to consider high-frequency ventilation. Except for short-term ventilator management of conditions with normal lungs, arterial access for blood gas determination is essential. Chronically intubated infants who are stable may be adequately managed by transcutaneous oxygen monitoring (pulse oximeter or transcutaneous oxygen sensor) plus infrequent capillary blood gas to monitor pH and P_{CO_2}.

Physical and Nutritional Needs

Temperature Regulation

Cold stress contributes significantly to a sick neonate's morbidity and mortality. Infants, especially premature infants, are at risk for cold stress due to their large surface area and lack of subcutaneous fat insulation. Concern for heat loss begins in the delivery room, where a newborn is exposed to a wet and cool environment. Although a fetus has a slightly higher temperature than maternal temperature, core temperature falls precipitously following birth. This drop can be slowed (but not eliminated) by rapidly and thoroughly drying the infant and placing him or her under a radiant warmer. It is also helpful to maintain the delivery room between 23.8° and 26.6° C (75° and 80° F) and to wrap the infant in warmed blankets for transport to the nursery.

Although newborn infants are especially prone to heat loss, they have accumulations of deep brown fat that provide a metabolic reservoir to generate heat. Utilizing brown fat and carbohydrate stores to maintain temperature, however, requires an increased metabolic rate, which is itself a significant stress. An infant may have a normal core temperature yet be under considerable metabolic stress trying to maintain that temperature. There is a narrow range of net environmental temperature that permits an infant to maintain normal body temperature while expending a minimum of energy. This is termed "neutral thermal environment" (NTE), and varies both with the infant's birthweight and age from birth.

Incubator temperature charts giving the proper NTE for incubators are available. One could empirically determine the proper incubator temperature by increasing the air temperature until the infant has a higher-than-normal core temperature, then backing off slightly. However, infants are prone to apnea in high air temperatures. Some incubators can be servo-controlled utilizing a skin probe that keeps the mean skin temperature in the normal range, approximating an appropriate NTE. However, this method of control allows wide swings in incubator temperature, which may produce apnea when high and cold stress when low. The overhead radiant warmer (in which the only way to control the heat is the servo skin

TABLE 7. **Endotracheal Tube Sizes**

Weight *(grams)*	Gestational Age	Size *(mm)*
<1000	<28	2.5
1000–2000	28–34	3.0
2000–3000	34–38	3.5
3000–4000	38–42	4.0
>4000	40–44	4.5

probe) has the advantage of being less prone to apnea if the probe is kept dry and insulated, and the infant's temperature is not raised by more than 0.5° C. Skin temperatures to maintain an NTE vary from 36.2°C for term infants to as high as 37.0° C for small prematures.

Parenteral Nutrition

Unstable infants should not be fed in the first few days of life, especially those with respiratory distress. However, it is important to attempt to provide optimal calories, protein, and other nutrients. This can be accomplished by utilizing parenteral nutrition, either via a central venous catheter or peripheral vein. We begin parenteral nutrition in premature infants immediately after stabilization of glucose and electrolytes, generally by the third day of life. Glucose is begun at whatever maintenance intravenous rate the parenteral nutrition is given and increased daily to 15 to 17 grams per kg per day, monitoring for hyperglycemia. Glucose concentrations above 13 to 15% cause small vein injury and frequent need to restart the IV. These high glucose concentrations should be administered via central line, where concentrations as high as 25% can be utilized. Protein is started at 0.5 to 1.0 gram per kg per day and gradually increased to 2.5 to 3.0 grams, monitoring for elevated BUN and acidosis. Fat (Intralipid) is provided, starting at 0.5 to 1.0 gram per kg per day and increasing to 2.5 to 3.0 grams. It is important to monitor serum triglyceride levels, as fat metabolism may vary. If an infant is septic, we decrease the fat intake to the minimal amount of 0.5 gram per kg per day to provide essential fatty acids while not impairing phagocytosis. Vitamins and trace elements should also be provided. For prolonged parenteral nutrition, calcium should be increased to 80 to 100 mg per kg per day and phosphorus to 40 to 50 mg per kg per day (a calcium:phosphorus ratio of 1.5:1 to 2.5:1 is optimal for bone growth). The caloric goal is 100 to 110 Cal per kg per day, although some infants may begin to gain weight adequately with as little as 90 Cal per kg per day. Postsurgical infants and those with bronchopulmonary dysplasia benefit from higher caloric intake.

Feeding High-Risk Infants

Sick or recovering infants may not tolerate oral feedings, and they, along with premature and growth-retarded infants, are at risk for NEC. We have found a combination of slowly progressive feeding volumes coupled with very close observation for feeding intolerance to reduce feeding-related morbidity significantly. Premature infants are begun at 40 mL per kg per day (half-strength formula or breast milk), and increased by 10 to 15 mL per kg each day (switching to full-strength formula by the 5th day). Small or sick premature infants may be fed at half that rate to prevent NEC or feeding intolerance. Infants weighing 1000 or more grams can be fed by intermittent gavage until they reach a developmental age of 33 to 34 weeks, when their breathing/ sucking/swallowing becomes well coordinated, following which nipple feedings may begin. Some infants under 1000 grams tolerate feedings better if fed by continuous gavage pump. The final volume goal is 150 mL per kg per day (providing 110 kilocalories per kg for 20 Cal per oz formula, or 120 Cal per kg for 24 Cal per oz premature formula). Volumes may be limited to 120 to 130 mL per kg for infants with bronchopulmonary dysplasia, or increased to 180 mL per kg for older, thriving infants. Breast milk fortifiers are usually necessary to provide premature infants with adequate electrolytes, calcium, and phosphorus.

COMMON NEONATAL DISEASES

Sepsis

This is a clinical syndrome of systemic illness accompanied by bacteremia occurring in the first month of life. The incidence of primary sepsis is 1 to 10 per 1000 live births. The mortality rate is 13 to 50%, with the highest rates seen in premature infants and those with fulminating disease. Three clinical situations may be encountered: early onset, late onset, and nosocomial disease.

Early-onset disease presents in the first 5 to 7 days of life and is usually multiple system fulminant illness with prominent respiratory symptoms. The infant is colonized with the pathogen in the perinatal period following chorioamnionitis. Several organisms, notably treponemes, viruses, *Listeria*, and probably *Candida* can be acquired hematogenously.

Late-onset disease may occur after 5 to 7 days of age. Although the organism may be acquired perinatally, these infants seldom have a history of obstetric complications, but usually have an identifiable focus of infection, most often meningitis.

Nosocomial sepsis occurs in high-risk neonates. Its pathogenesis is related to the underlying illness, invasive monitoring and therapy, and the flora in the NICU environment. It is often seen in premature infants.

Causative organisms are group B streptococci, *Escherichia coli*, staphylococci, enterococci, anaerobes, *Haemophilus influenzae*, *Mycoplasma*, and *Listeria monocytogenes*. The flora causing nosocomial sepsis varies in each nursery. Although *Staphylococcus epidermidis* predominates, *Staphylococcus aureus*, gram-negative rods (including *Pseudomonas*, *Klebsiella*, *Serratia*, and *Proteus*), and fungal organisms may also cause nosocomial infection.

Risk factors include prematurity, premature or prolonged (more than 24 hours) rupture of membranes, maternal chorioamnionitis, urinary tract infection, resuscitation at birth, and invasive procedures. Clinical presentation is nonspecific, such as temperature instability, lethargy, irritability, poor peripheral perfusion, cyanosis, pallor, mottling, jaundice, feeding intolerance, abdominal distention, vomiting or diarrhea, apnea, respiratory distress, acidosis, and hypo- or hyperglycemia.

The laboratory tests include total and differential white cell and platelet count along with blood culture from two sites (after the first day of life). Urine and cerebrospinal fluid (CSF) culture and counterimmunoelectrophoresis are done if the infant is over 7 days of age. Chest and abdominal radiographs are needed if the infant is symptomatic or has abnormal findings. Blood gas analysis may indicate metabolic acidosis, and coagulation studies may be abnormal.

The neonate with suspected sepsis must be treated immediately after appropriate diagnostic studies are performed. In suspected early- and late-onset sepsis, initial treatment is started with ampicillin and gentamicin or a cephalosporin. In suspected nosocomial infections, therapy is initiated with vancomycin (Vancocin) and gentamicin (Garamycin). Antibiotic sensitivity patterns direct further choice of antibiotics. The doses of selected antibiotics are listed in Table 8.

Hyperbilirubinemia

Jaundice is the most common symptom noted in neonates. Two of three full-term infants have a serum bilirubin level of greater than 5 mg per dL during the first few days of life, whereas most premature infants are jaundiced. This occurs most often due to "physiologic" jaundice because of hepatic immaturity, increased enterohepatic circulation, and decreased red cell survival. Physiologic jaundice usually peaks on day 2, 3, or 4 in full-term infants, and day 3 to 7 in preterm infants. It may last for 7 to 10 days and 3 to 4 weeks, respectively. Jaundice is usually considered nonphysiologic if the infant is jaundiced in the first 24 hours of life, the total serum bilirubin increases by more than 5 mg per dL per day or exceeds 12 mg per dL at any time, prolonged, the conjugated bilirubin exceeds 2 mg per dL, or the infant has symptoms or physical findings other than jaundice. Breast-fed infants may have higher levels of serum bilirubin.

Laboratory tests prior to phototherapy should include the mother's and infant's blood types, Coombs' test, HCT, peripheral smear, and reticulocyte count, along with total and conjugated serum bilirubin estimations.

Phototherapy is started in full-term infants at serum bilirubin levels of between 12 and 15 mg per dL. We use prophylactic phototherapy in premature infants weighing less than 1000 grams at birth, or at half the serum bilirubin level at which a neonate may potentially require exchange transfusion (to prevent kernicterus).

Infant of Diabetic Mother

Pregnant diabetic women have been classified alphabetically by Dr. White from A to R, according to the severity and duration of their diabetes, and this classification is also used to predict perinatal prognosis and define the management of their infants. The risk of complications is minimal in gestational diabetes or in Class A patients controlled by diet alone. If the mothers are insulin-dependent, the risk may be the same as in Class B, C, and D mothers. The most difficult maternal and fetal problems occur in women with renal, cardiac, or retinal disease. Sudden unexpected fetal death occurs in more than 5% of Class F (nephropathy) mothers. Women with Class H (cardiomyopathy) are at risk for cardiac failure and infarction. Women with Class R disease (malignant

TABLE 8. **Antibiotics for Neonatal Infection**

Postconceptual Age		Dose (IV or IM) *(mg/kg/dose)*	Interval
Ampicillin (For use in suspected sepsis and meningitis)			
Suspected sepsis	<1 week	50	q 12 h
Meningitis	<1 week	100	q 12 h
Suspected sepsis	>1 week	50	q 8 h
Meningitis	>1 week	100	q 8 h
Cefotaxime (For use with gram-negative meningitis and sepsis, e.g., *Escherichia coli, Haemophilus influenzae, Klebsiella,* and *Pseudomonas*)			
	Preterm infants <1 week	50	q 12 h
	Preterm infants >1 week	50	q 8 h
	Term infants <1 week	50	q 8 h
	Term infants >1 week	50	q 6 h
Gentamicin (Loading dose: 4 mg/kg/dose IV (preferred) or IM, *first dose only*. This includes anuric infants—one-time dose.)			
	<30 weeks	2.5	q 24 h
	30–37 weeks	2.5	q 18 h
	38–42 weeks	2.5	q 12 h
Vancomycin (For use with *Staphylococcus aureus* or *S. epidermidis* infection)			
	<29 weeks	18*	q 24 h
	30–36 weeks	15*	q 12 h
	37–44 weeks	10*	q 8 h
	>45 weeks	10*	q 6 h

*IV only.
Abbreviations: IV = intravenous; IM = intramuscular.
Modified from Koffler H: Care of the high-risk neonate. *In* Rakel RE: Conn's Current Therapy 1994. Philadelphia, WB Saunders, 1994, p 1025.

retinopathy) have a risk of vitreal hemorrhage or retinal detachment. Infants of mothers with Class H and Class R disease may be severely growth retarded or have intrauterine demise. Fetal macrosomia may be seen in gestational diabetics and in Class A, B, and C mothers, thus increasing their potential for birth trauma or primary cesarean section. Therefore, diabetic women should be educated about the need for adequate metabolic control before and during pregnancy. The goal is to achieve a fasting glucose below 100 mg per dL and a 2-hour postprandial level around 120 mg per dL. Glycosylated hemoglobin should be maintained within the normal range.

Specific problems in infants of diabetic mothers (IDM) are macrosomia, hypoglycemia, hypocalcemia, hypomagnesemia, respiratory distress syndrome, polycythemia, jaundice, poor feeding, congenital anomalies, cardiomyopathy, microcolon, and renal vein thrombosis.

Hypoglycemia (blood sugar less than 40 mg per dL) is seen in 30 to 40% of IDMs (within 1 to 2 hours of age) and is most common in macrosomic infants. Symptoms of hypoglycemia are lethargy, jitteriness, apnea, cyanosis, and seizures. Initially, most infants are asymptomatic. Hence, blood glucose is measured at birth, at one-half, 1, 2, 3, and 6 hours of age, and thereafter if indicated at 12, 24, and 48 hours, or more often if clinically indicated. Blood glucose screening is accomplished with capillary whole blood reagent strips (Dextrostix and Chemstrip). A screening blood glucose level of less than 40 mg per dL is confirmed by blood glucose determination in the clinical chemistry laboratory, and the infant is fed glucose water immediately. If the screening glucose is less than 30 mg per dL, or if the infant is symptomatic, a continuous intravenous infusion with 10% dextrose is started at 100 mL per kg per day and, if necessary, gradually increased to keep the blood glucose between 40 and 80 mg per dL. A minibolus of 2 to 4 mL per kg of 10 to 25% glucose should be given, followed by continuous infusion of 10% glucose if the infant is symptomatic. If there is difficulty in starting an IV, glucagon may be given in an emergency, but continuous intravenous glucose infusion must be started as soon as possible. When the infant tolerates oral feeding, the intravenous glucose should be gradually weaned.

Respiratory Distress

Respiratory distress in the newborn infant manifests as tachypnea, retraction of the chest wall, grunting, and often cyanosis. In the *full-term infant*, common pulmonary causes are pneumonia, transient tachypnea of the newborn, meconium aspiration, and persistent pulmonary hypertension of the newborn. Pneumothorax, other air leaks, and congenital diaphragmatic hernia must be excluded. In the premature infant, respiratory distress syndrome due to surfactant deficiency, pneumonia, septicemia, and patent ductus arteriosus are frequent causes of respiratory distress. To avoid error in the care of infants with respiratory distress, one should consider extrapulmonary disorders in addition to various respiratory diseases. One must rule out airway obstruction and nonpulmonary causes, such as hypovolemia, hyperviscosity (polycythemia), anemia, hypoglycemia, congenital heart disease, cerebral causes, metabolic acidosis, or the effects of drug withdrawal. Work-up of an infant with respiratory distress includes history, physical examination, and the following radiographic and laboratory tests: x-ray film of the chest, blood gases or Sa_{O_2} (pulse oximetry), HCT (central), and blood sugar estimation.

Respiratory Distress Syndrome

Respiratory distress syndrome (RDS) or hyaline membrane disease occurs in 0.5 to 1.0% of all deliveries and in approximately 10% of premature infants, with the greatest incidence in those born at a gestational age of less than 32 weeks. RDS results from primary deficiency or absence of pulmonary surfactant that is synthesized in the cytoplasmic lamellar bodies of the type II pneumocytes, which become prominent by 34 weeks of gestation. The surfactant, a complex lipoprotein rich in phosphatidylcholine, binds to the internal surface of the alveoli and lowers the surface tension at the air-liquid interphase, thus preventing the alveoli from collapsing at the end of expiration. In RDS, the resulting ventilation-perfusion mismatch is often worsened by asphyxia, which induces pulmonary vasoconstriction. Blood thus bypasses the lungs through the fetal pathway (patent ductus, foramen ovale), lowering pulmonary blood flow. The ensuing ischemia reduces lung metabolism and surfactant production.

RDS should be anticipated in infants born to mothers with premature labor, diabetes, bleeding, and perinatal asphyxia. Clinical signs include expiratory grunting (due to closure of the glottis), sternal and intercostal retractions (due to decreased lung compliance), nasal flaring, cyanosis, tachypnea, chest x-ray showing reticulogranular or ground-glass appearance plus air bronchograms, and blood gas findings of hypoxemia, hypercapnia, and metabolic acidosis.

Prevention remains the cornerstone in the management of RDS by (1) documenting pulmonary maturity in amniotic fluid, particularly prior to elective cesarean section; (2) prolonging pregnancy with bed rest and treatment of cervicitis, urinary tract infections, and incompetent cervix (by circlage), along with the use of tocolytic agents; and (3) inducing lung maturity with maternal administration of steroids and thyrotropin-releasing hormone. Therefore, whenever feasible, the mother in premature labor should be transported to a center experienced in the care of high-risk mothers and infants.

Likewise, treatment of infants with RDS should be undertaken only at a medical center with medical personnel (physicians, nurses, respiratory therapists, pharmacists, and social workers) trained and experienced in the care of such infants. If the infant is diagnosed with RDS, is less than 32 weeks of gestation, and requires more than 0.30 $F_{I_{O_2}}$, intratracheal surfactant should be administered as soon as the infant is resuscitated and stabilized, preferably within the first 2 hours of life. If an infant requires more than 0.40 FI_{O_2}, an arterial catheter should be placed to monitor blood gases and arterial pressure. Continuous pulse oximetry is used to prevent hypoxia and hyperoxia. Ventilatory assistance is used prudently with respiratory failure. Nasal continuous positive airway pressure (CPAP) may be used in infants greater than 32 weeks' gestation or birthweight more than 1500 grams; some centers treat infants with early CPAP or after administration of surfactant. Blood gases are monitored to keep the Pa_{O_2} between 50 and 70 torr, Pa_{CO_2} between 40 and 60 torr, and pH between 7.26 and 7.40. Other supportive measures include maintenance of body temperature, fluid and electrolyte balance, HCT greater than 45%, intravascular volume expansion, and antibiotics, along with supportive care of the parents and family.

Acute complications of RDS include alveolar rupture with air leak (diagnosed by transillumination and chest radiograph), patent ductus arteriosus, intracranial hemorrhage (diagnosed by cranial ultrasound), and infections. Long-term complications are bronchopulmonary dysplasia, retinopathy of prematurity, neurologic impairment, and familial psychopathology.

Patent Ductus Arteriosus

A left-to-right shunt through a *patent ductus arteriosus (PDA)* may become apparent during weaning of the infant from the respirator during the first 3 to 10 days of age. If blood-tinged secretions are observed with tracheal suctioning, or the infant develops acidosis or needs increasing ventilator support, one should strongly suspect PDA. The PDA may be "silent" or present clinically with widening of pulse pressure, bounding pulses, hyperdynamic precordium, systolic murmur, hypercapnia, or systemic hypoperfusion. Its presence may be confirmed by color Doppler echocardiography. It is treated with indomethacin and rarely with surgical ligation.

Bronchopulmonary Dysplasia

BPD is a chronic respiratory disease occurring most commonly in premature infants requiring prolonged oxygen and mechanical ventilation. BPD is defined as an oxygen requirement at a corrected gestational age of 36 weeks or more or at a chronologic age of 28 days, with chest x-ray findings of interstitial fluid, fibrosis, overdistention, and/or atelectasis.

Prevention starts with accepting relative hypercapnia and borderline oxygenation (to prevent barotrauma), and continues by facilitating early weaning of premature infants from the ventilator with aminophylline. Further preventive measures include the early use of corticosteroids and fluid restriction, along with treatment of PDA, infections, and nutritional deficiencies. Exposure to viral infection should be avoided and high RSV titer immunoglobulin should be considered during respiratory syncytial virus season.

Treatment consists of fluid restriction, diuretic therapy, bronchodilators, steroids, antibiotics for suspected infections, chest physical therapy, and judicious use of oxygen (monitored by pulse oximetry) and assisted ventilation.

Apnea in the Immature Infant

Apnea is defined as cessation of respiration lasting more than 15 to 20 seconds, or in association with symptoms such as cyanosis, bradycardia, hypotonia, or metabolic acidosis. Periodic breathing (short recurring pauses in respiration of 5 to 15 seconds), on the other hand, should be considered a normal pattern. The diagnosis of apnea of prematurity is considered after excluding infections, thermal instability, intracranial hemorrhage, seizures, metabolic disorders, maternal and neonatal drug use, gastroesophageal reflux (GER), and anemia. All premature infants at high risk for apnea should have continuous cardiorespiratory and pulse oximetry monitoring.

Treatment of apnea of prematurity consists of respiratory stimulants such as theophylline, caffeine, or doxapram, cutaneous stimulation, an apnea bed, nasal CPAP, and rarely, assisted ventilation.

If these infants have persistent apnea after a corrected gestational age of 36 weeks, they may be at an increased risk for sudden infant death and should be investigated thoroughly to exclude other causes such as GER. They may be sent home on theophylline and/or a home monitor (with all care providers trained in its use and in cardiopulmonary resuscitation). After discharge, infants with apnea should be managed in conjunction with physicians, respiratory therapists, and nurses experienced in their care.

Central Nervous System Hemorrhage and Injury

The various types of brain injuries encountered in the neonatal period are as follows:

Intraventricular Hemorrhage (IVH)

IVH occurs in premature infants below 34 weeks of gestation, with a 30% to 60% incidence in those born prior to 28 weeks. It usually occurs in the first week of life. The risk factors are immaturity, RDS, apnea, hypoxia, and hypercapnia, resulting in alteration in cerebral blood flow. Up to 50% to 60% of infants with IVH may be asymptomatic but the disease can be detected by cranial ultrasound, which is performed routinely in this group of infants. Anatomically, IVH is classified as germinal matrix hemorrhage (Grade I), IVH without distention (Grade II), IVH with ventricular distention (Grade III), and IVH with parenchymal bleeding (Grade IV). Clinical manifestations of IVH are nonspecific, such as apnea or bradycardia, hypo- or hyperglycemia, unexplained drop in hematocrit, seizures, or bulging anterior fontanelle. In our NICU, we attempt to prevent IVH by minimizing the risk factors and with the administration of indomethacin prophylactically within 6 to 12 hours of birth to premature infants requiring $F_{I_{O_2}}$ greater than 0.30. Cranial ultrasound studies are repeated weekly to assess the progress of IVH. Infants with uncomplicated (Grades I and II) IVH have good prognosis, whereas those with Grades III and IV usually have neurologic deficit. Hydrocephalus may occur in 10% to 30% of infants with grades II to IV IVH; and although it resolves spontaneously in most cases, may require surgical placement of a ventricular reservoir or a ventriculoperitoneal shunt.

Periventricular Leukomalacia (PVL)

PVL may occur in premature and full-term infants, either pre- or postnatally. Risk factors include chronic fetal distress (intrauterine growth rate) and decreased cerebral perfusion with associated hypotension. It is often associated with IVH. Anatomically, the ischemic necrosis of periventricular white matter is detected as echogenic density, whereas the cavitation and gliosis is visualized as a porencephalic cyst. Enlarged ventricles may be seen due to cerebral atrophy. Neurologic deficits may present as spastic diplegia with or without sensorineural and intellectual deficits.

Cerebral Infarction

Cerebral infarcts usually occur in full-term infants from arterial ischemia occurring either intrapartum or in the immediate postnatal period. They may also arise from maternal cocaine abuse, thromboembolism due to twin-twin transfusion, placental vascular anomalies, or disseminated intravascular coagulation (DIC). These infants usually present with focal seizures within a few days of birth, and the diagnosis is confirmed by either a computed tomography (CT) or magnetic resonance imaging (MRI) scan. The electroencephalogram (EEG) may be abnormal. They are managed with anticonvulsants and physical therapy.

Hypoxic-Ischemic Encephalopathy (HIE)

HIE occurs intrapartum or in the immediate postnatal period in post-term or full-term infants because of perinatal asphyxia. Pathologic findings are brain edema and cellular necrosis with or without hemorrhage. Clinically, they have seizures, altered sensorium, or both. EEG and brain scan are abnormal. Severe neurologic sequelae occur in up to 50% of survivors, with mental and motor handicap, epilepsy, or microcephaly.

Seizures

The tonic-clonic seizure pattern in the older infant is not seen in the neonate because of immaturity of the brain. The seizure patterns may be focal or multifocal clonic seizures, tonic, or myoclonic. However, about 50% of patients present with subtle manifestations such as apnea, tonic posturing, sucking, yawning or drooling, blinking or jerking of eyes, or changes in heart vital signs or Sa_{O_2}. Seizures must be differentiated from jitteriness, wherein the movement ceases if that extremity is held by the examiner.

The etiology consists of the central nervous system (CNS) causes just listed, congenital anomalies of the brain, metabolic problems (e.g., hypoglycemia, hypocalcemia, hypomagnesemia, hypo- and hypernatremia, hyperbilirubinemia, pyridoxine dependency, amino and organic acid disorders), meningitis and encephalitis, developmental problems (e.g., Sturge-Weber anomaly, Menkes' kinky hair disease, Zellweger's syndrome), drug-associated seizures, and hyperviscosity. Hence, persistent seizures must be thoroughly investigated. Management consists of anticonvulsant (generally phenobarbital and phenytoin [Dilantin]) and supportive therapy, treatment of the underlying disease, and genetic counseling when appropriate.

Necrotizing Enterocolitis

Necrotizing enterocolitis (NEC) is an acute inflammatory disease of the gastrointestinal tract, with the highest incidence noted in infants weighing less than 1500 grams or of less than 32 weeks' gestation. Risk factors include infants who are asphyxiated, hypotensive, and acidotic and have had umbilical vessel catheterization, sepsis, and a rapid increase in oral feedings.

Symptomatic infants may have feeding intolerance (residual feeds or emesis), abdominal distention, apnea, or temperature instability. Occult or frank bleeding may be noted, hence stools should be routinely examined for blood in premature infants. If not diagnosed early, perforation or extensive necrosis of the gut, sepsis, shock, DIC, or intraventricular hemorrhage may complicate its course. Abdominal radiographs (including a left lateral decubitus view) may show intramural gas, abnormal bowel gas patterns, edema, or free air in the peritoneal cavity.

Treatment consists of immediate stoppage of enteral feeds as soon as NEC is suspected, decompression of the gastrointestinal tract with low intermittent suction, broad-spectrum antibiotics after septic work-up, and use of blood and blood products and vasopressors as clinically indicated. Frequent abdominal radiographs to detect gut perforation and CBC with platelet count are performed, as well as careful abdominal examination to diagnose peritonitis and/or gut necrosis. Immediate surgical intervention by an experienced pediatric surgeon should be undertaken if gut perforation is suspected. Some infants with extensive necrosis, fulminant peritonitis, or intractable DIC also may benefit from excision of the necrotic bowel.

Prevention of NEC remains the best approach, and in many hospitals it is rarely seen because enteral feeding is introduced gradually in infants at risk for NEC, all stools are tested with Hematest for occult blood, and feedings are withheld when early warning signs develop.

Cardiac Problems

Neonatal cardiac problems may present clinically in several ways with the "six Cs": Cyanosis, Cardiac murmur, Congestive heart failure, Cardiac arrhythmias, Coincident with syndromes or congenital defects, and Circulatory collapse.

Central cyanosis needs immediate attention since it is a sign of severe cardiac, respiratory, or neurologic disease. Cyanosis from cardiac diseases is confirmed by administering 100% oxygen for 10 minutes (hyperoxia test) when it fails to increase arterial Po_2 to more than 150 torr. The "six Ts of neonatal cyanosis" represent the common anomalies; they are (1) Transitional circulation, (2) Transposition of great vessels, (3) Tetralogy of Fallot, (4) Tricuspid or pulmonary atresia with hypoplastic right ventricle (or single ventricle), (5) Truncus arteriosus, and (6) Total anomalous pulmonary venous return.

Persistent Pulmonary Hypertension of the Newborn (PPHN)

Persistent transitional circulation (commonly known as persistent fetal circulation or persistent pulmonary hypertension of the newborn) presents with cyanosis soon after birth and is characterized by a right-to-left shunt. The shunt may be at the level of the foramen ovale, patent ductus arteriosus, or lung (ventilation-perfusion mismatch) and occurs secondary to pulmonary hypertension. PPHN is often due to a variety of underlying pulmonary or pulmonary vascular bed disorders. These include aspiration syndromes (meconium, amniotic fluid, blood), pneumonia (group B beta-streptococcus, *Listeria*), pulmonary hypoplasia (primary or associated with congenital diaphragmatic hernia), polycythemia, chronic intrauterine asphyxia, or a cardiomyopathy. Common precipitating factors are acute asphyxia, metabolic acidosis, hypothermia, and hypoxia. All such infants must be immediately stabilized with oxygen and/or assisted ventilation to keep their Pa_{O_2} between 90 and 120 torr. An echocardiogram is performed to confirm the diagnosis of PPHN and rule out structural cyanotic heart diseases. Supportive therapy consists of correction of acidosis, hypoglycemia, hypothermia, and hypotension and use of antibiotics. Because of the high mortality, infants with suspected PPHN should be stabilized immediately and transferred to a regional tertiary center for further therapy, such as high-frequency ventilation, surfactant therapy (due to inactivation), inhaled nitric oxide, and/or extracorporeal membrane oxygenator support.

Congenital Cyanotic Heart Diseases

Diseases such as transposition of the great vessels, severe tetralogy of Fallot, and right heart lesions (pulmonary stenosis or atresia, tricuspid atresia) usually present early (most often within hours or days) when the patent ductus arteriosus begins to close as a result of extrauterine oxygenation. The infant develops cyanosis, or decreased peripheral perfusion with congestive failure or metabolic acidosis. Left-sided heart lesions such as aortic stenosis, coarctation of the aorta, and hypoplastic left heart syndrome present with respiratory distress, poor perfusion, or cyanosis during the third to seventh day of age and are often mistaken for sepsis. If necessary, intravenous prostaglandin E_1 (PGE_1) (Prostin VR) should be initiated to keep the ductus arteriosus open, at a dose of 0.025 to 0.05 µg per kg per minute. Side effects of PGE_1 include apnea, bradycardia, hyperthermia, flushing, and seizures. Hence, assisted ventilation should be available, and a cardiologist or neonatologist must be consulted prior to initiating this therapy. With the advent of level 2 ultrasound diagnosis in utero, the mother should be transferred for delivery at a regional perinatal-neonatal center.

SURGICAL EMERGENCIES

Congenital Diaphragmatic Hernia

The diagnosis of congenital diaphragmatic hernia (CDH) is considered in an infant with respiratory distress and cyanosis that gets worse with the infant crying or with mask and bag ventilation. These infants must be skillfully and quickly intubated and ventilated using low pressure and rapid rates, and the diagnosis must be confirmed immediately by a chest radiograph after placing a radiopaque feeding tube. In most patients, CDH occurs on the left side through the canal of Bochdalek and may present with scaphoid abdomen, barrel-shaped chest with decreased air entry on the left hemithorax, and the cardiac sounds shifted to the right side. The clinical signs of right-sided hernia are not so obvious, and thus diagnosis is often delayed and may be made by a chest radiograph. Often the diagnosis is made in utero by ultrasonography, permitting maternal transfer. The neonate or the mother should be transferred to a tertiary center with surgeons and neonatologists experienced in managing CDH patients and with facilities for ECMO, surfactant therapy, high-frequency ventilation, and inhaled nitric oxide therapy. In utero correction of CDH by surgeons at the University of California at San Francisco has had limited success.

Abdominal Wall Defects

These are often diagnosed in utero or are obvious after birth. An *omphalocele* represents herniation of the intra-abdominal contents through the umbilical ring. An omphalocele is usually covered by a membrane consisting of amnion and peritoneum. The defect may range from a small one contained within the umbilical cord to a large sac containing intestines and liver. Other congenital defects such as trisomy 13 or 18, Beckwith's syndrome, and exstrophy of the bladder may be associated with omphalocele in up to 50% of patients. *Gastroschisis* is a defect of the abdominal wall just lateral to the umbilicus and has no covering membrane. Approximately 15% of gastroschisis patients have associated anomalies, the commonest being intestinal atresia.

Initial management consists of passing a feeding tube and decompressing the gut with low intermittent suction, maintaining body temperature and fluid balance (to compensate for third-space losses), and covering exposed viscera with warm saline dressing. Infection is prevented by taking appropriate cultures and placing the infant on ampicillin and gentamicin (see Table 8). The infant, or preferably the mother, is transferred before delivery to a tertiary center with a pediatric surgeon. Primary closure of the defect is done, or if it is too large, it is reduced gradually over several days or weeks with the use of a silo. Postoperatively, the infant's cardiopulmonary status, intra-abdominal pressure (perfusion of lower extremities), clinical signs of accidental malrotation (following reduction), and urine output are closely monitored.

Gastrointestinal Obstruction

Obstruction of the gastrointestinal tract may occur anywhere from the proximal to the distal end. The diagnosis is often suspected antenatally due to polyhydramnios and confirmed by level 2 fetal ultrasound examination. Infants with tracheoesophageal fistula present soon after birth with excessive salivation, respiratory distress, cyanosis, or choking. The diagnosis is confirmed by a chest and abdominal radiograph after placing a radiopaque feeding tube, which usually coils in the upper blind esophageal pouch. Obstructions below the stomach may present with vomiting, abdominal distention, and failure to pass meconium or stools. The presence of bilious vomiting is considered an emergency. The diagnosis is confirmed by abdominal radiographs (anteroposterior and left lateral decubitus views). The infant is transferred to a regional tertiary center with a pediatric surgeon skilled in the care of such infants.

DISCHARGE PLANNING

Healthy Full-term Baby

It should be ensured that the baby is well and that the family can provide the basic physical needs of the infant and identify problems. Also, a specific plan is outlined for follow-up health care and parental support. With the recent emphasis on early discharge, these neonates should be followed closely for hyperbilirubinemia and cardiac diseases.

High-Risk Infants

When high-risk infants leave the NICU, they may be transferred either to a step-down unit, a community nursery, a chronic care facility, or most often, to their homes. Discharge planning is initiated early once the infant is stable. A comprehensive plan is delineated during weekly meetings in conjunction with the discharge planning nurse, physicians, nurse practitioners, social worker, nutritionist, developmentalist, home health agencies, early intervention programs, and the physician providing ongoing primary care. Community and social support systems should be arranged prior to discharge. Immunizations recommended by the American Academy of Pe-

diatrics and hearing and eye screenings are initiated before discharge. A copy of the discharge summary is provided to the primary care providers immediately after discharge, and the infant's major problems and plan of care are communicated with them directly.

NORMAL INFANT NUTRITION

method of
RONALD E. KLEINMAN, M.D.
Massachusetts General Hospital
Boston, Massachusetts

Infancy is characterized by extraordinary growth and development. During the first 12 months of life the birthweight may more than triple and length increases by 9 to 10 inches. Approximately 20% of the caloric intake is devoted to growth during the first year of life, compared with 1% to 2% in later years. Over the same period of time the infant goes from a state of total dependency to the beginnings of independent living. Yet, for much of this time the infant relies on a single source of nutrition to support all needs. Thus infancy is a period of nutritional vulnerability, and foods should be optimized to provide all the nutritional requirements to meet the infant's extraordinary needs. For this reason the Committee on Nutrition of the American Academy of Pediatrics recommends that infants be fed human milk or, as an alternative, infant formula for the entire first year of life. No other food is required for the first 4 to 6 months of life. At that time solid foods can be introduced one at a time to complement the nutrition supplied by the milk or formula.

Vitamin and mineral supplements are not necessary except for some breast-fed babies with dark skin or those with minimal exposure to sunlight who will require supplemental vitamin D at 10 μg per day. Iron supplements should be provided for all breast-fed infants at 4 to 6 months of age. Infants who are given prepared infant formulas fortified with iron require no additional iron supplement. One milligram of vitamin K is given to all babies at birth.

BREAST–FEEDING

It is now well established that human milk has significant benefits in addition to providing optimal nutrition. These include protection against upper respiratory tract and gastrointestinal infections, enhanced maturation of the gastrointestinal tract, a diminished risk of allergic reactions to cow milk proteins, and promotion of the psychological well-being of mother and infant. Parents should be encouraged to breast-feed, and health care providers should give adequate information to help them make an informed choice and, as well, support breast-feeding once it begins. In fact, the success of lactation depends in large part on the supportive attitude of professional personnel during prenatal visits as well as following delivery in the hospital. Because a short hospital stay may have a negative influence on nursing, information should be provided not only during the hospital stay but also following discharge. This requires availability by telephone of a physician, nurse, or breast-feeding instructor, an early home or office visit, and a visit within 14 days of discharge to answer questions and provide guidance in breast-feeding issues. Breast care advice should be provided, which includes avoiding soaps and alcohol, which may dry the breast. If there are very inverted nipples, then a shield placed inside the brassiere during the last months of pregnancy may help facilitate eversion of the nipples.

After delivery the mother should be offered the opportunity to nurse her infant as soon as possible. The infant is allowed to suckle at the first breast and then is repositioned on the second breast until the infant is satisfied and the breasts are emptied. Time to complete the suckling should be unrestricted, but generally it takes between 10 and 25 minutes. Infants will generally feed every 2 to 3 hours and by the end of the first week of life will urinate six times a day, passing a seedy yellow stool with each feeding over the next several months. The number of stools passed each day may decrease considerably by 2 to 3 months after birth.

Breast milk provides 67 to 70 kcal per dL with approximately 18 mEq per liter of sodium. The concentration of protein in breast milk decreases over a period of 2 weeks from approximately 3 grams per dL to 1.2 grams per dL, providing 7% to 8% of the total energy. Human milk differs from bovine milk in that the protein consists of 70% whey proteins and 30% casein; in bovine milk 82% of the protein is contributed by casein and 18% by whey proteins. Caseins are proteins with a low solubility in acid. The whey proteins remain in solution after acid precipitation. Thus, human milk provides lower concentrations of phenylalanine, tyrosine, and methionine and higher concentrations of taurine than cow milk. Fat provides 50% to 55% of the total energy of human milk and contains long-chain polyunsaturated fatty acids that are important in the development of central neural pathways. The remainder of the energy in milk is supplied by lactose.

Human milk contains a number of non-nutritive substances that are active in host defense and growth and maturation of the intestinal tract. These include secretory IgA, lactoferrin, lysozyme, oligosaccharides, and lymphocytes. The secretory antibodies in human milk reflect the mother's exposure to foreign antigens and, when transferred to the suckling infant, passively protect the infant against a variety of infectious diseases. This transfer of the mother's immune repertoire to her infant is also known as the enteromammary immune system. As a result of this, the incidence of gastrointestinal and respiratory diseases is decreased. There is also a marked decrease in the prevalence of necrotizing enterocolitis among breast-fed infants. It has not yet been definitively established that breast-feeding affects long-term health.

INFANT FORMULAS

The levels of nutrients in all infant formulas follow regulations established by the Food and Drug Administration. For many nutrients the minimal and maximal amounts are specified by FDA regulations that are similar to the recommendations of the Committee of Nutrition of the American Academy of Pediatrics. The Infant Formula Act of 1980 and its modifications of 1986 mandate quality control standards under which all infant formulas are manufactured. No single type of "milk-feeding" is suitable for all infants, and this is illustrated by the number of specialized formulas that have been developed to satisfy the requirements of infants with special needs. These include premature infants, infants with inherited metabolic deficiency disorders, infants with allergy to cow milk proteins, and infants with limitations of digestion or absorption.

Standard formulas for healthy infants are available in ready-to-use concentrated liquid and powdered forms. They contain cow milk proteins, which in some formulas have been adjusted to create a whey-predominant composition more similar to that of human milk. Lactose, vegetable oils, emulsifiers, and thickeners are added along with vitamins to complete the formula. The mineral content of these formulas is adjusted to suit the needs of human infants.

For those infants with intolerance to cow milk protein, soy formulas or formulas containing hydrolyzed proteins are useful. Goat milk has been used frequently for infants with cow milk intolerance. Goat milk is high in essential fatty acids and has a higher percentage of medium-chain triglycerides than standard infant formulas and cow milk. It is very low in folate. Its availability is limited, and infants who are truly allergic to cow milk are likely to be allergic to goat milk as well. For that reason the use of goat milk has diminished in favor of alternative commercially prepared infant formulas.

All formulas must contain a minimum of 1.5 mg per liter of iron. However, because of the substantial risks of iron deficiency, infants should be fed a formula fortified with higher levels of iron. Approximately 80% of infant formulas purchased today contain the higher levels of iron, which are considered iron-fortified formulas. The use of these formulas has led to a dramatic decrease in the prevalence of iron deficiency among infants in the United States.

SOLID FOODS

During the first 4 to 6 months of life, infants should be exclusively breast-fed if possible, or fed formula as an alternative. The introduction of solid foods begins at about 4 to 6 months of age when the infant has at least doubled the birthweight. At this time the infant should be able to sit with support and hold up its head, and be able to initiate sucking movements as the spoon touches the lips and then move the food to the back of the mouth for swallowing. Prior to the age of 4 months, a milk feeding can satisfy virtually all of the healthy infant's nutritional needs. After this time the need for extra calories and other nutrients increases and cannot be met by a single food. Infants should begin with a single-ingredient food and build to a variety of foods over the next 8 months. Thin pureed foods are introduced first, usually cereal, and then with continued physical development lumpier foods with more complex flavors can be introduced into the infant's diet. The introduction of egg white should be delayed until toward the end of the first year. With the introduction of solid foods, fats provide less of the total energy of the diet. During the second 6 months of life an infant generally receives between 30% and 40% of calories from fat. There should be no restrictions on the fat intake of infants and young children under the age of 2 years.

Whole cow milk should not be given during the first year of life. The mix of nutrients in cow milk is not optimal for the rapidly growing infant, with some nutrients such as calcium, phosphorus, protein, and sodium being present in concentrations too high and others such as zinc and iron in concentrations too low. The combination of human milk provided on demand or 16 to 32 ounces of infant formula per day along with solid foods provides a combination of nutrients that optimally support growth and development during infancy. Once whole cow milk is introduced, a full-fat milk should be provided, along with foods with a lumpy texture or soft foods cut into small pieces. This generally marks the end of the infancy period and transition into the toddler years.

DISEASES OF THE BREAST

method of
MONICA MORROW, M.D.
Northwestern University School of Medicine and
Northwestern Memorial Hospital
Chicago, Illinois

Breast cancer is the most common cancer in American women and the second most common cause of cancer death. It is estimated that in 1995 there were 46,240 new cases of breast cancer, and 46,000 deaths. In spite of this, the majority of breast complaints that bring women to physicians are due to benign breast disease or exaggerations of normal physiology. Benign disease is especially common in premenopausal women. The high level of breast cancer awareness among women makes the development of any breast problem a cause of extreme anxiety.

MANAGEMENT OF COMMON BREAST PROBLEMS

The most common breast complaints include pain, breast masses, nipple discharge, and an abnormal screening mammogram.

Breast Pain

Breast pain is an extremely common complaint but is a rare presenting symptom of breast cancer. Fewer than 10% of patients with cancer have pain as an associated symptom. In the past, breast pain was often dismissed as a sign of an unstable personality. However, a study comparing the incidence of psychoneurotic traits in women with breast pain and women with varicose veins identified no differences, and both groups scored significantly lower than female psychiatric outpatients.

The etiology of breast pain remains unclear but appears to be related to hormones, although no specific hormonal abnormalities have been identified. There are two common patterns of breast pain. Cyclic pain is the most frequent type; it usually consists of poorly localized pain that is often bilateral and frequently most severe in the upper outer quadrants of the breasts. The pain is described as heaviness, aching, and soreness and frequently radiates to the ipsilateral axilla and arm. Cyclic pain is typically maximal premenstrually and relieved with the onset of the menses, although pain of varying degree may persist throughout the cycle. The average age of women with cyclic mastalgia is 35 years. Cyclic mastalgia is characterized by a high rate of spontaneous remission.

Noncyclic mastalgia is unrelated to the menstrual cycle. It is more frequently unilateral and localized to a specific area than cyclic mastalgia, and it is often described as sharp, stabbing, or burning. Noncyclic mastalgia is most common in the fourth decade and is also seen after menopause.

A careful history detailing the character, location, intensity, and duration of breast pain is the first step in evaluation of the problem. Evidence of a relationship to the menstrual cycle should be sought, as well as a history of menstrual irregularity, emotional stress, or new medication, all of which have been reported to exacerbate mastalgia. A physical examination to exclude the presence of dominant breast masses should be done. Noncyclic breast pain may be due to benign breast lesions such as fibroadenoma, duct ectasia, or macrocysts. Breast pain due to these lesions responds well to excision of the fibroadenoma or ectatic ducts, or cyst aspiration. A mammogram is a routine part of the evaluation of women over 35 years of age with breast pain, but it is not indicated in younger women unless a dominant mass is present.

If the physical examination and mammogram fail to reveal evidence of breast neoplasia, the woman should be reassured that her pain is not due to a malignancy but is an exaggerated form of a normal physiologic process. In more than 90% of women, reassurance that mastalgia is not a sign of cancer and an explanation of its hormonal etiology is sufficient therapy. Women with breast pain should not be labeled as having "fibrocystic disease," since no histologic correlates of breast pain have been identified.

A variety of therapies have been proposed for breast pain, including caffeine restriction, diuretics, and vitamins B_6 and E. Randomized, placebo-controlled trials have not demonstrated a benefit for these treatments. The only drug approved by the Food and Drug Administration for the treatment of breast pain is the antigonadotropin danazol (Danocrine). However, the significant incidence of side effects (menstrual irregularity, acne, weight gain, hirsutism) makes this an unsatisfactory form of therapy for all but the most severe, activity-limiting breast pain.

Breast Masses

The determination of what constitutes a dominant mass is frequently difficult, particularly in the premenopausal woman. The normal glandular tissue of the breast is nodular, and this nodularity is usually most pronounced in the upper outer quadrant of the breast and the inframammary ridge area. Such nodularity, particularly when it waxes and wanes during the menstrual cycle, is a physiologic process and is not an indication of breast pathology. Dominant masses are characterized by their persistence throughout the menstrual cycle. They may be discreet or poorly defined, but they differ in character from the surrounding breast tissue and the corresponding area in the contralateral breast. The differential diagnosis of dominant breast masses includes macrocysts, fibroadenoma, prominent areas of fibrocystic change, fat necrosis, and carcinoma. If a dominant breast mass is palpated in a premenopausal woman, it should be aspirated to determine whether it is a cyst. Cysts are usually well demarcated from the surrounding breast tissue and are somewhat mobile and firm. Cysts that are very full are often quite hard and may be difficult to distinguish from solid masses by physical examination. Cysts require biopsy only if the aspirated fluid is bloody, the palpable abnormality does not resolve completely after the aspiration of fluid, or the same cyst recurs multiple times in a short time interval. The routine cytologic examination of cyst fluid is not indicated because of the low likelihood of carcinoma in the absence of the clinical findings just noted. In addition, the cytologic identification of atypical cells in cyst fluid is not uncommon, resulting in the clinical dilemma of a patient whose cyst resolves with aspiration, whose mammogram is normal, and who has a cytology report indicating the need for a biopsy.

Cysts may occur at any age but are particularly common in women in their forties and those who are perimenopausal. In postmenopausal women who are not taking exogenous estrogen, cysts are uncommon and should be regarded with a higher degree of suspicion than in the premenopausal years. Aspiration is still an appropriate first step, but a repeat examination 4 to 6 weeks postaspiration to check for recurrence of the cyst is essential. A dominant breast mass should not be dismissed as a cyst unless the diagnosis is documented by sonography or aspiration.

Noncystic masses in premenopausal women that are clearly different from the surrounding breast tissue require tissue sampling. Observation for one or two menstrual cycles is appropriate only for vague asymmetry or nodularity, when it is unclear that a dominant mass is present. A follow-up examination is also useful when the patient identifies a mass that the physician does not feel is clinically significant.

In postmenopausal women, clinical examination of the breasts is frequently easier due to atrophy of the nodular glandular elements. Benign breast problems causing palpable masses are less frequent in this age group and carcinoma is more common, so small areas of nodularity that might be observed in a premenopausal woman should be considered for prompt biopsy in a postmenopausal woman.

Mammography does not provide a diagnosis for palpable breast abnormalities. A mammogram should be obtained prior to a breast biopsy to evaluate the remainder of the breast tissue and define the extent of the palpable mass in case definitive cancer surgery is necessary. Between 15% and 20% of clinically evident breast cancers are not visualized on a mammogram, so a normal mammogram does not mean that a biopsy is not indicated.

Palpable breast masses may be diagnosed with fine needle aspiration (FNA) cytology, core-cutting needle biopsy, or excisional biopsy. A major controversy in the management of palpable breast masses is the attempt to avoid surgical biopsy by using physical examination, mammography, and FNA as a "triple test." If all three of these modalities indicate benign disease, reviews indicate that carcinoma is present in fewer than 4% of cases. However, for these statistics to apply, all elements of the triple test must be evaluable, and observation of lesions that are not seen on mammogram or those with cytologic aspirates insufficient for diagnosis is inappropriate. In addition, the accuracy of a clinical or mammographic diagnosis of a benign lesion is lowest in young women, the group in whom biopsy is most likely to be omitted. If a dominant mass is to be observed, a defined follow-up plan must be established to allow for the early detection of missed cancers. This approach should be employed only by clinicians experienced in the clinical evaluation of breast masses, and patients must be advised of the small, but real, risk that the diagnosis of cancer may be delayed. The management of the dominant breast mass is summarized in Figure 1.

Nipple Discharge

Nipple discharge is a common complaint but an uncommon sign of breast carcinoma. Three percent to 11% of women with carcinoma will have an associated nipple discharge. The likelihood of a nipple discharge being secondary to malignancy increases as patient age increases. In one study, 32% of women over age 60 years presenting with nipple discharge and no mass had carcinoma, compared with 7% of women under age 60 years with the same presenta-

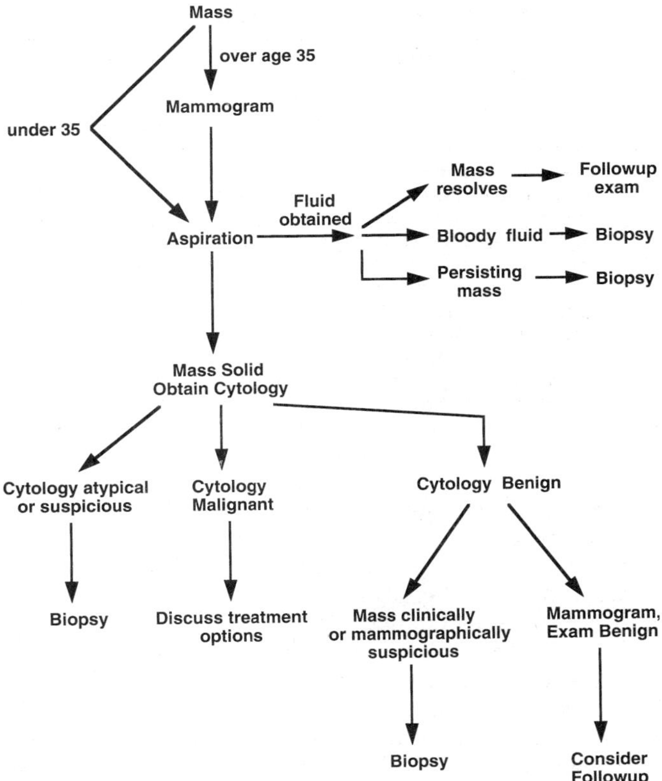

Figure 1. Management of dominant breast masses.

tion. The initial step in the evaluation of nipple discharge is to determine whether it is physiologic or pathologic. Discharges are classified as pathologic if they are spontaneous and localized to one duct. Pathologic discharges may be bloody or serous and are almost always unilateral. In contrast, physiologic discharges occur only with nipple compression, frequently originate from multiple ducts, and are often bilateral. This type of discharge may be clear, yellow, white, or dark green. If a physiologic discharge is present, a careful breast examination and a mammogram (in women over 35 years) should be obtained to exclude the presence of coexisting abnormalities. If these studies are normal, reassurance is the only therapy that is necessary. The clinical evaluation of a pathologic discharge should include testing the fluid for occult blood and identifying the quadrant of the breast from which the discharge originates. Although most discharges due to carcinoma contain blood, a nonbloody discharge that meets the other criteria of a pathologic discharge is an indication for a breast biopsy. Cytology is not usually useful in the evaluation of nipple discharge since the absence of malignant cells does not reliably exclude carcinoma, and a positive cytology result will not differentiate between intraductal and invasive carcinoma.

As part of the evaluation of a pathologic discharge, a mammogram should be obtained to look for nonpalpable masses, calcifications, or dilated ducts. When a discharge occurs in association with a mass, the mass should be biopsied. In the absence of a mass, a termi-

nal duct excision should be performed. The role of galactography in the management of nipple discharge is controversial.

Galactography may be useful in identifying lesions in the periphery of the breast that would not be removed with a standard terminal duct excision, or in minimizing the amount of the ductal system that is removed in women of childbearing age. However, galactography does not provide a definitive diagnosis for intraductal lesions and does not obviate the need for histologic sampling in women with pathologic discharges.

The Abnormal Screening Mammogram

Randomized trials have demonstrated that regular mammographic screening reduces breast cancer mortality by approximately 30%. The benefits of screening women age 50 years and older are clear. Controversy remains regarding whether screening is beneficial in women between the ages of 40 and 50 years. No single trial has shown a survival benefit in this age group, but a meta-analysis suggests that breast cancer mortality is reduced. When women under 50 years of age are screened, mammograms should be obtained annually. The major drawback to the use of routine screening mammography is the cost of surgical consultation and biopsy for the many subclinical, benign abnormalities that are identified. Mammography is a sensitive but nonspecific test, and only 30% of the mammographically generated biopsies reveal carcinoma. A complete radiologic evaluation prior to surgical referral will avoid many benign biopsies. The use of spot compression and magnification views and ultrasound will demonstrate that as many as 50% of equivocal abnormalities identified on a two-view screening mammogram are benign and do not require biopsy. The American College of Radiology has developed a standardized reporting terminology in which mammograms are classified into five groups (Table 1). A careful physical examination to ensure that no palpable abnormality is present is particularly important for lesions in categories 3 and 4, in which the presence of an associated clinical abnormality would be an indication for biopsy.

TABLE 1. **Classification of Mammographic Abnormalities by the American College of Radiology Breast Imaging Reporting and Data System (BIRADS)**

Category	Definition
1	Negative mammogram
2	Benign findings not suspicious for malignancy (ex-calcified fibroadenoma)
3	Probably benign finding. Short interval follow-up to ensure stability
4	Indeterminate abnormality. Biopsy should be considered. Includes lesions with risks of cancer ranging from 2% to 50%
5	Lesion suggestive of cancer that requires a biopsy

BIRADS = Breast Imaging Reporting and Data System (2nd ed, 1995).

In the past, the only available technique for the diagnosis of nonpalpable abnormalities was an excisional biopsy after needle localization. Imaging-guided percutaneous core biopsies, using either ultrasound or stereotaxis to localize nonpalpable lesions, are now available as an alternative to surgical excision. The core techniques appear to be more accurate for the diagnosis of mass lesions than of calcifications. Core biopsies are an ideal technique for the diagnosis of low-to-intermediate suspicion of mammographic abnormalities (BIRADS Category 4), resulting in cost savings by avoiding surgery while still allowing the early detection of cancers. The role of core biopsy in the management of highly suspicious mammographic abnormalities is less clear, since these lesions should be removed whether the biopsy is positive or negative. The successful application of a program of core biopsy is dependent on close cooperation between radiologists, surgeons, and pathologists.

RISK ASSESSMENT

Although many factors that influence the risk of breast cancer development have been identified, there is little consensus as to what constitutes a "high-risk" woman. The designation of a woman as high risk causes considerable anxiety for both the patient and her physician, and this concern may result in unnecessary physican visits, frequent mammography, and an excessive number of breast biopsies. The most common breast cancer risk factor is age. As shown in Table 2, half of a woman's risk of developing breast cancer occurs after the age of 65 years.

A family history of breast cancer is probably the most commonly recognized risk factor. It is now evident that there are two very different types of risk associated with a family history of breast cancer. Approximately 5% to 10% of breast cancer cases in this country are due to the inheritance of an abnormal gene from either maternal or paternal relatives. Genetically transmitted breast cancer should be suspected in women with multiple relatives with the disease, particularly at young ages, or when a history of breast and ovarian cancer is present. Mutations of the BRCA1, BRCA2, and P53 tumor suppressor gene have been shown to result in an 85% lifetime risk

TABLE 3. **Breast Cancer Risk Factors**

Factor	Relative Risk
Family History	
Mother or sister with breast cancer	1.2–3.0
Premenopausal	3.1
Postmenopausal	1.5
Premenopausal, bilateral	8.5–9.0
Hormonal	
Age at menarche <12	1.3
Nulliparity	1.5–3.0
First live birth after age 35	2.0–3.0
Age at menopause >55 yr	1.5–2.0
Benign Breast Disease	
Proliferative disease	1.5–2.0
Atypical hyperplasia	4.0–5.0
Lobular carcinoma in situ	6.9–12.0

of breast cancer development, and it is likely that additional genes will be identified in the future. In the absence of a genetic predisposition for breast cancer, the risk of cancer development is much lower, and rarely exceeds 30%.

Other factors that increase the risk of breast cancer development are summarized in Table 3. A major problem with risk evaluation has been the lack of knowledge of the interactions among risk factors. Gail and colleagues have developed a model that incorporates age at menarche, age at first live birth, number of first-degree relatives with breast cancer, and number of previous breast biopsies to provide an individualized risk estimate at different ages over a defined time interval. This model has been tested in two populations and found to be generally accurate for women undergoing regular mammographic screening. It is not a useful model for women with a strong family history of breast cancer, since it includes only first-degree relatives.

It is important to remember that the risk under discussion is the risk of breast cancer development. The risk of breast cancer death is approximately one third of the risk of developing the disease (see Table 2), and this must be pointed out to the patient. At present, the only available method of breast cancer prevention is the prophylactic mastectomy. Even bilateral prophylactic mastectomy does not provide 100% protection, although the precise risk of cancer development after the procedure is not known. The antiestrogen tamoxifen (Nolvadex)* is under study as a breast cancer preventive, but there is no indication for its use outside of a clinical trial at present.

DIAGNOSIS AND THERAPY OF BREAST CARCINOMA

Diagnosis and Staging

Breast carcinoma can be diagnosed by fine needle aspiration (FNA), core-cutting needle biopsy, or outpatient excisional biopsy. FNA and core biopsies have the advantage of being outpatient procedures that

TABLE 2. **Risk of Developing and Dying of Breast Cancer by Age**

Age *(years)*	Risk of Breast Cancer Development (%)	Risk of Breast Cancer Death (%)
20–40	0.49	0.09
35–55	2.53	0.56
50–70	4.67	1.04
65–85	5.48	1.01

Modified from Bilimoria M, Morrow M: The women at increased risk for breast cancer: Evaluation and management strategies. CA Cancer J Clin 45:263–278, 1995.

*Not FDA-approved for this indication.

are low cost and relatively painless. They allow a diagnosis of breast cancer without an incision on the breast, which maximizes the cosmetic outcome of definitive surgical therapy. Excisional biopsy allows a complete evaluation of the tumor size and its histologic characteristics before selecting a definitive local therapy. If a small margin of normal breast tissue is removed as part of the excisional biopsy, the procedure will often serve as the definitive lumpectomy.

A prebiopsy mammogram will allow evaluation of the index breast for breast-conserving therapy if cancer is identified. In addition, clinically occult contralateral carcinoma is detected mammographically in approximately 2.5% of patients.

The likelihood of identifying metastases in the asymptomatic patient is greatly influenced by the clinical stage of disease. The staging of breast cancer is described in Table 4. No metastatic work-up is needed for women with ductal carcinoma in situ. For asymptomatic patients with Stage 1 and 2 cancer, bone scans reveal disease in fewer than 5% of cases and are not indicated. The incidence of occult bony metastases in Stage 3 disease is considerably higher (approximately 20%), making bone scanning a worthwhile procedure. Liver imaging should be reserved for women with abnormal liver chemistries, hepatomegaly, or significant weight loss suggesting hepatic metastases. Serum tumor markers have not been shown to be useful preoperative tests in women with breast cancer. For the woman with Stages 1 and 2 breast cancer, bilateral mammography, a chest roentgenogram, a complete blood count, and liver chemistries are the only preoperative tests required.

TABLE 4. **Staging of Breast Cancer**

T_1	Tumor 2 cm or less
T_{1a}	0.5 cm or less
T_{1b}	>0.5 cm to 1 cm
T_{1c}	>1.0 cm to 2 cm
T_2	Tumor >2 cm to 5 cm
T_3	Tumor >5 cm
T_4	Tumor of any size involving chest wall or skin
N_0	No axillary nodal metastases
N_1	Metastasis to moveable ipsilateral axillary lymph nodes
N_2	Metastasis to ipsilateral axillary lymph nodes fixed to one another or to other structures
N_3	Metastases to ipsilateral internal mammary nodes
M_0	No distant metastasis
M_1	Distant metastasis (includes supraclavicular nodes)
Stage I	$T_1 \, N_0 \, M_0$
Stage IIA	$T_0 \, N_1 \, M_0$
	$T_1 \, N_1 \, M_0$
	$T_2 \, N_0 \, M_0$
Stage IIB	$T_2 \, N_1 \, M_0$
	$T_3 \, N_0 \, M_0$
Stage IIIA	$T_3 \, N_1 \, M_0$
	$T_0{-}T_3 \, N_2 \, M_0$
Stage IIIB	$T_4 \,$ any N $\, M_0$
	Any T $N_3 \, M_0$
Stage IV	Any T Any N M_1

NONINVASIVE BREAST CANCER

Lobular Carcinoma in Situ

Lobular carcinoma in situ (LCIS) is an incidental microscopic finding that cannot be identified clinically or by gross pathologic examination. LCIS is found in 0.8% to 8% of breast biopsies, and the frequency with which it is diagnosed appears to be increasing. LCIS was first described in 1941 as the anatomic precursor of invasive carcinoma. Subsequent information strongly suggests that LCIS is a risk factor for the development of breast cancer rather than a premalignant lesion.

Lobular carcinoma in situ is a disease of premenopausal women. It is usually multicentric and frequently bilateral. The risk of subsequent breast cancer development after a diagnosis of LCIS, approximately 1% per year, seems to persist indefinitely. However, subsequent carcinomas are equally distributed between the index and the contralateral breast, even when the LCIS is unilateral. Recognition of this fact has eliminated the use of mirror image biopsies in most centers. The amount of LCIS is not predictive of the risk of development of cancer, and infiltrating ductal carcinomas are the most common tumor type observed. The foregoing information suggests that most women with LCIS will not develop breast cancer, and that the risk of breast cancer development is equal in both breasts.

There are two options available for the women with LCIS. The first is careful observation, as would be carried out for any woman known to be at increased risk for breast cancer. In women unwilling to accept the risk of breast cancer development associated with this policy, prophylactic bilateral simple mastectomies, usually with immediate breast reconstruction, are another option. Radiotherapy has no role in the management of LCIS. It is unnecessary to obtain negative histologic margins in women who will be followed expectantly, since LCIS is known to be a diffuse lesion. To date efforts to identify features of LCIS associated with a higher likelihood of the development of malignancy have been unsuccessful.

Ductal Carcinoma in Situ

In contrast to LCIS, ductal carcinoma in situ (DCIS) has a variety of both clinical and mammographic presentations. Clinically, DCIS may present as a palpable mass, nipple discharge, or Paget's disease of the nipple. Microcalcifications are the most common mammographic presentation of DCIS, although mammographic masses may also be pure DCIS. The increased use of screening mammography has resulted in a dramatic increase in the number of cases of DCIS treated annually, and DCIS accounts for 30% to 50% of mammographically detected cancers in many reports.

In the past, mastectomy was the standard treatment for DCIS, and it was curative in 98% of cases. The increasing use of breast-conserving approaches for the treatment of invasive breast cancer, the increasingly frequent identification of microscopic DCIS by mammography, and the recognition that not all DCIS is an obligate precursor of invasive carcinoma have resulted in attempts to treat DCIS with excision alone or excision and radiotherapy. Current data on treatment with excision and radiotherapy indicate that 10% to 15% of patients will have breast cancer recurrences at 10 years. Half the recurrences are invasive carcinoma, resulting in a risk of death due to breast cancer in the 10-year interval of about 2% to 3%. In general, patients treated with excision alone have higher breast recurrence rates than patients treated with excision and irradiation, although the pattern of failure is unchanged (i.e., one half are invasive carcinoma). Some evidence indicates that when patients selected on the basis of small tumor size and low nuclear grade, using detailed mammographic and pathologic evaluation, are treated with excision alone, local failure rates are comparable to those seen with excision and irradiation. Definitive treatment recommendations for DCIS await improvements in our understanding of the natural history of the disease. Excision and irradiation is an appropriate option for the majority of patients with localized DCIS, regardless of grade or histologic type. Patients with extensive disease that cannot be encompassed by wide excision require mastectomy. Excision alone may be considered for very small, low-grade lesions, but careful lifetime follow-up is necessary, since the natural history of low-grade DCIS may be quite prolonged.

INVASIVE CARCINOMA, STAGES I AND II

The surgical therapy of invasive breast carcinoma changed dramatically in the past 20 years as our understanding of the biology of breast cancer has evolved. Current therapeutic options include modified radical mastectomy; breast-conserving therapy (BCT) consisting of lumpectomy, axillary dissection, and breast irradiation; and modified radical mastectomy with immediate reconstruction. Multiple prospective randomized trials have demonstrated no differences in survival for women with Stages 1 and 2 breast cancer treated by mastectomy and those treated with BCT.

The role of the physician is to identify contraindications to the various types of local therapy and to inform the patient of the risks and benefits of each of the treatments. Standard contraindications to BCT have been developed by a multidisciplinary group of surgeons, radiation oncologists, radiologists, and pathologists. Absolute contraindications to BCT are listed in Table 5. Relative contraindications include a large tumor-to-breast ratio, which precludes a cosmetically satisfactory excision, and the presence of collagen vascular diseases (especially scleroderma), which may be associated with severe reactions to radiation. The incidence of contraindications to BCT varies with tumor stage. BCT is feasible in

TABLE 5. **Contraindications to Breast-Conserving Therapy**

First- or second-trimester pregnancy
History of prior irradiation to breast region
Multiple gross tumors in separate quadrants of the breast
Diffuse indeterminate or suspicious microcalcifications

approximately 90% of patients with Stage 1 cancer and 75% of patients with Stage 2 cancer.

In performing a lumpectomy, the surgeon seeks to achieve a balance between a low incidence of breast cancer recurrence and a good cosmetic outcome. Routine resections of very large amounts of breast tissue (quadrantectomy) result in the lowest rates of local failure, but produce significant distortions in the appearance of the breast. The extent of surgical resection can be tailored for the individual patient by careful evaluation of the mammographic extent of tumor and knowledge of histologic tumor type. Patients with extensive intraductal carcinoma in association with invasive tumor, and those with infiltrating lobular carcinoma or mammographic evidence of multifocality, will often require wider resections to achieve negative margins. For the remainder, removal of a limited amount of breast tissue, with wider excision reserved for patients with positive margins after a conservative excision, is sufficient. Approximately 90% of patients treated with BCT rate their cosmetic outcome as excellent or good. The edema seen after BCT may require 1 to 2 years to resolve, and retraction develops slowly, but by 3 years the cosmetic appearance of the breast is stable.

A subgroup of patients who do not require radiotherapy after lumpectomy has not yet been identified. Four prospective randomized trials comparing excision alone to excision plus irradiation demonstrate a 75% to 98% reduction in the risk of breast recurrence in the irradiated group. At present, radiotherapy should be considered a standard part of BCT. Local recurrence in the breast occurs in about 8% of patients treated with BCT at 10 years, and the standard treatment of recurrence is completion mastectomy.

Breast Reconstruction After Mastectomy

Reconstruction may be done at the time of mastectomy or as a secondary procedure, but the possibility should be discussed prior to definitive surgery. The only true contraindication to immediate reconstruction is the presence of significant co-morbid conditions that would interfere with the patient's ability to tolerate a longer operative procedure. The patient's age, the need for adjuvant chemotherapy, and poor prognosis are not contraindications to reconstruction. Retrospective studies have shown that breast reconstruction does not impair the detection of local recurrence or increase its incidence. No delay in the time to initiating adjuvant chemotherapy has been noted in several studies of women undergoing immediate reconstruction. The advantages of immediate reconstruction include avoidance of an additional operative procedure, decreased psychological trauma, and improved coordination of the efforts of the oncologic and reconstructive surgeons to produce an optimal cosmetic result without compromising cancer care.

Reconstruction may be accomplished with implants, filled with either saline or silicone gel, or with myocutaneous flaps. The availability of adequate skin coverage, the size and shape of the patient's contralateral breast, the patient's cosmetic expectations, and the amount of surgery she is willing to undergo influence the choice of reconstuctive technique.

Adjuvant Systemic Therapy

The recognition that a substantial number of women with breast cancer are not cured by local therapy has resulted in the widespread use of chemotherapy and hormonal therapy in an effort to reduce the incidence of distant metastases. The effects of systemic therapy have been shown to be similar for both node-positive and node-negative breast cancer patients. A meta-analysis of 11,000 women receiving multidrug chemotherapy in randomized trials has demonstrated a 28% reduction in the risk of breast cancer death for women receiving chemotherapy. The antiestrogen tamoxifen reduces the risk of breast cancer death by 17%, with greater benefits seen with longer durations of therapy (24% reduction in risk when given for more than 2 years). The absolute benefit that a patient will receive from systemic therapy is dependent on her risk of breast cancer recurrence and death. For example, the patient with multiple positive axillary nodes who has a 60% risk of metastases will have her risk reduced by about one third, to 40%, with systemic treatment. The patient with a 1-cm cancer with negative nodes has only a 10% risk of relapse and will have only a 3% absolute benefit from the same treatment. Current recommendations for systemic therapy include the use of chemotherapy for node-positive premenopausal women, regardless of estrogen receptor status, and for node-positive postmenopausal women who are hormone receptor–negative. For node-positive postmenopausal women who are hormone receptor–positive, tamoxifen is the standard of therapy. The benefits of the combination of tamoxifen and chemotherapy in pre- and postmenopausal receptor-positive women are under study. The decision to use systemic therapy in node-negative women is based on an assessment of the risk of failure. Premenopausal high-risk patients (usually those with larger, high-grade tumors) receive chemotherapy, as do receptor-negative postmenopausal patients. Tamoxifen is used for good-risk, receptor-positive premenopausal women, and receptor-positive postmenopausal women in both good- and high-risk categories. In general, patients with a very low risk of relapse (tumors less than 1 cm in size) do not receive systemic treatment.

Locally Advanced Breast Cancer

The designation locally advanced breast cancer (LABC) encompasses a heterogeneous group of tumors that corresponds to Stage 3 as defined by the American Joint Cancer Committee (AJCC) staging system. Approximately 10% to 15% of breast cancer patients present with Stage 3 disease. The biologic diversity seen in this group makes the formation of a single treatment recommendation difficult. The goals of therapy for women with LABC are to maintain local control on the chest wall and to prolong survival.

In women with stage IIIA disease on the basis of large primary tumor size alone, modified radical mastectomy, followed by systemic adjuvant therapy, and irradiation of the chest wall and nodal areas are often the treatments of choice. In the presence of skin edema, ulceration, chest wall fixation, skin satellites, inflammatory carcinoma, or fixed axillary nodes, surgical resection as an initial therapeutic step is contraindicated. At most institutions a combined modality approach consisting of induction chemotherapy, mastectomy, radiotherapy, and further chemotherapy is employed. This approach has the potential benefits of prompt treatment of presumed systemic disease, reduction of the tumor burden before definitive local therapy, and the use of the response of the primary tumor as an in vivo chemosensitivity assay. Clinical response rates of 70% to 90% are reported after induction therapy, and pathologic complete remissions are seen in 5% to 10% of cases. In spite of this, high rates of systemic failure are still seen.

ENDOMETRIOSIS
method of
G. DAVID ADAMSON, M.D.
Fertility Physicians of Northern California
Palo Alto, California

Endometriosis is an enigmatic disease affecting about 7% of women of reproductive age—approximately 5 million Americans. Most of these women do not know that they have endometriosis, although many suffer significant symptoms ranging from pelvic pain to infertility. Because our understanding of the clinical presentation, diagnosis, and management of endometriosis has improved dramatically in the past few years, physicians can now provide better care for patients who suffer from this potentially debilitating disease.

DEFINITION

Endometriosis is the presence of endometrial tissue, consisting of endometrial glands and stroma, in ectopic locations. This tissue reacts to estrogen and progesterone. The usual location is in the pelvis, but endometriosis has also been found in omentum, small intestine, appendix, anterior abdominal wall, surgical scars, diaphragm, lung, urinary tract, and musculoskeletal and neural systems. The tissue can be very diverse histologically and can appear to be proliferative, secretory, or menstrual.

PREVALENCE AND INCIDENCE

The prevalence and incidence of endometriosis depend on the population of women being studied. The range is 1 to 50%, depending on the surgical series. It has been reported to occur in 10 to 15% of women undergoing diagnostic laparoscopy, 2 to 5% of women undergoing tubal sterilization, 30 to 40% of infertile women having laparoscopy, and 14 to 53% of women with pelvic pain.

PATHOPHYSIOLOGY

There are several theories about the pathogenesis of endometriosis, the most popular being retrograde menstruation through the fallopian tubes, metaplasia, activation of embryonic rests of müllerian tissue, hematogenous and lymphatic spread, or direct placement in wounds. Each of these and other possible etiologies may contribute variably to endometriosis in different patients. Altered immunity may also play a role. There are numerous factors that appear to affect whether a woman has this disease, the severity of the disease, symptoms, and response to treatment. These factors include genetics (an affected sister or mother doubles the risk), hormonal status (higher estrogen levels and prolonged heavy menses increase risk), lifestyle (low weight and smoking reduce risk by decreasing estrogen levels), contraceptive use (oral contraceptives possibly reduce progression of disease), obstetric history (pregnancy and lactation reduce risk), anatomic factors (cervical stenosis increases risk), treatment history (prior medical or surgical treatment reduces risk), race, and possibly exposure to environmental toxins, especially those that are estrogenic.

Endometriosis is thought to cause reproductive dysfunction by resulting in cyclic bleeding at the time of menses, which leads to an inflammatory reaction, fibrosis, and adhesions. This may cause distorted anatomy, endocrinopathies, altered pelvic physicochemical milieu, abnormally functioning immune system, interference with sperm function, and possibly an altered process of embryo implantation. Although there is almost certainly an association between endometriosis and infertility, a cause-effect relationship has been established only for moderate and severe conditions involving endometriomas, adhesions, and invasive disease.

CLINICAL PRESENTATION

Endometriosis presents primarily as pelvic pain in about 50% of patients, infertility in about 25%, pain and infertility in about 25%, and ovarian endometrioma in less than 5% of cases. There is also a large incidence of asymptomatic disease, from 1 to 40%. Endometriosis may occur anytime after puberty, including adolescence.

Pain symptoms of endometriosis often do not correlate well with severity of disease. Pain may occur as a result of secretion of irritating factors (e.g., histamine), adhesions that cause scarring or retraction, leaking endometriomas, compression of other visceral structures (e.g., bowel), compression of uterosacral nodules, and/or invasion of the urinary or gastrointestinal tract. Endometriosis may also be associated with intraluminal fallopian tube pathology. Studies overall do not support an association between endometriosis and increased spontaneous abortion rates.

Endometriosis lesions occur throughout the pelvis. They tend to be more common in the posterior cul-de-sac and the ovary than in the fallopian tubes. Endometriosis is almost certainly a progressive disease, but the rate of progression and the nature of lesions vary from patient to patient.

Adhesions develop as a result of the inflammatory process caused by long-standing endometriosis, with more extensive and dense adhesions developing over time. Complete cul-de-sac obliteration can result from long-standing invasive and adhesive disease.

DIAGNOSIS OF ENDOMETRIOSIS

The diagnosis of endometriosis is suggested by several symptoms, including dysmenorrhea, dyspareunia (especially with aching following coitus), dyschezia, dysuria, mittelschmerz, or focal or generalized pelvic pain. Hematuria and hematochezia may also be symptoms of endometriosis. About 30% of patients with endometriosis do not have any pain. Signs of endometriosis include tenderness or nodularity in the posterior cul-de-sac, especially on the uterosacral ligaments; anterior cul-de-sac nodularity; adnexal masses from endometriomas; and reduced mobility or fixation of the pelvis due to pelvic adhesions. The location of tenderness often corresponds to the location of the pain. Pelvic examination should be performed at the time of menses, because disease is more easily identified.

Ultrasonography may assist in the diagnosis of endometriosis by evaluating the adnexa for endometriomas and the uterus for myomas or adenomyosis. CA 125 is occasionally helpful for following the course of endometriosis after diagnosis and treatment, but the high false-positive and false-negative rates give it little utility in the initial diagnostic work-up.

Currently, the only definitive test for pelvic endometriosis is diagnostic laparoscopy. Biopsy of lesions is sometimes necessary to confirm the diagnosis of endometriosis and should always be performed if the surgeon is uncertain. Preoperative consultation with a gastroenterologist, urologist, general surgeon, or other specialist, as indicated, should be scheduled to ensure that laparoscopy produces maximal benefits for the patient.

The differential diagnosis includes pelvic inflammatory disease, ectopic pregnancy, adenomyosis, myoma, benign ovarian tumor, malignant ovarian tumor (rare), pelvic pain of undetermined etiology, and normal pelvis. It should be emphasized to patients that diagnosis requires laparoscopy but that endometriosis is not always found at laparoscopy, even when it has been suggested by the history, physical examination, and preoperative testing. The degree of pain frequently does not correlate with the extent of disease.

It has been estimated that the diagnosis of endometriosis is missed in more than 7% of patients, and the extent of disease is underestimated in as many as 50% of patients. Subtle lesions can be missed even by experienced laparoscopists. Other lesions such as old sutures, ovarian cancer, carbon deposits from prior laser surgery, and hemangiomas may look like endometriosis. The surgeon must recognize the classic powder burn or blueberry lesion; white scar tissue that may be older, less endocrinologically active disease; clear or slightly brown-colored papillary lesions; or strawberry or flamelike lesions of recently developed, highly active endometriosis. Peritoneal pockets may also be associated with endometriosis.

Indications for Laparoscopy

Indications for laparoscopy to diagnose endometriosis include infertility of more than 1 year duration without other symptoms, or possibly after 6 months if the patient has symptoms or is older than 35. Evaluation for other female factors and sperm quality should be performed before laparoscopy. Patients with pelvic pain that has not responded after 3 months of nonsteroidal anti-inflammatory drugs (NSAIDs) and/or 3 months of oral contraceptives are candidates for laparoscopy. A patient with an adnexal mass suspected of being an endometrioma should have laparoscopy if the lesion does not resolve by 3 months; laparoscopy should be performed sooner if there are concomitant symptoms such as pain or other factors that make surgery appropriate.

Contraindications

Contraindications to surgery include multiple repeat operations at short intervals to treat lesions. If appropriate surgery is performed, it is uncommon for endometriotic lesions to recur within a few months. Repeat surgery for adhesiolysis is indicated in selected patients, usually those with infertility. Repeat surgery is occasionally indicated after 1 to 2 years if symptoms recur and are not treatable with medical therapy. Laparoscopy may be repeated to perform gamete intrafallopian transfer (GIFT) in selected patients. Surgery should not be performed in patients with unacceptably high medical or surgical risks. Laparoscopy should not be performed in patients at high risk for bowel injury unless an open technique or a technique designed to avoid bowel injury is utilized. Laparotomy is an appropriate approach for many surgeons when laparoscopy is too hazardous or the surgeon does not have the requisite skills or facilities to perform operative laparoscopy.

MANAGEMENT OPTIONS

Managing a patient with endometriosis requires an evaluation of her reproductive goals. She may be a teenager desiring future pregnancy, a woman planning immediate pregnancy, or a woman who has completed her childbearing or does not desire future pregnancy. Patients may present with undiagnosed pelvic pain or pain associated with recurrence of endometriosis after prior treatment. The objectives of therapy are to remove or destroy implants, relieve symptoms, maintain or restore fertility, and avoid or delay recurrence of the disease. Several management options are available.

No Treatment. This includes expectant management and/or limited use of analgesics and NSAIDs. These may be especially helpful for women with dysmenorrhea associated with endometriosis.

Medical Treatment. Medical therapy can consist of oral contraceptives, progestins, danazol, or gonadotropin-releasing hormone (GnRH) agonists. Oral contraceptives can be given cyclically. Treatment lasts 3 to 6 months. Progestins (Provera 30 mg every day) alone suppress gonadotropin secretion and ovarian function but can be associated with breakthrough bleeding, mastalgia, bloating, weight gain, and depression. They may be useful in a few women who cannot tolerate oral contraceptives. Treatment is relatively inexpensive.

Danazol (Danocrine 200 to 400 mg twice a day) is an ethisterone derivative that functions primarily by suppressing follicle-stimulating hormone (FSH) and luteinizing hormone (LH) from the pituitary gland, thereby creating a hypoestrogenic state. However, danazol is also associated with androgenic side effects, including weight gain, vasomotor instability (hot flashes), muscle cramps, acne, edema, hirsutism, reduced breast size, vaginitis, and sweating. It is contraindicated during pregnancy and lactation and in women with undiagnosed abnormal genital bleeding or markedly impaired hepatic, renal, or cardiac function. These pharmacologic effects are reversed within 2 months of discontinuing treatment.

GnRH agonists are synthetic decapeptides. Nafarelin acetate (Synarel 200 μg nasal spray used twice a day) is a superactive, hydrophobic stimulatory analogue of GnRH that is 200 times more potent than naturally occurring GnRH and is delivered in a metered nasal spray pump. Leuprolide acetate (Lupron Depot) is usually given as a monthly 3.75-mg intramuscular injection. The GnRH agonists result in an initial stimulation of the pituitary gland, with release of FSH and LH and a consequent increase in serum estradiol levels to approximately 100 pg per mL. However, continued use of GnRH agonists leads to down-regulation and desensitization of the pituitary gland after 7 to 14 days and the inability to release FSH and LH. This produces hypoestrogenemia (estradiol less than 40 pg per mL) and resultant amenorrhea, which permits regression of endometriosis and relief of symptoms. The GnRH agonists do not have any known direct effects on the ovary. Treatment costs approximately $2000 for 6 months.

Side effects include hot flashes in about 90% of patients, decreased libido, vaginal dryness, headache, emotional lability, and insomnia. Cardiovascular and liver enzyme parameters showed favorable changes relative to danazol. The major concern with GnRH agonists is the loss of bone density, about 3 to 8%, which occurs over 6 months of drug therapy; a 2 to 3% loss persists about 1 year following treatment. The consensus of the Food and Drug Administration (FDA) and others is that this is not clinically significant in women who have no evidence of bone disease, and it is generally not necessary to perform an evaluation of bone density prior to initiating treatment. However, only one 6-month course of GnRH agonist is FDA-approved and recommended. Subsequent symptoms may be treated with oral contraceptives, danazol, and/or surgery. In selected patients, repeat GnRH agonist treatment for 3 to 6 months may be indicated if dual photon absorptiometry bone density is normal and the patient is fully informed of the risks.

Hot flashes can be effectively managed with norethindrone (Micronor) 3.5 mg per day. Higher doses of norethindrone may provide some protection against bone loss but have an unfavorable side-effect profile for liver and cardiovascular systems, and patients are often very symptomatic. Low doses of estrogen (Premarin 0.6 mg per day) have also been used as "add-back" therapy to reduce bone loss and show some promise. More recently, add-back therapy for 6 to 12 months with norethindrone 2.5 mg and alendronate 10 mg per day has been suggested, along with calcium 1000 mg per day. However, the long-term efficacy of such add-back therapy and its effect on the therapeutic efficacy of GnRH agonists are still being evaluated.

Surgical Treatment. Diagnostic laparoscopy provides a relatively safe and simple method of diagnosing endometriosis. When appropriate, operative laparoscopy enables treatment to be initiated and possibly completed at the same time. Surgical therapy is usually conservative, consisting of excision, laser vaporization, or electrosurgical fulguration of endometriosis. Adjunctive procedures such as salpingo-ovariolysis may also be performed. Occasionally, additional procedures for pain are indicated, including uterosacral nerve ablation; for severe midline dysmenorrhea, presacral neurectomy may be indicated. In cases of advanced disease, radical surgery comprising hysterectomy and/or bilateral salpingo-oophorectomy may be required. Laparoscopic treatment of endometriosis requires a surgeon who is familiar with the pathophysiology of endometriosis and can integrate this knowledge with surgical judgment and technique.

Medical and surgical treatment modalities sometimes have the same results, but surgical treatment completed at the time of diagnosis has a distinct advantage over medical therapy because of decreased time, cost, and side effects. The patient can also be spared a second operation (laparotomy) if operative laparoscopy can be performed at the time of diagnosis. Operative laparoscopy offers several advantages over laparotomy, primarily because of better visualization, less tissue trauma, and a much shorter recovery time. However, tactile sense is less than that which can be obtained digitally at laparotomy. It is important to give the patient the best operation possible in the particular surgeon's hands and not to compromise by performing a poor operation at laparoscopy.

Combined Treatments. Laparoscopic treatment of endometriosis can sometimes be combined with medical therapy involving danazol or GnRH agonists. The purpose of combined treatment is to improve treatment success or facilitate surgical procedures. Preoperative medical treatment suppresses ovulation so that functional cysts are not present or confused with endometriosis. Metastatic or extensive superficial disease is suppressed and becomes atrophic. The reduced vascularity in the pelvis may result in reduced inflammation and postoperative adhesions, although this has not been proved. There may be a slight reduction in endometrioma size. Other uses of GnRH agonists prior to surgery include reduction of symptoms, increased time for adequate preoperative evaluation, easier scheduling of surgery, and even delay or avoidance of surgery for a woman nearing menopause. Potential disadvantages of preoperative medical treatment include the changed appearance of endometriosis, which might make it more difficult to diagnose; drug cost and side effects; delay of diagnosis; and delay in attempting pregnancy. Postoperative medical treatment may be indicated if complete resection of disease has not been accomplished, for

treatment of microscopic or metastatic disease, or for treatment of pain. Preoperative or postoperative treatment is usually given for 2 to 6 months.

The approach to each patient must be individualized, depending on her symptoms, signs, age, type and extent of disease, and desire for fertility. Many patients prefer no treatment or medical treatment rather than surgery. However, surgery is often the most appropriate approach. Most patients prefer to retain as many of their reproductive organs as possible, but for some, oophorectomy and/or hysterectomy is a better option. Laparoscopy is generally the preferred surgical approach, but laparotomy may be appropriate in some cases, especially those requiring extirpation of large endometriomas, extensive enterolysis, enterostomy, or bowel resection. Alternatives to surgical treatment or medical treatment in combination with surgery, such as the use of GnRH agonists preoperatively to treat severe endometriosis, should be considered.

It is critical that physicians recognize the degree to which endometriosis can physically and emotionally disrupt patients' lives and that they provide comprehensive understanding and an empathetic management approach. Psychological support through information can be obtained from organizations such as the Endometriosis Association (414-355-2200), RESOLVE (617-623-1156), and the American Society of Reproductive Medicine (205-978-5000). Personal or group counseling may also be helpful, especially for patients with chronic pain. Some patients may seek nontraditional and unproven approaches to treatment, such as acupuncture, herbal medicine, special diets, and/or exercise. Management should focus on alleviation of symptoms and improved quality of life. A comprehensive evaluation of gastrointestinal, genitourinary, musculoskeletal, neurologic, and psychological systems may be indicated. Referral to a pain clinic may be helpful for further treatment, including biofeedback strategies, nerve blocks, psychotherapy, or other pain management techniques. A comprehensive long-range treatment approach needs to be individualized for each patient. A complete cure can sometimes be achieved only by total hysterectomy and bilateral salpingo-oophorectomy.

COMPARISON OF TREATMENT OUTCOMES

Pain

No treatment or mild analgesics or NSAIDs may be entirely appropriate for many young patients with minimal symptoms or for women who have just completed a course of medical treatment. Women who remain symptomatic with minimal or mild pain can frequently be treated successfully with cyclical oral contraceptives. For women who have persistent pain, endocrinologic treatment with progestins, danazol, or GnRH agonists have similar efficacy, with approximately 80 to 90% of patients obtaining significant relief.

In one study that is representative of those in the literature, nafarelin acetate (Synarel) at both high (400 μg twice a day) and low (200 μg twice a day) doses, as well as danazol (Danocrine 400 mg twice a day), provided significant relief of several types of pain associated with endometriosis during 6 months of daily treatment (Table 1). This beneficial effect persisted after discontinuation of drug treatment, but 6 months after treatment was completed, approximately two-thirds of patients had experienced a return of dysmenorrhea; pelvic pain was reported by about one-half and dyspareunia by about one-third of subjects. Dysmenorrhea returns with menses and, presumably, the cyclical release of endometrial prostaglandins. Generalized pelvic pain and dyspareunia may depend on the re-establishment of endometrial implants. Patients with severe disease or large endometriomas tend to have an earlier recurrence. Danazol and GnRH agonists should not be used in the treatment of endometriosis unless the diagnosis has been confirmed at laparoscopy.

Laparoscopy and laparotomy are also effective in the treatment of pelvic pain, with approximately 90% of patients showing significant clinical improvement following complete resection of disease. Approximately 90% of patients should have good symptom relief at 5 years and 50% at 10 years if the disease is completely resected.

Hysterectomy is the definitive treatment for patients with recurrent or intractable pain associated with endometriosis. In young women of reproductive age, removal of one or both ovaries is controversial, even though the ovaries are the most common site of endometrial implants and the growth of endometrial implants is driven by cyclical ovarian activity. An ovarian cystectomy for endometrioma is usually the most appropriate approach. If a hysterectomy is warranted, all remaining ovarian tissue should be removed at the same time.

Hysterectomy combined with oophorectomy for endometriosis results in a very high probability of "cure." There is a minimal recurrence rate in the range of 5 to 8%; this may be due to residual endometriosis, recurrent endometriosis, ovarian remnant syndrome, adhesions, or other nongynecologic problems. This recurrence rate may be reduced by meticulous resection of all endometriosis at the time of hysterectomy and oophorectomy. Studies to confirm that such an approach results in superior outcome have yet to be performed.

Infertility

For minimal and mild disease, no treatment, laparoscopy, and laparotomy result in equivalent 3-year estimated cumulative life-table pregnancy rates (Table 2). Likewise, no treatment or surgery is superior to medical treatment for minimal and mild endometriosis associated with infertility. Meta-analysis has also shown that there is no statistically significant difference in crude pregnancy rates between patients receiving no treatment and those receiving medical treatment (Figure 1). Therefore, no treatment is appropriate for selected young patients with minimal or mild disease and a short duration of infertility. Controlled ovarian hyperstimulation with clomiphene citrate (Clomid, Serophene) 150 mg every day from cycle days 3 to 7 or gonadotropins (Metrodin, Humegon) and intrauterine insemination probably improve pregnancy rates in this group.

Medical treatment for minimal and mild endometriosis results in negligible improvement in ultimate pregnancy rates and is associated with additional cost and undesirable side effects. Medical treatment

TABLE 1. **Reports of Specific Types of Pain in Patients with Laparoscopically Diagnosed Endometriosis Treated with Nafarelin Acetate or Danazol**

| | | Pain Reports | | | | | | | | |
| | | *Dysmenorrhea* | | | *Dyspareunia* | | | | *Pelvic* | |
Treatment	No.	ABSENT (%)	PRESENT (%)	No.	ABSENT (%)	PRESENT (%)	NOT REPORTED	No.	ABSENT (%)	PRESENT (%)
Nafarelin, 800 μg	45			26				40		
Admission		0	100		0	100	0		0	100
Treatment*		100	0		62	31	8		65	35
Post-treatment†		36	64		62	35	4		45	55
Nafarelin, 400 μg	45			31				37		
Admission		0	100		0	100	0		0	100
Treatment*		98	2		65	32	3		57	43
Post-treatment†		33	67		71	29	0		49	51
Danazol	34			23				28		
Admission		0	100		0	100	0		0	100
Treatment*		94	6		70	17	13		64	36
Post-treatment†		50	50		65	30	4		50	50

All subjects reported pain on admission.
*Treatment was continued for 6 months.
†Post-treatment period was 6 months follow-up.
From Adamson GD, Kwei L, Edgren RA: Pain of endometriosis: Effects of nafarelin and danazol therapy. Int J Fertil *39*:215–217, 1994.

TABLE 2. Estimated Cumulative Life-Table Pregnancy Rates by Treatment Group for Different Stages of Endometriosis

	Entire Patient Population						Endometriosis-Only Subset			
		No. Pregnant in 3 Years	Pregnant (%)				No. Pregnant in 3 Years	Pregnant (%)		
Treatment Group	No.		1 Year	2 Years	3 Years	No.		1 Year	2 Years	3 Years
Minimal/mild										
No treatment	15	10	53.3 ± 12.9*	66.7 ± 12.2	66.7 ± 12.2	13	9	61.5 ± 13.5	69.2 ± 12.8	69.2 ± 12.8
Medical treatment	44	20	26.5 ± 7.2	53.0 ± 8.9	62.3 ± 9.3	32	13	25.6 ± 8.4	47.7 ± 10.2	55.2 ± 11.2
Laparoscopy	241	122	43.6 ± 3.5	59.6 ± 3.8	67.8 ± 4.1	134	70	45.5 ± 4.7	60.4 ± 5.1	70.3 ± 5.4
Laparotomy	46	28	55.7 ± 7.9	65.6 ± 7.9	74.3 ± 8.1	13	6	38.0 ± 15.1	50.4 ± 16.4	64.5 ± 16.8
Moderate/severe†										
Laparoscopy	120	52	29.1 ± 4.5	50.8 ± 5.6	62.2 ± 6.2	48	25	32.2 ± 7.5	70.0 ± 9.0	82.0 ± 8.5
Laparotomy	102	37	23.8 ± 4.5	36.7 ± 5.3	44.4 ± 5.6	15	5	20.0 ± 10.3	26.7 ± 11.4	33.3 ± 12.2

*Values are estimates ± SE.

†Eleven patients treated nonsurgically have been excluded from the entire patient population. Three patients treated nonsurgically have been excluded from the endometriosis-only subset.

From Adamson GD, Hurd SJ, Pasta DJ, Rodriguez BD: Laparoscopic endometriosis treatment: Is it better? Fertil Steril *59*:35–44, 1993.

merely delays the possibility of pregnancy by the duration of the therapy. Medical therapy alone should never be used to treat minimal and mild endometriosis when the only symptom is infertility.

Preoperative medical therapy should be reserved for patients with severe symptoms, to facilitate surgery scheduling when necessary, or for patients with known severe disease when medical treatment may result in a better pelvic milieu for reconstructive surgery. It is unknown what, if any, effect preoperative medical treatment has on subsequent pregnancy rates. Postoperative medical treatment may be indicated for patients with severe refractory pelvic pain or in whom disease has not been completely extirpated, but it should be avoided whenever possible in infertility patients because of the inability to conceive while taking the medication. Postoperative medical treatment does not improve pregnancy rates (see Figure 1). Overall, the available data do not support the routine perioperative use of GnRH ago-

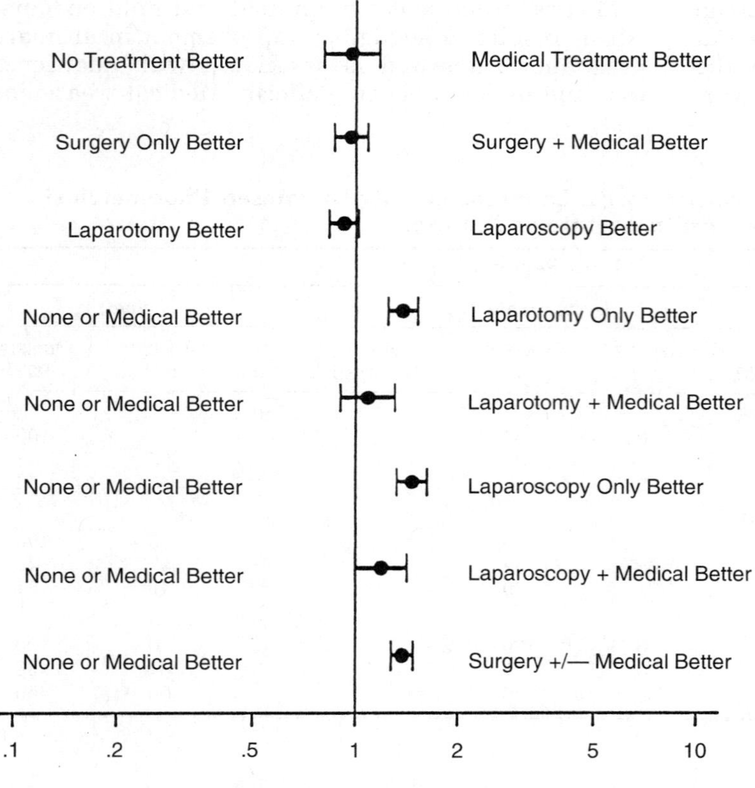

Figure 1. Summary of meta-analysis estimates of relative risk of pregnancy (point estimate and 95% confidence interval) after different endometriosis treatments. (From Adamson GD, Pasta DJ: Surgical treatments of endometriosis-associated infertility: Meta-analysis compared with survival analysis. Am J Obstet Gynecol *171*:1488–1505, 1994.)

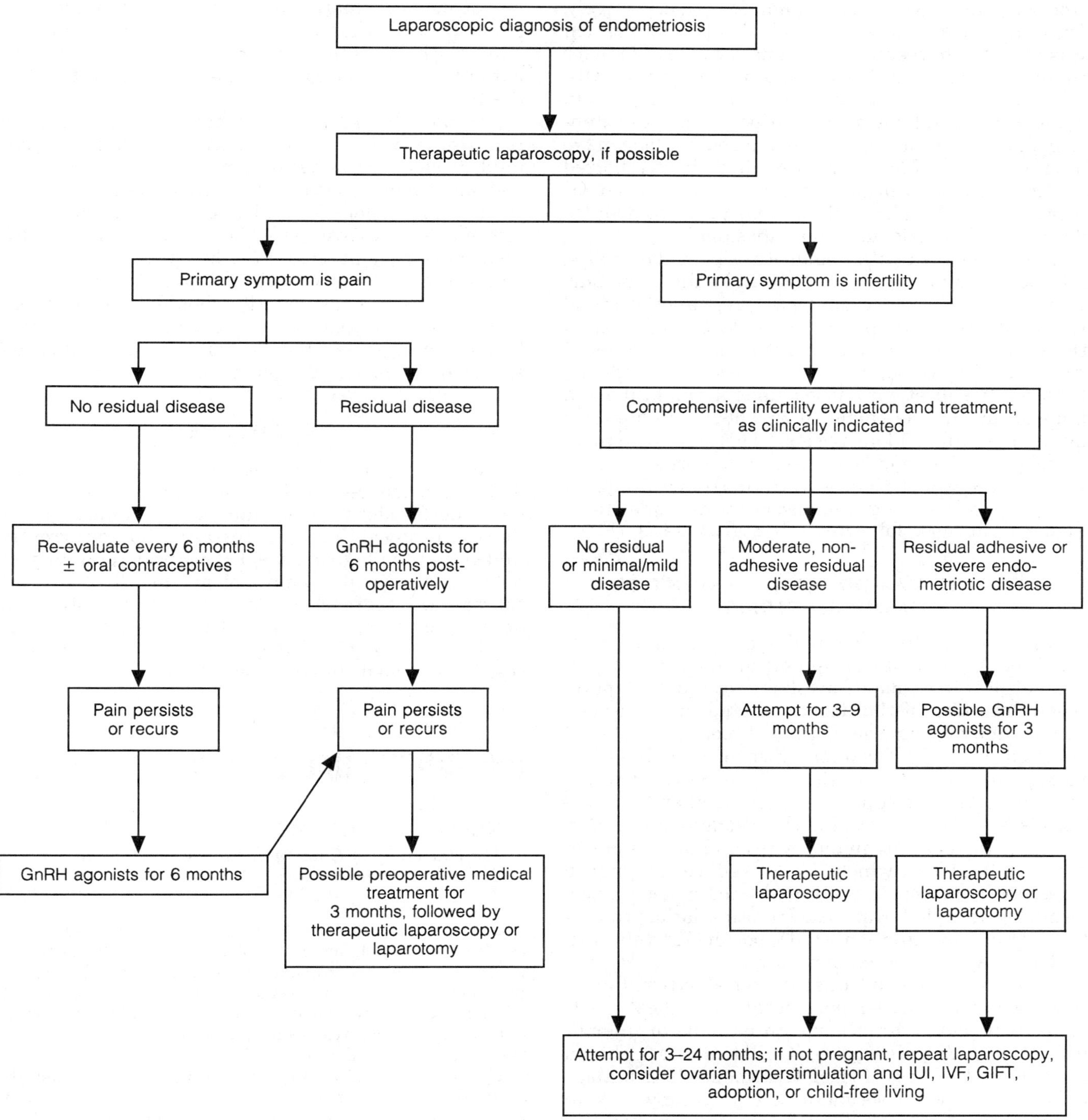

Figure 2. Postlaparoscopy management of endometriosis. (From Adamson GD: Laparoscopic treatment of endometriosis. *In* Adamson GD, Martin DC [eds]: Endoscopic Management of Gynecologic Disease. Philadelphia, Lippincott-Raven, 1995, pp 147–187.)

nists or other hormonal therapies, but these may be of value in selected patients.

A recent review of laparoscopic treatment of endometriosis reported that for those with minimal and mild disease, pregnancy rates after laparoscopic electrocoagulation were 64% and 52%, respectively. Treatment with carbon dioxide laser vaporization was reported to result in a pregnancy rate of 59% for those with minimal disease and 58% for those with mild disease. The author's experience is reflected in Table 2. It is not known whether patients with extensive and/or invasive peritoneal disease alone have pregnancy rates higher or lower than those reported in these studies. Surgical treatment is required for more advanced endometriosis with invasive nodular disease, endometriomas, and adhesions.

Infertile women with endometriosis can be treated at laparoscopy if the equipment and skill of the surgeon permit. In every analysis, pregnancy rates of the laparoscopy group were equal to or higher than those following other treatment options, whether it was in the entire population (n = 579), the endometriosis-only subset with at least one normal tube and fimbria and normal male (n = 258), patients with minimal or mild endometriosis, or patients with moderate or severe endometriosis. Furthermore, even when significant variables were controlled for, pregnancy rates following laparoscopy were equal to or higher than those following other treatments.

ALGORITHM FOR MANAGEMENT OF ENDOMETRIOSIS

Laparoscopy is required to diagnose endometriosis. Whether the patient's symptoms are pain or infertility, surgical treatment involving complete laparoscopic resection of the disease should be performed at the time of diagnosis if the surgeon is capable of doing so. The only exception is when the patient is a young woman with infertility as her only symptom and with extensive superficial peritoneal and/or ovarian disease. Treatment of such lesions has not been shown to increase pregnancy rates and may result in pelvic adhesions, which could reduce pregnancy rates, so laparoscopic treatment should not be performed. Controlled ovarian hyperstimulation and intrauterine insemination (IUI) postoperatively will probably increase pregnancy rates.

If the patient has adequate surgical extirpation of the disease, no further postoperative medical treatment is indicated for either pain patients or infertility patients. If pain recurs, GnRH agonists should usually be the first line of treatment. If a patient fails to conceive, a second-look laparoscopy at 6 to 24 months may be indicated, possibly with GIFT performed at the same time. If extensive endometriosis, adhesions, or tubal abnormalities are found, in vitro fertilization (IVF) should be considered.

If the patient does not have operative laparoscopy at the time of diagnosis or has incomplete resection of endometriosis and continues to have pain, she has the option of a repeat laparoscopy or laparotomy, most likely by a more experienced surgeon specializing in endometriosis, or the use of GnRH agonists or danazol for 3 to 6 months. GnRH agonists are generally preferred because of their more favorable side-effect profile. Failure to manage pain with surgical and/or medical treatment should result in referral to a pain specialist for a comprehensive approach to the pain. Such an option should be discussed with the patient at her first consultation and integrated into the treatment plan.

For infertility patients who have not had operative resection or with inadequate resection, minimal and mild disease (no adhesions, no invasive lesions, no endometriomas) needs no further treatment. Patients with moderate or advanced disease should be referred for laparoscopy or occasionally laparotomy. Medical treatment should not be used.

Infertile patients who do not conceive within approximately 3 to 24 months should have a repeat laparoscopy for treatment and/or assisted reproductive technologies such as ovarian hyperstimulation and IUI, and/or GIFT (Figure 2).

THE FUTURE

We have much to learn about endometriosis. More detailed evidence-based meta-analysis studies are being performed to help improve our clinical guidelines. It is hoped that basic research that is currently under way will give us a better understanding of $beta_3$ integrins and immunology and lead to new therapeutic approaches. An international study to determine the genetic basis of endometriosis is currently under way, and may lead to much more successful treatment in the years ahead.

DYSFUNCTIONAL UTERINE BLEEDING

method of
NEEOO W. CHIN, M.D.
The University of Cincinnati College of Medicine
Cincinnati, Ohio

Dysfunctional uterine bleeding (DUB) is defined as excessive, prolonged, irregular bleeding from the endometrium unrelated to any structural or systemic disease. It may normally occur in women at the beginning or end of their reproductive years. It is usually associated with anovulation, which results in unopposed estrogen stimulation to the endometrium.

The normal menstrual cycle occurs at regular intervals of 24 to 35 days. The average length of flow is 4 to 6 days but can be as few as 2 and as many as 7 days. A flow longer than 7 days warrants evaluation. The average blood loss during a menstruation is approximately 30 mL. A flow of 80 mL or more is considered abnormal and requires further work-up. It is difficult to quantify menstrual flow, and evaluation is needed when a patient perceives her menses as being abnormal.

Abnormal uterine bleeding can occur in the following patterns:

Amenorrhea: Absence of menses for 6 months or for longer than 3 of the patient's normal menstrual cycles

Intermenstrual bleeding: Bleeding that occurs between regular menstrual cycles

Menometrorrhagia: Excessive uterine bleeding occurring at irregular intervals

Menorrhagia: Profuse or prolonged bleeding occurring at regular intervals

Metrorrhagia: Irregular, acyclic bleeding occurring at frequent intervals

Oligomenorrhea: Bleeding in which the interval varies from 36 days to 6 months

Polymenorrhea: Bleeding that occurs at regular intervals of less than 21 days

There are four categories of dysfunctional bleeding:

1. *Estrogen withdrawal bleeding*. A type of bleeding that occurs after removal of both ovaries, radiation to the ovaries, chemotherapy, or discontinuation of estrogen therapy to a woman who has nonfunctioning ovaries. Occasionally, midcycle spotting may occur because of a decrease in estrogen that precedes ovulation.

2. *Estrogen breakthrough bleeding*. This type of bleeding is a result of low estrogen stimulation to the endometrium. Low levels of estrogen result in intermittent spotting and may produce a light, continuous flow. High levels of estrogen for prolonged periods of time result in extended lengths of amenorrhea, followed by acute, heavy bleeding with excessive blood loss.

3. *Progesterone withdrawal bleeding*. Removal of the corpus luteum or administration and then discontinuation of progesterone will result in endometrial sloughing. For progesterone withdrawal bleeding to occur, the endometrium must first be primed by estrogen. This type of withdrawal bleeding still occurs if estrogen therapy is continued after progesterone is withdrawn. Elevated estrogen levels of 10-fold to 20-fold may delay progesterone withdrawal bleeding.

4. *Progesterone breakthrough bleeding*. Occurs with an abnormally high progesterone-to-estrogen ratio. Continuous progesterone therapy without adequate estrogen replacement results in bleeding of variable duration. This is the type of bleeding that can be seen with contraception by means of long-acting progestin.

DIFFERENTIAL DIAGNOSIS

Diagnosis of DUB is made by exclusion. Other causes of uterine bleeding that must be considered before making the diagnosis are as follows:

Pregnancy-related events: Incomplete or threatened abortion, retained placenta, gestational trophoblastic neoplasia, ectopic pregnancy, placental polyp

Systemic diseases: Thyroid dysfunction, renal failure, cirrhosis, adrenal gland abnormalities, hyperprolactinemia

Anatomic lesions: Endometrial polyps, cervical polyps, uterine leiomyomata

Neoplasms: Endometrial hyperplasia, endometrial carcinoma, cervical carcinoma, estrogen-secreting ovarian tumors

Coagulopathies: von Willebrand's disease, prothrombin deficiency, platelet deficiency/dysfunction, factor V, VIII, or IX deficiency, leukemia

Nonuterine: Genital trauma, foreign body

Infection: Cervicitis, endometritis, vaginitis, vulvitis

LABORATORY EVALUATION

Laboratory evaluation may be helpful but is not necessary in all situations. Specific tests help exclude abnormal bleeding causes suggested by the history and physical examination.

Blood tests may include complete blood count with differential, quantitative beta human chorionic gonadotropin, thyroid function test, prolactin, clotting studies (prothrombin time, activated partial thromboplastin time, antithrombin III, protein C, protein S, fibrinogen, plasminogen), and liver and renal function tests.

Abnormalities of the uterus can be detected by vaginal or abdominal ultrasonography, hysterosalpingography, or hysteroscopy. Endometrial sampling should be considered in cases of abnormal uterine bleeding. Although not necessary in the premenarchal patient, it is often mandatory in the perimenopausal patient to exclude any premalignant or malignant condition. The age of the patient is not critical when considering an endometrial sampling, but the duration of the unopposed estrogen exposure is.

TREATMENT

When no organic pathology is found for the cause of the abnormal bleeding, medical therapy is preferred over surgery. Since anovulation is the most common cause of DUB, progestational therapy is usually the first line of therapy.

Medical Therapy

Progestational Agents. Medroxyprogesterone acetate (Provera), 10 mg per day for 10 days each month, will regulate and produce withdrawal bleeding in a cyclic fashion when the endometrium is estrogen primed. Progestins not only stop endometrial growth but also support and organize the endometrium such that sloughing occurs in an organized fashion. If contraception is required, an oral contraceptive can accomplish the same purpose.

When progestins are required to reverse a hyperplastic process, sampling of the endometrium is indicated. Resampling can be performed after 3 months of therapy. If hyperplasia continues or if atypia is found, further medical or surgical therapy with higher-dose progestin therapy and repeated endometrial sampling must be considered.

Estrogens. When there is insufficient tissue for progestational action, or if there has been prolonged intractable bleeding, then estrogen therapy is indicated to cause rapid growth of the endometrium. Estrogen also stimulates clotting at the capillary level.

Twenty-five milligrams of conjugated estrogen (Premarin) can be administered intravenously every 4 hours until the bleeding is under control or for a total of 12 hours. This can be followed by oral estrogens at a dose of 1.25 mg of conjugated estrogens (Premarin) or 2 mg of micronized estradiol (Estrace) every 4 hours for 24 hours, followed by one dose daily for 7 to 10 days. Medroxyprogesterone therapy should be given following the estrogen therapy or concomitantly. Following the course of estrogen therapy, a treatment cycle of a low-dose oral contraceptive may be used to induce a withdrawal bleed. To avoid further episodes of DUB the patient should consider the use of cyclic hormonal therapy.

When lesser bleeding occurs, use low-dose estrogen as add-back therapy when progestational atrophy occurs with oral contraceptives, medroxyprogesterone acetate (Depo-Provera) therapy, or levonorgestrel (Norplant) contraceptive.

Low-Dose Oral Contraceptives. When young anovulatory women experience prolonged unopposed estrogen stimulation resulting in endometrial build-up, severe, heavy bleeding can occur. A low-dose (less than 50 μg of estrogen) oral contraceptive pill can be effective in controlling both short- and long-term bleeding. One pill taken three times a day will often stop bleeding within 24 to 48 hours. This dosage is continued for 1 week, followed by 1 pill twice a day for 10 days, and finally a single pill a day for 21 days, which will be followed by a withdrawal bleed. The resultant withdrawal bleed will be less intense than that following intravenous estrogen therapy. If subsequent contraception is not desired, this regimen should be continued for approximately 3 months, and then the patient can be treated with monthly medroxyprogesterone as described previously.

Antiprostaglandins: (Nonsteroidal Anti-Inflammatory Drugs). These drugs inhibit the action of cyclooxygenase, which decreases certain members of the prostaglandin family. The mechanism of action of these drugs with DUB is activated through an alteration in the balance between the platelet proaggregating vasoconstrictor thromboxane A_2 and the antiaggregating vasodilator prostacyclin. Blood loss has been shown to be reduced by as much as 50%. This group of drugs should not be used in patients with aspirin intolerance, bronchial spastic pulmonary disease, peptic ulcer disease, and hepatic or renal disease.

Other Therapies. Some of the other methods used for DUB include antifibrinolytic agents, androgenic steroids, gonadotropin-releasing hormone (GnRH) analogues, ergot derivatives, desmopressin, and progestin intrauterine devices.

Surgical Therapies

Dilation and Curettage and Hysteroscopy. These are appropriate in women with DUB in whom medical management has failed or in perimenopausal women whose in-office endometrial biopsy was unsuccessful.

Hysterectomy. Occasionally hysterectomy is the proper treatment for DUB. There is a higher risk of morbidity and mortality, and the costs make it inappropriate as the first choice of management except in the most severe cases, as with failed medical management or endometrial hyperplasia with atypia.

Endometrial Ablation. In selected cases in whom no pathology exists and medical therapy is unsuccessful, combined with poor surgical candidates, endometrial ablation is an alternative therapy. Laser vaporization with the neodymium-YAG and roller ball coagulation are the techniques most widely used. The purpose of the ablation is to destroy the basal layers of the endometrium, preventing its regeneration. Ablation results in complete amenorrhea in about 50% of women, and 90% will have great reduction in their bleeding, but it is not 100% effective. The best results are accomplished when the endometrium has been first suppressed with a GnRH analogue, danazol, or medroxyprogesterone for about 4 to 6 weeks prior to the ablation. One concern is that obliteration of segments of the uterine cavity can allow isolated residual endometrial growth to progress to carcinoma without recognition. Long-term follow-up is needed to know whether this risk is real.

AMENORRHEA

method of
DAVID E. CARNOVALE, M.D., and
HOWARD A. ZACUR, M.D., Ph.D.
The Johns Hopkins University School of Medicine
Baltimore, Maryland

Amenorrhea, the absence of menses, may occur at various times during a woman's life. If it occurs prior to any episode of menstrual bleeding, it is classified as primary amenorrhea. Cessation of menses for 6 months in a woman who has had previous menstrual bleeding is called secondary amenorrhea. The medical evaluation for either situation follows a systematic approach based upon an understanding of the various etiologies that may be responsible. Because the causes of primary amenorrhea are also responsible for secondary amenorrhea, a simplified work-up may be created.

Certain anatomic and endocrinologic prerequisites are necessary in order for menstrual periods to take place. The anatomic and endocrinologic integrity of the hypothalamic-pituitary-ovarian axis must be intact and coexist with a functional end organ—i.e., the uterus—which communicates with a patent vagina.

When evaluating a patient with primary amenorrhea and normal external genitalia, it is useful to identify her as belonging to one of four diagnostic categories. These categories are based on the presence or absence of a uterus and whether or not breast development has occurred. The existence of a uterus establishes that normal anatomic development has occurred, whereas breast development indicates estrogen exposure, which presumes that the hypothalamic-pituitary-ovarian axis has functioned. The four categories identified are as follows:

  I. Breast development and uterus present
 II. Absent breast development and uterus present
III. Absent breast development and uterus absent
IV. Breast development present and uterus absent

By utilizing these four categories, a logical and systematic approach in evaluating patients with primary amenorrhea may be followed. Causes of primary amenorrhea with breast development and uterus present (category I) may also cause secondary amenorrhea. Each category and its management is discussed in detail.

I. BREAST DEVELOPMENT AND UTERUS PRESENT

It is estimated that approximately one third of patients with primary amenorrhea will present with a normal uterus and breast development. When both the uterus and breast development are present, it is necessary to know when to expect that menses will occur. The mean age of onset of menarche in the United States is 12.9 years, with a standard deviation of 1.2 years. One should initiate a work-up if menses has not occurred by age 16.5 (three standard deviations from the mean), or if 3 to 4 years have passed since the onset of breast development.

The work-up of these patients is approached in a manner similar to that for patients with secondary amenorrhea (Figure 1). A thorough history and physical examination should be obtained. Inquiries should be made about previous menstrual history if any, sexual developmental milestones, diet, exercise, weight gain or loss, stress, medication use, nipple discharge, and sexual activity. In all cases of secondary amenorrhea a pregnancy test should be obtained and also in cases of primary amenorrhea when the patient admits to being sexually active or the clinician otherwise feels that it is appropriate. As 25% of patients with primary amenorrhea who have breast development and a uterus present have been shown to have hyperprolactinemia and radiographic evidence of a prolactinoma, a serum prolactin level is obtained. Factors such as stress, diet, and time of day can increase serum prolactin levels. Preferably, blood for study should be obtained in the morning, with the patient fasting and under as little stress as possible. If the patient's prolactin level is truly elevated, then the thyroid-stimulating hormone (TSH) level also needs to be checked. Primary hypothyroidism with the resultant increase in thyrotropin-releasing hormone (TRH) stimulates pituitary prolactin secretion. Thyroid hormone replacement therapy can easily correct this disorder with resultant normalization of the prolactin level and resolution of the patient's amenorrhea. If the prolactin level is elevated and thyroid studies are normal, radiographic imaging either by computed tomography (CT) scan or magnetic resonance imaging (MRI) should be ordered to determine whether a pituitary lesion is present. MRI is superior in detecting and delineating such lesions and should be used if available. If a pituitary lesion is present, consultation with a reproductive endocrinologist and possibly a neurosurgeon is advisable.

In patients with both a uterus and breast development present and a normal prolactin level, the next

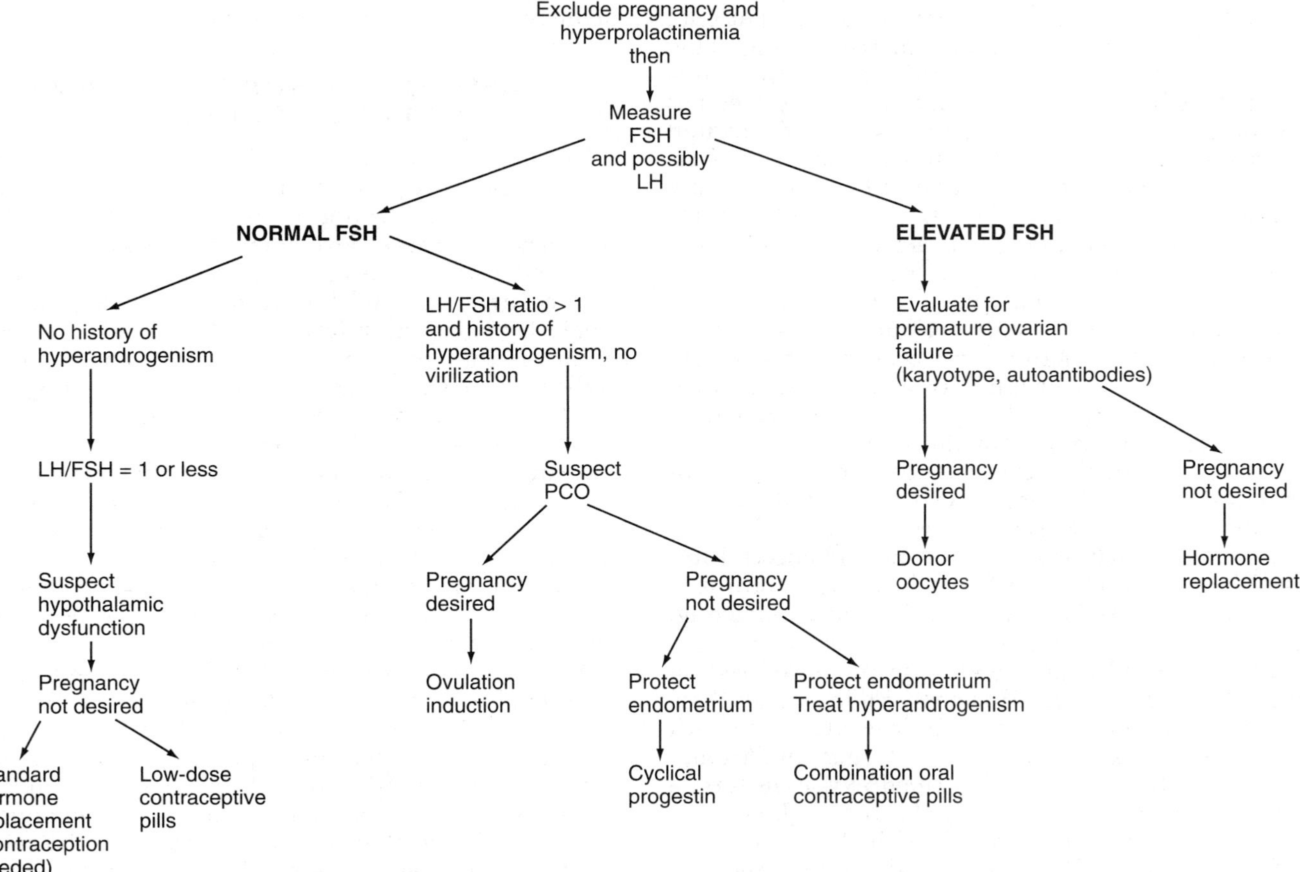

Figure 1. Evaluation of a patient with primary or secondary amenorrhea with breast development and uterus present. *Abbreviations:* FSH = follicle-stimulating hormone; LH = luteinizing hormone; PCO = polycystic ovarian syndrome.

step requires drawing blood for measurement of at least follicle-stimulating hormone (FSH) and, if possible, luteinizing hormone (LH). If the FSH level is within the normal or low-normal premenopausal range, the diagnostic categories of either hypothalamic dysfunction or functional ovarian hyperandrogenism, otherwise known as polycystic ovarian (PCO) syndrome, should be considered.

Hypothalamic dysfunction in this setting may be due to weight loss, stress, or medication use, or be idiopathic. Regardless of the initiating event, disrupted gonadotropin-releasing hormone (GnRH) release results, followed by altered LH and FSH release. In cases of hypothalamic dysfunction, the ratio of LH to FSH is usually less than 1 (when measured in mIU per mL), in contrast to ovulatory women in whom the value is approximately 1 prior to and following ovulation. An elevated LH-to-FSH ratio is observed normally at ovulation when the LH concentration greatly exceeds that of FSH. An increase in the amplitude and frequency in LH pulses may be detected in patients with PCO, resulting in an elevated basal concentration of LH producing a ratio of LH to FSH exceeding 1 and frequently reaching values of 2 or more.

Whether the cause of amenorrhea results from PCO or hypothalamic dysfunction, ovulation does not occur and progesterone secretion is lacking. To compensate for this deficit an oral progestin may be given cyclically (10 to 12 days each month) to PCO patients to induce sloughing of the endometrial lining. This regimen will consistently cause protective withdrawal bleeding for the PCO patient, but it does not provide contraception, nor will it reduce the elevated androgen levels commonly found in these patients. In contrast, oral contraceptive pill therapy (any brand) will protect the endometrium, provide contraception, and reduce androgenic activity. Should pregnancy be desired, clomiphene citrate (Clomid) induction of ovulation is usually very successful.

In patients suspected of hypothalamic dysfunction, cyclical progestin therapy will protect the endometrium if sufficient ovarian estrogen secretion is occurring. In some cases of hypothalamic dysfunction, the decline in pulsatile gonadotropin secretion is so great—e.g., anorexia nervosa, existence of hypothalamic lesions, or Sheehan's syndrome—that ovarian estradiol secretion is severely reduced, resulting in lack of stimulation or growth of the endometrial lining. When this occurs, administration of an oral progestin will not be followed by withdrawal bleeding. Persistence of hypoestrogenism in young women may result in reduced bone growth and increased risk of cardiovascular disease. Hormone replacement therapy should be given in this clinical situation, with conjugated estrogens, 0.625 to 1.25 mg taken daily by mouth. Cyclical progestin (medroxyprogesterone acetate [Provera]), 10 mg for 10 to 12 days each month, is also taken by mouth with the estrogen to protect the uterus. This regimen of hormone replacement should ultimately result in cyclical vaginal bleeding. If this does not occur, coexisting uterine

scarring should be considered (Asherman's syndrome). Since the regimen of hormone replacement just described will not inhibit spontaneous ovulation, patients should be counseled about contraceptive practices. Alternatively, low-dose combination oral contraceptive pills may also be prescribed to patients with hypothalamic dysfunction to provide contraception and adequate hormone replacement. When pregnancy is desired, human menopausal gonadotropin therapy is usually required to induce ovulation.

If the FSH measurement is reported as within the menopausal range in a woman with amenorrhea under 40 years of age, premature ovarian failure (POF) should be considered. Possible etiologies include autoimmune disease, genetic abnormalities, previous gonadal irradiation, and systemic chemotherapy.

A karyotype may be requested (particularly in the patient 35 years of age or younger) to identify genetic defects as the cause. When mosaicism with a Y chromosome is present, gonadectomy would be indicated to prevent malignant transformation. Other studies in patients with POF may include an autoimmune work-up to determine the presence of thyroid, adrenal, and/or ovarian antibodies. Although spontaneous resumption of ovulation is unlikely for these patients, it may still occur. Donor oocytes are almost always needed for patients who desire pregnancy. When pregnancy is not desired, hormonal replacement therapy should be provided.

II. ABSENT BREAST DEVELOPMENT AND UTERUS PRESENT

In one series of patients with primary amenorrhea, the largest group were those with absent breast development and a uterus present. In this category the lack of breast development indicates a hypoestrogenic state. This lack of estrogen may be secondary to either gonadal failure or lack of appropriate tropic hormone stimulation of the gonads. Gonadal failure is the most common cause of primary amenorrhea. Genetic defects account for the majority of these cases, with complete deletion of a sex chromosome—e.g., 45X (Turner's syndrome)—being the single most common chromosomal abnormality. Partial deletion of sex chromosome material and mosaicism involving a single sex chromosome may also lead to gonadal failure. These patients have fibrous tissue (streak gonads) in place of normal ovarian tissue. Extirpation of the gonads is not necessary unless a Y chromosome is present in the karyotype.

A rare cause of gonadal failure presenting in a patient without breast development but with a uterus is 17 alpha-hydroxylase deficiency with a 46XX karyotype. These patients lack an enzyme that prevents sex steroids from being produced and also prevents cortisol from being synthesized, leading to a state of elevated adrenocorticotropic hormone (ACTH) production. This results in excessive mineralocorticoid production (aldosterone) causing hypertension and hypokalemia. Glucocorticoid replacement normalizes ACTH levels and at the age of puberty, sex steroid replacement therapy should be administered to induce breast development and promote bone growth. Patients with gonadal failure are candidates for donor oocytes if pregnancy is desired.

In cases of gonadal failure, whether due to chromosomal, genetic, or enzymatic deficiencies, the picture will be one of hypergonadotropic (elevated LH and FSH) hypogonadism (lack of sex hormone production). The hypogonadism results in a menopause-like state. Some patients without breast development and uterus present have ovarian oocytes but lack appropriate ovarian hormonal stimulation, presumably as a consequence of absent or low FSH stimulation. When this occurs, a state of hypogonadotropic (low gonadotropin levels) hypogonadism exists. Because the ovaries do not produce estrogen, a menopause-like state also exists, but future pregnancy is possible. Etiologies seen with this scenario include anatomic lesions of the hypothalamus or pituitary, inadequate GnRH release, and isolated gonadotropin deficiency. Imaging of the hypothalamic-pituitary region by MRI should be ordered, even if prolactin levels are normal, to exclude a possible lesion.

To distinguish between the hypothalamus or pituitary as being responsible for the hypogonadotropic state, a GnRH stimulation test can be done. If the pituitary releases adequate LH after exogenous GnRH is administered, then it is assumed that the abnormality is at the level of the hypothalamus. If a negative response is seen, then the pituitary is the culprit. The test is performed by giving a 100-μg bolus of GnRH intravenously over 30 seconds. An LH level of 20 mIU per mL 30 minutes after the bolus is considered a positive response. If an initial negative response is obtained, then the pituitary should be primed with daily doses of GnRH for up to 10 days and the test repeated. The GnRH stimulation test is rarely indicated since a distinction between hypothalamic and pituitary lesions causing secondary amenorrhea is usually made from the history and imaging studies.

Isolated gonadotropin deficiency (negative GnRH test) can be associated with thalassemia major, retinitis pigmentosa, and mumps encephalitis, as well as with prepubertal hypothyroidism. If the etiology is believed to be at the hypothalamic level, then Kallman's syndrome should be ruled out by olfactory testing with substances such as coffee, tobacco, orange peel, or cocoa. Strenuous physical activity prior to the onset of puberty may also lead to a disruption of the hypothalamic-pituitary interaction. Such a patient could present with absent breast development, a normal uterus, and primary amenorrhea. For all patients with hypogonadotropic hypogonadism, hormone replacement therapy is indicated. For patients who desire pregnancy, a GnRH pump can be used for those with a functioning pituitary while human menopausal gonadotropins can be used to stimulate the ovaries directly in those with pituitary dysfunction.

III. ABSENT BREAST DEVELOPMENT AND ABSENT UTERUS

Individuals with no breast development and absent internal genitalia are rare. Their genotype is 46XY, and gonadal tissue may or may not be present. Three etiologies have been identified: 17 alpha-hydroxylase deficiency, 17,20-desmolase deficiency, and agonadism. In all three cases, factors are present that preclude normal sex hormone synthesis. Patients with either 17 alpha-hydroxylase or 17,20-desmolase deficiency have testes that produce müllerian-inhibiting factor (MIF), causing regression of the internal female structures during embryo development in utero. Unfortunately, testosterone production is insufficient to cause internal and external male genitalia to develop. Patients with agonadism, also known as vanishing testes syndrome, are believed to have had testes during fetal development which produced MIF, causing the absence of internal female genitalia, but these testes regressed (or vanished) before secreting testosterone.

In all three groups, gonadotropin levels are elevated and testosterone levels are in the female range. If abdominal testes are present, these should be removed. Estrogen replacement therapy should be given to induce breast development.

IV. BREAST DEVELOPMENT PRESENT AND UTERUS ABSENT

In the patient with breast development without a uterus, the two possible etiologies are androgen insensitivity syndrome (testicular feminization) and congenital absence of the uterus (Mayer-Rokitansky-Küster-Hauser syndrome). It is simple to determine which of the two is present in a particular patient. In the first instance the karyotype is 46XY with normal levels of testosterone for a male. Due to a receptor defect, male structures did not form despite normal testosterone levels. MIF production during fetal life caused regression of the internal female structures, while breast development occurred due to peripheral conversion of androgens to estrogens. These patients also lack normal terminal hair growth (axillary, pubic, and facial hair) due to the receptor defect to androgen, which aids in making the clinical diagnosis.

Congenital absence of the uterus is the second most common cause of primary amenorrhea, accounting for 15% of cases. These individuals are genetically and endocrinologically female with normal ovaries. They have normal development of secondary sexual characteristics, including axillary and pubic hair; however, they do not menstruate due to an absent uterus. A functional vagina may be absent or shortened, requiring either dilatation or surgery for satisfactory sexual intercourse. Urologic evaluation is indicated because of the 30 to 40% incidence of associated renal abnormalities. An increased incidence of skeletal, cardiac, and other congenital anomalies may also be seen. Oocytes from these patients may be obtained and through in vitro fertilization transferred as embryos to a surrogate carrier, allowing these patients and their partners to have their own genetic children.

EVALUATION

When evaluating amenorrhea, it is important to keep in mind that each patient will have specific needs depending on age, life situation, and previous menstrual function. These needs may arise because of physical and psychological limitations, coexisting medical disorders, or the desire to become pregnant. Primary amenorrhea may be particularly difficult for an adolescent to cope with. The type of hormonal replacement provided is as important psychologically as it is medically. For women who experience menopause (cessation of menses for 1 year) at ages when this may be expected to occur naturally (mean = 50, range of 43 to 57), hormone replacement therapy may be prescribed. Conjugated estrogen (Premarin) may be given orally as a 0.625-mg daily dose, as a 1- to 2-mg daily oral dose of micronized estradiol (Estrace), or as an estradiol patch (Estraderm). When estrogen is given to a woman with a uterus, a progestin (medroxyprogesterone acetate [Provera]) is also prescribed. Hormone replacement therapy given in this manner to menopausal women alleviates the symptoms of menopause—hot flashes and vaginal dryness—and also protects against bone loss and heart disease. A "menopausal state" (low estrogen) may exist in women under 40 years of age either because of premature loss of ovarian oocytes (hypergonadotropic hypogonadism) or because of a lack of ovarian stimulation (hypogonadotropic hypogonadism). Estrogens and progestins in the same doses as those given to menopausal women with onset at the normal age may be given to these younger women, but it has been customary to give higher estrogen doses. This is because these women "prematurely entered a menopausal state," and the expected ovarian estrogen production at this age is greater than that for the menopausal patient.

For a teenager, oral contraceptives may be used as hormone replacement. Low-dose pills are acceptable since it has been estimated that 0.625 mg of conjugated estrogen is roughly equivalent to 5 to 10 µg of ethinyl estradiol. Alternatively, 1.25 mg of conjugated estrogens may be used; however, this may cause embarrassment for some teenagers who may be teased about taking medications that older women usually receive.

It should be noted that in the medical literature a reduction in cardiovascular and osteoporotic risk with hormone replacement has been reported for postmenopausal women taking hormonal replacement. Comparable studies for younger women are lacking, but most authorities would still recommend hormone replacement for younger patients.

When evaluating patients with amenorrhea, it is important to remember that this is a multifactorial disorder that may represent either an underlying hypoestrogenic or euestrogenic state. Risks of developing osteoporosis or cardiovascular disease are important considerations to weigh in determining whether to use exogenous hormone replacement, but so is the risk of malignancy. It is incumbent on the practitioner to be familiar with all aspects of amenorrhea in order to evaluate and assist the patient in the management of this disorder.

DYSMENORRHEA

method of
ABRAHAM MORSE, M.D.
The Johns Hopkins Hospital
Baltimore, Maryland

and

VANESSA E. CULLINS, M.D., M.P.H.
The Johns Hopkins Bayview Medical Center
Baltimore, Maryland

Dysmenorrhea, or painful menstruation, affects more than half of all women of reproductive age. Severe pain with menses can be incapacitating and is estimated to result in 250,000 lost working days or roughly $2 billion in lost productivity annually. In addition, regardless of its effect on their work capacity, millions of women suffer needlessly from this usually easily and safely treated condition. Given the prevalence of dysmenorrhea, its morbidity and economic impact, and our ability to alleviate the problem with relatively simple medical interventions, all women of reproductive age should be questioned about this phenomenon when presenting to a primary care clinician.

Dysmenorrhea is typically divided into primary and secondary forms. Secondary dysmenorrhea is painful menstruation that is associated with visible, palpable, or radiologically identifiable pelvic pathology. Treatment of secondary dysmenorrhea is aimed at the underlying pathology (Table 1), whereas treatment of primary dysmenorrhea is based on our current biochemical and physiologic understanding of otherwise normal ovulatory menstruation. A complete discussion of the management of second-

TABLE 1. **Causes of Secondary Dysmenorrhea**

Endometriosis
Adenomyosis
Pelvic adhesive disease
Endometritis/salpingitis (pelvic inflammatory disease)
Endometrial/endocervical polyps
Uterine leiomyomas (fibroids)
Functional ovarian cysts
Outflow tract stenosis (congenital or acquired)
Intrauterine device
Pelvic congestion syndrome
Allen-Master syndrome
Cervical, endometrial, or ovarian neoplasm
Inflammatory bowel disease (may be exacerbated
   perimenstrually and thus occasionally presents as menstrually
   related pelvic pain)

Adapted from Dawood MY: Current concepts in the etiology and treatment of primary dysmenorrhea. Acta Obstet Gynecol Scand Suppl *138*:7–10, 1986. © 1986, Munksgaard International Publishers Ltd., Copenhagen, Denmark.

TABLE 2. **Characteristics of Primary Dysmenorrhea**

1. Crampy pain, sometimes associated with nausea and/or diarrhea
2. Pain beginning less than 12 hours before and usually not more than 12 hours after the onset of menstruation
3. Rarely lasts more than 3 to 5 days, and often only 1 to 2 days
4. Often begins with the first menstrual period and may improve after parturition

---

ary dysmenorrhea is beyond the scope of this chapter, but its diagnosis and treatment are discussed when there is overlap with the focus of the chapter—the treatment of primary dysmenorrhea.

Primary dysmenorrhea is painful menstruation in the absence of identifiable pelvic pathology. Although primary dysmenorrhea is technically a diagnosis of exclusion (i.e., the absence of any of the causes of secondary dysmenorrhea), there are several characteristic findings that help differentiate it from both secondary dysmenorrhea and the premenstrual syndrome (Table 2).

The etiology of primary dysmenorrhea remained obscure until the 1970s. At that time, the physiology of prostaglandins began to unfold; simultaneously, the pharmacology of nonsteroidal anti-inflammatory drugs (NSAIDs) as prostaglandin inhibitors was recognized.

Prior to the discovery of the physiologic basis for menstrual pain, dysmenorrhea was thought to be entirely psychosomatic. Complex psychological theories of its cause and treatment were advanced. Although it is now acknowledged that dysmenorrhea is "real," the symptoms associated with menstruation are often perceived as more disruptive when other life stressors are active. The psychosocial environment of a patient's menstrual complaints should always be an integral part of any assessment and treatment plan.

Current understanding of the pathogenesis of primary dysmenorrhea is based on the uterine effects of prostaglandin $F_{2\alpha}$ ($PGF_{2\alpha}$). Ovulation is a *sine qua non* for primary dysmenorrhea. During the follicular phase of the menstrual cycle (before ovulation), the levels of endometrial $PGF_{2\alpha}$ are low. During the late luteal phase, progesterone levels fall, the endometrial lining sloughs, and prostaglandins are released. The presence of high concentrations of $PGF_{2\alpha}$ leads to uterine contractions, local ischemia, and sensitization of nociceptive nerve endings in the myometrium. The result is the painful, crampy, lower abdominal pain that characterizes primary dysmenorrhea. It has been shown that women with primary dysmenorrhea have more $PGF_{2\alpha}$ in their menstruum than nondysmenorrheic women.

HISTORY AND PHYSICAL FINDINGS

The evaluation of a patient with painful menses begins with a detailed gynecologic and menstrual history:

1. A review of the patient's menstrual history (i.e., age of menarche, length and regularity of cycles, number of days of bleeding).
2. The relationship of her complaints to menarche and any changes in the quality of her menstrual pain after pregnancy.
3. The relationship of the pain to the onset of menses and the duration of her symptoms.
4. Any associated symptoms such as nausea, presyncope, diarrhea, palpitations, emotional lability, and dysphoria.

5. Any history of pelvic surgery, appendicitis, sexually transmitted diseases, or pelvic infections.
6. Any infertility issues.

The physician should inquire into the patient's psychosocial stressors and, most importantly, screen for domestic abuse. Both physical and sexual abuse survivors have a significantly higher incidence of pelvic pain of all types.

It is also important to differentiate menstrual symptoms from the premenstrual syndrome (see the applicable article for a more complete discussion). Symptoms of pain, emotional lability, and dysphoria that begin 2 to 7 days *before* the onset of menses should be distinguished from dysmenorrhea. The premenstrual syndrome does not usually respond to the same interventions (NSAIDs and oral contraceptives) that are effective in the treatment of dysmenorrhea.

Before embarking on symptomatic treatment of dysmenorrhea, it is important to first screen for malignancy with a Pap smear and breast and pelvic examinations. Sexually transmitted diseases should also be ruled out. The pelvic examination should rule out any significant adnexal masses and assess for causes of secondary dysmenorrhea (Table 3).

TREATMENT OF DYSMENORRHEA

The treatment of primary dysmenorrhea is directed at the reduction of uterine prostaglandin levels (Figure 1). This may be accomplished through direct inhibition of prostaglandin synthesis with NSAIDs, prevention of ovulation (usually with oral contraceptives), or reduction in the volume of endometrium through hormonal therapy (e.g., Depo-Provera), which causes endometrial atrophy.

If a woman has no contraindications to NSAIDs or low-dose oral contraceptive pills (<50 μg ethinyl estradiol with progestogen) and does not desire fertility, we advocate beginning therapy with NSAIDs (Table 4) *and* oral contraceptives. There have been few direct comparisons of NSAIDs and hormonal therapy or one versus both together, but we believe that there are several advantages to combination therapy:

TABLE 3. **Pelvic Examination Findings in Secondary Dysmenorrhea**

Condition	Findings
Adenomyosis	Tender, boggy, globular uterus
Endometriosis	Diffuse adnexal tenderness and lack of uterine mobility, especially a fixed, retroverted uterus; uterosacral nodularity and tenderness on rectovaginal examination
Pelvic adhesive disease	Lack of uterine and/or adnexal mobility; fixed, retroverted uterus; unusual thickness to the adnexa
Endometritis/pelvic inflammatory disease	Irregular, heavy bleeding; marked uterine, adnexal, and cervical motion tenderness
Fibroids	Enlarged uterus with irregular contours; calcified or pedunculated uterine masses

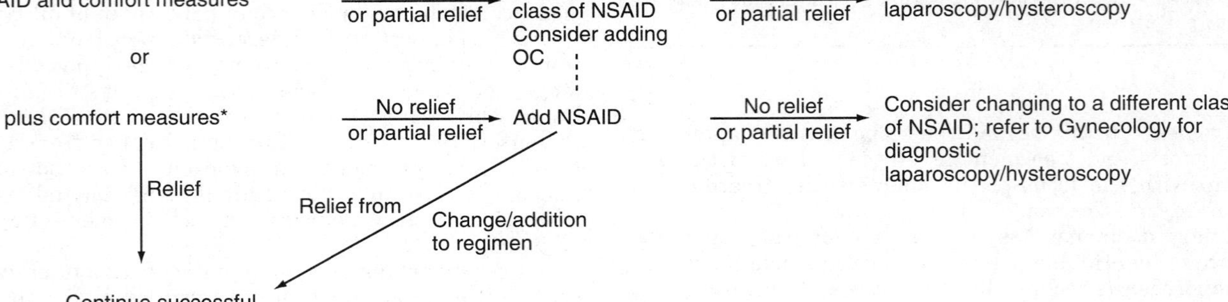

Figure 1. Treatment algorithm for primary dysmenorrhea. *Abbreviations*: NSAID = nonsteroidal anti-inflammatory agent; OC = oral contraceptive. (*Comfort measures include hot tea, warm baths, back massage, heating pad, rest.)

1. The two interventions work through different mechanisms.

2. NSAIDs should provide relief during the first cycle in which they are taken, whereas oral contraceptive pills may take several cycles to work.

3. If therapy is unsuccessful, the patient has failed conservative treatment, and referral to a gynecologist is indicated, thus eliminating one or more office visits required to add or change medical therapy.

Any low-dose oral contraceptive is acceptable. In general, a trial of at least 3 months of *continuous* oral contraceptives is necessary before the success or failure of the intervention can be adequately assessed. NSAIDs often provide relief with the next menstrual cycle. Analgesic response to NSAIDs can be idiosyncratic; therefore, switching at least once to a different class of nonsteroidals is recommended if there is no significant relief after one to two cycles. Rather than taking her NSAIDs on an as-needed basis, it may be efficacious for the patient to take NSAIDs continuously beginning with the first symptoms of menstruation. In addition to having some physiologic basis in the gate theory of nociception, continuous administration minimizes the extent to which the patient is forced to focus on her dysmenorrhea in order to decide when it has become "bad enough" to take her medicine. Patients should also

TABLE 4. Common NSAID Dosages for Treatment of Dysmenorrhea

Drug (by Class)	Brand Name	Dosage (mg)	Interval (h)
Phenylpropionic Acid			
Ibuprofen	Motrin, Advil, Nuprin	400–800	6
Naproxen	Naprosyn	250–375	6–8
Naproxen sodium	Anaprox, Aleve	220–550*	6–12
Ketoprofen	Orudis	50–75	6–8
Flurbiprofen	Ansaid	50	6
Oxaprozin	Daypro	600	24
Phenylacetic Acid			
Indomethacin	Indocin	25–50	6–8
Diclofenac potassium	Cataflam	50	8
Fenamate			
Mefenamic acid	Ponstel	250†	6
Oxicam			
Piroxicam	Feldene	20‡	24
Pyrroleacetic Acid			
Tolmetin	Tolectin	400	8

*Starting dose 550 mg followed by 275 mg every 6 to 8 h or 550 mg every 12 h.
†Starting dose 500 mg followed by 250 mg every 8 h.
‡Not a first line choice. Although therapeutic effect can be seen early, steady-state blood levels are not achieved for 7 to 12 days.
Adapted from Barnhart KT, Sondheimer SJ: Dysmenorrhea. *In* Rakel RE (ed): Conn's Current Therapy 1995. Philadelphia, WB Saunders, 1995, p 999.

be encouraged to try simple comfort measures such as heating pads, back massage, warm baths, and hot herbal tea.

It is worth noting that dysmenorrhea is a common complaint that leads women to consult complementary medical specialists such as acupuncturists, herbalists, homeopathists, and chiropractors. Some studies suggest that as many as a third of patients have tried complementary medical therapy at least once and are often embarrassed or defensive about informing their physicians of that fact. Patients should be encouraged to seek out any reputable therapeutic intervention and share their experiences with their physicians.

Not everyone with menstrual pain gains relief from medical therapy. Failure of a three-cycle trial of oral contraceptives and/or NSAIDs should lead to a repeat pelvic examination and probably referral to a gynecologist for consideration of a diagnostic laparoscopy and hysteroscopy. Among patients with a negative pelvic examination, endometriosis, pelvic adhesions, and submucous myomas are the most common treatable causes of refractory dysmenorrhea.

Approximately 20% of those with menstrual pain and no sign of pelvic pathology still have significant dysmenorrhea despite NSAID and oral contraceptive therapy. There is some evidence to suggest that leukotrienes and/or vasopressin play a role in dysmenorrhea in these women. Although the diagnosis and management of these few patients remain elusive, the vast majority of patients with dysmenorrhea can be managed with widely available medical therapies by the primary care physician.

PREMENSTRUAL SYNDROME

method of
JOSEPH F. MORTOLA, M.D.

Harvard Medical School
Boston, Massachusetts

Recent advances in elucidating the pathophysiology of premenstrual syndrome (PMS) have permitted the development of sound pharmacologic interventions for this previously treatment-resistant disorder. The earlier high failure rates of medical therapy for PMS can largely be attributed to improper diagnosis of the syndrome, overinclusion of patients with poorly characterized symptoms in controlled clinical trials, and underutilization of rigorous experimental methodology in studies of the efficacy of various therapies. Although presently no medications are approved by the U.S. Food and Drug Administration (FDA) for the treatment of PMS, extensive, well-designed studies have been conducted that can guide the clinician's treatment of the disorder. As a result, less proven nonpharmacologic modalities such as dietary modification, exercise regimens, and psychotherapy are more quickly supplanted by the use of medication. Prior to initiation of treatment, however, accurate diagnosis is required, particularly since PMS often mimics other disorders, including depression, anxiety disorders, and thyroid disease.

DIAGNOSIS

The prevalence of PMS is estimated to be 2.5% of women of reproductive age. Although prevalence rates of up to 80% have been reported, this is attributable to the inclusion of a large number of women with normal premenstrual symptoms, referred to as molimina, in the PMS population. Currently, diagnostic criteria are available that permit a more accurate assessment of women in need of medical intervention because of disabling disruption of social, vocational, and avocational performance (Table 1). Even with such strict diagnostic criteria, however, PMS is among the most common disorders in reproductive-age women.

Although more than 150 symptoms have been ascribed to PMS, careful statistical analysis in well-selected populations reveals the symptom constellation to be much more specific and well-defined. Only a select group of symptoms occurs selectively in the luteal phase of the menstrual cycle with sufficient frequency to merit inclusion in the syndrome. The most common of these symptoms are fatigue (92% of women with PMS), irritability (91%), depression (85%), breast tenderness, and bloated sensations in the abdomen or extremities. Appetite disturbance restricted to the luteal phase of the cycle is seen in 75% of women with PMS and is usually experienced as increased food cravings, particularly for carbohydrates. The other frequently noted behavioral symptoms include mood lability with alternating sadness and anger (81%), oversensitivity to trivial environmental events (69%), crying spells (65%), social withdrawal (65%), and difficulty concentrating (47%). Common physical symptoms also include acne (71%) and gastrointestinal upset (48%). Although less often observed, vasomotor flushes (18%), heart palpitations (13%), and dizziness (13%) occur more frequently in women with PMS than in women who do not suffer from the syndrome.

TABLE 1. **Diagnostic Criteria for Premenstrual Syndrome**

1. Presence of self-report of at least one of the following somatic *and* affective symptoms during the 5 days prior to menses in each of the three prior menstrual cycles:

Affective	**Somatic**
Depression	Breast tenderness
Angry outbursts	Abdominal bloating
Irritability	Headache
Anxiety	Swelling
Confusion	
Social withdrawal	

2. Relief of the above symptoms within 4 days of the onset of menses, without recurrence until at least cycle day 12.
3. Presence of the symptoms in the absence of any pharmacologic therapy, hormone ingestion, or drug or alcohol use.
4. Reproducibility of the symptoms during two cycles of prospective recording.
5. Presence of identifiable dysfunction in social or economic performance by one of the following criteria:
   Marital or relationship discord confirmed by partner
   Difficulties in parenting
   Poor work or school performance; poor attendance or tardiness
   Increased social isolation
   Legal difficulties
   Suicidal ideation
   Seeking medical attention for somatic symptoms

From Mortola JF, Girton L, Beck L, et al: Depressive episodes in premenstrual syndrome. Am J Obstet Gynecol *161*:1682, 1984.

None of the symptoms of PMS is unique to the disorder, and even presentation of the entire constellation of symptoms is less important in establishing the diagnosis than is the timing of the symptoms' occurrence with respect to the menstrual cycle. From the fourth day of menses until at least cycle day 12, symptoms, if they occur at all, are sporadic and no more common than would be expected in the general population. This criterion for the relatively symptom-free interval is applicable to most reproductive-age women, although women with menstrual cycles that are typically shorter than 26 days may have the onset of symptoms slightly earlier than day 12. The importance of prospectively documenting symptoms in establishing the diagnosis of PMS has been demonstrated in numerous studies. Validated symptom inventories such as the Calendar of Premenstrual Experiences (University of California, San Diego) are the most reliable methods of establishing the diagnosis (Figure 1). Prospective recording over the course of two menstrual cycles is optimal in order to assure reproducibility in the timing of symptoms. Scores on such inventories should reveal at least a twofold increase in total symptom severity during the last week of the menstrual cycle as compared with the second week.

In addition to the type of symptoms and their timing, several other criteria should be fulfilled in order to accurately diagnose PMS. These include the identifiable presence of socioeconomic difficulties and the absence of pharmacologic therapy with hormonal agents such as oral contraceptives.

DIFFERENTIAL DIAGNOSIS

The differential diagnosis of PMS includes a rather large number of medical and psychiatric disorders. Fortunately, the majority of these can be easily excluded by use of a prospective symptom calendar, history and physical examination, and simple laboratory investigation. In a study of 263 women presenting with the complaint of PMS, the use of oral contraceptives was found to confound the diagnosis in 10.6%. Early menopause was found in 10.2%. The most common disorders were depression and anxiety disorders, which were observed in 30.5%. These were easily identified by the absence of a symptom-free interval by either self-reporting or on prospective recording. Eating disorders were observed in 5.3%, and substance abuse disorders in 3.8%. Medical conditions, the most common of which were diabetes and thyroid disease, were found in 8.6%. Menstrual cycle irregularities were obtained by history in 16.6%. Because of the medical conditions and perimenopausal conditions that may present as PMS, laboratory evaluation should include serum glucose, thyroid-stimulating hormone, and follicle-stimulating hormone.

PATHOPHYSIOLOGY

PMS is a psychoneuroendocrine disorder that has recently been the subject of considerable scientific investigation. There is extensive evidence that the pathophysiologic basis of PMS is primarily the result of changes in central nervous system neurotransmitter economy that are induced by cyclical fluctuations in ovarian steroid (estrogen and progesterone) levels. There is currently a basis for implicating adrenergic, opioid, gamma-aminobutyric acid (GABA), and serotonin systems in the behavioral manifestations as well as the physical manifestations of PMS. Each of these neurotransmitter systems has been demonstrated to be influenced by estrogen and/or progesterone. The reason that women show different degrees of sensitivity to these ovarian steroid-induced neurotransmitter alterations, however, remains unknown. It is more likely that these differences in susceptibility are biologically endowed than that they are the result of environmental contingencies.

TREATMENT

Selective Serotonin Reuptake Inhibitors

Selective serotonin reuptake inhibitors (SSRIs)* are the first-line pharmacologic intervention for PMS. SSRIs are a novel class of antidepressants that act with relative specificity on the serotonergic system and hence differ from the majority of antidepressants, which have simultaneous effects on several neurotransmitter systems. Unlike SSRIs, classic antidepressants are remarkably ineffective in the treatment of PMS; in fact, they show even less efficacy in some studies than placebo. This is consistent with data that PMS and depression have distinct neuroendocrine manifestations.

Fluoxetine (Prozac) is the SSRI that has been most studied in PMS. It has been demonstrated in independent, double-blind, placebo-controlled studies to have a success rate of 90% in the 85% of patients who can tolerate the medication. This yields an overall response rate of 75%. The clinical demonstration of the efficacy of SSRIs in PMS is supported by the finding of differences in serotonin markers in women with PMS and fluctuations of serotonin levels during the menstrual cycle. The effective dose of fluoxetine is 20 mg daily. It is best taken in the morning, as it is generally an activating drug. In a minority of patients, it is sedating, and these individuals are best treated with an evening or bedtime regimen. Although it is safe to prescribe 60 to 80 mg per day in single or divided doses, the vast majority of patients respond to a 20-mg dose. Widely publicized reports of an increased risk of suicidal or homicidal behavior in patients who are on fluoxetine have been refuted in careful studies. Nonetheless, patient acceptance of the drug continues to be a problem. Reassurance that the earlier reports are unsubstantiated is often required. Recently, a small study suggested that fluoxetine administration in patients with PMS may be limited to the luteal phase. In clinical practice, the medication is started on day 14 of the menstrual cycle and continued until day 2 of the following cycle. This is a desirable method of initiating therapy, since smaller total monthly doses are required. Not infrequently, patients are unable to tolerate a full 20-mg dose of fluoxetine with either luteal-phase-only administration or full-cycle administration. In these patients, doses as small as 5 mg per day should be prescribed initially. Fluoxetine is available in a convenient elixir form for this purpose. In addition to fluoxetine, clinical trials have demonstrated the efficacy of other SSRIs, including sertraline and paroxetine. These are normally used as second-line inter-

---

*Not FDA-approved for this indication.

Name _________________________________ Month/Year _________ Age _________ Unit #_________________

Begin your calendar on the *first* day of your menstrual cycle. Enter the calendar date below the cycle day. Day 1 is your *first* day of bleeding. Shade the box above the cycle day if you have bleeding. ■ Put an X for spotting. ⊠

If more than one symptom is listed in a category, i.e., nausea, diarrhea, constipation, you do not need to experience all of these. Rate the most disturbing of the symptoms on the 1-3 scale.

Weight: Weigh yourself before breakfast. Record weight in the box below date.
Symptoms: Indicate the severity of your symptoms by using the scale below. Rate each symptom at about the same time each evening.

  0 = **None** (symptom not present) 2 = **Moderate** (interferes with normal activities)
  1 = **Mild** (noticeable but not troublesome) 3 = **Severe** (intolerable, unable to perform normal activities)

Other Symptoms: If there are other symptoms you experience, list and indicate severity.
Medications: List any medications taken. Put an X on the corresponding day(s).

	1	2	3	4	5	6	7	8	9	10	11	12	13	14	15	16	17	18	19	20	21	22	23	24	25	26	27	28	29	30	31	32	33	34	35	36	37	38	39	40
Bleeding																																								
Cycle Day	1	2	3	4	5	6	7	8	9	10	11	12	13	14	15	16	17	18	19	20	21	22	23	24	25	26	27	28	29	30	31	32	33	34	35	36	37	38	39	40
Date																																								
Weight																																								
SYMPTOMS																																								
Acne																																								
Bloatedness																																								
Breast tenderness																																								
Dizziness																																								
Fatigue																																								
Headache																																								
Hot flashes																																								
Nausea, diarrhea, constipation																																								
Palpitations																																								
Swelling (hands, ankles, breast)																																								
Angry outbursts, arguments, violent tendencies																																								
Anxiety, tension, nervousness																																								
Confusion, difficulty concentrating																																								
Crying easily																																								
Depression																																								
Food cravings (sweets, salts)																																								
Forgetfulness																																								
Irritability																																								
Increased appetite																																								
Mood swings																																								
Overly sensitive																																								
Wish to be alone																																								
Other Symptoms																																								
1. _______																																								
2. _______																																								
Medications																																								
1. _______																																								
2. _______																																								

Figure 1. Calendar of Premenstrual Experiences (COPE). (© University of California, San Diego; Department of Reproductive Medicine, Division of Reproductive Endocrinology.)

ventions because of the more extensive clinical information available on fluoxetine.

Approximately 15% of patients taking SSRIs experience side effects of sufficient severity or discomfort to warrant discontinuation of the drug. The most commonly reported side effects are agitation or insomnia, gastrointestinal disturbance and headache, and sexual dysfunction, which may include loss of libido, impotence, and anorgasmia. Each of these occurs with sufficient severity to require discontinuation of treatment in approximately 5% of patients. A larger percentage of patients experience these symptoms to lesser degrees.

The most commonly observed side effect of SSRIs is headache. This occurs in up to 20% of patients. Often the headaches resolve during the first 2 weeks of therapy. A variety of gastrointestinal complaints have been noted in up to 15% of patients on fluoxetine. These most commonly include nausea and diarrhea. Approximately 9% of patients on fluoxetine report marked anorexia. In patients with PMS, this has not been noted to a degree that warrants discontinuation of the drug. Rarely, hematologic disturbances, including anemia and thrombocytopenia, as well as alterations in liver enzymes have been observed in patients on SSRIs. These do not occur with sufficient frequency to mandate routine monitoring of asymptomatic patients.

The incidence of a decline in libido during treatment with SSRIs is reported to be approximately 2% in studies of depressed patients. However, this may be falsely low due to the already decreased libido that usually accompanies depression. In nondepressed patients, it appears that decreased libido is more commonly noted, particularly in women with PMS.

Although large doses of SSRIs given to animals have not been associated with birth defects, human studies are lacking. The use of fluoxetine in pregnant or breast-feeding patients should therefore be discouraged. Contraception is recommended for patients with PMS treated with SSRIs.

Benzodiazepines

At least two double-blind studies have demonstrated the efficacy of alprazolam (Xanax)* in the treatment of PMS. The usual dose is 0.25 mg four times a day during the luteal phase of the cycle. Occasionally, higher doses of 0.5 mg up to four times a day are required. Although efficacy has been demonstrated at these doses, clinically, many patients report significant improvement when the medication is taken during the luteal phase on an as-needed basis.

The side effect of greatest concern is alprazolam's addictive potential. This has prompted a number of clinicians to substitute other benzodiazepines for alprazolam in the treatment of PMS. Although there is a sound theoretical rationale to posit that other

benzodiazepines may have an efficacy similar to that of alprazolam based on their biochemical similarity, this has not been demonstrated in controlled studies. Moreover, although alprazolam may be more addictive than some other benzodiazepines, all agents in this class carry a substantial risk of addiction. For this reason, the use of benzodiazepines in PMS should be carefully restricted to luteal-phase administration in reliable patients. Addiction to alprazolam has not been reported when restricted to use during this prescribed interval.

Withdrawal symptoms similar to those observed with barbiturates have been noted on discontinuation of alprazolam prescribed on a daily basis. These can range from mild anxiety, dysphoria, and/or insomnia to more severe manifestations of muscle cramps, nausea, perspiration, and tremor. Withdrawal seizures have also been reported. Patients with underlying seizure disorders are not candidates for alprazolam because of the repeated alteration in the seizure threshold induced by the cyclical initiation and discontinuation of the drug.

In addition to addiction, three other side effects of alprazolam are frequently observed. Drowsiness occurs in up to 40% of patients. This symptom sometimes resolves after a period of weeks on the medication. Lowering the dose and using a more frequent dosing schedule are often successful in relieving this side effect. Approximately 5% of individuals on alprazolam have hypotension. Lightheadedness has also been reported in a similar number of individuals. Discontinuation of therapy is less commonly required in individuals experiencing the latter two side effects. A number of more idiosyncratic symptoms have been reported in patients on alprazolam. Among the most disturbing of these is paradoxic agitation. This usually resolves only by stopping the drug.

Administration of alprazolam has not been demonstrated to be safe in pregnancy and has been reported to cause lethargy in the infants of nursing mothers. Women on this agent for PMS should be instructed to use reliable methods of birth control.

GnRH Agonists*

In 1984, Muse and colleagues published the first results demonstrating a dramatic reduction of symptoms in women with PMS using daily injections of a gonadotropin-releasing hormone (GnRH) agonist. Since that time, several other reports using different GnRH agonists have confirmed these results. GnRH agonists cause pituitary desensitization to native GnRH, which is thought to be the result of internalization of the GnRH receptor. Depending on the potency of the agonist, the desensitization phase (termed down-regulation) requires 7 to 21 days. Once down-regulation has been established, it persists for as long as the agonist is administered. During down-regulation, luteinizing hormone (LH) and follicle-stimulating hormone (FSH) secretion by the pitu-

---

*Not FDA-approved for this indication.

*Not FDA-approved for this indication.

itary is substantially reduced. As a result, there is insufficient stimulation of the ovary for normal sex steroid production. Circulating estrogen levels are therefore in the postmenopausal range, and progesterone levels are similarly low.

The daily subcutaneous injection form of GnRH agonists is cumbersome for the patient. Administration of GnRH analogues may be associated with localized pain and irritation at the injection site. More recently, depot formulations of the compounds have become available. These are administered as monthly intramuscular injections. A nasal spray has also been formulated that is available for two- or three-times-a-day use. Although the nasal spray is less uncomfortable than subcutaneous administration, absorption may be somewhat more erratic, and patient reliability becomes a greater concern.

In women, the side effect profile of GnRH agonists is largely the result of hypoestrogenism. Most women on the medication experience significant hot flashes. These are generally classic postmenopausal hot flashes that last for minutes and tend to be more pronounced on the upper torso and face. The hot flashes tend to be most bothersome at the initiation of the down-regulation phase. In some women, they continue to be highly disturbing, but in others, their perceived severity decreases over weeks to months.

The acute menopausal syndrome includes emotional lability and insomnia in addition to hot flashes. In general, these symptoms tend to be less disturbing than the symptoms of severe PMS.

The long-term use of GnRH analogues is limited by the effects of chronic hypoestrogenism. The most pronounced of these is osteoporosis. As a result, use of GnRH analogues is limited to a period of 6 months unless accompanied by serial bone densitometry to demonstrate maintenance of bone integrity. There is also concern regarding the long-term consequences of negating the putative protective effect of estrogen on cardiovascular disease in women. Large epidemiologic studies are required to quantify this risk. Other symptoms of menopause, although not posing health risks, are also of concern when prescribing GnRH analogues. These include vaginal dryness, an increase in urinary tract symptoms, and a decrease in skin collagen content.

Given the association between breast and gynecologic cancers and ovarian function, there is a potential protective effect of long-term GnRH agonist administration on breast, ovarian, and endometrial carcinoma risk. Proof of this association also awaits large-scale epidemiologic studies.

In order to reverse the potential side effects of GnRH agonist administration, low-dose estrogen and progestin replacement therapy, similar to that used in postmenopausal women, has been advocated. Since almost all the short- and long-term side effects of the therapy are the result of this hypoestrogenism, this approach is based on a sound rationale. There is substantial evidence to suggest that this "add-back" therapy may maintain the majority of the beneficial effects of GnRH agonists on the symptoms of PMS.

TREATMENTS OF UNPROVEN EFFICACY

Progesterone*

Until recently, progesterone given in the form of vaginal or rectal suppositories was widely prescribed for PMS. This was based on uncontrolled studies. Progesterone has now been shown to be no more effective than placebo in treating PMS symptoms. Moreover, there is evidence that both the physical and the emotional symptoms of PMS may be progesterone induced. Thus, administration of progesterone commonly results in increased breast tenderness, bloating of the abdomen and extremities, and emotional lability. The use of progesterone in the treatment of PMS cannot be advocated.

Oral Contraceptives*

The success of treating PMS with oral contraceptive agents has not been consistent. For the most part, the side effects of oral contraceptive agents, including mood effects (particularly depression), water retention, and appetite changes, are precisely those that women with PMS experience. There appears to be a small percentage of women for whom oral contraceptives provide a preferable hormonal milieu to their endogenous estrogen and progesterone. In general, however, these agents are not effective in the treatment of PMS.

Vitamin B$_6$*

At least one placebo-controlled study of vitamin B$_6$ in PMS showed efficacy, although other studies failed to replicate these results. The efficacy of vitamin B$_6$ therapy in the syndrome is therefore controversial. At high doses (>600 mg per day), vitamin B$_6$ therapy has been associated with peripheral neuropathy. If this therapy is tried in PMS, patients must be cautioned against excess dosages.

Diet and Dietary Supplements

Multiple dietary supplements have been attempted in PMS, including magnesium, linoleic acid in the form of evening primrose oil, and multiple vitamin regimens. None of these has proved effective in treating PMS. Dietary restriction, such as the elimination of caffeine and chocolate, has not been demonstrated to be effective in PMS either.

DRUGS USED FOR SPECIFIC INDICATIONS

Premenstrual Migraines and Danazol

Although several reports have indicated the efficacy of danazol (Danocrine)* in PMS, since the advent of GnRH analogues, its use has been largely restricted to the treatment of premenstrual mi-

---

*Not FDA-approved for this indication.

graines. Danazol is a derivative of the synthetic androgen 17-alpha-ethinyl testosterone. As such, it possesses significant androgenic properties. Administration of danazol results in amenorrhea in a majority of women. The objective of therapy is to obtain the beneficial effects that occur secondary to this amenorrhea. The usual dose is 600 to 800 mg per day in divided doses. The side effect profile of danazol is considerable and is the result of both its androgenic activity and its antiestrogen properties. Acne and weight gain are commonly reported. Decreased breast size is a particularly disturbing complaint for many women. More rarely, overtly masculinizing side effects are noted, including deepening of the voice and clitoromegaly. Fluid retention on danazol therapy is particularly disturbing to women with PMS.

The antiestrogenic side effects, although better tolerated by most women than the androgen effects, can be quite bothersome. These are the same side effects observed with GnRH analogues and include hot flashes, vaginal dryness, and emotional lability. Although the osteoporosis that accompanies GnRH agonist therapy is less of a concern with danazol, the effects on lipid profiles are more worrisome. This is due to the combined adverse effects of hypoestrogenism and hyperandrogenism. For this reason, the use of danazol should be accompanied by monitoring of lipid profiles.

Danazol is contraindicated during pregnancy because of in utero female pseudohermaphroditism. There have also been reports of hepatotoxicity, manifested by increased liver function tests, while on danazol. Therefore, liver function studies should be monitored periodically in patients taking this drug. Taken together, approximately 80% of women on danazol experience side effects.

Based on the risk/benefit ratio, danazol is a poor choice for most patients with PMS. Overall, it is less efficacious and has many more side effects than GnRH analogues. Danazol may be somewhat more effective, however, in treating premenstrual migraines than are GnRH analogues. But because there are conventional, effective antimigraine medications with fewer side effects than danazol, danazol should not be considered a first-line agent even in premenstrual migraines.

Water Retention and Diuretics

Of the diuretics that have been used in PMS, spironolactone (Aldactone) has achieved the greatest popularity. This is largely the result of specific properties of this agent that are uniquely suited to hormonally based disorders. Spironolactone is an aldosterone inhibitor. As such, it shares considerable structural similarity with steroid hormones. Because of its steroidal properties and diuretic effects, spironolactone showed promise as an effective agent in the treatment of PMS. It was hypothesized that the inhibition of steroidogenesis seen with this agent might also improve hormonally related mood changes as well as

the physical symptoms of breast tenderness, water retention, and weight gain that accompany PMS. Overall, the results achieved with spironolactone have been disappointing, and it appears to be a mildly helpful agent at best. Nonetheless, because of its antisteroidal properties, it remains the diuretic most often chosen in the treatment of the water-retention symptoms of PMS.

Because of its aldosterone antagonist activity, spironolactone is a potassium-sparing diuretic. Patients should therefore be warned against taking potassium supplements while using this medication. Hypotensive effects are rarely observed in healthy young women.

Spironolactone has been associated with a number of side effects in women. They occur rarely, but when they do occur, gastrointestinal symptoms are the most common. Central nervous system side effects also occasionally occur, including drowsiness, lethargy, headache, and mental confusion. Because of its inhibition of steroid synthesis, irregular menses are not uncommon in patients taking spironolactone daily.

Many of the side effects of spironolactone have been noted with long-term daily administration. In general, adverse reactions are fewer when use is limited to the luteal phase of the cycle. Because spironolactone is now used primarily to treat the water-retention symptoms of PMS, therapy can be limited to short-term administration—usually for 7 to 10 days in the luteal phase of the cycle. Many of the agents that are most effective in treating overall PMS symptoms, particularly the mood and appetite disturbances, are less effective in relieving the water-retention symptoms of bloating and breast tenderness. In these cases, spironolactone provides a relatively safe adjunctive therapy.

Other diuretics have also been tried in PMS, with variable success in alleviating the water-retention symptoms. For the most part, these are reserved for spironolactone failures or those individuals with significant side effects from spironolactone. The most commonly used class of diuretics after spironolactone is the thiazides. Thiazide diuretics are often combined with an antikaliuretic agent such as triamterene. Even with these preparations, however, hypokalemia remains the major concern. Not uncommonly, diuretics are abused by women who become highly concerned about their weight. Particularly in women with PMS who are concerned about bloating, cautions about the overuse of diuretics should be stressed.

In addition to hypokalemia, thiazide diuretics are occasionally associated with anaphylactic responses, hematologic and central nervous system disturbances, and serious cardiac arrhythmias. Fortunately, these are rare events.

Overall, the side effect profile is better and the dosage tolerance range is higher with spironolactone than with thiazide diuretics. For this reason, as well as the potential for some beneficial effects exerted by its antisteroid properties, spironolactone remains the diuretic of choice for PMS. The use of more potent diuretics or low-dose thiazides in patients with PMS should be discouraged.

MENOPAUSE

method of
ROBERT W. REBAR, M.D.
College of Medicine, University of Cincinnati
Cincinnati, Ohio

Women often seek the advice of their physicians at the time of menopause regarding the possible benefits of so-called hormone replacement therapy (HRT) or estrogen replacement therapy (ERT). Although administration is not indicated for all postmenopausal women, the available evidence indicates that the benefits outweigh the risks for most women. Despite the apparent ability of estrogen to improve the quality of postmenopausal life for many women, most discontinue its use after only a short time. The reasons for stopping therapy are many but include the development of side effects, fear of cancer, intermittent uterine bleeding, and, for those without symptoms, failure to note any evidence of benefit. Because of such poor compliance, it is important to provide appropriate information to patients and to involve them in decisions regarding HRT. Treatment must clearly be individualized. Moreover, it is important to recognize that the recommendations outlined here may change as information about menopause and HRT continues to accumulate.

There is no question that exogenous estrogen replacement stops or diminishes hot flashes and night sweats and prevents or reverses atrophic genital changes. Exogenous estrogens also slow bone loss after menopause and decrease the frequency of osteoporotic fractures. Estrogens appear to have a protective effect against the development of atherosclerotic coronary artery disease as well.

It is the possibility of an increased risk of developing breast cancer that most frightens women about using HRT. At this point, the data are inconclusive, with some studies showing an increased risk and others failing to document any such tendency. Together, the data suggest that there may be a modest increase in the risk of developing breast cancer after many (more than 8 to 10) years of use. Despite large, ongoing prospective studies, it is unlikely that a definitive answer regarding breast cancer will be available soon, if ever. The sensitivity and the ability of epidemiologic methods to absolutely identify and quantify such modest increases in risk are limited. These findings should reassure clinicians and their patients regarding HRT and breast cancer risk, especially if HRT's ability to prevent atherosclerotic coronary artery disease is as great as it appears to be from retrospective studies. (an approximately 50% decrease in risk). These factors, all the other benefits

and risks of HRT, and the quality of life of the individual woman must be considered.

CONTRAINDICATIONS TO HRT

Regarded as absolute contraindications to exogenous estrogen are unexplained genital bleeding, active thromboembolic disease, impaired liver function, uncontrolled hypertension, porphyria, and estrogen-dependent cancer. Yet many clinicians now support the administration of exogenous estrogen to postmenopausal women with previously treated well-differentiated Stage I endometrial carcinoma and to those with a history of more advanced disease who have no evidence of recurrence 5 or more years after treatment. Even views about the administration of estrogens to women with a history of breast cancer are changing. There seems to be little point in withholding estrogen from women with widely disseminated breast cancer who suffer from the signs and symptoms of severe estrogen deficiency as well. Patients with a low risk of recurrence, including those more than 5 years from diagnosis without evidence of disease, those with ductal carcinoma in situ, those without any positive axillary nodes, those with tumor size less than 1 cm, those who are estrogen receptor negative, and those with well-differentiated (nuclear Grade I) tumors, might be especially good candidates for HRT if they are symptomatic. Obviously it would be prudent to attempt other approaches to control symptoms (discussed subsequently), and physicians need to support the individual patient in her decision to take or not take estrogen if other approaches are unsuccessful, particularly because the risk is unknown. Most studies examining the issue have failed to find an increased risk of breast cancer among estrogen users with a family history of breast cancer or a history of benign breast disease.

Relative contraindications to estrogen administration include diabetes mellitus, cholecystitis and cholelithiasis, pancreatitis, significant hypertriglyceridemia, endometriosis, leiomyomas, and migraine headaches. Although hyperinsulinemia, chronic hyperglycemia, insulin resistance, and diabetes mellitus are independent risk factors for cardiovascular disease morbidity and mortality and are direct causative factors for premature mortality from coronary artery disease, there is no evidence that HRT accelerates the progression of diabetes. In fact, estrogen may help prevent or retard atherosclerosis. Women with a history of endometriosis typically do well with low doses of estrogen but may benefit from continuous administration of a progestin with the estrogen. Most women with uterine fibroids do not experience any significant increase in tumor size with the low doses of estrogen administered to postmenopausal women. Convincing data indicate that at least some migraine headaches in women (i.e., menstrual migraines) are caused by estrogen withdrawal; in controlled trials, addition of estrogen at menses prevented the headaches. Thus, administering estrogen to postmenopausal migraine sufferers is not contraindicated and may reduce the frequency and severity of attacks. In the unlikely event that headaches worsen with estrogen therapy, consideration should be given to discontinuing the estrogen. Because migraine headaches may be due to fluctuations in circulating estrogen levels, consideration should be given to using a form of estrogen that produces relatively stable blood levels.

There is no absolute contraindication to administering estrogen to women with a past history of venous or arterial thromboembolism, but each patient must be considered individually. If the thromboembolism occurred many years earlier and was of a nonrecurring nature, such as following an auto accident or surgery, HRT should be safe. Individuals at high risk of recurrent thromboembolism may be treated with transdermal estrogen, as there is little effect on liver enzymes.

There appears to be no contraindication to providing estrogen to women with controlled hypertension. If a woman develops hypertension shortly after beginning therapy, it is wise to discontinue therapy to determine whether antihypertensive medications are required. HRT can be started again once the blood pressure has stabilized (with treatment, as necessary). Here, too, a transdermal form of estrogen may be used to decrease any estrogenic stimulation of hepatic synthesis of renin substrate, the mechanism by which estrogen is believed to elevate blood pressure in a small percentage of women.

PREPARATIONS OF ESTROGENS AND PROGESTINS

There are several types of estrogens. Naturally occurring estrogens—including estradiol (Estrace), estrone, and conjugated equine estrogens (Premarin), composed of several different estrogens, with estrone sulfate being the most abundant—are the estrogens usually provided for replacement therapy. Synthetic estrogens, including ethinyl estradiol and mestranol (present in combination oral contraceptive [OC] preparations), and nonsteroidal estrogens such as diethylstilbestrol (DES) usually are not used for ERT.

Estrogen can be administered in several different ways, but not all forms are currently available in the United States. Estrogens are most commonly prescribed as oral preparations, with conjugated equine estrogen being provided most frequently. A daily dose of 0.625 mg is generally effective in eliminating complaints in most postmenopausal women. Approximately equivalent oral alternatives include estropipate sulfate (Ogen) at a dose of 0.625 to 1.25 mg, which has less of an effect on renin substrate, and micronized estradiol (Estrace) at a dose of 1.0 mg. It is important to realize that 0.625 mg of conjugated estrogen is approximately equivalent to 5 µg of ethinyl estradiol (Estinyl). Considering that all the effects—and side effects—of estrogen are dose related and that the lowest dose of ethinylestradiol contained in any combination OC agent is 20 µg, the reason for using ERT in postmenopausal women rather than a combination OC is obvious. Conjugated equine estrogens can still be detected in the circulation 4 to 6 weeks after the last tablet is ingested; thus, missing one or a few days of therapy may not lead to the appearance of symptoms of estrogen deficiency. In contrast, estradiol is rapidly cleared from the circulation, and women may begin to complain of hot flushes after missing just a single tablet.

Transdermal patches of estradiol (Estraderm) allow direct absorption but must be worn as long as systemic levels of estrogen are desired, because the effect is not sustained. Transdermal estradiol has the advantage of producing much more constant levels of circulating estrone and estradiol than any of the oral preparations. As noted previously, it also has much less of an effect in inducing liver enzymes, because the "first-pass effect" in the liver, resulting in absorption through the gastrointestinal tract, is avoided. The most frequent side effect of transdermal patches is skin irritation. A patch of 0.05 mg transdermal estradiol is approximately equivalent to 0.625 mg of conjugated estrogen.

It is clear that both oral and transdermal forms of estrogen protect against the development of osteoporosis. Less clear is whether transdermal estradiol is as effective as oral forms of estrogen in protecting against cardiovascular disease. Transdermal estradiol appears to be less effective than oral estrogens in favorably altering the ratio of HDL- to LDL-cholesterol. But because it now appears that estrogens exert their apparent cardioprotective effects through a variety of mechanisms, and not just through an effect on HDL- and LDL-cholesterol, it is possible that transdermal estradiol is as effective as the oral forms of estrogen in protecting against cardiovascular disease.

Estrogens are absorbed even better from the vaginal mucosa than they are from the gastrointestinal tract. However, because it is difficult, if not impossible, to regulate the quantity of estrogen cream absorbed, such creams cannot be recommended for systemic therapy. It is fallacious to think that estrogen creams are not absorbed systemically; conversely, systemic estrogens affect the vaginal mucosa. It has been known for several years that estradiol tablets placed in the vagina lead to absorption of twice as much estrogen as when they are ingested orally. Here too, the "first-pass effect" is avoided; only in this situation are circulating levels of estradiol greater than those of estrone. Estradiol and estrone are interconvertible, and even when pure estradiol is administered, significant conversion to estrone occurs.

Long-acting injectable forms of estrogen cannot be recommended because of the extremely high circulating levels of estrogen achieved shortly after injection. Other forms of estrogen are currently under investigation, including vaginal rings containing estradiol, sublingual tablets, estradiol gels, and subcutaneous pellets.

Most postmenopausal women develop breast tenderness when estrogen is first administered. In all but a very small percentage of women, the tenderness abates in less than 4 weeks. If it does not, the dose of estrogen is probably too high for that patient. Individuals in whom symptoms of estrogen deficiency continue after 3 to 4 weeks of therapy probably require additional estrogen.

A few women continue to complain of symptoms of estrogen deficiency with even large doses of estrogens. In such circumstances, it is wise to change to a different preparation. Utilizing estrone sulfate or estradiol permits accurate measurement of circulating levels of estradiol to document the use of estrogen. For women who present on massive doses of estrogen, it may be necessary to discontinue therapy for 4 to 6 weeks and reinitiate estrogen therapy with a different preparation to eliminate the symptoms of estrogen deficiency. Perhaps the very large doses of estrogen down-regulate estrogen receptors and make therapy ineffective.

At the present time, progestin is administered only orally in the United States as part of HRT. The most commonly prescribed progestin is medroxyprogesterone acetate (MPA [Provera]), and the daily dose for which most data exist is 10 mg. This dose is not tolerated by as many as 25% of women; complaints include bloating, depression, acne, breast tenderness, and symptoms commonly associated with premenstrual tension. Beginning with a daily dose of 5 mg and increasing to a dose of 10 mg per day in women who have no complaints reduces the number of women who discontinue therapy. In some women with side effects, it may be necessary to reduce the daily dose to 2.5 mg of MPA. Norgestrel (Ovrette)* 150 to 500 μg and norethindrone and norethindrone acetate (Aygestin)* 1 to 5 mg are commonly used in Europe, but these 19-norsteroids lower the ratio of high-density to low-density lipoproteins more than MPA and are not commonly used in the United States. However, the effect on lipoproteins may not be significant with the use of lower doses, and 1 mg of norethindrone or norethindrone acetate appears to be sufficient to transform estrogen-stimulated endometrium to secretory. Unfortunately, norethindrone is available only in 0.35-mg tablets (for use as progestin-only contraceptive pills), and as 5-mg tablets, and norethindrone acetate is available only as scored 5-mg tablets. There should rarely, if ever, be any need to administer more than 2.5 mg daily. A 19-norsteroid may be tried in women who continue to complain of side effects with even 2.5 mg of MPA.

The use of oral micronized progesterone 200 to 300 mg daily is now under investigation. This preparation is well absorbed and has little effect on lipids. Unfortunately, data are insufficient to permit recommendation of this agent at this time. Lethargy and drowsiness have been the significant side effects.

TREATMENT REGIMENS

Although many regimens of hormone replacement are currently in use, none of them is really physio-

logic or "replacement." Estrogen should be given with a progestin to women with uteri to prevent endometrial hyperplasia. Estrogen can be given alone to women with prior hysterectomies to avoid the potential deleterious effects of progestins on lipoproteins. Some clinicians believe that it is advisable to administer both estrogen and progestin continuously to a woman who has had a hysterectomy and bilateral oophorectomy for endometriosis in order to prevent worsening of any remaining endometriosis.

Before beginning HRT, it is advisable to document estrogen deficiency. Generally, the smallest dose of estrogen needed to control the symptoms should be administered. Estrogen should always be prescribed for a limited time to ensure that the patient returns for regular evaluation.

For women with uteri, estrogen and progestin may be administered in one of two manners: cyclically or continuously. Although some clinicians administer the estrogen for only a portion of each month (i.e., for the first 25 days), I believe that it is preferable to administer the estrogen daily. Premenopausal women secrete estrogen every day. Estrogens with a relatively long half-life continue to exert their effects even on the occasional days when the patient forgets to take her medication, whereas if a short-acting estrogen is used, patients may quickly develop symptoms of estrogen deficiency (most commonly hot flashes and night sweats) during days when no medication is taken.

If the HRT is administered cyclically, the progestin can be administered for the first 12 to 14 days of the month. Available evidence indicates that a progestin must be administered for 12 or more days each month to maximize its effectiveness in preventing the development of endometrial hyperplasia. Because it is preferable to have a woman be compliant with the HRT, I am willing to reduce the dose of progestin as outlined previously, even in the absence of data regarding the effect on the prevention of endometrial hyperplasia.

Because it appears that the length of time that the progestin is administered is more important than the daily dose, trials are now under way in several parts of the world to determine how frequently the progestin must be administered. Published studies to date suggest that administering progestin for 2 weeks every 3 to 4 months may be sufficient to protect the endometrium. Because the vast majority of women given HRT in a cyclical fashion have withdrawal bleeding in response to the progestin, another presumed advantage to administering the progestin less frequently is less frequent menses. However, published reports also indicate that the incidence of unexpected spotting and bleeding is significantly increased in women taking the progestin every 3 months. Although I have no difficulty administering the progestin for the first 2 weeks of every other month to reliable patients and find that there is virtually no breakthrough bleeding, I am reluctant to recommend this practice for routine use in the absence of good data documenting efficacy. For

---

*Not FDA-approved for this indication.

women who have significant side effects when taking progestin, however, and for those who particularly dislike the bleeding, providing progestin every other month may be a reasonable option.

Continuous therapy with an estrogen and a progestin was suggested initially in an attempt to eliminate the bleeding that commonly occurs with cyclical therapy. The ideal ratio of estrogen to progestin has not yet been determined, and regimens commonly in use have been developed empirically. Irregular breakthrough bleeding is common in the majority of women utilizing continuous combined therapy for at least the first few months of therapy. Irregular bleeding is much less common among those women who are several years postmenopausal when they begin continuous combined therapy. As a consequence, many clinicians begin women on sequential therapy and then change them to continuous combined therapy after several years of hormone replacement. The likelihood of continuous amenorrhea increases with the months of therapy. Thus, clinicians need to be supportive of women who have bleeding during the first several months of therapy.

The major difficulty with continuous combined therapy for clinicians is deciding when and if to biopsy individuals who bleed. If menses were regular or absent or if a biopsy was performed prior to the institution of therapy, then there is little reason to biopsy any woman who bleeds during the first 6 months of therapy. Women who bleed after 6 or more months of amenorrhea while on therapy probably warrant biopsy. There should be no reason to biopsy any woman more frequently than every 6 months regardless of bleeding pattern.

There is no reason to measure circulating levels of either estrogen or gonadotropins in women receiving HRT. The patient serves as a bioassay and is the best indicator of whether the dose is appropriate. Moreover, gonadotropin levels are generally not completely suppressed even with pharmacologic quantities of exogenous steroids, perhaps because of the absence of inhibin secretion by the postmenopausal ovary. Young oophorectomized women may require larger doses of estrogen than do older women in order to eliminate symptoms of estrogen deficiency.

To minimize concerns about accelerated bone loss in postmenopausal and oophorectomized women, it is prudent to ensure that every patient ingests adequate calcium. It is recommended that estrogen-deficient women ingest 1.5 grams of elemental calcium and that premenopausal women and those on HRT ingest 1.0 gram of elemental calcium daily. Weight-bearing exercise should be encouraged, and patients should be advised to consume only moderate quantities of alcohol and to refrain from smoking cigarettes. Both drinking alcohol and smoking cigarettes have a detrimental effect on the rate of bone resorption.

When estrogens are contraindicated in women who suffer from hot flashes or are at risk of osteoporosis, progestin alone is one alternative. Daily doses of 20 to 40 mg of MPA or 40 to 80 mg of megestrol acetate (Megace) are required to alleviate symptoms. If pro-

gestins cannot be utilized, transdermal clonidine (Catapres-TTS)* 0.1 mg per 24 hours may reduce the frequency and severity of hot flashes but may be associated with significant postural hypotension. Any number of vaginal lubricants can be used to reduce vaginal dryness and dyspareunia.

Some clinicians agree that tamoxifen is a better choice than estrogen for symptomatic women with a history of breast cancer. This mixed estrogen agonist-antagonist has been shown to be more effective in preventing bone loss than placebo and to decrease total cholesterol and LDL-cholesterol and to increase triglycerides and (more variably) HDL-cholesterol. It is not clear that tamoxifen is as effective as estrogen in protecting against osteoporosis and cardiovascular disease. Moreover, about 25% of women develop vasomotor symptoms upon taking tamoxifen; those already having hot flashes develop worse symptoms with treatment.

Just how long HRT should be continued is unclear. Recent evidence indicates that estrogen must be provided for many years to provide long-term protection against osteoporosis. Whether estrogen can be stopped at an advanced age is uncertain. Theoretically, it seems logical to discontinue therapy when it no longer provides any benefit. For the present, however, I usually recommend therapy for the duration of a patient's life or until risks outweigh benefits. It is important to emphasize to the patient that recommendations may change from year to year as more knowledge is gained.

It is also reasonable to give HRT to women who are not yet postmenopausal but who complain of episodic symptoms of estrogen deficiency. Documenting intermittently elevated levels of follicle-stimulating hormone in such individuals lends further support to the use of estrogen. Cyclical HRT is often effective in eliminating the irregular menses common in such patients. They must be advised, however, that the dose of steroid administered may not be sufficient to block ovulation. It is important to provide contraception for perimenopausal women who are sexually active.

EVALUATING PATIENTS BEFORE AND DURING THERAPY

A careful history and a complete physical examination, including a Pap smear, should be performed before instituting HRT. Periodic mammograms are indicated in all women over the age of 40 years. Appropriate laboratory tests commonly include evaluation of fasting cholesterol and triglyceride levels at appropriate intervals and assessment of stool guaiac. Fasting blood sugars and electrolytes should be obtained as indicated. Liver function tests should be obtained in women with a past history of liver disease.

Pretreatment endometrial biopsies should be obtained in women with any irregular bleeding and in

---

*Not FDA-approved for this indication.

those at increased risk for endometrial hyperplasia and carcinoma. Women in this latter category include those with a family history of endometrial or breast carcinoma, as well as those who have a long history of amenorrhea or oligomenorrhea during the reproductive years or any history of alcoholism or hepatic disease. Endometrial biopsies are not routinely necessary prior to instituting HRT.

Women beginning HRT should be seen at frequent intervals, perhaps every 4 to 6 weeks, until an appropriate regimen has been established. Frequent visits instill confidence that the clinician is concerned with the patient's welfare and serve to reinforce the benefits and risks of HRT. Patients should be seen 4 to 6 weeks, 6 months, and 1 year after beginning therapy. They should be seen at least yearly thereafter.

A small percentage of women appear to be abnormally sensitive to estrogen and develop an increase in blood pressure shortly after beginning therapy. Estrogen should be discontinued in such patients to see if the hypertension resolves. If medications are required to control the hypertension, the estrogen can be started again after the blood pressure is controlled.

Periodic endometrial biopsies may be indicated in women who take less than 10 mg of MPA for less than 12 days each month. Biopsies are indicated in any woman on unopposed estrogen therapy for a prolonged period and in those with any history of abnormal bleeding on HRT. It has also been suggested that women on cyclical therapy who begin to bleed prior to the eleventh day of progestin require biopsy. The frequency at which biopsies should be performed is unclear and depends in part on the patient's and the physician's anxiety.

At least once a year, women on HRT should be reevaluated with blood pressure measurement, breast and pelvic examinations, Pap smear, and stool guaiac at a minimum. The interval at which mammography is indicated depends on the woman's age and her relative risk for breast cancer.

It is impossible to be dogmatic or rigid in recommending appropriate HRT. The patient must understand that recommendations will change with time. Never before have so many women lived so many productive years after the cessation of reproductive function. Such women warrant therapy that will improve the quality of their lives, and this need has focused attention on HRT.

VULVOVAGINITIS

method of
CHESNEY THOMPSON, M.D., and
JAMES A. McGREGOR, M.D., C.M.
University of Colorado Health Sciences Center
Denver, Colorado

Vaginal infections and other lower reproductive tract infections are among the most common reasons for consulting health care providers among women of reproductive age. Direct care of vaginal infections necessitates the expenditure of billions of dollars annually. Common complications of untreated vaginitis include pelvic inflammatory disease, postoperative pelvic infections, and preterm birth. Symptoms of vulvovaginitis include abnormal discharge, irritation, itching, odor, swelling, and soreness or pain, especially after intercourse. Some patients may not complain of symptoms despite the presence of florid discharge and other findings because of reticence regarding sexual matters or possibly because of the long-standing nature and acquired tolerance of some types of vaginitis.

In one study of nearly 400 female patients, objective evidence of vaginitis was found in 39%. The most common causes of vaginal complaints in family medicine and student health care clinics are bacterial vaginosis (35 to 50%), vaginal candidiasis (25%), and trichomoniasis (20%). Other infections (10%)—including primary genital herpes; bacterial infections with single organisms such as group B or A streptococcus, *Escherichia coli*, or *Staphylococcus aureus*; and a variety of less understood entities, including so-called vestibulitis, cytolytic vaginitis, and desquamative vaginitis—can cause "difficult to treat" vulvovaginitis syndromes. Mucopurulent endocervicitis (most commonly caused by *Chlamydia trachomatis*, *Neisseria gonorrhoeae*, group B streptococcus, and genital mycoplasmas) may also present with increased vaginal discharge and irritation. Infrequently, infections of Bartholin's gland, Skene's glands, endometrium, and the fallopian tubes can cause increased vaginal discharge and inflammation. Vaginal adenosis, retained foreign bodies, and allergic responses can also cause discharge and irritation. Summaries of the presentation, diagnosis, and suggested management of common vaginal infections are shown in Tables 1 to 4.

Lower genital tract infections are also increasingly recognized causes of morbidity and health care expenditures at the extremes of age. Vaginitis in newborns is most frequently caused by maternal vaginal microorganisms acquired during birth; vaginitis in children is frequently caused by microbial pathogens, including group A and B streptococcus and sometimes Enterobacteriaceae, *E. coli*, *Haemophilus influenzae*, *Salmonella* and *Shigella* species, and rarely *Enterobius vermicularis* (pinworm). Retained vaginal foreign bodies are associated with mixed aerobic and anaerobic microflora overgrowth. Bacterial vaginitis in postmenopausal women is most frequently caused by overgrowth of gastrointestinal microflora and/or bacterial vaginosis–associated organisms. Treatment of these infections commonly involves aerobic culture and specific treatment, along with systemic or topical estrogen treatment in estrogen-deficient women.

NORMAL VAGINAL FLORA

Characteristic groups of bacteria are normally present in the healthy vagina. *Lactobacillus* species normally account for more than 95% of vaginal microflora. These "healthy" hydrogen peroxide–producing lactobacilli, most importantly *Lactobacillus jensenii*, produce lactic acid as well as various antimicrobial factors that act to exclude or reduce colonization and possible infection with more pathogenic bacteria. "Healthy" lactobacilli attach avidly to vaginal squamous cells at low pH and exclude or "crowd out" other colonizing species. Usually 5 to 15 other species are recoverable in lesser concentrations, including other aerobic and anaerobic lactobacilli, *Gardnerella vaginalis* (less than 50%), and various aerobic and anaerobic bacteria, as well as *Mycoplasma hominis* (20 to 50%) and *Ureaplasma urealyticum* (50 to 75%) in sexually active women.

TABLE 1. **Presentation of the Three Most Common Causes of Vaginitis**

	Bacterial Vaginosis (BV)	Yeast	Trichomoniasis
Cause	Overgrowth of abnormal BV-associated bacteria	*Candida* yeast	*Trichomonas vaginalis* (parasite)
Vaginal discharge	Thin, milky white or gray	Thick, white, cheesy	Yellow, gray, green-tinged, creamy, purulent
Odor	Sometimes sharp or fishy, especially after intercourse	None	Musty or fishy
Vaginal itching, irritation	Mild or no symptoms	Itching, burning, sometimes intense	Wide variations from asymptomatic to intense itching, burning
Treatment	Antimicrobials, such as metronidazole, clindamycin pills, gels, or creams	Over-the-counter or prescription creams, suppositories, multidose or single-dose pills	Single-dose metronidazole for patient and sex partner(s)

Present understanding suggests that maintenance of healthy lactobacilli and low vaginal pH are mutually reinforcing factors that can reduce infections with various sexually transmitted bacteria, protozoa, and viruses, including HIV-1.

BACTERIAL VAGINOSIS

Bacterial vaginosis (BV) is the most common vaginal infection or condition found in women of reproductive age. It is best understood as a dramatic alteration of vaginal microecology that involves the replacement of healthy lactobacilli with massively (10,000 to 100,000-fold) increased populations of *G. vaginalis* and various characteristic anaerobic bacteria and genital mycoplasmas. Past names for this condition included *G. vaginalis* and *Haemophilus vaginalis* vaginitis. BV is common (12 to 25% in unselected populations) and can be found in children without any prior sexual exposure. Male sex partners

TABLE 2. **Diagnostic Features of Vaginal Infection in Reproductive-Age Women**

	Normal Vaginal Examination	Bacterial Vaginosis	Yeast Vaginitis	Trichomonal Vaginitis
Etiology	Uninfected; *Lactobacillus* predominant	Associated with *Gardnerella vaginalis*, various anaerobic bacteria, and mycoplasma	*Candida albicans* and other yeasts	*Trichomonas vaginalis*
Typical symptoms	None	Malodorous, slightly increased discharge	Vulvar itching and/or irritation	Profuse purulent discharge, vulvar itching
Discharge:				
Amount	Variable; usually scant	Moderate	Scant to moderate	Profuse
Color*	Clear or white	Usually white or gray	White	Purulent, yellowish
Consistency	Nonhomogeneous, floccular	Homogeneous, low viscosity	Clumped, adherent	Homogeneous
Inflammation of vulvar or vaginal epithelium	None	None	Erythema of vaginal epithelium, introitus; vulvar dermatitis common	Erythema of vaginal and vulvar epithelium; colpitis macularis (spot on cervix)
pH of vaginal fluid†	Usually ≤ 4.5	Usually ≥ 4.5	Usually ≤ 4.5	Usually ≥ 5.0
Amine ("fishy" or sharp) odor with 10% potassium hydroxide	None	Present	None	Common
Microscopy‡	Normal epithelial cells; lactobacilli predominate	Clue cells; few leukocytes; lactobacilli outnumbered by profuse mixed flora, nearly always including *G. vaginalis* plus anaerobic species on Gram's stain	Leukocytes, epithelial cells; yeast, mycelia, or pseudomycelia in up to 80%	Leukocytes; motile trichomonads seen in 80–90% of symptomatic patients, less often in the absence of symptoms

*Color of discharge is determined by examining vaginal discharge against the white background of a swab.

†pH determination is not useful if blood is present.

‡To detect fungal elements, vaginal fluid is digested with 10% potassium hydroxide prior to microscopic examination; to examine for other features, fluid is mixed (1:1) with physiologic saline. Gram's stain is also excellent for detecting yeasts and pseudomycelia and for distinguishing normal flora from the mixed flora seen in bacterial vaginosis but is less sensitive than the saline preparation for detection of *T. vaginalis*.

From Holmes KK, Mardh PA, Sparling PF, et al. (eds): Sexually Transmitted Diseases, 2nd ed. New York, McGraw-Hill, 1990. Reproduced by permission of The McGraw-Hill Companies.

TABLE 3. **Recommended Treatments for Common Causes of Vaginitis**

Cause	Generic Name	Trade Name	Dose	Route	Timing
Bacterial vaginosis	Metronidazole	Flagyl	500 mg	PO	bid × 7 days
		Flagyl	2 gm	PO	once
		MetroGel	5 gm 0.75%	Per vagina	bid × 7 days
	Clindamycin	Cleocin	300 mg	PO	tid × 7 days
		Cleocin Cream	5 gm 2.0%	Per vagina	qhs × 7 days
Yeast	Miconazole	Monistat	2% cream	Per vagina	qid × 7 days
		Monistat	1 100-mg suppository	Per vagina	qid × 7 days
		Monistat	1 200-mg suppository	Per vagina	qid × 3 days
	Clotrimazole	Gyne-Lotrimin, Mycelex	1% cream	Per vagina	qid × 7 days
			1 100-mg suppository	Per vagina	qid × 7 days
			2 100-mg suppositories	Per vagina	qid × 7 days
			1 500-mg suppository	Per vagina	qid × 1 day
	Butoconazole	Femstat	2% cream	Per vagina	qid × 3 days
	Terconazole	Terazol	0.4% cream	Per vagina	qid × 7 days
		Terazol	1 80-gm suppository	Per vagina	qid × 3 days
	Fluconazole	Diflucan	150 mg	PO	once
	Ketoconazole	Nizoral	400 mg	PO	qid × 3–7 days
	Nystatin	Mycostatin	100,000 U ointment	Per vagina	qid × 14 days
		Mycostatin	150,000 U tablet	Per vagina	qid × 15 days
	Boric acid		600-mg vaginal capsule	Per vagina	qid × 14 days
Trichomoniasis	Metronidazole	Flagyl	250 mg	PO	tid × 7 days
		Flagyl	2 gm	PO	once
	Clotrimazole	Gyne-Lotrimin, Mycelex	1% cream	Per vagina	qid × 7 days
			1 200-mg suppository	Per vagina	qid × 7 days
Atrophic vaginitis	Estrogen	Premarin	0.3–2.5 conjugated estrogen	Per vagina	qd
		Premarin	5 gm	Per vagina	q × 3 days
		Estrace	.05–.01 mg	Transdermal	q × 3 days
	Estradiol patch	Estraderm	1–2 mg, micronized estrogen	PO	qd
Bacterial vaginitis†	Clindamycin	Cleocin	2% cream	Per vagina	qhs × 7 days
	Ampicillin	—	500 mg	PO	qid × 7–10 days
	Metronidazole	Flagyl	500 mg	PO	bid
	Amoxicillin trihydrate; clavulanate potassium	Augmentin	250 mg	PO	tid
Vulvar dystrophy	Testosterone	—	2% cream	Topically	bid
Lichen sclerosus	Triamcinolone		0.01–0.025%	Topically	
Squamous cell hyperplasia	Crotamiton	Eurax	0.1% beta methasone valerate and crotamiton (7:3)		
Contact vulvovaginitis	Burow's solution	—	Diluted, 1:20	Applied	bid
	Fluocinolone	Synalar	0.1–0.025%	Topically	bid
	Hydrocortisone	—	1% cream	Topically	bid
	Triamcinolone	Aristocort, Kenalog	0.025–0.1%	Topically	bid
Herpes simplex virus	Acyclovir	Zovirax	200 mg	PO	5 × daily × 10 days
			400 mg	PO	qid for suppression
Human papilloma virus	Trichloroacetic acid	—	25–80%	Topically	once a week
	Podophyllin in benzoin	—	25%	Topically	once a week
	Podofilox	Condylox	0.5%		qd × 3d/wk × 4 wks
	5-fluorouracil	Efudex	0.5%		2 times a wk
Chlamydia	Azithromycin	Zithromax	1 gm	PO	once
	Tetracycline	—	500 mg	PO	qid × 7 days
	Doxycycline	Vibramycin	100 mg	PO	bid × 7 days
	Erythromycin base	—	500 mg	PO	qid × 7 days
	Erythromycin ethylsuccinate	—	800 mg	PO	qid × 7 days
	Clindamycin	Cleocin	450 mg	PO	qid × 14 days
	Sulfisoxazole	Gantrisin	500 mg	PO	qid × 10 days
	Ofloxacin	Floxin	300 mg	PO	bid × 7 days

Table continued on following page

TABLE 3. **Recommended Treatments for Common Causes of Vaginitis** *(Continued)*

Cause	Generic Name	Trade Name	Dose	Route	Timing
Neisseria gonorrhoeae	Ceftriaxone	Rocephin	250 mg	IM	once
	Cefixime	Suprax	400 mg	PO	once
	Spectinomycin	Trobicin	2 gm	IM	once
	Azithromycin	Zithromax	1 gm	PO	once‡
	Ciprofloxacin	Cipro	500 mg	PO	once
	Ofloxacin	Floxin	400 mg	PO	once
Ulcerative lichen planus (desquamative inflammatory vaginitis)	Clindamycin	Cleocin	2% cream	Intravaginal	qd
	Hydrocortisone	—	6–12 mg	Intravaginal	qd§
Psoriasis	Triamcinolone ointment	Aristocort, Kenalog	0.12–0.025%	Topically	bid
	Betamethasone valerate	Valisone	0.1%	Topically	bid
Seborrheic dermatitis	Hydrocortisone	—	1% cream	Topically	bid

*Supplement with progesterone if uterus is present.
†Treatment is based on the results of the culture.
‡Results in 96% cure rate.
§If refractory.

commonly harbor BV-associated microflora in the anterior urethra and possibly in the prostate gland. Despite this, sexual transmission of BV remains incompletely understood, and treatment of male partners with traditional antimicrobials has not been demonstrated to reduce recurrence. Predisposing factors include sexual activity, greater number of sexual partners, intrauterine device use, concurrent trichomoniasis, and African American ancestry.

Fully half of infected women are asymptomatic. The major complaint (50 to 75%) of symptomatic women is the presence of a homogeneous, sticky, milky, and sometimes malodorous (fishy or sharp smelling) white or gray discharge. The characteristic odor is caused by alkaline volatilization of amine byproducts of anaerobic bacterial metabolism, which is the basis for the "whiff test." This odor can be increased after coitus, menstruation, or douching due to a rise in vaginal pH. The discharge is characteristically thin and homogeneous and appears as if milk or cream had been poured into the vagina. Vulvovaginal itching and irritation are uncommon, and vaginal fluid polymorphonuclear cells are not commonly found during vaginal fluid wet-preparation examinations.

Diagnosis is readily confirmed at little expense by fulfilling three of four Amsell's criteria: (1) thin, homogeneous, adherent discharge; (2) elevated vaginal pH greater than 4.5; (3) a positive whiff test with potassium hydroxide; and (4) visualization of "clue cells" on wet-preparation microscopic examination. The positive predictive value of greater than 20% clue cells (desquamated vaginal cells densely speckled with small rod-shaped bacteria so as to obscure the borders of the cells) is approximately 85%. A whiff test is performed by mixing a dollop of vaginal fluid with several drops of 10% potassium hydroxide and noting a sharp but not necessarily unpleasant amine odor (90% specificity, 70% sensitivity). A vaginal pH over 4.5 is a sensitive test for both BV and trichomoniasis. These can be distinguished with wet-preparation microscopic examinations. BV and trichomoniasis can occur together. Each of these findings can be obscured by douching, coitus, menstruation, or use of vaginal medications.

Sequelae of BV are increasingly recognized as common and serious. The abundance of abnormal microflora and the virulence factors they produce (endotoxins, phospholipases, proteases, sialidases) are associated with the ascent and establishment of BV-associated microflora and inflammation in the endometrium and possibly fallopian tubes. Multiple studies show that BV is associated with ascending reproductive tract infection during pregnancy (preterm labor and birth, premature rupture of membranes, intra-amniotic fluid infection, postpartum endometritis, and postcesarean infection). Among nonpregnant women, there are increased risks of pelvic inflammatory disease (PID), post-termination endometritis, and infection following pelvic operations (hysterectomy, vaginal repair). Controlled trials show that women should be routinely screened and treated during antenatal care and possibly prior to any pelvic operation. Some authorities now suggest that screening for and treatment of BV (asymptomatic and symptomatic) be part of well woman care.

Treatment of BV (see Table 1) includes metronidazole (Flagyl), 500 mg orally twice a day for 7 days (preferred), or, alternatively, metronidazole, 2 grams orally once or clindamycin (Cleocin), 300 mg three times a day for 7 days, or topical treatment with metronidazole, 0.75% gel (MetroGel Vaginal), or clin-

TABLE 4. Potential Adverse Effects of Agents Used to Treat Vaginitis

Condition	Medication	Route	Precautions	Common Adverse Effects*	Occurrence (%)†
Trichomoniasis or bacterial vaginosis	Metronidazole‡, §	Oral	Disulfiram reaction with alcohol; potentiates anticoagulant effects; caution with high doses of lithium, drugs that decrease or increase microsomal enzymes	Nausea, headache Anorexia, vomiting Abdominal cramps Metallic taste *Candida* overgrowth (oral or vaginal use)	12 4‡ 40§ — 10‡
Bacterial vaginosis	Metronidazole	Vaginal	—	Vaginal yeast infection Abdominal cramps Nausea Metallic taste	6 3.4 2 1.7
	Clindamycin‖, ¶	Oral	Persons with history of colitis; possible interaction with neuromuscular blocking agents	Yeast vaginitis Metallic taste Abdominal cramps Nausea Vomiting Diarrhea	17‖ — — 10 — 4–6‖, ¶
	Clindamycin	Vaginal	Persons with history of colitis	Yeast vaginitis Vulvar irritation	11 6
Yeast vaginitis (candidiasis and other yeast vaginitis)	Miconazole	Vaginal	May weaken latex products	Burning Itching Irritation	2 2 2
	Clotrimazole, other topical antifungals	Vaginal	—	Burning, irritation	<1
	Fluconazole	Oral	Careful monitoring with terfenadine, cisapride, astemizole; interactions with oral hypoglycemics, coumarin-type anticoagulants, phenytoin, rifampin, theophylline; unstudied in pregnancy	Nausea Vomiting Abdominal pain Headache Diarrhea Skin rash	3.7 1.7 1.7 1.9 1.5 1.8
	Ketoconazole**, ††	Oral	Contraindicated with isoniazid, terfenadine; potentiates anticoagulant effects; interactions with phenytoin, rifampin, cyclosporine, methylprednisone, oral hypoglycemics; unstudied in pregnancy	Nausea/vomiting Pruritus Abdominal pain Transient elevations in liver enzymes	3** 2** 1** 10††

*Other adverse effects, including potentially serious effects that occurred in less than 1% of studied patients, are not listed here.

†Percentages cited in Physician's Desk Reference, 49th ed. Montauk, N.J. Medical Economics, 1995, unless otherwise noted.

‡Aubert JM, Sesta HJ: Treatment of vaginal trichomoniasis, single 2-gram dose of metronidazole as compared with a seven-day course. J Reprod Med 27:743, 1982.

§Swedberg J, Steiner JF, Deiss F, Steiner S, Drigger DA: Comparison of single-dose vs. one-week course of metronidazole for symptomatic bacterial vaginosis. JAMA 254:1046–1049, 1985.

‖McGregor JA, French JI, Parker R, Draper D, Patterson E, Jones W, Thorsgard K, McFee J: Prevention of premature birth by screening and treatment for common genital tract infections: Results of a prospective controlled evaluation. Am J Obstet 173:157–167, 1995.

¶Sweet RL, Gibbs RS: Antimicrobial agents. *In* Infectious Disease of the Female Genital Tract, 2d ed. Mitchell CW, ed. Baltimore, Williams & Wilkins, 1995.

**Heal RC, Brogden RN, Carmine A, et al: Ketoconazole: A review of its therapeutic efficacy in superficial and systemic fungal infection. Drugs 23:1, 1982.

††VanDerPas H, Peeters F, Janssens D, et al: Treatment of vaginal candidosis with oral ketoconazole. Eur J Obstet Gynecol Reprod Biol 14:399, 1983.

damycin, 2% cream once a day for 5 days. Clindamycin is safe during pregnancy. Although there is no evidence of fetal teratogenicity due to metronidazole in early pregnancy, vaginal gel provides only 4% of the systemic level and may provide a reasonable alternative to oral metronidazole early in pregnancy.

YEAST VAGINITIS

Yeasts are the second most frequent cause of vaginitis-associated complaints (20 to 40%) evaluated by primary care providers. It is estimated that up to 75% of reproductive-age women experience at least one episode of yeast-caused vulvovaginitis at some time during their lives. *Candida* species are the most common organisms identified in symptomatic women: *Candida albicans* represents at least 65% of isolates, and *C. tropicalis, glabrata,* and *krusei* are noted increasingly. *C. glabrata* is also known as *Torulopsis glabrata*. These non-*albicans* strains may be less susceptible to treatment with the topical imidazoles clotrimazole and miconazole, which are available over the counter. Predispositions to vulvovaginal candidiasis include diabetes mellitus, pregnancy, antibiotic treatment, use of high-dose oral contraceptives, immune suppression, and possibly constricting clothing. Women with symptomatic HIV infection can present with oral or esophageal candidiasis as well as repetitive or refractory vaginal yeast infection. Approximately 5% of women suffer recurrent candidiasis, possibly due to inadequate treatment, reinfection from the gastrointestinal tract or a sexual partner, or poorly characterized defects in mucosal immunity. Since up to 25% of women may be asymptomatic despite vaginal colonization with yeast species, other causes of vulvovaginal irritation should routinely be sought. Cultures for yeast identification and sensitivity testing (Sabouraud's media) are generally unnecessary outside of specialized clinics.

Symptoms of vulvovaginal candidiasis include intense itching and burning, which may worsen after intercourse or exercise. A thick, whitish, curdy, cottage cheese–like discharge is classically described, along with erythema of the vagina and the vulva. Florid cases may demonstrate a vulvar intertrigo appearance, with small blisters at the edge of vulvar erythema.

Diagnosis involves careful wet-preparation examination using both saline and 10% potassium hydroxide solutions overlaid by a cover slip. Multiple fields should be examined for pseudohyphae and budding yeast forms. Vaginal pH is characteristically less than or equal to 4.5. Since there may be multiple processes occurring, examination should include visual examination for trichomoniasis and a whiff test, in addition to pH and wet-preparation testing. Vaginal candidiasis and BV or trichomoniasis rarely occur together.

Treatment includes a 3- to 7-day course of topical imidazoles, including miconazole (Monistat), clotrimazole (Gyne-Lotrimin), butoconazole (Femstat), or terconazole (Terazol), as well as oral agents such as fluconazole (Diflucan) and ketoconazole (Nizoral), among other regimens. Recalcitrant candidiasis should be treated with longer (14-day) courses of topical agents or 2- or 3-day treatment with oral antifungal agents. Chronic suppressive treatment of recurring yeast vulvovaginitis includes daily topical imidazoles during the luteal phase, as well as intravaginal 600-mg boric acid gelatin capsules placed daily during the luteal phase (boric acid should be used only topically) or ketoconazole, 100 mg daily for up to 6 months. Avoidance of tight-fitting clothing and improved perineal hygiene are traditional recommendations. Treatment of sexual partners with topical imidazoles is popular in other countries but remains poorly studied. With the exception of ketoconazole and fluconazole, these treatment regimens are safe and effective during pregnancy.

TRICHOMONIASIS

This common vaginitis is caused by infestation with the flagellated protozoan *Trichomonas vaginalis*. It is estimated that over 3 million women are diagnosed with trichomoniasis yearly. Infection occurs in the vagina as well as the urethra and, occasionally, bladder trigone in both men and women. *T. vaginalis* is most frequently sexually transmitted; the protozoan can survive outside the body for several hours and may rarely be transmitted by fomites or contaminated water. Sexual partners are commonly (approximately 80%) infected and should be treated empirically even though they are asymptomatic to avoid reinfection and spread to future contacts. Neonates may acquire *T. vaginalis* infection from passage through the birth canal. Older children with trichomoniasis should be evaluated for possible sexual abuse.

Trichomoniasis is frequently asymptomatic in both women and men. Nonetheless, there may be a copious foamy or frothy off-white, purulent green, or yellow discharge present in 50 to 75% of infected women. There may be a fishy amine odor (positive whiff test) similar to that in BV after intercourse or douching. Vaginal itching, irritation, dyspareunia, and dysuria are common in symptomatic women. Vaginal examination shows copious, sometimes frothy or bubbly purulent discharge, with pooling in the postural fornix. The vagina is often erythematous, and the cervix may demonstrate punctate erythema (colpitis macularis).

The diagnosis is clinically established by visualization of motile trichomonads as well as a characteristic marked white blood cell response noted on the saline wet preparation. Similar to BV, whiff testing for amines with potassium hydroxide is positive, and pH is greater than 4.5. Motile or wiggling flagella distinguish the protozoa from slightly smaller leukocytes. Visualization of motile trichomonads is 100% specific but only 50 to 90% sensitive compared with culture (modified Diamond's media) or nucleic acid–based testing (polymerase chain reaction, amplification tests).

Effective treatment is limited to oral treatment with nitroimidazoles (metronidazole, 2 grams orally once a day or 500 mg orally twice a day for 7 days). Recent (prior 2 months) sexual partners should be treated similarly despite the absence of symptoms. Metronidazole may cause nausea, vomiting, and infrequently an Antabuse-like reaction if alcohol is taken during treatment. Despite multiple studies establishing the safety of metronidazole in early pregnancy and no evidence of embryo or fetal toxicity, there is a traditional resistance to using metronidazole in early pregnancy. If this is the case, topical clotrimazole suppositories twice daily for 7 days provide relief in 50% of women in the first trimester. Clotrimazole may also be used if there is a definite history of allergic reaction to metronidazole. Douching with povidone iodine solutions may also provide relief, if not cure (avoid use of iodine-containing douches in pregnancy). Metronidazole resistance is increasingly noted and may be overcome with high-dose regimens (similar to treatment of amebiasis: 750 mg to 1 gram orally three times a day for 3 to 7 days). Such high-dose regimens require specific counseling regarding adverse reactions. Partners should be similarly counseled, treated, and evaluated for cure.

OTHER CAUSES

Other causes of vaginitis are less frequent and less well characterized.

Atrophic Vaginitis. Atrophic vaginitis is due to absolute or relative estrogen deficiency. Estrogen-deficient vaginal tissue appears thin and poorly lubricated and is susceptible to local irritation, micro-trauma, and overgrowth with nonlactobacillus microflora. Wet-preparation microscopic examination characteristically shows scant material, with inadequately estrogenized parabasal cells (large nuclei) and few bacteria. Overgrowth with abnormal flora is associated with nonlactobacillus microbes and leukocytes on wet-preparation examination. Topical or oral estrogen replacement is usually effective; treatment of specific infections should be based on microscopic examination, pH, whiff testing, and selective use of aerobic cultures as necessary. "Hydrating" vaginal lubricants, such as Replens, can offer symptomatic relief to women who decline hormonal treatment.

Viral Vulvovaginitis. Viral vulvovaginitis is usually caused by primary or recurrent infection with herpes simplex virus type 1 or 2. The diagnosis is confirmed by clinical findings (clear or yellow vesicals or papules on an erythematous base) and virologic testing (culture, Tzanck smear, or nucleic acid testing). Treatment with antivirals (acyclovir [Zovirax], 200 mg five times daily for 7 days, or valacyclovir [Valtrex], 150 to 300 mg twice daily for 5 to 7 days) is usually effective. Partners should be counseled, and appropriate care providers should be notified if the patient is or becomes pregnant.

Genital infections with human papillomavirus (HPV) may be associated with vulvovaginal pruritus, clear mucoid discharge, and irritation, especially after coitus. Diagnosis is poorly characterized but includes visualization of verrucous or flat condylomata (warts). Flat condylomata can be visualized after local treatment with 5% acetic acid. Treatment may include eradication of visible warts (podophyllin, cryotherapy, or electrotherapy) and possibly treatment with several applications of 5% fluorouracil or trichloroacetic acid if simple supportive care, including sitz baths and local steroids, is not availing. Partners and pregnancy care providers should be counseled or informed.

Vulvovaginal dermatoses may cause severe vulvo-vaginal symptoms and may prove challenging to diagnose and treat. Vulvar dystrophies (lichen sclerosus, lichen planus, aphthous ulcers) are generally treated with topical steroids such as clobetasol propionate or fluocinonide (Lidex) ointment or cream. Patients with refractory complaints or findings should be referred for consultation, possible biopsy, and intensive therapy. Patients with so-called vestibulitis (erythematous, exquisitely tender vestibular glands) suffer from severe and refractory soreness and dyspareunia. Diagnosis is made by demonstrating focal marked tenderness of individual vestibular glands when touched by a cotton swab. Treatment is empirical and includes sitz baths and optimized perineal hygiene, avoidance of possibly irritating and sensitizing soaps and hygiene products, avoidance of tight-fitting clothes, and use of topical steroid (clobetasol propionate or fluocinonide ointment or cream).

So-called desquamative inflammatory vaginitis is characterized by findings of severe vaginal irritation, profuse purulent discharge, and often dramatic vaginal erythema. Recent studies show that this is most often caused by infection with group B streptococcus, which frequently responds to the use of 2% topical clindamycin for 14 days. Topical steroids provide rapid symptomatic relief. Possible genital tract neoplasia should always be considered in patients with refractory findings. Biopsy is required for diagnosis.

TOXIC SHOCK SYNDROME

method of
MARY-MARGARET ANDREWS, M.D., and
JEFFREY PARSONNET, M.D.
Dartmouth-Hitchcock Medical Center
Lebanon, New Hampshire

Toxic shock syndrome (TSS) is a clinical syndrome characterized by fever, an erythematous rash, hypotension, multiple organ-system dysfunction, and desquamation during convalescence. Strains of *Staphylococcus aureus* and group A streptococcus (*Streptococcus pyogenes*) may produce exotoxins leading to clinically similar diseases. Although these toxin-mediated diseases have a rich heritage spanning the last century, a formal case definition of staphylococcal TSS did not emerge until 1980, following a large outbreak of tampon- and menstruation-associated cases in the United States. The epidemiologic finding of a statistical association with a particular tampon brand and the resultant media attention cemented the association between TSS and tampon use in the minds of American physicians.

We now know that TSS may be a consequence of staphylococcal colonization or infection at anatomic sites other than the genitourinary tract, occurring in both males and females of all ages. Cases occur during menstruation both with and without tampon use, in association with barrier contraceptives such as the diaphragm and sponge, and following vaginal or cesarean delivery. TSS may also accompany staphylococcal infection of the skin (including surgical wounds), the upper or lower respiratory tract, and the musculoskeletal system.

ETIOLOGY AND PATHOGENESIS

Several staphylococcal toxins are capable of causing TSS, with TSS toxin–1 (TSST-1) being the most common. The staphylococcal enterotoxins, especially enterotoxin B, may serve as alternative TSS toxins in nonmenstrual cases. Development of TSS requires colonization or infection with a toxin-producing strain and an absence of antibody to the toxin. The TSS toxins are not true cytotoxins; rather, they are immunomodulators of a class known as "superantigens." TSST-1 exerts its effect by binding to cells that express Class II major histocompatibility complex (MHC) antigens, including monocytes and tissue macrophages, B lymphocytes, and activated endothelial cells. The TSST-1–Class II MHC complex then binds to a specific receptor on a subset of T cells, stimulating polyclonal lymphocyte expansion and the release of endogenous mediators of inflammation. The cascade of lymphocytes that follows is responsible for the clinical hallmark of TSS—capillary leak and multiple organ-system dysfunction caused by endothelial cell damage.

EPIDEMIOLOGY

TSS occurs when a person who lacks antibody to TSST-1 (or one of the alternative TSS toxins) becomes colonized or infected with a toxin-producing strain of *S. aureus*. TSS is primarily a disease of young people. Menstrual and contraceptive-related TSS occur most frequently among adolescents and young adults, but there appears to be a high incidence of nonmenstrual disease in the first decade of life. Epidemiologic studies of healthy children and adults have shown that the percentage of people with a protective level of antibody to TSST-1 increases with age. By age 10, approximately 50% of people have a protective antibody; by age 35, the seropositivity rate exceeds 90%. Seroconversion evidently follows colonization or minor infection with toxigenic strains of *S. aureus* (i.e., without TSS), thereby conferring protection against the disease.

Since the mid-1980s, the incidence of menstrual TSS has fallen substantially, from six to 12 cases per 100,000 adult women to one case per 100,000 women. The basis for this apparent decrease is uncertain but probably reflects changes in tampon composition and/or absorbency, heightened public awareness of the disease, and under-reporting. In contrast, the incidence of nonmenstrual cases has remained relatively constant, and such cases outnumber those of menstrual TSS.

Menstruation continues to be the most common risk factor for developing TSS, and tampon use further increases the risk. Menstruation itself brings about changes in the vaginal milieu, such as a neutral pH and dissolved oxygen, that are conducive to production of TSST-1 by toxigenic strains. Tampons and other intravaginal devices such as barrier contraceptives also introduce oxygen into the vagina, and this may be the principal mechanism by which they increase the risk. The usual signs of pyogenic infection are often lacking in TSS, so the diagnosis must be considered in any menstruating woman with suggestive symptoms. TSS may also occur in the setting of vaginal trauma or pelvic surgery.

TSS has been recognized in association with both vaginal and cesarean delivery. Symptoms may become manifest within hours to several days of delivery. Foul-smelling lochia or other evidence of endometritis may or may not be present. In addition to infection of the lower genitourinary tract, the surgical wound may provide a site for toxin-producing staphylococcal infection after cesarean delivery.

Infection of almost any mucosal, soft tissue, or visceral

TABLE 1. Case Definition of Toxic Shock Syndrome

Fever: temperature ≥38.9° C
Rash: typically a diffuse macular erythroderma
Hypotension: systolic blood pressure ≤90 mm Hg for adults or below fifth percentile by age for children below 16 years of age, orthostatic drop in diastolic blood pressure ≥ 15 mm Hg, orthostatic syncope, or orthostatic dizziness
Multisystem disease, consisting of three or more of the following:
  Gastrointestinal: vomiting or diarrhea at onset of illness
  Muscular: severe myalgias of creatine phosphokinase at least twice upper limit of normal
  Mucous membrane: vaginal, oropharyngeal, or conjunctival hyperemia
  Renal: blood urea nitrogen or creatinine at least twice the upper limit of normal, or pyuria (≥5 leukocytes per high-power field) in the absence of urinary tract infection
  Hepatic: total bilirubin or serum transaminase at least twice the upper limit of normal
  Hematologic: platelets ≤100,000/mm³
  Central nervous system: disorientation or alterations in consciousness without focal neurologic signs when fever and hypotension are absent
Desquamation: 1 to 2 weeks after onset of illness
Negative results on the following tests, if obtained: blood, throat, or cerebrospinal fluid cultures (blood culture may be positive for *S. aureus*); rise in titer to agents of Rocky Mountain spotted fever, leptospirosis, or rubeola

Reproduced with permission from Reingold AL, et al: Toxic shock syndrome surveillance in the United States, 1980 to 1981. Ann Intern Med *96* (part 2):875, 1982.

site with a toxigenic strain of *S. aureus* in the absence of antibody can result in nonmenstrual TSS. Males and females appear to be affected with equal frequency. Upper and lower respiratory tract infections that have been particularly associated with TSS include sinusitis (often with nasal packing), staphylococcal tracheitis in children, and postinfluenza staphylococcal infection of the lower respiratory tract in adults. Mere pharyngeal colonization with *S. aureus* may be sufficient to cause full-blown TSS. Skin and soft tissue infections are also frequently linked to TSS. Numerous cases have been reported in association with superinfection of existing skin lesions such as burns, lesions of varicella or herpes zoster, and surgical wounds. Diagnosis requires a high index of suspicion, as typical signs of infection may be lacking. Staphylococcal enterotoxin B is a relatively common cause of nonmenstrual TSS.

Recurrence of TSS is a well-recognized phenomenon. This was particularly common in the early years of disease recognition, when women at risk continued to use tampons and were not treated with an antistaphylococcal antibiotic. Fully two-thirds of women with a first episode of TSS fail to develop protective antibody within the ensuing 6 months, a phenomenon that may have a genetic basis or may be the consequence of the immunomodulating effects of the toxin. Nonmenstrual TSS is less likely to recur, but recurrences have been described.

CLINICAL MANIFESTATIONS

The case definition of TSS (Table 1) highlights most of its major clinical features. A temperature of greater than 38.9° C is characteristic. Within 48 hours of the onset of illness, another hallmark of the disease, a sunburn-like erythroderma, occurs. The rash may be evanescent and mistaken for the flush of fever. The rash is usually diffuse but may be limited to the face, extremities, or torso. There is frank hypotension or orthostatic signs or symptoms, such as dizziness upon standing. Symptoms of multiple organ-system involvement are nonspecific and include myalgias, vomiting, diarrhea, headache, and sore throat. Flu-like symptoms may predominate over the better known gastrointestinal symptoms of TSS. Physical examination may reveal pharyngitis or a strawberry tongue, conjunctival suffusion, rales, abdominal tenderness, peripheral edema, and altered mental status. The time course of the major clinical manifestations of TSS is shown in Figure 1.

Laboratory data also suggest multiple organ-system dysfunction. Leukocytosis (or leukopenia with a profound left shift) and thrombocytopenia are almost universal findings. Elevated prothrombin and partial thromboplastin times are often observed, but frank disseminated intravascular coagulation is not a common feature of TSS. Hypocalcemia and hypoalbuminemia almost always develop; their absence should prompt consideration of other diagnoses. Elevated blood urea nitrogen and creatinine and/or pyuria are seen in at least 70% of cases. Elevations in creatine phosphokinase may be severe enough to cause rhabdomyolysis with myoglobinuria.

Serious complications of TSS include adult respiratory distress syndrome requiring mechanical ventilation, hypotension that does not respond to fluid administration, and renal insufficiency, which may be severe enough to require dialysis. Peripheral gangrene may develop as a consequence of severe vasoconstriction.

Full-thickness desquamation is a late feature of TSS, with an onset between days 7 and 14 of illness. The face, palms, soles, and digits are most often involved. One-third of patients also experience a diffuse maculopapular rash several weeks after the onset of illness, and reversible alopecia and nail loss may occur after an interval of several months.

DIAGNOSIS

TSS remains a clinical diagnosis that requires fulfillment of established criteria. An awareness of the diverse epidemiologic settings and clinical manifestations of TSS is essential for early diagnosis. The abrupt onset of fever, rash, multiple organ-system dysfunction, or shock, particularly in a young, healthy host, should prompt consideration of TSS. Desquamation is not part of the initial clinical picture, and its absence should not dissuade one from considering the diagnosis of TSS. A menstrual and gynecologic history should always be obtained in evaluating patients with fever.

The laboratory evaluation of a patient with possible TSS should include a complete blood count, prothrombin and partial thromboplastin times, electrolytes, serum calcium and albumin, creatinine, liver function tests, and urinalysis. A chest x-ray and electrocardiogram should be obtained. The presence of myalgias should prompt an evaluation for rhabdomyolysis. Blood cultures should be obtained, as well as cultures of the genital or respiratory tract and any wounds, as appropriate.

The diagnostic criteria for TSS do not require isolation of *S. aureus*, but the diagnosis should be questioned if all cultures for the organism are negative. Because *S. aureus* may be considered normal flora when isolated from mucosal sites, the clinician must request that the microbiology laboratory identify all staphylococcal species "because of a suspicion of TSS."

The following specimens should be sent to reference labo-

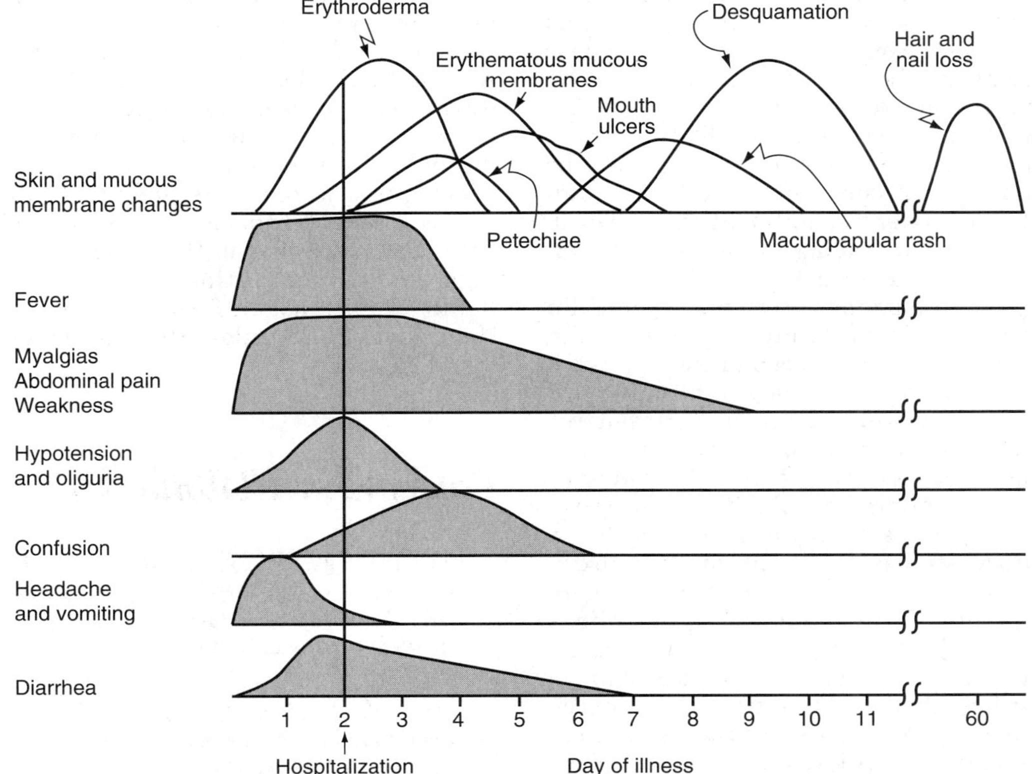

Figure 1. Composite drawing of major systemic, skin, and mucous membrane manifestations of toxic shock syndrome. (From Chesney PJ, et al: Clinical manifestations of toxic shock syndrome. JAMA *246*:741–748, 1981. Copyright 1981, American Medical Association.)

ratories in suspected cases of TSS: clinical isolates of *S. aureus*, for testing for TSST-1 production; and acute-phase serum, for testing for antibody to TSST-1. The utility of these tests in the setting of nonmenstrual TSS is less clear, as many cases are caused by other staphylococcal toxins. Although these tests are rarely useful early in disease management, they often provide confirmation of the diagnosis (e.g., if a TSST-1–positive strain is found in the absence of antibody). Furthermore, a convalescent-phase serum specimen may be useful in predicting the risk of recurrent disease.

Differential diagnostic considerations include other febrile illnesses associated with rash and/or hypotension. Examples include Kawasaki disease in children (especially under the age of 4), streptococcal TSS or scarlet fever, staphylococcal scalded skin syndrome, Rocky Mountain spotted fever, meningococcemia, severe allergic drug reactions, and viral illness with exanthems, such as measles or enterovirus infections.

THERAPY

Early consideration of the diagnosis of TSS is critical if therapy is to be started before the development of end-organ damage. Because the course of the illness can be difficult to predict, outpatient therapy should be considered for only the least ill and the most compliant of patients. An intensive care unit is desirable in the setting of persistent hypotension, hypoxemia, or oliguria. Invasive monitoring via pulmonary artery catheter placement, mechanical ventilation, and support with vasopressors may be required.

Several principles of management apply to all cases of TSS. First, any tampon or other nidus of infection should be removed or surgically drained without delay. Even wounds that do not appear overtly infected should be opened and cultured. Second, aggressive volume resuscitation should be undertaken; patients may require 5 to 10 liters over the first 24 hours. If necessary, vasopressors should be given to maintain organ perfusion, especially if pulmonary edema is a barrier to additional fluids. Third, a first-line antistaphylococcal antibiotic should be administered, usually intravenously.

Traditionally, beta-lactamase-resistant penicillin derivatives such as nafcillin (Unipen) and oxacillin (Prostaphlin), or first-generation cephalosporins such as cefazolin (Ancef), have been used to treat serious infections caused by *S. aureus*, because of their potent bactericidal activity in vitro. In actual practice, however, serum and tissue levels of beta-lactam antibiotics fall below the minimum inhibitory concentration (MIC) for *S. aureus* between antibiotic doses. Recent laboratory studies have shown that toxin-producing strains of *S. aureus* actually generate more toxin in the presence of subinhibitory concentrations of beta-lactam antibiotics than in the absence of an antibiotic. This finding correlates with the clinical observation, initially made with group A streptococci, that toxin-induced syndromes may progress despite the use of seemingly appropriate antibiotic regimens. Furthermore, when large inocula of *S. aureus* are present in infected tissues, many of the organisms

(those in stationary phase) express low levels of penicillin-binding proteins; hence, bacterial killing with beta-lactams may be impaired.

Based on these observations, as well as anecdotal clinical data, we suggest that clindamycin (Cleocin) may be the preferred antimicrobial agent for the treatment of TSS. Clindamycin and other inhibitors of protein synthesis have been shown to abort bacterial toxin synthesis in a fashion that is independent of bacterial inoculum or phase of bacterial growth. At most institutions, more than 90% of *S. aureus* strains are sensitive to this agent. A dose of 900 mg given intravenously every 8 hours is suggested, with no adjustment required for renal insufficiency. It is also acceptable, and well within standard practice, to treat with nafcillin or cefazolin, as clindamycin has not been proved to be more effective. Vancomycin (Vancocin) is an appropriate alternative empirical treatment for patients who are at increased risk for infection with methicillin-resistant *S. aureus* (MRSA), although the frequency with which TSS is caused by MRSA strains is low. Combination therapy with vancomycin and clindamycin is reasonable for critically ill patients until sensitivity results are available. A change to oral therapy is appropriate when the patient has stabilized, is afebrile, and can take oral medications. A 10- to 14-day course of antibiotics is recommended.

Anecdotal case reports and animal studies have suggested that high-dose intravenous immune globulin (IVIG [Gamimune N])* may be useful for the treatment of patients with severe or refractory cases of TSS. Commercially available preparations of IVIG are known to contain high levels of neutralizing antibody to TSST-1. We and others have treated patients with a single dose of 400 mg per kg, given as an intravenous infusion over 4 to 6 hours. Our practice has been to give IVIG to patients who have an undrainable focus of infection, who develop pulmonary edema, or who require vasopressors for the maintenance of renal perfusion or an acceptable blood pressure. The risks of such therapy are low, although its high cost can be justified only for seriously ill patients. We are not in favor of using steroids for the treatment of TSS unless there is evidence of adrenal insufficiency.

CHLAMYDIA TRACHOMATIS INFECTION

method of
JEFFREY F. PEIPERT, M.D., M.P.H.
*Brown University School of Medicine and
Women & Infants' Hospital*
Providence, Rhode Island

Chlamydia trachomatis infection is recognized as the most common bacterial sexually transmitted disease (STD) in the United States, with approximately 4 million cases

---

*Not FDA-approved for this indication.

annually. The sequelae of chlamydial infection include pelvic inflammatory disease (PID), infertility, chronic pelvic pain, ectopic pregnancy, and infection of the newborn. The public health and economic costs of chlamydial infection are staggering, with approximately $4 billion spent in 1992 for PID and its direct and indirect consequences. A large percentage of chlamydial infections are asymptomatic. Timely identification depends on a high index of suspicion and adequate screening of high-risk individuals. Recent technologic advances in new nonculture techniques for identifying chlamydial infections will enable clinicians to screen urine and offer treatment for infected individuals and their partners. In addition, single-dose antibiotics with long half-lives have been introduced to avoid problems with compliance and difficult side effects.

EPIDEMIOLOGY

The prevalence of genital chlamydial infection depends on the population studied and has ranged from 2 to 20%. With the exception of neonatal ocular infections and pneumonia, *C. trachomatis* is a genital tract pathogen transmitted through sexual contact. Risk factors for chlamydial infection are listed in Table 1 and include young age, presence of another STD such as *Neisseria gonorrhoeae* or *Trichomonas*, new or multiple sexual partners, nonwhite race, unmarried marital status, and possibly the use of oral contraceptives. It is unclear whether oral contraceptives are actually causal or whether this finding is a surrogate for sexual behavior. It is also possible that the identification of *C. trachomatis* is facilitated by oral contraceptive–induced cervical ectropion.

ORGANISM

The genus *Chlamydia* contains three species: *C. psittaci*, *C. pneumoniae*, and *C. trachomatis*. *C. trachomatis* parasitizes humans exclusively and is responsible for a variety of clinical syndromes, including pulmonary, ocular, enteric, and genital tract infections. *C. trachomatis* is divided into 17 different immunotypes on the basis of major antigenic differences in their outer membrane proteins. Immunotypes L1, L2, and L3 are responsible for the lymphogranuloma venereum (LGV) syndrome, and types A, B, Ba, and C are most commonly associated with trachoma. Genital infection is typically caused by types D through K, with D, E, and F immunotypes being by far the most common.

Chlamydia is an obligate intracellular parasite with a two-part life cycle. In the elementary body stage, the organism is metabolically inert and has a protective cell wall that enables it to survive extracellularly. In the reticulate body stage, the organism is found only intracellularly. During this stage, the organism lacks a cell wall and is metabolically active. It is during the reticulate body stage that active replication takes place. During the intracellular stage, chlamydia is an "energy parasite" as it efficiently makes use of the biochemical energy products provided by the host cell.

TABLE 1. **Demographic and Reproductive Risk Factors for Chlamydial Infection**

Young age	Lower socioeconomic status
Nonwhite race	Oral contraceptive use
Unmarried marital status	Presence of other sexually transmitted disease or bacterial vaginosis
Urban residence	Multiple sexual partners

PATHOPHYSIOLOGY

An elementary body binds to a cell surface to initiate the infection cycle. The elementary body enters the cytoplasm by endocytosis and is then surrounded by a membrane derived from the host cell but modified by the organism. A single phagosome is formed when multiple elementary bodies gain entry into a single cell and fuse. Within hours, the elementary body loses its cell wall and becomes metabolically active (reticulate body). At this point, the organism begins to replicate by binary fission. As replication occurs, the phagosome enlarges, filling the cytoplasm and displacing the cells nucleus. This expanding phagosome is referred to as an "inclusion." As the inclusion enlarges, glycogen is produced within it, which allows easy identification with iodine stains.

Columnar epithelial cells are the primary targets of the non-LGV immunotypes of *C. trachomatis*. These cells are present on the surfaces of the conjunctivae, urethra, endocervix, endometrium, and fallopian tubes. Acute chlamydial infection is characterized primarily by a polymorphonuclear cell response. Reinfection or chronic infections are characterized by a mononuclear cell response. Fibrosis often accompanies this chronic inflammatory mononuclear cell response and produces the long-term sequelae of chlamydial infection.

CLINICAL MANIFESTATIONS

C. trachomatis can cause urethritis, endocervicitis, endometritis or salpingitis (PID), or perihepatitis (Table 2). Between 15 and 25% of female sex partners of men infected with *C. trachomatis* have positive urethral cultures for *Chlamydia*. In addition, culturing both the urethra and the endocervix, rather than the endocervix alone, increases the percentage of culture-positive women by as much as 20%. Unexplained pyuria, culture-negative cystitis, and prolonged dysuria lasting greater than 7 to 10 days should raise the possibility of chlamydial urethritis.

The most common site of infection of *Chlamydia* in women is the endocervix. Most of these infections are asymptomatic and are usually detected by routine screening (see "Diagnosis"). The presence of green or yellow mucopus on the endocervical swab (cotton swab test) or 10 or more polymorphonuclear leukocytes (PMNs) noted on oil-immersion field in a Gram's stain is presumptive evidence for endocervical chlamydial infection. Other clinical findings associated with chlamydial endocervicitis include cervical friability, edema, erythema, the presence of other STDs or bacterial vaginosis, and a marked increase in inflammatory cells noted on saline preparation of vaginal secretions (leukorrhea).

Chlamydia is an important cause of upper genital tract infection in women. Histologic evidence of endometritis may be present in approximately 50% of women with mucopurulent cervicitis and almost all women with salpingitis. How often *C. trachomatis* is recovered from the endometrium or fallopian tube is determined by the technique used for recovery (swab, brush, or biopsy) and the method of detection (see "Diagnosis"). Detection of *C. trachomatis* also varies by patient population under investigation. The clinical presentation of chlamydial PID is more indolent and less severe than gonococcal PID. The major presenting complaints include pain and abnormal vaginal discharge. However, the diagnosis of upper genital tract chlamydial infection should be considered with complaints of dyspareunia, abnormal uterine bleeding, dysuria, and back pain. For further details about the clinical presentation, diagnosis, and treatment of PID, see page 1113.

TABLE 2. **Clinical Spectrum of Chlamydial Infection in Women**

Diagnosis	Clinical Criteria	Laboratory Criteria	
		Presumptive	*Confirmatory*
Urethritis	Dysuria, frequency, and/or urgency >7 days	Pyuria, no bacteria (negative culture)	*Chlamydia* culture or nonculture test
Endocervicitis	Mucopus present on cotton swab test (mucopurulent cervical discharge); cervical edema or erythema; easily induced cervical bleeding (friability); hypertrophic ectropion	Cervical Gram's stain with ≥10 PMNs/hpf	*Chlamydia* culture or nonculture test
Pelvic inflammatory disease	Abdominal tenderness, cervical motion tenderness, and adnexal tenderness (unilateral or bilateral); evidence of lower genital tract infection	Cervical mucopus, leukorrhea	Laparoscopy demonstrating tubal edema, erythema, and purulent exudate; histologic evidence of endometritis; positive culture or nonculture test from the upper genital tract
Perihepatitis	Right upper quadrant pain or tenderness associated with salpingitis or PID	Cervical mucopus, leukorrhea, possible abnormal LFTs associated with PID	Laparoscopy demonstrating "violin-string" adhesions from liver to anterior abdominal wall

Abbreviations: PMNs = polymorphonuclear leukocytes; hpf = high-power field; LFTs = liver function tests; PID = pelvic inflammatory disease.

C. trachomatis has also been shown to be a common cause of perihepatitis associated with PID, known as Fitz-Hugh–Curtis syndrome. Organisms presumably follow the flow of peritoneal fluid to the diaphragm and right upper quadrant and have been recovered on liver biopsies performed at laparoscopy. Recent studies suggest that perihepatitis is now more commonly caused by *C. trachomatis* than by *N. gonorrhoeae.*

Complications of chlamydial genital tract infections in women include tubal infertility, ectopic pregnancy, and chronic pelvic pain. Swedish studies have demonstrated that after one episode of PID, the rate of infertility is 11%. With two episodes, the rate doubles to 23%, and after three or more episodes, the rate of infertility is greater than 50%. Support for chlamydia as an etiologic agent has been demonstrated with serologic studies that showed that infertile women with fallopian tube scarring were more likely to have *C. trachomatis*–specific antibodies than infertile women without tubal scarring. Serologic studies have also linked *C. trachomatis* infection with ectopic pregnancy. Most women with tubal-factor infertility or ectopic pregnancy do not give a history of prior PID. It is believed that many of these women have had subclinical tubal infection or "silent PID" (PID without pain), which may be explained by the indolent course of *C. trachomatis* infection. Animal data support this concept and have demonstrated that chronic and/or recurrent chlamydial infection causes tubal scarring.

Serologic, epidemiologic, and animal studies have led to the concept that *C. trachomatis* commonly infects the fallopian tubes, which only occasionally causes clinically apparent, symptomatic disease. More often, the infection causes a low-grade chronic inflammatory process that evades diagnosis and treatment. Clinicians must have a high level of suspicion to increase the sensitivity of diagnosing *C. trachomatis* infection in women.

Lymphogranuloma venereum is an uncommon disease in the United States, with only a few hundred cases reported annually. Although the primary infection may be in the endocervix, rectal mucosa, or keratinized epithelium of the external genitalia, clinical evidence of the primary lesion is apparent in less than 5% of cases. The most common clinical presentation of LGV is enlarged, painful inguinal lymph nodes, which are usually unilateral. In approximately one-third of cases, a "groove sign" is present, which is formed from enlarged nodes above and below the inguinal ligament. The lymph nodes are often quite tender and may form buboes. In the absence of effective therapy, the buboes may break down to form chronically draining cutaneous sinuses.

DIAGNOSIS

Culture has traditionally been considered the "gold standard" for the diagnosis of *C. trachomatis* infection. Unfortunately, the organism grows inefficiently in vitro, and several steps are necessary to optimize its isolation rates. In addition, special precautions must be taken to properly collect and transport clinical specimens to achieve reliable *Chlamydia* culture results.

Nonculture-based diagnostic tests for *Chlamydia* include the direct fluorescent antibody (DFA) test, the enzyme immunoassay (EIA), nucleic acid probes, and amplification techniques. DFA tests are highly dependent on the skill and dedication of the microbiologist. The EIA has an objective end point for a positive test and may be less prone to interobserver variation. Nucleic acid probes (e.g., GenProbe) initially suffered from poor sensitivity (60 to 83%), but recent modifications have resulted in significant improvement. Polymerase chain reaction (PCR) and ligase chain reaction (LCR) are amplification techniques that are extremely sensitive. One study evaluating 500 women noted a sensitivity of GenProbe and culture of 65 and 86%, respectively, compared with 95% by PCR. DNA amplification techniques are now approved to detect *C. trachomatis* infection from male urine, and approval to test for *Chlamydia* in female urine is pending. PCR and LCR may be the tests of choice in the future for the diagnosis of *C. trachomatis.*

TREATMENT

The treatment of uncomplicated urethral, endocervical, or rectal chlamydia in nonpregnant women is

TABLE 3. **Treatment of Uncomplicated Chlamydial Infections in Nonpregnant Women**

Medication	Dose	Route	Frequency
First-Line Therapy			
Doxycycline (Vibramycin)	100 mg	Orally	bid for 7 days
Azithromycin (Zithromax)	1 gm	Orally	Single dose, once
Alternatives			
Ofloxacin (Floxin)*	300 mg	Orally	bid for 7 days
Erythromycin base	500 mg	Orally	qid for 7 days
Erythromycin ethylsuccinate	800 mg	Orally	qid for 7 days
Sulfisoxazole†	500 mg	Orally	qid for 10 days

*Ofloxacin is not recommended for treating adolescents less than 17 years of age nor for pregnant women.

†The efficacy of sulfisoxazole is inferior to that of other regimens.

listed in Table 3. Doxycycline is still the recommendation of the Centers for Disease Control and Prevention (CDC), but azithromycin (Zithromax) offers the advantage of a single oral dose. With recent price reductions for azithromycin, many clinicians consider this the agent of choice when treating uncomplicated chlamydial infection. Other alternatives include ofloxacin (Floxin), erythromycin, and sulfisoxazole.

In the obstetric population, doxycycline and ofloxacin are not recommended. The CDC first-line agent is erythromycin base 500 mg orally four times a day for 7 days. Alternatives are listed in Table 4 and include erythromycin ethylsuccinate and amoxicillin. Erythromycin estolate is contraindicated during pregnancy, since drug-related hepatotoxicity can result. Azithromycin is not a CDC-recommended agent in pregnancy. However, several recent studies have demonstrated its safety and excellent tolerance and efficacy in the obstetric population. Azithromycin is listed as a category "B" drug in pregnancy according to the *Physician's Desk Reference* and may be considered an alternative for the treatment of uncomplicated chlamydia in pregnancy.

Doxycycline (100 mg orally twice a day for 21 days) is also the preferred treatment for LGV. Alternatives include either erythromycin or sulfisoxazole 500 mg orally four times a day for 21 days.

TABLE 4. **Treatment of Chlamydial Infections in Pregnancy**

Medication	Dose	Route	Frequency
First-Line Therapy			
Erythromycin base	500 mg	Orally	qid for 7 days
Azithromycin (Zithromax)	1 gm	Orally	Single dose, once
Alternatives			
Erythromycin base	250 mg	Orally	qid for 14 days
Erythromycin ethylsuccinate	800 mg	Orally	qid for 7 days
Erythromycin ethylsuccinate	400 mg	Orally	qid for 14 days
Amoxicillin*	500 mg	Orally	tid for 7–10 days

Note: Erythromycin estolate is contraindicated during pregnancy, since drug-related hepatotoxicity can result.

*Recommended if erythromycin is not tolerated.

Prevention strategies include primary prevention, or efforts to prevent chlamydial infection, and secondary prevention, targeted at preventing complications among persons infected with chlamydia. Primary prevention includes behavioral changes that reduce the risk of acquiring chlamydia, such as reducing the number of sexual partners, delaying first intercourse, selecting partners carefully, and using barrier methods of contraception. In addition, primary prevention includes screening and treating persons with genital chlamydial infection before they infect sex partners and, for pregnant women, before they infect their babies. Screening often targets high-risk populations such as adolescents, persons with multiple sexual partners, and individuals with other STDs. Secondary prevention strategies attempt to prevent complications among persons infected with chlamydia. This includes early identification of chlamydial infections in women with signs of mucopurulent cervicitis or urethral syndrome, treating partners of men with infection, and early diagnosis of ascending infection.

Routine test of cure is not currently recommended for first-line treatment regimens. However, when alternative therapies are used or if poor compliance with medication is suspected, retesting may be informative. If a nonculture method is employed for follow-up testing, at least 3 to 4 weeks should pass after antimicrobial therapy due to prolonged antigen shedding, resulting in a high rate of false-positives. Clinicians should consider screening for other STDs in all cases, and sex partners of infected women should be treated to avoid reinfection.

PELVIC INFLAMMATORY DISEASE

method of
EDWIN M. THORPE, JR., M.D., and
FRANK W. LING, M.D.
University of Tennessee
Memphis, Tennessee

Pelvic inflammatory disease (PID) is associated with substantial morbidity and is fatal in some instances. The Centers for Disease Control and Prevention (CDC) estimates that more than 1 million new cases of PID are diagnosed each year. Approximately 25% of women with PID experience one or more serious, long-term sequelae. Of the major sequelae, the two that most seriously threaten reproductive health are involuntary infertility and ectopic pregnancy. PID is an important risk factor for chronic pelvic pain, a common complaint among gynecologic patients. Other sequelae include dyspareunia, pelvic adhesions, pyosalpinx, inflammatory residua, and tubo-ovarian abscess. Many women with acute PID require surgical intervention and removal of reproductive organs. The resultant psychological consequences are often devastating. The economic consequences of PID are staggering. When the direct costs related to inpatient and outpatient treatment and management of sequelae are factored, over

$4 billion is spent annually. This article outlines diagnostic criteria and treatment guidelines and provides an overview for prevention strategies.

DIAGNOSIS

PID is underdiagnosed. During the past 20 years, a complaint of severe lower abdominal pain accompanied by high fever and often an elevated white blood cell count was viewed as the classic presentation of PID. More recently, information from patients with laparoscopic-confirmed cases indicates that the sensitivity of using temperature elevation is only about 34%, and an elevated white blood cell count is not a significant predictor of PID.

Currently, the diagnosis of PID remains challenging because of the wide variation in presenting signs and symptoms. Some patients have mild signs and symptoms such as abnormal uterine bleeding, dyspareunia, or abnormal vaginal discharge that are not readily recognized as PID. Some women with PID are asymptomatic. Laparoscopy may be used to verify the diagnosis of salpingitis, but it is difficult to justify this procedure for a patient who has only mild or atypical symptoms and signs. Because of the difficulty of the diagnosis and serious consequences of untreated PID, the CDC intentionally chose a low diagnostic threshold. It defines PID on the basis of three clinical findings: lower abdominal tenderness, cervical motion tenderness, and adnexal tenderness. These criteria can be used to diagnose PID, provided there are no competing diagnoses, such as urinary tract infection, ectopic pregnancy, ovarian accidents, or gastroenteritis. Routine criteria include an oral temperature greater than 38° C, abnormal cervical or vaginal discharge, elevated sedimentation rate or C-reactive protein, and laboratory documentation of gonococcal or chlamydial infection. More elaborate criteria for increasing diagnostic specificity include histopathologic evidence of endometritis on endometrial biopsy, tuboovarian abscess on ultrasound or computed tomography (CT) scan, and laparoscopic abnormalities consistent with PID.

TREATMENT GUIDELINES

Treatment encompasses not only the selection of an antimicrobial agent but also whether therapy should take place in the hospital or in an outpatient setting, the optimal duration of therapy, and the role of adjuvant therapy. Selection of antimicrobial therapy must take into account the role of anaerobic bacteria and the use of monotherapy versus combination therapy. The treatment guidelines recommended by the CDC in 1993 provide two options for patients requiring hospitalization and two for outpatient therapy.

Inpatient Regimens

Inpatient regimen A is a combination of cefoxitin (Mefoxin) 2 grams intravenously every 6 hours or cefotetan (Cefotan) 2 grams intravenously every 12 hours plus intravenous or oral doxycycline (Vibramycin) 100 mg every 12 hours. This regimen should be continued for at least 48 hours after the patient demonstrates significant clinical improvement, after which doxycycline 100 mg orally twice daily should

be continued for a total of 14 days of therapy. Inpatient regimen B is a combination of intravenous clindamycin (Cleocin) 900 mg every 8 hours and intravenous or intramuscular gentamicin, 2 mg per kg of body weight loading dose, followed by 1.5 mg per kg maintenance dose. These should be continued for 48 hours after improvement. Therapy is then continued with either oral clindamycin 450 mg every 6 hours or oral doxycycline 100 mg every 12 hours to complete a total of 14 days of therapy. The presence of tuboovarian abscess has prompted many health providers to use clindamycin rather than doxycycline for continued therapy because of its greater efficacy against anaerobic organisms. Limited data, including at least one clinical trial, support the use of other inpatient regimens. These include ampicillin/sulbactam (Unasyn) 3.0 grams intravenously every 6 hours, plus doxycycline 100 mg intravenously or orally every 12 hours and ofloxacin (Floxin) 400 mg intravenously every 12 hours, plus metronidazole (Flagyl) 500 mg intravenously every 6 hours or clindamycin (Cleocin) 900 mg intravenously every 8 hours.

Outpatient Regimens

The current CDC guidelines recommend two outpatient regimens. Regimen A includes intramuscular cefoxitin 2.0 grams plus oral probenecid (Benemid) 500 mg given in a single dose concurrently, or intramuscular ceftriaxone (Rocephin) 250 mg or another parenteral third-generation cephalosporin such as ceftizoxime (Cefizox) or cefotaxime (Claforan). This is followed by twice-daily oral doxycycline 100 mg for 14 days. A concern with regimen A is that one dose of either cefoxitin or ceftriaxone does not give effective long-term coverage for anaerobic organisms. If anaerobic organisms are considered to have an important role in the pathogenesis of PID, then every recommended regimen should include an agent active against these bacteria. Regimen B, which is a new addition to the recommended guidelines, consists of 14 days of treatment with oral ofloxacin 400 mg every 12 hours plus either oral metronidazole 500 mg twice daily or oral clindamycin 450 mg every 6 hours. Ofloxacin has a broad spectrum of activity and excellent microbiologic activity against common pathogens in PID, including *Neisseria gonorrhoeae, Chlamydia trachomatis,* and *Ureaplasma urealyticum.*

PREVENTION

PID is preventable. Through patient education and recognition of the early signs of infection, primary care providers can greatly decrease the spread of *N. gonorrhoeae* and *C. trachomatis.* Additional preventive measures include early detection through screening, effective treatment, and treatment of sex partners. Unless PID is detected early, effective treatment is not possible. The challenge for providers and decision makers is to decrease the incidence of PID and its sequelae.

UTERINE LEIOMYOMA

method of
CHARLES C. CODDINGTON, M.D., and
MARK WAYNE AUSTIN, M.D.
Eastern Virginia Medical School
Norfolk, Virginia

Uterine leiomyomas are the most common solid pelvic tumors in women, noted in as many as 50% of postmortem examinations; however, clinically, they may be present in only 25 to 30% of women. They occur most often in nulliparous single black women of reproductive age. Uterine fibroids are responsive to estrogen stimulation and may grow rapidly during pregnancy. Their growth can cause dystocia, or they may begin to degenerate, resulting in significant pain, as well as the possibility of premature labor. Other symptoms depend on the size, number, and location of these tumors. Some of the more common symptoms are irregular uterine bleeding, pelvic pressure or pain, urinary frequency or incontinence, and decreased fertility. Patients present with multiple symptoms.

The role of uterine leiomyomas in the etiology of infertility is under study. It is obvious that if the myoma enlarges and occludes the fallopian tube, this will affect fertility. Other more subtle etiologies are altered sperm transport, variable hormone response of the underlying endometrium, and disruption of nidation. Even in the absence of symptoms, there is concern that once the tumor becomes enlarged, it may obscure more serious disease, such as ovarian cancer. These concerns have diminished recently with the advent and widespread application of ultrasonography.

Only rarely are these tumors malignant. In one study of 13,000 specimens, only 2.9% were malignant. In a more recent study of patients of reproductive age, only 1% of 800 specimens were malignant. Sarcomatous changes suggestive of malignancy appear to be more common in submucosal tumors. A malignant diagnosis is made at histology with greater than 10 mitotic figures per 10 high-power fields.

Evidence regarding the cause of uterine leiomyomas supports the central tenet of tumor biology—that most human tumors are cytogenetically abnormal clones of cells derived from a single progenitor cell that underwent mutation. Glucose-6-phosphate dehydrogenase (G6PD) isoenzyme analysis of multiple fibroids demonstrates monoclonality. Chromosomal analysis demonstrates abnormal karyotypes, with chromosomes 7, 12, and 14 most frequently affected. This alteration of genetics may play a role in the tumor growth pattern.

Leiomyomas are estrogen-sensitive tumors, and estrogen may play a pivotal role in the oncogenesis of fibroids. Estrogen regulates the frequency of mitosis in myometrial cells and thus influences the rate at which somatic mutations are propagated. Several studies have demonstrated increased concentrations of estradiol in leiomyomas as compared with adjacent myometrium, perhaps as a consequence of decreased 17-β-OH-dehydrogenase activity. Other studies have identified more estrogen receptors in the myomatous tissue as compared with adjacent tissues.

Recently, it has been noted that growth factors are also important. There appears to be more insulin-like growth factor I (IGF-I) in the myomas as compared with adjacent myometrium, and epidermal growth factor (EGF) was found to be increased in fibroids, but only during the luteal phase of the menstrual cycle. Cellular studies by Wilson demonstrated that hormones (estradiol, progesterone) by themselves did not alter the growth of myoma cells versus myometrium, but when EGF was added, there was an enhancement of growth as measured by 3H-thymidine inclusion. It seems clear that growth-promoting steroid hormones act through peptide growth factors to affect tissue growth.

The treatment for uterine leiomyomas varies greatly, depending on the patient's age, symptoms, and desires. Obviously, if a patient is older, has completed childbearing, and has troublesome symptoms, a hysterectomy might be the most reasonable alternative. Indications for consideration of myomectomy are as follows: (1) reproductive age, desiring to maintain reproductive potential; (2) a rapidly enlarging pelvic mass in a young woman; (3) persistent irregular bleeding; (4) lack of fertility with an otherwise normal evaluation; and (5) a persistent pelvic mass that is larger than 8 cm. Contraindications for myomectomy include presence of malignancy, pregnancy, extensive tubal disease, and age greater than 45 years. A preoperative evaluation should include a search for the causes of infertility if this is the presenting complaint. A hysterosalpingogram can delineate the involvement of the endometrial surface. Any operative report from prior laparoscopy or prior surgery may be helpful in determining the condition of the fallopian tubes, ovaries, and fimbria.

The decision to proceed with myomectomy is based on a risk/benefit analysis. Potential complications include emergency hysterectomy, formation of surgical adhesions, and surgical morbidity, including infection and transfusion. There is a 10 to 15% risk of regrowth of the tumors. In 18 reports of 1202 infertile patients operated on and receiving no further therapy, 40% conceived postoperatively, but there were no controls in these reports. Furthermore, in seven reports in which information was available regarding first-trimester fetal loss, it was noted that surgical therapy for leiomyoma improved fetal salvage from 59 to 81% and decreased fetal loss in the second trimester from 41 to 19%.

Medical therapy for uterine leiomyomas has existed for many years but is usually regarded as an adjunct to surgical therapy. Goodman first reported using progesterone therapy to suppress leiomyomas. In 1966, medroxyprogesterone was used and elicited degenerative changes in leiomyomas. Danazol resulted in only a 20% reduction in volume. Recently, gonadotropin-releasing hormone (GnRH) analogues have been used to induce a hypoestrogenic state. Freeman and colleagues studied the use of depot leuprolide acetate and demonstrated a significant reduction in myoma size over a 3- to 6-month period. However, after the medication was discontinued, the myoma size increased to 81% of its original volume within 1 year. Since prolonged hypoestrogenism and the attendant risk of osteoporosis and breast disease are obviously not options, a combination of GnRH analogue and surgery seems most reasonable. Benefits of combination therapy include decreased blood loss at the time of either myomectomy or hysterectomy, decreased blood loss in the menorrhagic patient to allow time for autologous blood donation, and conversion from abdominal to transvaginal approach in the case of hysterectomy. One report suggested that 2 months of therapy is as effective as 3 months. Also, a period of "coast" after the last dose may make it easy to establish tissue planes. Ideally surgery should be scheduled 5 weeks after the second dose of GnRH agonist, usually Lupron Depot 3.75 mg. Laparoscopy with current techniques may not allow complete removal of myomas nor reapproximation of tissue.

When myomectomy is performed and fertility is desired, great care must be taken to reduce the formation of surgical adhesions. In addition to the usual surgical techniques of meticulous hemostasis, gentle tissue handling, and keeping peritoneal surfaces moist, barrier methods are recommended. Both Interceed and Gore-Tex have been used with success when applied over the uterine incision during myomectomy. Interceed has the advantages of quick, easy application and complete absorption. Gore-Tex was marginally better than Interceed for adhesion prevention in the monkey model but is difficult to apply and must be removed surgically.

Other conservative methodologies are available to patients with smaller leiomyomas (≤3 cm). These include endoscopic resection of submucosal tumors, which can be performed with pelviscopy and/or laser therapy. Somewhat larger pedunculated tumors have been removed via morcellation or a colpotomy incision. With further advances in instrumentation, more therapeutic procedures will be performed utilizing endoscopy in conjunction with laser or electrosurgical energy.

CANCER OF THE ENDOMETRIUM

method of
THOMAS W. BURKE, M.D.

*University of Texas M. D. Anderson Cancer
  Center
Houston, Texas*

Endometrial carcinoma consistently affects 35,000 to 40,000 women in the United States annually, making it the most common gynecologic malignancy. However, annual deaths from this tumor average only about 6000—fewer

than those reported for either ovarian or cervical cancer. Endometrial cancers develop within the glandular epithelium of the uterus. About 90% of cases are typical endometrial adenocarcinomas; these are further subdivided into grades based on the amount of solid tumor growth. Two-thirds of women with typical endometrial adenocarcinomas have Grade 1 (well-differentiated) tumors; the remaining third have more aggressive Grade 2 or 3 lesions. Several uncommon, variant cell types constitute the other 10% of cases of endometrial carcinoma. These include papillary serous carcinoma, papillary endometrioid carcinoma, adenosquamous carcinoma, and clear cell carcinoma. Variant tumors are known for their aggressive clinical behavior and frequently demonstrate rapid growth, early dissemination, and poor response to therapy. Rarely, cancers of the uterine fundus arise from mesenchymal tissues (leiomyosarcoma, endometrial stromal sarcoma, other sarcomas) or contain mixtures of epithelial and mesenchymal elements (malignant mixed müllerian tumor). Such tumors, which account for only 5% of uterine malignancies, have a poor overall prognosis and a propensity for hematogenous dissemination to lung, liver, and brain.

EPIDEMIOLOGY AND HORMONE USE

A number of epidemiologic risk factors for the development of endometrial carcinoma have been identified (Table 1). Most of these revolve around the concept of chronic exposure to either endogenous or exogenous estrogen. Prolonged periods of anovulation, hormone-secreting tumors, peripheral conversion of adrenal steroids to estrogen by fat cells, and oral intake of unopposed estrogen can all produce chronic stimulation of the endometrium that ultimately results in malignant transformation. For instance, in early schedules of postmenopausal hormone replacement, the prescribed daily estrogen intake produced a clear-cut increase in endometrial cancer among continuous estrogen users. Current techniques for postmenopausal hormone replacement that combine estrogen with either cyclical or daily progestin avoid this risk while also relieving menopausal symptoms, maintaining cardiac function, and conserving bone density. The breast cancer risk associated with hormone replacement therapy is unclear, but if an increased risk exists, it is small. There have been reports of endometrial cancers developing in a few women who used the antiestrogen tamoxifen to suppress breast cancer. More data are needed to adequately assess the impact of long-term tamoxifen use, but preliminary data suggest that the cancer risk it imposes is probably not much greater than that for the general population. Some risk factors, such as diabetes mellitus and hypertension, do not readily fit into the estrogen stimulation hypothesis of

TABLE 1. **Risk Factors for Endometrial Cancer**

Feature	Increased Risk
Chronic anovulation	2×
Nulliparity	2×
Late menopause	3×
Estrogen-producing tumor	2×
Unopposed exogenous estrogen intake	6–8×
Postmenopause	4–8×
White race	2×
Diabetes mellitus	3×
Hypertension	1–2×
Obesity	3×
Prior pelvic irradiation	8×

endometrial carcinogenesis. Nevertheless, they have been consistently reported as independent risk factors in multiple studies.

PRESENTATION, DIAGNOSIS, AND EVALUATION

Endometrial lesions typically have an initial polypoid growth phase during which the tumor projects into the uterine cavity. As portions of the tumor outgrow their blood supply, necrosis and hemorrhage occur. This becomes evident to the patient as either postmenopausal bleeding or, for premenopausal women, menometrorrhagia. About 90% of women with endometrial carcinoma present with abnormal vaginal bleeding. Because this symptom is regarded as ominous by both the woman and her physician, a prompt diagnosis is usually obtained. A correctly obtained outpatient endometrial biopsy should provide adequate tissue for diagnosis. The biopsy technique must ensure passage of the biopsy instrument completely into the uterine cavity and should include multiple passes to avoid missing a small tumor. An operative dilatation and curettage may be necessary for a few women with cervical stenosis, an uncertain diagnosis, or inadequate tissue from outpatient biopsy. Because precise diagnostic criteria are difficult to apply to fragmented specimens, minor discrepancies between biopsy and final surgical specimens are common. Although some women have malignant cells detectable on cervical cytology smears, the Pap smear should not be used to make or exclude the diagnosis of endometrial cancer. Rarely, patients present with symptoms of advanced disease, such as an abdominal mass, ascites, pleural effusion, lymphadenopathy, bone metastasis, or brain metastasis. The diagnosis may be suggested by diagnostic studies or biopsy of a distant metastatic site; nevertheless, an endometrial biopsy should also be done to confirm the site of origin. A limited pretreatment evaluation that includes a physical examination, endometrial biopsy, laboratory studies, chest radiograph, and electrocardiogram is adequate for most cases. Additional diagnostic studies should be done in women with symptoms that suggest metastatic disease and in women with coexisting medical conditions that might limit or preclude surgery.

SURGICAL THERAPY, STAGING, AND RISK ASSESSMENT

Definitive surgical resection by total abdominal hysterectomy with bilateral salpingo-oophorectomy is the primary treatment for women with endometrial cancer. Removal of the uterus provides potentially curative resection of the tumor as well as important prognostic information. Additional staging biopsies are obtained to detect or confirm extrauterine spread. These include peritoneal cytology, omental biopsy, biopsy of visible or palpable abnormalities, and biopsy of pelvic and para-aortic lymph nodes. Although some gynecologists perform staging procedures in all cases of endometrial cancer, we limit staging biopsies to those women thought to be at risk for extrauterine spread. Prognostic factors for endometrial cancer are well established and can be grouped into uterine and extrauterine categories. Important uterine factors include cell type, histologic grade, depth of myometrial invasion, extension to the cervix, and presence of lymph-vascular space invasion. Extrauterine features that point to a poor prognosis are spread to the adnexal structures, positive peritoneal cytology, peritoneal metastasis, and lymph node metastasis. Based on the histopathologic results of the hysterectomy and staging laparotomy, the patient is assigned to one of the surgical stage categories (Table 2). Occasional patients are poor candidates for surgical therapy because of advanced disease or severe medical illness. Radiation therapy can provide excellent control of extensive pelvic disease and can often be curative when the tumor is confined to the uterus.

ADDITIONAL TREATMENT FOR HIGH–RISK CASES

Women with biopsy-proven extrauterine disease (surgical Stages III and IV) are at particularly high risk for tumor recurrence and death from disease. Additional postoperative treatment is generally recommended for such cases, but there is no consensus as to which therapy is most appropriate. Options include some form of irradiation, cytotoxic chemotherapy, or hormonal manipulation. Because prospective comparative treatment data are not available, selection of a specific therapeutic modality is often individualized based on disease location and physician bias. Whole pelvic or extended-field external beam irradiation can be considered for patients whose disease has metastasized to the adnexa or regional nodes and can be incorporated within the treatment field. Patients whose tumors have spread within the abdominal cavity can be treated with whole abdominal irradiation, although our preference is to use systemic chemotherapy. Progestational agents can be considered in women with advanced tumors that are positive for steroid hormone receptors.

A similar list of adjuvant therapy options is available for patients with high-risk Stage I and II tumors. Randomized trials evaluating the adjuvant use of pelvic irradiation or progestin have failed to demonstrate a survival advantage for treated patients.

TABLE 2. **Surgical Staging of Uterine Fundal Tumors**

Stage I		**Confinement to the uterine fundus**
	IA	Invasion of the endometrium only
	IB	Invasion of less than half of the myometrial thickness
	IC	Invasion of more than half of the myometrial thickness
Stage II		**Extension to the cervix**
	IIA	Invasion of the endocervical glands only
	IIB	Invasion of the cervical stroma
Stage III		**Regional spread**
	IIIA	Involvement of the uterine serosa or adnexa, or positive peritoneal cytology
	IIIB	Vaginal metastases
	IIIC	Spread to pelvic or para-aortic lymph nodes
Stage IV		**Bulky pelvic disease or distant spread**
	IVA	Invasion of the mucosa of the bladder or rectosigmoid
	IVB	Distant metastases

Experience with adjuvant chemotherapy is limited but warrants further study, since many women with recurrent endometrial cancer have disseminated disease. Many gynecologists recommend local vaginal cuff irradiation to reduce the incidence of isolated vaginal vault failures. Such therapy is probably effective but has little survival impact, because isolated vaginal recurrence is not common. Patients with low-grade, superficially invasive tumors confined to the uterus rarely develop recurrent cancer and require no therapy beyond surgery.

DETECTION AND TREATMENT OF RECURRENT DISEASE

Following the completion of primary therapy, patients enter a surveillance phase. Most recurrences are clinically evident within 3 years of treatment. Over half of women who develop recurrent disease are symptomatic; physical examination or radiographic studies can then be targeted to confirm the diagnosis. Many of the remaining patients with treatment failure are asymptomatic and have their recurrences detected by scheduled physical examination. The routine use of diagnostic imaging studies is not recommended for surveillance. Serial monitoring of serum CA 125 levels may be useful in some patients, especially those with extrauterine disease. Tumor recurrence should be pathologically confirmed. This can be accomplished by direct biopsy of accessible sites or fine-needle aspiration from deep tissue sites. Currently, we evaluate patients 6 and 12 months after the completion of therapy and annually thereafter. Any patient who develops symptoms of recurrence is seen and evaluated immediately.

Some patients with isolated vaginal apex recurrences can be cured with irradiation or radical surgery. However, the treatment of women with more distant sites of failure is largely palliative. Hormonal therapy can be given to women with well-differentiated or receptor-positive tumors. Occasional long-term responses can be obtained. Systemic chemotherapy can be attempted in other cases. Active drugs include doxorubicin (Adriamycin), cisplatin (Platinol), carboplatin (Paraplatin), and paclitaxel (Taxol). Response rates to single agents are roughly 30%, but response duration tends to be short.

OUTCOME

Fortunately, most women with endometrial cancer present with well-differentiated tumors confined to the uterus. Patients with Stage I, low-risk tumors have an excellent prognosis and a 5-year disease-free survival of 95% or better. In contrast, the survival of women in the high-risk categories is only 50 to 60%, and survival of those with Stage IV disease is less than 10%. Because of their poorer prognosis, these subgroups provide an ideal population on which to test and evaluate new therapy. Selecting such patients for adjuvant and adjunctive treatment minimizes the overtreatment of low-risk women and limits the morbidity of additional therapy to those patients most likely to develop recurrent cancer (Figure 1).

CARCINOMA OF THE CERVIX UTERI

method of
KATHERINE A. O'HANLAN, M.D.
Stanford University School of Medicine
Stanford, California

Worldwide, cervical carcinoma is the most common cancer among women. This cancer and the precancerous changes of the cervix are now largely viewed as a spectrum of sexually transmitted disease, given the initiating role of the venereally transmitted human papillomavirus (HPV), which is identified in over 90% of cases worldwide. Although the Pap test has been confirmed as a cost-effective screening device, it is underutilized in nonindustrialized countries, as well as in developed countries. In the United States, cervical cancer is variably the sixth leading cause of cancer death, trailing lung, breast, colorectal, ovarian, and endometrial malignancies.

RISK FACTORS

An estimated 20 to 30 million Americans carry HPV, yet little attention is paid to this epidemic. Only 30% of HPV infections are clinically recognizable as genital warts; fully 70% of HPV infections are subclinical and without symptoms. Because HPV is considered the etiologic agent for cervical cancer, this epidemic represents a major health problem for women.

The risk factors for cervical dysplasia and cervical carcinoma fall into three categories: the exposure to *initiating* HPV, the exposure to cancer-*promoting* agents, and the health of one's *immune system*. Venereal exposure to HPV at an early age (first intercourse during teenage years) increases the risk of HPV being incorporated into the meta-

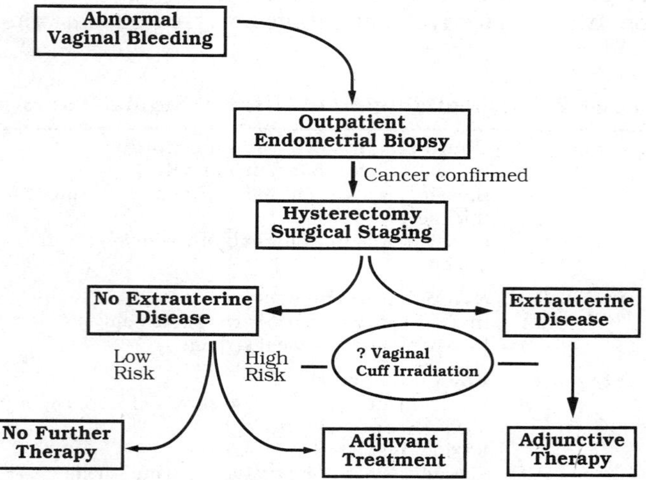

Figure 1. Schematic representation of the sequences for diagnostic and treatment decisions in women with endometrial carcinoma. This approach minimizes overtreatment of low-risk cases and focuses adjuvant and adjunctive therapy on those patients at greatest risk for treatment failure.

plastic cell genome. The greater the number of lifetime sexual partners, the greater the probability of exposure to HPV. Intercourse with males who have had multiple partners, a sexually transmitted disease, penile carcinoma, or a prior mate with cervical carcinoma significantly increases exposure to HPV. HPV prevalence among women with lower levels of education and lower income has also been observed. Although the use of oral contraceptives has been implicated as a risk factor for cervical carcinoma, detailed studies suggest that it is not the hormonal influence that imparts risk but rather the fact that oral contraceptive users have more sexual experiences and are less likely to use spermicidal creams. Such creams have a virucidal effect.

Cancer-promoting risk factors include cigarette smoking, herpes simplex virus infection, and poor nutrition. Poor nutrition and low intake of antioxidant fruits and vegetables have been associated with a higher risk for developing cervical dysplasia and carcinoma. In one study, healthy controls had higher levels of vitamin A and folic acid than did cervical cancer patients.

Immune suppression due to intrinsic immune suppressive disorders, human immunodeficiency virus (HIV) infection, transplant medication, or chronic steroid use increases the risk for HPV infection and predisposes to the development of premalignant cervical dysplasias and cervical cancer.

PREVENTION AND RISK MODIFICATION

Techniques that reduce exposure to HPV, reduce exposure to cancer promoters, and enhance immune status can prevent HPV infection and reduce cancer rates. Monogamy or celibacy and consistent use of barrier contraceptive methods are critical in reducing rates of cervical carcinoma. Condom use, which effectively reduces HIV transmission, should be encouraged among all individuals at risk. Establishment of dysplasia prevention programs predicated on reducing male and female factors known to increase risk, encouragement of screening for all women, and the use of patient education to reduce the practice of high-risk sexual behaviors are necessary. Many acquired immune deficiency syndrome (AIDS) and sex education programs have significant effects on adolescent sexual risk-taking behavior—delaying the initiation of intercourse, reducing the frequency of intercourse, reducing the number of sexual partners, or increasing the use of condoms or other contraceptives. Such programs have the potential to reduce exposure to unintended pregnancy and sexually transmitted diseases, including HPV infection. These programs should be replicated widely in U.S. schools.

Clinical prevention programs should include obtaining a history of the male partner's genital warts, hygiene, smoking, number of sexual partners, and practice (or not) of safe sexual behaviors. Although limited available data suggest that dysplasia is less common among lesbians than among heterosexual women, transmission of HPV among lesbians and bisexual women has been documented. Safer sex techniques should be used by all individuals, including lesbians.

The Pap smear has been shown to effectively diagnose the noninvasive precursors of cervical carcinoma. Treatment of the precursor lesions by laser ablation, freezing, or surgical excision can prevent the development of cervical malignancy. The Pap smear has reduced cervical cancer rates to less than one-quarter of the rate half a century ago. However, patient noncompliance, inadequate sample collection, and inaccurate pathologic interpretation are the most common causes of failure of early detection. Pap testing should be performed yearly, starting either at age 18 or during the year of first coitus. Women with none of the risk factors for cervical carcinoma who have had three normal yearly Pap smears can reduce their testing frequency to once every 3 years.

Closer surveillance of high-risk women, such as those with HIV, those on immune suppressive medications, and those with immune suppressive diseases, is indicated. Vitamin A and folic acid supplementation may offer some protective effect.

Substance abuse, including cigarettes, drugs, and alcohol, confers a significantly lower success rate for dysplasia treatment and a poorer survival from carcinoma than that observed for non–substance abusers. Women with dysplasia should be cautioned to discontinue all substance abuse.

SYMPTOMS

Irregular or postmenopausal bleeding and a new discharge are the most common symptoms experienced by over 90% of patients. The bleeding can be an exaggeration of the menstrual cycle duration or intensity, or it can occur after physical perturbation, such as sexual activity or douching. Discharges can range from profuse nonodorous mucus to foul, watery, and purulent. Any new bleeding or discharge in a postmenopausal woman requires gynecologic work-up to rule out an occult malignancy in the reproductive tract.

DIAGNOSIS

Examination of a cervix with primary carcinoma usually immediately reveals an exophytic friable lesion, but occasionally, only cervical erythema or ectropion is observed, with Pap smear data similarly showing only inflammatory atypia. Occult endocervical carcinoma, endometrial carcinoma, or even fallopian tube or ovarian carcinoma can present in this subtle fashion. A biopsy of any suspicious change of the ectocervix or endocervix and a detailed pelvic examination, with emphasis on the rectovaginal portion, should be performed. Further work-up consisting of endocervical curettage, endometrial suction aspiration, and possibly CA 125 with transvaginal sonography is indicated.

PATHOPHYSIOLOGY

Cervical dysplasia is considered a clonogenic event, starting in most cases at the squamocolumnar junction at the basement membrane and replacing the normal epithelium. Left untreated, locally invasive growth proceeds through the basement membrane into the stroma, expanding the cervix with an exophytic mass or, with endophytic growth, resulting in a classic barrel-shaped cervix. Once invasion into the stroma is deeper than 3.0 mm, the tumor can gain access to the lymphatic ducts and spread to the pelvic nodes in up to 15% of cases (Stage I). Growth in the cervical stroma proceeds with cancer cells spreading in either or both of two directions: superficially along the cervical epithelium and down the vaginal wall, or interstitially along fascial planes, resulting in direct spread laterally into the parametrium (Stage II). This advance of tumor growth enables more cells to gain access to the lymphatics, resulting in about 30% of patients having positive pelvic lymph nodes. Further growth into the parametrium typically blocks the ureter as it encroaches toward the bony pelvic sidewall (Stage III) and is associated with about 60% lymph node positivity. Distant spread of cancer is possible, with rare patients exhibiting growth into the bladder, rectum, liver, lung, or brain (Stage IV).

Approximately 85% of cervical carcinomas are squamous in origin, with the majority being large cell nonkeratinizing. Adenocarcinoma constitutes 10% of cervical malignancies and offers a slightly lower survival, possibly because its frequently endophytic growth pattern means that it can take longer for symptoms to develop. Small cell carcinoma of neuroendocrine origin and other rare histotypes occur in only 3 to 5% of cases.

The important favorable prognostic features of cervical carcinoma include younger age, lower stage, smaller lesion size, absence of lymphatic ductal and nodal involvement, lower grade of differentiation, minimal depth of invasion in the cervical stroma, and nonsmoking status.

STAGING

The staging schema for cervical carcinoma replicates the natural history of the disease. Standards for staging have been defined and are maintained by an international board of cooperative gynecologists, the Federation Internationale Gynecologic Obstetrica (FIGO), which last revised the standards in 1994 (Table 1). Only physical examination findings and widely available radiographic tests (the intravenous pyelogram and chest x-ray) are permitted to be used in assigning the FIGO stage. Lymphangiogram is also permitted in staging but is rarely used. Cystoscopy and proctoscopy typically have limited value and are thus omitted in early-stage, small-lesion cases, but they are necessary and occasionally positive in more advanced disease. Findings from more sophisticated or invasive radiographic investigations, such as computed tomography (CT) or magnetic resonance imaging (MRI), can sometimes provide clinically useful information, but they cannot be used to assign or to change a patient's FIGO stage. Once the FIGO stage has been assigned, it does not change.

THERAPY

Therapy for early invasive cervical carcinoma is based on the standard set by the Committee on Nomenclature of the Society of Gynecologic Oncologists in 1974, which defined *microinvasive carcinoma* of the cervix as neoplastic invasion of the stroma in one or more places to a maximum of 3.0 mm, with no lymphatic or blood vessel involvement. The working assumption about microinvasive carcinoma is that there is only negligible risk of spread beyond the cervix; therefore, only local, nonradical therapy is needed. Thus, no patients in whom either lymphatic or vascular channel involvement is observed are treated with conservative therapy for *microinvasion*.

The diagnosis, staging, and treatment planning for microinvasive cervical carcinoma are undertaken following an adequate cone biopsy with pathologically clear endocervical, ectocervical, and deep stromal margins. A small biopsy or endocervical curettage is not adequate to rule out the presence of a deeply invasive disease process or to ensure the safety of conservative therapy. Likewise, a simple hysterectomy is not performed to diagnose, stage, and treat because, in most cases, it is unnecessary; in others, it is inadequate therapy. Treatment by conservative observation, simple hysterectomy, or radical hysterectomy is determined only after detailed pathologic analysis of the cone specimen.

TABLE 1. **FIGO Staging of Carcinoma of the Cervix**

Preinvasive Carcinoma

Stage O   Carcinoma in situ, intraepithelial carcinoma.

Invasive Carcinoma

Stage I*   Carcinoma strictly confined to the cervix (extension to the corpus should be disregarded).

    Ia   Invasive cancer identified only microscopically. All gross lesions even with superficial invasion are stage Ib cancers. Invasion is limited to measured stromal invasion* with maximum depth of 5.0 mm and no wider than 7.0 mm.

    Ia1   Measured invasion of stroma no greater than 3.0 mm in depth and no wider than 7.0 mm.

    Ia2   Measured invasion of stroma greater than 3 mm and no greater than 5 mm and no wider than 7 mm. *The depth of invasion should not be more than 5 mm taken from the base of the epithelium, either surface or glandular, from which it originates. Vascular space involvement, either venous or lymphatic, should not alter the staging.

    Ib   Clinical lesions confined to the cervix or preclinical lesions greater than stage Ia.

    Ib1   Clinical lesions no greater than 4.0 cm in size.

    Ib2   Clinical lesions greater than 4 cm in size.

Stage II   The carcinoma extends beyond the cervix but has not extended to the wall. The carcinoma involves the vagina, but not the lower third.

    IIa   No obvious parametrial involvement.

    IIb   Obvious parametrial involvement.

Stage III   Either the carcinoma has extended to the pelvic wall (on rectal examination, there is no cancer-free space between the tumor and the pelvic wall) or the tumor involves the lower third of the vagina. This stage includes all cases with hydronephrosis or nonfunctioning kidney.

    IIIa   No extension to the pelvic wall; involvement of only the lower third of the vagina.

    IIIb   Extension to the pelvic wall and/or hydronephrosis or nonfunctioning kidney.

Stage IV   The carcinoma has extended beyond the true pelvis or has clinically involved the mucosa of the bladder or rectum. A bullous edema as such does not permit a case to be allotted to Stage IV.

    IVa   Spread of the growth to adjacent organs, confirmed by biopsy.

    IVb   Spread to distant organs.

*The diagnosis of Stage Ia1 and Ia2 is based on microscopic examination of removed tissue, preferably a cone, which includes the entire lesion. Vascular space involvement, either venous or lymphatic, does not change the staging but must be recorded, because it may affect treatment decisions in the future.

Stage Ia1

Lesions in which invasion is only minimally microscopically evident can be treated with a cone biopsy only and conservatively followed with endocervical and ectocervical Pap testing every 3 months for 2 years. There is no need for hysterectomy in patients who have Stage Ia1 disease and negative margins. If a margin is involved with only dysplasia that is clearly distant from the invasive process, further local ablational therapy is needed in about one third of cases as determined by a follow-up Pap smear in 3 months. However, if there is a dysplastic margin that is in the vicinity of the invasive focus, a repeat cone biopsy or local excisional therapy is indicated.

Management of Stage Ia1 disease is individualized, based on the depth of invasion. In those patients whose lesions have less than 3 mm of invasion and who do not have high-risk histology or lymphatic space involvement, an adequate cone biopsy is sufficient if fertility is desired or if hysterectomy is considered a high-risk procedure. This subset of patients requires close observation, consisting of clinical examinations every 3 months for the next 2 years that include separate endocervical and ectocervical assessments. Otherwise, a simple extrafascial hysterectomy can be performed.

Patients in Stage Ia1 with lymph-vascular space invasion should be treated with a radical hysterectomy and bilateral pelvic lymphadenectomy. A Type II radical hysterectomy in which the ureter is mobilized laterally for a medial parametrial dissection can be performed because there is a lower rate of morbidity compared with the Type III radical hysterectomies in which the parametrium is ligated far laterally. Because the ovaries are almost never involved by cervical squamous or adenocarcinoma, oophorectomy should be performed only if there are independent indications.

Stages Ia2, Ib, and IIa

Primary surgical therapy is generally reserved for slender patients who are good medical risks for radical pelvic surgery and have small lesions less than 4 cm in maximal diameter. Typically, a Type III radical hysterectomy with bilateral radical pelvic lymphadenectomy and low para-aortica lymph node sampling are performed. If the patient is not an ideal medical risk for surgery, radical pelvic radiation should be provided. The total minimum dose of 85 Gy at point A and 65 Gy to the lateral pelvic nodes should be delivered by external beam to sterilize the region and shrink the primary disease so that high-dose brachytherapy can then eradicate residual disease at the primary site. The surgery or radiation needs to be performed by a specialist in gynecologic oncology or radiation oncology who is trained and experienced in treating pelvic cancers. When the surgeon or radiation therapist is less than optimally experienced, the surgery is usually less than radical, and the dose of radiation is usually less than maximal, sacrificing cure rates either way.

The surgery is performed through a midline or Maylard incision. Laparoscopic approaches are not standard therapy at this writing. If grossly enlarged pelvic nodes are identified at laparotomy, the procedure should be terminated in favor of the equally curative pelvic radiotherapy. Completing the radical hysterectomy in such cases does not add to the cure rate but adds significantly to the postoperative incidence of leg edema and long-term bowel or bladder dysfunction. More importantly, it is useful to leave the uterus in place to serve as a conduit for the intracavitary brachytherapy portion of the radiotherapy, which critically boosts the parametrial dose by some 1500 cGy.

Should the final pathology report reveal two or more positive pelvic nodes or parametrial or vaginal margin involvement or proximity, pelvic radiotherapy is indicated. Patients with larger (>4 cm) Stage I lesions or a large, barrel-shaped cervix are more likely to have either positive pelvic lymph nodes or microscopic parametrial disease. Recently, the Radiation Therapy Oncology Group reported a significant 10% improvement in overall survival at 10 years but no difference in disease-free survival for patients with Stage Ib bulky disease or Stage IIb disease who received pelvic plus para-aortic irradiation. Patients who had a complete response had a lower incidence of subsequent distant failure and a better salvage even if they later failed locally. At this writing, patients with bulky Stage Ib disease are treated preoperatively with pelvic radiotherapy and a single intracavitary implant to shrink the cervical tumor, followed by an extrafascial hysterectomy and para-aortic node sampling. Chemotherapy may prove useful if it is given concurrently with the radiation as a sensitizer. Current trials are awaiting follow-up data to confirm the utility of the addition of hysterectomy.

Any patient who is not an ideal surgical candidate should be treated with definitive external beam pelvic radiotherapy, followed by two intracavitary implants to optimize the probability of central disease control. Ongoing research to optimize survival probability is looking at the use of interstitial needle insertion for patients with irregular parametrial residual disease after external beam radiation. The addition of chemosensitizers to postoperative radiotherapy for women with high-risk disease is also being studied.

More than 85% of cervical carcinomas are of the squamous variety. The majority of the remainder are adenocarcinomas. Although some studies have suggested a worse prognosis for this latter histotype, it must be recognized that the commonly found endophytic growth pattern of adenocarcinomas may allow the tumor to reach a greater size prior to detection of the development of symptoms in comparison to exophytic or squamous cell carcinomas of a similar stage. Adenocarcinoma is not more radioresistant than squamous cell carcinoma. Elevated carcinoembryonic antigen, CA 19-9, and CA 125 may provide tumor markers for patients with invasive adenocarcinoma or squamous cell cervical carcinoma.

Stages IIb to IVa

Radiation therapy is the mainstay of therapy for any large or advanced cervical carcinoma. Survival from advanced cervical carcinoma has nearly doubled in the last 2 decades because of advances in radiation dosing and machinery. Although FIGO staging is entirely clinical, a CT scan of the abdomen is performed on patients with disease beyond the cervix to tailor the radiation therapy to provide precise dose delivery and to maximize survival. Distant disease must also be ruled out by examining the aortic nodal chain first. In patients with no suspicious aortic adenopathy by CT, further evaluation to rule out occult adenopathy is performed by extraperitoneal or laparoscopic para-aortic lymph node sampling. A retroperitoneal approach to pretherapy surgical staging and the absence of previous surgery are associated with a reduced incidence of subsequent complications of radiation therapy. If the aortic nodes are radiographically suspicious for spread of disease, a fine-needle aspiration is used to confirm disease presence, and a CT scan of the chest should be obtained to examine the mediastinum and lungs. If mediastinal or lung disease is histologically confirmed, treatment should proceed as described for Stage IVb.

Patients with negative aortic nodes and nonbulky pelvic nodes are treated with whole pelvic four-field external beam radiation and one or two intracavitary or interstitial applications of cesium. High-dose intracavitary radiation therapy for carcinoma of the uterine cervix has gradually found wider acceptance. However, treatment results have been equivalent for high-dose and low-dose techniques, with a slightly higher complication rate for the high-dose group. Hydroxyurea (Hydrea) has a proven advantage as a radiosensitizer in therapy for advanced disease, given at a dose of 80 mg per kg orally twice weekly during radiotherapy. Cisplatin (Platinol) and 5-fluorouracil have been added to radiation treatments both as sensitizers and for their cytocidal effect on distant disease; however, the latter effect has been disappointing, and 5-fluorouracil may not offer any advantage over cisplatin alone. It remains unclear which of the various regimens has the best therapeutic index, but cooperative group trials are ongoing.

Extended field radiotherapy involves the traditional pelvic field, but the superior field margin is moved from the L4–5 interspace to the L3–4 interspace. It appears to benefit patients who have bulky disease in the pelvic nodes. With histologically confirmed aortic nodes, the radiation field from the L4–5 interspace should be narrowed superiorly and extended to the level of the diaphragm. Currently, there is no evidence that resection of bulky aortic or pelvic nodes offers a survival advantage. Microscopic and macroscopic metastases both confer a 5-year survival of about 12%, with most patients failing distantly.

Rectovaginal fistulas may develop during or after completion of pelvic radiotherapy, especially in patients with bulky parametrial or central disease. Fecal diversion by end colostomy offers control and can be done with minimal interruption of the radiotherapy. Vesicovaginal fistulas can develop in patients with anterior spread of tumor along the vesicouterine septum. Percutaneous nephrostomies can divert the urinary stream, although they are not always effective. Formation of a new bladder should usually be delayed until completion of radiotherapy, once local disease control has been ascertained.

Stage IVb

The goal in patients with distant metastases or recurrent disease is palliative. Combination chemotherapy trials using bleomycin, cisplatin, and ifosfamide offer an overall tumor response rate of over 60%, but cures are rare. Rapid-course high-dose external beam pelvic radiotherapy, with or without systemic chemosensitizing chemotherapy, can be given, depending on the patient's desire. Urinary or fecal diversion should be performed in the least invasive manner possible in an attempt to alleviate specific symptoms.

Recurrent Disease

Recurrent disease develops in nearly half of women with cervical carcinoma and carries a poor prognosis. Most recurrences become clinically apparent within the first 2 years after therapy. Therefore, follow-up clinical examinations and tumor marker assessment are indicated every 3 months for the initial 2 years, and every 4 to 6 months until 5 years after therapy. Yearly post-treatment chest x-ray has been advocated but does not offer a survival advantage.

Site, timing, and size of recurrence are important predictors of successful therapy, with small apical cervical lesions presenting after 1 year carrying the best prognosis. Prior to beginning any new therapy, a thorough evaluation of the extent of the recurrence is essential. MRI has the highest resolution of neoplastic lesions in a radiated field and should be routinely performed.

Patients initially treated by radical hysterectomy with pelvic recurrence should have pelvic radiotherapy with a sensitizer and should be considered for extended-field radiation. Patients with recurrent disease previously treated with radiotherapy, even after a radical hysterectomy, are evaluated for exenterative surgery.

The mortality rate from exenteration is 3 to 5%, with a surgical morbidity rate over 60%. Five-year survival rates from the institutions where exenterations are frequently performed are as high as 60%. Therefore, careful patient selection for this morbid procedure is necessary. Preoperative evaluation with pelvic and abdominal MRI, chest x-ray, bone scan, and occasionally lymphangiogram and directed fine-needle aspiration is indicated. Patients whose disease appears clinically and radiographically localized to the central pelvis should be explored for exenteration. Parametrial fixation of the central tumor does not preclude successful exenteration, as many of these patients have lateral planes of dissection free of tumor. Some surgeons have had some success using intraoperative radiation therapy for close or positive lateral pelvic margins. However, large (≥5 cm) recurrences, lateral pelvic wall disease, hydroureter, bladder or rectal involvement, and nodal disease remain poor prognostic indicators, reducing survival probabilities to 15 to 30%.

Careful intra- and retroperitoneal exploration is performed, with intraoperative examination of peritoneal cytology in patients with adenocarcinoma. Up to 60% of these patients are found to have intraperitoneal or distant disease and do not qualify for exenteration. If the recurrence is confined to the pelvis, the exenteration proceeds, with removal of the bladder, the upper or total vagina, and, depending on the anatomy of the postsurgical pelvis and the recurrence, the rectum. Total pelvic exenteration can now be performed in conjunction with simultaneous neovagina and genitourinary and gastrointestinal reconstruction, with minimal morbidity. The development of the continent urinary diversion, with primary reanastomosis of the rectosigmoid, helps make such extensive surgery less disfiguring and disabling.

A subset of patients has been identified with such small central recurrences that only radical hysterectomy was performed. In these few cases, cure rates similar to those for exenteration were observed. Urinary fistula was one complication that occurred more frequently because the bladder was irradiated. Further research is ongoing, focusing on selecting patients for less radical procedures, minimizing operative morbidity, and maximizing postoperative functional and cosmetic effects while maintaining the highest possible survival rates.

CERVICAL CARCINOMA DURING PREGNANCY

Cervical carcinoma presenting during pregnancy requires individualized treatment decisions, based on the stage of the pregnancy and the size and stage of the tumor at diagnosis. Small lesions identified early in pregnancy can sometimes be observed during the gestation, planning a combined delivery and radical extirpation or delayed radiation therapy. Larger lesions and higher-stage tumors should usually proceed to radiotherapy, focusing on the survival of the mother.

PROGNOSIS

Overall, about half of patients with cervical carcinoma are cured. The 5-year survival rates for patients with early, small lesions are about 90%. However, the survival is 75% for all Stage I patients, because some Stage I cancers are large or have nodal metastases. Stage II tumor, invading the parametrium or upper vagina, confers a 5-year survival of 55%. Once the tumor spreads outward to the sidewall or ureter or down the vagina (Stage III), about 35% survive. Less than 5% are cured with disease invading the bladder or rectum or with distant spread (Stage IV).

NEOPLASMS OF THE VULVA

method of
DALE BROWN, JR., M.D.
Houston, Texas

Both benign and malignant neoplasms are found in the vulva. Inspection of the vulva and vagina with the use of a hand magnifying glass allows the clinician to inspect the vulva in greater detail. The use of a colposcope may also be of value. Vulvar biopsies should be liberally performed in the office setting, because adequate therapy is based on an accurate diagnosis. Excision biopsy is the ideal method for treating small discrete lesions. The Keyes cutaneous punch biopsy instrument can be utilized for biopsy of large or widespread skin lesions. A 4-mm instrument is adequate in most cases.

The biopsy tissue specimen should be oriented on a small piece of filter paper or paper towel before being placed into a fixative solution. This allows for proper orientation of the tissue when the sections are cut. Tangential cutting occasionally leads to an erroneous diagnosis. Changes often seen in human papillomavirus (HPV) infection or intraepithelial neoplasia may be highlighted by washing the vulva with 4 to 5% acetic acid. This often turns the mucosal lesions acetowhite after the application of the solution. The use of 1% toluidine blue stain (a nuclear protein stain) may also be helpful in selecting a biopsy site in widespread lesions. Liberal washing of the vulva with 1% toluidine blue and then washing with 1% acetic acid after the toluidine blue has been given adequate time to dry can direct the practitioner to locations for biopsy. Lesions such as invasive and intraepithelial carcinomas retain the blue color after being washed with the acetic acid. Unfortunately, the dye may be retained on any ulcerative site. When a thick keratin layer covers the surface of intraepithelial or invasive carcinoma, the dye is not retained.

BENIGN TUMORS OF THE VULVA

The vulva may be affected by a wide spectrum of benign, solid, and cystic tumors. Classification of these tumors is based on the tissue of origin, embryologic derivation, morphologic findings, or gross appearance. An easy and useful classification of benign vulvar tumors devised by Fredrich and Kaufman is presented in Table 1.

If the diagnosis of a benign tumor is apparent on gross inspection and the patient is not experiencing any adverse symptoms or discomfort, no treatment is necessary. If the clinician is not absolutely sure of the exact nature of the tumor, a biopsy should be obtained.

Benign Solid Tumors

Acrochordons (often called fibroepithelial polyps), along with fibromas, lipomas, and neurofibromas, are the most common benign solid tumors affecting the vulva. Benign solid tumors may also arise in the Bartholin and vestibular glands. Wide excision of the tumor with appropriate anesthesia, either in the office or in the hospital, should be performed when the diagnosis is uncertain or the tumor is symptomatic and causing discomfort. Wide local excision with primary closure of the defect is all that is necessary. Prepubertal females have been found to have interlabial masses that histologically reveal benign ureteral polyps and pigmented apocrine hamartomas.

Benign Cystic Tumors

Epidermal inclusion cysts and developmental cysts of the urogenital sinus, paramesonephric duct, meso-

TABLE 1. Classification of Benign Vulvar Tumors

Benign Solid Tumors	Benign Cystic Tumors
Epidermal origin	Epidermal origin
Condyloma acuminatum	Epidermal inclusion cyst
Molluscum contagiosum	Pilonidal cyst
Acrochordon	Epidermal appendage origin
Seborrheic keratosis	Sebaceous cyst
Nevus	Hidradenoma
Epidermal appendage origin	Fox-Fordyce disease
Hidradenoma	Syringoma
Sebaceous adenoma	Embryonic remnant origin
Basal cell carcinoma	Mesonephric (Gartner's) cyst
Mesodermal origin	Paramesonephric (müllerian) cyst
Fibroma	Urogenital sinus cyst
Lipoma	Cyst of canal of Nuck (hydrocele)
Neurofibroma	Adenosis
Leiomyoma	Cyst of supernumerary mammary glands
Granular cell myoblastoma	Dermoid cyst
Hemangioma	Bartholin's gland origin
Pyogenic granuloma	Duct cyst
Lymphangioma	Abscess
Bartholin's and vestibular gland origin	Urethral and paraurethral origin
Adenofibroma	Paraurethral (Skene's duct) cyst
Mucous adenoma	Urethral diverticula
Urethral origin	Miscellaneous origin
Caruncle	Endometriosis
Prolapse of the urethral mucosa	Cyst lymphangioma
	Liquefied hematoma

nephric duct, and ectopic mammary glandular tissue are the most common cystic tumors involving the vulva. These tumors can be left untreated if they are asymptomatic and the clinician is confident of the diagnosis. Again, if the diagnosis is in doubt or if the patient has symptoms related to the mass, local excision is indicated and is usually adequate therapy.

Hidradenoma, an epidermal appendage origin tumor, is commonly confused with a primary or metastatic adenocarcinoma of the vulva. This tumor can easily be excised as an office procedure using local anesthesia. The histopathology reveals the characteristic pattern of the tumor as well as the absence of nuclear atypia and multilayering of cells.

Cystic Bartholin's duct tumors, both simple cysts and abscesses, may be seen in approximately 2% of gynecologic patients. Occlusion of the duct usually occurs near the opening of the main duct into the vestibule, therefore, the cyst is usually unilocular. Occasionally, one or more loculi lie deep in the main cyst. Unless symptomatic, Bartholin's duct cysts can be left untreated. Most patients with small cysts have no symptoms, although occasionally mild discomfort is experienced with sexual intercourse. Marsupialization is indicated when the cyst causes discomfort and pressure with ambulation and/or coital activity. The incision for marsupialization should be located medial enough so that the new orifice is close to the original opening of the Bartholin duct into the vestibule. The incision should extend through the wall of the cyst. After evacuation of its contents, the lining of the cyst is sewn to the mucosal and skin surfaces with interrupted fine, absorbable sutures (Vicryl 3-0 or 4-0).

An acute Bartholin abscess may occur in the pres-

ence of a previous Bartholin's duct cyst or may arise primarily. Cultures of Bartholin's abscesses reveal a wide spectrum of organisms. Cultures for gonococcal organisms should be performed in sexually promiscuous females. Most abscesses, especially if they are recurrent, develop as a result of a nongonococcal infection of the fluid contents of a Bartholin cyst. Varying degrees of pain and tenderness over the affected gland are the chief symptoms. The rapidity of development and the extent of involvement depend on the size of the infected cyst and the virulence of the infectious agent. Unilateral swelling over the site of the infected gland, erythema of the overlying skin, and frequently edema of the surrounding labia are present. The abscess is a palpable and extremely tender fluctuant mass. An acute Bartholin abscess requires immediate treatment. Local application of hot, wet dressings or sitz baths may enhance spontaneous drainage within 72 hours. Incision and drainage can be accomplished in a physician's office with local anesthesia. Use of the Word catheter—an inflatable, bulb-tipped, closed catheter for marsupialization—is an effective and proficient method for outpatient treatment. After appropriate anesthesia of the skin with 1% lidocaine (Xylocaine) or an appropriate local anesthetic, a small stab wound incision is made into the abscess cavity close to the hymenal ring. The contents of the abscess are evacuated, and any loculization can be broken with the use of a hemostat. After the catheter is inserted, the small balloon is inflated with 2 mL of saline. The distal end of the catheter is then placed into the vaginal vault. The catheter should be left in place at least 4 to 6 weeks, during which time the balloon may be deflated partially. It takes approximately 6 weeks for adequate epithelialization to be accomplished for the formation of a new ostium. While the catheter is in place, the patient may continue with normal activities, including coital activity, without difficulty.

MALIGNANT NEOPLASMS OF THE VULVA

The cause of vulvar malignancy (Table 2) remains unknown, but it seems to be multifactorial. HPV alone is not sufficient for malignant transformation. Primary among cofactors may be the patient's own immune competence, including conditions of local immune deficiency. The International Society for the Study of Vulvovaginal Diseases has classified intraepithelial neoplastic disorders of the vulvar skin and mucosa as follows:

1. Squamous (may include changes resulting from HPV infection)
   A. Vulvar intraepithelial neoplasia (VIN-1) (mild dysplasia)
   B. VIN-2 (moderate dysplasia)
   C. VIN-3 (severe dysplasia, carcinoma in situ)
2. Other
   A. Paget's disease
   B. Melanoma (level one)

VIN

VIN is more frequently diagnosed in younger patients. Whereas the incidence of VIN-3 has markedly increased, the incidence of invasive carcinoma has remained stable. The largest increase has occurred in white women under the age of 35. Carcinoma in situ or VIN-3 has a peak onset in the fourth decade. Several factors may contribute to the increased incidence of this disease and its occurrence in younger age groups. The heightened awareness of neoplasia by physicians and the liberal use of biopsy to obtain

TABLE 2. **Malignant Tumors of the Vulva**

Epithelial tumors of the skin and mucosa
  Squamous cell origin
    Squamous cell carcinoma
    Verrucous cell carcinoma
  Basal cell carcinoma
  Melanoma
  Adenocarcinoma
    Paget's disease
    Skin appendage
Malignant tumors of the urethra
Bartholin's gland carcinoma
  Squamous cell carcinoma
  Adenocarcinoma
  Adenoid cystic carcinoma
  Adenosquamous carcinoma
  Transitional cell carcinoma
Carcinoma and sarcoma of ectopic breast tissue
Soft tissue sarcomas
  Embryonal rhabdomyosarcoma
  Leiomyosarcoma
  Malignant fibrous histiocytoma
  Epithelial sarcoma

an accurate diagnosis have been contributing factors in its more frequent diagnosis. The association of high-risk types of HPV (such as 16, 18, 31, 33, 35, and 39) with the development of lower genital tract neoplasia is now well accepted. It has been postulated that possibly two forms of invasive squamous cell carcinoma of the vulva are seen. One is observed in younger women who smoke, whose lesions morphologically resemble the changes seen with intraepithelial neoplasia, and whose tumors have a high association with HPV infection. The other type of cancer is seen more often in older women with a more well-differentiated type of squamous cell carcinoma who do not smoke and whose lesions are infrequently associated with HPV infection.

The diagnosis of VIN must be established by biopsy before treatment is undertaken. A high index of suspicion and several biopsies are appropriate, especially in lesions that are not very focal. VIN is frequently a multifocal disease, with the posterior half of the vulva being the area most often affected.

Because the biologic potential of VIN remains uncertain, conservative therapy is appropriate. The treatment should be individualized on the basis of the location and extent of the lesion. Additionally, the presence or absence of factors increasing the risk for occult invasive cancer should be considered. Wide excision of the intraepithelial neoplasia is more appropriate than a total vulvectomy for unifocal lesions. When wide local excision is selected as the method of treatment, the entire lesion should be surgically removed, including a tissue margin of 1 to 1.5 cm beyond the limits of the lesion. Frozen sections should be taken from the peripheral margins of the excised tissue to be certain that no residual disease is present. When disease persists along the margins of the excised tissue, more skin and mucosa must be excised until the margins are disease free. Recurrence of disease is related to the presence or absence of free margins. Because the disease may have widespread multifocal involvement, shallow "skinning" procedures that remove the full thickness of the epithelium of the labia majora, labia minora, and clitoris but preserve the underlying connective tissues may be used. Often the defect can be closed primarily, but occasionally it is necessary to use a skin graft to adequately cover the denuded vulvar surfaces. When disease extends into the anal canal, it is necessary to remove the anal mucosa up to the level of the pectinate line. The rectal mucosa can then be undermined and pulled down to cover the defect.

Laser therapy for ablation of VIN is appropriate in selected cases. An occult invasive carcinoma must be excluded from adequate biopsies because of the loss of tissue for histologic interpretation. Lesions demonstrating thickening of the tissues or those that appeared ulcerative are best treated by excision rather than by laser. Ablation by the laser to a depth of 1 to 3 mm, including the zone of thermal necrosis, and a surrounding 0.5 to 1 mm of normal tissue should be sufficient to destroy most epidermal lesions without skin appendage involvement. Deeper tissue destruction is necessary if the initial biopsy showed involvement of adjacent hair follicles or sebaceous glands. The ablation should be carried to a depth of 3 mm to remove any possible disease that extends down into the superficial skin appendages. Ablation to a depth of 1 mm is adequate on mucosal surfaces. Because of the significant postoperative discomfort and the time involved, we prefer not to use the carbon dioxide laser in treating extensive VIN.

Topical chemotherapy with 5% fluorouracil cream (Efudex)* has produced a response in approximately 50% of cases in which it has been used, although recurrence has been noted. There is significant morbidity because of local irritation, ulceration, and denudation accompanying its use. Possible reduction of morbidity can be accomplished by weekly application over several months.

Paget's Disease

Paget's disease is primarily an intraepithelial disease that tends to recur locally and has a minimal propensity to invade. About 10 to 15% of patients have an associated invasive adenocarcinoma. Paget's disease may also be related to primary carcinoma of the rectum, especially when it involves the perianal region, urethra, or bladder. Chanda reported that 12% of women with Paget's disease of the vulva had an associated concurrent underlying internal malignancy. He observed that perianal Paget's disease was associated with digestive tract carcinoma.

Paget's cells are of epidermal origin and represent aberrant differentiation of the epidermal multifocal stem cells. Large cells containing clear vacuolated cytoplasm are characteristic of Paget's cells. The intraepidermal migration of Paget's cells may be confused with invasive carcinoma. Histochemical stains yield positive reactions for acid or neutral intracellular mucopolysaccharides in characteristic Paget's cells, this clearly distinguishes them from cells of even more unusual superficial amelanotic melanoma. Monoclonal antibodies have also been applied in distinguishing the cells of Paget's disease from those of intraepithelial squamous cell carcinoma and melanoma. Such monoclonal antibodies as KA-4 and GCDFP-15 can be used to distinguish the cells of Paget's disease from those of other intraepithelial disorders.

Paget's disease of the vulva occurs most often in white postmenopausal women. The appearance of the disease is variable. Typically, it appears as a red or bright-pink desquamative eczematoid area with scales and crust scattered over the surface. The borders appear slightly elevated and sharply demarcated.

Treatment encompasses wide excision of a margin of at least 2 cm from the initial definition of the lesion. Because of the need to exclude an underlying skin appendage carcinoma, a greater depth of subcutaneous tissue should be removed. There is also the possibility of intraepidermal migration of Paget's cells deep in the epidermis or somewhat removed from the apparent margins of the tumor. The margins should be evaluated by examination of frozen sections; otherwise, the frequency of recurrence will be high. The corrected survival rate for all patients, including those with associated underlying adenocarcinoma, is approximately 90%. In about 20% of cases, intraepidermal occurrences have been reported following total excision.

INVASIVE NEOPLASMS OF THE VULVA

Invasive malignancies of the vulva are responsible for 1 to 4% of all female cancers. The most common of the malignant tumors is squamous cell carcinoma, which accounts for 90% of vulvar malignancies. Most invasive carcinomas arise in a unifocal manner, presenting with signs of ulceration, friability, or induration of the surrounding tissues. Although invasive squamous cell carcinoma is seen in association with vulvar dystrophies such as lichen sclerosis, vulvar dystrophy is not considered a high-risk premalignant entity. The likelihood of such a patient developing invasive carcinoma of the vulva is less than 5%. The patient may be asymptomatic or complain of pruritus, bleeding, discharge, or associated pain. The diagnosis is confirmed by biopsy.

Treatment depends on the stage of the disease (Table 3). Surgical staging approved by the International Federation of Gynecology and Obstetrics (FIGO) includes assessment of node involvement. The pattern of lymphatic dissemination from the primary lesion seems to be an orderly progression through the superficial inguinal nodes to the deep inguinal nodes. The cancer may then spread to the contralateral groin nodes, the deep pelvic nodes, or both. In the treatment of invasive squamous cell carcinoma, the clinical status of the inguinal nodes provides prognostic criteria regarding the risk of pelvic metastasis. Because as many as 25% of patients may have occult metastases with no palpable nodes or nonsuggestive palpable nodes, a patient must be adequately evaluated for the presence of distant me-

TABLE 3. **FIGO Staging System for Carcinoma of the Vulva**

Stage 0	Carcinoma in situ; intraepithelial carcinoma.
Stage I	Tumor confined to the vulva and/or perineum; 2 cm or less in greatest dimension; nodes are not palpable.
Stage II	Tumor confined to the vulva and/or perineum; more than 2 cm in greatest dimension; nodes are not palpable.
Stage III	Tumor of any size with adjacent spread to the lower urethra and/or the vagina, or the anus; and/or unilateral regional lymph node metastasis.
Stage IVA	Tumor invades any of the following: upper urethra, bladder mucosa, rectal mucosa, or pelvic bone, and/or bilateral regional node metastasis.
Stage IVB	Any distant metastasis, including pelvic lymph nodes.

*Not FDA-approved for this indication.

tastases prior to the formation of a treatment plan. Preoperative bone scan and computed tomography (CT) scan of the pelvis, along with chest x-ray, should be used to search for enlarged lymph glands, especially in those individuals with Stage III or IV disease. Radical vulvectomy with bilateral femoroinguinal lymph node dissection remains the treatment of choice for advanced disease, but this is no longer true of localized disease. Treatment is individualized and based on the knowledge of the natural spread of vulvar carcinoma.

Treatment of Stage I. With a tumor that is superficially invasive, less than 2 cm in diameter, and limited to one side of the vulva and does not involve the clitoris, urethra, vagina, or anus, treatment may consist of a hemipelvectomy and ipsilateral inguinal lymphadenectomy. This allows preservation of cosmetic appearance and sexual function. It is associated with decreased postoperative morbidity. At least a 2- to 3-cm margin of normal skin should be removed surrounding the tumor, and the subcutaneous fat should be excised down to the fascia. Ipsilateral groin dissection should be performed through a separate incision; if the contralateral nodes are positive, they should be removed, or the groin should be treated with external radiation. Additionally, the deep pelvic nodes should receive external beam therapy. Whenever an invasive carcinoma is a midline lesion, bilateral inguinofemoral lymph node dissection should be performed.

Treatment of Stage II. The treatment plan formulated for Stage I lesions can also be used in the treatment of Stage II disease. When the lesion is of significant size, it may be necessary to perform a complete vulvectomy to enable an adequate margin of normal skin to be obtained. A separate groin incision should be utilized for removal of the superficial and femoral nodes.

Treatment of Stage III. Depending on the extent of the tumor, if the urethra and vagina are involved, portions of both should be removed along with the vulvectomy specimen. Allowance should be made for at least a 2-cm margin of normal tissue. When the anus is involved with the tumor, an abdominal perineal resection, with removal of the anal canal, may be necessary. Additionally, bilateral inguinal and femoral node dissections should be performed through separate incisions. Occasionally, preoperative radiotherapy may be used to decrease the size of a large lesion, to allow for less extensive surgery. It may be necessary to form a full-thickness skin flap using gracilis muscle to cover large vulvar defects.

Treatment of Stage IV. Treatment of Stage IV depends on the presence or absence of distant metastasis. Local palliative excision or radiation therapy, alone or together, may be utilized. In the absence of distant metastasis, the treatment plan is managed as previously described for Stage III disease.

VERRUCOUS CARCINOMA

Verrucous carcinoma, a much less common carcinoma, locally invades the vulvar tissue without the development of metastases. If infection occurs in association with verrucous carcinoma, the microscopic picture may be confusing and lead to an erroneous diagnosis of advanced squamous cell carcinoma. The verrucous lesions are thick neoplasms that invade and compress broad areas of relatively well-differentiated squamous cells with "pushing" margins. Notable is the condyloma of the Buschke-Löwenstein exophytic tumor. HPV type 6 has been implicated in its development. Treatment consists of wide local excision. Recurrences may occur if the margins are involved by the neoplasm. Rarely is groin lymph node dissection necessary. Radiation therapy is contraindicated, because radiation frequently transforms verrucous carcinoma into an aggressive neoplasm that may metastasize. Recurrence connotes a poor prognosis.

MELANOMA

It has been stated that approximately 8% of all melanomas occur on the vulva. Very infrequently does melanoma occur as a primary lesion. Melanomas that occur on the vulva require careful inspection and prophylactic excision of all darkly pigmented lesions of the vulva. Early diagnosis is crucial if cure is to be obtained. Prognostic factors consist of tumor thickness (Table 4), inguinal node metastases, and older age at diagnosis. The diagnosis is established by biopsy, and microstaging is determined following excision of the neoplasm. Radical local excision is the preferred treatment. A low-risk patient with a nonulcerative tumor less than 1 mm thick and without clinical evidence of inguinal lymph node metastases can be treated by wide local excision with a 2- to 3-cm margin. Those patients with an ulcerative lesion or a depth greater than 1 mm should receive a wide radical excision with ipsilateral inguinofemoral lymph node removal. Groin node dissection serves as a prognostic rather than a therapeutic procedure, because once regional lymph node involvement has occurred, the prognosis is extremely poor regardless of additional adjunctive therapy.

BARTHOLIN'S GLAND CARCINOMA

A rare malignancy that must be considered in the differential diagnosis of a labial mass is Bartholin's gland carcinoma. The etiology remains unknown, and no optimal plan of treatment has been established. Tentative diagnosis is based on the cytologic

TABLE 4. **Levels of Melanoma**

Clark's Levels	Breslow's Levels (Modified)
1. Intraepithelial	<0.76 mm
2. Extends into papillary dermis	0.76–1.49 mm
3. Fills papillary dermis	1.50–2.49 mm
4. Extends into reticular dermis	2.50–3.00 mm
5. Extends into subcutaneous fat	>4 mm

findings and location of the tumor. The skin over the neoplasm should be intact. Histologic evidence of Bartholin's glands' structures should be contiguous to the tumor. Treatment presently consists of radical vulvectomy and bilateral inguinofemoral lymph node dissection.

CLEAR-CELL HIDRADENOCARCINOMA

Clear-cell hidradenocarcinoma is a rare malignant tumor that occurs primarily on the vulva with metastatic disease. Most often it is found on the trunk, head, and extremities. The origin may be from mammary ectopic tissue in the vulva or from vulvar skin adnexa. Because of the tumor's tendency to spread profusely into surrounding soft tissues, as well as to inguinal lymph nodes, treatment is similar to that of basal cell carcinoma of the vulva.

BASAL CELL CARCINOMA

Basal cell carcinomas occur most frequently in white females over 50 years of age. The lesions are solitary and ulcerative, with a slightly elevated margin at the periphery. The most common location is the anterior two-thirds of the labia majora. Very rarely do these tumors metastasize; thus, simple wide excision is curative in most cases. Those tumors that do metastasize manifest several features that distinguish them from most of the nonmetastasizing tumors: vaginal bleeding at presentation; involvement of the subcutaneous fat, urethra, and vagina; advanced clinical stage; tumor thickness greater than 1 cm; and a pattern of growth characterized by indurated plaques of thickened dermal fibrous tissue surrounded by a pinkish or purplish halo.

SOFT TISSUE SARCOMA

Soft tissue sarcomas are extremely rare and usually appear as a rapidly enlarging and painful mass. The prognosis is variable, depending on the biologic character of the individual sarcoma, but may be related to hematogenous metastasis. Even though radical vulvectomy and lymph node groin dissection yield the lowest incidence of recurrent disease, many patients do not survive very long. Most tumors are related to the leiomyosarcoma group; however, the prognosis for all sarcomas depends on the biologic character of the individual sarcoma. Radiotherapy is of little use in the management of most vulvar sarcomas.

THROMBOEMBOLIC DISEASE IN PREGNANCY

method of
GENO J. MERLI, M.D., and
ROSEMARIE A. LEUZZI, M.D.
Jefferson Medical College, Thomas Jefferson University Hospital
Philadelphia, Pennsylvania

Deep venous thrombosis (DVT) and pulmonary embolism (PE) are major causes of maternal morbidity and mortality during pregnancy. The incidence of deep venous thrombosis in pregnancy is 0.5% to 0.7%, which increases to 1.4% when superficial thrombophlebitis is included. The incidence of PE has been reported to be 0.3% to 1.2%, with the overall incidence of deep vein thrombosis and pulmonary embolism between 0.3% and 1.2% for all pregnancies. This increased risk of thrombosis is related to stasis, intimal injury, and hypercoagulability. Progesterone causes a decrease in venous tone, thereby increasing lower extremity venous capacitance. These factors, along with impaired venous outflow due to compression of the inferior vena cava by the gravid uterus, contribute to stasis in the lower extremities. Intimal injury may result from the trauma of delivery; hypercoagulability is secondary to an increase of clotting factors during pregnancy. The hematologic changes of pregnancy, assessment of DVT/PE, treatment modalities, and complications of these therapies are presented here.

HEMATOLOGIC CONSIDERATIONS

Pregnancy alters the coagulation system in preparation for birth and placental separation to prevent excessive peripartum blood loss. Table 1 describes each of the clotting factors that are affected by pregnancy. In addition there is a decrease in the activity of the fibrinolytic system, although this returns to normal within a few hours of delivery. Table 1 does not represent all the data on clotting factors in pregnancy but the best available at this time.

The platelet count does not change significantly during normal pregnancy, but it appears that there is a small decrement in the platelet count near term. In the postpartum period, the platelet count may increase in reaction to the hemostatic challenge of delivery. Although platelet counts of less than 150×10^9 per liter are considered thrombocytopenia in nonpregnant adults, counts of less than 100×10^9 per liter constitute thrombocytopenia in pregnancy.

The intrinsic inhibitors of coagulation are affected differently by gestation. Antithrombin III (AT-III) levels do not appreciably decrease, except in the presence of preeclampsia, acute fatty liver of pregnancy, disseminated intravas-

TABLE 1. **Pregnancy and the Clotting System**

Changes	Factors
Increased	I, II, V, VII, VIII, IX, X, XII, fibrinogen
Very little change	Protein C, AT-III, platelets
Significantly decreased	Protein S
Decreased fibrinolysis	Increased PAI-1, PAI-2

Abbreviations: AT-III = antithrombin III; PAI = plasminogen activator inhibitor.

cular coagulation (DIC), acute infections, and thrombosis. Protein C levels are not significantly affected by pregnancy whereas protein S levels are significantly decreased.

Fibrinolysis appears to be impaired during pregnancy but rapidly returns to normal in the postpartum period. This dampening of the fibrinolytic system during pregnancy is believed to be related to the increased plasminogen activator inhibitor-2 (PAI-2) from the placenta and a threefold increase in the endothelium-derived plasminogen activator inhibitor-1(PAI-1). Despite these changes, fibrinolysis continues to occur, as evidenced by the presence of fibrin degradation products and D-dimer fragments throughout pregnancy.

DIAGNOSIS OF THROMBOEMBOLISM IN PREGNANCY

The clinical diagnosis of DVT/PE is difficult during pregnancy since leg edema and dyspnea are common throughout the gestational period. The left lower extremity has a disproportionately higher incidence of DVT, most likely secondary to compression by the gravid uterus and the anatomy of the iliac vein and artery. Women undergoing cesarean section have a 3 to 16 times higher incidence of DVT when compared with normal vaginal deliveries. Since the history and physical examination are at best 50% reliable, noninvasive or invasive testing is indicated when there is an acute onset of painful, progressive lower extremity swelling that has not improved with elevation and rest.

Noninvasive Testing

Compression ultrasound, also known as venous imaging or duplex ultrasonography, is a sensitive and specific test for proximal deep vein thrombosis involving the femoral and popliteal veins. The specificity decreases for small calf vein thrombosis below the popliteal bifurcation. This is most likely secondary to the smaller diameter of the calf vessels and the inability to observe the cardinal sign of noncompressibility. At present no large prospective studies assess the predictive value of compression ultrasound in pregnancy.

Impedance plethysmography (IPG) measures changes in electrical resistance following acute blood volume changes caused by proximal obstruction to venous flow, using pneumatic cuff obstruction to flow. The procedure is performed with the patient in the lateral recumbent position to avoid proximal occlusion by the gravid uterus. Its sensitivity and specificity are high for proximal vein thrombosis. Impedance plethysmography has been studied in a large group of consecutive pregnant patients. The patients with negative initial studies underwent serial IPGs. No therapy was rendered if testing remained negative. This approach requires frequent studies, which may be a problem for long-term care. At present, IPG is being replaced by compression ultrasound as the optimal study for assessing proximal vein thrombosis.

Invasive Testing

Venography remains the "gold standard" for assessing lower extremity thrombotic disease. This study consists of six to seven spot films and 1 minute of fluoroscopy for each leg. The estimated fetal radiation exposure for unilateral unshielded venography is 0.314 rad. A limited study with abdominal shielding exposes the fetus to less than 0.050 rad. Less than 5 rads of in utero radiation exposure is associated with a low risk of embryopathy.

Pulmonary angiography, the "gold standard" for pulmonary embolism, is completed via the brachial or femoral route, resulting in different radiation exposure dosages to the fetus because of the fluoroscopy time over the abdomen. This study consists of 21 to 31 spot films coned to one lung, with 2 to 5 minutes of fluoroscopy time. Pulmonary angiography via the brachial approach exposes the fetus to less than 0.050 rad and the femoral route allows 0.221 to 0.375 rad.

The reluctance to perform ventilation/perfusion (V/Q) lung scans is related to the radiation exposure from the radiopharmaceuticals used for the studies. The perfusion portion of the studies is completed using technetium macroaggregates of human albumin (^{99m}Tc-MAA). These microspheres are metabolized in the liver and spleen of the reticuloendothelial system. The standard dose of 3 millicuries (mCi) of ^{99m}Tc-MAA exposes the fetus to 0.018 rad. The employment of lower doses of ^{99m}Tc-MAA, such as 1.0 to 2 mCi, will provide good-quality images with a lesser fetal exposure of 0.006 and 0.012 rad, respectively. For ventilation scans, 1 mCi of xenon-133 (^{133}xe) per liter of air with 3 minutes of rebreathing results in a fetal absorbed dose of 0.004 rad. When Tc-DTPA is used as the inhaled agent, the fetal exposure rate is 0.007 to 0.035 rad. On the other hand, inhaled ^{99m}Tc sulfur colloid (SC) has less radiation exposure to the fetus since the agent does not leave the lung. The fetal absorption dose would be 0.001 to 0.005 rad. As in the non-pregnant state, V/Q results other than normal or high probability should be investigated by pulmonary angiography when the lower extremities are negative for DVT.

MANAGEMENT OF THROMBOEMBOLIC DISEASE

Heparin Therapy
(Table 2)

Patients developing an acute deep vein thrombosis or pulmonary embolism during pregnancy are treated with constant infusion heparin via the weight-based or high-dose methods of administration. Whichever regimen of dosing is selected, the goal of treatment is the rapid attainment of a therapeutic activated partial thromboplastin time (APTT) to prevent thrombus propagation and recurrent thromboembolic events.

A constant infusion of heparin is maintained for a full 7 days of therapy, after which time conversion to adjusted-dose subcutaneous heparin is initiated. Heparin may then be self-administered subcutaneously every 12 hours to achieve a 6-hour postmorning dose APTT of 1.5 times the patient's baseline value. This latter method was reported to be as effective as warfarin in preventing recurrent thrombotic events in nonpregnant patients. A very important point about the adjusted-dose regimen is that once the dose of heparin achieves a therapeutic APTT of 1.5 times the patient's baseline, no further adjustments are required nor APTTs obtained unless bleeding is clinically suspected. We realize that the adjusted-dose method was not evaluated in pregnant patients; therefore, we recommend that an APTT be obtained

TABLE 2. **Heparin Therapy in Pregnancy**

High-Dose Regimen

1. Bolus 5000 U, IV push if APTT < 45 sec (Note: If APTT > 45 sec, do not bolus and begin therapy with infusion)
2. Continuous infusion at a rate of 1200–1300 U/h; obtain APTT 6 h after starting infusion
3. Target APTT: 55–75 sec
   a. If APTT is in target range: continue heparin infusion at initial dose
   b. If APTT is low (<55 sec): bolus 5000 U IV, then increase infusion by 200 U/h to achieve target APTT
   c. If APTT > 99 sec
      1. Decrease infusion rate by 200 U/h and recheck APTT in 6 h
      2. Stop infusion for 1 h, restart infusion at 200 U less per h, then recheck in 6 h
4. APTT required every 6 h after change in dosage until APTT is within desired range

Weight-Adjusted Regimen

1. Bolus heparin 80 U/kg, IV push
2. Heparin continuous infusion at a rate of 18 U/kg/h; obtain APTT 6 hr after initiation of heparin therapy
3. Target APTT: 46–70 sec
   a. If APTT < 35 sec, give 80 U/kg bolus, then increase infusion rate by 4 U/kg/h
   b. If APTT 35–45 sec, give 40 U/kg bolus, then increase infusion rate by 2 U/kg/h
   c. If APTT is in target range of 46–70 sec, no change needed
   d. If APTT 71–90 sec, decrease infusion rate by 2 U/kg/h
   e. If APTT > 90 sec, hold infusion for 1 h, then decrease infusion rate by 3 U/kg/h
4. PTT required every 6 h after change in dosage until APTT is within desired range

Abbreviation: APTT = activated partial thromboplastin time.

once every 2 weeks for appropriate dosage adjustments. For those patients with a prolonged APTT secondary to lupus anticoagulant, anti-Xa levels should be obtained and maintained between the range of 0.2 and 0.4 U per mL.

An issue for clinicians is the duration and methods of treating thromboembolic disease with respect to the trimester of pregnancy. Patients developing DVT or PE in the first or second trimester are maintained on adjusted-dose subcutaneous heparin until delivery, after which this regimen is resumed for 4 to 6 weeks. Warfarin, which is not excreted in the breast milk, may be substituted during the postpartum period if subcutaneous heparin dosing is not desired. Third-trimester thromboembolic events are approached with a strategy based on the event point during the trimester. DVT or PE in the seventh or eighth month is treated as noted earlier, but the prophylaxis for recurrence in the postpartum period is extended beyond the 4- to 6-week window to include the full duration of prophylaxis for recurrence chosen by the clinician (i.e., 3 to 6 months).

Thromboembolic episodes in the ninth month are of greater concern since there is inadequate time for clot endothelialization and vessel wall adherence as the time of delivery approaches. Thromboses developing within 2 weeks of delivery have a greater potential for embolization in the peridelivery period if anticoagulation is not resumed either secondary to

bleeding or to C-section. In this case, inferior vena caval filter placement may be the best therapeutic option. These recommendations are based on the best clinical judgment, since there are no controlled trials to support these approaches.

Thrombolytic Therapy
(Table 3)

Pregnancy is a relative contraindication for the use of thrombolytic therapy because of the risk of maternal and fetal hemorrhagic complications. Despite this risk, pregnant patients presenting with pulmonary embolism associated with hypoxia and hemodynamic compromise or extensive lower extremity thrombosis with threatened limb viability will require thrombolysis. This form of therapy, which includes streptokinase, urokinase, and tissue plasminogen activator, reduces clot burden and reestablishes circulatory integrity.

In the world's literature there are 172 reported cases of the use of thrombolytic therapy in pregnancy, including cases of deep vein thrombosis, pulmonary embolism, thrombosed prosthetic valves, axillary clots, and cerebral emboli. These reports documented the use of thrombolytic therapy predominantly in the second and third trimester of pregnancy. Of concern with the use of these agents is the risk of maternal bleeding in the intrapartum and/or postpartum period, as well as the risk of fetal hemorrhage and pregnancy loss rate. Thrombolytics given in the peripartum period have a higher incidence of bleeding than constant-infusion heparin. The overall pregnancy loss rate was 5.8% in the 172 patients reported. This included spontaneous abortion, abruptio placentae, intrauterine fetal death, and maternal death. There were no reported congenital anomalies with this form of therapy.

Despite the bleeding risks, the use of thrombolytic

TABLE 3. **Thrombolytic Therapy in Pregnancy**

Streptokinase* (Kabikinase, Streptase)

1. Prep patient with acetaminophen, 1 gm, and diphenhydramine, 50 mg, PO, 1 h prior to infusion (reduces chills, rigors, fever)
2. Loading dose 250,000 U IV
3. Maintenance 100,000 U/h; check thrombin time in 4 h; if range (2 to 5 × normal) not achieved, then bolus 250,000 U and continue maintenance infusion; recheck thrombin time again and continue cycle until the desired thrombin time is obtained (24 h for PE and 48–72 h for DVT)

Urokinase* (Abbokinase)

1. Prep patient with acetaminophen, 1 gm, and diphenhydramine, 50 mg, PO, 1 h prior to infusion (reduces chills, rigors, fever)
2. Loading dose 4400 U/kg
3. Maintenance 4400 U/kg/h (12 h for PE and 24–48 h for DVT)

Tissue Plasminogen Activator* (Activase)

1. 100 mg IV over 2 h (approved only for PE)

*After terminating thrombolytic therapy, restart heparin without bolus at 1000 U/h, adjusting the dose to the desired APTT.

agents in life-threatening situations is indicated. The regimens listed in Table 5 are recommendations for use in the treatment of thrombotic disorders.

Mechanical Modalities

Inferior vena caval filters are indicated in patients with acute thrombosis unable to receive or maintain anticoagulants because of bleeding or adverse reactions. Inferior vena caval filter placement has been reported to be safe and effective in preventing fatal pulmonary embolism in pregnant patients. This intervention requires an inferior vena cavagram to assess the anatomy, size, and presence of thrombosis. The approach can be either through the femoral or jugular route, with final filter placement below the renal veins. Small pulmonary emboli approximately 2 to 3 mm in size may occur despite caval interruption, but they are not usually clinically significant.

PREVENTION OF DEEP VEIN THROMBOSIS/PULMONARY EMBOLISM
(Table 4)

Pregnant patients with a previous history of DVT or PE have been shown to have a 7% to 30% risk of recurrent disease both antepartum and postpartum. These patients may receive active prophylaxis with heparin or clinical surveillance with or without noninvasive testing. The recommended regimens for prophylaxis remain controversial because of lack of controlled trials for this patient population.

TABLE 4. **Deep Vein Thrombosis/Pulmonary Embolism: Heparin Prophylaxis: Pregnancy and Previous DVT/PE**

Antepartum	Postpartum
1. 5000 U SC q 12 h*	5000 U SC q 12 h or warfarin, INR 2:3 for 4 to 6 wk
2. 5000 U SC q 12 h, adjusting the dose based on maintaining a heparin level of 0.1–0.2 U/ml*	Same
3. 5000 U SC q 12 h for 1st and 2nd trimesters; third trimester, adjust dose to achieve a 6-h APTT of 1.5 × patient baseline *OR* 10,000 U SC q 12 h throughout pregnancy unless the heparin level is > 0.3 IU/ml†	Same
4. 7500 or 10,000 U SC q 12 h throughout or surveillance up to delivery then prophylaxis with heparin 5000 U SC q 12 h‡	Same

*American College of Chest Physicians, 1955.
†British Society for Haematology Guidelines, 1992.
‡Maternal and Neonatal Haemostasis Working Party of the Haemostasis Task Force, 1992.
Abbreviation: INR = International Normalized Ratio.

The regimen supported by the American College of Chest Physicians conference guidelines on antithrombotic therapy consists of subcutaneous heparin, 5000 units every 12 hours, as a safe and effective method for preventing peripartum DVT. Higher-dose regimens have been recommended based on the greater neutralization of heparin by platelet factor IV as well as increases in heparin-binding proteins, blood volume, glomerular filtration rate, and placental degradation by heparinase. Two regimens have been proposed based on these principles:

1. British Society for Haematology Guidelines, 1992: Heparin 5000 units subcutaneously every 12 hours for the first and second trimesters, then adjust the dose to prolong the 6-hour postmorning dose APTT to 1.5 times the patient's baseline, or 10,000 units every 12 hours throughout pregnancy unless the heparin level is greater than 0.3 IU per mL.

2. Maternal and Neonatal Haemostasis Working Party of the Haemostasis Thrombosis Task Force, 1992: A woman with a single episode of DVT/PE and no thrombophilia or risk factors should receive careful antenatal surveillance with prophylaxis intrapartum and 6 weeks postpartum, or heparin 7500 to 10,000 units every 12 hours throughout pregnancy.

These regimens should be discontinued 6 to 8 hours prior to delivery and restarted 6 to 8 hours postpartum or when the patient is hemostatically stable. If heparin cannot be reinstituted during the immediate postpartum period, external pneumatic compression sleeves may be used as a prophylactic modality after the lower extremities have been shown noninvasively to be free of clot. At this time warfarin therapy (International Normalized Ratio 2:3) may be considered as an alternative to heparin during the 4- to 6-week postpartum period.

SPECIAL CASES
Congenital and Acquired Hypercoagulable States

Protein C and Protein S Deficiency

The incidence of thromboembolic events in pregnant patients with protein C deficiency has been reported to be 7% antepartum and 19% in the postpartum period. In addition, it must be remembered that the levels of protein C are not significantly altered during pregnancy.

Protein S levels significantly decrease during pregnancy, making the risk of potential thrombosis of concern. The incidence of DVT in pregnant protein S–deficient patients has been reported to be 17% in the postpartum period. The risk has varied during the antepartum period, with some studies showing an increased risk while others have documented a very low risk.

Patients with protein C and protein S deficiency who are on permanent warfarin therapy for previous thrombotic episodes should have this treatment discontinued and adjusted-dose heparin initiated for the duration of the pregnancy. In the postpartum period, warfarin can be reinstituted with appropriate heparin cross-over. Protein C– and S–deficient patients without a previous history of thromboembolic events should receive prophylaxis as noted earlier. Prophylaxis should be continued in the postpartum period for 4 to 6 weeks. If warfarin is to be used in the postpartum period, concomitant heparin must be used initially because of the short half-life of protein C and protein S and the risk of warfarin skin necrosis.

Antithrombin III Deficiency

The levels of antithrombin III do not change appreciably during pregnancy, but retrospective studies show the incidence of thromboembolic events in patients not receiving prophylactic therapy to be 40% to 70%. Thrombotic events occur throughout pregnancy and the early postpartum, with a predominant number in the first trimester.

Patients with antithrombin III deficiency who are on permanent warfarin therapy for previous thrombotic episodes should have this treatment discontinued and adjusted-dose heparin initiated for the duration of the pregnancy (see section on Management of DVT/PE). Since heparin decreases antithrombin III levels, high doses of heparin may be required to achieve the desired anticoagulation level. Patients requiring greater than 40,000 units of heparin per day may be treated with prophylactic biweekly doses of antithrombin III concentrate. This will help in reducing the amount of heparin required. In addition, antithrombin III concentrate (50 to 70 U per kg loading dose followed by 20 to 30 U per kg per day maintenance) should be used during labor and delivery to maintain an antithrombin III level of 80% and reduce heparin dosing during these periods. Postpartum warfarin is restarted with the appropriate heparin cross-over.

Antithrombin III–deficient patients without a previous history of thromboembolic events should be treated with adjusted-dose heparin. Treatment should be continued into the postpartum period for 4 to 6 weeks. Antithrombin III concentrate should be used in the peripartum period, as noted earlier. If warfarin is to be used as the postpartum prophylactic therapy of choice, concomitant heparin must be used initially. One small study advocated the use of heparin until the 16th week of gestation followed by warfarin to week 36, with the reinstitution of heparin for delivery and the postpartum period. As recommended earlier, the risk/benefits of warfarin use during pregnancy should be taken into consideration.

Antiphospholipid Antibodies
(Table 5)

Women with antiphospholipid antibodies have a greater risk of thrombosis and pregnancy loss. The management of these patients during pregnancy focuses on the prevention of thromboembolic events that may result in fetal loss as well as maternal morbidity and mortality. A number of regimens have

TABLE 5. **Management Strategies for Special Thrombotic Disorders in Pregnancy**

Condition	Regimen
Antiphospholipid Antibodies	
> 1 pregnancy loss	ASA* (81 mg) plus prednisone (40 mg) *or* ASA (81 mg) plus heparin* *or* ASA (81 mg)
0 or 1 pregnancy loss	Heparin 5000 U SC q 12 h for 2nd and 3rd trimester
With previous DVT	Adjusted-dose heparin as in Table 4†
Without previous DVT	Heparin 5000 U SC q 12 h throughout pregnancy and postpartum; clinical surveillance with periodic IPG or CUS

*ASA: The original work had 80 mg.

†Heparin: 10,000 U SC q 12 h until a viable fetus is documented, then adjust the dose by the 6-hr APTT to achieve a normal range or to the prolonged baseline level.

Abbreviations: IPG = impedance plethysmography; CUS = compression ultrasound.

been evaluated in small trials but to date there are no large clinical trials assessing treatment modalities.

Regimens that have been evaluated include acetylsalicylic acid (ASA 81 mg) alone or in combination with prednisone (40 mg per day), or unfractionated heparin (10,000 U subcutaneously every 12 hours and adjust dose) and intravenous gamma globulin. In one study, 20 patients were randomized to receive ASA (81 mg) plus prednisone (40 mg per day) or ASA (81 mg) plus heparin (10,000 U subcutaneously every 12 hours). Fetal survival was the same in both groups, but the patients treated with prednisone were found to have a higher rate of premature rupture of membranes, preterm delivery, preeclampsia, and increased maternal morbidity. A second randomized trial concluded that ASA (81 mg) was as effective as but safer than ASA plus prednisone. Pregnant women with antiphospholipid antibodies and multiple pregnancy losses should receive either ASA plus prednisone, ASA plus heparin, or ASA alone. Patients with antiphospholipid antibodies on permanent warfarin therapy for previous thrombotic episodes should have this treatment discontinued and adjusted-dose heparin initiated for the duration of the pregnancy. In the postpartum period warfarin can be reinstituted with appropriate heparin cross-over. Patients with antiphospholipid antibody, without a previous history of thromboembolic events and 0 or 1 pregnancy loss, should receive prophylaxis with low-dose aspirin during the second and third trimester. Prophylaxis should be continued in the postpartum period for 4 to 6 weeks. Finally, patients with antiphospholipid antibodies, no previous thromboembolic events, and no pregnancy loss may receive heparin (5000 U subcutaneously every 12 hours) or clinical surveillance with impedance plethysmography or compression ultrasound. These prophylactic regimens must be carried out for 4 to 6 weeks postpartum.

Superficial Thrombophlebitis

Pregnant patients developing greater saphenous superficial thrombophlebitis below the knee should be treated conservatively with moist heat application four times per day and aspirin or acetaminophen for pain. Minimal ambulation is advised until improvement in signs and symptoms is noted. If the greater saphenous superficial thrombophlebitis extends above the knee or presents initially at this site, a compression ultrasound study should be performed to assess for propagation into the saphenofemoral junction. Thrombus located in this position has a greater risk for embolization because of its proximal location in the deep venous system. Full anticoagulation should be instituted.

Septic Pelvic Vein Thrombophlebitis

Septic pelvic vein thrombophlebitis (SPVT) is a serious complication of postpartum endometritis and occurs in approximately 0.1% of pregnancies. It is more common after cesarean sections. Patients present with a postpartum fever and pelvic tenderness that does not respond to adequate intravenous antibiotic therapy covering aerobic and anaerobic organisms. Septic pulmonary emboli occur in approximately 30% of untreated patients. Imaging techniques such as ultrasound, computed tomography (CT), and magnetic resonance imaging (MRI) have been shown to be helpful in confirming the diagnosis, but there have not been any trials assessing their sensitivity or specificity. These patients should be treated with full anticoagulation concomitant with antibiotics for 10 days. Full anticoagulation for 3 months is recommended if pulmonary embolization has occurred. Some investigators believe that there is no proved benefit to treating SPVT for 3 months similar to the therapy recommended for deep vein thromboses. We recommend 3 months of warfarin or adjusted-dose heparin therapy. There are no controlled trials supporting these recommendations.

Ovarian Vein Thrombosis

Acute ovarian vein thrombosis occurs in 1 of every 4000 deliveries. Clinical signs and symptoms presenting 2 to 3 days postpartum include severe adnexal pain (right more common than left) which may radiate into the flank, or a deep tender mass lateral to the uterus, and fever. These symptoms are often associated with endometriosis. CT scan and ultrasound will assist in confirming the clinical findings. More recently, MRI has been shown to be helpful in evaluating ovarian vein thrombosis, but the costs are higher compared with the aforementioned studies. These patients should be treated with full anticoagulation for 10 days, like the patients with SPVT. We recommend 3 months of anticoagulation with warfarin or adjusted-dose heparin. There are no controlled trials to support these recommendations.

COMPLICATIONS OF ANTICOAGULANTS DURING PREGNANCY

Osteoporosis

Asymptomatic osteopenia secondary to heparin has been documented in 17% to 36% of patients using this agent for thromboembolic prophylaxis during pregnancy. These initial studies used radiologic evidence for osteopenia, documenting late-onset disease. The more recent protocols used dual photon bone densitometry, which is a more sensitive study for detecting early-onset osteopenia. Symptomatic fractures occur in less than 2% of pregnant woman with heparin-induced osteopenia. The mechanism of these bony changes is currently unknown. In addition, none of the studies was able to demonstrate a risk for osteopenia based on dose and duration of heparin treatment. Currently, all these changes appear to be reversible, but larger and longer trials need to be completed to adequately address this issue.

Fetal and Maternal Issues

Heparin does not pose a problem for the fetus since it does not cross the placenta. The only possible concern would be bleeding at the uteroplacental junction. On the other hand, warfarin does cross the placenta and has the potential for both bleeding and teratogenicity.

Warfarin used in the first trimester (6 to 12 weeks) has been associated with chondromalacia punctata (stippled epiphyses, nasal and limb hypoplasia). In the second and third trimester, reports of central nervous system abnormalities, including dorsal midline dysplasia, midline cerebellar atrophy, and ventral midline dysplasia manifested by optic atrophy and hemorrhage, have been associated with warfarin. Finally, spontaneous abortion and stillbirth are increased with this agent.

Warfarin and heparin are safe for use in women who breast-feed their children. Neither drug is found in breast milk and neither is a risk for the fetus.

NEW AGENTS FOR THROMBOEMBOLIC PROPHYLAXIS AND TREATMENT

Recently, low-molecular-weight heparins were approved for DVT/PE prophylaxis in orthopedic and abdominal surgery. These new heparins have more specific binding to factor Xa, are better absorbed, have a longer half-life, and cause less bleeding than standard heparin. At present, only case reports of their safety and efficacy during pregnancy have appeared in the literature. For the treatment of DVT in the nonpregnant population, low-molecular-weight heparins have also been shown to be as effective and safe given subcutaneously as constant-infusion standard heparin. A number of studies using low-molecular-weight heparins for prophylaxis or treatment during pregnancy are in progress. At present, we do not recommend their use during pregnancy.

CONTRACEPTION

method of
CATHERINE L. DEAN, M.D., M.P.H.
Washington University School of Medicine
St. Louis, Missouri

Two thirds of American women have at least one unintended pregnancy by the time they reach menopause. Despite readily available contraceptives, more than one half of the nearly 6 million pregnancies annually in the United States are unintended. Fifty percent of women presenting with unintended pregnancy report they were using contraception at the time they conceived. Thus, it is essential that health care providers understand the reasons contributing to the surprisingly high lifetime failure rate of contraception in order to reduce the number of unintended pregnancies.

DETERMINANTS OF CONTRACEPTIVE CHOICE

A woman's choice of a contraceptive method is key in determining her risk for future unintended pregnancy. The health care provider's role in counseling women is critical in providing all the necessary information needed to make the best choice. The ideal contraceptive is a balance between effectiveness, ease of compliance, safety (real or perceived), reversibility (or permanence), and personal acceptability. Moreover, the woman must understand that all contraceptive methods, even when used correctly, can fail and result in pregnancy.

The health care provider can further assist the woman with her choice by informing her of any non-contraceptive health benefits (Table 1). Protection against sexually transmitted diseases (STDs) is a critical noncontraceptive benefit for women at risk. The simultaneous use of two contraceptive methods can add protection against STDs and lower the risk of contraceptive failure.

Effectiveness

Many women are not aware of the differing levels of effectiveness between various contraceptive methods. One needs to remember that just as contraceptives fail women, women sometimes fail to use contraceptives correctly each time. Thus, the failure rate of any given contraceptive applies to women in general, not to any one individual. For example, the diaphragm has an 18% first-year failure rate. That failure rate would be lower with a 40-year-old woman with biologically declining fertility who rarely has intercourse, compared with a 20-year-old woman in her reproductive prime who has frequent intercourse.

Ease of Compliance

Contraceptive methods that are compliance-independent are permanent sterilization, implants, long-acting injectables, and intrauterine devices (IUDs). These methods require differing amounts of medical intervention, from one-time implementation, as with sterilization, to relatively infrequent maintenance (varying between 3 months and 10 years). Because of their ease of use, failure rates are low and are rarely due to user error.

Contraceptive methods that are compliance-dependent are pills, all barrier methods, spermicides, withdrawal, periodic abstinence, and the lactational amenorrhea method (LAM). The pill is intercourse-independent and requires strict compliance: A woman must take the pill at the same time every day. The woman has to assess honestly whether she can remember to take her pill correctly because inconsistent use is associated with high failure rates. All the barrier and spermicide methods are intercourse-dependent. The woman has to consider her

TABLE 1. **Noncontraceptive Benefits of Major Methods of Contraception**

Contraceptive Method	Noncontraceptive Benefits
Sterilization	None known
Levonorgestrel implant (Norplant), medroxyprogesterone acetate (Depo-Provera), progestin-only pills	May protect against PID; decreased anemia; reduced menstrual pain and blood loss; lactation not affected; decreased risk of endometrial and ovarian cancer
IUD	Copper IUD, none known; progestin IUD may decrease menstrual blood loss and pain
Combined oral contraceptive pill	*Decreases* ovarian cancer, endometrial cancer, PID, benign breast disease, dysmenorrhea, ectopic pregnancies; *increases* menstrual regularity, bone density
Male condom	Protects against STDs; delays premature ejaculation
Female condom	Protects against STDs
Diaphragm, cervical cap	Protects somewhat against STDs
Spermicide	Protects against STDs
Periodic abstinence, withdrawal	None known
Lactational amenorrhea method	Provides excellent nutrition for infant during first 6 months

Abbreviations: PID = pelvic inflammatory disease; STD = sexually transmitted disease; IUD = intrauterine device.

sexual lifestyle, and whether she will have the needed method at hand each time intercourse occurs. Withdrawal requires trust in the partner and complete ejaculatory control. Periodic abstinence and LAM both require the woman to monitor her reproductive cycle and abstain or use another method during potentially fertile times.

Safety

Generally, contraception is safe for most women. However, certain women should not use specific contraceptive methods, particularly in the presence of certain medical conditions. Specific safety considerations are discussed in the sections on methods.

More important is to differentiate between real safety considerations and misconceptions. A woman will not use a method that she fears. If the health care provider cannot educate her and her support system as to the safety of a given method *to their satisfaction*, another method should be chosen.

Personal Acceptability

Only the woman can decide, for her own specific set of reasons, what methods are most acceptable for her. These reasons generally change over time. Partner acceptance is important as well. She may prefer a barrier method that her partner does not like. She may want a method that is quickly reversible under her control. It is important that she understands it is acceptable to change her mind and try a different method. The cost of the method may limit her choice. Many women use one method while saving money for another method. Finally, the desire for future fertility, if any, is an important consideration in choosing a contraceptive method.

SURGICAL STERILIZATION

One third of reproductive-age women in the United States rely on sterilization as their contraceptive method, making this the most popular method. Twenty-five percent of women have had a tubal ligation, and 11% of women depend on their partner's vasectomy. These methods are highly effective, with failure rates of less than 1%. Both male and female sterilization are low-risk surgical procedures, making sterilization much safer than pregnancy, in terms of morbidity and mortality. Couples must be carefully counseled as to the intended permanence of these methods, since reversal procedures are expensive and unreliable. The first-year failure rate for tubal ligation is 0.4%, and for vasectomy, 0.15%.

COMPLIANCE-INDEPENDENT REVERSIBLE METHODS

Levonorgestrel Implant

Levonorgestrel implant (Norplant) is the first contraceptive in this new drug delivery system approved by the Food and Drug Administration (FDA). This implant system consists of six Silastic rods containing the progestin levonorgestrel; they are placed just under the skin in the upper inner arm. The implants slowly release the hormone, which then inhibits ovulation, suppresses the endometrium, and thickens cervical mucus. Norplant is effective for 5 years, with failure rates equal to sterilization in the first 2 years of use. The overall failure rate is 3 per 1000. When the implant is removed, fertility returns almost immediately.

Contraindications to this implant system are pregnancy, undiagnosed abnormal vaginal bleeding, most antiseizure medications, active pulmonary emboli or thrombophlebitis, and breast cancer. The most significant side effect is menstrual disturbances, which all women should be counseled to expect. Most women like the method, with 85% of women continuing to use it after 1 year.

Medroxyprogesterone Acetate Injectable

Medroxyprogesterone acetate (Depo-Provera) (DMPA) 150 mg intramuscularly provides 12 weeks of contraception with a 2-week grace period. DMPA inhibits ovulation, thickens cervical mucus, and suppresses the endometrium. The effectiveness is similar to that of the levonorgestrel implant, and contraindications to its use are generally the same. DMPA also causes menstrual disturbances but is more likely to cause amenorrhea after 6 months of use. Of key significance, a return of fertility could be delayed up to 18 months after cessation.

Intrauterine Devices

The copper IUD (ParaGard T 380A) is FDA-approved for 10 years of use, and Progestasert, the progesterone IUD, is FDA-approved for 1 year of use. Studies from the Centers for Disease Control and Prevention have confirmed that IUDs are very safe in the appropriately screened patient, that is, a woman who is in a mutually monogamous relationship. Although there is a slightly increased risk of infection related to insertion for the first few months, there is no additional risk of infection from the IUD itself. However, if the woman should contract an STD, the STD infection is likely to be severe when an IUD is in place, often leading to tubal damage and subsequent infertility. This is why patient selection is crucial. Unfortunately, IUDs remain underutilized in the United States. The highly publicized Dalkon Shield litigation has created many negative perceptions concerning the IUD. With public health education, women in the United States are now gradually choosing the IUD as their contraceptive method. IUDs are highly effective and have a "typical use" first-year failure rate of 0.8% for the copper IUD (ParaGard T 380A) and 2% for the Progestasert System.

COMPLIANCE–DEPENDENT REVERSIBLE METHODS

Oral Contraceptives

Oral contraceptives remain the number one reversible contraceptive choice of women in the United States. The most commonly used pill is the combined estrogen and progestin pill used for 21 days, with a 7-day pill-free interval. The "mini-pill," progestin only, is used much less frequently and must be taken daily.

Although the new lower-dose pills are much safer than the original formulations, there are still some women who should not use the pill. Fortunately, this list continues to decrease with increased knowledge about the current pill formulations. Major contraindications include thrombophlebitis or thromboembolism (current or past), stroke, coronary heart disease, breast cancer, other estrogen-dependent cancer, current impaired liver function, benign hepatic adenoma or liver cancer, smoking past the age of 35, and pregnancy. Women with the following conditions may be able to use the pill with extreme caution and close follow-up: hypertension (medication-controlled), controlled diabetes mellitus, migraine headaches that start after pill use, sickle cell disease (SS) or sickle C (SC) disease, active gallbladder disease, Gilbert's disease (congenital hyperbilirubinemia), age over 50 years, and lactation.

The reduced hormonal content of current pills has also decreased undesirable side effects. The most common side effects are breakthrough bleeding and amenorrhea. Both can generally be corrected by changing pill formulations. Women need to be warned of these side effects so they do not stop using the pill before seeking medical care.

The oral contraceptive pill has many noncontraceptive benefits summarized in Table 1. Oral contraceptives are highly effective when used correctly and have a "typical use" first-year failure rate of 3%.

Barrier or Spermicide Methods

Male Condom

Condoms are the second most popular reversible contraceptive method in the United States. Latex condoms have been shown to protect against STDs and are now widely promoted for use in addition to most other contraceptive methods for safer sexual practices. Condoms are available in various sizes, lubricated or nonlubricated, with or without spermicide, with or without a reservoir tip, and in a variety of textures and colors. Lambskin condoms are available for those with latex allergies but are not as effective at infection prevention. Condoms have a "typical use" first-year failure rate of 12% when used alone. Efficacy is increased when they are used with a vaginal spermicide.

Female Condom

The Reality female condom consists of a polyurethane sheath containing two flexible rings. One ring is inside and serves as an insertion guide and internal anchor. The second larger ring serves as an external anchor. The interior sheath is prelubricated with a silicone-based lubricant. It does not contain spermicide and cannot be used with a male condom. The female condom is available over the counter, is disposable, and is intended for only one use. The female condom protects against STDs and pregnancy. The "typical use" first-year failure rate of the female condom used alone is 21%.

Diaphragm

The diaphragm is the first female contraceptive method ever used in the United States. The diaphragm must be fitted by a health care provider, and the woman must be taught proper placement. Spermicide is placed in the cap and around the rim at the time of insertion, and the diaphragm may be inserted up to 6 hours before intercourse. The diaphragm must remain in place for at least 6 hours after intercourse. Repeated intercourse needs to be preceded with additional spermicide placed by an applicator. The diaphragm should not be left in place for more than 24 hours because of the possible risk of toxic shock syndrome. Some women cannot be properly fitted with a diaphragm, particularly in the presence of a cystocele. The "typical use" first-year failure rate is 18%.

Cervical Cap

The Prentif cavity rim cervical cap fits snugly on the cervix and is held in place by suction. It must be fitted by a health care provider, and the woman must be taught proper placement. All the previous caveats regarding the diaphragm also apply to the cervical cap, except the cap may be worn for up to 48 hours, and additional spermicide with repeated intercourse is not needed. Some women cannot be fitted with the cap. The "typical use" first-year failure rate is 18% in nulliparous women and 36% in parous women.

Foam, Suppositories, Jellies, Film

Vaginal spermicides are available in a variety of formats. They have been shown to reduce the transmission of STDs such as gonorrhea and chlamydial infection. The effect of spermicide on human immunodeficiency virus (HIV) infection without a condom is unclear. Nonoxynol 9 is the active agent in most spermicidal products. Octoxynol is also available in the United States. Spermicides are necessary with vaginal barrier methods such as the diaphragm and cervical cap. Spermicides are much more effective when used with a condom than when used alone. When used alone, the "typical use" first-year failure rate of spermicides is 21%.

Behavioral Methods

Withdrawal

Withdrawal and condoms are the only two male reversible contraceptive methods. Withdrawal depends on trust and absolute ejaculatory control. Withdrawal can be used with other methods to further improve contraceptive efficacy. When no other contraceptive method is available, withdrawal can significantly reduce conception rates. When used alone, the "typical use" first-year failure rate is 18%.

Periodic Abstinence

Fertility awareness methods are used to prospectively predict ovulation and thereby allow the couple to abstain from intercourse during the "unsafe" time of the cycle. Highly motivated women with regular cycles can achieve low failure rates. Women with irregular cycles are poor candidates for these methods. The "typical use" first-year failure rate is 20%.

Lactational Amenorrhea Method

Women who are exclusively breast-feeding generally do not ovulate for the first 6 months. However, if during the first 6 months weaning begins, if the infant's diet is supplemented, or if menses return, other forms of contraception should be initiated. Clinical studies estimate a "perfect use" 6-month failure rate of 0.7%.

Emergency Contraception

Emergency contraception can dramatically reduce unintended pregnancy from unprotected intercourse. Condoms can break, diaphragms can be dislodged or forgotten, and rape continues to occur.

Hormonal Method

The use of higher-dose combined oral contraceptive pills within 72 hours of a single episode of unprotected intercourse during the midcycle is highly effective in preventing pregnancy. The best-known regimen is 100 micrograms of ethinyl estradiol and 1.0 mg of norgestrel (two Ovral tablets) taken immediately and two more tablets taken in 12 hours. Transient nausea and vomiting is a common side effect with this method. Clinical studies indicate emergency contraceptive pill treatment reduces the risk of pregnancy by 75%.

Postcoital Intrauterine Device Insertion

Insertion of the ParaGard copper IUD within 5 to 7 days after unprotected midcycle intercourse is also a highly effective contraceptive method, with the resulting pregnancy rate less than 1%.

ALCOHOLISM

method of
HENRY R. KRANZLER, M.D.
University of Connecticut Health Center
Farmington, Connecticut

Alcohol consumption occurs along a continuum, with no sharp demarcation between "moderate" drinking and "problem" drinking. Increases in either average alcohol consumption or frequency of intoxication are associated with an increase in medical and psychosocial problems. Acute consequences tend to vary with the amount consumed per occasion. Many of the medical consequences, such as hepatic cirrhosis, occur only with chronic alcohol use. Although the most visible group of people affected by alcohol problems are those who have developed a syndrome of alcohol dependence (i.e., alcoholics), a more numerous group consists of early problem drinkers who, although they may not be dependent on alcohol, are either at risk or have already experienced alcohol-related problems.

Early problem drinking and alcoholism are particularly prevalent among medical patients, psychiatric patients, and individuals in the criminal justice system. Although most common among young and middle-aged males, it is important to remember that females and the elderly may also drink heavily and may benefit from interventions aimed at reducing or stopping drinking.

GENERAL ASSESSMENT

Despite alcoholics' tendency to deny their alcohol-related problems, adequate assessment procedures *can* yield a valid alcohol history. A complete alcohol history should include specific questions concerning average alcohol consumption; maximal consumption per drinking occasion; frequency of heavy drinking occasions; and drinking-related problems, such as social (e.g., problems with family members, friends, or people at work), legal (e.g., driving while intoxicated), psychiatric (e.g., mood or anxiety symptoms), and medical problems (e.g., alcoholic gastritis or pancreatitis). A comprehensive assessment provides the basis for an individualized plan of treatment.

The AUDIT (Alcohol Use Disorders Identification Test) questionnaire (Figure 1) identifies a broad range of heavy drinking and may be used to organize the alcohol use history or as a self-report questionnaire. For those patients in whom the AUDIT shows evidence of hazardous drinking (i.e., indicated by a score of $\geq$ 8), further inquiry and intervention to reduce risk are warranted. In quantifying a patient's drinking, it is useful to think in terms of a standard drink: 12 ounces of beer, 4 ounces of wine, 2

The writing of this article was supported by grants P50-AA03510, and K20-AA00143 (to HRK) from the National Institute on Alcohol Abuse and Alcoholism.

ounces of fortified wine, or 1 ounce of whiskey or other spirits. Males who drink more than 4 standard drinks in a day or 16 drinks per week and females who drink more than 3 standard drinks in a day or 12 drinks per week are at risk of alcohol-related problems. In addition, some patients should not drink at all, including women who are pregnant, trying to conceive, or nursing; people who plan to drive or engage in activities that require attention; individuals whose medications may interact with alcohol; and heavy drinkers who cannot keep their drinking to a moderate level.

A thorough medical and psychiatric assessment should also be conducted in patients being seen for alcohol problems. Although alcoholism may show no physical or laboratory abnormalities early in its course, as it progresses, it is widely manifested throughout most organ systems. The cardiovascular, gastrointestinal, and central and peripheral nervous systems are particularly vulnerable to alcohol-related pathology. Foremost among the psychiatric problems that occur among alcoholics are depressive and anxiety symptoms, suicidal risk, and abuse of other drugs.

There are a number of potentially life-threatening conditions for which alcoholics are at increased risk. The presence of any of the following requires immediate attention: acute alcohol withdrawal (with the potential for seizures and delirium tremens), serious medical or surgical disease (e.g., acute pancreatitis, bleeding esophageal varices), and serious psychiatric illness (e.g., psychosis, suicidal intent). In the presence of any of these emergent conditions, acute stabilization should be the first priority of treatment.

Laboratory tests, particularly those related to hepatic function (e.g., serum transaminases and gamma-glutamyl transpeptidase [GGTP]), can be used as objective indicators of heavy drinking and, together with physical findings, can provide tangible evidence of the need for treatment. In addition, the alcohol breath test provides a reliable and inexpensive method for assessing recent alcohol consumption. Although these indicators have limited sensitivity, they can be used to impress upon the patient the need to reduce or discontinue drinking. They may also be used to monitor progress following interventions for heavy drinking.

EVALUATION AND TREATMENT OF ALCOHOL WITHDRAWAL

It is important that the physician ask in detail about the patient's drinking during the preceding 24 to 48 hours and, if possible, measure the breath alcohol concentration. Early signs and symptoms of alcohol withdrawal (Table 1) are usually evident within 12 to 24 hours of the patient's last drink. In patients who have recently consumed alcohol, evaluating the potential for alcohol withdrawal is largely dependent on a prior history of alcohol withdrawal. Patients with no evidence of withdrawal after 72 or more

World Health Organization

AUDIT

Please place a mark in the box next to your answer. One standard drink equals approximately one 12-oz glass of beer; one 4-oz glass of wine; one 2-oz glass of sherry or port; or one ounce of spirits. *Note:* **the average light beer is about half the strength of normal beer.**

1 How often do you have a drink containing alcohol?
☐ never (0)   ☐ monthly or less (1)   ☐ 2 to 4 times a month (2)   ☐ 2 to 3 times a week (3)   ☐ 4 or more times a week (4)

2 How many standard drinks containing alcohol do you have on a typical day when you are drinking?
☐ 1 or 2 (0)   ☐ 3 or 4 (1)   ☐ 5 or 6 (2)   ☐ 7 to 9 (3)   ☐ 10 or more (4)

3 How often do you have six or more drinks on one occasion?
☐ never (0)   ☐ less than monthly (1)   ☐ monthly (2)   ☐ weekly (3)   ☐ daily or almost daily (4)

4 How often during the last year have you found that you were not able to stop drinking once you had started?
☐ never (0)   ☐ less than monthly (1)   ☐ monthly (2)   ☐ weekly (3)   ☐ daily or almost daily (4)

5 How often during the last year have you failed to do what was normally expected from you because of drinking?
☐ never (0)   ☐ less than monthly (1)   ☐ monthly (2)   ☐ weekly (3)   ☐ daily or almost daily (4)

6 How often during the last year have you needed a drink in the morning to get yourself going after a heavy drinking session?
☐ never (0)   ☐ less than monthly (1)   ☐ monthly (2)   ☐ weekly (3)   ☐ daily or almost daily (4)

7 How often during the last year have you had a feeling of guilt or remorse after drinking?
☐ never (0)   ☐ less than monthly (1)   ☐ monthly (2)   ☐ weekly (3)   ☐ daily or almost daily (4)

8 How often during the last year have you been unable to remember what happened the night before because you had been drinking?
☐ never (0)   ☐ less than monthly (1)   ☐ monthly (2)   ☐ weekly (3)   ☐ daily or almost daily (4)

9 Have you or someone else been injured as a result of your drinking?
☐ no (0)   ☐ yes, but not in the last year (2)   ☐ yes, during the last year (4)

10 Has a relative, a friend, a doctor or other health worker been concerned about your drinking or suggested you cut down?
☐ no (0)   ☐ yes, but not in the last year (2)   ☐ yes, during the last year (4)

Figure 1. (Adapted from Babor TF, De La Fuente JR, Saunders J, and Grant M: The Alcohol Use Disorders Identification Test: Guidelines for use in primary health care. WHO Publication no. 89.4. Geneva, World Health Organization, 1989; and Saunders JB, Aasland OB, Babor TF, De La Fuente JR, and Grant M: Development of the Alcohol Use Disorders Identification Test (AUDIT); WHO Collaborative Project on Early Detection of Persons with Harmful Alcohol Consumption-II. Addiction, *88*:791–804, 1993. All rights to this questionnaire are reserved by the World Health Organization. However, this questionnaire may be freely reproduced or translated but not for sale or use in conjunction with commercial purposes.)

hours of not drinking are unlikely to experience serious alcohol withdrawal. However, drinking during this period may mask withdrawal symptoms.

Mild to moderate alcohol withdrawal generally requires no medical treatment or can safely be treated in an outpatient setting. The safety of ambulatory detoxification is increased when a dependable individual (e.g., a family member) is available to monitor the patient's progress. Moderate to severe alcohol withdrawal has the potential for serious medical consequences, including seizures. The presence of withdrawal symptoms such as frequent vomiting, hallucinations, or disorientation requires prompt attention, preferably in an inpatient setting. Irrespective of the treatment setting, attention to the patient's rehabilitation needs is also important, since detoxification alone does little to prevent relapse to heavy drinking.

Treatment of alcohol withdrawal usually involves a tapering dose of one of the benzodiazepines, all of which are cross-dependent with alcohol. Although

benzodiazepines are not lethal when taken alone in overdose, their combination with other brain depressants, including alcohol, is dangerous. Consequently, in the ambulatory setting, it may be preferable to use shorter-acting benzodiazepines, such as lorazepam (Ativan) or oxazepam (Serax). Although longer-acting benzodiazepines require less frequent dosing, they

TABLE 1. **Signs and Symptoms of Alcohol Withdrawal**

Early (beginning during the first day of abstinence *or* reduced drinking)		
Tremor	Nausea	Vomiting
Irritability	Tachycardia	Weakness
Insomnia	Hallucinosis	Seizures
Late (beginning after the first day of abstinence *or* reduced drinking)		
Tremor	Delusions	Sleeplessness
Agitation	Tachycardia	Fever
Confusion	Hallucinosis	Sweating

yield long-lived active metabolites that may interact with alcohol consumed during detoxification or accumulate when hepatic function is impaired.

Dietary and metabolic conditions that are common in heavy drinkers should also be evaluated in patients undergoing detoxification. Thiamine and other B vitamin deficiencies can generally be repleted with oral supplements. Electrolyte disturbances resulting from vomiting or diarrhea may occur during heavy drinking or alcohol withdrawal. When present, significant electrolyte disturbances require hospitalization, as do recurrent seizures.

PSYCHOSOCIAL TREATMENT

The available evidence suggests that any treatment for alcoholism is better than no treatment. As many as two-thirds of patients treated demonstrate improvement, which is roughly double the improvement seen in patients not receiving treatment. The extent to which physicians choose to provide counseling varies. Some refer nearly all heavy drinkers for specialized treatment; others may opt to provide counseling in the office setting, either by identifying a particular nurse to serve in that role or by devoting physician time to it.

Among heavy drinkers without evidence of alcohol-related harm, an intervention aimed at the reduction of drinking may suffice. Under these circumstances, patients should be told that their drinking puts them at risk for health problems, similar to high blood pressure or a high cholesterol level. This report should be delivered with the seriousness associated with a significant health problem but without the use of such labels as alcoholic, alcoholism, abuse, and so forth. Concern expressed in this fashion is generally well received by patients.

Among patients with significant alcohol dependence, there are a variety of associated disabilities, so it is necessary to address both the excessive drinking *and* the problems related to it. The physician should begin with an objective review of the patient's drinking, based on the results of the AUDIT and subsequent assessment. Current drinking patterns should be compared with safe practices. Specific health and safety information should be provided. The benefits of reduced drinking or abstinence should be discussed, with specific reference to the potential for reducing any of the health risks or problems the patient is experiencing. The patient should also be helped to identify the causes, triggers, and occasions for heavy drinking. Establishing a goal of either abstinence or a specific level of reduced drinking is often helpful, although abstinence is the preferred goal for patients with particularly high levels of alcohol consumption and related problems. In this case, however, a trial of reduced drinking may be necessary to convince the patient of the need for total abstinence.

Specific coping skills and aids that may be offered to assist the patient include establishing a diary of drinking occasions, identifying feelings and external events that accompany the desire to drink, and keeping track of the number of drinks consumed. Consuming food with alcohol, diluting hard liquor, or waiting between drinks of alcohol are ways that people can pace their drinking. Planning ahead for risky drinking situations (e.g., weddings, weekend get-togethers) may allow patients to decide whether to drink on those occasions, what limits to set, whether to ask a friend to help monitor drinking, or whether to avoid the situation. Developing regular exercise programs, cultivating social activities and relationships that are alcohol-free, and designating alcohol-free days help some people adopt healthier habits.

The effectiveness of a plan is enhanced if the physician can work directly with the patient in developing it. The patient should be encouraged to describe the plan to the physician and to provide regular updates concerning progress in achieving goals. Regular follow-up visits should be scheduled in an effort to underscore the importance of the patient's efforts and to monitor the effectiveness of those efforts.

Patients may find that attendance at Alcoholics Anonymous (AA) may help achieve abstinence. However, not all people are willing to endorse the emphasis on spirituality and a disease model of alcoholism that requires lifelong abstinence as the only means to recovery, both of which are essential elements of AA. Familiarity with AA will help clinicians identify those patients who might reasonably be expected to benefit from this approach. Open discussion of the 12-step approach with the patient prior to referral, and monitoring the patient's response to the meetings attended, should increase the benefit that the patient derives from a referral to AA.

Alcoholism creates major stress on the family system by threatening health, interpersonal relations, and the economic functioning of family members. Since there is a strong association between healthy family functioning and positive outcome following alcoholism treatment, efforts to involve family members in treatment may yield direct benefits both for the patient and for family members. This can be accomplished by the physician's counseling family members and by referring them to Al-Anon, a 12-step program for the family members of alcoholics.

PHARMACOTHERAPY

There is growing interest in the use of medications as adjuncts to psychosocial treatment of early problem drinkers and alcoholics. Two medications are currently approved for the treatment of alcohol dependence. In the presence of alcohol, disulfiram (Antabuse), given in a single daily dose of 125 to 500 mg, produces an aversive reaction. Potential side effects of disulfiram include drowsiness, lethargy, peripheral neuropathy, hepatotoxicity, and hypertension. However, in the absence of substantial efforts to enhance medication compliance, controlled studies have shown the drug to be no more efficacious than placebo in the maintenance of sobriety.

The opioid antagonist naltrexone (ReVia) has recently been shown to be efficacious as an adjunct to psychosocial treatment of alcoholism. Naltrexone, 50 mg per day, was well tolerated and resulted in significantly less craving for alcohol, fewer drinking days, and fewer drinks per drinking day than placebo. Use of this medication in the absence of psychosocial treatment has not been evaluated and is not recommended. Adverse effects associated with naltrexone include transient nausea, anxiety, insomnia, headaches, and muscle aches. Elevated hepatic transaminase levels have been observed in a limited number of subjects treated with the drug, but only in high doses (300 mg per day, or roughly six times the recommended daily dosage). The duration of treatment is best determined in discussion with the patient, but a minimum of 2 to 3 months to help establish reduced drinking or abstinence is warranted. A longer period of therapy may prove useful with some patients.

In addition, a variety of medications have been employed in an effort to improve outcomes in alcoholics by treating co-morbid psychiatric symptoms and disorders. The use of these medications (e.g., antidepressants) in alcoholics requires careful consideration of the added potential for adverse effects attributable to co-morbid medical disorders and the pharmacokinetic effects of acute and chronic alcohol consumption. Bearing these caveats in mind, indications for the use of these medications in alcoholics are similar to those for nonalcoholic populations and can be arrived at only through careful psychiatric diagnosis.

Harmful drinking is a chronic condition in which relapses are not uncommon. Once patients who need treatment are identified and initial efforts have been made to engage them in treatment, the physician is in a good position to promote and help maintain change. A variety of treatment approaches are available, many of which lend themselves readily to the primary care setting. Ongoing efforts by the physician, together with the patient, can produce lasting, clinically meaningful benefits.

DRUG ABUSE

method of
EDWARD JAROSZEWSKI, M.D.

Hartford Hospital
Hartford, Connecticut

Drug abuse is pervasive in every socioeconomic, ethnic, and religious culture. Although alcohol clearly remains the main substance of abuse, the use and abuse of recreational drugs remains a major problem for the medical community. The statistics from the Hartford Hospital Psychiatric Emergency Room over the past four years reveal a startling and frightening pattern. The total number of patients remained approximately 2700, but the diagnosis of a co-morbid substance abuse problem increased from 50% in 1991 to an astonishing 85% in 1994. Alcohol was the drug of abuse in about 50% of all cases. Crack cocaine, heroin,

and benzodiazepine abuse constitutes the bulk of the rest, with episodic endemic use of hallucinogens and inhalants.

Acute mental status changes are a very common diagnostic problem in the emergency setting and are part of a multiorganic system toxic syndrome—the toxidrome. The differential is extremely broad and includes trauma, metabolic disturbances, infection, neuroanatomic and neurophysiologic abnormalities, as well as drug intoxication or withdrawal. A complete medical examination with accurate vital signs is imperative. Blood should be drawn to check complete blood counts, glucose, electrolytes, blood urea nitrogen, creatinine, and, on occasion, liver function and thyroid function studies. If indicated, an electrocardiogram, arterial blood gases, computer tomographic scan of the head, and a lumbar puncture should be considered. Urine and serum toxicology screens can be very helpful but are occasionally deceiving. It is imperative that medical personnel in a given hospital be familiar with the type of toxicology screening offered in that setting. False-positives and false-negatives can be a problem, leading to erroneous diagnoses and treatments. Table 1 shows some of the problems associated with the EMIT (enzyme-multiplied immunosorbent technology) system used commonly in many hospitals across the United States.

The EMIT is one of a variety of immunoassays available for the detection of drugs. Antibodies are generated to a representative class antigen. The detection of this or antigenically similar substances is dependent on competition for antibody binding between unlabeled drugs from the patient sample and labeled drugs (antigens) provided in the test kit. In the case of the EMIT, the enzyme-labeled antigen will compete with a drug in the urine for binding to the antibody. If there is little or no drug of this type present in the sample, the enzyme/antigen complex will bind to the antibody. This large complex inhibits the action of the enzyme (glucose-6-phosphate dehydrogenase) by preventing substrate access to the action site. Thus the rate of product formation is low and the EMIT reading is low. Conversely, if there is a lot of drug, the enzyme/antigen complex will be free of antibody binding, yielding a greater reaction time and higher readings. The assay is semiquantitative; for example, one can differentiate larger amounts of drugs in the urine from near-threshold concentrations.

The EMIT suffers from a lack of both specificity and sensitivity. The antibodies for these tests were derived against single substances (e.g., amitriptyline for the tricyclics), but dissimilar antidepressants (e.g., diphenhydramine) will yield a positive result.

TABLE 1. **Potential Problems with Enzyme-Multiplied Immunosorbent Technology**

	Detects	Poor Detection
Amphetamines	D-amphetamine Methamphetamine Pseudoephedrine Ephedrine Phenylpropanolamine	MDMA
Narcotics	Morphine Codeine Heroin Hydrocodone	Oxycodone Meperidine Methadone Fentanyl
Benzodiazepines	Alprazolam Diazepam Oxazepam Triazolam	Chlordiazepoxide Lorazepam Clonazepam

Abbreviation: MDMA = 3,4-methylene dioxyamphetamine.

Similarly, the opioid and benzodiazepine assay screens are not sensitive enough. The opioid screen does well with some semisynthetic opioids such as hydrocodone, but not with others (e.g., oxycodone), except in high concentrations.

COCAINE

Cocaine is an alkaloid extracted from the leaves of coca shrubs that are indigenous to South America. It has become perhaps the drug that is responsible for the second greatest number of emergency department visits (alcohol is first). The visits are prompted by both the toxidrome and withdrawal states.

Cocaine may be taken in many forms, including intranasal (insufflation), free basing (crack cocaine), and intravenous abuse (often with heroin, called "speed balling"). Intranasal use is associated with a more prolonged "high" or "rush," with intravenous use second and free basing third, causing a considerable high or rush that is very short-lived. For this reason crack cocaine has an enormous recidivist rate in terms of long-term treatment.

Acute cocaine use causes its effects by blocking presynaptic re-uptake primarily of dopamine and also norepinephrine and serotonin. This creates the toxidrome (Table 2) that is divided into two phases. The first is that of euphoria, grandiosity, hyperalertness, and anxiety, which eventually can lead to paranoid ideation and visual, auditory, or tactile hallucinations. These tactile hallucinations are called "cocaine bugs." Treatment of this toxidrome is generally symptomatic, with use of benzodiazepines, e.g., lorazepam (Ativan), 2 mg orally, sublingually, intramuscularly, or intravenously for anxiety states (which is why alprazolam [Xanax] is commonly abused, as the anxiety is not a welcome side effect). If hallucinations or paranoia become part of the toxi-

drome, small doses of haloperidol (Haldol), 5 mg orally or intramuscularly every hour, will make the patient more comfortable. Because cognition is impaired, I do not believe that talking with a patient is very helpful in calming anxiety and/or paranoia.

The second phase of acute cocaine intoxication does pose some medical emergencies. One must always keep in mind for all drugs that abusers do not always know how potent their drug is and therefore may accidentally overdose. Large doses of cocaine can depress cardiac conduction and contractility and can cause atrial and ventricular arrhythmias as well as myocardial infarction without evidence of coronary artery disease. It is likely that hypertension (with or without vasculitis) secondary to cocaine is a prominent cause of cerebral vascular accidents in the young. Seizures, albeit uncommon sequelae, are often difficult to manage. Hyperthermia caused by both central and peripheral effects and combativeness can lead to extreme rhabdomyolysis. Hydration, alpha-adrenergic blocking drugs, and benzodiazepines are generally considered the treatments of choice. Acidification of the urine may help excrete the cocaine faster but runs the risk of creating more renal failure and therefore is not recommended.

Chronic use of cocaine has been associated with a schizophreniform psychosis that is very difficult to distinguish from paranoid schizophrenia. Paranoid delusions and auditory, visual, and tactile hallucinations are very common. Dangerousness to self or others is the clinical problem. This psychotic state will dissipate in one to two days, but patients (particularly free basers) who abuse at least an "eight ball" (an eighth of an ounce of cocaine) per day may have lingering psychotic symptoms for over a week even when hospitalized in secure and calm environments.

The other common presentation for cocaine abuse is the withdrawal state. It is common for many to "crash" and become extremely dysphoric and even suicidally depressed. It appears that many in the medical profession believe that these people are simply coming in to sleep off the withdrawal effects (see Table 2), but it would be foolhardy to believe that they are not an extreme suicide risk for up to 48 hours. I have tried to decrease the dysphoria and cravings with dopamine agonists such as amantadine (Symmetrel),* bromocriptine (Parlodel),* and pergolide (Permax)* with little success, likely secondary to the down-regulation of postsynaptic dopamine receptors. Those patients who remain suicidally depressed after 48 to 72 hours should be carefully evaluated for chronic dysthymia or major depression by a psychiatrist.

TABLE 2. **Stimulants (Cocaine and Amphetamines)**

Toxidrome

Phase 1	Euphoria
	Insomnia
	Anorexia
	Mydriasis
	Hypertension
	Tachycardia
	Diaphoresis
	Hallucinations
	Paranoia
	Cocaine bugs
	Schizophreniform psychosis
Phase 2	Hyperthermia
	Arrhythmias
	Myocardial infarction
	Rhabdomyolysis
	Seizures
	Coma

Withdrawal

	Hypersomnia
	Hyperphagia
	Unmasking of underlying psychopathology
	Suicidal ideation cravings

AMPHETAMINES

Amphetamines are not nearly as abused now as cocaine except perhaps for certain areas of the West Coast. They include methylphenidate (Ritalin), dextroamphetamine (Dexedrine), and pemoline (Cylert).

---

*Not FDA-approved for this indication.

They are a group of compounds related structurally to dopamine and norepinephrine. The toxidrome of the intoxicated state is shown in Table 2.

As with cocaine, there are various routes of administration, including oral, insufflation, intravenous, and smokable forms. Oral amphetamines are used for enhancing job or athletic performance and weight loss. Most patients will experience anxiety as a side effect, but there are certainly cases of paranoia and hallucinatory psychosis even from slightly higher than "therapeutic" doses. Insufflation of amphetamine (particularly "crystal meth") is very similar to that of cocaine and has a higher degree of addiction than oral use.

Intravenous users of amphetamines and smokable forms (particularly "Ice," the long-acting smokable form) certainly are at the highest risk for contracting psychiatric and medical problems. These complications should be treated in the same fashion as cocaine intoxication. As is the case with cocaine withdrawal, amphetamine withdrawal will likely lead to dysphoria and/or suicidal ideation (see Table 2). The same precautions should be taken as discussed for cocaine.

DESIGNER STIMULANT DRUGS

"Ecstasy," "E," "Adam," and "ETC" are street names for the amphetamine analogue 3,4-methylene dioxymethamphetamine (MDMA). Its cousin, 3,4-methylene dioxyethamphetamine (MDME) ("Eve"), is much less common. Recently, MDMA has proved to be the drug of choice for "rave parties," which are clandestine all-night dance parties usually found in large cities in the United States. Prior to that, MDMA was used and abused for a "nonaddictive, benign high" and even for stimulating people in psychotherapy. However, the drug has proved to be far from benign.

The common effects of MDMA at therapeutic doses are tremor, bruxism, insomnia, diaphoresis, and euphoria. But at higher doses MDMA has been associated with many deaths by induction of cardiac arrhythmias, seizures, intracerebral hemorrhage, disseminated intravascular coagulation (DIC), and hyperthermia. Treatment of overdose consists of providing a clear airway. Agitation and seizures should be treated with benzodiazepines (e.g., diazepam [Valium], 5 to 10 mg intravenously). The necessity of immediate reduction of temperature is imperative as the severity and duration of hyperthermia appear to be the most important prognosticators of morbidity and mortality. Ice packs, cooling blankets, and infusion of ice-cold saline intravenously can be utilized. Severe metabolic acidosis may occur, and therefore sodium bicarbonate and glucose insulin therapy should be initiated to prevent cardiac arrhythmias.

NARCOTICS

Sydenham wrote in 1680, "Among the remedies which it has pleased Almighty God to give to man to relieve his sufferings, none is so universal and so efficacious as opium." Clearly drugs related to opium have been a major medical miracle for many and a major medical problem for others. Although most medical personnel are aware of the street "junkies" who arrive in the emergency room, many are not aware of the "regular citizens" who are addicted to narcotics (sometimes iatrogenically). Also, there is a growing concern among some physicians of the naïveté of college students who are recreationally snorting high-grade heroin in the false belief they will not become addicted. The usual presentation of narcotic abuse is the overdose situation. Although this could be a suicide attempt, accidental overdoses are common. The percentage of heroin in a particular area may be increased by a factor of two- or threefold to attract "new customers." Even long-term intravenous users who are aware of an increasing percentage might overdose as they attempt to "cut" the drug themselves.

The narcotics are divided into two major categories: (1) natural, e.g., opium, morphine, and heroin, and (2) synthetic, e.g., fentanyl ("China White"), meperidine (Demerol), 1-methyl-4-phenyl-1,2,3,6-tetrahydropyridine (MPTP), 1-methyl-4-phenyl propionoxy-piperidine tetrahydropyridine (MPPP), and methadone.

Narcotics can be used orally, by insufflation, intravenously, or in smokable form. The user's euphoria depends on the dose and the route of administration. Symptoms are analgesia, drowsiness, and respiratory depression (Table 3). The table shows that there is a difference in the natural vs. meperidine in terms of the toxidrome. Pinpoint pupils are the rule for the natural opioids whereas normal or even mydriasis may occur with meperidine. Meperidine overdoses are often accompanied by seizures. Treatment generally is to provide a patent airway with ventilation as well as to administer naloxone (Narcan). Note that the synthetic opioids may need larger doses of naloxone than the natural ones. Also note that because

TABLE 3. **Narcotics**

	Toxidrome	Withdrawal
Natural	Euphoria	(8 to 12 h after last dose)
	Miosis	
	Analgesia	Rhinorrhea
	Sedation	Piloerection
	Respiratory depression	Nausea
		Agitation
		Abdominal cramps
		Muscular cramps
Synthetic		
Meperidine (Demerol)	Same except no miosis	Same except 3 to 5 h after last dose
		Seizures
Fentanyl (Sublimaze)	Same except for marked muscle rigidity	Same except for less than 3 h after last dose
Methadone (Dolophine)	Same except no euphoria	Same except 36 to 48 h after last dose

many often use "speed balls," the sedative effect of the opioid will be reversed, uncovering the agitation of cocaine. In addition, the natural opioids have an antipsychotic effect for some individuals, and thus the reversal may uncover a psychotic state.

Withdrawal symptoms are different for the natural vs. synthetic opioids, especially the time frames. In the case of heroin and morphine, lacrimation, rhinorrhea, yawning, and diaphoresis appear about 4 to 8 hours after the last dose. As the syndrome progresses, anorexia, piloerection ("goose flesh"), restlessness, and irritability appear after 12 to 24 hours. Abdominal and muscular cramping follows in 1 to 2 days.

The meperidine withdrawal syndrome may begin 3 to 5 hours after the last dose. The peak intensity occurs in 8 to 12 hours. Craving is much more intense than with heroin and morphine, and the cramping and restlessness may be far more intense.

The withdrawal of methadone is very similar to that of heroin, but symptoms do not occur for 36 to 48 hours after the last dose. The peak intensity may not be reached for 3 to 4 days, and the entire abstinent syndrome may last 3 to 4 weeks. This is why the controversy over methadone maintenance exists: it is more prolonged to recover from methadone dependence than from shorter-acting narcotics. However, it is clear that in two groups of patients methadone maintenance is necessary: (1) People with pre-existing endocarditis or human immunodeficiency virus (HIV) disease, i.e., those who need to avoid further use of needles, will likely need long-term methadone maintenance; (2) Pregnant women need to be on methadone for the entire pregnancy. It appears that the withdrawal can cause multiple birth defects, particularly of the neural tube.

ANTICHOLINERGICS

Abuse of anticholinergics ranges from eating the seeds or smoking the leaves of the plant *Datura stramonium* (jimson weed) to antiparkinsonian drugs, e.g., benztropine (Cogentin), antihistamines (Benadryl), and tricyclic antidepressants—especially amitriptyline (Elavil) and doxepin (Sinequan).

The atropinic effects will produce euphoria and excitement as well as delirium with concomitant visual hallucinations. There is marked mydriasis, increased pulse, and increased blood pressure. The mnemonic "mad as a hatter, dry as a bone, red as a beet, blind as a bat" applies. Elevated temperatures, seizures, and arrhythmias occur with larger doses of atropinic compounds. Treatment consists of protecting the airway and administering charcoal and a cathartic. Because these drugs markedly decrease gastrointestinal motility, decontamination may be a benefit for many hours after the ingestion.

Arrhythmias that do not respond to beta blockers might require physostigmine, a reversible anticholinesterase. The initial adult dose is 0.5 to 2 to 3 mg by very slow intravenous push over approximately 3 to 5 minutes. However, its use has been associated with

TABLE 4. **Benzodiazepines**

Chlordiazepoxide (Librium)	Temazepam (Restoril)
Diazepam (Valium)	Triazolam (Halcion)
Clorazepate (Tranxene)	Oxazepam (Serax)
Halazepam (Paxipam)*	Prazepam (Centrax)
Lorazepam (Ativan)	Midazolam (Versed)
Flurazepam (Dalmane)	Alprazolam (Xanax)
Clonazepam (Klonopin)	Quazepam (Doral)

*Not available in the United States.

seizures (usually if given too quickly) and the syndrome of cholinergic crisis, consisting of severe bradycardia, miosis, salivation, bronchospasm, and laryngospasm. Clinical judgment must be used to determine the risk-benefit ratio if physostigmine is indicated in any individual case.

SEDATIVE HYPNOTICS

Sedative hypnotics include the benzodiazepines and the barbiturates and their congeners. Because of the fall in barbiturate use and abuse in recent years, I will primarily deal with benzodiazepines.

The benzodiazepines exert their influence primarily on the gamma-aminobutyric acid (GABA) system. That receptor is now known to have at least three parts: Omega 1, Omega 2, and Omega 3. These parts are responsible for the different actions of the drug, including sedation, anxiolytic activity, and anticonvulsant activity.

Chlordiazepoxide (Librium) was discovered in the late 1950s, and thus began the introduction of many congeners (Table 4). In recent years, alprazolam (Xanax) has became one of the largest selling drugs in the United States. As has been noted before, alprazolam is commonly abused with other drugs, especially the stimulants.

The toxidrome of benzodiazepines includes sedation, slurred speech, ataxia, disinhibition, and occasionally violence, especially when mixed with other drugs. In elderly people, the decreased excretion of the drug often leads to delirium (Table 5). In the overdose situation, the usual procedures are indicated even though death from single-drug benzodiaz-

TABLE 5. **Benzodiazepines**

Toxidrome	Slurred speech
	Sedation
	Euphoria
	Disinhibition
	Ataxia
	Delirium in elderly people
Withdrawal	Tremor
	Nausea
	Diaphoresis
	Irritability
	Tachycardia
	Hypertension
	Hallucinations
	Paranoia
	Seizures

epine overdoses is rare. However, single-drug over-doses are generally not the rule for most suicides. Flumazenil (Mazicon) rapidly reverses central nervous system (CNS) depression of benzodiazepines but seems to have fallen out of favor, likely due to the fact that suicidal overdoses are commonly multidrug.

The withdrawal state of benzodiazepines looks very much like that of alcohol except in time frame. The shorter-acting ones, lorazepam (Ativan) and oxazepam (Serax), can occur in 1 to 2 days, whereas longer-acting ones, diazepam (Valium) and chlordiazepoxide (Librium), may be delayed 3 to 4 days. Signs and symptoms include tremor, irritability, nausea, diaphoresis, and abdominal pain. Severe cases include symptoms similar to severe alcohol withdrawal e.g., hallucinations (auditory, visual, or tactile), paranoia, and seizures. Withdrawal is treated with other benzodiazepines, with the addition of carbamazepine (Tegretol) or valproic acid (Depakote) in severe cases.

The withdrawal state of alprazolam (Xanax) is somewhat different. Because of its short half-life, people can experience severe restlessness and tremor 8 to 12 hours after the last dose. But of more concern is the high rate of seizures in the first day of withdrawal. It is clear that suspected withdrawal from alprazolam must be much more aggressively treated than that from other benzodiazepines, using a combination of longer-acting benzodiazepines and carbamazepine.

PHENCYCLIDINE PIPERIDINE

Phencyclidine (PCP) was synthesized in 1957 and was originally intended for use as an intravenous anesthetic. However, 10% to 20% of patients exhibited extreme agitation, delirium, muscular rigidity, and seizures. It was then used as a veterinary anesthetic from 1965 to 1978. By 1979, all legal manufacturing ceased.

PCP was reportedly first used as a street drug circa 1967 in San Francisco as the "PeaCePill." However, it developed a bad reputation because of "bad trips" and violent behavior of the user. Some time later, it was found that by smoking it, one could titrate the negative effects somewhat, and now it is most commonly mixed with marijuana or tobacco and then smoked.

The toxidrome of PCP includes euphoria, disinhibition, grandiosity, elimination of pain, and altered perception of time and space. Attraction to water, as part of the delusional system, can lead to drowning by misadventure. Cerebellar effects include dizziness, ataxia, slurred speech, and nystagmus. Extreme violent behavior with demonstration of extreme strength is very prominent and most likely responsible for the enforced visits to the emergency department via the police.

Most patients with acute PCP intoxication require triple leather restraints as well as haloperidol (Haldol), 5 to 10 mg intramuscularly, with lorazepam (Ativan), 1 to 4 mg intravenously. Chlorpromazine (Thorazine) may delay the metabolism of PCP and is

thus contraindicated. The use of ascorbic acid, 1000 mg intramuscularly, was advocated in San Francisco. In a small portion of patients the intoxicated state was shortened noticeably. The patient should be kept in restraints for at least 18 hours, keeping in mind that there can be 5- to 10-minute lucid periods every few hours, and then the deliriform psychosis abruptly returns. The patient may then revert quickly to a very violent psychotic state.

Continuous use of PCP leads to tolerance and withdrawal symptoms consisting of anxiety and suicidal depression. A long-acting PCP compound called "illy" may cause more withdrawal symptoms when chronically used.

HALLUCINOGENS

Hallucinogenic plants have been ingested for thousands of years. Some religions still use them. For example, Native Americans of the Southwest still use peyote cactus (containing mescaline). The most popular hallucinogen for recreational abusers has been D-lysergic acid diethylamide (LSD).

LSD causes blurred vision, paresthesias, nausea, and euphoria in a few minutes after ingestion. After 1 to 2 hours, there are visual distortions and altered body image. Hyperacusis often occurs, as well as hallucinations, particularly visual ones. These may be quite simple in nature or extremely complex and may be quite beautiful or grotesque and frightening. "Bad trips" have led to self-destructive activity, suicide, and homicide. Symptoms usually last from 8 to 16 hours, but "flashbacks" are common for those who have ingested 10 or more "hits." Flashbacks are typically pseudohallucinations. "Light trailings," one of the most common type, are comet-like trailings of light that follow a moving object.

Treatment is generally supportive but may require lorazepam (Ativan), 1 to 2 mg orally or intravenously, and/or haloperidol, 2 to 5 mg orally or intramuscularly.

LSD, mescaline, and psilocybin differ in potency and duration of action, but their effects are indistinguishable although many users will state that the hallucinations of LSD are more difficult to "control," i.e., retain some degree of reality testing. Withdrawal symptoms do not occur.

INHALANTS

The abuse of inhalants is a worldwide problem, especially for children and adolescents. Generally speaking, their use is a product of socioeconomic problems and psychological deprivation. In very poor areas, people cannot afford other recreational drugs. Thus, there has been a large increase in the abuse of solvents. A tremendous variety of substances may be used, including aerosols, cleaning fluids, glues, lighter fluid, refrigerants, marker pens, gasoline, and paint remover. Substances are usually sniffed or "huffed" from a plastic bag or saturated rag.

Despite their variety, the toxidromes are somewhat

similar for all inhalants. Immediate effects include euphoria, excitement, sedation, lightheadedness, and delirium with visual and auditory hallucinations, as well as slurred speech and ataxia. Distortions of space and time are common. The effects of the acute intoxication may last 15 to 45 minutes. Sudden death may occur from suffocation in a plastic bag or from cardiac arrhythmias. There are many reported cases of irreversible damage to the central nervous system, liver, kidney, and bone marrow.

Treatment for the acute intoxication is generally supportive and symptom-specific (e.g., arrhythmias). Although most inhalants do not produce a withdrawal state, there are a few reported cases of toluene withdrawal that mimic alcohol withdrawal.

ANXIETY DISORDERS

method of
MANUEL E. TANCER, M.D., and
THOMAS W. UHDE, M.D.
Wayne State University School of Medicine
Detroit, Michigan

Anxiety is one of the most common symptoms seen by physicians. Anxiety can be a symptom of a wide range of medical conditions (Table 1), can be a side effect of a variety of medications (Table 2), or can be due to intoxication or withdrawal from medications and substances of abuse (Table 3). It is therefore essential that the symptom of anxiety be carefully evaluated by detailed history, physical examination, and appropriate laboratory evaluation. It is essential that a patient's age and gender be considered in formulating a differential diagnosis and planning a diagnostic work-up. For example, a 20-year-old person with paroxysmal chest pain is much less likely to be having ischemic cardiac pain than a 50-year-old with hypertension (although now cocaine intoxication must be considered in the differential).

A careful history of ethanol and drug use is essential in the evaluation of complaints of anxiety. Many anxious patients report using ethanol to alleviate their symptoms. However, ethanol use can also cause anxiety symptoms, as can withdrawal from ethanol in dependent patients. Use of benzodiazepines in the long-term or chronic treatment of anxiety symptoms in patients with histories of ethanol and/or drug abuse or dependence is cautioned and should be con-

TABLE 2. Medications and Substances Associated with Anxiety Symptoms

Corticosteroids
Antihypertensives
Lidocaine
Birth control pills
Selective serotonin re-uptake inhibitors
Analgesics containing caffeine
Nonsteroidal anti-inflammatory agents
Cocaine
Alcohol
Hallucinogens (PCP/LSD)
Marijuana

Abbreviations: PCP = phencyclidine piperidine; LSD = lysergic acid diethylamide.

sidered only when a careful risk-benefit analysis has been performed.

Caffeine, one of the most widely consumed psychoactive drugs, can cause symptoms of anxiety and arousal, so a thorough caffeine use history is also important. Most commonly consumed in coffee, tea, chocolate, and carbonated soft drinks, caffeine can also be found in several over-the-counter analgesic compounds. Reduction or elimination of caffeine can sometimes be an effective therapeutic intervention.

In addition to the organic causes of anxiety summarized in Tables 1 to 3, complaints of anxiety symptoms are common manifestations of an acute or subacute psychosocial stress, such as marital discord or job-related stress. Furthermore, anxiety symptoms can be prominent features in some psychiatric disorders, such as major depression, personality disorders, or schizophrenia. Finally, anxiety may be an integral feature of one of the nine anxiety disorder syndromes defined by the *Diagnostic and Statistical Manual for Mental Disorders*, fourth edition (DSM-IV).

The National Comorbidity Study reported a 17.2% 12-month and 24.9% lifetime prevalence of anxiety disorders in the general population. Of note, only a minority (11.5%) of the demographically representative individuals with a psychiatric disorder had sought mental health attention for their difficulties over the past 12 months.

Many patients present with features or symptoms of more than one anxiety disorder. Most clinical trials, on the other hand, limit participation to carefully screened patients who fulfill strict inclusion/exclusion criteria. Results from published treatment trials might not generalize to clinical samples.

Cognitive-behavioral treatment of anxiety disorders is based on the conceptual theories of several researchers. The assumption made in the cognitive

TABLE 1. Organic Syndromes Associated with Anxiety Symptoms

Endocrinopathies	Cardiorespiratory
Cushing's disease	Ischemic chest pain
Pheochromocytoma	Chronic pulmonary emboli
Hypothyroidism	Respiratory distress
Hyperthyroidism	

TABLE 3. Medications and Substances in Which Withdrawal Is Associated with Anxiety Symptoms

Corticosteroids	Cocaine
Beta blockers	Alcohol
Caffeine	Hallucinogens (PCP/LSD)
Opiates	Marijuana

treatment of anxious patients is that negative experiences lead to the beliefs (cognitive set) that certain objects, places, or situations are somehow dangerous, threatening, or shameful, and negative or unpleasant interactions can be reduced only by avoiding these objects, places, or situations altogether or by behaving in a perfect, or overcontrolled, manner.

Cognitive-behavioral therapy (CBT) can be conducted individually or in groups. It involves identifying patients' distorted cognitions and "automatic thoughts," dichotomous thinking (black or white), and catastrophic notions associated with the feared or avoided place, object, or situation. Once these thoughts are identified, more realistic appraisals of situations are taught. Some patients require some relaxation training or other techniques to deal with the anxiety symptoms. A fear hierarchy is developed with the most terrifying situations confronted last. Exposure is the major feature of the behavioral component of the treatment. Exposure occurs first in imagination, then in role play situations, and finally, in real, anxiety-provoking situations. This treatment involves a commitment from the patient to do homework and to fill out logs of automatic thoughts and reactions to different situations, and the motivation to place himself or herself in uncomfortable situations. Cognitive-behavioral approaches, with syndrome-specific modifications, appear to be effective in the treatment of most anxiety disorders. The exceptions are obsessive-compulsive disorder and specific phobias, in which variants of exposure therapy (without a cognitive focus) are the most widely used psychotherapeutic approach.

Both pharmacologic and behavioral and cognitive-behavioral treatments are effective in groups of patients suffering from anxiety disorders. There are patients who respond to one form of treatment but not the other; unfortunately, there are few pretreatment predictors of who these individuals are. Few studies have systematically examined the efficacy of combined treatments on outcome. If an anxiety disorder patient is not clinically improved after 6 to 8 weeks of treatment using one treatment modality, a reassessment of the patient and a shift in treatment modalities is probably warranted.

The essential diagnostic features for the nine DSM-IV Anxiety Disorders are listed in Table 4. Several significant changes from the DSM third revised

TABLE 4. **Essential Diagnostic Features for DSM-IV Anxiety Disorders***

Panic Disorder with and Without Agoraphobia	Recurrent paroxysmal panic attacks Initially spontaneous or "out of the blue" Distress about another attack Avoidance of places associated with attacks
Social Phobia	Marked distress or embarrassment or humiliation in situations involving performance, interaction, or being the focus of attention No spontaneous panic attacks Excessive/unreasonable fear
Specific Phobia	Marked and persistent fear that is excessive or unreasonable, cued by presence or anticipation of a specific object or situation (e.g., snakes, heights, flying, or seeing blood) Excessive/unreasonable fear
Obsessive-Compulsive Disorder	Recurrent obsessions (intrusive thoughts that increase or cause anxiety) and Recurrent compulsions (thoughts or behaviors [rituals] which decrease anxiety) Excessive or unreasonable Time-consuming ($>$1h/d)
Post-Traumatic Stress Disorder	Exposure to traumatic event in which the person experienced, witnessed, or was confronted with events that involved actual or threatened death or serious injury, or a threat to the physical integrity of self or others, and the person's response involved intense fear, helplessness, or horror There must also be evidence of re-experiencing the trauma, persistent avoidance of stimuli associated with the trauma, and persistent symptoms of increased arousal Symptoms persisting at least 30 d
Acute Stress Disorder	Exposure to traumatic event in which the person experienced, witnessed, or was confronted with events that involved actual or threatened death or serious injury, or a threat to the physical integrity of self or others, and the person's response involved intense fear, helplessness, or horror There must also be evidence of re-experiencing the trauma, persistent avoidance of stimuli associated with the trauma, and persistent symptoms of increased arousal Symptoms persisting at least 2 d and less than 4 wk
Generalized Anxiety Disorder	Excessive worry and anxiety, more days than not, for greater than 6 mo Difficulty controlling the worry Symptoms of arousal or tension
Anxiety Disorder Due to General Medical Condition	Prominent anxiety which is felt to be directly related to a medical condition or drug or substance ingestion (e.g., caffeine, corticosteroids, theophylline)
Anxiety Disorder Not Otherwise Specified	Prominent anxiety but not meeting criteria for a specific disorder

*Note that all diagnoses require "significant interference with the person's normal routine, occupational (or academic) functioning, or usual social activities or relationships" in addition to syndrome-specific criteria.

edition have been made. The changes will be discussed separately under the individual anxiety disorders. Panic disorder is being covered in its own section and will not be discussed here.

SOCIAL PHOBIA

Social phobia is characterized by interactional, social, or performance dread, avoidance, or impairment in function. The most common phobic situation is speaking in public. Recent epidemiologic surveys place the 12-month prevalence of social phobia at 7.9% of the general population. The minority of people meeting diagnostic criteria for social phobia have sought professional help for their problem. The impact of social phobia on people is often discounted because of the high frequency of discomfort in public speaking situations. Social phobia is associated with high rates of distress and increased rates of co-morbid substance abuse. Social phobia has an earlier age of onset than panic disorder. Patients with social phobia often have panic attacks during the phobic situations but not "out of the blue." Also, flushing or blushing is a symptom reported more frequently by patients with social phobia than by panic disorder patients. The primary change in social phobia diagnostic conventions under DSM-IV is the inclusion of individuals under 18 years of age. Social phobic subjects have been divided into "generalized" and "specific" subtypes, depending on the variety of situations causing phobic and/or avoidant symptoms. There are hints of different pharmacologic response patterns in the two groups. A recent family study has found a markedly increased familial clustering of generalized, but not specific, social phobia subtypes.

Pharmacotherapy trials in social phobia have undergone an explosion over the past few years (Table 5). No drug has been designated as safe and effective by the Food and Drug Administration (FDA) for the treatment of social phobia. Monoamine oxidase inhibitors, selective serotonin re-uptake inhibitors, high-potency benzodiazepines, and the serotonin-3 receptor antagonist ondansetron have been shown to be more effective than placebo in double-blind, placebo-controlled trials in patients with social phobia. Although beta blockers are often used in clinical practice in the treatment of "stage fright," two double-blind trials have shown that daily beta-adrenergic blockade is no better than placebo in the treatment of social phobia. Controlled studies of "as needed" beta blockers in patients with specific and predictable social phobic symptomatology are needed. As with panic disorder, the optimal duration of treatment is not known.

SPECIFIC PHOBIA

Specific phobias are the irrational or excessive fears of objects, places, or situations. The 12-month prevalence is 8.8% and lifetime prevalence is 11.3% of the population. To meet the criteria for a phobia, there must be social or occupational impairment or excessive distress by having the fear. The most common specific phobias are to animals (e.g., spiders, rats, snakes) or to situations (e.g., closed places, heights). Exposure or desensitization therapy is the treatment of choice for specific phobias. There are no controlled trials indicating a role for pharmacotherapy. Nevertheless, many patients use alcohol as a self-medication when flying, despite studies showing that alcohol ingestion actually delays the effects of exposure treatment. One type of specific phobia, namely "blood-injection-injury," is familial and associated with prominent vasovagal symptoms. Little research has been conducted on this subtype, and there is no consensus as to the most effective treatment.

OBSESSIVE-COMPULSIVE DISORDER

Obsessions are intrusive thoughts that increase or cause anxiety symptoms, whereas compulsions are repetitive thoughts or behaviors that, initially at least, reduce anxiety. Obsessive-compulsive disorder (OCD) symptoms may develop gradually or suddenly. One percent to 2% of the general population suffers from OCD. The age of onset is variable, and both acute and insidious symptom onset have been reported.

Positron emission tomography studies reveal an increase in orbitofrontal cortex and cingulate gyrus blood flow or glucose metabolic rates in OCD patients. Some patients with OCD also suffer from Tourette's syndrome or simple tic disorder. Medications indicated by the FDA for the treatment of OCD include clomipramine, fluoxetine, and fluvoxamine (Table 6). Although the medications can make a clinically significant reduction in OCD symptoms, many patients remain moderately impaired by residual symptoms. This has led several groups to examine

TABLE 5. **Drugs for the Treatment of Social Phobia**

Drug	Dose Range	Efficacy	FDA Approved
Phenelzine (Nardil)	30–90 mg/d	+ + +	No
Fluvoxamine (Luvox)	150 mg/d	+ +	No
Alprazolam (Xanax)	1.5–6 mg/d	+ +	No
Clonazepam (Klonopin)	1.0–4 mg/d	+ +	No
Ondansetron (Zofran)	0.25 mg bid	+	No

+ + + = Several double-blind, placebo-controlled trials; + + = One double-blind, placebo-controlled trial or several case series; + = One double-blind, placebo-controlled trial with little clinical efficacy or several case reports.

TABLE 6. **Drugs for the Treatment of Obsessive-Compulsive Disorder**

Drug	Dose (mg/24 h)	Efficacy	FDA Approved
Clomipramine (Anafranil)	150–250	+ + +	Yes
Fluoxetine (Prozac)	20–80	+ + +	Yes
Fluvoxamine (Luvox)	100–300	+ + +	Yes
Sertraline (Zoloft)	50–200	+	No
Paroxetine (Paxil)	20–50	+	Yes

+ + + = Several double-blind, placebo-controlled trials; + = One double-blind, placebo-controlled trial with little clinical efficacy or several case reports.

potentiation strategies or combined treatment strategies. Lithium,* clonazepam,* buspirone,* and neuroleptics potentiation has been tried with limited success. In severe cases, psychosurgery, specifically anterior cingulotomy, has been reported to alleviate symptoms. The behavioral therapy that has been most widely studied and used in the treatment of OCD is exposure plus response prevention. Treatment requires both exposure to feared objects, situations, or places and the prevention of rituals. Though effective, this treatment requires tremendous commitment from patients and an experienced therapist.

POST-TRAUMATIC STRESS DISORDER

PTSD is arguably the most heterogeneous anxiety disorder, in that a wide range of traumatic experiences, such as incest, rape, fires, and accidents, can result in PTSD. The age at onset of the trauma, the duration, its intensity, and the premorbid function of the individual have an impact on the presentation, severity, and prognosis of the disorder. Symptoms of PTSD are organized into three groups: persistent re-experiencing of the traumatic event, persistent avoidance or numbing, and persistent hyperarousal, all persisting for at least 30 days after the traumatic event. DSM-IV criteria delete the need for stressors to be "outside the range of normal human experience," which was not reliable, and replaced the criteria so that subjects had to experience the trauma with intense fear, helplessness, or horror. Also, the proviso of clinically significant distress or impairment was required in all the anxiety diagnostic sets. Frequently, substance abuse or major depression complicates the presentation and treatment of patients suffering from PTSD. Both psychotherapeutic and pharmacologic interventions have been reported to benefit some individuals with PTSD. There is no FDA-approved pharmacotherapy of PTSD. Although double-blind placebo-controlled trials have included tricyclic antidepressants, monoamine oxidase inhibitors, and the selective serotonin re-uptake inhibitors, no single agent is uniformly effective in the treatment of the three domains (re-experiencing, numbing/avoidance, or hyperarousal). Trials of the opiate antagonist naltrexone* have been made. While these medications have given symptomatic relief, most patients remain symptomatic. The role of combination psychotherapy and pharmacotherapy deserves further investigation.

ACUTE STRESS DISORDER

This is a new diagnostic category under DSM-IV. It is used to describe transient symptoms that develop after an acute stressor. The stress is comparable to that causing PTSD, but the symptoms do not persist after 30 days. Psychological treatments are focused on affect regulation and controlled or focused thinking about the traumatic event. No medication is approved for this indication, although a wide range of medications have been used for symptom relief.

GENERALIZED ANXIETY DISORDER

Generalized anxiety disorder (GAD) has a 12-month prevalence of 3.1% and a lifetime prevalence of 5.1%. The Criterion A for the diagnosis of generalized anxiety disorder has been changed so that excessive anxiety and worry, rather than unrealistic worries (DSM-III-R), are required. The anxiety must also be difficult for the subject to control. The 18-item

*Not FDA-approved for this indication.

TABLE 7. **Drugs for the Treatment of Generalized Anxiety Disorder**

Drug	Dose (mg/24 h)	Efficacy	FDA Approved
Buspirone (Buspar)	15–60	+ + +	Yes
Diazepam (Valium)	4–40	+ +	Yes
Alprazolam (Xanax)	1.5–4	+ + +	Yes
Clorazepate (Tranzene)	15–60	+ +	Yes
Doxepin (Sinequan)	75–200	+	Yes for "psychoneurotic anxiety"

+ + + = Several double-blind, placebo-controlled trials; + + = One double-blind, placebo-controlled trial or several case series; + = One double-blind, placebo-controlled trial with little clinical efficacy or several case reports.

symptom list has been reduced to six items. The DSM-III-R diagnosis of Overanxious Disorder of Childhood has been incorporated into GAD in DSM-IV. Six months of symptoms are required for the diagnosis to be made, thereby making GAD, by definition, a chronic disorder.

Benzodiazepines and the serotonin 1a receptor antagonist buspirone (Buspar) are approved by the FDA for the treatment of GAD (Table 7). In addition, some older, sedating antidepressants such as doxepin are FDA-indicated for the treatment of "psychoneurotic anxiety" (Table 7). Patients who have previously been treated with a benzodiazepine appear to demonstrate less efficacy following buspirone therapy than patients with no prior benzodiazepine treatment, although more recent studies do not confirm this clinical observation.

OTHER DISORDERS

The DSM-IV includes two final anxiety diagnoses, Anxiety Disorder Due to [General Medical Condition] and Anxiety Disorder Not Otherwise Specified. In the former, the anxiety is a "direct physiologic consequence" of the medical condition (including substance-induced anxiety disorder) and causes significant distress or impairment. Anxiety Disorder Not Otherwise Specified is a category for anxious or phobic individuals who do not meet the diagnostic criteria for any specific anxiety disorder, or meet exclusion criteria—such as a patient with Parkinson's disease who is socially phobic secondary to embarrassment about the tremor.

BULIMIA NERVOSA

method of
RICHARD L. PYLE, M.D.
University of Minnesota
Minneapolis, Minnesota

DIAGNOSIS

Bulimia nervosa is an eating disorder recognized as a significant problem with considerable psychosocial and medical morbidity. Bulimia nervosa is one of three eating disorders identified by specific diagnostic criteria in the *Diagnostic and Statistical Manual for Psychiatric Disorder* (DSM-IV), the other two being anorexia nervosa and binge-eating disorder. The diagnostic criteria for bulimia nervosa are listed in Table 1.

Anorexia nervosa differs from bulimia nervosa in that it is manifested by (1) refusal to maintain body weight at or above a minimally normal weight for age and height; (2) intense fear of gaining weight or becoming fat even though underweight; (3) disturbance in the way in which one's body weight or shape is experienced; and (4) in postmenarchal women, amenorrhea, i.e., the absence of at least three consecutive menstrual cycles, assuming that menstrual cycles are not induced by estrogens. There are two basic types of anorexia nervosa in DSM-IV: the restricting type and the binge-eating-purging type, in which the individual

engages in binge eating or purging behavior, i.e., self-induced vomiting or laxative or diuretic abuse.

Binge-eating disorder is a more recent diagnostic category and resembles very closely the diagnostic criteria for the original DSM-III Bulimia diagnosis. The diagnostic description includes (1) recurrent episodes of binge eating as defined in Table 1, and (2) binge-eating episodes associated with at least three of the following: (a) eating more rapidly than normal, (b) eating until feeling uncomfortably full, (c) eating large amounts of food when not feeling physically hungry, (d) eating alone because of being embarrassed by how much one is eating, and (e) disgust, guilt, or depression after overeating. In addition, these patients experience marked distress regarding binge eating. To meet diagnostic criteria, patients need to binge eat, on the average, at least twice a week for 6 months.

CLINICAL FEATURES

Clinical characteristics of bulimia nervosa are described in Table 2. Binge eating associated with bulimia nervosa is usually accompanied by self-induced vomiting on at least a daily basis. Our studies have indicated that an average of 14 hours a week is spent in binge eating, with an average binge size of 3500 calories. There is, however, considerable variability, and some patients may consume up to 30,000 calories in a 24-hour period. Self-induced vomiting is present in 90% of the cases. The patients usually experience weight gain after initial weight loss because of increased binge size. As the vomiting becomes more difficult or less effective, patients may turn to laxatives (5% to 10%) or ipecac (3%). Additional methods of purging include diuretic abuse (15%), use of enemas (7%), and chewing and spitting out food, which occurs in about two thirds of the patients. Over one fourth of women may experiment with the dangerous practice of ipecac ingestion to induce vomiting.

MEDICAL COMPLICATIONS

Medical complications are commonly found in bulimia nervosa, including elevated amylase levels and salivary

TABLE 1. **Diagnostic Criteria for Bulimia Nervosa**

1. Recurrent episodes of binge eating. An episode of binge eating is characterized by both of the following:
   a. Eating, in a period of time (e.g., within any 2-h period), an amount of food that is definitely larger than most people would eat during a similar period of time and under similar circumstances, and,
   b. A sense of lack of control over eating during the episode (e.g., a feeling that one cannot stop eating or control what or how much one is eating)
2. Recurrent inappropriate compensatory behavior in order to prevent weight gain, such as self-induced vomiting; misuse of laxatives, diuretics, or other medications; fasting; or excessive exercise
3. The binge eating and inappropriate compensatory behaviors both occur, on average, at least twice a wk for 3 mo
4. Self-evaluation is unduly influenced by body shape and weight
5. The disturbance does not occur exclusively during episodes of anorexia nervosa
   a. Specific type:
      (1) *Purging type:* If person regularly engages in self-induced vomiting or the misuse of laxatives or diuretics
      (2) *Nonpurging type:* The person uses other inappropriate compensatory behaviors, such as fasting or excessive exercise, but does not regularly engage in self-induced vomiting or the misuse of laxatives or diuretics

TABLE 2. **Clinical Characteristics of Bulimia Nervosa**

Demographic

Median age at onset, 18 years
Female-to-male ratio, 20:1
Prevalence of 1% to 4% of females at risk (those aged 15 to 30 years)
Premorbid adjustment frequently described as either obsessive-compulsive or impulsive
Previous history of anorexia nervosa in 15% to 25%
Apparently, a familial relationship to *affective disorders, obesity,* and *alcoholism*
Significantly *higher risk of drug abuse* problems compared with the general population (about 25%)

Clinical Picture

Alternating *binges and fasts* in 100% of patients; patients often do not eat normally at other times
Self-induced *vomiting* present in about 90% (and more than 50% of those who self-induce vomiting do so on at least a daily basis)
Laxative abuse (66%)

gland swelling, which often are more pronounced during major shifts in the frequency of bingeing and/or vomiting. Dental complications are quite common and include erosion of enamel with frequent cavities. Fluid and electrolyte balance is disturbed and is associated with life-threatening hypokalemia. In addition, dehydration, alkalosis, and hypochloremia are common. Thyroid function is altered, and low triiodothyronine levels and impaired thyrotropin-releasing hormone responsiveness are often found.

TREATMENT

The first treatment goal is to *stabilize the eating pattern.* Frequently, if patients start eating more regularly, many of the associated symptoms seen with bulimia, such as depression and interpersonal problems, will diminish in intensity. The most important treatment plan component is to encourage the patient to accept a stable weight and to agree not to attempt further weight reduction until eating behavior is stabilized.

Experimental evidence is accumulating that antidepressants have both antibulimic and antidepressant features. The selective serotonin re-uptake inhibitors have been effective, most notably fluoxetine (Prozac)* in doses of up to 60 mg per day in the morning, taken after breakfast. The response is apparently bimodal at both 20- and 60-mg doses. Consequently, the initial 20-mg dose should be increased at the usual rate of every 3 weeks until the effective dose is reached.

Behavioral treatment approaches that focus on the behavior rather than the underlying issues appear to be most useful, either in individual or group settings. Cognitive-behavioral therapy appears to be the treatment of choice. Dealing with competing psychological issues, such as a history of physical or sexual abuse, should be de-emphasized until the eating behavior is stabilized. For those patients who abuse alcohol, chemical dependency treatment is indicated since it

---

*Not FDA-approved for this indication.

is difficult to focus on normalizing the eating behavior if alcohol abuse is occurring.

Role of Family Physician in Treatment of Bulimia Nervosa

Family physicians have a major role to play in the treatment of bulimia nervosa. Medical evaluation is one of the most important aspects of treatment. A careful history and complete physical examination should be performed, along with appropriate laboratory work that includes electrolytes, complete blood count, urinalysis, blood urea nitrogen, glucose, and serum amylase, and liver, renal, and thyroid function. All are helpful adjuncts to treatment, with serum electrolytes being the most important laboratory values to assess.

In addition to monitoring physical problems, dental referral is often indicated, along with education about appropriate dental hygiene for patients with bulimia nervosa. Patients are often conscientious and brush their teeth thoroughly each time they vomit. Because the enamel is damaged, the brushing often causes problems to the remaining enamel. Patients should be encouraged to rinse the mouth with sodium bicarbonate to reduce the acid damage immediately after inducing vomiting.

The family physician and the dietitian may also play important roles in stabilizing eating behavior. Patients believe that normal food intake will cause major weight gain, and they often complain of having a low metabolic rate. We encourage patients to plan meals a day in advance and eat only foods on their meal plan. They are instructed not to rely on either external or internal cues for eating behavior, but only to follow the meal plan. Normalizing eating behavior requires that patients take sufficient calories each day to avoid the urge to binge eat (usually 13 to 15 kilocalories per pound of ideal weight per day, depending on age and exercise level). Meals need to be frequent enough so that hunger is reduced, although we would prefer to have patients achieve a goal of eating three meals a day without snacks. Overweight patients who need to reduce calories after the eating disorder is stabilized should have a gradual decrease in calories consisting of 10 calories per pound of present weight to prevent relapse to binge eating. Patients need to be encouraged to introduce sufficient variety into their diet so that food cravings do not develop. Most important is the need to have sufficient satiety (fat) exchanges to prolong satiety and support enzyme system function.

In addition to prescribing and monitoring antidepressant medications, the family physician has a role in promoting services in the community that will be helpful to eating-disordered individuals. These should include professional individual or group psychotherapy, emphasizing cognitive-behavioral techniques; self-help groups consisting of exbulimic patients; and in smaller communities, general support groups for women. All of these have been found to be of value in reducing relapse.

Bulimia nervosa is a disabling, surreptitious illness, which, if suspected by the family physician, may be diagnosed early in its course and be more likely to respond to appropriate treatment.

DELIRIUM

method of
BENJAMIN LIPTZIN, M.D., and
STEPHEN MUELLER, M.D.
Baystate Medical Center, Springfield, and Tufts
*   University School of Medicine*
Boston, Massachusetts

Delirium is a generalized disorder of brain functioning that can have serious consequences. Key features (as described in the American Psychiatric Association *Diagnostic and Statistical Manual of Mental Disorders*, fourth edition) include a disturbance of consciousness with impaired ability to maintain or shift attention, a change in cognition (memory deficit, disorientation, language disturbance), perceptual disturbances (hallucinations, misinterpretations), development of symptoms over a short period of time (hours to days), fluctuation in mental status over the course of the day, and evidence that the disturbance is caused by a medical condition or substance/medication intoxication or withdrawal. Associated features include disturbance of the sleep-wake cycle, altered psychomotor behavior (ranging from agitated to lethargic), impaired judgment, emotional disturbances (anxiety, fear, irritability, apathy), and paranoia.

The disorder is most common in general hospital settings, particularly in elderly patients. Some studies have found the prevalence to be as high as 80% in elderly medical/surgical patients. Symptoms may develop over several hours or over several days. Once the symptoms appear, they may persist for days or weeks, even when the presumed underlying causes have been treated. Hospitalized patients with delirium often have a longer hospital stay or a higher probability of dying during the hospitalization or over the next 12 months. A new onset of delirium is often the first sign of acute illness (e.g., infection, dehydration, or myocardial infarction) in an elderly patient.

Despite its importance, delirium often goes undetected by physicians and nurses, especially when the patient is quietly confused rather than agitated, combative, paranoid, or hallucinating. The key differential diagnosis is that of dementia. Delirious patients can present with severe cognitive impairments, including disorientation to time and place, poor memory, and inability to give a coherent history. If the onset is acute or the patient is cognitively intact at some point during the day, delirium should be assumed rather than dementia. Even in demented patients, a rapid change in cognitive status is probably due to a superimposed delirium and not to a worsening of the dementia. Elderly patients who present acutely with psychotic features such as delusions or hallucinations should also be assumed to have a delirium unless they have a past history of schizophrenia, mania, psychotic depression, or delusional disorder.

EVALUATION

Careful observation and history taking is the key to making the diagnosis of delirium. Patients should be asked orientation questions (person, place, date), as well as questions about recent history and reason for hospitalization. Patients may seem pleasant and cooperative but give a rambling, incoherent story and have no idea that they are sick and in a hospital. Questions about living situation and family can also be useful. As part of a standardized mental status examination, the patient should also be asked to perform serial 7 subtractions (or to spell "world" backward) and to recall three objects after a 5-minute delay. One useful tool to assess cognitive function quickly is the Mini-Mental State Examination.

The patient should be observed for restlessness, suspiciousness, somnolence, hyperalertness, labile mood, belligerence, or distractibility. Even if a patient seems completely intact, one should talk to the nursing staff and read any written notes about the patient's behavior over the previous 48 hours. Any abnormalities should be checked with family members to determine whether they were present before the acute illness that led to hospitalization. Delirium is a final common pathway for many different disorders (Table 1), and these need to be systematically inquired about through history taking, physical examination, and laboratory evaluation.

Prescribed and nonprescribed medications (including alcohol) frequently lead to delirium in an older person who has reduced metabolism of the drug or increased sensitivity to its effects because of age or drug–disease or drug–drug interactions. If no obvious medication is causing the delirium, it is necessary to evaluate each organ system carefully. Often multiple pathologies will be uncovered, and it will not be obvious that any one was the specific cause of the delirium.

In addition to a standard laboratory assessment that includes a complete blood count, chemistry profile, and urinalysis, if the clinical history warrants it, other sources of infection should be sought (including human immunodeficiency virus) and a chest radiograph and electrocardiogram obtained. Blood gases and oxygen saturation may be

TABLE 1. **Causes of Delirium**

Drug intoxication
  Psychotropic drugs
    Antidepressants, sedative/hypnotics, anxiolytics,
      neuroleptics, lithium
  Other prescribed medications:
    Cardiac: Digitalis, antiarrhythmics, antihypertensives
    GI: Cimetidine, ranitidine, famotidine
    Anti-inflammatory agents
    Narcotic analgesics
  Over-the-counter drugs: Alcohol, antihistamines

Drug withdrawal
  Alcohol, sedatives/hypnotics/anxiolytics

Metabolic disorders
  Hypoxia, hypoglycemia, and hyperglycemia, fluid/electrolyte
    imbalance, acid-base imbalance, kidney failure, hepatic
    failure, anemia, vitamin deficiencies, endocrinopathies

Cardiovascular disorders
  Congestive heart failure, myocardial infarction, cardiac
    arrhythmia, shock

CNS disorders
  Head trauma, seizures, cerebrovascular diseases, infections,
    space-occupying lesions (tumor, subdural hematoma,
    abscess)

Infections

Sleep deprivation

Postoperative states

helpful. If a specific central nervous system disorder is suspected, a careful neurologic examination should be done and an electroencephalogram, computed tomography or magnetic resonance scan, and lumbar puncture should be considered.

TREATMENT
(Table 2)

Discovering the underlying medical cause for the delirium and reversing it, if possible, is the key to treating the delirious patient. Until that can be accomplished, the patient needs to be closely observed in a safe environment, usually a hospital. Whatever the underlying etiology, general supportive measures can be helpful. The patient should be kept in a quiet room with lights on in the daytime and a night light after bedtime. Stimulation should not be excessive, but some gentle music or television program may be soothing. Orientation cues, such as a calendar or clock, should be visible. Sensory impairments should be corrected with eyeglasses or a hearing aid. Family members should be encouraged to spend time with the patient for reassurance and orientation. Staff interventions should be carefully explained in a firm but caring manner. Patients should be encouraged to do as much for themselves and be as active as possible. Physical restraints should be used only if the patient is unsupervised and at risk of falling or is pulling out intravenous lines or other tubes.

In the quietly confused patient, the preceding interventions, along with careful monitoring, may be sufficient to get the patient safely through the episode of delirium. The highly agitated or psychotic patient may need pharmacologic intervention. In a delirium due to withdrawal from alcohol or other central nervous depressants, standard detoxification should be done. If the patient is clearly psychotic, a neuroleptic can be used. The butyrophenones are preferable to most phenothiazines since the latter have anticholinergic effects that can cause delirium. Haloperidol (Haldol), 0.5 to 5 mg, can be given orally, intramuscularly, or intravenously every 4 hours, up to a maximum of 20 mg per day, and titrated to the patient's response. The drug should be tapered over several days as the delirium resolves. If sedation is required, short-acting benzodiazepines, such as lorazepam (Ativan), 0.25 to 2 mg depending on the patient's size or frailty, can be given at bedtime or every 4 hours if needed up to a maximum of 8 mg per day. A benzodiazepine sometimes worsens delirium or increases agitation.

TABLE 2. **Management of Delirium**

Hospitalization unless mild
Careful monitoring
Consultations: psychiatric, geriatric, neurologic
Physiologic support: adequate hydration, adequate nutrition,
    treatment of underlying illness
Environmental support
Supportive nursing care
Psychotropic drugs: short-acting benzodiazepine, neuroleptic

MOOD (AFFECTIVE) DISORDERS
method of
RUSTIN BERLOW, M.D., and
HAGOP S. AKISKAL, M.D.
University of California, San Diego
La Jolla, California

Mood disorders are characterized by pathologically depressed mood, irritability, or inappropriate elation. These disorders have a lifetime prevalence of 15% (rates being higher in women), with a strong tendency to recur, and they result in considerable morbidity and mortality. The social burden of mood disorders has been estimated to be 43 billion dollars (U.S. data for 1991), comparable to the cost of major physical disorders like hypertension, diabetes, lung disease, and arthritis. Using careful inquiry based on mood pathology, a physician can distinguish between everyday changes in mood and clinical problems that require assessment and treatment. When mood disorders are caused by general medical problems or substance abuse (and withdrawal), this is termed a *secondary* mood disorder; in this case, the therapy will be first directed to the primary disorder. The five subtypes of *primary* mood disorders include bipolar I and II, cyclothymia, dysthymia, and major (unipolar) depression.

Treatment may include psychoeducation and lifestyle changes (sleep hygiene, diet, exercise, and light exposure), other types of counseling or practical psychotherapy, and antidepressant or mood-stabilizing medications. Severe depression and psychotic or suicidal depression (or mania) may require hospitalization, antipsychotic medications, and electroconvulsive therapy (ECT).

Untreated or inadequately treated depression (or mania) often leads to scholastic failure, serious handicaps at work, disruption of relationships, and sometimes to suicide. Proper diagnosis and treatment can lead to prolonged remissions, offering the opportunity for normal functioning. Since depression is prevalent in general medical settings, all physicians must participate in this effort.

SECONDARY MOOD DISORDERS
General Medical Conditions Causing Mood Syndromes

Before the diagnosis of a primary mood disorder can be made, one must rule out underlying medical conditions and substance use. How much should the clinician investigate before declaring the problem a primary mood disorder? How cost-effective would it be to do exhaustive series of laboratory tests on every patient? This depends on the clinical index of suspicion and several patient factors, such as lack of family history of mood disorders, first age of onset above 40 years, and associated symptoms suggestive of medical illness. The most common underlying medical conditions include endocrinologic (especially thyroid disease), neurologic (most often stroke but also multiple sclerosis and other degenerative diseases), and neoplastic (notably lymphatic, gastrointestinal, and gynecologic). Findings on physical examination should be used to confirm the need for laboratory tests, but lack of physical findings does not rule out the presence of an underlying medical condition as the cause of the depression.

Standard laboratory investigation includes (but is not limited to) complete blood count (CBC) (anemia and white cell malignancy), chemistry panel with electrolytes, B_{12} and folate, and protein/albumin (malnutrition), as well as liver function tests (malignancy and hepatitis). Human immunodeficiency virus (HIV) testing should be considered for highly moody or depressed patients with HIV risk factors. Thyroid function tests provide the highest yield because of the high incidence of thyroid problems, especially among women with mood disorders. Drugs commonly used in medicine and psychiatry can also trigger depression in vulnerable individuals (Table 1).

Substance-Induced Mood Disorder

Often patients claim that they drink or use drugs to treat their pain, anxiety, or depression. Mood complaints are such a common part of the natural history of substance use (and withdrawal) that this claim cannot be evaluated until the patient is cautiously withdrawn from alcohol and drugs.

The patient who presents with concurrent substance use and mood problems needs to stop using the drug(s) and tolerate the continued withdrawal depression (and/or anxiety) for at least 30 days before antidepressant or mood-stabilizing therapy is considered. If drugs and alcohol are the primary problem, abstinence alone will eventually lead to reduction of the affective symptoms. Helpful goals to discuss with the patient include the need to get and maintain a high level of motivation, learning to recognize and cope with relapse signs, and rebuilding a life free of substance use. Twelve-step programs are a source of valuable education and support for the motivated substance user. Diagnosis of mood disorder should be considered if, after withdrawal, mood symptoms escalate or persist beyond one month. Family history for mood disorders and past history for unmistakable mood episodes unrelated to drugs or alcohol also point toward the diagnosis of an independent primary mood disorder.

PRIMARY MOOD DISORDERS

Depression

Depression was formerly called "melancholia" (a term now reserved for severe forms), a word derived from Greek, meaning "black bile." The ancient notion implied a chemical etiology that still has not been discovered. Much evidence, however, supports a dysregulation in monoamine (dopamine, norepinephrine, and serotonin) neurotransmitter systems. Limbic neuroendocrine dysfunction is suggested by redistribution of REM sleep to the earlier part of the night, abnormalities in ACTH, dexamethasone and thyrotropin challenge tests, and blunted melatonin response to different lighting conditions. Brain imaging studies have extended the neuroanatomic substrate to include

TABLE 1. Pharmacologic Agents Commonly Precipitating Depression

Progesterone-containing contraceptives
Corticosteroids
Most antihypertensive agents
Amphetamine (and cocaine) withdrawal
Sedative use and alcohol withdrawal
Phenothiazine neuroleptics
Cimetidine
Indomethacin
Thallium; mercury
Cycloserine
Chemotherapeutic agents (e.g., vincristine, vinblastine, amphotericin B, interferon)

TABLE 2. Clinical Manifestations of Depressive Illness

Emotional-Cognitive	Neurovegetative
Depressed mood	Anhedonia (inability to experience pleasure)
Negative ruminations	
Memory impairment	Decreased sex drive
Poor concentration	Middle and late insomnia
Low self-esteem	Appetite loss
Excessive guilt	Slowed or agitated movement
Hopelessness	Fatigue
Helplessness	Feeling worse in the morning (diurnal variation)
Suicidal ideation	

the subcortical and the frontal areas (especially the left frontal lobe). The term "depression" is most relevant to pathology in these areas, which are known to depress activity, drive, and positive emotions. Recurrent forms of the disease are highly familial. Studies of serotonin in the cerebrospinal fluid (CSF) have shown differences, but specific genetic findings have not yet been identified. Clinical manifestations divide into emotional-cognitive and neurovegetative (Table 2), such as guilt, autonomously depressed mood (nothing cheers up the patient), insomnia, anorexia, and agitation. An alternative depressive presentation is *atypical depression*, in which there is hypersomnia, hyperphagia, a feeling of "leaden paralysis," and mood reactivity (good things typically cheer up a patient, and disappointment can make mood instantly worse). Distinguishing everyday sadness from the symptom of depressed mood must be done in the context of the patient's history and family history. For an episode of major depression, the patient must exhibit the signs and symptoms listed in Table 2 (2 to 3 items from each column) sustained for several weeks. It is important to determine whether there is occupational or social impairment and whether the mood problem is very distressing to the patient. Again, pathologic depression involves a mood problem that is persistent, impairing, or troublesome (suicide and psychosis are clearly pathologic).

Anxiety symptoms (such as sweating, palpitations, worrying, groundless fears, obsessions of wrongdoing) often accompany depression and almost always resolve as the depression lifts and generally do not require independent treatment. Psychotic symptoms like hallucinations or delusions need rapid psychiatric evaluation about the need for hospitalization. Likewise, if a patient is having active suicidal thoughts or has attempted suicide, emergency psychiatric consultation is prudent.

Depressive illness, which occurs in about 7% to 8% of the population, typically pursues its course with episodes from which the patient makes full (60%) or partial (30%) recovery; even when chronic (10%), the episode of illness begins at a definite point in time preceded by long periods of freedom from depression.

In what has recently been termed "*dysthymia*," the illness begins insidiously in juvenile years and pursues a low-grade, fluctuating course, without sustained remission; if major depression episodes are superimposed ("double depression"), they resolve quickly, with the patient returning to the dysthymic baseline. These patients are frequent users of the general medical sector, presenting with chronic symptoms of lack of energy, low drive, sleep complaints, inability to function at work or in school, not enjoying life, feeling empty and dissatisfied, not understanding the purpose of existence, and feeling sentenced to life in order to suffer. This list gives a flavor of the type of presenting lifelong complaints that in the past led to misdiagnosis of character neurosis.

Studies of neurophysiology have revealed altered circadian redistribution of REM sleep to the first part of the night, suggesting close links to melancholia. Moreover, family histories are often full of major affective disorder, leading to the conclusion that dysthymia is a variant of primary affective illness (3% of the population). As expected, current pharmacologic trials have elicited responses to antidepressant medication.

Mania

Mania is thought by some to be the opposite of depression. Indeed, mania does exhibit such symptoms as elation (or elevated mood), increased energy (often with decreased need for sleep), and grandiosity. Nearly a third of the episodes of mania, however, are characterized by increased energy but unpleasantly excited (dysphoric) mood. This may be either irritability or anxious or depressed mood and often is a mixture. This mixture with excitement is known as a mixed state, a more recalcitrant form of mania. Mania is often an extremely destructive event in a patient's life, because the patient is typically unaware of being ill. Often the patient is brought in by others for whom the mania is disruptive.

A lack of insight into the problem often delays treatment until well after much damage has been done. Problems usually involve sex (infidelity, promiscuity, or unprotected sex) or money (e.g., wild spending sprees and unwise investments). A decreased need for sleep often precedes the episode by a few days to weeks. Laboratory studies have shown that manic switches are often preceded by decreased REM sleep. Sleep deprivation, antidepressant medications, or stimulant use appear to trigger some manic episodes.

Psychotic symptoms like hallucinations or delusions are relatively common. A patient with mania, especially a first episode, needs rapid psychiatric evaluation for a mood stabilizer, neuroleptics, and often psychiatric hospitalization.

Mania (or dysphoric mania) characteristically pursues a recurrent course, alternating with major depressive episodes (*bipolar I*). This accounts for slightly under 1% of the population and conforms to what classically has been termed "manic-depressive illness." A more prevalent variant of this disease is *bipolar II* (2 to 3%), characterized by major depressions and a milder form of excitement known as hypomania. These typically occur at the tail end of a depression (up to a week or so) and manifest in intense well-being, high energy, confidence; psychotic overactivity, grandiose delusions, and hallucinations are absent. Bipolar II is often seasonal (depression in fall-winter and hypomania in the spring). The disability in bipolar II is due to the repeated episodes of depression; the hypomania itself can be associated with greater goal-directing activity and achievement.

In a third form termed "cyclothymia," subjects alternate between minidepressions of a few days and brief hypomania occurring since adolescence or early adulthood. Though 10% to 20% of the patients are artistically inclined, these individuals nonetheless often suffer from lifelong instability in their love or family life, as well as their vocational life, owing to their unstable and changing mood states. These patients often consult primary care physicians for various complaints like fatigue, insomnia, and complications of substance abuse.

Cyclothymia often coexists with bipolar II. These highly labile patients are particularly prone to experience rapid cycles of depression (more than four per year). Other bipolar II patients without cyclothymia experience one major depression every few years.

TREATMENT OF MOOD (AFFECTIVE) DISORDERS

Psychotherapy

Medications and psychotherapy have been the main treatments for mood disorders. Psychotherapy refers to counseling conducted by a trained psychotherapist (e.g., M.D., Ph.D., social worker with special training, marriage or family therapist). Psychotherapy varies in its effectiveness depending on the method, the therapist, and severity of the disorder. Most therapists use a combination of techniques, or an "eclectic approach." Among the schools of psychotherapy (of which there are many), most fall into the categories of psychodynamic, interpersonal, or cognitive-behavioral. Psychodynamic psychotherapy (freudian and others), which attempts to delve into developmentally based characterologic dispositions to depression, has not been demonstrated to be effective for mood disorders, but the aforementioned two other types of psychotherapy—interpersonal and cognitive-behavioral—have shown in well-controlled studies to be as effective as medication in mild depression.

Interpersonal (ITP) therapy is available in a few select areas and is used extensively as a research tool. It is best considered as a *practical* application of dynamic principles that bypass developmental vicissitudes and instead focus on the current psychological context of depression, such as bereavement, other interpersonal losses, role reversal, and social deficits, all of which prevent an individual from benefiting from environmental contingencies to begin life anew after depression. Providing social support and supportive therapy constitutes an important component of the interpersonal approach.

Cognitive-behavioral therapy (CBT) is offered throughout the country as well as in inexpensive workbooks that a patient can read and benefit from, even in the absence of formal therapy. The emphasis here is on providing hope and encouragement to surmount the barrier of negative thinking and emotion that prevents the depressed individual from engaging in potentially rewarding activities that, in turn, would elevate the individual's sense of self-esteem and overall outlook on life. Most psychiatrists who treat depression successfully utilize the principles of IPT and CBT, even if they do not formally profess to do so. These therapies are often used conjointly with medication in moderate depression (even if the superiority of their *joint* efficacy has not been consistently demonstrated).

These psychotherapeutic principles apply to unipolar patients. Specific psychotherapeutic approaches in more severe depressives (suicidal, agitated, or psychotic) are lacking and must be considered contraindicated (i.e., they often lead to worsening of the depressive condition). Formal psychotherapies are obviously impossible in mania and typically useless in hypomania. These patients, however, do benefit from psychoeducational approaches.

Psychopharmacotherapy

SSRIs (selective serotonin re-uptake inhibitors) are the mainstay of current antidepressant therapy. Fluoxetine (Prozac), sertraline (Zoloft), paroxetine (Paxil), and fluvoxamine (Luvox) are the SSRIs available in the United States. Improvements over previous antidepressants are tolerability (93% to 95% vs. 75% to 80% for tricyclics), which therefore brings better compliance; and safety in overdose.

Antidepressants, especially the SSRIs, are helpful in depressive spectrum disorders, premenstrual accentuation of mood problems, panic disorder, social phobia, obsessive-compulsive disorder (OCD), bulimia, and migraine.

SSRIs are the agents of first choice unless there has been prior failure, unacceptable sexual side effects, or depression. All SSRIs seem to be equally effective. The physician should start with low doses: fluoxetine, 10 mg; sertraline, 25 mg; paroxetine, 10 mg. Double the dose in 4 to 10 days as tolerated. Elderly patients should be kept on the low dose.

Fluoxetine is often activating, is usually taken in the morning, and may be preferable in lethargic (slowed-down) depression. It also has a long half-life, which is an advantage if compliance is uncertain. If someone forgets 2 days of fluoxetine, there will probably be no effect; however, with sertraline or paroxetine, relapse can begin in 2 to 4 days. Agitation and akathisia (a feeling of restlessness and need to move) are sometimes reported. They may be relieved by lowering the dose or switching to another SSRI.

Sertraline is usually neither activating nor sedating. It has few side effects and is generally thought to be "gentler." Side effects may include diarrhea (actually, questioning may reveal only loose stools) and headache.

Paroxetine is sedating and usually taken at bedtime. It thus may have an edge for more anxious patients with panic attacks. Side effects often include nausea and vomiting.

Fluvoxamine is FDA indicated only for obsessive-compulsive disorder, but it is widely used also as an antidepressant. In Europe it has been available and used since 1983. Experience there and multiple well-controlled clinical trials have shown it to be as effective as the tricyclics and other SSRIs. Early studies reported more side effects, but these studies were done with large doses. At lower doses (100 to 150 mg), it appears to have equivalent tolerance and effectiveness to the other agents.

All the SSRIs have sexual side effects (30% of patients); these include decreased libido, decreased genital sensitivity, delayed orgasm, and inability to experience an orgasm (secondary anorgasmia). Lowering the dosage may reduce the sexual problems. In well-stabilized patients, omission of a day's dose may permit adequate sexual activity.

Bupropion (Wellbutrin) is an excellent option if sexual side effects from SSRIs are unacceptable, if there is concurrent attention deficit hyperactivity, or if depression is part of bipolar II. It is believed to be a "dopaminergic" agent and should be avoided if there is a history of psychosis. It is contraindicated in bulimics because of possible seizures. The main side effect is agitation. Available in 75- or 100-mg tablets, bupropion is given in a starting dose of 75 or 100 mg twice or thrice a day, then increased by one tablet to 300 to 450 mg. Single doses should not exceed 225 mg.

Venlafaxine (Effexor) is active at norepinephrine and serotonin receptors. In this respect it is like the tricyclic antidepressants (TCAs), but unlike them, it does not cause the anticholinergic and histaminic side effects of dry mouth, sedation, and orthostatic hypotension. In rare cases (2% to 3%), it may *increase* blood pressure, which should be monitored. Side effects of venlafaxine are common but less so if the dose is started very, very low (one half of a 37.5-mg tablet twice daily). Venlafaxine appears to be more effective in refractory and hospitalized melancholic depressives.

Nefazodone (Serzone) is a trazodone analogue, and trazodone is actually one of nefazodone's metabolites. Like trazodone, it is sedating. However, unlike trazodone, it has not to date been associated with priapism. Like bupropion, nefazodone is a good alternative for patients who can not tolerate SSRIs because of sexual dysfunction.

Tricyclic antidepressants are less used than in the past, due to the risk of overdose and bothersome side effects. The efficacy of these agents is not in doubt, and many physicians still hold the view that they are more robust than the newer medications, especially in severely depressed patients. Desipramine (Norpramin, available in 25- and 50-mg doses; give 25 to 50 mg orally every morning, increase by 25 to 50 mg every 3 days to 200 to 300 mg) and nortriptyline (Pamelor, available in 10- and 25-mg doses; start at 10 to 25 mg and increase by 10 to 25 mg every 3 days to 50 to 150 mg) are preferred for their relatively few side effects and low toxicity.

Insomnia may be caused by any of these agents, but it is usually a manifestation of the depression itself. Encouraging good sleep hygiene is the first step, but addition of a second agent is often helpful. Other antidepressants are often used to facilitate sleep and probably have an additive antidepressant effect. Trazodone (Desyrel) (available as 50- and 100-mg tablets, sig: 50 to 200 mg at bedtime or as needed at bedtime) and amitriptyline (Elavil) (available as 25-, 50-, and 100-mg tablets, sig: 25 to 100 mg at bedtime or as needed at bedtime—do not dispense more than 1000 mg to a patient with suicidal ideation) are commonly used. They can be judiciously combined with activating SSRIs such as fluoxetine. Nonantidepressants are sometimes used with good hypnotic effect, including diphenhydramine (Benadryl) (available at 25 and 50 mg, sig: 25 to 50 mg at bedtime or as needed at bedtime) and zolpidem (Ambien) (10-mg tablets, 5 to 20 mg at bedtime or as needed at bedtime). Except for hospital patients, chloral hydrate is usually avoided due to rapid development of tolerance. Benzodiazepines (diazepam [Valium], alprazolam [Xanax], lorazepam [Ativan], and others) are used infrequently due to (1) disruption of sleep architecture, (2) abuse potential, and (3) risk of further depressing mood.

The relapse rate for SSRIs is high (30%), but patients respond well (quickly and substantially) to a dose increase. Adding a tricyclic antidepressant is an alternative; lithium may be helpful if there is bipolar disease in the family. Switching to a different SSRI is also an option; failure or relapse with one SSRI does not predict poor response to another one. Mood disorder experts often use monoamine oxidase inhibitors (MAOIs) such as phenylzine (Nardil), 45 to 75 mg per day, and tranylcypromine (Parnate), 20 to 40 mg per day, especially for those with atypical or *reverse* neurovegetative signs.

Clinicians using MAOIs must guard against drug and food interactions. The most dangerous are interactions with meperidine (Demerol), antihypertensive agents, TCAs and SSRIs, sympathomimetic amines, and tyramine-containing foods and beverages. Four to five weeks must elapse between an MAOI and use of these agents; otherwise a dangerous hypertensive crisis could occur. If one does, it is best treated with chlorpromazine (Thorazine),* 50 mg orally or intramuscularly, or nifedipine (Procardia), 10 mg sublingually.

Dysthymia is best managed with SSRIs in relatively high doses (e.g., fluoxetine, 20 to 40 mg per day; sertraline, 100 to 150 mg per day; paroxetine, 30 to 50 mg per day). Thyroid augmentation (e.g. levothyroxine [Synthroid], 0.2 mg, and others) is not generally useful in major depression but can benefit 15% to 20% of the dysthymics.

Time Course of Treatment of Depression

Initial Phase. The first 2 to 8 weeks of treatment is when major relief from mood symptoms is expected. Psychoeducation and support are important in this phase to maximize the benefit realized from the medications. Thus, reassurance is needed in the early phase (2 to 4 weeks) when transient side effects (headache, gastrointestinal upset, and sedation) need to be endured. Because benefits have not been seen, pessimism regarding future improvement occurs; side effects can be uncomfortable, and motivation to continue to take the antidepressant may waver. Encouraging the patient to comply is often vital to successful outcome.

Continuation Phase. This is counted from that point in time when significant improvement has been achieved and any residual symptoms have equilibrated. This phase lasts 2 to 6 months and needs to be accompanied by education regarding the illness to facilitate a better adjustment to life stressors. Monthly medication visits help the physician assess any change, the need for dose adjustment, side effects, or manic symptoms.

Taper and Termination. For those with a first episode or infrequent episodes, the antidepressant can be tapered (after 4 to 9 months' maintenance) over a 2- to 4-week period, depending on the dose. Recurrence of some depressive symptoms may occur; if such symptoms persist over two weeks or lead to functional impairment, or if the patient requests it, a return to pharmacotherapy is advised.

For patients with frequent episodes, dysthymia, and double depression, antidepressants are used indefinitely.

The Suicidal Patient

Faced with a depressed patient, the physician must inquire about suicidal intent; this inquiry *does not* precipitate suicide. A neutral question like "Does it seem like life isn't worth living?" is a good entry. If the answer is yes, ask: "Have you been thinking about killing yourself?" Plan and intent are critical issues. If a patient's plan is to take an overdose of pills, it is good to ascertain what is available at home or elsewhere; tricyclic antidepressants like amitriptyline (Elavil) and doxepin (Sinequan) are particularly lethal in overdose. If the patient's plan is by gunshot — is there a gun available? "Do you think you really might do it?" is a good start to explore the topic of intent. If the answer is no, a verbal (or written) contract can be entered into wherein the patient agrees to call or make an emergency appointment if intent develops.

Suicidal ideation must be taken very seriously in any patient, but especially in men, in psychotic patients with command suicidal auditory hallucinations, in elderly retired men living alone who have had personal or financial reverses, in those who have been diagnosed with a terminal illness, and in depressed individuals with substance or alcohol abuse. Hopelessness elicited on the mental status examination is an important predictor of suicide.

Hospitalization

Acutely suicidal patients, psychotic and stuporous depressives, and those with physical debilitation or serious concurrent medical disease should be managed on an inpatient unit. Electroconvulsive therapy (ECT) should also be preferably administered on an inpatient basis and is generally the most effective treatment for all such depressives, with rapid (within 1 to 2 weeks) remission in over 90%. ECT can be unilateral or bilateral; there is less memory loss and less effectiveness if unilateral. There is no evidence that ECT per se causes permanent brain damage. The mortality rate with ECT is one per 3500 courses—infinitely less than that of severe depression. ECT is contraindicated in patients with increased intracranial pressure or fractures and in those who cannot receive the medications necessary for its safe administration. ECT is the treatment of choice for psychotic depression and depression refractory to medication.

---

*Not FDA-approved for this indication.

The antipsychotic medications usually do not work immediately but require a period of 2 days to a few weeks. The neuroleptics thioridazine (Mellaril), 50 to 200 mg per day, or thiothixene (Navane), 2 to 10 mg per day, are commonly used, often combined with one of the tricyclic antidepressant drugs given slightly under standard dosages. In view of the risk for tardive dyskinesia, it is preferable either to use the neuroleptic in the lower-dose range or to resort to monotherapy with a higher dose of the antidepressant as soon as possible.

Treatment of Bipolar Spectrum Disorders

Mania is usually treated by psychiatrists because of the need for hospitalization and the necessity for intensive and expert pharmacotherapy. Because of this and other complexities, bipolar illness, especially if severe, is best treated by psychiatrists. However, because the illness interfaces with other medical diseases, all physicians must have a working knowledge of the complex pharmacology of bipolar spectrum conditions.

Mood Stabilizers (Thymoleptics)

Lithium Therapy. Lithium has been used widely for bipolar disorder. It is effective in the acute manic episode and also in preventing recurrence. Because considerable medical and pharmacologic sophistication is required in the safe and competent use of this salt (especially in the presence of concurrent medical conditions), all physicians must be familiar with certain aspects of lithium therapy even if they are not primarily involved in treating patients with mood disorder.

LABORATORY EVALUATION. In young, physically healthy subjects, preparation for lithium therapy should include medical history, system review, physical examination including weight, and laboratory studies including CBC, urinalysis, serum creatinine, electrolytes, and thyroid-stimulating hormone (TSH). In the presence of cardiac disease, a baseline electrocardiogram (ECG) should be obtained, and an electroencephalogram (EEG) should be performed if brain disease is suspected. If there is a history of renal disease, thorough evaluation of baseline kidney function (especially creatinine clearance, 24-hour urine volume, and urine concentration test) is mandatory.

Although mania is thought of as a manifestation of bipolar illness, the physician must first consider two possibilities: (1) substance abuse (notably stimulants like cocaine or amphetamines), and (2) medical-neurologic conditions as listed in Table 3. Given rigorous clinical indications for lithium therapy, concurrent medical diseases do not necessarily contraindicate its use; however, slow dosage build-up should preferably be initiated during a relatively stable phase of the medical disease; greater medical vigilance is advised, including lower initial dose of lithium (e.g., 150 to 300 mg per day) and frequent determination of blood levels that should be kept at the

TABLE 3. **Common Causes of Symptomatic Manias**

Pharmacologic	Corticosteroids
	Levodopa, bromocriptine, cocaine, amphetamines, methylphenidate (Ritalin)
	Most antidepressants
Infectious	General paresis (tertiary syphilis)
	Influenza
	St. Louis encephalitis
	AIDS/HIV disease
Endocrine	Hyperthyroidism
Collagen-vascular	Systemic lupus erythematosus
	Rheumatic chorea
Neurologic	Multiple sclerosis
	Huntington's chorea
	Head trauma
	Complex partial seizures (temporal lobe)
	Diencephalic tumors
	Stroke (esp. right frontal)

lower range (0.3 to 0.7 mEq per liter). The same remarks generally apply to geriatric patients. While lower levels are less associated with side effects, they have also been shown to be less likely to prevent manic episodes.

Lithium is rapidly and completely absorbed from the gastrointestinal tract and peaks in the serum in about 1.5 to 4.5 hours, depending on whether standard (Lithobid or Eskalith, 300 mg) or slow-release forms (Eskalith CR, 450 mg) are used. Its half-life varies from 24 to 36 hours; steady state is reached in about 4 days. Lithium is not protein-bound and is excreted through the kidneys. Acutely ill patients with bipolar disorder have a high tolerance for lithium and retain it during the first 10 days, while excreting sodium; a regular diet is recommended. Postpubertal patients with bipolar disorder who have excellent glomerular function require higher doses to achieve the same level of serum equilibrium. In healthy subjects who achieve good episode prevention, serum (12 hours after the last dose) and serum creatinine levels every 3 months are generally sufficient; thyroid indices must be obtained at least once a year.

MANIC AND MIXED PHASES. Despite impending, or actual, social catastrophes resulting from their poor judgment, hypomanic and manic patients have a remarkable capacity to convince physicians and attorneys that they are not ill. It is therefore crucial that the physician stay firm in the decision to obtain hospital admission for acutely ill manic patients.

After lithium work-up, lithium carbonate is started at 300 mg orally twice daily, and the dosage is increased over a 7- to 10-day period until a serum level of 0.8 to 1.2 mEq per liter is reached; some patients require levels as high as 1.5 mEq per liter before a response is seen. In patients who refuse to take pills, lithium citrate syrup (Cibalith-S), 5 to 10 mL (8 to 16 mEq of lithium) three times daily, can be administered mixed with a juice. Because of the 4- to 15-day latency before the onset of action, especially in those with precarious fluid balance, it may be necessary to start a treatment with an intramuscular neuroleptic, such as trifluoperazine (Stelazine), thiothixene (Navane), or haloperidol (Haldol), 5 to 10 mg two to three times daily, until the psychotic frenzy is under control; intramuscular lorazepam (Ativan), 1 to 2 mg two to four times daily, can be used synergistically, and often reduces the need for large neuroleptic doses. Lithium can be added once the psychotic acceleration is brought under control. In view of rare reports of neurotoxicity with a neuroleptic-lithium combination, it is desirable to discontinue the neuroleptic as soon as behavioral control of the mania is achieved.

Lithium therapy for a first manic episode should be continued for about 6 months. This also generally applies to mania precipitated by drugs (e.g., exogenous steroids) or by medical disease (e.g., systemic lupus erythematosus) when removal of the offending chemical or adequate medical control, respectively, often fails to bring remission of the manic state.

Control of the sleep-wake cycle can be very helpful in re-establishing a normal mood. The acutely manic patient may feel rested with as little as 1 to 4 hours of sleep. Inducing more sleep can accelerate the return to baseline. This can be done with neuroleptics (such as chlorpromazine, 50 to 500 mg, or thioridazine, 25 to 250 mg), benzodiazepines (clonazepam [Klonopin], 1 to 4 mg at bedtime), or other agents such as zolpidem (Ambien), 5 to 10 mg at bedtime.

Depression complicated by psychosis usually requires a mid- to high-potency neuroleptic (perfenazine, 4 to 12 mg per day, or thiothixene, 5 to 20 mg per day), and it should be tapered quickly when the psychotic symptoms begin to resolve. The same is generally true for mixed states. Agitated depression in the bipolar patient is a mixed state until proved otherwise. Irritability, anger, and decreased sleep are often misinterpreted as a depressed phase and inappropriately treated with antidepressants that may paradoxically make the patient worse (feel "revved" up, nervous, restless); this may be also mistaken for akathisia (especially in neuroleptic-treated patients) or anxiety (it is important to ask about specific anxiety symptoms to differentiate the two, since anxiety is common in bipolar episodes).

Carbamazepine (Tegretol). Carbamazepine's activity in bipolar patients is broader than that of lithium, since it is more effective in mixed, rapid cycling, and fulminant psychotic forms of mania. These usages, although supported by clinical studies in many countries, have not been subjected to the FDA approval process. Dosing usually starts at 200 mg twice daily and increases, with serum levels checked every week, until stable (maximum, 12 µg per mL), then every four weeks and thereafter every 3 to 6 months. This close monitoring is because carbamazepine induces its own hepatic metabolism, which may lead to recurrence of symptoms due to decreased blood levels.

Common side effects include sedation, GI upset, dizziness, depressed mood, blurred vision, headaches, rash, and increased white count on the CBC. A rare complication is aplastic anemia, which occurs in fewer than 1 in 10,000 cases. For this reason, CBC should be ordered at baseline and every time a carbamazepine blood level is drawn. Also, the patient should be instructed to report any fever, cough, sore throat, or symptom of infection. Elevated liver function tests have been seen, but whether this is clinically relevant is unclear. Many who use this compound also obtain baseline liver function tests and repeat them in 1, 3, 6, and 12 months.

Valproate. In its divalproex form (Depakote), this anticonvulsant is the second FDA-approved agent for mania. It offers several advantages over lithium (and carbamazepine), being safer in overdose, and less blunting to the bipolar temperament. Like carbamazepine, valproate appears effective for a broad spectrum of bipolar presentations, especially mixed states and rapid cycling (including unstable bipolar II patients).

The starting dose is usually 250 mg two or three times daily, increased to a total of 1 to 2 grams per day in divided doses. Blood levels may be monitored, with a maximum of 120 µg per mL, until improvement is achieved or until side effects warrant a reduction. Some clinicians start with a loading dose of 2 grams per day over 3 to 5 days until high levels are obtained; this is reported to hasten the antimanic response time and potentially reduce hospital stay.

Although valproic acid is often substituted as the generic form and appears to be effective as well, it has a significantly higher incidence of gastric upset and discontinuation due to side effects. When cost is a major consideration, we try valproic acid and then, if needed, switch to the better-tolerated divalproex (Depakote).

Aside from gastric complaints from the "generic" form, other side effects common to both include sedation, benign tremor, transient hair loss, and vivid dreaming. Acute pancreatitis is rare, and reversible thrombocytopenia is seen at higher doses. Elevations in liver function tests (LFTs) are not uncommon, and some clinicians monitor baseline and repeat LFTs (see Carbamazepine); whether this is needed is unproved. Deaths due to hepatotoxicity have been reported *in children*, at very high doses, and with concomitant medications, casting doubt on the possibility of a causal relationship.

Overall, valproic acid and especially divalproex are a major advance in the pharmacotherapy of bipolar disorder (Table 4).

Combination Therapy. If one agent is not benefiting the patient, another is usually tried (previously lithium first, then divalproex, but recently divalproex as first-line). If neither is adequate to reduce symptoms to a safe level, another is added. Usually the second is not used in high doses nor are blood levels needed since the dose is low (lithium, 300 to 600 mg per day, or valproic acid, 500 to 750 mg per day).

The combination of two mood stabilizers is also used to avoid the need for high doses. It is believed by some that low levels of two agents may be safer and better tolerated than high doses of one. The effectiveness of this has not been proved in well-

TABLE 4. **Clinical Pharmacology of Mood Stabilizers**

	Dose	Blood Level	LD$_{50}$	Clinical Spectrum of Effectiveness
Lithium	300 mg bid to 2400 mg/d	0.5–1.2 mEq/L	low	narrow
Carbamazepine (Tegretol)	200 mg bid to 1200 mg/d	4–12 µg/mL	low	broad
Valproic acid (divalproex)	250 mg bid to 2000 mg/d	50–120 µg/mL	high	broad

controlled trials, but we have seen it work well in many cases. The atypical neuroleptic clozapine (Clozaril, 25 to 200 mg) has been used in refractory manic, mixed, or cycling forms. In view of the risk for agranulocytosis, we recommend that such use be limited to experienced clinical psychopharmacologists. Bipolar patients refractory to all pharmacotherapy often respond to ECT.

Treatment of Depression in Bipolar Patients

Depression in bipolar disorder can be extraordinarily severe and very refractory to treatment, which is a source of frustration for the clinician as well as the patient. A dearth of carefully performed studies has left a void in our knowledge on this topic. We do know that ECT may be particularly useful and that use of antidepressant medication often helps. The mood stabilizer—especially lithium—should be maintained, and the patient should be cautioned not to discontinue it.

Different antidepressants have been reported to have different characteristics. Tricyclics have been reported to cause an increase in the rate of bipolar cycles, from perhaps once every 1 to 2 years to a more frequent rate of 4 to 8 times per year ("rapid cycling"). This is particularly true for female bipolar II patients, who are prone to rapid cycling. SSRIs such as fluoxetine, sertraline, and especially paroxetine may be effective but in fewer patients and to a lesser extent than in unipolar depressives. Bupropion has been reported to have a more stabilizing effect and be less likely to switch a patient into excitement.

What to do? The best thing is to avoid antidepressants in milder bipolar episodes. Severe episodes require neuroleptics and/or ECT. Moderate depressive episodes might preferably be treated with bupropion, paroxetine, or the MAOI tranylcypromine (Parnate) in relatively small doses and for no more than a few weeks—and always in conjunction with a mood stabilizer. Thyroid augmentation is often helpful in bipolar II female patients. Lamotrigine (Lamictal) is being used experimentally in refractory bipolar depressives, again to be entrusted to the hands of sophisticated psychopharmacological clinicians.

Intense, well-focused, goal-directed behavior is often observed in bipolar II, but some patients are quite distractible and this, coupled with their restless behavior, may be mislabeled as attention deficit disorder without regard to their childhood course or functioning between acute phases during "normal" periods. Treatment with stimulants, ironically, may be effective since stimulants tend to regularize or "entrain" the sleep-wake cycle. The danger of making bipolar disorder worse or producing psychosis with stimulants militates against this use and reinforces the importance of proper diagnosis. In bipolar patients with a credible childhood history of ADHD, bupropion (Wellbutrin) with a mood stabilizer (e.g., divalproex) is often preferable.

SCHIZOPHRENIA

method of
HERBERT Y. MELTZER, M.D.
Vanderbilt University School of Medicine
Nashville, Tennessee

and

S. HOSSEIN FATEMI, M.D., PH.D.
University of Minnesota School of Medicine
Minneapolis, Minnesota

Schizophrenia is a brain disease of unknown etiology that afflicts 1% of the adult population. It is generally accepted that schizophrenia is a syndrome rather than a single disease. From a historical perspective, Emil Kraepelin, in 1896, first identified an early onset and deteriorating lifelong form of psychosis, which he called dementia praecox to distinguish it from a remitting-relapsing psychosis, of manic-depressive illness. Eugen Bleuler, in 1911, considered disorganization of thought processes and loss of normal affect as the central concept and suggested that disturbances in four primary areas were central to the disease process which he labeled schizophrenia: loose associations, flat affect, autism, and ambivalence. Recently, the cognitive disturbance of schizophrenia has again been emphasized as the critical factor in the etiology, course, and response to treatment.

EPIDEMIOLOGY

The onset of schizophrenia is gender dependent: between 15 and 25 years for males and 21 and 26 years for females. The prevalence of the disease does not vary across ethnic groups but may be higher in lower socioeconomic classes. The mortality rate from natural causes is approximately twice as high in schizophrenics compared with the general population. The suicide rate in schizophrenia is 9% to 13%.

ETIOLOGY

There is increasing evidence that schizophrenia is a neurodevelopmental disorder and that the vulnerability to schizophrenia may begin during brain development in utero. Perinatal complications may also contribute to its etiology. Postmortem neuropathologic studies have demonstrated abnormalities in various cortical areas as well as the hippocampus, some of which are thought to have arisen during the second trimester of development. However, the frequency of these changes, their specificity for schizophrenia, as well as their behavioral consequences, if any, are unknown. Neuroimaging studies have demonstrated large ventricles and increased prefrontal cortical prominence, indicating loss of cortical mass. Magnetic resonance imaging (MRI) studies have provided evidence for decreased size of the thalamus as well.

There is substantial evidence for a genetic contribution to schizophrenia. The concordance rate for dizygotic and monozygotic twins is 13% and 55%, respectively, indicating that the heritability of schizophrenia is approximately 90%. There is no evidence to support a single major gene in schizophrenia. Rather, a complex group of genetic factors may be involved, including some genes that include multiple trinucleotide repeats.

COURSE OF ILLNESS

The appearance of psychotic symptoms is usually preceded by a period of behavioral and cognitive changes lasting from weeks to several years. This is generally referred to as the prodrome. One or more of the following changes may be noted during this period: increased withdrawal, anxiety, aggression, personality changes, loss of interest in sex, depression, decreased ability to concentrate, diminished school performance, magical thinking, and so on. However, some patients have a rather dramatic appearance of delusions and hallucinations over a period of a few weeks. This is generally in individuals who are experiencing some major environmental stress. Prognosis is better in patients with a rapid onset of florid psychotic symptoms compared with those individuals who have a more insidious onset and have more negative rather than positive or disorganization symptoms in the initial stages of the illness.

In most patients, the initial positive symptoms respond to treatment, as will be discussed. However, negative symptoms and cognitive dysfunction may be prominent even at the very early stages of the illness. Social and work function are seriously compromised in most patients. A recent survey of intermediate long-term outcome (3 or more years) in schizophrenia indicated that only 30% to 40% of patients with schizophrenia treated with conventional antipsychotic agents have a good outcome as indicated by no or mild positive symptoms and work or social function within the normal range. This percentage has been only slightly increased since the introduction of typical antipsychotic drugs.

COST OF ILLNESS

Schizophrenia is one of the most costly illnesses in the world because of its high prevalence and because it begins at an early age, devastates the patient's ability to support himself or herself, does not have an extremely high mortality rate, and engenders high-cost interventions such as hospitalization, emergency room visits, and in some societies, a high incidence of incarceration. The latter is usually for minor crimes such as vagrancy or substance abuse rather than violent crimes, although most definitely incidents of violence are committed by patients with this illness.

In the United States, a 1990 survey of schizophrenia identified indirect and direct costs of approximately 20 billion dollars each. Direct costs are mainly due to hospital-

ization and nursing home costs (80%), outpatient and rehabilitation costs (17%), and drug costs (3%). The cost of drug treatment has increased slightly as a percentage of the total as new, meritorious patented drugs have been widely introduced and the availability of hospitalization has decreased. On the other hand, outpatient costs, especially for community housing and support services, have also increased. Indirect costs are due to loss of earned income and Social Security disability payments.

TREATMENT OF SCHIZOPHRENIA

Following a presumptive diagnosis of schizophrenia and exclusion of various medical, neurologic, and drug/substance-induced psychoses, a patient should be started on antipsychotic medication either in a hospital setting or on an outpatient basis, depending on the nature of the symptomatology as well as many other considerations. Antipsychotic medications are generally classified as either "typical" or "atypical." Atypical antipsychotic agents are so called because they produce fewer extrapyramidal symptoms (EPS) than the typical antipsychotic drugs but have equal or possibly greater efficacy to treat either positive, negative, or disorganization symptoms, or some combination thereof. Whereas the typical neuroleptic drugs have almost invariably been found to have equal efficacy but qualitatively different side effect profiles other than EPS, the atypical antipsychotic drugs appear to differ significantly in both efficacy and side effect profiles.

The prototypical atypical antipsychotic drug is clozapine (Clozaril), about which the most is known, since it has been in clinical use since 1969. Risperidone (Risperdal) is the only other atypical antipsychotic drug that is currently approved for use in the United States and many other countries. Whereas clozapine does not produce significant EPS in any patient and is even well tolerated by patients with Parkinson's disease, risperidone, although superior to typical neuroleptic drugs with regard to causing EPS, produces dose-dependent EPS and has been reported to produce severe motor impairment in some but not all patients with Parkinson's disease.

Three other atypical antipsychotic agents are likely to be approved for use in the United States in 1996 or early 1997. These are quietepine (Seroquel),* olanzapine,* and sertindole.* At clinically effective doses, these drugs produce fewer EPS than do the typical neuroleptic drugs but, as is the case with risperidone, they do cause EPS in some patients. There are virtually no data comparing these agents with each other, with risperidone, or with clozapine. Therefore, it is hazardous at this point to conclude which of these agents is closest to clozapine with regard to freedom from EPS. This will be discussed in more detail subsequently.

The important point is that there are significant differences between the atypical antipsychotics with regard to EPS, other side effects, and probably efficacy as well. Therefore, clinicians will generally find

---

*Not yet approved for use in the United States.

it useful to become familiar with all these agents as they are approved and enter the clinic.

Typical Neuroleptics

The standard drug treatment for schizophrenia has, until recently, been the typical neuroleptic drugs. They are believed to act by antagonism of dopamine D_2 receptors. These agents are effective in reducing positive symptoms and disorganization in about 60% to 90% of schizophrenic patients, with the response rate diminishing over time as some patients become refractory to them. These drugs do not markedly influence negative symptoms. Indeed, they may cause the so-called secondary negative symptoms, i.e., withdrawal and anergia, that may be secondary to EPS. They have little efficacy in reducing the cognitive impairment present in schizophrenia, which includes deficits in attention, executive function, working, and semantic and storage memory. Indeed, some of the more anticholinergic of these agents, such as thioridazine and chlorpromazine, have sometimes been reported to worsen memory impairment. All typical neuroleptics also cause tardive dyskinesia. Numerous studies show that patients are frequently noncompliant with these agents. About 50% of patients will discontinue treatment with these agents within six months of discharge from hospital unless family members, case managers, and community treatment teams make a major effort to keep patients in treatment.

These agents are generally given orally in the United States and must be taken indefinitely by most patients to prevent relapse. A recent meta-analysis of neuroleptic withdrawal studies indicated that 50% of patients will relapse within six months after withdrawal. However, many patients will relapse within days to weeks if medication is removed. This is partially a function of how recently they have experienced an acute psychotic episode. Long-acting parenteral forms of haloperidol (Haldol), 25 to 200 mg, and fluphenazine (Prolixin), 12.5 to 50 mg, are available. These provide effective control of positive symptoms for 2 to 4 weeks in most patients, depending on the dose and individual responsivity. Compliance is better with this route of administration, especially if the drug is given by visiting nurses or in special clinics with an active outreach program to remind patients of their next visit.

Most of these agents are available in generic form so that the cost may be $25 to $50 per month. The long-acting injectable forms may cost as much as $100 per month, not counting the costs of the clinic or home visit. The new antipsychotic drugs, which are not available in generic form, are much more expensive. Since cost-effectiveness data for these agents are limited, the use of the typical neuroleptic drugs remains by far the most frequent form of treatment, but there is increasing evidence to support a much greater use of the atypical antipsychotic drugs as first-line treatment as well as for all cases of neuroleptic-resistant or -intolerant patients.

Table 1 provides a list of the major classes of antipsychotic drugs and specific examples of each type. The typical neuroleptic drugs are classified as low, medium, or high potency, depending on dose range. There is an inverse relationship between potency and frequency of EPS.

Table 2 lists the new generation of atypical agents, and Table 3 presents other concepts of antipsychotic agents.

TABLE 1. **Classes of Antipsychotic Agents**

Class		Potency	Daily Dose Range (mg)	Chlorpromazine Equivalent	EPS	Anticholinergic Side Effects
I	**Phenothiazines**					
	Chlorpromazine (Thorazine)	low	200–1200	100	low	↓ /high
	Fluphenazine (Prolixin)	high	1–20	2	high	low
	Fluphenazine decanoate	high	12.5–50 q 1–4 weeks, IM	—	high	low
	Perphenazine (Trilafon)	medium	8–32	10	high	medium
	Thioridazine (Mellaril)	low	200–700	100	low	high
	Trifluoperazine (Stelazine)	high	6–20	5	↓ /high	low
II	**Butyrophenone**					
	Haloperidol (Haldol)	high	5–20	2	high	low
	Haloperidol decanoate	high	25–200 q 4 weeks, IM	25	medium	low
III	**Dibenzodiazepine**					
	Clozapine (Clozaril)	low	200–900	75	absent	↑ /high
IV	**Dibenzoxapine**					
	Loxapine (Loxitane)	medium	40–100	10	↑ /medium	medium
V	**Indole**					
	Molindone (Moban)	medium	50–225	10	↑ /medium	medium
VI	**Diphenylbutylpiperidine**					
	Pimozide (Orap)	high	1–10	1	high	↑ /medium
VII	**Thioxanthene**					
	Thiothixene (Navane)	high	6–30	5	high	low
VIII	**Benzisoxazole**					
	Risperidone (Risperdal)	low	2–10	0.6–1	low	low

TABLE 2. **New Generation of Atypical Antipsychotic Agents****

5-HT₂/D₂ Antagonists	Selective D₂ Agonists
Iloperidone	Amisulpride
Melperone	Sulpride
Olanzapine	
Quietepine (Seroquel)	
Sertindole	
Ziprasidone	
Zotepine	

*Not available in the United States.

For acute oral treatment, the most commonly used antipsychotic drugs in the United States are haloperidol in doses of 5 to 20 mg per day, fluphenazine, 5 to 15 mg per day, thioridazine (Mellaril), 200 to 700 mg per day, and perphenazine (Trilafon), 16 to 48 mg per day. Numerous studies indicate that the lower doses are as effective as the higher doses in most patients and are better tolerated. Generally 1 to 6 weeks of treatment are required to ascertain whether patients will respond to these agents; during that time it is important to keep the dose low to minimize EPS. A frequent clinical error is to keep raising the dose during this period rather than allowing adequate time for the medication to take effect. However, if there is severe agitation, sleeplessness, excitability, aggression toward staff or others, it is reasonable to increase the dose in small increments and then reduce it later as the indication for the higher dose subsides. For pharmacokinetic as well as pharmacodynamic reasons, there will always be some patients who require more medication than others. Short-acting parenteral forms of haloperidol and chlorpromazine are often used to achieve rapid control of highly agitated or violent patients. There is no evidence that so called rapid tranquilization, in which frequent intramuscular injections of these agents are given, achieves more effective control than oral medication.

Lower doses of the neuroleptic agents have been shown to occupy striatal D₂ dopamine receptors fully. Presumably, the same is the case for mesolimbic dopamine receptors, the likely site of their antipsychotic action. Therefore, higher doses of these agents are unlikely to be more effective. If higher doses are used during the acute phase, these can generally be decreased toward the 5 to 10 mg per day haloperidol equivalent dose during maintenance treatment. If signs of impending relapse appear, the dose should again be raised. Monitoring plasma levels of these agents is not generally recommended.

TABLE 3. **Other Concepts of Antipsychotic Agents**

D₃ agonists or antagonists
D₄ antagonists
D₂ partial agonists
Selective 5-HT₂A antagonists
Glutamate receptor–stimulating agents (D-cycloserine, glycine)

Because all these agents produce EPS, it is generally useful to administer an antiparkinsonian agent when significant EPS emerge. Some clinicians prefer to use antiparkinsonian drugs prophylactically, but that will result in some patients receiving them unnecessarily. Anticholinergics such as trihexyphenidyl (Artane), biperiden (Akineton), procyclidine (Kemadrin), and benztropine (Cogentin) are the most commonly used agents, but amantadine and antihistaminic agents such as diphenhydramine are sometimes employed. Continued use of antiparkinsonian agents throughout the maintenance period is often unnecessary. Akathisia, a syndrome characterized by agitation and restlessness, is a form of EPS that responds better to beta-adrenergic receptor antagonists such as propranolol or pindolol.

Neuroleptic malignant syndrome is a rare side effect of these agents. It is characterized by muscular rigidity, fever, autonomic instability and increased serum creatine kinase activity. Discontinuation of the neuroleptic and treatment with muscle relaxants and dopaminomimetic agents is necessary to prevent a sometimes fatal outcome. A switch to risperidone or possibly clozapine may be indicated after recovery from the neuroleptic malignant episode.

Maintenance treatment with an antipsychotic drug is generally necessary for all schizophrenic patients. It may be possible for patients who have had only one or two psychotic episodes to discontinue neuroleptic drugs for an extended period of time before another acute episode recurs.

Signs of emergent tardive dyskinesia (TD) should be watched for during the maintenance period. Usually these are mild and will be reversible if the agents are stopped. However, this may not be feasible because of the severity of psychosis. Should TD symptoms be moderate to severe, substitution of clozapine or possibly risperidone for the typical neuroleptic drug would be the treatment of choice. Increasing the dose of neuroleptic would ordinarily suppress most of the symptoms of TD, but this is not the recommended approach because of the possibility of causing greater TD.

Risperidone (Risperdal)

Risperidone has been found in multicenter trials with schizophrenic inpatients to be more effective than haloperidol in decreasing total psychopathology and positive and negative symptoms, although usually at some intermediate doses only, e.g., 6 mg per day. In this dose range, it also produced fewer EPS, and patients required fewer antiparkinsonian agents. Higher doses produced significant EPS and less effect on psychopathology, possibly due to excessive dopamine receptor blockade. Risperidone has a greater affinity for serotonin (5-HT)₂A than D₂ dopamine receptors and at lower doses would be expected to leave a significant proportion of D₂ receptors free to respond to dopamine. There is no evidence yet that risperidone is effective in a significant proportion of patients who fail to have an adequate response to typical neuroleptic drugs. Similarly, there is no evidence that risperidone can improve cognitive function. The potential for risperidone to cause TD is not yet established. It is possible that chronic administration of low doses of risperidone would have some advantage over typical neuroleptic drugs in this regard.

There are, as yet, no cost-effective studies of risperidone that would determine whether the advantages noted in clinical trials are present in clinical practice and justify the increased cost. A year's supply of risperidone may cost between $2500 and $4000, depending on the dose. The difference between this and the cost of a generic neuroleptic may be easily offset by smaller hospitalization or crisis intervention costs. It is also unclear whether risperidone reduces the indirect costs of schizophrenia, including family burden. There is no evidence yet that the lower EPS potential of risperidone will lead to greater compliance, but this seems like a realistic possibility. Risperidone would definitely be a reasonable choice for patients who respond to typical neuroleptics with a reduction in positive symptoms but who have troublesome EPS and secondary negative symptoms. There is also some evidence that risperidone is effective in suppressing the symptoms of established TD. Side effects of risperidone other than EPS include akathisia, weight gain, sexual dysfunction, decreased libido, and galactorrhea. Unlike clozapine, risperidone increases serum prolactin levels. There is no evidence that risperidone has any increased risk of causing agranulocytosis.

Clozapine (Clozaril)

Clozapine is the only antipsychotic drug that has been shown in controlled clinical trials to be effective in reducing positive and negative symptoms in patients who fail to respond to typical neuroleptic drugs. It also produces almost no EPS, including akathisia. It has been used in several hundred thousand patients in Western countries for periods as long as 17 years with no definite cases of TD being reported. These remarkable advantages, and others to be described, must be considered in light of its ability to cause granulocytopenia or agranulocytosis in 1% of patients. This has led to clozapine being approved in the United States only for patients with schizophrenia who have failed to respond adequately to typical neuroleptic drugs or who are intolerant of typical neuroleptic drugs because of EPS or TD. Just what is an adequate response to an antipsychotic agent should be left to the judgment of the patient, the family, and mental health workers. Poor work function and residual negative symptoms may be considered a poor response, even if mild positive symptoms are present.

Agranulocytosis during clozapine treatment generally occurs within 4 to 18 weeks after initiating treatment but can occur rarely at later times. Weekly monitoring of white cell counts is required in the United States on an indefinite basis. When the white cell count falls below 3000 mm^3, clozapine should be stopped and not restarted. If agranulocytosis has

developed, granulocyte colony–stimulating factor or some other growth factors can be used to hasten the recovery process. Hospitalization to prevent or treat sepsis is essential. To date, the death rate from clozapine due to agranulocytosis has been about 1 per 10,000 patients. Clozapine can also cause leukocytosis and eosinophilia in the early stages. Other side effects of clozapine include sedation, weight gain, major motor seizures, treatment-emergent obsessive-compulsive disorder, hypersalivation, tachycardia, hypotension, hypertension, stuttering, neuroleptic-malignant syndrome, urinary incontinence, constipation, and hyperglycemia. These side effects can generally be managed by dose reduction.

The dose of clozapine ranges from 200 to 900 mg per day for most patients. It must be titrated slowly with a starting dose of 25 mg per day. The average dose is 400 to 500 mg per day. Plasma levels of 350 to 400 ng per mL are more likely to be associated with clinical response than lower levels.

Clozapine has been shown to be effective in reducing depression and suicidal ideation. The latter effect leads to a major decrease in overall mortality despite the slight increase due to agranulocytosis. Four studies have reported that clozapine can improve some aspects of cognitive function, especially verbal fluency, attention, and recall memory. This appears to be unrelated to its lack of effect on motor function. Several cost-effectiveness studies have indicated that the cost of clozapine ($3000 to $5000 per year plus monitoring costs) is offset by decreased need for hospitalization. Clozapine has also been shown to improve work function and quality of life, which leads to the conclusion that a premium price is justified for some patients.

Olanzapine,* Sertindole,* and Quietepine*

These three agents could be approved for use in the United States during 1996 or 1997. Like risperidone and clozapine, they are potent 5-HT$_{2A}$ and relatively weaker D$_2$ antagonists, although it is by no means certain that this is the major reason that these agents produce fewer EPS than typical neuroleptic drugs. Their affinities vary for other types of dopamine, serotonin, acetylcholine, and noradrenergic receptors. Some combination of these actions may contribute to their atypical properties and should lead to significant differences among them. All three drugs appear to produce fewer EPS than typical neuroleptic drugs. Head-to-head comparisons of multiple doses of these agents with each other and risperidone will be needed truly to compare these agents. Cost-effectiveness studies will also be needed to determine whether these agents justify premium prices. Based upon the clinical trials reported to date, this is a real possibility. It is likely that decreased negative symptoms and EPS, improvement in quality of life, work capacity, and decreased indirect costs including family burden will be significant in this regard. Olanzapine appears to be effective on a once-a-day sched-

---

*Not available in the United States.

ule (dose of 10 or 15 mg per day), whereas quietepine may require twice- or three-times-a-day administration. No parenteral form for any of these agents is available at this time. None of the three agents increases serum prolactin levels. Head-to-head comparisons among these drugs, clozapine, risperidone, and typical neuroleptics are urgently needed.

Psychosocial Treatment

In addition to drug treatment, patients with schizophrenia frequently benefit from group therapy, social skills training, activity therapy, vocational support, and family support. The defect in cognition and social function characteristic of this illness is only partially ameliorated by drug treatment alone, even the novel agents. These psychosocial treatments can frequently make the difference in the quality of life and compliance with treatment that leads to less hospitalization and less long-term impairment.

The research reported was supported in part by USPHS MH 41684, GCRC MO1RR00080 and the National Alliance for Research on Schizophrenia and Depression (NARSAD), as well as grants from the Elisabeth Severance Prentiss and John Pascal Sawyer Foundations and Stanley Foundation. H.Y.M. is the recipient of USPHS Research Career Scientist Award MH 47808. The secretarial assistance of Ms. Lee Mason is greatly appreciated.

PANIC DISORDER

method of
SCOTT W. WOODS, M.D., and
ANDREW W. GODDARD, M.D.
Yale University School of Medicine
New Haven, Connecticut

Panic disorder is a common psychiatric condition which when untreated usually runs a chronic course, often with considerable attendant disability. Current treatments are quite effective. The illness has previously been described under a number of historical synonyms, including agoraphobia with panic attacks, anxiety neurosis, hyperventilation syndrome, cardiac neurosis, and neurasthenia. The key pathologic feature is the presence of recurrent panic attacks. Panic attacks, sometimes called anxiety attacks, are characterized by a sudden surge of intense anxiety or fear accompanied by a variety of physical sensations, lasting typically less than 30 minutes. The physical sensations can suggest the possibility of pathology in nearly any body system. Common physical symptoms include palpitations, chest pain, dyspnea, dizziness, flushing, sweating, and abdominal cramping. Severe attacks are quite disturbing, comparing roughly in the distress they produce to the passage of a kidney stone in patients who have experienced both. The patient is frequently motivated to seek medical consultation, often in the emergency setting, generally with the fear that the attack symptoms reflect a life-threatening illness such as myocardial infarction, cardiac arrhythmia, pulmonary embolus, or stroke.

Epidemiology studies typically find panic disorder prevalence rates around 2%, making it one of the common illnesses. Women are twice as often affected as men. The disorder generally has onset with an initial, severe, well-remembered attack between the late teens and early thirties. Stressful life events are common near the time of onset. There is evidence for an early childhood prodrome consisting of shyness and avoidance of novelty, but most patients remember themselves as "normal" prior to the first attack. After onset, attack frequency varies from one or so a month to several daily. At some point after the first attack, other features of the illness often appear, including anxiety in anticipation of future attacks, avoidance of situations associated with attacks (agoraphobia), and not infrequently alcohol and drug abuse. Agoraphobia can become so severe that patients lose jobs or become housebound. Depression is frequently co-morbid. The etiology of panic disorder has yet to be established. The illness runs strongly in families, with most patients having at least one affected first-degree relative. Research evidence points toward pathology in brain norepinephrine, serotonin, benzodiazepine-GABA, and/or cholecystokinin chemical systems. There is no clinically accepted laboratory test to confirm the diagnosis.

TREATMENT

Panic disorder generally runs a chronic course when untreated, with disability varying from slight to incapacitating. Although panic usually responds quite well to medication treatment, behavioral therapies, or their combination, community practice surveys find that most patients receive no treatment and those who do seldom receive treatment adequate to produce remission. The goal of treatment should be complete suppression of panic attacks, phobic disability, and depression. This goal is achievable for the large majority of patients. Partially responding patients should continue to receive vigorous treatment, including higher medication doses, medication combinations, and behavior therapy–medication combinations as needed.

Antidepressant Treatment

Several antidepressants are known to be effective for panic disorder (Table 1). These include the tricy-

TABLE 1. **Medications Effective in Panic Disorder**

Generic Name	Brand Name	Drug Class	Initial Dose (mg)	Target Dose (mg)	Time to Response
imipramine†	Tofranil*	TCA	10 q d	150 q d	2–8 wk
desipramine†	Norpramin*	TCA	10 q d	150 q d	2–8 wk
clomipramine†	Anafranil	TCA	25 q d	150 q d	2–8 wk
fluoxetine†	Prozac	SSRI	5 q d	20 q d	2–8 wk
sertraline†	Zoloft	SSRI	25 q d	100 q d	2–8 wk
paroxetine†	Paxil	SSRI	10 q d	20 q d	2–8 wk
fluvoxamine†	Luvox	SSRI	25 q d	150 q d	2–8 wk
alprazolam	Xanax*	BZ	0.5 tid	1 qid	first few d
clonazepam†	Klonopin	BZ	0.25 bid	1 bid	first few d
lorazepam†	Ativan*	BZ	1 tid	2 qid	first few d

*Generic preparation available.
†Not FDA-approved for this indication.
Abbreviations: TCA = tricyclic antidepressants; SSRI = selective serotonin re-uptake inhibitors; BZ = benzodiazepines.

TABLE 2. **Medications Probably Not Effective in Panic Disorder**

Generic Name	Brand Name	Class
trazodone	Desyrel	antidepressant
bupropion	Wellbutrin	antidepressant
buspirone	BuSpar	anxiolytic
propranolol	Inderal	beta blocker

clics imipramine,* desipramine,* and clomipramine,* the selective serotonin re-uptake inhibitors (SSRIs) fluoxetine,* sertraline,* paroxetine,* and fluvoxamine,* as well as the nowadays rarely used MAO inhibitors (not shown in Table 1). These medications appear to be roughly equivalent in efficacy, although the effectiveness of the SSRIs has been established more recently. The serotonin-norepinephrine re-uptake inhibitor venlafaxine* (Effexor) also shows promise in open clinical trials. Antidepressant medications are effective for panic disorder regardless of whether depression is co-morbid with the panic.

Several available medications have been reported to be not effective or equivocally effective in panic disorder. These include the antidepressants trazodone* and bupropion,* the antigeneralized anxiety drug buspirone,* and the commonly utilized beta blocker propranolol* (Table 2).

The tricyclics and the SSRIs are the medication treatments of first choice for panic disorder. The generic-available tricyclics are inexpensive, while SSRI therapy typically costs $2 per day or more. The side effect profile of the SSRIs (nausea, headache, insomnia, orgasmic failure) is generally more acceptable to patients than the side effect profile of the tricyclics (dry mouth, sedation, constipation, weight gain). All these medications typically require a few weeks to work.

For panic disorder, the starting dose for all these medications should be lower than the eventual target dose, necessitating dose titration. The low initial doses are necessary for panic disorder because panic patients are sensitive, in the first week or so of treatment, to anxiogenic side effects of these medications, which can include a brief initial increase in panic attack frequency. The target dose should generally be reached in two to three weeks. Response is typically observed a few weeks later. Doses higher than the target doses listed in Table 1 are often helpful in resistant cases.

Longer-term side effects, if any, are most often easily managed. Many side effects diminish with continued treatment. The dry mouth seen with tricyclics generally responds to gums or mints or dose reduction, the constipation to bulking agents, the sedation to placement of the entire daily dose at bedtime, and weight gain to dietary discretion. Nausea and headache with the SSRIs often require dose reduction. Insomnia often responds to trazodone, 50 to 200

mg at bedtime, and orgasmic failure to dose reduction or yohimbine, up to 5.4 mg three times a day, or buspirone, up to 10 mg three times a day.

Treatment discontinuation as a rule should not be attempted until an asymptomatic period of six months or more has been achieved. Discontinuation is accomplished by dose tapering over 1 to 2 weeks. Relapse is not uncommon but generally responds to retreatment. As panic disorder is a chronic illness, many patients may require long-term treatment.

Benzodiazepine Treatment

Several benzodiazepines are known to be effective for panic disorder (see Table 1). Diazepam (Valium) has also been shown to be effective in panic disorder but is generally less acceptable to patients and families. The effective benzodiazepine dose for panic disorder is generally somewhat higher than that used for temporary situational anxiety or chronic generalized anxiety (Table 1). Antipanic relief is achieved very quickly.

The initial use of benzodiazepines should generally be reserved for the few patients in whom a rapid antipanic response is clinically urgent, or alternative medications were poorly tolerated. Benzodiazepines induce physical dependence, and discontinuation can lead to a precipitated withdrawal syndrome, even after only a few weeks at modest doses. In panic patients the withdrawal syndrome can be difficult to distinguish from the original panic symptoms. Benzodiazepine discontinuation is best achieved by a slow taper over several weeks to several months. Alprazolam is probably more prone to withdrawal symptoms than are other commonly used benzodiazepines because of its relatively shorter half-life.

One often sees patients who appear to be receiving a long-term antipanic benefit from chronic benzodiazepine prescription. These patients only rarely increase their dose and seldom if ever resort to nonmedical benzodiazepine use unless there has been a history of abuse of other substances in the past. Reasonable but not heroic efforts should be made to stabilize such patients on nonbenzodiazepine alternatives and then initiate a slow taper.

Behavioral Treatment

Cognitive-behavioral psychotherapeutic techniques are known to be effective for panic disorder, either alone or in combination with medication. The relative effectiveness of behavioral therapies compared with medication has not been clearly established, either for short-term or long-term treatment outcomes. Patients should be invited to choose among behavior therapies, medication, or their combination based on personal preferences and the availability of trained providers. Effective techniques for panic attacks include breathing retraining, cognitive restructuring, and interoceptive desensitization. Breathing retraining teaches patients to prevent some of the more severe symptoms of panic attacks

---

*Not FDA-approved for this indication.

by avoiding hyperventilation. Cognitive restructuring teaches patients to identify and banish catastrophic thoughts triggered by the initial symptoms of a panic attack that contribute to the rapid symptom escalation. In interoceptive desensitization, patients induce early panic attack symptoms, such as dizziness induction by spinning in a swivel chair, to gradually more intense levels until high levels of the symptom can be tolerated without provoking an attack. Other behavioral techniques directed at phobic avoidance, such as gradual, systematic exposure to phobic situations, are best employed if needed after panic attacks have been eliminated by other treatments.

Physical and Chemical Injuries

BURNS

method of
DAVID G. GREENHALGH, M.D.
Shriners Burns Institute
Cincinnati, Ohio

Burns are a very common injury, with estimates of at least two million individuals per year being burned severely enough to require medical attention. Seventy thousand of these burn victims require hospitalization, and approximately five thousand people die every year in the United States from burn injury.

The physician orchestrates much of the care and the surgeon performs skin grafts, but an entire team approach is necessary to optimize the chances of survival and to reduce scar formation on an extensively burned patient. Burn centers have highly skilled nursing staffs, knowledgeable occupational and physical therapists, and the means for providing the prolonged support that is necessary for optimizing the functional and cosmetic results after a burn injury. Patients with small burn injuries simply need to be followed to determine whether they will heal within 2 to 3 weeks. Whether in a small community hospital or a large medical center, the initial care of the burn injured patient, is extremely valuable for improving the chances of the patient's survival and ultimate outcome.

It is estimated that up to 90% of burns are completely preventable, and the role of the caregiver should always be to try to educate people about the prevention of such injuries. Simple measures, such as lowering the temperature of a hot water heater, can prevent a majority of the burn injuries that are seen in emergency departments.

TREATMENT

At the Scene

First, stop the burning process. The patient should be carefully checked for smoldering clothes and covered with dry, clean sheets. There is a great tendency to cover the burned areas with cool, wet dressings because it is felt that the cool temperature will stop the burning process in the skin, and the cool dressings may help the pain. After a minute or two, cooling has no effect. We stress that cool, wet dressings should never be used because the benefit of cooling the burn is almost always gone by the time caregivers arrive at the scene. We have received several patients with temperatures as low as 31° to 32° C as a result of being wrapped in wet dressings. Even if the wet dressing is warm, by the time the patient arrives at the care facility, the dressings have cooled the patient significantly.

While the patient's clothing is being removed, one should also remember that any constricting jewelry such as rings should also be removed, because significant swelling can lead to constriction of the distal blood flow. Any patient who has suffered a chemical burn needs to be immediately stripped and washed with copious amounts of fluid. There should be no attempt to find an antidote since that is time wasted that should be spent diluting the chemical. Moreover, an exothermic reaction can occur to produce heat while neutralizing the agent. In patients who have sustained electrical injuries, the first priority is not to electrocute any of the rescuing party. Emergency medical personnel are highly skilled in these procedures; other individuals should not attempt to rescue someone in contact with electricity.

Emergency medical personnel should also attempt to get a history of what occurred at the scene. Being informed regarding a patient's history of being found unconscious in a smoke-filled room or of a patient jumping from a third floor window can be valuable in guiding emergency physicians to look for smoke inhalation or for fractures from a fall.

Immediate Care

Burn patients should be treated like any other trauma patient. A brief history of the incident should be obtained while the ABCs—airway, breathing, circulation—are being attended to. Wise burn surgeons always say forget the burn injury and examine the patient for other signs of trauma. The patient should have an entire body survey just like any other trauma victim.

Airway

Patients with burns to greater than 25% to 30% of the total body surface area (TBSA) tend to develop swelling throughout the entire body. Edema may occur in the glottic region, leading to loss of the airway. Once the patient starts to develop symptoms of glottic stenosis, intubation becomes quite difficult. Any patient with a burn larger than 50% should be considered a candidate for endotracheal intubation. Those patients with total head and face burns along with burns inside the mouth may be prone to developing significant edema in the glottic region. Not all burns to the face require endotracheal intubation. Those patients with superficial flash burns to the face with minimal burns elsewhere will usually do fine, despite swelling around the eyes and lips. It is also important to remember that the maximal edema in the face and glottic region will occur at approximately 24 hours. If there is a question of whether to intubate someone at the scene, especially with a small burn, one almost always has time to bring the patient to a special care facility where intubation can be performed in a controlled fashion. Once the patient is intubated, the endotracheal tube should be left in place for 3 to 4 days, when generalized edema has resolved. An air leak is usually a good sign that the edema has resolved enough for extubation.

Smoke Inhalation

The special concern for breathing in the burn patient is smoke inhalation. The diagnosis of smoke inhalation can be quite difficult; however, a history is very important. Any patient who has been in a smoke-filled, closed space should be suspected of having smoke inhalation. Carbonaceous sputum may help but is not clearly diagnostic. Of immediate concern is the potential for hypoxia. Most people who die in house fires actually die from the smoke inhalation, or more specifically, hypoxia. Fire consumes the oxygen so that people in smoke-filled rooms lie in a hypoxic environment and, in essence, suffocate. Patients who are found unconscious but alive at the scene are at risk for hypoxic brain injury.

Carbon monoxide poisoning is quite common in patients found in smoke-filled rooms. Carbon monoxide binds to hemoglobin with an affinity 200 times that of oxygen. In other words, in a room filled with 0.1% carbon monoxide, there will be equal binding between oxygen and carbon monoxide for hemoglobin (20% for both). It should be remembered that many of our tests for oxygen saturations and arterial blood gases will not reveal the extent of tissue hypoxia since oximeters do not detect carboxyhemoglobin, and the P_{O_2} is simply the partial pressure of oxygen dissolved in serum. One must obtain a carboxyhemoglobin level in order to get an estimate of carbon monoxide poisoning. Levels less than 10% are not a problem; this level may be found in heavy smokers. At 20%, most people develop headache, nausea, vomiting, and a loss of manual dexterity. Confusion and lethargy set in at approximately 30%, and electrocardiographic changes showing cardiac ischemia may be detected. Patients at these levels become confused and do not realize that their life is in danger. Between 40% and 60%, patients lapse into coma, and above 60% patients routinely expire. It is important to remember that levels of 40% to 50% may be obtained within 2 to 3 minutes in a house fire.

Since carbon monoxide is reversibly bound to the heme pigments (hemoglobin and myoglobin) and to enzymes of the metabolic pathway, the treatment is to increase oxygen delivery. The half-life of carboxyhemoglobin is approximately 4 to 5 hours for patients breathing room air. Giving a patient 100% oxygen reduces the half-life to 45 to 60 minutes. All patients suspected of having inhalation injury should receive 100% oxygen by mask or, if appropriate, endotracheal tube, until assessment of carboxyhemoglobin levels has been performed. The treatment of patients with hyperbaric oxygen is hotly disputed. Hyperbaric oxygen may reduce the half-life to 20 to 30 minutes; however, most patients have acceptable carboxyhemoglobin levels after sitting in the emergency department for an hour or two.

It is important to understand two other components of smoke inhalation that commonly occur after burn injury. Burn patients are prone to acute respiratory distress syndrome as a result of their injury and pulmonary insult. These problems usually occur at about 24 to 48 hours. True smoke inhalation, however, results from the toxic chemicals and particulate matter of smoke settling in the lungs. Initial evaluation of the patient is not very helpful in the diagnosis of the severity of inhalation injury. Initial chest radiograph has little value, and initial arterial blood gases, if abnormal, may help with the diagnosis of inhalation injury. One of the earliest indicators is an abnormally low P/F ratio (Pa_{O_2} divided by the fraction of inspired oxygen [Fi_{O_2}]). A ratio of 400 to 500 is normal; however, those patients with a ratio of less than 300 are at risk for a prolonged course of pulmonary support. Unfortunately, changes in P/F ratios usually do not occur until after completion of burn shock resuscitation. Inhalation injury leads to a sloughing of the bronchiolar and bronchial mucosa, which can cause distal atelectasis and an increased risk for pneumonia. These problems are not usually manifest for several days. In the meantime, aggressive pulmonary toilet and support are required.

Circulation

Any injury, including burns, leads to a local inflammatory response that produces edema in the injured area. Unfortunately, when a burn becomes larger than 25% TBSA, the local mediators released at the site of injury spill into the systemic circulation, and the patient develops a systemic response to injury. The entire body tends to swell from an increase in vascular permeability. In simpler terms, there is a massive "third space" fluid loss that must be replaced in order to prevent shock. Clearly, not all burn injuries require formal resuscitation, but to determine which patients need intravenous hydration, one must have an idea of the severity of burn injury. Since the systemic response does not occur in burns of less than 25% TBSA, many patients can be treated without a formal resuscitation if they have superficial burns and relatively small surface area involvement. The question of whether to resuscitate someone formally is quite simple; one must follow the physiologic response of each patient. If the patient is not making adequate urine or has significant changes in hemodynamics, then he or she must be resuscitated. The key point is that one must treat the patient, see how she or he responds, and not depend solely on formulas.

The severity of a burn injury is dependent on:

(1) the total body surface area involved,
(2) the depth of injury,
(3) the presence of an inhalation injury,
(4) the presence of concomitant injuries,
(5) the presence of predisposing conditions,
(6) the age of the patient.

A rough idea of the extent of the body surface area involved can be estimated by using the "rule of nines." The body can be divided into several areas of 9%, with the head and each arm being 9%. The anterior trunk, posterior trunk, and legs are each 18%. This leaves 1% for the genitalia. The rule of nines applies only to adults, since young children have a larger body surface area in the head when compared with the legs. Most emergency departments and burn units rely on more specific Lund-Browder diagrams, in which the burn injury is drawn on each involved section of the body and then totaled to give a percentage for the burn injury.

For burn shock resuscitation, the larger the percentage of burn, the more fluids will be required. The most commonly used formula for estimating the initial burn shock resuscitation, called the Parkland or Baxter formula, estimates the fluid requirements to be 4 mL per kg per % burn, with half the total volume being given in the first 8 hours and the other half being required in the next 16 hours. Since the patient is losing serum through the leaking capillaries, one should use the most physiologic solution, lactated Ringer's, for replacement. It is extremely important to remember that formulas give only a rough estimate of the fluid requirements, since those patients with more superficial burns require less, and those with deeper burns require more, fluids for an equal-size burn. Fluid requirements are even further increased after an inhalation injury. Once the fluid requirements have been calculated, one should initiate fluid resuscitation at that rate. After this point, all adjustments of the fluid administration should be based on the physiologic response of the patient. Urine output should be 0.5 mL per kg per hour (roughly 30 to 50 mL per hour) for adults or 1 mL per kg per % burn for small children. For children less than 2 years, the burn resuscitation calculation should include an estimate of the basal fluid requirements.

Immediately after a burn injury, albumin also leaks, so giving a colloid is a waste since large molecules such as albumin are lost into the interstitium. We occasionally will add 1 ampule (50 mEq) of sodium bicarbonate ($NaHCO_3$) to each liter of lactated Ringer's in order to give a slightly hypertonic solution. Once the patient develops a base excess, however, the sodium bicarbonate is removed. Some studies suggest that even greater hypertonic sodium (3% NaCl) solutions may assist with initial burn shock. After about 12 hours, the capillary leak starts to close, and we will often add 25% albumin at a rate of 5 to 10 mL per hour to help with resuscitation by increasing plasma oncotic pressure.

The resuscitative fluid rate is cautiously decreased while maintaining urine output at 0.5 to 1 mL per kg per hour. Increasing fluid rates to produce excessive urine output is not necessary and may lead to needless edema. Burn shock lasts approximately 24 hours. Upon completion, the capillary leak syndrome stops, and the patient needs only daily maintenance fluids. We usually calculate the maintenance fluid based on basal requirements (1500 × body surface area, or 2000 × body surface area for small children) plus evaporative losses ([25 + % burn] × body surface area for adults, or [35 + % burn] × body surface area for children). When the intravenous rate has decreased to maintenance level, then the fluid is switched over to a maintenance fluid of $D_5$0.45 normal saline with added potassium chloride. Once the patient reaches the maintenance fluid rate, urine output is driven by breakdown products of the hypermetabolic response. Usually, urine output tends to remain at 2 to 4 mL per kg per hour because of this osmotic diuresis. If one adjusts fluid rates to maintain a urine output of 30 to 50 mL per hour, then the patient will become dehydrated. We keep the total fluids at the calculated maintenance rate and make adjustments based on blood urea nitrogen (BUN) levels. Again, it is important to remember that all the burn formulas are only rough estimates of how fast to initiate the burn shock resuscitation. Once initiated, the fluid rate should be titrated to the physiologic response of the patient.

Depth of Injury

The second factor affecting the severity of injury is related to the depth of the burn injury. The classic description of first-, second-, third-, and fourth-degree burns is an anatomic one based on the depth of injury related to the skin anatomy. A *first-degree burn* has not penetrated the basal layer of the epithelium. In essence, the epithelium has not been breached. These injuries are typified by sunburns and essentially need little care, except possibly for a moisturizer. They will heal spontaneously without scarring.

A *second-degree burn* extends from beneath the basal layer of the epithelium to, but not through, the entire dermis. Epithelial cells lining the dermal adnexa (such as hair follicles and sweat glands) remain viable and migrate to cover the surface of the wound. The more superficial second-degree burns tend to blister, are moist, blanch easily, are extremely tender, and heal within 2 to 3 weeks. Superficial wounds heal more rapidly because most of the hair follicles and other adnexa persist, allowing for multiple points of re-epithelialization. The more hair follicles, the more rapidly the wound heals. Areas with high concentrations of skin adnexa such as in the scalp will heal very rapidly because little distance needs to be traveled between the hair follicles in order to re-epithelialize the surface. As a second-degree burn becomes deeper, fewer and fewer adnexa remain, and a greater distance must be traveled by the epithelium to resurface the wound. The longer the wound remains open, the more granulation tissue forms and the greater the potential for scarring. Studies have clearly shown that if a second-degree burn requires greater than 2 to 3 weeks to heal, then the risk for scarring increases. The current philosophy is to not allow deeper second-degree burns to re-epithelialize totally; instead, these wounds require skin grafts for optimal functional and cosmetic results.

A *third-degree burn* extends completely beneath the dermis and into the fat. In other words, the entire skin has been destroyed. These wounds can have multiple colors, with the classic presentation being the whitish to tan color of burn eschar. There is no blanching, and the wounds tend to be less tender than the second-degree burns because the dermal plexus of nerves has been destroyed. Color can be confusing since these burn injuries may be red and can be found beneath a blister. Except for very small third-degree burns, which heal by contraction and re-epithelialization, these deeper injuries must be treated with skin grafts. A *fourth-degree burn* extends into muscle or bone and requires treatment in a specialized burn center.

There has been a great deal of discussion about how to distinguish a second-degree from a third-degree burn. These exercises are unnecessary since the treatment of burn injury can be greatly simplified if one classifies burns based on their healing and scarring potential. If a burn heals in 2 to 3 weeks, minimal scarring will result. If a burn is not clearly superficial or deep, or is what we call "indeterminate depth," it should be treated conservatively with a topical antimicrobial ointment to determine whether it heals. Those burn injuries that take longer than 2 to 3 weeks to heal lead to significant functional and cosmetic deformities if allowed to heal completely. These injuries should be treated with a skin graft.

Our philosophy with outpatient burn wound treatment has become quite simple and relatively inexpensive. Any burn injury that is clearly quite small (10% to 15%) and does not involve an important functional area can be treated at home in a very simple and inexpensive way. We teach families and patients to use regular soap and tap water. Sterile technique is unnecessary, and gloves are not needed. Gloves are used in emergency departments and burn centers because of concern about the transfer of infection from one patient to another. We use a nonsticky dressing (Adaptic, Johnson and Johnson Medical, Inc., Arlington, Texas) with an inexpensive antimicrobial ointment, such as Bacitracin. In essence, the goal is to minimize bacterial overgrowth and to keep the wound moist for optimal epithelialization. Except for the face, light wraps over the injured area are required, and if a lower extremity is involved, an Ace wrap certainly helps with swelling while allowing for ambulation. Faces are left open after treatment with an antimicrobial ointment. The patient should be encouraged to move all extremities actively, since aggressive early mobilization minimizes edema and helps minimize future range of motion problems.

If the burn wound is too large for the patient to be discharged, or if the social situation requires admission, the treatment is the same and is taught to family members or other caregivers so that when the family is comfortable with doing the care, the patient can be discharged. It is not necessary for the patient to remain in the hospital for the entire 2 to 3 weeks while waiting for the burn injury to heal. This treatment philosophy has been very successful, and the infection rate has been near zero. Even in those patients who have sizeable burn injuries that require hospitalization, we will still wait 2 to 3 weeks to ascertain whether indeterminate burns heal before grafting. Once a superficial burn has re-epithelialized, Bacitracin and Adaptic should be stopped. Prolonged use of Bacitracin will ultimately lead to a rash that may be related to fungal overgrowth. The rash is easily treated by allowing the wound to dry in the air. Moisturizing creams are required after a burn has healed, since the natural moisturizers (oil glands) of the skin fail to function for several weeks. A moisturizer should be massaged into the wound until it disappears and the wound no longer appears dry. All patients should also be evaluated by a therapist who can assess the patient's need for outpatient therapy to ensure return of normal range of motion. Any patient who develops thickening of the burn wound may require pressure garments.

For those patients whose burn wounds have not healed in 2 to 3 weeks, skin grafting should be performed. We believe in placing whole sheets of split-thickness skin over the area to produce the optimal cosmetic and functional result. We have used sheets of skin to cover burns as large as 55% TBSA. For larger burns, meshed grafts may be required. Relatively small skin grafts may be performed on an outpatient basis, again minimizing the cost of burn care. Those patients requiring extensive grafts or needing coverage of face or hand burns clearly must be treated in a burn center.

Compartment Syndromes

Once edema becomes generalized, one must be aware of the likelihood of compartment syndromes. This is especially true for patients with circumferential third-degree extremity burns. Full-thickness burns are inelastic, but the patient still develops a generalized edema. In other words, swelling occurs beneath a constricting burn. If the pressure inside the compartment becomes greater than 30 mmHg, lymphatic emptying stops and venous return is impaired. This increase in pressure stops all blood flow to the muscle in the compartment, leading to the potential destruction of the muscle in the extremity. It is a common belief that if the patient has distal pulses, then circulation to the muscle is intact. One must remember that it only requires a pressure of approximately 30 mmHg to stop all blood flow to the muscle, whereas the artery flowing through the compartment will not be obstructed until pressure greater than the systolic blood pressure has been achieved. In other words, loss of the pulse is the last sign of a compartment syndrome, and usually pulse disappears after many hours of muscle ischemia. We have performed many fasciotomies in children with distal pulses and have found necrotic muscle.

Measuring compartment pressures is quite easy. One must simply connect a needle to the pressure tubing used for an arterial line. The needle is then inserted into the compartment, and if the pressure is greater than 30 mmHg, then the patient should undergo an escharotomy. Even after escharotomies, the subfascial compartment should be checked, and if pressure is greater than 30 mmHg, a fasciotomy should be performed. Escharotomies may seem severe, but most of the time escharotomies are performed through third-degree burns that ultimately require grafting, and the escharotomy scar is rarely visible. Simple escharotomy or fasciotomy can save the muscle and even prevent an amputation.

Another site of compartment syndrome that is often not considered is the intra-abdominal compartment. Patients with circumferential abdominal and chest wounds may end up having restriction of respiratory excursion, leading to an increase in P_{CO_2}. An increase in intra-abdominal pressure greater than 30 mmHg may lead to hemodynamic instability and complete cessation of urine output. Abdominal and chest escharotomies usually lead to improvement. We have also relieved increased intra-abdominal pressures by placing intraperitoneal catheters to drain fluid and have even performed laparotomies for emergency relief. These severe measures have led to survival in otherwise terminal situations.

Other Considerations

One must always make sure that the patient has adequate tetanus prophylaxis after a burn injury. Control of pain after a burn injury is best carried out by the intravenous route. No medicine should be given intramuscularly or subcutaneously, since perfusion of these areas is very erratic. The patient may require multiple doses of narcotic intramuscularly with minimal response, and once perfusion of the muscle returns, the patient may develop complications of narcotic overdose. One must also remember that those patients with burns greater than 20% TBSA have an increased metabolic rate that requires nutritional supplementation. Aggressive feeding has been one of the great advances in burn care. We will place a nasoduodenal feeding tube during burn shock and start feeding within hours of injury. Early feeding has been well tolerated even in those patients with severe burn injuries.

Patients with burns to the face should have the eyes assessed. Corneal abrasions are not uncommon after burn injury, especially those involving flash burns. Most patients with burn injuries to the face and corneal abrasions develop swelling that leads to closure of the eyelids. This forced eyelid closure is an excellent physiologic treatment of corneal abrasions. If more severe injury occurs, ophthalmologic consultation may be necessary.

As with any severe injury, psychosocial support is important. The support of a social services department is of great value in this situation.

Transfer Criteria

Such treatments as whirlpools may help clean the patient but they do not accelerate the healing of a deep second- or third-degree burn. Those patients with nonhealing burns of greater than 2 weeks' duration need to undergo expeditious excision and grafting procedures. To help with making the decision, the American Burn Association has developed criteria for transfer to a burn center. All burns that are greater than 20% TBSA should be referred to a burn center. Since the young and old tend to have more problems, the American Burn Association states that patients with burns greater than 10% TBSA and ages less than 10 and greater than 50 years should be referred to a burn center. The American Burn Association also states that third-degree burns greater than 5% TBSA fit the criteria for transfer. All burns involving the face, hands, feet, major joints, genitalia, and perineum should also be cared for by burn specialists. Special burns that should also be referred include electrical injuries, chemical burns, inhalation injuries, or circumferential burns of the extremities or chest. Similarly, patients sustaining burns that are associated with pre-existing diseases or concurrent trauma are better dealt with in a burn center. Burn care requires not only the healing of the burn wound but also the management of the scar, which can take a year or more of aggressive follow-up and therapy.

Chemical Burns

Chemical burns are usually the result of industrial accidents, use of drain cleaners, or occasionally assault. The damaging effects of a chemical burn often persist until the agent's actions are neutralized. The chemical should be diluted with copious irrigation, and no attempt to neutralize the agent should be undertaken. Acid burns tend to be more limited and, in essence, "tan" the skin to create a barrier at the burn injury site. Alkali injuries tend to progress more deeply since the alkali combines with the lipids of the cell membranes to dissolve the skin until the alkali is neutralized by the tissue buffers. In a few instances a specific neutralizing agent should be sought, such as for a hydrochloric acid burn. These injuries, however, should all be treated at a burn center.

Electrical Burns

Electrical burns create varying types of tissue damage. A common injury results from the extreme heat that is generated from the flash of an electrical explosion. These injuries are, in essence, thermal burns, and should be treated as such. The classic electrical injury occurs as current flows through the body. The body acts as a resistor, with those tissues that have the greatest amount of resistance creating greater amounts of heat. The smaller the size of the body part, the more intense the heat that is produced and the less the heat is dissipated. Therefore, distal extremities are frequently damaged to a greater extent than the trunk. Electrical injuries can be the most devastating injury that one may see, and frequently the burn on the surface is only the tip of the iceberg.

All patients injured with high voltage current (greater than 1000 volts) should be evaluated for compartment syndromes, especially in the forearms, and often require formal fasciotomies. Exploration of the extremities for necrotic muscle is usually required in these patients. The wounds require multiple procedures to re-examine the tissue, since there is a tendency for progression of necrosis with time. Since the injury involves destruction of large amounts of muscle, myoglobinuria is not an uncommon finding. Myoglobin can lead to renal failure and needs to be treated if present in large amounts. It is a good rule of thumb that if the urine appears to be colored from myoglobin (appears red or tea-colored), increased fluids should be administered to dilute out the pigment. The usual treatment for myoglobinuria involves administration of a large volume of fluid to produce a urine output of greater than 100 mL per hour for adults or 2 mL per kg per hour for children. Frequently, an increased intravenous fluid rate is all that is required for elimination of myoglobin. Correction of acidosis should also be a goal, and adding $NaHCO_3$ may be helpful. Occasionally, mannitol may need to be given to help initiate diuresis. The usual dose is 12.5 grams followed by another 12.5 grams in 30 to 45 minutes.

Electrical injuries may produce damage to structures away from the obvious site of injury. One must be aware that viscera may be involved; however, frequent examinations of the patient lead to the diagnosis. Damage to nervous structures is not uncommon, and the patient should have a complete neurologic examination. Patients occasionally develop neurologic problems and should have neurologic follow-up. Patients who suffer electrical injury also may develop cataracts and should be checked closely for these changes. The heart is also very sensitive to the electrical stimulation. Patients coming in contact with low voltage tend to develop fibrillation, and if these patients are resuscitated by immediate CPR and other life-sustaining procedures, they frequently will have no sequelae. Those patients coming into contact with very high voltage, greater than 1000 volts, tend to have cardiac standstill and, with time, their heart will regain function. Patients sustaining contact with greater than 440 volts should be monitored for cardiac arrhythmias for 24 hours.

DISTURBANCES DUE TO HIGH ALTITUDE SICKNESS

method of
DAVID ROMERO-ALVIRA, Ph.D., M.D., and
ENRIQUE ROCHE, Ph.D.
Hospital Miguel Servet
Zaragoza, Spain

PATHOPHYSIOLOGIC BACKGROUND

The main feature of altitude is that barometric and partial oxygen pressures decrease as altitude increases. Since partial oxygen pressure is instrumental in achieving oxygen saturation of hemoglobin, the result of reaching high altitudes is that the amount of oxygen bound to hemoglobin and consequently distributed to the body tissues decreases. This condition is known as hypoxia.

Adaptive short- and long-term mechanisms operate to compensate for this oxygen deficit. It is believed that the failure of these adaptive mechanisms leads to the manifestation of altitude-related disorders. These mechanisms include:

1. An increase in pulmonary hypertension as a result of increased tachypnea. This phenomenon is exaggerated by physical exercise associated with alpinism. In some instances, the high arterial pressure cannot be compensated for in certain areas of the lung, producing local pulmonary edema.

2. Increased cardiac rhythm to supply more oxygen to the tissues. In some cases, this cannot occur because pulmonary hypertension is accompanied by systemic vasodilatation. In other words, the right ventricle is working against hypertension and the left ventricle against hypotension. The result is the production of hypovolemia, with alterations in hemoconcentration, ionic and blood pH, calcium overload, and general myocardial dysfunction.

A similar situation occurs in fetal hemodynamics. The fetus has a very high vascular pulmonary resistance and an arterial oxygenation similar to that found in a person on the top of Mount Everest. This high resistance changes the blood flux through the foramen ovale and ductus arteriosus, alleviating the pressure and allowing the development of fetal life. In addition, part of the fetal adaptation to low oxygenation is due in part to the presence of an isoform of hemoglobin called hemoglobin F.

3. Blood alkalosis resulting from hyperventilation during exercise, with a concomitant reduction of carbon dioxide partial pressure in the alveoli. Excessive pulmonary and blood alkalosis may lead to lassitude, poor judgment, and loss of consciousness.

4. Increased production of 2,3-bisphosphoglycerate. This compound makes oxygen available to the tissues by decreasing the affinity for oxygen for hemoglobin.

5. Stimulation of erythropoietin synthesis and secretion to increase the number of red blood cells, thus favoring a greater oxygen supply to the tissues.

6. A twofold increase in the plasma level of endothelin has been described in healthy alpinists. This peptide binds to specific receptors located in endothelial cells and induces contractile effects in the vascular system through the activation of calcium channels in order to favor blood supply to the skin. This increase is linked to the high pressure present in the pulmonary arteries. Both changes are reversible by oxygen administration.

7. Other hormonal and metabolic changes favoring metabolic energy production.

Although the molecular mechanisms underlying the impaired adaptive changes to altitude are poorly defined, it has been established that hypoxia, as a result of exposure to high altitude, may lead to an increased production of toxic oxygen derivative species: oxygen free radicals. In this respect, antioxidative strategies have been successful in treatment of hypoxic-related disorders by reducing the levels of oxygen free radicals. Therefore, we suggest that similar strategies could be useful in the treatment of altitude sickness.

RELATIONSHIP BETWEEN OXIDATIVE STRESS AND HYPOXIA

Little attention has been given to the role of oxidative stress in altitude-related disorders. We believe that there is a strong correlation between the adaptation to high altitude and the balance between pro-oxidative/antioxidative mechanisms in the body, as demonstrated by the following observations:

1. Enhanced activity of oxidative enzymes and mitochondrial content and a disruption of the mitochondrial electron transport chain during hypoxic conditions have been described. These situations favor the production of oxygen free radicals and related pro-oxidant substances. Oxygen free radicals are able to react with biologic macromolecules such as proteins, nucleic acids, and lipids, producing alterations in cellular activities, mutations, and lipid peroxides, respectively. This results in acute cell dysfunction and altered cell homeostasis.

2. The anaerobiosis accompanying hypoxia produces a rapid depletion of cellular energy stores such as adenosine triphosphate (ATP) and creatine phosphate. The ATP depletion leads to changes in the potassium currents through potassium channels at the arterial level, producing vasodilatation and vasoconstriction as well as changes in calcium homeostasis. The molecular mechanisms by which acute alveolar hypoxia produces pulmonary hypertension have yet to be well established. The clinical evidence indicates that low partial oxygen pressure in systemic vascular beds produces vasodilatation while causing vasoconstriction in the pulmonary vascular beds. Both phenomena have been attributed to the activity of ATP-dependent potassium channels, which are abundant in systemic arteries. The hypoxia due to low partial oxygen pressure depletes the ATP levels. This increases the potassium current and produces vasodilatation in systemic vascular beds. However, the opposite occurs in the pulmonary arteries and carotid bodies, producing vasoconstriction. The hypoxia leads to closure of the potassium channels, membrane depolarization, and calcium entry via voltage-dependent channels. The fetus undergoes a similar event of pulmonary hypertension in the uterus. However, the foramen ovale and ductus arteriosus can derive blood from the pulmonary system for the systemic beds.

3. In addition, products resulting from ATP degradation, such as xanthine and hypoxanthine, increase in the bloodstream. These products are eliminated by the xanthine dehydrogenase/oxidase system. The dehydrogenase form operates in normal aerobic conditions and uses NAD^+ as an electron acceptor when oxidizing xanthine to uric acid. However, in hypoxic conditions, the release of calcium from intracellular stores and the overproduction of oxygen free radicals can transform the dehydrogenase into the oxidase isoform. The transformation mechanism implies the proteolytic cleavage of the enzyme by calpains (calcium-dependent proteases) and the oxidation of amino acid residues by oxygen free radicals. The oxidase isoform preferentially uses oxygen rather than NAD^+. Upon reoxygenation, xanthine is oxidized to uric acid by xanthine oxidase, forming the superoxide radical. In this respect, reoxygenation occurs very often at high altitude, where alpinism exercise and temperature changes can produce situations of ischemia-reperfusion in some tissues.

4. The release of iron from proteins such as hemoglobin, myoglobin, and ferredoxin can increase oxidative stress through Fenton-related mechanisms, producing free radicals that can participate in protein and membrane lipid

TABLE 1. **Manifestations of High-Altitude Exposure**

Pathology	Characteristics	Symptoms
AH	Following rapid exposure to 5500 m	Mental deterioration, collapse
AMS	Occurs at moderate altitude (2500–3000 m) Autolimited process Very common	Anorexia, hyperventilation, oliguria, proteinuria, resting tachycardia, headache, nausea, vomiting, sleeping disturbances, and lethargy Central nervous system alterations similar to those in excessive alcohol intake
CMS	Affects people living in mountainous regions	Mental deterioration, asthenia, apathy, pulmonary hypertension, thrombophlebitis, polycythemia (hematocrit around 65%), and congestive cardiac insufficiency
HAPE	Appears between 6 and 96 h (65% of cases at 3500–4000 m and 35% of cases at more than 4500 m) Very dangerous situation; life-threatening	Resting dyspnea, tachycardia, dry cough, light fever, chest pain, night dyspnea with orthopnea, nausea, and tachypnea Progression to pulmonary edema, increased dyspnea, cyanosis, cough, and hemoptysis
HACE	Occurs at 5000–5500 m Very rare Continuation of AMS Life-threatening	Confusion, headache, hallucinations, stupor, papillary edema, ataxia Affected precise motion (fingers, hands, and eyes), progressive dazzled state
ARP	Can occur below 5000 m Altered catabolism at more than 5000 m (40% decrease in muscle blood flux, 15% decrease in muscle mass, and 35% decrease in muscle protein)	Retinal hemorrhage, thrombophlebitis, embolism, facial or peripheral edema Sickle cell anemia crisis (if predisposition) Visual and auditory hallucinations, paranoid delusions, altered sense of reality and danger

See abbreviations in the text.

TABLE 2. **Strategies for Different Forms of Altitude Sickness**

Pathology	Strategies
AMS	Early symptoms: Rest
	When produced by rapid ascension to high altitude: (1) Descend to a lower altitude; (2) oral rehydration (IV if necessary)
CMS	Decrease altitude
	Long stay at sea level
HAPE	Rest
	Rapidly descend to a lower altitude
	Oxygen administration (Ventimask 40–50%)
	Furosemide (Lasix), 40 mg IV
	If morphine is required, administer carefully because it depresses respiratory function
	Naloxone (Narcan)* IV is a good alternative to morphine
	Digitalis and platelet antiaggregants for complete arrhythmia caused by atrial fibrillation
	Hyperbaric chamber (if available)
HACE	Rest
	Rapid descent to a lower altitude
	Oxygen administration (Ventimask 40–50%)
	Betamethasone (Celestone), 4 mg IV q 4 h†
	10% mannitol solution IV
	Evaluation of serum levels of K^+, Mg^{2+}, Cl^-, Na^+ and hydration state
	Hyperbaric chamber (if available)
ARP	Early identification of the problem and specific treatment
	Warning signal for future disturbances

*Not FDA-approved for this indication.
†Exceeds dosage recommended by the manufacturer.
See abbreviations in the text. These strategies, classically applied by physicians to treat these disorders, are related to antioxidative strategies.

peroxidation. Therefore, it is important to use chelating agents in cases of overloading or hemolytic episodes.

5. Blood catecholamines are also oxidized during hypoxia, yielding superoxide radical. Activation of neutrophils can also be observed in affected areas, leading to local inflammatory reactions and to the production of oxy-

TABLE 3. **Preventive Recommendations (Prophylaxis)**

Slow acclimatization
Start with a maximal altitude of 3000 m, reached by train, car, or plane.
Good physical training and conditioning
Nutritional status in good condition
No physical problems (as listed in Table 4)
No daily ascensions above 3000 m: 300–400 m/d until 5000 m, then 150–200 m/d from 5500 m
Maintain an abundant and regular intake of liquids. Green tea infusion is recommended for antioxidative properties
Absolutely no alcohol consumption. Ethanol ingested at more than 28 gm is a strong oxidant
Avoid strenuous efforts, which induce lipid peroxidation
Absolutely no smoking
Avoid sedatives (they aggravate hypoxemia) and pro-oxidative agents
Try sleeping at an altitude below that reached during the day
Ingestion of acetazolamide (Diamox), 250 gm tid, starting 24 h before the ascension
Avoid hematomas or treat them with anti-inflammatory agents containing antioxidants
Do not treat headaches with acetaminophen (an oxidative agent that causes glutathione depletion)
Avoid ingestion of complexes containing multiple vitamins and minerals. Usually they possess low doses of iron, copper, and vitamin C that behave as pro-oxidants

gen free radicals. Finally, it is noteworthy that under hypoxic conditions there is a depletion of the body antioxidants.

FORMS OF ALTITUDE ILLNESS; TREATMENT AND PREVENTION

Altitude sickness can be manifested in several different forms: (1) acute hypoxia (AH), (2) acute mountain sickness (AMS), (3) chronic mountain sickness (CMS), or Monge's disease, (4) high-altitude pulmonary edema (HAPE), (5) high-altitude cerebral edema (HACE), and (6) altitude-related problems

TABLE 4. **Some Diseases Related to Oxidative Stress***

Acetaminophen toxicity	Lead intoxication
Aging	Lipofuscinosis
AIDS (acquired immunodeficiency syndrome)	Myocardiopathies
Amyloidosis	Neurofibromatosis
Arrhythmia	Oxygen and ozone toxicity
Arteriosclerosis	Pancreas diseases
Betalipoproteinemia	Parkinson's disease
Cancer	Peptic ulcer
Cataract formation	Phagocytic activity
Collagen diseases	Pulmonary dysplasia
Contact dermatitis	Mitral valve prolapse
Coronary risk factor (produced by cholesterol auto-oxidation)	Retina degeneration
Damage induced by oxidative contaminants	Rheumatoid arthritis
Damage produced by smoking (emphysema, asthma)	Sickle cell anemia
Dementia (some types such as Alzheimer's, etc.)	Stunned and hibernated myocardium
Diabetic disorders	Tissue damage induced by carbon tetrachloride
Granulomatosis	Tissue damage produced by endo- and neurotoxins
High blood pressure	Tissue damage produced by sun/ionizing radiation
Hydroxydopamine toxicity	Ulcerative colitis
Inflammatory-related processes	Vasculitis
Ischemic cardiopathy (coronary heart disease)	Wegener's granulomatosis

*These medical situations are related, directly or indirectly, to oxidative stress. Exposure to high altitudes, which is also related to oxidative stress pathologies, may seriously aggravate these disorders in affected individuals.

TABLE 5. **Future Considerations for High-Altitude Sickness***

Improvement of previous nutritional status and lifestyle, focusing on:
Elimination of circumstances that induce oxidative stress:
Avoid alcohol consumption and smoking entirely
Avoid prolonged exposure to ultraviolet and ionizing radiations
Avoid extreme efforts
Reduction of ingestion of meat and its derivatives; vegetable proteins are preferable
Adjustment of the caloric intake to the physical environment and degree of activity (diet rich in carbohydrates)
Reduction of the ingestion of total fat, especially saturated; monounsaturated fat (i.e., olive oil) is preferable
Increased ingestion of fruits and vegetables
Frequent infusions of green tea (rich in polyphenols); avoid dehydration-hemoconcentration
Increased consumption of antioxidative vitamins (i.e., beta-carotenes, C, and E) and oligoelements (i.e., selenium and zinc)
Development of the use of antioxidative strategies, mainly avoiding iatrogenic situations, focusing on the following antioxidants:
Albumin
Superoxide dismutase, allopurinol (Xyloprim)†
Polarized solutions (glucose-insulin and potassium)
Calcium antagonists
N-Acetyl cysteine (Mucomyst)†
Chelating agents of transition metals
Plasma reposition
Endothelin antagonists (PD 147953, PD 145065, BQ 123)‡

*Subject to further research.
†Not FDA-approved for this indication.
‡These are all investigational drugs in the United States, possibly not antioxidants.

(ARP). The main characteristics and symptoms of each form are shown in Table 1.

Treatment depends on the form of the disease (Table 2). Usually, the best solution is to reach a lower altitude for two reasons: (1) lower altitudes facilitate the equilibration of oxygen partial pressure within the tissues; and (2) for practical reasons, this allows a medical team to easily reach the patient for treatment.

Nonetheless, prophylaxis and early diagnosis are the best treatment for altitude sickness (Table 3). Generally, this implies good physical training under medical supervision during the preparatory season. The training programs should be adapted to the objective and the altitude to be reached. In addition, a balanced diet rich in fruits and vegetables, important sources of antioxidants, is strongly recommended during the preparation phase.

In planning a nutritional strategy once on location (in the mountains), one must take into account the difficulties in the carrying and conservation of certain meals. In this respect, certain infusions (such as green tea rich in polyphenolic antioxidants), lyophilized preparations, and nutritional supplements (under medical supervision) are extremely useful. We recommend frequent intakes of carbohydrate-rich meals, vitamins A, C, E, and selenium (antioxidants), as well as frequent ingestions of liquids and electrolytes (at least 3 to 5 liters per day in some instances) for good hydration. Vegetable protein and lipid-rich

meals should be eaten twice a day and with moderation. Avoid pro-oxidative habits such as alcohol consumption and smoking. It is also important to perform gradual ascensions that permit the body to develop the biochemical changes necessary for adaptation to high altitude. Finally, alpinism is not advisable for individuals suffering from certain pathologies such as those listed in Table 4.

A better knowledge of the molecular mechanisms operating in altitude sickness is essential in order to design therapeutic strategies to treat this pathology. Presently, prevention and early diagnosis are the best way to avoid altitude-related disorders. Further scientific and clinical research are needed to answer the still-unknown questions about altitude sickness and related disorders (Table 5).

DISTURBANCES DUE TO COLD

method of
MARIE-DENISE SCHALLER, M.D.,
DAMIEN TAGAN, M.D., and
CLAUDE H. PERRET
University Hospital
Lausanne, Switzerland

ACCIDENTAL HYPOTHERMIA

Etiology

Human beings as homeotherms try to maintain their body temperature constant, despite variations in the surroundings. Their thermoregulatory mechanisms can be briefly summarized as follows: In the presence of cold, thermoreceptors within the skin are activated, a local immediate reflex vasoconstriction is elicited, and impulses are sent to the thalamus through the dorsal root of the spinal cord. The ensuing sympathetic nervous system activation enhances further peripheral vasoconstriction in an attempt to decrease heat loss, increases heart rate and cardiac output, and induces a vasodilatation in the muscles, in order to preserve heat. Muscle shivering can increase the metabolic rate up to fivefold and thus enhance heat production. All these defense reactions against cold are rapidly set in gear, in contrast to the much slower heat production following thyroid gland activation. As a result, temperature in the superficial zone of the body (skin and subcutaneous tissue) may drop to nearly environmental temperature, the goal being the maintenance of a central body or core temperature of around 36° to 37° C. Whenever heat loss exceeds heat production or conservation, hypothermia develops.

Accidental hypothermia is defined as an unintentional decrease of central body temperature below 35° C. It can develop either in individuals with excellent thermoregulatory function who are faced with extreme climatic conditions ("maximal defense" hypothermia), or in patients presenting with one or several alterations in thermoregulation ("minimal defense" hypothermia). To appreciate climatic conditions better, one has to remember that heat is dissipated by conduction (transfer of heat by direct contact), convection (transfer of particles of air heated on the body surface), radiation (transfer by nonparticulate means), and water evaporation. Thus, heat loss is markedly increased during immersion in cold water (thermal conductivity being 32 times higher than in air); with the convective effect of wind; or from radiation from unprotected body areas—the head, for instance.

Accidental hypothermia can be secondary to snow avalanche accident, immersion in cold water, prolonged exposure to cold after an accident (fall in a crack, in a cave), or without accident while practicing sports (swimming, skiing, mountaineering, climbing, speleology), or while working outdoors (Table 1). Victims are usually healthy and physically well-trained individuals. Deficient housing associated with poverty, natural disasters, or war is another risk factor.

Whereas it is easy to make this diagnosis in a patient rescued in snow or water during cold season, there is a danger that hypothermia will be overlooked when developing in a mild or moderate climate. Failure to recognize this condition may occasionally prove fatal owing to incorrect monitoring and inappropriate therapy. This can happen with thermoregulation dysfunction (see Table 1). Numerous drugs, either used for self-poisoning or therapy, can induce hypothermia. Intoxication with tricyclic agents, phenothiazines, and barbiturates, among others, alters thermoregulation while affecting central nervous system and cardiovascular functions. The same is true for alcohol, which produces peripheral vasodilatation and central nervous system depression. In addition, narcotized or hallucinating patients behave inappropriately and can stay for a prolonged time outdoors in cold, windy, and wet weather without any protection. Endocrine dysfunction, namely hypothyroidism and hypopituitarism or hypoglycemia, can lead to hypothermia. Lesions in the central nervous system such as from stroke, trauma, tumor, hemorrhage, and other less frequent diseases can interfere with thermoregulatory centers. The same is true for spinal cord transection, trauma, and tumor: Peripheral cold transmission to neurologic centers is impaired as well as muscle shivering below

the medullary lesion. In extensive burns or erythroderma, heat loss is limited only by surrounding temperature and humidity. The extremes of life are at particular risk: In the neonate, the unfavorable surface to body weight ratio explains the increased difficulty of preserving heat. Altered thermoreceptor function, decreased subcutaneous tissue and muscle mass, and impaired shivering capacity, frequently associated with autonomic dysfunction and lower cardiac output, explain the propensity of elderly people to develop hypothermia. All debilitating conditions (heart failure, sepsis, malnutrition) can be associated with hypothermia.

Clinical Findings (Table 2)

Accidental hypothermia is usually classified as mild (35° to 32° C), moderate (32° to 28° C) and severe (below 28° C). With temperature drop, there is a progressive decrease in all organ functions. Enzymatic and biochemical reactions are depressed or abolished. Oxygen consumption decreases, reaching 50% of initial values at 30° C and 10% at 20° C.

In *mild hypothermia*, there is an increase in heart rate, blood pressure, and respiratory rate, a progressive subileus and increased diuresis due to cold, marked muscle shivering, and gradual exhaustion.

In *moderate hypothermia*, apathy, ataxia, and dysarthria develop. Confusion and hallucinations are responsible for strange behavior, such as undressing in cold weather or fighting the rescue team. Shivering ability disappears around 30° C. Bradycardia succeeds initial tachycardia. Cardiac output decreases as the temperature drops below 30° C. On ECG, the QT, QRS, and PQ intervals augment progressively.

In *severe hypothermia*, the patient is in a coma and is hypotonic, with areactive dilated pupils. Shock, oliguria, and a low respiratory rate are noticed. Atrial fibrillation or flutter, premature ventricular beats, and the pathognomonic Osborne (J) waves are common findings. By 28° C, the danger is great for ventricular fibrillation to occur. Around 20° C and below, the skin appears pale and livid; the patient may be hypertonic, rigid, and comatose, with dilated, fixed pupils, or in cardiorespiratory arrest, with no activity recorded either on electrocardiogram or electroencephalogram. At this stage, it is impossible to differentiate between hypothermia and death, on a clinical basis.

Laboratory Studies

Blood tests may reveal hemoconcentration (following cold diuresis and third space and capillary leakage), with high hematocrit, hemoglobin, and protein concentration. Platelet dysfunction and disseminated intravascular coagulation have been observed at 28° C. High blood glucose levels are common, attributable to stress and impaired response to insulin. Hypokalemia, secondary to cellular shifts, is usual. Blood gas analysis—which we recommend for practical purposes measuring at 37° C, without correction for temperature—may first disclose respiratory alkalosis, followed by respiratory or sometimes mixed acidosis. High creatine kinase activity secondary to rhabdomyolysis can be found. Specific tests for the precise etiology of hypothermia should be performed.

Prognosis

Prognostic factors include advanced age, underlying diseases, duration of cold exposure, and circumstances and

---

TABLE 1. **Risk Factors for Accidental Hypothermia**

I. Normal thermoregulatory mechanisms:
  a. Snow avalanche accident
  b. Immersion in cold water
  c. Prolonged cold exposure
  d. Deficient housing

II. Altered thermoregulatory mechanisms:
  a. Acute drug intoxication (barbiturates, tricyclic agents, methaqualone, etc.)
  b. Acute intoxication with alcohol, ethylene glycol, etc.
  c. Medication side effects (general anesthetics, phenothiazines, etc.)
  d. Endocrine dysfunction
    Hypothyroidism
    Hypoglycemia
    Hypopituitarism
  e. Central nervous system disorders
    Hemorrhage, trauma, tumor
    Parkinson's disease
  f. Spinal cord injury
    Trauma
    Tumor
    Hemorrhage
  g. Skin disorders
    Extensive burns
    Erythroderma
  h. Extremes of life
    Newborn
    Premature baby
    Elderly
  i. Miscellaneous
    Sepsis
    Heart failure
    Malnutrition
    Anorexia nervosa

III. I + II:
  a. Cold exposure after trauma, with associated thermoregulation alteration (shock, spinal cord injury, etc.)
  b. Cold exposure after acute alcohol intoxication

TABLE 2. **Clinical Signs of Accidental Hypothermia**

	Mild	Moderate	Severe	
	35° C	32° C	28° C	20° C
Cardiovascular function				
Heart rate	↑	↓		No pulse
Blood pressure	↑		↓ Shock	
Cardiac output		↓	↓	
ECG	Normal	QT, QRS, PQ prolongation	Atrial fibrillation Osborne (J) wave Ventricular fibrillation	Asystole Ventricular fibrillation
Respiratory function				
Respiratory rate	↑		↓	Respiratory arrest
Neurologic function				
Consciousness	Normal	Apathy Confusion Hallucinations Dysarthria	Coma	
Speech				
Muscles	Shivering	No shivering		
Pupils	Normal		Fixed, dilated	
EEG	Normal		Theta, delta waves ↓	No activity
Urine output	↑			Anuria
Gastrointestinal tract	Subileus	Ileus	Ileus	Ileus
Pancreas function		——— Progressive	decrease ————→	
Liver function		——— Progressive	decrease ————→	
Coagulation			Possible disseminated intravascular coagulation	

severity of hypothermia. Until recently, there were no generally accepted biologic and clinical criteria precluding resuscitation and a rewarming attempt. At present, the demonstration of extreme hyperkalemia (higher than 10 mmol per liter) appears to be the only index to differentiate between severe hypothermia and death.

MANAGEMENT OF ACCIDENTAL HYPOTHERMIA

The first step is to make the diagnosis and to confirm it by measuring the patient's temperature. The thermometer should be a precise tool, able to record very low temperatures. Central temperature is measured by rectal, esophageal, or tympanic probes or by central venous or pulmonary artery catheters. Tympanic recordings are supposed to be close to the brain temperature, whereas esophageal and central blood vessel readings reflect the heart situation. Inserting a probe 6 to 8 cm into the rectum lessens the influence of cold venous return from the legs. However, temperatures recorded with this practical and commonly used method are about 0.5° to 1° C *below* heart temperature. Measuring temperature at two different sites simultaneously can be worthwhile. Continuous monitoring of temperature, heart rate, respiratory rate, and blood pressure is imperative.

Therapy is aimed at elimination of hypothermia-aggravating factors, support of vital functions, and rewarming.

Elimination of Hypothermia-Aggravating Factors

The patient should be removed from the cold, protected from wind, and placed in a dry environment with wet clothing removed. If present, hypoglycemia ought to be corrected. Specific treatment of the etiology is mandatory when feasible, as in the case of sepsis, heart failure, hypothyroidism, and so on.

Cardiovascular and Respiratory Support

Vital functions should be sustained by nonspecific means during hypothermia correction. As a basic principle, one should avoid drug administration. Drug efficacy is frequently blunted or unknown in this temperature range. Prolonged half-life, rebound, and toxic effects following rewarming could be dangerous. Supplemental oxygen is administered either by nasal prongs, masks, or mechanical ventilation, in order to meet increased needs during rewarming. Hypotension, when due to hypovolemia, can be reversed with volume expansion. Atrial fibrillation or flutter should not be treated by antiarrhythmic agents with unknown efficacy and pharmacokinetics: They usually disappear with rewarming. The same is true for ventricular premature beats. Blunted efficacy of electrical defibrillation for ventricular fibrillation in deep hypothermia has been reported. However, this should not prevent one from attempting defibrillation in this situation, keeping in mind that ventricular fibrillation in *very deep* hypothermia will resolve either spontaneously or following countershock during rewarming. One should be especially cautious when the core temperature reaches 28° C.

Owing to a particular heart irritability, rough mobilization of the patient or insertion of a central venous catheter can induce ventricular fibrillation. In such conditions, bretylium tosylate (5 to 10 mg per kg intravenously) is the antiarrhythmic of choice. In contrast, lidocaine has not been proved useful. In the presence of ventricular fibrillation, asystole, or electromechanical dissociation, cardiac compressions are performed at a rate of 50 per minute. The efficacy of this technique is questionable in very severe hypothermia (temperature below 20° C), if one considers heart muscle and thorax rigidity. The risk of converting profound bradycardia into ventricular fibrillation is not a contraindication for cardiopulmonary resuscitation in pulseless hypothermic patients. Before recommending dopamine, an adrenergic agent with a presumed potent thermogenic effect, more data should be available. Insulin should not be administered to treat hyperglycemia. Correction of hypokalemia on a clinical basis would lead to dangerous hyperkalemia after rewarming. In brief, hypotension, shock, arrhythmias, acidosis, metabolic alterations, and coma should be corrected by the only specific measure—i.e., rewarming.

Rewarming

Methods

Rewarming may occur spontaneously by the patient's own heat production (*passive rewarming*) or following the application of heat either directly to the body surface (*active external*) or to different internal organs or systems (*active internal*) (Table 3). When using heating cradles, heated beds or blankets, or a hot bath, the superficial zone is rewarmed first, leading to cutaneous vasodilatation, enhanced return of cold blood to the heart, further decrease in core temperature (i.e., "afterdrop"), and shock due to peripheral vasodilatation and persistence of low cardiac output and heart rate. Arrhythmias and irreversible shock may prove fatal. Moreover, resuscitation of an immersed patient may be hazardous. Rewarming shock could be theoretically minimized by volume expansion under Swan-Ganz catheter monitoring. However, considering the risk of arrhythmias during central venous catheter insertion, the difficulty in interpreting cardiac filling pressures in the absence of established physiologic values in this setting, and the risk of pulmonary edema due to possible alveolar

capillary wall dysfunction, use of this technique should be restricted. To avoid afterdrop and rewarming shock, the core should be rewarmed before the shell.

Several methods are available for internal active rewarming. Administration of heated (to 46° C) humidified air through a face mask or an orotracheal tube achieves *airways rewarming* and hence can increase core temperature by 0.5° C per hour. Even if heat gain is low, this procedure is easy to use and prevents further respiratory heat loss. The efficacy of continuous or intermittent *gastric warm irrigation* is not very different. Colonic lavage, with even lower effects and possible electrolyte imbalance, is thus discarded. Tracheal intubation should always precede gastric lavage. *Peritoneal* or *pleural irrigation* with warm (40° to 42° C) fluid results in faster rewarming rates, up to 5° C per hour. Continuous irrigation is performed through two intraperitoneal catheters or two thoracostomy tubes. Precise fluid balance should be ensured. Indeed, pleural lavage is rarely used due to the risks of mediastinal displacement, respiratory failure, and trauma and lung perforation during tube insertion. Trauma or recent surgery are contraindications for the involved body cavity lavage.

Continuous arteriovenous or *venovenous rewarming* techniques have proved useful. Blood flows from a catheterized femoral artery through a warming device back to a central vein. In the warming device, hot water (40° C) separated from the blood by highly conductive layers is pumped in a countercurrent direction. These methods are effective and technically feasible in most intensive care units. In addition, if anticoagulation is contraindicated, they can be run with minimal heparinization.

Rewarming rates with *cardiopulmonary bypass* are the highest (up to 10° C per hour) and can be precisely controlled. Another advantage of this method is that it provides both an optimal hemodynamic support and oxygenation during rewarming.

Proposed Rewarming Protocol (Figure 1)

When *mild hypothermia* supervenes in a patient without impairment of consciousness and stable cardiovascular and respiratory functions, passive rewarming is sufficient. It can be accelerated by warm drinks, heated infusions, and insulated blankets over the trunk. In *moderate hypothermia*, muscle shivering progressively decreases, and thermogenesis is impaired. Air rewarming is a useful adjunct to the foregoing measures. However, if the patient is comatose or develops respiratory failure, orotracheal intubation and mechanical ventilation are mandatory, even if hypothermia is mild. The presumed increased risk of ventricular fibrillation induced by tracheal intubation has not been confirmed. In this situation, gastric lavage is a useful adjunctive method. An increase of 0.5° to 1° C per hour is expected. In case of failure or in the presence of cardiovascular instability, a more active internal rewarming, such as peritoneal lavage or continuous arteriovenous or venove-

TABLE 3. **Rewarming Methods**

A. Passive rewarming
Spontaneous
B. Active external
Heat applied directly to the surface of the body
(heated blankets or beds, heating cradles, warm bath)
C. Active internal
Airways: heated, humidified air (↑ 0.5°C/h)
Gastrointestinal tract: gastric lavage (↑ 0.5°–1°C/h), colonic
lavage
Pleural irrigation: heated (40°–42°C) fluid through
thoracostomy tubes (up to 5°C/h)
Peritoneal lavage: heated (40°C) fluid (up to 5°C/h)
Extracorporeal shunt (hemodialysis, arteriovenous, or
venovenous) rewarming
Cardiopulmonary bypass: precise and rapid rewarming (up to
10°C/h) with optimal cardiovascular support and
oxygenation

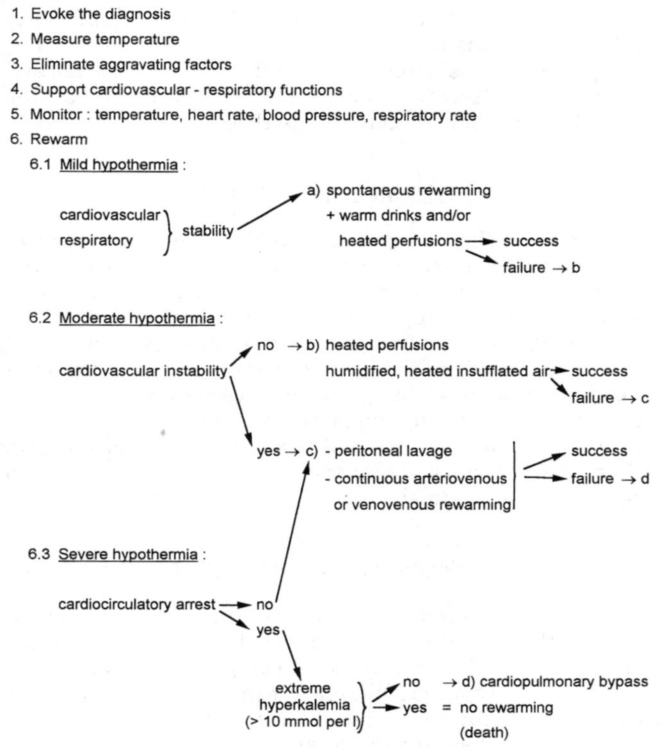

Figure 1. Management of accidental hypothermia.

nous rewarming, is indicated. In *severe hypothermia*, in the absence of cardiocirculatory arrest, peritoneal lavage and extracorporeal shunt are the methods of choice. In the presence of cardiorespiratory arrest, cardiopulmonary bypass must be preferred. In our opinion, the verified demonstration of extremely high plasma potassium levels (higher than 10 mmol per liter) in a clinically dead individual is a sufficient reason to stop therapy.

FROSTBITE

Frostbite is localized cold injury, most commonly involving fingers, toes, nose, ears, and cheeks. During cold exposure, tissues may freeze, ice crystals form, and cells dehydrate. Marked local vasoconstriction and blood hyperviscosity result in hypoperfusion, microthrombosis, and anoxia, worsening further tissue injury. Wind and humidity enhance the effects of cold.

Clinical Findings

With *first-degree frostbite*, the skin is pale and cyanotic. There is little or no edema; sensitivity is decreased. By definition, recovery is complete. *Superficial second-degree frostbite* is characterized by cyanosis, erythema, and substantial edema with development of clear fluid vesicles. Anesthesia is common. Recovery is slow, with long-lasting cold hypersensitivity. *Deep second-degree lesions* are recognized by pronounced and persistent cyanosis, marked

edema, and hematic blebs. As a rule, necrosis is limited to the derma. Persistent altered sensitivity may ensue. It is difficult to differentiate this stage from *third-degree frostbite*, which includes the development of deep tissue necrosis. Involvement of muscles and bones leads to permanent sequelae and amputation. Demarcation limits appear late in the evolution, usually after 45 days, justifying the surgical maxim: "Frostbite in January, amputate in July."

Treatment of Frostbite (Table 4)

Prehospital

Cold and humidity exposure should be discontinued as soon as possible. No rewarming should be undertaken if there is a risk of refreezing, which would markedly enhance initial lesions. Special attention is paid to avoid trauma. Rubbing the extremities does not augment local blood flow but may in fact aggravate tissue injury. Exposure to a campfire, footwarmer, oven heat, or engine exhaust, representing temperatures higher than 50° C, may be catastrophic, superimposing burning injury to cold lesions. Soaking the extremities in warmed water and protecting the skin surface with loose clothing is appropriate therapy, provided cold exposure does not recur. Immediate referral to a medical center is mandatory.

In Hospital

If frostbite is associated with moderate or severe accidental hypothermia, hypothermia should be treated first. Rapid rewarming in a 32° to 41° C warmed water bath is the preferred thawing method. Gradual and spontaneous rewarming at room temperature or delayed thawing using cold water, snow, and massage are not recommended. Prolonged hospitalization is required for second- and third-degree frostbite.

Correction of dehydration, hemodilution, infusion of low-molecular-weight dextran, antiaggregants, and anticoagulation with heparin have all been proposed to improve microcirculation. Vasodilators and sympatholytic agents have also been prescribed for the same indication. Sympathectomy is a common practice, although the benefits regarding tissue preservation have not been definitively proved. Nonsteroidal anti-inflammatory agents are administered to

TABLE 4. **Frostbite Treatment**

Prehospital
Interrupt cold exposure
Avoid trauma
Avoid thaw-refreeze-thaw
In hospital
Rewarm rapidly in 32°–41°C waterbath
Improve microcirculation
Avoid infection, trauma
Repeat warm baths (whirlpool)
Do not proceed to early surgical amputation

inhibit production of prostaglandins, especially thromboxane, which has been demonstrated to be markedly elevated in frostbite blisters. For the same reason, local application of aloe vera is of interest. Blister débridement or fluid aspiration is recommended before regular application of aloe vera. Baths in warmed and antiseptic water, for 30 minutes, should be repeated twice a day. The extremities should be placed in a raised position, in sterile sheets. Great care must be taken to prevent infection and avoid trauma. Antibiotics are not routinely prescribed. Tetanus vaccine booster is recommended, according to the patient's immunization state. Morphine is frequently required to relieve severe pain during rewarming.

All aggravating factors should be corrected as quickly as possible: surgical fixation of dislocated fractures, fasciotomy in the compartment syndrome. This is in contrast with the surgical amputation of necrotized extremities, which should be delayed for several weeks in order to avoid tissue loss maximally. However, in the presence of uncontrolled infections or sepsis, surgical amputation must be performed immediately.

IMMERSION FOOT

Prolonged exposure to water, even when not especially cold (as while working or bathing for hours in water, in shipwreck survivors, and in soldiers standing in trenches) induces a lower extremity injury, immersion foot. The extremity is cold, slightly swollen, discolored, numb, and hyperemic. Management consists in careful drying of the feet, progressive mild rewarming, and placement in an upright position.

OPHTHALMIC INJURIES

Freezing of the corneas causes blurred vision and severe pain. Eyelid closure and local warmth application, for example by one's own hand, may suffice. To prevent a recurrence, protection from the cold and snow goggles are recommended. In severe forms, sequelae may require corneal transplantation.

DISTURBANCES DUE TO HEAT

method of
MICHAEL P. WAINSCOTT, M.D.
*University of Texas Southwestern Medical
   Center
Dallas, Texas*

The spectrum of heat illness encompasses a broad range from heat cramps to life-threatening heat stroke. Deaths from all causes of heat illness increase during heat waves. The summer of 1995 brought a record heat wave that generated an estimated 750 deaths in the United States, including 500 deaths in Chicago. These are reasonable data, in spite of the fact that mortality statistics for hyperthermia are difficult to obtain due to the lack of uniformity in defining deaths related to hyperthermia.

Hyperthermia is a temperature in excess of the normal range of 36° C (96.8° F) to 37.5° C (99.5° F). Temperatures above 41° C (105.8° F) may be life threatening.

THERMOREGULATION

Control for thermoregulation resides within the hypothalamus, which stimulates cutaneous vasodilation and sweating via the autonomic nervous system in response to elevation of blood temperature. Blood flow to the skin may increase 20-fold. Cooling normally occurs by transfer of heat from the skin via radiation, convection, and evaporation. As the ambient temperature exceeds the body's temperature, a rise in body temperature may occur in response to radiation and convection of heat from the environment. When the humidity rises, the body's ability to cool via evaporation is diminished.

PREDISPOSING FACTORS

Many factors predispose to heat illness, often by impairing thermoregulation (Table 1). Heat production within the body increases as a result of exercise, drugs such as sympathomimetics, fever, exertional states such as drug-induced agitation, and muscular rigidity states such as malignant hyperthermia and neuroleptic malignant syndrome. Drugs such as sympathomimetics impede the body's ability to lose heat. Hot, humid environments with little air movement both outside and inside buildings play a key role in the development of environmental heat illness. Lack of acclimatization (the physiologic process by which a person adapts to work/recreation in a hot environment) is another factor. Dehydration increases body temperature at rest and limits sweating because of volume depletion. Cardiovascular disease (CV) or medications used to treat CV disease have an impact on cardiac output and decrease the ability of the body to meet the increased circulatory demand of hyperthermia.

The infant and young child are more susceptible to heat illness through underdeveloped thermoregulatory mechanisms and their increased surface area-to-mass ratios. Elderly people are at increased risk because of decreased cardiac reserve, medications, decreased sweating, and poor physical conditioning. Obese patients are also less tolerant of heat. Heavy clothing or external equipment limits cooling mechanisms, as do skin diseases such as scleroderma, psoriasis, and burn scarring.

A host of medications and drugs of abuse may predispose to heat illness, including diuretics, medications with anticholinergic effects, neuroleptics, beta blockers, calcium channel blockers, alcohol, and cocaine.

TABLE 1. **Predisposing Factors for Heat Illness**

Increased heat production
Hot, humid, windless environment
Lack of acclimatization or physical conditioning
Dehydration
Cardiovascular disease
Extremes of age
Obesity
Inappropriate clothing or external equipment
Skin diseases
Medications/drugs of abuse

MINOR HEAT ILLNESS

Heat edema is a self-limited condition, typically found in nonacclimated individuals following a prolonged period of inactivity, such as sitting in a car or bus. Edema occurs in the feet, ankles, and hands. Some researchers feel that increased aldosterone and antidiuretic hormone may play a role. Once other causes such as right-sided heart failure are ruled out, treatment is reassurance and support. Activity is not usually limited. Diuretics are of no benefit. The edema usually resolves in a few days as the patient becomes more acclimated, but it may last up to 6 weeks.

Heat cramps occur in heavily exercised muscles, most frequently the calves, thighs, and shoulders. Typically these patients sweated profusely and replaced fluid and sodium losses only with water. Treatment includes stretching the affected muscles for rapid relief of the muscle cramp, followed by consumption of sodium-containing solutions, such as commercially available electrolyte drinks, or even a saltwater solution of 1 teaspoon of salt in a quart of water. Salt tablets may be irritating to the gastric lining. More severe cases may require intravenous infusion of saline solution.

Heat tetany presents as carpopedal spasm and paresthesias following periods of intense heat stress, resulting from hyperventilation. Reducing the heat stress and managing the hyperventilation alleviate symptoms.

Heat syncope is a variant of orthostatic syncope, resulting from postural hypotension. Peripheral vasodilation and volume depletion predispose to postural hypotension. Treatment consists of evaluation for other causes of syncope, oral or intravenous hydration, and rest. Hospitalization is seldom needed.

Prickly heat is also known as heat rash, lichen tropicus, or miliaria rubra. It is a red, maculopapular, pruritic rash found on skin covered by clothing. Sweat gland pores become occluded and secondarily infected, most frequently with *Staphylococcus aureus*. Treatment is directed at decreasing time in hot environments, avoidance of talcum or baby powder, use of antihistamines for itching, and wearing loose-fitting clothing. Washing with chlorhexidine (Hibiclens) two or three times a day is useful, or the agent may be applied as a light cream or lotion. Skin desquamation can be accomplished using a 1% solution of salicylic acid three times a day, though care should be taken with large areas of skin involvement to avoid salicylate toxicity. Oral antibiotics such as cephalexin (Keflex) may be used to treat the *S. aureus* infection.

HEAT EXHAUSTION

Heat exhaustion is a relatively common disorder in patients exposed to high ambient temperature who do not adequately replace fluid and electrolyte losses. It is different from heat cramps in that the patient now has systemic symptoms, which may include fatigue, headache, dizziness, weakness, nausea, vomiting, and lightheadedness. The patient may complain of muscle cramps or syncope.

Clinical evaluation may reveal diaphoresis, orthostatic hypotension, and tachycardia. Temperature may be normal or elevated up to 40° C (104° F). Mental status is normal. If mental status changes are present the patient must be treated as a heatstroke patient. It can be difficult to distinguish severe heat exhaustion from the early phases of heatstroke, and the latter is presumed when the diagnosis is in doubt.

Classic descriptions of heat exhaustion suggest two types: water depletion heat exhaustion, in which fluid replacement does not keep up with fluid losses, and salt depletion heat exhaustion, which occurs more slowly and fluids are replaced with inadequate volume and too little salt. It is far more practical to consider heat exhaustion patients as being somewhere in between these classic descriptions. All patients with heat exhaustion are suffering from volume depletion, with electrolyte disturbances based on fluid and electrolyte intake vs. losses.

In addition to rest and removal of the patient to a cool environment, treatment is directed at volume replacement, usually with intravenous saline solution. Further decisions regarding electrolyte management can be made on the basis of laboratory studies. Elevated blood urea nitrogen and hemoconcentration are common. Though uncommon, severe hypernatremia associated with extremely limited fluid intake may be seen and must be treated slowly to avoid cerebral edema.

Heat exhaustion patients are monitored by vital signs, symptom relief, and urine output. Hospitalization is usually not necessary unless there are complicating conditions, such as impaired renal function, major electrolyte disturbances, underlying illness, injuries, or extremes of age.

HEATSTROKE WITH HIGH AMBIENT TEMPERATURE

The classic definition of heatstroke requires temperature elevated above 41° C (105.8° F), altered mental status, and anhidrosis or lack of sweating. One problem with this definition is that the lack of sweating is not a reliable indicator since patients with heat stroke may still be sweating. In addition, because cooling may have been begun by emergency medical personnel, the first recorded temperature may be below 41° C (105.8° F). As organ temperatures reach 42° C (107.6° F), enzyme denaturation, protein coagulation, cell dysfunction, lipid liquefaction, and tissue damage begin to occur. Cell injury depends on the maximum temperature reached and the duration of exposure. *A more useful operational definition of heatstroke includes a temperature greater than 41° C (105.8° F) and mental status changes.*

Two epidemiologically distinct types of heatstroke associated with high ambient temperatures are described: exertional and nonexertional. Patients with *exertional heatstroke* are typically young people who exercised or exerted themselves intensely in a hot, humid environment. Predisposing factors include sedentary lifestyle, recent diarrheal or febrile illness, obesity, inappropriate clothing or gear, volume depletion, sleep deprivation, drugs of abuse (such as amphetamines or cocaine), and medications that impair thermoregulation. Sweating is frequently present. Major metabolic disturbances occur, including lactic acidosis, respiratory alkalosis (from hyperventilation), hypoglycemia, hypocalcemia, hypokalemia (from aldosterone effect) or hyperkalemia (from muscle cell damage and renal failure), and hypophosphatemia (from renal injury). Other complications include highly elevated creatinine kinase (CK), aspartate aminotransferase (AST), and lactate dehydrogenase (LDH) levels, rhabdomyolysis with associated myoglobinuric renal failure, hepatic necrosis, and disseminated intravascular coagulation.

Patients with *nonexertional heatstroke* are usually elderly or chronically ill, and sedentary. Elderly patients have diminished cardiac output, decreased ability to sweat, and decreased ability to vasoregulate. They may have impaired awareness of their surroundings and of the development of heat illness. These patients are also frequently on medications that predispose them to heat illness because of negative effects on cardiac output (beta blockers) or on sweating (anticholinergics), or because of volume depletion (diuretics). Other patients predisposed to heat illness include those with cardiac disease, peripheral vascular disease, diabetes, skin disorders, and cognitive impairment. Nonexertional heatstroke may be indolent in its onset and have significant volume depletion. Acute renal failure is less common with nonexertional heatstroke, but it remains no less life-threatening.

In both types of heatstroke, by definition, central nervous system dysfunction is present. Patients may present with confusion, bizarre behavior, combativeness, hallucinations, delirium, stupor, seizures, and coma. Ataxia may be a manifestation of acute cerebellar injury. The duration of coma is a predictor of death.

Regardless of the type or etiology of heatstroke, treatment is the same. Interventions are made for problems with the airway, breathing, or circulation. Oxygen therapy is initiated. Cardiac and pulse oximetry monitors are placed. Intravenous access is obtained, and isotonic solutions such as normal saline are started. Body temperature is recorded using thermometers capable of measuring temperatures above 41° C (105.8° F). Glass thermometers are not recommended because of potential injury to a patient with altered mental status and agitation. A Foley catheter is inserted into the bladder to monitor urine output.

It is critical that patients with heatstroke are quickly recognized and cooled. Clothing should be removed and the patient rapidly cooled to 39° C (102.2° F). Ice water immersion is the classic method used to cool these patients. The patient's trunk and extremities are immersed while the head remains above water. The technique provides rapid cooling and is noninvasive. It does limit access to the patient and should not be used if defibrillation or other resuscitative procedures are anticipated. Shivering occurs quickly and can be controlled using diazepam (Valium),* which is given intravenously in 2- to 5-mg increments titrated to the patient's response. Diazepam has no effect on thermoregulation. Chlorpromazine (Thorazine)* is no longer recommended for shivering due to its anticholinergic effects that may have an impact on thermoregulation.

Another popular cooling method is evaporative cooling, using tepid water continuously applied by spray bottles or sponged onto the skin, and fans. This is better tolerated than ice water immersion by the conscious patient. Shivering is treated the same as mentioned earlier. Theoretically, this method causes less vasoconstriction than ice water immersion. Studies evaluating cooling rates show ice water immersion cools very rapidly, and a number of studies demonstrate good survival rates with this technique. Literature on survival rates using the evaporative cooling technique is more limited, but one study showed a dramatic impact on survival using the technique on pilgrims to Mecca. Comparison studies on survival rates for the two techniques are not available. Many researchers, however, suggest weighing the ease of utilizing evaporative cooling (with appropriate equipment) against the difficulties with ice water immersion. There is considerable support now for using the evaporative cooling technique.

Ice packs may be placed in strategic locations, such as the groin and axillae, if ice water immersion is not utilized. Cold gastric lavage may be used if the patient's airway is protected. Cold colonic lavage is not generally recommended. Cold peritoneal lavage provides rapid core cooling but is limited by the experience of the physician.

Complications of heatstroke should be anticipated. Dextrose should be administered if the patient is hypoglycemic. Renal function must be monitored. Rhabdomyolysis is classically treated with fluids, alkalinization of the urine, and mannitol. Alkalinization of the urine may cause large shifts in calcium and potassium and tetany. Arterial blood gas measurements of oxygen and carbon dioxide tensions and pH can be corrected for temperature, but the clinical significance of this correction is debatable. Antipyretics such as salicylates and acetaminophen are not useful since the thermoregulatory setpoint in the hypothalamus is unchanged. Dantrolene is also not recommended for exertional and nonexertional heatstroke when muscular rigidity is not present. Patients with heatstroke should be admitted to an intensive care setting. Patients who are no longer hyperthermic on arrival to the hospital should be admitted for observation and monitored for complications.

---

*Not FDA-approved for this indication.

HEATSTROKE WITHOUT HIGH AMBIENT TEMPERATURE

Excessive muscular activity or rigidity may cause heatstroke, even when ambient temperatures are not elevated. Severe extrapyramidal rigidity with or without fever may predispose to severe hyperthermia and associated lethal medical complications. Neuroleptic malignant syndrome (NMS), serotonin syndrome, and malignant hyperthermia are all associated with heatstroke. Agitated states may lead to heatstroke in the absence of elevated ambient temperatures. These include drug-induced delirium and agitation (typically due to cocaine, amphetamine, or phencyclidine) with intense muscular activity; poisonings (salicylates, monoamine oxidase inhibitors, anticholinergic agents); status epilepticus; advanced parkinsonism; withdrawal from alcohol (delirium tremens) or sedative hypnotic agents; and thyrotoxicosis.

Neuroleptic malignant syndrome (NMS) is a rare disorder associated with use of neuroleptic agents. Controversy exists about the etiology of heatstroke in these patients—agitation and muscular rigidity versus central dopamine-blocking effects of neuroleptic agents on thermoregulation. Some workers feel it may be a combination of both. NMS occurs within the first 4 weeks (and sometimes longer) after initiation of neuroleptics, though most commonly in the first week. Patients present with severe hyperthermia, muscular rigidity, altered mental status, and autonomic instability. Elevation of CK, metabolic acidosis, hypoxemia, and hypocalcemia are common. Hyponatremia or hypernatremia, renal failure, and coagulopathies may also be present. Resolution occurs in 5 to 10 days following discontinuation of neuroleptics. Respiratory failure and cardiac arrest are the most common causes of death.

Lethal catatonia (or fatal catatonia) is another rare syndrome of hyperthermia, first described in the 1800s. These patients were in very hot asylum environments, were frequently dehydrated, and commonly treated with scopolamine as a sedative. These cases most certainly were due to exertional heatstroke brought on by manic hyperactivity and not caused by a rare form of hyperthermia.

Malignant hyperthermia is an extremely rare autosomal dominant syndrome that results in muscular rigidity, fever, and autonomic dysfunction in the presence of certain anesthetic agents. It is due to altered calcium regulation in the sarcoplasmic reticulum.

The *serotonin syndrome* is a recently recognized syndrome that usually occurs soon after increasing the dose of a potent serotonin agonist such as a selective serotonin re-uptake inhibitor or monoamine oxidase inhibitor, or after the addition of a second serotonergic agent such as lithium or meperidine (Demerol). It is characterized by altered mental status (agitation, anxiety, confusion, coma); hyperthermia; abnormal neuromuscular activity (tremors, shivering, myoclonus, hyperreflexia, rigidity — especially in the lower extremities); salivation and diarrhea; tachycardia; and mild hypertension. Ventricular tachycardia, hypotension, severe hyperthermia, and seizures have been reported.

Treatment of heatstroke without high ambient temperature is the same as for other forms of heatstroke. The top priority is to cool the patient rapidly at the same time that problems with airway, breathing, and circulation are identified and managed. Identification of underlying causes should be undertaken and specific treatments started, such as diazepam (Valium) for delirium tremens or seizure activity. Dopamine agonists such as bromocryptine (Parlodel)* and amantadine (Symmetrel)* are suggested treatments for NMS, but data on the efficacy of these agents is limited and anecdotal. Both are oral agents and therefore are not recommended for critical patients. Dantrolene (Dantrum)* is a nonspecific muscle relaxant that inhibits calcium release from the sarcoplasmic reticulum of skeletal muscle and has been anecdotally reported to be effective in treating malignant hyperthermia and NMS. It is given intravenously in the critical care setting. Diazepam (Valium) is also effective in the treatment of neuromuscular rigidity. Dantrolene (Dantrum) is not recommended for treatment of the common forms of heatstroke without rigidity. Some case reports suggest that serotonin antagonists such as benzodiazepines, cyproheptadine (Periactin),* propranolol (Inderal, Inderide),* and methysergide (Sansert)* may be useful in the treatment of the serotonin syndrome.

PREVENTION

Prevention of heat illness is focused on high-risk groups and situations. The work or play environment both inside and outside buildings can create a high-risk environment for the development of heatstroke. Elderly patients and their caretakers should be educated to limit activity on hot, humid days and given information on potential adverse effects of their medications. Parents of infants and small children should be warned of the dangers of prolonged heat exposure. Persons living in the higher stories of multistory buildings are also at higher risk. Air conditioning, proper acclimatization (usually around 2 weeks), adequate hydration, avoidance of alcohol and drugs of abuse, appropriate clothing/gear, and limiting exercise in hot, humid environments are important factors in the prevention of environmental heat stroke, especially exertional heatstroke. Finally, patients with agitation or rigidity are predisposed to hyperthermia and heatstroke and should receive aggressive intervention with sedation and temperature monitoring.

---

*Not FDA-approved for this indication.

SPIDER BITES AND SCORPION STINGS

method of
RICHARD F. CLARK, M.D.
San Diego Regional Poison Center
San Diego, California

Although there are 10 families of arthropods, very few have envenomation apparatuses large or advanced enough to pierce human skin. Of those capable of human envenomation, spiders and scorpions are perhaps feared most by humans. Folklore has largely contributed to much of this distinction, since the American Association of Poison Control Centers has recorded over 50,000 envenomations by these arachnids in this country over the past five years, with only one questionable resulting fatality. However, significant morbidity can occur from bites or stings from some varieties of these insects. A much greater problem in the United States is Hymenoptera-induced anaphylaxis, leading to several deaths each year.

LATRODECTUS

There are 50 American spider species with fangs capable of human envenomation. In North America, the most commonly implicated species are *Latrodectus*, or widow spiders, and *Loxosceles*, or brown spiders. There is at least one variety of *Latrodectus* in each state, and all can inflict a bite resulting in the same characteristic signs and symptoms. Female *Latrodectus* are usually large black spiders, the most common of which, *Latrodectus mactans*, has a characteristic red hourglass on her abdomen. Other species can be shades of brown or even red. The male is smaller and incapable of human envenomation. These spiders are not aggressive and only bite when threatened. They reside mostly in dark areas around garages, wood piles, and basements. Most bites occur to the extremities after clothing containing the spider is mistakenly worn.

Latrodectus venom is one of the world's most potent neurotoxins, thought to act at neuronal endplates, causing the nonspecific release of neurotransmitters such as acetylcholine and norepinephrine. The bite site is immediately painful, and most victims develop a pathognomonic "target lesion" during the first several hours after envenomation. Target lesions appear as a small, central, punctate red bite site surrounded by a blanched area and a peripheral rim of erythema. Diaphoresis may be present over the bite site or be localized to a distant area. Systemic symptoms such as hypertension, tachycardia, nausea, and vomiting may be present. The most characteristic symptom of *Latrodectus* envenomation is pain. Pain may be immediate or begin soon after the bite and is usually localized to the area or extremity of the bite. Depending on the severity, pain may remain localized, or it may spread to include the back, chest, or abdomen, often waxing and waning. Although many victims describe cramping of muscles, physical examination almost never exhibits extremity rigidity, and significant rhabdomyolysis is rare. Symptoms generally resolve in 24 to 48 hours without treatment. Necrosis of tissue generally does not occur.

Latrodectus envenomation can be divided into mild, moderate, or severe. Mild envenomations (Grade 1) are characterized by pain localized to the bite site and are treated effectively with oral analgesics. Moderate and severe cases (Grades 2 and 3) display extension of pain to sites distant from the bite as well as a variety of systemic symptoms and may require parenteral therapy. Although some patients may respond to intravenous calcium, our experience with this therapy has been disappointing. For moderate and most severe envenomations, we recommend liberal administration of parenteral opioid analgesics, such as morphine, combined as needed with a sedative such as diazepam. Many of these individuals will require hospital admission for repeated administration.

For severe *Latrodectus* envenomations exhibiting unrelenting generalized pain, or those with significant systemic symptoms such as hypertension, or when the patient is also pregnant, we recommend consideration of *Latrodectus*-specific antivenin. This antivenin is equine derived and should not be used in patients with allergies to horses or horse serum, or in individuals with multiple medical or environmental allergies. Skin testing is required before administration, but a negative test does not absolutely eliminate the possibility of an allergic reaction. We usually infuse the antivenin in 100 mL of saline, and one vial is often sufficient. Symptoms frequently resolve within 30 to 60 minutes of infusion and do not return. A second vial may be administered if there is no effect after the first, but alternate etiologies for the pain should be sought if relief is not attained after the second vial. Most patients can be discharged after 2 or 3 hours of observation following successful relief of pain with the antivenin, but they should be warned about the possibility of horse serum allergy in the future, as well as about the infrequent occurrence of delayed hypersensitivity or serum sickness (rash, myalgias, arthralgias) up to 7 days after the infusion.

LOXOSCELES AND NECROTIC ARACHNIDISM

Many different varieties of spiders have been implicated in causing necrotic skin lesions (known as necrotic arachnidism), including *Tegenaria, Lycosa, Phidippus,* and *Araneus*. Among the most fabled is *Loxosceles*. The most commonly encountered species of this group in the United States is *L. reclusa*, also known as the brown recluse, or fiddle back spider (for the violin-shaped marking on its cephalothorax). *Loxosceles* are timid, short-haired, and often inconspicuous, preferring dark areas of buildings; they bite only when threatened. *Loxosceles* spiders are found extensively across North America, but some of the most significant bites are inflicted by South

American species that have been transplanted to this country. *Loxosceles* venom is mostly cytotoxic, but patients with severe envenomations can also exhibit nausea, vomiting, fever, chills, and rarely disseminated intravascular coagulation. Hemolysis is occasionally reported, more commonly in children.

The bite from *Loxosceles* may not be immediately painful, but within 1 to 2 hours may become tender, with a gradually developing area of necrosis. A blister with some underlying necrosis may form over the bite site, and in most cases the lesion remains small and begins to heal in 2 to 3 days. Rarely, extensive necrosis can occur, requiring frequent débridement and occasionally skin grafting. No laboratory test is available to diagnose necrotic arachnidism. A complete blood count may aid in identifying the infrequent case of coagulopathy or hemolysis. Treatment for necrotic arachnidism is supportive; there are no antivenins. Good wound care is paramount, and antibiotics should be started if secondary infection is noted. Although elaborate therapies such as hyperbaric oxygen, dapsone, corticosteroids, and cyproheptadine have been suggested for limiting necrosis in severe necrotic arachnidism, animal studies evaluating these therapies have not demonstrated any greater efficacy than conventional wound care and débridement alone.

SCORPIONS

Several species of scorpions are found in North America. These arachnids are generally nocturnal and are common throughout the warmer parts of the southern United States. All are capable of stinging humans. Most species found in the United States cause little more than localized pain similar to that seen following Hymenoptera envenomation. Cytotoxicity or inflammation does not occur from scorpion venom, and the exact site of the sting may not be readily apparent. Only *Centruroides exilicauda*, found throughout Arizona, New Mexico, and parts of Texas and California, possesses venom potent enough to cause systemic toxicity.

C. exilicauda venom can open sodium channels on neurons, causing prolonged and excessive firing of axons, and may lead to abnormal activity along motor, sensory, and autonomic fibers. Systemic symptoms following a sting from this scorpion can be pronounced and extremely variable. Immediate onset of pain and tingling in the stung extremity is usually noted, which may become generalized. In severe cases, cranial nerve and somatic motor dysfunction may develop, leading to abnormal eye movements, blurred vision, loss of control of pharyngeal muscles, and drooling, occasionally resulting in respiratory compromise. Excessive somatic muscle activity may present as restlessness or uncontrollable jerking of the extremities, with severe cases at times mixed with generalized seizure activity. Nausea, vomiting, and tachycardia can be present in significant envenomations. Symptoms usually last 24 to 48 hours. Cardiac dysfunction, pulmonary edema, and bleeding

disorders can be seen with stings from Asian and African scorpions such as *Buthus, Tityus*, and *Androctonus* but are not found following envenomation by scorpions native to the United States.

Treatment of scorpion envenomation should consist of liberal use of analgesics and sedatives. Antihistamines, such as diphenhydramine, and barbiturates have been used by some clinicians with success. A *Centruroides*-specific antivenin is available only in Arizona; it is produced from goat serum. The antivenin is administered similarly to *Latrodectus* antivenin after skin testing, and one or two vials are usually sufficient to reverse all signs of toxicity. There may be up to a 60% incidence of serum sickness after *Centruroides* antivenin administration, which can be effectively treated with antihistamines and tapered corticosteroids.

SNAKEBITE

method of
CRAIG S. KITCHENS, M.D.
*University of Florida and Veterans Affairs
    Medical Center
Gainesville, Florida*

The combination of fear of snakes and the unfamiliarity of most physicians with the management of snakebite often leads to an unnecessary perception of danger on the part of practitioners. The physician should keep in mind that there are approximately 10,000 poisonous snakebites in the United States every year, and approximately 10 victims die; accordingly, the chances of a patient surviving are statistically overwhelming. In the past, treatment was often empirical or even shrouded by folklore. Because survival is statistically near certain, various therapies, including alcohol, ice therapy, electric shock therapy, or even no therapy, appeared to be efficacious. Treatment has now evolved from this disorganized state into a much more scientifically supported therapeutic regimen based on the availability of antivenin and the accumulation and reproducibility of several large studies published in reputable scientific literature. Morbidity and mortality can be minimized by appropriate therapy in conjunction with sound medical care.

This article discusses the diagnosis and treatment of patients bitten by North American poisonous snakes. In the United States, approximately 95% of poisonous snakebites involve pit vipers (family Crotalidae), which comprise multiple species of rattlesnakes as well as water moccasins and copperheads. Approximately 1 to 2% of all U.S. snakebites involve coral snakes (family Elapidae). A final 2 to 3% of snakebites are inflicted by exotic snakes that are either housed appropriately in zoos or kept, increasingly inappropriately, as pets. Treatment of persons bitten by exotic snakes is beyond the scope of this article.

It is of prime importance to know the species of offending snake, because prognosis and treatment are both heavily dependent on this information. Although additional undue risk should not be assumed by either the victim or others, identification of the snake is important, and it should be brought (either dead or alive) to the treatment facility, if possible. The species of snake is more important in terms of outcome than its size. Primary care practitioners and emergency room personnel should have at least a modicum of knowledge regarding poisonous snakes indigenous to the treatment area. For instance, in my locale in Florida, offending snakes vary from the pygmy rattlesnake *(Sistrurus miliaris),* whose bites have resulted in no recorded human deaths, to the eastern diamondback rattlesnake *(Crotalus adamanteus),* which accounts for the majority of deaths from snakebite in this country.

The majority of victims of snakebite are males ranging in age from adolescence to young adulthood. In my own series of approximately 400 patients, only 15 to 20% of all snake envenomations were truly accidental, with approximately 80% resulting from a combination of altered mental status from alcohol or other mind-altering substances and surprisingly stupid behavior. In fact, more victims knew the snake was poisonous than otherwise. Presumably, alcohol and other mind-altering substances lead to the bad combination of an increased sense of machismo and, unfortunately, a decreased reaction time, which often results in envenomation.

Because toxicology, prognosis, and treatment are dependent on whether the snake is a pit viper or a coral snake, the discussion that follows is divided between those two families.

CORAL SNAKE ENVENOMATION

Although coral snake *(Micrurus fulvius)* envenomation involves only 1 to 2% of all cases of North American snake envenomation, the neurotoxicity secondary to the snake's venom accounts for morbidity and mortality far in excess of frequency alone. Coral snakes are indigenous to the entire southeastern quadrant of the United States and can be surprisingly numerous, even in well-developed urban areas. A small and secretive snake, it has difficulty poisoning people because it lacks the envenomation apparatus characteristic of the pit viper family.

The morbidity and mortality of coral snake envenomation are due to neurotoxicity. Patients envenomated by this colorful snake may exhibit few or no symptoms for 8 to 24 hours and then develop an explosive progression of neurotoxicity, both local (paresthesias and dysesthesias in the bitten extremity) and central (cranial nerve paralysis, including apnea). Although data are inconclusive, it appears from collected cases that prior to the availability of effective antivenin, at least 50% of documented cases resulted in respiratory paralysis and death. This mortality has plummeted to near zero with the development in the 1960s of effective antivenin and respiratory support in intensive care units.

Key in the management of coral snake envenomation is recognition that local manifestations of coral snake envenomation are nil. Failure to realize this is a major and common pitfall. In contrast to pit viper envenomation, there is no swelling, no discoloration, and very little local pain, even with major cases of envenomation. The volume of venom injected is very small, and the venom is not composed of proteolytic enzymes, which account for the swelling, pain, and discoloration seen in pit viper bites. Accordingly, patients who have sustained even major envenomation

by a coral snake may be regarded as not having been envenomated because of the lack of local symptoms and the delay in neuropathic symptoms. These facts, coupled with the extremely high mortality in untreated cases, lead to the axiom that therapy should be aggressive in cases of even suspected coral snake envenomation.

There are three key indications for initiating antivenin therapy in coral snake envenomation: (1) proof that the snake involved was a coral snake; (2) history that the snake "hung on" and had to be forcibly extracted or flung off, often resulting in the sensation of layers of Velcro being separated; and (3) the presence of minute fang marks that may not even be visible unless pressure is applied, which results in the expression of small drops of blood through the skin, indicating access to the circulatory system. If any two of these three are present, therapy is warranted (Table 1).

The most common signs and symptoms in coral snake envenomation are paresthesias, nausea, vomiting, and euphoria. As the neurotoxin progresses centrally, patients experience diplopia, dyspnea, altered mental status, respiratory collapse, and generalized muscle flaccidity. Routine laboratory studies are not required for coral snake victims, as neither tissue destruction nor coagulopathy results.

In cases evidencing two or three of the treatment criteria, 5 vials of Wyeth antivenin for *Micrurus fulvius* are promptly administered after a nonreactive skin test. More severe cases or cases involving progressive neuropathy may require another 10 to 15 vials in the first 24 hours. Because cranial nerve paralysis is common in advanced envenomation by the coral snake, attention must be paid to the distinct possibility of aspiration pneumonia, which may be the most common secondary effect of the snakebite. Elective intubation to protect the airway may be in order for patients with progressive symptoms. With prompt therapy, symptoms may not be expressed. When symptoms are present before antivenin is given, reversal is usually complete in 3 to 6 days. No long-term sequelae have been noted.

PIT VIPER ENVENOMATION

Pit vipers comprise approximately 20 species of rattlesnakes that are spread throughout the continental United States. These snakes are chiefly encountered in nonresidential areas. Camping, back-

TABLE 1. **Therapy of Coral Snake Bite**

Assume coral snake envenomation with any two of these three:
 Positively identified coral snake
 History of snake "hanging on"
 Small fang marks through which blood can be expressed
Skin test and, if negative, administer 5 vials coral snake antivenin over 1–2 h. Repeat up to 20 vials for severe or progressive neurologic symptoms
Observe for and be prepared to protect against paralysis

packing, and other outdoor recreational activities bring humans into the snake's habitat. All pit vipers have a "pit" (an infrared heat-seeking organ) roughly halfway between the nose and each eye, as well as an efficient system for envenomation, which includes large venom sacs. This accounts for the unusually large appearance of their heads. Pit vipers have large hollow fangs through which the venom is injected into the victim. This venom has evolved as an offensive device to help snakes digest prey; it only inadvertently serves as a defensive weapon against larger animals.

Pit viper venom is extremely complex, containing a broad range of proteolytic enzymes to digest protein, fat, connective tissue, nucleic acids, and other biologic material. It also contains numerous small peptides, which may account for the autonomic symptoms observed, such as tachycardia, diaphoresis, diarrhea, and vomiting. There is a tremendous variability in the nature of this complex poison not only between species of pit vipers but also within species or within the same specimen observed over time. The variability of venom may account for the variability of signs and symptoms in pit viper envenomation.

Emergency treatment of the patient in the field involves prompt evacuation of the victim to a facility equipped to handle medical emergencies. Time should not be spent with local manipulation of the wound. If the snake can be apprehended and brought in without further danger, this will aid caregivers in diagnosis and treatment.

Highly characteristic of pit viper envenomation is the immediate pain, swelling, and discoloration of the bite site. Swelling occurs nearly immediately and is due to the dissolution of tissue. Discoloration often results from local hemorrhage and destruction of vessels. The pain is often likened to the intense, acute pain experienced from blunt trauma, such as slamming one's hand or fingers in a car door. The initial local tissue destruction resulting from pit viper envenomation begins nearly immediately and cannot be reversed by any treatment modality. As venom travels proximally through both the bloodstream and the lymphatic system, swelling progresses proximally; this progression may be either slow or alarmingly rapid. The rate of progression over time is key in distinguishing minor from moderate snake envenomations. Mild envenomation is characterized by local swelling, even of a marked degree, but not rapid proximal progression; moderate envenomation results in much more notable proximal progression, such as a doubling of the volume of swollen tissue every hour or so. Swelling, pain, and discoloration are characteristically noted within minutes of the snakebite, but occasionally may not be seen until after an hour or so. Lack of any local symptoms indicates either a bite by a nonpoisonous snake or a bite from a pit viper that was not accompanied by envenomation. These so-called dry bites constitute up to 20% of all snakebites and must be appreciated, as no systemic therapy is warranted in such fortunate victims.

Paradoxically, envenomation may be associated with very few local signs but severe systemic toxicity, including nausea, vomiting, hypertension or hypotension, bradycardia or tachycardia, diaphoresis, fasciculations, and cardiovascular collapse. This is best explained by envenomation in a muscular site having a rich vascular supply that allows the venom prompt access into the circulation, resulting directly in systemic poisoning and short-circuiting local manifestations.

Table 2 depicts the grades of envenomation of pit viper bites. The concept of grades is important, because it dictates prognosis and treatment (in contrast to coral snake bite, where even the possibility of envenomation is almost always treated with antivenin). Approximately 50% of pit viper bites are best treated with antivenin. Currently available antivenin is not recommended for milder bites, as the indications are less pronounced and the side effects of antivenin cannot be dismissed lightly. Commercially available antivenin is prepared from horse serum and is therefore antigenic. Up to 10% of patients have mild to moderate allergic symptoms (hives or wheezing) with the intravenous administration of an-

TABLE 2. **Grades of Severity of Envenomation by Pit Vipers**

Grade	Frequency	Findings	Antivenin Vials in First 12 Hours
No envenomation	15–20%	No local, systemic, or laboratory abnormalities 2 h after bite	0
Minimal envenomation	20–40%	Local and slowly progressive swelling without systemic or laboratory abnormalities	0
Moderate envenomation	20–40%	Rapidly progressive local swelling; systemic symptoms of nausea, vomiting, diarrhea, diaphoresis, fasciculation, moderate hypotension, and moderate hemostatic abnormalities, but without bleeding	4–8
Severe envenomation	5–10%	Severe systemic symptoms as above plus severe hypotension and lethargy; severe hemostatic abnormalities and possible bleeding	12–40

tivenin, whereas approximately 0.5% have major immediate reactions, including anaphylaxis. An additional 50% may develop signs and symptoms of serum sickness (rash, arthralgias, and fever) 1 to 2 weeks following administration of antivenin.

I do not treat patients with no or minimal envenomation with antivenin. Severe envenomation nearly always requires antivenin treatment, as do approximately half the patients who have moderate envenomation. Treatment with antivenin is advisable in uncertain cases when patients are at the extremes of age or have co-morbid illnesses.

Antivenin is the mainstay of treatment in moderate to severe envenomation by pit vipers. Antivenin testing should be done prior to treatment, as described in the package insert. Unfortunately, the accuracy of sensitivity testing is not good; anaphylaxis can occur following negative tests, and positive tests do not absolutely predict an allergic reaction. Testing should not be done on patients unless the therapeutic intent is to treat the patient, as skin testing itself can result in sensitization to horse serum. Patients who are bitten by poisonous snakes are more likely than the general population to be bitten again.

Table 3 provides various treatment suggestions. One of the most common and regrettable errors is failure to practice modern resuscitative medicine. Hypotension should be treated with aggressive fluid administration through at least one large intravenous site. Tetanus prophylaxis status should be determined and managed appropriately. Patients should be observed and treated in a closely monitored environment such as an emergency room or an intensive care unit until they are stable (usually 24 to 48 hours). If the decision has been made to treat with antivenin, skin testing should be implemented. If any tourniquets were in place prior to the patient's

TABLE 3. **Therapy of Pit Viper Envenomation**

DO:	▶ practice good resuscitation medicine
	▶ use standard tetanus prophylaxis
	▶ observe patient in a monitored environment (ER, ICU)
	▶ decide whether to use antivenin and then skin test
	▶ administer antivenin with crash cart and assistants nearby
	▶ release any tourniquets that might have been placed
	▶ prescribe antibiotics for "dirty" or manipulated wounds
	▶ serially examine bite site for viability
	▶ rarely (1–5%) surgically release anatomic compartment syndrome
	▶ rarely (1–5%) employ blood component therapy
DO NOT:	▶ skin test without intention to administer antivenin
	▶ use ice, tourniquets, or corticosteroids
	▶ cover, hide, or conceal bitten extremity
	▶ surgically "explore" wounds
	▶ send patients to surgery without vigorous fluid, electrolyte, and antivenin resuscitation

arrival at the emergency room, these tourniquets should not be released until antivenin has been administered. The administration of antibiotics is reserved for "dirty" wounds, which may result from manipulation of the wound site.

Laboratory evaluation should include coagulation studies (prothrombin time, partial thromboplastin time, thrombin time, and fibrin degradation products), a complete blood count and platelet count, and a chemistry battery that includes electrolytes and tests for renal and hepatic function.

The bitten extremity should be examined frequently to ascertain that neurovascular integrity remains intact despite swelling and pain. The leading edge of swelling and the circumference of the limb can be serially monitored to determine the rate of advancement. Darkened skin or bleb formation at the bite site are neither unusual nor ominous. The extremity should be placed in an anatomically neutral position, with slight elevation above the plane of the body. The extremity should be cleansed but not bandaged, as serial observation is key to good management.

Surgery is required in approximately 1 to 5% of patients, chiefly for those bitten in anatomically defined closed compartments such as the anterior lateral compartment of the lower leg or the palm of the hand. Other bites, although accompanied by impressive swelling, generally do not compromise viability of the extremity. Prior to surgery, resuscitation must be performed, including aggressive fluid administration, correction of hematologic and chemical abnormalities to the extent possible, and the administration of intravenous antivenin.

Coagulation abnormalities are often more impressive than important. Defibrination is common in rattlesnake bites, and occasionally one observes significant thrombocytopenia. Bleeding, however, is unusual, so these laboratory findings are usually not corrected unless the patient is bleeding or is being prepared for surgery or an invasive procedure. Heparin has no role. Platelets are best supplied by infusion of platelet concentrates, and cryoprecipitate (approximately 10 units) is the component of choice to resupply fibrinogen. Spontaneous correction usually occurs 6 to 12 hours after antivenin therapy if no blood products are administered.

Upon determination that antivenin is indicated, 4 to 8 vials of Wyeth polyvalent Crotalidae antivenin are mixed in 1 liter of crystalloid. Therapy is initiated at not more than 1cc per minute for 3 to 5 minutes; the remaining fluid is administered over the next hour. In severe envenomation, this may be repeated several times, up to a total of 40 vials in the first 12 hours.

Patients typically arrive in an emergency room from 30 minutes to 2 hours after the event. About 10 to 30 minutes is needed to determine the severity of the poisoning. Once the decision to institute antivenin treatment is made, it takes another 15 to 30 minutes for skin testing and interpretation. At the time the decision is made to administer antivenin, the first vials of antivenin should be prepared, as it often requires 30 minutes to go into solution. Ideally, antivenin administration commences within 60 to 90 minutes of the patient's arrival in the emergency room. Almost all antivenin should be infused in the first 12 hours, and usually no antivenin is administered after 24 hours following the bite.

Efficacy of the antivenin is demonstrated by a slowing or cessation of progressive swelling, although regression of swelling should not be immediately anticipated. Efficacy is also demonstrated by correction of metabolic and hematologic abnormalities, as well as a prompt reduction in systemic symptoms such as hypotension, diaphoresis, fasciculation, nausea, vomiting, and diarrhea.

Swelling typically resolves after 2 to 3 days, and full normal function of the extremity returns soon thereafter. A mild serum sickness may occur in up to 50% of patients treated with antivenin but is readily controlled with nonsteroid anti-inflammatory agents. Long-term sequelae are not noteworthy, although the risk of another encounter with a snake is likely.

UNDERWATER MEDICINE

method of
W. ROBERT LANGE, M.D., M.P.H., and
MAUREEN MORIARTY-SHEEHAN, R.N.,
C.A.N.P.

Johns Hopkins School of Medicine
Baltimore, Maryland

TRAUMA

Underwater injuries run the gamut from seemingly minor problems to life-threatening conditions. Even though the majority of such injuries involve incidental superficial wounds, it is important to remember one's ABCs when dealing with underwater injuries. Airways must be maintained, and breathing must be assured; an accident victim must not drown as a consequence of an underwater accident. Nor should the victim exsanguinate before reaching safety and more definitive aid, so circulation must also be preserved, remembering that extraneous blood in the water might be an invitation for additional trouble.

Underwater injuries should be regarded as contaminated wounds that must be thoroughly cleaned, vigorously irrigated with saline and/or hydrogen peroxide, adequately débrided, and appropriately explored. Wounds from coral and sea urchin spines are particularly prone to slow healing and scar tissue or granuloma formation. Foreign body material, including residual portions of marine life, may be difficult to detect but must be removed. Such wounds may require scrubbing with a soft brush or rough washcloth to remove embedded particles.

Antibiotic management should be tailored to the circumstances. Minor injuries should not be ignored and may need nothing more than a thorough cleaning and a topical antibiotic ointment for 4 to 5 days. More serious injuries necessitate more aggressive antibiotic coverage. Trauma leading to hospitalization requires treatment with intravenous penicillin or a third-generation cephalosporin. Nonhospitalized trauma patients should receive a broad-spectrum fluoroquinolone, such as ciprofloxacin (Cipro). More serious injuries, particularly bite wounds, should be packed open with delayed primary closure. The need for tetanus prophylaxis must be considered. Since clostridial organisms have been cultured from the mouths of larger predator fish, tetanus toxoid and even tetanus immune globulin may be selectively indicated.

COMMON FORMS OF DERMATITIS

Aquatic dermatology covers a multitude of conditions (bite and sting injuries are addressed later). Swimmer's itch is a condition associated with freshwater bathing, the result of exposure to cercariae (schistosome larvae), which attach to the epidermis and subsequently die. The condition produces a generalized pruritus and is prevented by brisk towel drying after freshwater swimming. It is treated with antipruritics and topical steroids.

Seabather's eruption, associated with saltwater immersion, is being recognized more often. Although prevalent in warmer waters such as in Florida and the Caribbean, cases as far north as Long Island have been described. The condition is characterized by an intensely pruritic vesicular or maculopapular rash of skin surfaces covered by swimwear. The rash typically begins within 24 hours of exposure, and pressure areas where swimwear hugs the skin are more prone to occurrence. Although previously attributed to so-called sea lice, the larva of the thimble jellyfish is now considered to be the cause. April through July is the high-risk season. Most cases resolve spontaneously with symptomatic therapy, but protracted cases may require steroid treatment. Delayed occurrences have been reported.

Swimmer's ear is the result of three factors: moisture, warmth, and microbial contamination. Predisposing factors include excess cerumen, underlying dermatitis, and so-called surfer's ear. It is a painful and pustular infection, and *Pseudomonas* species are typically involved. An irrigation solution of alcohol and vinegar is effective treatment. Pustular debris may be removed with peroxide lavage. Facilitating drainage from the external auditory canal following immersion can prevent the condition, and drying can be further promoted through the judicious use of a hairdryer after swimming.

BITE INJURIES

Fish

The majority of marine-related bite injuries involve what are generally considered to be docile fish and human carelessness. Divers who inappropriately handle or feed fish and fishermen who inattentively handle captured prey are typical victims. Most wounds are minor and need nothing more than the usual first-aid measures described earlier. The potential for infection is generally the greatest concern.

Some fish are more imposing and subsequently more dangerous, based on their sheer size. In his text *Dangerous Marine Animals,* Halstead states that large groupers and other members of the sea bass family may attain a length in excess of 12 feet and weigh upwards of 1000 pounds. These naturally curious fish are ravenous feeders and may appear aggressive because of their boldness. These fish possess sharp teeth that are in proportion to their size. In popular diving spots, some fish have become accustomed to being fed by divers, so close encounters are common, and bites may occur. Larger fish naturally inflict larger bites.

Despite the rarity of attacks, shark bite injuries are still a major concern. Worldwide, there are approximately 2 dozen attacks on humans per year, with the tiger shark, not the great white, most commonly involved. Based on size and feeding habits, a shark bite generally results in severe trauma. Sharks that feed on marine mammals often engineer an attack designed to inflict severe initial trauma and exsanguination, with the shark returning to feed after the prey has bled to death. Consequently, initial care must include both drowning avoidance and bleeding control, including the use of a tourniquet when indicated. Not all shark bites produce mortal injuries, but these wounds tend to be severe and require extensive medical management and coverage for infection.

Barracuda are generally inquisitive and not a threat; however, in some regions of the Caribbean, this fish is allegedly more feared than the shark. In recent years, there have been reports of giant barracuda actually jumping into small boats and biting the occupants. The reasons for such behavior are not understood, but these fish are not instinctively aggressive toward humans. Management is the same as that for a shark bite.

The moray eel is another fish worthy of specific comment. As with other large bottom feeders, these fish have become accustomed to human presence and to being hand-fed by divers in some areas. Although not aggressive, they may bite if handled or if a careless hand gropes within a moray's lair. Once a bite is inflicted, a moray may not release its grip until the victim is dead. As a result, the danger of drowning is real. Bites tend to be deep and jagged, and because the moray's teeth are coated with a bacteria-rich mucus, wound infection is to be expected.

Sea Snakes

Sea snakes have been described as the most abundant reptile on earth. Although not found along U.S. coasts or within Atlantic or Caribbean waters, they have been reported in the Gulf of California. These highly venomous reptiles, which possess one of the most potent venoms known, generally reside in the tropical Pacific and Indian Oceans.

Most bites result from extricating a snake that has become entangled in a fishing net, but during mating season, these reptiles become somewhat aggressive and territorial. Even though the fangs are relatively short and the mechanics of mouth opening interfere with effective biting, the teeth can penetrate a diver's wet suit. A small bite with minimal envenomization can be fatal. Not all bites involve envenomization, and fatality rates in the range of 30% have been described.

The venom is a potent neurotoxin, similar to that of the cobra, and the bite may be painless. An ascending paralysis, including cranial nerve involvement, is the typical clinical picture. Difficulties with vision, chewing, swallowing, and speech are common. Treatment involves immobilization of the affected extremity and the administration of an antivenin product. Even though specific sea snake antivenin is supplied through Commonwealth Laboratories in Australia, immediate availability can be a problem. Land snake antivenin can be administered, employing either tiger snake fraction or a polyvalent product containing krait fraction. Four or more ampules may be required. Hospitalization and intensive care are indicated, and assisted ventilation is often required. Renal shutdown is a risk, and dialysis is often indicated.

STING INJURIES
Jellyfish

There are over 200 species of jellyfish capable of inflicting sting injury, and despite popular opinion, the real coelenterate nuisances do not reside within U.S. coastal waters. The true threats are sea wasps, including the box jellyfish, which reside in Indo-Pacific waters. A sting results in immediate excruciating pain, the rapid development of shock, and the possibility of death within as little as 10 minutes. There is a Caribbean sea wasp whose sting may be sufficiently severe to require acute hospitalization, and a Chesapeake Bay variety that is less lethal. A specific sea wasp antivenin is available from Commonwealth Laboratories and is reserved for the Pacific variety. Experimentally, the calcium channel antagonist verapamil has been shown to block the reaction to the toxin, but its value under field conditions is unclear.

For U.S. physicians, the Portuguese man-of-war, whose tentacles may trail up to 100 feet, represents the most pressing challenge. The toxin induces histamine release and prostaglandin-induced vasodilatation. Consequently, its sting can produce systemic symptoms, including shock, and the risk of drowning is the most immediate threat. Treatment requires intravenous hydration and volume expanders, as indicated. Painful muscle spasms can be relieved with intravenous diazepam (5 to 10 mg) and 10% calcium gluconate (10 mL). Pain may require meperidine.

The topical treatment of jellyfish sting has been the subject of considerable debate. Because the stinging nematocysts release a proteinaceous toxin, the use of meat tenderizer (papain) for enzymatic deactivation has been investigated. The benefit is considered to be too little too late, and other treatment modalities should be pursued. The sting should not be treated with fresh water, as the hypotonic solution will induce further nematocyst discharge. A saltwater rinse is the best immediate treatment, taking care that the rinsing solution does not contain additional jellyfish. The topical administration of alcohol was previously considered an effective stinging deactivator, but this agent is now thought to promote nematocyst firing and is no longer recommended. Presently, vinegar is considered the best topical remedy for immediate first aid of a jellyfish sting, and the initial soaking should last 30 minutes. If vinegar is not available, any residual tentacles should be dried with the topical application of fine dry sand, salt, or talcum powder and then gently scraped away. After cleaning the sting site, the topical administration of a steroid cream should be continued for 5 days. Analgesics are usually required.

Other Invertebrate Stings

Fire coral, which is not a true coral, is present throughout tropical waters. The stinging cells of fire coral appear as fine hairlike filaments protruding from the main body of the structure. Contact produces an immediate burning pain; untreated, the discomfort usually resolves within several hours. Contact also produces a contact skin reaction that subsides within 24 hours, although chronic skin discoloration may persist for many weeks. Treatment consists of the local application of vinegar, followed by topical and/or systemic steroids. Sea anemone sting presents in a similar fashion and is managed in a similar manner.

Sea urchins are ubiquitous, and puncture wounds are common among divers and waders. In addition to acute toxicity resembling an insect sting, there is the risk of urchin spines breaking off below skin level, leading to foreign body and infectious complications. Injuries are also prone to tissue staining. The toxins are heat-sensitive, and immersion of the affected extremity in hot water (50° C) for 30 to 60 minutes produces deactivation and pain relief. Removal of broken spines is often more problematic, but because they are radiopaque, radiographic visualization can assist débridement. Spines do not dissolve from immersion in various chemical baths as was once believed.

A variety of sponges can release a toxin when handled. Local pain and burning, redness, and swelling are common reactions. This toxin is not inactivated by heat, which may actually worsen the symptoms, and cooling often helps. Symptoms typically subside over several days.

Sea cucumbers can produce a bothersome dermatitis if handled. Severe ocular symptoms, including blindness, can result if the toxin gets too close to the eye. Sea cucumbers can be lethal if eaten, as the toxin reportedly possesses potent cardioglycoside activity. Management of dermatitis includes removal of residual toxin by hot soapy water and the topical application of a corticosteroid preparation. Ocular symptoms require ophthalmic consultation and intraocular steroids.

Venomous octopi exist in tropical waters, and the Australian blue-ringed octopus is best known among toxic species. Typically shy, these creatures are a risk only if handled. Potent neurotoxins, including tetrodotoxin (see "Puffer Fish Poisoning"), that are capable of inducing respiratory paralysis can be injected with the bite. The toxin is not heat-sensitive, there is no antivenin available, and treatment is supportive.

A variety of other stinging invertebrates, including starfish, cone shells, and bristle worms, possess a heat-sensitive toxin. Again, immediate hot-water immersion followed by foreign body removal, appropriate wound care, and symptomatic management are indicated.

Vertebrate Stings

Even though close to 300 fish species are known to be venomous, the stingray is the best known. The sting typically occurs when the fish is accidentally stepped on by waders, although careless fishermen are also at risk. When provoked, the fish thrashes its tail upward, driving the stinging barb into the flesh, with subsequent infusion of the venom. The stinging apparatus may be left impaled in the tissue. Most symptoms are localized to the sting site, although some systemic complaints attributable to the gastrointestinal tract or neuromuscular system may occur. If the sheath of the stinging barb is still embedded, it should be carefully removed without squeezing more venom into the wound. Again, the toxin is heat-sensitive, so immersion in water as hot as can be tolerated results in toxin deactivation and symptom relief. The wound should then be cleaned as previously described.

Many of the fish capable of producing sting injuries also possess a heat-sensitive toxin, including scorpion fish, zebra fish (lion fish), stinging catfish, and stonefish. Management is the same as that for the stingray.

INFECTIONS

In approaching infectious disease, conditions can be categorized either by location (local, systemic, enteric) or by class of causative organism (viral, bacterial, parasitic). This section takes the latter approach.

Viral

The viral burden within the seas and the concomitant threat of human disease have not been adequately studied. Nevertheless, viral illness is regularly transmitted through infected seafood, generally via shellfish harvested from sewage-contaminated waters. Hepatitis A has been transmitted via raw clams and oysters, as well as by steamed shellfish that has been inadequately cooked or inappropriately handled. Most authorities recommend not eating raw shellfish. Hepatitis A vaccine is indicated for adventurous eaters as well as adventurous travelers.

Another viral illness associated with shellfish that produces a nonspecific gastroenteritis involves the Norwalk agent (and Norwalk-like agents such as the Snow Mountain agent). Following ingestion and an incubation period of 24 to 48 hours, nausea, vomiting, abdominal cramps, diarrhea, and headache are typical features. The illness is usually self-limited and of short duration—2 to 60 hours. Treatment is symptomatic.

Bacterial

Marine-associated trauma produces a contaminated wound, and bite injuries typically involve both aerobes and anaerobes, including *Vibrio* and *Clostridium* organisms. Trauma management, including antibiotic guidelines, has already been described.

Noncholera vibrios, particularly *Vibrio vulnificus,* deserve particular comment. This latter facultative anaerobe is widely distributed along U.S. coasts and is highly prone to infect wounds and rapidly progress to severe septicemia. It can also be transmitted from raw and undercooked shellfish, and certain patient groups are at increased risk. Although it is generally recommended that raw shellfish be avoided, the following patient groups should clearly abstain because of the risk of *V. vulnificus:* those with chronic liver disease (alcoholism, hemochromatosis, cancer, viral hepatitis, thalassemia major), impaired immune function (AIDS, cancer, steroid therapy), diabetes mellitus, or gastrointestinal disorders (low gastric acid levels).

Specific comment is also in order regarding *Pseudomonas,* the notorious cause of hospital-acquired infection. This organism can produce a folliculitis in association with whirlpool bath and hot-tub immersion. Malaise, chills, and low-grade fever, in association with a pustular skin rash over the lower abdomen, buttocks, or inner thighs, is a typical presentation. The condition has even been associated with public swimming pools and water slides, and inadequate water treatment and crowding are common factors. No specific antibiotic treatment is required, but steroids should definitely be avoided. Swimmer's ear, as already mentioned, is frequently associated with *Pseudomonas.*

Parasitic

Although a variety of parasitic conditions and organisms can be associated with the aquatic environment, including amoebic meningoencephalitis and *Diphyllobothrium latum* (fish tapeworm), this discussion is limited to issues surrounding sushi (or, more accurately, sashimi)—specifically, anisakiasis (herring worm disease). Although raw fish can be a vector for anisakiasis as a result of ascarid larva contamination, evidence suggests that the vast majority of reputable sushi restaurants serve conscientiously prepared, safe cuisine. Home-prepared dishes and those from restaurants not specializing in sushi are more problematic.

Although relatively rare, the incidence of anisakiasis is on the increase in the United States, and there is vast under-reporting. Raw salmon is the most common vehicle. Severe, sudden epigastric distress within 1 to 12 hours of consuming raw seafood should raise concern regarding the possibility of this condition. Upper gastrointestinal endoscopy is valuable in establishing the diagnosis and can be useful in subsequent treatment for worm removal. Thiabendazole 25 mg per kg twice daily for 3 days is also therapeutic if the worms remain localized to the stomach or upper intestinal lumen.

INTOXICATIONS

Ciguatera Fish Poisoning

Ciguatera is considered the most common marine intoxication. Dinoflagellates producing ciguatera toxins bloom as a result of ecologic damage to tropical and semitropical reef ecosystems. A variety of neurotoxins are produced that are subsequently passed up the food chain. Grouper, snappers, jacks, and barracuda are the most common species associated with the condition in the United States and Caribbean. In the South Pacific, moray eel are also incriminated. The toxins are heat-stable and are not inactivated by cooking or freezing.

These toxins produce a variety of symptoms, with nonspecific gastrointestinal complaints (nausea, abdominal cramps, and diarrhea) often occurring within hours of consumption. Cardiovascular findings (hypotension and bradycardia) may be evident, but the most enduring complaints are neurologic and include pruritus, headache, and paresthesias of the extremities and circumoral region. Cold-to-hot temperature-reversal dysesthesia and symptom worsening following alcohol consumption are classic features.

Symptoms typically last for 1 to 2 weeks but may persist for months or even years. Acute symptoms appear to be ameliorated by the intravenous administration of mannitol (1 gram per kg body weight piggyback over 30 to 60 minutes), but management of chronic symptoms is more difficult. Prevention involves avoidance of certain fish portions (organ meat), fish size (over 6 pounds), and fish species, particularly in highly endemic areas.

Scombroid Fish Poisoning

This type of toxicity is the result of consuming certain dark-meat fish (e.g., tuna, bonito, wahoo, dolphin, bluefish) that have been improperly handled following capture. Inadequate refrigeration allows bacterial decomposition of histidine to histamine. Although the clinical picture is that of an allergic reaction, it is a toxic syndrome rather than a hypersensitivity and is mediated by high levels of histamine in the fish (>50 mg per 100 grams). Reactions are more common and more severe in patients medicated with isoniazid (INH). Nausea, vomiting, flushing, itching, and even urticaria are common manifestations. The condition is short-lived, and treatment with antihistamine preparations facilitates relief.

Puffer Fish Poisoning

This condition is the result of eating puffer fish (fugu) containing the neurotoxin tetrodotoxin. It is uncommon in the United States, and toxicity can lead to respiratory paralysis. The condition has a relatively high fatality rate, and there is no specific antidote. Treatment is supportive, and prevention entails avoidance of puffer fish.

Shellfish Toxicities

Paralytic shellfish poisoning is the result of consuming shellfish contaminated with the neurotoxin saxitoxin. It is often associated with a "red tide" bloom, particularly during the warmer months. Severe symptoms can occur within 30 to 60 minutes of shellfish consumption. Paresthesias can progress rapidly to paralysis. Treatment consists of induced vomiting, activated charcoal, fluid management, and supportive care, including assisted ventilation when indicated.

Neurotoxic shellfish poisoning is a less severe toxicity that is managed in a similar fashion. In some coastal regions, particularly the southeastern United States, the toxin can be aerosolized in the surf, leading to upper airway symptoms, including cough, and conjunctival irritation. These symptoms are short-lived and require no specific treatment.

This listing is not complete, and other shellfish toxicities such as diarrheic shellfish poisoning and mussel toxicity mediated by domoic acid can occur. All require supportive management.

ACUTE POISONINGS

method of
HOWARD C. MOFENSON, M.D.,
THOMAS R. CARACCIO, PHARM.D., and
JOSEPH GREENSHER, M.D.
Long Island Regional Poison Control Center
East Meadow, New York

BASIC MANAGEMENT OF POISONINGS

The severity of the manifestations of acute poisoning exposures varies greatly with the age and intent of the victim. Accidental poisoning exposures make up 80 to 85%
of all poisoning episodes and are most frequent in children under 5 years of age. Many of these episodes are actually ingestions of relatively nontoxic substances that require minimal medical care. Intentional poisonings constitute 10 to 15% of poisonings, and often these patients require the highest standards of medical and nursing care and the occasional use of sophisticated equipment for recovery. Suicide attempts represent a significant number of these poisonings, and the use of toxic substances is often involved. The majority of the drug-related suicide attempts involve a central nervous system (CNS) depressant, and "coma management" is vital to the treatment.

Sixty percent of patients who take a drug overdose do so with their own prescribed medication and 15% with drugs prescribed for relatives. The top poisoning categories for all ages are over-the-counter analgesics, sedative-hypnotics, benzodiazepines, cleaning agents and petroleum products, alcohol and controlled substances, pesticides, tricyclic antidepressants, plants, carbon monoxide, and opioids.

ASSESSMENT AND MAINTENANCE OF VITAL FUNCTIONS

Upper airway obstruction is the most common cause of death in intoxicated patients outside the hospital. Any patient who is comatose and has absent protective airway reflexes is able to tolerate an endotracheal tube (cuffed for those over the age of 7 to 9 years) and should have it inserted as soon as possible.

Ventilation is required if the respiratory rate and depth are inadequate.

The circulatory status is best assessed by the blood pressure and heart rate and rhythm. The circulatory clinical status and tissue perfusion may be inferred from the skin temperature, the return of color after pressure blanching (capillary filling), and the urine output. Intra-arterial blood pressure measurements are essential for adequate monitoring.

If the circulation fails to improve after adequate ventilation and oxygenation, a 15- to 20-cm elevation of the foot of the bed may aid by increasing the venous return to the heart. A fluid challenge also may improve the circulatory status if hypovolemia is the cause. If these measures fail, plasma expanders and similar products may be required. As a last resort, vasopressors may be needed. If these measures fail to produce a response, a central venous pressure or pulmonary artery wedge pressure (PAWP) line should be inserted to monitor for heart failure and fluid overload.

The level of consciousness of all intoxicated patients should be assessed and the time of assessment recorded. The Glasgow Coma Score used in head trauma is not useful in intoxications because alcohol, depressant drugs, and hypotension may give falsely lowered scores. The Reed Coma Scale is preferred (Table 1).

PREVENTION OF ABSORPTION AND REDUCTION OF LOCAL DAMAGE

Ocular exposure should be immediately treated with water or saline irrigation for 20 minutes with

TABLE 1. **Level of Consciousness (Reed Coma Scale)**

Stage	Conscious Level	Pain Response	Reflexes	Respiration	Circulation
0	Asleep	Normal	Normal	Normal	Normal
1	Coma	Decreased	Normal	Normal	Normal
2	Coma	None	Normal	Normal	Normal
3*	Coma	None	None	Normal	Normal
4†	Coma	None	None	Abnormal	Abnormal

*Patients in Stages 3 and 4 require intubation and placement in an intensive care unit.
†Patients in Stage 4 need intervention to sustain life.

eyelids fully retracted. Neutralizing chemicals should not be used. All caustic and corrosive injuries should be evaluated by an ophthalmologist.

Dermal exposure is treated immediately with rinsing, not a forceful flushing in a shower, which might result in deeper penetration of the toxic substance. The skin should be rinsed with copious amounts of water for at least 30 minutes. Shampooing of the hair, cleansing of the fingernails and navel, and irrigation of the eyes are necessary in an extensive exposure. The clothes may have to be discarded. Leather goods are irreversibly contaminated and must be abandoned. Caustic (alkali) exposures often require hours of irrigation until the "soapy" feeling of the burn is gone. Dermal absorption may occur with pesticides, hydrocarbons, and cyanide.

Injected exposures to drugs and toxins or those introduced by envenomation may require a lymphatic restricting band and early suction. (See Antidotes 4 through 6 in Table 4.)

Inhalation exposure to toxic substances is treated by immediately removing the victim from the contaminated environment.

Gastrointestinal exposure is the most common route of poisoning, and an estimate of what, when, and how much of the toxic substance was ingested must be made. If there is a possibility of potential intoxication, gastrointestinal decontamination is performed rather than waiting for symptoms to develop.

Gastrointestinal Decontamination

To decrease gastrointestinal absorption, emesis should be induced or gastric aspiration and lavage performed. Neither of these methods is completely effective; each removes only 30 to 50% of the ingested substance. They are recommended up to 1 hour postingestion; however, there are few indications for induced emesis in the emergency department in an adult because it delays the administration of activated charcoal, which is more effective.

Emesis

Contraindications

Relative contraindications to the induction of emesis are (1) petroleum distillate ingestion of high-viscosity agents, (2) ingestions of agents that are likely to rapidly produce coma (short-acting barbiturates) or convulsions (propoxyphene, camphor, isoniazid, strychnine, tricyclic antidepressants) in less than 30 minutes and therefore may predispose to aspiration during emesis, and (3) prior significant vomiting.

Absolute contraindications to the induction of emesis are (1) caustic (alkali) or corrosive (acid) ingestions, (2) convulsions, because of the danger of aspiration and possible induction of laryngospasm, (3) coma, because of the possibility of aspiration with the loss of protective airway reflexes, (4) the absence of a cough reflex—an absence of the gag reflex is not a reliable indication of a lack of airway protection because a number of healthy people lack gag reflexes, (5) hematemesis, in which vomiting may produce additional damage, (6) age under 6 months, because of immature protective airway reflexes, (7) foreign bodies—emesis is ineffective and risks obstruction or aspiration, and (8) the absence of bowel sounds (when no bowel sounds are present, gastric lavage is preferred).

Inducing Emesis

Syrup of ipecac is the preferred agent but never fluid extract of ipecac, which is too potent, or salt water, which has produced fatal hypernatremia. It is not recommended that emesis be induced at home in children younger than 1 year of age; however, emesis can be performed in a medical facility under supervision when indicated. The dose of syrup of ipecac in the 6- to 9-month-old infant is 5 mL; in the 9- to 12-month-old, 10 mL; and in the 1- to 12-year-old, 15 mL. In children over 12 years and in adults, the dose is 30 mL. The dose may be repeated *once* if the child does not vomit in 15 to 20 minutes. The vomitus should be inspected for remnants of pills or toxic substances, and the appearance and odor should be noted.

Apomorphine is a parenteral emetic that must be freshly prepared. Its use is fraught with complications, although it produces more rapid onset of emesis than syrup of ipecac. We do not recommend its use in the cooperative patient. Naloxone (Narcan) should be available to reverse CNS depression.

Gastric aspiration and lavage may be preferable to the induction of emesis in cooperative adolescents or adults because a large tube can be introduced through the oral cavity. Contraindications to gastric aspiration and lavage in intoxicated patients are (1) caustic (alkali) and corrosive (acid) ingestions, because of the risk of esophageal perforation, (2) uncontrolled convulsions, because of the danger of aspiration and injury during the procedure, (3) ingestions of petroleum distillate products, (4) coma or absent protective airway reflexes, which require the insertion of an endotracheal tube to protect against aspiration, (5) significant cardiac dysrhythmias, which should be controlled first, and (6) hematemesis, which may be a relative contraindication.

The best results with gastric aspiration and lavage are obtained with the largest possible orogastric tube that can be reasonably passed (nasogastric tubes are not large enough for this purpose). In adults, a large-bore orogastric Lavacuator hose or a No. 42 French Ewald tube should be used; in children, a No. 22–28 French orogastric-type tube.

The amount of fluid used varies with the patient's age and size, but in general, aliquots of 150 to 200 mL per lavage are used in adolescents or adults and 5 mL per kg or 50 to 100 mL per lavage in children younger than 5 years of age.

Continuous gastric suction has been used for substances that have an enterohepatic recirculation or are actively secreted into the gastrointestinal tract, such as tricyclic antidepressants (imipramine [Tofranil]) and local anesthetics such as mepivacaine (Carbocaine) (Table 2).

Activated charcoal is produced by combustion of organic material in the absence of air until the carbon particle is formed. There are few relative contraindications to the use of activated charcoal: (1) it should not be administered before, concomitantly with, or shortly after syrup of ipecac because it may adsorb the ipecac and interfere with its emetic properties, (2) it should not be given before, concomitantly with, or shortly after oral antidotes unless it has been proved not to interfere significantly with their absorption, (3) it does not effectively adsorb caustics and corrosives and may produce vomiting or cling to the esophageal or gastric mucosa and falsely appear as a burn on endoscopy, (4) it should not be given if there are no bowel sounds, and (5) it should not be given if the location of the nasogastric tube cannot be confirmed (because of the potential for charcoal lung). Activated charcoal has no absolute contraindications, but it does not effectively adsorb alcohols, boric acid, caustics, corrosives, cyanide, metals, and drugs insoluble in aqueous acid solution (Table 3).

Table 2. **Substances with Enterohepatic Recirculation**

Chloral hydrate
Colchicine
Digitalis preparations (digoxin, digitoxin)
Glutethimide
Halogenated hydrocarbons (DDT derivatives)
Isoniazid
Methaqualone
Nonsteroidal anti-inflammatory drugs
Phencyclidine
Phenothiazines
Phenytoin
Salicylates
Tricyclic antidepressants

Table 3. **Substances Poorly Adsorbed by Activated Charcoal**

C—caustics and corrosives
H—heavy metals (arsenic, iron, lead, lithium, mercury)
A—alcohols (ethanol, methanol) and glycols (ethylene glycols)
R—Rapid onset or absorption (cyanide and strychnine)
C—chlorine and iodine
O—other substances insoluble in water
A—aliphatic and poorly adsorbed hydrocarbons
L—laxatives (sodium, magnesium, sorbitol)

Activated charcoal is a stool marker, indicating that the toxin has passed through the gastrointestinal tract and that no further significant absorption from the original ingestion will occur.

The dose of activated charcoal is 1 gram per kg per dose orally, with a minimum of 15 grams. The usual adolescent and adult dose is 60 to 100 grams. It is administered as a slurry mixed with water or by orogastric tube. A continuous nasogastric drip of activated charcoal, 0.25 gram per kg per hour, is an alternative in children. It should not be mixed with milk, marmalade, or starch because these interfere with charcoal's adsorptive action. Charcoal is administered with a cathartic initially. Subsequently, cathartics should be given every 24 hours.

Activated charcoal may be administered orally every 4 hours as long as bowel sounds are present, and it may be especially beneficial in intoxications that have an enterohepatic recirculation (see Table 2). Repeated dosing with oral activated charcoal has been shown to increase the clearance of many drugs without allowing enterohepatic recirculation (see later discussion of individual poisonings).

Catharsis is used to hasten the elimination of any remaining toxin in the gastrointestinal tract. Cathartics are relatively contraindicated (1) when ileus is indicated by an absence of bowel sounds, (2) in intestinal obstruction or evidence of intestinal perforation, and (3) in cases with a pre-existing electrolyte disturbance. Magnesium sulfate (Epsom salts) is contraindicated in renal failure; sodium sulfate (Glauber's salts) in heart failure or diseases requiring sodium restriction. Magnesium sulfate or sodium sulfate is administered in doses of 250 mg per kg per dose as 20% solutions. The adolescent and adult dose is 30 grams. In adults, sorbitol is given at 2.8 mL per kg to a maximum of 214 mL of a 70% solution. The cathartic should be given with the initial dose of activated charcoal. Sorbitol should be used with caution in children younger than 3 years of age and is not recommended in children under 1 year of age.

Dilutional treatment is indicated for the immediate management of caustic and corrosive poisonings but is otherwise not useful. Contraindications to dilution are (1) an inability of the patient to swallow, resulting in aspiration of the diluting fluid and (2) signs of upper airway obstruction, esophageal perforation, and shock. The administration of large quantities of diluting fluid—above 30 mL in children and 250 mL in adults—may produce vomiting, re-exposing the vital tissues to the effects of local damage and possible aspiration.

Neutralization has not been proved to be scientifically effective.

In whole-bowel irrigation, bowel-cleansing solutions of polyethylene glycol with electrolytes are used. It may be indicated with ingestions of substances that are poorly adsorbed by activated charcoal, such as iron, lithium, or sustained-release preparations. The procedure has been used successfully with iron overdose when abdominal radiographs reveal incomplete emptying of excess ingested iron. There are additional implications in other ingestions, e.g., body packing of illicit drugs, such as cocaine and heroin. The procedure is to administer, orally or by nasogastric tube, the solution (GoLYTELY or Colyte), 0.5 liter per hour in children younger than 5 years of age and 2 liters per hour in adolescents and adults. The end point is reached when the rectal effluent is clear. This takes approximately 2 to 4 hours. These measures should not be used if there is extensive hematemesis, ileus, or signs of bowel obstruction, perforation, or peritonitis.

USE OF ANTIDOTES

Antidotes are available for only a relatively small number of poisons. An available antidote should be administered only after the vital functions have been established. Table 4 summarizes the commonly used antidotes and their indications and methods of administration. Most informational, so-called first aid measures and antidotes on commercial product labels are notorious for their inaccuracy; it is preferable to contact the Regional Poison Control Center rather than follow the recommendations on these labels.

ENHANCEMENT OF ELIMINATION

The medical methods of the elimination of absorbed toxic substances are diuresis, dialysis, hemoperfusion, exchange transfusion, plasmapheresis, enzyme induction, and inhibition. Methods of increasing urinary excretion of toxic chemicals and drugs are being studied extensively, but the other modalities have not been well evaluated.

In general, these methods are needed in only a minority of instances and should be reserved for life-threatening circumstances or when a definite benefit is anticipated.

Diuresis

Diuresis increases the renal clearance of compounds that are partially reabsorbed in the renal tubules. Forced-fluid diuresis is based on the principle that it will shorten exposure to reabsorption at the distal renal tubules. The risks of diuresis are fluid overload, with cerebral and pulmonary edema, and disturbances in acid-base and electrolyte balance. Failure to produce a diuresis may imply prere-

nal or renal failure. If renal failure is present, dialysis should be considered.

Osmotic diuresis is meant to increase the osmotic gradient and prevent reabsorption from the proximal loop and distal tubules. Mannitol is used to initiate this type of diuresis, and then fluids are added in sufficient amounts to produce a diuresis similar to forced-fluid diuresis.

Acid and alkaline diuresis is based on the principle that inhibition of reabsorption of certain toxic agents can be encouraged by adjusting the urinary pH so the substance is maintained in its ionized form, which interferes with its passage back into the blood. Electrolyte and acid-base monitoring are necessary. Hypokalemia and hypocalcemia are frequent complications. Acid diuresis is accomplished by using ammonium chloride (Antidote 2, Table 4). Although it may enhance the elimination of weak bases, such as amphetamines and fenfluramine (Pondimin), it is not recommended. Ammonium chloride is contraindicated if rhabdomyolysis is present. Alkaline diuresis with sodium bicarbonate can be used in the therapy of weak acids, such as salicylates, and long-acting barbiturates, such as phenobarbital (Antidote 39, Table 4).

Dialysis

Dialysis is the extrarenal means of removing certain toxins from the body and can substitute for the kidney when renal failure occurs. Dialysis is never the first measure instituted; however, it may be lifesaving later in the course of a severe intoxication. It is needed in only a small minority of intoxicated patients (Table 5). Peritoneal dialysis is only one-twentieth as effective as hemodialysis. It is easier to use and less hazardous to the patient but also less reliable in removing the toxin; thus it is seldom used. Hemodialysis is the most effective means of dialysis but requires experience with sophisticated equipment. The patient-related criteria for dialysis are anticipated prolonged coma and the likelihood of complications, renal impairment, and deterioration despite careful medical management. Most dialyzable substances have a volume of distribution (Vd) of less than 1 liter per kg and protein binding of less than 50%.

Hemoperfusion

Hemoperfusion is the extracorporeal exposure of the patient's blood to an adsorbing surface (charcoal or resin). This procedure has extended extracorporeal removal to a large range of substances that were formerly either poorly dialyzable or nondialyzable. Hemoperfusion may be used for agents that have high protein binding, low aqueous solubility, and poor distribution in the plasma water. In these cases, hemodialysis is relatively ineffective. Hemoperfusion has proved useful in glutethimide intoxication, barbiturate overdose even with short-acting barbiturates, and intoxication with theophylline, tricyclic anti-

Text continued on page 1206

TABLE 4. **Antidotes***

Medication	Indications	Comments
1. *N-Acetylcysteine* (NAC, Mucomyst, Mead Johnson). Glutathione precursor that prevents accumulation and helps detoxify acetaminophen metabolites. **Dose:** *Adult,* 140 mg/kg PO of 5% solution as loading dose, then 70 mg/kg PO q 4 h for 17 doses as maintenance dose. *Child,* same as for adult. **Packaged:** 10 and 20% solution in 4-, 10-, and 30-mL vials.	Acetaminophen toxicity. Most effective within first 8 h (to make more palatable, administer through a straw inserted into closed container of citrus juice). **AR:** Stomatitis, nausea, vomiting. See Acetaminophen in text. The full course of therapy is required in any patient whose level falls in the toxic range.	IV preparation experimental.‡ The dose of NAC should be repeated if the patient vomits within 1 h after administration. Methods to stop vomiting of the NAC are: (a) placement of a tube in the duodenum, (b) slow administration over 1 h, (c) ½ h before NAC dose use metoclopramide (Reglan), 1 mg/kg IV over 15 min (max dose 10 mg) q 6 h; infants 0.1 mg/kg/dose IM, IV. Droperidol (Inapsine), 1.25 mg IV; for extrapyramidal reactions, use diphenhydramine (Benadryl) (see 19).
2. **Ammonium chloride.**	Not recommended.	
3. **Amyl nitrate.**	See 14, Cyanide antidote kit.	
4. **Antivenin,** black widow spider (*Latrodectus mactans).* **Dose:** 1–2 vials infused over 1 h. **Packaged:** 6000 U/vial with 2.5 mL of sterile water and 1 mL of horse serum 1:10 dilution.	Envenomation by black widow spider or by any *Latrodectus* spp producing severe symptoms. Most healthy adults survive with supportive care. Antivenin is used in elderly or infants or if there is underlying medical condition causing hemodynamic instability. **AR:** Same as for 5, Antivenin polyvalent because derived from horse serum.	Preliminary sensitivity test. Supportive care alone is standard management.
5. **Antivenin polyvalent** for Crotalidae (pit vipers), Wyeth, IV only. **Dose:** Depends on degree of envenomation: minimal: 5–8 vials; moderate: 8–12 vials; severe: 13–30 vials. Dilute in 500–2000 mL of crystalloid solution and start IV at slow rate, increasing after first 20 min, if no reaction occurs. **Packaged:** 1 vial (10 mL) of lyophilized serum, 1 vial of (10 mL) bacteriostatic water for injection, 1 vial (1 mL) of normal horse serum.	Venoms of crotalids (pit vipers) of North and South America. **AR:** Anaphylactic shock reaction occurs within 30 min. Serum sickness usually occurs 5–44 days after administration. It may occur in <5 days, especially in those who have received horse serum products in past. Signs and symptoms include fever, edema, arthralgia, nausea, and vomiting, as well as pain and muscle weakness.	Consider consulting with Regional Poison Control Center and herpetologist. Administer IV. Preliminary sensitivity test. Never inject in fingers, toes, or bite site.
6. **Antivenin,** North American coral snake, Wyeth, IV only. **Dose:** 3–5 vials (30–50 mL) by slow IV injection. First 1–2 mL should be injected over 3–5 min. **Packaged:** 1 vial of antivenin, 10 mL. 1 vial of bacteriostatic water (10 mL) for injection.	*Micrurus fulvius* (Eastern coral snake); *Micrurus tenere* (Texas coral snake). **AR:** Anaphylaxis (sensitivity reaction). Usually 30 min after administration. Signs and symptoms: Flushing, itching, edema of face, cough, dyspnea, cyanosis. Neurologic manifestations—usually involve the shoulders and arms. Pain and muscle weakness are frequently present, and permanent atrophy may develop.	Same as for Antivenin polyvalent for Crotalidae. Will not neutralize the venom of *Micrurus euryxanthus* (Arizona or Sonoran coral snake).
7. **Atropine** (various manufacturers). Antagonizes cholinergic stimuli at muscarinic receptors. **Dose:** *Adult,* initial dose 2–4 mg IV. Dose every 10–15 min as necessary until cessation of secretions. Severe poisoning may require doses up to 2000 mg. *Child,* initial dose of 0.02 mg/kg to a max of 2 mg every 10–15 min as necessary until cessation of secretions. Use preservative-free atropine if infusion. **Packaged:** 0.3 mg/mL; 0.4 mg/mL in 0.5-, 1-, 20-, and 30-mL vials; 1 mg/mL in 1- and 10-mL vials.	Carbamate and organophosphate insecticide poisonings. Rarely needed in cholinergic mushroom intoxication (*Amanita muscaria, Clitocybe, Inocybe* spp). Lack of signs of atropinization confirms diagnosis of cholinesterase inhibition. **AR:** Flushing and dryness of skin, blurred vision, rapid and irregular pulse, fever, and loss of neuromuscular coordination. **Diagnostic Test:** *Child:* 0.01 mg/kg IV. *Adult:* 1 mg total.	If cyanosis, establish respiration first because atropine in cyanotic patients may cause ventricular fibrillation. If severe signs of atropinization, may correct with physostigmine in doses equal to one-half dose of atropine. If symptomatic, administer until the end point of drying secretions and clearing of lungs. Hallucinations, flushing of the skin, dilated pupils, tachycardia, and elevation of the body temperature are not end points and do not preclude atropine administration. Maintain atropinization for 12–24 h, then taper dose and observe for relapse.

*This is for information purposes and is not intended to substitute for independent judgment. It is always advisable to review the package insert for the most up-to-date information. Contact Regional Poison Control Center for additional details on use.

†This dose may exceed the manufacturer's recommended dose.

‡Investigational drug in the United States.

§Not FDA-approved for this indication.

Abbreviations: AR = adverse reaction to antidotes; MP = monitoring parameters; FDA = U.S. Food and Drug Administration; Conc = concentration; ECG = electrocardiogram; TIBC = total iron-binding capacity; G6PD = glucose-6-phosphate dehydrogenase; CNS = central nervous system; GI = gastrointestinal; AV = atrioventricular; EEG = electroencephalogram; RBC = red blood count; CBC = complete blood count.

Table continued on following page

TABLE 4. **Antidotes*** *Continued*

Medication	Indications	Comments
		Atropine has been administered successfully by IV infusion, although this method has not received FDA approval. **Dose:** Place 8 mg of atropine in 100 mL D5W or saline. Conc = 0.08 mg/mL. Dose range = 0.02–0.08 mg/kg/h or 0.25–1 mL/kg/h. Severe poisoning may require supplemental doses of IV atropine intermittently in doses of 2–4 mg until drying of secretions occurs.
8. **BAL** (British antilewisite; dimercaprol).	See 17, Dimercaprol.	
9. **Bicarbonate.**	See 39, Sodium bicarbonate.	
10. **Botulism antitoxin,** Connaught Medical Research Labs. **Dose:** *Adult,* 1 vial IV stat, then 1 vial IM, repeat in 2–4 h if symptoms appear in 12–24 h. *Child,* check with state health department.	Prevention or treatment of botulism.	Contact local or state health department for full management guidelines.
11. **Calcium disodium edetate** (EDTA, Disodium versenate, Riker). **Dose:** *Adult,* max 4 gm. *Child,* max 1 gm. Moderate toxicity: IM or IV, 50 mg/kg/day for 3–5 days. Severe toxicity: IV or IM, 75 mg/kg/day for 4–5 days. Dose divided into 3–6 doses daily. Dilute 1 gm in 250–500 mL saline or D5W, infuse over 4 h bid for 5–7 days. For lead levels over 69 μg/dL or if symptoms of lead poisoning or encephalopathy: Add BAL alone initially, 4 mg/kg, then combination BAL and EDTA at different sites. EDTA dose: 12.5 mg/kg IM. (See "Lead" in text for latest recommendations.) Modify dose in renal failure. **Packaged:** 200 mg/mL ampules.	For chelation of cadmium, chromium, cobalt, copper, lead, magnesium, nickel, selenium, tellurium, tungsten, uranium, vanadium, and zinc poisoning. **AR:** 1. Thrombophlebitis. 2. Nausea, vomiting. 3. Hypotension. 4. Transient bone marrow suppression. 5. Nephrotoxicity, reversible tubular necrosis (particularly in acid urine). 6. Fever 4–8 h after infusion. 7. Increased prothrombin time.	Hydrate first and establish renal flow. Avoid plain sodium EDTA because hypocalcemia may result. Procaine 0.25–1 mL of 0.5% for each mL of IM EDTA to reduce pain. Do not use EDTA orally. Limit use to 7 days (otherwise loss of other ions and cardiac dysrhythmias may occur). **MP:** Calcium levels, urinalysis, renal profile, erythrocyte protoporphyrin, blood lead, and liver profile. Contraindicated in iron intoxication, hepatic impairment, and renal failure.
12. (A) **Calcium gluconate** 10%. **Dose:** IV 0.2–0.5 mL/kg of elemental calcium up to max 20 mL (2 gm) over 10–15 min with continuous ECG monitoring. Titrate to adequate response. **Packaged:** 10% solution in 10-mL vial.	Calcium channel blocker poisoning, e.g., nifedipine (Procardia), verapamil (Calan), diltiazem (Cardizem). It improves blood pressure but does not affect dysrhythmias. Hypocalcemia as result of poisonings. Black widow spider envenomation.	Repeat dose as needed. Monitor calcium levels. Contraindicated with digitalis poisoning.
(B) **Calcium chloride.** **Dose:** IV 0.2 mL/kg up to max 10 mL (1 gm) with continuous IV monitoring. Titrate to adequate response. Rate should not exceed 2 mL/min.	Hydrofluoric acid (HF) exposure (if irrigation with cool water fails to control pain). **AR:** IV bradycardia, asystole, necrosis with extravasation.	Infiltration with calcium gluconate should be considered if HF exposure results in immediate tissue damage and erythema and pain persist after adequate irrigation.
(C) **Infiltration of calcium gluconate.** **Dose:** Infiltrate each cm² of affected dermis and subcutaneous tissue with about 0.5 mL of 10% calcium gluconate using a 30-gauge needle. Repeat as needed to control pain. **Packaged:** 10% solution in 10-mL vial.		
(D) **Calcium gel:** 3.5 gm USP calcium gluconate powder added to 5 oz of water-soluble lubricating jelly.	Dermal exposure of HF less than 20%.	Gel must have direct access to burn area; if pain persists, calcium gluconate injection may be needed. Placing loose-fitting surgical glove over gel when fingers are involved helps to keep preparation in contact with burn area.

*This is for information purposes and is not intended to substitute for independent judgment. It is always advisable to review the package insert for the most up-to-date information. Contact Regional Poison Control Center for additional details on use.

†This dose may exceed the manufacturer's recommended dose.

‡Investigational drug in the United States.

§Not FDA-approved for this indication.

Abbreviations: AR = adverse reaction to antidotes; MP = monitoring parameters; FDA = U.S. Food and Drug Administration; Conc = concentration; ECG = electrocardiogram; TIBC = total iron-binding capacity; G6PD = glucose-6-phosphate dehydrogenase; CNS = central nervous system; GI = gastrointestinal; AV = atrioventricular; EEG = electroencephalogram; RBC = red blood count; CBC = complete blood count.

TABLE 4. **Antidotes*** *Continued*

Medication	Indications	Comments
13. Chemet.	See 42, Succimer.	
14. Cyanide antidote kit, Lilly. Nitrite-induced methemoglobin attracts cyanide off cytochrome oxidase, and thiosulfate forms nontoxic thiocyanate. **Doses:** *Adult,* amyl nitrite. Have patient inhale for 30 s of every min. Use new ampule every 3 min. Reapply until sodium nitrite can be given. Then inject IV 300 mg (10 ml of 3% solution of sodium nitrite) over 20 min. Alternative: IV infusion, 300 mg in 50–100 mL of 0.9% saline over 20 min. Then inject 12.5 gm (50 mL of 25% solution) of sodium thiosulfate over 20 min. *Child,* use following chart for children's dosage. **Packaged:** 2- to 10-mL ampules sodium nitrite injection; 2- to 50-mL ampules sodium thiosulfate injection; 0.3-mL amyl nitrite inhalant.	Cyanide poisoning. **AR:** Hypotension, methemoglobinemia.	*Note:* If child is given adult dose of sodium nitrite, fatal methemoglobinemia may result. Do not use methylene blue for methemoglobinemia in cyanide therapy. Observe for hypotension and have epinephrine available. Cyanide kits should have amyl nitrite changed annually. Administer oxygen 100% between inhalations of amyl nitrite. Monitor hemoglobin, arterial blood gases, methemoglobin concentration (nitrite given to obtain methemoglobin level of 25%). Some add nitrite ampule to resuscitation bag.

Chart should be used to determine dose of sodium nitrite and sodium thiosulfate in children on basis of hemoglobin concentration on left. Average child with normal hemoglobin requires 0.33–0.39 mL/kg of sodium nitrite up to 10 mL over 20 min.

Hemoglobin (gm)	*Initial Child Dose of Sodium Nitrite 3% (mL/kg) (do not exceed 10 mL)*	*Initial Child Dose of Sodium Thiosulfate (mL/kg) (do not exceed 12.5 gm)*
8	0.22 (6.6 mg/kg)	1.10
10	0.27 (8.7 mg/kg)	1.35
12	0.33 (10 mg/kg)	1.65
14	0.39 (11.6 mg/kg)	1.95

If signs of poisoning reappear, repeat above procedure at one-half above doses. Each agent should be given at rate of over 20 min.

Medication	Indications	Comments
15. Deferoxamine mesylate (DFOM, Desferal, Ciba). Has remarkable affinity for ferric iron and chelates it. **Therapeutic dose:** *Adult,* 90 mg/kg† IM or IV q 8 h to maximum of 1 gm per injection; may repeat to maximum of 6 gm in 24 h. *Child,* same as adult. IV administration can be given by slow infusion at rate not exceeding 15 mg/kg/h. **Packaged:** 500 mg/ampule (powder).	DFOM is useful in treatment of symptomatic iron poisoning or cases where serum iron is greater than 500 µg/dL. If DFOM challenge test is positive, it is not definite indication that therapy is necessary in asymptomatic patient. Oral DFOM is not recommended. Iron intoxication. Therapeutic—see dose in left column. *Diagnostic trial:* Give deferoxamine, 50 mg/kg IM (up to 1 gm). If serum iron exceeds TIBC, unbound iron is excreted in urine, producing "vin rosé" color of chelated iron complex in the urine (pink-orange). However, may be negative with high serum iron exceeding TIBC. **AR:** Flushing of skin, generalized erythema, urticaria, hypotension, and shock may occur. Blindness has occurred rarely in patients receiving long-term, high-dose DFOM therapy. Continuous infusions of DFOM over 24 h have produced severe pulmonary manifestations such as adult respiratory distress syndrome. Contraindicated in patients with renal disease or anuria.	Therapy is usually continued until serum iron <100 µg/dL, or when positive "vin rosé" urine turns clear, or when patient is asymptomatic. Therapy is rarely required over 24 h. Establish good renal flow. To be effective, DFOM should be administered in first 12–16 h. In mild to moderate iron intoxication or shock, IV route only. Monitor serum iron levels, urine output, and urine color.
16. Diazepam (Valium, Roche). **Dose:** *Adult,* 5–10 mg IV (max 20 mg) at rate of 5 mg/min until seizure is controlled. May be repeated 2 or 3 times. *Child,* 0.1–0.3 mg/kg up to 10 mg IV slowly over 2 min. **Packaged:** 5 mg/mL; 2- and 10-mL vials.	Any intoxication that provokes seizures when specific therapy is not available, e.g., amphetamines, phencyclidine (PCP) use, barbiturate and alcohol withdrawal. Chloroquine poisoning. **AR:** Confusion, somnolence, coma, hypotension.	Intramuscular absorption is erratic. Establish airway and administer 100% oxygen and glucose.

*This is for information purposes and is not intended to substitute for independent judgment. It is always advisable to review the package insert for the most up-to-date information. Contact Regional Poison Control Center for additional details on use.

†This dose may exceed the manufacturer's recommended dose.

‡Investigational drug in the United States.

§Not FDA-approved for this indication.

Abbreviations: AR = adverse reaction to antidotes; MP = monitoring parameters; FDA = U.S. Food and Drug Administration; Conc = concentration; ECG = electrocardiogram; TIBC = total iron-binding capacity; G6PD = glucose-6-phosphate dehydrogenase; CNS = central nervous system; GI = gastrointestinal; AV = atrioventricular; EEG = electroencephalogram; RBC = red blood count; CBC = complete blood count.

Table continued on following page

TABLE 4. **Antidotes** * *Continued*

Medication	Indications	Comments
17. **Dimercaprol** (Bal, Hynson, Westcott, & Dunning). **Dose:** Recommendations vary; contact Regional Poison Control Center. Prevents inhibition of sulfhydryl enzymes. Given deep IM only. *For severe lead poisoning*—see 11, Calcium disodium edetate. *For mild arsenic or gold poisoning*—2.5 mg/kg q 6 h for 2 days, then q 12 h on third day, and once daily thereafter for 10 days. *For severe arsenic or gold poisoning*—3–5 mg/kg q 6 h for 3 days, then q 12 h thereafter for 10 days.† *For mercury poisoning*—5 mg/kg initially, followed by 2.5 mg/kg 1 or 2 times daily for 10 days. **Packaged:** 100 mg/mL 10% in oil in 3-mL ampules.	For chelation of antimony, arsenic, bismuth, chromates, copper, gold, lead, mercury, and nickel. **AR:** 30% of patients have reactions: fever (30% of children), hypertension, tachycardia, may cause hemolysis in G6PD deficiency patients. Doses greater than recommended may cause various adverse effects: nausea, vomiting, headache, chest pain, tachycardia, and hypertension.	Contraindicated in instances of hepatic insufficiency, with exception of postarsenic jaundice. Should be discontinued or used only with extreme caution if acute renal insufficiency is present. Monitor blood pressure and heart rate (both may increase), urinalysis, qualitative urine excretion of heavy metal. Contraindicated in iron, silver, uranium, selenium, and cadmium poisoning.
18. **Dimercaptosuccinic acid** (DMSA).	See 42, Succimer.	
19. **Diphenhydramine** (Benadryl, Parke-Davis). Antiparkinsonian action. **Dose:** Adult, 10–50 mg IV over 2 min. *Child,* 1–2 mg/kg IV up to 50 mg over 2 min. Max in 24 h: 400 mg. **Packaged:** 10 mg/mL in 10- and 30-mL vials. 50 mg/mL in 1-, 5-, 10-, and 30-mL vials. Capsules, tablets 25 and 50 mg. Elixir, syrup 12.5 mg/5 mL.	Used to treat extrapyramidal symptoms and dystonia induced by pheno-thiazines and related drugs. **AR:** Fatal dose, 20–40 mg/kg. Dry mouth, drowsiness.	Continue with oral diphenyhydramine, 5 mg/kg/day to 25 mg 3 times a day for 72 h, to avoid recurrence.
20. **EDTA.**	See 11, Calcium disodium edetate.	
21. **Ethanol** (ETOH). Competitively inhibits alcohol dehydrogenase. **Dose:** *Loading*—administer 7.6–10.0 mL/kg of 10% ETOH in D5W over 30 min IV or 0.8–1.0 mL/kg 95% ETOH PO in 6 oz of orange juice over 30 min. While administering loading dose, start maintenance. *Maintenance:* Volume of 10% ETOH needed IV or 95% oral solution (not in dialysis). See chart on maintenance dose, below. If patient is on dialysis, add 91 mL/h in addition to regular maintenance dose. See comments to prepare 10% solution if not commercially available. **Packaged:** 10% ethanol in D5W 1000 mL; 95% ethanol. May be given as 50% solution orally.	Methanol, ethylene glycol poisoning. Ethanol infusion therapy may be started in cases of suspected methanol and ethylene glycol poisoning presenting with increased anion gap and osmolal gap, or if urine shows crystalluria of ethylene glycol poisoning or hyperemia of optic disk of methanol intoxication. **AR:** CNS depression, hypoglycemia.	Monitor blood ethanol 1 h after starting infusion and q 4–6 h. Maintain blood ethanol concentration of 100–200 mg/dL. Monitor blood glucose, electrolytes, blood gases, urinalysis, and renal profile at least daily. Continue infusion until safe concentration of ethylene glycol or methanol is reached. Ethanol-induced hypoglycemia may occur. Dialysis, preferably hemodialysis, should be considered in severe intoxication not controlled by ethanol alone. To prepare 10% ethanol for infusion therapy: Remove 100 mL from 1 L of D5W and replace with 100 mL of tax-free bulk absolute alcohol after passing through 0.22-μm filter; 50-mL vials of pyrogen-free absolute ethanol for injection are available from Aper Alcohol Company, Shelbyville, KY, telephone 800-456-1017, or American Reagent, Shirley, NY, telephone 800-645-1706.

Maintenance Dose

Patient Category	mL/kg/h using 10% IV	mL/kg/h using 50% oral
Nondrinker	0.83	0.17
Occasional drinker	1.40	0.28
Alcoholic	1.96	0.39

Medication	Indications	Comments
22. **Fab** (antibody fragment, Digibind). **Dose:** Average dose used during clinical testing was 10 vials. Dosage details are specified by manufacturer. It should be administered by IV route over 30 min. Calculate on basis of body burden either by known amount ingested or by serum digoxin concentration.	Toxicity due to digoxin, digitoxin, oleander tea, with following: 1. Imminent cardiac arrest or shock. 2. Hyperkalemia >5.5 mEq/L. 3. Serum digoxin >10 ng/mL at 6–12 h postingestion in adults. 4. Life-threatening dysrhythmias. 5. Ingestion over 10 mg in adults or 4 mg in child (0.3 mg/kg). 6. Bradycardia or second- or third-degree heart block unresponsive to atropine.	Contact Regional Poison Control Center. Preliminary sensitivity test. Administer through a 0.22-μm filter. Fab causes a rise in measured bound digoxin but a fall in free digoxin. 40 mg binds 0.6 mg of digoxin.

*This is for information purposes and is not intended to substitute for independent judgment. It is always advisable to review the package insert for the most up-to-date information. Contact Regional Poison Control Center for additional details on use.

†This dose may exceed the manufacturer's recommended dose.

‡Investigational drug in the United States.

§Not FDA-approved for this indication.

Abbreviations: AR = adverse reaction to antidotes; MP = monitoring parameters; FDA = U.S. Food and Drug Administration; Conc = concentration; ECG = electrocardiogram; TIBC = total iron-binding capacity; G6PD = glucose-6-phosphate dehydrogenase; CNS = central nervous system; GI = gastrointestinal; AV = atrioventricular; EEG = electroencephalogram; RBC = red blood count; CBC = complete blood count.

Medication	Indications	Comments
Calculation of Dose of Fab: 1. Known amount ingested multiplied by bioavailability (0.8) = body burden. Body burden divided by 0.6 = number of vials. 2. Known serum digoxin (obtained 6 h postingestion) multiplied by Vd (5.6 L/kg) and weight in kg divided by 1000 = body burden. Body burden divided by 0.6 = number of vials.		
23. **Flumazenil** (Romazicon, Roche Labs), Benzodiazepine (BZP) receptor antagonist. **Dose:** 1. *Management of BZP overdose:* (Caution) 0.2 mg (2 mL) IV over 30 sec; may repeat after 30 s with 0.3 mg (3 mL). Further doses of 0.5 mg over 30 s. If no response in 5 min and max of 5 mg, cause of sedation is unlikely to be BZP. 2. *Reversal of conscious sedation or in general anesthesia:* 0.2 mg (2 mL) IV over 15 s; may repeat in 45 s. Doses may be repeated at 60-s intervals to max dose of 1 mg (10 mL). If resedation, repeated doses may be administered at 20-min intervals to max 1 mg (0.2 mg/min). Max 3 mg should be given in any 1 h. **Packaged:** 0.1 mg/mL in 5- and 10-mL multiple-use vials.	1. Reversal of sedative effects of BZP general anesthesia. 2. Sedation with BZP for procedures. 3. Caution in management of overdose. **AR:** Convulsions, dizziness, injection site pain, increased sweating, headache, and abnormal or blurred vision (3–9%).	Not treatment for hypoventilation. Caution with overdose. Flumazenil is not recommended for cyclic antidepressant poisoning, or if patient has seizures or increased intracranial pressure. Flumazenil has been associated with seizures in long-term benzodiazepine use or dependency.
24. **Folic acid.**	See 28, Leucovorin.	
25. **Folinic acid.**	See 28, Leucovorin.	
26. **Glucagon.** Works by stimulating production of cyclic adenyl monophosphate. **Dose:** 50–150 μg/kg over 1 min IV followed by a continuous infusion of 1–5 mg/h in dextrose. Then taper over 5–12 h. 2 mg of phenol per 1 mg of glucagon. 50 mg is the maximum amount of phenol recommended; therefore, toxicity may result when high doses of glucagon are used. **Packaged:** 1-mg (1-U) vial with 1-mL diluent with glycerin and phenol; also in 10-mL size.	Beta blocker, quinidine, and calcium channel blocker intoxication. **AR:** Glucagon is generally well tolerated—most frequent reactions are nausea, vomiting.	Do not dissolve the lyophilized glucagon in the solvent packaged with it when administering IV infusion because of possible phenol toxicity. Use D5W, not 0.9% saline. Effects of single dose observed in 5–10 min and last for 15–30 min. A constant infusion may be necessary to sustain desired effects.
27. **Labetalol hydrochloride** (Normodyne, Schering; Trandate, Glaxo). Nonselective beta and mild alpha blocker. **Dose:** IV 20 mg over 2 min. Additional injections of 40 or 80 mg can be given at 10-min intervals until desired supine blood pressure is achieved. Max dose 300 mg. Alternative: Slow IV infusion: 200 mg (40 mL) is added to 160 or 250 mL of D5W and given at 2 mg/min. Titrate infusion according to response. **Packaged:** Solution 5 mg/mL in 20 mL.	Hypertensive crises secondary to cocaine. **AR:** GI disturbances, orthostatic hypotension, bronchospasm, congestive heart failure, AV conduction disturbances, and peripheral vascular reactions.	Concomitant diuretic enhances therapeutic response. Patient should be kept in supine position during infusion. **MP:** Monitor blood pressure during and after administration.
28. **Leucovorin.** **Dose:** For methanol poisoning: 1 mg/kg up to 50 mg IV q 4 h for 6 doses. For methotrexate overdose, see comments. **Packaged:** 3 mg/mL (1 mL), 5 mg/mL (1 and 5 mL), 50 mg/vial.	1. **Methanol poisoning§:** Active form of folic acid used to enhance metabolism of formic acid in animals to carbon dioxide and water. 2. **Methotrexate (MTX) overdose:** Supplies tetrahydrofolate cofactor, which is blocked by methotrexate. **AR:** Allergic sensitization.	For MTX overdose, initial dose can be given IV or IM in MTX equivalent dose up to 75 mg. If MTX blood level is measured 6 h postingestion and is above 10^{-8} molar or is unavailable, give 12 mg q 6 h after MTX level is below 10^{-8} molar. Alternatively, if GI function is adequate, may give orally 10 mg/m^2 q 6 h until MTX levels are lowered to less than 10^{-8} molar. Leucovorin in doses of 5–15 mg/day PO has also been recommended to counteract hematologic toxicity from folic acid antagonists such as trimethoprim and pyrimethamine.

*This is for information purposes and is not intended to substitute for independent judgment. It is always advisable to review the package insert for the most up-to-date information. Contact Regional Poison Control Center for additional details on use.

†This dose may exceed the manufacturer's recommended dose.

‡Investigational drug in the United States.

§Not FDA-approved for this indication.

Abbreviations: AR = adverse reaction to antidotes; MP = monitoring parameters; FDA = U.S. Food and Drug Administration; Conc = concentration; ECG = electrocardiogram; TIBC = total iron-binding capacity; G6PD = glucose-6-phosphate dehydrogenase; CNS = central nervous system; GI = gastrointestinal; AV = atrioventricular; EEG = electroencephalogram; RBC = red blood count; CBC = complete blood count.

Table continued on following page

TABLE 4. **Antidotes*** *Continued*

Medication	Indications	Comments
29. **Methylene blue.** Methylene blue reduces ferric ion of methemoglobin to ferrous ion of hemoglobin. **Dose:** *Adult,* 0.1–0.2 mL/kg of 1% solution (1–2 mg/kg) over 5 min IV. Max adults 7 mg/kg. *Child,* same as adults. Max infants 4 mg/kg. May repeat in 1 h if necessary. Repeat only once. **Packaged:** 1% 10-mL ampules.	Methemoglobinemia. **AR:** GI (nausea, vomiting), headache, hypertension, dizziness, mental confusion, restlessness, dyspnea, hemolysis, blue skin, blue urine, burning sensation in vein when IV dose exceeds 7 mg/kg. Treatment is unnecessary unless methemoglobin is over 30% or respiratory distress is present.	Saliva, urine, and other body fluids may turn blue. Contraindications: Renal insufficiency, cyanide poisoning when sodium nitrite is used to induce methemoglobinemia; in G6PD-deficiency patients. Monitor hemolysis, methemoglobin level, and arterial blood gases. Avoid extravasation because of local necrosis.
30. **Naloxone** (Narcan). Pure opioid antagonist. **Dose:** *Adult,* 0.4–2.0 mg IV and repeat at 3-min intervals until respiratory function is stable. Before excluding opioid intoxication on basis of lack of naloxone response, minimum of 2 mg in child or 10 mg in adult should be administered. *Child,* initial dose is 0.1 mg/kg IV. **Packaged:** 0.02 mg/mL, 0.4 mg/mL ampule, 10-mL multidose vial.	1. Comatose (not just lethargic) patient. 2. Ineffective ventilation or adult respiratory rate <12. 3. Pinpoint pupils. 4. Circumstantial evidence of opioid intoxication, e.g., known drug abuser, track marks, opioid paraphernalia. **AR:** Relatively free of adverse reactions. Rare reports of pulmonary edema. Should be administered with caution in pregnancy.	Naloxone infusion therapy should be used if large initial dose was required, repeated boluses are necessary, or long-acting opiate is involved. In infusion therapy initial response dose is administered every hour and may need to be boostered in ½ h after starting. Infusion may be tapered after 12 h of therapy. Naloxone infusion: calculate daily fluid requirements, add initial response dose of naloxone multiplied by 24 to solution. Divide fluid by 24 h for naloxone infusion rate/h. Does not cause CNS depression. Routes: IV and endotracheal are preferred routes. Pentazocine (Talwin), dextramethorphan, propoxyphene (Darvon), and codeine may require larger doses.
31. **Nicotinamide,** various manufacturers. **Dose:** *Adult,* 500 mg IM or IV slowly, then 200–400 mg q 4 h. If symptoms develop, the frequency of injections should be increased to q 2 h (max 3 gm/day). *Child,* One-half suggested adult dose. **Packaged:** 100 mg/mL: 2-, 5-, 10-, and 30-mL vials; 25- and 50-mg tablets.	Vacor poisoning: phenylurea pesticide intoxication. *Note:* Vacor 2% is now available only to professional exterminators. 0.5% Vacor is available to general public and can be toxic to children if swallowed. **AR:** Large doses—flushing, pruritus, sensation of burning, nausea, vomiting, anaphylactic shock.	Nicotinamide is most effective when given within 1 h of ingestion. Do not use niacin or nicotinic acid in place of nicotinamide. Monitor liver profile.
32. **Oxygen** 100%. **Dose:** *Adult,* 100% oxygen by inhalation or 100% oxygen in hyperbaric chamber at 2–3 atm. *Child,* Same as adult.	Carbon monoxide or cyanide exposure, methemoglobinemia. Any inhalation intoxication.	The t½ of carboxyhemoglobin is 240 min in room air 21% oxygen; if patient is hyperventilated with 100% oxygen, t½ of carboxyhemoglobin is 90 min; in chamber at 2 atm, t½ is 25–30 min.
33. **Pancuronium bromide** (Pavulon, Organon). Nondepolarizing (competitive) blocking agent. **Dose:** *Adults and children,* initially, 0.1 mg/kg IV; for intubation, 0.1 mg/kg IV, repeated as required (generally every 40–60 min).† **Packaged:** Solution 1 mg/mL in 10 mL. 2 mg/mL in 2- and 5-mL containers.	Neuromuscular blocking agent. Used for intubation and seizure control, acts in 2 min, lasts 40–60 min. **AR:** Main hazard is inadequate postoperative ventilation. Tachycardia and slight increase in arterial pressure may occur due to vagolytic action.	Required dose varies greatly, and a peripheral nerve stimulator aids in determining appropriate amount. Should monitor EEG, because motor effect may be abolished without decreasing electrical discharge from brain.
34. **D-Penicillamine** (Cuprimine, Merck; Depen, Wallace Labs). Effective chelator and promotes excretion in urine. **Dose:** *Adults,* 250 mg 4 times daily PO for up to 5 days for long-term (20–40 days) therapy; 30–40 mg/kg/day in children. Max 1 gm/day. For chronic therapy, 25 mg/kg/day in 4 doses. **Packaged:** 125- and 250-mg capsules.	For chelation of heavy metals: arsenic, cadmium, chromates, cobalt, copper, lead, mercury, nickel, and zinc. **MP:** Routine urinalysis, white blood count differential, hemoglobin determination, direct platelet count, renal and hepatic profiles. Collect 24-h urine, quantify for heavy metal. **AR:** Leukopenia (2%); thrombocytopenia (4%); GI—nausea, vomiting, diarrhea (17%); anaphylactic shock, fever, rash, lupus syndrome, renal and hepatic injury.	This is not considered standard therapy for lead poisoning after chelation therapy. May produce ampicillin-like rash, allergic reactions, neutropenia, and nephropathy. Contraindication: hypersensitivity to penicillin.

*This is for information purposes and is not intended to substitute for independent judgment. It is always advisable to review the package insert for the most up-to-date information. Contact Regional Poison Control Center for additional details on use.

†This dose may exceed the manufacturer's recommended dose.

‡Investigational drug in the United States.

§Not FDA-approved for this indication.

Abbreviations: AR = adverse reaction to antidotes; MP = monitoring parameters; FDA = U.S. Food and Drug Administration; Conc = concentration; ECG = electrocardiogram; TIBC = total iron-binding capacity; G6PD = glucose-6-phosphate dehydrogenase; CNS = central nervous system; GI = gastrointestinal; AV = atrioventricular; EEG = electroencephalogram; RBC = red blood count; CBC = complete blood count.

TABLE 4. **Antidotes*** *Continued*

Medication	Indications	Comments
35. **Physostigmine salicylate** (Antilirium, O'Neil). Cholinesterase inhibitor; a diagnostic trial is not recommended. **Dose:** *Adult,* 1–2 mg IV over 2 min; may repeat every 5 min to max dose of 6 mg. *Child,* IV, 0.5 mg (0.02 mg/kg) over paralysis, 2 min to max dose of 2 mg q 30–60 min if symptoms recur.† Once effect is accomplished, give lowest effective dose. **Packaged:** 1 mg/mL in 2-mL ampule.	Not advised for use in diagnostic testing or for routine use in treating anticholinergic effects. Reserve for life-threatening complications. **AR:** Death may result from respiratory paralysis, hypertension or hypotension, bradycardia or tachycardia or asystole, hypersalivation, respiratory difficulties or convulsions (cholinergic crisis).	Do not consider for toxicities due to the following: antidepressants, amoxapine, maprotiline, nomifensine, bupropion, trazodone, imipramine. IV administration should be at a slow controlled rate, not more than 1 mg/min. Rapid administration can cause adverse reactions.
36. **Pralidoxime chloride** (2-PAM, Protopam, Ayerst). Cholinesterase reactivator; acts by removing phosphate. **Dose:** *Adult,* 1–2 gm IV infused in 100–250 mL saline IV over 15–30 min. Repeat in 1 h if needed. Repeat q 8–12 h when needed; if toxicity is severe, can give 0.5 gm/h infusion. *Child,* 25–50 mg/kg IV over 30 min. No faster than 10 mg/kg/min. Max 12 gm/24 h. **Packaged:** 1 gm/20-mL vials.	Organophosphate insecticide (OPI) poisoning. Not usually needed in carbamate insecticide poisoning. Most effective if started in first 24 h before bonding of phosphate. **AR:** Rapid IV injection has produced tachycardia, muscle rigidity, transient neuromuscular blockade. IM: conjunctival hyperemia, subconjunctival hemorrhage, especially if concentrations exceed 5%. Oral: nausea, vomiting, diarrhea, malaise.	Should be used only after initial treatment with atropine. Draw blood for RBC cholinesterase level before giving 2-PAM. Use of 2-PAM may require reduction in dose of atropine. End point is absence of fasciculations and return of muscle strength. **MP:** Monitor renal profile and reduce dose accordingly. t½: 1–2 h. Reversal of OPI effects at 4 µg/mL of 2-PAM. Start early because "aging" of PO_4 on acetylcholinesterase makes it more difficult to reverse.
37. **Protamine sulfate.** **Dose:** 1 mg neutralizes 90–115 U of heparin, max dose 50 mg IV over 5 min at 10 mg/mL. **Packaged:** 5 mL (50 mg); 25 mL (250 mg).	Heparin overdose. **AR:** Rapid administration causes anaphylactoid reactions.	**MP:** Monitor thromboplastin times. Doses of up to 200 mg have been tolerated over 2 h in adult.
38. **Pyridoxine** (Vitamin B₆). Gamma–amino acid agonist. **Dose:** *Unknown amount ingested:* 5 gm over 5 min IV. *Known amount:* add 1 gm of pyridoxine for each gram of INH ingested IV over 5 min. **Packaged:** 50 and 100 mg/mL; 10 and 30 mL.	Isoniazid (INH), monomethyl hydrazine mushrooms. **AR:** Unlikely owing to the fact that vitamin B₆ is water-soluble. However, nausea, vomiting, somnolence, and paresthesia have been reported from chronic high doses; up to 52 gm IV and up to 357 mg/kg have been tolerated.	Pyridoxine is given as 5–10% solution IV mixed with water. It may be repeated every 5–20 min until seizures cease. Some administer pyridoxine over 30–60 min. **MP:** Correct acidosis, monitor liver profile, acid-base parameters. Lethal dose of pyridoxine in animals is 1 gm/kg.
39. **Sodium bicarbonate.** **Dose:** IV 1–3 mEq/kg as needed to keep pH 7.5 (generally 2 mEq/kg q 6 h). When alkalinization is desired to correct acidosis to pH of 7.3, use 2 mEq/kg to raise pH 0.1 unit. **Packaged:** 50 mL and 50-mEq ampule.	To promote urinary alkalinization for salicylates, phenobarbital (weak acids with low Vd and excreted in urine unchanged). To correct severe acidosis. To promote protein binding and supply sodium ions to Purkinje cells in cyclic antidepressant intoxication. **AR:** Large doses in patients with renal insufficiency may cause metabolic alkalosis. In patients with ketoacidosis, rapid alkalinization with sodium bicarbonate may result in clouding of consciousness, cerebral dysfunction, seizures, hypoxia, and lactic acidosis.	Alkaline diuresis. Assessment of need for bicarbonate should be based on both blood and urine pH. Maintain blood pH at 7.5. Keep urinary output at 3–6 mL/kg/h. May use diuretic to enhance diuresis. Potassium is necessary to produce alkaline diuresis. Monitor electrolytes, calcium, pH of both urine and blood, arterial blood gases.
40. **Sodium nitrite.**	See 14, Cyanide antidote kit.	
41. **Sodium thiosulfate.**	See 14, Cyanide antidote kit.	
42. **Succimer** (DMSA, Chemet, McNeil Consumer Products). **Dose:** 10 mg/kg or 350 mg/m² q 8 h for 5 days, then 10 mg/kg or 350 mg/m² q 12 h for 14 more days (see following chart). Therapy course lasts 19 days. **Packaged:** 100-mg capsule.	For chelation in children only when blood lead is >45 µg/dL. **AR:** Rashes, nausea, vomiting, an elevation of serum transaminases occur in 6–10% of patients.	Minimum of 2 weeks between courses is recommended unless venous lead indicates need for more prompt therapy. Patients who have received Ca-EDTA or BAL may use succimer after an interval of 4 weeks. In young children capsule can be opened and sprinkled on soft food. Monitor venous lead before therapy, on day 7, and weekly for rebound. Monitor following tests: CBC, platelets, ferritin, liver.

*This is for information purposes and is not intended to substitute for independent judgment. It is always advisable to review the package insert for the most up-to-date information. Contact Regional Poison Control Center for additional details on use.

†This dose may exceed the manufacturer's recommended dose.

‡Investigational drug in the United States.

§Not FDA-approved for this indication.

Abbreviations: AR = adverse reaction to antidotes; MP = monitoring parameters; FDA = U.S. Food and Drug Administration; Conc = concentration; ECG = electrocardiogram; TIBC = total iron-binding capacity; G6PD = glucose-6-phosphate dehydrogenase; CNS = central nervous system; GI = gastrointestinal; AV = atrioventricular; EEG = electroencephalogram; RBC = red blood count; CBC = complete blood count.

Table continued on following page

TABLE 4.　**Antidotes*** *Continued*

Medication	Indications	Comments

Pediatric Dosing Chart

Weight (lb)	Weight (kg)	Dose (mg)	No. of Capsules
18–35	8–15	100	1
36–55	16–23	200	2
56–75	24–34	300	3
76–100	35–44	400	4
>100	>45	500	5

Medication	Indications	Comments
43. **Vitamin K** (AquaMEPHYTON, Merck). Promotes hepatic biosynthesis of prothrombin and other coagulation factors. Competitive antagonist of warfarin. It may be administered orally in absence of vomiting. **Dose:** *Adult,* 2.5–10 mg IV, depending on potential for hemorrhage. Oral dose is 15–25 mg/day. Severe bleeding, 5–25 mg slow IV push. Rate 1 mg/min. Repeat q 4–8 h depending on prothrombin time. *Child,* 1–5 mg IV may be given orally when vomiting ceases at dose of 5–10 mg/day. **Packaged:** 2 mg/mL in 0.5-mL ampules. 2.5- or 5-mL vials. Child oral dose 5–10 mg.	Overdose of warfarin (Coumadin) or superwarfarins, salicylate intoxication.	Fatalities from anaphylactic reaction have been reported after IV route. It takes 24 h for vitamin K to be effective. Need for further vitamin K is determined by prothrombin time. If bleeding is severe, fresh blood or plasma transfusion may be needed.

*This is for information purposes and is not intended to substitute for independent judgment. It is always advisable to review the package insert for the most up-to-date information. Contact Regional Poison Control Center for additional details on use.

†This dose may exceed the manufacturer's recommended dose.

‡Investigational drug in the United States.

§Not FDA-approved for this indication.

Abbreviations: AR = adverse reaction to antidotes; MP = monitoring parameters; FDA = U.S. Food and Drug Administration; Conc = concentration; ECG = electrocardiogram; TIBC = total iron-binding capacity; G6PD = glucose-6-phosphate dehydrogenase; CNS = central nervous system; GI = gastrointestinal; AV = atrioventricular; EEG = electroencephalogram; RBC = red blood count; CBC = complete blood count.

depressants, or chlorophenothane (DDT). Activated charcoal cartridges are the primary type of hemoperfusion that is currently available. In general, supportive care is all that is required. Analysis of studies with hemodialysis and hemoperfusion does not indicate that they reduce morbidity or mortality substantially except in certain cases (Table 6).

SUPPORTIVE CARE, OBSERVATION, AND THERAPY OF COMPLICATIONS

The comatose patient is on the threshold of death and must be stabilized initially by establishing an airway. Intubation should be accomplished in any comatose patient.

An intravenous line should be inserted in all comatose patients, and blood should be collected for appropriate tests, including toxicologic analysis (10 mL of clotted blood, initial gastric aspirate, 100 mL of urine). The initial management of the comatose patient should include the administration of 100% oxygen, 100 mg of thiamine intravenously, 50% glucose as an intravenous bolus, and 2 to 10 mg of naloxone intravenously. Other causes associated with coma and mimicking intoxications should be eliminated by examination and laboratory tests (trauma, infection, cerebrovascular accident, hypoxia, and endocrine-metabolic causes).

Pulmonary edema complicating poisoning may be cardiac or noncardiac in origin. Fluid overload during forced diuresis may cause the cardiac variety, particularly if the drugs used have an antidiuretic effect (opioids, barbiturates, and salicylates). Some toxic agents produce increased pulmonary capillary permeability, and other agents may cause a massive sympathetic discharge resulting in neurogenic pulmonary edema (opioids and salicylates). Management consists of minimizing fluid administration and administering diuretics and oxygen. If renal failure is present, dialysis may be necessary. The noncardiac type of pulmonary edema occurs with inhaled toxins, such as ammonia, chlorine, and oxides of nitrogen, or with drugs, such as salicylates, opioids, paraquat, and intravenous ethchlorvynol (Placidyl). This type does not respond to cardiac measures, and oxygen with intensive respiratory management using mechanical ventilation with positive end-expiratory pressure (PEEP) is necessary.

Hypotension and circulatory shock may be caused by heart failure due to myocardial depression, hypovolemia (fluid loss or venous pooling), a decrease in peripheral vasculature resistance (adrenergic blockage), or a loss of vasomotor tone caused by CNS depression.

Renal failure may be due to tubular necrosis as a result of hypotension, hypoxia, or a direct effect of the poison (e.g., salicylate, paraquat, acetaminophen, carbon tetrachloride) on the tubular cells. With he-

TABLE 5. **Dialysis: Indications and Contraindications**

Immediate Consideration of Dialysis: Life-Threatening Toxicities

Ethylene glycol with refractory acidosis
Methanol with refractory acidosis and levels consistently over 50 mg/dL
Lithium levels consistently elevated over 4 mEq/L
Amanita phalloides

Severe Toxicities Due to Dialyzable Drugs (Stage 3 or Higher on Reed Coma Scale)

Alcohol*	Iodides
Ammonia	Isoniazid*
Amphetamines	Meprobamate
Anilines	Paraldehyde
Antibiotics	Potassium*
Barbiturates* (long-acting)	Quinidine
Boric acid	Quinine
Bromides*	Salicylates*
Calcium	Strychnine
Chloral hydrate*	Thiocyanates
Fluorides	(Certain other drugs also dialyzable)

Conditions Requiring Dialysis for General Supportive Therapy

Uncontrollable metabolic acidosis or alkalosis
Uncontrollable electrolyte disturbance, particularly sodium or potassium
Overhydration
Renal failure
Hyperosmolality not responding to conservative therapy
Marked hypothermia
Stage 3 or higher on Reed Coma Scale

Dialysis Contraindicated on Pharmacologic Basis Except for Supportive Care: Nondialyzable Drug Toxicities

Antidepressants (tricyclic and monoamine oxidase inhibitors)
Antihistamines
Barbiturates (short-acting)
Belladonna alkaloids
Benzodiazepines (Valium, Librium)
Digitalis and derivatives
Hallucinogens
Meprobamate (Equanil, Miltown)
Methyprylon (Noludar)
Opioids (heroin, Lomotil)
Phenothiazines (Thorazine, Compazine)
Phenytoin (Dilantin)

*Most useful.

---

moglobinuria or myoglobinuria, hemoglobin or myoglobin may precipitate in the renal tubules and produce renal failure.

Cerebral edema in intoxicated patients is produced by hypoxia, hypercapnia, hypotension, hypoglycemia, and drug-impaired capillary integrity. Computed tomography (CT) may aid in diagnosis. Therapy consists of correction of the arterial blood gas and metabolic abnormalities and the hypotension. Reduction of the increased intracranial pressure may be accomplished by giving 20% mannitol, 0.5 gram per kg, infused over a 30-minute period, and hyperventilation to reduce the Pa_{CO_2} to 25 mmHg. The head should be elevated, and intracranial pressure monitoring should be considered. Fluid administration should be minimized.

Seizures are caused by many substances, such as amphetamines, camphor, chlorinated hydrocarbon insecticides, cocaine, isoniazid, lithium, phencyclidine, phenothiazines, propoxyphene, strychnine, and tricyclic antidepressants, and by drug withdrawal from ethanol and sedative hypnotics. Recurring or protracted seizures require intravenous diazepam (Valium) and phenytoin (Dilantin) and, if seizure persists, a neuromuscular blocking agent and assisted ventilation.

Cardiac dysrhythmias occur with poisoning. A wide QT interval occurs with phenothiazines, and a wide QRS complex occurs with tricyclic antidepressants, quinine, or quinidine overdose. Digitalis, cocaine, cyanide, propranolol, theophylline, and amphetamines are among the more frequent toxic causes of dysrhythmias. Correction of metabolic disturbances and adequate oxygenation correct some of the dysrhythmias; others may require antidysrhythmic drugs or a cardiac pacemaker or cardioversion.

Metabolic acidosis with an increased anion gap is seen with many agents in overdose. There is a mnemonic by which to remember these agents: MUD PILES (*m*ethanol, *u*remia, *d*iabetic ketoacidosis, *p*araldehyde and *p*henformin, *i*ron and *i*soniazid, *l*actic acidosis, *e*thylene glycol and *e*thanol, and *s*alicylate, *s*tarvation, and *s*olvents such as toluene). Assessment of the arterial blood gases, serum electrolytes, and plasma osmolality may be a clue to the etiologic agent. Intravenous sodium bicarbonate may be needed when the pH is below 7.1 if there is adequate ventilation.

Hematemesis can be produced by caustics and corrosives, iron, lithium, mercury, phosphorus, arsenic, mushrooms, plant poisons, fluoride, and organophosphates. Therapy consists of fluid and blood replacement and iced saline lavage if there is no esophageal

TABLE 6. **Plasma Concentrations Above Which Removal by Extracorporeal Means May Be Indicated**

Drug	Plasma Concentration (mg/dL)*	Method of Choice
Phenobarbital	10	HP>HD
Other barbiturates	5	HP
Glutethimide	4	HP
Methaqualone	4	HP
Salicylates	80	HD>HP
Ethchlorvynol	15	HP
Meprobamate	10	HP
Trichloroethanol	5	HP
Paraquat	0.1	HP>HD
Theophylline	6 (chronic)	HP
	10 (acute)	
Methanol	50	HD
Ethylene glycol	Unknown	HD
Lithium	4 mEq/L	HD
Ethanol	500	HD

*1 mg/dL = 10 µg/mL.
Abbreviations: HP = hemoperfusion; HD = hemodialysis.
Modified from Haddad L, Winchester JF (eds): Clinical Management of Poisoning and Drug Overdose. Philadelphia, WB Saunders Co, 1983, p 162.

damage. Although controversial, antacids, H_2 blockers, sucralfate, or misoprostol may be used.

TOXICOKINETICS FOR THE PRACTICING PHYSICIAN

Toxicokinetics is clinical pharmacokinetics from the viewpoint of the toxicologist. Pharmacokinetics is a mathematic description of what the body does to a drug. Knowledge of the toxicokinetics of a specific toxic agent allows the physician to plan a rational approach to the definitive management of the intoxicated patient after the vital functions have been stabilized.

The LD_{50} (the lethal dose for 50% of experimental animals) and the MLD (the minimal lethal dose) are seldom relevant in human intoxications but indicate potential toxicity of the substance. Protein binding of toxic agents influences the volume distribution, elimination, and action of the drug. Diuresis and dialysis are usually reserved for drugs with less than 50% protein binding. The "therapeutic blood range" for a drug is the range of drug concentrations at which the majority of the treated population can be expected to receive therapeutic benefit. The "toxic blood range" is the range of drug concentrations at which this majority would be expected to have toxic manifestations. The drug range values are not absolute. Blood concentrations are a quantitative aid in determining whether more specific measures need to be instituted in correlation with the clinical manifestations. The "apparent Vd" is the percentage of body mass in which the drug is distributed. It is determined by dividing the amount absorbed by the blood concentration. When a substance has a large Vd (above 1 liter per kg), as do most lipid-soluble chemicals, and is concentrated in the body fat, it is not available for diuresis, dialysis, or exchange transfusion. Elimination routes of detoxification allow the physician to make therapeutic decisions, such as using ethanol to interfere with the metabolism of methanol and ethylene glycol into more toxic metabolites. Urine identification is usually qualitative and allows only the identification of an agent.

Never manage a poisoned patient solely by laboratory tests, and always treat according to the manifestations of poisoning, not the laboratory test results. The laboratory toxicology analyst should be given whatever historical information is available so that the agent can be sought and identified as rapidly as possible. Toxicologic analysis is like a mini-research project, unlike most other laboratory tests. Specimens for toxicologic analysis require the patient's name, the date, the time of exposure, the time the specimen was drawn, any therapeutic drugs administered, the patient's manifestations, and other relevant data. The toxicologic specimens that should be obtained for analysis are (1) vomitus or initial gastric aspiration, (2) blood, 10 mL (ask the analyst about the type of container and anticoagulant), and (3) urine, 100 mL. Acetaminophen plasma concentrations should be assessed in all suicide attempts.

COMMON POISONS AND THERAPY

Abbreviations Used in the Following List of Common Poisons

$t\frac{1}{2}$	=	half-life (time required for blood level to drop by 50% of original value)
Vd	=	volume of distribution (liters per kg)
TLV	=	threshold limit value in air
TWA	=	time-weighted average
PPM	=	parts per million in air and water
ECG	=	electrocardiogram
CPK	=	creatine phosphokinase
PEEP	=	positive end-expiratory pressure
EEG	=	electroencephalogram
BUN	=	blood urea nitrogen
EDTA	=	ethylenediaminetetraacetic acid

Conversion Factors

1 gram	= 1000 milligrams (mg)
1 milligram (mg)	= 1000 micrograms (μg)
1 microgram (μg)	= 1000 nanograms (ng)
Standard International Units:	
1 mole	= mol wt in grams per liter
1 millimole	= mol wt in mg per liter
1 micromole	= mol wt in μg per liter
Blood levels:	
1 microgram per milliliter (mL)	= 100 μg per dL
	= 1 mg per liter
	= 1000 ng per mL
100 milligrams per deciliter (dL)	= 0.1 gram per dL
	= 1000 mg (1 gram) per liter
	= 1 mg per mL

Acetaminophen (APAP, Tylenol). *Toxic dose*: Child, 3 grams or more; adult, 7.5 grams or more. Liver toxicity, 140 mg per kg. *Toxicokinetics*: Absorption time, 0.5 to 1 hour. Vd, 0.9 liter per kg. *Route of elimination*: Liver. Draw peak blood level after 4 hours in overdose. *Manifestations*: First 24 hours: malaise, nausea, vomiting, and drowsiness, followed by latent period of 24 hours to 5 days; then hepatic symptoms, disturbances in clotting mechanism, and renal damage. *Management*: (1) Activated charcoal may be given when *N*-acetylcysteine (NAC) therapy is contemplated. In these circumstances, separate activated charcoal from NAC administration by 1 to 2 hours. (2) Give NAC for a toxic overdose (Antidote 1, Table 4). Start and give a full course if a toxic dose has been ingested or if blood concentrations are above the toxic line on the nomogram shown in Figure 1. (3) In this instance, a saline sulfate cathartic is preferred to sorbitol. Treat at 50% APAP plasma levels of nomogram if the patient has a history of alcoholism or is taking enzyme-inducer medication, e.g., anticonvulsants. *Laboratory aids*: APAP level, optimally at 4 to 6 hours. Plot levels on the nomogram in Figure 1 as a guide for treatment. Monitor liver and renal profiles daily.

Acids. See Caustics and Corrosives.

Alcohols

1. ETHANOL (grain alcohol). *Manifestations*: Blood ethanol levels over 30 mg per dL produce euphoria; over 50, incoordination and intoxication; over 100,

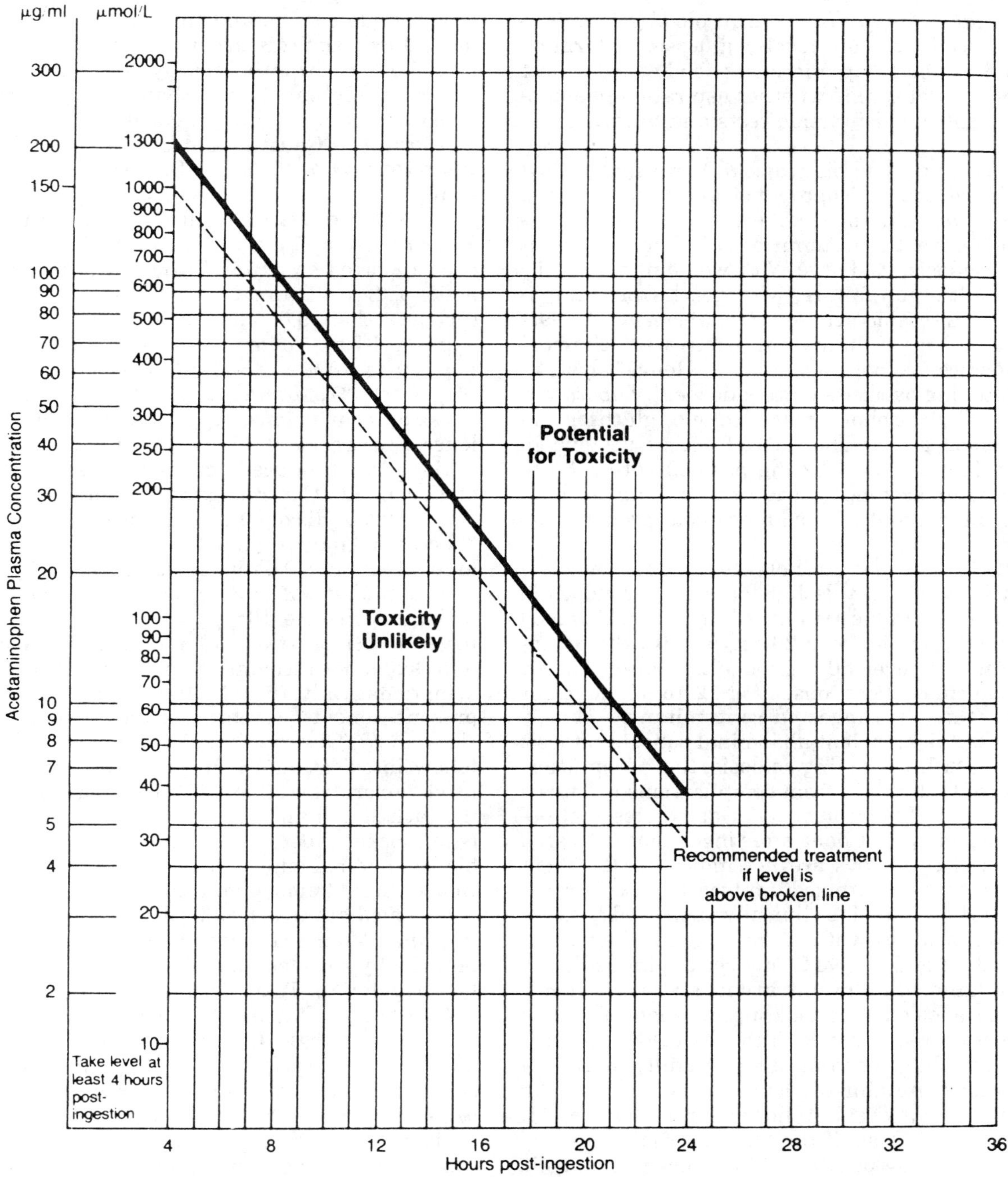

Figure 1. Nomogram for acetaminophen intoxication. Start *N*-acetylcysteine therapy if levels and time coordinates are above the lower line on the nomogram. Continue and complete therapy even if subsequent values fall below the toxic zone. The nomogram is useful only in acute, single ingestions. Serum levels drawn before 4 hours may not represent peak levels. (From Rumack BH, Matthew H: Acetaminophen poisoning and toxicity. Reproduced by permission of Pediatrics, Vol. 55, Page 871, Copyright 1975.)

ataxia; over 300, stupor; and over 500, coma. Levels of 500 to 700 mg per dL may be fatal. Chronic alcoholic patients tolerate higher levels, and the correlation may not be valid. *Management*: (1) Gastrointestinal decontamination. Caution: The rapid onset of CNS depression may preclude the induction of emesis. Activated charcoal and cathartics are not indicated. (2) Give 0.25 gram per kg of dextrose, 50%, intravenously if the blood glucose level is less than 60 mg per dL. (3) Thiamine, 100 mg intravenously, if chronic alcoholism is suspected, to prevent Wernicke-Korsakoff syndrome. (4) Hemodialysis is indicated in severe cases when conventional therapy is ineffective (rarely needed). (5) Treat seizures with diazepam (Valium) followed by phenytoin (Dilantin) if the patient is unresponsive. (6) Treat withdrawal with hydration and chlordiazepoxide (Librium) or diazepam. Large doses of sedatives may be required for delirium tremens. *Laboratory aids*: Arterial blood gases, electrolytes, blood ethanol levels, glucose; determine anion and osmolar gap and check for ketosis. Chest radiograph to determine whether aspiration pneumonia is present. Liver function tests and bilirubin levels.

2. ISOPROPANOL (rubbing alcohol). Normal propyl alcohol is related to isopropanol but is more toxic. *Manifestations*: Ethanol-like intoxication with acetone odor to breath, acetonuria, acetonemia without systemic acidosis, gastritis. With worsening acidosis, there is multiorgan failure, with death from complications of intractable acidosis. *Management*: (1) Gastrointestinal decontamination. Activated charcoal and cathartics are not indicated. (2) Hemodialysis in life-threatening overdose (rarely needed). *Laboratory aids*: Isopropyl alcohol levels, acetone, glucose, and arterial blood gases. The lack of excess acetone in the blood (normal 0.3 to 2 mg per dL) within 30 to 60 minutes or acetone in the urine within 3 hours excludes the possibility of significant isopropanol exposure.

3. METHANOL (wood alcohol). *Toxic dose*: One teaspoonful is potentially lethal for a 2-year-old child and can cause blindness in an adult. The toxic blood level of methanol is above 20 mg per dL, the potentially fatal level over 50 mg per dL. *Manifestations*: Metabolism may delay onset for 12 to 18 hours or longer if ethanol is ingested concomitantly. Hyperemia of optic disk, violent abdominal colic, blindness, and shock. With worsening acidosis, there is multiorgan failure, with death from complications of intractable acidosis. *Management*: (1) Gastrointestinal decontamination up to 1 hour after ingestion. Activated charcoal and cathartics are not indicated. (2) Treat acidosis vigorously with sodium bicarbonate intravenously. (3) If methanol is clinically suspected because of metabolic acidosis, with an anion gap if the methanol concentration is above 20 mg per dL, immediately initiate ethanol therapy intravenously or by mouth to produce a blood ethanol concentration of 100 to 150 mg per dL (Antidote 21, Table 4). (4) Folinic acid and folic acid have been used successfully in animal investigations. Administer leucovorin, 1 mg per kg up to 50 mg IV every 4 hours for six doses. (5) Consider hemodialysis if the blood methanol level is greater than 50 mg per dL or if significant metabolic acidosis or visual or mental symptoms are present. *Note*: The ethanol dose has to be increased during dialysis therapy. (6) Continue therapy (ethanol and hemodialysis) until the blood methanol level is pref-

erably undetectable and there is no acidosis and no mental or visual disturbances. This often requires 2 to 5 days. (7) Ophthalmology consultation. *Laboratory aids*: Methanol and ethanol levels, electrolytes, glucose, and arterial blood gases.

Alkali. See Caustics and Corrosives.

Amitriptyline (Elavil). See Tricyclic Antidepressants.

Amphetamines (diet pills, various trade names). *Toxicity*: Child, 5 mg per kg; adult, 12 mg per kg has been reported as lethal. *Toxicokinetics*: Peak time of action is 2 to 4 hours. t½—8 to 10 hours in acid urine (pH less than 6.0) and 16 to 31 hours in alkaline urine (pH 7.5). *Route of elimination*: Liver, 60%; kidney, 30 to 40% at alkaline urine pH; at acid urine pH, 50 to 70%. *Manifestations*: Dysrhythmias, hyperpyrexia, convulsions, hypertension, paranoia, violence. *Management*: (1) Gastrointestinal decontamination. Avoid induced emesis because of rapid onset of action. (2) Control extreme agitation or convulsions with diazepam (Valium). Chlorpromazine (Thorazine) may be dangerous if ingestion is not pure amphetamine. (3) Treat hypertensive crisis with nitroprusside at 0.3 to 2 mg per kg per minute; maximal infusion rate 10 μg per kg per minute; should never last more than 10 minutes. (4) Acidification diuresis is not recommended. (5) Treat hyperpyrexia symptomatically. (6) If focal neurologic symptoms are present, consider cerebrovascular accident. Obtain a CT scan. (7) Observe for suicidal depression that may follow intoxication. (8) In life-threatening agitation, use haloperidol (Haldol). (9) Significant life-threatening tachydysrhythmia may respond to the alpha and beta blocker labetalol (Normodyne; Antidote 27, Table 4) or other appropriate antidysrhythmic agents. In a severely hemodynamically compromised patient, use immediate synchronized cardioversion. *Laboratory aids*: Monitor for rhabdomyolysis (CPK), myoglobinuria, hyperkalemia, and disseminated intravascular coagulation. Toxic blood level, 10 μg per dL.

Aniline. See Nitrites (NO_2) and Nitrates (NO_3).

Anticholinergic Agents. Examples are antihistamines: hydroxyzine (Atarax), diphenhydramine (Benadryl); antipsychotics (neuroleptics): phenothiazines (Thorazine); antidepressant drugs (tricyclic antidepressants): imipramine (Tofranil); antiparkinsonian drugs: trihexyphenidyl (Artane), benztropine (Cogentin); over-the-counter sleep, cold, and hay fever medicines (methapyrilene); ophthalmic products (atropine); plants: jimsonweed (*Datura stramonium*), deadly nightshade (*Atropa belladonna*), henbane

TABLE 7. **Toxicokinetics of Anticholinergic Agents**

Drug	Potential Fatal Dose	Time to Peak Effect	Volume of Distribution (L/kg)	t½ (h)	Excretion Route
Atropine	Child: 10–20 mg; adult: 100 mg	1–2 h, may be prolonged in overdose	2.3	2–3	Renal (30–50%); hepatic (50–70%)
Diphenhydramine	Child: 25 mg/kg; adult: 2–8 gm	2 h, may be prolonged in overdose	3.3–6.8	3–10	98% hepatic

TABLE 8. **Anticonvulsants**

Drug	Peak Time of Action (Steady State)	Volume of Distribution (L/kg)	t½ (h)	Route of Elimination (%)	Protein Binding (%)	Blood Level (µg/mL)	Comment*
Carbamazepine (Tegretol)	8–24 h (2–4 days)	1.0	18–54	Liver (98)	70	Therapeutic, 4–10	Related to tricyclic antidepressants, can cause dysrhythmias
Ethosuximide (Zarontin)	24–48 h (5–8 days)	0.8	36–55	Liver (80–90)	0	Therapeutic, 40–100	
Phenytoin (Dilantin)	PO, 6–12 h; IV, 1 h (5–10 days)	1.0	24; varies in toxic doses: zero-order kinetics	Liver (95)	90	Therapeutic, 10–20; toxic, 20–30; nystagmus only, 30–40; ataxia, 40+; coma, convulsions	Dysrhythmias with parenteral use only
Primidone (Mysoline)	?3–4 days	0.6	Parent, 3–12; metabolites, 30–36	Liver	60	Therapeutic, 6–12 primidone and 15–40 phenobarbital (PB); toxic, over 50 primidone and over 40 PB (see Barbiturates)	Metabolized to active metabolites phenylethylmalonamide and PB; overdose gives white crystals in urine†
Valproic acid (Depakene)	?1–2 days	0.4	5–15	Liver (80–100)	84–96	Therapeutic, 50–100	Produces nausea and vomiting, changes in liver function
Clonazepam (Klonopin)	?		20–60	Liver (98)	90	Therapeutic, 20–70 ng/mL	
Phenobarbital (Luminal)	3–6 h	0.75	50–120	Liver	30	Therapeutic, 15–40	

*Manifestations: The major manifestations of these agents are depression of consciousness and respiratory depression. Other significant manifestations are mentioned in this column.

†Primidone produces whorls of shimmering white crystals in the urine from precipitation of intact primidone in massive overdose.

(Hyoscyamus niger); and antispasmodic agents for the bowel (atropine). *Toxicokinetics*: See Table 7. *Manifestations*: Anticholinergic signs—hyperpyrexia, dilated pupils, flushing of skin, dry mucosa, tachycardia, delirium, hallucinations, coma, and convulsions. *Management*: (1) Gastrointestinal decontamination up to 12 hours postingestion. *Note*: Use caution with emesis if treating a diphenhydramine overdose because of rapid onset of action and seizures. (2) Control seizures with diazepam (Valium). (3) Control ventricular dysrhythmias with lidocaine (Xylocaine). (4) Physostigmine (Antilirium; Antidote 35, Table 4) for life-threatening anticholinergic effects refractory to conventional treatments. (5) Relieve urinary retention by catheterization to avoid reabsorption. (6) Treat cardiac dysrhythmias only if tissue perfusion is not adequate or if the patient is hypotensive. (7) Control hyperpyrexia by external cooling. No antipyretics.

Anticonvulsants. See Table 8. *Toxic dose*: Specific anticonvulsant blood levels and the clinical manifestations indicate toxicity. In general, the ingestion of five times the therapeutic dose is expected to have the potential for toxicity. *Management*: (1) Gastrointestinal decontamination up to 12 hours postingestion. Repeated doses of activated charcoal shorten t½ of carbamazepine, phenobarbital, primidone, phenytoin, and possibly others. Naloxone (Narcan) (Antidote 30, Table 4) may improve valproic acid–induced coma. (2) Monitor specific anticonvulsant blood levels. (3) The effectiveness of hemoperfusion and dialysis has not been established.

Antidepressants. See Tricyclic Antidepressants.

Antifreeze. See Alcohols (Methanol) and Ethylene Glycol.

Antihistamines (H₁-Receptor Antagonists). See Anticholinergic Agents. Newer nonsedating long-acting preparations—terfenadine (Seldane) and astemizole (Hismanal)—may produce prolonged QT intervals and torsades de pointes. In patients who have impaired hepatic function or are receiving cimetidine, ketoconazole, or macrolide antibiotics, the metabolism of terfenadine and astemizole may be inhibited. All children who ingest these newer nonsedating antihistamines or adults who ingest more than the therapeutic dose require close cardiac monitoring for 24 hours. Gastrointestinal decontamination is advised.

Arsenic and Arsine Gas. *Toxic dose*: In humans, the inorganic arsenic trioxide toxic dose is 5 to 50 mg; the potential fatal dose is 120 mg or 1 to 2 mg per kg. Sodium arsenite is nine times more toxic than arsenic trioxide. Organic arsenic is less toxic. The maximal allowable concentration for prolonged exposure is 0.05 PPM. See Table 9. Humans are more sensitive than rodents to arsenic. Acute poisoning results from accidental ingestion of arsenic-containing pesticides. (Ant traps sold in some states contain arsenic.) *Toxicokinetics*: Arsenates are water-

TABLE 9. **Comparative Acute Toxicities of Some Common Arsenicals**

Arsenic Compound	Lethal Dose
Arsenate	5–50 mg/kg
Arsenites	<5 mg/kg
Arsenic trioxide (insoluble)	120 mg total
Arsenic trioxide (soluble)*	13 mg total

*Nine times as toxic as insoluble form.

soluble and arsenite is lipid-soluble. The soluble forms of arsenic are rapidly absorbed by inhalation and ingestion. Arsenic crosses the placenta and can cause fetal damage. Distributes into spleen, liver, kidneys. *Excretion*: In urine, 90%. After acute ingestion, it takes 10 days to clear a single dose; after chronic ingestion, up to 70 days. *Arsine gas*: Forms when active hydrogen comes in contact with arsenic. This may occur when zinc, antimony, lead, or iron is contaminated with arsenic and comes in contact with acid. This causes arsine inhalation intoxication characterized by a latent period of 2 to 48 hours and a triad of abdominal pain, jaundice (due to hemolysis), and hematuria. *Manifestations*: Arsenic intoxication produces gastroenteritis, neurologic and cardiac abnormalities, subsequent renal involvement. A garlic odor to the breath may be a clue. Smaller doses

and prolonged low-level exposure produce subacute (stomatitis) and chronic (peripheral neuropathy) symptoms. *Management*: (1) Gastrointestinal decontamination. Activated charcoal is ineffective. Cathartics are not advised because of the potential for diarrhea. Follow with abdominal radiographs because arsenic is radiopaque. Consider whole-bowel washout if usual methods fail to remove arsenic. (2) Intravenous fluids to correct dehydration and electrolyte deficiencies. (3) Treat shock with oxygen, blood, and fluids as needed. (4) In severe cases, administer BAL (dimercaprol) (Antidote 17, Table 4). (5) In chronic poisoning, D-penicillamine (Antidote 34, Table 4) may be used to chelate arsenic. Therapy should be continued in 5-day cycles until the urine arsenic level is less than 50 μg per liter. (6) Treat liver and renal impairment. (7) Hemodialysis is effective in acute

TABLE 10. **Features of Barbiturates***

Feature	Long-Acting (LAB)	Intermediate-Acting (IAB)	Short-Acting (SAB)
Duration (h)	>8	3–8	<3
Medical use	Anticonvulsants	Sedative hypnotics	
t½ (h)	>50	<50	<50
DEA	Schedule IV	Schedule II	Schedule II

Feature	Barbital	Phenobarbital†	Amobarbital	Pentobarbital	Secobarbital
Trade name	Veronal	Luminal	Amytal	Nembutal	Seconal
Slang name	—	Purple hearts	Blues	Yellows	Red devils
pKa	7.8	7.24	7.9	7.96	7.9
Elimination route	Renal 20% Hepatic 80%	Renal 30% Hepatic 70%	Hepatic 98%	Hepatic >90%	Hepatic >90%
Onset IV (min)	22	12	—	0.1	0.1
Onset oral	1 h	20–60 min	13–30 min	15–30 min	10–30 min
Peak conc oral (h)	12–18	6–18	3–4	2–4	1–2
Protein-bound (%)	6	20–40	40–60	40–65	40–60
Oral Doses					
Fatal dose (gm)	10	8	5	3	3
(mg/kg)	75	65	40	50	30
Toxic dose (mg/kg)	>10	10	>6	>6	>6
Adult nontolerant (mg)	—	300	200–300	200–300	200
Therapeutic dose (mg/kg)	2–6	2–6	2–6	2–6	6
Adult dose (mg)	300–500	100–200	100–200	100–200	100–200
Blood Concentrations					
Therapeutic (μg/mL)	5–8	15–40	5–6	1–5	1–5
Toxic (μg/mL)	>30	>40	10–30	>10	>10
Lethal‡ (μg/mL)	>300	>100	>50	>35	>35
Duration (h)	16	6–8	6	6	6
Elimination t½ (h)	56–96	50–120	15–40	15–30	22–29
Volume of distribution (L/kg)	—	0.75	0.5	0.65	1.5
Availability					
Capsule (mg)	—	16	65, 200	50, 100	50, 100
Tablet (mg)	—	16, 32, 65, 100	15, 30, 50, 100	—	100
Elixir (mg/5 mL)	—	15, 20	—	20	—
Suppository (mg)	—	—	—	30, 60, 120, 200	—

Manifestations

Low dose: Euphoria, ataxia, incoordination, nystagmus on lateral gaze
High dose: Flaccid coma, hypotension, respiratory depression, pulmonary edema (particularly with the short-acting barbiturates), subcutaneous bullae (6%), dermatographia

---

*Classification into long-, intermediate-, and short-acting has no relationship to the duration of coma.
†The t½ in children is approximately 50% of adult.
‡These levels are not absolute, and tolerance occurs.
Abbreviations: DEA = Drug Enforcement Agency; conc = concentration; t½ = half-life.

poisoning and can be used concurrently with chelation therapy in severe cases, especially if renal failure develops. (8) Arsine intoxication is treated by exchange transfusion and hemodialysis if renal failure occurs. BAL is ineffective. *Laboratory aids*: Blood arsenic and 24-hour urine arsenic levels. Excessive exposure is indicated by a level of 50 μg per liter of arsenic in urine, but persons whose diets are rich in seafood may excrete larger amounts. View values over 50 μg per day with suspicion. Monitor ECG and renal function. A blood arsenic level above 1.0 mg per liter is toxic, and one of 9 to 15 mg per liter is potentially fatal (false values occur in inexperienced laboratories).

Aspirin. See Salicylates.

Atropine. See Anticholinergic Agents.

Barbiturates. See Table 10. *Management*: (1) Gastrointestinal decontamination. Avoid emesis in short-acting barbiturate intoxications. Activated charcoal and a cathartic in repeated doses have been shown to reduce the serum half-life of phenobarbital and increase the nonrenal clearance by over 50%. Give every 4 hours while the patient is comatose. (2) Supportive and symptomatic care is all that is necessary in the majority of cases. (3) Alkalinization with sodium bicarbonate, 2 mEq per kg intravenously during the first hour, followed by sufficient sodium bicarbonate (Antidote 39, Table 4) to keep the urinary pH at 7.5 to 8.0, enhances the excretion of long-acting barbiturates. Alkalinization is not useful for short-acting barbiturate intoxication. Forced diuresis should be used with caution because of fluid overload. At present, alkalinization without diuresis is advocated. (4) In severe cases that do not respond to conservative measures, consider hemodialysis and hemoperfusion. (5) Treat any bulla as a local second-degree skin burn. (6) Give intensive care monitoring to the comatose patient. *Treatment of withdrawal: In an emergency*, use thiopental (Pentothal) or diazepam (Valium) intravenously. If the patient is stable, pentobarbital is given orally and the patient examined after 1 hour for signs of intoxication (nystagmus, slurred speech, and ataxia). If none is present, the dose is repeated every 3 hours until these signs develop. This is the stabilizing dose; the patient is maintained on this dose for 72 hours and then changed to phenobarbital, 30 mg substituted for each 100 mg of pentobarbital. The phenobarbital is tapered, decreasing by 10% or 30 mg every 3 to 5 days. *Laboratory aids*: Emergency plasma barbiturate concentrations rarely alter management.

Benzene. See Hydrocarbons.

Benzodiazepines (BZPs). See Table 11. *Toxicity*: Low toxic potential. More than 500 mg has been ingested without respiratory depression. Benzodiazepines have an additive effect with sedatives, such as alcohol and barbiturates. Most patients intoxicated with benzodiazepines alone recover within 24 hours. Many of these agents have active metabolites with a long plasma t½, so performance in skilled tasks, such as driving, may be impaired. Withdrawal may be delayed. *Manifestations*: CNS depression. Deep coma leading to respiratory depression suggests the presence of other drugs. *Management*: (1) Gastrointestinal decontamination. (2) Supportive and symptomatic care. (3) Flumazenil (Romazicon) is a recently approved specific benzodiazepine antagonist. It is not a treatment for hypoventilation and should be used with caution in overdose cases because of dependency and seizures (Antidote 23, Table 4). (4) Withdrawal, if it occurs, is treated with a long-acting benzodiazepine on a tapering schedule. *Laboratory aids*: Document benzodiazepines in urine. Quantitative blood levels are not useful.

Bleach. Household bleaches are 4 to 6% sodium hypochlorite. Commercial types are 10 to 20%. *Manifestations*: Difficulty in swallowing; pain in mouth, throat, chest, or abdomen. General household strength bleach does not produce burns; commercial strength bleach may. Inhalation of gases produced by mixing chlorine bleach with acids (toilet bowl cleaner and rust removers—chlorine gas) or with household ammonia (chloramine gas) causes irritation of mucous membranes, eyes, and upper respiratory tract. *Management*: (1) Ingestion—(a) Avoid gastrointestinal decontamination procedures. Dilute with small amounts of water or milk. Avoid acids. (b) Use esophagoscopy only if unusually large amounts have been ingested, the patient is symptomatic, or the product was stronger than the average household bleach. (2) Inhalation—remove from contaminated area. Observe for pulmonary edema. (3) Ocular exposure requires immediate gentle irrigation with water for at least 15 minutes, followed by fluorescein dye stain to detect any damage.

Botulism. See the article "Food-Borne Illness" in Section 2.

Brake Fluid. See Ethylene Glycol.

Calcium Channel Blockers. Used in treatment of effort angina, supraventricular tachycardia, and hypertension. See Table 12. *Manifestations*: Hypotension, bradycardia within 1 to 5 hours, CNS depression, and gastric distress. Manifestations are delayed after the ingestion of slow-release preparations. *Management*: (1) Gastrointestinal decontamination. If long-acting preparation, consider whole-bowel washout. If patient is symptomatic, obtain a cardiac consult. May need pacemaker. (2) Treat hypotension and bradycardia with positioning, fluids, and calcium gluconate or chloride (Antidote 12B, Table 4). Dopamine or norepinephrine may be used if necessary. If calcium fails, use sodium bicarbonate, glucagon, or both (Antidote 26, Table 4). (3) Heart block—may respond to intravenous calcium (Antidote 12B, Table 4) or atropine sulfate, 0.5 to 1 mg, if no response. (4) Ventricular pacing may be required in the severely intoxicated patient. (5) Patients receiving digitalis run the risk of toxicity and should be carefully monitored. (6) Extracorporeal washout measures are generally not considered to be useful. *Laboratory aids*: Specific drug levels, blood sugar and calcium, ECG.

Camphor (external analgesic rubs, Vicks VapoRub 4.8%, Campho-Phenique 11%). Many camphorated oil products were removed from the marketplace in

TABLE 11. **Benzodiazepines (BZPs)**

Drug	Oral Dosage Range	Time to Peak Oral Plasma Level (h)	t½ (h)	Major Active Metabolites (t½ in h)	Elimination Rate
Anxiolytics					
Diazepam (Valium)	6–40 mg/day	1–2	14–100	Desmethyldiazepam (50–100 h)	Slow
Chlordiazepoxide (Librium, Libritabs, various others)	15–100 mg/day	2–4	5–30	Desmethylchlordiazepoxide, demoxepam, desmethyldiazepam (50–100 h)	Slow
Clorazepate (Tranxene)	15–60 mg/day	1–2.5	1.1–2.9	Desmethyldiazepam (50–100 h)	Slow
Prazepam (Centrax)	20–60 mg/day	6	0.6–2	3-Hydroxyprazepam, desmethyldiazepam (50–100 h)	Slow
Halazepam (Paxipam)	50–160 mg/day	1–3	1.6–5.3	*N*-3-Hydroxyhalazepam, desmethyldiazepam (50–100 h)	Slow
Oxazepam (Serax)	30–120 mg/day	1–2	8–25	None	Rapid to intermediate
Lorazepam (Ativan)	2–6 mg/day	2–5	10–20	None	Intermediate
Alprazolam (Xanax)	0.75–4 mg/day	0.7–1.6	6–26	α-Hydroxyalprazolam	Intermediate
Hypnotics					
Flurazepam (Dalmane)	15–60 mg	0.5–2	50–100	Desalkylflurazepam (t½ = 50–100 h)	Slow
Midazolam (Versed)	5–30 mg/day IV	0.3–0.8	1.2–12.3	None	—
Flunitrazepam (Robypnol—investigational, Roche)	1–2 mg	<1	0.5–2	7-Aminoflunitrazepam (t½ = 23 h), *N*-desmethyl-flunitrazepam (t½ = 31 h)	—
Temazepam (Restoril)	15–30 mg	2–3	10–20	None	Intermediate
Triazolam (Halcion)	0.125–0.5 mg	0.5–1.5	2–5	α-Hydroxytriazolam	Rapid
Quazepam (Doral)	7.5–15 mg	1–2	>39	2-Oxoquazepam *N*-desalkylflurazepam	Intermediate
Estazolam (ProSom)	1–2 mg	1–2	12–15	1-Oxoestazolam	Intermediate
Anticonvulsants					
Clonazepam (Klonopin)	1.5–20 mg/day	1–4	18–50	None	—
Zolpidem* (Ambien)	5–20 mg/day	2	1.5–2.5	None	Rapid

*Not a benzodiazepine chemically but an imidazopyridine that is a selective benzodiazepine-1 receptor agonist.

September 1982. Five milliliters of camphorated oil (20% camphor) equals 1 gram of camphor. *Toxicity*: More than 10 mg per kg by ingestion may cause seizures. Adult, 5 grams has been fatal; child, 1 gram. *Toxicokinetics*: Time to onset of manifestations, 5 to 90 minutes. Readily and rapidly absorbed through the skin, mucous membranes, and gastrointestinal tract, and crosses the placenta. *Route of elimination*: Rapidly metabolized in liver to glucuronide form, which is excreted in urine. Pulmonary excretion causes a distinctive odor on the breath. *Manifestations*: Nausea, vomiting, and burning epigastric pain. Seizures may occur suddenly and without warning within 5 minutes of ingestion. Apnea and vision disturbances may occur. *Management*: Medical evaluation and admission should be considered for ingestion of over 50 mg per kg or over 3000 mg. (1) Induction of emesis is contraindicated because of early seizures. (2) Remove residual drug by gastric lavage. (3) Administer activated charcoal and a saline cathartic. Avoid giving oils or alcohol. (4) Treat seizures with intravenous diazepam (Valium). (5) Treat apnea with respiratory support.

Carbon Monoxide (CO). This is an odorless gas produced from incomplete combustion; it is found also as an in vivo metabolic breakdown product of methylene chloride (paint removers). Observe for the symptoms described in Table 13. Contrary to popular belief, the skin rarely shows a cherry-red color in the living patient. *Toxicokinetics*: CO is rapidly absorbed through the lungs. The rate of absorption is directly related to alveolar ventilation. Elimination occurs through the lungs. The t½ in room air equals 5 to 6 hours; in 100% oxygen, 90 minutes; in hyperbaric oxygen, 20 minutes. The nomogram pictured in Figure 2 can be used to decide quickly whether serious

TABLE 12. **Kinetics of the Calcium Channel Blockers**

Parameter	Nifedipine	Verapamil	Dilti-azem	Nicardipine	Nimodipine	Felodi-pine*	Amlodi-pine	Bepridil	Isradi-pine
Class	Dihydro-pyridine	Phenylal-kylamine	Benzothia-zepine	Dihydro-pyridine	Dihydro-pyridine	Dihydro-pyridine	Dihydro-pyridine	Dihydro-pyridine	Dihydro-pyridine
Trade name	Procardia	Calan, Isoptin	Cardizem	Cardene	Nimotop	Plendil	Norvasc	Vascor	DynaCirc
Preparations	10-, 20-mg cap	40-, 80-, 120-mg tab	30-, 60-, 90-, 120-mg tab	20-, 30-mg cap	30-mg cap	None	2.5-, 5-, 10-mg tab	200-, 300-, 400-mg tab	2.5-, 5-mg cap
Slow-release preparation	30-, 60-, 90-mg cap	120-, 180-, 240-mg tab	60-, 90-, 120-, 180-, 240-, 300-mg tab	30-, 45-, 60-mg cap	None	5-, 10-mg tab	See above	None	None
Bioavail-ability (%)	65–70	20–30	40	35	3–30	20	60–65	60	17
Mean toxic dose	340 mg	3.2 gm	? rare toxicity	NA	NA	NA	NA	NA	NA
Serious toxic dose	Lowest 200 mg	40 mg/kg child 2–3 gm adult	Up to 300 mg well tolerated by adults	NA	NA	NA	NA	NA	NA
Dose range (mg/day)	30–120	120–480	90–360	60–120	60–360	5–30	2.5–10	200–400	2.5–15
Max daily dose (mg/day)	—	—	—	—	—	—	10	400	20
Onset of action (min)									
Oral	<20	30–120	<15	<20	<20	—	—	—	—
IV	<1	<3	<1	—	—	—	—	—	—
SL	3–5	—	—	—	—	—	—	—	—
Peak action									
Oral	30–90 min	60–90 min	30–60 min	60 min	60 min	2.6–6 h	6–9	2–3	2–3
SL	20 min	—	—	—	—	—	—	—	—
Sustained	—	4–8 h	3–4 h	—	—	—	—	—	—
Peak blood conc (min)	30–60	90–120	120–180	60	NA	NA	—	—	—
t½ (h)	3–6	6–12	4–9	8	1–8	24	35–50	33–42	5–10.7
Duration (h)	4–12	6–12	—	4–6	NA	—	24	24	12
Protein binding (%)	92–98	90–99	70–85	>95	>95	NA	98	99	97
Volume of distribution (L/kg)	1–5	4.5–7	3–5	NA	—	—	21	8	3
Elimination	Renal 50–70%	Hepatic 60–65%	Renal 70–80%	Hepatic	—	—	Hepatic	Hepatic	Hepatic
Metabolite	Inactive	Active mild norverapa-mil	Active 50% parent diacetyl-diltiazem	NA	NA	NA	Pyridine deriv. (not active)	17 metabo-lites (one active)	None active

*Anonymous: Felodipine—another calcium channel blocker for hypertension. Med Lett *33*:115–116, 1991.
Abbreviations: cap = capsules; tab = tablets; NA = no available information; SL = sublingual; conc = concentration.

TABLE 13. **Progression of Signs and Symptoms with Carbon Monoxide (CO) Exposure**

CO in Atmosphere (PPM)	Duration of Exposure (h)	Saturation of Blood (%)	Signs and Symptoms
Up to 0.01	Indefinite	1–10	None
0.01–0.02	Indefinite	10–20	Tightness across forehead, slight headache, dilatation of cutaneous vessels
0.02–0.03	5–6	20–30	Headache, throbbing temples
0.04–0.06	4–5	30–40	Severe headache, weakness and dizziness, nausea and vomiting, collapse, leukocytosis
0.07–0.10	3–4	40–50	Above, plus increased tendency to collapse and syncope, increased pulse and respiratory rate
0.11–0.15	1.5–3	50–60	Increased pulse and respiratory rate, syncope, Cheyne-Stokes respirations, coma and intermittent convulsions
0.16–0.30	1–1.5	60–70	Coma with intermittent convulsions, depressed heart action and respirations, death possible
0.50–1.00	1–2	70–80	Weak pulse, depressed respirations, respiratory failure, death

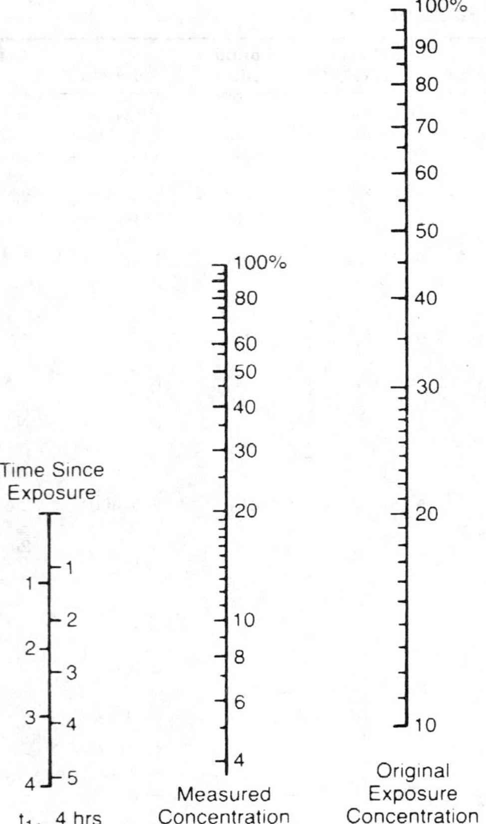

Figure 2. Nomogram for calculating carboxyhemoglobin concentration at time of exposure. The time since exposure is given on two scales to allow for the effects of previous oxygen administration on the half-life (t½) of carboxyhemoglobin (left-hand scale assumes a t½ of 3 hours). *Note*: The nomogram assumes a t½ of carboxyhemoglobin of 4 hours in a subject breathing room air. Most patients will not have received supplementary oxygen before admission, and at best this will have been administered via a face mask, giving a maximal fractional inspired oxygen concentration of 50 to 60% with little effect on carboxyhemoglobin elimination. The scale on the left side of the time column makes allowances for prior oxygen supplements by assuming a short t½ of 3 hours. The nomogram may help decide quickly whether serious carbon monoxide intoxication is likely to have occurred and may help select patients at high risk who need early management in the intensive care unit. The nomogram may be an oversimplification because patients usually are not resuscitated with constant concentrations of oxygen, and many patients may hyperventilate, thus changing elimination characteristics. (Redrawn from Clark CJ, Campbell D, Reid WH: Blood carboxyhaemoglobin and cyanide levels in fire survivors. Lancet *1*[8234]:1332–1335, © by The Lancet Ltd, 1981.)

CO intoxication is likely to have occurred and to select patients at high risk or who need early management in the intensive care unit or need hyperbaric oxygen. *Management*: (1) Remove the patient from contaminated area and expose to fresh air. Establish vital functions. (2) Give 100% oxygen to all patients until the carboxyhemoglobin level falls to 5% or less. Assisted ventilation may be necessary. The exposed pregnant woman should be kept in 100% oxygen for several hours after the carboxyhemoglobin level is zero because carboxyhemoglobin concentrates in the fetus and oxygen is needed five times longer

to ensure elimination of CO from fetal circulation. CO or hypoxia may be teratogenic. (3) Monitor arterial blood gases and carboxyhemoglobin levels. Determine carboxyhemoglobin level at time of exposure by using nomogram. *Note*: A near-normal carboxyhemoglobin level does not rule out significant CO poisoning. (4) Only if pH is below 7.1 after correction of hypoxia and adequate ventilation, give sodium bicarbonate to correct acidosis. (5) Indications for 100% oxygen and, if possible, therapy with hyperbaric oxygen—(a) carboxyhemoglobin level higher than 25%, (b) carboxyhemoglobin level higher than 15% in a child or in a patient with cardiovascular disease, (c) carboxyhemoglobin level higher than 10% in a pregnant woman (and monitor fetus), (d) abnormal or ischemic chest pain or ECG abnormality, (e) abnormal chest radiograph, (f) presence of hypoxia, myoglobinuria, or abnormal renal function, or (g) history of unconsciousness, syncope, or neuropsychiatric symptoms. The most important indication for the hyperbaric chamber is a history of unconsciousness. A list of hyperbaric oxygen chambers can be obtained by contacting a Regional Poison Control Center. (6) Treat seizures with intravenous diazepam (Valium). (7) Monitor ECG, chest radiograph, and serum CPK and lactate dehydrogenase levels. (8) Treat cerebral edema with elevation of the patient's head, minimizing intravenous fluid and hyperventilation; if needed, give mannitol and monitor intracranial pressure. (9) Re-evaluate after recovery for neuropsychiatric sequelae. *Laboratory aids*: Arterial blood gases show metabolic acidosis and normal oxygen tension but reduced oxygen saturation, as measured by a co-oximeter.

Carbon Tetrachloride. See Hydrocarbons.

Caustics and Corrosives. Common acid substances are hydrochloric acid, sulfuric acid (battery acid), carbolic acid (phenol), nitric acid, oxalic acid, hydrofluoric acid, and aqua regia (mixture of hydrochloric and nitric acids). These are used as cleaning agents. Common alkaline substances are sodium or potassium hydroxide (lye), sodium hypochlorite (bleach [Chlorox]), sodium carbonate (nonphosphate detergents), potassium permanganate, ammonia, electric dishwasher agents, cement, and flat disk batteries. *Manifestations*: Dysphagia, drooling, pain in the throat or abdomen. Esophageal or gastric perforation, chest or abdominal pain, and peritoneal irritation may occur. *Toxicity*: Acids produce mucosal coagulation necrosis. They usually do not penetrate deeply (exception: hydrofluoric acid). The gastric mucosa is the primary site of injury. Alkalis produce liquefaction necrosis and saponification and penetrate deeply. Oropharyngeal and esophageal damage by solids is more frequent than that by liquids. Liquids are more likely to produce gastric damage. *Toxic dose*: Potential fatal dose of concentrated acid or alkali is 5 mL. The absence of oral burns does not exclude the possibility of esophageal burns (seen in 10 to 15% of patients). *Management*: (1) Dilute with milk or water immediately up to 30 mL in children or 250 mL in adults. Neutralization with acidic or alkaline agents is contraindicated. Dilute only if patient can swallow. Contraindications to dilution are an inability to swallow and signs of respiratory distress, shock, or esophageal perforation. (2) Gastrointestinal decontamination is contraindicated. In acid ingestions, however, some authorities advocate nasogastric intubation and aspiration in the early postingestion phase. The patient should receive only intravenous fluids after dilution until surgical consultation is obtained. Dermal and ocular decontamination should be carried out. (3) Endoscopy at 12 to 48 hours postingestion may be indicated to assess the severity of burn. (4) Steroids are controversial. (5) Antibiotics are not useful prophylactically. (6) Barium swallow may be necessary at 10 days to 3 weeks to assess the severity of damage. (7) Esophageal dilatation may need to be performed at 2- to 4-week intervals if evidence of stricture is found. (8) Interposition of the colon may be necessary if dilatation fails to provide an adequate-sized esophagus. (9) Inhalation management requires immediate removal from the environment, and clinical, radiographic, and arterial blood gas evaluation when appropriate. Oxygen and respiratory support may be required.

Chloral Hydrate. See Sedative Hypnotics, Nonbarbiturate.

Chlordane. See Organochlorine Insecticides.

Chlordiazepoxide (Librium). See Benzodiazepines.

Chlorine Gas. Chlorine gas is a yellow-greenish gas with an irritating odor, used in bleach, in the manufacture of plastics, and for water purification. Exposure usually results from transportation mishaps, industrial accidents, chemistry experiments, the mixing of household cleaners with bleach containing hypochlorite, and accidental release around swimming pools. Its density is greater than that of air, and an odor is detected at concentrations of less than 0.04 to 0.2 PPM. Chlorine acts as an oxidizing agent and also reacts with tissue water to form hypochlorous and hydrochloric acids and to generate free oxygen radicals. *Toxic dose*: The threshold limit value is less than 1 PPM, but mild mucous irritation occurs in some patients; 30 PPM produces choking and chest pain; 60 PPM produces pulmonary edema; 400 PPM for 30 minutes is lethal; and 1000 PPM is fatal in a few minutes. *Management*: (1) Remove the patient from the contaminated environment and stabilize vital functions. Use decontamination procedures for dermal and ocular contamination as indi-

cated. Protect rescue personnel with breathing apparatus. There are patients who have responded to nebulized 3.75% sodium bicarbonate (4 mL) (prepared by diluting 2 mL of 7.5% intravenous sodium bicarbonate with 2 mL of saline). *Classification*: If patient is symptomless or presents with a cough that clears up in less than 1 hour, advise rest for 12 hours and ask the patient to report if symptoms occur; no vigorous exercise for 24 hours. If symptoms persist beyond the period of exposure, admit to hospital and treat with bronchodilators (use aerosol beta agonists and theophylline, not epinephrine) and humidified oxygen. Noncardiac pulmonary edema is treated with PEEP; corticosteroids are controversial; furosemide (Lasix) may be used. For conjunctival irritation, use copious water irrigation and fluorescein stain for corneal damage. For dermal burns, use copious water irrigation and conventional treatment of burns. *Laboratory aids*: Chest radiograph (may not reflect damage for 24 hours), arterial blood gases, cardiac monitor for dysrhythmias.

Chlorpromazine (Thorazine). See Phenothiazines and Other Major Neuroleptics.

Clinitest Tablets. See Caustics and Corrosives.

Cocaine (benzoylmethylecgonine). *Toxic dose*: The potential fatal dose is 1200 mg, but death has occurred with 20 mg parenterally. *Toxicokinetics*: See Table 14. *Manifestations*: Hypertension, convulsions, hyperthermia, and cardiac dysrhythmias. *Management*: Supportive care. Avoid the induction of emesis or gastric lavage because of the rapid onset of action of cocaine. Blood pressure and thermal monitoring. Control anxiety, convulsions, and life-threatening dysrhythmias with diazepam (Valium). Lidocaine (Xylocaine) is controversial. Nitroprusside infusion, 0.5 to 10 µg per kg per minute, may be used for severe hypertension. Avoid propranolol (Inderal). Labetalol intravenously (Normodyne; Antidote 27, Table 4) has been used to control life-threatening hypertension and tachycardia but has been shown to increase the mortality in mice given cocaine. Most cases of hypertension and tachycardia are transient and can be managed without drugs or careful titration of benzodiazepines. A nonthreatening environment to reduce all sensory stimuli and protect the patient from injury is required. Apply precautions against suicide attempts and monitor the fetus if the patient is pregnant. The management of the "body packer" and "body stuffer" is to administer repeated doses of activated charcoal (except plastic vials), se-

TABLE 14. Pharmacotoxicokinetics of Cocaine

Type	Route	Time to Onset of Action	Peak	$t^{1/2}$	Possible Fatal Dose (Adult)
Hydrochloride	Insufflation	1–5 min	15–60 min	60–75 min	750–800 mg
	Ingested	Delayed	50–90 min	Sustained	1.4 gm
	IV	30–120 s	5–11 min	60–90 min	20–800 mg
Coca paste	Smoked	—	—	Not known	—
Crack and free base	Smoked	(Fastest) 5–10 s	5–11 s	Up to 20 min	Not known

cure venous access, and have drugs readily available for treating life-threatening manifestations until contraband is passed in the stool. Surgical removal may be indicated if the material does not pass the pylorus. Endoscopy may be used to remove hard plastic vials, but not the bags, containing crack. Whole-body irrigation may be useful if plastic vials or bags were ingested.

Codeine. See Opioids.

Corrosives. See Caustics and Corrosives.

Cyanide. See Table 15. Hydrocyanic acid and sodium and potassium salts act rapidly and are extremely poisonous. The acid is extremely volatile, producing cyanide, which has a distinctive odor of bitter almonds and can produce death within minutes after inhalation. Cyanide interferes with the cytochrome oxidase system. *Classes of cyanides and derivatives*: (1) Hydrogen cyanide and simple salts in large doses produce death in 15 minutes. (2) Halogenated cyanides, such as cyanogen chloride, produce irritant and vesicant gases that may cause pulmonary edema. (3) Nitriles, such as acrylonitrile and acetonitrile (artificial-nail removers). (4) Residential fires. (5) Cyanides are used as fumigants (hydrogen cyanide), in synthetic rubber (acrylonitrile), in fertilizers (cyanamide), in metal refining (salts), and in the home in some silver and furniture polishes. (6) Cyanide in the seeds of fruit stones is harmful only if the capsule is broken. *Manifestations*: Seizures, stupor, cardiac dysrhythmias, pulmonary edema, lactic acidemia, decreased arterial venous oxygen difference. Bright red venous blood. *Management*: Attendants should not administer mouth-to-mouth resuscitation. (1) Immediately, 100% oxygen. If cyanide was inhaled, remove the patient from the contaminated atmosphere. (2) Cyanide antidote kit (Antidote 14, Table 4). Use antidote only if certain of diagnosis or residential fires involving plastics, urethane, or upholstery plus (a) significant toxicity (impairment of consciousness), (b) manifestations not corrected by oxygen and out of proportion to carboxyhemoglobin level, and (c) lactic acidosis and bright red venous blood with high or normal Pa_{O_2}. (3) Gastrointestinal decontamination by gastric lavage. *No syrup of ipecac.* Activated charcoal is used but is not very effective (1 gram binds only 35 mg of cyanide). (4) Treat seizures with intravenous diazepam (Valium). (5) Correct acidosis. (6) Other antidotes: In Europe, dicobalt edetate, 600 mg, is used intravenously, followed by 300 mg if the response is not satisfactory. Hydroxocobalamin (vitamin B_{12a}) is a useful antidote but must be given immediately after exposure in large doses. Dose: 1800 mg of vitamin B_{12} per dL of potassium cyanide (KCN) is usually required (forms cyanocobalamin [vitamin B_{12}]).

DDT and Derivatives. See Organochlorine Insecticides.

Desipramine (Norpramin, Pertofrane). See Tricyclic Antidepressants.

Diazepam (Valium). See Benzodiazepines.

Digitalis Preparations. See Table 16. *Manifestations*: Manifestations may be delayed 9 to 18 hours.

TABLE 15. **Sources of Cyanide and Their Toxicity**

Plants Containing Cyanide Glycosides		
Common Name	*Part of Plant**	*Botanical Name*
Apple	Seeds	*Malus* spp
Apricot	Seeds	*Prunus armeniaca*
Arrow grass		*Triglochin* spp
Bamboo	Sprouts, stems	Tribe Bambuseae
Bermuda grass		*Cynodon dactylon*
Bird's-foot trefoil		*Lotus corniculatus*
Bitter almond	Seeds	*Prunus amygdalus amara*
Blackhorn, sloe		*Prunus spinosa*
Calabash tree		*Crescentia cujete*
Cassava	Beans and roots	*Manihot esculenta*
Catclaw		*Acacia greggi*
Cherry laurel		*Prunus laurocerasus*
Chokecherry		*Prunus virginiana*
Cotoneaster		*Cotoneaster* spp
Cycad nut		*Zamia pumila*
Elderberry	Leaves and shoots	*Sambucus* spp
Eucalyptus		*Eucalyptus chladocalyx*
False sago palm		*Cycas circinalis*
Flax		*Linus usitatissimum*
Hyacinth bean	Bean	*Dolichos lablab*
Hydrangea	Leaves and bulb	*Hydrangea* spp
Jetbead		*Rhodotypos tetrapetala*
Johnson grass		*Sorghum halepense*
Lima bean		*Phaseolus lunatus* (not in United States)
Mountain mahogany		*Cercocarpus montanus*
Passionflower (African)		*Adenia volkensii*
Peach	Seed	*Prunus persica*
Pear	Seeds	*Pyrus communis*
Plains bahia		*Bahia oppositifolia*
Plum	Seed	*Prunus domestica*
Poison suckleya		*Suckleya suckleyana*
Queen's delight		*Stillingia syvatica*
Sudan grass		*Sorghum* spp
Velvet grass		*Holcus lanatus*
Vetch	Seed	*Vicia sativa*

*In most cases, cyanide is distributed throughout the plant.

Hydrogen Cyanide Liberated from Samples of Carcinogenic Glycosides	
Sample	*HCN (mg/gm/ or mL)*
Laetrile (amygdalin)*	
Sigma	55.9
Tablet yellow	400
Kemdalin	14.1
Apricot seeds	2.92
Peach seeds	2.60
Apple seeds	0.61

*Laetrile is a 500-mg tablet for oral use, which is 6% cyanide by weight.

Forms of Cyanide and Their Toxicity	
Product	*Toxicity (Potential Lethal Dose)*
Hydrocyanic acid	50 mg (1.0 mg/kg)
Potassium or sodium cyanide	150–300 mg (2 mg/kg)
Ferriferrocyanide (Prussian blue)	50 gm
Sodium nitroprusside	5 mg/kg causes toxicity
Bitter almonds	
Oil	2 oz
Almonds	50–60 (each contains 0.001 gm of cyanide)
Pulp	240 gm
Apricot seeds	
Wild	100 gm of moist seeds = 217 mg of cyanide
Cultivated	100 gm of seeds = 8.7 mg of cyanide

TABLE 16. **Toxicity and Kinetics of Common Digitalis Preparations**

Characteristics	Digoxin	Digitoxin
Trade name	Lanoxin	Crystodigin
Loading dose (LD) over 18–24 h	Varies with age	Varies with age
Premature infant (mg/kg)	0.005	—
Child <10 years (mg/kg)	0.020–0.060	<2 yr 0.025–0.040
Child >10 years (mg/kg)	0.010–0.015	>2 yr 0.020–0.040
Total adult (mg)	0.5–7.5	0.8–1.4
Maintenance dose (MD) (% of LD)	23–35	10
Total adult (mg)	0.125–0.50	0.05–0.20
Toxic dose		
Child (mg/kg)	0.3	NA
Normal adult (mg)	2	3–5
Adult fatal dose (mg)	10–20	3–10
Gastrointestinal absorption (%)	50–80	90–100
Tablet bioavailability (%)	60–75	—
Capsule bioavailability (%)	95	—
Elixir bioavailability (%)	85	—
Onset oral (min)	15–30	25–120
Peak IV (h)	1.5–6	4–12
Peak oral (h)	3–6	4–12
Duration of action	3–6 days	2–3 wk
Protein bound (%)	25	>90
Volume of distribution (L/kg)		
In neonate	7.5–10	—
In infants and children	16	—
In adults	5–8	0.6
Fetal plasma concentrations equal maternal concentrations		
$t\frac{1}{2}$		
In premature infants (h)	37–170	—
In neonates (h)	35–69	—
In infants (h)	19–35	—
In adults	26–45 h (1½ days)	6–8 days or longer
Shorter $t\frac{1}{2}$ in overdose (h)	6–22	—
Elimination (%)	Renal 75	Liver 80
Active metabolite	None	8% converted digoxin
Plasma concentration should be measured 6–8 h after last dose		
Therapeutic plasma concentration (ng/mL)	0.5–2	15–30
Toxic plasma concentration	>4 ng/mL; varies	>35 ng/mL
There is considerable overlap between therapeutic and toxic ranges		
Normal blood concentrations do not exclude toxicity		
Serious toxic concentration (ng/mL)	>10	—
Healthy children tolerate high concentrations better than adults		
Enterohepatic recirculation (%)	Up to 14	30
Availability		
Capsules (mg)	0.05, 0.1, 0.2	—
Tablets (mg)	0.125, 0.25, 0.50	0.05, 0.1, 0.15, 0.2
Elixir (mg/mL)	0.05	0.05

SI conversion factor: ng/ml × 1.281 = mmol/L.
Abbreviation: NA = not available.
From Clinical Data Handbook 1988, pp 472–474; AMA Drug Evaluations. Chicago, AMA, 1986, pp 425–427.

Abdominal pain, nausea, vomiting, diarrhea, dysrhythmias, heart block, CNS depression, colored-halo vision. No dysrhythmia on ECG is characteristic of digitalis toxicity. *Management*: (1) Gastrointestinal decontamination. Avoid ipecac syrup; it may increase the vagal effect if the patient is symptomatic. Repeated doses of activated charcoal may interrupt enterohepatic recirculation. Gastric lavage may increase vagal effect. Pretreat with atropine 0.01 mg per kg if symptomatic. (2) Treat hemodynamically unstable ventricular dysrhythmias with Fab (antibody fragment [Digibind], Antidote 22, Table 4). Antidysrhythmic agents and a pacemaker should be used only when Fab therapy fails. Phenytoin (Dilan-

tin) and lidocaine (Xylocaine) also may be administered for ventricular dysrhythmias. Magnesium sulfate, 20 mL of 20% intravenously given slowly over 20 minutes, has been useful for malignant ventricular dysrhythmias, such as torsades de pointes. (3) Treat bradycardia and second- and third-degree atrioventricular block with atropine or low-dose phenytoin, 25 mg per dose intravenously in adults. If patient is unresponsive, use Fab (see Table 4). Insertion of a pacemaker should be seriously considered. Avoid isoproterenol, which causes dysrhythmias. External pacing may be needed. (4) Treat hyperkalemia (above 5.5 mEq per liter) with Fab (antibody fragment; see Table 4). Avoid calcium. Hemodialysis is the treatment of choice for severe or refractory hyperkalemia. (5) Direct current countershock may cause life-threatening dysrhythmias. (6) Specific Fab antibody fragments (see Table 4) have been used if cardiac arrest or shock is imminent; the dose is 10 mg in an adult, 4 mg (or over 0.3 mg per kg) in a child, or lower (0.2 mg per kg) in an adolescent. Fab is also given for hyperkalemia (serum potassium >5.5 mEq per liter), serum digoxin toxicity (>10 ng per mL in adults or >5 ng per mL in children) at 6 to 8 hours postingestion, or life-threatening dysrhythmias. Contact Poison Control Center for calculation of Fab or use package insert. *Laboratory aids*: Monitor ECG and potassium and digitalis levels. Draw blood for digoxin levels 6 to 8 hours postingestion, as well as when it is given by the intravenous route. An endogenous digoxin-like substance that cross-reacts with most common immune assay antibodies, with values as high as 4.1 ng per mL, has been reported in newborns, patients with chronic renal failure, and patients with abnormal immune globulin levels. The bound digoxin blood concentrations rise after the use of Fab, but the free (usually unmeasured) digoxin level falls.

Diphenhydramine (Benadryl). See Anticholinergic Agents.

Doxepin (Sinequan, Adapin). See Tricyclic Antidepressants.

Ethchlorvynol (Placidyl). See Sedative Hypnotics, Nonbarbiturate.

Ethyl Alcohol. See Alcohols.

Ethylene Glycol (solvent, antifreeze). *Toxic dose*: Death has occurred after a 60-mL ingestion of 95% ethylene glycol; fatal dose is 1.4 mL per kg of 100% solution. The TLV is 50 PPM. *Toxicokinetics*: Time of onset, 30 minutes to 12 hours for CNS and metabolic abnormalities to occur (Phase I). Twelve to 36 hours postingestion, cardiopulmonary depression (Phase II). In Phase III (2 to 3 days postingestion), renal failure occurs. The t½ is 3 hours (during ethanol therapy this is prolonged to 17 hours). Urine oxalate or monohydrate crystals may be seen 4 to 8 hours postingestion but are not always present. *Management*: (1) Gastrointestinal decontamination up to 30 minutes postingestion. Activated charcoal and cathartics are not indicated. (2) Treat seizures with intravenous diazepam (Valium). Exclude hypocalcemia and treat if necessary. (3) Correct acidosis with intravenous sodium bicarbonate. (4) Initiate ethanol therapy to block metabolism (Antidote 21, Table 4) if the blood ethylene glycol level is higher than 20 mg per dL, or if the patient is symptomatic or acidotic with an increased anion gap or osmolar gap. Ethanol should be administered intravenously or orally to produce a blood ethanol concentration of 100 to 150 mg per dL. (5) Early hemodialysis is indicated if the ingestion was large; if the blood ethylene glycol level is greater than 50 mg per dL; if severe acid-base or electrolyte abnormalities occur despite conventional therapy; or if renal failure occurs. (6) Thiamine (100 mg per day) and pyridoxine (50 mg four times daily) have been recommended for 48 hours but have not been extensively studied. (7) Continue therapy (ethanol and hemodialysis) until the plasma ethylene glycol level is below 10 mg per dL, the acidosis has cleared, the creatinine level is normal, and the urinary output is adequate. *Laboratory aids*: Complete blood count, electrolytes, urinalysis (look for oxalate ["envelope"] and monohydrate ["hemp seed"] crystals), and arterial blood gases. Obtain ethylene glycol and ethanol levels, plasma osmolarity (use freezing point depression method). Calcium, creatinine, and BUN studies. An ethylene glycol level of 20 mg per dL is usually toxic (levels are very difficult to obtain). The oral mucosa and urine will appear fluorescent under Wood's light if ethylene glycol is present. Propylene glycol, a vehicle in many liquid and intravenous medications (phenytoin, diazepam), may produce spurious ethylene glycol levels.

Flurazepam (Dalmane). See Benzodiazepines.

Fluoxetine (Prozac). *Toxic dose*: greater than 3.5 mg per kg in children. Over 1800 mg has produced seizures in adults. Adult fatal dose, 6 grams. *Manifestations*: Minimal risk of cardiovascular or neurologic complications. *Toxicokinetics*: See Table 31. *Management*: See Tricyclic Antidepressants.

Glutethimide (Doriden). See Sedative Hypnotics, Nonbarbiturate.

Hallucinogens

1. LSD (lysergic acid diethylamide). *Toxic dose*: equal to or greater than 35 µg. Street doses are typically 50 to 300 µg. *Toxicokinetics*: Peak effect, 1 to 2 hours. Duration, 12 to 24 hours. t½, 3 hours. Route of elimination, hepatic.

2. MORNING GLORY SEEDS *(Rivea corymbosa* or *Ipomoea)*. These have one-tenth the potency of LSD.

3. MESCALINE/PEYOTE (trimethoxyphenethylamine, or the toxic principle of *Lophophora williamsii*). *Toxic dose*: equal to or greater than 5 mg per kg. Each button of mescaline contains 45 mg (4 to 12 produce symptoms). *Toxicokinetics*: Peak effect, 4 to 6 hours. Duration, 14 hours.

4. PSILOCYBIN. Similar in effect to LSD but short-acting. Peak effect, 90 minutes. Duration, 5 to 6 hours.

5. NUTMEG *(Myristica)*. *Toxic dose*: 5 to 15 grams (1 to 3 nutmegs). Peak effect, 3 to 6 hours. Duration, up to 60 hours.

6. MARIJUANA *(Cannabis sativa)* (Δ^9-tetrahydrocannabinol, THC). One joint equals 500 mg of marijuana; when the plant is smoked, 50% is destroyed. *Toxicokinetics*: Time of onset, 2 to 3 minutes (smoked). Duration, 2 to 3 hours. t½, 28 to 47 hours (shorter for chronic user). *Note*: 1% of the metabolite can be detected in urine up to 2 weeks after use. *Manifestations*: Visual illusions, sensory perceptual distortions, depersonalization, and derealization. *Management*: "Talk-down" technique.

7. INHALANTS. Nitrites (amyl and isobutyl nitrite) act immediately; aromatic hydrocarbon in airplane model glues, plastic cements (benzene, toluene, xylene)—see Hydrocarbons; Nitrous Oxide.

8. TRYPTAMINE DERIVATIVES (DMT, *N*-dimethyltryptamine; DET, diethyltryptamine; DPT, dipropyltryp-

tamine). Rapid onset of action, but duration is only 1 to 2 hours.

9. STP OR DOM (2,5-dimethoxy-4-methylamphetamine). Acts like LSD but lasts 72 hours or longer.

10. MDA (3-methoxy-4,5-ethylenedioxyamphetamine). Related to amphetamine, produces a mild LSD-like reaction lasting 6 to 10 hours ("love pill").

See also Alcohols, Amphetamines, Anticholinergic Agents, Barbiturates, Cocaine, Opioids, Phencyclidine, Phenothiazines and Other Major Neuroleptics, and Tricyclic Antidepressants.

Haloperidol (Haldol). See Phenothiazines and Other Major Neuroleptics.

Heroin. See Opioids.

Hydrocarbons

1. PETROLEUM DISTILLATES. Gasoline (petroleum spirit), 2 to 5% benzene; kerosene (coal oil, kerosene, jet aviation fuel No. 1, charcoal lighter fluid); petroleum naphtha (cigarette lighter fluid, ligroin, racing fuel); petroleum ether (benzin); turpentine (pine oil, oil of turpentine); and mineral spirits (Stoddard solvent, white spirits, varsol, mineral turpentine, petroleum spirit). *Manifestations*: Materials aspirated during the process of ingestion may produce pneumonitis. Hypoxia associated with aspiration, not absorption, is the cause of CNS depression. It is *unlikely* that a child accidentally or an adult during siphoning of gasoline would ingest a sufficient quantity to warrant the induction of emesis.

2. AROMATIC HYDROCARBONS. *Benzene*, a solvent used in manufacturing dyes, phenol, and nitrobenzene, has a TLV of 10 PPM by inhalation according to the Occupational Safety and Health Administration (OSHA). The National Institute for Occupational Safety and Health (NIOSH) value is 1 PPM. The adult ingested toxic dose is 15 mL. Chronic exposure may cause leukemia. A level of 200 PPM is fatal in 5 minutes. *Toluene*, used in manufacturing TNT, has an OSHA TLV of 200 PPM by inhalation; the NIOSH figure is 100. The adult ingested toxic dose is 50 mL. *Styrene* has an OSHA TLV of 100 PPM by inhalation. *Xylene*, used in the manufacture of perfumes, has an OSHA TLV of 100 PPM by inhalation. The adult ingested toxic dose is 50 mL. *Manifestations*: Asphyxiation, CNS depression, defatting dermatitis, and aspiration pneumonitis. A bite into a tube of household plastic cement by a young child does not warrant the induction of emesis. Ingestion of hydrocarbon with a benzene fraction over 5% may warrant induction of emesis.

3. ALIPHATIC HALOGENATED HYDROCARBONS. See Table 17 for common examples. *Manifestations*: Myocardial sensitization and irritability, hepatorenal toxicity, and CNS depression. Dichloromethane may be converted into carbon monoxide in the body. Trichloroethylene concentrates in the fetus (pregnant women should not be exposed) and causes a disulfiram (Antabuse) reaction ("degreaser's flush") when associated with the ingestion of ethanol. The decision to induce emesis must be based on the toxicity of the agent.

4. DANGEROUS ADDITIVES. Dangerous additives to the hydrocarbons, such as heavy metals, nitrobenzene, aniline dyes, insecticides, and demothing agents, may warrant the induction of emesis.

5. HEAVY HYDROCARBONS. These have high viscos-

TABLE 17. **Common Examples of Aliphatic Halogenated Hydrocarbons**

	Estimated Toxic Dose (Ingested 100%)*	TLV–TWA (PPM ACGIH)	Synonym(s)
1,2-Dichloromethane†	0.3 mL/kg,† one swallow adult, lethal >0.5 mL/kg	1	Methylene chloride
1,2-Dichloroethylene	150–200 mL toxic in adults or large intentional ingestion	200	Acetylene dichloride
1,2-Dichloropropane	0.3 mL/kg toxic, one swallow	75	Propylene dichloride
Tetrabromoethane	1 mL/kg toxic, several swallows	—	Acetylene tetrabromide
Tetrachloroethane	0.3 mL/kg toxic, one swallow	1	Acetylene tetrachloride
Tetrachloroethylene	1 mL/kg toxic, several swallows	50	Perchloroethylene
Tetrachloromethane	0.3 mL/kg toxic, one swallow	5	
1,1,1-Trichloroethane	5.0 mL/kg fatal, 150–200 mL toxic in adults or large intestinal ingestion	350	Methyl chloroform, Triethane, Glamorene Spot Remover, Scotchgard Typewriter fluid
Trichloroethylene	0.3 mL/kg toxic, >one swallow	50	Vapor degreaser, typewriter correction fluid, fire retardant
Trichloromethane	0.3 mL/kg toxic, one swallow	10	Cleaning agent, fumigant, insecticide
1,1,2-Trichloro-1,2,2-fluoroethane	>200 mL? toxic adult		
1,1,2-Trichloroethane	0.5 mL/kg toxic, >2.0 mL/kg lethal	10	Vinyl trichloride
Carbon tetrachloride	3–5 mL total amount Lethal 4 mL total	2	

*Estimated fatal dose assumes pure 100% of the halogenated hydrocarbon in the ingested product. At this dose it is recommended that medical evaluation be sought. A *swallow* in 2-year-old is approximately 5 mL (0.3 mL/kg), in adult, 15–20 mL. *Larger intentional amount* is 120–150 mL in adults. The decision for medical evaluation should be based on the most toxic substance present at concentrations exceeding 10 to 20%.

†Amount of methylene chloride in a single Christmas tree bubbling fluid light (0.5 mL) is nontoxic if ingested by small children.

Abbreviations: ACGIH = American Conference of Government Industrial Hygienists; PPM = part per million; TLV = threshold limit value for 8-hour workday; TWA = time-weighted average concentration for normal workday and 40-hour workweek to which nearly all workers may be repeatedly exposed.

ity, low volatility, and minimal absorption, so emesis is unwarranted. Examples are asphalt (tar), machine oil, motor oil (lubricating oil, engine oil), diesel oil (engine fuel, home heating oil), petrolatum liquid (mineral oil, suntan oils), petrolatum jelly (Vaseline), paraffin wax, transmission oil, cutting oil, and greases and glues.

6. PRODUCTS TREATED AS PETROLEUM DISTILLATES. Essential oils (e.g., turpentine, pine oil) are treated as petroleum distillates. Mineral seal oil (signal oil), found in some furniture polishes, is a heavy, viscous oil that *never* warrants emesis; it can produce severe pneumonia if aspirated. It has minimal absorption. *Management*: Dermal decontamination. Removal from the environment in inhalation.

FIRST AID TREATMENT. See Table 18. *The use of activated charcoal, oils, and cathartics is not advised in petroleum distillate ingestions. General management*: (1) In the asymptomatic patient: observe several hours for the development of respiratory distress. (2) In the symptomatic patient: supportive respiratory care for respiratory distress. Bronchospasm may be treated with intravenous aminophylline. Avoid epinephrine. Monitor ECG; arterial blood gases; liver, pulmonary, and renal function; serum electrolytes; serial radiographs. Observe for signs of intravascular hemolysis and disseminated intravascular coagulation. If cyanosis that does not respond to oxygen is present or the arterial Pa_{O_2} is normal, suspect methemoglobinemia that may require therapy with methylene blue. Steroids have not been shown to be beneficial. Antimicrobial agents are not useful in prophylaxis. (Fever or leukocytosis may be produced by the chemical pneumonitis itself.) It is not necessary to treat pneumatoceles. Most infiltra-tions resolve spontaneously in 1 week except for lipoid pneumonia, which may last up to 6 weeks.

Imipramine (Tofranil). See Tricyclic Antidepressants.

Iron. The iron content of some preparations appears in Table 19. *Toxic dose*: Range, 20 to 60 mg per kg or greater of elemental iron. Dose requiring induction of emesis, equal to or greater than 20 mg per kg. The potential fatal dose is 180 mg per kg (600 mg of elemental iron). *Toxicokinetics*: Absorption occurs chiefly in the small intestine. For excretion there is no normal route except blood loss or gastrointestinal desquamation. *Manifestations*: Phase I—mucosal injury possibly with hematemesis (1 to 6 hours postingestion). Phase II—patient appears improved (2 to 24 hours). Phase III—cardiovascular collapse and severe metabolic acidosis (12 to 48 hours). Phase IV—hepatic injury associated with jaundice (2 to 4 days). Phase V—sequelae of intestinal stricture and obstruction or anemia (2 to 6 weeks). Patients asymptomatic for 6 hours rarely develop serious intoxication manifestations. *Management*: (1) Gastrointestinal decontamination. Emesis should be induced in ingestions of elemental iron that are over 20 mg per kg. Emesis should be followed by gastric lavage in an adult or in a child who has ingested a chewable or liquid preparation. The solution to be used for lavage is saline 0.9% or 1 to 1.5% sodium bicarbonate to form ferrous carbonate salts, which are poorly absorbed. One hundred milliliters of this solution should be left in the stomach (prepared by dilution of a sodium bicarbonate ampule with saline). The use of deferoxamine (Desferal Mesylate) in the gastrointestinal tract is not recommended. The use of diluted Fleet Enema

---

TABLE 18. **Initial Management of Hydrocarbon Ingestions**

Symptoms	Contents	Amount	Initial Management
None	Petroleum distillate only	Any amount	None
None	Heavy hydrocarbon	Any amount	None*
	Mineral seal oil		None
None	Petroleum distillate with dangerous additive (heavy metals, pesticide)	Depends on toxicity of additive	Gastric lavage with small-bore tube
	Aromatic hydrocarbons	>1 mL/kg	
	Halogenated hydrocarbons†		
	A. Very toxic compounds	>0.3 mL/kg	Gastric lavage
	B. Moderately toxic compounds	>0.5 mL/kg	Gastric lavage
	C. Low-toxicity compounds	>1.0 mL/kg	Gastric lavage
	D. Christmas tree bubbling light	Nontoxic	None
Loss of protective airway reflexes, coma, seizures	Petroleum distillate with dangerous additive, aromatic, or halogenated hydrocarbons	Same as aromatic or halogenated hydrocarbons above	Endotracheal tube before gastric lavage

*Emesis may be necessary if machine oil contains triorthocresyl phosphate (TOCP), which causes weakness, sensory impairment, and "partially reversible damage to the spinal cord."

†Amounts of halogenated hydrocarbons ingested assume 100% of product.

A. More than one swallow in adult or 0.3 mL/kg in a child of 100% of 1,2-dichloromethane (methylene chloride), 1,2-dichloropropane (propylene dichloride), tetrachloroethane (acetylene tetrachloride), tetrachloromethane, trichloroethylene, tetrachloroethylene, trichloromethane, or tetrabromoethane (acetylene tetrabromide).

B. Several swallows in an adult or 0.5 mL/kg in a child of 100% 1,2-dichloroethane (ethylene dichloride), 1,2-dichloroethylene (acetylene dichloride), 1,1,2-trichloroethane (vinyl trichloride), tetrabromoethane, tetrachloroethylene (perchloroethylene), or 1,1,2,2-tetrachloroethylene.

C. A large intentional ingestion in an adult (150–200 mL) or over 1 mL/kg in a child of 100% 1,2-dichloroethylene, tetrachloromethane, 1,1,1,-trichloroethane (methyl chloroform), or 1,1,2-trichloro-1,2,2,-fluoroethane.

D. The amount of dichloromethane (methylene chloride) in a single Christmas tree bubbling fluid light (0.5 mL) is nontoxic if ingested by small children.

TABLE 19. **Iron Content of Some Preparations**

Iron Salt	Elemental Iron Content (%)	Average Tablet Strength (mg)	Elemental Iron/ Tablet (mg)	Average FeSO$_4$, Strength (mg)
Ferrous sulfate (hydrous)	20	300	60	Drp 75/0.6 mL
	20	SR 160	32	Syp 90/5 mL
	20	195	39	Solu 125/mL
	20	325	65	Elxr 220/5 mL
Ferrous sulfate (dried)	30	200	60	
	30	SR 160	48	
Ferrous gluconate	12	320	36	Elxr 320/5 mL
Ferrous fumarate	33	200	67	
	33	SR 324	107	Drp 45.0/6 mL
	33	Chewable 100	33	Susp 100/5 mL

Abbreviations: SR = slow release; Drp = dropper; Syp = syrup; Solu = solution; Elxr = elixir; Susp = suspension.

(mono- and dibasic sodium phosphate) solution risks severe hypertonic phosphate poisoning. Activated charcoal is not recommended. (2) Postlavage abdominal radiograph—if significant amounts of residual radiopaque material are present, consider whole-bowel irrigation with polyethylene glycol solution first. Removal by endoscopy or surgery may also be required because coalesced tablets have produced hemorrhagic infarction and perforation peritonitis. (3) Diagnostic chelation test—deferoxamine not reliable. (4) Indications for chelation therapy with deferoxamine are serum iron levels over 500 mg per dL or systemic signs of intoxication independent of the serum iron level. Chelation should be performed within 12 to 18 hours to be effective (Antidote 15, Table 4). *Laboratory aids*: Serum iron levels correlate with the clinical course. Iron levels that are below 350 mg per dL when taken at 2 to 6 hours predict an asymptomatic course; levels of 350 to 500 are associated with mild gastrointestinal symptoms (rarely serious); and levels greater than 500 suggest the possibility of serious Phase III manifestations. Draw blood for serum iron (SI) before administering deferoxamine because it interferes with analysis. Total iron-binding capacity is not necessary. An SI at 8 to 12 hours is useful to exclude delayed absorption from a bezoar or sustained-release preparation. White blood cell counts greater than 15,000 per μL, blood glucose levels over 150 mg per dL, radiopaque material present on abdominal radiograph, vomiting, and diarrhea predict iron levels greater than 300 mg per dL. Monitor complete blood counts, blood glucose, serum iron, stools, and vomitus for occult blood; electrolytes; acid-base balance; urinalysis and urinary output; liver function tests; BUN; and creatinine. Obtain type and match of blood in severe cases. Abdominal radiographs. Follow-up is necessary for sequelae in significant intoxications—gastrointestinal series for intestinal strictures and anemia secondary to blood loss. Patients who develop fever or toxic symptoms after iron overdose should have blood and stool cultures checked for *Yersinia enterocolitica.*

Isoniazid (INH, Nydrazid). This is an antituberculosis drug frequently used in suicide attempts by Native Americans and Eskimos. *Mechanism of toxicity*: It produces pyridoxine deficiency (doubles excre-

tion of pyridoxine). *Toxic dose*: 1.5 grams, 35 to 40 mg per kg, produces convulsions; severe toxicity is seen at 6 to 10 grams; at 200 mg per kg it is an obligatory convulsant. *Toxicokinetics*: Absorption is rapid, with a peak in 1 to 2 hours (clinical symptoms may start in 30 minutes). The Vd is 0.6 liter per kg. It passes the placenta and into breast milk at 50% of the maternal serum level. Not protein-bound. Elimination is by the liver, which produces a hepatotoxic metabolite, acetylisoniazid. t½—Slow acetylators (2 to 4 hours) (50% of blacks and whites) may develop peripheral neuropathy. Fast acetylators (0.7 to 2 hours) (90% of Asians and a majority of patients with diabetes) may develop hepatitis. Excreted unchanged, 10 to 40%. *Major toxic manifestations*: Visual disturbances, convulsions (≥90% with one or more seizures), coma, resistant severe acidosis (due to lactate secondary to hypoxia, convulsions, and metabolic blocks). *Management*: (1) Control seizures with large doses of pyridoxine, 1 gram for each gram of isoniazid ingested (Antidote 38, Table 4). If the dose ingested is unknown, give at least 5 grams of pyridoxine intravenously. Diazepam (Valium) is given and works synergistically to control seizures. (2) Correct acidosis with fluids and sodium bicarbonate (pyridoxine may spontaneously correct the acidosis). (3) After the patient is stabilized, or if asymptomatic, gastrointestinal decontamination procedures may be carried out, keeping in mind the rapid onset of convulsions. Asymptomatic patients should be observed for 4 hours. (4) Hemodialysis is rarely needed but may be used as an adjunct for uncontrollable acidosis and seizures. Hemoperfusion has not been adequately evaluated. Diuresis is ineffective. *Laboratory aids*: Isoniazid toxic levels are above 10 to 20 μg per mL. Monitor the blood glucose (often hyperglycemia), electrolytes (often hyperkalemia), bicarbonate, arterial blood gases, liver function tests, BUN, and creatinine. If convulsions persist obtain an EEG. Monitor the temperature closely (often hyperpyrexia).

Isopropyl Alcohol. See Alcohols.

Kerosene. See Hydrocarbons.

Lead. *Acute* lead poisoning is rare. *Acute toxic dose*: 0.5 gram in children. *Management*: (1) Gastrointestinal decontamination. (2) Supportive care, including measures to deal with the hepatic and renal failure and intravascular hemolysis. (3) EDTA in all severe cases if lead levels confirm absorption. *Chronic* lead poisoning occurs most often in children 6 months to 6 years of age who are exposed in their environment and in adults in certain occupations. *Chronic toxic dose*: Determined by blood lead level and clinical findings. A level of 10 µg per dL or over is the threshold of concern in children; 40 µg per dL or over in adult workers; 30 µg per dL or over for those planning pregnancy. Medical removal from work at 60 µg per dL. *Toxicokinetics*: Absorption—10 to 15% of the ingested dose is absorbed in adults; in children up to 40% is absorbed with iron deficiency anemia. Inhalation absorption is rapid and complete. Vd—95% present in bone. In blood, 95% is in red blood cells. t½—35 days; in bone, 10 years. The major elimination route for inorganic lead is renal. Organic lead is metabolized in the liver to inorganic lead; 9% is excreted in the urine per day. *Manifestations of acute symptoms of chronic lead poisoning* (ABCDE): Anorexia, apathy, anemia; behavior disturbances; clumsiness; developmental deterioration; and emesis. Manifestations of encephalopathy are remembered by the mnemonic PAINT: *P*, persistent forceful vomiting; *A*, ataxia; *I*, intermittent stupor and lucidity; *N*, neurologic coma and convulsions; *T*, tired and lethargic. In adults, one may see peripheral neuropathies and "lead gum lines." *Management*: (1) Gastrointestinal decontamination with enemas if radiopaque foreign bodies are noted. Do not delay therapy until clear. (2) Remove from exposure. For children, see Table 20. Dimercaptosuccinic acid, a derivative of dimercaprol (BAL), is an oral agent approved by the FDA for chelation only in children with venous blood lead levels of over 45 µg per dL. The recommended dose is 10 mg per kg every 8 hours for 5 days, then every 12 hours for 14 days (Antidote 42, Table 4). *Laboratory aids*: (1) Provocation mobilization test—500 mg of EDTA per m² of body surface area for one dose given deeply intramuscularly with 0.5% procaine diluted 1:1; collect the urine for 8 hours. If the ratio of micrograms excreted in the urine to milligrams of Ca-EDTA administered is greater than 0.6, there is an increased lead body burden, and chelation should be carried out. (2) Evaluate complete blood count, levels of serum iron, or ferritin; repeat blood lead levels and erythrocyte protoporphyrin. (3) Flat plate of the abdomen and long bone radiographs (knees usually). (4) Renal function tests. (5) Monitor electrolytes, serum calcium, phosphorus, blood glucose.

Lindane. See Organochlorine Insecticides.

Lithium (Eskalith, Lithane). Most cases of intoxication have occurred as therapeutic overdoses. The toxic dose is determined by serum levels, although intoxication has occurred with levels in the therapeutic range. *Toxicokinetics*: Absorption is rapid, with complete peaking in 1 to 4 hours. Vd is 0.5 to 0.9 liter per kg. It is not protein-bound. The t½ therapeutically is 18 to 24 hours. The kidney excretes 89 to 98% unchanged, one-third to two-thirds in 6 to 12 hours. Excretion is decreased in the presence of hyponatremia and dehydration. The cerebrospinal fluid concentration is one-half the plasma concentration. The breast milk level is 50% of the maternal serum level—toxic to the nursling. *Manifestations*: The first sign of toxicity may be diarrhea. Fine tremor of hands, lethargy, weakness, polyuria and polydipsia, goiter and hypothyroidism, and fasciculations are side effects. Severe toxicity is manifested by ataxia, impaired mental state, coma, and seizures (limbs held in hyperextension with eyes open in "coma vigil"). Cardiovascular manifestations are dysrhythmias, hypotension, flat T waves, and an increased QT interval. *Management*: (1) Gastrointestinal decontamination may not be useful after 2 hours because of rapid absorption. In slow-release preparations, decontamination may be useful up to 24 hours postingestion. Activated charcoal is not indicated. Sodium polystyrene sulfonate (Kayexalate), 60 mL orally four times a day, is useful in preventing absorption. Determine serum sodium level before administration because this agent may aggravate existing hypernatremia. (2) Hospitalize if intoxication is suspected because seizures may occur unexpectedly. (3) Restore normothermia and fluid and electrolyte balance, particularly sodium. If diabetes insipidus is present, an infusion of sodium may cause hypernatremia. Current evidence supports saline infusion as enhancing excretion of lithium. An infusion of 1 to 2 liters of 0.89% saline (adults) or 20 mL per kg (children) should be started to correct fluid and electrolyte deficits. When fluid deficits are corrected, administer 0.45% saline. (4) Hemodialysis is the treatment of choice for severe intoxication. Lithium is the most dialyzable toxin known. Long runs should be used until the lithium level is less than 1 mEq per liter because of extensive re-equilibration rebound. Monitor levels every 4 hours after dialysis. Dialysis may have to be repeated. Expect a time lag in neurologic recovery. If hemodialysis is not available or delayed, peritoneal dialysis can be used but is less effective. (5) Monitor ECG. Refractory dysrhythmias may be treated with magnesium sulfate and sodium bicarbonate. (6) Avoid thiazides and spironolactone diuretics, which increase lithium levels. *Laboratory aids*: Lithium level determinations should be performed every 2 to 4 hours. Although they do not always correlate with the manifestations at low levels, they are predictive in severe intoxications. Levels of 0.6 to 1.2 mEq per liter are usually therapeutic. Levels over 4.0 mEq per liter are usually severely toxic. Other tests to be monitored are complete blood count (lithium causes leukocytosis), renal function, thyroid, ECG, and electrolytes. Factors that predispose to lithium toxicity are febrile illness, sodium depletion, concomitant drugs (thiazide and spironolactone diuretics), impaired renal function, advanced age, and fluid loss in vomiting and diarrheal illness.

Lomotil (Diphenoxylate and Atropine). See Opioids and Anticholinergic Agents.

LSD (Lysergic Acid Diethylamide). See Hallucinogens.

TABLE 20. **Choice of Chelation Therapy Based on Symptoms and Blood Lead Concentration**

Clinical Presentation	Treatment	Comments
Symptomatic Children		
Acute encephalopathy	BAL,* 450 mg/m²/24 h CaNa₂-EDTA, 1500 mg/m²/24 h	BAL, 75/m² q 4 h After 4 h, start infusion of EDTA or use IM q 4 h† Duration, 5 days Interrupt therapy for 2 days If blood Pb > 70 μg/dL, BAL and EDTA for 5 more days; EDTA alone if blood Pb = 45–69 μg/dL Other cycles depend on blood Pb rebound
Blood Pb > 70 μg/dL	BAL, 300 mg/m²/24 h CaNa₂-EDTA, 1000 mg/m²/24 h Do not use CaNa₂-EDTA alone if symptomatic	BAL, 50 mg/m² q 4 h After 4 h, start infusion of EDTA or use IM q 4 h† Duration, 5 days Interrupt therapy for 2 days Discontinue BAL in 3 days if blood Pb < 50 μg/dL; BAL and EDTA for 5 more days if blood Pb > 50 μg/dL Other cycles depend on blood Pb rebound
Asymptomatic Children		
BEFORE TREATMENT, MEASURE VENOUS BLOOD LEAD		
Blood Pb > 70 μg/dL	BAL, 300 mg/m²/24 h CaNa₂-EDTA, 1000 mg/m²/24 h	BAL 50 mg/m² IM q 4 h After 4 h, start infusion of EDTA or use IM q 4 h Duration, 5 days Discontinue BAL in 3 days if blood Pb < 50 μg/dL Give second course of EDTA if blood Pb > 45 μg/dL within 5 days Other cycles depend on blood Pb rebound
Blood Pb = 45–69 μg/dL‡	CaNa₂-EDTA, 1000 mg/m²/24 h or DMSA	EDTA, IM q 4 h or IV Duration, 5 days Give second course of EDTA if blood Pb > 45 μg/dL within 7–14 days; wait 5–7 days before giving second course If lead exposure controlled, give single IV or IM dose on outpatient basis Other cycles depend on blood Pb rebound
Blood Pb = 25–44 μg/dL	CaNa₂-EDTA, 1000 mg/m²/24 h	Provocation, EDTA test Duration, 5 days IM or IV Provocation test periodically
Guidelines for Chelation of Excess Lead in Adults		
INORGANIC LEADS§		
Symptomatic Cases		
Acute encephalopathy	BAL-EDTA	Same as for children
Abdominal pain, weakness, and colic	BAL-EDTA	Course for 3–5 days followed by oral penicillamine until urine Pb < 500 μg/24 h or 2 months, whichever less
Painless peripheral neuropathy	D-Penicillamine	For 1–2 months If blood lead > 100 μg/dL, BAL-EDTA first course 3–5 days, followed by oral penicillamine
Asymptomatic Cases		
Blood Lead Concentration (μg/dL)		
100	BAL-EDTA	
80–100	Penicillamine alone	
40–79 and EP > 60	Provocation test	
ORGANIC LEAD	No chelation therapy	

Note: OSHA requires that workers be removed from the work environment when lead levels exceed 50 μg/dL and until they are below 40 μg/dL.

*Dimercaprol.
†Some physicians prefer to give EDTA IM to avoid large fluid volumes in high intracranial pressure.
‡DMSA may be used.
§Data from Rempel D: The lead exposed worker. JAMA 262:532–534, 1989. Copyright 1989, American Medical Association.
Abbreviations: BAL = British antilewisite; Blood Pb = venous blood lead concentration; CaNa₂ = calcium disodium; DMSA = 2,3-dimercaptosuccinic acid; EDTA = ethylenediaminetetraacetic acid; EP = erythrocyte protoporphyrin.
Modified from Piomelli S, Rosen JF, Chisolm JJ Jr, Graef JW: Management of childhood lead poisoning. J Pediatr 105(4):527, 1984, and CDC Prevention of Childhood Lead Poisoning. Atlanta, CDC, 1991.

Marijuana. See Hallucinogens.

Meperidine (Demerol). See Opioids.

Meprobamate (Equanil, Miltown). See Sedative Hypnotics, Nonbarbiturate.

Mercury. *Management*: (1) Inhalation of elemental mercury—remove from exposure. (2) Ingestion of mercuric salt—gastrointestinal decontamination. Do not induce emesis. A protein solution such as egg white or 5% salt-poor albumin can be given to reduce salt to mercurous ion (less toxic). Activated charcoal does absorb mercuric chloride. (3) Chelating agents (do not use Ca-EDTA because of nephrotoxicity): dimercaprol (BAL) enhances mercury excretion through the bile as well as the urine and is the first choice if renal impairment from the mercury exists (Antidote 17, Table 4). Alternatives are penicillamine (Antidote 34, Table 4) and *N*-acetyl-DL-penicillamine (investigational use). Use of BAL in methyl mercury intoxication increases the brain mercury level and appears to be contraindicated; penicillamine and its analogue should be used (decreases mercury levels in brain). Another chelator, 2,3-dimercaptosuccinic acid, holds promise of less toxicity and more specific therapy.* (4) Monitor fluid and electrolyte levels, renal function, hemoglobin levels. Obtain blood and urine mercury levels (consult the laboratory for proper collection technique and containers). (5) Hemodialysis early in the symptomatic patient is useful. (6) Newer but not established approaches are use of polythiol resin to bind the methyl mercury excreted in the bile; heat and sauna treatment to increase mercury excretion through perspiration; and a regional dialyzer system using L-cysteine. (7) Surgical excision of *local injection sites*. *Laboratory aids*: (1) Blood levels are below 2 to 4 μg per dL and urine levels below 10 to 20 μg per liter in 90% of the adult population. Levels above 4 μg per dL in blood and 20 μg per liter in urine probably should be considered abnormal. Blood levels are not always reliable after the first few hours. Exposed industrial workers' urine levels are 150 to 200 μg per liter. (2) In asymptomatic patients with urine levels under 300 μg per liter, a chelating challenge with BAL or penicillamine may bring a significant increase that may aid in establishing the diagnosis. (3) Approximately 150 μg per liter of mercury in urine is equivalent to 3.5 μg per dL in blood. (4) Methyl mercury is excreted mainly through the feces, so urine mercury would not be a reliable measurement. (5) Mercury is also excreted in the sweat and saliva. The parotid fluid level is approximately two-thirds that of the blood. Because the hair is porous, it may absorb mercury from the atmosphere; however, hair concentrations of 400 to 500 μg per gram are likely to be associated with neurologic symptoms. Radiographs of the abdomen for ingestion and chest radiographs for injections may be helpful in showing radiopaque material.

Methadone. See Opioids.

Methanol. See Alcohols.

---

*Not FDA-approved for this purpose.

Methaqualone. See Sedative Hypnotics, Nonbarbiturate.

Methyprylon (Noludar). See Sedative Hypnotics, Nonbarbiturate.

Narcotic Analgesics. See Opioids.

Neuroleptics. See Phenothiazines and Other Major Neuroleptics.

Nitrites (NO₂) and Nitrates (NO₃). These are readily available in both inorganic and organic forms. Organic nitrates used for angina pectoris are listed in Table 21. Inorganic nitrates have more toxicologic importance in small infants in vegetables (carrots, spinach, beets) and preservatives used in meat products and contaminated well water. *Potential fatal doses*: Nitrite, 1 gram; nitrate, 10 grams; nitrobenzene, 2 mL; nitroglycerin, 0.2 gram; and aniline dye (pure), 5 to 30 grams. *Toxicokinetics*: Time to onset of action of nitroglycerin sublingually is 1 to 3 minutes, with a time to peak action of 3 to 15 minutes and a duration of 20 to 30 minutes. Other routes have a slower onset (2 to 5 minutes) and longer duration of action (1.5 to 6 hours). Nitrites are potent oxidizing agents converting ferrous to ferric iron in the hemoglobin molecule, which cannot carry oxygen. Normally humans have 0.7% methemoglobin, which is converted by methemoglobin reductase into oxygen-carrying hemoglobin. *Route of elimination*: Liver detoxification by dinitration. *Toxic manifestations* depend on the level of methemoglobinemia. At 10%, "chocolate cyanosis" occurs; at 10 to 20%, headache, dizziness, and tachypnea occur; and at 50%, mental alterations are present and coma and convulsions may occur. Headache, flushing, and sweating are due to the vasodilatory effect; hypotension, tachycardia, and syncope may also occur. Severe hypoxia may produce pulmonary edema and encephalopathy. Levels above 50% produce metabolic acidosis and ECG changes; cardiovascular collapse occurs at levels of 70%. *Management*: (1) Dermal decontamination, if indicated. Aniline dyes may be removed with 5%

TABLE 21. **Organic Nitrates for Angina Pectoris**

Drug and Route	Trade Name	Time to Onset of Action (min)	Duration (h)
Nitroglycerin			
Oral	Many	Varies	4–6
Sublingual	Many	1–3	¼–½
2% ointment	Nitro-Bid	15	3–6
Transdermal	Nitrol		
	Nitro-Dur	30	2–4
Isosorbide dinitrate	Isordil		
Sublingual		1–3	1.3–3
Oral		2–5	4–6
Chewable		2–5	2–3
Timed release		Varies	—
Isosorbide mononitrate	ISMO	1–2	6–12
Pentaerythritol tetranitrate, oral	Peritrate	2–5	3–5
Erythrityl tetranitrate, oral	Cardilate	2–5	4–6

acetic acid (vinegar). (2) Gastrointestinal decontamination if ingested. (3) Hypotension can be treated by the Trendelenburg position and fluid challenge. Vasoconstrictors (dopamine or norepinephrine) are rarely needed. (4) Methylene blue (Antidote 29, Table 4) is indicated for methemoglobin levels above 30%, dyspnea, metabolic acidosis (lactic acidosis), or an altered mental state. (5) Oxygen, 100%, or a hyperbaric chamber should be used in symptomatic patients if methylene blue fails or is not effective, e.g., as in chlorate intoxication or glucose-6-phosphate dehydrogenase deficiency. *Laboratory aids*: Methemoglobin levels, arterial blood gases. Blood has a chocolate-brown appearance and fails to turn red on exposure to oxygen. Methemoglobin levels and oxygen saturation should be measured by co-oximeter, not by pulse oximetry.

Nortriptyline (Aventyl, Pamelor). See Tricyclic Antidepressants.

Opioids (Narcotic Opiates). See Table 22. The major metabolic pathway differs for each opioid, but they are 90% metabolized in the liver. Patients should be observed for CNS and respiratory depression and hypotension. Pulmonary edema is a potentially lethal complication of mainlining (intravenous use). *Manifestations*: All opiate agonists produce miotic pupils (except meperidine [Demerol] and diphenoxylate-atropine [Lomotil] early), respiratory and CNS depression, physical dependence, and withdrawal symptoms. *Management*: (1) Supportive care, particularly an endotracheal tube and assisted ventilation. (2) Gastrointestinal decontamination up to 12 hours postingestion, because opiates delay gastric emptying time, but this is of no benefit if overdose is by injection. Convulsions occur rapidly with propoxyphene (Darvon) and codeine overdose, and this may be an indication not to use an emetic for gastrointestinal decontamination in this drug overdose. (3) Naloxone (Narcan) (Antidote 30, Table 4) may be given in bolus intravenous doses and by continuous drip. Naloxone must be titrated against the clinical response and precipitation of withdrawal in narcotic addicts. It should be repeated as often as necessary, because the effects of many opioids in overdose can last 24 to 48 hours, whereas the action of naloxone lasts only 2 to 3 hours. *Larger doses are needed for buprenorphine, codeine, designer drugs, dextromethorphan, diphenoxylate, methadone, pentazocine, and propoxyphene.* (4) Pulmonary edema does not respond to naloxone, and the patient needs respiratory supportive care. Fluids should be given cautiously in opioid overdose because these agents stimulate the antidiuretic hormone effect and pulmonary edema is frequent. (5) *If the patient is comatose, give 50% glucose* (3 to 4% of comatose narcotic overdose patients have hypoglycemia). (6) *If the patient is agitated,* consider hypoxia rather than withdrawal and treat as such. (7) *Observe for withdrawal* signs and symptoms (nausea, vomiting, cramps, diarrhea, dilated pupils, rhinorrhea, piloerection). If these occur, stop naloxone.

Opioid Addict Withdrawal Score. Signs and symptoms of withdrawal are diarrhea, dilated pupils, gooseflesh, hyperactive bowel sounds, hypertension, insomnia, lacrimation, muscle cramps, restlessness, tachycardia, and yawning. Each sign or symptom is given 0, 1, or 2 points, depending on the severity. A score of 1 to 5 is mild; 6 to 10, moderate; and 11 to 15, severe. Seizures are unusual in withdrawal. They indicate severity regardless of the rest of the score.

TABLE 22. **Opioids (Narcotic Opiates)***

Drugs		Equivalent IM		Time to Peak Action (h)	t½ (h)	Duration of Action (h)	Potential Toxic Dose (mg)
Generic	*Trade*	*Dose† (mg)*	*Oral† (mg)*				
Alphaprodine‡	Nisentil	40–60	—	—	2	1–2	—
Butorphanol	Stadol	2	—	0.5–1.0	3	2.5–3.5	—
Camphorated tincture of opium	Paregoric	—	25 mL	—	—	4–5	—
Codeine	Various	120	200	—	3	4–6	800
Diacetylmorphine	Heroin	5	60	—	0.5	3–4	100
Diphenoxylate	Lomotil	—	10	Delayed by atropine	2.5	14	300
Fentanyl	Sublimaze	0.1–0.2	—	0.5	4–6	0.5–2	—
Hydrocodone	Hycodan	5–10	5–10	—	3.8	3–4	100
Hydromorphone	Dilaudid	1.5	6.0	0.5–1.5	2–3	2–4	100
Meperidine	Demerol	50–100	75–100	0.5–1	2–5	3–4	1000
Methadone	Dolophine	10.0	20	2–4	22–97	4–12	120
Morphine	Various	10.0	60	0.3–1.5	2–3	3–4	200
Nalbuphine	Nubain	10.0	—	0.5–1.0	3–4	3–4	—
Oxycodone	Percodan	—	15	—	—	3–4	—
Oxymorphone	Numorphan	1.0	—	1	2–3	4–5	—
Pentazocine	Talwin	—	30–60	1	2–6	3–4	—
Propoxyphene	Darvon	—	65–100	2–4	8–24	2–4	500

*"Ts and blues" are a combination of pentazocine (Talwin) and tripelennamine (Pyribenzamine) used intravenously. Pentazocine now has naloxone added to it to counter this abuse. Innovar is fentanyl plus droperidol, used as an IV anesthetic.
†Dose equivalent to 10 mg of morphine.
‡Not available in the United States.

Management: Mild withdrawal is treated with diazepam (Valium) orally, 10 mg every 6 hours; moderate withdrawal, with intramuscular diazepam; and severe withdrawal, with diazepam and diphenoxylate-atropine for the diarrhea. Methadone orally may be used, 20 to 40 mg every 12 hours, decreased by 5 mg every 12 hours. When 10 mg is reached, add diphenoxylate-atropine. Clonidine (Catapres), 6 μg per kg every 6 hours, can be used with informed consent. (This is an unlisted use of clonidine; the manufacturer states that relief from withdrawal symptoms has been reported with 0.8 mg per day.) *Laboratory aids*: For acute overdose obtain levels of blood gases, blood glucose, and electrolytes; chest radiographs; and ECG. Blood opioid levels confirm the diagnosis but are not useful for making a therapeutic decision. For drug abusers, consider testing for hepatitis B, syphilis, and human immunodeficiency virus (HIV) antibody (HIV testing usually requires consent).

PROPOXYPHENE (Darvon). *Manifestations*: Onset may be as early as 30 minutes after ingestion. Convulsions occur early. Patients may develop diabetes insipidus, pulmonary edema, and hypoglycemia. *Elimination*: Metabolism is 90% by demethylation in the liver. Peak plasma level 1 to 2 hours after oral dose. The t½ is 1 to 5 hours. As little as 10 mg per kg has caused symptoms, and 35 mg per kg has caused cardiopulmonary arrest. Therapeutic blood level is less than 200 μg per mL. *Treatment* (in addition to the general management): (1) Emesis can be dangerous because of the rapid onset of seizures. (2) Indications for naloxone are respiratory depression, seizure activity, coma, and miotic pupils. Signs of naloxone effect are dilatation of pupils, increased rate and depth of respirations, reversal of hypotension, and improvement of obtunded or comatose state. Larger doses of naloxone are often required and can be continued as an infusion of the initial response dose every hour. (3) Naloxone and intravenous glucose should be tried first to control seizures. If these fail, diazepam may be tried.

Organochlorine Insecticides (DDT derivatives). See Table 23 for a listing of these agents. The *toxic dose* varies greatly. For chlorophenothane (DDT), 200 to 250 mg per kg is fatal; 16 mg per kg causes seizures. For methoxychlor, 500 to 600 mg per kg is fatal. For chlordane, 200 mg per kg is fatal (chlordane house air guidelines are below 5 μg per m³; the occupational TLV is 500 μg per m³). These insecticides interfere with axon transmission of nerve impulses. Metabolism varies; they resist degradation in human tissue and the environment. They accumulate in adipose tissue; the elimination route is via the liver. *Manifestations*: CNS stimulation, convulsions, late respiratory depression, and increased myocardial irritability usually develop within 1 to 2 hours and may last for 1 week or more. Endrin produces liver toxicity with a guarded prognosis. Chronic exposure causes liver and kidney damage. *Management*: (1) Dermal decontamination; discard contaminated leather goods. Protect personnel. Gastrointestinal decontamination, no oils. Emesis can be dangerous, owing to rapid onset of seizures. Many of these agents are dissolved in petroleum distillates, presenting an aspiration hazard. (2) No adrenergic stimulants (epinephrine) should be used because of myocardial irritability. (3) Cholestyramine, 4 grams

TABLE 23. **Organochlorine Pesticides (DDT Derivatives)**

Chemical Name	Trade Name	Toxicity Rating	Fatal Dose (Adult)	Elimination Time	Comment
Endrin	Hexadrin	Highest	NA	Hours–days	Banned
Lindane	1% in Kwell; Benesan; Isotox; Gamene	Moderate to high	10 gm	Hours–days	Scabicide; general garden insecticide
Endosulfan	Thiodan	Moderate	NA	Hours–days	
Benzene hexachloride	BHC, HCH	Moderate	NA	Weeks–months	Banned, produces porphyria (cutanea tarda)
Dieldrin	Dieldrite	High	3 gm	Weeks–months	Banned in 1974
Aldrin	Aldrite	High	3 gm	Weeks–months	Banned in 1974
Chlordane (10% is heptachlor)	Chlordan	High	3 gm	Weeks–months	Restricted in 1979; termiticide
Toxaphene	Toxakil Strobane-T	High	2 gm	Hours–days	
Heptachlor	—	Moderate	NA	Weeks–months	Malignancy in rats; banned in 1976
Chlorophenothane	DDT	Moderate	NA	Months–years	Banned in 1972
Mirex	—	Moderate	NA	Months–years	Banned; red anticide
Chlordecone	Kepone	Moderate	NA	Months–years	Tidewater, Virginia, contamination
Methoxychlor	Marlate	Low	600 mg/kg	Hours–days	
Ethylan	Perthane	Low	NA	Hours–days	
Dicofol	Kelthane	Low	NA	Hours–days	
Chlorbenzilat	Acaraben	Low	NA	Hours–days	Banned

Abbreviation: NA = not available.

every 8 hours, has been reported to increase the fecal excretion. (4) Anticonvulsants, if needed.

Organophosphate and Carbamate Insecticides (OPIs). These may cause (1) irreversible inhibition of cholinesterase, either direct (tetraethyl pyrophosphate [TEPP]) or delayed (parathion or malathion), or (2) reversible inhibition of cholinesterase (carbamates). Examples of OPIs are listed in Table 24. Absorption is by all routes. The onset of acute toxicity is usually before 12 hours and always before 24 hours, unless the agents are absorbed by the dermal route or are liquid-soluble (fenthion), which may delay onset for 24 hours. Inhalation produces intoxication within minutes. *Toxic manifestations*: Garlic odor of the breath or gastric contents or from the container that the OPI is stored in. Miosis and muscle twitching are helpful clues to acute OPI poisoning. Early, cholinergic crisis—cramps, diarrhea, excess secretion, bronchospasms, bradycardia. Later, sympathetic and nicotine effects occur—twitching, fasciculations, weakness, tachycardia and hypertension, and convulsions. CNS effects are anxiety, confusion, emotional lability, and coma. Delayed respiratory paralysis and neurologic disorders have been described. *Management*: (1) Basic life support and decontamination with careful protection of personnel. (2) Atropine (Antidote 7, Table 4), if patient is symptomatic, every 10 to 30 minutes until drying of secretions and clearing of lungs occur. Maintain for 12 to 24 hours, then taper the dose and observe for relapse.

TABLE 24. **Examples of Common Organophosphate Insecticides (OPIs)**

Common Name	Trade Name(s)	EFD (gm/70 kg)	LD_{50} (mg/kg)
Agricultural Products (25–50% formulations, highly toxic; LD_{50} is 1–40 mg/kg)			
Azinphos-methyl	Guthion	0.2	10.0
Chlortriphos	Calathion		
Demeton*	Systox		1.5
Disulfoton*	Di-Syston	0.2	12.0
Ethyl-nitrophenyl-thiobenzene PO_4	EPN		
Fonofos	Dyfonate		
Methamidophos†	Monitor		
Mevinphos	Phosdrin	0.15	
Monocrotophos	Azodrin		21.0
Octamethyldiphosphoramide	OMPA, Schradan		
Parathion	Thiophos	0.10	2.5
Ethyl parathion	Parathion		
Methyl parathion	Dalf		
Phorate	Thimet		
Terbufos	Counter		
Tetraethyl pyrophosphate	TEPP, Tetron	0.05	1.5
Animal Insecticides (moderately toxic; LD_{50} is 40–500 mg/kg)			
Chlorfenvinphos (tick dip)	Supona, Dermaton		
Coumaphos	Co-ral		
DEF	DeGreen		
Dichlorvos‡	DDVP, Vapona		46
Dimethoates§	Cygon, De-fend		>500
Fenthion‖	Baytex		40
Leptophos	Phosvel		
Phosmet	Imidan		
Ronnel	Korlan		
Trichlorfon	Dylox	10.0	
Household and Garden Pest Control (1–2% formulations, low toxicity; LD_{50} is 200–1400 mg/kg)			
Acephate¶	Orthene		>1000
Bromophos**			>1000
Chlorpyrifos** (toxic dose is 300 mg/kg)	Lorsban, Dursban, Pyrinex		>500
Dimpylate*††	Spectracide, Diazinon	25.0	>400
Dichlorvos‡‡	DDVP, Vapona (plastic strip)		
Malathion	Cythion	60.0	1375
Merphos	Folex		>1000
Temephos	Abate		<2000

*Most OPIs degrade in the environment in a few days to nontoxic radicals. These may be taken up by plants and fruits.
†Delayed neuropathy.
‡Found in flea collars and No-Pest Strips.
§t½ is <24 h.
‖Long-acting.
¶t½ is 1–6 days.
**Some authors classify this as moderately toxic; t½ is 27 h.
††In rats, t½ is 12 h.
‡‡Some authors classify this as moderately toxic.
Abbreviations: EFD = estimated fatal dose; common lawn chemical has 14.3%; LD_{50} = dose that is fatal in 50% of animals.

(3) Intravenous pralidoxime (2-PAM) is required after atropinization (Antidote 36, Table 4). It should be given early. Its use may require reduction in the dose of atropine. (4) Careful dermal and gastrointestinal decontamination when patient is stable. (5) Suction secretions until atropinization drying is achieved. Intubation and assisted ventilation may be needed. (6) *Do not* use morphine, aminophylline, phenothiazine, or reserpine-like drugs or succinylcholine. *Laboratory aids*: Draw blood for red blood cell cholinesterase determination before giving pralidoxime. Levels are usually more than 90% depressed for severe symptoms. A postexposure rise of 10 to 15% determined after at least 10 to 14 days without exposure is important in the diagnosis. Monitor chest radiographs, blood glucose, arterial blood gases, ECG, blood coagulation status, liver function, and urine for the metabolite alkyl phosphate *p*-nitrophenol. *Note*: If the diagnosis is probable, do not delay therapy until it is confirmed by laboratory tests. Atropine is both a diagnostic and a therapeutic agent. A test dose of 1 mg in adults and 0.01 mg per kg in children may be administered parenterally. In the presence of severe cholinesterase inhibition, the patient fails to develop signs of atropinization.

PROPHYLAXIS. It is not medically advisable to administer atropine or pralidoxime prophylactically to workers exposed to organophosphate pesticides.

CARBAMATES (esters of carbonic acid). Carbamates cause reversible carbamylation of acetylcholinesterase. Pralidoxime is usually not indicated in the management, but atropine may be required. The major differences from OPIs are that (1) toxicity is less and of shorter duration, (2) they rarely produce overt CNS effects because of poor penetration, and (3) cholinesterase returns to normal rapidly, so blood values are not useful in confirming the diagnosis. Some common examples of carbamates are ziram, aldicarb (Temik) (taken up by plants and fruit), Matacil (aminocarb, carazol), Vydate (oxamyl), Isolan, carbofuran (Furadan), methomyl (Lannate; Nudrin), mexacarbate (Zectran), and methiocarb (Mesural). These agents are all highly toxic. Moderately toxic are propoxur (Baygon) and carbaryl (Sevin). Some of these agents may be formulated in wood alcohol and have the added toxicity of methyl alcohol.

Paradichlorobenzene. See Hydrocarbons.

Paraquat and Diquat. Paraquat is a quaternary ammonia herbicide rapidly inactivated in the soil by clay particles. Nonindustrial preparations of 0.2% are unlikely to cause serious intoxications. *Toxic dose*: Commercial preparations such as Gramoxone 20% are very toxic; one mouthful has produced death. Systemic absorption in the course of occupational use is apparently minimal. Paraquat on marijuana leaves is pyrolyzed to nontoxic dipyridyl. *Toxicokinetics*: "Hit and run" toxin. Less than 20% is absorbed. The peak is 1 hour postingestion. *Route of elimination*: Kidney. Most of the dose is eliminated in the first 40 hours; it is detected in urine for 15 days. The Vd is over 500 liters per kg. *Manifestations*: Local corrosive effect on skin and mucous membranes.

Acute renal failure in 48 hours (often reversible). Pulmonary effects in 72 hours are progressive, and oxygen aggravates the pulmonary fibrosis. Diquat does not produce effects on the lungs but produces convulsions and gastrointestinal distention. Longterm exposure may cause cataracts. Chlormequat's target organ is the kidney. *Management*: (1) Gastrointestinal decontamination despite corrosive effects should be done cautiously with a nasogastric tube. Repeated doses of activated charcoal are recommended. Dermal and ocular decontamination as needed. (2) Hemodialysis and hemoperfusion may be carried out in tandem. Hemoperfusion with charcoal alone, if started within 2 hours after ingestion, may be effective; if started after 2 hours, however, the results are poor. Continue hemoperfusion until blood paraquat levels cannot be detected. (3) Diuresis may be of value but consider the risk of fluid overload. (4) Niacin and vitamin E have not been effective. (5) Avoid oxygen unless absolutely necessary (Pa_{O_2} below 60 mmHg) because this aggravates fibrosis. Some use hypoxic air, FI_{O_2} 10 to 20%. (6) Corticosteroids may help prevent adrenocortical necrosis. (7) Sepsis often develops within 7 to 10 days and should be treated appropriately. *Laboratory aids*: Blood levels above 2 µg per mL at 4 hours or above 0.10 µg per mL at 24 hours are usually fatal. Blood level testing and advice may be obtained from ICI America, 1-800-327-8633. Monitor renal, liver, and pulmonary functions and chest radiographs. Urine test for paraquat exposure—alkalinization and sodium dithionite give an intense blue-green color in exposure.

Parathion. See Organophosphate and Carbamate Insecticides.

Pentazocine (Talwin). See Opioids.

Perphenazine. See Phenothiazines and Other Major Neuroleptics.

Petroleum Products. See Hydrocarbons.

Phencyclidine (angel dust, PCP, peace pill, hog). This is the "drug of deceit" because it is substituted for many other drugs, such as tetrahydrocannabinol (THC) and mescaline. There are now at least 38 analogues. Smoking may give cyanide poisoning. Improper mixing has caused explosions. *Toxic dose*: Two to 5 mg smoked or "snorted" produces drunken behavior, agitation, and excitement. Five to 10 mg produces stupor, coma, and myoclonus convulsions. Ten to 25 mg smoked, snorted, or taken orally results in prolonged coma and respiratory failure. It is usually fatal over 25 mg (250 ng per mL blood concentration). *Toxicokinetics*: Weak base. Rapidly absorbed when smoked, insufflated nasally, or ingested and secreted into stomach gastric juice. Absorbed in alkaline intestine, but ion trapping takes place in acid gastric media. $t\frac{1}{2}$ is 30 to 60 minutes. Lipophilic drug with extensive Vd. The onset of action if smoked is 2 to 5 minutes (peak in 15 to 30 minutes); orally, 30 to 60 minutes. The duration at low doses is 4 to 6 hours, and normality returns in 24 hours. At large overdoses, coma may last 6 to 10 days (waxes and wanes). An adverse reaction in overdose occurs in 1 to 2 hours. *Route of elimination*: By liver metabolism

(50%). Urinary excretion of conjugates and free PCP. *Manifestations*: Sympathomimetic, cholinergic, cerebellar. Observe for violent behavior, paranoid schizophrenia, self-destructive behavior. Clues to diagnosis are bursts of horizontal, vertical, and rotary nystagmus, coma with eyes open. *Management* (avoid overtreatment of mild intoxications): (1) Gastrointestinal decontamination up to 4 hours postingestion, but this may not be effective because PCP is rapidly absorbed. Insert nasogastric tube into stomach for administration of activated charcoal every 6 hours because PCP is secreted into the stomach even if it is smoked or snorted. (2) Protect patient and others from harm. "Talk down" is usually ineffective. Low sensory environment. Diazepam (Valium) may be used orally or intramuscularly in the uncooperative patient. (3) For behavioral disorders and toxic psychosis—diazepam. (4) Seizures and muscle spasm—control with diazepam, 2.5 mg, up to 10 mg (Antidote 16, Table 4). (5) Dystonia reaction—diphenhydramine (Benadryl) intravenously (Antidote 19, Table 4). (6) Hyperthermia—external cooling. (7) Hypertensive crisis (dopaminergic)—use nitroprusside, 0.3 to 2 μg per kg per minute. Maximal infusion rate—10 μg per kg per minute; should never last more than 10 minutes. (8) Acid diuresis ion trapping (controversial). Ammonium chloride use is not recommended because of rhabdomyolysis and the danger of myoglobin precipitation in the renal tubules (Antidote 2, Table 4). (9) Avoid phenothiazines in the acute phase of intoxication because they lower the convulsive threshold. May be needed later for psychosis. *Laboratory aids*: (1) Elevation of the CPK level is a clue to the amount of rhabdomyolysis occurring and the chance of development of myoglobinuria. Values up to 20,000 U have been reported. (2) Test urine for myoglobin and pigmented casts. Test urine with orthotoluidine; a positive test without red blood cells on microscopic examination suggests myoglobinuria. (3) Monitor urine and blood pH and urinary output if acidifying patient. (4) Measure PCP level. (5) Evaluate BUN, ammonia, electrolytes, blood glucose levels (20% of patients have hypoglycemia). (6) Test for PCP in gastric juice; levels are 40 to 50 times higher than in blood. *Complications*: Rhabdomyolysis, myoglobinuria, and renal failure. Dopaminogenic hypertensive crisis, cerebrovascular accident, encephalopathy, and malignant hyperthermia. Schizophrenic paranoid psychosis (induced in chronic users or precipitated in acute users). Loss of memory for months. Delayed toxicity and "flashbacks" occur. Teratogenic cases have been reported. Children have been intoxicated from inhalation in a room where adults were smoking PCP. PCP-induced depression and suicide have been reported.

Phenobarbital. See Barbiturates.

Phenothiazines and Other Major Neuroleptics. Phenothiazines are represented by aliphatic compounds: chlorpromazine (Thorazine), promethazine (Phenergan), promazine (Sparine), triflupromazine (Vesprin), methoxypromazine (Tentone)*; piperazine compounds (dimethylamine series): acetophenazine (Tindal), fluphenazine (Prolixin), prochlorperazine (Compazine), perphenazine (Trilafon), trifluoperazine (Stelazine); and piperidine compounds: mesoridazine (Serentil), thioridazine (Mellaril), pipamazine (Mornidine).* Nonphenothiazines are the thioxanthines: chlorprothixene (Taractan), thiothixene (Navane); butyrophenones: haloperidol (Haldol), droperidol (Inapsine); dibenzoxazepines: loxapine (Loxitane); and dihydroindolones: molindone (Moban). These have pharmacologic properties similar to those of the phenothiazines. See Table 25. *Manifestations*: If patient is asymptomatic, monitor vital signs and ECG for at least 6 to 12 hours. Clues to phenothiazine overdose are miosis, tremor, hypotension, hypothermia, respiratory depression, radiopaque pills on radiograph of abdomen, and increased QT waves on the ECG. Anticholinergic actions are also present. Major problems are respiratory depression, myocardial toxicity (quinidine-like), neurogenic hypotension (antidopaminogenic), and idiosyncratic reaction, which may occur at therapeutic levels. Idiosyncratic reaction consists of opisthotonos, torticollis, orolingual dyskinesis, and oculogyric crisis (painful upward gaze) and can be mistaken for a psychotic episode. Extrapyramidal crisis is frequent in children and women. Malignant neuroleptic syndrome may occur. It is characterized by hyperthermia, muscle rigidity, and autonomic dysfunction. Death is usually due to cardiac effects. Phenothiazines are metabolized by the liver into many metabolites. Some remain in the body longer than 6 months. *Management*: (1) Gastrointestinal decontamination. Avoid emesis. If symptoms are already present, many of these agents have antiemetic action, so lavage may be required. Always provide gastric lavage to comatose patients after the airway is protected regardless of the time of ingestion because of inhibition of gastric motility. (2) Extrapyramidal signs (idiosyncratic reaction) can be treated with diphenhydramine (Benadryl) (Antidote 19, Table 4), or benztropine (Cogentin), 1 to 2 mg intravenously slowly. Symptoms recur, and these drugs should be continued orally for 5 to 7 days. *This is not the treatment of overdose*, only of the idiosyncratic reaction. (3) Monitor ECG for dysrhythmias and treat with antidysrhythmic agents. Avoid quinidine, procainamide, or disopyramide (Norpace). Treat the membrane depressant effects with intravenous sodium bicarbonate. (4) Hypotension is treated with the Trendelenburg position or fluid challenge or both. Vasopressors are used only if these fail. Dopamine (Intropin) should *not* be used to treat the hypotension because these drugs are antidopaminogenic. If a pressor agent is needed, use norepinephrine (levarterenol, Levophed). (5) Treat neuroleptic malignant syndrome by discontinuing the offending agent, reducing the patient's temperature with external cooling, and correcting any metabolic imbalance. Dantrolene and bromocriptine are agents that have been shown to be useful pharmaco-

---

*Not available in the United States.

TABLE 25. **Pharmacokinetics of Phenothiazines and Related Compounds**

Medication	Metabolism	Dose Equivalent (mg)	Absorption	Volume of Distribution (L/kg)	t½ (h)	Therapy
Aliphatic Type						
Moderate cardiotoxic and hypotensive effects; low sedation; moderate extrapyramidal effects; moderate anticholinergic effects						
Chlorpromazine (Thorazine) (high sedation)	Hepatic	100	Rapid	10–20	16–30	PO: child, 2 mg/kg/24 h; max <12 years old, 75 mg/24 h; adult, 200–2000 mg/24 h
Promethazine (Phenergan)	Hepatic	25	Rapid	—	12	PO: child, 0.5–1.0 mg/kg/dose; adult, 12.5–25 mg/dose (25–200 mg/24 h)
Piperazine						
Least cardiotoxic and hypotensive effects; very high extrapyramidal effects; moderate anticholinergic effects						
Prochlorperazine (Compazine)	Hepatic	15	Slow	10–35	8–12	PO: child, 0.1 mg/kg/dose (not <2 years old); adult, 10 mg/dose
Fluphenazine HCl (Prolixin) (injectable decanoate salt)	Hepatic	2	Rapid	—	2–12 (6.8–9.6 days)	PO: adult, 2.5–10 mg/24 h
Piperidine						
Highest cardiotoxic and hypotensive effects; low extrapyramidal effects; high anticholinergic effects						
Thioridazine (Mellaril) (high sedation)	Hepatic	100	Slow	3.5	26–36	PO: child, 1 mg/kg/24 h (not <3 years old); adult, 150–300 mg/24 h
Butyrophenone						
Low cardiotoxic and hypotensive effects; low sedation; very high extrapyramidal effects; very low anticholinergic effects						
Haloperidol (Haldol)	Hepatic	2–15	Rapid	20–30	12–22	PO: child, 0.1 mg/kg/24 h; adult, 20–100 mg/24 h
Droperidol (Inapsine)	Hepatic	2.5–10	NA	Large	2.2	IM/IV: child, 0.1–1.5 mg/kg/dose; adult, 2.5–10 mg/dose
Thioxanthene						
Low cardiotoxic and hypotensive effects; low sedation; high extrapyramidal effects; low anticholinergic effects						
Thiothixene (Navane)	Hepatic	2	NA	Large	34	PO: child, 0.25 mg/kg/24 h; adult, 16–60 mg/24 h (max, 60 mg)
Dibenzoxazepine						
Low cardiotoxic and hypotensive effects; low sedation; high extrapyramidal effects; low anticholinergic effects						
Loxapine (Loxitane)	Hepatic	15	NA	Large	3–4	PO: adult, initially 10 mg bid to max of 50 mg
Dihydroindolones						
Molindone (Moban)	Hepatic	10	Rapid	Large	1.5	PO: adult, initially 50–75 mg/24 h increased up to 225 mg

Peak levels occur mainly 1–4 h postingestion, and these drugs have enterohepatic recirculation. The pharmacokinetics of most phenothiazines resemble those of chlorpromazine. See pharmacokinetics for details.
Abbreviation: NA = not available.

logic adjuncts for the management of this syndrome. (6) Treat hypothermia or hyperthermia with external physical measures (not drugs). (7) Physostigmine should be avoided because it can produce seizures and cardiac toxicity. *Laboratory aids*: A ferric chloride test of urine can confirm exposure to phenothiazines if there is a sufficient blood level. Blood levels are *not* useful in management. A radiograph of the abdomen is useful to detect undissolved tablets, which may be radiopaque. Monitor arterial blood gases, renal and hepatic function, and levels of electrolytes and blood glucose for creatine kinase and myoglobinemia in neuroleptic malignant syndrome.

Phenylpropanolamine (PPA). See Amphetamines.

Primidone. See Anticonvulsants.

Propoxyphene. See Opioids.

Propranolol and Beta Blockers. Some of these agents available in the United States at this time are listed in Table 26. Beta blockers generally act as negative cardiac inotropes and chronotropes, although some have partial agonist activity with the opposite effect. *Toxic dose*: Varies considerably. *Toxicokinetics*: Time to peak action is 1 to 2 hours orally; the effects last 24 to 48 hours. In drugs with long half-lives, e.g., nadolol, it may take many days to

TABLE 26. **Pharmacokinetic Properties of Beta Blockers**

Drug Name	Solubility and Absorption (%)	Plasma t½ (h)	Elimination Route	Time to Peak Concentration	Protein Binding (%)	Volume of Distribution (L/kg)	Beta$_1$ Cardiac Selective
Acebutolol* (Sectral) Dose: 400–800 mg MDD: 800 mg TPC: 200–2000 ng/ mL	Moderate, lipid (90)	3–4, metabolite diacetolol	Hepatic, active metabolite	—	26	1.2	+
Alprenolol* (Aptin,† Betapin; Betacard) Dose: 200–800 mg MDD: 800 mg TPC: 50–200 ng/mL	Lipid (10)	3.1	Hepatic	1–3	85	3.4	—
Atenolol (Tenormin) Dose: 50–100 mg MDD: 100 mg TPC: 200–500 ng/mL	Water (46–62)	6–9	Renal, 95%	2–4	3–10	0.7	+
Betaxolol (Betoptic, Kerlone) Dose: 1 drop in eye twice daily MDD: Not available	Water (70–90)	12–22	Hepatic, 3–12%	—	50–60	4.9–13	+
Bisoprolol (Zebeta) Dose: 5–20 mg	Water (82–94)	9–12	Renal, 50%	3–4	30	2.9	+
Carteolol (Cartrol) Dose: 2.5–10 mg MDD: 40 mg	Lipid (84)	6–11	Renal, 60%	1–3	15	NA	—
Esmolol (Brevibloc) Dose: IV 50–500 µg/ kg/min (loading dose) MDD: 300 µg/kg/min	Water	9 min	Hepatic, plasma esterases	—	55	3.4	+
Labetalol (Normodyne, Trandate) Dose: 400–800 mg MDD: 1–2 gm	Water (50)	6–8	Hepatic, 95% Blocks alpha (weakly) and beta activity	—	50	11	—
Levobunolol (Betagan) Dose: Ophthalmic: 1 drop twice daily, 0.5%, 1%	Water (100)	6.1	Hepatic	—	—	—	—
Metoprolol (Lopressor) Dose: 50–100 mg MDD: 450 mg TPC: 50–100 ng/mL	Lipid (>95)	3–4	Hepatic	1–2	10	5.6	+
Nadolol (Corgard) Dose: 40–320 mg MDD: 320 mg TPC: 20–400 ng/mL	Water (15–25)	14–23	Renal, 70%	3–4	25	2.1	—
Oxprenolol (Trasicor)‡ Dose: 80–320 mg MDD: 480 mg TPC: 80–100 ng/mL	Lipid (70–95)	1.5–3	Hepatic	1–2	80	1.5	—
Penbutolol (Levatol) Dose: 20–80 mg MDD: 80 mg	Lipid (100)	4–8	Hepatic	1–1.5	80–90	0.5	—
Pindolol* (Visken) Dose: 20–60 mg MDD: 60 mg TPC: 50–150 ng/mL	Lipid (>90)	3–4	Hepatic, 60%; renal, 40%	1.25	57	2.0	—
Practolol* (Eraldin)‡ Dose: 25–600 mg MDD: 800 mg TPC: 1500–5000 ng/ mL	No longer available in United States because of adverse reactions						+
	Water (100)	6–8	Renal	3	40	—	
Propranolol (Inderal) Dose: 40–160 mg MDD: 480 mg TPC: 50–100 ng/mL	Lipid (100) (70% first pass)	2–3	Hepatic; renal (<1%), active hydroxy metabolite	1.5	90–95	3.6	—
Sotalol (Betapace) Dose: 80–320 mg MDD: 480 mg TPC: 500–4000 ng/ mL	Prolongs QT and may produce torsades de pointes						—
	Water (70)	5–13	Renal	2–3	54	0.7	

Table continued on following page

TABLE 26. **Pharmacokinetic Properties of Beta Blockers** *Continued*

Drug Name	Solubility and Absorption (%)	Plasma t½ (h)	Elimination Route	Time to Peak Concentration	Protein Binding (%)	Volume of Distribution (L/kg)	Beta₁ Cardiac Selective
Timolol§‖ Dose: 20 mg (Blocadren); ophthalmic (Timoptic, 0.25%, 0.5%), 1 drop twice daily MDD: 60 mg TPC: 5–10 ng/mL	Lipid (>90)	3–5	Hepatic, 80%; renal, 20%	4–5	<10	5.5	—

*Partial agonists.
†Investigational drug in the United States.
‡Not available in the United States.
§Substantial first pass.
‖Mitochondrial calcium protection during ischemia.
Abbreviations: MDD = maximal daily dose; TPC = therapeutic plasma concentration; NA = not available.

recover from overdose toxicity (Table 26). *Manifestations*: Observe for bradycardia and hypotension. Fat-soluble drugs have greater intensity of CNS effects. Partial agonists may initially produce tachycardia and hypertension (oxprenolol, pindolol). ECG changes include differing degrees of atrioventricular conduction delay or frank asystole. May cause hypoglycemia. *Management*: (1) Gastrointestinal decontamination with gastric lavage and activated charcoal and cathartic. Before gastric lavage, treatment with atropine, 0.01 mg per kg for a child and 0.5 mg for an adult, has been suggested to decrease the vagal effect in patients with bradycardia or significant intoxications. Avoid induced emesis because of early onset of seizures and vagal stimulation. Asymptomatic patients may be discharged after 12 to 24 hours of observation. (2) Treat hypoglycemia (frequent in children) and hyperkalemia. (3) Control convulsions. (4) Cardiovascular manifestations: Bradycardia—if patient is hemodynamically stable and asymptomatic, no therapy. If patient is unstable (hypotension or atrioventricular block), use atropine, glucagon, isoproterenol, and pacemaker. Ventricular tachycardia or premature beats—use lidocaine (Xylocaine), phenytoin (Dilantin), or overdrive pacing. Myocardial depression and hypotension—correct dysrhythmias; institute Trendelenburg positioning and fluids. Monitor with a PAWP catheter. If low cardiac output with low PAWP, give more fluids. If low cardiac output with normal PAWP, use glucagon (Antidote 26, Table 4). Avoid quinidine, procainamide, and disopyramide (Norpace). Glucagon is probably the drug of choice because it works through an adenyl cyclase mechanism not affected by the beta blockers. It is given as a bolus and may be continued as an infusion (Antidote 26, Table 4). If bronchospasm is present, give aminophylline. Hemodialysis or hemoperfusion for low-volume distribution drugs that are low–protein binding and water-soluble (nadolol, atenolol, and sotalol), particularly with evidence of renal failure. If hypoglycemia is present, give intravenous glucose. *Laboratory aids*: Monitor blood glucose, potassium, ECG, PAWP. Toxic blood level of propranolol is over 2 μg per mL.

Quinidine and Quinine (antidysrhythmic and antimalarial agents). *Toxic dose*: Quinidine in child, 60 mg per kg; in adult, 2 to 8 grams. Quinine, 15 mg per kg in child; 1 gram in adult. *Toxicokinetics*: There is 95 to 100% absorption, with peak action in 2 to 6 hours. The t½ is 3 to 4 hours (quinidine gluconate, 8 to 12 hours). Large Vd. Metabolized predominantly by the liver. *Manifestations*: Cinchonism (headache, nausea, vomiting, tinnitus, deafness, diplopia, dilated pupils). Myocardial depression, dysrhythmias, ECG changes—widening of PR and QT intervals and QRS complexes. Rashes and flushing. Hemolysis in glucose-6-phosphate dehydrogenase deficiency. Dementia reported. Quinidine produces more cardiovascular damage, and quinine produces more ocular damage. *Management*: (1) Obtain an immediate cardiac consultation. Electrophysiologic support of the heart should be readily available. (2) Gastrointestinal decontamination. Avoid emesis because of rapid onset of seizures and coma. (3) Monitor ECG and liver function. (4) May need antidysrhythmic drugs (but avoid Class IA antidysrhythmics), and pacemaker and alkalinization. Treat torsades de pointes in adults with magnesium sulfate, 2 grams intravenously over 2 to 3 minutes. *Laboratory aids*: Quinidine—therapeutic level 2 to 6 μg per mL. Toxic greater than 8 μg per mL. Fatal greater than 16 μg per mL. Quinine—therapeutic level 7 μg per mL. Toxic greater than 10 μg per mL.

Salicylates. *Toxic dose*: 150 mg per kg or 7.5 to 10 grams. See Table 27. Methyl salicylate (oil of wintergreen)—1 mL equals 1.4 grams of salicylate. One teaspoonful equals 21 adult aspirins. *Toxicokinetics*: Plasma concentration is significant in 30 minutes and peaks in 1 to 2 hours but may be delayed 6 hours or more in overdose with enteric-coated, sustained-release preparations or concretions. The t½ is 3 to 6 hours (therapeutic) to 12 to 36 hours (toxic). Urine pH influences urine salicylate elimination. *Manifestations of acute ingestion* (see Table 27): The

TABLE 27. **Quantities of Aspirin Ingested: Deposition and Manifestations***

Category	Amount Ingested (mg/kg)	Toxicity Expected	Gastrointestinal Decontamination	Manifestations Anticipated
Nontoxic	<150	No	No	None
Mild intoxication	150–200	Yes	Yes (ECF)	Vomiting, tinnitus, mild hyperventilation
Moderate intoxication	200–300	Yes	Yes (ECF)	Hyperpnea, lethargy, or excitability
Severe intoxication	300–500	Yes	Yes (ECF)	Coma, convulsions, severe hyperpnea
Very severe intoxication	>500	Yes	Yes (ECF)	Potentially fatal

*See toxic dose section for gastrointestinal decontamination.
Abbreviation: ECF = emergency care facility.

metabolic disturbance in adults and older children is usually respiratory alkalosis; in children younger than 5 years of age, the initial respiratory alkalosis usually changes to metabolic or mixed metabolic acidosis and respiratory alkalosis, with acidosis predominating within a few hours. *Management*: Do not wait for a 6-hour salicylate level to start treatment of symptomatic patients. If hemodialysis may be required, suggest an immediate consult with a nephrologist. (1) Gastrointestinal decontamination is useful up to 12 hours postingestion because some factors delay absorption (food, enteric-coated tablets, other drugs), pylorospasm may delay emptying, and concretions may form. Activated charcoal should be administered every 4 hours until stools are black. Concretions may be removed by lavage, whole-body irrigation, endoscopy, or gastrostomy. (2) Intravenous fluid should be given as recommended in Table 28. Alkalinization (Antidote 39, Table 4) enhances salicylate excretion. Potassium is essential to produce adequate alkalinization. Monitor both the urine and blood pH. Do not use the urine pH alone to assess the need for alkalinization. (3) Fluid retention can be treated with mannitol (20%), 0.5 gram per kg over 30 minutes, or furosemide (Lasix), 1 mg per kg intravenously. (4) Hyperpyrexia should be treated with external cooling. (5) Patients with abnormal bleeding or hypoprothrombinemia need vitamin K, 10 to 50 mg intravenously, and, if bleeding continues,

fresh blood or platelet transfusion (Antidote 43, Table 4). (6) Hemodialysis is indicated if there is persistent acidosis (pH 7.0) and lack of response to fluid or alkali in 6 hours; if serum salicylate levels are initially greater than 160 mg per dL or greater than 100 to 120 mg per dL at 6 hours postingestion (do *not* use the salicylate level as the sole criterion for dialysis); or if the patient has coma and uncontrollable seizures, congestive heart failure, acute renal failure, progressive deterioration despite good management. Lower levels such as 30 to 60 μg per mL may be an indication for hemodialysis in chronic salicylism with altered mental status. (7) Chronic toxicity is usually a more severe intoxication because of the cumulative pharmacokinetics of salicylates. Management needs are outlined in Table 29. *Laboratory aids*: The metabolic acidosis of salicylism has a moderately elevated anion gap. Hyperglycemia or hypoglycemia may exist. Serum salicylate levels used in conjunction with the Done nomogram (Figure 3) are useful predictors of expected severity following *acute single ingestions*. The Done nomogram is *not* useful in chronic intoxications or in methyl salicylate, phenyl salicylate, or homomethyl salicylate ingestions. The salicylate level for use in the Done nomogram should be obtained 6 hours postingestion. Before 6 hours, levels in the toxic range should be treated, and patients with levels below the toxic range should be retested if a potentially toxic dose is

TABLE 28. **Recommendations for Fluid Management for Moderate or Severe Salicylism***

Purpose	Rate (mL/kg/h)	Duration (h)	Na	K	Cl	HCO₃	Glucose (%)
				Electrolyte Concentration (mEq/L)			
Volume expansion	20	0.5–1.0	100	0	77	23	5–10
Administered as 0.45% saline with 23 mEq/L NaHCO₃							
Hydration Ongoing losses Alkalinization	4–8	Until therapeutic blood serum concentration is 30 mg/dL	56	40	56	1–2 mEq/kg child; 50–100 mEq adult	5–10
Administered as 0.33% saline and NaHCO₃ to obtain urine pH 7.5–8.0, blood pH 7.5							
				mEq/kg/day			
Maintenance	2–6	—	3	2	4		

*For severe acidosis (pH <7.15), may require 1–2 mEq/kg of sodium bicarbonate every 1–2 h. Usual fluid loss is 200–300 mL/kg, but carefully monitor for fluid overload. Potassium may be needed in excess of 40 mEq/L when alkalinizing.

TABLE 29. **Management of Chronic Salicylate Intoxication**

Classification	Urine pH	Blood pH	Hydration	NaHCO$_3$ (mEq/L)	Potassium (mEq/L)
Mild	Alkaline	Alkaline	Yes	Yes*	20
Moderate	Acid†	Alkaline	Yes	pH 7.5†	40
Severe	Acid	Acid	Yes	pH 7.5	40‡
					80§

*Bicarbonate administered to keep blood pH at 7.5 and urine pH at 7.5–8.0.
†Paradoxical acid urine and alkaline blood indicate potassium depletion.
‡Normal serum potassium and electrocardiogram (ECG).
§Low serum potassium and/or abnormal ECG indicate potassium deficiency.

ingested. Monitor urine output, urine pH, electrolytes, arterial blood gases, blood glucose, prothrombin time, renal function, serum salicylate level, and urine salicylate with the ferric chloride test. Arterial blood pH should be kept at 7.5. *Prognosis*: Persistent vigorous treatment of salicylate ingestion is essential because recovery has occurred despite decerebrate rigidity.

Sedative Hypnotics, Nonbarbiturate. See Table 30. *Management*: Primarily supportive (especially intubation and ventilator therapy with continuous positive airway pressure for adult respiratory distress syndrome) with the use of hemoperfusion or hemodialysis in patients who are severely intoxicated and fail to respond to good supportive care and whose intoxication is life-threatening. Avoid emesis because of rapid onset of convulsions, apnea, and coma. (1) *Chloral hydrate* management includes cautious gastrointestinal decontamination. Avoid the use of epinephrine and catecholamines that may produce dysrhythmias. Propranolol (Inderal), 0.1 mg per kg in 1-mg increments, appears to be more effective than lidocaine (Xylocaine) for ventricular dysrhythmias. Charcoal hemoperfusion may effectively remove chloral hydrate and its metabolite in patients who fail to respond and have potentially fatal plasma levels (20 μg per mL or higher). Hemodialysis may be ineffective because of lipid solubility. (2) *Ethchlorvynol* management includes gastrointestinal decontamination up to several hours postingestion. Charcoal hemoperfusion is the best method of extracorporeal removal when other measures fail in a life-threatening situation (ingestion of over 10 grams or 100 mg per kg, with serum levels of over 100 μg per mL in the first 12 hours or 70 μg per mL after 12 hours in patients with prolonged life-threatening coma). External rewarming if temperature is below 32° C (89.6° F). (3) *Glutethimide* management includes gastrointestinal decontamination up to 24 hours postingestion. Concretions may form. Charcoal hemoperfusion appears to be the best method of extracorporeal removal in life-threatening protracted coma when the patient has ingested over 10 grams and has a serum level of over 30 μg per mL. Treat hyperthermia with external cooling. (4) *Meprobamate* management includes gastrointestinal decontamination up to several hours postingestion, with charcoal hemoperfusion in prolonged coma with life-threatening complications. Concretions may form in the stomach and may require whole-bowel irrigation, endoscopy, or surgical removal. (5) *Methaqualone* management includes gastrointestinal decontamination up to 12 hours postingestion. Forced diuresis, dialysis, and hemoperfusion are not indicated. Fatalities are rare. (6) *Methyprylon* management includes gastrointestinal decontamination and may require treatment of the hypotension with vasopressors of the alpha-adrenergic variety—e.g., levarterenol (norepinephrine, Levophed). The hypotension usually does not respond to position or fluids alone. This is a dialyzable drug, but dialysis usually is not necessary. Fatalities are rare.

Strychnine. Primarily available as a rodenticide and component of cathartics and "tonics." Adulterant

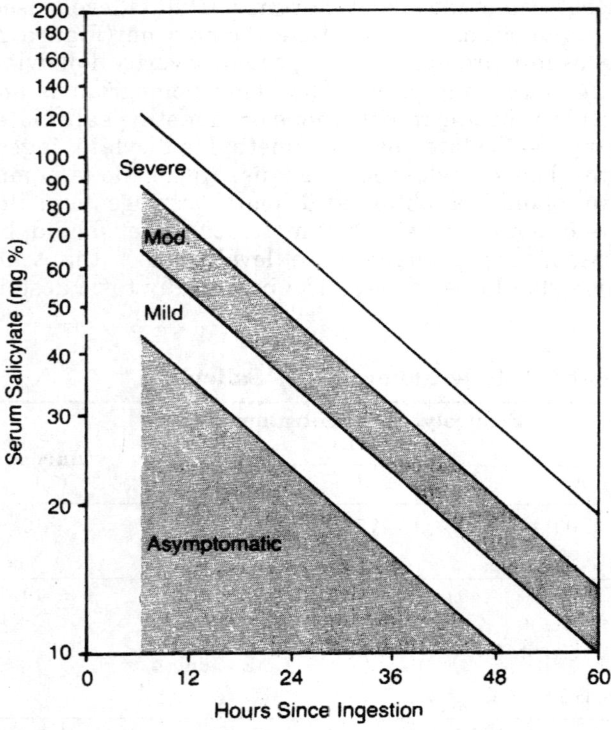

Figure 3. The Done nomogram for salicylate intoxication. For limitations of use, see *Laboratory aids*. (Redrawn from Done A: Salicylate intoxication: Significance of measurements of salicylate in blood in cases of acute ingestion. Reproduced by permission of Pediatrics, Vol. 26, Page 800, Copyright 1960.)

TABLE 30. **Nonbarbiturate Sedative Hypnotic Drugs**

Drug	Absorption and Toxic Dose	Time to Peak Effect (h)	Volume of Distribution (L/kg)	Protein Binding (%)	Elimination Route	Serum $t\frac{1}{2}$ (h)	Toxic Level (µg/mL)	Manifestations and Comment*
Chloral hydrate (Noctec)	Rapid TD, 2 gm FD, 4–10 gm	1–2	0.75–0.9	40	Hepatic 90% to active metabolite trichloroethanol (TCE)	4–8 min; TCE: 8–12 h	100 (80 TCE— very toxic)	Pear-like odor, dysrhythmias (especially ventricular), hepatotoxicity, irritant to mucosa of GI tract, ARDS, radiopaque capsules
Ethchlorvynol (Placidyl)	Rapid TD, 2.5 gm FD, 10–25 gm	1–2	3–4	35–50	Hepatic 90%	10–25 in OD over 100	20–80	Prolonged coma up to 200 h, apnea, hypothermia, pulmonary edema, pink gastric aspirate, pungent odor
Glutethimide (Doriden) (highest mortality of all sedative hypnotics, 14%)	Slow, erratic TD, 5 gm FD, 10 gm	6	Large, 2–2.7	50	Hepatic 98% to toxic metabolite 4-hydroxyglutarimide	10–40 in OD over 100	20–80	Prolonged, cyclic comas up to 120 h, anticholinergic signs, convulsions, recurrent apnea, hyperthermia
Meprobamate (Equanil, Miltown)	Rapid TD, 10–20 gm FD, 10–20 gm	4–8	10	20	Hepatic 90%	6–16	30–100	Coma, convulsions, pulmonary edema, apnea, concretions in stomach
Methaqualone (Quaalude, "love drugs")	Rapid TD, 800 mg FD 3–8 gm	1–3	2–6	80	Hepatic 90%	10–40	8–10	Hypertonia, hyperreflexia, convulsions, apnea, acts "drunk," bleeding tendencies
Methyprylon (Noludar)	Rapid TD, 3 gm FD, 8–20 gm	2–4	1–2	—	Hepatic 97%	3–6 in OD over 50	30	Hyperactive, coma lasts 30 h, miosis, persistent hypotension, pulmonary edema, mortality rare

*Comment includes other features besides the typical manifestations of all these agents—coma, respiratory depression, psychological and physiologic withdrawal, hypotension, hypothermia (except glutethimide hyperthermia).

Abbreviations: TD = toxic dose; FD = fatal dose; OD = overdose; ARDS = adult respiratory distress syndrome; GI = gastrointestinal.

of "street drugs," particularly marijuana and cocaine. *Toxic dose*: 5 to 10 mg; fatal in doses of 15 to 30 mg. *Toxicokinetics*: Rapid absorption. Manifestations may occur within 15 to 30 minutes. Low protein binding. Hepatic metabolism, which appears to be saturable. Twenty percent is excreted in urine. Has been found in the urine up to 48 hours after a 700-mg dose. *Manifestations*: Interferes with postsynaptic neurotransmitter inhibition by glycine. Hyperacusis is often the first sign. Mild cases—facial stiffness (trismus and risus sardonicus). Moderate cases—extensor muscle thrusts. Severe cases—tetanic convulsions with opisthotonos. Death occurs within 1 to 3 hours after ingestion. The prognosis for recovery improves if the patient survives beyond 5 hours. The complications of intoxication are lactic acidosis, hyperthermia, rhabdomyolysis and renal damage from precipitation of myoglobin in the renal tubules, and death from hypoxia. *Management*: (1) Emesis is contraindicated because of rapid absorption and the early onset of seizures. Gastric aspiration and lavage may be used after the seizures are controlled. Activated charcoal should be given and repeated. (2) Control convulsions with diazepam (Valium) or phenobarbital. (3) Supportive care for respiratory depression. (4) Acid diuresis and dialysis do not appear to be justified on the basis of available studies. (5) Paralysis with assisted ventilation is useful.

Tear Gas (lacrimators). CS (chlorobenzylidine), "riot control"; CN powder (chloroacetophenone, 1%); Mace (chloroacetophenone). *Management*: Dermal and ocular decontamination. Protect attendants from contamination. Ophthalmic evaluation. Oxygen therapy may be needed for dyspnea and respiratory distress.

Theophylline. *Toxic dose*: Acute, single dose greater than 10 mg per kg yields mild toxicity. Greater than 20 mg per kg, moderate manifestations. *Toxicokinetics*: Absorption is complete. Peak levels occur within 60 minutes after ingestion of liquid preparations; 1 to 3 hours after regular tablets; and 3 to 10 hours after slow-release preparations. Vd, 0.3 to 0.7 liter per kg. Protein binding, 15 to 40%. The $t\frac{1}{2}$ varies: 3.5 hours average in a child and 4.5 hours in an adult (range from 3 to 9 hours). In neonates and young infants the drug's half-life is much longer. Overdose increases the $t\frac{1}{2}$. *Elimination*: Hepatic metabolism, 90% (demethylation and oxidation); 8 to 10% is excreted unchanged in the urine. *Manifestations*: Acute toxicity generally correlates with blood levels; chronic toxicity does not. From 10 to 20 µg per mL is the therapeutic range, but mild gastrointestinal toxicity may occur in some. From 20 to 40 µg per mL is moderate toxicity, with gastrointestinal and CNS stimulation. Over 50 µg per mL, seizures and dysrhythmias may occur, but they may also occur at lower levels and without gastrointestinal symptoms. Children tolerate higher serum levels. Chronic intoxication is more serious and difficult to treat. Many factors increase theophylline concentration. *Management*: (1) Gastrointestinal decontamination in acute overdose, up to 4 hours with regular preparations and up to 8 to 12 hours with slow-release preparations. Test aspirate or vomitus for blood. Give activated charcoal every 4 hours until serum theophylline levels are less than 20 µg per mL. Do not induce emesis if hematemesis exists. If there is intractable vomiting, administer the antiemetic metoclopramide (Reglan), 0.4 mg per kg per dose intravenously (maximum, 0.5 mg per kg per 24 hours) in infants and children, and 10 mg slowly over 15 minutes every 6 to 8 hours in adults. Alternative: droperidol (Inapsine), 2.5 mg intravenously or 0.05 to 0.1 mg per kg per dose every 6 to 8 hours if needed. Both drugs may cause extrapyramidal symptoms. Ondansetron is not recommended because it inhibits metabolism of theophylline. (2) Monitor ECG, obtain theophylline levels every 4 hours until they remain in the therapeutic range of 10 to 20 µg per mL. (3) Control seizures with diazepam (Valium). If coma, convulsions, or vomiting exists, intubate immediately. (4) Hypotension is treated with fluid challenge and, if this fails, vasopressors. (5) Hematemesis is managed with saline lavage and blood replacement if needed. (6) Charcoal hemoperfusion is the management of choice in life-threatening convulsions, dysrhythmias, hematemesis, or intractable vomiting refractory to conventional measures. It is recommended for acute intoxications with serum theophylline concentrations of 70 to 100 µg per mL, or with chronic overdoses with drug levels of 40 to 60 µg per mL, especially if the patient has risk factors that increase serum levels, e.g., age younger than 6 months or older than 60 years, liver disease, heart failure, viral infections, pneumonia, fever greater than 38.9° C (102° F); medications: macrolide antibiotics, oral contraceptives, cimetidine, beta blockers, carbamazepine, and caffeine. Differences in slow-release preparations from regular preparations: few or no gastrointestinal symptoms with high levels; peak concentration times may be 10 to 24 hours postingestion; and onset of seizures may occur 10 to 12 hours postingestion. *Laboratory aids*: Monitor theophylline levels, check for occult blood in vomitus and stools, monitor vital signs and hemoglobin and hematocrit (for hemorrhage). Monitor cardiac, renal, and hepatic function, electrolytes, blood glucose, arterial blood gases, and acid-base balance.

Toluene. See Hydrocarbons.

Tranquilizers. See Sedative Hypnotics, Nonbarbiturate.

Trichloroethylene. See Hydrocarbons.

Tricyclic Antidepressants (TCADs). See Table 31. These agents are generally rapidly absorbed from the gastrointestinal tract, but absorption may be prolonged in overdose owing to anticholinergic action. Their bioavailability has considerable variation among patients, and they are highly bound to plasma and tissue proteins. Protein binding decreases with decreasing pH. The Vd is large, usually 10 to 20 liters per kg. The TCADs are metabolized primarily in the liver. *N*-Demethylation of the tertiary amines yields the active secondary amine metabolites; hydroxylation gives rise to inactive metabolites. Forty

percent is excreted in the feces and only 3% in the urine unchanged. The t½ varies from 9 to 198 hours. In an overdose, the t½ may be much longer. Tricyclic tertiary amines (metabolized to active metabolites) are amitriptyline (Elavil), imipramine (Tofranil), and doxepin (Sinequan, Adapin). Tricyclic secondary amines (metabolized to nonactive metabolites) are desipramine (Norpramin, Pertofrane), protriptyline (Vivactil), and nortriptyline (Pamelor). Tricyclic dibenzoxazepine (metabolized to a major metabolite) is amoxapine (Asendin). *Manifestations*: The onset of action varies from less than 1 hour to 12 hours after ingestion. The phases of intoxication are (1) consciousness with dry mouth, mydriasis, ataxia, increased deep tendon reflexes, and changes in the ST segment; (2) Stages I and II coma with hypertension, tachycardia above 160, mydriasis, and supraventricular tachycardia; and (3) Stages III and IV coma with hypotension, heart rate under 120, respiratory depression, tonic-clonic seizures, and ventricular dysrhythmias. The CNS effects occur early, and seizures are common. *Cardiovascular toxicity* is frequent in the serious poisonings and results from anticholinergic effects, sympathomimetic activity (by blocking reuptake of catecholamines), quinidine activity, catecholamine depletion, and alpha-adrenergic blockade. Cardiotoxic effects include cardiac dysrhythmias, hypertension, hypotension, and pulmonary edema.

Toxic dose: The TCADs have a narrow margin of safety. In a child a 375-mg dose and in adults as little as 500 to 750 mg have been fatal. The following dosages may serve as a guide to the degree of imipramine toxicity: Less than 10 mg per kg produces light coma, mydriasis, and tachycardia and has a good prognosis. At 20 mg per kg, Stage III manifestations are produced. At 30 mg per kg, fatalities may result. At 50 mg per kg, the mortality rate is increased. Over 70 mg per kg is rarely survived. Relative adult dosage equivalents may serve as a guide: amitriptyline, 100 mg; amoxapine, 125 mg; desipramine, 75 mg; doxepin, 100 mg; imipramine, 75 mg; maprotiline (Ludiomil), 75 mg; nortriptyline, 50 mg; and trazodone (Desyrel), 200 mg (see Table 31). Therapeutic blood levels are in the range of 50 to 170 ng per mL. If the QRS interval is less than 0.10 second for 6 hours, the prognosis is good. If it is greater than 0.10 second, seizures may occur, and if it is over 0.16 second, serious dysrhythmia may occur. In general, most antidepressants possess anticholinergic activity. The tricyclics produce dysrhythmias, hypotension, and seizures. The tetracyclics (amoxapine, maprotiline) produce convulsions that may result in rhabdomyolysis and renal dysfunction. The new agents trazodone and fluoxetine (Prozac) appear to have mild sedative effects and cardiotoxicity, although orthostatic hypotension, vertigo, and priapism have been reported. Bupropion (Wellbutrin) is a phenylaminoketone antidepressant that produces dose-related seizures. Nomifensine (Merital) was withdrawn in 1986 because of reports of hemolytic anemia associated with it. *Management*: (1) Maintenance of vital functions. If the patient is asympto-

TABLE 31. **Kinetics of Cyclic Antidepressants**

Anti-depressant (Trade Name)	Absorption	Time to Peak Effect (h)	Volume of Distribution (L/kg)	t½ (h)	Protein Binding (%)	Elimination	Toxic Level (ng/mL)	Availability	Therapeutic Plasma Level (Range) (ng/mL)	Usual Dose	
										Adult (total daily dose) (mg)	Child (mg/kg/24 h)
TRICYCLIC TERTIARY AMINES (METABOLIZED TO ACTIVE METABOLITES)											
Amitriptyline (Elavil)	Slow	2–12	8–10	15–19	82–96	Hepatic	>500	Tab 10, 25, 75, 100, 150 mg	50–250	75–300	1.5–2.0
Imipramine (Tofranil)	Rapid (29–77%)	1–2	5–20	8–16	76–96	Hepatic	>500	Tab 10, 25, 50 mg; Cap 75, 100, 125, 150 mg	150–250	75–300	3–7
Doxepin (Sinequan, Adapin)	Rapid, complete	2–4	20	15–19	95	Hepatic	>150	Cap 25, 50, 75, 100, 150 mg	150–250	75–300	—
Trimipramine (Surmontil)	Rapid	2	NA	NA	Large	Renal		Cap 25, 50, 100 mg	100–200	75–300	—
TRICYCLIC SECONDARY AMINES (METABOLIZED TO NONACTIVE METABOLITES)											
Desipramine (Norpramin, Pertofrane)	Rapid, incomplete	4–6	28–60	18–28	73–92	Hepatic	>500	Tab 10, 25, 50, 100, 150 mg; Cap 10, 50 mg	125–300	75–300	—
Protriptyline (Vivactil)	Slow	NA	NA	NA	>90	Hepatic	NA	Tab 5, 10 mg	70–260	20–60	—
Nortriptyline (Aventyl)	Slow (46–77%)	7–8	21–57	50–150	93–95	Hepatic	>500	Cap 10, 25, 75 mg	50–150	75–150	1.5–2.0
TETRACYCLIC DIBENZOXAZEPINES (METABOLIZED TO MAJOR METABOLITES)											
Amoxapine (Asendin)	Rapid	1.5	Large	8–30	90	Renal and hepatic	NA	Tab 25, 50, 100, 150 mg	200–600	150–600	—
Maprotiline (Ludiomil)	Slow	8–24	13–22	27–58	88	Hepatic	>300	Tab 25, 50, 75 mg	200–600	75–300	—
TRIAZOLOPYRIDINES											
Trazodone (Desyrel)	Rapid	0.5–2	NA	4–13	89–95	Hepatic	NA	Tab 50, 100, 150 mg	800–1600	50–600	
UNCLASSIFIED OR BICYCLICS (METABOLIZED TO ACTIVE METABOLITES)											
Fluoxetine (Prozac)	Rapid	4–6	14–102	24–96	94	Hepatic	>400	Cap 20 mg; syrup 20 mg/5 mL, 4-oz bottles	NA	20–80	
Norfluoxetine (active metabolite) peak 76 h, t½ 5–7 days											
DIBENZAZEPINES											
Clomipramine* (Anafranil)	Rapid	3–5	12	21	98	Hepatic	500	Cap 25, 50, 75 mg	—	25–200	—
Dimethylclomipramine (DM) (primary active metabolite) t½ 54–77 h											
AMINOKETONES											
Bupropion (Wellbutrin)	Rapid 5–20% bioavailability	2	NA	8–24	80	Hepatic	NA	Tab 75, 100 mg	—	200–450 tid	—
Several active metabolites relate to toxicity											

*Available to psychiatrists free of charge to treat patients: 1-800-842-2422 (Med Lett *30*:102–104, 1988).
Abbreviations: Toxic level = toxic serum concentration; NA = not available; Tab = tablets; Cap = capsules.

matic, there should be vascular access, and cardiac monitoring should continue for at least 6 hours from admission or 8 to 12 hours postingestion. All children should be observed closely for 24 hours in an intensive care unit. If patient is symptomatic, obtain cardiac consultation and monitor in an intensive care unit until the patient is asymptomatic and shows no ECG abnormalities for at least 72 hours. (2) Gastrointestinal decontamination (omit emesis) if the patient is alert. Intact pills have been recovered by lavage up to 18 hours after ingestion. Suspected patients should have ECG monitoring. (3) Activated charcoal initially with a cathartic. No more than two doses of activated charcoal are advised. (4) Control seizures with intravenous diazepam (Valium). Intravenous phenytoin (Dilantin) may be added in patients with seizures not responding to diazepam alone. If not immediately successful, consider an aggressive approach to airway management and rapid-sequence intubation with paralysis by short nonpolarizing neuromuscular blockers such as vecuronium. (5) Cardiovascular complications of TCAD intoxication, including a QRS complex of over 0.14 second, ventricular tachycardia, severe conduction blocks, hypotension, or seizures, should *first* be treated by alkalinization of blood with sodium bicarbonate to a pH of 7.5 to 7.55 (Antidote 39, Table 4). Administer sodium bicarbonate 1 mEq per kg undiluted as a bolus and repeated twice a few minutes apart. If it does not affect cardiotoxicity, an infusion of sodium bicarbonate may follow to keep blood pH at 7.5 to 7.55 but not higher. Monitor serum sodium, potassium, and blood pH because fatal alkalemia and hypernatremia have been reported. Continuous infusion of bicarbonate by itself is of limited usefulness in TCAD intoxication because of its delayed onset. The combination of hyperventilation and sodium bicarbonate has produced fatal alkalemia. Alkalinization increases the protein binding of the TCAD. Serum potassium levels should be monitored because a sudden increase in blood pH can aggravate or precipitate hypokalemia. Specific cardiovascular complications should be treated as follows:

Hypotension—norepinephrine (Levophed), a predominantly alpha-adrenergic drug, is preferred over dopamine. (Hypertension that occurs early rarely requires treatment.) *Serious conduction defects* are best managed with phenytoin, and patients may need a temporary transvenous pacemaker. *Sinus tachycardia* usually does not require treatment except for alkalinization. *Supraventricular tachycardia* with hemodynamic instability requires synchronized cardioversion, 0.25 to 1.0 watt-second per kg, after sedation. *Ventricular tachycardia*—after alkalinization and phenytoin, intravenous lidocaine (Xylocaine) (for one dose only) may be required for persistent ventricular tachycardia. Synchronized cardioversion may be needed if lidocaine fails. *Ventricular fibrillation* should be treated with direct current countershock. *Torsades de pointes* is treated with intravenous magnesium sulfate 20%, 2 grams over 2 to 3 minutes, followed by a continuous infusion of 5 to 10 mg per minute of isoproterenol, lidocaine, phenytoin, and bretylium and atrial or ventricular overdrive pacing to shorten the QT interval. *Laboratory aids*: Arterial blood gases with blood pH, ECG, serum electrolytes, BUN and creatinine, serum phenytoin level, and urine output; and, in severe cases, central venous pressure, PAWP, or both should be monitored.

Turpentine. See Hydrocarbons.

Xylene. See Hydrocarbons.

Appendices and Index

REFERENCE INTERVALS FOR THE INTERPRETATION OF LABORATORY TESTS

method of
WILLIAM Z. BORER, M.D.
Thomas Jefferson University Hospital
Philadelphia, Pennsylvania

Most of the tests performed in a clinical laboratory are quantitative in nature—that is, the amount of a substance present in blood or serum is measured and reported in terms of concentration, activity (e.g., enzyme activity), or counts (e.g., blood cell counts). The laboratory must provide reference values to assist the clinician in the interpretation of laboratory results. These reference ranges specify the physiologic quantities of substance (concentrations, activities, or counts) to be expected in healthy individuals. Deviation above or below the reference range may be associated with a disease process, and the severity of the disease process may be associated with the magnitude of the deviation. Unfortunately, a sharp demarcation between physiologic and pathologic values rarely exists, and the transition between these two is often gradual as the disease process progresses.

The terms "normal" and "abnormal" have been used to describe the laboratory values that fall inside or outside the reference range, respectively. Use of these terms is now discouraged because it is virtually impossible to define normality and because "normal" may be confused with the statistical term "gaussian." Reference ranges are established from statistical studies in groups of healthy volunteers. Although these study subjects must be free of disease, they may have lifestyles or habits that result in subtle variations in their laboratory values. Examples of these variables include diet, body mass, exercise, and geographic location. Age and gender may also affect reference values. When the data from a large cohort of healthy subjects fit a gaussian distribution, the usual statistical approach is to define the reference limits as two standard deviations above and below the mean. By definition, the reference range excludes the highest and the lowest 2.5% of the population. Nongaussian distributions are handled by different statistical methods, but the result is similar in that the reference range is defined by the central 95% of the population. In other words, the odds are 1 in 20 that a healthy individual will have a laboratory result that falls outside the reference range. If 12 laboratory tests are performed, the odds increase to about 1 in 2 that at least one of the results is outside the reference range. This means that all healthy individuals are likely to have a few laboratory results that are unexpected. The clinician must then integrate these data with other clinical information such as the history and physical examination to arrive at the appropriate clinical decision. The reference range for many tests (especially enzyme and immunochemical measurements) will vary with the method used. It is important that each laboratory establish reference ranges appropriate for the methods it employs.

SI UNITS

During the 1980s, a concerted effort was made to introduce SI units (le Système International d'Unités). The rationale for conversion to SI units is sound. Laboratory data are scientifically more informative when the units are based on molar concentration rather than mass concentration. For example, the conversion of glucose to lactate and pyruvate or the binding of a drug to albumin is more easily understood in units of molar concentration. Another example is illustrated as follows:

Conventional Units
1.0 gram of hemoglobin
Combines with 1.37 mL of oxygen
Contains 3.4 mg of iron
Forms 34.9 mg of bilirubin

SI Units
4.0 mmol of hemoglobin
Combines with 4.0 mmol of oxygen
Contains 4.0 mmol of iron
Forms 4.0 mmol of bilirubin

TABLE 1. **Base SI Units**

Property	Base Unit	Symbol
Length	meter	m
Mass	kilogram	kg
Amount of substance	mole	mol
Time	second	s
Thermodynamic temperature	kelvin	K
Electric current	ampere	A
Luminous intensity	candela	cd
Catalytic amount	katal	kat

TABLE 2. **Derived SI Units and Non-SI Units Retained for Use with the SI**

Property	Unit	Symbol
Area	square meter	m^2
Volume	cubic meter	m^3
	liter	L
Mass concentration	kilogram/cubic meter	kg/m^3
	gram/liter	g/L
Substance concentration	mole/cubic meter	mol/m^3
	mole/liter	mol/L
Temperature	degree Celsius	$°C = °K - 273.15$

TABLE 3. **Standard Prefixes**

Prefix	Multiplication Factor	Symbol
yocto	10^{-24}	y
zepto	10^{-21}	z
atto	10^{-18}	a
femto	10^{-15}	f
pico	10^{-12}	p
nano	10^{-9}	n
micro	10^{-6}	μ
milli	10^{-3}	m
centi	10^{-2}	c
deci	10^{-1}	d
deca	10^{1}	da
hecto	10^{2}	h
kilo	10^{3}	k
mega	10^{6}	M
giga	10^{9}	G
tera	10^{12}	T

The international use of SI units would also enhance the standardization of nomenclature to facilitate global communication of medical and scientific information. The units, symbols, and prefixes employed in the International System are shown in Tables 1, 2, and 3.

Unfortunately, problems have arisen with the implementation of SI units in the United States. Their introduction in 1987 prompted many medical journals to report laboratory values in both SI and conventional units in anticipation of complete conversion to SI units in the early 1990s. The lack of a coordinated effort toward this goal has forced a retrenchment on the issue. Physicians continue to think and practice using laboratory results expressed in conventional units and few, if any, American hospitals or clinical laboratories exclusively use SI units. It is not likely that complete conversion to SI units will occur in the foreseeable future, yet most medical journals will probably continue to publish both sets of units. For this reason the tables of reference ranges in this Appendix are given in both conventional units and SI units.

TABLES OF REFERENCE VALUES

Some of the values included in the tables have been established by the Clinical Laboratories at Thomas Jefferson University Hospital in Philadelphia and have not been published elsewhere. Other values have been compiled from the sources cited herein. These tables are provided for information and educational purposes only. They are intended to complement data derived from other sources, including the medical history and physical examination. Users must exercise individual judgment when employing the information provided in this Appendix.

Reference Values for Hematology

	Conventional Units	SI Units
Acid hemolysis (Ham test)	No hemolysis	No hemolysis
Alkaline phosphatase, leukocyte	Total score 14–100	Total score 14–100
Cell counts		
Erythrocytes		
Males	4.6–6.2 million/mm³	$4.6–6.2 \times 10^{12}$/L
Females	4.2–5.4 million/mm³	$4.2–5.4 \times 10^{12}$/L
Children (varies with age)	4.5–5.1 million/mm³	$4.5–5.1 \times 10^{12}$/L
Leukocytes, total	4500–11,000/mm³	$4.5–11.0 \times 10^{9}$/L
Leukocytes, differential counts*		
Myelocytes	0%	0/L
Band neutrophils	3–5%	$150–400 \times 10^{6}$/L
Segmented neutrophils	54–62%	$3000–5800 \times 10^{6}$/L
Lymphocytes	25–33%	$1500–3000 \times 10^{6}$/L
Monocytes	3–7%	$300–500 \times 10^{6}$/L
Eosinophils	1–3%	$50–250 \times 10^{6}$/L
Basophils	0–1%	$15–50 \times 10^{6}$/L
Platelets	150,000–400,000/mm³	$150–400 \times 10^{9}$/L
Reticulocytes	25,000–75,000/mm³ (0.5–1.5% of erythrocytes)	$25–75 \times 10^{9}$/L
Coagulation tests		
Bleeding time (template)	2.75–8.0 min	2.75–8.0 min
Coagulation time (glass tube)	5–15 min	5–15 min
D-Dimer	<0.5 µg/mL	<0.5 mg/L

Reference Values for Hematology *Continued*

	Conventional Units	SI Units
Factor VIII and other coagulation factors	50–150% of normal	0.5–1.5 of normal
Fibrin split products (Thrombo-Welco test)	<10 µg/mL	<10 mg/L
Fibrinogen	200–400 mg/dL	2.0–4.0 g/L
Partial thromboplastin time (PTT)	20–35 s	20–35 s
Prothrombin time (PT)	12.0–14.0 s	12.0–14.0 s
Coombs' test		
Direct	Negative	Negative
Indirect	Negative	Negative
Corpuscular values of erythrocytes		
Mean corpuscular hemoglobin (MCH)	26–34 pg/cell	26–34 pg/cell
Mean corpuscular volume (MCV)	80–96 µm³	80–96 fL
Mean corpuscular hemoglobin concentration (MCHC)	32–36 g/dL	320–360 g/L
Erythrocyte sedimentation rate (ESR)		
Wintrobe		
Males	0–5 mm/h	0–5 mm/h
Females	0–15 mm/h	0–15 mm/h
Westergren		
Males	0–15 mm/h	0–15 mm/h
Females	0–20 mm/h	0–20 mm/h
Haptoglobin	20–165 mg/dL	0.20–1.65 g/L
Hematocrit		
Males	40–54 mL/dL	0.40–0.54
Females	37–47 mL/dL	0.37–0.47
Newborns	49–54 mL/dL	0.49–0.54
Children (varies with age)	35–49 mL/dL	0.35–0.49
Hemoglobin		
Males	13.0–18.0 g/dL	8.1–11.2 mmol/L
Females	12.0–16.0 g/dL	7.4–9.9 mmol/L
Newborns	16.5–19.5 g/dL	10.2–12.1 mmol/L
Children (varies with age)	11.2–16.5 g/dL	7.0–10.2 mmol/L
Hemoglobin, fetal	<1.0% of total	<0.01 of total
Hemoglobin A$_{1C}$	3–5% of total	0.03–0.05 of total
Hemoglobin A$_2$	1.5–3.0% of total	0.015–0.03 of total
Hemoglobin, plasma	0.0–5.0 mg/dL	0.0–3.2 µmol/L
Methemoglobin	30–130 mg/dL	19–80 µmol/L

*Conventicnal units are percentages; SI units are absolute counts.

Reference Values* for Clinical Chemistry (Blood, Serum, and Plasma)

	Conventional Units	SI Units
Acetoacetate plus acetone		
Qualitative	Negative	Negative
Quantitative	0.3–2.0 mg/dL	30–200 µmol/L
Acid phosphatase, serum (Thymolphthalein monophosphate substrate)	0.1–0.6 U/L	0.1–0.6 U/L
ACTH (see Corticotropin)		
Alanine aminotransferase (ALT, SGPT), serum	1–45 U/L	1–45 U/L
Albumin, serum	3.3–5.2 g/dL	33–52 g/L
Aldolase, serum	0.0–7.0 U/L	0.0–7.0 U/L
Aldosterone, plasma		
Standing	5–30 ng/dL	140–830 pmol/L
Recumbent	3–10 ng/dL	80–275 pmol/L
Alkaline phosphatase (ALP), serum		
Adult	35–150 U/L	35–150 U/L
Adolescent	100–500 U/L	100–500 U/L
Child	100–350 U/L	100–350 U/L
Ammonia nitrogen, plasma	10–50 µmol/L	10–50 µmol/L
Amylase, serum	25–125 U/L	25–125 U/L
Anion gap, serum, calculated	8–16 mEq/L	8–16 mmol/L
Ascorbic acid, blood	0.4–1.5 mg/dL	23–85 µmol/L

Table continued on following page

Reference Values* for Clinical Chemistry (Blood, Serum, and Plasma) *Continued*

	Conventional Units	SI Units
Aspartate aminotransferase (AST, SGOT), serum	1–36 U/L	1–36 U/L
Base excess, arterial blood, calculated	0 ± 2 mEq/L	0 ± 2 mmol/L
β-carotene, serum	60–260 μg/dL	1.1–8.6 μmol/L
Bicarbonate		
Venous plasma	23–29 mEq/L	23–29 mmol/L
Arterial blood	21–27 mEq/L	21–27 mmol/L
Bile acids, serum	0.3–3.0 mg/dL	0.8–7.6 μmol/L
Bilirubin, serum		
Conjugated	0.1–0.4 mg/dL	1.7–6.8 μmol/L
Total	0.3–1.1 mg/dL	5.1–19.0 μmol/L
Calcium, serum	8.4–10.6 mg/dL	2.10–2.65 mmol/L
Calcium, ionized, serum	4.25–5.25 mg/dL	1.05–1.30 mmol/L
Carbon dioxide, total, serum or plasma	24–31 mEq/L	24–31 mmol/L
Carbon dioxide tension (P_{CO_2}), blood	35–45 mmHg	35–45 mmHg
Ceruloplasmin, serum	23–44 mg/dL	230–440 mg/L
Chloride, serum or plasma	96–106 mEq/L	96–106 mmol/L
Cholesterol, serum or EDTA plasma		
Desirable range	<200 mg/dL	<5.20 mmol/L
LDL cholesterol	60–180 mg/dL	1.55–4.65 mmol/L
HDL cholesterol	30–80 mg/dL	0.80–2.05 mmol/L
Copper	70–140 μg/dL	11–22 μmol/L
Corticotropin (ACTH), plasma, 8 A.M.	10–80 pg/mL	2–18 pmol/L
Cortisol, plasma		
8:00 A.M.	6–23 μg/dL	170–630 nmol/L
4:00 P.M.	3–15 μg/dL	80–410 nmol/L
10:00 P.M.	<50% of 8:00 A.M. value	<50% of 8:00 A.M. value
Creatine, serum		
Males	0.2–0.5 mg/dL	15–40 μmol/L
Females	0.3–0.9 mg/dL	25–70 μmol/L
Creatine kinase (CK), serum		
Males	55–170 U/L	55–170 U/L
Females	30–135 U/L	30–135 U/L
Creatine kinase MB isoenzyme, serum	<5% of total CK activity	<5% of total CK activity
	<5% ng/mL by immunoassay	<5% ng/mL by immunoassay
Creatinine, serum	0.6–1.2 mg/dL	50–110 μmol/L
Estradiol-17β, adult		
Males	10–65 pg/mL	35–240 pmol/L
Females		
Follicular phase	30–100 pg/mL	110–370 pmol/L
Ovulatory phase	200–400 pg/mL	730–1470 pmol/L
Luteal phase	50–140 pg/mL	180–510 pmol/L
Ferritin, serum	20–200 ng/mL	20–200 μg/L
Fibrinogen, plasma	200–400 mg/dL	2.0–4.0 g/L
Folate, serum erythrocytes	2.0–9.0 ng/mL	4.5–20.4 nmol/L
	170–700 ng/mL	385–1590 nmol/L
Follicle-stimulating hormone (FSH), plasma		
Males	4–25 mU/mL	4–25 U/L
Females, premenopausal	4–30 mU/mL	4–30 U/L
Females, postmenopausal	40–250 mU/mL	40–250 U/L
γ-glutamyltransferase (GGT), serum	5–40 U/L	5–40 U/L
Gastrin, fasting, serum	0–110 pg/mL	0–110 mg/L
Glucose, fasting, plasma or serum	70–115 mg/dL	3.9–6.4 nmol/L
Growth hormone (hGH), plasma, adult, fasting	0–6 ng/mL	0–6 μg/L
Haptoglobin, serum	20–165 mg/dL	0.20–1.65 g/L
Immunoglobulins, serum (see Reference Values for Immunologic Procedures)		
Insulin, fasting, plasma	5–25 μU/mL	36–179 pmol/L
Iron, serum	75–175 μg/dL	13–31 μmol/L
Iron binding capacity, serum		
Total	250–410 μg/dL	45–73 μmol/L
Saturation	20–55%	0.20–0.55
Lactate		
Venous whole blood	5.0–20.0 mg/dL	0.6–2.2 mmol/L
Arterial whole blood	5.0–15.0 mg/dL	0.6–1.7 mmol/L
Lactate dehydrogenase (LD), serum	110–220 U/L	110–220 U/L
Lipase, serum	10–140 U/L	10–140 U/L
Lutropin (LH), serum		
Males	1–9 U/L	1–9 U/L
Females		
Follicular phase	2–10 U/L	2–10 U/L
Midcycle peak	15–65 U/L	15–65 U/L
Luteal phase	1–12 U/L	1–12 U/L
Postmenopausal	12–65 U/L	12–65 U/L

Reference Values* for Clinical Chemistry (Blood, Serum, and Plasma) *Continued*

	Conventional Units	SI Units
Magnesium, serum	1.3–2.1 mg/dL	0.65–1.05 mmol/L
Osmolality	275–295 mOsm/kg water	275–295 mOsm/kg water
Oxygen, blood, arterial, room air		
Partial pressure (Pa$_{O_2}$)	80–100 mm Hg	80–100 mm Hg
Saturation (Sa$_{O_2}$)	95–98%	95–98%
pH, arterial blood	7.35–7.45	7.35–7.45
Phosphate, inorganic, serum		
Adult	3.0–4.5 mg/dL	1.0–1.5 mmol/L
Child	4.0–7.0 mg/dL	1.3–2.3 mmol/L
Potassium		
Serum	3.5–5.0 mEq/L	3.5–5.0 mmol/L
Plasma	3.5–4.5 mEq/L	3.5–4.5 mmol/L
Progesterone, serum, adult		
Males	0.0–0.4 ng/mL	0.0–1.3 mmol/L
Females		
Follicular phase	0.1–1.5 ng/mL	0.3–4.8 mmol/L
Luteal phase	2.5–28.0 ng/mL	8.0–89.0 mmol/L
Prolactin, serum		
Males	1.0–15.0 ng/mL	1.0–15.0 µg/L
Females	1.0–20.0 ng/mL	1.0–20.0 µg/L
Protein, serum, electrophoresis		
Total	6.0–8.0 g/dL	60–80 g/L
Albumin	3.5–5.5 g/dL	35–55 g/L
Globulins		
Alpha$_1$	0.2–0.4 g/dL	2.0–4.0 g/L
Alpha$_2$	0.5–0.9 g/dL	5.0–9.0 g/L
Beta	0.6–1.1 g/dL	6.0–11.0 g/L
Gamma	0.7–1.7 g/dL	7.0–17.0 g/L
Pyruvate, blood	0.3–0.9 mg/dL	0.03–0.10 mmol/L
Rheumatoid factor	0.0–30.0 IU/mL	0.0–30.0 kIU/L
Sodium, serum or plasma	135–145 mEq/L	135–145 mmol/L
Testosterone, plasma		
Males, adult	300–1200 ng/dL	10.4–41.6 nmol/L
Females, adult	20–75 ng/dL	0.7–2.6 nmol/L
Pregnant females	40–200 ng/dL	1.4–6.9 nmol/L
Thyroglobulin	3–42 ng/mL	3–42 µg/L
Thyrotropin (hTSH), serum	0.4–4.8 µIU/mL	0.4–4.8 mIU/L
Thyrotropin-releasing hormone (TRH)	5–60 pg/mL	5–60 ng/L
Thyroxine (FT$_4$), free, serum	0.9–2.1 ng/dL	12–27 pmol/L
Thyroxine (T$_4$), serum	4.5–12.0 µg/dL	58–154 nmol/L
Thyroxine-binding globulin (TBG)	15.0–34.0 µg/mL	15.0–34.0 mg/L
Transferrin	250–430 mg/dL	2.5–4.3 g/L
Triglycerides, serum, after 12-hr fast	40–150 mg/dL	0.4–1.5 g/L
Triiodothyronine (T$_3$), serum	70–190 ng/dL	1.1–2.9 nmol/L
Triiodothyronine uptake, resin (T$_3$RU)	25–38%	0.25–0.38
Urate		
Males	2.5–8.0 mg/dL	150–480 µmol/L
Females	2.2–7.0 mg/dL	130–420 µmol/L
Urea, serum or plasma	24–49 mg/dL	4.0–8.2 nmol/L
Urea nitrogen, serum or plasma	11–23 mg/dL	8.0–16.4 nmol/L
Viscosity, serum	1.4–1.8 × water	1.4–1.8 × water
Vitamin A, serum	20–80 µg/dL	0.70–2.80 µmol/L
Vitamin B$_{12}$, serum	180–900 pg/mL	133–664 pmol/L

*Reference values may vary depending on the method and sample source used.

Reference Values for Therapeutic Drug Monitoring (Serum)

	Therapeutic Range	Toxic Concentrations	Proprietary Names
Analgesics			
Acetaminophen	10–20 µg/mL	>250 µg/mL	Tylenol
			Datril
Salicylate	100–250 µg/mL	>300 µg/mL	Aspirin
			Bufferin
Antibiotics			
Amikacin	25–30 µg/mL	Peak >35 µg/mL	Amikin
		Trough >10 µg/mL	

Table continued on following page

Reference Values for Therapeutic Drug Monitoring (Serum) *Continued*

	Therapeutic Range	Toxic Concentrations	Proprietary Names
Chloramphenicol	10–20 µg/mL	>25 µg/mL	Chloromycetin
Gentamicin	5–10 µg/mL	Peak >10 µg/mL Trough >2 µg/mL	Garamycin
Tobramycin	5–10 µg/mL	Peak >10 µg/mL Trough >2 µg/mL	Nebcin
Vancomycin	5–10 µg/mL	Peak >40 µg/mL Trough >10 µg/mL	Vancocin
Anticonvulsants			
Carbamazepine	5–12 µg/mL	>15 µg/mL	Tegretol
Ethosuximide	40–100 µg/mL	>150 µg/mL	Zarontin
Phenobarbital	15–40 µg/mL	40–100 ng/mL (varies widely)	Luminal
Phenytoin	10–20 µg/mL	>20 µg/mL	Dilantin
Primidone	5–12 µg/mL	>15 µg/mL	Mysoline
Valproic acid	50–100 µg/mL	>100 µg/mL	Depakene
Antineoplastics and Immunosuppressives			
Cyclosporine	50–400 ng/mL	>400 ng/mL	Sandimmune
Methotrexate, high dose, 48 hr	Variable	>1 µmol/L 48 hr after dose	Mexate Folex
Tacrolimus (FK-506), whole blood	3–10 µg/L	>15 µg/L	Prograf
Bronchodilators and Respiratory Stimulants			
Caffeine	3–15 ng/mL	>30 ng/mL	
Theophylline (Aminophylline)	10–20 µg/mL	>20 µg/mL	Elixophyllin Quibron
Cardiovascular Drugs			
Amiodarone (Obtain specimen more than 8 h after last dose)	1.0–2.0 µg/mL	>2.0 µg/mL	Cordarone
Digitoxin (Obtain specimen 12–24 h after last dose)	15–25 ng/mL	>35 ng/mL	Crystodigin
Digoxin (Obtain specimen more than 6 h after last dose)	0.8–2.0 ng/mL	>2.4 ng/mL	Lanoxin
Disopyramide	2–5 µg/mL	>7 µg/mL	Norpace
Flecainide	0.2–1.0 ng/mL	>1 ng/mL	Tambocor
Lidocaine	1.5–5.0 µg/mL	>6 µg/mL	Xylocaine
Mexiletine	0.7–2.0 ng/mL	>2 ng/mL	Mexitil
Procainamide	4–10 µg/mL	>12 µg/mL	Pronestyl
Procainamide plus NAPA	8–30 µg/mL	>30 µg/mL	
Propranolol	50–100 ng/mL	Variable	Inderal
Quinidine	2–5 µg/mL	>6 µg/mL	Cardioquin Quinaglute
Tocainide	4–10 ng/mL	>10 ng/mL	Tonocard
Psychopharmacologic Drugs			
Amitriptyline	120–150 ng/mL	>500 ng/mL	Elavil
Bupropion	25–100 ng/mL	Not applicable	Triavil Wellbutrin
Desipramine	150–300 ng/mL	>500 ng/mL	Norpramin Pertofrane Tofranil
Imipramine	125–250 ng/mL	>400 ng/mL	Janimine
Lithium (Obtain specimen 12 h after last dose)	0.6–1.5 mEq/L	>1.5 mEq/L	Lithobid
Nortriptyline	50–150 ng/mL	>500 ng/mL	Aventyl Pamelor

Reference Values for Clinical Chemistry (Urine)

	Conventional Units	SI Units
Acetone and acetoacetate, qualitative	Negative	Negative
Albumin		
Qualitative	Negative	Negative
Quantitative	10–100 mg/24 hr	0.15–1.5 µmol/day
Aldosterone	3–20 µg/24 hr	8.3–55 nmol/day
δ-Aminolevulinic acid (δ-ALA)	1.3–7.0 mg/24 hr	10–53 µmol/day
Amylase	<17 U/hr	<17 U/hr

Reference Values for Clinical Chemistry (Urine) *Continued*

	Conventional Units	SI Units
Amylase/creatinine clearance ratio	0.01–0.04	0.01–0.04
Bilirubin, qualitative	Negative	Negative
Calcium (regular diet)	<250 mg/24 hr	<6.3 nmol/day
Catecholamines		
Epinephrine	<10 μg/24 hr	<55 nmol/day
Norepinephrine	<100 μg/24 hr	<590 nmol/day
Total free catecholamines	4–126 μg/24 hr	24–745 nmol/day
Total metanephrines	0.1–1.6 mg/24 hr	0.5–8.1 μmol/day
Chloride (varies with intake)	110–250 mEq/24 hr	110–250 mmol/day
Copper	0–50 μg/24 hr	0.0–0.80 μmol/day
Cortisol, free	10–100 μg/24 hr	27.6–276 nmol/day
Creatine		
Males	0–40 mg/24 hr	0.0–0.30 mmol/day
Females	0–80 mg/24 hr	0.0–0.60 mmol/day
Creatinine	15–25 mg/kg/24 hr	0.13–0.22 mmol/kg/day
Creatinine clearance (endogenous)		
Males	110–150 mL/min/1.73m²	110–150 mL/min/1.73m²
Females	105–132 mL/min/1.73m²	105–132 mL/min/1.73m²
Cystine or cysteine	Negative	Negative
Dehydroepiandrosterone		
Males	0.2–2.0 mg/24 hr	0.7–6.9 μmol/day
Females	0.2–1.8 mg/24 hr	0.7–6.2 μmol/day
Estrogens, total		
Males	4–25 μg/24 hr	14–90 nmol/day
Females	5–100 μg/24 hr	18–360 nmol/day
Glucose (as reducing substance)	<250 mg/24 hr	<250 mg/day
Hemoglobin and myoglobin, qualitative	Negative	Negative
Homogentisic acid, qualitative	Negative	Negative
17–Hydroxycorticosteroids		
Males	3–9 mg/24 hr	8.3–25 μmol/day
Females	2–8 mg/24 hr	5.5–22 μmol/day
5–Hydroxyindoleacetic acid		
Qualitative	Negative	Negative
Quantitative	2–6 mg/24 hr	10–31 μmol/day
17–Ketogenic steroids		
Males	5–23 mg/24 hr	17–80 μmol/day
Females	3–15 mg/24 hr	10–52 μmol/day
17–Ketosteroids		
Males	8–22 mg/24 hr	28–76 μmol/day
Females	6–15 mg/24 hr	21–52 μmol/day
Magnesium	6–10 mEq/24 hr	3–5 mmol/day
Metanephrines	0.05–1.2 ng/mg creatinine	0.03–0.70 mmol/mmol creatinine
Osmolality	38–1400 mOsm/kg water	38–1400 mOsm/kg water
pH	4.6–8.0	4.6–8.0
Phenylpyruvic acid, qualitative	Negative	Negative
Phosphate	0.4–1.3 g/24 hr	13–42 mmol/day
Porphobilinogen		
Qualitative	Negative	Negative
Quantitative	<2 mg/24 hr	<9 μmol/day
Porphyrins		
Coproporphyrin	50–250 μg/24 hr	77–380 nmol/day
Uroporphyrin	10–30 μg/24 hr	12–36 nmol/day
Potassium	25–125 mEq/24 hr	25–125 mmol/day
Pregnanediol		
Males	0.0–1.9 mg/24 hr	0.0–6.0 μmol/day
Females		
Proliferative phase	0.0–2.6 mg/24 hr	0.0–8.0 μmol/day
Luteal phase	2.6–10.6 mg/24 hr	8–33 μmol/day
Postmenopausal	0.2–1.0 mg/24 hr	0.6–3.1 μmol/day
Pregnanetriol	0.0–2.5 mg/24 hr	0.0–7.4 umol/day
Protein, total		
Qualitative	Negative	Negative
Quantitative	10–150 mg/24 hr	10–150 mg/day
Protein/creatinine ratio	<0.2	<0.2
Sodium (regular diet)	60–260 mEq/24 hr	60–260 mmol/day
Specific gravity		
Random specimen	1.003–1.030	1.003–1.030
24-hour collection	1.015–1.025	1.015–1.025
Urate (regular diet)	250–750 mg/24 hr	1.5–4.4 mmol/day
Urobilinogen	0.5–4.0 mg/24 hr	0.6–6.8 μmol/day
Vanillylmandelic acid (VMA)	1.0–8.0 mg/24 hr	5–40 μmol/day

Reference Values for Toxic Substances

	Conventional Units	SI Units
Arsenic, urine	<130 μg/24 hr	<1.7 μmol/day
Bromides, serum, inorganic	<100 mg/dL	<10 mmol/L
Toxic symptoms	140–1000 mg/dL	14–100 mmol/L
Carboxyhemoglobin, blood	% Saturation	Saturation
Urban environment	<5%	<0.05
Smokers	<12%	<0.12
Symptoms		
Headache	>15%	>0.15
Nausea and vomiting	>25%	>0.25
Potentially lethal	>50%	>0.50
Ethanol, blood	<0.05 mg/dL <0.005%	<1.0 mmol/L
Intoxication	>100 mg/dL >0.1%	>22 mmol/L
Marked intoxication	300–400 mg/dL 0.3–0.4%	65–87 mmol/L
Alcoholic stupor	400–500 mg/dL 0.4–0.5%	87–109 mmol/L
Coma	>500 mg/dL >0.5%	>109 mmol/L
Lead, blood		
Adults	<25 μg/dL	<1.2 μmol/L
Children	<15 μg/dL	<0.7 μmol/L
Lead, urine	<80 μg/24 hr	<0.4 μmol/day
Mercury, urine	<30 μg/24 hr	<150 nmol/day

Reference Values for Cerebrospinal Fluid

	Conventional Units	SI Units
Cells	<5/mm³; all mononuclear	<5 × 10⁶/L, all mononuclear
Glucose	50–75 mg/dL (20 mg/dL less than in serum)	2.8–4.2 mmol/L (1.1 mmol less than in serum)
IgG		
Children under 14	<8% of total protein	<0.08% of total protein
Adults	<14% of total protein	<0.14 % of total protein
IgG index $\left(\dfrac{\text{CSF/serum IgG ratio}}{\text{CSF/ serum albumin ratio}}\right)$	0.3–0.6	0.3–0.6
Oligoclonal banding on electrophoresis	Absent	Absent
Pressure, opening	70–180 mmH₂O	70–180 mmH₂O
Protein, total	15–45 mg/dL	150–450 mg/L
Protein electrophoresis	Albumin predominant	Albumin predominant

Reference Values for Tests of Gastrointestinal Function

	Conventional Units		Conventional Units
Bentiromide	6-hr urinary arylamine excretion greater than 57% excludes pancreatic insufficiency	Maximum (after histamine or pentagastrin)	
β-Carotene, serum	60–250 ng/dL	Males	9.0–48.0 mmol/hr
Fecal fat estimation		Females	6.0–31.0 mmol/hr
Qualitative	No fat globules seen by high-power microscope	Ratio: basal/maximum	
		Males	0.0–0.31
Quantitative	<6 g/24 hr (>95% coefficient of fat absorption)	Females	0.0–0.29
Gastric acid output		Secretin test, pancreatic fluid	
Basal		Volume	>1.8 mL/kg/hr
Males	0.0–10.5 mmol/hr	Bicarbonate	>80 mEq/L
Females	0.0–5.6 mmol/hr		
		D-Xylose absorption test, urine	>20% of ingested dose excreted in 5 hr

Reference Values for Immunologic Procedures

	Conventional Units	SI Units
Complement, serum		
C3	85–175 mg/dL	0.85–1.75 g/L
C4	15–45 mg/dL	150–450 mg/L
Total hemolytic (CH_{50})	150–250 U/mL	150–250 U/mL
Immunoglobulins, serum, adult		
IgG	640–1350 mg/dL	6.4–13.5 g/L
IgA	70–310 mg/dL	0.70–3.1 g/L
IgM	90–350 mg/dL	0.90–3.5 g/L
IgD	0.0–6.0 mg/dL	0.0–60 mg/L
IgE	0.0–430 ng/dL	0.0–430 µg/L

Lymphocyte Subsets, Whole Blood, Heparinized

Antigen	Cell Type	Percentage	Absolute
CD3	Total T cells	56–77	860–1880
CD19	Total B cells	7–17	140–370
CD3 and CD4	Helper-inducer cells	32–54	550–1190
CD3 and CD8	Suppressor-cytotoxic cells	24–37	430–1060
CD3 and DR	Activated T cells	5–14	70–310
CD2	E rosette T cells	73–87	1040–2160
CD16 and CD56	Natural killer (NK) cells	8–22	130–500

Helper/suppressor ratio: 0.8–1.8.

Reference Values for Semen Analysis

	Conventional Units	SI Units
Volume	2–5 mL	2–5 mL
Liquefaction	Complete in 15 min	Complete in 15 min
pH	7.2–8.0	7.2–8.0
Leukocytes	Occasional or absent	Occasional or absent
Spermatozoa		
Count	60–150 $\times$ 10^6/mL	60–150 $\times$ 10^6/mL
Motility	>80% motile	>0.80 motile
Morphology	80–90% normal forms	>0.80–0.90 normal forms
Fructose	>150 mg/dL	>8.33 mmol/L

REFERENCES

AMA Drug Evaluations, Annual. Chicago, American Medical Association, 1994.

Bick RL (ed): Hematology—Clinical and Laboratory Practice. St. Louis, Mosby–Year Book, 1993.

Borer WZ: Selection and use of laboratory tests. *In* Tietz NW, Conn RB, Pruden EL (eds): Applied Laboratory Medicine. Philadelphia, WB Saunders Co, 1992, pp 1–5.

Campion EW: A retreat from SI units. N Engl J Med *327*:49, 1992.

Friedman RB, Young DS: Effects of Disease on Clinical Laboratory Tests, 2nd ed. Washington, DC, AACC Press, 1989.

Henry JB: Clinical Diagnosis and Management by Laboratory Methods, 18th ed. Philadelphia, WB Saunders Co, 1991.

Hicks JM, Young DS: DORA 1992–1993: Directory of Rare Analyses. Washington, DC, AACC Press, 1992.

Jacobs DS, Kasten BL, Demott WR, Wolfson WL: Laboratory Test Handbook, 2nd ed. Baltimore, Williams & Wilkins Co, 1990.

Kaplan LA, Pesce AJ: Clinical Chemistry—Theory, Analysis, and Correlation, 2nd ed. St. Louis, CV Mosby, 1989.

Kjeldsberg CR, Knight JA: Body Fluids—Laboratory Examination of Amniotic, Cerebrospinal, Seminal, Serous, and Synovial Fluids, 3rd ed. Chicago, ASCP Press, 1993.

Laposata M: SI Unit Conversion Guide. Boston, New England Journal of Medicine Books, 1992.

Scully RE, McNeely WF, Mark EJ, McNeely BU: Normal reference laboratory values. N Engl J Med *327*:718–724, 1992.

Speicher CE: The Right Test—A Physician's Guide to Laboratory Medicine, 2nd ed. Philadelphia, WB Saunders Co, 1993.

Tietz NW (ed): Clinical Guide to Laboratory Tests, 2nd ed. Philadelphia, WB Saunders Co, 1990.

Wallach J: Interpretation of Diagnostic Tests—A Synopsis of Laboratory Medicine, 5th ed. Boston, Little, Brown, and Co, 1992.

Young DS: Determination and validation of reference intervals. Arch Pathol Lab Med *116*:704–709, 1992.

Young DS: Effects of Drugs on Clinical Laboratory Tests, 3rd ed. Washington, DC, AACC Press, 1990.

Young DS: Implementation of SI units for clinical laboratory data. Ann Intern Med *106*:114–129, 1987.

DRUGS APPROVED IN 1995

compiled by
DIRK LUCAS, PHARM.D., B.C.P.S.
University of Houston College of Pharmacy
Houston, Texas

Generic Name	Trade Name (Manufacturer)	Dosage	Average Dosage Range	FDA Rating*	Approved Use
acarbose	Precose (Bayer)	50- and 100-mg tablets	50–100 mg three times daily	1–S	Type II diabetes mellitus
alendronate sodium	Fosamax (Merck)	10- and 40-mg tablets	10 mg daily (osteoporosis); 40 mg daily (Paget's disease)	1-P	Osteoporosis; Paget's disease
azelaic acid	Azelex (Allergan)	20% cream, 30-gram tube	Apply to affected areas twice daily	1-S	Acne vulgaris
bicalutamide	Casodex (Zeneca)	50-mg tablet	50 mg daily	1-S,E,H	Advanced prostate cancer
carvedilol	Coreg (SmithKline Beecham)	6.25-, 12.5-, and 25-mg tablets	6.25–25 mg twice daily	1-S	Hypertension
ceftibuten	Cedax (Schering)	40-mg capsules; 90 mg/5 mL and 180 mg/5 mL oral suspension in 30-, 60-, and 120-mL bottles	Adults: 400 mg daily; children: 9 mg/kg daily	1-S	Pharyngitis/tonsillitis; acute and chronic bronchitis; otitis media; skin infections
cetirizine hydrochloride	Zyrtec (Pfizer)	5- and 10-mg tablets	5–10 mg daily	1-S	Allergic rhinitis
dexrazoxane	Zinecard (Pharmacia Upjohn)	250 and 500 mg and single use vials	dexrazoxane: doxorubicin ratio of 10:1	1-P,E,H,V	Cardiomyopathy associated with doxorubicin
dirithromycin	Dynabac (Bock; Lilly)	250-mg tablets	500 mg daily	1-S	Mild-to-moderate respiratory tract and skin infections
ibutilide fumarate	Corvert (Pharmacia & Upjohn)	0.1 mg/mL IV solution, 10-mL vials	0.1 mL/kg over 10 minutes	1-S	Atrial fibrillation/flutter
lamivudine	Epivir (Glaxo Wellcome)	150-mg tablets	150 mg twice daily	1-P,AA,E,H	HIV infection
lansoprazole	Prevacid (Abbott)	15- and 30-mg capsules	15–60 mg daily	1-S	Duodenal ulcer, erosive esophagitis, Zollinger-Ellison syndrome
losartan potassium	Cozaar (Merck)	25- and 50-mg tablets	25–100 mg daily	1-S	Hypertension
moexipril hydrochloride	Univasc (Schwarz)	7.5- and 15-mg tablets	7.5–30 mg daily	1-S	Hypertension
mycophenolate mofetil	CellCept (Roche)	250-mg capsules	1 gram twice daily	1-P	Prophylaxis of organ rejection
nalmefene hydrochloride	Revex (Ohmeda)	100 µg/mL, 1-mL ampules and 1 mg/mL, 2-mL ampules	0.25 µg/kg at 2- to 5-minute intervals; 0.5 mg/70 kg (overdose)	1-S	Complete or partial reversal of opioid effects; known or suspected opioid overdose
nisoldipine	Sular (Zeneca)	10-, 20-, 30-, and 40-mg extended-released tablets	20–40 mg daily	1-S	Hypertension
porfimer sodium	Photofrin (QuadraLogic Technologies)	75-mg vials	2 mg/kg per treatment course	1-P,V	Esophageal cancer
riluzole	Rilutek (Rhone-Poulenc Rorer)	50-mg tablets	50 mg twice daily	1-P,V	Amyotrophic lateral sclerosis

Generic Name	Trade Name (Manufacturer)	Dosage	Average Dosage Range	FDA Rating*	Approved Use
saquinavir mesylate	Invirase (Roche)	200-mg capsules	600 mg three times daily	1-P,AA,E,H	HIV infection
sevoflurane	Ultane (Abbott)	250-mL bottles	0.5–3.0% by vaporization	1-S	General anesthesia
tramadol hydrochloride	Ultram (Ortho-McNeil)	50-mg tablets	50–100 mg every 4 to 6 hours	1-S	Moderate to moderately severe pain

*Ratings:
- 1   New molecular entity.
- 4   Combination product.
- E   Treatment for life-threatening or severely debilitating illnesses.
- H   Accelerated approval.
- P   Priority review, therapeutic gain.
- S   Standard review, substantially equivalent.
- V   Orphan drug.
- AA Treatment for acquired immunodeficiency syndrome (AIDS) and/or its complications.

TOP 200 DRUGS PRESCRIBED IN THE UNITED STATES

compiled by
DIRK LUCAS, Pharm.D., B.C.P.S.
University of Houston College of Pharmacy
Houston, Texas

Rank*	Generic Name	Brand Name (Manufacturer)	Cost Index†
1.	conjugated estrogens	Premarin (Wyeth-Ayerst)	$
2.	amoxicillin	Trimox (Apothecon)	$
3.	levothyroxine	Synthroid (Knoll)	$$
4.	amoxicillin	Amoxil (SmithKline Beecham)	$$
5.	ranitidine	Zantac (Glaxo Wellcome)	$$$
6.	digoxin	Lanoxin (Glaxo Wellcome)	$
7.	nifedipine	Procardia XL (Pfizer)	$$$
8.	enalapril	Vasotec (Merck)	$$
9.	fluoxetine	Prozac (Dista)	$$$$
10.	albuterol	Proventil inhaler (Schering)	$$
11.	diltiazem	Cardizem CD (Hoechst Marion Roussel)	$$$
12.	hydrocodone/acetaminophen	(Watson)	$
13.	sertraline	Zoloft (Roerig)	$$$$
14.	warfarin	Coumadin (DuPont)	$
15.	amoxicillin/clavulanate	Augmentin (SmithKline Beecham)	$$$
16.	amoxicillin	(Biocraft)	$
17.	triamterene/hydrochlorothiazide	(CibaGeneva)	$
18.	lisinopril	Zestril (Stuart)	$$
19.	acetaminophen/codeine	(Lemmon)	$
20.	ciprofloxacin	Cipro (Bayer)	$$$
21.	propoxyphene/acetaminophen	(Mylan)	$
22.	clarithromycin	Biaxin (Abbott)	$$$$
23.	furosemide	(Mylan)	$
24.	penicillin-VK	Veetids (Apothecon)	$
25.	albuterol	Ventolin Inhaler (Glaxo Wellcome)	$$
26.	omeprazole	Prilosec (Astra Merck)	$$$$

Continued on following page

Rank*	Generic Name	Brand Name (Manufacturer)	Cost Index†
27.	amlodipine	Norvasc (Pfizer)	$$$
28.	loratadine	Claritin (Schering)	$$$
29.	lovastatin	Mevacor (Merck)	$$$$
30.	ethinyl estradiol/norethindrone	Ortho-Novum 7/7/7 (Ortho)	$$$
31.	captopril	Capoten (Bristol-Myers Squibb)	$$
32.	medroxyprogestrone	Provera (Upjohn)	$$
33.	paroxetine	Paxil (SmithKline Beecham)	$$$$
34.	ibuprofen	IBU (Knoll)	$
35.	cephalexin	(Biocraft)	$
36.	insulin	Humulin N (Lilly)	$
37.	terazosin	Hytrin (Abbott)	$$$
38.	alprazolam	(CibaGeneva)	$
39.	phenytoin	Dilantin (Parke-Davis)	$
40.	acetaminophen/codeine	(Purepac)	$
41.	famotidine	Pepcid (Merck)	$$$
42.	ethinyl estradiol/levonorgestrel	Triphasil (Wyeth-Ayerst)	$$$
43.	terfenadine	Seldane (Hoechst Marion Roussel)	$$$
44.	nabumetone	Relafen (SmithKline Beecham)	$$$$
45.	simvastatin	Zocor (Merck)	$$$$
46.	potassium chloride	K-Dur (Key)	$$
47.	amitriptyline	(Mylan)	$
48.	clonazepam	Klonopin (Roche)	$$$
49.	cefaclor	(Mylan)	$$
50.	acyclovir	Zovirax capsules (Glaxo Wellcome)	$$
51.	azithromycin	Zithromax (Pfizer)	$$$$
52.	estradiol	Estrace (Mead Johnson)	$
53.	beclomethasone	Vancenase AQ (Schering)	$$$
54.	lisinopril	Prinivil (Merck)	$$
55.	cefuroxime axetil	Ceftin (Glaxo Wellcome)	$$$$
56.	cephalexin	(Apothecon)	$
57.	erythromycin	Ery-Tab (Abbott)	$
58.	pravastatin	Pravachol (Bristol-Myers Squibb)	$$$$
59.	ethinyl estradiol/desogestrel	Ortho-Cept (Ortho)	$$$
60.	trimethoprim/sulfamethoxasole	(Biocraft)	$
61.	hydrocodone/acetaminophen	(Qualitest)	$
62.	zolpidem	Ambien (Searle)	$$$$
63.	estradiol	Estraderm (CibaGeneva)	$$$
64	levothyroxine	Levoxyl (Daniels)	$
65.	nizatidine	Axid (Lilly)	$$$
66.	etodolac	Lodine (Wyeth-Ayerst)	$$$
67.	atenolol	(Mylan)	$
68.	cefprozil	Cefzil (Bristol Lab)	$$$
69.	ipratropium bromide	Atrovent (Boeringer Ingelheim)	$$$
70.	alprazolam	Xanax (Upjohn)	$$$
71.	verapamil	Calan SR (Searle)	$$$
72.	glyburide	(Copley)	$
73.	prednisone	Deltasone (Upjohn)	$$
74.	oxycodone/acetaminophen	Roxicet (Roxane)	$
75.	nitroglycerin	Nitrostat (Parke-Davis)	$

Rank*	Generic Name	Brand Name (Manufacturer)	Cost Index†
76.	triamterene w/hydrochlorothiazide	Dyazide (SmithKline Beecham)	$$
77.	propoxyphene/acetaminophen	(Lemmon)	$
78.	benazepril	Lotensin (CibaGeneva)	$$
79.	lorazepam	(Mylan)	$
80.	diclofenac sodium	Voltaren (CibaGeneva)	$$$
81.	oxaprozin	Daypro (Searle)	$$$$
82.	cefadroxil	Duricef (Mead Johnson)	$$$
83.	verapamil	(Goldline)	$
84.	cisapride	Propulsid (Janssen)	$$
85.	betamethasone/clotrimazole	Lotrisone (Schering)	$$
86.	ethinyl estradiol/desogestrel	Desogen (Organon)	$$$
87.	prednisone	(Schein)	$
88.	furosemide	Lasix (Hoechst Marion Roussel)	$$
89.	cimetidine	(Mylan)	$$
90.	insulin syringe	(Becton Dickinson)	$
91.	insulin	Humulin 70/30 (Lilly)	$
92.	triamcinolone acetonide	Azmacort (Rhone-Poulenc Rorer)	$$
93.	quinapril	Accupril (Parke-Davis)	$$
94.	hydrochlorothiazide	(Zenith)	$
95.	medroxyprogesterone	Cycrin (ESI)	$$
96.	buspirone	BuSpar (Mead Johnson)	$$$$
97.	medroxyprogesterone	(Greenstone)	$
98.	loratidine/pseudoephedrine	Claritin-D (Schering)	$$$$
99.	trimethoprim/sulfamethoxasole	(Mutual)	$
100.	lorazepam	(Purepac)	$
101.	naproxen	(Mylan)	$
102.	ketoconazole	Nizoral-external (Janssen)	$$
103.	beclomethasone	Beconase AQ (Glaxo Wellcome)	$$$
104.	propoxyphene/acetaminophen	Darvocet-N 100 (Lilly)	$$
105.	ethinyl estradiol/norgestrel	Lo/Ovral (Wyeth-Ayerst)	$$$
106.	terfenadine/pseudoephedrine	Seldane-D (Hoechst Marion Roussel)	$$$$
107.	tretinoin	Retin-A (Ortho Derm)	$$$$
108.	methylphenidate	(M D Pharm)	$
109.	loracarbef	Lorabid (Lilly)	$$$$
110.	alprazolam	(Greenstone)	$
111.	pentoxifylline	Trental (Hoechst Marion Roussel)	$$$
112.	nifedipine	Adalat (Bayer)	$$
113.	tramadol	Ultram (Ortho-McNeil)	$$$$
114.	neomycin/polymyxin/hydrocortisone	(Schein)	$
115.	potassium chloride	Klor-Con (Upsher-Smith)	$$
116.	atenolol	(Lederle)	$
117.	potassium chloride	(Ethex)	$
118.	timolol	Timoptic (Merck)	$$
119.	ethinyl estradiol/levonorgestrel	Tri-Levlen (Berlex)	$$
120.	fluconazole	Diflucan (Pfizer)	$$$$
121.	glipizide	Glucotrol XL (Pfizer)	$$
122.	glyburide	Glynase PresTabs (Upjohn)	$$$
123.	ethinyl estradiol/norethindrone	Ortho-Novum (Ortho)	$$
124.	cefixime	Suprax (Lederle)	$$$$

Continued on following page

Rank*	Generic Name	Brand Name (Manufacturer)	Cost Index†
125.	fluvastatin	Lescol (Sandoz)	$$
126.	doxazosin	Cardura (Pfizer)	$$$
127.	carbamazepine	Tegretol (Basel)	$$
128.	glipizide	(Mylan)	$
129.	valproic acid	Depakote (Abbott)	$$$
130.	metoprolol tartrate	Lopressor (Geigy)	$$
131.	gemfibrozil	(Warner Chilcott)	$
132.	nitrofurantoin	Macrobid (Procter & Gamble)	$$
133.	diazepam	(Mylan)	$
134.	cefaclor	Ceclor (Lilly)	$$$
135.	ibuprofen	Children's Motrin (McNeil)	$$
136.	cyclobenzaprine	(Mylan)	$
137.	glyburide	Diabeta (Hoechst Marion Roussel)	$$$
138.	nitroglycerin	Nitro-Dur (Key)	$$$
139.	ketorolac tromethamine	Toradol (Roche)	$$$
140.	doxycycline	(Zenith)	$
141.	albuterol oral liquid	(Lemmon)	$
142.	atenolol	Tenormin (Zeneca)	$$
143.	glyburide	Micronase (Upjohn)	$$$
144.	cephalexin	(Zenith)	$
145.	sumatriptan	Imitrex (Cerenex)	$$$
146.	propoxyphene/acetaminophen	Propacet (Lemmon)	$
147.	hydrocodone/acetaminophen	Lorcet (UAD)	$$
148.	indapamide	Lozol (Rhone-Poulenc Rorer)	$$$
149.	temazepam	(Mylan)	$
150.	promethazine	Phenergan (Wyeth-Ayerst)	$$
151.	verapamil	Verelan (Lederle)	$$
152.	metoprolol tartrate	(Mylan)	$
153.	metoprolol tartrate	(CibaGeneva)	$
154.	ramipril	Altace (Hoechst Marion Roussel)	$$
155.	insulin	Humulin R (Lilly)	$
156.	terconazole	Terazol (Ortho)	$$$
157.	theophylline	Theo-Dur (Shering)	$
158.	albuterol nebulization solution	(Warrick)	$
159.	methylprednisolone	(Duramed)	$
160.	diltiazem	Dilacor XR (Rhone-Poulenc Rorer)	$$
161.	mupirocin	Bactroban (SmithKline Beecham)	$$$$
162.	erythromycin stearate	(Abbott)	$$
163.	nortriptyline	(Schein)	$
164.	methylphenidate	Ritalin (CibaGeneva)	$$$
165.	atenolol	(CibaGeneva)	$
166.	ofloxacin	Floxin (Ortho)	$$$
167.	glipizide	Glucotrol (Pfizer)	$$
168.	ethinyl estradiol/ethynodiol diacetate	Demulen (Searle)	$$$
169.	cyclobenzaprine	(Schein)	$
170.	salmeterol	Serevent (Glaxo Wellcome)	$$$
171.	beclomethasone	Vanceril (Schering)	$$$
172.	dicyclomine HCl	(Rugby)	$
173.	astemizole	Hismanal (Janssen)	$$$

Rank*	Generic Name	Brand Name (Manufacturer)	Cost Index†
174.	ethinyl estradiol/norethindrone/ferrous fumarate	Loestrin Fe (Parke-Davis)	$$
175.	trimethoprim/sulfamethoxasole	Cotrim D.S. (Lemmon)	$
176.	tetracycline	Sumycin (Apothecon)	$
177.	ibuprofen	Children's Advil (Wyeth-Ayerst)	$$
178.	hydrocodone w/acetaminophen	Vicodin (Knoll)	$$
179.	sucralfate	Carafate (Hoechst Marion Roussel)	$$$
180.	venlafaxine	Effexor (Wyeth-Ayerst)	$$$
181.	guaifenesin/phenylpropanolamine	(Duramed)	$
182.	amoxicillin	(Warner Chilcott)	$
183.	glyburide	(Greenstone)	$
184.	promethazine/codeine	(Barre)	$
185.	penicillin-VK	(Mylan)	$
186.	doxycycline	(Mutual)	$
187.	erythromycin base	(Abbott)	$
188.	metoprolol	Toprol XL (Astra)	$$
189.	ampicillin	Principen (Apothecon)	$
190.	carisoprodol	(Schein)	$
191.	acetaminophen w/codeine	Tylenol w/Codeine (McNeil)	$$
192.	cephalexin	(Barr)	$
193.	one touch test strip	(Lifescan)	$$
194.	mometasone furoate	Elocon (Schering)	$$$$
195.	triamcinolone acetonide	Nasacort (Rhone-Poulenc Rorer)	$$
196.	hydrocodone/acetaminophen	Lorcet Plus (UAD)	$$
197.	aspirin/caffeine/butalbital/codeine	Fiorinal w/Codeine (Sandoz)	$$
198.	diazepam	Valium (Roche)	$$$
199.	ketoprofen	Oruvail (Wyeth-Ayerst)	$$
200.	erythromycin	PCE (Abbott)	$$

*The ranking is based on the total number of prescriptions for all strengths of drugs dispensed in United States community pharmacies.

†This is a comparison of relative cost of drugs in a given therapeutic class. Less expensive drugs are noted by "$" and the more expensive drugs in the class as "$$$$." The relative cost is based on average wholesale price (AWP). The cost index is not an absolute indicator of cost; for example, drugs listed as "$$$$" will not be exactly four times as expensive as drugs listed as "$."

NOMOGRAM FOR THE DETERMINATION OF BODY SURFACE AREA OF CHILDREN AND ADULTS

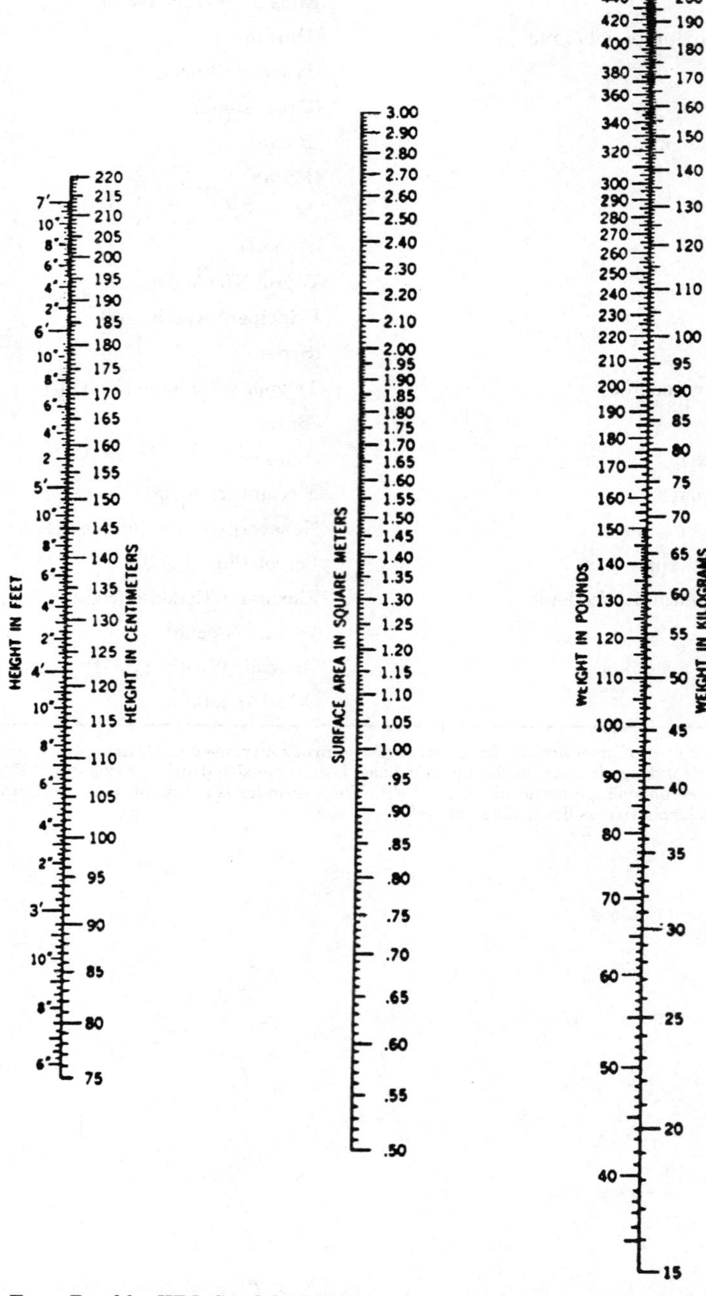

From Boothby WM, Sandiford RB: Boston Med Surg J *185*:337, 1921.

Index

Note: Page numbers followed by (t) refer to tables; page numbers in *italics* refer to illustrations.

ISBN 0-7216-8674-5

𝓔nhance your medical library with these exceptional references... Try them FREE for 30 days!

Order extra copies for hospital, office, or colleagues!

Rakel
Conn's CURRENT THERAPY 1997: Latest Approved Methods of Treatment for the Practicing Physician

NEW Vol.!

Plug into the pulse of medicine! Delivers more than 1,000 therapies for over 300 medical conditions. *"A good curbside consult from someone you trust...A tour de force...A good value."* (*Archives of Family Medicine,* review of previous volume)

Dec. 1996. Over 1355 pp. Illustd. **Order #W8674-5/SCONN***

> ** For your convenience, when you purchase a volume of this book, you will be entered as a subscriber to future volumes and automatically will be sent and billed for subsequent volumes. You may examine each new volume for 30 days, and may return it within that time period for full credit. You also may cancel an upcoming volume or your subscription at any time by calling 1-800-545-2522.*

Dorland's ILLUSTRATED MEDICAL DICTIONARY, 28th Edition

Unlock the gold! *"Carries on an impressive tradition of accuracy, clarity, and conciseness going back to the early years of the century...Users...will find...the same amiable and authoritative guide they have come to respect and trust."* (*JAMA*)

1994. 1974 pp. 382 ills. (24 in 2-color) **Order #W2859-1.**

Rakel
Saunders MANUAL OF MEDICAL PRACTICE

This master key to everyday practice clearly outlines common symptoms, diseases, treatments, and procedures. By simply scanning the material, you'll find the direction you need to recognize and understand a disorder, develop a diagnosis, and plan a successful management strategy.

1996. 1287 pp. 388 ills. (118 in 2-color) **Order #W5192-5.**

Bennett & Plum
Cecil TEXTBOOK OF MEDICINE, 20th Edition

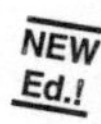

NEW Ed.!

Diagnose and treat the full range of conditions with the 20th Edition of this easy-to-use classic! *"A complete, well-written, authoritative source of information on all aspects of internal medicine."* (*Journal of Family Practice,* review of last edition) Organized by disease and group for at-a-glance review.

Feb. 1996. 2287 pp. 1256 tables, 1330 figs. (170 full-color plates, 635 in 2-color) 2-volume set: **Order #W3573-3.** Single volume: **Order #W3561-X.**

Braunwald
HEART DISEASE: A Textbook of Cardiovascular Medicine, 5th Edition

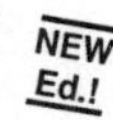

NEW Ed.!

"Will prove immensely useful to all of us faced with 'the awesome task of learning and remaining current in this dynamic field.' Highly recommended." (*Chest,* review of previous edition) 21 new chapters and 22 new expert contributors bring you the state of the art in this field!

Sept. 1996. Over 2140 pp. Over 1070 ills. (48 in full color) Single volume. **Order #W5666-8.**

Behrman, Kliegman & Arvin
Nelson TEXTBOOK OF PEDIATRICS, 15th Edition

"This classic text has undergone a rather thorough and improved revision...Giv[es] thorough coverage to virtually every topic encountered in the field of pediatric and adolescent medicine...Most highly recommended...A very worthwhile purchase." (*Emergency and Office Pediatrics*)

1996. 2245 pp. 1622 ills. (49 in full color) **Order #W5578-5.**

For faster service, **call toll-free 1-800-545-2522** (8:30 to 7:00 Eastern Time) and mention **DM#37629**... or **FAX** your order **FREE** to **1-800-874-6418.**
Available from your bookstore or the publisher.

𝓨es!

Please send me the books checked below. If not completely satisfied, I may return the book(s) with the invoice within 30 days at absolutely no risk.

☐ W8674-5/SCONN* Please enroll me as a **Conn's CURRENT THERAPY** series subscriber. I will receive future volumes upon publication.
    ☐ W8674-5 Send me _______ copies of **Rakel: Conn's CURRENT THERAPY 1997.**
☐ W2859-1 **Dorland's ILLUSTRATED MEDICAL DICTIONARY, 28th Edition**
☐ W5192-5 **Rakel: Saunders MANUAL OF MEDICAL PRACTICE**
☐ W3573-3 **Bennett & Plum: Cecil TEXTBOOK OF MEDICINE, 20th Edition** 2-volume set
    ☐ W3561-X **Bennett & Plum, 20th Edition** Single volume
☐ W5666-8 **Braunwald: HEART DISEASE: A Textbook of Cardiovascular Medicine, 5th Edition** Single volume
☐ W5578-5 **Behrman, Kliegman & Arvin: Nelson TEXTBOOK OF PEDIATRICS, 15th Edition**
☐ Bill me later—plus shipping and the applicable sales tax for my area
☐ Charge my credit card (SAVE SHIPPING) ☐ VISA ☐ MC ☐ AmEx

Card # _ _ _ _ /_ _ _ _ /_ _ _ _ /_ _ _ _ Exp. date _ _ /_ _

Add the applicable sales tax for your area. Make checks payable to **W.B. SAUNDERS COMPANY. Staple this to your purchase order to expedite delivery.**

Name ____ Address ____

City ________________________ State ________ Zip ____________ Telephone (________)________________

© **W.B. SAUNDERS COMPANY** 1996. *Professional references may be tax-deductible.* Offer valid in USA only. Printed in USA.

C#14263

DM#37629

BUSINESS REPLY MAIL
FIRST CLASS MAIL   PERMIT NO. 7135   ORLANDO, FL

POSTAGE WILL BE PAID BY ADDRESSEE

BOOK ORDER FULFILLMENT DEPT.

WB SAUNDERS COMPANY
A Division of Harcourt Brace & Company
6277 SEA HARBOR DR
ORLANDO FL 32821-9816

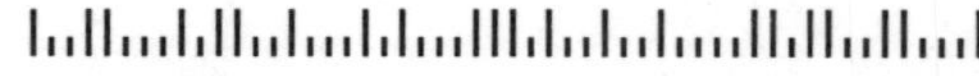